ANDREOLI and CARPENTER'S
CECIL Essentials of
MEDICINE
7th Edition

Editor-in-Chief

Thomas E. Andreoli, M.D., M.A.C.P., F.R.C.P. (Edin.), Sc.D. (hon.), Docteur (hon.), Professor (hon.), M.D. (hon.)
Distinguished Professor
Department of Internal Medicine
Department of Physiology and Biophysics
University of Arkansas College of Medicine
Little Rock, Arkansas

ANDREOLI and CARPENTER'S
CECIL Essentials of
MEDICINE

Seventh Edition

Editors

Charles C.J. Carpenter, M.D., M.A.C.P.
Professor of Medicine
Brown Medical School
Director, Brown University AIDS Center
Providence, Rhode Island

Robert C. Griggs, M.D., F.A.C.P., F.A.A.N.
Edward A. and Alma Vollertsen Rykenboer Professor of Neurophysiology
Chair, Department of Neurology
Professor of Medicine, Pathology and Laboratory Medicine, and Pediatrics
University of Rochester School of Medicine and Dentistry
Rochester, New York

Ivor J. Benjamin, M.D., F.A.C.C., F.A.H.A.
Professor of Medicine
Christi T. Smith Chair for Cardiovascular Research
Chief, Division of Cardiology
University of Utah School of Medicine
Salt Lake City, Utah

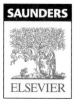

SAUNDERS

ELSEVIER

SAUNDERS
ELSEVIER

1600 John F. Kennedy Blvd.
Ste 1800
Philadelphia, PA 19103-2899

ANDREOLI AND CARPENTER'S CECIL ESSENTIALS OF MEDICINE

ISBN-13: 978-1-4160-2933-5
ISBN-10: 1-4160-2933-8

Library of Congress Cataloging-in-Publication Data

Andreoli and Carpenter's Cecil essentials of medicine / editor-in-chief, Thomas E. Andreoli; editors, Charles C.J. Carpenter, Robert C. Griggs, and Ivor J. Benjamin.—7th ed.
    p. ; cm.
Rev. ed. of: Cecil essentials of medicine, c2004
Includes bibliographical references and index.
ISBN 1-4160-2933-8
    1. Internal medicine.   I. Andreoli, Thomas E., 1935–   II. Carpenter, Charles C.J. (Charles Colcock J.)
III. Cecil, Russell L. (Russell La Fayette), 1881–1965.   IV. Cecil essentials of medicine.   V. Titles: Essentials of medicine.
[DNLM: 1. Internal Medicine. WB 115 A559 2007]
RC46.C42 2007
616—dc22

                                                                                    2006045276

Cover: Hemoglobin subunit: Phantatomix / Photo Researchers, Inc.; False-color (computer graphics) photograph of a resin cast of the human bronchial tree, the network of airways serving both lungs: Alfred Pasieka / Photo Researchers, Inc.; DNA: Dr. A. Lesk, MRC-LMB / Photo Researchers, Inc.; Osteoarthritis of foot, X-ray: DR P. MARAZZI / Photo Researchers, Inc.

Acquisitions Editor: James Merritt
Developmental Editor: Rebecca Gruliow
Publishing Services Manager: Linda Van Pelt
Project Manager: Melanie Peirson Johnstone
Design Direction: Steven Stave

Printed in Canada

Last digit is the print number: 9 8 7 6 5 4 3 2 1

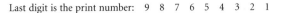

Dedication

Charles C.J. Carpenter

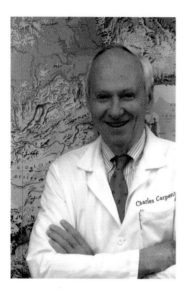

Charles C.J. Carpenter, Professor of Medicine at Brown University, was one of the founding Editors of *Cecil Essentials of Medicine*. He was also one of the major contributors articulating the concept that the founding Editors and all subsequent Editors have adhered to, namely, to provide a concise readable textbook for students of medicine of all ages. This Seventh Edition of *Cecil Essentials*, now titled *Andreoli and Carpenter's Cecil Essentials of Medicine*, will be Chuck's last effort with *Essentials*, and so the Editors, with great delight, are privileged to honor him, not only by naming the title of the book permanently in his name, but also in dedicating this Edition of *Essentials* to Chuck Carpenter.

Chuck is a remarkably splendid human being. His photograph defines precisely the nature of the man: a gentle man, a gentleman, implacably warm and generous in spirit and behavior.

As an academician, Chuck has excelled. He trained in Internal Medicine at Johns Hopkins where he served as Chief Resident for the late A. McGehee Harvey. Subsequently, he became Chair of Medicine at Case Western Reserve University, 1973–1986. For excellence as a Chair, he will receive, in 2007, the Robert H. Williams Distinguished Chair of Medicine Award conferred by the Association of American Physicians. Chuck then became Professor of Medicine at Brown University, 1986–present. He is currently Director of the Brown Center for AIDS Research.

Chuck's academic career includes far more contributions than one can list in this dedication. But some major themes warrant particular consideration.

In his early faculty years, he worked on fluid and electrolyte balance, and was among the first to identify angiotensin II as the principal stimulator to aldosterone secretion.

He made seminal contributions to understanding the pathophysiology of cholera and cholera-like syndromes in clinical and experimental studies which contributed to the development of oral rehydration therapy for secretory diarrheas in developing countries, most notably in the Indian Subcontinent.

Almost immediately following the appearance of AIDS, Chuck involved himself heavily, both experimentally and clinically, in the diagnosis and treatment of AIDS and in humane care for patients afflicted with AIDS. About 20 years ago, he developed a unique program in which Brown University faculty assumed the care for all persons living with HIV/AIDS in the Rhode Island prison system.

Chuck is an exceptional teacher recognized, among other ways, by the Distinguished Teacher Award from the American College of Physicians. He is a superb clinician versed in all aspects of Internal Medicine. He has therefore been honored as a Master of the American College of Physicians, and has received more encomia than virtually anyone in academic medicine.

It has been my genuine privilege to work with Chuck Carpenter, a dear friend. I know I speak for all of the Editors when I say that we will miss you, Chuck, and that replacing you with an individual having your assets and talents will be a singularly difficult task.

Thomas E. Andreoli

Editor-in-Chief

Lead Authors and Contributors

Section I: Introduction to Molecular Medicine

Lead Author
Ivor J. Benjamin, M.D.
Professor of Medicine
Christi T. Smith Chair for Cardiovascular Research
Chief, Division of Cardiology
University of Utah School of Medicine
Salt Lake City, Utah
ivor.benjamin@hsc.utah.edu

Section II: Evidence-Based Medicine

Lead Author
Susan S. Beland, M.D.
Associate Professor of Internal Medicine
Director, Division of General Internal Medicine
University of Arkansas College of Medicine
Little Rock, Arkansas
BelandSusanS@uams.edu

Contributor
Sara G. Tariq, M.D.
Assistant Professor of Medicine
Division of General Internal Medicine
University of Arkansas for Medical Sciences
Little Rock, Arkansas
TariqSaraG@uams.edu

Section III: Cardiovascular Disease

Lead Author
Ivor J. Benjamin, M.D.
Professor of Medicine
Christi T. Smith Chair for Cardiovascular Research
Chief, Division of Cardiology
University of Utah School of Medicine
Salt Lake City, Utah
ivor.benjamin@hsc.utah.edu

Contributors
David A. Bull, M.D.
Professor
Division of Cardiothoracic Surgery
University of Utah School of Medicine
Salt Lake City, Utah
Bull@hsc.utah.edu

Saurabh Gupta, M.D.
Division of Cardiology
University of Utah School of Medicine
Salt Lake City, Utah
Saurabh.Gupta@hsc.utah.edu

Mohamed H. Hamdan, M.D.
Associate Chief, Division of Cardiology
Professor of Internal Medicine
Division of Cardiology
University of Utah Health Sciences Center
Nora Eccles Harrison Cardiovascular Research and
Training Institute
University of Utah
Salt Lake City, Utah
Mohamed.Hamdan@hsc.utah.edu

L. David Hillis, M.D.
Professor and Vice Chair
James M. Wooten Chair in Cardiology
Department of Internal Medicine
University of Texas Southwestern Medical Center
Dallas, Texas
leslie.hillis@utsouthwestern.edu

Richard A. Lange, M.D.
E. Cowles Andrus Professor of Cardiology
Chief, Clinical Cardiology
Department of Medicine–Cardiology
Johns Hopkins University
School of Medicine
Baltimore, Maryland
rlange3@jhmi.edu

Dean Y. Li, M.D., Ph.D.
Associate Professor of Internal Medicine
University of Utah School of Medicine
Director, Vascular Biotherapeutics Center
University of Utah
Salt Lake City, Utah
dean.li@hhmbh.utah.edu

Sheldon E. Litwin, M.D.
Professor of Internal Medicine
Director of Cardiac Imaging
Division of Cardiology
University of Utah
Salt Lake City, Utah
Sheldon.Litwin@hsc.utah.edu

Christopher J. McGann, M.D.
Assistant Professor of Cardiology
Division of Cardiology
University of Utah School of Medicine
Salt Lake City, Utah
chris.mcgann@hsc.utah.edu

Ronald G. Victor, M.D.
Professor of Internal Medicine
Division of Hypertension
University of Texas Southwestern Medical Center
at Dallas
Dallas, Texas
Ronald.Victor@UTSouthwestern.edu

Wanpen Vongpatanasin, M.D.
Associate Professor of Internal Medicine
The University of Texas Southwestern Medical Center
at Dallas
Dallas, Texas
Vongpatanasin@UTSouthwestern.edu

Kevin J. Whitehead, M.D.
Assistant Professor
Division of Cardiology
University of Utah School of Medicine
Salt Lake City, Utah
Kevin.whitehead@hsc.utah.edu

Section IV: Pulmonary and Critical Care Medicine

Lead Author
Kenneth L. Brigham, M.D.
Professor of Medicine
Vice-Chairman for Research, Department of Medicine
Director, Center for Translational Research in the Lung
Associate Director for Research, McKelvey Lung
Transplantation Center
Emory University School of Medicine
Whitehead Biomedical Building
Emory University School of Medicine
Atlanta, Georgia
kbrigha@Emory.edu

Contributors
Jesse Roman, M.D.
Associate Professor
Department of Medicine Division
Director, Pulmonary, Allergy and Critical Care Medicine
Emory University School of Medicine
Atlanta, Georgia
jroman@emory.edu

Bonnie S. Slovis, M.D., M.S.H.S.
Assistant Professor of Medicine
Department of Medicine, Division of Allergy,
Pulmonology, and Critical Care
Vanderbilt University
Director, Pulmonology Patient Care Center
Vanderbilt University Medical Center
Nashville, Tennessee
bonnie.slovis@vanderbilt.edu

Section V: Renal Disease

Lead Author
Sudhir V. Shah, M.D.
Professor of Internal Medicine
Director, Division of Nephrology
University of Arkansas College of Medicine
Little Rock, Arkansas
ShahSudhirV@uams.edu

Contributors
Sameh R. Abul-Ezz, M.D.
Associate Professor of Internal Medicine
Division of Nephrology
University of Arkansas College of Medicine
Little Rock, Arkansas
AbulezzSamehR@uams.edu

Muhammad G. Alam, M.D.
Assistant Professor of Medicine
UAMS Division of Nephrology
University of Arkansas for Medical Sciences
Little Rock, Arkansas
alammuhammadg@uams.edu

Thomas E. Andreoli, M.D.
Distinguished Professor
Department of Internal Medicine
Department of Physiology and Biophysics
University of Arkansas College of Medicine
Little Rock, Arkansas
AndreoliThomasE@uams.edu

Michelle W. Krause, M.D.
Assistant Professor
Department of Internal Medicine
University of Arkansas for Medical Sciences
Little Rock, Arkansas
KrauseMichelleW@uams.edu

Jayant Kumar, M.D.
Assistant Professor of Medicine
UAMS Division of Nephrology
University of Arkansas for Medical Sciences
Little Rock, Arkansas
kumarjayant@uams.edu

Didier Portilla, M.D.
Associate Professor of Medicine
Department of Internal Medicine
University Hospital
Internal Medicine-Nephrology
University of Arkansas for Medical Sciences
Staff Physician, Internal Medicine and Nephrology
Central Arkansas Veterans Hospital
Little Rock, Arkansas
portilladidier@uams.edu

Robert L. Safirstein, M.D.
Vice Chairman of Internal Medicine
University of Arkansas for Medical Sciences
Little Rock, Arkansas
SafirsteinRobertL@uams.edu

Patrick D. Walker, M.D.
Professor of Pathology
University of Arkansas for Medical Sciences
Director, Neuropathology Associates
Little Rock, Arkansas
walkerpd@kidneybx.com

Section VI: Gastrointestinal Disease

Lead Author
M. Michael Wolfe, M.D.
Professor of Medicine
Director, Division of Gastroenterology
Boston University School of Medicine
Boston, Massachusetts
michael.wolfe@bmc.org

Contributors
Charles M. Bliss, Jr., M.D.
Assistant Professor of Medicine
Boston University Medical School
Staff Physician, Medicine/Gastroenterology
Boston Medical Center
Boston, Massachusetts
charles.bliss@bmc.org

Francis A. Farraye, M.D.
Associate Professor of Medicine and Epidemiology
Boston University School of Medicine
Boston, Massachusetts
charles.bliss@bmc.org

Christopher S. Huang, M.D.
Instructor of Medicine
Boston University School of Medicine
Boston, Massachusetts
cshuang@bu.edu

Brian C. Jacobson, M.D., M.P.H.
Assistant Professor of Medicine
Associate Director of Endoscopy
Gastroenterology Section
Boston University Medical Center
Boston, Massachusetts
brian.jacobson@bmc.org

David R. Lichtenstein, M.D.
Brigham & Women's Hospital
Boston, Massachusetts
davidL@bu.edu

Robert C. Lowe, M.D.
Boston Medical Center
Section of Gastroenterology
Boston, Massachusetts
RoLowe@bu.edu

Daniel S. Mishkin, M.D., C.M.
Instructor of Medicine
Boston University School of Medicine
Boston, Massachusetts
damishki@bu.edu

Jaime A. Oviedo, M.D.
Instructor of Medicine, Section of Gastroenterology
Boston University School of Medicine
Boston Medical Center
Boston, Massachusetts
JOviedo@bu.edu

Lawrence J. Saubermann, M.D.
Assistant Professor of Medicine and Staff Physician
Department of Gastroenterology
Boston University Medical Center
Boston, Massachusetts
Lawrence.saubermann@bmc.org

Elihu M. Schimmel, M.D.
Professor of Medicine
Boston University School of Medicine
Staff Physician, Gastroenterology
VA Boston Healthcare System
Boston, Massachusetts
Elihu.schimmel@med.va.gov

Paul C. Schroy III, M.D., M.P.H.
Associate Professor of Medicine
Boston University School of Medicine
Director, Clinical Research
Section of Gastroenterology
Boston Medical Center
Boston, Massachusetts
pschroy@bu.edu

Satish K. Singh, M.D.
Boston University School of Medicine
Department of Medicine
Boston, Massachusetts
singhsk@bu.edu

Chi-Chuan Tseng, M.D.
Associate Professor of Medicine
Boston University School of Medicine
Boston, Massachusetts
ethan@bu.edu

Section VII: Diseases of the Liver and Biliary System

Lead Author
Michael B. Fallon, M.D.
Associate Professor of Medicine
Division of Gastroenterology and Hepatology
University of Alabama School of Medicine
Birmingham, Alabama
mfallon@uab.edu

Contributors
Gary A. Abrams, M.D.
UAB Liver Center
Department of Medicine
University of Alabama at Birmingham
Birmingham, Alabama
gabrams@uab.edu

Miguel R. Arguedas, M.D.
UAB Liver Center
Department of Medicine
University of Alabama at Birmingham
Birmingham, Alabama
Arguedas@uab.edu

Joseph R. Bloomer, M.D.
Department of Medicine
University of Alabama at Birmingham
Birmingham, Alabama
jbloomer@uab.edu

Rudolf Garcia-Gallont, M.D.
Hospital Roosevelt
Guatemala City, Guatemala

Brendan M. McGuire, M.D.
UAB Liver Center
Department of Medicine
University of Alabama at Birmingham
Birmingham, Alabama
bmcguire@uab.edu

Aasim M. Sheikh, M.D.
Assistant Professor
UAB Liver Center
Department of Medicine
University of Alabama at Birmingham
Birmingham, Alabama
asheikh@uab.edu

Shyam Varadarajulu, M.D.
Assistant Professor of Medicine
University of Alabama at Birmingham
School of Medicine
Birmingham, Alabama
svaradar@uabmc.edu

Section VIII: Hematologic Disease

Lead Author
Nancy Berliner, M.D.
Arthur and Isabel Bunker Associate Professor of
Medicine and Genetics
Yale University School of Medicine
New Haven, Connecticut
Nancy.Berliner@yale.edu

Contributors
Jill Lacy, M.D.
UAMS Division of Nephrology
University of Arkansas for Medical Sciences
Little Rock, Arkansas
Jill.Lacy@yale.edu

Henry M. Rinder, M.D.
Associate Professor
Department of Laboratory Medicine and Internal
Medicine (Hematology)
Yale University
New Haven, Connecticut
henry.rinder@yale.edu

Michal G. Rose, M.D.
Assistant Professor
Medical Oncology
Yale Cancer Center
New Haven, Connecticut
Michal.Rose@yale.edu

Stuart Seropian, M.D.
Department of Internal Medicine and Oncology
Yale University School of Medicine
New Haven, Connecticut
stuart.seropian@yale.edu

Richard Torres, M.D.
Department of Laboratory Medicine
Yale University School of Medicine
New Haven, Connecticut
Richard.Torres@yale.edu

Eunice S. Wang, M.D.
Research Assistant Professor, Leukemia Service
Departments of Medicine and Immunology
Roswell Park Cancer Institute
New York, New York
Eunice.Wang@roswellpark.org

Section IX: Oncologic Disease

Lead Authors
Christopher E. Desch, M.D.[†]
Virginia Cancer Institute
Richmond, Virginia
CDESCH@aol.com
cdesch@gems.vcu.edu

Jennifer J. Griggs, M.D.
University of Michigan
Ann Arbor, Michigan
jengrigg@med.umich.edu

Contributors
Barbara A. Burtness, M.D.
Medical Science Division
Fox Chase Cancer Center
Philadelphia, Pennsylvania
Barbara.Burtness@fccc.edu

Alok A. Khorana, M.D.
Assistant Professor of Medicine
James P. Wilmot Cancer Center
University of Rochester
Rochester, New York
alok_khorana@urmc.rochester.edu

Section X: Metabolic Disease

Lead Author
Reed E. Pyeritz, M.D., Ph.D.
Professor of Medicine
Chief, Division of Medical Genetics
University of Pennsylvania School of Medicine
Philadelphia, Pennsylvania
reed.pyeritz@uphs.upenn.edu

[†]deceased

Contributor
David G. Brooks, M.D., Ph.D.
Medical Genetics Division
Maloney Building
University of Pennsylvania
Philadelphia, Pennsylvania
david.brooks@merck.com

Section XI: Endocrine Disease

Lead Author
Glenn D. Braunstein, M.D.
Professor of Medicine
UCLA School of Medicine
Chair, Department of Medicine
Cedars-Sinai Medical Center
Los Angeles, California
braunstein@cshs.org

Contributors
Philip S. Barnett, M.D., Ph.D.
Cedars-Sinai Medical Center
Pituitary Center
Los Angeles, California
Philip.Barnett@cshs.org

Theodore C. Friedman, M.D.
Department of Endocrinology
Cedars-Sinai Medical Center
Los Angeles, California
friedmantc@csmc.edu

Vivien S. Herman-Bonert, M.D.
Associate Clinical Professor
Clinical Coordinator
UCLA School of Medicine
Los Angeles, California
vivien.bonert@cshs.org
bonertv@cshs.org

Section XII: Women's Health

Lead Author
Anne L. Taylor, M.D.
Professor of Medicine
Associate Dean for Faculty Affairs
University of Minnesota School of Medicine
Minneapolis, Minnesota
Taylo135@umn.edu

Contributors
Sharon S. Allen, M.D., Ph.D.
Professor
Department of Family Medicine and Community Health
University of Minnesota Cancer Center
Minneapolis, Minnesota
allen001@umn.edu

Karyn D. Baum, M.D.
Associate Professor of Medicine
University of Minnesota Medical School
Minneapolis, Minnesota
kbaum@umn.edu

Sally L. Hodder, M.D.
Executive Vice Chair, Department of Medicine
Professor of Medicine
Division of Infectious Disease
University of Medicine & Dentistry of New Jersey
Newark, New Jersey
hoddersa@umdnj.edu

Nancy L. Raymond, M.D.
Associate Professor
Department of Psychiatry
University of Minnesota
Minneapolis, Minnesota
raymo002@umn.edu

Section XIII: Men's Health

Lead Author
Joseph A. Smith, Jr., M.D.
Professor and Chair
Department of Urologic Surgery
Vanderbilt University School of Medicine
Nashville, Tennessee
joseph.smith@mcmail.vanderbilt.edu

Contributors
Douglas F. Milam, M.D.
Associate Professor of Urologic Surgery
Department of Urologic Surgery
Vanderbilt Medical Center
Vanderbilt University
Nashville, Tennessee
doug.milam@vanderbilt.edu

Jonathan S. Starkman, M.D.
Instructor of Urologic Surgery
Vanderbilt University School of Medicine
Nashville, Tennessee
jonathan.s.starkman@vanderbilt.edu

Section XIV: Diseases of Bone and Bone Mineral Metabolism

Lead Author
Andrew F. Stewart, M.D.
Professor of Medicine
Chief, Division of Endocrinology and Metabolism
University of Pittsburgh School of Medicine
Pittsburgh, Pennsylvania
stewarta@pitt.edu

Contributors
Susan L. Greenspan, M.D.
Professor of Medicine
University of Pittsburgh
Pittsburgh, Pennsylvania
greenspans@msx.dept-med.pitt.edu

Mara J. Horwitz, M.D.
University of Pittsburgh
Division of Endocrionology
Pittsburgh, Pennsylvania
Horwitz@pitt.edu

G. David Roodman, M.D., Ph.D.
University of Pittsburgh
Division of Endocrinology
Pittsburgh, Pennsylvania
roodmangd@msx.upmc.edu

Section XV: Musculoskeletal and Connective Tissue Disease

Lead Author
Robert W. Simms, M.D.
Associate Professor of Medicine
Arthritis Center
Boston University School of Medicine
Boston, Massachusetts
rsimms@bu.edu

Contributor
Peter A. Merkel, M.D., M.P.H.
Massachusetts General Hospital
Arthritis Unit
Boston, Massachusetts
pmerkel@bu.edu

Section XVI: Infectious Disease

Lead Author
Charles C.J. Carpenter, M.D.
Professor of Medicine
Brown University School of Medicine
Director, Lifespan/Tufts/Brown Center for AIDS Research
The Miriam Hospital
Providence, Rhode Island
ccjc@lifespan.org

Contributors
Keith B. Armitage, M.D.
Associate Professor of Medicine
Division of Infectious Diseases
Case Western Reserve University
University Hospitals of Cleveland
Cleveland, Ohio
keith.armitage@case.edu

Curt G. Beckwith, M.D.
Assistant Professor of Medicine
Division of Infectious Diseases
Brown Medical School
Providence, Rhode Island
cbeckwith@lifespan.org

David B. Blossom, M.D.
Division of Infectious Disease
Case Western Reserve University
School of Medicine
Cleveland, Ohio
David_Blossom@hotmail.com

David A. Bobak, M.D.
Associate Professor of Medicine
Division of Infectious Diseases
Case Western Reserve University
University Hospitals of Cleveland
Cleveland, Ohio
david.bobak@case.edu

Scott A. Fulton, M.D.
Assistant Professor of Medicine
Division of Infectious Diseases
Case Western Reserve University
University Hospitals of Cleveland
Cleveland, Ohio
sxf24@case.edu

Christoph Lange, M.D.
Head of Clinical Infectious Diseases
Medical Clinic of Borstel Research Center
Borstel, Germany
clange@fz-borstel.de

Michael M. Lederman, M.D.
Scott R. Inkley Professor of Medicine
Director, Center for AIDS Research
Case Western Reserve University
Cleveland, Ohio
lederman.michael@clevelandactu.org

Michelle V. Lisgaris, M.D.
Assistant Professor of Medicine
Division of Infectious Diseases
Case Western Reserve University
University Hospitals of Cleveland
Cleveland, Ohio
mvl@case.edu

Benigno Rodríguez, M.D.
Assistant Professor of Medicine
Case Western Reserve University
Cleveland, Ohio
rodriguez.benigno@clevelandactu.org

Robert A. Salata, M.D.
Professor and Vice-Chair
Department of Medicine
Chief, Division of Infectious Diseases
Case Western Reserve University
University Hospitals of Cleveland
Cleveland, Ohio
ras7@case.edu

Gopala K. Yadavalli, M.D.
Assistant Professor of Medicine
Division of Infectious Diseases
Case Western Reserve University
Louis B. Stokes VAMC
Cleveland, Ohio
gxy6@case.edu
gopala.yadavalli@case.edu

Section XVII: Bioterrorism

Lead Author
Robert W. Bradsher, Jr., M.D.
Professor and Vice-Chair for Education
Department of Internal Medicine
Director, Division of Infectious Diseases
University of Arkansas College of Medicine
Little Rock, Arkansas
BradsherRobertW@uams.edu

Section XVIII: Neurologic Disease

Lead Author
Robert C. Griggs, M.D.
Edward A. and Alma Vollertsen Rykenboer Professor of
Neurophysiology
Chair, Department of Neurology
University of Rochester School of Medicine and Dentistry
Rochester, New York
Robert_Griggs@urmc.Rochester.edu

Contributors
Timothy J. Counihan, M.D., M.R.C.P.I.
Assistant Professor of Neurology
University of Rochester School of Medicine and Dentistry
Rochester, New York
timothy_counihan@urmc.rochester.edu

Jennifer J. Griggs, M.D.
University of Michigan
Ann Arbor, Michigan
jengrigg@med.umich.edu

Frederick J. Marshall, M.D.
Assistant Professor of Neurology
University of Rochester School of Medicine and Dentistry
Attending Physician, Neurology
Strong Memorial Hospital
Chief, Geriatric Neurology Unit
Montroe Community Hospital
Rochester, New York
fmarshall@mct.rochester.edu

Roger P. Simon, M.D.
Graduate Faculty
Department of Molecular and Cell Biology
Oregon State University
Director and Robert Stone Dow Chair of Neurobiology
Research
RS Dow Neurobiology Laboratories
Legacy Research
Portland, Oregon
rsimon@downeurobiology.org

Maria J. Sunseri, M.D.
Assistant Professor of Neurology
University of Pittsburgh
Pittsburgh, Pennsylvania
mjsunseri@msn.com

Section XIX: The Aging Patient

Lead Author
Hal H. Atkinson, M.D.
Assistant Professor of Internal Medicine
Sticht Center on Aging
Medical Director, Acute Care for the Elderly Unit
Program Director, Geriatric Fellowship Training
Wake Forest University School of Medicine
Winston-Salem, North Carolina
hatkinso@wfubmc.edu

Contributor
Leslie E. Sutton, M.D.
Wake Forest University
School of Medicine
Winston-Salem, North Carolina
lsutton@wfubmc.edu

Section XX: Substance Abuse

Lead Author
L. David Hillis, M.D.
Professor of Internal Medicine
Division of Cardiology
University of Texas Southwestern Medical School
Dallas, Texas
Leslie.Hillis@utsouthwestern.edu

Contributor
Richard A. Lange, M.D.
E. Cowles Andrus Professor of Cardiology
Chief, Clinical Cardiology
Department of Medicine-Cardiology
Johns Hopkins University
School of Medicine
Baltimore, Maryland
rlange3@jhmi.edu

Preface

This Seventh Edition of *Andreoli and Carpenter's Cecil Essentials of Medicine* retains the fundamental nature of *Essentials*, that is, to provide a concise but comprehensive and fully updated treatise on medicine for students of medicine at all levels of their careers. But *Essentials* has also undergone significant transformations in the Seventh Edition.

This is Dr. Carpenter's last term as Editor. Chuck was one of the founding Editors and this Seventh Edition is therefore dedicated to him. The Dedication speaks for itself. Second, Joseph Loscalzo has rotated off the Board of Editors, being replaced by a towering figure in Cardiology and Molecular Biology, Ivor J. Benjamin, M.D., F.A.C.C., F.A.H.A., Professor of Medicine, the Christi T. Smith Chair for Cardiovascular Research, and Chief of the Division of Cardiology at the University of Utah School of Medicine.

As noted above, the goals of the book are to be current, to be compact, and to be understandable by students of medicine of all ages. This new Edition takes advantage of computer-based technology to augment the hard copy Edition of the book. The book will remain an entity in its own right; the same version of the book will also appear, *in toto*, on the Internet.

At the same time, we wish to provide extensive supplementary material on the Internet version of the book, from which the readers will, we hope, benefit substantially. As an example, in Section V, Renal Disease, Chapter 28, Glomerular Diseases, in the text one will find in color the symbol (**Web Figs. 1-27**). The icon, which will be present both in the hard copy of the book as well as on the Internet version, will direct the reader to a series of illustrations (**Web Figs. 1-27**) of the glomerulopathies in the Internet version of *Essentials*. The Editors believe that this kind of material is central to understanding modern medicine, but space limitations constrain inserting all of the material in the text. The Web figures in *Essentials VII* contain abundant examples of this kind of supplementary material, including heart sounds, bronchoscopy videos, gastrointestinal endoscopy studies, and movement disorders. It is our hope that, in this manner, the supplemental material will enrich the amount of information available to readers of *Essentials*, without having enlarged the book significantly.

Finally, as in previous Editions, the book makes abundant use of four-color illustrations, tabular material, and, particularly, algorithms for evaluating the functions of different systems and the diseases of those systems. And as in prior Editions, the material in *Essentials* has been updated thoroughly and reviewed extensively by all of the Editors.

We thank James T. Merritt, Senior Acquisitions Editor, Medical Education, of Elsevier, Inc., and particularly, Rebecca Gruliow, Managing Editor, Global Medicine, Elsevier, Inc. Both Jim and Rebecca contributed, in a very significant way, to the concepts, design and preparation of the Seventh Edition of *Essentials*. Finally, we thank our very able secretarial staff, Ms. Clementine M. Whitman (Little Rock); Ms. Barbara S. Bottone (Providence); Ms. Shirley E. Thomas (Rochester); and Ms. Linda J. Moore (Salt Lake City).

The Editors

Contents

Section I

Introduction to Molecular Medicine

Cecil

Andreoli and Carpenter's
Essentials of Medicine

Molecular Basis of Human Disease

Ivor J. Benjamin

Medicine has evolved dramatically over the last century from a healing art in which standards of practice were established on the basis of personal experience, passed on from one practitioner to the next, to a rigorous intellectual discipline steeped in the scientific method. The scientific method, a process that tests the validity of a hypothesis or prediction through experimentation, has led to major advances in the fields of physiology, microbiology, biochemistry, and pharmacology. These advances served as the basis for the diagnostic and therapeutic approaches to illness in common use by physicians through most of the twentieth century. Since the 1980s, the understanding of the molecular basis of genetics has expanded dramatically, and advances in this field have identified new and exciting dimensions for defining the basis of *conventional* genetic diseases (e.g., sickle cell disease), as well as the basis of complex genetic traits (e.g., hypertension). The molecular basis for the interaction between genes and environment has also begun to be defined. Armed with a variety of sensitive and specific molecular techniques, contemporary physicians can now begin not only to understand the molecular underpinning of complex pathobiologic processes, but they can also identify individuals at risk for common diseases. Understanding modern medicine therefore requires an understanding of molecular genetics and the molecular basis of disease. This introductory chapter offers an overview of this complex and rapidly evolving topic and attempts to summarize the principles of molecular medicine that will be highlighted in specific sections throughout this text.

Deoxyribonucleic Acid and the Genome

All organisms possess a scheme to transmit the essential information of the species through successive generations. A double-stranded, linear polymer of deoxyribonucleic acid (DNA) that constitutes the genome of the organism encodes this information. In the human genome, approximately 6×10^9 nucleotides, or 3×10^9 pairs of nucleotides, associate in the double helix. All of the specificity of DNA is determined by the base sequence, and this sequence is stored in complementary form in the double-helical structure, which facilitates correction of sequence errors and provides a mechanistic basis for replication of the information during cell division. Each DNA strand serves as a template for replication, which is accomplished by the action of DNA-dependent DNA polymerases that unwind the double-helical DNA and copy each single strand with remarkable fidelity.

In human cells, 23 pairs of chromosomes are present, each pair of which contains a unique sequence and therefore unique genetic information. All cell types except for gametocytes contain this duplicate, diploid number of genetic units, one half of which is referred to as a *haploid number*. The genetic information contained in chromosomes is separated into discrete functional elements known as *genes*. A gene is defined as a unit of base sequence that usually encodes a specific polypeptide sequence. New evidence suggests that small, noncoding RNAs play critical roles in expression of this essential information. An estimated 30,000 genes are present in the human haploid genome, and these are interspersed among regions of sequence that do not code for protein and whose function is as yet unknown. For example, non-coding RNAs (e.g., tRNA, rRNA, other small RNAs) act as components of enzyme complexes such as the ribosome and spliceosome. The average chromosome contains 3000 to 5000 genes, and these range in size from approximately 1 kilobase (kb) to 2 Mb.

Ribonucleic Acid Synthesis

Transcription, or ribonucleic acid (RNA) synthesis, is the process for transferring information contained in nuclear DNA to an intermediate molecular species known as messenger ribonucleic acid (mRNA) (**Web Fig. 1–1**). Two biochemical differences distinguish RNA from DNA: (1) the polymeric backbone is made up of ribose rather than deoxyribose sugars linked by phosphodiester bonds, and (2)

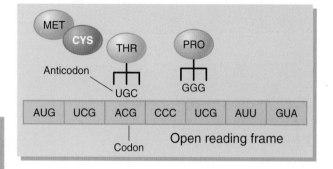

Figure 1–1 Transcription. Genomic DNA is shown with enhancer and silencer sites located 5′ upstream of the promoter region, to which RNA polymerase is bound. The transcription start site is shown downstream of the promoter region, and this site is followed by exonic sequences interrupted by intronic sequences. The former sequences are transcribed *ad seriatim* (i.e., one after another) by the RNA polymerase.

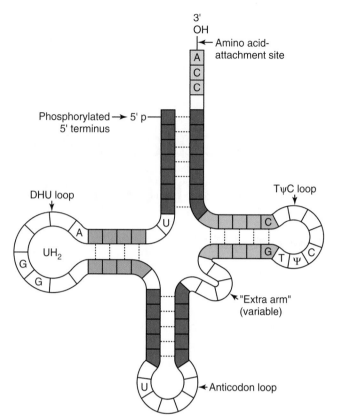

Figure 1–2 Translation. The open-reading frame of a mature mRNA is shown with its series of codons. tRNA molecules are shown with their corresponding anticodons, charged with their specific amino acid. A short, growing polypeptide chain is depicted. A = adenine; C = cytosine; CYS = cysteine; G = guanine; MET = methionine; PRO = proline; THR = threonine; U = uracil.

the base composition is different in that uracil is substituted for thymine. RNA synthesis from a DNA template is performed by three types of DNA-dependent RNA polymerases, each a multisubunit complex with distinct nuclear location and substrate specificity. RNA polymerase I, located in the nucleolus, directs the transcription of genes encoding the 18S, 5.8S, and 28S ribosomal RNAs, forming a molecular scaffold with both catalytic and structural functions within the ribosome. RNA polymerase II, located in the nucleoplasm instead of the nucleoli, primarily transcribes precursor mRNA transcripts and small RNA molecules. The carboxyl-terminus of RNA polymerase II is uniquely modified with a 220-kd protein domain, the site of enzymatic regulation by protein phosphorylation of critical serine and threonine residues. All transfer RNA (tRNA) precursors and other ribosomal RNA (rRNA) molecules are synthesized by RNA polymerase III in the nucleoplasm.

RNA polymerases are synthesized from precursor transcripts that must first be cleaved into subunits before further processing and assembling with ribosomal proteins into macromolecular complexes. Ribosomal architectural and structural integrity is derived from the secondary and tertiary structures of rRNA, which assume a series of folding patterns containing short duplex regions. Precursors of tRNA in the nucleus undergo the removal of the 5′ leader region, splicing of an internal intron sequences, and modification of terminal residues.

Precursors of mRNA are produced in the nucleus by the action of DNA-dependent RNA polymerase II, which copies the *antisense* strand of the DNA double helix to synthesize a single strand of mRNA that is identical to the *sense* strand of the DNA double helix in a process called *transcription* (Fig. 1–1). The initial, immature mRNA first undergoes modification at both the 5′ and 3′ ends. A special nucleotide structure called the *cap* is added to the 5′ end, which functions to increase binding to the ribosome and enhance translational efficiency. The 3′ end undergoes modification by nuclease cleavage of approximately 20 nucleotides, followed by the addition of a length of polynucleotide sequence containing a uniform stretch of adenine bases, the so-called poly A tail that stabilizes the mRNA.

In addition to these changes that uniformly occur in all mRNAs, other more selective modifications can also occur. Because each gene contains both exonic and intronic sequences and the precursor mRNA is transcribed without regard for exon-intron boundaries, this immature message must be edited in such a way that splices all exons together in appropriate sequence. The process of splicing, or removing intronic sequences to produce the mature mRNA, is an exquisitely choreographed event that involves the intermediate formation of a spliceosome, a large complex consisting of small nuclear RNAs and specific proteins, which contains a loop or lariat-like structure that includes the intron targeted for removal. Only after splicing, a catalytic process requiring ATP hydrolysis, has concluded is the mature mRNA able to transit from the nucleus into the cytoplasm, where the encoded information is translated into protein.

Alternative splicing is a process for efficiently generating multiple gene products often dictated by tissue specificity, developmental expression, and pathologic state. Gene splicing allows the expression of multiple isoforms by expanding the repertoire for molecular diversity. An estimated 30% of genetic diseases in humans arise from defects in splicing. The resulting mature mRNA then exits the nucleus to begin the process of *translation* or conversion of the base code to polypeptide (Fig. 1–2). Alternative splicing pathways (i.e.,

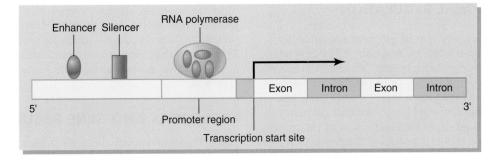

Figure 1–3 Secondary structure of tRNA. The structure of each tRNA serves as an adapter molecule that recognizes a specific codon for the amino acid to be added to the polypeptide chain. About one half the hydrogen-bonded bases of the single chain of ribonucleotides are shown paired in double helices like a cloverleaf. The 5' terminus is phosphorylated, and the 3' terminus contains the hydroxyl group on an attached amino acid. The anticodon loop is typically located in the middle of the tRNA molecule. UH$_2$ = dihydrouridine; ψ = pseudouridine; U = uracil; G = guanine; C = cytocide; T = ribothymidine. (Modified from Berg JM, Tymoczko JL, and Strayer JL: Berg, Tymoczko and Stryer's Biochemistry, 5th ed, New York: WH Freeman Co., 2006)

alternative exonic assembly pathways) for specific genes also serve at the level of transcriptional regulation. The discovery of catalytic RNA, the capacity for self-directed internal excision and repair, has advanced the current view that RNA per se serves both as a template for translation of the genetic code and, simultaneously, as an enzyme (please see section on "Transcription Regulation" later in this chapter).

Protein synthesis, or translation of the mRNA code, occurs on ribosomes, which are macromolecular complexes of proteins and rRNA located in the cytoplasm. Translation involves the conversion of the linear code of a triplet of bases (i.e., the codon) into the corresponding amino acid. A four-base code generates 64 possible triplet combinations ($4 \times 4 \times 4$), and these correspond to 20 different amino acids, many of which are encoded by more than one base triplet. To decode mRNA, an adapter molecule (tRNA) recognizes the codon in mRNA via complementary base pairing with a three-base anticodon that it bears; in addition, each tRNA is charged with a unique amino acid that corresponds to the anticodon (Fig. 1–3).

Translation on the mRNA template proceeds without punctuation of the nonoverlapping code with the aid of rRNA on an assembly machine, termed *ribosomes*–essentially a polypeptide polymerase. At least one tRNA molecule exists for each 20 amino acids, although degeneracy in the code expands the number of available tRNA molecules, mitigates the chances of premature chain termination, and ameliorates the potential deleterious consequences of single-base mutations. The enzymatic activity of the ribosome then links amino acids through the synthesis of a peptide bond, releasing the tRNA in the process (**Web Fig. 1–2**).

Consecutive linkage of amino acids in the growing polypeptide chain represents the terminal event in the conversion of information contained within the nuclear DNA sequence into mature protein (DNA → RNA → protein). Proteins are directly responsible for the form and function of an organism. Thus, abnormalities in protein structure or function brought about by changes in primary amino acid sequence are the immediate precedent cause of changes in phenotype, adverse forms of which define a disease state.

Inhibition of RNA synthesis is a well-recognized mechanism of specific toxins and antibiotics. Toxicity from the ingestion of the poisonous mushroom (*Amanita phalloides*), for example, leads to the release of the toxin α-amanitin, a cyclic octapeptide that inhibits the RNA Pol lI and blocks elongation of RNA synthesis. The antibiotic actinomycin D binds with high affinity to double-helical DNA and intercolates between base pairs, precluding access of DNA-dependent RNA polymerases and the selective inhibition of transcription. Several major antibiotics function through inhibition of translation. For example, the aminoglycoside antibiotics function through the disruption of the mRNA-tRNA codon–anticodon interaction, whereas erythromycin and chloramphenicol inhibit peptide bond formation.

Control of Gene Expression
OVERVIEW

The timing, duration, localization, and magnitude of gene expression are all important elements in the complex tapestry of cell form and function governed by the genome. Gene expression represents the flow of information from the DNA template into mRNA transcripts and the process of translation into mature protein.

Four levels of organization involving transcription factors, RNAs, chromatin structure, and epigenetic factors are increasingly recognized to orchestrate gene expression in the mammalian genome. Transcriptional regulators bind to specific DNA motifs that positively or negatively control the expression of neighboring genes. The information contained in the genome must be transformed into functional units of either RNA or protein products. How DNA is packed and modified represents additional modes of gene regulation by disrupting the access of transcription factors from DNA-binding motifs. In the postgenomic era, the challenge is to understand the architecture by which the genome is organized, controlled, and modulated.

Transcription factors, chromatin architecture, and modifications of nucleosomal organization make up the major mechanisms of gene regulation in the genome.

TRANSCRIPTIONAL REGULATION

The principal regulatory step in gene expression occurs at the level of gene transcription. A specific DNA-dependent RNA polymerase performs the transcription of information contained in genomic DNA into mRNA transcripts. Transcription begins at a proximal (i.e., toward the 5′ end of the gene) transcription start site, containing nucleotide sequences that influence the rate and extent of the process (see Fig. 1–1). This region is known as the *promoter region* of the gene and often includes both an element of sequence rich in adenine and thymine (the TATA box) and other sequence motifs within approximately 100 bases of the start site. These regions of DNA that regulate transcription are known as *cis*-acting regulatory elements. Some of these regulatory regions of promoter sequence bind proteins known as *trans*-acting factors, or transcription factors, which are themselves encoded by other genes. The *cis*-acting regulatory sequences to which transcription factors bind are often referred to as *response elements*. Families of transcription factors have been identified and are often described by unique aspects of their predicted protein secondary structure, including helix-turn-helix motifs, zinc-finger motifs, and leucine-zipper motifs. Transcription factors make up an estimated 3% to 5% of the protein-coding products of the genome.

In addition to gene-promoter regions, enhancer sites are distinct from promoter sites in that they can exist at distances quite remote from the start site, either upstream or downstream (i.e., beyond the 3′ end of the gene), and without clear orientation requirements. *Trans*-acting factors bind to these enhancer sites and are believed to alter the tertiary structure or conformation of the DNA in a manner that facilitates the binding and assembly of the transcription-initiation complex at the promoter region, perhaps in some cases by forming a broad loop of DNA in the process. Biochemical modification of select promoter or enhancer sequences, such as methylation of CpG-rich sequences, can also modulate transcription; methylation typically suppresses transcription. The terms *silencer* and *suppressor* elements refer to *cis*-acting nucleotide sequences that reduce or shut off gene transcription and do so through association with *trans*-acting factors that recognize these specific sequences.

Regulation of transcription is a complex process that occurs at several levels; importantly, the expression of many genes is regulated to maintain high basal levels, which are known as *housekeeping* or constitutively expressed genes. They typically yield protein products that are essential for normal cell function or survival and thus must be maintained at a specific steady-state concentration under all circumstances. Many other genes, in contrast, are not expressed or are only modestly expressed under basal conditions; however, with the imposition of some stress or exposure of the cell to an agonist that elicits a cellular response distinct from that of the basal state, the expression of these genes is induced or enhanced. For example, the heat shock protein genes encoding *stress proteins* are rapidly induced in response to diverse pathophysiologic stimuli (e.g., oxidative stress, heavy metals, inflammation) in most cells and organisms. The increased heat shock protein expression is complementary to the basal level of heat shock proteins whose functions as molecular chaperones play key roles during protein synthesis to prevent protein misfolding, increase protein translocation, and accelerate protein degradation. These adaptive responses often mediate changes in phenotype that are homeostatically protective to the cell or organism.

MICRORNAS AND GENE REGULATION

Less is currently known about the determinants of translational regulation than is known about transcriptional regulation. The recent discovery and identification of small RNAs (21 to 24 mer), termed *microRNAs* (miRNA), adds further complexity to the regulation of gene expression within the eukaryotic genome. First discovered in worms over 10 years ago, miRNAs are conserved noncoding strands of RNA that bind to the 3′-untranslated regions of target mRNAs, enabling gene silencing of protein expression at the translational level. Gene-encoding miRNAs exhibit tissue-specific expression and are interspersed in regions of the genome unrelated to known genes.

Transcription of miRNAs proceeds in multiple steps from sites under the control of an mRNA promoter. RNA polymerase II transcribes the precursor miRNA, termed *primary miRNA* (primiRNA), containing 5′ caps and 3′ poly (A) tails. In the nucleus, the larger primiRNAs of 70 nucleotides form an internal hairpin loop, embedding its miRNA portion that undergoes recognition and subsequent excision by double stranded RNA-specific ribonuclease, termed *Drosha*. Gene expression is silenced by the affect of miRNA on nascent RNA molecules targeted for degradation (**Web Fig. 1–3**).

Because translation occurs at a fairly invariant rate among all mRNA species, the stability or half-life of a specific mRNA also serves as another point of regulation of gene expression. The 3′-untranslated region of mRNAs contains regions of sequence that dictate the susceptibility of the message to nuclease cleavage and degradation. Stability appears to be sequence specific and, in some cases, dependent on *trans*-acting factors that bind to the mRNA. The mature mRNA contains elements of untranslated sequence at both the 5′ and 3′ ends that can regulate translation.

Beginning in the organism's early development, miRNAs may facilitate much more intricate ways for the regulation of gene expression as have been shown for germ-line production, cell differentiation, proliferation, and organogenesis. Because recent studies have implicated the expression of miRNAs in brain development, cardiac organogenesis, colonic adenocarcinoma, and viral replication, this novel mechanism for gene silencing has potential therapeutic roles for congenital heart defects, viral disease, neurodegeneration, and cancer.

CHROMATIN REMODELING AND GENE REGULATION

Both the size and complexity of the human genome with 23 chromosomes, ranging in size between 50 and 250 megabases (Mb), pose formidable challenges for transcription factors to exert the specificity of DNA-binding properties in gene regulation. Control of gene expression also takes place in diverse types of cells often with exquisite temporal and spatial specificity throughout the life span of the organism. In eukaryotic cells, the genome is highly organized into densely packed nucleic acids DNA- and RNA-protein structures, termed *chromatin*. The building blocks of chromatin are called *histones*, a family of small basic proteins that occupy one half of the mass of the chromosome. Histones derive their basic properties from the high content of basic amino acids, arginine, and lysine. Five major types of histones–H1, H2A, H2B, H3, and H4–have evolved to form complexes with the DNA of the genome. Two pairs each of the four types of histones form a protein core, the histone octomer, which is wrapped by 200 bp of DNA to form the nucleosome (Fig. 1–4). The core proteins within the nucleosomes have protruding amino terminal ends, exposing critical lysine and arginine residues for covalent modification. Further DNA condensation is achieved as higher order structure is imparted on the chromosomes. The nucleosomes are further compacted in layered stacks with a left-handed superhelix resulting in negative supercoils that provide the energy for DNA-strand separation during replication.

Condensation of DNA in chromatin precludes the access of regulatory molecules such as transcription factors. Reversal of chromatin condensation, on the other hand, typically occurs in response to environmental and other developmental signals in a tissue-dependent manner. Relaxation of chromatin structure at promoter sites undergoing active transcription that become susceptible to enzymatic cleavage by nonspecific DNAase I are called *hypersensitive sites*. Transcription factors on promoter sites may gain access by protein-protein interactions to enhancer elements containing tissue-specific proteins at remote sites, several thousand bases away, resulting in transcription activation or repression.

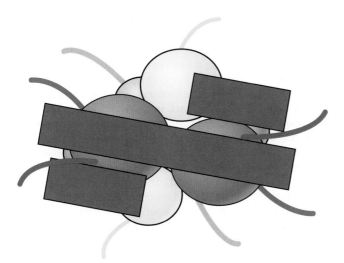

Figure 1–4 Schematic representation of a nucleosome. Rectangular blocks represent the DNA strand wrapped around the core that consists of eight histone proteins. Each histone has a protruding tail that can be modified to repress or activate transcription. (Adapted from Modified from Berg JM, Tymoczko JL, and Strayer JL: Berg, Tymoczko and Stryer's Biochemistry 5th ed, New York: WH Freeman Co., 2006)

EPIGENETIC CONTROL OF GENE EXPRESSION

Complex regulatory networks revolve around transcription factors, nucleosomes, chromatin structure, and epigenetic markings. Epigenetics refers to heritable changes in gene expression without changes in the DNA sequence. Such examples include DNA methylation, gene silencing, chromatin remodeling, and X chromosome inactivation. This form of inheritance involves the alterations in gene function without changes in DNA sequence. Chemical marking of DNA methylation is both cell-specific and developmentally regulated. Methylation of the 5′ CpG dinucleotide by specific methyl transferases, which occurs in 70% of the mammalian genome, is another mechanism of gene regulation. Steric hindrance from the bulky methyl group of 5′ methylcytosine precludes occupancy by transcription factors that stimulate or attenuate gene expression. Most genes are found in CpG islands, reflecting sites of gene activity across the genome.

In an analogous manner, modifications of histone by phosphorylation, methylation, ubiquination, and acetylation are transmitted and reestablished in an inheritable manner. It is conceivable that other epigenetic mechanisms do not involve genomic modifications of DNA. For example, modification of the gene encoding the estrogen receptor α has been implicated in gene silencing at ^{5m}C sites of multiple downstream targets in breast cancer cells. Powerful new approaches are being developed to examine feedback and feed-forward loops in transmission of epigenetic markings.

The concept that dynamic modifications (e.g., DNA methylation and acetylation) of histones or epigenesis contribute, in part, to tumorigenic potential, progression has already been translated into current therapies. Histone acetyltransferases (HATs) and histone deacetyltransferases (HDACs) play antagonistic roles in the addition and removal of acetylation in the genome. Furthermore, genome-wide analysis of HATs and HDACs is beginning to provide important insights into complex modes of gene regulation. Several inhibitors of histone deacetylases, with a range of biochemical and biologic activities, are being developed and tested as anticancer agents in clinical trial. Phase I clinical trials have suggested these drugs are well tolerated. In general, the inhibition of deacetylase remodels chromatin assembly and reactivates transcription of the genome. Because the mechanisms of actions of HDACs extend to apoptosis, cell-cycle control, and cellular differentiation, current clinical trials are seeking to determine the efficacy of these novel reagents in the drug compendium for human cancers.

Genetic Sequence Variation, Population Diversity, and Genetic Polymorphisms

A stable, heritable change in DNA is defined as a *mutation*. This strict contemporary definition does not depend on the functional relevance of the sequence alteration and implicates a change in primary DNA sequence. Considered in historical context, mutations were first defined on the basis of identifiable changes in the heritable phenotype of an organism. As biochemical phenotyping became more precise in the mid-twentieth century, investigators demonstrated that many proteins exist in more than one form in a population, and these forms were viewed as a consequence of variations in the gene coding for that protein (i.e., allelic variation). With advances in DNA-sequencing methods, the concept of mutation evolved from one that could be appreciated only by identifying differences in phenotype to one that could quite precisely be defined at the level of changes in the structure of DNA. Although most mutations are stably transmitted from parents to offspring, some are genetically lethal and thus cannot be passed on. In addition, the discovery of regions of the genome that contain sequences that repeat in tandem a highly variable number of times (tandem repeats) suggests that some mutations are less stable than others. These tandem repeats are further described later in this section.

The molecular nature of mutations is quite varied (Table 1–1). A mutation can involve the deletion, insertion, or substitution of a single base, all of which are referred to may occur as *point mutations.* Substitutions can be further classified as *silent* when the amino acid encoded by the mutated triplet does not change, as *missense* when the amino acid encoded by the mutated triplet changes, and as *nonsense* when the mutation leads to premature termination of translation (stop codon). On occasion, point mutations can alter the processing of precursor mRNA by producing alternate

splice sites or eliminating a splice site. When a single- or double-base deletion or insertion occurs in an exon, a frameshift mutation results, usually leading to premature termination of translation at a now in-frame stop codon. The other end of the spectrum of mutations includes large deletions of an entire gene or a set of contiguous genes; deletion, duplication, and translocation of a segment of one chromosome to another; or duplication or deletion of an entire chromosome. Such chromosomal mutations play a large role in the development of many cancers.

Each individual possesses two alleles for any given gene locus, one from each parent. Identical alleles define homozygosity and nonidentical alleles define heterozygosity for any gene locus. The heritability of these alleles follows typical Mendelian rules. With a clearer understanding of the molecular basis of mutations and of allelic variation, their distribution in populations can now be analyzed quite precisely by following specific DNA sequences. Differences in DNA sequences studied within the context of a population are referred to as *genetic polymorphisms,* and these polymorphisms underlie the diversity observed within a given species and among species.

Despite the high prevalence of benign polymorphisms in a population, the occurrence of harmful mutations is comparatively rare because of selective pressures that eliminate the most harmful mutations from the population (lethality) and the variability within the genomic sequence to polymorphic change. Some portions of the genome are remarkably stable and free of polymorphic variation, whereas other portions are highly polymorphic, the persistence of variation within which is a consequence of the functional benignity of the sequence change. In other words, polymorphic differences in DNA sequence between individuals can be divided into those producing no effect on phenotype, those causing benign differences in phenotype (i.e., normal genetic variation), and those producing adverse consequences in phenotype (i.e., mutations). The last group can be further subdivided into the polymorphic mutations that alone are able to produce a functionally abnormal phenotype such as monogenic disease (e.g., sickle cell anemia) and those that alone are unable to do so but in conjunction with other mutations can produce a functionally abnormal phenotype (complex disease traits [e.g., essential hypertension]).

Polymorphisms are more common in noncoding regions of the genome than they are in coding regions, and one common type of these involves the tandem repetition of short DNA sequences a variable numbers of times. If these tandem repeats are long, then they are termed *variable number tandem repeats* (STR); if these repeats are short, they are termed *short tandem repeats.* During mitosis, the number of tandem repeats can change, and the frequency of this kind of replication error is high enough to make alternative lengths of the tandem repeats common in a population. However, the rate of change in length of the tandem repeats is low enough to make the size of the polymorphism useful as a stable genotypic trait in families. In view of these features, polymorphic tandem repeats are quite useful in determining the familial heritability of specific genomic loci. Polymorphic tandem repeats are sufficiently prevalent along the entire genomic sequence, enabling them to serve as genetic markers for specific genes of interest through an analysis of their linkage to those genes during crossover and

Table 1–1	**Molecular Basis of Mutations**
Type	**Examples**
Point Mutations	
Deletion	α-Thalassemia, polycystic kidney disease
Substitution	
Silent	Cystic fibrosis
Missense	Sickle cell anemia, polycystic kidney disease, congenital long QT syndrome
Nonsense	Cystic fibrosis, polycystic kidney disease
Large Mutations (Gene or Gene Cluster)	
Deletion	Duchenne's muscular dystrophy
Insertion	Factor VIII deficiency (hemophilia A)
Duplication	Duchenne's muscular dystrophy
Inversion	Factor VIII deficiency
Expanding triplet	Huntington's disease
Very Large Mutation (Chromosomal Segment or Chromosome)	
Deletion	Turner's syndrome (45,X)
Duplication	Trisomy 21
Translocation	XX male [46X, t(X;Y)]*

*Translocation onto an X chromosome of a segment of a Y chromosome that bears the locus for testicular differentiation.

recombination events. Analyses of multiple genetic polymorphisms in the human genome reveal that a remarkable variation exists among individuals at the level of the sequence of genomic DNA (genotyping). Single-nucleotide polymorphism (SNP), the most common variant, differs by a single base between chromosomes on any given stretch of DNA sequence (Fig. 1–5). From genotyping of the world's representative population, 10 million variants (one site per 300 bases) are estimated to make up 90% of the common SNP variants in the population with the rare variants making up the remaining 10%. With each generation of a species, the frequency of polymorphic changes in a gene is 10^{-4} to 10^{-7}. Thus, in view of the number of genes in the human genome, between 0.5% and 1.0% of the base sequence of the human genome is polymorphic. In this context the new variant can be traced historically to the surrounding alleles on the chromosomal background present at the time of the mutational event. A haplotype is a specific set or combination of alleles on a chromosome or part of a chromosome (see Fig. 1–5). When parental chromosomes undergo crossover, new *mosaic* haplotypes, containing additional mutations, are created from such recombinations. SNP alleles within haplotypes can be co-inherited in association with other alleles in the population, termed *linkage disequilibrium* (LD). The association between two SNPs will decline with increasing distance, enabling patterns of LD to be decided from the proximity of nearly SNPs. Conversely, a few well-selected SNPs are often sufficient to predict the location of other common variants in the region.

Haplotypes associated with a mutation are expected to become common by recombination in the general population over thousands of generations. In contrast, genetic mapping with LD departs from traditional Mendelian genetics by using the entire human population as a large family tree without an established pedigree. Of the possible 10 million variants, the International HapMap Project and the Perlegen private venture have deposited over 8 million variants comprising the public human SNP map from over 341 people representing different population samples. The SNPs distributed across the genome of unrelated individuals provide a sufficiently robust sample set for statistical associations to be drawn between genotypes and modest phenotypes. A mutation can now be defined as a specific type of allelic polymorphism that causes a functional defect in a cell or organism.

The causal relationship between monogenic diseases with well-defined phenotypes that co-segregate with the disease requires only a small number of affected individuals compared with unaffected control individuals. In contrast, complex disorders (e.g., diabetes, hypertension, cancer) will necessitate the combinatorial effects of environmental factors and genes with subtle effects. Only through searching for variations in genetic frequency between patients and the general population can the causation of disease be discerned. In the postgenomic era, gene mapping entails the statistical association with the use of LD and high-density genetic maps that span thousands to 100,000 base pairs. To enable comprehensive association studies to become routine in clinical practice, inexpensive genotyping assays and denser maps with all common polymorphisms, must be linked to all possible manifestations of the disease. Longitudinal studies of the HapMap and Perlegen cohorts will determine the effects of diet, exercise, environmental factors, and family history on future clinical events. Without similar approaches on securing adequate sample sizes and datasets, the promise of genetic population theory will not overcome the inherent limitations of linking human sequence variation with complex disease traits.

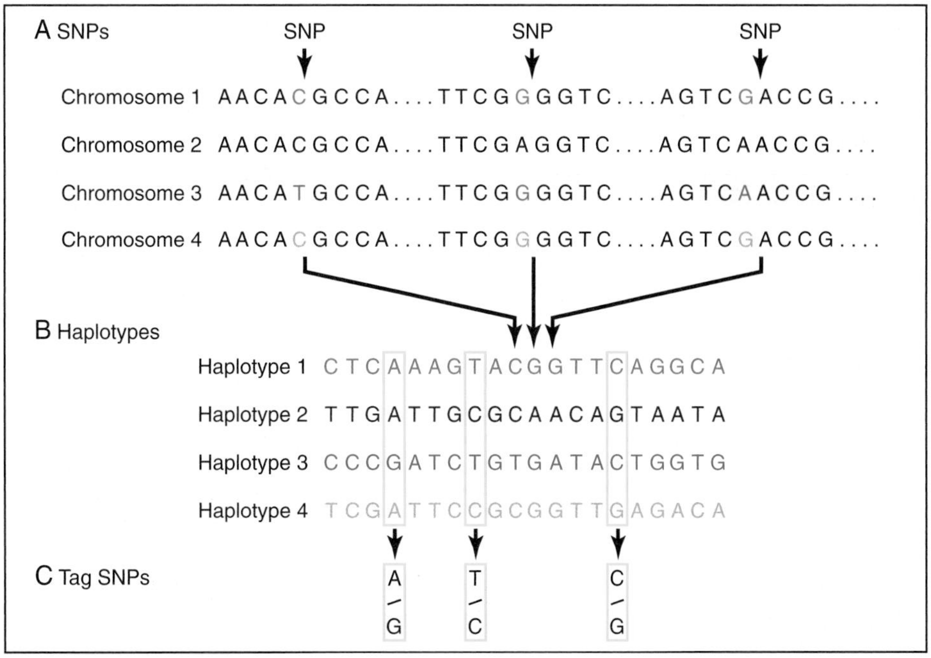

Figure 1–5 Single nucleotide polymorphisms (SNPs), Haplotypes, and Tag SNPs. A stretch of mostly identical DNA on the same chromosome is shown from four different individuals. A SNP refers to the variation of the three bases shown in DNA region. The combination of nearby SNPs defines a haplotype. Tag SNPs are useful tools shown *(panel C)* for genotyping four unique haplotypes from the 20 haplotypes *(panel B)*. (Adapted from International HapMap Consortium: The International HapMap Project. Nature Dec 18;426(6968):789–96, 2003.)

Gene Mapping and the Human Genome Project

The process of gene mapping involves identifying the relative order and distance of specific loci along the genome. Maps can be of two types: genetic and physical. Genetic maps identify the genomic location of specific genetic loci by a statistical analysis based on the frequency of recombination events of the locus of interest with other known loci. Physical maps identify the genomic location of specific genetic loci by a direct measurement of the distance along the genome at which the locus of interest is located in relation to one or more defined markers. The precise location of genes on a chromosome is important for defining the likelihood that a portion of one chromosome will interchange, or cross over, with the corresponding portion of its complementary chromosome when genetic recombination occurs during meiosis (Fig. 1–6).

During meiotic recombination, genetic loci or alleles that have been acquired from one parent interchange with those acquired from the other parent to produce new combinations of alleles, and the likelihood that alleles will recombine during meiosis varies as a function of their linear distance from one another in the chromosomal sequence. This recombination probability or distance is commonly quantitated in centimorgans (cM): 1 cM is defined as the chromosomal distance over which there is a 1% chance that two alleles will undergo a crossover event during meiosis. Crossover events serve as the basis for mixing parental base sequences during development and, thereby, promoting genetic diversity among offspring. Analysis of the tendency for specific alleles to be inherited together indicates that the recombination distance in the human genome is approximately 3000 cM.

Identifying the gene or genes responsible for a specific disease phenotype polygenic disease phenotype requires an understanding of the topographic anatomy of the human genome, which is inextricably linked to interactions with the environment. The Human Genome Project, first proposed in 1985, represented an international effort to determine the complete nucleotide sequence of the human genome, including the construction of its detailed genetic, as well as physical and transcript maps with identification and characterization of all genes. This foray into *large-scale biology* was championed by Nobel Laureate James Watson as the defining moment in his lifetime for witnessing the path from the double helix to the sequencing of 3 billion bases of the human genome, paving the way for understanding human evolution and harnessing the benefits for human health.

Among the earliest achievements of the Human Genome Project were the development of 1 cM-resolution maps, each containing 3000 markers and the identification of 52,000 sequenced tagged sites (STS). For functional analysis on a genome-wide scale, major technologic advances such as high-throughput oligonucleotide synthesis, normalized and subtracted complementary DNA (cDNA) libraries, and DNA micro-arrays were developed. In 1998, the Celera private venture proposed a similar goal as the Human Genome Project using a revolutionary approach, termed *shotgun sequencing,* to determine the sequence of the human genome (**Web Movie 1–1**). The shotgun sequencing method was designed for random large-scale sequencing and subsequent alignment of sequenced segments using computational and mathematic modeling. In the end, The Human Genome Project, in collaboration with the Celera private venture, produced a refined map of the entire human genome in 2001.

Because of the differences in genomic sequence that arise as a consequence of normal biologic variations or sequence polymorphisms, the resulting restriction fragment length polymorphisms (RFLPs) differ among individuals and are inherited according to Mendelian principles. These polymorphisms can serve as genetic markers for specific loci in the genome. One of the most useful types of RFLPs for localization of genetic loci within the genome is that produced by tandem repeats of sequence. Tandem repeats arise through *slippage* or stuttering of the DNA polymerase during replication in the case of STRs; longer variations arise through unequal crossover events. STRs are distributed throughout the genome and are highly polymorphic. Of importance is that these markers have two different alleles at

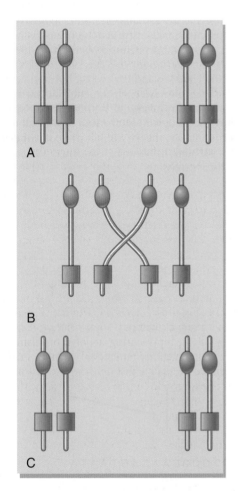

Figure 1–6 Crossing over and recombination. *A,* Two haploid chromosomes are shown, one from each parent *(red and blue)* with two genomic loci denoted by the circles and squares. *B,* Crossing over of one haploid chromosome from each parent. *C,* Resulting recombination of chromosomal segments now redistributes one haploid locus *(denoted by squares)* from one diploid pair to another.

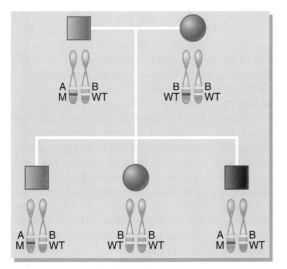

Figure 1–7 Linkage analysis. Analysis of the association (genomic contiguity) of a mutation *(M)* and a polymorphic allelic marker *(A)* shows close linkage in that the mutation segregates with the A allele, whereas the wild-type gene locus *(WT)* associates with the B allele.

each locus that are derived from each parent; thus, the origins of the two chromosomes can be discerned through this analysis.

The use of highly polymorphic tandem repeats that occur throughout the genome as genomic markers has provided a basis for mapping specific gene loci through establishing the association or linkage with select markers. Linkage analysis is predicated on a simple principle: The likelihood that a crossover event will occur during meiosis decreases the closer the locus of interest is to a given marker. The extent of genetic linkage can be ascertained for any group of loci, one of which may contain a disease-producing mutation (Fig. 1–7).

Identifying Mutant Genes

Deducing the identity of a specific gene sequence believed to cause a specific human disease requires that mutations in the gene of interest be identified. If the gene believed to be responsible for the disease phenotype is known, then its sequence can be determined by conventional cloning and sequencing strategies, and the mutation can be identified. A variety of techniques are currently available for detecting mutations. Mutations that involve insertion or deletion of large segments of DNA can be detected by Southern blot, in which the isolated DNA is annealed to a radioactively labeled fragment of cDNA sequence. Prior incubation of the DNA with a specific restriction endonuclease cleaves the DNA sequence of interest at specific sites to produce smaller fragments that can be monitored by agarose gel electrophoresis. Shifts in mobility on the gel in comparison with wild-type sequence become apparent as a function of changes in the molecular size of the fragment. Alternatively, the polymerase chain reaction (PCR) can be used to identify mutations (**Web Movie 1–2**).

In this approach, small oligonucleotides (20 to 40 bases in length), which are complementary to regions of DNA that bracket the sequence of interest and one complementary to each strand of the double-stranded DNA, are synthesized and serve as primers for the amplification of the DNA sequence of interest. These primers are added to the DNA solution. The temperature of the solution is increased to dissociate the individual DNA strands and is then reduced to permit annealing of the primers to their complementary template target sites. A thermostable DNA polymerase is included in the reaction to synthesize new DNA in the 5′-to-3′ direction from the primer annealing sites. The temperature is then increased to dissociate duplex structures, after which it is reduced, enabling another cycle of DNA synthesis to occur. Several temperature cycles (usually up to 40) are used to amplify progressively the concentration of the sequence of interest, which can be identified as a PCR product by agarose gel electrophoresis with a fluorescent dye. The product can be isolated and sequenced to identify the suggested mutation.

If the gene is large and the site of the mutation is unknown (especially if it is a point mutation), then other methods can be used to identify the likely mutated site in the exonic sequence. One commonly used approach involves scanning the gene sequence for mutations that alter the structural conformation of short complexes between parent DNA and PCR products, leading to a shift in mobility on a nondenaturing agarose gel (i.e., single-strand conformational polymorphism). A single-base substitution or deletion can change the conformation of the complex in comparison with wild-type complexes and yield a shift in mobility. Sequencing this comparatively small region of the gene then facilitates precise identification of the mutation.

When the gene believed to cause the disease phenotype is unknown, when its likely position on the genome has not been identified, or when only limited mapping information is available, a candidate gene approach can be used to identify the mutated gene. In this strategy, potential candidate genes are identified on the basis of analogy to animal models or by analysis of known genes that map to the region of the genome for which limited information is available. The candidate gene is then analyzed for potential mutations. Regardless of the approach used, mutations identified in candidate genes should always be correlated with functional changes in the gene product because some mutations could be functionally silent, representing a polymorphism without phenotypic consequences. Functional changes in the gene product can be evaluated through the use of cell-culture systems to assess protein function by expressing the mutant protein through transiently transfecting the cells with a vector that carries the cDNA coding for the gene of interest and incorporating the mutation of interest. Alternatively, unique animal models can be developed in which the mutant gene is incorporated in the male pronucleus of oocytes taken from a super-ovulating impregnated female. This union produces an animal that over expresses the mutant gene; that is, it produces a transgenic animal or an animal with more than the usual number of copies of a given gene or an animal in which the gene of interest is disrupted and the gene product is not synthesized (i.e., a gene *knock-out* animal or an animal with one half [heterozygote] or none [homozygote] of the usual number of a given gene).

MOLECULAR DIAGNOSTICS

The power of molecular techniques extends beyond their use in defining the precise molecular basis of an inherited disease. By exploiting the exquisite sensitivity of PCR to amplify rare nucleic acid sequences, it is possible to diagnose rapidly a range of infectious diseases for which unique sequences are available. In particular, infections caused by fastidious or slow-growing organisms can now be rapidly diagnosed, similar to the case for *Mycobacterium tuberculosis.* The presence of genes conferring resistance to specific antibiotics in microorganisms can also be verified by PCR techniques. The sequencing of the entire genome of organisms such as *Escherichia coli, M. tuberculosis,* and *Treponema pallidum* now offers unparalleled opportunities to monitor the epidemiologic structures of infections, follow the course of acquired mutations, tailor antibiotic therapies, and develop unique gene-based therapies (vide infra) for infectious agents for which conventional antibiotic therapies are ineffective or marginally effective.

The application of molecular methods to human genetics has clearly revolutionized the field. Through the use of approaches that incorporate linkage analysis and PCR, simple point mutations can be precisely localized and characterized. At the other end of the spectrum of genetic changes that underlie disease, chromosomal translocations, deletions, or duplications can be identified by conventional cytogenetic methods. Large deletions that can incorporate many kilobase pairs and many genes can now be visualized with fluorescent *in situ* hybridization (FISH), a technique in which a segment of cloned DNA is labeled with a fluorescent tag and hybridized to chromosomal DNA. With the deletion of the segment of interest from the genome, the chromosomal DNA fails to fluoresce in the corresponding chromosomal location.

Advances in molecular medicine have also revolutionized the approach to the diagnosis and treatment of neoplastic diseases, as well as the understanding of the mechanisms of carcinogenesis. According to current views, a neoplasm arises from the clonal proliferation of a single cell that is transformed from a regulated, quiescent state into an unregulated growth phase. DNA damage accumulates in the parental tumor cell as a result of either exogenous factors (e.g., radiation exposure) or heritable determinants. In early phases of carcinogenesis, certain genomic changes may impart intrinsic genetic instability that increases the likelihood of additional damage. One class of genes that becomes activated during carcinogenesis is oncogenes, which are primordial genes that normally exist in the mammalian genome in an inactive (proto-oncogene) state but, when activated, promote unregulated cell proliferation through activation of specific intracellular signaling pathways.

Molecular methods based on the acquisition of specific tumor markers and unique DNA sequences that result from oncogenetic markers of larger chromosomal abnormalities (i.e., translocations or deletions that promote oncogenesis) are now broadly applied to the diagnosis of malignancies. These methods can be used to establish the presence of specific tumor markers and oncogenes in biopsy specimens, to monitor the presence or persistence of circulating malignant cells after completion of a course of chemotherapy, and to identify the development of genetic resistance to specific chemotherapeutic agents. In addition, through the use of conventional linkage analysis and candidate-gene approaches, future studies will enable the identification of individuals with a heritable predisposition to malignant transformation. Many of these specific topics are discussed in later chapters.

The advent of *gene chip* technologies or expression arrays has revolutionized molecular diagnostics and has begun to clarify the pathobiologic structures of complex diseases. These methods involve labeling the cDNA generated from the entire pool of mRNA isolated from a cell or tissue specimen with a radioactive or fluorescent marker and annealing this heterogeneous population of polynucleotides to a solid-phase substrate to which many different polynucleotides of known sequence are attached. The signals from the labeled cDNA strands bound to specific locations on the array are monitored, and the relative abundance of particular sequences are compared with those from a reference specimen. Using this approach, micro-array patterns can be used as molecular fingerprints to diagnose a particular disease (i.e., type of malignancy and its susceptibility to treatment and prognosis), as well as to identify the genes whose expression increases or decreases in a specific disease state (i.e., identification of disease-modifying genes).

Of course, many other applications of molecular medicine techniques are available, in addition to these applications in infectious diseases and oncology. Molecular methods can be used to sort out genetic differences in metabolism that may modulate pharmacologic responses in a population of individuals *(pharmacogenomics),* address specific forensic issues such as paternity or criminal culpability, and approach epidemiologic analysis on a precise genetic basis.

GENES AND HUMAN DISEASE

Human genetic diseases can be divided into three broad categories: (1) those that are caused by a mutation in a single gene (e.g., monogenic disorders, Mendelian traits); (2) those that are caused by mutations in more than one gene (e.g., polygenic disorders, complex disease traits); and (3) those that are chromosomal in nature (Table 1–2). In all three groups of disorders, environmental factors can contribute to the phenotypic expression of the disease by modulating gene expression or unmasking a biochemical abnormality that has no functional consequences in the absence of a stimulus or stress. Classic monogenic disorders include sickle cell anemia, familial hypercholesterolemia, and cystic fibrosis. Importantly, these genetic diseases can be exclusively produced by a single specific mutation (e.g., sickle cell anemia) or by any one of several mutations (e.g., familial hypercholesterolemia, cystic fibrosis) in a given family (Pauling paradigm). Interestingly, some of these disorders evolved to protect the host. For example, sickle cell anemia evolved as protection against falciparum malaria and cystic fibrosis developed as protection against cholera. Examples of polygenic disorders or complex disease traits include type 1 (insulin-dependent) diabetes mellitus, atherosclerotic cardiovascular disease, and essential hypertension. A common example of a chromosomal disorder is the presence of an extra chromosome 21 (trisomy 21). The overall frequency of monogenic disorders is approximately 1%. Approximately

Table 1–2	**Molecular Basis of Mutations**	

Type	Examples
Monogenic Disorders	
Autosomal dominant	Polycystic kidney disease 1, neurofibromatosis I
Autosomal recessive	β-Thalassemia, Gaucher is disease
X-linked	Hemophilia A, Emery-Dreifuss muscular dystrophy
One of multiple mutations	Familial hypercholesterolemia, cystic fibrosis
Polygenic Disorders	
Complex disease traits	Type I (insulin-dependent) diabetes, essential hypertension, atherosclerotic disease, cancer

60% of these include polygenic disorders, which includes those with a genetic substrate that develops later in life. Approximately 0.5% of monogenic disorders include chromosomal abnormalities. Importantly, chromosomal abnormalities are frequent causes of spontaneous abortion and malformations.

Contrary to the view held by early geneticists, few phenotypes are entirely defined by a single genetic locus. Thus monogenic disorders are comparatively uncommon; however, they are still useful as a means to understanding some basic principles of heredity. Monogenic disorders are of three types: autosomal dominant, autosomal recessive, and X-linked. *Dominance* and *recessiveness* refer to the nature of the heritability of a genetic trait and correlate with the number of alleles affected at a given locus. If a mutation in a single allele determines the phenotype, then the mutation is said to be dominant; that is, the heterozygous state conveys the clinical phenotype to the individual. In contrast, if a mutation is necessary at both alleles to determine the phenotype, then the mutation is said to be recessive; that is, only the homozygous state conveys the clinical phenotype to the individual. Dominant or recessive mutations can lead to either a loss or a gain of function of the gene product. If the mutation is present on the X chromosome, then it is defined as X-linked (which in males can, by definition, be viewed only as dominant); otherwise, it is autosomal. The importance of identifying a potential genetic disease as inherited by one of these three mechanisms is that, if one of these patterns of inheritance is present, the disease must involve a single genomic abnormality that leads to an abnormality in a single protein. Classically identified genetic diseases are produced by mutations that affect coding (exonic) sequences. However, mutations in intronic and other untranslated regions of the genome occur that may disturb the function or expression of specific genes. Examples of diseases with these types of mutations include myotonic dystrophy and Friedreich's ataxia.

An individual with a dominant monogenic disorder typically has one affected parent and a 50% chance of trans-

mitting the mutation to his or her offspring. In addition, men and women are equally likely to be affected and equally likely to transmit the trait to their offspring. The trait cannot be transmitted to offspring by two unaffected parents. In contrast, an individual with a recessive monogenic disorder typically has parents who are clinically normal. Affected parents, each heterozygous for the mutation, have a 25% chance of transmitting the clinical phenotype to their offspring but a 50% chance of transmitting the mutation to their offspring (i.e., producing an unaffected carrier).

Notwithstanding the clear heritability of common monogenic disorders (e.g., sickle cell anemia), the clinical expression of the disease in an individual with a phenotype expected to produce the disease may vary. *Variability in clinical expression* is defined as the range of phenotypic effects observed in individuals carrying a given mutation. *Penetrance* refers to a smaller subset of individuals with variable clinical expression of a mutation and is defined as the proportion of individuals with a given genotype who exhibit any clinical phenotypic features of the disorder. Three principal determinants of variability in clinical expression or incomplete penetrance of a given genetic disorder can occur. They are (1) environmental factors, (2) the effects of other genetic loci, and (3) random chance. Environmental factors can modulate disease phenotype by altering gene expression in several ways, including their action on transcription factors (e.g., transcription factors that are sensitive to cell redox state [nuclear factor κB]) or *cis*-elements in gene promoters (e.g., folate-dependent methylation of CpG rich regions); or by post-translationally modifying proteins (e.g., lysine oxidation). That other genes can modify the effects of disease-causing mutations is a reflection of the overlay of genetic diversity on primary disease phenotype. Numerous examples exist of the effects of these so-called *disease-modifying genes* producing phenotypic variations among individuals with the identical primary disease-causing mutations *(gene-gene interactions)* and the effects of disease-modifying genes interacting with environmental determinants to alter phenotype further *(gene-environment interactions)*. These interactions are clearly important in polygenic diseases; gene-gene and gene-environment interactions can modify the phenotypic expression of the disease. Among patients with sickle cell disease, for example, some patients experience painful crises, whereas others exhibit acute chest syndrome; still other presentations include hemolytic crises.

Genetic disorders affecting a unique pool of DNA, mitochondrial DNA, have been identified. Mitochondrial DNA is unique in that it is inherited only from the mother. In addition, mutations in mitochondrial DNA can vary among mitochondria within a given cell and within a given individual (heteroplasmy). Examples of genetic disorders based in the mitochondrial genome are the Kearns-Sayre syndrome and Leber's hereditary optic neuropathy. The list of known mitochondrial genomic disorders is growing rapidly, and mitochondrial contributions to a large number of common polygenic disorders may also exist.

MOLECULAR MEDICINE

A principal goal of current molecular strategies is to restore normal gene function to individuals with genetic mutations. Methods to do so are currently primitive, and a number of obstacles must be surmounted for this approach to be successful.

The principal problems are that to deliver a complete gene into a cell is not easy, and persistent expression of the new gene cannot be ensured because of the variability in its incorporation in the genome and the consequent variability in its regulated expression. Many approaches have been used to date, but none has been completely successful. They include the following: (1) packaging the cDNA in a viral vector, such as an attenuated adenovirus, and using the cell's ability to take up the virus as a means for the cDNA to gain access to the cell; (2) delivering the cDNA by means of a calcium phosphate–induced perturbation of the cell membrane; and (3) encapsulating the cDNA in a liposome that can fuse with the cell membrane and thereby deliver the cDNA.

Once the cDNA has been successfully delivered to the cell of interest, the magnitude and durability of expression of the gene product are important variables. The magnitude of expression is determined by the number of copies of cDNA taken up by a cell and the extent of their incorporation in the genome of the cell. The durability of expression appears to be dependent partly on the antigenicity of the sequence and protein product.

Notwithstanding these technical limitations, gene therapy has been used to treat adenosine deaminase deficiency successfully, which suggests that the principle on which the treatment is based is reasonable. Clinical trials of gene therapy have slowed considerably after unexpected deaths were widely reported in both the scientific and lay media. Efforts on other genetic disorders and as a means to induce expression of a therapeutic protein (e.g., vascular endothelial cell growth factor to promote angiogenesis in ischemic tissue) are ongoing.

Understanding the molecular basis of disease leads naturally to the identification of unique disease targets. Recent examples of this principle have led to the development of novel therapies for diseases that have been difficult to treat. Imatinib, a tyrosine kinase inhibitor that is particularly effective at blocking the action of the bcr-abl kinase, is quite effective for the treatment of chronic-phase chronic myelogenous leukemia. Monoclonal antibody to tumor necrosis factor-α (infliximab) or soluble tumor necrosis factor-α receptor (etanercept) are prime examples of *biologic modifiers* that are effective in the therapy of chronic inflammatory disorders, including inflammatory bowel disease and rheumatoid arthritis. This approach to molecular therapeutics is rapidly expanding and holds great promise for improving the therapeutic armamentarium for a variety of diseases.

Beyond cancer-related categories (e.g., DNA, RNA repair), gene expression arrays have provided additional interactions of regulatory pathways of clinical interest. The limitation of gene expression profile using micro-arrays, which does not account for post-transcriptional and other post-translational modifications of protein-coding products, will likely be overcome by approaches and advances in proteomics. Such processes by signaling networks tend to amplify or attenuate gene expression on time scales lasting between seconds to weeks. Much work still remains to improve current knowledge about the pathways that initiate and promote tumors. The basic pathways and nodal points of regulation will be identified for rational drug design and target from mechanistic insights gleaned from expression profiling of cultured cell lines, from small animal models of human disease, and from human samples. Although accounting for tissue heterogeneity and variation among different cell types, the new systems' approach for incorporating genomic and computational appears particularly promising to decipher the pathways that promote tumorigenesis. In turn, biologists and clinicians will use information derived from these tools to understand the events that promote survival, proangiogenesis, and immune escape, all of which may confer metastatic potential and progression.

What potential diagnostic tools are available to establish genetic determinants of drug response? Genome-wide approaches from the Human Genome Project in combination with micro-arrays, proteomic analysis, and bioinformatics will identify multiple genes encoding drug targets (e.g., receptors). Similar high throughput screening should provide insights into the predisposition to adverse effects of outcomes from treatments that are linked to genetic polymorphisms. The future of pharmacogenetics is to know all the factors that influence adverse drug effects. In this way, the premature abandonment of special drug classes can be avoided in favor of rational drug design and therapy.

Many hurdles must be overcome for pharmacogenetics to become more widespread and to be integrated into medical practice. Current approaches of trial and error in medical practice are well engrained on the parts of physicians. In addition, the allure for blockbuster drugs by the pharmaceutical industry warrants a new model for approaching individualized doses. New training for physicians in molecular biology and genetics should complement clinical pharmacogenomic studies that determine efficacy in an era of evidence-based medicine. Pharmacogenetic polymorphisms, unlike other clinical variables such as renal function, need only a single test, ideally as a newborn. Polygenic models of therapeutic optimization still face hurdles that reduce the chances for abuse of genetic information and additional costs. On the other hand, SNP haplotyping has the potential to identify genetically similar subgroups of the population and to randomize therapies based on more robust genetic markers. On a population level, genomic variability is much greater within than among distinct racial and ethnic groups.

Both therapeutic efficacy and host toxicity are influenced by the patient's specific disease, age, renal function, nutritional status, and other co-morbid factors. New challenges will be posed for the selection and guide to drug therapy for patients with cancer, hypertension, and diabetes. It is conceivable that treatment of multisystem disorders (e.g., metabolic syndrome) might be derived from novel therapeutics based on individual, interacting, and complementary molecular pathways.

Prospectus for the Future

The concept of personalized medicine will be realized from the functional and analytical phenotyping that aids diagnosis and treatment based on the individual's genome and disease profile. An important future challenge will be the extraction of biologically meaningful data of direct clinical relevance to diagnosis, prognosis, therapeutic response, and, ultimately, prevention.

What are the functional consequences of genome occupancy and modification in health and disease? Computational analyses will play an increasing role in understanding cancer pathogenesis and the mechanisms of disease. Information about the hierarchy of cellular functions is being coupled with powerful approaches to derive different yet complementary perspectives about molecular mechanisms. Micro-array analysis has already provided new classes of hematologic diseases and prognostic factors in breast cancer. Experimental approaches are already underway to reduce tumorigenesis into discrete modules of regulatory networks and biologic processes. A catalog of listed genes that change with tumor type, for example, should not be equated with prognosis, therapeutic response, or adverse outcomes. How to move diagnostic tools using micro-arrays and gene expression profiles into clinical decision making will be the focus of research programs in translational and clinical outcomes.

References

Acharya MR, Sparreboom A, et al: Rational development of histone deacetylase inhibitors as anticancer agents: A review. *Mol Pharmacol* 68(4): 917–932, 2005.

Collins FS, Green ED, et al: A vision for the future of genomics research. *Nature* 422(6934):835–847, 2003.

Evans WE, McLeod HL: Pharmacogenomics: Drug disposition, drug targets, and side effects. *N Engl J Med* 348(6):538–549, 2003.

Hinds DA, Stuve LL, et al: Whole-genome patterns of common DNA variation in three human populations. *Science* 307(5712):1072–1079, 2005.

Krause DS, Van Etten RA: Tyrosine kinases as targets for cancer therapy. *N Engl J Med* 353(2):172–187, 2005.

van Steensel B: Mapping of genetic and epigenetic regulatory networks using microarrays. *Nat Genet* 37 Suppl:S18–S24, 2005.

Zamore PD, Haley B: Ribo-gnome: Rhe big world of small RNAs. *Science* 309(5740):1519–1524, 2005.

Section II

Evidence-Based Medicine

Evidence-Based Medicine, Quality of Life, and the Cost of Medicine

Sara G. Tariq

Susan S. Beland

The diagnosis and treatment of individual patients involve clinical experience and skills on the part of the physician and knowledge of scientific information obtained through clinical trials. In the past, most of the daily practice was based on informal learning and a tradition of knowledge transferred from experienced clinicians to trainees and colleagues. Increasingly, however, this informal technique is being supplanted by rigorous analysis of the scientific underpinnings of clinical logic. Electronic databases and Internet technology enable collation and dissemination of information to help identify which techniques are supported by clinical trials. *Evidence-based medicine* has evolved over the last decade and stresses the use of the best-available evidence from published research as the foundation for clinical decision making. This foundation, in addition to clinical expertise and a respect for patient preference, will aid the physician in providing optimal outcomes and a quality of life for the patient. However, the development of new techniques in medicine, often at great cost, can strain the ability of a society to fund and provide such services. Critical appraisal of both new and traditional diagnostic and treatment modalities is thus needed.

Critical Appraisal of the Literature

Being cognizant of the types of evidence is crucial to practice evidence-based medicine. Research studies can be divided into two major categories: primary and secondary (Table 2–1).

Primary studies can have a number of designs. In *randomized controlled studies* participants in the trial are randomly allocated to one intervention or another. Both groups are followed for a specified period and analyzed in terms of specific outcomes defined at the outset of the study. This type of study allows rigorous assessment of a single variable in a defined patient group, has a prospective design that potentially eradicates bias by comparing two otherwise similar groups, and allows for meta-analysis. However, these studies are expensive and time consuming. Results of randomized controlled trials can have enormous impact on the practice of medicine, as exemplified by the Women's Health Initiative randomized controlled trial. This study was designed to assess the risks and benefits for postmenopausal hormone use in healthy women. However, the trial was stopped early because of an increased incidence of breast cancer, coronary heart disease, stroke, and thromboembolic disease in the hormone-treated group. *Cohort studies* have two or more groups of participants selected on the basis of differences in their exposure to a particular agent. The participants are prospectively followed to see how many in each group develop a disease or other specific outcome. A well-known example is the Framingham Heart Study that enrolled 5200 participants in 1948 and followed them forward in time to examine the progression and risk factors for heart disease. The data provided from the Framingham Study have helped clinicians understand the development and progression of heart disease and its risk factors. As with randomized trials, cohort studies are time consuming. *Case-control studies* involve patients with a particular disease or condition who are identified and matched with control

Table 2–1	**Types of Research Studies**
Primary Studies	**Secondary Studies**
Randomized control	Meta-analyses
Case control	Clinical practice guidelines
Cohort studies	Decision analysis
Cross sectional	Cost-effectiveness analysis
Case series	
Case report	

Table 2–2	**Requirements of Screening Tests**

- Prevalence of disease must be sufficiently high.
- Disease must have significant morbidity and mortality rates.
- Effective treatment must be available.
- Improved outcomes from early diagnosis and treatment must be present.
- Test should have good sensitivity and specificity parameters.
- Test should carry acceptable risks and be cost effective.

patients. The control participants can be patients with another disease or individuals from the general population. The validity of these retrospective studies depends on careful selection of the control group. For example, the impact of risk factors for men and women was recently evaluated in The CARDIO 2000 Study. The authors evaluated 848 hospitalized patients after their first episode of acute coronary syndrome and used 1078 age- and gender-matched controls. The data revealed that women experiencing their first event were significantly older than men. *Case reports* describe the medical history of a single patient. When medical histories of more than one patient with a particular condition are described together to illustrate one aspect of the disease process, the term *case series* is used.

Secondary (integrative) studies attempt to summarize and draw conclusions from primary information. Meta-analyses use statistical techniques to combine and summarize the results of primary studies. By combining the results from many trials, meta-analyses are able to estimate the magnitude of the effect of an intervention or risk factor, as well as evaluate previously unanswered questions by performing subgroup analyses. The use of meta-analysis has provoked some controversy. Some investigators believe that meta-analyses may be as reliable as randomized controlled trials, whereas others believe that the technique should be used only as an alternate to randomized trials. However, in the absence of a large randomized controlled study, a meta-analysis of multiple smaller studies may be the best source of information to answer a specific question.

Clinical practice guidelines attempt to summarize diagnostic and treatment strategies for common clinical problems to assist the physician with specific circumstances. They are usually published by medical organizations, such as the American College of Physicians, and government agencies, such as the Agency for Health Care Policy and Research.

Decision analysis uses the results of primary studies to generate probability trees to aid both health professionals and patients in making choices about clinical management. *Cost-effectiveness analysis* evaluates whether a particular course of action is an effective use of resources.

Testing in Medical Practice

Screening tests are performed on asymptomatic healthy people to detect occult disease and should meet the criteria listed in Table 2–2. Screening tests are most useful when a high prevalence of disease is present in the population and the test has adequate sensitivity and specificity parameters. When applied to a disease with low prevalence, a test with low specificity would have an unacceptable number of false-positive results, which would lead to further procedures that are often invasive and expensive.

Diagnostic tests are used to determine the cause of illness in symptomatic persons and can be helpful in *patient management* by evaluating the severity of disease, determining prognosis, detecting disease recurrence, or selecting appropriate medications or other therapies. When considering diagnostic tests, the physician should weigh the potential benefits against the risks and expense.

When comparing the efficacy of a new diagnostic test, the critical issues are the following: (1) Does the new test have something to offer that the currently accepted test does not? (2) Does the new test provide additional information that alters the *post-test probability,* which is the likelihood that a patient who has a positive test has the disease? Comparing the post-test probability with the *pre-test probability* before ordering the test, which is the clinical assessment of diagnostic possibilities, is also important.

Values for some pre-test probabilities have been published, but more often they are derived from the physician's clinical experience and are influenced by the practice setting. For instance, an obese African-American woman from the rural South is experiencing fatigue, blurry vision, and frequent vaginal yeast infections, and she has a strong family history of diabetes. Based on these features, she would have a high pre-test probability for type 2 diabetes mellitus. If a new diagnostic test is available for the diagnosis of diabetes, then a comparison could be made on the post-test probabilities expected from the standard test (fasting blood glucose) and the new test. Ideally, the new test would offer greater diagnostic accuracy.

Sensitivity and *specificity* are important parameters to consider when evaluating a diagnostic test. Sensitivity is an index of the diagnostic test's ability to detect the disease when it is present. Specificity is the ability of the diagnostic test to identify correctly the absence of the disease. These parameters are calculated by the use of a 2×2 table (Table 2–3). An additional value, the *likelihood ratio,* which uses both sensitivity and specificity, gives an even better indication of the test's performance. A high positive likelihood ratio indicates a high likelihood of the presence of disease,

Table 2–3	**Schematic Outcomes of a Diagnostic Test (2× 2 Table)**	
Test Result	**Disease Present**	**Disease Absent**
Positive	True positive (*a*)	False positive (*b*)
Negative	False negative (*c*)	True negative (*d*)

Positive predictive value (true-positive rate) = *a*/(*a* + *b*)
Negative predictive value (false-positive rate) = *d*/(*c* + *d*)
Sensitivity = *a*/(*a* + *c*). Patients with the disease who have a positive test
Specificity = *d*/(*b* + *d*). Patients without the disease who have a negative test

whereas a high negative likelihood ratio identifies the absence of disease.

Positive likelihood ratio:
$$= \frac{\text{Sensitivity (probability that test is positive in diseased patients)}}{1 - \text{Specificity (probability that test is positive in nondiseased patients)}}$$

Negative likelihood ratio:
$$= \frac{1 - \text{Sensitivity (probability that test is negative in diseased patients)}}{1 - \text{Specificity (probability that test is negative in nondiseased patients)}}$$

After determining the validity of the diagnostic test, its applicability to the patient in question and whether the test is affordable and accurate in a particular setting should be ascertained. If the diagnostic test requires special devices or skills that are not available in the practice facility, then the results provided can be inaccurate. Most importantly, an assessment should be made about whether the test will change the management offered or decrease the need for the use of other tests.

Evaluating Evidence About Treatment

One of the most common problems facing physicians is the need to assess the validity of new treatments being developed, as well as validity of traditional treatments that have been used for years. For example, how long after discharge from the hospital should treatment with antimicrobial agents continue for the patient who had been hospitalized for pneumonia? What is the value of plasmapheresis in thrombotic thrombocytopenic purpura? The first step in evaluating prospective treatments is to assess whether the information is derived from a properly conducted randomized controlled study. Every patient who enters the trial must be accounted for at the end of the study. The patients who are lost to follow-up often have different outcomes. If the conclusion of the trial does not change after accounting for the lost patients, then validity is added to the study. Another point to consider is whether patients were analyzed in their original randomized groups even if they did not undergo the intervention in question. This is termed an *intention-to-treat analysis*. A description of whether both groups were treated differently regarding other interventions (e.g., co-interventions) should be included.

Assessing the importance of the data provided is the next step. This includes a number of simple statistical calculations applied to the available results. The first is *relative risk reduction* (RRR):

$$\text{RRR} = \frac{\begin{array}{c}\text{Incidence of outcome in}\\ \text{control group} - \text{Incidence}\\ \text{of outcome in study group}\end{array}}{\text{Incidence of outcome in control group}}$$

For example, the Diabetes Control and Complications Trial investigated the effect of tight control of blood glucose in patients with type 1 diabetes on the development and progression of long-term complications. The study involved more than 1400 patients, with one half randomized to intensive treatment and one half to conventional therapy. In this study, 3.4% of the patients in the conventional group and 2.2% in the intensive group developed microalbuminuria, which is a 35% decrease in the occurrence of microalbuminuria in the primary prevention group:

$$\text{RRR} = \frac{0.034 - 0.022}{0.034} \times 100 = 35\%$$

The greater the RRR, the more effective the therapy. However, the RRR does not take into account the baseline risk of the patients entering the trial and thus does not differentiate between large and small effects.

The significance of RRR is discussed on the web site (see **Web text 2–1**).

Calculating the *absolute risk reduction* (ARR), which gives the absolute difference in rates between the two groups, is another way of assessing the outcome. The ARR is defined as the number (X) that had the ill effect in the control group minus the number (Y) in the treatment group (i.e., ARR = $X - Y$). Using the previous example, the ARR for the development of microalbuminuria is $0.034 - 0.022 = 0.012$, or 1.2%. Another valuable calculation is the *number needed to treat*, which represents the number of patients who need to be treated to prevent a single outcome event and is the inverse of the ARR (i.e., $1/[X - Y]$). The lower the number needed to treat, the more clinically relevant is the treatment. Again, using the example, to prevent 1 patient from developing microalbuminuria, 83 patients with diabetes would have to be treated with intensive therapy ($1/[X - Y] = 1/0.012 = 83$). From this example, what seems like a large RRR of 35% actually translates to a relatively small (although significant) number of patients who benefited from intensive treatment.

As before, assessment of the applicability of this information to a particular patient should be made by taking into account whether the patient in question has the same characteristics of the patients included in the study. Evidence of side effects, cause, or value of a particular clinical sign in diagnosis can be assessed along these same lines.

Table 2–4	**Worldwide Websites**

- Cochrane Collaboration—One of the major organizations involved in evidence-based medicine (*hiru/mcmaster.ca/cochrane/default.htm*)
- MD Consult—Comprehensive medical information service (*www.mdconsult.com*)
- Centers for Disease Control and Prevention (*www.cdc.gov*)
- National Institutes of Health (*www.nih.gov*)
- Up to date—Comprehensive clinical information web site that is constantly updated (*www.uptodate.com*)
- Student Consult—Provides access to full standard texts online. (*www.studentconsult.com*)

Internet in Clinical Practice

The use of computer systems for disseminating medical information has increased exponentially. Numerous worldwide web sites offer high-quality medical news, information about practice guidelines, on-line textbooks and journals, and information about evidence-based medicine. In addition, many government sites offer up-to-date information (e.g., Centers for Disease Control and Prevention, National Institutes of Health). Table 2–4 lists some of these sites.

Including the Patient in the Decision Process

Searching for the best evidence and applying it have the ultimate goal of providing better patient care. The process should also involve informing the patient of the available options and offering options based on good evidence. Effective communication, geared toward your patient's level of health literacy, is crucial to ensure that your patient makes an informed decision. Using a certain therapy or implementing a diagnostic test may be inconvenient, or the patient may develop a certain side effect that he or she is not willing to accept. Involvement of the patient in the decision-making process requires good communication and adequate resources for patient education.

Quality of Life

Health care in the millennium has changed significantly. An increasing number of patients survive illnesses that used to be fatal, and many patients have multiple co-existing illnesses. Assessing clinical improvement to a given treatment covers only one aspect of the clinician's success. For example, although survival is an important outcome for patients with cancer, overall quality of life is fundamental. A patient can have improvement in disease-free survival without having a significant change in quality of life, and vice versa. Quality of life represents a subjective concept that is defined by the subjective perception of the patient, and includes physical, emotional, social, and cognitive functions; and the disease symptoms and side effects of a given treatment or interven-

tion. For example, in examining the efficacy of a drug for post-chemotherapy anemia, it would not only be important to know whether the hemoglobin rises appropriately, but also to know whether the patient subjectively has more energy and is able to perform the normal duties of life.

Quality of life is more commonly becoming a defined outcome measure in clinical trials. An increasing number of studies have been conducted in which health-related quality of life is either the primary or secondary endpoint. Hopefully, clinicians can then take the information gained from these data and apply it in a holistic manner to optimize patient care.

COST OF MEDICINE

The practice of medicine has significantly changed over the past 30 years. The cost of medicine has risen astronomically, and it is the duty of the physician to be cognizant of this in daily practice. Health-care spending is growing much faster than the rest of the economy. Rising hospital expenses reflect many factors, including the demand for new medications and technology, as well as the aging population. Physicians can contribute to the reduction of costs by being aware of medication prices and the appropriate use of tests.

The pharmaceutical industry has been accused of contributing to medical inflation. The industry spends more than $11 billion annually on promotion and marketing, and $8,000 to $13,000 per physician each year. They employ 1 drug representative for every 11 physicians in the United States. The average price of drugs rose almost 50% between 1992 and 2000. Literature suggests that the gifts and perks physicians receive from the pharmaceutical representatives have a major influence on their practices and prescribing habits. Caution is recommended when analyzing data from pharmaceutical representatives, taking into account the inherent bias that exists regarding the medication they are marketing. The medical profession is responsible for providing the best care possible for patients, and barriers to this care arise when a gift or amenity accepted from a pharmaceutical representative obscures the judgment of appropriate and cost-effective care. Generic drugs should be prescribed whenever possible. Studies have shown that if physicians substitute generic drugs for the brand name, then the potential national savings would be up to 5.9 billion dollars annually. In addition, all medical schools should stress the use of generic drugs to students and residents.

The use of tests is the second area in which physicians must be prudent when it comes to cost. The routine ordering of expensive and unnecessary tests has become part of the medical culture, but they can never take the place of a thorough history and physical examination. Evidence-based medicine is an important tool to use when deciding whether a certain diagnostic test is needed to help in the care of a patient. The risks and benefits of each test that is ordered must be weighed against the costs. For example, asymptomatic patients who are concerned about ovarian cancer may want their physician to order a pelvic ultrasound. The prudent physician will know that the prevalence of ovarian cancer is low in the population and thus the literature does not support the routine use of pelvic ultrasound as a screening tool. Therefore, a pelvic ultrasound is not a cost-effective test for screening ovarian cancer in all female patients.

These are two ways in which physicians can take an active role in helping reduce the cost of medical care in this nation, but the problem is clearly larger than this. Physicians will need to find a balance between being cost conscious and maintaining high-quality patient care as the medical field continues to expand.

Prospectus for the Future

Challenges to be met:
- Medical schools need to expand the teaching of evidence-based medicine to students and physicians in training.
- Risks and benefits of screening tests need to be better defined (e.g., use of computed tomography in the diagnosis of early lung cancer versus risk of radiation exposure).

- To affect the cost of medicine, the overuse of technology (e.g., computed tomography for every patient with abdominal pain) needs to be addressed from the standpoint of evidence-based medicine.
- Finally, a government-sponsored program is imperative to ensure universal health coverage for United States' citizens.

References

Bhat SK: The cost of medicine, Ann Intern Med 139:74–75, 2003.

Bottomley A: The cancer patient and quality of life, Oncologist 7:120–125, 2002.

Diabetes Control and Complications Trial Research Group: The effect of intensive treatment of diabetes on the development and progression of long-term complications in insulin-dependent diabetes mellitus, N Engl J Med 329:977–986, 1993.

Hall, WJ: The ethical dilemma of accepting gifts from drug makers, ACP-ASIM Observer, December, 2001.

Potential savings from substituting generic drugs for brand-name drugs: Medical expenditure panel survey, 1997–2000, Ann Intern Med 142:891–897, 2005.

Sacket D: Evidence-based medicine, 2nd ed, Oxford, 2000, Churchill Livingstone, pp. 13–29.

Writing Group for the Women's Health Initiative Investigators: Risks and benefits of estrogen plus progestin in healthy postmenopausal women, JAMA 288:321–333, 2002.

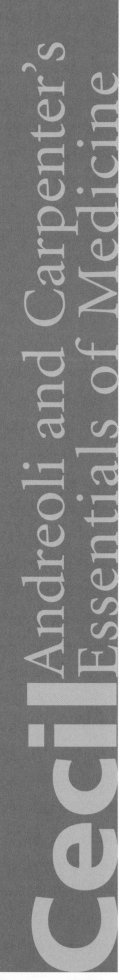

SECTION III

Cardiovascular Disease

Cecil

Andreoli and Carpenter's Essentials of Medicine

Structure and Function of the Normal Heart and Blood Vessels

Dean Y. Li

Ivor J. Benjamin

Gross Anatomy

The heart is composed of four chambers, two atria and two ventricles, which form two separate pumps arranged side by side and in series (Fig. 3–1). The atria are low-pressure capacitance chambers that mainly function to store blood during ventricular contraction (systole) and then fill the ventricles with blood during ventricular relaxation (diastole). The two atria are separated by a thin interatrial septum. The ventricles are high-pressure chambers responsible for pumping blood through the lungs and to the peripheral tissues. Because the pressure generated by the left ventricle is greater than that generated by the right, the left ventricular myocardium is thicker than the right. The two ventricles are separated by the interventricular septum, which is a membranous structure at its superior aspect and a thick, muscular structure at its medial and distal portions.

The atrioventricular (AV) valves separate the atria and ventricles. The mitral valve is a bileaflet valve that separates the left atrium and ventricle. The tricuspid valve is a trileaflet and separates the right atrium and ventricle. Strong chords (chordae tendineae) attach the ventricular aspects of these valves to the papillary muscles of their respective ventricles. These papillary muscles are extensions of normal myocardium that project into the ventricular cavities and are important for optimal valve closure. The semilunar valves separate the ventricles from the arterial chambers: the aortic valve separates the left ventricle from the aorta, and the pulmonic valve separates the right ventricle from the pulmonary artery. These valves do not have chordae. Rather, they are fibrous valves whose edges coapt closely, thus allowing for adequate valve closure. Each of the four valves is surrounded by a fibrous ring, or annulus, that forms part of the structural support of the heart. When open, the valves allow free flow of blood across them and into the adjacent chamber or vessel. When closed, the valves effectively prevent the backflow of blood into the preceding chamber.

The thin, double-layered pericardium surrounds the heart. The visceral pericardium is adherent to the heart and constitutes its outer surface, or *epicardium.* This outer surface is separated from the parietal pericardium by the pericardial space, which normally contains less than 50 mL of fluid. The parietal pericardium has attachments to the sternum, vertebral column, and diaphragm that serve to stabilize the heart in the chest. Normal pericardial fluid lubricates contact surfaces and limits direct tissue-surface contact during myocardial contraction. In addition, the normal pericardium modulates interventricular interactions during the cardiac cycle.

Circulatory Pathway

The circulatory system is composed of two distinct and parallel vascular networks, arterial and venous networks, which interconnect via capillary beds of the distal target organs (see Fig. 3–1). Deoxygenated blood drains from peripheral tissues and enters the right atrium through the superior and inferior venae cavae. Blood draining from the heart itself enters the right atrium through the coronary sinus. This blood mixes in the right atrium during ventricular systole and then flows across the tricuspid valve and into the right ventricle during ventricular diastole. When the right ventricle contracts, blood is ejected across the pulmonic valve and into the main pulmonary artery, which then bifurcates into the left and right pulmonary arteries as these branches enter their respective lungs. After multiple bifurcations, blood flows into the pulmonary capillaries, where carbon dioxide is exchanged for oxygen across the alveolar-capillary membrane. Oxygenated blood then drains from the lungs into the

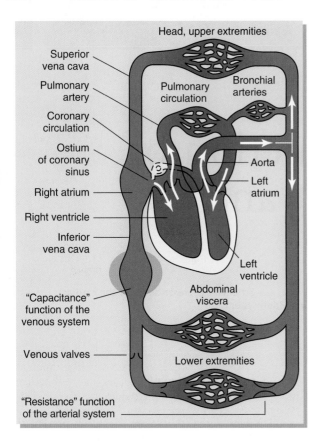

Figure 3–1 Schematic representation of the systemic and pulmonary circulatory systems. The venous system contains the greatest amount of blood at any one time and is highly distensible, accommodating a wide range of blood volumes (high capacitance). The arterial system is composed of the aorta, arteries, and arterioles. Arterioles are small muscular arteries that regulate blood pressure by changing tone (resistance).

four pulmonary veins, which empty into the left atrium. During ventricular diastole, the blood flows across the open mitral valve and into the left ventricle. With ventricular contraction, the blood is ejected across the aortic valve and into the aorta and is subsequently delivered to the various organs, where oxygen and nutrients are exchanged for carbon dioxide and metabolic wastes.

The heart itself receives blood through the left and right coronary arteries (Fig. 3–2). These are the first arterial branches of the aorta and originate in outpouchings of the aortic root called the *sinuses of Valsalva*. The left main coronary artery originates in the left sinus of Valsalva and is a short vessel that bifurcates into the left anterior descending (LAD) and the left circumflex (LCx) coronary arteries. The LAD travels across the surface of the heart in the anterior interventricular groove toward the cardiac apex. It supplies blood to the anterior and anterolateral left ventricle through its diagonal branches and to the anterior two thirds of the interventricular septum through its septal branches. The LCx traverses posteriorly in the left AV groove (between the left atrium and left ventricle) and supplies blood to the lateral aspect of the left ventricle through obtuse marginal branches, as well as gives off branches to the left atrium. The right coronary artery (RCA) originates in the right sinus of Valsalva and courses down the right AV groove to a point where the left and right AV grooves and the inferior interventricular groove meet, the *crux* of the heart. The RCA gives off atrial branches to the right atrium and acute marginal branches to the right ventricle. The blood supply to the diaphragmatic and posterior aspects of the left ventricle varies. In 85% of individuals, the RCA bifurcates at the crux into the posterior descending coronary artery (PDA), which travels in the inferior interventricular groove to supply blood to the inferior left ventricular wall and inferior third of the interventricular septum and to the posterior left ventricular (PLV) branches, which supply the posterior left ventricle.

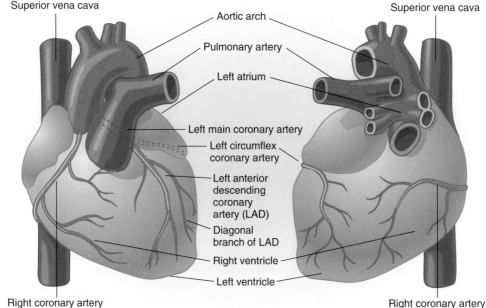

Figure 3–2 Major coronary arteries and their branches.

This course is termed a *right dominant circulation.* In 10% of individuals, the RCA terminates before reaching the crux and the LCx supplies the PLV and PDA. This course is termed a *left dominant circulation.* In the remaining individuals, the RCA gives rise to the PDA and the LCx gives rise to the PLV in a so-called *co-dominant circulation.* The blood supply to the sinoatrial (SA) node may originate from the RCA (60%) or the LCx (40%), whereas the dominant artery supplies the AV node. An understanding of coronary artery anatomy and distribution of blood supply enables the clinician to define the location of coronary artery disease based on history, physical and noninvasive tests such as electrocardiography (ECG), echocardiography, and radionuclide ventriculography. Small vascular channels, called *collateral vessels,* interconnect the normal coronary arteries. These vessels are nonfunctional in the normal myocardium because no pressure gradient develops across them. However, in the setting of severe stenosis or complete occlusion of a coronary artery, the pressure in the vessel distal to the stenosis decreases and a gradient develops across the collateral vasculature, resulting in flow through the collateral vessel. The development of collateral vasculature is directly related to the severity of the coronary stenosis and may be stimulated by ischemia, hypoxia, and a variety of growth factors. Over time, these vessels may reach up to 1 mm in luminal diameter and are almost indistinguishable from similarly sized, normal coronary arteries.

The majority of the venous drainage from the heart occurs through the coronary sinus, which runs in the AV groove and empties into the right atrium. A small amount of blood from the right side of the heart drains directly into the right atrium through the thebesian veins and small anterior myocardial veins.

Conduction System

The electrical impulse that initiates cardiac contraction originates in the SA node, a collection of specialized pacemaker cells measuring 1 to 2 cm in length located high in the right atrium between the superior vena cava and the right atrial appendage (Fig. 3–3). The impulse then spreads through the atrial tissue through preferential internodal tracts, ultimately reaching the AV node. This structure consists of a meshwork of cells located at the inferior aspect of the right atrium between the coronary sinus and the septal leaflet of the tricuspid valve.

The AV node provides the only normal electrical connection between the atria and ventricles. After an electrical impulse enters the AV node, conduction transiently slows and then proceeds to the ventricles by means of the His-Purkinje system. The bundle of His extends from the AV node down the membranous interventricular septum to the muscular septum, where it divides into the left and right bundle branches. The right bundle branch is a discrete structure that extends along the interventricular septum and enters the moderator band on its way toward the anterolateral papillary muscle of the right ventricle. The left bundle branch is less distinct; it consists of an array of fibers organized into an anterior fascicle, which proceeds toward the anterolateral papillary muscle of the left ventricle, and a posterior fascicle, which proceeds posteriorly in the septum

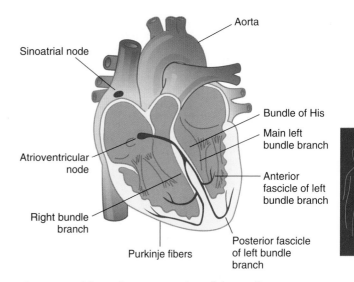

Figure 3–3 Schematic representation of the cardiac conduction system.

toward the posteromedial papillary muscle. Both the right and the left bundle branches terminate in Purkinje cells, which are large cells with well-developed intercellular connections that allow for the rapid propagation of electrical impulses. These impulse-generating cells then directly stimulate myocytes.

Neural Innervation

The normal myocardium is richly innervated by the autonomic nervous system. Sympathetic nerve terminals are located throughout the atria and ventricles, where an increase in sympathetic activity results in increased force of myocardial contraction. The parasympathetic system innervates the atria by means of the vagus nerve but has few projections to the ventricles. The SA and AV nodes are densely innervated by both sympathetic and parasympathetic neurons, allowing for neural regulation of the heart rate (HR). Increases in sympathetic tone lead to an increase in the HR and shortened conduction time through the AV node. Increases in parasympathetic tone lead to decreases in the HR and slower conduction through the AV node.

Myocardium

Cardiac tissue (myocardium) is composed of several cell types that together produce the organized contraction of the heart. Specialized myocardial cells make up the cardiac electrical system (conduction system) and are responsible for the generation of an electrical impulse and organized propagation of that impulse to cardiac muscle fibers (myocytes), which, in turn, respond by mechanical contraction. Atrial and ventricular myocytes are specialized, branching muscle cells connected end-to-end by intercalated discs. These thickened regions of the cell membrane (sarcolemma) aid in the transmission of mechanical tension between cells. The sarcolemma has functions similar to those of other cell membranes, including maintenance of ionic gradients, propagation of electrical impulses, and provision of

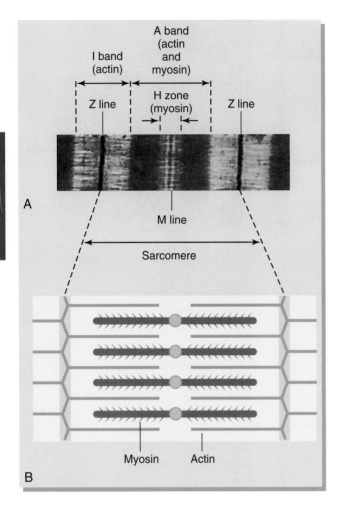

Figure 3–4 *A,* Sarcomere as it appears under the electron microscope. *B,* Schematic of the location and interaction of actin and myosin.

Muscle Physiology and Contraction

Contraction of myocytes begins with electrical depolarization of the sarcolemma, resulting in an influx of calcium into the cell through channels in the T tubules (Fig. 3–5). This initial calcium entry stimulates the rapid release of large amounts of calcium from the sarcoplasmic reticulum into the cell cytosol. The calcium then binds to the calcium-binding troponin subunit (troponin C) on the actin filaments of the sarcomere, resulting in a conformational change in the troponin-tropomyosin complex. This change facilitates the actin-myosin interaction, which results in cellular contraction. As the wave of depolarization passes, the calcium is rapidly and actively resequestered in the sarcoplasmic reticulum, where it is stored by various proteins, including calsequestrin, until the next wave of depolarization occurs. Calcium is also extruded from the cytosol by various calcium pumps in the sarcolemma. The force of myocyte contraction can be regulated by the amount of free calcium released into the cell by the sarcoplasmic reticulum. More calcium allows for greater actin-myosin interaction, producing a stronger contraction.

The energy for myocyte contraction is derived from adenosine triphosphate (ATP), which is generated by oxidative phosphorylation of adenosine diphosphate (ADP) in the abundant mitochondria of the cell. ATP is required both for calcium influx and for force generation by actin-myosin interaction. During contraction, ATP promotes dissociation of myosin from actin, thereby permitting the sliding of thick filaments past thin filaments as the sarcomere shortens. Under normal circumstances, fatty acids are the preferred energy source, although glucose can also be used as a substrate. These substrates must be constantly delivered to the heart through the bloodstream because minimal energy is stored in the heart itself. Myocardial metabolism is aerobic and thus requires a constant supply of oxygen. Under ischemic or hypoxemic conditions, glycolysis and lactate may serve as a source of ATP, although in insufficient quantities to sustain the working heart.

receptors for neural and hormonal inputs. In addition, the sarcolemma is intimately involved with the coupling of myocardial excitation and contraction through small transverse tubules (T tubules) that extend from the sarcolemma into the intracellular space. The myocytes contain several other organelles: the nucleus; the multiple mitochondria responsible for generating the energy required for contraction; an extensive network of intracellular tubules called the *sarcoplasmic reticulum,* which functions as the major intracellular storage site for calcium; and the myofibrils, which are the contractile elements of the cell. Each myofibril is made up of repeating units called *sarcomeres,* which are, in turn, composed of overlapping thin actin filaments and thick myosin filaments and their regulatory proteins troponin and tropomyosin (Fig. 3–4).

Circulatory Physiology and the Cardiac Cycle

The cardiac cycle is a repeating series of contractile and valvular events during which the valves open and close in response to pressure gradients between different cardiac chambers (Fig. 3–6). This cycle can be divided into systole, the period of ventricular contraction, and diastole, the period of ventricular relaxation. With the onset of ventricular contraction, the pressure in the ventricles increases and exceeds that in the atria, at which time the AV valves close. Intraventricular pressure continues to rise, initially without a change in ventricular volume (isovolumic contraction), until the intraventricular pressures exceed the pressures in the aorta and pulmonary artery, at which time the semilunar valves open and ventricular ejection of blood occurs. With the onset of ventricular relaxation, the pressure in the ventricles falls until the pressure in the arterial chambers exceeds that in the ventricles, and the semilunar valves close. Ventricular relaxation continues, initially without a change in ventricular volume (isovolumic relaxation). When the pressure in the ventricles falls below the pressure in the atria, the AV valves open and a rapid phase of ventricular filling occurs as blood in the atria empties into the ventricles. At the end of diastole, active atrial contraction augments ventricular filling. This augmentation is particularly important

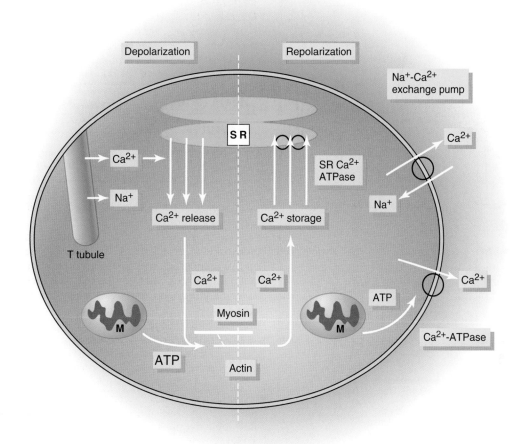

Figure 3–5 Calcium dependence of myocardial contraction. Electrical depolarization of the myocyte results in an influx of Ca^{2+} into the cell through channels in the T tubules. This initial phase of calcium entry stimulates the release of large amounts of Ca^{2+} from the sarcoplasmic reticulum (SR). The Ca^{2+} then binds to the troponin-tropomyosin complex on the actin filaments, resulting in a conformational change that facilitates the binding interaction between actin and myosin. In the presence of adenosine triphosphate (ATP), the actin-myosin association is cyclically dissociated as the thick and thin filaments slide past each other, resulting in contraction. During repolarization, the Ca^{2+} is actively pumped out of the cytosol and sequestered in the SR. *M,* Mitochondrion.

in patients with poor ventricular function or stiff ventricles and is lost in patients with atrial fibrillation.

In the absence of valvular disease, no impediment to the flow of blood exists from the ventricles to the arterial beds and the systolic arterial pressure rises sharply to a peak. During diastole, the arterial pressure gradually falls as blood flows distally and elastic recoil of the arteries occurs. This response contrasts with the pressure response in the ventricles during diastole, in which pressure gradually increases as blood enters the ventricles from the atria. Atrial pressure can be directly measured in the right atrium, whereas occluding a small pulmonary artery branch and measuring the pressure distally (the pulmonary capillary *wedge* pressure) is often used to obtain left atrial pressure indirectly. An atrial pressure tracing is shown in Figure 3–6 and is composed of several waves. The *a wave* represents atrial contraction. As the atria subsequently relax, the atrial pressure falls and the *x descent* is noted on the pressure tracing. The *x* descent is interrupted by a small *c wave,* which is generated as the AV

valve bulges toward the atrium during ventricular systole. As the atria fill from venous return, the *v wave* is seen, after which the *y descent* appears as the AV valves open and blood from the atria empties into the ventricles. The normal ranges of pressures in the various cardiac chambers are shown in Table 3–1.

CARDIAC PERFORMANCE

The amount of blood ejected by the heart each minute is referred to as the cardiac output (CO) and is the product of the stroke volume (SV) (SV = Amount of blood ejected with each ventricular contraction) and the HR:

$$CO = SV \times HR$$

The cardiac index is the CO divided by the body surface area; it is measured in liters per minute per square meter and is a way of normalizing CO to body size. The normal CO at rest

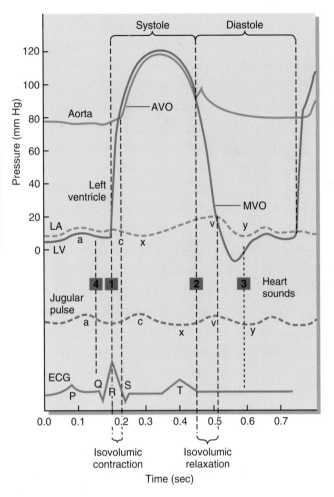

Figure 3–6 Simultaneous electrocardiogram (ECG) and pressure tracings obtained from the left atrium (LA), left ventricle (LV), and aorta, and the jugular venous pressure during the cardiac cycle. For simplification, right-sided pressures have been omitted. Normal right atrial pressure closely parallels that of the left atrium, and right ventricular and pulmonary artery pressures are timed closely with their corresponding left-sided heart counterparts; they are reduced only in magnitude. The normal mitral and aortic valve closure precedes tricuspid and pulmonic valve closure, respectively, whereas valve opening reverses this order. The jugular venous pulse lags behind the right atrial pulse.

During the course of one cardiac cycle, the electrical events (ECG) initiate and therefore precede the mechanical (pressure) events and the latter precedes the auscultatory events (heart sounds) they themselves produce. Shortly after the P wave, the atria contract to produce the *a* wave; a fourth heart sound may succeed the latter. The QRS complex initiates ventricular systole, followed shortly by LV contraction and the rapid buildup of LV pressure. Almost immediately, LV pressure exceeds LA pressure, closing the mitral valve and producing the first heart sound. After a brief period of isovolumic contraction, LV pressure exceeds aortic pressure and the aortic valve opens (AVO). When the ventricular pressure once again falls below the aortic pressure, the aortic valve closes to produce the second heart sound and terminate ventricular ejection. The LV pressure decreases during the period of isovolumic relaxation until it drops below LA pressure and the mitral valve opens (MVO). A period of rapid ventricular filling commences, during which a third heart sound may be heard. (See text for a discussion of the jugular venous pulse.)

Table 3–1	Normal Values for Common Hemodynamic Parameters	
Heart Rate		**60–100 Beats/Min**
Pressures		
Central venous		≤9 mm Hg
Right atrial		≤9 mm Hg
Right ventricular		
Systolic		15–30 mm Hg
End-diastolic		≤9 mm Hg
Pulmonary arterial		
Systolic		15–30 mm Hg
Diastolic		3–12 mm Hg
Pulmonary capillary wedge		≤12 mm Hg
Left atrial		≤12 mm Hg
Left ventricular		
Systolic		100–140 mm Hg
End-diastolic		3–12 mm Hg
Aortic		
Systolic		100–140 mm Hg
Diastolic		60–90 mm Hg
Resistance		
SVR		800–1500 dynes-sec/cm^{-5}
PVR		30–120 dynes-sec/cm^{-5}
Cardiac output		4–6 L/min
Cardiac index		2.5–4.0 L/min

PVR = pulmonary vascular resistance; SVR = systemic vascular resistance.

is 4 to 6 L/min, although this value can increase fourfold to sixfold during strenuous exercise as a result of increases in HR (chronotropic) and SV (inotropic).

The SV is a measure of the mechanical function of the heart and is affected by preload, afterload, and contractility (Table 3–2). *Preload* is the volume of blood in the ventricle at the end of diastole and is primarily a reflection of venous return. Within limits, as the preload increases, the ventricle stretches and the ensuing ventricular contraction becomes more rapid and forceful. This phenomenon is known as the Frank-Starling relationship. Because ventricular volume is not easily measured, ventricular filling pressure (ventricular end-diastolic pressure, atrial pressure, or pulmonary capillary wedge pressure) is frequently used as a surrogate measure of preload. Two major means can manipulate the preload in a clinical setting. The first means is to modulate volume status: intravenous fluids to increase preload and diuretics to decrease preload. The second is to regulate vascular tone: nitroglycerin to diminish preload.

Afterload is the force against which the ventricles must contract to eject blood. The arterial pressure is often used as a practical measure of afterload; although, in truth, the intraventricular pressure, the size of the ventricular cavity, and the thickness of the ventricular walls (Laplace's law)

Table 3–2 Factors Affecting Cardiac Performance

Preload (left ventricular diastolic volume)	Total blood volume Venous (sympathetic) tone Body position Intrathoracic and intrapericardial pressures Atrial contraction Pumping action of skeletal muscle	
Afterload (impedance against which the left ventricle must eject blood)	Peripheral vascular resistance Left ventricular volume (preload, wall tension) Physical characteristics of the arterial tree (elasticity of vessels or presence of outflow obstruction)	
Contractility (cardiac performance independent of preload or afterload)	Sympathetic nerve impulses Circulating catecholamines Digitalis, calcium, other inotropic agents Increased heart rate or post-extrasystolic augmentation	Increased contractility
	Anoxia, acidosis Pharmacologic depression Loss of myocardium Intrinsic depression	Decreased contractility
Heart rate	Autonomic nervous system Temperature, metabolic rate	

determine afterload. Thus, afterload is increased in the setting of systemic hypertension or stenosis of the aortic valve but may be equally increased in the setting of ventricular dilation or ventricular hypertrophy. Some antihypertensive drugs such as angiotensin-converting enzyme (ACE) inhibitors and hydralazine reduce blood pressure by reducing afterload.

Contractility, or inotropy, although difficult to define, represents the force of ventricular contraction independent of loading conditions. For example, an increase in contractility results in a stronger ventricular contraction even when the preload and afterload are kept constant. Direct stimulation from adrenergic nerves in the myocardium and circulating catecholamines released from the adrenal glands can alter contractility under normal conditions. Several medications have important positive inotropic effects that can be exploited clinically, including digoxin and the sympathomimetic amines (e.g., epinephrine, norepinephrine, dopamine). Other medications, many of them antihypertensive medications, (e.g., β-blockers, calcium-channel antagonists) have negative inotropic effects and can decrease the strength of ventricular contraction.

Overall ventricular systolic function is frequently quantified by the ejection fraction, which is the ratio of the SV to the end-diastolic volume, that is, the fraction of blood in the ventricle ejected with each ventricular contraction. The normal ejection fraction is approximately 60% and can be measured by invasive (contrast ventriculography) or noninvasive (echocardiography or radionuclide ventriculography) methods.

Clearly, systolic contraction is an important component of ventricular function; however, ventricular diastolic relax-

ation (lusitropy) also plays an important role in overall cardiac performance. Impaired relaxation (diastolic dysfunction), as occurs with ventricular hypertrophy or ischemia, results in a stiff, noncompliant ventricle, leading to impaired ventricular filling and an increased ventricular pressure for any given diastolic volume.

PHYSIOLOGY OF THE CORONARY CIRCULATION

The heart is an aerobic organ requiring a constant supply of oxygen to maintain normal function. Under normal conditions, the supply of oxygen delivered to the heart is closely matched to the amount of oxygen required by the heart (the myocardial oxygen consumption [Mvo_2]). The main determinants of Mvo_2 are HR, contractility, and wall stress. The wall stress, as determined by Laplace's law, is directly related to the systolic pressure and the heart size:

$$\text{Wall stress} = (\text{pressure} \times \text{radius})/(2 \times \text{wall thickness})$$

Thus, the Mvo_2 parallels changes in HR, blood pressure, contractility, and heart size. In general, oxygen delivery to an organ can be augmented by either increasing blood flow or increasing oxygen extraction from the blood. For all practical purposes, the oxygen extraction by the heart is maximal at rest, and thus increases in coronary blood flow must meet increases in Mvo_2.

Because of the compression of intramyocardial blood vessels during systole, the majority of coronary flow occurs during diastole. Therefore, diastolic pressure is the major pressure driving the coronary circulation. An important implication of this fact is that tachycardia, which primarily shortens the duration of diastole, results in reduced time for coronary flow, which occurs despite the increase in Mvo_2 associated with increased HR. The systolic pressure has little affect on coronary blood flow except insofar as changes in blood pressure lead to changes in Mvo_2.

Regulation of coronary blood flow occurs primarily through changes in coronary vascular resistance. In response to a change in Mvo_2, the coronary arteries can dilate or constrict to allow for appropriate changes in coronary flow. Additionally, in the range of coronary perfusion pressures of 60 to 130 mm Hg, coronary blood flow is held constant by the process of autoregulation of the coronary arteries. This regulation of arterial resistance occurs at the level of the arterioles and is mediated by several factors. As ATP is metabolized during increased myocardial activity, adenosine is released and acts as a potent vasodilator. Decreased oxygen tension and increased carbon dioxide, as well as acidosis and hyperkalemia, all develop during increased myocardial metabolism and may also mediate coronary vasodilation.

The coronary arteries are innervated by the autonomic nervous system, and activation of sympathetic or parasympathetic neurons alters coronary blood flow by affecting changes in vascular tone. Parasympathetic innervation occurs through the vagus nerve and, through the neurotransmitter acetylcholine, results in vasodilation. Sympathetic neurons use norepinephrine as a neurotransmitter and may have opposing effects on the coronary vasculature. Stimulation of α-receptors results in vasoconstriction, whereas stimulation of β-receptors leads to vasodilation.

The ability of the coronary vasculature to mediate changes in blood flow through changes in vascular tone depends in large part on an intact, normally functioning endothelium. The endothelium produces several potent vasodilators, including endothelium-derived relaxing factor (EDRF) and prostacyclin. EDRF is likely to be nitric oxide or a compound containing nitric oxide and is released by the endothelium in response to acetylcholine, thrombin, ADP, serotonin, bradykinin, platelet aggregation, and an increase in shear stress. The latter stimulus accounts for the dilation of the coronary arteries in response to increases in blood flow in the setting of increases in Mvo_2 (the so-called flow-dependent vasodilation).

Vasoconstricting factors, most notably endothelin, are also produced by the endothelium and also are likely to play a role in regulating vascular tone. The balance of these vasodilator and vasoconstriction factors may be important in conditions such as coronary vasospasm. Aside from influencing vascular tone, the endothelium has several other functions that have important implications for blood flow and tissue perfusion. These include maintenance of a non-thrombotic surface through inhibition of platelet activity, control of thrombosis and fibrinolysis, and modulation of the inflammatory response of the vasculature. Disturbances in these normal properties of the endothelium (*endothelial dysfunction*) are likely to play an important role in the pathophysiologic conditions of coronary atherosclerosis and thrombosis.

PHYSIOLOGY OF THE SYSTEMIC CIRCULATION

The walls of the aorta and large arteries are rich in elastic fibers. With the ejection of blood during ventricular systole, these fibers allow the arteries to stretch and subsequently recoil, resulting in the gradual delivery of blood to the periphery. The larger arteries branch to become progressively smaller arteries and then to arterioles, the terminal regulatory branches of the arterial tree. The arterioles function as *resistance vessels,* owing to the presence of muscular sphincters and control the flow of blood to the capillary systems. The arterioles themselves are under dual regulatory control: (1) centrally through the autonomic nervous system, and (2) locally by means of conditions in the immediate vicinity of the blood vessels. Both sympathetic and parasympathetic fibers innervate the vascular system. Stimulation of the α-adrenergic system results in vasoconstriction, whereas β-adrenergic or vagal stimulation results in vasodilation. Locally, low partial pressure of oxygen (Po_2), high partial pressure of carbon dioxide (Pco_2), and acidosis result in vasodilation by directly causing relaxation of arteriolar sphincters. The systemic vascular resistance (SVR) is a measure of total vascular tone and is defined as the pressure drop across the peripheral capillary beds divided by the blood flow across the beds. In practice, this is calculated as the mean arterial pressure minus the right atrial pressure divided by the cardiac output and is normally in the range of 800 to 1500 dynes-sec/cm^5.

Blood leaves the arterioles and flows into the capillary systems, where oxygen and nutrients are delivered to cells and carbon dioxide and metabolic wastes are removed. The deoxygenated blood then drains into peripheral veins, which contain valves to prevent backflow. These veins have thinner walls than arteries and function as *capacitance vessels;* they are able to accommodate a significantly larger volume of blood than the arterial system. With the aid of the pumping action of skeletal muscles and the respiratory motion of the chest wall, blood returns to the right atrium. This venous return can be altered by constriction or dilation of the peripheral veins. In addition to the venous drainage, a rich system of lymphatic vessels helps drain excess interstitial fluid from the periphery. The various lymphatic vessels drain into the thoracic duct and, subsequently, into the left brachiocephalic vein.

PHYSIOLOGY OF THE PULMONARY CIRCULATION

Similar to the systemic circulation, the pulmonary circulation consists of a branching network of progressively smaller arteries, arterioles, capillaries, and veins. The pulmonary capillaries are separated from the alveoli by a thin alveolar-capillary membrane through which gas exchange occurs. Carbon dioxide thus diffuses from the capillary blood into the alveoli, and oxygen diffuses from the alveoli into the blood. The flow of blood to various lung segments is regulated by several factors, the most important being the Po_2 in the alveoli. In this manner, blood is shunted toward well-ventilated lung segments and away from poorly ventilated segments. As a result of the extensive nature of the pulmonary capillary system and the distensibility of the pulmonary vasculature, the resistance across the pulmonary system (the pulmonary vascular resistance) is approximately one tenth that of the systemic circulation. Owing to these features, the pulmonary system is able to tolerate significant increases in blood flow with little or no rise in pulmonary pressure. Thus, intracardiac shunts (e.g., atrial septal defects) may be associated with normal pulmonary pressure.

The lung receives a dual blood supply. The pulmonary artery accounts for the vast majority of pulmonary blood flow; however, the lungs also receive oxygenated blood through the bronchial arteries. These vessels supply oxygen to the lung itself and drain into the bronchial veins. The bronchial veins drain partly into the pulmonary veins; thus a small amount of deoxygenated blood normally enters the systemic circulation and accounts for a physiologic right-to-left shunt. In the normal setting, this shunt is insignificant, accounting for only 1% of the total systemic blood flow.

Cardiovascular Response to Exercise

The response of the heart to exercise is multifaceted and involves many of the previously discussed mechanisms of circulatory control (Table 3–3). In anticipation of exercise, neural centers in the brain stimulate vagal withdrawal and an increase in sympathetic tone, resulting in an increase in HR and contractility (thus an increase in CO) before exercise ever starts. With exercise, sympathetic venoconstriction, augmented pumping action of skeletal muscles, and increased respiratory movements of the chest wall all result in an increase in venous return to the heart. Through the Frank-Starling relationship, this increase in venous return results in an increase in contractility, thus augmenting CO. Sympathetic activation may also increase contractility; however, the majority of the increase in CO during exercise (up to four to six times the normal rate) is a consequence of an increase in the HR. The peak HR that can be achieved is dependent on age and can be estimated by the following formula: maximal HR = (220 − age) ± 10 to 12 beats/min.

Local factors in exercising muscle cause arteriolar dilation, resulting in increased flow to the capillary beds. This vasodilation results in decreased resistance to flow, and therefore the SVR decreases with exercise. Despite this change in resistance, the systolic blood pressure rises, owing to the augmented CO and to sympathetic vasoconstriction, which leads to the preferential shunting of blood away from nonexercising vascular beds. The diastolic blood pressure, by contrast, generally remains constant during exercise. The

pulmonary system is able to tolerate the increased flow with only small increases in pulmonary pressure. The increases in HR and contractility result in a significant increase in Mvo_2 (up to 300%), and coronary blood flow subsequently increases.

Various types of exercises have different effects on the circulatory system. The response described in this text occurs with isotonic exercises, such as running or biking. With isometric exercises, such as weight lifting, the predominant response is an increase in blood pressure, owing to an increase in peripheral vasoconstriction.

Table 3–3	**Physiologic Responses to Exercise**
Increased heart rate	Increased sympathetic stimulation
Increased stroke volume	Decreased parasympathetic stimulation
Increased contractility	Increased sympathetic stimulation
Increased venous return	Sympathetic-mediated venoconstriction
	Pumping action of skeletal muscles
	Decreased intrathoracic pressure with deep inspirations
	Arteriolar vasodilation in exercising muscle
Decreased afterload	Arteriolar vasodilation in exercising muscle (mediated chiefly by local metabolites)
Increased blood pressure	Increased cardiac output
	Vasoconstriction (sympathetic stimulation) on nonexercising vascular beds
Increased O_2 extraction	Shift in oxyhemoglobin dissociation curve as a result of local acidosis

Prospectus for the Future

Recent years have witnessed an explosion in the growth of basic knowledge governing normal heart development and function of the circulatory system. New insights about the molecular switches and factors that promote the formation of heart chambers and blood vessels are unraveling the genetic basis for unusual causes of congenital heart disease. Similarly, the recent discovery of specific growth factors with properties for angiogenesis and neural guidance is stimulating possible therapeutic approaches for cardiac regeneration and repair for acquired cardiac illnesses. With increasing refinement in this basic knowledge, future milestones appear on the horizon for diagnosis, early treatment, and even prevention of cardiovascular diseases.

References

Berne RM, Levy MN: Physiology, Updated Edition, 5th edition with Student Consult Access, IV, The Cardiovascular System, St Louis: Elsevier, 2004.

Guyton AC, Hall JE: Textbook of Medical Physiology, St. Louis: Elsevier, 2005.

Chapter 4

Evaluation of the Patient with Cardiovascular Disease

Sheldon E. Litwin

Ivor J. Benjamin

History

As with diseases of most organ systems, the ability of the physician to diagnose diseases of the cardiovascular system is in large part dependent on eliciting and interpreting the patient's clinical history. A thorough history can enable the physician to identify a patient's symptoms as characteristic of a specific cardiovascular disorder or to suggest that symptoms are unlikely to be caused by cardiovascular disease. In addition, a complete history will reveal the presence of other systemic diseases that may have cardiovascular manifestations, identify existing risk factors that may be modified to prevent the future development of cardiovascular disease (see Chapter 9), enable the selection of appropriate further diagnostic testing (see Chapter 5), and allow the assessment of functional capacity and extent of cardiovascular disability. The patient should be asked about prior medical conditions, including childhood illnesses (e.g., rheumatic fever), as well as intravenous drug use, which may lead to the development of valvular heart disease. Several cardiovascular disorders are inherited (e.g., hypertrophic cardiomyopathy, Marfan syndrome, long QT syndrome), and a thorough family history may bring this potential to the examiner's attention.

The classic symptoms of cardiac disease include precordial discomfort or pain, dyspnea, palpitations, syncope or presyncope, and edema. Although characteristic of heart disease, these symptoms are nonspecific and may also occur as a result of diseases of other organ systems (e.g., musculoskeletal, pulmonary, renal, gastrointestinal). Furthermore, some patients with established cardiovascular disease may be asymptomatic or have atypical symptoms.

Chest pain is a frequent symptom and may be a manifestation of cardiovascular or noncardiovascular disease (Tables 4–1 and 4–2). Full characterization of the pain with regard to quality, quantity, frequency, location, duration, radiation, aggravating or alleviating factors, and associated symptoms may help distinguish among various causes. Reversible myocardial ischemia caused by obstructive coronary artery disease commonly results in episodic chest pain or discomfort during exertion or stress (angina pectoris). Patients frequently deny having pain and, instead, describe a discomfort in their chest. Sometimes they will refer to the discomfort as a *squeezing, tightening, pressing,* or *burning* sensation or as a *heavy weight* on their chest, and they will sometimes clench their fist over their chest while describing the discomfort (Levine's sign). Anginal discomfort is classically located substernally or over the left chest. It frequently radiates to the epigastrium, neck, jaw, or back and down the ulnar aspect of the left arm. Radiation to the right chest or arm is less common, whereas radiation above the jaw or below the epigastrium is not typical of cardiac disease. Angina is usually brought on by either physical or emotional stress, is mild to moderate in intensity, lasts 2 to 10 minutes, and resolves with rest or sublingual administration of nitroglycerin. It may occur more frequently in the morning, in cold weather, after a large meal, or after exposure to environmental factors, including cigarette smoke, and is frequently accompanied by other symptoms, such as dyspnea, diaphoresis, nausea, palpitations, or lightheadedness. Patients frequently report a stable pattern of angina that is predictably reproducible with a given amount of exertion. Unstable angina occurs when a patient reports a significant increase in the frequency or severity of angina or when angina occurs with progressively decreasing exertion or at rest. When anginal-type pain occurs mainly at rest, it may be of a noncardiac origin, or it may reflect true cardiac ischemia resulting from coronary spasm (Prinzmetal's or variant angina). The pain of an acute myocardial infarction may be similar to angina, although the former is usually more severe and prolonged (>30 min).

Table 4–1   Cardiovascular Causes of Chest Pain

Condition	Location	Quality	Duration	Aggravating or Alleviating Factors	Associated Symptoms or Signs
Angina	Retrosternal region: radiates to or occasionally isolated to neck, jaw, shoulders, arms (usually left), or epigastrium	Pressure, squeezing, tightness, heaviness, burning, indigestion	<2–10 min	Precipitated by exertion, cold weather, or emotional stress; relieved by rest or nitroglycerin; variant (Prinzmetal's) angina may be unrelated to exertion, often early in the morning	Dyspnea; S_3, S_4, or murmur of papillary dysfunction during pain
Myocardial infarction	Same as angina	Same as angina, although more severe	Variable; usually longer than 30 min	Unrelieved by rest or nitroglycerin	Dyspnea, nausea, vomiting, weakness, diaphoresis
Pericarditis	Left of the sternum; may radiate to neck or left shoulder, often more localized than pain of myocardial ischemia	Sharp, stabbing, knifelike	Lasts many hours to days; may wax and wane	Aggravated by deep breathing, rotating chest, or supine position; relieved by sitting up and leaning forward	Pericardial friction rub
Aortic dissection	Anterior chest; may radiate to back, interscapular region	Excruciating, tearing, knifelike	Sudden onset, unrelenting	Usually occurs in setting of hypertension or predisposition, such as Marfan syndrome	Murmur of aortic insufficiency; pulse or blood pressure asymmetry; neurologic deficit

The pain of acute pericarditis is usually sharper than anginal pain, is located to the left of the sternum, and may radiate to the neck or left shoulder. In contrast to angina, the pain may last hours, typically worsens with inspiration, and improves when the patient sits up and leans forward; it may be associated with a pericardial friction rub. Acute aortic dissection produces severe, sharp, *tearing* pain that radiates to the back and may be associated with asymmetric pulses and a murmur of aortic insufficiency. Pulmonary emboli may produce the sudden onset of sharp chest pain that is worse on inspiration, is associated with shortness of breath, and may have an associated pleural friction rub, especially if a pulmonary infarction is present. A multitude of noncardiac conditions may also produce chest pain (see Table 4–2). The clinical history and physical examination findings will often help distinguish these causes from ischemic chest pain.

Dyspnea, an uncomfortable, heightened awareness of breathing, is commonly a symptom of cardiac disease. Patients with decreased left ventricular function may exhibit significant abnormalities of the aortic or mitral valves or decreased myocardial compliance (i.e., left ventricular

hypertrophy, acute ischemia), left ventricular diastolic, and/or left atrial pressure increases transmitted through the pulmonary veins to the pulmonary capillary system, producing vascular congestion. This congestion results in exudation of fluid into the alveolar space and impairs gas exchange across the alveolar-capillary membrane, producing the subjective sensation of dyspnea. Dyspnea frequently occurs on exertion; however, in patients with severe cardiac disease, it may be present at rest. Patients with heart failure commonly sleep on two or more pillows because the augmented venous return that occurs on assuming the recumbent position produces an increase in dyspnea (orthopnea). In addition, these patients report awakening 2 to 4 hours after the onset of sleep with dyspnea (paroxysmal nocturnal dyspnea), which is likely caused by the central redistribution of peripheral edema in the supine position.

Dyspnea may be associated with diseases of the lungs or chest wall and is also seen in anemia, obesity, deconditioning, and anxiety disorders. In addition, the sudden onset of dyspnea, with or without chest pain, may be present with pulmonary emboli. Dyspnea is frequently difficult to

Table 4–2 Noncardiac Causes of Chest Pain

Condition	Location	Quality	Duration	Aggravating or Alleviating Factors	Associated Symptoms or Signs
Pulmonary embolism (chest pain often not present)	Substernal or over region of pulmonary infarction	Pleuritic (with pulmonary infarction) or angina-like	Sudden onset (min to hr)	Aggravated by deep breathing	Dyspnea, tachypnea, tachycardia; hypotension, signs of acute right ventricular heart failure, and pulmonary hypertension with large emboli; pleural rub; hemoptysis with pulmonary infarction
Pulmonary hypertension	Substernal	Pressure; oppressive	—	Aggravated by effort	Pain usually associated with dyspnea; signs of pulmonary hypertension
Pneumonia with pleurisy	Located over involved area	Pleuritic	—	Aggravated by breathing	Dyspnea, cough, fever, bronchial breath sounds, rhonchi, egophony, dullness to percussion, occasional pleural rub
Spontaneous pneumothorax	Unilateral	Sharp, well localized	Sudden onset; lasts many hours	Aggravated by breathing	Dyspnea; hyperresonance and decreased breath and voice sounds over involved lung
Musculoskeletal disorders	Variable	Aching, well localized	Variable	Aggravated by movement; history of exertion or injury	Tender to palpation or with light pressure
Herpes zoster	Dermatomal distribution	Sharp, burning	Prolonged	None	Vesicular rash appears in area of discomfort
Esophageal reflux	Substernal or epigastric; may radiate to neck	Burning, visceral discomfort	10–60 min	Aggravated by large meal, post-prandial recumbency; relief with antacid	Water brash
Peptic ulcer	Epigastric, substernal	Visceral burning, aching	Prolonged	Relief with food, antacid	—
Gallbladder disease	Right upper quadrant; epigastric	Visceral	Prolonged	Spontaneous or following meals	Right upper quadrant tenderness may be present
Anxiety states	Often localized over precordium	Variable; location often moves from place to place	Varies; often fleeting	Situational	Sighing respirations; often chest wall tenderness

distinguish cardiac from pulmonary causes by history alone, because both may produce resting or exertional dyspnea, orthopnea, or cough. Wheezing and hemoptysis are classically results of pulmonary disease, although they are also frequently present in the patient with pulmonary edema resulting from left ventricular dysfunction or mitral stenosis. True paroxysmal nocturnal dyspnea is, however, more specific for cardiac disease. In patients with coronary artery disease, dyspnea may be an *anginal equivalent;* that is, the dyspnea is the result of ischemia and occurs in a pattern consistent with angina but in the absence of chest discomfort.

Palpitation refers to the subjective sensation of the heart beating. Patients may describe a *fluttering* or *pounding* in the chest or a feeling that their heart *races* or *skips a beat.* Some people feel post-extrasystolic beats as a painful or uncomfortable sensation. Common arrhythmic causes of palpitations include premature atrial or ventricular contractions, supraventricular tachycardia, ventricular tachycardia, and sinus tachycardia. Occasionally, patients report palpitations even when no rhythm disturbance is noted during monitoring, as occurs commonly in patients with anxiety disorders. The pattern of palpitations, especially when correlated to the pulse, may help narrow the differential diagnosis: Rapid, regular palpitations are noted with supraventricular tachycardia or ventricular tachycardia; rapid, irregular palpitations are noted with atrial fibrillation; and *skipped beats* are noted with premature atrial or ventricular contractions.

Syncope is the transient loss of consciousness resulting from inadequate cerebral blood flow and may be the result of a variety of cardiovascular diseases (see Chapter 10). True syncope must be distinguished from primary neurologic causes of loss of consciousness (i.e., seizures) and metabolic causes of loss of consciousness (e.g., hypoglycemia, hyperventilation). Cardiac syncope occurs after an abrupt decrease in cardiac output, as may occur with acute myocardial ischemia, valvular heart disease (aortic or mitral stenosis), hypertrophic obstructive cardiomyopathy, left atrial tumors, tachyarrhythmias (ventricular, or less commonly supraventricular, tachycardias), or bradyarrhythmias (e.g., sinus arrest, atrioventricular block, Stokes-Adams attacks). Reflex vasodilation or bradycardia may also result in syncope (vasovagal syncope, carotid sinus syncope, micturition syncope, cough syncope, or neurocardiogenic syncope), as may acute pulmonary embolism and hypovolemia. Because global, or at the very least bilateral, cortical ischemia is required to produce syncope, it rarely occurs as a result of unilateral carotid artery disease. However, syncope is occasionally the result of bilateral carotid artery disease and can also occur when disease of the vertebrobasilar system results in brainstem ischemia. In up to 50% of patients, the cause of a syncopal episode cannot be determined; however, in the cases in which a cause is determined, the most important factor in establishing the diagnosis is obtaining an accurate history of the event.

Edema is a nonspecific symptom that commonly accompanies cardiac disease, as well as renal disease (e.g., nephrotic syndrome), hepatic disease (e.g., cirrhosis), and local venous abnormalities (e.g., thrombophlebitis, chronic venous stasis). When edema occurs as a result of cardiac disease, it reflects an increase in venous pressure. This increased pressure alters the balance between the venous hydrostatic and oncotic forces, resulting in extravasation of fluid into the extravascular space. When this process occurs as a result of elevated left-sided heart pressure, pulmonary edema results, whereas elevated right-sided heart pressure results in peripheral edema. Characteristically, the peripheral edema of heart failure is *pitting;* that is, an indentation is left in the skin after pressure is applied to the edematous region. The edema is exacerbated by long periods of standing, is worse in the evening, improves after lying down, and may first be noted when a patient has difficulty in fitting into his or her shoes. The edema may shift to the sacral region after a patient lies down for several hours. When visible edema is noted, it is usually preceded by a moderate weight gain (i.e., 5 to 10 lb), indicative of volume retention. As heart failure progresses, the edema may extend to the thighs and involve the genitalia and abdominal wall, and fluid may collect in the abdominal (ascites) or thoracic (pleural effusion) cavities. Anasarca with ascites should raise suspicion for constrictive pericarditis because this disease may progress very slowly and insidiously.

Cyanosis is an abnormal bluish discoloration of the skin resulting from an increase in the level of reduced hemoglobin in the blood and, in general, reflects an arterial oxygen saturation of 85% or less (normal arterial oxygen saturation ≥95%). Central cyanosis exhibits as cyanosis of the lips or trunk and often reflects right-to-left shunting of blood caused by structural cardiac abnormalities (e.g., atrial or ventricular septal defects) or pulmonary parenchymal or vascular disease (e.g., chronic obstructive pulmonary disease, pulmonary embolism, pulmonary arteriovenous fistula). Peripheral cyanosis may occur because of systemic vasoconstriction in the setting of poor cardiac output or may be a localized phenomenon resulting from venous or arterial occlusive or vasospastic disease (e.g., venous or arterial thrombosis, arterial embolic disease, Raynaud's disease). When cyanosis occurs in childhood, it usually reflects congenital heart disease with right-to-left shunting of blood.

A myriad of *other symptoms,* many of them nonspecific, may occur with cardiac disease. Fatigue frequently occurs in the setting of poor cardiac output or may occur secondary to the medical therapy of cardiac disease from overdiuresis, aggressive blood pressure lowering, or use of β-blocking agents. Nausea and vomiting frequently occur during an acute myocardial infarction and may also reflect intestinal edema in the setting of right ventricular heart failure. Anorexia and cachexia may occur in severe heart failure. Positional fluid shifts may result in polyuria and nocturia in patients with edema. In addition, epistaxis, hoarseness, hiccups, fever, and chills may reflect underlying cardiovascular disease.

Many patients with significant cardiac disease are asymptomatic. Patients with coronary artery disease frequently have periods of asymptomatic ischemia that can be documented with ambulatory electrocardiographic (ECG) monitoring. Furthermore, nearly one third of patients who suffer an acute myocardial infarction are unaware of the event. This silent ischemia appears to be more common in older adults and in patients with diabetes. Patients may also be asymptomatic despite having severely depressed ventricular function; this usually bespeaks a chronic, slowly progressive process. Reduced exercise capacity may only be seen during provocative testing. Similarly, recent findings show that a high percentage of episodes of atrial fibrillation are unrecognized by patients.

Assessment of Functional Capacity

In patients with cardiac disorders, their ability or inability to perform various activities (functional status) plays an important role in determining their extent of disability, deciding when to institute various therapies or interventions, and assessing their response to therapy, as well as determining their overall prognosis. The New York Heart Association Functional Classification is a standardized method for the assessment of functional status (Table 4–3) and relates functional capacity to the presence or absence of cardiac symptoms during the performance of *usual activities*. The Canadian Cardiovascular Society has provided a similar classification of functional status specifically in patients with angina pectoris. These tools are useful in that they allow a patient's symptoms to be classified and then compared with their symptoms at a different point in time.

Physical Examination

EXAMINATION OF THE JUGULAR VENOUS PULSATIONS

The examination of the neck veins allows for estimation of the right atrial pressure and for identification of the venous waveforms. The right internal jugular vein is used for this examination because it more accurately reflects right atrial pressure than the external jugular or left jugular vein. With the patient lying at a 45-degree angle (higher in patients with elevated venous pressure, lower in patients with low venous pressure) with his or her head turned to the left, the vertical distance from the sternal angle (angle of Louis) to the top of the venous pulsation can be determined. Because the right

atrium lies approximately 5 cm vertically below the sternal angle, distention of the internal jugular vein 4 cm above the sternal angle reflects a right atrial pressure of 9 cm of water (H_2O). The right atrial pressure is normally 5 to 9 cm H_2O and is increased with congestive heart failure, tricuspid insufficiency or stenosis, and restrictive or constrictive heart disease. With inspiration, negative intrathoracic pressure develops, venous blood drains into the thorax, and the normal venous pressure falls; the opposite is true with expiration. This pattern is reversed (Kussmaul's sign) in the setting of right ventricular heart failure, constrictive pericarditis, or restrictive myocardial disease. With right ventricular heart failure, the elevated venous pressure results in passive congestion of the liver. Pressure applied over the liver for 1 to 3 minutes in this setting results in an increase in the jugular venous pressure (hepatojugular reflux).

The normal waveforms of the venous pulsation consist of the *a*, *c*, and *v* waves and the *x* and *y* descents; these waveforms are shown in Figure 4–1A and reflect events in the right side of the heart. The *a* wave results from atrial contraction. Subsequent atrial relaxation results in a decrease in the right atrial pressure, which is seen as the *x* descent. This descent is interrupted by the *c* wave, generated by the bulging of the tricuspid valve cusps into the right atrium during ventricular systole. As the atrial pressure increases owing to venous return, the *v* wave is generated. This wave is normally smaller than the *a* wave and is followed by the *y* descent as the tricuspid valve opens and blood flows from the right atrium to the right ventricle during diastole.

Abnormalities of the venous waveforms reflect underlying structural, functional, or electrical abnormalities of the heart (see Fig. 4–1B through G). The *a* wave increases in any condition in which greater resistance to right atrial emptying occurs (e.g., tricuspid stenosis, right ventricular hypertrophy or failure, pulmonary hypertension). *Cannon a waves* are seen when the atrium contracts against a closed tricuspid valve, as occurs with complete heart block, with junctional or ventricular rhythms, and occasionally with ventricular pacemakers. The *a* wave is absent in atrial fibrillation. In tricuspid regurgitation, the *v* wave is prominent and may merge with the *c* wave (*cv* wave), thus diminishing or eliminating the *x* descent altogether. The *y* descent is attenuated in tricuspid stenosis, owing to the impaired atrial emptying. In pericardial constriction and restrictive cardiomyopathy, as well as in right ventricular infarction, the *y* descent becomes rapid and deep, and the *x* descent may also become prominent (*w* waveform). In pericardial tamponade, the *x* descent is prominent, but the *y* descent is diminished or absent.

EXAMINATION OF THE ARTERIAL PULSE

The arterial blood pressure can be measured with the use of a sphygmomanometer. The cuff is applied to the upper arm, rapidly inflated to 30 mm Hg above the anticipated systolic pressure, and then slowly deflated (= 3 mm Hg/sec) while listening for the sounds produced by blood entering the previously occluded brachial artery (Korotkoff sounds). The pressure at which the first sound is heard (usually a clear, tapping sound) represents the systolic pressure. Diastolic pressure occurs at the point at which the Korotkoff sounds disappear. Normally, the pressure in both arms is the same

Table 4–3	**Classification of Functional Status**	
Class I	Uncompromised	Ordinary activity does not cause symptoms.* Symptoms only occur with strenuous or prolonged activity.
Class II	Slightly compromised	Ordinary physical activity results in symptoms; no symptoms at rest.
Class III	Moderately compromised	Less than ordinary activity results in symptoms; no symptoms at rest.
Class IV	Severely compromised	Any activity results in symptoms; symptoms may be present at rest.

*Symptoms refer to undue fatigue, dyspnea, palpitations, or angina in the New York Heart Association classification and refer specifically to angina in the Canadian Cardiovascular Society classification.

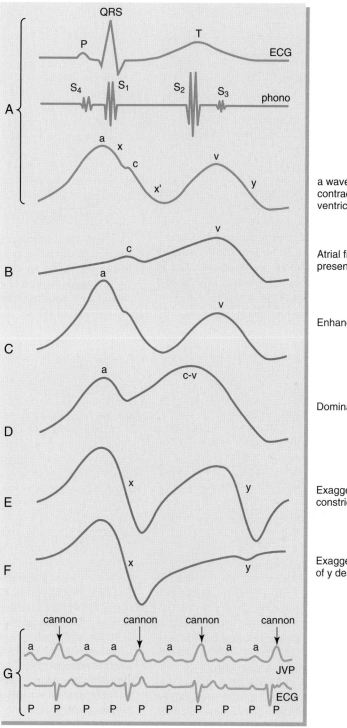

Figure 4–1 Normal and abnormal jugular venous pulse tracings. *A,* Normal jugular pulse tracing with simultaneous ECG and phonocardiogram. *B,* Loss of the *a* wave in atrial fibrillation. *C,* Large *a* wave in tricuspid stenosis. *D,* Large *c-v* wave in tricuspid regurgitation. *E,* Prominent *x* and *y* descents in constrictive pericarditis. *F,* Prominent *x* descent and diminutive *y* descent in pericardial tamponade. *G,* Jugular venous pulse tracing and simultaneous ECG during complete heart block demonstrating *cannon a waves* occurring when the atrium contracts against a closed tricuspid valve during ventricular systole.

(approximately 120/70 mm Hg), and the systolic pressure in the legs is 10 to 20 mm Hg higher. Asymmetric arm pressures can result from atherosclerotic disease of the aorta, aortic dissection, and stenosis of the innominate or subclavian arteries. Coarctation of the aorta and severe atherosclerotic disease of the aorta or the femoral or iliac arteries can result in a lower blood pressure in the legs than in the arms. Aortic insufficiency is frequently associated with a leg pressure greater than 20 mm Hg higher than the arm pressure (Hill's sign). Use of a cuff that is too small for a patient's arm

will result in erroneously high pressure measurements. Similarly, a cuff that is too large results in erroneously low measurements.

The arterial examination should include assessments of the carotid, radial, brachial, femoral, popliteal, posterior tibial, and dorsalis pedis pulses, although the carotid artery pulse most accurately reflects the central aortic pulse. The rhythm, strength, contour, and symmetry of the pulses should be noted. The normal arterial pulse (Fig. 4–2A) rises rapidly to a peak in early systole, plateaus, and then falls. The

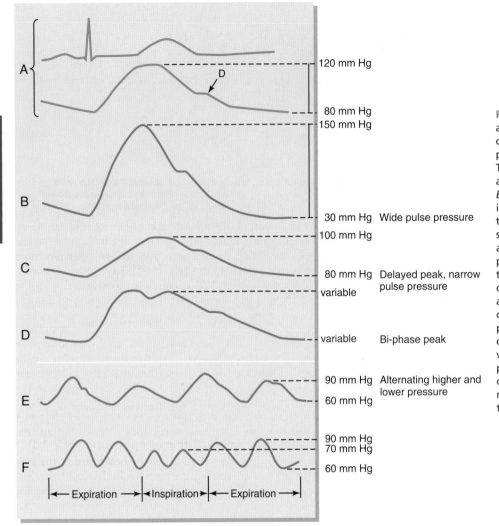

120 mm Hg

80 mm Hg
150 mm Hg

30 mm Hg   Wide pulse pressure

100 mm Hg

80 mm Hg   Delayed peak, narrow
variable   pulse pressure

variable   Bi-phase peak

90 mm Hg   Alternating higher and
60 mm Hg   lower pressure

90 mm Hg
70 mm Hg
60 mm Hg

←— Expiration —→|←Inspiration→|←— Expiration —→|

Figure 4–2 Normal and abnormal carotid arterial pulse contours. *A,* Normal arterial pulse with simultaneous ECG. The dicrotic wave *(D)* occurs just after aortic valve closure. *B,* Wide pulse pressure in aortic insufficiency. *C,* Pulsus parvus et tardus (small amplitude with a slow upstroke) associated with aortic stenosis. *D,* Bisferious pulse with two systolic peaks, typical of hypertrophic obstructive cardiomyopathy or aortic insufficiency, especially if concomitant aortic stenosis is present. *E,* Pulsus alternans, characteristic of severe left ventricular failure. *F,* Paradoxic pulse (systolic pressure decrease of >10 mm Hg with inspiration), most characteristic of cardiac tamponade.

descending pressure wave is interrupted by the dicrotic notch, related to aortic valve closure. This normal pattern is altered in a variety of cardiovascular disease states (see Fig. 4–2*B* through *F*). The amplitude of the pulse increases in aortic insufficiency, anemia, pregnancy, and thyrotoxicosis and decreases in conditions such as hypovolemia, tachycardia, left ventricular failure, and severe mitral stenosis. Aortic insufficiency results in a *bounding* pulse (Corrigan's pulse or water-hammer pulse), owing to an increased pulse pressure (the difference between systolic and diastolic pressure), and is accompanied by a multitude of abnormalities in the peripheral pulses that reflect this increased pulse pressure. Aortic stenosis characteristically results in an attenuated carotid pulse with a delayed upstroke (pulsus parvus et tardus) and may be associated with a palpable thrill over the aortic area (the carotid shudder). A bisferious pulse is commonly felt in the presence of pure aortic regurgitation and is characterized by two systolic peaks. The first peak is the percussion wave, resulting from the rapid ejection of a large volume of blood early in systole; the second peak is the tidal wave, a reflected wave from the periphery. This bifid pulse may also be noted in hypertrophic cardiomyopathy in which the initial rapid upstroke of the pulse is cut short by the

development of a left ventricular outflow tract obstruction, resulting in a fall in the pulse. The reflected wave again produces the second impulse. In severe left ventricular dysfunction, the intensity of the pulse may alternate from beat to beat *(pulsus alternans),* and in atrial fibrillation, the pulse intensity is variable. With inspiration, negative intrathoracic pressure is transmitted to the aorta and the systolic pressure normally decreases by up to 10 mm Hg. Pulsus paradoxus is an exaggeration of this normal inspiratory fall in systolic pressure and is characteristically seen with pericardial tamponade, although it may also occur as a result of severe obstructive lung disease, constrictive pericarditis, hypovolemic shock, and pregnancy.

Atherosclerotic disease of the peripheral vascular system frequently accompanies coronary atherosclerosis; therefore, the presence of peripheral vascular disease warrants a search for symptoms or signs of coronary artery disease and vice versa. When atherosclerosis occurs in a peripheral artery to the lower extremity and impairs blood flow distally, the patient may complain of intermittent cramping in the buttocks, thigh, calf, or foot (claudication). Severe peripheral vascular disease may result in digital ischemia or necrosis, without or with associated erectile dysfunction (Leriche's syndrome). The peripheral pulses should be palpated and the abdominal aorta assessed for enlargement in all cardiac patients; a pulsatile, expansile, periumbilical mass suggests the presence of an abdominal aortic aneurysm. With significant stenosis of the peripheral vasculature, the distal pulses may be diminished or absent, and the blood flow through the stenotic artery may be audible (a *bruit*). With normal aging, the elastic arteries lose their compliance, and this change in physical property may obscure abnormal findings.

EXAMINATION OF THE PRECORDIUM

Inspection and palpation of the precordium may yield valuable clues as to the existence of cardiac disease. Chest wall abnormalities should be noted, such as pectus excavatum, which may be associated with Marfan syndrome or mitral valve prolapse, pectus carinatum, which may be associated with Marfan syndrome, and kyphoscoliosis (occasionally a cause of secondary pulmonary hypertension and right ventricular heart failure). The presence of visible pulsations in the aortic (second right intercostal space and suprasternal notch), pulmonic (third left intercostal space), right ventricular (left parasternal region), and left ventricular (fourth to fifth intercostal space and left midclavicular line) regions should be noted and will help direct the palpation of the heart. Retraction of the left parasternal area may be seen with severe left ventricular hypertrophy, and systolic retraction of the chest wall at the cardiac apex or left axilla (Broadbent's sign) is characteristic of constrictive pericarditis.

Precordial palpation is best performed with the patient supine or in the left lateral position, with the examiner standing to the patient's right side. In this position, firm placement of the examiner's right hand over the patient's lower left chest wall places the fingertips over the region of the cardiac apex and the palm over the region of the right ventricle. The normal cardiac apical impulse is a brief, discrete impulse (approximately 1 cm) located in the fourth to fifth intercostal space in the left midclavicular line generated as the left ventricle strikes the chest wall during early systole. In a patient with a structurally normal heart, the apex is the point of maximal impulse (PMI) of the heart against the chest wall. Enlargement of the left ventricle results in lateral displacement of the apical impulse, whereas chronic obstructive pulmonary disease may result in inferior displacement of the PMI. Volume overload states, such as aortic insufficiency and mitral regurgitation, produce ventricular enlargement primarily from dilation and result in a hyperdynamic apical impulse; that is, the impulse is brisk and increased in amplitude. Pressure overload states, such as aortic stenosis and long-standing hypertension, produce ventricular enlargement primarily from hypertrophy. In this setting, the apical impulse is sustained, and atrial contraction is frequently detected (a palpable S_4). Hypertrophic cardiomyopathy characteristically produces a double or triple apical impulse. Left ventricular aneurysms produce an apical impulse that is larger than normal and dyskinetic.

The right ventricular impulse is not normally palpable. When an impulse is felt over the left parasternal region, it usually reflects right ventricular hypertrophy or dilation. Aortic aneurysms may be palpable (or visible) in the suprasternal notch or the second right intercostal space. Pulmonary hypertension may produce a palpable systolic impulse in the left third intercostal space and may also be associated with a palpable pulmonic component of the second heart sound (P_2). Harsh murmurs originating from valvular or congenital heart disease may be associated with palpable vibratory sensations (thrills), as can occur with aortic stenosis, hypertrophic cardiomyopathy, and ventricular septal defects.

Auscultation
TECHNIQUE

Auscultation of the heart should ideally be performed in a quiet room with the patient in a comfortable position and the chest fully exposed. Certain heart sounds are better heard with either the bell or diaphragm of the stethoscope. Low-frequency sounds are best heard with the bell applied to the chest wall with just enough pressure to form a seal. As more pressure is applied to the bell, low-frequency sounds are filtered out. High-frequency sounds are best heard with the diaphragm firmly applied to the chest wall. In a patient with a normally situated heart, four major zones of cardiac auscultation are assessed. Aortic valvular events are best heard in the second right intercostal space. Pulmonary valvular events are best heard in the second left interspace. The fourth left interspace is ideal for auscultating tricuspid valvular events, and mitral valvular events are best heard at the cardiac apex or PMI. Because anatomic abnormalities, both congenital and acquired, can alter the location of the heart in the chest, the auscultatory areas may vary among patients. For instance, in patients with emphysema, the heart is shifted downward, and heart sounds may be best heard in the epigastrium. In dextrocardia, the heart lies in the right hemithorax, and the auscultatory regions are reversed. Additionally, auscultation in the axilla or supraclavicular areas or over the thoracic spine may be helpful in some settings, and having the patient lean forward, exhale, or perform various maneuvers may help accentuate particular heart sounds (Table 4–4).

NORMAL HEART SOUNDS

The two major heart sounds heard during auscultation are termed S_1 and S_2. These heart sounds are high-pitched sounds originating from valve closure (**Web Sounds normal**). S_1 occurs at the onset of ventricular systole and corresponds to closure of the atrioventricular valves. It is usually perceived as a single sound, although occasionally its two components, M_1 and T_1, corresponding to closure of the mitral and tricuspid valves, respectively, can be heard. M_1 occurs earlier, is the louder of the two components, and is best heard at the cardiac apex. T_1 is somewhat softer and heard at the left lower sternal border. The second heart sound results from closure of the semilunar valves. The two components, A_2 and P_2, originating from aortic and pulmonic valve closure, respectively, can be easily distinguished. A_2 is usually louder than P_2 and is best heard at the right upper sternal border. P_2 is loudest over the second left intercostal space. During expiration, the normal S_2 is perceived as a single event. However, during inspiration, the augmented venous return to the right side of the heart and the increased capacitance of the pulmonary vascular bed result in a delay

Table 4–4 Effects of Physiologic Maneuvers on Auscultatory Events

Maneuver	Major Physiologic Effects	Useful Auscultatory Changes
Respiration	↑ Venous return with inspiration	↑ Right heart murmurs and gallops with inspiration; splitting of S_2 (see Fig. 4–3)
Valsalva (initial ↑ BP, phase I; followed by ↓ BP, phase II)	↓ BP, ↓ venous return, ↓ LV size (phase II)	↑ HCM ↓ AS, MR MVP click earlier in systole; murmur prolongs
Standing	↑ Venous return ↑ LV size	↑ HCM ↓ AS, MR MVP click earlier in systole; murmur prolongs
Squatting	↑ Venous return ↑ Systemic vascular resistance ↑ LV size	↑ AS, MR, AI ↓ HCM MVP click delayed; murmur shortens
Isometric exercise (e.g., handgrip)	↑ Arterial pressure ↑ Cardiac output	↑ Gallops ↑ MR, AI, MS ↓ AS, HCM
Post PVC or prolonged R-R interval	↑ Ventricular filling ↑ Contractility	↑ AS Little change in MR
Amyl nitrate	↓ Arterial pressure ↑ Cardiac output ↓ LV size	↑ HCM, AS, MS ↓ AI, MR, Austin Flint murmur MVP click earlier in systole; murmur prolongs
Phenylephrine	↑ Arterial pressure ↑ Cardiac output ↓ LV size	↑ MR, AI ↓ AS, HCM MVP click delayed; murmur shortens

↑ = increased intensity; ↓ = decreased intensity; AI = aortic insufficiency; AS = aortic stenosis; BP = blood pressure; HCM = hypertrophic cardiomyopathy; LV = left ventricle; MR = mitral regurgitation; MS = mitral stenosis; MVP = mitral valve prolapse; PVC = premature ventricular contraction; R-R = interval between the R waves on an electrocardiogram.

in pulmonic valve closure. In addition, the slightly decreased venous return to the left ventricle results in slightly earlier aortic valve closure. Thus, *physiologic splitting* of the second heart sound, with A_2 preceding P_2 during inspiration, is a normal respiratory event.

Occasionally, additional heart sounds may be heard in normal individuals. A third heart sound (see later discussion) can be heard in normal children and young adults, in whom it is referred to as a *physiologic S_3*; it is rarely heard after the age of 40 years in healthy individuals (**Web Sound S_3**).

A fourth heart sound (S_4) is generated by forceful atrial contraction and is rarely audible in normal young individuals but is fairly common in older individuals (**Web Sound S_4**).

A murmur is an auditory vibration usually generated either by abnormally increased flow across a normal valve or by normal flow across an abnormal valve or structure. *Innocent* murmurs are always systolic murmurs, are usually soft and brief, and are by definition not associated with abnormalities of the cardiovascular system. They arise from flow across the normal aortic or pulmonic outflow tracts and are present in a large proportion of children and young adults. Murmurs associated with high-flow states (e.g., pregnancy, anemia, fever, thyrotoxicosis, exercise) are not considered innocent, although they are not usually associated with structural heart disease. These are termed *physiologic murmurs*, owing to their association with altered physiologic states. Diastolic murmurs are never *innocent* or *physiologic*.

ABNORMAL HEART SOUNDS

Abnormalities of S_1 and S_2 relate to abnormalities in their intensity (Table 4–5) or abnormalities in their respiratory splitting (Table 4–6). As noted, splitting of the S_1 is normal but not frequently noted. This splitting becomes more apparent with right bundle branch block or with Ebstein's anomaly of the tricuspid valve, owing to delay in closure of

Table 4–5   Abnormal Intensity of Heart Sounds

	S_1	A_2	P_2
Loud	Short PR interval Mitral stenosis with pliable valve	Systemic hypertension Aortic dilation Coarctation of the aorta	Pulmonary hypertension Thin chest wall
Soft	Long PR interval Mitral regurgitation Poor left ventricular function Mitral stenosis with rigid valve Thick chest wall	Calcific aortic stenosis Aortic regurgitation	Valvular or subvalvular pulmonic stenosis
Varying	Atrial fibrillation Heart block	—	—

Table 4–6   Abnormal Splitting of S_2

Single S_2	Widely Split S_2 with Normal Respiratory Variation	Fixed Split S_2	Paradoxically Split S_2
—	Right bundle branch block	Atrial septal defect	Left bundle branch block
Pulmonic stenosis	Left ventricular pacing	Severe right ventricular dysfunction	Right ventricular pacing
Systemic hypertension	Pulmonic stenosis	—	Angina, myocardial infarction
Coronary artery disease	Pulmonary embolism	—	Aortic stenosis
Any condition that can lead to paradoxical splitting of S_2	Idiopathic dilation of the pulmonary artery Mitral regurgitation Ventricular septal defect	—	Hypertrophic cardiomyopathy Aortic regurgitation

the tricuspid valve in these conditions (**Web Sound Ebstein**). The intensity of S_1 is determined in part by the opening state of the atrioventricular valves at the onset of ventricular systole. If the valves are still widely open, as may occur with tachycardia or a short P-R interval, S_1 will be accentuated. Conversely, in the presence of a long P-R interval, the mitral valve drifts toward a closed position before the onset of ventricular systole, and the subsequent S_1 is soft. The intensity of S_1 may vary in the presence of Mobitz type I heart block, atrioventricular dissociation, and atrial fibrillation when the relationship between atrial and ventricular systole varies. In mitral stenosis with a pliable valve, the persistent pressure gradient at the end of diastole keeps the mitral valve leaflets relatively open and results in a loud S_1 at the onset of systole. In severe mitral stenosis, when the mitral valve is heavily calcified and has decreased leaflet excursion, S_1 becomes faint or absent (Figs. 4–3 and 4–4).

S_2 may be loud in systemic hypertension, owing to accentuated aortic valve closure (loud A_2), or in pulmonary hypertension, owing to accentuated pulmonic valve closure (loud P_2). When the aortic or pulmonary valves are stenotic, the force of valve closure is decreased, thus A_1 and P_2 become soft or inaudible. In this setting, S_2 may appear to be single; in the setting of aortic stenosis, prolonged left ventricular ejection narrows the normal splitting of S_2; and with severe aortic stenosis, S_2 may become absent altogether as prolonged ejection and its accompanying murmur obscure P_2. Wide splitting of the S_2 with normal respiratory variation occurs when either pulmonic valve closure is delayed (e.g., right bundle branch block, pulmonic stenosis) or aortic valve closure occurs earlier owing to more rapid ejection of left ventricular volume (e.g., mitral regurgitation, ventricular septal defect). Fixed splitting of S_2 without respiratory variation is characteristic of atrial septal defects and also occurs with right ventricular failure (**Web Sounds ASD**). Paradoxic splitting of S_2 is a reversal of the usual closure sequence of the aortic and pulmonic valves (i.e., P_2 precedes A_2). In this setting, a single S_2 with inspiration and splitting of S_2 with expiration can be heard. This circumstance occurs most commonly when delay occurs in closure of the aortic valve resulting from either delay in electrical conduction to the left ventricle (e.g., left bundle branch block) or prolonged mechanical contraction of the left ventricle (e.g., aortic stenosis, hypertrophic cardiomyopathy).

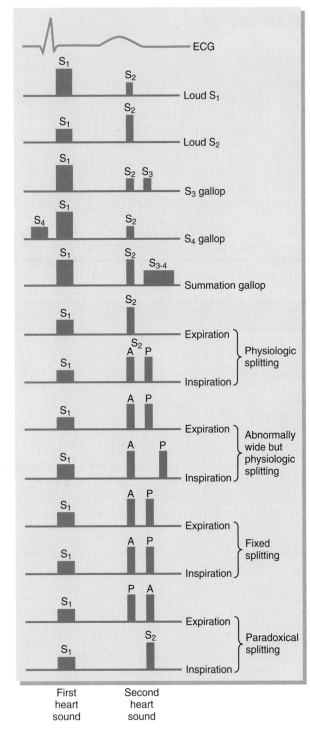

Figure 4–3 Abnormal heart sounds can be related to abnormal intensity, abnormal presence of a gallop rhythm, or abnormal splitting of S_2 with respiration.

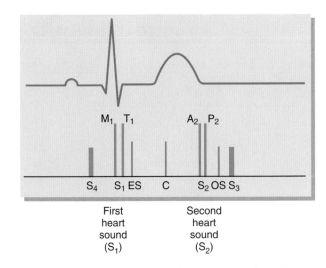

Figure 4–4 The relationship of extra heart sounds to the normal first (S_1) and second (S_2) heart sounds. S_1 is composed of the mitral (M_1) and tricuspid (T_1) closing sounds, although it is frequently perceived as a single sound. S_2 is composed of the aortic (A_2) and pulmonic (P_2) closing sounds, which are usually easily distinguished. A fourth heart sound (S_4) is soft and low pitched and precedes S_1. A pulmonic or aortic ejection sound *(ES)* occurs shortly after S_1. The systolic click *(C)* of mitral valve prolapse may be heard in mid systole or late systole. The opening snap *(OS)* of mitral stenosis is high pitched and occurs shortly after S_2. A tumor plop or pericardial knock occurs at the same time and can be confused with an OS or an S_3, which is lower in pitch and occurs slightly later.

The third heart sound, S_3 (also called the *ventricular diastolic gallop*), is a low-pitched sound occurring shortly after A_2 in mid diastole and heard best at the cardiac apex with the patient in the left lateral position. A pathologic S_3 is distinguished from a physiologic S_3 by age or the presence of underlying cardiac disease. It is frequently heard with ventricular systolic dysfunction from any cause and likely results either from blood entering the ventricle during the rapid filling phase of diastole or from the impact of the ventricle against the chest wall. Maneuvers that increase venous return accentuate S_3, and maneuvers that decrease venous return make the S_3 softer. An S_3 can also be heard in hyperdynamic states, where it likely results from rapid early diastolic filling. The left ventricular S_3 is best noticed at the cardiac apex, whereas the right ventricular S_3 is heard best at the left lower sternal border and increases in intensity with inspiration. The timing of the S_3 is similar to the sound generated by atrial tumors *(tumor plop)* and constrictive pericarditis *(pericardial knock)* and can also be confused with the *opening snap* of a stenotic mitral valve.

The fourth heart sound, S_4 (also called the *atrial diastolic gallop*), is best heard at the cardiac apex with the bell of the stethoscope. It is a low-pitched sound originating from the active ejection of blood from the atrium into a noncompliant ventricle and is therefore not present in the setting of atrial fibrillation. S_4 is commonly heard in patients with left ventricular hypertrophy from any cause (e.g., hypertension, aortic stenosis, hypertrophic cardiomyopathy) or acute myocardial ischemia and in hyperkinetic states. Frequently, the S_4 is also palpable at the cardiac apex. S_3 and S_4 are occasionally present in the same patient. In the presence of tachycardia or a prolonged PR interval, the S_3 and S_4 may merge to produce a summation gallop.

The opening of normal cardiac valves is not audible. However, abnormal valves may produce opening sounds. In the presence of a bicuspid aortic valve or in aortic stenosis with pliable valve leaflets, an *ejection sound* is audible as the leaflets open to their maximal extent. A similar ejection sound may originate from a stenotic pulmonic valve, and in this case, the ejection sound decreases in intensity with inspiration. These ejection sounds are high pitched, occur early in systole, and are frequently followed by the typical ejection murmur of aortic or pulmonic stenosis. Ejection sounds are also heard with systemic or pulmonary hypertension, the exact mechanism of which is not clear.

Ejection sounds heard in mid systole to late systole are referred to as systolic *clicks* and are most commonly associated with mitral valve prolapse. As the redundant mitral valve prolapses and reaches its maximal superior displacement, it produces a high-pitched click. Several clicks may be heard as various parts of the redundant valve prolapse (**Web Sound MVP**). Frequently, the click is followed by a mitral regurgitant murmur. Maneuvers that decrease venous return cause the clicks to occur earlier in systole and the murmur to become longer (see Table 4–4).

The opening of abnormal mitral or tricuspid valves can also be heard in the presence of rheumatic valvular stenosis, when the sound is referred to as an *opening snap* (**Web Sounds MS**). The *snap* is heard only if the valve leaflets are pliable and is generated as the leaflets abruptly dome during early diastole. The interval between S_2 and the opening snap is of diagnostic importance: As the stenosis worsens and the atrial pressure increases, the mitral valve opens earlier in diastole, and the interval between the S_2 and the opening snap shortens.

MURMURS

As stated previously, murmurs are a series of auditory vibrations generated when either abnormal blood flow across a normal cardiac structure or normal flow across an abnormal cardiac structure results in turbulent flow. These sounds are longer than the individual heart sounds and can be described by their location, intensity, frequency (pitch), quality, duration, and timing in relation to systole or diastole. The intensity of a murmur is graded on a scale of 1 to 6 (Table 4–7). In general, murmurs of grade 4 or greater are associated with a palpable thrill. The loudness of a murmur does not necessarily correlate with the severity of the underlying abnormality. For instance, flow across a large atrial septal defect is essentially silent, whereas flow across a small ventricular septal defect is frequently associated with a loud murmur (**Web Sound VSD**). Higher-frequency murmurs correlate with a higher velocity of flow at the site of turbulence. Important to note are the pattern or configuration of the murmur (e.g., crescendo, crescendo-decrescendo, decrescendo, plateau) (Fig. 4–5) and the quality of the murmur (e.g., harsh, blowing, rumbling), as well as the location of maximal intensity and the pattern of radiation of the murmur. Various physical maneuvers may help clarify the nature of a particular murmur (see Table 4–4).

Table 4–7	**Grading System for Intensity of Murmurs**
Grade 1	Barely audible murmur
Grade 2	Murmur of medium intensity
Grade 3	Loud murmur, no thrill
Grade 4	Loud murmur with thrill
Grade 5	Very loud murmur; stethoscope must be on the chest to hear it; may be heard posteriorly
Grade 6	Murmur audible with stethoscope off the chest

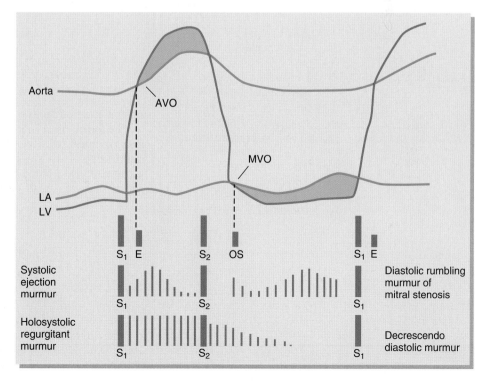

Figure 4–5 Abnormal sounds and murmurs associated with valvular dysfunction displayed simultaneously with left atrial *(LA)*, left ventricular *(LV)*, and aortic pressure tracings. AVO = aortic valve opening; E = ejection click of the aortic valve; MVO = mitral valve opening; OS = opening snap of the mitral valve. The shaded areas represent pressure gradients across the aortic valve during systole or mitral valve during diastole, characteristic of aortic stenosis and mitral stenosis, respectively.

Murmurs can be divided into three categories—(1) systolic, (2) diastolic, and (3) continuous (Table 4–8)—and can result from abnormalities on the right or left side of the heart, as well as the great vessels. Right-sided murmurs may become significantly louder after inspiration, owing to the resulting augmentation of venous return, whereas left-sided murmurs are relatively unaffected by respiration. Systolic murmurs can be further divided into ejection-type murmurs and regurgitant murmurs. Ejection murmurs reflect turbulent flow across the aortic or pulmonic valve (**Web Sounds AS and PS**). They begin shortly after S_1, increase in intensity as the velocity of flow increases, and subsequently decrease in intensity as the velocity falls (crescendo-decrescendo). Examples of ejection-type murmurs include innocent murmurs and the murmurs of aortic sclerosis, aortic stenosis, pulmonic stenosis, and hypertrophic cardiomyopathy. Innocent murmurs and aortic sclerotic murmurs are short in duration and do not radiate (Web Sound benign murmur). The duration of aortic or pulmonic stenotic murmurs varies depending on the severity of the stenosis (compare Web Sound AS-early and AS-late). With more severe stenosis, the murmur becomes longer, and the time to peak intensity of the murmur lengthens (i.e., early-, mid-, and late-peaking murmurs). The murmur of aortic stenosis is usually harsh, radiates to the carotid arteries, and at times may radiate to the cardiac apex (Gallavardin phenomenon). The murmur of hypertrophic cardiomyopathy may be confused with aortic stenosis, but it does not radiate to the carotids, and it is the only ejection murmur that becomes louder with decreased venous return. Mitral regurgitation associated with mitral valve prolapse may also show this response, but it is not a typical ejection murmur.

The classic regurgitant systolic murmurs of mitral (MR) and tricuspid regurgitation (TR) last throughout all of systole (holosystolic), are plateau in pattern, and terminate at S_2 (**Web Sound MR**). With acute MR, the murmur may be limited to early systole and may be somewhat decrescendo in pattern. When MR is secondary to mitral valve prolapse,

Table 4–8 Classification of Heart Murmurs

Timing	Class	Description	Characteristic Lesions
Systolic	Ejection	Begins in early systole; may extend to mid or late systole Crescendo-decrescendo pattern Often harsh in quality Begins after S_1 and ends before S_2	Valvular, supravalvular, and subvalvular aortic stenoses Hypertrophic cardiomyopathy Pulmonic stenosis Aortic or pulmonary artery dilation Malformed but nonobstructive aortic valve ↑ Transvalvular flow (e.g., aortic regurgitation, hyperkinetic states, atrial septal defect, physiologic flow murmur)
	Holosystolic	Extends throughout systole* Relatively uniform in intensity	Mitral regurgitation Tricuspid regurgitation Ventricular septal defect
	Late	Variable onset and duration, often preceded by a nonejection click	Mitral valve prolapse
Diastolic	Early	Begins with A_2 or P_2 Decrescendo pattern with variable duration Often high pitched, blowing	Aortic regurgitation Pulmonic regurgitation
	Mid	Begins after S_2, often after an opening snap Low-pitched *rumble* heard best with bell of stethoscope Louder with exercise and left lateral position Loudest in early diastole	Mitral stenosis Tricuspid stenosis ↑ Flow across atrioventricular valves (e.g., mitral regurgitation, tricuspid regurgitation, atrial septal defect)
	Late	Presystolic accentuation of mid-diastolic murmur	Mitral stenosis Tricuspid stenosis
Continuous	—	Systolic and diastolic components "machinery murmurs"	Patent ductus arteriosus Coronary atrioventricular fistula Ruptured sinus of Valsalva aneurysm into right atrium or ventricle Mammary souffle Venous hum

*Encompasses both the first and second heart sounds.

it starts in mid systole to late systole and is preceded by a mitral valve click. Ventricular septal defects may also result in holosystolic murmurs, although a small muscular ventricular septal defect may have a murmur limited to early systole.

Early-diastolic murmurs result from aortic or pulmonic insufficiency and are decrescendo in pattern. The duration of the murmur reflects chronicity: A short murmur is heard in acute aortic insufficiency or mild insufficiency, whereas chronic aortic insufficiency may produce a murmur throughout diastole. A Graham Steell murmur denotes a pulmonic insufficiency murmur in the setting of pulmonary hypertension. Mid-diastolic murmurs classically result from mitral or tricuspid stenosis, are low pitched, and are referred to as *diastolic rumbles.* Similar murmurs may be heard with obstructing atrial myxomas or in the presence of augmented diastolic flow across an unobstructed mitral or tricuspid valve, as occurs with an atrial or ventricular septal defect or with significant MR or TR. Severe, chronic aortic insufficiency may also produce a diastolic rumble, owing to premature closure of the mitral valve (Austin Flint murmur). Late-diastolic murmurs reflect presystolic accentuation of the mid-diastolic murmurs, owing to augmented mitral or tricuspid flow after atrial contraction.

Continuous murmurs are murmurs that last throughout all of systole and continue into at least early diastole. These murmurs are referred to as *machinery murmurs* and are generated by continuous flow from a vessel or chamber with high pressure into a vessel or chamber with low pressure. A patent ductus arteriosus produces the classic continuous murmur (**Web Sound PDA**).

OTHER CARDIAC SOUNDS

Pericardial rubs occur in the setting of pericarditis. These rubs produce coarse, scratching sounds heard best at the left sternal border with the patient leaning forward and holding his or her breath at end expiration. The classic rub has three components corresponding to atrial systole, ventricular systole, and ventricular diastole, although frequently only one or two of the components are audible (**Web Sound pericardial rubs**). Localized irritation of the surrounding pleura may result in an associated pleural friction rub (pleuropericardial rub), which varies with respiration.

Continuous venous murmurs, or venous *hums,* are almost universally present in children. They are also frequent in adults, especially during pregnancy or in the setting of thyrotoxicosis or anemia. These murmurs are best heard at the base of the neck with the patient's head turned to the opposite direction and can be eliminated by gentle pressure over the vein.

PROSTHETIC HEART SOUNDS

Prosthetic valves produce characteristic auscultatory findings. Porcine or bovine bioprosthetic valves produce heart sounds that are similar to native valve sounds; however, because these valves are smaller than the native valves that they replace, they almost always have an associated murmur (systolic ejection murmur when placed in the aortic position and diastolic rumble when placed in the mitral position). Mechanical valves result in crisp, high-pitched sounds related to valvular opening and closure. With ball-in-cage valves (e.g., Starr-Edwards valves, the opening sound is louder than the closure sound. With all other mechanical valves (e.g., Björk-Shiley valves, St. Jude valves), the closure sound is louder. These valves also produce an ejection-type murmur. Listening for all of the expected prosthetic sounds in patients with prosthetic valves is important because dysfunction of these valves may first be suggested by a change in the intensity or quality of the heart sounds or the development of a new or changing murmur.

Prospectus for the Future

Thanks to advances in chip technology, the essential art of cardiac auscultation is making a resurgence with the use of the computerized heart sound phonocardiography. Students and experienced practitioners alike will be able to use an algorithm for predicting left ventricular dysfunction based on the characteristics of the S_3 and S_4 heart sounds and biomarkers of disease compensation and progression. Personal digital assistants (PDAs), smartphones, and other technologies will make inroads for more accurate diagnosis during initial screening evaluation and bedside management of patients with cardiovascular disease.

References

Goldman L, Ausiello D: Cecil Textbook of Medicine, 22nd ed, Part VIII, Cardiovascular Disease. Philadelphia, WB Saunders, 2004.

Perloff JK: Physical Examination of the Heart and Circulation, 3rd ed. Philadelphia, WB Saunders, 2000.

Chapter 5

Diagnostic Tests and Procedures in the Patient with Cardiovascular Disease

Sheldon E. Litwin

Chest Radiography

The chest radiograph is an integral part of the cardiac evaluation and gives valuable information regarding structure and function of the heart, lungs, and great vessels. A routine examination includes posteroanterior and lateral projections (Fig. 5–1).

In the posteroanterior view, cardiac enlargement may be present when the transverse diameter of the cardiac silhouette is greater than one half of the transverse diameter of the thorax. The heart may appear falsely enlarged when it is displaced horizontally, such as with poor inflation of the lungs, and if the film is an anteroposterior projection, which magnifies the heart shadow. Left atrial enlargement is suggested when the left-sided heart border is straightened or bulges toward the left. In addition, the main bronchi may be widely splayed, and a circular opacity or *double density* within the cardiac silhouette may be seen. Right atrial enlargement may be present when the right-sided heart border bulges toward the right. Left ventricular enlargement results in downward and lateral displacement of the apex. A rounding of the displaced apex suggests ventricular hypertrophy. Right ventricular enlargement is best assessed in the lateral view and may be present when the right ventricular border occupies more than one third of the retrosternal space between the diaphragm and thoracic apex.

The aortic arch and thoracic aorta may become dilated and tortuous in patients with severe atherosclerosis, longstanding hypertension, and aortic dissection. Dilation of the proximal pulmonary arteries may occur when pulmonary pressures are elevated and pulmonary vascular resistance is increased. Disease states associated with increased pulmonary artery flow and normal vascular resistance, such as atrial or ventricular septal defects, may result in dilation of the proximal and distal pulmonary arteries.

Pulmonary venous congestion secondary to elevated left ventricular heart pressures results in redistribution of blood flow in the lungs and prominence of the apical vessels. Transudation of fluid into the interstitial space may result in fluid in the fissures and along the horizontal periphery of the lower lung fields (Kerley's B lines). As venous pressures further increase, fluid collects within the alveolar space, which early on collects preferentially in the inner two thirds of the lung fields, resulting in a characteristic *butterfly* appearance.

Fluoroscopy or plain films may identify abnormal calcification involving the pericardium, coronary arteries, aorta, and valves. In addition, fluoroscopy can be instrumental in evaluating the function of mechanical prosthetic valves.

Specific radiographic signs of congenital and valvular diseases are discussed in their respective sections.

Electrocardiography

The electrocardiogram (ECG) represents the electrical activity of the heart recorded by skin electrodes. This wave of electrical activity is represented as a sequence of deflections on the ECG (Fig. 5–2). The horizontal scale represents time such that, at a standard paper speed of 25 mm/sec, each small box (1 mm) represents 0.04 seconds and each large box (5 mm) represents 0.20 seconds. The vertical scale represents amplitude (10 mm = 1 mV). The heart rate can be estimated by dividing the number of large boxes between complexes (R-R interval) into 300.

In the normal heart, the electrical impulse originates in the sinoatrial (SA) node and is conducted through the atria. Given that depolarization of the SA node is too weak to be detected on the surface ECG, the first, low-amplitude deflection on the surface ECG reflects atrial activation and is

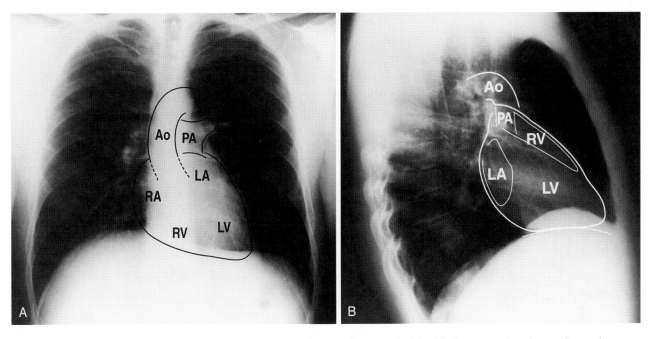

Figure 5–1 Schematic illustration of the parts of the heart, whose outlines can be identified on a routine chest radiograph. *A*, Posteroanterior chest radiograph. *B*, Lateral chest radiograph. Ao = aorta; LA = left atrium; LV = left ventricle; PA = pulmonary artery; RA = right atrium; RV = right ventricle.

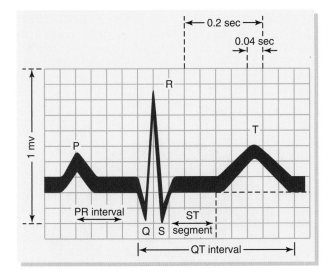

Figure 5–2 Normal electrocardiographic (ECG) complex with labeling of waves and intervals.

termed the *P wave*. The interval between the onset of the P wave and the next rapid deflection (QRS complex) is known as the PR interval and primarily represents the time taken for the impulse to travel through the atrioventricular (AV) node. The normal PR segment ranges from 0.12 to 0.20 seconds. A PR interval greater than 0.20 seconds defines AV nodal block.

Once the wave of depolarization has moved through the AV node, the ventricular myocardium is depolarized in a sequence of four phases. First, the interventricular septum depolarizes from left to right. This phase is followed by depo-larization of the right ventricle and inferior wall of the left ventricle, then the apex and central portions of the left ventricle, and, finally, the base and the posterior wall of the left ventricle. Ventricular depolarization results in a high-amplitude complex on the surface ECG known as the QRS complex. The first downward deflection of this complex is the Q wave, the first upward deflection is the R wave, and the subsequent downward deflection is the S wave. In some individuals, a second upward deflection may be present after the S wave and is termed *R prime* (R′). Normal duration of the QRS complex is less than 0.10 seconds. Complexes greater than 0.12 seconds are usually secondary to some form of interventricular conduction delay.

The isoelectric segment after the QRS complex is the ST segment and represents a brief period during which relatively little electrical activity occurs in the heart. The junction between the end of the QRS complex and the beginning of the ST segment is the J point. The upward deflection after the ST segment is the T wave and represents ventricular repolarization. The QT interval, which reflects the duration and transmural gradient of ventricular depolarization and repolarization, is measured from the onset of the QRS complex to the end of the T wave. The QT interval varies with heart rate, but, for rates between 60 and 100 beats/min, the normal QT interval ranges from 0.35 to 0.44 seconds. For heart rates outside this range, the QT interval can be corrected by the formula:

$$QT_c = QT \text{ (sec)}/\text{R-R interval}^{1/2} \text{ (sec)} \qquad (1)$$

In some individuals, a U wave (of varying amplitude) may be noted after the T wave, the cause of which is unknown.

The standard ECG consists of 12 leads: six limb leads (I, II, III, aVR, aVL, and aVF) and six chest or precordial leads

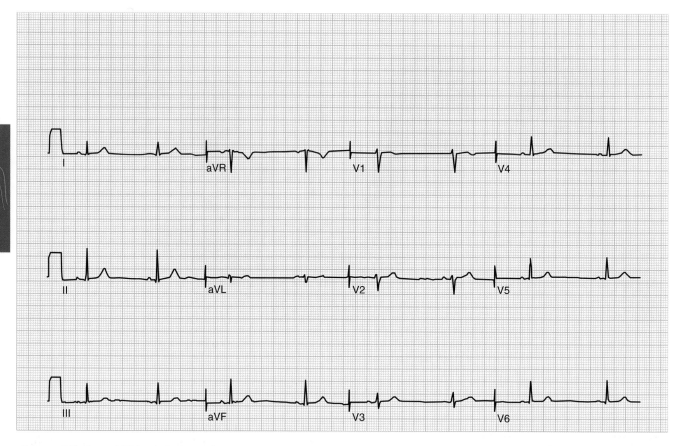

Figure 5–3 Normal 12-lead electrocardiogram.

(V_1 to V_6) (Fig. 5–3). The electrical activity recorded in each lead represents the direction and magnitude (vector) of the electrical force as seen from that particular lead position. Electrical activity directed toward a particular lead is represented as an upward deflection, and an electrical impulse directed away from a particular lead is represented as a downward deflection. Although the overall direction of electrical activity can be determined for any of the waveforms previously described, the mean QRS axis is the most clinically useful and is determined by examining the six limb leads. Figure 5–4 illustrates Einthoven's triangle and the polarity of each of the six limb leads of the standard ECG. Skin electrodes are attached to both arms and legs, with the right leg serving as the ground. Leads I, II, and III are bipolar leads and represent electrical activity between two leads: Lead I represents electrical activity between the right and left arms (left arm positive), lead II between the right arm and left leg (left leg positive), and lead III between the left arm and left leg (left leg positive). Leads aVR, aVL, and aVF are designated the augmented leads. With these leads, the QRS will be positive or have a predominant upward deflection when the electrical forces are directed toward the right arm for aVR, left arm for aVL, and left leg for aVF. These six leads form a hexaxial frontal plane of 30-degree arc intervals. The normal QRS axis ranges from −30 to +90 degrees. An axis more negative than −30 defines left-axis deviation, and an axis greater than +90 defines right-axis deviation. In general,

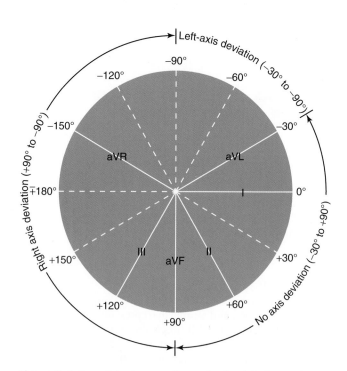

Figure 5–4 Hexaxial reference figure for frontal plane axis determination, indicating values for abnormal left and right QRS axis deviations.

a positive QRS complex in leads I and aVF suggests a normal QRS axis between 0 and 90 degrees.

The six precordial leads (V_1 to V_6) are attached to the anterior chest wall. Electrical activity directed toward these leads results in a positive deflection on the ECG tracing. Leads V_1 and V_2 are closest to the right ventricle and interventricular septum, and leads V_5 and V_6 are closest to the anterior and anterolateral walls of the left ventricle. Normally, a small R wave occurs in lead V_1 reflecting septal depolarization and a deep S wave reflecting predominantly left ventricular activation. From V_1 to V_6, the R wave becomes larger (and the S wave smaller) because the predominant forces directed at these leads originate from the left ventricle. The transition from a predominant S wave to a predominant R wave usually occurs between leads V_3 and V_4. Right-sided chest leads are used to look for evidence of right ventricular infarction. ST segment elevation in V_{4R} has the best sensitivity and specificity for making this diagnosis. Some groups have advocated the use of posterior leads to increase the sensitivity for diagnosing lateral and posterior wall infarction or ischemia (areas that are often deemed to be *electrically silent* on traditional 12-lead ECGs).

Abnormal Electrocardiographic Patterns

CHAMBER ABNORMALITIES AND VENTRICULAR HYPERTROPHY

The P wave is normally upright in leads I, II, and F; inverted in aVR; and biphasic in V_1. Left atrial abnormality (defined as enlargement, hypertrophy, or increased wall stress) is characterized by a wide P wave in lead II (0.12 second) and a deeply inverted terminal component in lead V_1 (1 mm). Right atrial abnormality is present when the P waves in the limb leads are peaked and 2.5 mm or more in height.

Left ventricular hypertrophy may result in increased QRS voltage, slight widening of the QRS complex, late intrinsicoid deflection, left-axis deviation, and abnormalities of the ST-T segments (Fig. 5–5). Multiple criteria with variable sensitivity and specificity for detecting left ventricular hypertrophy are available. The most frequently used criteria are given in Table 5–1.

Right ventricular hypertrophy is characterized by tall R waves in leads V_1 through V_3; deep S waves in leads I, aVL, V_5, and V_6; and right-axis deviation. In patients with chronically elevated pulmonary pressures, such as with chronic lung disease, a combination of ECG abnormalities reflecting a right-sided pathologic condition may be present and include right atrial abnormality, right ventricular hypertrophy, and right-axis deviation. In patients with acute pulmonary embolus, ECG changes may suggest right ventricular strain and include right-axis deviation; incomplete or complete right bundle branch block; S waves in leads I, II, and III; and T wave inversions in leads V_1 through V_3.

INTERVENTRICULAR CONDUCTION DELAYS

The ventricular conduction system consists of two main branches, the right and left bundles. The left bundle further divides into the anterior and posterior fascicles. Conduction block can occur in either of the major branches or in the fascicles (Table 5–2).

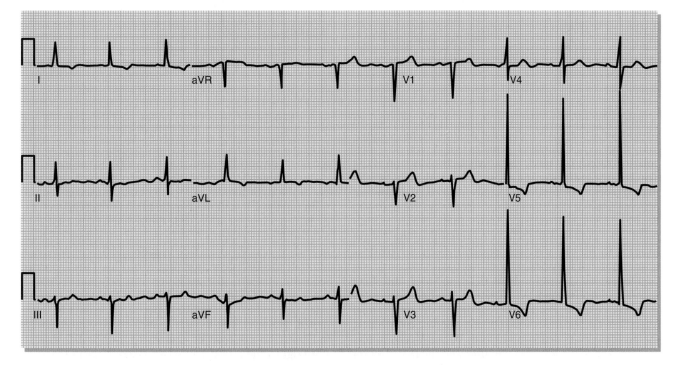

Figure 5–5 Left ventricular hypertrophy as seen on an electrocardiographic (ECG) recording. Characteristic findings include increased QRS voltage in precordial leads (deep S in lead V_2 and tall R in lead V_5) and down-sloping ST depression and T wave inversion in lateral precordial leads (*strain* pattern) and leftward axis.

Table 5–1

Electrocardiographic Manifestations of Atrial Abnormalities and Ventricular Hypertrophy

Left Atrial Abnormality

P wave duration ≥0.12 sec
Notched, slurred P wave in leads I and II
Biphasic P wave in lead V_1 with a wide, deep, negative
  terminal component

Right Atrial Abnormality

P wave duration ≤0.11 sec
Tall, peaked P waves of ≥2.5 mm in leads II, III, and aVF

Left Ventricular Hypertrophy

Voltage criteria
R wave in lead aVL ≥12 mm
R wave in lead I ≥15 mm
S wave in lead V_1 or V_2 + R wave in lead V_5 or V_6 ≥35 mm
Depressed ST segments with inverted T waves in the lateral
  leads
Left axis deviation
QRS duration ≥0.09 sec
Left atrial enlargement

Right Ventricular Hypertrophy

Tall R waves over right precordium (R:S ratio in lead V_1 > 1.0)
Right axis deviation
Depressed ST segments with inverted T waves in V_1–V_3
Normal QRS duration (if no right bundle branch block)

Table 5–2

Electrocardiographic Manifestations of Fascicular and Bundle Branch Blocks

Left Anterior Fascicular Block

QRS duration ≤0.1 sec
Left axis deviation (more negative than −45 degrees)
rS pattern in leads II, III, and aVF
qR pattern in leads I and aVL

Right Posterior Fascicular Block

QRS duration ≤0.1 sec
Right axis deviation (+90 degrees or greater)
qR pattern in leads II, III, and aVF
rS pattern in leads I and aVL
Exclusion of other causes of right axis deviation (chronic
  obstructive pulmonary disease, right ventricular
  hypertrophy)

Left Bundle Branch Block

QRS duration ≥0.12 sec
Broad, slurred or notched R waves in lateral leads (I, aVL, V_5,
  and V_6)
QS or rS pattern in anterior precordium leads (V_1 and V_2)
ST-T wave vectors opposite to terminal QRS vectors

Right Bundle Branch Block

QRS duration ≥0.12 sec
Large R′ wave in lead V_1 (rsR′)
Deep terminal S wave in lead V_6
Normal septal Q waves
Inverted T waves in leads V_1 and V_2

Fascicular block results in a change in the sequence of ventricular activation but does not prolong overall conduction time (QRS duration remains <0.10 second). Left anterior fascicular block is a relatively common ECG abnormality and is sometimes associated with right bundle branch block. This conduction abnormality is present when extreme left-axis deviation occurs (more negative than −45 degrees); when the R wave is greater than the Q wave in leads I and aVL; and when the S wave is greater than the R wave in leads II, III, and aVF. Left posterior fascicular block is uncommon but is associated with right-axis deviation (>90 degrees); small Q waves in leads II, III, and aVF; and small R waves in leads I and aVL. The ECG findings associated with fascicular blocks can be confused with myocardial infarction. For example, with left anterior fascicular block, the prominent QS deflection in leads V_1 and V_2 can mimic an anteroseptal myocardial infarction, and the rS deflection in leads II, III, and aVF can be confused with an inferior myocardial infarction. Similarly, the rS deflection in leads I and aVL in left posterior fascicular block may be confused

with a high lateral infarct. The presence of abnormal ST and T wave segments and pathologic Q waves (see "Myocardial Ischemia and Infarction" later) are helpful findings to differentiate myocardial infarction from a fascicular block.

In left bundle branch block, depolarization proceeds down the right bundle, across the interventricular septum from right to left, and then to the left ventricle. Characteristic ECG findings include a wide QRS complex (0.12 second); a broad R wave in leads I, aVL, V_5, and V_6; a deep QS wave in leads V_1 and V_2; and ST depression and T wave inversion opposite the QRS deflection (Fig. 5–6). Given the abnormal sequence of ventricular activation with left bundle branch block, many ECG abnormalities, such as Q wave myocardial infarction and left ventricular hypertrophy, cannot be interpreted. However, left bundle branch block almost always indicates the presence of underlying myocardial disease. With right bundle branch block, the interventricular septum depolarizes normally from left to right, and therefore the initial QRS deflection remains unchanged. As a result, ECG abnormalities such as Q wave myocardial infarction can still

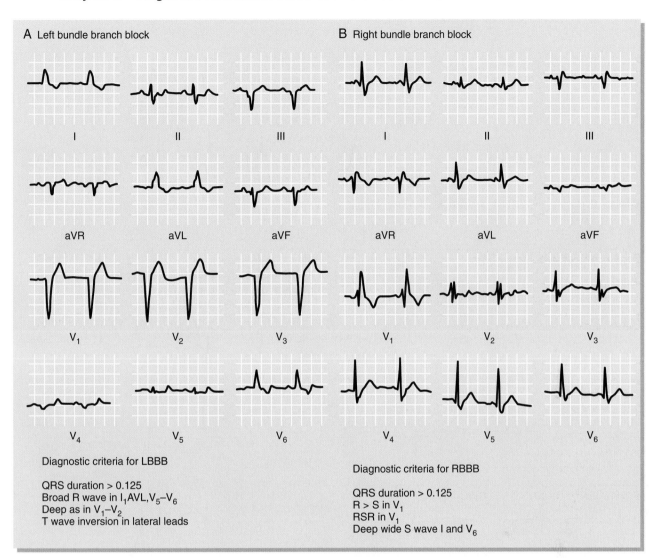

A Left bundle branch block

B Right bundle branch block

Diagnostic criteria for LBBB

QRS duration > 0.125
Broad R wave in I,AVL,V$_5$–V$_6$
Deep as in V$_1$–V$_2$
T wave inversion in lateral leads

Diagnostic criteria for RBBB

QRS duration > 0.125
R > S in V$_1$
RSR in V$_1$
Deep wide S wave I and V$_6$

Figure 5–6 *A,* Left bundle branch block. *B,* Right bundle branch block. Criteria for bundle branch block are summarized in Table 5–2.

be interpreted. After septal activation, the left ventricle depolarizes, followed by the right ventricle. The ECG is characterized by a wide QRS complex; a large R′ wave in lead V$_1$ (R-S-R′); and deep S waves in leads I, aVL, and V$_6$, representing delayed right ventricular activation (see Fig. 5–6). Although right bundle branch block may be associated with underlying cardiac disease, it may also appear as a normal variant.

MYOCARDIAL ISCHEMIA AND INFARCTION

Myocardial ischemia and infarction may be associated with abnormalities of the ST segment, T wave, and QRS complex. Myocardial ischemia primarily affects repolarization of the myocardium and is often associated with horizontal or down-sloping ST segment depression and T wave inversion. These changes may be transient, such as during an anginal episode or an exercise stress test, or may be long lasting in the setting of unstable angina or myocardial infarction. T

wave inversion without ST segment depression is a nonspecific finding and must be correlated with the clinical setting. Localized ST segment elevation suggests more extensive myocardial injury and is often associated with acute myocardial infarction (Fig. 5–7). Vasospastic or Prinzmetal's angina may be associated with reversible ST segment elevation without myocardial infarction. ST elevation may occur in other settings not related to acute ischemia or infarction. Persistent, localized ST segment elevation in the same leads as pathologic Q waves is consistent with a ventricular aneurysm. Acute pericarditis is associated with diffuse ST segment elevation and PR depression. Diffuse J point elevation in association with upward-coving ST segments is a normal variant common among young men and is often referred to as *early repolarization.*

The presence of a Q wave is one of the diagnostic criteria used to verify a myocardial infarction. Infarcted myocardium is unable to conduct electrical activity, and therefore electrical forces will be directed away from the surface electrode overlying the infarcted region, resulting in

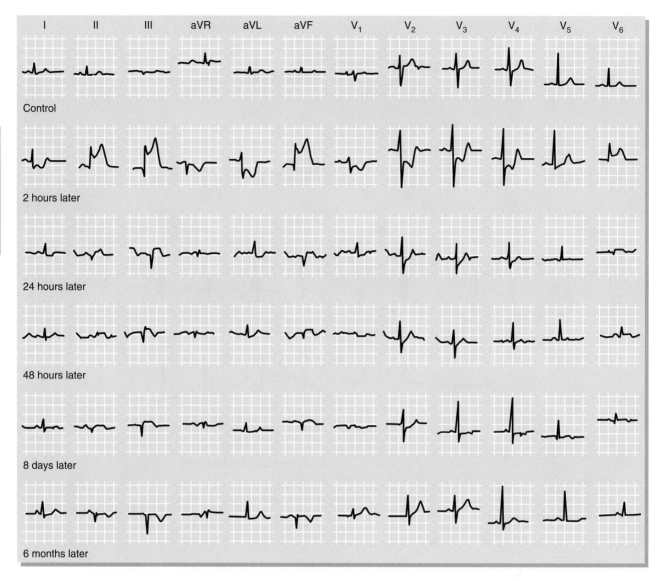

Figure 5–7 Evolutionary changes in a posteroinferior myocardial infarction. Control tracing is normal. The tracing recorded 2 hours after onset of chest pain demonstrated development of early Q waves, marked ST segment elevation, and hyperacute T waves in leads II, III, and aVF. In addition, a larger R wave, ST segment depression, and negative T waves have developed in leads V_1 and V_2. These are early changes indicating acute posteroinferior myocardial infarction. The 24-hour tracing demonstrates evolutionary changes. In leads II, III, and aVF, the Q wave is larger, the ST segments have almost returned to baseline, and the T wave has begun to invert. In leads V_1 to V_2, the duration of the R wave now exceeds 0.04 seconds, the ST segment is depressed, and the T wave is upright. (In this example, ECG changes of true posterior involvement extend past lead V_2; ordinarily, only leads V_1 and V_2 may be involved.) Only minor further changes occur through the 8-day tracing. Finally, 6 months later, the ECG illustrates large Q waves, isoelectric ST segments, and inverted T waves in leads II, III, and aVF and large R waves, isoelectric ST segment, and upright T waves in leads V_1 and V_2, indicative of an *old* posteroinferior myocardial infarction.

a Q wave on the surface ECG. Knowing which region of the myocardium each lead represents enables the examiner to localize the area of infarction (Table 5–3). A pathologic Q wave has a duration of greater than or equal to 0.04 seconds and/or a depth one fourth or more the height of the corresponding R wave.

Not all myocardial infarctions will result in the formation of Q waves. In addition, small R waves can return many weeks to months after a myocardial infarction.

Abnormal Q waves, or *pseudoinfarction,* may also be associated with nonischemic cardiac disease, such as ventricular pre-excitation, cardiac amyloidosis, sarcoidosis, idiopathic

or hypertrophic cardiomyopathy, myocarditis, and chronic lung disease.

ABNORMALITIES OF THE ST SEGMENT AND T WAVE

A number of drugs and metabolic abnormalities may affect the ST segment and T wave (Fig. 5–8). Hypokalemia may result in prominent U waves in the precordial leads and prolongation of the QT interval. Hyperkalemia may result in tall, peaked T waves. Hypocalcemia typically lengthens the QT interval, whereas hypercalcemia shortens it. A commonly

Table 5–3 Electrocardiographic Localization of Myocardial Infarction

Infarct Location	Leads Depicting Primary Electrocardiographic Changes	Likely Vessel* Involved
Inferior	II, III, aVF	RCA
Septal	V_1, V_2	LAD
Anterior	V_3, V_4	LAD
Anteroseptal	V_1–V_4	LAD
Extensive anterior	I, aVL, V_1–V_6	LAD
Lateral	I, aVL, V_5–V_6	CIRC
High lateral	I, aVL	CIRC
Posterior[†]	Prominent R in V_1	RCA or CIRC
Right ventricular[‡]	ST elevation in V_1 and, more specifically, V_4R in setting of inferior infarction	RCA

*This is a generalization; variations occur.
[†]Usually in association with inferior or lateral infarction.
[‡]Usually in association with inferior infarction.
CIRC = circumflex artery; LAD = left anterior descending coronary artery; RCA = right coronary artery.

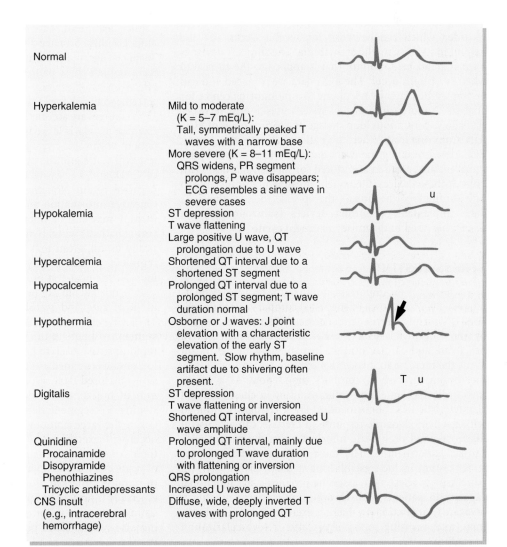

Figure 5–8 Metabolic and drug influences on the electrocardiographic (ECG) recording.

Normal

Hyperkalemia
Mild to moderate
(K = 5–7 mEq/L):
Tall, symmetrically peaked T
waves with a narrow base
More severe (K = 8–11 mEq/L):
QRS widens, PR segment
prolongs, P wave disappears;
ECG resembles a sine wave in
severe cases

Hypokalemia
ST depression
T wave flattening
Large positive U wave, QT
prolongation due to U wave

Hypercalcemia
Shortened QT interval due to a
shortened ST segment

Hypocalcemia
Prolonged QT interval due to a
prolonged ST segment; T wave
duration normal

Hypothermia
Osborne or J waves: J point
elevation with a characteristic
elevation of the early ST
segment. Slow rhythm, baseline
artifact due to shivering often
present.

Digitalis
ST depression
T wave flattening or inversion
Shortened QT interval, increased U
wave amplitude

Quinidine
Procainamide
Disopyramide
Phenothiazines
Tricyclic antidepressants
Prolonged QT interval, mainly due
to prolonged T wave duration
with flattening or inversion
QRS prolongation
Increased U wave amplitude

CNS insult
(e.g., intracerebral
hemorrhage)
Diffuse, wide, deeply inverted T
waves with prolonged QT

used cardiac medication, digoxin, often results in diffuse, scooped ST segment depression. Minor or *nonspecific* ST segment and T wave abnormalities may be present in many patients and have no definable cause. In these instances, the physician must determine the significance of the abnormalities based on the clinical setting.

Several excellent **websites** containing examples of normal and abnormal ECGs are available.

Long-Term Ambulatory Electrocardiographic Recording

Ambulatory ECG (Holter monitoring) is a widely used, noninvasive method to evaluate cardiac arrhythmias and conduction disturbances over an extended period and to detect electrical abnormalities that may be brief or transient. With this approach, ECG data from two to three surface leads are stored on a tape recorder that the patient wears for a minimum of 24 to 48 hours. The recorders have both patient-activated event markers and time markers so that any abnormalities can be correlated with the patient's symptoms or time of day. These data can then be printed in a standard, real-time ECG format for review.

For patients with intermittent or rare symptoms, an event recorder, which can be worn for several weeks, may be helpful in identifying the arrhythmia. The simplest device is a small, hand-held monitor that is applied to the chest wall when symptoms occur. The ECG data are recorded and can be transmitted later by telephone to a monitoring center for analysis. A more sophisticated system uses a wrist recorder that allows continuous loop storage of 4 to 5 minutes of ECG data from one lead. When the patient activates the system, ECG data preceding the event and for 1 to 2 minutes after the event are recorded and stored for further analysis. With both of these devices, the patient must be physically able to activate the recorder during the episode to store the ECG data. Implantable recording devices (subcutaneous) are sometimes used to diagnose infrequent events.

STRESS TESTING

Stress testing is an important noninvasive tool for evaluating patients with known or suggested coronary artery disease (CAD). During exercise, the increased demand for oxygen by the working skeletal muscles is met by increases in heart rate and cardiac output. In patients with significant CAD, the increase in myocardial oxygen demand cannot be met by an increase in coronary blood flow. As a result, myocardial ischemia may occur, resulting in chest pain and characteristic ECG abnormalities. These changes, combined with the hemodynamic response to exercise, can give useful diagnostic and prognostic information in the patient with cardiac abnormalities. The most frequent indications for stress testing include establishing a diagnosis of CAD in patients with chest pain, assessing prognosis and functional capacity in patients with chronic stable angina or after a myocardial infarction, evaluating exercise-induced arrhythmias, and assessing for ischemia after a revascularization procedure.

The most common form of stress testing uses continuous ECG monitoring while the patient walks on a treadmill. With each advancing stage, the speed and incline of the belt increases, thus increasing the amount of work the patient performs. Exercise testing may also be performed using a bicycle or arm ergometer. The stress test is deemed adequate if the patient achieves 85% of his or her maximal heart rate, which is equal to 220 minus the patient's age. Indications for stopping the test include fatigue, severe hypertension (>220 mm Hg systolic), developing worsening angina during exercise, developing marked or widespread ischemic ECG changes, significant arrhythmias, or hypotension. The diagnostic accuracy of stress testing is improved with adjunctive echocardiography or radionuclide imaging. Contraindications to stress testing include unstable angina, acute myocardial infarction, poorly controlled hypertension (blood pressure >220/110 mm Hg), severe aortic stenosis (valve area <1.0 cm^2), and decompensated congestive heart failure. In the era of reperfusion therapy (thrombolytic and/or percutaneous interventions), for acute coronary syndromes or acute MI, little role exists for the predischarge submaximal stress test that was commonly used in the past.

The diagnostic accuracy of the exercise test is dependent on the pre-test likelihood of CAD in a given patient, the sensitivity and specificity of the test results in that patient population, and the ECG criteria used to define a positive test. Clinical features that are most useful at predicting important angiographic coronary disease before exercise testing include advanced age, male sex, and the presence of typical (vs. atypical) anginal chest pain. The diagnostic accuracy and cost effectiveness of exercise testing is best in patients with an intermediate risk for CAD (30% to 70%) and when ischemic ECG changes are accompanied by chest pain during exercise. Exercise testing is less cost effective in diagnosing CAD in a patient with classic symptoms of angina because a positive test will not significantly increase the post-test probability of CAD, and a negative test would likely represent a false-negative result. Nonetheless, prognostic information and objective information about the efficacy of pharmacologic therapy may still be obtained. Similarly, exercise testing in young patients with atypical chest pain may not be diagnostically useful, given that an abnormal test result will likely represent a false-positive test and will not significantly increase the post-test probability of CAD.

The normal physiologic response to exercise is an increase in heart rate and systolic and diastolic blood pressures. The ECG will maintain normal T wave polarity, and the ST segment will remain unchanged or, if depressed, will have a rapid upstroke back to baseline. An ischemic ECG response to exercise is defined as (1) 1.5 mm of up-sloping ST depression measured 0.08 seconds past the J point, (2) at least 1 mm of horizontal ST depression, or (3) 1 mm of downsloping ST segment depression measured at the J point. Given the large amount of artifact on the ECG that may occur with exercise, these changes must be present in at least three consecutive depolarizations. Other findings suggestive of more extensive CAD include early onset of ST depression (6 minutes); marked, down-sloping ST depression (2 mm), especially if present in more than five leads; ST changes persisting into recovery for more than 5 minutes; and failure to increase systolic blood pressure to 120 mm Hg or more or a sustained decrease of 10 mm Hg or more below baseline.

The ECG is not diagnostically useful in the presence of left ventricular hypertrophy, left bundle branch block, Wolff-Parkinson-White syndrome, or chronic digoxin therapy. In these instances, nuclear or echocardiographic imaging may be helpful in demonstrating signs of ischemia. In patients who are unable to exercise, pharmacologic stress testing with myocardial imaging has been shown to have sensitivity and specificity for detecting CAD equal to those of exercise stress imaging. Intravenous dipyridamole and adenosine are coronary vasodilators that result in increased blood flow in normal arteries without significantly changing flow in diseased vessels. The resulting heterogeneity in blood flow can be detected by nuclear imaging techniques and the regions of myocardium supplied by diseased vessels identified. Another commonly used technique to evaluate for ischemia is dobutamine-stress echocardiography. Dobutamine is an inotropic agent that increases myocardial oxygen demand by increasing heart rate and contractility. The echocardiogram is used to monitor for ischemia, which is defined as new or worsening wall motion abnormalities during the infusion. Demonstrating improvement in wall thickening with low-dose dobutamine can also assess myocardial viability of abnormal segments (i.e., segments that are hypokinetic or akinetic at baseline).

ECHOCARDIOGRAPHY

Echocardiography is a widely used, noninvasive technique in which sound waves are used to image cardiac structures and evaluate blood flow. A piezoelectric crystal housed in a transducer placed on the patient's chest wall produces ultrasound waves. As the sound waves encounter structures with different acoustic properties, some of the ultrasound waves are reflected back to the transducer and recorded. Ultrasound waves emitted from a single, stationary crystal produce an image of a thin slice of the heart (M-mode),

which can then be followed through time. Steering the ultrasound beam across a 90-degree arc multiple times per second creates two-dimensional imaging (Fig. 5–9). Transthoracic echocardiography is safe, simple, fast, and relatively inexpensive. Hence it is the most commonly used test to assess cardiac size, structure, and function. The development of three-dimensional echocardiographic imaging techniques offers great promise for more accurate measurements of chamber volumes and mass, as well as the assessment of geometrically complex anatomy and valvular lesions (**Web Fig. 5–1** shows a three-dimensional image).

Doppler echocardiography allows assessment of both direction and velocity of blood flow within the heart and great vessels. When ultrasound waves encounter moving red blood cells, the energy reflected back to the transducer is altered. The magnitude of this change (Doppler shift) is represented as velocity on the echocardiographic display and can be used to determine if the blood flow is normal or abnormal (Fig. 5–10). In addition, the velocity of a particular jet of blood can be converted to pressure using the modified Bernoulli equation ($\Delta P \cong 4v^2$). This process allows for the assessment of pressure gradients across valves or between chambers. Color Doppler imaging allows visualization of blood flow through the heart by assigning a color to the red blood cells based on their velocity and direction (Fig. 5–11, **Web Fig. 5–2**). By convention, blood moving away from the transducer is represented in shades of blue, and blood moving toward the transducer is represented in red. Color Doppler imaging is particularly useful in identifying valvular insufficiency and abnormal shunt flow between chambers. Recently, the use of Doppler techniques to record myocardial velocities or strain rates has provided a great deal of insight into myocardial function and hemodynamics.

Two-dimensional echocardiography and Doppler echocardiography are often used in conjunction with exercise or pharmacologic stress testing. Although variability

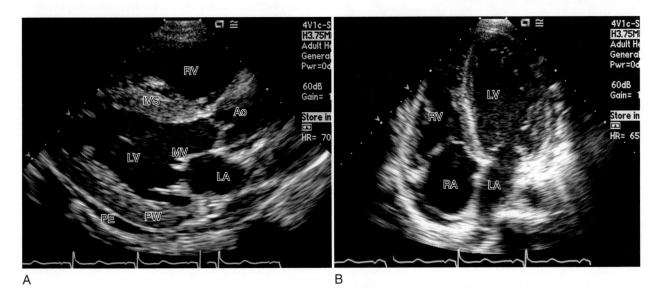

A   **B**

Figure 5–9 Portions of standard two-dimensional echocardiograms (*A,* parasternal long-axis view; *B,* apical four-chamber view) showing the major cardiac structures. Ao = aorta; IVS = interventricular septum; LA = left atrium; LV = left ventricle; MV = mitral valve; PE = pericardial effusion; PW = posterior LV wall; RV = right ventricle. See **Web Figure 5–3** for a moving image of a two-dimensional echocardiogram. (Image courtesy Sheldon E. Litwin, MD, Division of Cardiology, University of Utah.)

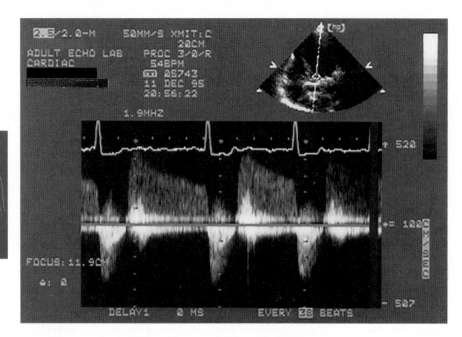

Figure 5–10 Doppler tracing in a patient with aortic stenosis and regurgitation. The velocity of systolic flow is related to the severity of obstruction.

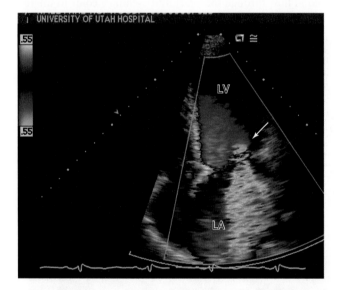

Figure 5–11 Color Doppler recording demonstrating severe mitral regurgitation. The regurgitant jet seen in the left atrium *(LA)* is represented in blue because blood flow is directed away from the transducer. The yellow components are the mosaic pattern traditionally assigned to turbulent or high velocity flow. The arrow points to the hemisphere of blood accelerating proximal to the regurgitant orifice (proximal isovelocity surface area [PISA]). The size of the PISA can be used to help grade the severity of regurgitation. LA = left atrium; LV = left ventricle. See **Web Figure 5–2** for a dynamic echocardiographic image in a patient with mitral regurgitation. (Image courtesy Sheldon E. Litwin, MD, Division of Cardiology, University of Utah.)

occurs among studies, the sensitivity of stress echocardiography is apparently slightly lower, but the specificity is slightly higher, compared with myocardial perfusion imaging with nuclear tracers. The overall cost effectiveness of stress echocardiography is estimated to be significantly better than nuclear perfusion imaging because of the lower cost.

The development of ultrasound contrast agents composed of microbubbles that are small enough to transit through the pulmonary circulation has greatly improved the ability to use ultrasound to image obese patients, patients with lung disease, and those with otherwise difficult acoustic windows (Fig. 5–12, **Web Fig. 5–3** shows a dynamic contrast echocardiographic image). These agents are also being developed as molecular imaging agents by complexing the bubbles to compounds that can selectively bind to the target site of interest (i.e., clots, neovessels).

Transesophageal echocardiography (TEE) allows two-dimensional and Doppler imaging of the heart through the esophagus by having the patient swallow a gastroscope mounted with an ultrasound crystal within its tip. Given the close proximity of the esophagus to the heart, high-resolution images can be obtained, especially of the left atrium, mitral valve apparatus, and aorta. TEE is particularly useful in diagnosing aortic dissection, endocarditis, prosthetic valve dysfunction, and left atrial masses (Fig. 5–13, **Web Fig. 5–4**).

MAGNETIC RESONANCE IMAGING

Magnetic resonance angiography or imaging (MRI) is an increasingly used noninvasive method of studying the heart and vasculature, especially in patients who have contraindications to standard contrast angiography (Fig. 5–14). Magnetic resonance angiography has become particularly popular in the evaluation of cerebral, renovascular, and lower extremity arterial disease. MRI offers significant advantages over other imaging techniques for the characterization of different tissues (e.g., muscle, fat, scar). The presence of delayed gadolinium contrast enhancement within the myocardium is characteristic of scar or permanently damaged tissue (**Web Fig. 5–5**).

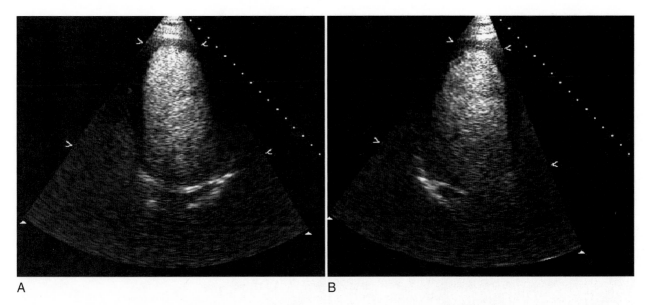

Figure 5–12 Echocardiogram enhanced with intravenous ultrasound contrast agent (*A*, apical four-chamber view; *B*, apical long-axis view). Highly echo-reflectant microbubbles make the left ventricular cavity appear white, whereas the myocardium appears dark. See **Web Figure 5–3** for a dynamic image of echocardiographic contrast. (Image courtesy Sheldon E. Litwin, MD, Division of Cardiology, University of Utah.)

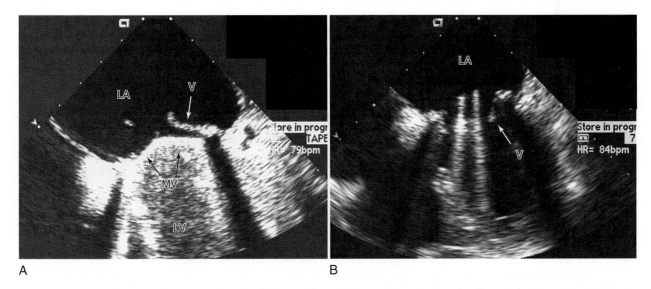

Figure 5–13 Transesophageal echocardiogram demonstrating the presence of a vegetation adherent to the ring of a bi-leaflet tilting disc mitral valve prostheses (*A*, systole, leaflets closed with vegetation seen in left atrium; *B*, diastole, leaflets open, vegetation prolapsing into left ventricle). Transesophageal echocardiography is the diagnostic test of choice for assessing prosthetic mitral valves because the esophageal window allows unimpeded views of the atrial surface of the valve. LA = left atrium, LV = left ventricle, MV = prosthetic mitral valve discs, V = vegetation. See **Web Figure 5–4** for a dynamic transesophageal echocardiographic image. (Image courtesy Sheldon E. Litwin, MD, Division of Cardiology, University of Utah.)

NUCLEAR CARDIOLOGY

Radionuclide imaging of the heart allows quantification of left ventricular size and systolic function, as well as myocardial perfusion. With radionuclide ventriculography, the patient's red blood cells are labeled with a small amount of a radioactive tracer (usually technetium-99m). Left ventricular function can then be assessed by one of two methods. With the first-pass technique, radiation emitted by the tagged red blood cells as they initially flow though the heart

is detected by a gamma camera positioned over the patient's chest. With the gated equilibrium method, or multigated acquisition (MUGA) method, the tracer is allowed to achieve an equilibrium distribution throughout the blood pool before count acquisition begins. This second method improves the resolution of the ventriculogram. For both techniques, the gamma camera can be gated to the ECG, allowing for determination of the total emitted end-diastole counts (EDC) and end-systole counts (ESC). Left ventricular ejection fraction (LVEF) can then be calculated as:

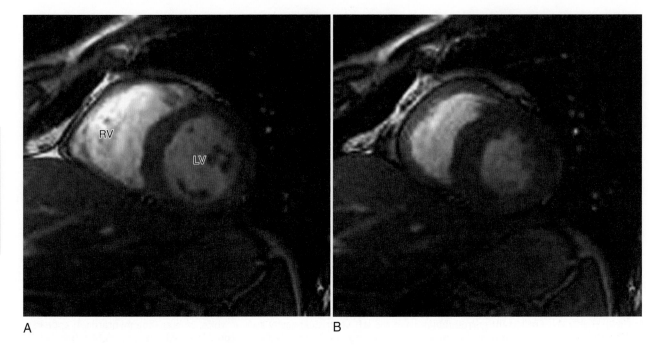

A   B

Figure 5–14 Cardiac magnetic resonance imaging (MRI) showing short axis views of the left ventricle *(LV)* and right ventricle *(RV)* in diastole *(A)* and systole *(B)*. Excellent spatial resolution and clear distinction between myocardial tissue and blood are evident. (Images courtesy of Chris McGann, MD, Division of Cardiology, University of Utah.) See **Web Figure 5–5** for a dynamic cardiac MRI image. (Web image courtesy Sheldon E. Litwin, MD, Division of Cardiology, University of Utah.)

$$LVEF = (EDC - ESC)/EDC \qquad (2)$$

If scintigraphic information is collected throughout the cardiac cycle, then a computer-generated image of the heart can be displayed in a cinematic fashion, allowing for the assessment of wall motion.

Myocardial perfusion imaging is usually performed in conjunction with exercise or pharmacologic (vasodilator) stress testing. Persantine, or more commonly adenosine, is used as the coronary vasodilator. Each agent can increase myocardial blood flow by four- to fivefold. Adenosine is more expensive, but has the advantage over persantine of a very short half-life. Newer adenosine-like agents with reduced side effect profiles are being investigated. Technetium-99m sestamibi is the most frequently used radionuclide and is usually injected just before completion of the stress test. Tomographic (single-photon emission computed tomography [SPECT]) images of the heart are obtained for qualitative and quantitative analyses at rest and after stress. In the normal heart, radioisotope is relatively equally distributed throughout the myocardium. In patients with ischemia, a localized area of decreased uptake will occur after exercise but partially or completely fill in at rest (redistribution). A persistent defect at peak exercise and rest (fixed defect) is consistent with myocardial infarction or scarring. However, in some patients with apparently fixed defects, repeat rest imaging at 24 hours or after re-injection of a smaller quantity of isotope will demonstrate improved uptake, indicating the presence of viable, but severely ischemic, myocardium. The use of new approaches such as combined low-level exercise and vasodilators, prone imaging, attenuation correction, and computerized data analysis has improved the quality and reproducibility of the data from these studies.

Myocardial perfusion imaging may also be combined with ECG-gated image acquisition to allow for simultaneous assessment of ventricular function and perfusion. Not only can LVEF be quantitated with this technique, but also regional wall motion can be assessed to help rule out artifactual perfusion defects (**Web Fig. 5–6**).

Positron-emission tomography (PET) is a noninvasive method of detecting myocardial viability by the use of both perfusion and metabolic tracers. In patients with left ventricular dysfunction, the presence of metabolic activity in a region of myocardium supplied by a severely stenotic coronary artery suggests viable tissue that may regain more normal function after revascularization (Fig. 5–15). PET is less widely available than conventional SPECT imaging; however, PET offers improved spatial resolution because of the higher energy of the isotopes used for this type of imaging.

CARDIAC CATHETERIZATION

Cardiac catheterization is an invasive technique in which fluid-filled catheters are introduced percutaneously into the arterial and venous circulation. This method allows for the direct measurement of intracardiac pressures and oxygen saturation and, with the injection of a contrast agent, visualization of the coronary arteries, cardiac chambers, and great vessels. Cardiac catheterization is generally indicated when a clinically suggested cardiac abnormality requires confirmation and its anatomic and physiologic importance needs to be quantified. In the current era, coronary angiog-

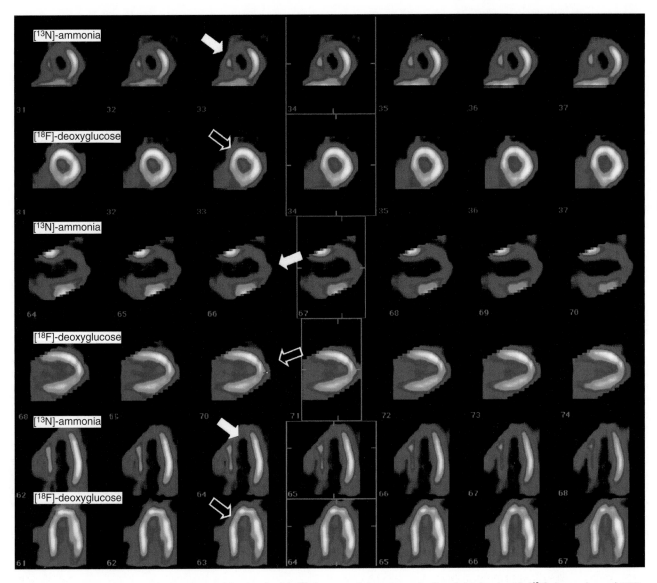

Figure 5–15 Resting myocardial perfusion (obtained with [^{13}N]-ammonia) and metabolism (obtained with [^{18}F]-deoxyglucose) PET images of a patient with ischemic cardiomyopathy. The study demonstrates a perfusion-metabolic mismatch (reflecting hibernating myocardium) in which large areas of hypoperfused *(solid arrows)* but metabolically viable myocardium *(open arrows)* are involving the anterior, septal, and inferior walls and the left ventricular apex. See **Web Figure 5–6** for a dynamic image obtained with cardiac SPECT imaging. (Courtesy of Marcelo F. Di Carli, MD, Brigham and Women's Hospital, Boston, MA.)

raphy for the diagnosis of CAD is the most common indication for this test. Noninvasive testing compared with catheterization is safer, cheaper, and equally effective in the evaluation of most valvular and hemodynamic questions. Most often, catheterization will precede some type of beneficial intervention, such as coronary artery angioplasty, coronary bypass surgery, or valvular surgery. Although cardiac catheterization is generally safe (0.1% to 0.2% overall mortality rate), procedure-related complications such as vascular injury, renal failure, stroke, and myocardial infarction can occur.

An important objective during the cardiac catheterization is to document the filling pressures within the heart and great vessels. This task is accomplished through use of fluid-filled catheters that transmit intracardiac pressures to a transducer that displays the pressure waveform on an oscilloscope. During a right ventricular heart catheterization, pressures within the right atrium, right ventricle, and pulmonary artery are routinely measured in this manner. The catheter can then be advanced further until it *wedges* in the distal pulmonary artery. The transmitted pressure measured in this location originates from the pulmonary venous system and is known as the pulmonary capillary wedge pressure. In the absence of pulmonary venous disease, the pulmonary capillary wedge pressure reflects left atrial pressure and, similarly, if no significant mitral valve pathologic condition exists, reflects left ventricular diastolic pressure. A more direct method of obtaining left ventricular filling pressures is to advance an arterial catheter into the left ventricular cavity. With these two methods of obtaining intracardiac pressures, each chamber of the heart can be assessed and the gradients across any of the valves determined (Fig. 5–16).

Cardiac output can be determined by one of two widely accepted methods: the Fick oxygen method and the indicator dilution technique. The basis of the Fick method is that total uptake or release of a substance by an organ is equal to the product of blood flow to that organ and the concentration difference of that substance between the arterial and venous circulation of that organ. If this method is applied to the lungs, then the substance released into the blood is oxygen; if no intrapulmonary shunts exist, then pulmonary blood flow is equal to systemic blood flow or cardiac output. Thus the cardiac output can be determined by the following equation:

Cardiac output = oxygen consumption/(arterial oxygen
                content − venous oxygen content)   (3)

Oxygen consumption is measured in milliliters per minute by collecting the patient's expired air over a known period while simultaneously measuring oxygen saturation in a sample of arterial and mixed venous blood (arterial and venous oxygen content, respectively, measured in milliliters per liter). The cardiac output is expressed in liters per minute and then corrected for body surface area (cardiac index). The normal range of cardiac index is 2.6 to 4.2 L/min/m^2. Cardiac output can also be determined by the indicator dilution technique, which most commonly uses cold saline as the indicator. With this method, cold saline is injected into the blood, and the resulting temperature change *downstream* is monitored. This action generates a curve in which temperature change is plotted over time, and the area under the curve represents cardiac output.

Detection and localization of intracardiac shunts can be performed by sequential measurement of oxygen saturation in the venous system, right side of the heart, and two main pulmonary arteries. In patients with left-to-right shunt flow, an increase in the oxygen saturation, or *step-up,* will occur as one sample from the chamber where arterial blood is mixing with venous blood. By using the Fick method for calculating blood flow in the pulmonary and systemic systems, the shunt ratio can be calculated. Noninvasive approaches have large supplanted catheterization laboratory assessment of shunts.

Left ventricular size, wall motion, and ejection fraction can be accurately assessed by injecting contrast into the left ventricle (left ventriculography). Aortic and mitral valve insufficiency can be qualitatively assessed during angiography by observing the reflux of contrast medium into the left ventricle and left atrium, respectively. The degree of valvular stenosis can be determined by measuring pressure gradients across the valve and determination of cardiac output (Gorlin formula).

The coronary anatomy can be defined by injecting contrast medium into the coronary tree. Atherosclerotic lesions appear as narrowings of the internal diameter (lumen) of the vessel. A hemodynamically important stenosis is defined as 70% or more narrowing of the luminal diameter. However, the hemodynamic significance of a lesion can be underestimated by coronary angiography, particularly in settings in which the atherosclerotic plaque is eccentric or elongated.

Biopsy of the ventricular endomyocardium can be performed during cardiac catheterization. With this technique, a bioptome is introduced into the venous system through the right internal jugular vein and guided into the right ventricle by fluoroscopy. Small samples of the endocardium are then taken for histologic evaluation. The primary indication for endomyocardial biopsy is the diagnosis of rejection after cardiac transplantation and documentation of cardiac amyloidosis; however, endomyocardial biopsy may have some use in diagnosing specific etiologic agents responsible for myocarditis.

RIGHT VENTRICULAR HEART CATHETERIZATION

A right ventricular heart catheterization can be performed at the bedside with a balloon-tipped pulmonary artery (Swan-Ganz) catheter. This technique allows for serial measurements of right atrial, pulmonary artery, and pulmonary capillary wedge pressures, as well as cardiac output by thermodilution (Fig. 5–17). Such measurements may be useful in monitoring the response to various treatments, such as diuretic therapy, inotropic agents, and vasopressors (Table 5–4). The pulmonary artery catheter is most useful in the critically ill patient for assessing volume status and differentiating cardiogenic from noncardiogenic pulmonary edema. Notably, however, several papers have suggested no improvements in outcomes of critically ill patients in whom pulmonary artery catheterization was performed. Improvements in noninvasive imaging techniques have made the pulmonary artery catheter much less important in diagnosing cardiac conditions, such as pericardial tamponade, constrictive pericarditis, right ventricular infarction, and ventricular septal defect.

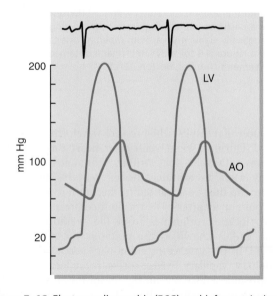

Figure 5–16 Electrocardiographic (ECG) and left ventricular (LV) and aortic (AO) pressure curves in a patient with aortic stenosis. A pressure gradient occurs across the aortic valve during systole.

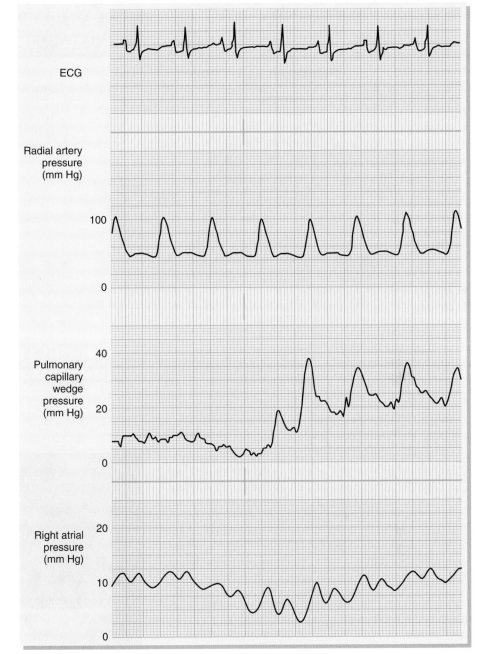

Figure 5–17 Electrocardiographic (ECG) and Swan-Ganz flotation catheter recordings. The left portion of tracing three was obtained with the balloon inflated, yielding the pulmonary arterial wedge pressure. The left portion of tracing three was recorded with the balloon deflated, depicting the pulmonary arterial pressure. In this patient, the pulmonary arterial wedge pressure (left ventricular filling pressure) is normal and the pulmonary artery pressure is elevated because of lung disease.

OTHER DIAGNOSTIC PROCEDURES

Similar to MRI, new applications of computed tomography (CT) have greatly advanced our ability to diagnose cardiovascular disease noninvasively. Great vessel morphology and chamber size can be accurately assessed with both of these methods and, in contrast to echocardiography, they are not limited by the presence of lung disease or chest wall deformity. However, obesity and the presence of prosthetic materials (i.e., mechanical valves) will still affect image quality with these modalities. These tests are most frequently used to diagnose aortic aneurysm and acute aortic dissection and pulmonary embolism. They are also sensitive methods for defining congenital abnormalities and detecting pericardial thickening associated with constrictive pericarditis. Ultrafast

CT (contrast medium–enhanced electron beam CT) provides complete cardiac imaging in real time and is a highly accurate noninvasive method for quantifying left ventricular volume and ejection fraction. MRI offers similar accuracy without radiation exposure (see Fig. 5–14). However, the presence of permanent cardiac pacemakers is a contraindication to MRI. Given the radiation exposure, lack of portability and expense, cardiac CT is not yet routinely used in clinical practice for the purposes of assessing left ventricular function. Electron beam and multidetector CT can visualize and quantitate the extent of coronary artery calcification. Although coronary artery calcification is a sensitive marker for the presence of significant CAD in some individuals, many older patients have such calcification without significant stenoses. In contrast, young patients may have

Table 5–4 Differential Diagnosis Using a Bedside Balloon Flow-Directed (Swan-Ganz) Catheter

Disease State	Thermodilution Cardiac Output	PCW Pressure	RA Pressure	Comments
Cardiogenic shock	↓	↑	nl or ↓	↑ Systemic vascular resistance
Septic shock (early)	↑	↓	↓	↑ Systemic vascular resistance; myocardial dysfunction can occur late
Volume overload	nl or ↑	↑	↑	—
Volume depletion	↓	↓	↓	—
Noncardiac pulmonary edema	nl	nl	nl	—
Pulmonary heart disease	nl or ↑	nl	↑	↑ PA pressure
RV infarction	↓	↓ or nl	↑	—
Pericardial tamponade	↓	nl or ↑	↑	Equalization of diastolic RA, RV, PA, and PCW pressure
Papillary muscle rupture	↓	↑	nl or ↑	Large v waves in PCW tracing
Ventricular septal rupture	↑	↑	nl or ↑	Artifact caused by RA → PA sampling of higher in PA than RA; may have large v waves in PCW tracing

↑ = increased; ↓ = decreased; nl = normal; PA = pulmonary artery; PCW = pulmonary capillary wedge; RA = right atrium; RV = right ventricle.

high-grade noncalcified (soft) plaques that are missed by calcium scoring alone. Very recently, both ultrafast CT and MRI have also been shown to be useful methods of assessing the extent of CAD (Fig. 5–18). However, at the current time, coronary angiography remains the *gold standard* for localizing and quantifying the severity of CAD. Rapid improvements in both MRI and CT technology may lead to major shifts in diagnostic testing strategies in the near future. Some advocates of cardiac CT have proposed the use of this test for the *triple rule out* in patients with acute chest pain—namely, the ability to diagnose pulmonary embolism, aortic dissection, and coronary artery disease with one imaging study. Formal evaluation of this hypothesis still needs to be performed.

NONINVASIVE VASCULAR TESTING

Assessment for the presence and severity of peripheral vascular disease is an important component of the cardiovas-

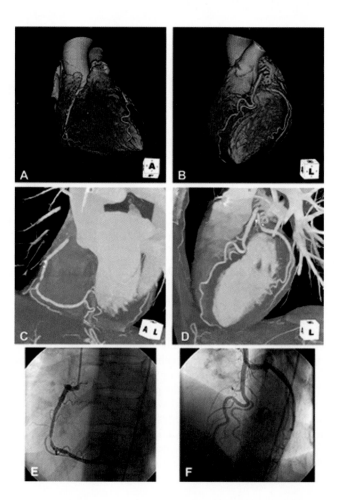

Figure 5–18 Computed tomographic (CT) coronary angiography compared with conventional x-ray contrast angiography. *A* and *B*, volume-rendering technique demonstrating stenosis of the right coronary artery and normal left coronary artery; *C* and *D*, Maximum intensity projection of the same arteries demonstrating severe soft plaque in the right coronary artery with superficial calcified plaque; *E* and *F*, Invasive angiography of the same arteries. (Reproduced from Raff GL, Gallagher MJ, O'Neill WW, et al: Diagnostic accuracy of noninvasive coronary angiography using 64-slice spiral computed tomography. J Am Coll Cardiol 46:552, 2005, with permission from Elsevier, Inc.)

cular evaluation. Comparison of the systolic blood pressure in the upper and lower extremities is one of the simplest tests to detect the presence of hemodynamically important arterial disease. Normally, the systolic pressure in the thigh is similar to that in the brachial artery. An ankle-to-brachial pressure ratio (ankle-brachial index) of less than or equal to 0.9 is abnormal. Patients with claudication usually have an index ranging from 0.5 to 0.8, and patients with rest pain have an index less than 0.5. In some patients, measuring the ankle-brachial index after treadmill exercise may be helpful in identifying the importance of borderline lesions. During normal exercise, blood flow increases to the upper and lower extremities and decreases in peripheral vascular resistance, whereas the ankle-brachial index remains unchanged. In the presence of a hemodynamically significant lesion, the increase in systolic blood pressure in the arm is not matched by an increase in blood pressure in the leg. As a result, the ankle-brachial index will decrease, the magnitude of which is proportional to the severity of the stenosis.

Once significant vascular disease in the extremities has been identified, plethysmography can be used to determine the location and severity of the disease. With this method, a pneumatic cuff is positioned on the leg or thigh and, when inflated, temporarily obstructs venous return. Volume changes in the limb segment below the cuff are converted to a pressure waveform, which can then be analyzed. The degree of amplitude reduction in the pressure waveform corresponds to the severity of arterial disease at that level.

Doppler ultrasound uses reflected sound waves to identify and localize stenotic lesions in the peripheral arteries. This test is particularly useful in patients with severely calcified arteries, in whom pneumatic compression is not possible and ankle-brachial indices are inaccurate. In combination with real-time imaging (duplex imaging), this technique is useful in assessing specific arterial segments and bypass grafts for stenotic or occlusive lesions.

Prospectus for the Future

Multidisciplinary teams consisting of cardiologists, cardiac surgeons, vascular surgeons, and radiologists will replace existing and traditional approaches for the evaluation and management of patients with cardiac disease. Such collaboration will foster efficiency and rapid advances for improvements for patient care, education, and research within a seamless, integrated environment. Career opportunities within organizations with the supporting infrastructure for cardiac imaging will likely realize the promise for patient-oriented, team-based cardiovascular medicine.

References

Cheitlin MD, Armstrong WF, Aurigemma GP, et al: ACC/AHA/ASE 2003 guideline update for the clinical application of echocardiography—summary article: A report of the American College of Cardiology/American Heart Association Task Force on Practice Guidelines (ACC/AHA/ASE Committee to Update the 1997 Guidelines for the Clinical Application of Echocardiography). J Am Soc Echocardiogr 16:1091–1110, 2003.

Eagle KA, Berger PB, Calkins H, et al: ACC/AHA guideline update for perioperative cardiovascular evaluation for noncardiac surgery--executive summary: A report of the American College of Cardiology/American Heart Association Task Force on Practice Guidelines (Committee to Update the 1996 Guidelines on perioperative Cardiovascular Evaluation of Noncardiac Surgery) Circulation 105:1257–1267, 2002.

Gibbons RJ, Abrams J, Chatterjee K, et al: ACC/AHA 2002 guideline update for the management of patients with chronic stable angina--summary article: A report of the American College of Cardiology/American Heart Association Task Force on Practice Guidelines (Committee on the Management of Patients With Chronic Stable Angina). Circulation 107:149–158, 2003.

Gibbons RJ, Balady GJ, Bricker JT, et al: ACC/AHA 2002 guideline update for exercise testing--summary article: A report of the American College of Cardiology/American Heart Association Task Force on Practice Guidelines (Committee to Update the 1997 Exercise Testing Guidelines). J Am Coll Cardiol 40:1531–1540, 2002.

Klein C, Nekolla SG: Assessment of myocardial viability with contrast-enhanced magnetic resonance imaging: Comparison with positron emission tomography. Circulation 105:162–167, 2002.

Morey SS: ACC and AHA update guidelines for coronary angiography. American College of Cardiology. American Heart Association. Am Fam Physician 60:1017–1020, 1999.

Raff GL, Gallagher MJ, O'Neill WW, et al: Diagnostic accuracy of noninvasive coronary angiography using 64-slice spiral computed tomography. J Am Coll Cardiol 46:552–557, 2005.

Sandham JD, Hull RD, Brant RF, et al: A randomized, controlled trial of the use of pulmonary artery catheters in high-risk surgical patients. N Engl J Med 348:5–14, 2003.

Chapter **6**

Heart Failure and Cardiomyopathy

Sheldon E. Litwin

Ivor J. Benjamin

The syndrome of heart failure occurs when an abnormality of cardiac function results in failure to provide adequate blood flow to meet the metabolic needs of the body's tissues and organs or in an excessive rise in cardiac filling pressures. In most cases, myocardial dysfunction causes impaired ventricular filling, as well as emptying. Heart failure can result from a large number of heterogeneous disorders (Table 6–1). Idiopathic cardiomyopathy is defined as a primary abnormality of myocardial tissue in the absence of occlusive, valvular, or systemic disease. However, in the clinical setting, the term *cardiomyopathy* is often used to refer to myocardial dysfunction that is the result of a known genetic, cardiac, or systemic disease. These *secondary* cardiomyopathies may be related to a significant number of disorders, but in the United States, they are most often the result of ischemic heart disease. Ventricular dysfunction can also result from excessive pressure overload, such as with long-standing hypertension or aortic stenosis, or volume overload, such as aortic insufficiency or mitral regurgitation. Diseases that result in infiltration and replacement of normal myocardial tissue, such as amyloidosis, are rare causes of heart failure. Hemochromatosis can cause a dilated cardiomyopathy that is believed to result from iron-mediated mitochondrial damage. Diseases of the pericardium, such as chronic pericarditis or pericardial tamponade, can impair cardiac function without directly affecting the myocardial tissue. Long-standing tachyarrhythmias have been associated with myocardial dysfunction that is often reversible. In addition, an individual with underlying myocardial or valvular disease may develop heart failure with the acute onset of an arrhythmia. Finally, multiple metabolic abnormalities (e.g., thiamine deficiency, thyrotoxicosis), drugs (e.g., alcohol, doxorubicin), and toxic chemicals (e.g., lead, cobalt) can damage the myocardium.

Forms of Heart Failure

Heart failure can be classified as predominantly left or right sided, high output or low output, and acute or chronic. High-output failure is an uncommon disorder that can occur with severe anemia, vascular shunting, or thyrotoxicosis. This failure results when the heart is unable to meet the abnormally elevated metabolic demands of the peripheral tissues even though cardiac output is elevated. Fluid retention is a common component of this syndrome. Low-output failure is much more common than high-output failure and is characterized by insufficient forward output, particularly during times of increased metabolic demand. Cardiac dysfunction may predominantly affect the left ventricle, as with a large myocardial infarction, or the right ventricle, as with an acute pulmonary embolus; however, in many disease states, both ventricles will be impaired (biventricular heart failure). *Acute heart failure* usually refers to the situation in which an individual who was previously asymptomatic develops heart failure signs and/or symptoms following an acute injury to the heart, such as myocardial infarction, myocarditis, or rupture of a heart valve. *Chronic heart failure* refers to an individual whose symptoms have developed over a long period, most often when pre-existing cardiac disease is present. However, a patient with myocardial dysfunction from any cause may be well compensated for long periods and then develop heart failure symptoms only after an acute insult, such as an arrhythmia or infection.

The severity of heart failure symptoms does not correlate closely with the usual clinical measures of cardiac function (i.e., left ventricular ejection fraction [LVEF]), although the LVEF is a good prognostic marker. This situation likely reflects the fact that ventricular filling pressures are a more important determinant of symptoms than myocardial function *per se*. Heart failure may occur in the setting of a

Table 6–1 Causes of Congestive Heart Failure and Cardiomyopathy

Coronary Artery Disease

Acute ischemia
Myocardial infarction
Ischemic cardiomyopathy with hibernating myocardium

Idiopathic

Idiopathic dilated cardiomyopathy*
Idiopathic restrictive cardiomyopathy
Peripartum

Pressure Overload

Hypertension
Aortic stenosis

Volume Overload

Mitral regurgitation
Aortic insufficiency
Anemia
Atrioventricular fistula

Toxins

Ethanol
Cocaine
Doxorubicin (Adriamycin)
Methamphetamine

Metabolic-Endocrine

Thiamine deficiency
Diabetes
Hemochromatosis
Thyrotoxicosis
Obesity
Hemochromatosis

Infiltrative

Amyloidosis

Inflammatory

Viral myocarditis

Hereditary

Hypertrophic
Dilated

*Genetic bases for these cardiomyopathies have been identified in a large number of individual patients and families. The majority of the mutations have been found in cardiac contractile or structural proteins.

reduced or preserved ejection fraction (EF). Recent data suggest that when sensitive methods for assessing myocardial function (i.e., tissue velocity or strain rate imaging) are used, changes are usually detected in both systolic and diastolic function in patients with heart failure (even when the EF is normal or near normal). Importantly, the predisposing conditions for heart failure (e.g., hypertension, advanced age, coronary artery disease, renal dysfunction) are similar, the prognosis is similar, and the efficacies of various medical treatments for heart failure are similar, irrespective of whether the LVEF is preserved or reduced.

ACUTE PULMONARY EDEMA

In patients with the acute onset of pulmonary edema, initial management should be directed at improving oxygenation and providing hemodynamic stability. These patients commonly have marked elevation of blood pressure, cardiac ischemia, and worsening mitral regurgitation as contributing factors to the pulmonary edema. Standard therapy includes supplemental oxygen and an intravenous loop diuretic. Sublingual or intravenous nitroglycerin helps reduce preload through venodilation and may provide symptomatic relief in patients with ischemic and nonischemic ventricular dysfunction. Intravenous morphine acts in a similar manner but must be used with caution, given its depressive effects on respiratory drive. In patients with hypertensive urgency, severe hypertension, or congestive heart failure related to aortic or mitral regurgitation, an arterial vasodilator, such as nitroprusside, may be helpful in reducing afterload.

Evaluation of the patient's response to treatment requires frequent assessments of blood pressure, heart rate, end-organ perfusion, and oxygen saturation. In patients with persistent hypoxia or respiratory acidosis, mechanical ventilation may be necessary for support. Pulmonary artery catheterization may be helpful in documenting filling pressures, cardiac output, and peripheral vascular resistance and in monitoring the response to therapy. In patients with refractory pulmonary edema, an inotropic agent or an intra-aortic balloon pump may be necessary.

DIASTOLIC DYSFUNCTION

Slowed relaxation of the left ventricle and/or increased chamber stiffness impair ventricular filling and may contribute to elevated left ventricular, left atrial, and pulmonary venous pressures. Diastolic filling abnormalities contribute to heart failure symptoms in most patients with reduced left ventricular function. However, some patients with a diagnosis of heart failure have normal or *nearly normal* EF. These patients have been commonly labeled as having *diastolic heart failure.* As described earlier in this chapter, newer imaging techniques have revealed that most of these patients also have a component of systolic dysfunction as well. Thus the term *heart failure with preserved EF* is now being used more frequently.

Relaxation abnormalities are present in most patients over the age of 65 and are almost universal after age 75; however, the vast majority of such patients do not have heart failure. Thus, isolated abnormalities of left ventricular relaxation are apparently not sufficient to directly cause heart failure in the absence of other predisposing conditions.

In patients with a variety of cardiovascular diseases, relaxation abnormalities appear at earlier ages than would otherwise be expected. As of this writing, no therapeutic agents that specifically target impaired relaxation have been developed. β-Agonists (dobutamine) and phosphodiesterase inhibitors (milrinone) have potent lusitropic effects (improve relaxation); however, they also directly increase contractility and enhance myocyte calcium cycling. Chronic β-blocker therapy is associated with parallel improvements in systolic and diastolic function, even though both of these may actually deteriorate during the early phases of treatment. Although calcium channel blockers have been proposed as therapy for diastolic abnormalities, little evidence supports their use for this purpose. Moreover, calcium entry into cardiac myocytes via L-type calcium channels occurs almost exclusively during systole; thus the theoretical basis for their use is also not firm. In general, all therapies that result in improved systolic function also tend to improve diastolic function, or at least diastolic filling pressures.

RESYNCHRONIZATION THERAPY

Interventricular conduction delays, demonstrated as a prolonged QRS duration, are a common complication in patients with heart failure and have been associated with reduced exercise capacity and a poor long-term prognosis. Biventricular pacing or resynchronization therapy results in more normal ventricular contraction and has been associated with an improvement in cardiac output and LVEF. Biventricular pacing may have a beneficial effect on left ventricular remodeling by reducing left ventricular volume, left ventricular mass, and severity of mitral regurgitation. Clinically, these hemodynamic and structural changes have translated into an improvement in exercise duration, functional capacity, and quality of life. Biventricular pacing has also been shown to reduce mortality. Unfortunately, up to 30% of patients undergoing biventricular pacemaker placements do not respond favorably to the treatment. At present, this therapy is generally reserved for patients with severe heart failure and a widened QRS complex who remain symptomatic despite optimal pharmacologic therapy. Intense research efforts are underway to identify with increased accuracy the patients who are likely to derive the greatest benefit. Efforts are currently focused on the quantification of mechanical asynchrony using tissue Doppler imaging.

Adaptive Mechanisms in Heart Failure

A large number of compensatory changes occur in the cardiovascular and renal systems to maintain adequate blood flow to the vital organs of the body in the setting of myocardial dysfunction. These changes include increases in left ventricular volume and pressure through the Frank-Starling mechanism, ventricular remodeling, and neurohormonal activation.

In the normal heart, increasing the stroke volume or heart rate can augment cardiac output. Stroke volume is dependent on the contractile state of the myocardium, left

ventricular filling (preload), and resistance to left ventricular emptying (afterload). According to the Frank-Starling law (Fig. 6–1), stroke volume can be increased with minimal elevation in left ventricular pressure as long as contractility is normal and outflow is not impeded. In the failing heart with depressed intrinsic contractility (Fig. 6–2, curve A), larger increases in filling pressures are required to produce similar increases in stroke volume. When left ventricular diastolic pressure approaches 20 to 25 mm Hg, the hydrostatic pressure in the pulmonary capillaries exceeds the oncotic pressure, and pulmonary edema may ensue. Both depressed myocardial contractility and increased chamber stiffness can lead to pulmonary congestion through similar mechanisms.

The failing heart may also undergo changes in left ventricular size, shape, and mass to maintain adequate forward flow. This process is known as *remodeling* and occurs in response to myocyte loss, such as after a myocardial infarction, or to hemodynamic overload, such as aortic or mitral valve insufficiency. The initial response to increased cardiac stress or load is usually hypertrophy of the viable myocytes. If the increase occurs mainly in cell length, then ventricular dilation is the predominant form of remodeling (usually seen in volume overload or myocardial infarction). The eccentric pattern of remodeling helps maintain cardiac output but occurs at the expense of increased ventricular wall stress. If the myocytes predominantly increase in width (as in the setting of pressure overload), then the heart will tend to thicken with maintenance of cavity volume. This form of remodeling, usually referred to as *concentric hypertrophy,* will tend to reduce wall stress but may do so at the expense of increased filling pressures. If the extent of hypertrophy is inadequate to normalize wall stress, then a vicious cycle is established. Overstretching of the myocytes can lead to an increase in myocyte death, ventricular dilation, development of a spheric left ventricular cavity, and further elevation in wall stress.

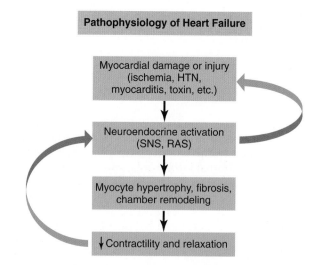

Figure 6–1 Schematic diagram illustrating the progressive nature of left ventricular dysfunction that can occur following an initial cardiac insult. Attenuation of the neurohumoral activation (or blockade of the downstream effects) may interrupt the positive feedback and slow or reverse the progression of heart failure.

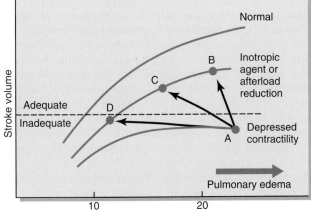

Figure 6–2 Normal and abnormal ventricular function curves. When the left ventricular end-diastolic pressure acutely rises above 20 mm Hg (A), pulmonary edema often occurs. The effect of diuresis or venodilation is to move leftward along the same curve, with a resultant improvement in pulmonary congestion with minimal decrease in cardiac output. The stroke volume is poor at any point along this depressed contractility curve; thus, therapeutic maneuvers that would raise it more toward the normal curve would be necessary to improve cardiac output significantly. Unlike the effect of diuretics, the effect of digitalis or arterial vasodilator therapy in a patient with heart failure is to move the patient into another ventricular function curve intermediately between the normal and depressed curves. When the patient's ventricular function moves from A to B by the administration of one of these agents, the left ventricular end-diastolic pressure may also decrease because of improved cardiac function; further administration of diuretics or venodilators may shift the patient further to the left along the same curve from B to C and eliminate the risk of pulmonary edema. A vasodilating agent that has both arteriolar and venous dilating properties (e.g., nitroprusside) would shift this patient directly from A to C. If this agent shifts the patient from A to D because of excessive venodilation or administration of diuretics, then the cardiac output may fall too low, even though the left ventricular end-diastolic pressure would be normal (10 mm Hg) for a normal heart. Thus, left ventricular end-diastolic pressures between 15 and 18 mm Hg are usually optimal in the failing heart to maximize cardiac output but avoid pulmonary edema.

The mechanical changes are triggered, in part, by activation of several neurohormonal systems. The renin-angiotensin-aldosterone system helps maintain cardiac output via expansion of intravascular volume by promoting retention of sodium and water. Stimulating arterial vasoconstriction through the actions of angiotensin II enhances tissue perfusion. In addition, release of vasopressin will promote free water absorption by the kidney. The sympathetic nervous system helps maintain tissue perfusion by increasing arterial tone, as well as increasing heart rate and ventricular contractility.

Although adaptive in the short term, activation of these systems is associated with several deleterious effects, including elevation in ventricular filling pressures, depression of stroke volume secondary to an increase in peripheral vascular resistance, and stimulation of myocardial hypertrophy

and left ventricular remodeling. These maladaptive changes are ultimately responsible for many of the signs and symptoms associated with congestive heart failure and provide the rationale for treatment.

Countering these effects, and in response to the increase in ventricular filling pressures, the myocardial cells secrete atrial natriuretic peptide and brain natriuretic peptide (BNP). The plasma concentration of both of these hormones has been shown to increase in patients with heart failure. The measurement of serum BNP or its precursors has proved to be clinically useful in the diagnosis of heart failure. Although endogenous natriuretic peptides promote salt and water excretion by the kidneys and result in arterial vasodilation, they are relatively ineffective at reversing the maladaptive changes associated with the powerful renin-angiotensin and sympathetic nervous systems.

Evaluation of Patients with Heart Failure

The history and physical examination are integral parts of the diagnosis of heart failure and the determination of its underlying or precipitating cause. One of the cardinal manifestations of left ventricular heart failure is dyspnea, which is related to elevation in pulmonary venous pressure. In patients with chronic heart failure, shortness of breath initially occurs only with exertion but may progress to occur at rest. Cardiac dyspnea is often worsened by the recumbent position (orthopnea) when increased venous return further elevates pulmonary venous pressure. Paroxysmal nocturnal dyspnea occurs after several hours of sleep and is probably caused by central redistribution of edema. If cardiac output is low but left ventricular filling pressures are normal, then the patient may complain primarily of fatigue resulting from diminished blood flow to the exercising muscles. In some instances, heart failure is slow to progress, and the patient may unknowingly restrict his or her activities. Thus, the history should include an assessment not only of the patient's symptoms, but also of his or her level of activity (functional capacity). Many patients will complain of peripheral edema, usually involving the lower extremities. The edema commonly worsens during the day and decreases overnight with elevation of the legs. In patients with severe, longstanding heart failure, the edema can involve the thighs and abdomen, and ascites may develop. Importantly, peripheral edema often does not have a cardiac cause.

Many of the physical findings of heart failure are related to the neurohormonal changes that help compensate for the reduced cardiac output. An increased heart rate may be present as a result of increased sympathetic tone. The pulse pressure may be narrowed secondary to peripheral vasoconstriction and low stroke volume. If left ventricular filling pressures are elevated, then crackles may be heard on auscultation of the lung fields. Elevation in right-sided filling pressures will result in distended neck veins. If the liver is also congested, then firm pressure applied to the right upper quadrant will cause the jugular veins to become further engorged (hepatojugular reflux). Palpation of the precordium may reveal left ventricular enlargement. An early-diastolic third heart sound (S₃) or gallop suggests elevated atrial pressure and increased ventricular chamber stiffness.

The sound results from rapid deceleration of the passive component of blood flow from the atrium into the noncompliant ventricle. An S_3 can be generated from the left or right ventricle. A fourth heart sound (S_4) suggests an increased atrial contribution to left ventricular filling but is not specific for heart failure. The murmurs of both mitral and tricuspid regurgitation are common in patients with congestive heart failure and may become accentuated during an acute decompensation. As stated earlier, peripheral edema is a common finding on physical examination and may be related to elevation in venous pressure and/or increased sodium and water retention. In bedridden patients, the edema may predominantly be in the presacral region.

The electrocardiogram in patients with congestive heart failure is not specific, but it may provide insight into the cause of the cardiac dysfunction, such as prior myocardial infarction, left ventricular hypertrophy, or significant arrhythmias. The chest radiograph may show chamber enlargement and signs of pulmonary congestion (Fig. 6–3). Treatment of heart failure will result in improvement of the vascular congestion on the chest radiograph, but these changes may lag 24 to 48 hours behind clinical improvement. Certain blood chemistries may be altered in the patient with heart failure. The serum sodium concentration may be low, owing to increased water retention with activation of the renin-angiotensin system. The use of potent diuretics is almost always partially responsible for the hyponatremia. Renal function may be impaired secondary to intrinsic kidney disease and/or reduced perfusion secondary to renal artery vasoconstriction and low cardiac output. Hepatic congestion is common with right ventricular heart failure and may result in elevated liver enzyme levels.

Because many of the signs and symptoms of heart failure may also occur with pulmonary disease, differentiating between these two disease processes may be difficult. Initial therapy will often be directed at both potential pulmonary and cardiac causes until further testing can be performed. Echocardiography is arguably the central means for diagnostic testing in patients with suspected heart failure. This test is fast, safe, portable, and allows for noninvasive assessments of chamber sizes, systolic function, valvular function, both right and left ventricular filling pressures, and quantification of stroke volume or cardiac output. Documentation of heart size, wall thickness, and ventricular function will have important therapeutic implications in most patients (Fig. 6–4). Rapid measurement of the plasma concentration of BNP provides objective and complementary data to aid in the diagnosis of heart failure in the patient with dyspnea. Clinical studies have shown that plasma levels of BNP are elevated in patients with symptomatic left or right ventricular dysfunction but are usually normal in patients with dyspnea secondary to noncardiac causes. Unfortunately, a relatively large indeterminate range exists in which the test is not helpful. Advanced age and renal dysfunction also reduce the utility of the test, particularly if the BNP concentration is mildly elevated.

An important point to note is that pulmonary edema may also be secondary to noncardiac causes, such as sepsis, certain pulmonary infections, drug toxicity, or neurologic injury. This syndrome, termed *adult respiratory distress syndrome*, can be differentiated from cardiogenic pulmonary edema by the presence of a low or normal pulmonary capillary wedge pressure. Peripheral edema may also occur in disease states other than congestive heart failure. Renal disease, especially nephrotic syndrome, cirrhosis, and severe venous stasis disease, may be associated with peripheral edema.

Treatment

Treatment of congestive heart failure should be directed not only at relieving the patient's symptoms, but also at treating

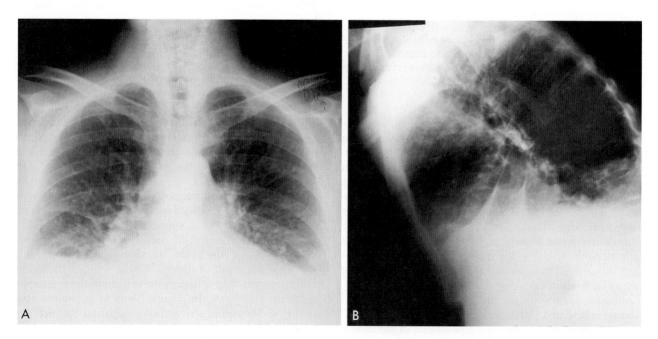

Figure 6–3 *A,* Posteroanterior chest radiograph showing cardiomegaly. *B,* Lateral chest radiograph showing pulmonary vascular congestion typical of pulmonary edema.

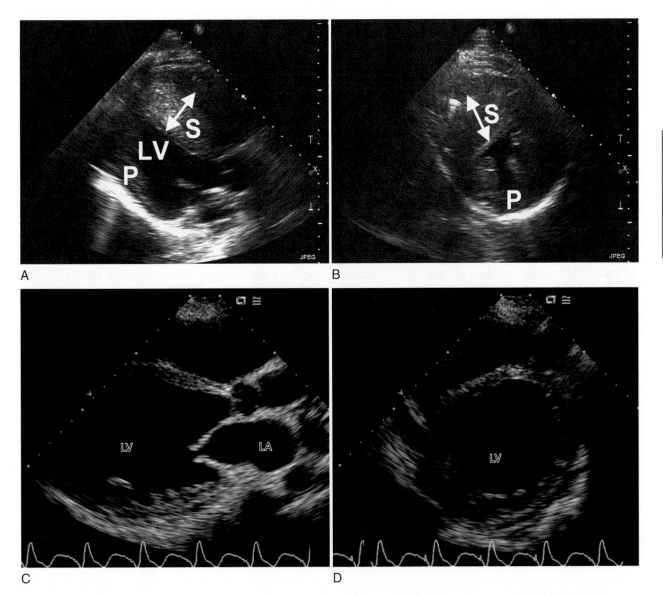

Figure 6–4 Echocardiographic examples of hypertrophic cardiomyopathy seen in long axis *(A)* and short axis *(B)* views. Note normal size of left ventricular *(LV)* cavity and marked thickening of interventricular septum *(S)* compared to posterior wall *(P)*. In contrast, similar views in a patient with dilated cardiomyopathy *(C, D)* reveal a markedly enlarged left ventricular cavity with diffuse wall thinning.

the underlying or precipitating causes (Table 6–2) and preventing progression. Patients should be educated about the importance of compliance with medical therapy, as well as dietary salt and fluid restriction. Rhythm disturbances, such as atrial fibrillation, may precipitate congestive heart failure and may require specific therapy. Treatment of active coronary artery disease, hypertension, or valvular disease may relieve heart failure symptoms. In addition, correction of concomitant medical problems may help stabilize heart function.

NONPHARMACOLOGIC TREATMENT

All patients with heart failure should be instructed to restrict sodium intake to approximately 2 g/day. Fluid intake should also be limited to avoid hyponatremia. Weight reduction in the obese patient helps reduce the workload of the failing heart. Although a growing body of data suggests that a higher body mass index may paradoxically have protective effects in patients with heart failure, each condition is an independent risk factor for increased morbidity and mortality of cardiac disease. A supervised exercise cardiac rehabilitation program can help reduce heart failure symptoms and improve functional capacity in select patients.

PHARMACOLOGIC TREATMENT

Diuretics

Salt and water retention is common in congestive heart failure secondary to activation of the renin-angiotensin-aldosterone system. Diuretics help promote renal excretion of sodium and water and provide rapid relief of pulmonary congestion and peripheral edema. Loop diuretics, such as

Table 6–2	**Precipitants of Heart Failure**

Dietary (sodium and fluid) indiscretion
Noncompliance with medications
Development of cardiac arrhythmia
Anemia
Uncontrolled hypertension
Superimposed medical illness (pneumonia, renal dysfunction)
New cardiac abnormality (acute ischemia, acute valvular insufficiency)

furosemide, are the preferred agents in the treatment of symptomatic heart failure. In patients who are refractory to high doses of these agents, diuretics that block sodium absorption at different sites within the nephron may be beneficial (i.e., thiazide-type diuretics). Spironolactone is an aldosterone antagonist with weak diuretic effects that has been shown to reduce hospitalizations for heart failure and cardiac mortality in patients with severe (New York Heart Association class III or IV) heart failure.

Notably, diuretic therapy will lower intracardiac filling pressures and thus cardiac output through the Frank-Starling mechanism. In most patients, this change is well tolerated. However, in some patients, the reduced cardiac output will result in decreased renal perfusion and a rise in the blood urea nitrogen and creatinine levels.

Vasodilators

A large number of vasodilators have been shown to reverse the peripheral vasoconstriction that occurs in congestive heart failure. The most important group of vasodilator agents is the angiotensin-converting enzyme (ACE) inhibitors. These agents help relieve heart failure symptoms, in part, by blocking production of angiotensin II and reducing afterload. In addition, ACE inhibitors have been shown to reduce mortality in patients with both symptomatic and asymptomatic left ventricular dysfunction. The major side effects of ACE inhibitors include hypotension, hyperkalemia, and azotemia. Cough may occur in approximately 10% of patients and is related to increased bradykinin levels associated with ACE inhibitor use.

Hydralazine in combination with oral nitrates has also been shown to reduce mortality in patients with symptomatic congestive heart failure, although not to the degree of ACE inhibitors. This combination provides an alternative to the patient who is ACE-inhibitor intolerant or may require additional therapy for blood pressure control. In addition, recent prospective studies reveal that the combination of hydralazine and nitrates was more beneficial than ACE inhibitors in the African-American population.

A newer class of agents, the angiotensin II–receptor antagonists, prevents the binding of angiotensin II to its receptor. This action has the theoretical advantage of blocking the effects of angiotensin II produced in the bloodstream, as well as at the tissue level. In addition, the angiotensin II-receptor blockers do not interfere with bradykinin metabolism and therefore are not associated with cough. Several studies comparing ACE inhibitors to

angiotensin II blockers suggest that these two classes of agents are equally effective in reducing morbidity and mortality in patients with heart failure. The current guidelines for the management of chronic heart failure, however, recommend that angiotensin II–receptor blockers be reserved for patients who are intolerant of ACE inhibitors.

The negative inotropic effects of the calcium channel blockers and their activation of the sympathetic nervous system make these agents less attractive in the treatment of patients with congestive heart failure. In particular, several studies have shown worsening of heart failure symptoms in patients treated with nifedipine. Other calcium channel blockers, such as diltiazem, have been shown to relieve symptoms and increase functional capacity without a deleterious effect on survival in patients with idiopathic dilated cardiomyopathy. Amlodipine has been studied in patients with both ischemic and nonischemic cardiomyopathy and also has not been associated with an increased cardiac morbidity and mortality. In addition, patients with nonischemic cardiomyopathy treated with amlodipine may have a modest survival benefit. Further studies with these agents are necessary before general recommendations regarding their use in patients with heart failure can be made.

Inotropic Agents

Inotropic agents help relieve heart failure symptoms by increasing ventricular contractility. The oldest and most commonly used agent in this class is digoxin, which has been associated with symptomatic improvement in heart failure in patients with systolic dysfunction. However, a recent trial found no significant improvement in survival among patients randomized to digoxin compared with patients treated with placebo. A small reduction in hospitalizations and in death secondary to heart failure was observed, but this was counterbalanced by a slight increase in death secondary to arrhythmias. In general, digoxin therapy should be considered in the patient with left ventricular systolic dysfunction who remains symptomatic after treatment with an ACE inhibitor and a diuretic. No evidence has been found that digoxin should be administered to the patient with asymptomatic left ventricular dysfunction. In addition, digoxin may be harmful in patients with infiltrative cardiomyopathies, such as amyloidosis.

Several other classes of oral inotropic agents have been evaluated for treatment of congestive heart failure, such as flosequinon, milrinone, vesnarinone, and xamoterol. All of these agents have been associated with increased mortality with long-term use. More recently, promising data have emerged involving the calcium-sensitizing agent levosimendan. This class of agents has the theoretical advantage of not increasing calcium fluxes into the myocyte; therefore, they should be less arrhythmogenic and have a more favorable energetic effect.

β-Blockers

As previously discussed, many of the symptoms associated with heart failure are related to activation of several neurohormonal systems, including the sympathetic nervous system. Release of catecholamines may initially help maintain blood pressure and cardiac output but, in the long term, may induce further myocardial injury. To date, long-term use of three different β-blockers—metoprolol, bisoprolol, and carvedilol—have been shown in clinical trials to improve LVEF and survival in patients with symptomatic left ventricular dysfunction. Of these agents, carvedilol is unique in that it is also an antioxidant and an α-blocker, additional properties that may be beneficial in patients with heart failure. Data from clinical trials comparing the efficacy of metoprolol to carvedilol in patients with heart failure have recently been reported. These data suggest superior effects of carvedilol; however, controversy about the experimental design has limited widespread adoption of a single agent. Therapy with one of the aforementioned β-blockers should be strongly considered in all patients who have been stabilized on an ACE inhibitor, digoxin, and a diuretic but remain symptomatic (New York Heart Association classes II to IV). β-Blockers also appear to be effective in patients who are not taking ACE inhibitors. β-Blocker therapy is generally withheld from patients with acutely decompensated heart failure and/or significant volume overload. Gradual up titration of the dose improves the ability to tolerate these drugs, which are intrinsically negatively inotropic.

Anticoagulation

Thrombosis and thromboemboli occur in patients with left ventricular remodeling and congestive heart failure secondary to stasis of blood, intracardiac thrombi, and atrial arrhythmias. Although long-term warfarin therapy remains controversial, certain patients may benefit from its use, including patients with chronic atrial fibrillation or flutter, patients with definite mural thrombi noted by echocardiography or ventriculography, and patients in sinus rhythm with LVEF less than 20%. In the general heart failure population, prevention of thromboembolism is roughly balanced by increased bleeding risks.

Refractory Heart Failure

Despite adequate medical therapy, many patients with congestive heart failure will fail to have significant reduction in their symptoms. In these instances, therapy with intravenous inotropic agents for 24 to 96 hours, sometimes with hemodynamic monitoring (Swan-Ganz catheter), may be necessary to stabilize the patient. One commonly used agent is dobutamine, which enhances contractility of the heart and reduces peripheral vasoconstriction through stimulation of β_2-receptors. Milrinone is an intravenous phosphodiesterase inhibitor that has similar effects on contractility and afterload. Administration of these agents will often promote diuresis, especially when given concomitantly with intravenous loop diuretics. In patients with markedly elevated systemic vascular resistance, the use of intravenous vasodilators, such as sodium nitroprusside, can significantly reduce afterload and improve cardiac output. A newly available agent, nesiritide, is a recombinant form of human BNP that has been shown to reduce systemic and pulmonary vascular resistance, increase cardiac output, and promote diuresis comparable to standard inotropic agents and vasodilators. Although nesiritide is less likely to provoke serious dysrhythmias as compared with dobutamine, recent data have questioned the safety profile and efficacy of nesiritide. Until further studies document safety, nesiritide is not a first-line agent.

If the previously mentioned measures fail to produce a satisfactory diuretic response, then dopamine given in doses ranging from 2 to 5 mcg/kg/min may facilitate sodium and water excretion by stimulating renal dopaminergic receptors. If heart failure is accompanied by hypotension, then higher doses of dopamine may be necessary. With doses of more than 5 mcg/kg/min, dopamine can increase heart rate and peripheral vascular resistance through stimulation of β_1- and α-receptors. Although this dose range of dopamine may help stabilize blood pressure, the increase in afterload may have further deleterious effects on the failing heart. In addition, dopamine may provoke arrhythmias that may lead to further hemodynamic instability. If hypotension persists despite dopamine doses greater than 15 mcg/kg/min, then mechanical assist devices, such as the intra-aortic balloon pump, should be considered as a means to stabilize the patient.

In patients who cannot be weaned from pharmacologic or mechanical support, or in ambulatory patients with severe functional impairment refractory to medical therapy, cardiac transplantation should be considered as a means to improve symptoms and prolong survival (see Chapter 12).

Cardiovascular Assist Devices

The most commonly used mechanical support device is the intra-aortic balloon pump. This device can be inserted percutaneously through the femoral artery and advanced into the descending thoracic aorta. Inflation of the balloon occurs during diastole such that perfusion pressure in the proximal aorta and coronary arteries is enhanced. Deflation, which occurs just before the onset of systole, greatly reduces aortic impedance and thus significantly reduces afterload. This device is particularly useful in stabilizing patients with severe coronary disease before percutaneous or following surgical revascularization. In addition, this device may provide hemodynamic support in patients with severe mitral regurgitation or acquired ventricular septal defect before surgical repair. In patients with refractory congestive heart failure, the intra-aortic balloon pump may serve as a temporizing measure until cardiac transplantation can be performed.

In addition to the intra-aortic balloon pump, several ventricular assist devices are available that provide hemodynamic support. These devices can be placed percutaneously, but most commonly are implanted through a sternotomy incision. They can be used to support either ventricle. Blood is collected from the right atrium, left atrium, or the left ventricular apex into an extracorporeal reservoir and then actively pumped back into the pulmonary or systemic circulation by the assist device. These units were initially intended to provide hemodynamic support for several days to weeks (most often a *bridge* to transplantation in the patient who is critically ill). Because of the success with these devices and the limited availability of donor hearts, assist devices are now being implanted as *destination* therapy. The pump is placed within the peritoneum, and portable battery packs allow the patient to ambulate. Newer left ventricular–assist devices, as well as total artificial hearts, are currently undergoing clinical investigation as permanent cardiac replacement therapy.

Prospectus for the Future

External Containment Devices

In patients with left ventricular dysfunction, cardiac remodeling characterized by progressive ventricular chamber dilation and wall thinning can lead to elevation in wall stress and activation of neurohormonal mechanisms that further impair myocardial function. Experimental devices that passively contain the heart have been shown, in animal models, to reduce ventricular cavity size and improve myocardial responsiveness to β-adrenergic stimulation without impairing left ventricular filling or interfering with coronary blood flow. Randomized trials evaluating the efficacy of these devices in patients with end-stage cardiomyopathy are currently underway.

Mitral Valve Repair

Mitral regurgitation contributes to the progression of heart failure in a large number of patients. However, the majority of patients with severe heart failure are deemed to be poor surgical candidates. Several new and exciting percutaneous approaches to mitral valve repair are being explored as ways to treat some of these patients.

Cell-Based Therapies

Permanent loss of myocytes is the final common pathway in most forms of heart failure. Presently, some experimental data support the notion that implantation of cells into the failing heart might effectively regenerate new cardiac muscle. Skeletal myoblasts, bone marrow derived progenitor cells, and embryonic stem cells are all undergoing testing in both animals and humans. Although many types of transplanted cells are able to contract, ineffective formation of gap junctions and hence ineffective electrical continuity between the transplanted cells and the existing myocardial syncytium continue to be obstacles.

References

Burkhoff D, Maurer MS, Packer M, et al: Heart failure with a normal ejection fraction: Is it really a disorder of diastolic function? Circulation 107:656–658, 2003.

Cleland JG, Daubert JD, Erdmann E, et al: The effect of cardiac resynchronization on morbidity and mortality in heart failure. N Engl J Med 352:1539–1549, 2005.

Dokainish H, Zoghbi WA, Lakkis NM, et al: Optimal noninvasive assessment of left ventricular filling pressures: A comparison of tissue Doppler echocardiography and B-type natriuretic peptide in patients with pulmonary artery catheters. Circulation 109:2432–2439, 2004.

Poole-Wilson PA, Swedberg K, Cleland JG, et al: Comparison of carvedilol and metoprolol on clinical outcomes in patients with chronic heart failure in the Carvedilol Or Metoprolol European Trial (COMET): Randomised controlled trial. Lancet 362:7–13, 2003.

Rose EA, Gelijns AC, Moskowitz AJ, et al: Long-term mechanical left ventricular assistance for end-stage heart failure. N Engl J Med 345:1435–1443, 2001.

Taylor AL, Ziesche S, Yancy C, et al: Combination of isosorbide dinitrate and hydralazine in blacks with heart failure. N Engl J Med 351:2049–2057, 2004.

Young JB, Abraham WT, Smith AL, et al: Combined cardiac resynchronization and implantable cardioversion defibrillation in advanced chronic heart failure: The MIRACLE ICD trial. JAMA 289:2685–2694, 2003.

Congenital Heart Disease

Kevin J. Whitehead

Dean Y. Li

Approximately 0.8% of all live births are complicated by congenital cardiac abnormalities, not including infants with bicuspid aortic valve and mitral valve prolapse (see Chapter 8), which are more prevalent (2% and 2.4%, respectively). Congenital heart disease is a major cause of infant morbidity and mortality. As a result of advances in pediatric cardiology and cardiothoracic surgery, approximately 85% of infants born with congenital heart disease can be expected to survive into adulthood. In turn, adults with congenital heart disease represent a large and growing population that is encountered more frequently in clinical practice. An equal number of adults and children live with congenital heart disease, with an estimated 800,000 adult patients in the United States alone.

Most cases of congenital heart disease occur sporadically, without a known specific cause. Genetic abnormalities are responsible for a proportion of cases and may contribute to cases occurring sporadically as well. Environmental factors are also known to cause congenital heart disease. An increased incidence is found in children of patients with congenital heart disease, with a higher risk for mothers than for fathers. In most cases, the nature of the parent's defect does not predict the lesion in affected offspring.

The size and nature of the congenital defect often determine the onset of symptoms. Normal physiologic changes in cardiovascular hemodynamics at birth can prompt presentation. Symptoms can develop shortly after birth when transition from fetal to adult circulation represents a new dependence on biventricular circulation with a pulmonary circuit. The isolated pulmonary and systemic circulations of D-transposition of the great arteries become apparent on closure of the last fetal connections between circuits, the ductus arteriosus and the foramen ovale. In other conditions, the primary lesion results in changes that delay presentation until such compensatory mechanisms fail. Hypertrophy of the morphologic right ventricle in L-transposition of the great arteries is sufficient to compensate for systemic vascular resistance and maintain normal perfusion for years with symptoms often developing when the systemic ventricle fails. Still other lesions may develop in adulthood when degenerative changes, such as stenosis of a previously well-functioning bicuspid aortic valve, are superimposed on an initial lesion. Some congenital defects may go undetected throughout life (e.g., small atrial septal defects [ASDs], whereas some may resolve spontaneously (small muscular ventricular septal defects [VSDs]). Many adult patients with congenital heart disease will have already undergone palliative or reparative surgical procedures and will have subsequent care directed at residual defects and sequelae of such procedures. This chapter focuses on the most common congenital abnormalities observed in adults, including those that develop in adulthood and those for which surgical correction during infancy and childhood permits survival into adulthood.

Septal Defects

ATRIAL SEPTAL DEFECTS

ASDs are some of the most common congenital defects, representing 10% to 17% of cases with a higher prevalence in women (60%). Defects are classified according to their location in the interatrial septum. The most common ASD (60%), the ostium secundum defect, involves the fossa ovalis. Ostium primum defects (20%) involve the atrioventricular junction and are at one end of the spectrum of atrioventricular septal defects (or endocardial cushion defects). Primum ASDs are usually associated with a cleft mitral valve and mitral regurgitation. In rare cases, primum ASD can be associated with a large VSD and a single atrioventricular (AV) valve, forming an AV septal defect. Sinus venosus defects are located in the superior septum and may be associated with partially anomalous pulmonary venous drainage into the superior vena cava or right atrium.

In patients with uncomplicated ASDs (e.g., with normal pulmonary vascular resistance), oxygenated blood shunts from the left to the right atrium. The magnitude of the shunting is determined by the size of the defect and the compliance of the left and right ventricles. Small ASDs accommodate the increased blood flow in the right atrium without sequelae and no significant hemodynamic compromise of the right heart. If the defect is large, then the right atrium and right ventricle dilate to accommodate the increased volume of shunted blood (Fig. 7–1). Pressure in the pulmonary artery increases secondary to the increased volume of blood; however, with the exception of extremely large, long-standing defects, pulmonary vascular resistance usually remains normal.

Most patients with ASD are asymptomatic until adulthood, when symptoms such as fatigue, dyspnea, and poor exercise tolerance develop, secondary to right ventricular dysfunction. Older patients may decompensate when acquired heart disease leads to a rise in left ventricular filling pressures and more blood is shunted from the left atrium to the already volume-overloaded right heart. Patients with ASD are prone to atrial fibrillation, especially after 50 years of age. Irreversible pulmonary vascular obstruction resulting in right-to-left shunting and cyanosis (Eisenmenger syndrome) is uncommon and occurs infrequently (>5% of patients with ASDs). The presence of an ASD may be heralded by a paradoxical embolus traversing the defect, resulting in stroke or transient ischemic attack.

A prominent right ventricular pulsation may be heard on physical examination, along the left sternal border secondary to a dilated, hyperdynamic right ventricle (Table 7–1). The S2 sound is widely split and fixed. Wide splitting occurs because right ventricular volume overload results in a prolonged ejection period and delayed closure of the pulmonic valve. Fixed splitting results from a lack of respiratory variation in right ventricular filling with variation in the left-to-right shunt, compensating for varying venous return. An ejection-quality murmur that increases with inspiration is commonly heard at the left sternal border and is secondary to increased blood flow across the pulmonic valve. If severe pulmonary vascular obstruction develops, the P2 sound becomes loud, the splitting of S2 narrows, and a right ventricular gallop may be heard.

The diagnosis of ASD is usually made with two-dimensional and color Doppler echocardiography. In particular, transesophageal imaging allows for excellent visualization of the interatrial septum, as well as associated congenital defects such as anomalous pulmonary veins,

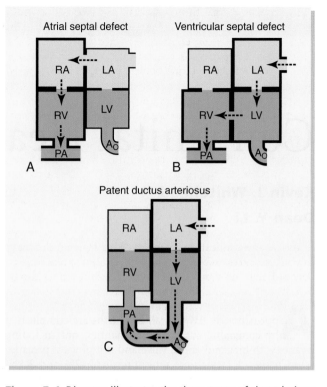

Figure 7–1 Diagram illustrates the three types of shunt lesions that commonly survive until adulthood and their effects on chamber size. *A,* Uncomplicated atrial septal defect (ASD) demonstrating left-to-right shunt flow across the interatrial septum and resulting in dilation of the right atrium (RA), right ventricle (RV), and pulmonary artery (PA). *B,* Uncomplicated ventricular septal defect (VSD), resulting in dilation of the RV, left atrium (LA), and left ventricle (LV). *C,* Uncomplicated patent ductus arteriosus, resulting in dilation of the LA, LV, and PA. (From Liberthson RR, Waldman H: Congenital heart disease in the adult. In Kloner RA [ed]: The Guide to Cardiology, 3rd ed. Greenwich, Conn: Le Jacq Communications, 1991, pp 24–47. Copyright ©1991 by Le Jacq Communications, Inc.)

Table 7–1	**Findings in Uncomplicated Shunt Lesions**		
Type	**Physical Findings**	**Electrocardiogram**	**Chest Radiograph**
Atrial septal defect	Parasternal RV impulse Widely and fixed split S2 Ejection murmur across pulmonic valve	Right bundle branch block Left axis deviation with ostium primum defect	Large pulmonary artery Increased pulmonary markings
Ventricular septal defect	Hyperdynamic precordium Holosystolic left parasternal murmur, with or without thrill	LV and RV hypertrophy	Cardiomegaly Prominent pulmonary vasculature
Patent ductus arteriosus	Hyperdynamic apical impulse Continuous machinery-like murmur	LV hypertrophy	Prominent pulmonary artery Enlarged LA and LV

LA = left atrium; LV = left ventricle; RV = right ventricle.

VSDs, and abnormalities of the mitral leaflets. This technique provides additional information pertaining to right ventricular size and function and the degree of shunt flow. Cardiac catheterization is needed to assess and define the shunt fraction (Qp/Qs ratio) to measure pulmonary arterial pressures and to estimate pulmonary vascular resistance. Concomitant coronary artery disease can be identified by angiography in adults older than 40 years who are contemplating surgical repair.

Once diagnosed, ASDs should be closed without delay. The presence of cardiac enlargement by chest x-ray studies or right ventricular enlargement by echocardiography, the elevation of pulmonary artery pressure, or a shunt fraction of 2:1 or greater should prompt referral for closure, even in the absence of symptoms. Defects less than 8 mm in diameter are rarely significant. Significant pulmonary hypertension is a contraindication to ASD closure. When pulmonary arterial pressures exceed two thirds of systemic pressure, evidence of ongoing significant left-to-right shunt must also be present or the reversibility of pulmonary hypertension with the administration of vasodilators or oxygen must be administered to justify the increased risk of closure.

Percutaneous device closure of a secundum ASD is an acceptable alternative to surgical closure and is becoming the preferred intervention for this condition. A sufficient rim of tissue is required for successful device deployment. Short- and intermediate-term results with the Amplatzer closure device have been excellent. The long-term results remain unknown, and patients who have received such devices should continue to receive close follow-up care. Primum and sinus venosus defects should be surgically closed.

Because a significant ASD should be closed, closure before the age of 25 years is expected to convey a mortality benefit. Closure before the age of 40 years of age is expected to decrease the long-term risk of atrial arrhythmias. After the fourth decade, symptoms are usually significantly improved after surgical repair. However, some degree of right ventricular dysfunction may persist. Antibiotic prophylaxis for infective endocarditis is not required for small ASDs or patent foramen ovale or after ASD closure.

VENTRICULAR SEPTAL DEFECT

VSD is a common congenital abnormality in newborns and is present in approximately 1 in 500 normal births. Because nearly 50% of VSDs close spontaneously during childhood and most large defects are surgically corrected at an early age, this defect is rarely encountered in adults. VSDs are classified according to their location within the interventricular septum. Most isolated VSDs involve the membranous (80%) or muscular (5% to 20%) portion of the interventricular septum and often close spontaneously during childhood if small. Less common types of VSD involve the atrioventricular canal, which is often associated with ostium primum ASDs, along with mitral and tricuspid leaflet abnormalities. Such congenital defects are common in patients with Down syndrome. High (supracristal) membranous VSDs are located beneath the aortic annulus and often lead to aortic valvular incompetence.

In patients with uncomplicated VSDs, oxygenated blood from the left ventricle is shunted across the defect into the right ventricle. If the defect is small, then right ventricular size and function are normal and pulmonary vascular resistance does not increase. If the defect is large, however, the right ventricle dilates to accommodate the increased volume and pulmonary blood flow increases (see Fig. 7–1). If the condition is uncorrected, then pulmonary vascular obstruction may develop and may lead to pulmonary artery hypertension, reversal of the interventricular shunt, and systemic desaturation and cyanosis (Eisenmenger syndrome).

The clinical course of a patient with VSD depends on the size of the defect. Most small defects spontaneously close, or if still present in adulthood, they are usually not associated with any significant hemodynamic complications. Large defects are usually detected and repaired during infancy. Affected individuals with uncorrected defects who survive to adulthood may have signs and symptoms of right-sided ventricular heart failure. If pulmonary vascular obstruction with Eisenmenger physiologic symptoms develops, cyanosis and clubbing of the fingers may be present. All patients with VSD (or repaired VSD with residual shunt flow) are at risk of bacterial endocarditis that usually involves the right ventricular outflow tract.

On physical examination, the patient with an uncomplicated VSD has a hyperdynamic precordium and a palpable thrill along the left sternal border (see Table 7–1). The murmur is usually holosystolic and is best heard at the left sternal border. In general, small defects are associated with loud murmurs because of the significant pressure gradient between the left and the right ventricles. As pulmonary hypertension develops and left-to-right shunt flow decreases, the murmur may soften and a loud P2 sound may be present.

Two-dimensional and Doppler echocardiography are useful in diagnosing VSDs, as well as in assessing right ventricular size and function and associated cardiac abnormalities. Cardiac catheterization is often necessary before surgical repair to document the severity of shunt flow and to determine pulmonary artery pressure and pulmonary vascular resistance. Documentation involves identifying a rise in oxygen content in blood that is sampled from the right ventricle and pulmonary artery compared with blood from the right atrium. Patients with Eisenmenger syndrome and net right-to-left shunt flow are not surgical candidates. Surgical closure of the VSD with sutures or a prosthetic patch is recommended for patients with left-to-right shunt flow greater than 2:1 without evidence of irreversible pulmonary hypertension.

Valvular Defects

CONGENITAL AORTIC STENOSIS AND BICUSPID AORTIC VALVE

Congenital left ventricular outflow obstruction may occur at the valvular, subvalvular, or supravalvular level. Valvular stenosis is most often secondary to a bicuspid aortic valve, which is present in approximately 2% of the population and occurs more frequently in men than in women. Associated cardiovascular abnormalities can occur in less than or equal to 20% of affected persons and include coarctation of the aorta and descending coronary artery (PDA). Bicuspid aortic valves rarely cause significant obstruction during infancy and early childhood. However, their abnormal structure results in turbulent flow that leads to leaflet injury and a thickening, calcification, and, ultimately, narrowing of the orifice.

Although a few patients with bicuspid aortic stenosis remain asymptomatic throughout life, most affected individuals develop symptoms during the fifth and sixth decades of life. As with acquired aortic stenosis, chest pain, syncope, and congestive heart failure are the most frequent symptoms. Complications of bicuspid aortic valves include sudden death, which may occur during periods of rest or exertion, and infective endocarditis, which can lead to significant aortic regurgitation. Less commonly, aortic regurgitation is the predominant abnormality associated with a bicuspid aortic valve.

The physical examination of a patient with a stenotic bicuspid aortic valve is similar to that of the patient with acquired aortic stenosis and is usually characterized by an ejection-quality murmur at the left sternal border (Table 7–2). If the leaflets are still pliable, then an early systolic ejection click may be appreciated as the leaflets open. The decrescendo diastolic murmur of aortic insufficiency may also be present, as may typical signs of significant aortic regurgitation.

The diagnosis of bicuspid aortic valve and the determination of degree of stenosis and/or regurgitation are usually made by two-dimensional and Doppler echocardiography. (Treatment of patients with significant obstruction or insufficiency is outlined in Chapter 8.) Children and young adults with significant stenosis may have improvement with percutaneous valvuloplasty, especially when calcification of the valve cusps is minimal. In older adults or those patients with significant leaflet calcification, aortic valve replacement remains the treatment of choice. Endocarditis prophylaxis is required for all patients with bicuspid aortic valves, whether the valve functions normally, is stenotic, or is regurgitant.

Other causes of congenital left ventricular outflow tract obstruction are much less common. *Subaortic stenosis* is often first diagnosed in adulthood and is characterized by the presence of a discrete, fibrous diaphragm that encircles the left ventricular outflow tract between the mitral annulus

Table 7–2	**Findings in Select Uncomplicated, Unrepaired Cardiac Defects**		
Type	**Physical Findings**	**Electrocardiogram**	**Chest Radiogram**
Congenital aortic stenosis	Decreased carotid upstroke Sustained apical impulse Single S_2, S_4 Systolic ejection murmur	LV hypertrophy	Post-stenotic aortic dilation Prominent LV
Coarctation of aorta	Delayed femoral pulses Reduced blood pressure in lower extremities Findings associated with bicuspid aortic valve	LV hypertrophy	Post-stenotic aortic dilation Prominent ascending aorta LV enlargement
Pulmonic valve stenosis	RV lift Pulmonic ejection sound Systolic ejection murmur at left sternal border RV S_4, widely split S_2, soft P_2	RV hypertrophy RA abnormality	Post-stenotic dilation of the main or left pulmonary artery RA and RV enlargement
Tetralogy of Fallot	Usually cyanotic Possible clubbing Prominent ejection murmur at left sternal border Soft or absent P_2	RV hypertrophy RA abnormality	Boot-shaped heart Small pulmonary artery Normal pulmonary vasculature
Ebstein's anomaly	Acyanotic or cyanotic Increased jugular venous pressure Prominent *v* wave Systolic murmur at sternal border, increases with inspiration	RA abnormality Right bundle branch block PR prolongation Ventricular pre-excitation	Enlarged RA Normal pulmonary vasculature

LV = left ventricle; PR = pulse rate; RA = right atrium; RV = right ventricle.

and the basal interventricular septum. Patients with this defect have a characteristic outflow murmur but not the systolic ejection click appreciated in patients with bicuspid aortic valves. *Supravalvar aortic stenosis* (SVAS) is a rare form of outflow obstruction characterized by varying degrees of ascending aortic root stricture. Loss-of-function mutations in the extracellular matrix protein, elastin, are responsible for smooth muscle hypertrophy in SVAS, which is a generalized arteriopathy most commonly affecting the sinotubular junction of the ascending aorta but also affecting the pulmonary and other systemic arteries. This abnormality is usually diagnosed in childhood and is often part of a syndrome with hypercalcemia and multiple skeletal, vascular, and developmental abnormalities. Nonsyndromic cases also occur in both sporadic and familial forms. Endocarditis prophylaxis is required for subvalvar or supravalvar aortic stenosis.

PULMONIC VALVE STENOSIS

Pulmonic valve stenosis is the most common cause of obstruction to right ventricular outflow and usually occurs as an isolated congenital lesion. Fusion of the pulmonary leaflets creates the pressure-overloaded state and results in right ventricular hypertrophy. Some patients develop discrete hypertrophy of the infundibulum beneath the pulmonic valve, further contributing to outflow obstruction.

Unless the valve is severely stenotic at birth, most affected persons live a normal life until adolescence or young adulthood. The development of symptoms depends on the severity of the stenosis and right ventricular function. Patients with mild-to-moderate stenosis are usually asymptomatic and rarely have complications associated with the defect. Patients with moderate-to-severe obstruction often exhibit progressive fatigue and dyspnea. If right ventricular dysfunction occurs, then symptoms and signs of right-sided ventricular heart failure may be present.

On physical examination, the patient with severe stenosis has a right ventricular lift on palpation of the precordium (see Table 7–2). The S1 sound is usually normal and is followed by an opening click that becomes louder with expiration. The P2 sound becomes softer and is delayed as the severity of the stenosis increases. The characteristic murmur of pulmonic stenosis is a systolic ejection murmur heard best at the left upper sternal border, which increases with inspiration. As with aortic stenosis, a late-peaking murmur indicates more severe stenosis. A prominent jugular venous *a* wave and right-sided S4 sound may also be present in patients with severe obstruction to right ventricular outflow.

For asymptomatic patients with mild pulmonic stenosis, therapy is limited to endocarditis prophylaxis. Patients with moderate stenosis (peak gradient >50 mm Hg) are likely to develop symptoms and require intervention over time and should be treated even in the absence of symptoms. Patients with severe obstruction (peak gradient >80 mm Hg) also require intervention. In children and adults with isolated pulmonic stenosis, percutaneous balloon valvuloplasty is a suitable therapeutic option that offers results comparable with those achieved with surgery. Balloon valvuloplasty is unlikely to relieve obstruction from significant infundibular stenosis in which case surgical repair is preferred. Repair of the valve involves separation of the fused commissures and resection of the infundibulum if significant hypertrophy is present. Valve replacement is rarely necessary.

OTHER VALVULAR DEFECTS

Ebstein's anomaly is a rare condition (0.5% of patients with congenital heart disease) characterized by apical displacement of the tricuspid valve into the right ventricle. As a result, the basal portion of the right ventricle forms part of the right atrium and leaves a small functional right ventricle. The tricuspid leaflets are often dysplastic and may partially adhere to the interventricular septum or right ventricular free wall, often with significant tricuspid regurgitation. The degree of right ventricular dysfunction depends on the size of the *functioning* right ventricle and the severity of the tricuspid regurgitation. Ebstein's anomaly frequently develops in adulthood. A patent foramen ovale or ostium secundum ASD is present in more than 50% of patients and may result in right-to-left shunt flow as right atrial pressure increases. Supraventricular arrhythmias are common in those with Ebstein's anomaly, as is ventricular pre-excitation associated with Wolff-Parkinson-White syndrome.

Diseases of the Aorta
COARCTATION OF THE AORTA

Coarctation of the aorta is a fibrotic narrowing of the aortic lumen usually located distal to the left subclavian artery in the region of the ligamentum (ductus) arteriosus. The defect is more common in men than in women (2:1) and represents 5% to 8% of all congenital heart defects. Approximately 25% to 50% of patients have an associated bicuspid aortic valve. The most common extracardiac abnormality is an aneurysm of the circle of Willis (present in 3% to 5% of patients).

Coarctation produces obstruction to left ventricular outflow and results in a rise in blood pressure in the proximal aorta and great vessels relative to the distal aorta and lower extremities. The development of left ventricular hypertrophy helps maintain normal stroke volume in the presence of increased afterload. Most cases of coarctation are diagnosed in infancy or childhood, during which a high mortality rate is observed for severe coarctation that has not been repaired. Occasional cases of mild coarctation will remain undiagnosed until adulthood, when a work-up for secondary causes of hypertension may reveal the abnormality. A coarctation should be excluded in all young patients with hypertension. If the condition is left untreated, then more than two thirds of patients will develop left ventricular dysfunction and congestive heart failure by the fourth decade of life. Other complications include aortic dissection or rupture, stroke secondary to chronic hypertension, or spontaneous rupture of cerebral aneurysms. As such, patients with coarctation can be considered to have a generalized arteriopathy. Endocarditis involving the coarctation or the associated bicuspid aortic valve is a dangerous complication.

Clinically, most patients with coarctation have upper extremity hypertension with forceful carotid and upper

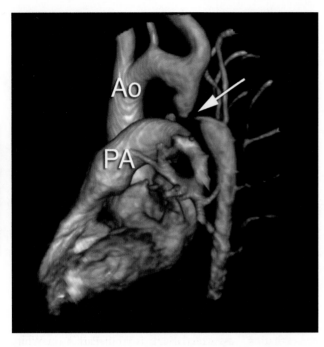

Figure 7–2 Three-dimensional reconstruction of cardiac magnetic resonance image (MRI) from a patient with uncorrected coarctation of the aorta. The coarctation *(arrow)* of the descending thoracic aorta *(Ao)* occurs in close proximity to the pulmonary artery *(PA)* in the expected location of the ligamentum arteriosus. Prominent intercostal arterial collaterals are observed.

extremity pulses (Fig. 7–2, see also Table 7–2). The pulses in the lower extremities are typically weak and delayed relative to the carotid upstroke. An ejection-quality murmur may be heard if a bicuspid aortic valve is present. A systolic murmur originating from the coarctation is typically heard over the left upper back. Older adults may have findings of heart failure.

The diagnosis of coarctation may be made by two-dimensional and Doppler echocardiography. Echocardiography may be the only study required for diagnosis in infants and children. However, in adults, magnetic resonance imaging and cardiac catheterization are the preferred methods for defining the location of the coarctation and the anatomy of the arch vessels. Surgical repair in adults is recommended at the time of diagnosis, although only approximately 50% of patients become normotensive after the procedure. Restenosis of the aorta may occur postoperatively, although in many instances this recurrent stenosis may be dilated using percutaneous techniques. A new or unusual headache in a patient with coarctation should prompt an evaluation for berry aneurysms. Endocarditis prophylaxis is recommended for the remainder of the patient's life, regardless of prior repair.

PATENT DUCTUS ARTERIOSUS

The ductus arteriosus functionally closes several hours after birth and anatomically closes within 4 to 8 weeks thereafter. PDA is more common in infants who are premature or who are born at a high altitude. PDA is also more common in women than in men, and it may be associated with other cardiac abnormalities such as coarctation and VSD.

A persistent communication between the aorta and pulmonary artery is the result of the failure of the ductus arteriosus to close. The hemodynamic consequences of this communication depend on the size of the ductus. If the defect is small, then pulmonary artery resistance remains normal and blood flows from left-to-right from the aorta to the pulmonary circulation. Most patients with small PDAs are asymptomatic and survive into adulthood without developing significant hemodynamic complications. When the ductus is large, blood flow through the pulmonary circulation and returning to the left side of the heart is significantly increased, resulting in left ventricular volume overload and pulmonary congestion (see Fig. 7–1). Persistence of a large PDA may result in elevated pulmonary vascular resistance with Eisenmenger physiologic symptoms. When pulmonary vascular resistance exceeds systemic vascular resistance, shunt flow reverses and passes from right to left. Such patients have cyanosis of the lower extremities with clubbing of the toes, whereas the upper extremities are usually normal in color without evidence of clubbing of the fingers. This differential cyanosis is secondary to shunting of poorly oxygenated blood from the pulmonary artery to the aorta distal to the left subclavian artery, whereas well-oxygenated blood from the left ventricle is supplied to the head and upper limbs. The increased volume and pressure load on the right ventricle can precipitate right-sided ventricular heart failure.

The characteristic physical examination finding of uncomplicated PDA is a loud, continuous, machinery-like murmur best heard in the left infraclavicular region (see Table 7–2). If the PDA is small, then the peripheral pulses remain normal. A hemodynamically significant PDA also has a continuous murmur, but it is typically associated with bounding pulses and a wide pulse pressure. The left ventricle may be enlarged, and signs of pulmonary congestion may be present. An Eisenmenger PDA is characterized by the loss of the continuous murmur, signs of pulmonary hypertension, and differential cyanosis and clubbing.

The diagnosis of PDA is usually confirmed with two-dimensional and Doppler echocardiography, at which time the size of the shunt and the pulmonary pressures can be estimated. Oximetry should be performed on both fingers and toes. Cardiac catheterization is usually performed at the same time as percutaneous closure for further confirmation. Evidence for reversibility of pulmonary hypertension at cardiac catheterization is reassuring. Closure of the PDA is indicated in all cases except in those patients with silent PDAs, found only by a screening examination and without audible murmur, and in those individuals with large PDAs associated with severe, irreversible pulmonary vascular disease.

Percutaneous device closure is the preferred intervention in most centers, particularly if calcification of the duct is present. Surgery is reserved for the PDA that is too large for percutaneous closure or with distorted anatomy such as a ductal aneurysm or after endarteritis. Surgical complications include recurrent laryngeal or phrenic nerve injury and thoracic duct damage. All patients with known PDA should receive endocarditis prophylaxis.

Cyanotic and Other Complex Conditions

TETRALOGY OF FALLOT

Tetralogy of Fallot is the most common cyanotic congenital heart lesion in adults and represents 10% of all congenital heart defects. It may be exhibited to the physician before or, more commonly, after corrective or palliative surgery (see Table 7–2). Tetralogy is the result of a malalignment of the aorticopulmonary septum that divides the truncus arteriosus into the aorta and pulmonary artery during development, resulting in deviation of the aorta anteriorly toward the pulmonary artery. The four components of tetralogy are the following: (1) overriding of the aorta in relation to the ventricular septum; (2) right ventricular outflow obstruction, which may be valvular, subvalvular, supravalvular, or a combination of all three; (3) membranous VSD; and (4) right ventricular hypertrophy. The VSD is usually large and allows free communication between the right and left ventricles. The presence of right ventricular outflow obstruction is protective, preventing volume and pressure overload of the pulmonary circulation, which would result in fixed pulmonary hypertension. The degree of right-to-left shunt flow depends on the degree of right ventricular outflow obstruction. If pulmonic stenosis is mild, then right-to-left shunt flow is minimal, and the patient remains acyanotic (pink tetralogy). More commonly, the pulmonic stenosis is severe, and a large volume of poorly oxygenated blood is shunted into the systemic circulation with resulting cyanosis. The degree of cyanosis is worsened with exercise, when the fall in systemic vascular resistance increases the degree of right-to-left shunt flow. Tetralogy may also be associated with ASD, muscular VSD, right aortic arch, and other coronary anomalies. A chromosomal deletion (22q11) is found in 15% of cases, particularly in those with associated anomalies. Such a deletion implies a higher risk of transmission of congenital heart disease to offspring.

Surgical correction of tetralogy is usually performed during infancy or childhood and involves relief of right ventricular obstruction and patch closure of the VSD. After reparative surgery, patients are at risk for residual pulmonary stenosis or regurgitation, which may lead to right ventricular enlargement and dysfunction and tricuspid regurgitation. Aortic insufficiency is common after repair and may become clinically significant. Residual VSDs, aneurysms of the right ventricular outflow tract, and sustained arrhythmias are also recognized complications. Arrhythmias may be supraventricular or ventricular, may signify hemodynamic impairment, and may contribute to an increased risk of sudden death. Prolongation of the QRS duration (to >180 ms) on the surface electrocardiographic (ECG) study is a marker for increased risk of ventricular tachycardia and sudden death.

Palliative surgery may have been performed in childhood to improve pulmonary blood flow. Occasionally, patients may elect not to undergo complete repair. Such palliation involves the creation of a shunt between the systemic and pulmonary circulation (e.g., subclavian artery to ipsilateral pulmonary artery [Blalock-Taussig shunt]), which results in increased pulmonary blood flow and improved oxygenation of the systemic blood. A variety of palliative shunts have been used for this purpose. Although such procedures often result in long-term palliation of hypoxia, several complications can occur. Patients may outgrow their shunts, or the shunts may spontaneously close and may lead to progressive cyanosis. If the shunt is too large, then the increased volume of blood into the pulmonary circulation and left heart may result in pulmonary congestion and progress to irreversible pulmonary vascular obstruction. In patients surviving to adulthood, corrective surgery should still be undertaken, but the operative risk is higher secondary to the presence of right ventricular dysfunction.

All patients with tetralogy, even if the condition has been surgically corrected, should receive endocarditis prophylaxis.

COMPLETE TRANSPOSITION OF THE GREAT ARTERIES

Complete transposition (also known as D-transposition) represents 5% to 7% of congenital heart disease and is the most common cyanotic congenital heart disease in the newborn. It is characterized by abnormal ventriculoarterial connections with the aorta arising from the right ventricle and the pulmonary artery arising from the left. The circulation is thus two circuits in parallel. This anatomy can support fetal development, but serious consequences result on closure of the foramen ovale and ductus arteriosus shortly after birth, at which point the systemic and pulmonary circuits are separated and oxygenated blood no longer mixes with the systemic circulation. Uncorrected D-transposition has a 90% mortality rate in the first year of life. Associated defects include VSD, left ventricular outflow tract (subpulmonic) stenosis, and coarctation of the aorta.

The first successful palliative procedure for D-transposition was the atrial switch procedure (e.g., Mustard or Senning procedures) in which the venous return is baffled to the contralateral ventricle to achieve two circuits in series. These procedures result in excellent short- and mid-term outcomes. Complications include failure of the systemic right ventricle, tricuspid regurgitation, sinus node dysfunction, tachyarrhythmias, and baffle leaks or obstruction. Progressive ventricular failure should prompt consideration of heart transplantation.

In the 1980s, the arterial switch procedure supplanted the Mustard and Senning procedures. This technically challenging procedure restores normal anatomy by attaching the aorta to the left ventricle and the pulmonary artery to the right ventricle with reimplantation of the coronary arteries into the neo-aorta. Few patients with the arterial switch procedure have yet to become adults, but similar favorable mid-term outcomes have been noted, relative to the Mustard and Senning procedures.

CORRECTED TRANSPOSITION OF THE GREAT ARTERIES

Inversion of the ventricles and abnormal positioning of the great arteries characterize congenital-corrected transposition of the great arteries (L-transposition). In this anomaly, the anatomic right ventricle lies on the left and receives oxygenated blood from the left atrium. Blood is ejected into an anteriorly displaced aorta. The anatomic left ventricle lies on the right and receives venous blood from the right atrium and ejects it into the posteriorly displaced pulmonary artery. This condition is not generally cyanotic and is quite uncommon, representing 0.5% of those with congenital heart disease.

The clinical course of patients with corrected transposition depends on the severity of other intracardiac anomalies. When the abnormality is an isolated lesion, many individuals survive into adulthood without symptoms. In some persons, the systemic ventricle (anatomic right ventricle) may fail, and pulmonary congestion may result. Associated anomalies include atrioventricular nodal block, VSD, and Ebstein's anomaly.

SINGLE VENTRICLE AND FONTAN OPERATION

A variety of anatomic defects can functionally result in a single ventricle supporting both the pulmonary and systemic circulation. As such, tricuspid atresia, double-inlet left ventricle with VSD, and large atrioventricular septal defect (among others) may all have similar consequences to the patient. The cardiac output is directed in common to both the aorta and the pulmonary artery, with the balance between the two circulatory beds determined by the degree of outflow tract obstruction. If outflow obstruction is equal, then the lower pulmonary vascular resistance will tend to favor pulmonary flow, thus the ideal single ventricle will have some degree of pulmonary outflow obstruction to prevent the development of fixed pulmonary hypertension. Patients with univentricular hearts who are not repaired have a poor prognosis, with a median survival of 14 years of age. Most patients have cyanosis and functional limitations and would benefit from palliative surgery.

The goal with palliation is to optimize pulmonary blood flow without volume loading the ventricle. In suitable patients, the Fontan procedure can offer improved functional status and relieve cyanosis. The Fontan procedure and its modifications connect all systemic venous return to the pulmonary artery without an intervening ventricular pump. This can be accomplished by anastomosis of the right atrium to the pulmonary arteries, separate connections between the superior vena cava and the adjacent right pulmonary artery, and the inferior vena cava through a graft to the left pulmonary artery or a tunnel connecting the vena cava and anastomosed to the pulmonary artery. The Fontan procedure separates the two circulations and provides relief of cyanosis without providing a volume load on the left ventricle or a pressure load on the pulmonary arteries. Complications include thrombosis, obstruction, or leaks in the Fontan circuit, ventricular dysfunction, arrhythmias, hepatic dysfunction, and protein-losing enteropathy. Patients with poor ventricular function or intractable protein-losing enteropathy after the Fontan procedure should be considered for transplantation.

EISENMENGER SYNDROME

In 1897, Victor Eisenmenger first described the clinical and pathologic features of a patient with fixed pulmonary hypertension resulting from a large VSD. In 1958, Paul Wood used the term *Eisenmenger complex* to describe the combination of a large VSD with systemic pulmonary pressures and a reversed or bidirectional shunt. The same pulmonary pathologic condition can result from a large shunt at any level, and the term *Eisenmenger syndrome* was suggested to describe pulmonary hypertension with reversed or bidirectional shunting at any level. Thus a VSD, a PDA, or an ASD could all result in Eisenmenger physiologic characteristics. The defect size generally exceeds 1.5 cm in diameter for VSD, with approximately one half that diameter for PDA and twice that diameter for ASD. Large surgical shunts can also lead to Eisenmenger syndrome.

Most patients with Eisenmenger syndrome survive to adulthood, with complications generally occurring from the third decade onward. The prognosis is better than that for patients with other causes of pulmonary hypertension such as primary pulmonary hypertension.

Complications include hyperviscosity syndrome, hemorrhage or thrombosis, arrhythmias and sudden death, endocarditis and cerebral abscess, ventricular dysfunction, hyperuricemia and gout, and renal impairment, among others. Hyperviscosity syndrome results from excessive erythrocytosis driven by increased erythropoietin in response to chronic hypoxia. Symptoms include headache, myalgias, and altered mentation. Many patients can tolerate a high hematocrit level with mild or no symptoms, and phlebotomy should not be undertaken simply in response to the hematocrit level. Excessive phlebotomy can lead to iron deficiency. Iron-deficient erythrocytes are less distensible and result in higher blood viscosity for any given hematocrit level, with microcytosis being the strongest independent predictor for cerebrovascular events.

Patients with Eisenmenger syndrome have achieved a delicate balance, and management of such patients should respect that balance. Prevention of complications is the preferred strategy. Influenza inoculations, endocarditis prophylaxis, and an avoidance of inappropriate phlebotomy are the mainstays of management. Extreme caution should be exercised with noncardiac surgery to avoid precipitous changes in vascular resistance that may lead to cardiovascular collapse. Sterilization is preferred because oral contraceptives can aggravate the risk of thrombosis. Specialized care is usually required with pregnancy, considering the high risk to both the mother and the fetus.

Other Conditions

Congenital anomalies of the coronary arteries are not uncommon and may be asymptomatic or associated with myocardial ischemia. The left circumflex or left anterior descending artery may arise from the right sinus of Valsalva and is usually not associated with abnormalities of myocardial perfusion. Either coronary artery may arise from the right sinus and may pass between the pulmonary trunk and aorta. This abnormality may result in myocardial ischemia, infarction, or sudden death in young adults, especially during exertion. Coronary artery fistulas with drainage into the right ventricle, vena cava, or pulmonary vein may be associated with myocardial ischemia if a significant amount of coronary blood flow is shunted into the venous system. Diagnosis of these abnormalities is made by coronary angiography.

Prospectus for the Future

The growing population of patients with successful outcomes after intervention for congenital heart disease is posing new challenges during adulthood. The increasing prevalence of genetic studies must be linked to genetic counseling. Early prenatal diagnoses that are linked to specific molecular defects will engender therapeutic strategies *in utero*. Genetic epidemiologic studies will provide important insights about the influences of the *in utero* environment on the subsequent susceptibility and risk factors for heart disease during adulthood.

References

Deanfield J, Thaulow E, Warnes C, et al: Management of grown up congenital heart disease, Eur Heart J 24:1035, 2003.

Gatzoulis MA, Webb GD, Daubeney PEF: Diagnosis and Management of Adult Congenital Heart Disease, Philadelphia: Elsevier, 2003.

Therrien J, Dore A, Gersony W, et al: Canadian Cardiovascular Society Consensus Conference 2001 update: Recommendations for the management of adults with congenital heart disease—Part I. Can J Cardiol 17:940, 2001.

Therrien J, Gatzoulis M, Graham T, et al: Canadian Cardiovascular Society Consensus Conference 2001 update: Recommendations for the management of adults with congenital heart disease—Part II. Can J Cardiol 17:1029, 2001.

Therrien J, Warnes C, Daliento L, et al: Canadian Cardiovascular Society Consensus Conference 2001 update: Recommendations for the management of adults with congenital heart disease—Part III. Can J Cardiol 17:1135, 2001.

Webb GD, Williams RG: Care of the adult with congenital heart disease, J Am Coll Cardiol 37: 1166, 2001.

Chapter 8

Acquired Valvular Heart Disease

Sheldon E. Litwin

Aortic Stenosis

Aortic stenosis can be congenital or acquired in origin (Table 8–1). The most common congenital cardiac abnormality affects the bicuspid aortic valve. Significant narrowing of the orifice usually occurs during middle age after years of turbulent flow through the valve results in leaflet injury, thickening, and calcification. Rheumatic aortic stenosis results from fusion of the leaflet commissures and is usually associated with mitral valve disease. The most common cause of aortic stenosis in adults is degenerative or senile aortic stenosis, which usually occurs in patients older than the age of 65 years. Aortic stenosis is more common in men than it is in women.

In patients with aortic stenosis, the outflow obstruction gradually increases over many years, resulting in left ventricular hypertrophy. This response allows the left ventricle to generate and maintain a large pressure gradient across the valve without a reduction in stroke volume. However, left ventricular hypertrophy often results in increased diastolic chamber stiffness because greater intracavitary pressure is required to maintain left ventricular filling. Systolic dysfunction may also occur as a result of changes in expression of myocyte contractile and calcium-cycling proteins.

Patients with severe aortic stenosis may be asymptomatic for many years despite the presence of severe obstruction. The cardinal symptoms associated with aortic stenosis are angina, syncope, and congestive heart failure. Angina can occur in the absence of epicardial coronary artery disease because of the increased oxygen demand of the hypertrophied ventricle and decreased coronary blood flow secondary to elevated left ventricular diastolic pressure. Syncope may result from transient arrhythmias but more commonly occurs with exertion when cardiac output is insufficient to maintain arterial pressure in the presence of exercise-induced peripheral vasodilation. Dyspnea may result from increased filling pressures associated with the noncompliant, hypertrophied left ventricle or may signal the onset of systolic dysfunction. Once patients with severe

aortic stenosis develop symptoms, the prognosis is poor unless surgical correction is undertaken. Previous studies have shown that the mean survival rate after the onset of symptoms is approximately 2 years in patients with heart failure, 3 years in patients with syncope, and 5 years in patients with angina (Fig. 8–1).

On physical examination, the patient with aortic stenosis may have a laterally displaced, sustained apical impulse secondary to left ventricular hypertrophy (Table 8–2). An audible or palpable S_4 may also be present if the patient is in sinus rhythm. Decreased mobility of the aortic cusps may cause the A_2 component of S_2 to be soft or absent. The murmur of aortic stenosis is a harsh, crescendo-decrescendo murmur that is best heard over the right upper sternal border and often radiates to the neck. As the obstruction increases, the *peak* of the murmur occurs later in systole. If left ventricular dysfunction develops, then the murmur may decrease in intensity secondary to a reduction in stroke volume. The carotid impulse is often diminished in intensity and delayed (i.e., *pulsus parvus et tardus*) (see Chapter 4), although in older adults these changes may be present secondary to intrinsic vascular disease in the absence of significant aortic stenosis.

The principal electrocardiographic finding in aortic stenosis is left ventricular hypertrophy. Heart block may develop as a result of calcification from the aortic valve extending into the conducting system. Echocardiography is the most important diagnostic test and is useful to determine the cause of the aortic stenosis and to quantitate the degree of obstruction. The mean transvalvular gradient and valve area can be measured and calculated using Doppler techniques. Patients with severe stenosis will often undergo cardiac catheterization both to confirm the presence of severe aortic stenosis and to determine whether concomitant coronary artery disease is present. A valve area less than or equal to $0.7\,cm^2$ defines critical aortic stenosis (normal valve area is $3\,cm^2$) and is usually associated with a mean transvalvular gradient of more than $50\,mm\,Hg$ when normal left ventricular function is present. It should be noted that in

Table 8–1 Major Causes of Valvular Heart Disease in Adults

Aortic Stenosis

Bicuspid aortic valve
Rheumatic fever
Degenerative stenosis

Aortic Regurgitation

Bicuspid aortic valve
Aortic dissection
Endocarditis
Rheumatic fever
Aortic root dilation

Mitral Stenosis

Rheumatic fever

Mitral Regurgitation

Chronic

Mitral valve prolapse
Left ventricular dilation
Posterior wall myocardial infarction
Rheumatic fever
Endocarditis

Acute

Posterior wall or papillary muscle ischemia
Papillary muscle or chordal rupture
Endocarditis
Prosthetic valve dysfunction

Tricuspid Regurgitation

Functional (annular) dilation
Tricuspid valve prolapse
Endocarditis

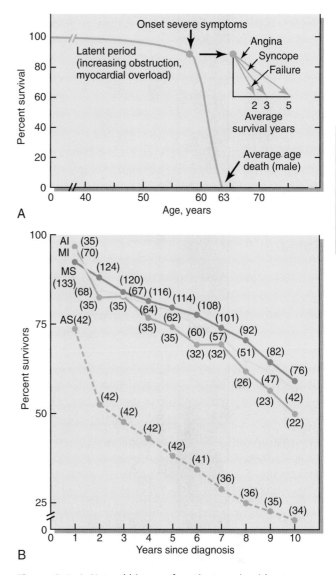

Figure 8–1 *A,* Natural history of aortic stenosis without surgical therapy. *B,* Natural history of mitral and aortic valve disease in an era when surgical therapy was not widely available. Survival rates in 42 patients with aortic stenosis *(AS, orange circles with dotted line)*, 35 patients with aortic insufficiency *(AI, orange circles with solid line)*, and 133 patients with mitral insufficiency *(MI, yellow circles with solid line)*. Clinical course in AI, MS *(red circles with dotted line)*, and MI is similar with a 5-year survival rate of ~80% and a 10-year survival rate of ~60%. Patients with AS have a worse prognosis with 5- and 10-year survival rates of ~40 and 20%, respectively. (Part *A* from Ross J Jr, Braunwald E: Aortic stenosis. Circulation 38[Suppl V]:61, 1968. Copyright © 1968 American Heart Association. Part *B* from Rapaport E: Natural history of aortic and mitral valve disease, Am J Cardiol 35:221–227, 1975.)

patients with reduced systolic function, the mean gradient might be low despite the presence of severe aortic stenosis. Moreover, symptoms are often present with valve areas of 0.7 to 1.0 cm^2.

Treatment in most adults with symptomatic aortic stenosis is surgical replacement of the valve. The operative risk and prognosis are best in patients with preserved left ventricular systolic function. However, surgery should still be considered in patients with left ventricular dysfunction because relief of the obstruction can result in significant clinical and hemodynamic improvement. Advanced age is associated with higher operative morbidity but is not a contraindication to surgical therapy. Balloon aortic valvuloplasty is a percutaneous technique in which a balloon

catheter is positioned across the aortic valve. Inflation results in fracture and/or separation of the fused and calcified cusps. This procedure is most effective in young patients with noncalcified congenital aortic stenosis and is rarely used in adult patients with calcific aortic stenosis because of significant complications and a high restenosis rate (~30% at 6 months).

Table 8-2   Characteristic Physical, Electrocardiographic, and Chest Radiographic Findings in Chronic Acquired Valvular Heart Disease

Physical Findings*		Electrocardiogram	Radiograph
Aortic stenosis	Pulsus parvus et tardus (may be absent in older patients or in patients with associated aortic regurgitation); carotid *shudder* (coarse thrill) Ejection murmur radiates to base of neck; peaks late in systole if stenosis is severe Sustained but not significantly displaced LV impulse A_2 decreased, S_2 single or paradoxically split S_4 gallop, often palpable	LV hypertrophy Left bundle branch block is also common Rare heart block from calcific involvement of conduction system	LV prominence without dilation Post-stenotic aortic root dilation Aortic valve calcification
Aortic regurgitation	Increased pulse pressure Bifid carotid pulses Rapid pulse upstroke and collapse LV impulse hyperdynamic and displaced laterally Diastolic decrescendo murmur; duration related to severity Systolic flow murmur S_{3G} common	LV hypertrophy, often with narrow deep Q waves	LV and aortic dilation
Mitral stenosis	Loud S_1 OS S_2–OS interval inversely related to stenosis severity S_1 not loud, and OS absent if valve heavily calcified Signs of pulmonary arterial hypertension	Left atrial abnormality Atrial fibrillation common RV hypertrophy pattern may develop if associated pulmonary arterial hypertension is present	Large LA: double-density, posterior displacement of esophagus, elevation of left main stem bronchus Straightening of left heart border as a result of enlarged left appendage Small or normal-sized LV Large pulmonary artery Pulmonary venous congestion

	Physical findings	ECG	Chest radiograph
Mitral regurgitation	Hyperdynamic LV impulse S₃ Widely split S₂ may occur Holosystolic apical murmur radiating to axilla (murmur may be atypical with acute mitral regurgitation, papillary muscle dysfunction, or mitral valve prolapse)	Left atrial abnormality LV hypertrophy Atrial fibrillation	Enlarged LA and LV Pulmonary venous congestion
Mitral valve prolapse	One or more systolic clicks, often midsystolic, followed by late systolic murmur Auscultatory findings dynamic Symptoms may include tall thin habitus, pectus excavatum, straight back syndrome	Often normal Occasionally ST segment depression and/or T wave changes in inferior leads	Depends on degree of valve regurgitation and presence or absence of those abnormalities
Tricuspid stenosis	Jugular venous distention with prominent α wave if sinus rhythm Tricuspid OS and diastolic rumble at left sternal border; may be overshadowed by concomitant mitral stenosis Tricuspid OS and rumble increased during inspiration	Right atrial abnormality Atrial fibrillation common	Large RA
Tricuspid regurgitation	Jugular venous distention with large regurgitant (systolic) wave Systolic murmur at left sternal border, increased with inspiration Diastolic flow rumble RV S₃ increased with inspiration Hepatomegaly with systolic pulsation	RA abnormality; findings are often related to cause of the tricuspid regurgitation	RA and RV are enlarged; findings are often related to cause of the tricuspid regurgitation

*Findings are influenced by the severity and chronicity of the valve disorder.
ECG = electrocardiogram; LA = left atrium; LV = left ventricle; OS = opening snap; RA = right atrium; RV = right ventricle.

Aortic Regurgitation

Aortic regurgitation (AR) may be secondary to primary disease of the aortic leaflets, aortic root, or both (see Table 8–1). Abnormalities of the aortic leaflets may be secondary to rheumatic disease, congenital abnormalities, endocarditis, or use of certain anorexigenic drugs. In addition, AR is commonly a consequence of degenerative and bicuspid aortic stenosis. An aortic root pathologic condition associated with annular and root dilation may result in separation and/or prolapse of the leaflets.

With chronic AR, the left ventricle must accommodate the normal inflow from the left atrium in addition to the aortic regurgitant volume. As a result, the left ventricle dilates and hypertrophies to maintain normal effective forward flow and to minimize wall stress. As the AR progresses, these changes in left ventricular size and wall thickness may be insufficient to maintain normal left ventricular filling pressures, and irreversible myocyte damage may occur. As a result, the left ventricle will dilate further and systolic function and effective stroke volume will decrease.

Clinically, patients with chronic, severe AR may be asymptomatic for long periods secondary to the compensatory changes in the left ventricle. When symptoms do develop, they are primarily related to an elevation in left ventricular filling pressures and include dyspnea on exertion, orthopnea, and paroxysmal nocturnal dyspnea. Many patients will describe chest or head pounding secondary to the hyperdynamic circulation. If effective cardiac output is reduced, then the patient may complain primarily of fatigue and weakness. As with aortic stenosis, angina may occur in patients with AR even in the absence of epicardial coronary artery disease secondary to elevated left ventricular filling pressures and reduced coronary perfusion pressure.

On physical examination, patients with severe AR have a widened pulse pressure (difference between the systolic and diastolic pressures) as a result of the runoff of blood back into the left ventricle (see Table 8–2). The arterial pulse is usually bounding, with a rapid upstroke and quick collapse (Corrigan's disease or water-hammer pulse) (see Chapter 4). The cardiac impulse is hyperdynamic and is displaced laterally and inferiorly. The murmur of AR is a high-pitched, decrescendo diastolic murmur best heard at the lower left sternal border with the patient sitting up and leaning forward. Asking the patient to hold his or her breath at end expiration while the hands are held behind the head may also improve the ability to auscultate the murmur of AR. A systolic ejection murmur is often heard secondary to increased forward flow across the aortic valve. An S_3 gallop may be present, especially if the patient has developed symptoms of heart failure. A low-pitched, diastolic murmur (Austin Flint murmur) may be heard at the apex and confused with the murmur of mitral stenosis (MS). This sound is thought to be secondary to the incomplete opening of the mitral leaflets (functional MS) secondary to elevated left ventricular filling pressures or impingement of the AR jet on the anterior mitral leaflet.

The natural history of chronic AR is varied. Many patients with moderate-to-severe AR will remain asymptomatic for many years and generally have a favorable prognosis. Other patients may have progression of AR severity and develop left ventricular dysfunction and symptoms of congestive heart failure. Echocardiography is the primary tool to monitor the progression of disease and optimize the timing of surgery. Prior studies have shown that patients at high risk are those with left ventricular end-systolic diameters greater than 50 mm or an ejection fraction of less than 50%. Surgery is usually recommended before developing this degree of left ventricular enlargement or dysfunction. Therefore patients with known moderate-to-severe AR should be monitored regularly with noninvasive testing to detect early signs of cardiac (i.e., left ventricular) decompensation.

Treatment of patients with moderate-to-severe AR theoretically should include vasodilator therapy, such as nifedipine or angiotensin-converting enzyme (ACE) inhibitors, because these agents unload the left ventricle. Although some published data suggest that these agents may slow the progression of myocardial dysfunction and delay the need for surgery, more recent data do not support that contention.

Valve replacement surgery should be considered in symptomatic patients and those with evidence of significant left ventricular enlargement or left ventricular systolic dysfunction. In patients with reduced left ventricular ejection fraction of short duration (14 months), valve replacement usually results in significant improvement in ventricular function. If left ventricular dysfunction has been present for a prolonged period, then permanent myocardial damage may occur. Although such patients should not be excluded from surgery, their long-term prognosis remains poor.

As compared with chronic AR, acute AR is a medical emergency that often requires immediate surgical intervention. The causes of acute AR include infective endocarditis, traumatic rupture of the aortic leaflets, aortic root dissection, and acute dysfunction of a prosthetic valve. Acute AR is the result of hemodynamic instability because the left ventricle is unable to dilate to accommodate the increased diastolic volume, resulting in decreased effective forward flow. Left ventricular and left atrial pressures rise quickly, leading to pulmonary congestion.

Patients with acute AR often exhibit symptoms and signs of cardiogenic shock. The patient is usually pale with cool extremities as a result of peripheral vasoconstriction. The pulse is weak and rapid, and the pulse pressure is normal or decreased. The murmur of acute AR is low pitched and short because of rapid equilibration of aortic and left ventricular pressures during diastole. An S_3 gallop is often present. Echocardiography is useful to assess AR severity and to determine its cause and can be quickly performed at the bedside in the patient who is acutely ill.

The medical treatment of acute AR includes vasodilator therapy and diuretics if the blood pressure is stable. In patients who are hemodynamically compromised, inotropic support and vasopressors may be necessary. For most patients with acute AR, urgent valve replacement remains the treatment of choice. Intra-aortic balloon counterpulsation is relatively contraindicated because it may worsen AR severity.

Mitral Stenosis

MS occurs when thickening and immobility of the mitral leaflets impede flow from the left atrium to the left ventricle. Rheumatic fever is by far the most common cause of MS.

Rarely, congenital abnormalities, connective tissue disorders, left atrial tumors, and overly aggressive surgical repair of a regurgitant valve may lead to obstruction of the mitral valve. Two thirds of patients with MS are women. The pathologic changes that occur with rheumatic MS include fusion of the leaflet commissures and thickening, fibrosis, and calcification of the mitral leaflets and chordae. These changes occur over many years before dysfunction becomes hemodynamically important.

The initial hemodynamic change that occurs with MS is an elevated left atrial pressure created by obstruction to left ventricular inflow (Fig. 8–2). This pressure change is transmitted back to the pulmonary venous system and may result in pulmonary congestion. Initially, this change may only occur at more rapid heart rates, such as with exercise or atrial arrhythmias, when higher left atrial pressures develop during the shortened diastolic period. As the MS becomes more severe, left atrial pressure remains elevated even at normal heart rates, and symptoms related to elevated pulmonary venous pressures may be present at rest. Chronic elevations in pulmonary venous pressures may lead to an increase in pulmonary vascular resistance and pulmonary arterial pressures. If the MS is not corrected, then irreversible changes in the pulmonary vasculature may occur, and signs and symptoms of right ventricular heart failure may develop. In contrast, left ventricular filling pressures are usually normal or low with mild-to-moderate MS. As the stenosis becomes severe, filling of the left ventricle is impaired and stroke volume and cardiac output are reduced.

Patients with MS of rheumatic origins usually become symptomatic during the third or fourth decade of life. Dyspnea, orthopnea, and atrial fibrillation are the most common symptoms. Some patients may have sudden hemoptysis secondary to rupture of the dilated bronchial veins (pulmonary apoplexy) or blood-tinged sputum associated with pulmonary edema. Peripheral embolism from left atrial thrombus may also occur even in the absence of atrial fibrillation. In long-standing, severe MS, patients may develop peripheral edema secondary to elevated right ventricular pressures and right ventricular dysfunction. Compression of the left recurrent laryngeal nerve from a severely dilated left atrium may result in hoarseness (Ortner's syndrome).

On physical examination, S_1 is loud early in the course of MS because the leaflets remain fully open throughout diastole and then quickly close (see Table 8–2). As the leaflets become more calcified and immobile, S_1 will become softer or completely absent. The opening snap is a high-pitched sound after the S_2 and reflects the abrupt mitral valve opening. As the MS becomes more severe, the interval between the S_2 and opening snap becomes shorter because left atrial pressure exceeds left ventricular pressure earlier in diastole. The characteristic low-pitched rumbling murmur of MS is best heard at the left ventricular apex with the patient in the left lateral decubitus position. The murmur is loudest in early diastole when rapid ventricular filling occurs. If sinus rhythm is present, then the murmur may increase in intensity after atrial contraction (presystolic accentuation). In some patients the murmur may only be heard at times of increased blood flow through the mitral valve, such as after exercise. If pulmonary artery pressures are elevated, then a palpable P_2 may be detected at the upper left sternal border. On auscultation, the pulmonic component of S_2 is prominent and a right ventricular gallop may be present.

Echocardiography is the most useful tool for pathologic assessment of the mitral apparatus, as well as the severity of the stenosis. The characteristic rheumatic deformity observed with two-dimensional imaging is doming (i.e., *hockey stick* deformity) of the anterior mitral valve leaflet, which is secondary to fusion of the commissures and tethering of the leaflet tips (Fig. 8–3). In addition, the mobility of the leaflets and the extent of valvular calcification can be assessed and used to determine treatment options. Doppler techniques allow calculation of the mitral valve area and the transvalvular gradient. Transesophageal echocardiography is a useful tool for studying the mitral apparatus and examining the left atrium for thrombus before percutaneous valvuloplasty.

The severity of MS and associated hemodynamic changes can also be evaluated with cardiac catheterization. Measurements of the cardiac output and transvalvular gradient can be used to calculate the valve area by means of the Gorlin formula. A normal mitral valve area is 4 to 6 cm², and critical MS is defined as a valve area less than 1 cm².

Patients with mild-to-moderate MS can usually be managed medically. Heart rate control is imperative in these patients because more rapid rates reduce the length of the diastolic filling period. This is especially true in patients with atrial fibrillation, in whom loss of atrial contraction may further reduce left ventricular filling. Anticoagulant therapy is indicated for patients with atrial fibrillation and for those patients with sinus rhythm who have had prior embolic events or who have moderate-to-severe MS. Diuretics are

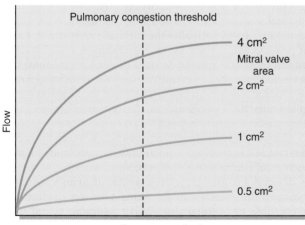

Figure 8–2 Graphic illustration of the relationship between the diastolic gradient across the mitral valve and the flow through the mitral valve. As the mitral valve becomes more stenotic, the pressure gradient across the mitral valve must increase to maintain flow into the left ventricle. When the mitral valve area is 1.0 cm² or less, the flow rate into the left ventricle cannot be significantly increased, despite a significantly elevated pressure gradient across the mitral valve. (Adapted from Wallace AG: Pathophysiology of cardiovascular disease. In Smith LH Jr, Thier SO [eds]: The International Textbook of Medicine, vol 1. WB Saunders, 1981, p 1192.)

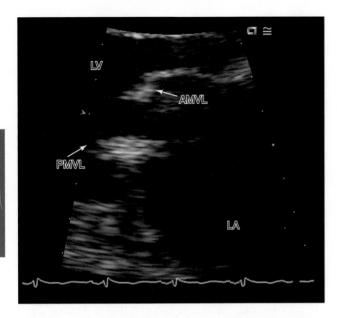

Figure 8–3 Example of *hockey stick* deformity of mitral valve in chronic rheumatic heart disease as visualized by echocardiography. Tips of anterior mitral valve leaflet (AMVL) are tethered, thus restricting opening of the valve. Posterior mitral valve leaflet (PMVL) is thickened and has reduced mobility. Left atrium (LA) is characteristically enlarged.

useful in relieving pulmonary congestion and signs of right ventricular heart failure. All patients should be instructed on the importance of endocarditis prophylaxis. Prophylaxis against recurrent bouts of rheumatic fever may be used in patients less than 30 years of age.

Patients with severe symptoms (New York Heart Association classes III through IV) and moderate-to-severe MS should be considered for a percutaneous or surgical intervention. Percutaneous balloon valvuloplasty is a new technique in which a balloon catheter positioned across the mitral valve is quickly inflated, resulting in separation of the fused cusps. Optimal short- and long-term results are obtained in patients with pliable, noncalcified leaflets and chords, minimal mitral regurgitation (MR), and no evidence of left atrial thrombus. A surgical option in this same group of patients is open mitral valve commissurotomy. With direct visualization of the mitral valve, the surgeon is able to débride the valve, separate the fused cusps, and remove left atrial thrombi. Although the valve remains abnormal, this procedure is associated with a low operative mortality and a good hemodynamic result and may spare the patient from a valve replacement for many years. If mitral commissurotomy is not an option, then valve replacement with a bioprosthetic or mechanical prosthesis can be performed.

Mitral Regurgitation

MR can result from abnormalities of the mitral leaflets, annulus, chordae, or papillary muscles (see Table 8–1). The most common leaflet abnormality resulting in chronic MR is myxomatous degeneration of the mitral valves. This condition results in mitral valve prolapse (MVP), which progresses as the chordae become elongated or rupture

(Fig. 8–4). Both acute and chronic rheumatic fever may also cause MR.

With chronic MR, the left ventricle dilates to compensate for the increased regurgitant volume. However, in contrast to aortic insufficiency, the increased volume is ejected into the low-pressure left atrium. Thus left ventricular wall stress and pressure remain normal for a significant period. If the left atrium dilates sufficiently to accommodate the increased volume, then left atrial and pulmonary venous pressures will remain normal. As the MR progresses, myocyte damage may occur, resulting in further left ventricular dilation, an elevation in diastolic filling pressures, and a reduction in left ventricular systolic function. As left atrial and pulmonary venous pressures increase, pulmonary congestion may occur.

Patients with chronic compensated MR are usually asymptomatic and have normal functional capacity. When symptoms do occur, left ventricular systolic function is sometimes depressed. Patients may initially complain of fatigue and dyspnea with exertion secondary to reduced cardiac output and elevation in pulmonary venous pressures. If the MR remains untreated, pulmonary hypertension and right ventricular heart failure may occur.

MR characteristically produces a holosystolic murmur best heard at the apex and radiating to the axilla and back (see Table 8–2). If an eccentric, anteriorly directed jet of MR is present, then an ejection-quality murmur may be present and confused with an aortic outflow murmur. If the MR is secondary to MVP, then a midsystolic click may be present, followed by a late systolic murmur. MR associated with rheumatic mitral disease may be accompanied by heart sounds typical of MS.

Echocardiography is the primary noninvasive method for defining mitral valve pathologic evaluation and assessing left ventricular size and function. Doppler techniques are useful in grading the severity of MR. Quantitative echocardiographic measures of MR severity are predictive of long-term survival, even in patients who are asymptomatic. Mitral valve repair appears to normalize the survival curves in this group of patients. MR can also be assessed during cardiac catheterization by estimating the amount of contrast medium that is ejected into the left atrium during left ventriculography. In addition, left ventricular size and systolic function can be quantitated, filling pressures can be measured, and the coronary anatomy can be defined.

The medical treatment of patients with compensated chronic MR is afterload reduction with vasodilator therapy, such as ACE inhibitors or hydralazine. The timing of surgery is difficult because the development of symptoms often indicates the presence of left ventricular dysfunction and irreversible myocardial damage. In addition, mitral valve replacement with disruption of the chordal apparatus often results in further left ventricular dilation and decline in systolic function.

Echocardiographic parameters that identify patients at risk for a poor response to mitral valve replacement are a left ventricular end-diastolic diameter greater than 70 mm, an end-systolic diameter greater than 45 mm, and a low-normal or reduced left ventricular ejection fraction. Patients with known MR should be followed with yearly studies to monitor left ventricular function and size so that surgery can be performed *before* irreversible myocyte damage and left ventricular remodeling occur. The development of either

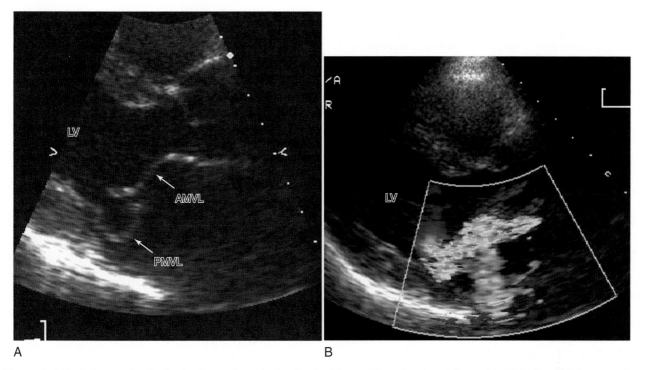

Figure 8–4 Typical example of mitral valve prolapse is visualized with transthoracic echocardiography. *A*, Prolapse of the posterior mitral valve leaflet (PMVL) behind the mitral valve annular plane results from lengthening and rupture of chordae tendineae. In this patient a highly eccentric *(blue)* jet of moderate-to-severe mitral regurgitation is observed *(B)*.

atrial fibrillation or pulmonary hypertension may be indications for earlier surgical intervention, even if left ventricle size and function are still normal.

In many patients the mitral valve may be repaired, thus avoiding many of the potential complications associated with valve replacement. With this surgery, sections of redundant leaflet can be excised, leaflets débrided, and chordae shortened. A prosthetic ring (annuloplasty) can be sewn into the mitral annulus to reduce the size of the orifice and increase the degree of leaflet coaptation. The advantage of this procedure is that preservation of the mitral apparatus helps maintain normal left ventricular geometry and function. In addition, long-term anticoagulation is not necessary in most patients in sinus rhythm. Valve repair is generally not indicated if the mitral valve is heavily calcified or disrupted secondary to papillary muscle disease or endocarditis. In these instances, valve replacement is the procedure of choice.

Based on excellent surgical outcomes and long-term durability, mitral valve repair is the procedure of choice in all patients in whom it is technically feasible. Severe MR, even in the absence of symptoms or left ventricular dysfunction, may be an appropriate reason for surgical intervention. A variety of percutaneous mitral valve repair techniques are in development.

Acute severe MR is often a life-threatening condition that can result from a variety of papillary muscle, chordal, and leaflet abnormalities (see Table 8–1). Patients with acute MR usually become severely ill because the left atrium does not dilate to accommodate the regurgitant volume. As a result, left atrial and pulmonary venous pressures abruptly increase, resulting in pulmonary congestion. In addition, the decreases in stroke volume and cardiac output result in an increase in systemic vascular resistance and, as a consequence, an

increase in the severity of MR. Patients usually exhibit pulmonary edema and signs of cardiogenic shock. On auscultation, the MR murmur is often a soft, low-pitched sound in early systole, resulting from rapid equilibration of left ventricular and left atrial pressures. Afterload reduction with either an intravenous vasodilator, such as nitroprusside, or an intra-aortic balloon pump may help stabilize the patient before urgent valve replacement surgery. Ischemia of the posterior wall and/or papillary muscles may cause acute but transient MR.

Mitral Valve Prolapse

MVP is reported to be present in approximately 1% to 3% of the population. Although MVP can be observed in all ages and in both sexes, epidemiologic studies suggest that the prevalence is greater in women than it is in men. In some patients, MVP is inherited as an autosomal dominant trait with variable penetrance.

MVP is present when superior displacement in ventricular systole of one or both mitral valve leaflets exists across the plane of the mitral annulus toward the left atrium (see Fig. 8–4). Primary or classic MVP occurs when myxomatous degeneration of the mitral valve occurs without evidence of systemic disease. Secondary MVP is also characterized by myxomatous degeneration of the mitral apparatus but in the presence of a recognizable systemic or connective tissue disease, such as Marfan syndrome or systemic lupus erythematosus. Functional MVP results from structural abnormalities of the mitral annulus or papillary muscles or reduced left ventricular volume, but the mitral leaflets are anatomically normal.

Most patients with MVP are asymptomatic. Although a variety of nonspecific symptoms have been associated with MVP (e.g. chest pain, palpitations, dizziness, anxiety [MVP syndrome]), the frequency of these symptoms is no different from the general population. MVP may be associated with varying degrees of MR. MR severity is probably the main determinant of long-term complications. The characteristic physical examination finding in MVP is the midsystolic click, followed by a late systolic murmur (see Table 8–2). The auscultatory findings of MVP are subtle and are greatly affected by changes in left ventricular volume. Maneuvers that reduce left ventricular volume will result in prolapse of the redundant leaflets early in systole; as a result, the click will occur early in systole and the MR murmur will sound more holosystolic. If left ventricular volume is increased, then the click will be heard late in systole, followed by a short systolic murmur. The diagnosis of MVP is usually confirmed by echocardiography, which allows examination of the mitral apparatus and determination of the MR severity.

Most patients with mild prolapse and insignificant MR are asymptomatic and require no specific intervention. Endocarditis prophylaxis is generally recommended only if mild or greater MR exists. However, in some individuals the MR may progress to such a degree that serial examinations and echocardiograms are necessary to monitor MR severity and left ventricular function. Middle-aged and older men and patients with asymmetric prolapse are at highest risk for developing complications from MVP, such as severe MR and endocarditis. MR that acutely worsens may be related to rupture of the chordae tendineae. Sudden death in the absence of hemodynamically significant MR is rare.

Patients with MVP and evidence of structural leaflet abnormalities and/or significant MR should receive endocarditis prophylaxis. Symptomatic arrhythmias should be treated as discussed in Chapter 10. For patients with severe MR, mitral valve repair or replacement may be indicated as discussed earlier (see "Mitral Regurgitation").

Tricuspid Stenosis

Tricuspid stenosis is most often rheumatic in origin and is usually associated with mitral and/or aortic disease. Other rare causes include carcinoid syndrome, congenital valve abnormalities, and leaflet tumors or vegetations.

Similar to MS, tricuspid stenosis is more common in women than it is in men and tends to be a slowly progressive disease. Patients generally exhibit symptoms and signs of right ventricular heart failure, such as fatigue, abdominal bloating, and peripheral edema. On physical examination, a prominent jugular venous *a* wave may be present if the patient is in sinus rhythm and may be confused with an arterial pulsation. In addition, a palpable pre-systolic pulsation coinciding with atrial contraction may be felt on palpation of the liver. On auscultation, the findings of tricuspid stenosis may not be detected secondary to the presence of mitral and aortic valve disease. However, an opening snap may be audible at the left sternal border, followed by a soft, high-pitched diastolic murmur. In contrast to MS, the murmur of tricuspid stenosis is shorter in duration and accentuated with inspiration.

Tricuspid stenosis can be diagnosed by echocardiography or right ventricular catheterization. Because the right heart is a low-pressure system, the mean gradient across the tricuspid valve may be quite small (5 mm Hg) yet still clinically important.

Tricuspid Regurgitation

Tricuspid regurgitation (TR) is most often secondary to dilation of the right ventricle and tricuspid annulus that may occur with right ventricular heart failure of any cause. Other causes include endocarditis, carcinoid syndrome, congenital abnormalities, and chest wall trauma.

In the absence of pulmonary hypertension, TR is usually well tolerated. However, if right ventricular dysfunction is present, then patients will usually have symptoms of right ventricular heart failure. On physical examination, the jugular veins are distended and a prominent *v* wave is usually present. Hepatic congestion is common and often associated with a palpable systolic pulsation. The murmur of TR is high-pitched and pansystolic and is best heard along the sternal border. Maneuvers that increase venous return, such as inspiration or leg rising, accentuate the murmur and are helpful in differentiating TR from MR or aortic outflow tract murmurs. If the TR is acute, then the murmur is usually soft and present only during early systole.

TR related to pulmonary hypertension and right ventricular dysfunction will usually significantly improve with treatment of the underlying cause. Repair of the tricuspid annulus (annuloplasty) may restore tricuspid valve competence in patients with persistent symptoms despite treatment. In individuals with a primary leaflet pathologic condition, tricuspid valve replacement may be necessary.

Pulmonic Stenosis and Regurgitation

Pulmonic stenosis is most often congenital in origin and is discussed further in Chapter 7. Rheumatic deformity of the pulmonic valve is rare and not usually associated with hemodynamically important obstruction.

Pulmonic regurgitation is most often the result of dilation of the annulus secondary to pulmonary hypertension of any cause. Symptoms are usually related to the primary disease and in most cases are secondary to right ventricular heart failure. In this setting, the murmur of pulmonic regurgitation is a high-pitched, blowing murmur best heard at the second left intercostal space (Graham Steell murmur). In the absence of pulmonary hypertension, the murmur is usually low pitched and occurs late in diastole. Treatment is usually directed at the underlying cause of the pulmonary hypertension. Rarely and usually in the setting of congenital or previously repaired pulmonic valve disease, the valve will need to be replaced because of intractable right ventricular heart failure.

Multivalvular Disease

Multivalvular disease is common, especially in patients with rheumatic heart disease and in the older adult population. Often, regurgitant lesions, such as TR and pulmonic regurgitation, are the result of another valve lesion, such as MS in association with pulmonary hypertension. In general, symptoms are most often related to the most proximal valve lesion. However, the severity of each individual lesion may be difficult to assess clinically, and therefore careful evaluation with echocardiography and right and left ventricular heart catheterization is necessary to assess valve function before any planned surgery. Failure to correct all significant valvular lesions may result in a poor clinical outcome. Double valve replacement is associated with a higher operative and long-term mortality than single valve replacement.

Rheumatic Heart Disease

Acute rheumatic fever (ARF) is the sequela of group A β-hemolytic streptococcal infection. The disease is thought to be secondary to an abnormal immunologic response to the streptococcal infection. ARF usually occurs in children 4 to 9 years of age, with boys and girls being equally affected. Although the prevalence of this disease has significantly decreased in the United States over the past several decades, it still poses a major health care problem in many developing nations, and endemic outbreaks have been identified even in the United States.

ARF is characterized by a diffuse inflammation of the heart (pancarditis). An exudative pericarditis is common and often results in fibrosis and obliteration of the pericardial sac. Constrictive pericarditis is rare. The myocardium is often infiltrated with lymphocytes, and areas of necrosis may occur. The characteristic histologic finding in the myocardium is the Aschoff body, which is a confluence of monocytes and macrophages surrounded by fibrous tissue. Valvulitis is characterized by verrucous lesions on the leaflet edge, which are composed of cellular infiltrates and fibrin. The mitral valve is most frequently involved, followed by the aortic valve. Involvement of the tricuspid or pulmonic valve is rare. Valvulitis can be recognized by the presence of a new insufficiency murmur. Aortic stenosis and MS do not occur for many years, when progression of the fibrosis results in restricted leaflet mobility.

The presentation of ARF is usually an acute, febrile illness 2 to 4 weeks after a streptococcal pharyngitis infection. Because the diagnosis of ARF cannot be made by laboratory tests alone, guidelines based on the symptoms and a physical examination have been established (modified Jones criteria) (Table 8–3). A diagnosis of ARF can be made if two major, or one major and two minor, criteria are present after a recent, documented streptococcal pharyngitis infection. Major criteria include evidence of carditis (e.g., pleuritic chest pain, friction rub, heart failure, MR), polyarthritis, chorea, erythema marginatum, and subcutaneous nodules. Minor criteria include fever, arthralgia, and a history of rheumatic fever or known rheumatic heart disease.

Once the diagnosis is established, a course of therapy with penicillin is indicated to eradicate the streptococcal infection. Salicylates are effective for the treatment of fever and arthritis. Corticosteroids and immunosuppressive therapy have not been proved beneficial in the management of the carditis. Heart failure should be treated with standard therapy.

Recurrent attacks of rheumatic fever are common, especially during the first 5 to 10 years after the primary illness. Rheumatic fever prophylaxis should be continued during this period, and for 10 years in patients with a high

Table 8–3	**Revised Jones Criteria**

Major Criteria

Carditis (pleuritic chest pain, friction rub, heart failure)
Polyarthritis
Chorea
Erythema marginatum
Subcutaneous nodules

Minor Criteria

Fever
Arthralgia
Previous rheumatic fever or known rheumatic heart disease

exposure rate to streptococcal infection (e.g., health care professionals, childcare workers, military recruits). Patients with significant rheumatic heart disease should receive prophylaxis indefinitely, considering the high rate of recurrence in these individuals. The recommended therapy for prophylaxis is an intramuscular injection of 1.2 million units of benzathine penicillin monthly. Alternatively, oral penicillin or erythromycin may be used. Noncompliance with these agents reduces the effectiveness of this mode of therapy.

Prosthetic Heart Valves

Two types of artificial heart valves are available for use in the atrioventricular and aortic positions: mechanical valves (tilting disk and bi-leaflet) and tissue valves (bioprostheses) (Fig. 8–5). The mechanical valves have a favorable hemodynamic profile and are extremely durable. However, mechanical valves carry a high thromboembolic risk and require long-term anticoagulation. Bioprosthetic use is less likely to be complicated by thromboembolic disease, but the durability of the valve is significantly less than with mechanical valves, especially in young patients. The type of prosthesis used in a particular patient is dependent on multiple factors, including the patient's age, suitability for long-term anticoagulation, and valve position.

Replacement of a diseased valve with an artificial valve results in a new set of potential risks and complications with the prosthesis. All valve prostheses result in some degree of stenosis because the effective valve orifice is smaller than that of the native valve. Thrombosis or calcification of the prosthetic valve can result in prosthetic dysfunction and hemodynamically important stenosis. Prosthetic valve insufficiency can result from peri-valvular leaks in the area of the sewing ring. With bioprosthetic valves, deterioration of the prosthetic valve leaflets can lead to valve insufficiency and stenosis. Hemolysis is a frequent complication of the older mechanical valves (e.g., ball-cage, disk-cage) and can occur with present-day prostheses if turbulent flow associated with prosthetic valve dysfunction exists, especially regurgitation. Endocarditis remains a potential complication in all patients with prosthetic valves. The guidelines for endocarditis prophylaxis are provided later (see Section on Endocarditis).

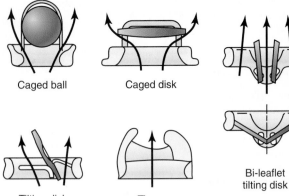

Caged ball   Caged disk

Tilting disk   Tissue

Bi-leaflet
tilting disk

Figure 8–5 Designs and flow patterns of major categories of prosthetic heart valves: caged ball, caged disk, tilting disk, bi-leaflet tilting disk, and bioprosthetic (tissue) valves. Whereas flow in mechanical valves must course along both sides of the occluder, bioprostheses have a central flow pattern. (From Schoen FJ, Titus JL, Lawrie GM: Bioengineering aspects of heart valve replacement. Ann Biomed Eng 10:97–128, 1982; Schoen FJ: Pathology of cardiac valve replacement. In Morse D, Steiner RM, Fernandez J [eds]: Guide to Prosthetic Cardiac Valves. New York, Springer-Verlag, 1985, p 208. Copyright © 1985 Springer-Verlag.)

Evaluation of prosthetic valve function is best performed with two-dimensional and Doppler echocardiographic techniques. Transesophageal echocardiography is particularly useful in studying prosthetic valves when thrombosis or endocarditis is suggested. Mechanical valves can be assessed with fluoroscopy to determine whether leaflet excursion is normal.

Endocarditis Prophylaxis

Patients with valvular heart disease and prosthetic heart valves are at increased risk for developing endocarditis (Table 8–4) (see Chapter 100). The role of antibiotic prophylaxis is to prevent infection of the abnormal valve during procedures that are associated with transient bacteremia (Table 8–5). The flora commonly found in the part

Table 8–4	**Cardiac Conditions in Which Antibiotic Prophylaxis Is Recommended**

Prosthetic heart valves
Previous bacterial endocarditis
Rheumatic and other acquired valvular dysfunctions
Most congenital cardiac malformations
Hypertrophic cardiomyopathy
Mitral valve prolapse with mitral regurgitation (and most patients with leaflet thickening)

Table 8–5	**Dental and Surgical Procedures in Which Endocarditis Prophylaxis Is Recommended**

Dental procedures known to induce gingival bleeding, including professional cleaning
Tonsillectomy and/or adenoidectomy
Surgery involving intestinal or respiratory mucosa
Sclerotherapy for esophageal varices
Cystoscopy
Gallbladder surgery
Urinary tract surgery if urinary tract infection is present
Incision and drainage of infected tissue
Vaginal hysterectomy

of the body being instrumented determines the choice of antibiotics. All patients with known valve disease or prosthetic heart valves should carry a card indicating the nature of their valve lesion and the type of endocarditis prophylaxis recommended.

Prospectus for the Future

Infectious disease such as ARF as the principal cause of acquired valvular heart disease will continue to decline worldwide. For isolated mitral valvular stenosis, for example, percutaneous approaches by a skilled operator will become the standard and the preferred treatment modality over a surgical procedure. Aortic and mitral regurgitation caused by degenerative and other acquired diseases will create the major morbidity and mortality rates with advancing age.

References

ACC/AHA guidelines for the management of patients with valvular heart disease. A report of the American College of Cardiology/American Heart Association. Task Force on Practice Guidelines. J Am Coll Cardiol 32:1486–1588, 1998.

Freed LA, Levy D, Levine RA, et al: Prevalence and clinical outcome of mitral-valve prolapse. N Engl J Med 341:1–7, 1999.

Enriquez-Sarano M, Avierinos JF, Messika-Zeitoun D, et al: Quantitative determinants of the outcome of asymptomatic mitral regurgitation. N Engl J Med 352:875–883, 2005.

Freeman RV, Otto CM: Spectrum of calcific aortic valve disease: Pathogenesis, disease progression, and treatment strategies. Circulation. 111:3316–3326, 2005.

Zoghbi WA, Enriquez-Sarano M, Foster E, et al: Recommendations for evaluation of the severity of native valvular regurgitation with two-dimensional and Doppler echocardiography. J Am Soc Echocardiogr 16:777–802, 2003.

Coronary Heart Disease

Richard A. Lange

L. David Hillis

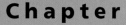

Epidemiology

Coronary heart disease (CHD) is the leading cause of death in the industrialized world. Apart from its influence on mortality, it causes substantial morbidity, disability, and loss of productivity. With improvements in diagnosis, prevention, and treatment, the mortality rate from CHD has declined gradually over the past several decades. Nonetheless, 1.2 million people have a myocardial infarction (MI) or fatal cardiac event each year in the United States alone. Nearly one half of all deaths in industrialized nations and 25% of those in developing countries are due to CHD. By the year 2020, CHD is predicted to surpass infectious disease as the world's leading cause of death and disability.

Pathophysiology of Atherosclerosis

In the industrialized world, atherosclerosis often begins in the early decades of life. One in six American teenagers dying accidentally has pathologic evidence of coronary atherosclerosis. Several processes contribute to the initiation and progression of atherosclerosis, including accumulation of lipoproteins, endothelial injury, and inflammation.

In the early phase of atherosclerosis, small lipoprotein particles penetrate the vascular endothelium, where they are oxidized and coalesce into aggregates in the intimal layer. This process is accelerated at sites of endothelial injury, which may be caused or accelerated by hypertension, hypercholesterolemia, cigarette smoking, or excessive sheer forces. The accumulation of intimal lipid aggregates stimulates the expression of adhesion molecules (e.g., intracellular adhesion molecule-1, vascular cell adhesion molecule-1, selectins) on the luminal surface of the endothelial cells, thereby enabling them to bind circulating monocytes (e.g., macrophages). The adherent monocytes intercalate between the endothelial cells into the intimal layer in response to chemokines and cytokines produced by endothelial and medial smooth muscle cells. The intimal monocytes ingest the lipoprotein aggregates to become lipid-filled monocytes, or *foam cells*. Aggregates of these foam cells make up the earliest visible evidence of atherosclerosis, or the *fatty streak*.

Foam cells replicate and release pro-inflammatory mediators, thereby perpetuating the local inflammatory process with resultant lesion progression. In addition, they release enzymes that cause endothelial denudation. Because the endothelium is involved in the control of vascular tone through its production of vasodilating substances such as prostacyclin and nitric oxide (e.g., endothelium-derived relaxing factor) and thrombosis, injury to these cells impairs vasodilation and creates a local prothrombotic state. Circulating platelets adhere to sites of endothelial injury and release growth factors, which stimulate the migration and proliferation of smooth muscle cells and fibroblasts from the media. This leads to formation of a fibrous cap over the lipid-rich core.

As lipids continue to accumulate in the foam cells, they undergo necrosis and leave a remnant lipid pool in the core of the plaque. Metalloproteinase enzymes (e.g., collagenase, gelatinase) released by macrophages and mast cells in the plaque degrade collagen and extracellular matrix proteins adjacent to the lipid pool, whereas cytokines (e.g., interferon-α) released by T lymphocytes inhibit the formation of collagen by vascular smooth muscle cells. This combination of increased collagen degradation and decreased collagen production creates a vulnerable plaque, which is predisposed to fissure or rupture. Such vulnerable plaques have a lipid-laden core and a thin, weakened fibrous cap. When the thin fibrous cap fissures or ruptures, highly thrombogenic collagen and lipid are exposed to circulating blood with resultant adhesion of platelets and formation of an intraluminal thrombus. Activated platelets release substances (e.g., thromboxane, serotonin) that promote vasoconstriction and thrombus propagation. When the extent of platelet aggregation and thrombosis is sufficient to impair blood flow (partially or completely), an acute coronary event (unstable angina, non–ST-segment elevation myocardial infarction [NSTEMI] or ST-segment elevation myocardial infarction [STEMI]) occurs.

When the atherosclerotic plaque is covered with a thick fibrous cap, rupture is less likely, but the plaque may

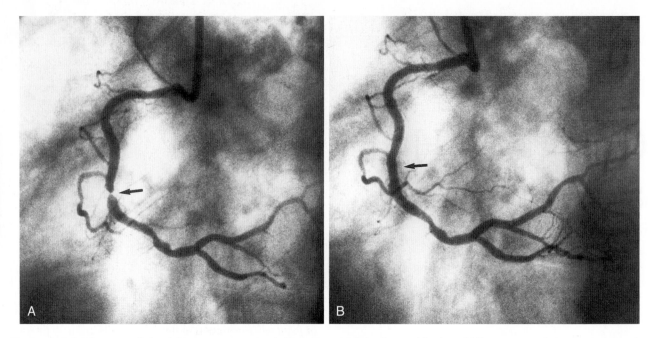

Figure 9–1 Angiograms of the right coronary artery. *A,* Discrete stenosis is observed in the middle segment of the artery *(arrow).* *B,* Same artery is shown after successful balloon angioplasty of the stenosis and placement of an intracoronary stent.

gradually increase in size. As it increases, the coronary arterial lumen is compromised and blood flow is impaired (Fig. 9–1). The hemodynamic significance of plaque is determined by the length and severity of the luminal narrowing; in general, a 70% decrease in the luminal diameter of a coronary artery limits blood flow in the presence of increased myocardial oxygen demands (e.g., exercise, emotional excitement), leading to the clinical condition of exertional angina. A 90% decrease in luminal diameter is sufficient to limit flow even when myocardial oxygen demands are normal.

Risk Factors

Several risk factors for the development of atherosclerosis have been identified (Table 9–1). Nonmodifiable risk factors include (1) advanced age, (2) male sex, and (3) family history of premature atherosclerosis. The prevalence of coronary artery disease (CAD) increases with age. At any given age, the prevalence is higher in men than in women. On average, the clinical manifestations of CAD become evident about 10 years later in women than in men. A family history of premature atherosclerosis (occurring in men before age 55 and in women before age 65) increases the risk of atherosclerosis in an individual, likely as a result of environmental factors (e.g., dietary habits, cigarette smoking) and a genetic predisposition to the disease.

Other risk factors are modifiable, and their treatment may decrease the risk of atherosclerosis. These modifiable risk factors include hyperlipidemia, hypertension, diabetes mellitus, the metabolic syndrome, cigarette smoking, obesity, physical activity, and alcohol intake. Finally, markers associated with an increased incidence of CAD include lipoprotein(a), hyperhomocysteinemia, C-reactive protein (CRP), and coronary arterial calcification.

Lipids play a central role in the atherosclerotic process, and elevated levels of cholesterol, primarily low-density lipoprotein (LDL) cholesterol, are associated with accelerated atherosclerosis. High-density lipoprotein (HDL) cholesterol, by contrast, functions as a protective agent, and its serum level is inversely related to the risk of CAD. Elevated triglycerides are often associated with reduced levels of HDL cholesterol and are an independent risk factor for CAD. Large trials of lipid-lowering therapy have demonstrated the effectiveness of cholesterol reduction in the primary and secondary prevention of CAD.

Hypertension, defined as a systolic arterial pressure greater than 140 mm Hg or a diastolic pressure greater than 90 mm Hg, increases the risk of CAD. The risk increases proportionally with the extent of blood pressure elevation, and proper treatment of hypertension reduces the risk.

Diabetes mellitus increases both the risk of developing CAD and the mortality associated with it. Although CAD is the leading cause of death in adult patients with diabetes, tight glycemic control has not been shown to reduce the risk. Diabetes mellitus often co-exists with other risk factors, including dyslipidemia (elevated triglycerides level, low HDL level), hypertension, and obesity. This grouping of risk factors has been termed the *metabolic syndrome,* and its presence identifies a person at increased risk of having or developing atherosclerotic disease.

Cigarette smoking has adverse effects on the lipid profile, clotting factors, and platelet function, and it is associated with a twofold to threefold increase in the risk for CAD. Cessation of smoking reduces the excess risk of a coronary event by 50% within the first 1 to 2 years of quitting.

Obesity, defined as a body mass index >30 kg/m², is often associated with other risk factors (e.g., hypertension, dyslipidemia, glucose intolerance); in addition, obesity appears to be an independent risk factor for CAD. The

Table 9–1   Risk Factors and Markers for Coronary Artery Disease

Nonmodifiable Risk Factors

Age
Male sex
Family history of premature coronary artery disease

Modifiable Independent Risk Factors

Hyperlipidemia
Hypertension
Diabetes mellitus
Metabolic syndrome
Cigarette smoking
Obesity
Sedentary lifestyle
Heavy alcohol intake

Markers

Elevated lipoprotein(a)
Hyperhomocysteinemia
Elevated high-sensitivity C-reactive protein (hsCRP)
Coronary arterial calcification detected by electron-beam
    computed tomography (EBCT) or multidetector computed
    tomography (MDCT)

distribution of body fat is important, with abdominal adiposity posing a substantially greater risk for CAD in both men and women.

Multiple observational studies have demonstrated an inverse relationship between the amount of physical activity and the risk of CAD. Although the ideal duration, frequency, and intensity of such physical activity have not been determined, numerous studies have shown that exercise is beneficial in healthy patients and those with or at risk for CAD.

Moderate alcohol intake (1 to 2 drinks daily) is associated with a reduction in the risk of cardiovascular events; in contrast, heavy intake increases cardiovascular mortality.

Lipoprotein(a) consists of LDL cholesterol linked to an apo(a) molecule. It has a homologic structure with plasminogen and interferes with the generation of plasmin, thereby creating a predisposition to thrombosis.

Elevated levels of homocysteine are associated with an increased risk of coronary, cerebral, and peripheral vascular disease. Hyperhomocysteinemia can be treated effectively with dietary folate supplementation. However, such treatments have not been shown to reduce the incidence of stroke or cardiovascular events in patients with elevated serum homocysteine levels.

CRP, a marker of inflammation, may indicate or contribute to an increased propensity for plaque rupture and thrombosis. Elevated serum CRP levels—when measured with the new high-sensitivity assays (i.e., high-sensitivity CRP [hsCRP])—strongly correlate with the risks of MI,

stroke, peripheral arterial disease, and sudden cardiac death. Levels of hsCRP <1 mg/L are associated with a low risk of vascular events; levels of 1 to 3 mg/L pose an intermediate risk; levels >3 mg/L create a high risk.

Coronary arterial calcification is a prominent feature of coronary atherosclerosis, and it correlates with the presence and severity of CAD. Electron-beam computed tomography (EBCT) or multidetector computed tomography (MDCT) can accurately quantify coronary calcification, thereby serving as screening tests for CAD in asymptomatic patients. Currently, the usefulness of EBCT or MDCT and CRP in the clinical setting is poorly defined. However, the finding of coronary calcification or elevated hsCRP levels in patients without known CAD or risk factors for CAD may identify those who warrant aggressive risk factor modification.

Nonatherosclerotic Causes of Cardiac Ischemia

Although atherosclerosis is the most common disease affecting the coronary arteries, several nonatherosclerotic processes may produce myocardial ischemia or MI. Embolization from infective endocarditis, mural thrombi in the left atrium or ventricle, prosthetic valves, intracardiac tumors, or paradoxical emboli from the venous system across an atrial or a ventricular septal defect may compromise coronary blood flow, leading to myocardial ischemia or MI. Chest wall trauma may result in coronary arterial dissection or thrombosis. Aortic dissection can propagate to the aortic root and occlude a coronary artery at its origin. Coronary arterial dissection may occur spontaneously during pregnancy or with connective tissue disorders such as Marfan syndrome or Ehlers-Danlos syndrome.

Several forms of arteritis may involve the coronary arteries, including syphilis, Takayasu's arteritis, polyarteritis nodosa, systemic lupus erythematosus, and giant-cell arteritis. These syndromes may result in obstruction, occlusion, or thrombosis of the coronary arteries. Kawasaki disease, a mucocutaneous lymph node syndrome, is a systemic disease of children that causes coronary vasculitis with resultant coronary aneurysms. Spontaneous in situ coronary thrombosis may occur in the setting of hematologic disorders (e.g., polycythemia vera, disseminated intravascular coagulation, sickle cell anemia, paroxysmal nocturnal hemoglobinuria). Congenital coronary anomalies may cause myocardial ischemia. Spontaneous coronary spasm (e.g., Prinzmetal's vasospastic angina) with or without underlying CAD may cause myocardial ischemia or, rarely, MI. Cocaine use may result in myocardial ischemia or MI through several mechanisms, including coronary vasospasm, thrombosis, and accelerated atherosclerosis. An occasional patient treated with sumatriptan for migraine headaches or paclitaxel for cancer may experience MI in the absence of CAD.

In 10% to 20% of patients with suggested angina, coronary angiography reveals normal epicardial coronary arteries. In some of these individuals, microvascular or small vessel disease, the *syndrome X*, has been implicated. The small resistance vessels in these patients, which are not visualized angiographically, appear to have reduced vasodilatory capability. This dysfunction may lead to myocardial ischemia, as evidenced by exercise-related abnormalities on echocardiographic or nuclear scintigraphic studies. Some patients respond to treatment with common anti-anginal medications; although, in general, these drugs are less effective in patients with syndrome X than in those with atherosclerotic CAD.

Finally, myocardial ischemia may result when significant increases in the demand for myocardial oxygen exceed oxygen supply. Such an oxygen supply-demand imbalance may occur on occasion in individuals with thyrotoxicosis, aortic stenosis, aortic insufficiency, tachyarrhythmias, or sepsis. Diminished oxygen supply may occur as a result of acute blood loss, hypotension, severe anemia, or carbon monoxide poisoning.

Pathophysiology and Consequences of Myocardial Ischemia

In the normal myocardium, a balance between myocardial oxygen supply and demand is present at rest and during physical exertion or emotional excitement. In response to an increase in oxygen demand, an appropriate increase in oxygen supply maintains adequate tissue oxygenation. When oxygen demands increase in the setting of limited oxygen supply, myocardial ischemia results. At rest, the myocardium extracts most of the oxygen that is delivered to it via the coronary arteries. As a result, any increase in myocardial oxygen demand, as a result of an increase in heart rate, wall stress, or contractility, must be accompanied by a concomitant proportional increase in myocardial blood flow. Regulation of coronary blood flow occurs at the level of the arterioles and is dependent on autonomic tone and an intact, functioning endothelium.

Endothelial dysfunction secondary to atherosclerosis impairs the ability of the coronary arterioles to dilate when oxygen demands increase. In addition, when a flow-limiting stenosis is present in an epicardial coronary artery, the arterioles distal to the stenosis may already be maximally or nearly maximally dilated in the resting state. The inability of the arterioles to dilate and increase coronary arterial flow during periods of increased demand (e.g., decreased coronary vasodilator reserve) results in a supply-demand mismatch with resultant ischemia and the clinical pattern of stable angina.

When myocardial oxygen supply cannot meet oxygen demand, myocardial ischemia occurs. This ischemia, in turn, initiates a series of pathophysiologic events. Regional hypoxia causes anaerobic glycolysis, lactate production, intracellular acidosis, and disordered calcium homeostasis. These intracellular changes induce abnormalities in myocardial relaxation, leading to reduced compliance and contraction, which cause regional wall motion abnormalities. Finally, electrocardiographic (ECG) evidence of ischemia (i.e., ST-segment depression or elevation) occurs, and angina pectoris ensues.

If myocardial ischemia is transient, then the duration of the resultant mechanical dysfunction may be short. In contrast, more prolonged ischemia may produce myocardial stunning, hibernation, or even an MI. Myocardial stunning refers to a prolonged period (e.g., hours, days) of reversible myocardial dysfunction after an ischemic event. Hibernation occurs in the setting of chronic ischemia when oxygen delivery is adequate to maintain myocardial viability but inadequate to maintain normal function. The clinical importance of the hibernating state is that restoration of blood flow to the involved myocardium results in improved mechanical function.

Because of limited energy expenditure, conduction tissue is more resistant to ischemia than contractile tissue. Nevertheless, ischemia may result in altered ionic transport, altered autonomic tone, and injury to the conduction system, resulting in a variety of ischemia-induced arrhythmias and conduction abnormalities.

Angina Pectoris

For many years, patients with chronic, stable angina pectoris were believed to develop myocardial ischemia because of a transient increase in myocardial oxygen demand as a result of physical exertion or emotional excitement in the setting of limited oxygen supply caused by fixed atherosclerotic CAD. Angina of effort was thought to be a problem of excessive oxygen demand with limited oxygen supply. However, some patients with chronic, stable angina may develop myocardial ischemia because of dynamic coronary vasoconstriction in the setting of fixed atherosclerotic CAD. Such *inappropriate coronary vasoconstriction* has been shown to occur during exposure to cold, while under mental stress, and during isometric or isotonic exercise, as well as while smoking cigarettes. In short, chronic, stable angina is a syndrome of both increased myocardial oxygen demands in the setting of limited supply and dynamic reductions in myocardial oxygen supply, most of which are induced by common, everyday events.

The patient with exertional angina pectoris (Table 9–2) usually complains of a retrosternal pressure or dull ache during physical exertion, as well as while eating, during exposure to cold, or with emotional excitement. Other adjectives that the patient may use to describe the chest discomfort include "viselike," "constricting," "crushing," "heavy," and "squeezing." In many patients, the retrosternal pain radiates to the jaw, neck, and left shoulder and arm. Dyspnea often accompanies exertional angina pectoris and may be associated with diaphoresis and nausea. Although its duration varies considerably from one patient to another, the episode usually lasts 3 to 10 minutes. On occasion, however, it may linger for as long as 30 minutes. It is typically relieved by sublingual nitroglycerin within 1 to 5 minutes.

At a time when the patient is not experiencing angina, the physical examination is usually normal. During an episode of chest discomfort, the patient may become somewhat pale and diaphoretic and the respiratory rate and effort may increase. The heart rate and systemic arterial pressure are usually greater than at rest. Pulmonary congestion (e.g., rales at both bases posteriorly) may be evident. On auscultation of the heart, an S_4 is usually audible as a result of decreased left ventricular compliance, and a transient S_3 may be present if left ventricular systolic dysfunction occurs. In an occasional patient, ischemia-induced papillary muscle dysfunction will cause a murmur of mitral regurgitation to be audible at the cardiac apex. As the episode of angina resolves,

Table 9–2	**Angina Pectoris**			
Type	**Pattern**	**ECG**	**Abnormality**	**Medical Therapy**
Stable	Stable pattern, induced by physical exertion, exposure to cold, eating, emotional stress Lasts 5–10 min Relieved by rest or nitroglycerin	Baseline often normal or nonspecific ST-T changes Signs of previous MI ST-segment depression during angina	≥70% Luminal narrowing of one or more coronary arteries from atherosclerosis	Aspirin Sublingual nitroglycerin Anti-ischemic medications*
Unstable	Increase in anginal frequency, severity, or duration Angina of new onset or now occurring at low level of activity or at rest May be less responsive to sublingual nitroglycerin	Same as stable angina, although changes during discomfort may be more pronounced Occasional ST-segment elevation during discomfort	Plaque rupture with platelet and fibrin thrombus, causing worsening coronary obstruction	Aspirin Anti-ischemic medications Heparin or LMWH Glycoprotein IIb/IIIa inhibitors Statin
Prinzmetal's or variant angina	Angina without provocation, typically occurring at rest	Transient ST-segment elevation during pain Often with associated AV block or ventricular arrhythmias	Coronary artery spasm	Calcium channel blockers Nitrates

AV = atrioventricular; ECG = electrocardiography; LMWH = low–molecular-weight heparin.

the pulmonary rales, S_3, and systolic murmur may quickly disappear.

Three noninvasive techniques have been used to demonstrate transient episodes of myocardial ischemia in the patient with exertional angina pectoris. (1) During exercise-induced or spontaneous chest pain, the ECG usually shows ST-segment depression that is reflective of subendocardial ischemia, which resolves within minutes of the pain's disappearance (Fig. 9–2). (2) During episodes of angina, global left ventricular systolic function may decline, and segmental wall motion abnormalities may develop. These abnormalities can be observed with two-dimensional echocardiography, magnetic resonance imaging, or gated blood-pool scintigraphy. The assessment of regional abnormalities and systolic function using two-dimensional echocardiography performed during exercise or intravenous dobutamine infusion is a particularly useful technique for detecting myocardial ischemia. As with the ECG alterations, these segmental wall motion abnormalities may resolve within minutes after relief of pain or they may linger for hours. (3) Myocardial perfusion may be assessed during exercise-induced angina by the intravenous injection of a radioactive tracer, such as thallium-201 or technetium sestamibi, followed by imaging with the appropriate equipment.

EVALUATION OF THE PATIENT WITH ANGINA

For the patient in whom the cause of chest pain is unclear, stress testing may help clarify the diagnosis by reproducing the patient's symptoms and demonstrating objective evidence of ischemia. Submitting the patient to exercise or pharmacologic stress provides an opportunity to assess the evidence of ischemia through the evaluation of ECG abnormalities (e.g., routine stress testing), perfusion defects (e.g., radionuclide imaging), or segmental wall motion abnormalities (e.g., echocardiography). As with all diagnostic tests, the predictive value of exercise testing is influenced by the pre-test probability that the patient has CAD. For example, in the patient with a high pre-test probability of having CAD, a positive test is highly predictive, whereas a test with negative results has a high likelihood of being falsely negative. Conversely, in the individual with a low likelihood of having CAD, a negative test is highly predictive, but a positive test result has a high likelihood of being falsely positive.

Stress testing may also be useful in the patient with chronic stable angina for the determination of exercise capacity, documentation of the effectiveness of medications, and risk stratification (i.e., identifying patients at risk for CAD in whom more aggressive therapies may be warranted) (Fig. 9–3).

In a patient with a normal resting ECG, routine stress testing with ECG monitoring is usually sufficient. However, in patients with baseline ECG abnormalities (e.g., nonspecific ST-segment abnormalities, left ventricular hypertrophy, left bundle branch block [LBBB], or ventricular pre-excitation) and in patients taking digoxin, the specificity of exercise-induced ST-T wave changes is diminished. In these individuals, echocardiographic or nuclear scintigraphic imaging improves both the sensitivity and the specificity of stress testing, albeit at substantially increased cost. Exercise-induced ECG changes in women are less specific than in men; for this reason, many physicians perform exercise testing with imaging in all women. Several prognostic

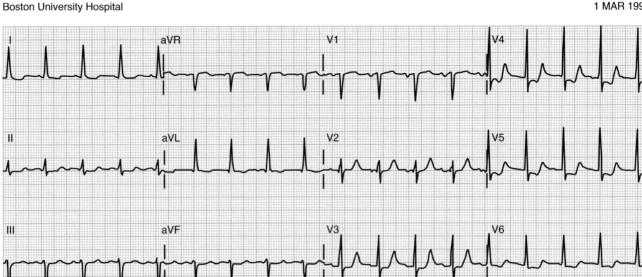

A

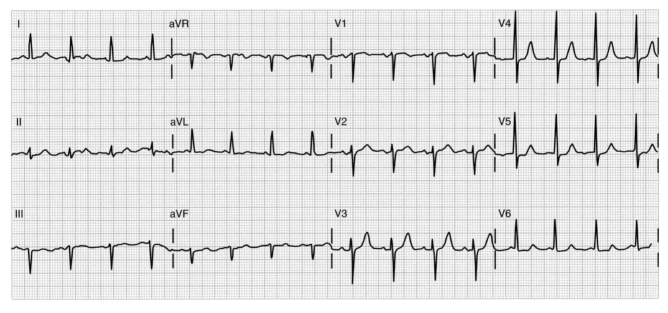

B

Figure 9–2 Electrocardiogram obtained during angina (*A*) and after the administration of sublingual nitroglycerin and subsequent resolution of angina (*B*). During angina, transient ST-segment depression and T-wave abnormalities are present.

markers associated with a poor clinical outcome have been identified in the patient undergoing routine stress testing; these include (1) ischemic ECG changes (ST-segment depression) that occur early in exercise, in multiple leads, or persist for several minutes after the completion of exercise; and (2) an associated decrease (rather than the normal increase) in blood pressure levels.

In patients whose baseline ECG is sufficiently abnormal to preclude an adequate analysis of it during exercise, the standard exercise test may be combined with radionuclide perfusion imaging or an echocardiographic assessment of left ventricular global and segmental function. When stress testing is combined with imaging, the sensitivity for detecting CAD is approximately 90%, which is somewhat greater than that achieved with standard ECG-guided exercise testing. The specificity is about 80%, and the predictive value is approximately 90%.

When a radionuclide stress perfusion imaging study is performed, a radioactive tracer, such as thallium-201, technetium-99m sestamibi, or technetium-99 tetrofosmin, is immediately administered intravenously before exercise is terminated. Because the radioactive tracer is distributed to

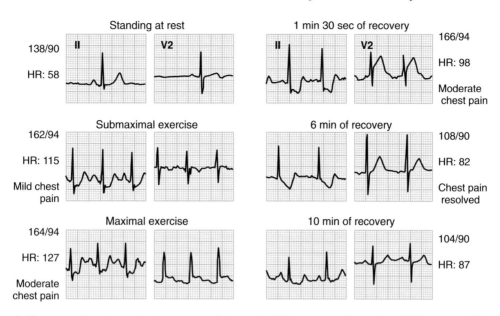

Figure 9–3 Treadmill exercise test demonstrates a markedly ischemic ECG response. The resting ECG is normal. The test was stopped when the patient developed angina at a relatively low workload, accompanied by ST-segment depression in lead II and ST-segment elevation in lead V2. These changes worsened early in recovery and resolved after administration of sublingual nitroglycerin. Only leads II and V2 are shown; however, ischemic changes were seen in 10 of the 12 recorded leads. Severe atherosclerotic disease of all three coronary arteries was documented at subsequent cardiac catheterization.

the myocardium in proportion to coronary arterial blood flow, segments of myocardium that become ischemic during exercise have decreased uptake of the radioactive tracer relative to normally perfused areas of myocardium. Within 4 hours of the injection of thallium, approximately 50% of it is redistributed throughout the myocardium, which results in a *filling in* of areas that were hypoperfused at peak exercise. Unlike thallium, technetium sestamibi and tetrofosmin do not redistribute to areas that were ischemic. The presence and extent of exercise-induced perfusion abnormalities provide prognostic information. Patients with a normal stress perfusion study—with or without CAD—have an extremely low risk of future cardiac events (<1% per year), whereas those with an abnormal stress perfusion study have an event rate of approximately 7% annually, the risk in correlation with the magnitude of the perfusion defect(s).

When exercise induces ischemia, global left ventricular systolic function may decline and regional wall motion abnormalities may develop. These changes can be observed with two-dimensional echocardiography, magnetic resonance imaging, or gated equilibrium blood-pool scintigraphy (e.g., radionuclide ventriculography, multigated acquisition [MUGA] scanning). The extent of wall motion abnormalities correlates with the extent of CAD and the risk of future cardiac events.

For patients who are able to ambulate, exercise stress is preferable to pharmacologic stress because it provides more physiologic information. In patients who are nonambulatory or have very limited exercise capacity, pharmacologic stress may provide similar diagnostic information, but it cannot yield information regarding exercise capacity or the hemodynamic response to exercise. A vasodilator (dipyridamole or adenosine) or an intravenous inotropic agent (dobutamine) is typically administered to perform a pharmacologic stress test. With the former, blood flow in unobstructed coronary arteries increases to a greater extent than in obstructed arteries, and this can be detected with perfusion imaging. In contrast, dobutamine infusion increases myocardial contractility—and hence myocardial oxygen demand—and is combined with radionuclide perfusion or echocardiographic imaging to assess the presence of perfusion defects or regional wall motion abnormalities.

As previously noted, EBCT has been used for the detection of CAD. The absence of calcification on computed tomography (CT) strongly correlates with the absence of hemodynamically significant coronary atherosclerosis. In contrast, the presence of coronary calcification is diagnostic of coronary atherosclerosis, although the extent of luminal diameter narrowing cannot be predicted by the extent of calcification. Newer multidetector CT machines can actually visualize coronary arterial stenoses in addition to detecting coronary calcification. Their roles in the detection and management of CAD are evolving.

Cardiac catheterization with coronary angiography allows visual assessment of the extent and severity of CAD. The anatomic information obtained must be interpreted in light of functional information (e.g., stress testing) because the anatomic severity of a given coronary stenosis does not necessarily correlate with its physiologic significance. Coronary angiography is invasive and is associated with a small risk. Nonetheless, the risk-benefit analysis of catheterization favors the procedure in many patients with angina (Table 9–3).

MEDICAL MANAGEMENT OF STABLE ANGINA

The approach to the management of the patient with angina involves (1) risk factor modification and lifestyle changes to slow or to arrest the progression of CAD and thrombosis, (2) pharmacotherapy to prevent or to relieve angina, and (3)

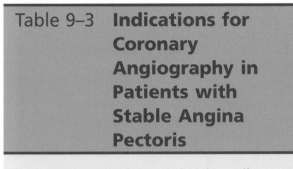

Table 9–3	**Indications for Coronary Angiography in Patients with Stable Angina Pectoris**

- Unacceptable angina despite medical therapy (for consideration of revascularization)
- Noninvasive testing results with at-risk features
- Angina or risk factors for CAD in the setting of depressed left ventricular systolic function
- For diagnostic purposes in the individual in whom the results of noninvasive testing are unclear

CAD = coronary artery disease.

Table 9–4	**Goals of Risk Factor Modification**

Risk Factor	Goal
Dyslipidemia	
Elevated LDL cholesterol level	
Patients with CAD or CAD equivalent[a]	LDL <70 mg/dL
Without CAD, ≥two risk factors[b]	LDL <130 mg/dL (or <100 mg/dL[c])
Without CAD, none or one risk factor[b]	LDL <160 mg/dL
Elevated TG	TG <200 mg/dL
Reduced HDL cholesterol level	HDL >40 mg/dL
Hypertension	Systolic blood pressure <130 mm Hg Diastolic blood pressure <85 mm Hg
Smoking	Complete cessation
Obesity	<120% of ideal body weight for height
Sedentary lifestyle	30–60 min moderate intensity activity (e.g., walking, jogging, cycling, rowing) five times per week

[a]CAD equivalents include diabetes mellitus, noncoronary atherosclerotic vascular disease, or >20% 10-year risk of a cardiovascular event as predicted by the Framingham risk score.
[b]Risk factors include cigarette smoking, blood pressure ≥140/90 mm Hg or on antihypertensive medication, HDL cholesterol level <40 mg/dL, family history of premature coronary atherosclerosis (e.g., man ≤45 years; woman ≤55 years).
[c]Target of 100 mg/dL should be strongly considered for men ≥60 years of age and individuals with a high burden of subclinical atherosclerosis (>75th percentile of patient's age and sex for coronary calcification), hsCRP >3 mg/dL, or metabolic syndrome.
CAD = coronary artery disease; CRP = C-reactive protein; HDL = high-density lipoprotein; hsCRP, high sensitivity C-reactive protein; LDL = low-density lipoprotein; TG = triglycerides.

revascularization to improve symptoms or prognosis or both. In addition, concurrent medical conditions (e.g., anemia, congestive heart failure, chronic obstructive pulmonary disease, hyperthyroidism) that may precipitate or worsen angina should be corrected, if possible.

Control of hypertension, diabetes mellitus, hyperlipidemia, and smoking cessation are important in controlling the progression of disease in patients with coronary atherosclerosis. Guidelines for aggressive risk factor reduction have been established (Table 9–4). Patients should be instructed on dietary changes; an evaluation by a nutritionist may be helpful.

All patients with known or suggested CAD should be placed on antiplatelet therapy (e.g., aspirin, 81 to 325 mg daily; clopidogrel, 75 mg daily for patients allergic to aspirin) unless a contraindication to antiplatelet therapy is present. These agents decrease the rates of MI and death in patients with angina or previous MI. In addition, they may decrease the risk of MI in individuals without suggested CAD but with multiple risk factors. Angiotensin-converting enzyme (ACE) inhibitors should be prescribed to patients with CAD who have diabetes mellitus or left ventricular systolic dysfunction unless contraindicated. Although exercise is often limited by angina, regular activity at a level that is tolerated should be encouraged. Isometric exercise, such as weight lifting and high-intensity activities especially in the cold (e.g., skiing, shoveling snow) are not advisable. However, many patients with stable angina may perform vigorous activities, including moderate physical exertion at work.

As previously noted, the pathophysiologic characteristics of angina are one of supply-demand mismatch. Therefore its therapy is directed at correcting the mismatch by decreasing myocardial oxygen demands or augmenting myocardial oxygen supply or both. Nitrates, β-blockers, and calcium channel blockers are among the pharmacologic options most commonly used for the control of symptoms in patients with chronic stable angina (Table 9–5). They appear to be of similar efficacy in controlling anginal symptoms. When a single agent fails to control angina, combination therapy is usually effective. Unlike aspirin and lipid-lowering therapy,

none of these agents has been convincingly shown to decrease mortality in patients with CAD.

Nitrate preparations have been used in the medical management of exertional angina for many years. The effect of nitrates is mediated through relaxation of vascular smooth muscle. Dilation of arterioles reduces systemic vascular resistance and therefore afterload. Nitrates have a more pronounced effect on the venous system, whereas venodilation results in venous pooling, decreased venous return, and therefore decreased preload. The arteriolar and venodilatory effects substantially reduce myocardial oxygen demands, thereby decreasing angina. In addition, nitrates augment coronary blood flow by dilating epicardial coronary arteries (although this effect is minimal in extensively diseased arteries) and increasing blood flow through collateral vessels. Several formulations are available. Sublingual nitroglycerin tablets or oral spray is effective for the acute treatment of anginal episodes and as prophylactic therapy before an activity that is likely to provoke angina. Topical nitroglycerin ointment and oral preparations are effective for the chronic management of stable angina, whereas intravenous nitroglycerin is appropriate for patients with unstable angina and acute MI. The chronic use of nitrates results in tolerance, an

Table 9–5 Medications for Angina Pectoris

Drug Class	Examples	Anti-anginal Effect	Physiologic Side Effects	Comments
Nitroglycerin	Sublingual Topical Intravenous Oral	Decreased preload and afterload Coronary vasodilation Increased collateral blood flow	Headache Flushing Orthostasis	Tolerance develops with continuous use
β-Adrenergic blocking agents	Metoprolol Atenolol Propranolol Nadolol	Decreased heart rate Decreased blood pressure Decreased contractility	Bradycardia Hypotension Bronchospasm Depression	May worsen heart failure and AV conduction block; avoid in vasospastic angina
Calcium channel blocking agents	Phenylalkylamine (verapamil) Benzothiazepine (diltiazem)	Decreased heart rate Decreased blood pressure Decreased contractility Coronary vasodilation	Bradycardia Hypotension Constipation with verapamil	May worsen heart failure and AV conduction
Calcium channel blocking agents	Dihydropyridines (nifedipine, amlodipine)	Decreased blood pressure Coronary vasodilation	Hypotension, reflex tachycardia Peripheral edema	Short-acting nifedipine associated with increased risk of cardiovascular events

AV, Atrioventricular.

effect that can be minimized by allowing for a daily nitrate-free period; for example, removing topical nitrate preparations during sleeping hours or prescribing oral nitrates that avoid around the clock administration.

β-Adrenergic blocking drugs are competitive inhibitors of catecholamine β-receptors. They decrease myocardial oxygen demands by reducing heart rate, blood pressure, and contractility. These agents are effective in controlling anginal symptoms (especially exercise-induced symptoms), and they decrease mortality and reinfarction in survivors of MI. β-Blockers differ in their lipid solubility, duration of action, and β-receptor selectivity. $β_1$-Receptors predominate in the heart, where they mediate increases in heart rate, contractility, and atrioventricular (AV) conduction. $β_2$-Receptors predominate in the vascular and bronchial smooth muscle. Blockade of $β_1$-receptors produces several beneficial cardiac effects, whereas $β_2$-receptor blockade may induce bronchospasm and peripheral vasoconstriction. Atenolol and metoprolol are $β_1$ selective at low doses; however, at the moderate-to-high doses often used in clinical practice, all β-blockers lose their selectivity. Because β-blockers may worsen underlying conduction system abnormalities, they should be used with caution in patients with conduction system dysfunction. In addition, these agents may result in a mild increase in the triglyceride level and a mild decrease in the HDL cholesterol level.

Calcium ions play a critical role in myocardial and vascular smooth muscle contraction and in the genesis of the cardiac action potential (see Chapter 10). Blocking these effects with a calcium antagonist results in a decrease in heart rate, myocardial contractility, and peripheral arterial vasodilation, all of which decrease myocardial oxygen demands. In addition, coronary vasodilation occurs, resulting in augmented oxygen supply. Three major classes of calcium antagonists are available, and the specific agent of choice should be individualized for the particular patient. The dihydropyridine medications (e.g., nifedipine, amlodipine) predominantly cause vasodilation with little or no effect on heart rate, contractility, or AV conduction. In fact, the vasodilation may lead to a reflex tachycardia. The phenylalkylamine medications (e.g., verapamil) reduce heart rate, slow AV conduction, depress contractility, and have less of an effect on peripheral vascular tone than the dihydropyridine medications. They may not be tolerated in patients with depressed ventricular systolic function or underlying conduction system disease. The benzothiazepine medications (e.g., diltiazem) have less vasodilatory action than the dihydropyridine medications and less myocardial suppressant action than the phenylalkylamine medications.

REVASCULARIZATION IN PATIENTS WITH ANGINA

In patients for whom medical therapy does not effectively control anginal symptoms and in patients considered to be clinically at risk (e.g., unstable angina, angina associated with heart failure, poor exercise capacity) or by noninvasive testing (e.g., depressed left ventricular systolic function, at-risk stress test results), revascularization plays an important therapeutic role. Several modalities for coronary revascularization exist, including surgical revascularization (e.g., coronary artery bypass grafting [CABG]) and catheter-based percutaneous techniques (e.g., percutaneous transluminal coronary angioplasty [PTCA]) and related interventional techniques.

With advances in equipment and increasing operator experience, percutaneous revascularization can now be achieved with high success rates and at relatively low risk. More than 1 million percutaneous coronary revascularization procedures are performed each year in the United States alone. With PTCA, a high-pressure inflation of a distensible balloon is performed at the site of coronary arterial narrowing with resultant enlargement of the lumen. Balloon inflation causes denudation of the endothelial surface, fracture of the atherosclerotic plaque, and disruption of the vessel intima. The vessel lumen can be successfully dilated in greater than 90% of cases. In 2% to 5% of patients undergoing PTCA, the coronary arterial injury is severe, and, as a result, the artery occludes abruptly. Such patients are usually treated with intracoronary stenting or urgent CABG to prevent acute MI. In patients in whom PTCA is initially successful, about 50% develop restenosis at the site of balloon dilation within 1 to 6 months of the angioplasty. Of the patients who develop restenosis, about 50% experience recurrent angina, and the remainder are asymptomatic. Restenosis is a complex process involving elastic recoil of the artery, vascular remodeling, and hyperplasia of the vascular intima. It is not prevented by the administration of antiplatelet agents, anticoagulant drugs, or anti-anginal medications.

Over the past decade, intracoronary stenting has become the most widely used percutaneous coronary intervention. The stent—a cylindric, expandable metal structure available in varying diameters and lengths—is mounted on an angioplasty balloon. When the balloon is positioned at the site of the stenosis and inflated to expand the stent, the stent becomes embedded in the arterial wall. Subsequently, the balloon is deflated and removed, but the stent maintains its expanded cylindric configuration, thereby acting as a scaffold to maintain vessel patency. In this way, stenting results in a greater increase in luminal size than can be achieved with balloon angioplasty alone (see Fig. 9–1B). Stents can be used to treat PTCA-related coronary arterial dissections, thereby avoiding the need for urgent CABG. In comparison with balloon angioplasty, stenting is associated with a reduced incidence of abrupt closure (approximately 1% to 2%) and restenosis (approximately 20% to 25%), thereby explaining why it is the procedure of choice in more than 90% of percutaneous coronary interventions. At the same time, stenting may not be the procedure of choice in small coronary arteries (luminal diameter <2.5 mm) because the incidence of abrupt closure and restenosis in these arteries is high. The person in whom intracoronary stenting has been performed should receive aspirin indefinitely and clopidogrel for 2 to 4 weeks to prevent thrombosis. During the weeks after stent deployment, the stent becomes endothelialized, at which time it is no longer thrombogenic or subject to abrupt closure.

Recently, stents have been coated with antiproliferative drugs (e.g., sirolimus [Rapamycin], paclitaxel [Taxol]), which are extremely effective in preventing restenosis. The incidence of restenosis is 5% to 10% when a drug-eluting stent is used for coronary revascularization. The person who receives a drug-eluting stent should receive aspirin indefinitely and clopidogrel for at least 6 months. The antiproliferative agent that coats the stent delays the process of endothelialization; as a result, these stents are subject to thrombosis and abrupt closure for months after their placement.

Other percutaneous interventional techniques that have a limited role in coronary revascularization include rotational and directional atherectomy; thrombectomy; brachytherapy, which is the application of local radiation therapy to treat restenosis after stenting; and coronary laser therapy.

Studies performed in the 1970s and 1980s established the effectiveness of CABG for the control of anginal symptoms and, in some patients, offered an improvement in survival when compared to anti-anginal medical therapy. Harvesting a segment of saphenous vein or radial artery and anastomosing it to the ascending aorta (proximally) and the distal portion of the diseased coronary artery (distally) is performed with CABG. Alternatively, the internal mammary artery can be dissected free from the pleural surface and its distal end anastomosed to a diseased coronary artery. These procedures effectively bypass the sites of atherosclerotic narrowing, thereby allowing blood to flow freely to the myocardium perfused by the diseased artery. Whenever possible, the mammary artery is used because its long-term patency is superior to that of venous or radial arterial conduits. Experienced surgeons perform CABG with a peri-operative mortality rate of 1% to 2%, a stroke rate of 1% to 2%, and a peri-operative MI rate of 5% to 10%.

CABG improves survival (when compared with medical therapy) in patients with >50% luminal diameter narrowing of the left main coronary artery or narrowing of all three major epicardial coronary arteries in conjunction with mildly or moderately depressed left ventricular systolic function (e.g., ejection fraction, 35% to 50%). In addition, CABG improves long-term survival in patients with a narrowing of two or three epicardial coronary arteries and normal left ventricular systolic performance, provided that the proximal portion of the left anterior descending coronary artery is significantly narrowed.

In the short term (within 1 to 2 years of the procedure), those having percutaneous coronary intervention are more likely than those undergoing surgery to require anti-anginal medications or a subsequent revascularization procedure largely because of the incidence of symptomatic restenosis after successful percutaneous coronary revascularization. Because of the progressive decline of graft patency between 5 and 10 years postoperatively, the benefits of surgery over percutaneous revascularization are less apparent in the long term. Small, randomized studies comparing the two approaches to revascularization in patients with multivessel CAD and preserved left ventricular systolic function (e.g., ejection fraction >0.50%) demonstrate no difference in mortality after 1 to 5 years of follow-up, except in patients with diabetes, who fare better with CABG. Recently, however, larger observational studies showed that CABG is associated with higher long-term survival than stenting in patients with multivessel CAD.

Unfortunately, neither percutaneous nor surgical revascularization techniques halt the underlying atherosclerotic process, and new stenoses may develop at previously uninvolved sites in native coronary arteries and in the bypass grafts. Within 10 years of CABG, approximately 50% of saphenous vein grafts are occluded; the rate is substantially lower with internal mammary grafts. Aspirin should be administered immediately after CABG and continued thereafter because it improves graft patency. If a stenosis develops in a bypass graft, then percutaneous revascularization is often effective. In addition, repeat CABG is possible, although the surgical risks are higher than with the first procedure.

VARIANT ANGINA

In 1959, Prinzmetal and colleagues described a group of patients with *variant* angina. These patients usually experienced chest pain at rest rather than with physical exertion or emotional excitement, and the ECG recorded during chest pain showed ST-segment elevation rather than depression, which resolved as the pain subsided (Fig. 9–4). On occasion, episodes of chest discomfort were accompanied by varying degrees of AV block or ventricular ectopy, but MI was uncommon. Patients with variant angina did not often have the usual risk factors for atherosclerosis, although cigarette smoking was frequent. Subsequent angiographic studies demonstrated that variant angina is the result of coronary arterial spasm, which may occur either at the site of an atherosclerotic plaque or in the setting of angiographically normal coronary arteries.

During cardiac catheterization, coronary vasospasm may be provoked by the intracoronary infusion of acetylcholine. In addition, methacholine, a parasympathomimetic agent, has been used to induce coronary arterial spasm, similar to the arterial spasm in response to exposure to cold (e.g., cold pressor test), the production of a significant alkalosis (e.g., vigorous hyperventilation during the intravenous infusion of an alkalotic buffer solution), and histamine administration.

Calcium channel blockers, alone or in combination with long-acting nitrate preparations, are highly effective in patients with coronary arterial spasm. They are the treatment of choice for patients with variant angina. β-Blockers are contraindicated in patients with vasospastic angina because blockade of the vasodilatory effects of β₂-receptor stimulation may result in unopposed α-adrenergic vasoconstriction. For the rare patient who has continued episodes of coronary arterial spasm despite maximal medical therapy, intracoronary stenting may be performed.

Acute Coronary Syndromes

The term *acute coronary syndrome* encompasses the clinical syndromes of unstable angina, non–ST-segment elevation myocardial infarction (NSTEMI), and ST-segment elevation myocardial infarction (STEMI). Patients with unstable angina and with NSTEMI are usually indistinguishable by history, physical examination, and ECG findings. The distinction between these two groups is made only after the results of the serum cardiac enzyme analyses are available.

The patient with unstable angina or NSTEMI may develop myocardial ischemia or MI via several mechanisms. Most commonly, these individuals have subendocardial ischemia or necrosis as a result of decreased coronary blood flow, which is due to platelet aggregation or a partially occlusive intracoronary thrombus at the site of an ulcerated atherosclerotic plaque. In addition, concomitant platelet-mediated coronary arterial vasoconstriction at the site of plaque ulceration may occur. Alternatively, the patient may develop myocardial ischemia or MI because of an increase in myocardial oxygen demand that cannot be met by an appropriate increase in coronary blood flow. In some individuals, the coronary blood flow cannot appropriately increase because of severe CAD. In those without CAD,

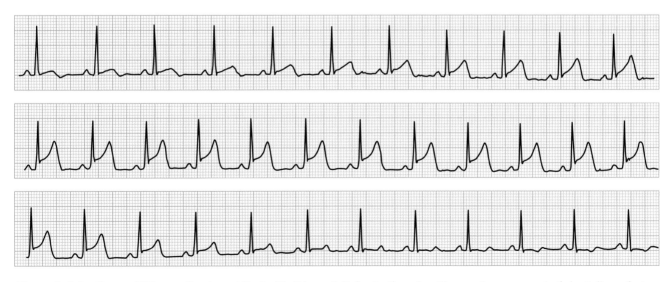

Figure 9–4 Continuous ECG recording in a patient with Prinzmetal's (variant) angina. The spontaneous onset of chest discomfort began during the *top strip*, accompanied by transient ST-segment elevation. By the *bottom strip*, several minutes later, both discomfort and ST-segment elevation have resolved.

subendocardial ischemia or infarction may occur solely as a result of significantly augmented myocardial oxygen demands in the setting of a normal supply (e.g., uncontrolled hypertension, thyrotoxicosis) or a decrease in myocardial oxygen delivery (e.g., profound anemia, hypoxemia).

The patient with unstable angina pectoris usually complains of retrosternal chest pain similar in character and consistency to that of the patient with stable, exertional chest pain. In contrast to the patient whose angina is stable, however, these individuals usually report that their anginal frequency, severity, or duration has worsened, and they may report pain at rest. Furthermore, the patient may note that nitroglycerin is ineffective or less effective in relieving the chest pain.

On physical examination, the patient may exhibit no visible or audible abnormalities at a time when he or she is pain free. During an episode of chest pain, however, the patient may become anxious, diaphoretic, and dyspneic. The heart rate often increases, although bradycardia may occur secondary to enhanced vagal tone or transient AV block and most commonly with inferior wall ischemia or infarction. On auscultation of the heart, an S_4 may be audible as a result of decreased left ventricular compliance. An S_3 may be present if left ventricular systolic dysfunction occurs, and a systolic murmur of mitral valve papillary muscle dysfunction may be appreciated. Evidence of pulmonary congestion is often present and may reflect an elevated left ventricular filling pressure as a result of decreased left ventricular compliance or systolic dysfunction. If a large area of myocardium is involved and left ventricular systolic dysfunction ensues, then frank pulmonary edema may occur.

For the patient who is experiencing chest pain, an ECG should be immediately obtained because it is frequently diagnostic of myocardial ischemia or MI and is important in determining the appropriate treatment plan. STEMI, previously referred to by the pathologically inaccurate term, *transmural infarction,* or by the term, *Q wave myocardial infarction,* refers to an acute coronary syndrome in which ST-segment elevation (e.g., $\geq 1\,mV$ in concordant limb leads, $\geq 2\,mV$ in concordant precordial leads) is present on the surface ECG. These infarctions are the result of complete thrombotic occlusion of a coronary artery and may first be exhibited on the ECG by symmetrically peaked or hyperacute T waves. These peaked T waves resolve after several minutes as the characteristic ST-segment elevation develops (Fig. 9–5).

NSTEMI, previously termed *subendocardial infarction* or *non–Q wave myocardial infarction,* and unstable angina occur as a result of a subtotally occlusive thrombus or a thrombus that was initially totally occlusive but not sustained, enabling partial or complete lysis to occur within minutes to hours of its formation. They are associated with ST-segment depression or T wave inversions (or both) on the surface ECG (Fig. 9–6).

In one fourth to one half of patients with acute MI, the first ECG does not demonstrate typical ST-segment changes. In this situation, serial ECGs should be obtained to increase the diagnostic yield. If acute MI is suggestive but the initial ECG does not confirm the diagnosis, then demonstration of new regional wall motion abnormalities with echocardiography may be helpful in confirming the diagnosis.

Myocardial necrosis results in the release of certain intracellular enzymes into the blood. Their appearance in the blood allows the identification of myocardial necrosis, and their quantitation over a number of hours allows for the estimate of its amount. Because 20% of patients with acute MI have atypical or no symptoms (i.e., *silent* MI) and the initial ECG is nondiagnostic in up to 50% of patients, serologic identification of myocyte necrosis has become an important diagnostic tool. Several serum markers have been identified (Fig. 9–7).

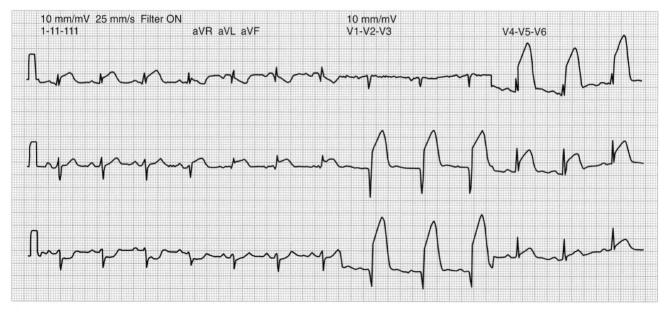

Figure 9–5 Acute anterolateral MI. Leads I, aVL, and V_2 to V_6 demonstrate ST-segment elevation. Reciprocal ST-segment depression is seen in leads II, III, and aVF. Deep Q waves have developed in leads V_2 and V_3.

Boston University Hospital

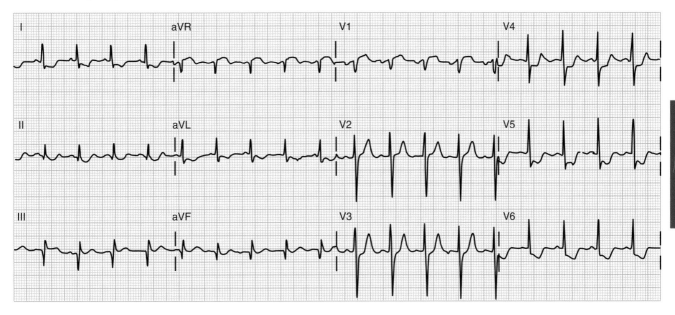

Figure 9–6 Marked ST-segment depression in a patient with prolonged chest pain is the result of an acute non–ST-segment elevation MI (NSTEMI). Between 1 and 3 mm of ST-segment depression is seen in leads I, aVL, and in V$_4$ to V$_6$. The patient is known to have had a previous inferior MI.

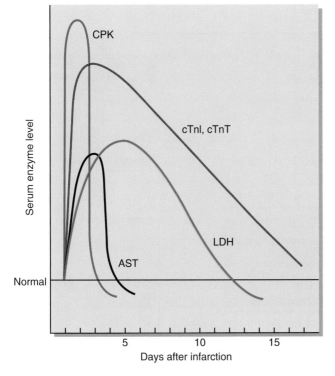

Figure 9–7 Typical time course for the detection of enzymes released after MI. *AST,* Serum aspartate aminotransferase; *CPK,* creatine kinase; *cTnI,* cardiac troponin I; *cTnT,* cardiac troponin T; *LDH,* lactate dehydrogenase.

Creatine kinase (CK) and its myocardial-specific isoenzyme, creatine kinase muscle band (CK-MB), are detectable in the blood within 3 to 6 hours of the onset of MI. They reach their peak concentration at 24 hours and return to normal within 48 hours. Although CK-MB is relatively specific for cardiac injury, it may be elevated in subjects with extensive skeletal muscle injury or disease, chronic renal disease, or hypothyroidism.

Troponins I and T are regulatory proteins involved in the interaction of cardiac actin and myosin. Because they are not present to any extent in other organs and are not detectable in blood under normal circumstances, an increase in their serum concentration is more specific and sensitive for myocyte necrosis than an increase in the concentration of other enzymes. After cardiac injury, the serum troponin concentration begins to rise within 4 to 6 hours and remains elevated for 7 to 10 days. False-positive elevations of troponin T, but not troponin I, have been observed in patients with renal failure. The presence of heterophilic antibodies or fibrin may interfere with the assay for troponin I and give false-positive results. The former is found in 3% of the general population and a high percentage of patients with autoimmune disease; the latter may be found in blood that has been heparinized. Because serum troponin concentration is an extremely sensitive measure of myocardial necrosis, such elevations are sometimes observed in patients with myocardial necrosis as a result of increased myocardial oxygen demands in the absence of epicardial CAD (i.e., subjects with a significantly elevated heart rate or blood pressure, pulmonary embolism, hypoxemia).

TREATMENT OF UNSTABLE ANGINA AND NSTEMI

Unstable angina and NSTEMI may be clinically indistinguishable with ECG studies. They are differentiated only by the presence of serologic evidence of myocardial necrosis. Accordingly, the initial treatment of these patients is similar and includes (1) hospital admission with serial assessment of ECGs and sequential measurements of cardiac enzymes; (2) aggressive anti-anginal, antiplatelet, and antithrombotic therapy; and (3) identification of the patient at increased risk of having recurrent ischemia, MI, or death who may benefit from revascularization. With optimal medical therapy, the 1-year mortality rate of patients with unstable angina or NSTEMI is 3% to 5% (Fig. 9–8).

Rest for 24 to 48 hours with continuous ECG monitoring, analgesics, and supplemental oxygen therapy are frequently prescribed. Sublingual nitroglycerin should be given initially, and intravenous nitroglycerin should be administered if recurrent chest pain occurs. In the absence of a contraindication, β-blockers should be promptly instituted because they decrease heart rate and blood pressure levels and left ventricular contractility, thereby reducing myocardial oxygen demand. The calcium antagonists, verapamil or diltiazem, may be useful for the patient who fails to respond to nitrates and β-blockers, as well as for the patient with a contraindication to β-blockers. However, calcium antagonists should not be used in the patient with known depressed left ventricular systolic function or with evidence of pulmonary vascular congestion on physical examination or chest x-ray studies. Because dihydropyridine calcium antagonists (e.g., nifedipine, amlodipine) may cause a reflex tachycardia with a resultant worsening of angina, they should be avoided unless they can be used in combination with a β-blocker.

As noted, enhanced platelet aggregation and partial coronary arterial occlusion by platelet-rich thrombus play important pathophysiologic roles in most patients with unstable angina or NSTEMI. Aspirin has been shown to decrease mortality and rates of recurrent MI in these patients. Accordingly, the patient without a contraindication should receive oral aspirin, 80 to 325 mg daily. The addition

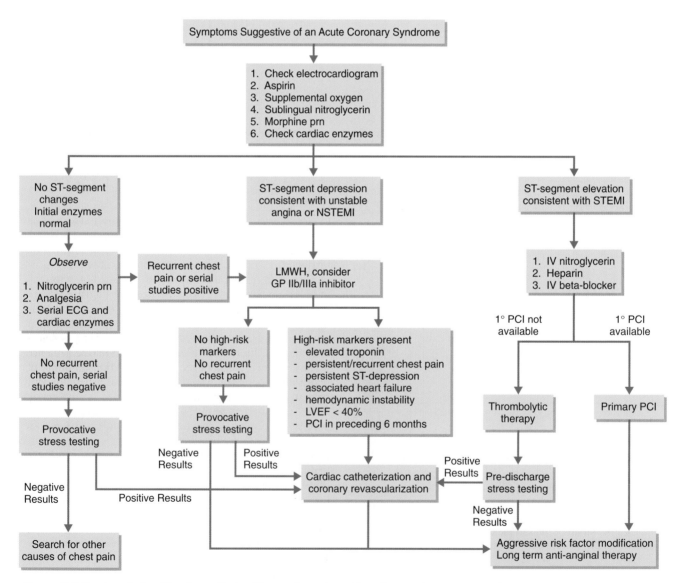

Figure 9–8 Treatment algorithm for patients with symptoms suggestive of an acute coronary syndrome.

of oral clopidogrel or an intravenous glycoprotein IIb/IIIa inhibitor (e.g., tirofiban, eptifibatide) provides more effective platelet inhibition, thereby reducing the risk of recurrent ischemia or infarction. If clopidogrel is administered, then it is continued for 3 to 12 months. If a glycoprotein IIb/IIIa inhibitor is used, then it is infused for 48 to 96 hours. These agents are typically used in patients who have at-risk features predictive of a subsequent cardiac event or in whom percutaneous revascularization is planned.

Heparin, unfractionated or low–molecular-weight, is given concomitantly with antiplatelet therapy. If unfractionated heparin is used, then it is usually infused for 48 hours. Enoxaparin, a low–molecular-weight heparin, may be used instead of unfractionated heparin. It is administered subcutaneously twice daily and continued until hospital discharge. Unlike unfractionated heparin, it does not require monitoring of its anticoagulant effects by serially measuring the activated partial thromboplastin time. In patients considered to be at risk for a subsequent cardiac event, low–molecular-weight heparin is superior to unfractionated heparin in preventing recurrent ischemia. Thrombolytic therapy has not been shown to be beneficial for the treatment of individuals with unstable angina or NSTEMI. In these patients, in fact, it may be detrimental (Table 9–6).

Many physicians choose to treat patients with unstable angina or NSTEMI with heparin for 2 to 3 days to allow for plaque stabilization. With aggressive medical therapy, 80% to 90% of these patients become and remain pain free. Because the patient with persistent or recurrent chest pain despite the previously described measures is at increased risk of MI and death, more aggressive management is warranted. If chest pain continues despite maximal medical therapy, then intra-aortic balloon counterpulsation may be instituted, and urgent coronary angiography followed by revascularization should be considered.

For the patient with unstable angina or NSTEMI who promptly and completely responds to medical therapy, subsequent evaluation should be aimed at determining the patient's risk for a subsequent cardiac event. The patient deemed to be at low risk might undergo exercise or pharmacologic stress testing. The patient considered to be high risk for subsequent events should receive maximal antiplatelet therapy with aspirin and a glycoprotein IIb/IIIa inhibitor, low–molecular-weight heparin, and coronary angiography within 4 to 48 hours, followed by revascularization with percutaneous intervention or CABG, if indicated. Patients most likely to benefit from this approach are those with elevated serum cardiac enzyme values or those with three or more at-risk variables, including the following: (1) age 65 years or older, (2) at least three risk factors for atherosclerosis, (3) a previously documented coronary arterial stenosis of 50% or greater, (4) ECG ST-segment deviation at the time of hospital arrival, (5) at least two anginal episodes in the 24 hours before hospitalization, or (6) use of aspirin during the 7 days before hospitalization.

Urgent coronary angiography should be performed in the patient with continued or recurrent chest pain despite optimal medical therapy or hypotension or severe heart failure during medical therapy. Elective angiography should be considered for the patient with an acute coronary syndrome and any of the following risk factors: (1) previous angioplasty or CABG, (2) congestive heart failure or depressed left ventricular systolic function, (3) life-threatening ventricular arrhythmias, (4) recurrent low-threshold ischemia, or (5) exercise or pharmacologic stress testing that indicates a high likelihood of severe CAD. Based on coronary anatomy, the experience of the medical personnel, the presence of co-existing medical conditions, and the preferences of the patient, a recommendation for percutaneous or surgical revascularization can be made.

TREATMENT OF ST-SEGMENT ELEVATION MYOCARDIAL INFARCTION

Numerous studies have shown that coronary thrombosis is the cause of most STEMIs. Postmortem studies have demonstrated that 85% to 95% of patients dying of STEMI have a fresh thrombotic occlusion of a large epicardial coronary artery, and angiographic studies performed within several hours of the onset of STEMI have shown a similar incidence of total occlusion. After as little as 15 to 20 minutes of coronary occlusion, irreversible cellular injury and necrosis ensue. The subsequent extent of myocardial injury is determined by the duration of coronary occlusion, the presence or absence of collateral vessels, and the amount of myocardium perfused by the infarct-related artery. Prompt restoration of antegrade flow in the infarct-related artery minimizes the extent of myocardial necrosis. In arteries with gradually developing stenoses, sufficient collateral vessels may develop to prevent irreversible myocardial injury even with complete arterial occlusion. In contrast, if acute plaque rupture and thrombotic occlusion occur at the site of a previously nonobstructive stenosis, then collateral circulation does not have sufficient time to develop, and extensive infarction ensues. With infarction of 20% to 25% of the left ventricle, congestive heart failure usually ensues. With infarction of 40% or more of the left ventricle, cardiogenic shock usually develops (Fig. 9–9).

In the patient with suggested acute MI, a 12-lead ECG should be performed within minutes of the patient's arrival,

---

Table 9–6	**Selection Criteria for Thrombolytic Therapy in Acute Myocardial Infarction**

1. Chest pain consistent with acute myocardial infarction
2. Electrocardiographic changes:
   a. ST-segment elevation ≥1 mm in two or more contiguous limb leads or ≥2 mm in two or more contiguous precordial leads
   b. New or presumed new left bundle branch block
   c. ST-segment depression with prominent R wave in leads V_2 and V_3 if believed to represent posterior infarction
3. Time from onset of symptoms: <12 hours
4. Age:
   <75 years: definite benefit
   >75 years: benefit less clear

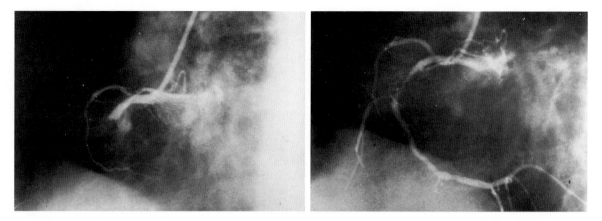

Figure 9–9 Right coronary artery angiogram in a patient with acute inferior MI. The *left panel* demonstrates total occlusion of the right coronary artery. The *right panel* depicts restoration of flow 90 minutes after the intravenous administration of tissue-type plasminogen activator (t-PA).

and serum cardiac enzymes levels should be assessed. If ST-segment elevation in contiguous ECG leads or LBBB is present, subsequent care should be focused on sedation and pain relief, prompt restoration of antegrade flow in the occluded infarct-related coronary artery, and prevention or treatment of immediate and late complications.

A large-bore intravenous line should be introduced for the administration of fluids and medications, and supplemental oxygen should be initiated. Intravenous morphine sulfate should be used to relieve chest pain and to decrease sympathetic stimulation. However, it should be given cautiously because it may cause hypotension, respiratory depression, or bradycardia. The usual dose is 2 to 5 mg every 5 to 10 minutes until chest pain is relieved; systemic arterial pressure should be monitored carefully during its administration. The patient should be kept on bed rest for the first 24 to 48 hours of hospitalization. Intravenous nitroglycerin should be administered to patients with continued chest pain, congestive heart failure, or systemic arterial hypertension. The nitroglycerin infusion should be initiated at 5 to 10 mcg /min and gradually increased until a 10% reduction in systolic arterial pressure in normotensive patients or a 25% to 30% reduction in systolic arterial pressure in hypertensive patients is realized. Nitroglycerin should be avoided in the patient suggested as having right ventricular infarction because a nitroglycerin-induced reduction in preload may cause profound systemic arterial hypotension. The patient with acute MI should receive oral aspirin, 160 to 325 mg, immediately and then daily thereafter because of its effectiveness in reducing mortality. If aspirin is contraindicated (i.e., the occasional patient with a true aspirin allergy), then clopidogrel, 75 mg daily, should be initiated.

Restoration of antegrade flow in the occluded infarct-related artery within 12 hours of pain onset reduces morbidity and mortality. This reduction can be accomplished mechanically with a primary percutaneous coronary intervention or with a pharmacologic intervention using a thrombolytic agent. In general, the restoration of antegrade flow should be attempted with whichever of these can be accomplished safely and expeditiously because a delay in reperfusion increases the extent of myocardial damage and mortality.

A β-blocker should be administered unless contraindicated (i.e., heart rate <60 beats per minute, systolic arterial pressure <100 mm Hg, congestive heart failure or peripheral hypoperfusion, second- or third-degree AV block, severe obstructive lung disease, asthma). In the patient with acute MI, a β-blocker can be administered either within minutes to hours of admission or later (i.e., beyond this time). Intravenous β-blockade, initiated immediately, decreases the incidence of recurrent ischemia and reinfarction. The β-blockers most often used in this setting are metoprolol and atenolol. Each is administered as three 5-mg boluses at 2- to 5-minute intervals to achieve a resting heart rate of <70 beats/min. Oral β-blockade, initiated within several days of MI and continued indefinitely reduces the risk of nonfatal reinfarction and cardiovascular mortality by 20% to 25% when compared with placebo. The specific β-blockers shown to exert this beneficial effect are propranolol, timolol, metoprolol, and atenolol. Although the mechanisms by which β-blockers exert their beneficial effect are not completely understood, they appear to have an anti-arrhythmic and anti-ischemic influence. For the patient in whom β-blockers are contraindicated, verapamil may decrease the incidence of reinfarction and mortality. However, the other calcium antagonists are not beneficial, and the dihydropyridine agents actually increase mortality.

In the patient with congestive heart failure or depressed left ventricular systolic function (ejection fraction <0.40%) without systemic arterial hypotension, the administration of an ACE inhibitor improves outcome. Randomized, placebo-controlled trials have demonstrated that ACE inhibitor therapy with captopril, enalapril, ramipril, trandolapril, or zofenopril begun 24 hours to 16 days after MI limits left ventricular dilation, improves left ventricular ejection fraction, reduces the incidence of reinfarction and heart failure, and improves short- and long-term survival. In two large trials, the administration of ACE inhibitors within 1 day of hospitalization reduced short-term mortality. The recommended initial regimens include captopril (initial dose, 6.25 mg, increased every 6 to 8 hours to a maximum of 50 mg 3 times daily as long as the systolic arterial pressure is >90 to 100 mm Hg); enalapril (initial dose, 2.5 mg/day, gradually increased to 20 mg twice daily), or lisinopril (initial dose 2.5 mg/daily, increased to a maximum of 10 mg/day). ACE inhibitors should not be administered to patients with systemic arterial hypotension (systolic pressure <90 to 100 mm Hg), an allergy to ACE inhibitors, renal failure, a history of bilateral renal arterial stenosis, previous worsening of renal failure with ACE inhibitors, or pregnancy.

During the hours after the initiation of the therapies previously described, the patient should be closely observed for the development of complications related to the MI. Systemic arterial hypotension during the early hours of infarction may be due to intravascular volume depletion, right ventricular infarction, severe left ventricular systolic dysfunction, medications (most notably morphine or nitroglycerin), bradycardia, or tachyarrhythmia. Less commonly, a mechanical complication (e.g., left ventricular free-wall rupture, ventricular septal defect, papillary muscle rupture with resultant mitral regurgitation) can occur within hours of the onset of MI.

Reperfusion Therapy

In patients with STEMI, early restoration of blood flow to the jeopardized myocardium can limit necrosis, improve left ventricular function, and reduce mortality. This can be mechanically accomplished with primary percutaneous intervention or pharmacologically with a thrombolytic agent. If a cardiac catheterization facility is accessible and experienced physicians and personnel can quickly perform primary percutaneous coronary intervention (i.e., within 90 minutes of the patient's arrival), then it is the preferred method of restoring antegrade flow in most patients. On the other hand, if primary percutaneous coronary intervention is not immediately available or the delay in transporting the patient to a catheterization facility would be inordinately long, then thrombolytic therapy should be given. Primary percutaneous coronary intervention is particularly preferable in patients with a contraindication to thrombolytic therapy, in cardiogenic shock, or older than 70 years.

Thrombolytic therapy is very effective in restoring infarct-related artery patency. It should be administered to the patient with STEMI who seeks medical attention at a center without catheterization facilities or appropriately experienced personnel, as well as to the patient with a condition that would make catheterization inappropriate (i.e., allergy to radiographic contrast material, severe renal insufficiency, severe peripheral vascular disease). In the United States, five thrombolytic agents are currently approved for use in patients with STEMI (Table 9–7): (1) streptokinase, (2) anistreplase (anisoylated plasminogen streptokinase activator complex [APSAC]), (3) alteplase (tissue plasminogen activator [t-PA]), (4) reteplase plasminogen activator (r-PA), and (5) tenecteplase tissue plasminogen activator (TNK-tPA). Although slight differences in their effectiveness and bleeding complications have been reported, the choice of agent is less important than the timely decision to administer it.

Streptokinase (1.5 million units) is given as a 1-hour infusion. Rarely, the recipient may experience an acute allergic reaction. Although its administration is frequently associated with mild hypotension, the drop in systemic arterial pressure is rarely of sufficient magnitude to warrant interruption of the infusion. Because antibodies to streptokinase develop within days of its administration, it should not be given to patients who have previously received it or who have had a recent streptococcal infection. APSAC is derived from and has the same limitations as streptokinase, but it is significantly more costly. As a result, it is seldom used.

T-PA and its derivatives r-PA and TNK-tPA are much more expensive than streptokinase and are associated with a

Table 9–7	Dosing Regimens of Commonly Used Thrombolytic Agents
Thrombolytic Agent	**Dosing Regimen**
PA (alteplase)	15 mg bolus IV, followed by 0.75 mg/kg body weight (not to exceed 50 mg) over 30 min, followed by 0.5 mg/kg (not to exceed 35 mg) over 60 min
r-PA (reteplase)	Two 10 U IV boluses, given 30 min apart
TNK-tPA (tenecteplase)	Single bolus IV 0.5 mg/kg (dose rounded to the nearest 5 mg, ranging from 30 to 50 mg)
Streptokinase	1.5 million U IV over 60 min

IV = intravenous; PA = plasminogen activator; r-PA = reteplase plasminogen activator; TNK-tPA = tenecteplase tissue plasminogen activator; U = units.

slightly higher rate of intracranial hemorrhage (0.7% versus 0.5%, respectively). However, they are also more *clot specific* in that they do not cause a generalized fibrinolytic state and are more effective at lysing older thrombi (e.g., those associated with an MI > 4 hours duration). T-PA and its derivatives do not elicit an antibody response or hypotension. T-PA is given as an initial bolus or *front-loaded*, followed by a 90-minute infusion (15 mg as a bolus, another 50 mg infused over 30 minutes, and the remaining 35 mg infused over the next 60 minutes). r-PA is administered as a double bolus (two 10-unit boluses delivered 30 minutes apart), and TNK-tPA is administered as a single bolus (0.5 mg/kg to a maximum of 50 mg). Although r-PA and TNK-tPA are somewhat more likely than t-PA to restore early patency of the infarct-related artery, the mortality rate with these three agents is similar.

Overall, thrombolytic therapy decreases short-term mortality in subjects with STEMI by about 20%. Angiographic studies comparing thrombolytic regimens demonstrate that restoration of blood flow in the infarct-related artery is faster and more complete with t-PA than with streptokinase, and this translates into a modestly decreased mortality rate with t-PA, especially when it is given in a front-loaded fashion. Specifically, in the GUSTO trial, t-PA was associated with a statistically significant 1% absolute reduction in mortality when compared with streptokinase. The majority of this benefit occurred in patients less than 70 years of age within 4 hours of the onset of an anterior STEMI. In older patients, in patients over 4 hours after symptom onset, and in those with an MI in a territory other than the anterior wall, the mortality difference between these two agents was negligible.

The contraindications to thrombolytic therapy are listed in Table 9–8; they identify those with an unacceptably high risk of bleeding complications. The most catastrophic potential complication of thrombolytic therapy is intracranial hemorrhage. This risk is substantially increased in patients

Table 9–8 Contraindications to Thrombolytic Therapy in Acute Myocardial Infarction

Absolute

Aortic dissection
  Acute pericarditis
  Any active bleeding*
  Previous cerebral hemorrhage
  Intracranial neoplasm
  Cerebral aneurysm or arteriovenous malformation
  Recent cerebrovascular accident (within 3 months)

Relative

Bleeding diathesis or coagulopathy
Major surgery, puncture of a noncompressible vessel, or head
  or major body trauma within previous 2 weeks
Nonhemorrhagic stroke or gastrointestinal hemorrhage
  within 6 months
Proliferative retinopathy
Severe uncontrolled hypertension (systolic blood pressure
  >180 mm Hg or diastolic blood pressure >95 mm Hg)
Prolonged cardiopulmonary resuscitation
Pregnancy

*Does not include menstrual bleeding.

Table 9–9 Complications of Acute Myocardial Infarction

Mechanical

Left ventricular failure
Right ventricular failure
Cardiogenic shock
Structure
Free-wall rupture
Ventricular septal defect
Papillary muscle rupture with acute mitral regurgitation

Electrical

Arrhythmias
Bradyarrhythmias
Ventricular ectopy
Tachyarrhythmias (ventricular, supraventricular)
Sudden cardiac death
Conduction abnormalities
First-, second-, and third-degree atrioventricular blocks
Bundle branch and fascicular blocks

with a history of hemorrhagic stroke, uncontrolled hypertension, body weight under 70 kg, and over 65 years of age.

Aspirin is an obligatory adjunct to thrombolysis; its use is associated with an additive benefit on mortality and a decrease in recurrent ischemic events. Intravenous heparin administered for 48 hours is necessary to maintain patency of the infarct-related artery after successful thrombolysis when a t-PA is administered but not with streptokinase. Low–molecular-weight heparin may be slightly more effective than unfractionated heparin as adjunctive therapy after successful thrombolysis. Its use is associated with a higher rate of vessel patency and a lower rate of reocclusion, leading to fewer episodes of recurrent ischemia and infarction, albeit with a somewhat increased risk of hemorrhagic complications.

COMPLICATIONS

The complications of MI may be electrical or mechanical in cause (Table 9–9).

Arrhythmias and Conduction Abnormalities

Cardiac arrhythmias may occur in patients with acute coronary syndromes. Those that cause symptoms or hemody-namic compromise almost always warrant treatment, whereas those who do not often can be managed expectantly. Although most of these arrhythmias are a direct result of the ischemic process, other reversible aggravating factors, such as electrolyte disturbances, hypoxemia, and medication toxicity, must be excluded.

Premature ventricular complexes, ventricular couplets, and nonsustained ventricular tachycardia (VT) occur frequently in the peri-infarction period. Although such ectopy can be effectively suppressed with anti-arrhythmic agents, treatment is not warranted in the absence of symptoms or hemodynamic compromise. The presence of frequent ventricular ectopy does not predict the development of more malignant arrhythmias, and empiric therapy of such ectopy is associated with an increased mortality rate. Accelerated idioventricular rhythm, or *slow VT*, often occurs after successful reperfusion; it does not require treatment.

Over the past several decades, mortality in hospitalized patients with acute MI has substantially declined in large part because of the early recognition and treatment of lethal arrhythmias. Because most deaths from acute MI occur as a result of sustained VT or ventricular fibrillation (VF), these rhythm disturbances should be treated with immediate electrical defibrillation (150 to 360 joules), after which administering intravenous anti-arrhythmic medications (e.g., lidocaine, amiodarone, procainamide) is reasonable for 24 to 48 hours. Sustained but hemodynamically stable VT can be treated initially with anti-arrhythmic agents with electrical cardioversion held in reserve. In the absence of electrolyte abnormalities, polymorphic VT is usually a marker of recurrent or persistent ischemia, and aggressive anti-ischemic treatment is warranted. When sustained VT or VF occurs in the first 48 hours after MI, it does not portend the same poor prognosis as it does when it occurs later.

Transient supraventricular tachyarrhythmias may occur in patients with acute MI, with sinus tachycardia and atrial fibrillation being the most common. The cause of sinus tachycardia (e.g., anxiety, fever, anemia, hypoxemia, hypovolemia, pulmonary vascular congestion, thyrotoxicosis,) should be promptly identified and corrected. If atrial fibrillation is accompanied by a rapid ventricular response, with resultant ongoing ischemia or hemodynamic compromise, then electrical shock cardioversion should be considered. In the patient with atrial fibrillation and a rapid ventricular response, intravenous β-blockers or amiodarone are usually effective for controlling the ventricular response, provided no contraindications to their use exist. Calcium channel-blocking agents are also effective but should be avoided in the patient with heart failure. (These arrhythmias are discussed at length in Chapter 10.)

Bradyarrhythmias may complicate acute MI. The most common bradyarrhythmia is sinus bradycardia, which is observed in 20% to 25% of patients with acute MI and is more common in those with inferior than anterior MI. In patients with inferior MI, sinus bradycardia is often associated with hypotension caused by increased vagal tone as a result of stimulation of vagal afferent fibers in the inferoposterior portion of the left ventricle (Bezold-Jarisch reflex). Unless accompanied by hemodynamic instability, sinus bradycardia should be simply observed. If treatment is necessary, then intravenous atropine (0.5 to 2 mg) should be administered, aiming for a heart rate of 60 beats/min and a resolution of symptoms. Temporary pacing is rarely required.

Ischemia and infarction can result in transient or permanent injury to the conduction system. Varying degrees of AV block may occur in patients with acute MI. Ischemia of the AV node can result in first-degree or Mobitz type II second-degree (Wenckebach phenomenon) AV block. These rhythms are most often associated with inferior MI; they are transient, do not adversely affect survival, and do not require treatment unless the ventricular rate is sufficiently slow to produce syncope, congestive heart failure, or angina. Mobitz type II second-degree AV block is a rare complication of acute MI (1% of cases) and usually results from injury to the His-Purkinje system in the setting of an extensive anterior MI. It often is associated with progression to complete or third-degree AV block and is an indication for temporary transvenous or transcutaneous pacing in anticipation of implantation of a permanent pacemaker. Complete or third-degree AV block may occur with inferior or anterior MI. When it occurs in the setting of an inferior MI, the block is usually at the level of the AV node. It is associated with a stable escape rhythm and tends to be transient, although it may take up to 2 weeks to resolve. As a result, treatment with only a temporary and not a permanent pacemaker is usually required. In contrast, when complete AV block occurs in the setting of an anterior MI, the His-Purkinje system is usually involved. The block is usually permanent, and a permanent pacemaker should be implanted.

Block in one or more branches of the conduction system may occur with acute MI and is more common with anterior than with inferior infarction. Patients with isolated left anterior or left posterior fascicular block or right bundle branch block (RBBB) do not require specific therapy. Conversely, temporary pacing is suggested in patients with new bifascicular blocks (e.g., LBBB or RBBB with left anterior or left posterior fascicular block) because progression to complete heart block is common. If bifascicular block persists after an MI, a permanent pacemaker should be placed.

Pump Failure

Patients who die of cardiac failure after acute MI have extensive myocardial necrosis with loss of at least 40% of the functioning left ventricular muscle mass, either as a consequence of new infarction or a combination of old and new infarctions.

The patient with an acute MI and no evidence on physical examination or chest x-ray studies of left ventricular failure has an excellent prognosis, with only a 2% to 5% in-hospital mortality rate (Killip class I). The individual with some evidence of pulmonary vascular congestion (e.g., basilar rales, S_3, radiographic evidence of pulmonary venous congestion) is classified as Killip class II and has a short-term mortality rate of 10% to 15%. In the patient with overt pulmonary edema evidenced on physical examination or chest x-ray studies, mortality rate is 20% to 30% (Killip class III). Finally, the patient with cardiogenic shock is said to be Killip class IV and has a mortality rate of 50% to 60% even with maximal therapy. In these individuals, infarction is associated with systemic arterial hypotension and diminished peripheral perfusion, as manifested by mental confusion, cold and clammy skin, peripheral cyanosis, and oliguria. Hemodynamically, the systemic arterial systolic pressure is <90 mm Hg, the cardiac index is <1.8 L/min/m^2, the systemic arteriolar resistance is greatly increased (>2000 dynes/sec/cm^5), and the left ventricular filling pressure is elevated (>20 mm Hg). The reduced systemic arterial pressure further diminishes coronary arterial perfusion pressure, thereby increasing myocardial ischemia. The low cardiac output and systemic arterial pressure induce an intense sympathetic discharge that produces peripheral vasoconstriction, further decreasing tissue perfusion and causing a systemic lactic acidosis, which depresses myocardial function. In response to a reduced cardiac output, the heart rate increases, thereby increasing myocardial oxygen demand. As left ventricular filling pressure rises, subendocardial perfusion is further compromised. In short, the hemodynamic and metabolic consequences of cardiogenic shock cause worsening myocardial ischemic injury, which, in turn, leads to worsening left ventricular dysfunction. A cycle of severe hemodynamic impairment and deteriorating myocardial oxygenation is established.

The therapy of the patient with an acute MI and resultant left ventricular dysfunction depends on the extent of such dysfunction. The normotensive individual with symptoms and signs of Killip class II congestive heart failure (i.e., mild orthopnea, basilar rales, S_3) usually responds to bed rest, salt restriction, a loop diuretic, and low-dose vasodilator therapy with an ACE inhibitor. Additional therapy with digitalis or other inotropic agents is not usually necessary nor is invasive hemodynamic monitoring. The management of the patient with more severe heart failure (Killip class III or IV) should be based on a careful assessment of hemodynamic variables obtained with a balloon-tipped flotation catheter in the pulmonary artery and an intra-arterial cannula. Adequate oxygenation should be ensured by continuous pulse oximetry with supplemental oxygen or ventilator support as needed. Placement of a urinary catheter enables the urine output to be assessed accurately, and endotracheal intubation and assisted ventilation may reduce the work of breathing and improve tissue oxygenation. Intravenous furosemide should be administered in an attempt to reduce the pulmonary capillary wedge pressure in the range of 18 to 20 mm Hg; this appears to be the optimal preload in the setting of acute MI. In the normotensive individual, vasodilator therapy with nitroglycerin should be instituted to reduce afterload, increase cardiac output, and lower left ventricular filling pressure. The resultant decrease in left ventricular wall stress reduces myocardial oxygen requirements, improves subendocardial perfusion, and helps relieve ischemia. Nitroglycerin should be administered to avoid an excessive reduction in systemic arterial pressure, which may compromise myocardial perfusion, while keeping pulmonary capillary wedge pressure in the range of 18 to 20 mm Hg. The patient with heart failure and hypotension or an inadequate response to diuretics and vasodilators (i.e., cardiac output <1.8 to 2.0 L/min/m², pulmonary capillary wedge pressure >20 mm Hg) should be treated with intravenous inotropic agents (e.g., dopamine or dobutamine, depending on the systemic arterial pressure). If the patient is normotensive or only mildly hypotensive, then dobutamine is the preferred inotropic agent. Dopamine should be reserved for the patient with more severe hypotension because it may increase pulmonary capillary wedge pressure.

In the patient with severe heart failure or cardiogenic shock, a careful search for a potentially correctable cause should be undertaken. Two-dimensional and color Doppler echocardiography, which can rapidly be performed at the bedside, will allow the clinician to determine whether the shock is due to extensive left ventricular dysfunction or a mechanical problem, such as acute mitral regurgitation, acute ventricular septal defect, extensive right ventricular infarction, or a contained rupture of the left ventricular free wall (see "Mechanical Complications").

Patients with shock who are examined within the first few hours of the onset of MI should be considered for immediate reperfusion therapy. Thrombolytic agents appear to be less effective in opening the occluded infarct-related artery in the patient with cardiogenic shock, and these agents have not convincingly exerted a beneficial effect in such patients. Conversely, early coronary revascularization within 12 hours of the onset of cardiogenic shock, accomplished percutaneously or surgically, has been shown to improve in-hospital and 1-year survival when applied to patients under 75 years of age. For the patient 75 years or older with cardiogenic shock after acute MI, early revascularization does not improve the short- or long-term outcome.

By reducing afterload and increasing myocardial perfusion pressure, intra-aortic balloon counterpulsation may be effective in stabilizing the patient with cardiogenic shock. Although initial hemodynamic improvement in this setting may be dramatic, balloon counterpulsation alone probably does not improve the poor prognosis associated with cardiogenic shock. Rather, counterpulsation should be considered a supportive measure in patients with potentially reversible abnormalities before cardiac catheterization, cardiac surgery, or, in some cases, cardiac transplantation.

Right Ventricular Infarction

Right ventricular infarction usually occurs in association with inferior MI because the blood supply to both of these areas usually comes from the right coronary artery. The presence of a concomitant right ventricular infarction substantially increases the mortality of an inferior MI. Right ventricular MI results in the clinical picture of hypotension, clear lungs (i.e., normal pulmonary capillary wedge pressure), and prominent jugular venous distension. In the absence of hemodynamic measurements, right ventricular infarction may be confused with hypovolemia, pulmonary embolism, or cardiac tamponade. In fact, the patient with acute right ventricular failure may have a prominent *y* descent in the atrial pressure tracing (Fig. 9–10), a Kussmaul's sign, and pulsus paradoxus, all of which mimic pericardial tamponade. Demonstrating ST-segment elevation in the right precordial leads (e.g., >0.1 mV elevation in V_4R) confirms the diagnosis of right ventricular infarction. For this reason, a right-sided precordial ECG should be obtained in all patients with inferior MI. The treatment of hypotension in the patient with right ventricular infarction often requires rapid intravascular volume repletion and inotropic agents (e.g., dobutamine). Diuretic and vasodilator (e.g., nitroglycerin) therapy should be avoided because they may provoke hypotension in this setting. If the patient can be supported during the first few days of hemodynamic

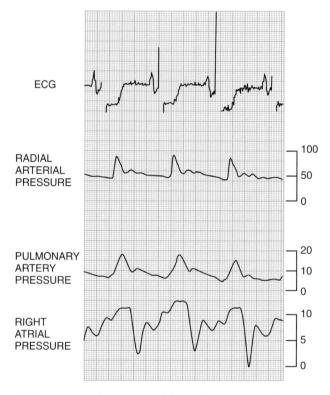

Figure 9–10 Electrocardiographic (ECG), arterial, and Swan-Ganz bedside catheter recordings in a patient with right ventricular infarction. Hypotension is present, and cardiac output, estimated by thermodilution (*not shown*), is reduced. The pulmonary arterial pressures are normal, whereas the right atrial pressure is elevated, and it demonstrates a prominent *y* descent.

instability, then considerable improvement in right ventricular function often occurs.

Mechanical Complications

Mechanical complications of acute MI include papillary muscle rupture, ventricular septal defect, and ventricular free-wall rupture. Patients with these complications frequently experience hemodynamic collapse 3 to 5 days after acute MI. These complications are associated with very high mortality rates; they account for approximately 15% of the mortality from acute MI. Thrombolytic therapy appears to hasten the appearance of these complications but does not clearly increase their incidence.

Papillary muscle rupture results in acute mitral regurgitation. The resultant sudden increase in left atrial volume causes a significantly elevated left atrial pressure, with resultant pulmonary edema. Papillary muscle rupture occurs most commonly with inferior MI because the posteromedial papillary muscle usually has a single source of blood supply from the right coronary artery. Conversely, the anterolateral papillary muscle has a dual blood supply. A loud, apical holosystolic murmur is usually audible, although an occasional patient with severe mitral regurgitation has no audible murmur. The diagnosis may be rapidly confirmed with transthoracic echocardiography or right-heart ventricular catheterization, with the latter demonstrating large *v* waves in the pulmonary capillary wedge tracing in the absence of an oxygen *step-up* in the right ventricle.

An acute ventricular septal defect may occur after anterior or inferior MI. On physical examination a harsh holosystolic murmur is audible at the left lower sternal border, which may be difficult to differentiate from acute mitral regurgitation; this murmur is often accompanied by a palpable thrill. The diagnosis can be confirmed by obtaining blood samples from each of the cardiac chambers during right-heart ventricular catheterization and by demonstrating a higher oxygen saturation in the samples obtained from the right ventricle or pulmonary artery than those obtained from the right atrium (e.g., oxygen *step up*). Specifically, an increase in oxygen saturation of >6% between the right atrium and pulmonary artery strongly suggests the presence of a ventricular septal defect with concomitant left-to-right shunting. Doppler echocardiography also allows visualization of left-to-right shunting of blood through the ventricular septal defect.

Treatment of acute papillary muscle rupture or ventricular septal defect includes inotropic agents, vasodilators, and intra-aortic balloon counterpulsation. These temporizing measures help prepare the patient for urgent cardiac surgery to repair the ventricular septal defect or replace the mitral valve.

Free-wall rupture of the left ventricle almost always results in hemopericardium, cardiac tamponade, and electromechanical dissociation. Survival is uncommon and depends on prompt recognition and emergent surgical repair. In an occasional patient, a pseudoaneurysm, or false aneurysm, develops when free-wall rupture occurs, so that the rupture is confined by the adherent pericardium, organized thrombus, and hematoma. Because the wall of the pseudoaneurysm contains no myocardium, it may rupture at a later date. The pseudoaneurysm maintains continuity with the left ventricular cavity through a narrow connecting orifice (e.g., neck). In contrast, a true aneurysm represents an area of infarcted myocardium that has become thinned and dilated through a process of ventricular remodeling. True aneurysms have a wide orifice or neck, their walls always contain some myocardial elements, and they rarely rupture. Pseudoaneurysms should undergo prompt surgical resection because of the risk for rupture. Conversely, a true aneurysm does not require surgical resection.

Prospectus for the Future

1. New methods are needed to identify patients at risk for CAD using genomics and/or proteomics and to treat them (e.g., raising HDL level, lowering hsCRP level, targeting antiplatelet therapy) to reduce cardiac events.
2. Evaluation is needed to compare the efficacy and safety of drug-eluting stents (e.g., rapamycin, tacrolimus, taxol) with CABG for patients needing coronary revascularization.
3. Development of regional cardiac centers is necessary to provide reperfusion therapy for patients with acute MI who enter a hospital that does not have a catheterization laboratory.
4. Examination of the usefulness of facilitated reperfusion strategies (e.g., administration of full- or partial-dose thrombolytic therapy) is needed before primary percutaneous coronary intervention.

References

Antman EM, Anbe DT, Armstrong PW, et al: ACC/AHA guidelines for management of patients with ST-elevation myocardial infarction. Circulation 110:588–636, 2004.

Braunwald E, Antman EM, Beasley JW, et al: ACC/AHA 2002 guideline update for the management of patients with unstable angina and non–ST-segment elevation myocardial infarction—summary article. J Am Coll Cardiol 40:1366–1374, 2002.

Eagle KA, Guyton RA, Davidoff R, et al: ACC/AHA 2004 guideline update for coronary artery bypass graft surgery. Circulation 110: e340-e437, 2004.

Gibbons RJ, Abrams J, Chatterjee K, et al: ACC/AHA 2002 guideline update for the management of patients with chronic stable angina. Circulation 107:149–158, 2002.

Gibler WB, Cannon CP, Blomkalns AL, et al: Practical implementation of the guidelines for unstable angina/non–ST-segment elevation myocardial infarction in the emergency department. Circulation 111:2699–2710, 2005.

Klocke FJ, Baird MG, Lorell BH, et al: ACC/AHA/ASNC guidelines for the clinical use of cardiac radionuclide imaging. Circulation 108:1404–1418, 2003.

Lauer M, Froelicher ES, Williams M, et al: Exercise testing in asymptomatic adults: A statement for professionals from the American Heart Association Council on Clinical Cardiology. Circulation 112:771–776, 2005.

Scanlon PJ, Faxon DP, Audet AM, et al: ACC/AHA guidelines for coronary angiography. J Am Coll Cardiol 33:1756–1824, 1999.

Smith SC Jr, Dove JT, Jacobs AK, et al: ACC/AHA guidelines for percutaneous coronary interventions. J Am Coll Cardiol 37:2215–2239, 2001.

Chapter 10

Cardiac Arrhythmias

Mohamed H. Hamdan

Cardiac Action Potential and Normal Conduction

The electrical activity of a single cardiac cell can be recorded with the aid of a microelectrode and demonstrates that the resting potential of a myocyte is −80 to −90 mV. This resting potential is maintained by the accumulation of potassium inside the cell and the removal of sodium from the cell by the energy-requiring sodium-potassium adenosine triphosphatase (Na^+,K^+-ATPase). When a cardiac myocyte is depolarized to below threshold level (threshold potential), an action potential is produced by a complex series of ionic shifts (Fig. 10–1A). The action potential can be divided into five phases. Phase 0 is the rapid initial depolarization and is mediated by an increased permeability of the sarcolemma to sodium ions. This phase is followed by phase 1, an early, rapid, repolarization resulting from the movement of potassium out of the cell. The plateau phase (phase 2) of the action potential is mainly determined by the inward movement of calcium ions but also by the movement of sodium, chloride, and potassium ions. Phase 3 constitutes the repolarization phase of the action potential and is the result of the movement of potassium ions out of the cell. Phase 4 of the action potential represents the outward flow of potassium and the inward flow of sodium and results in the gradual depolarization of the cell from resting to threshold potential (see Fig. 10–1B). During the action potential and shortly thereafter, a period occurs during which an adequate depolarizing stimulus fails to elicit an action potential. This period is termed the *absolute refractory period* and is most closely related to the duration of phase 3 of the action potential.

The appearance of the action potential of sinus and atrioventricular (AV) nodal cells is different from that of the typical myocyte. The normal resting potential of these cells is higher (−60 mV), the initial upstroke of depolarization is slower and calcium dependent, and the phase 4 depolarization is highly pronounced (see Fig. 10–1B). The slope of the phase 4 depolarization determines the rate at which a cell will spontaneously depolarize (automaticity) until it reaches threshold potential, thus generating an action potential that is then propagated to surrounding cells. The sinus node usually has the fastest phase 4 depolarization and thus functions as the normal pacemaker of the heart, producing a rate of contraction (heart rate) of 60 to 100 beats/min. If the sinus node fails, the AV node has the next fastest pacemaker rate (approximately 50 beats/min). The ventricular myocytes have slow phase 4 depolarization and produce a heart rate of 30 to 40 beats/min if higher pacemakers fail. When a lower pacemaker focus appropriately fires in the setting of slowing of the higher focus, the firing is termed an *escape beat* (if single) or an *escape rhythm* (if sustained).

The autonomic nervous system has important effects on the generation and propagation of cardiac impulses. The sinus and AV nodes are the most richly innervated regions of the heart and are most affected by changes in autonomic tone. Sympathetic stimulation, either directly from sympathetic nerve endings in the heart or indirectly by means of circulating catecholamines, increases the heart rate by increasing the rate of phase 4 depolarization and also increases intercellular conduction velocity. Parasympathetic stimulation has the opposite effects. Vagal tone is, in part, controlled by the baroreceptors of the carotid sinus and aortic arch and responds to increases in blood pressure by increasing vagal output, with a resulting decrease in heart rate and AV nodal conduction velocity.

The normal cardiac impulse starts at the sinoatrial node, passes through the atria to the AV node, where it slows, and then continues down the His-Purkinje system to the ventricular myocardium, where the wave of depolarization terminates because no further tissue exists to depolarize. Further conduction occurs only after a new impulse is formed in the sinoatrial node.

Cardiac Arrhythmias

Cardiac arrhythmias result from disorders of (1) *impulse formation* and/or (2) *impulse conduction.* Disorders of impulse formation include enhanced or abnormal automaticity and triggered activity. Disorders of impulse conduction include conduction block with or without re-entry (defined later). One or more of the previously

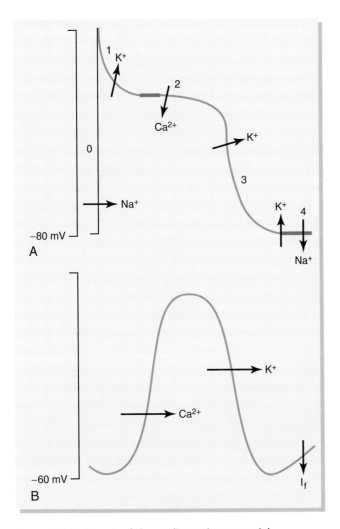

Figure 10–1 Genesis of the cardiac action potential.
A, Ventricular action potential with predominant ionic
currents. *B*, Sinus node action potential with predominant
ionic currents. See text for details. Ca^{2+} = calcium;
1_f = hyperpolarization-activated current; K^+ = potassium;
mV = millivolt; Na^+ = sodium.

described electrophysiologic mechanisms can explain most
cardiac arrhythmias.

DISORDERS OF IMPULSE FORMATION

Cardiac depolarization is driven by the sinus node (normal
pacemaker), which is located in the high right atrium along
the cristae terminalis. This waveform propagates down the
AV node and His-Purkinje system, resulting in synchronized
activation of both ventricles. Subsidiary pacemakers with a
lower discharge rate are mainly present in the AV junction
and the His-Purkinje system. These pacemakers do not reach
threshold because of overdrive suppression by the sinus
node. However, under certain conditions, such as sinus node
slowing or conduction block, these pacemaker sites may
become active and discharge at their normal rate.

Enhanced automaticity refers to pacemaker cells discharging at a rate faster than their normal rate. By definition, these
cells have intrinsic automaticity (slow response type of

action potential; see Fig. 10–1*B*), but under certain conditions (partial depolarization, decrease in threshold, or
increase in the slope of phase 4), the automaticity rate is
enhanced. *Abnormal automaticity* refers to spontaneous
depolarization resulting in impulse formation in cardiac
tissues that lack intrinsic automaticity (fast response type of
action potential; see Fig. 10–1*A*). Under certain conditions,
these cells may show spontaneous automaticity, resulting in
premature depolarizations, which, if repetitive, can lead to
tachycardia. Singular premature atrial or ventricular depolarizations may arise by this mechanism. Some sustained
rhythms, including ectopic atrial tachycardia, accelerated
junctional or idioventricular rhythms, and some forms of
ventricular tachycardia (VT), may also result from increased
automaticity. Ischemia, digoxin, methylxanthine toxicity,
electrolyte abnormalities, and high catecholamine states are
well-known causes of abnormal and enhanced automaticity.

Triggered activity means impulse initiation caused by
afterdepolarizations. Afterdepolarizations are oscillations in
membrane potentials that occur after the upstroke of the
action potential. If the amplitude is large enough to reach
threshold, afterdepolarizations can generate a subsequent
action potential. By definition, afterdepolarizations must be
preceded by at least one action potential, thus the term triggered activity. They do not occur spontaneously but, rather,
are triggered by prior activation of the heart. When afterdepolarizations occur during repolarization, they are called
early afterdepolarizations (EADs). EADs are usually exacerbated by hypokalemia or potassium-channel blockade or
drugs and may be catecholamine driven or provoked by a
critical heart rate. EADs may also occur spontaneously in
patients with congenital long QT syndrome (LQTS). When
afterdepolarizations occur after full repolarization, they are
called *delayed afterdepolarizations* (DADs). DADs are more
pronounced at fast heart rates, are facilitated by intracellular calcium overload, and account for the mechanism underlying most digoxin-toxic rhythms. They are usually caused
by ischemia, catecholamines, and digitalis.

DISORDERS OF IMPULSE CONDUCTION

Disorders of impulse conduction include conduction block
with or without *reentry*. Reentry is the most common mechanism of arrhythmogenesis. During reentry, a depolarization
propagates in one direction while blocking in adjacent tissue,
returns to depolarize the area not initially excited, and, if
successful, will travel around repeating its course. Therefore,
three criteria are needed for reentry to be present: (1) two
available pathways, (2) unidirectional block in one and (3)
conduction delay in the other with return excitation. Based
on these general concepts, three types of reentry have been
described: (1) anatomic, (2) functional (leading circle or
reentry), and (3) reentry by reflection. Describing these
mechanisms in detail is not the purpose of this chapter;
however, it should be emphasized that the presence of a discrete anatomic obstacle (such as a scar) is not always needed
for reentry, given that conduction delay and block can be
caused by many factors, including differences in refractoriness, ischemia, fibrosis, electrolyte abnormalities, and drug
toxicity. An example of reentry in which two distinct pathways are present is provided in Figure 10–2. Pathway A conducts rapidly but has a relatively long refractory period.

Pathway B conducts slowly but has a relatively short refractory period. In the usual state (see Fig. 10–2A), an impulse enters the two pathways by means of a proximal common pathway. Conduction occurs rapidly down pathway A and, after reaching the distal common pathway, continues distally and proceeds retrograde up pathway B until it intercepts the slow antegrade impulse traveling down this pathway and is extinguished. The surface electrocardiogram (ECG) may appear normal, without evidence of the dual pathways. If a premature depolarization occurs, it also enters the two pathways through the proximal common pathway. If it occurs early enough, it is unable to conduct down pathway A because of the long refractory period of this path (see Fig. 10–2B). The impulse therefore travels down pathway B, which has the short refractory period, and reaches the distal common pathway, where it continues distally. However, because pathway B conducts relatively slowly, by the time the impulse reaches the distal aspect of pathway A, this path is no longer refractory, and the impulse rapidly conducts in a retrograde direction up pathway A, reenters the loop by means of pathway B, and conducts retrograde up the proximal common pathway. If the reentrant circuit is in the AV node, the resulting surface ECG demonstrates a premature complex, initiating a tachycardia, and retrograde P waves may be seen.

Reentry can occur at any point along the normal conduction system, including the sinoatrial node, the AV node, and atrial or ventricular myocardium. It may occur in a small focus of cardiac tissue such as the AV node (a micro-reentrant circuit) or involve anatomically distinct pathways such as bypass tracts (a macro-reentrant circuit).

As stated previously, cardiac arrhythmias are the result of disorders in impulse formation and/or impulse conduction with reentry being the most common underlying mechanism. Clinically, cardiac arrhythmias can be divided into three categories: (1) premature beats, (2) bradyarrhythmias (slow heart rates), and (3) tachyarrhythmias (fast heart rates).

I. Premature Beats

ATRIAL PREMATURE COMPLEXES

An atrial premature complex (APC) is defined as a premature activation of the atria arising from a site other than the sinus node. APCs appear on the surface ECG as P waves with morphologic characteristics different from those of the sinus P wave occurring before the anticipated sinus beat (Fig. 10–3A). An APC may conduct with a short, normal, or prolonged PR interval, or it may not conduct at all. The PR interval is determined by the site of origin and the degree of prematurity. If conducted, an APC may be associated with either a normal or a wide (aberrant) QRS complex. Distinguishing aberrant APCs from ventricular premature depolarizations may be difficult. The presence of a full compensatory pause (RR interval surrounding the APC = twice sinus cycle length) suggests lack of sinus node resetting, thus favoring a ventricular rather than an atrial site of origin. Because the right bundle branch has a longer refractory period than the left bundle branch, an early APC is more likely to conduct with right bundle branch block (RBBB) aberrancy. When nonconducted, an APC may produce only

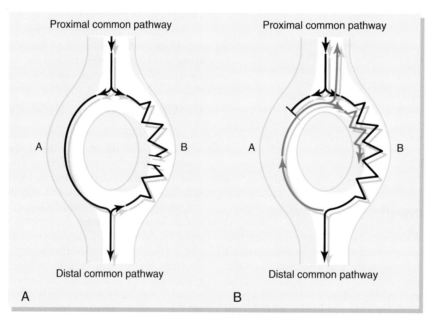

Figure 10–2 Mechanism of reentry. Reentry requires two distinct pathways with disparate conductive and repolarizing properties. *A,* An impulse enters the two pathways and conducts rapidly down pathway A and slowly down pathway B. When the impulse reaches the distal common pathway, it proceeds distally, as well as traveling retrograde up pathway B, where it is extinguished, owing to collision with the antegrade depolarization in this pathway. *B,* A premature depolarization enters the pathways but is blocked in pathway A, owing to the long refractory period of this pathway. The impulse travels down pathway B (slow conducting and rapidly repolarizing) to the distal common pathway, where it proceeds distally as well as traveling up pathway A, which by then is fully repolarized and able to conduct in a retrograde fashion, allowing the impulse to reenter the loop and produce the reciprocating rhythm.

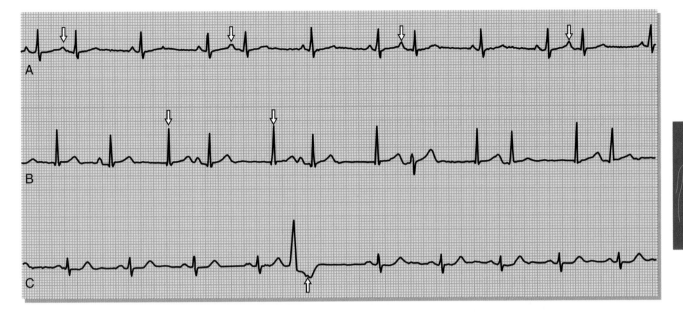

Figure 10–3 Premature complexes. *A,* Atrial premature complexes (APCs) with a trigeminal rhythm. An atrial premature beat occurs after every two sinus beats. Note the presence of a P wave *(arrows)* preceding the QRS complex with a long PR interval caused by decremental conduction in the AV node. The QRS complex is narrow because the origin of the impulse is supraventricular. *B,* Junctional premature complexes (JPCs) *(arrows)*. JPCs often conduct in a retrograde fashion, resulting in a P wave that is buried in the QRS complex. Similar to APCs, the QRS complex is narrow because the origin of the impulse is supraventricular. *C,* Ventricular premature complexes (VPCs). Note the wide QRS morphology and the presence of a retrograde P wave. PVCs might conduct retrograde resulting in a P wave that follows the QRS.

as a small deformity on the T wave followed by a pause. The pause is the result of sinus node resetting, which is common with APCs regardless whether conducted or not.

Twenty-four hour Holter studies have shown that APC frequency increases with age. APCs occur in patients with normal hearts but appear to be more frequent in patients with structural heart disease such as chronic renal failure and chronic pulmonary disease. APCs have been shown to increase in the early stages of a myocardial infarction (MI), with a subsequent decrease in frequency after 10 days. This characteristic may be related to atrial ischemia, increased filling pressures, or the increased-catecholamine state often seen during MI. APCs also appear to be frequent in the setting of pericarditis.

The most common symptoms include palpitations, or the sensation of skipped beats. Dizziness and heart failure–like symptoms might occur in the setting of atrial bigeminy with nonconducted atrial premature beats. Therapy is aimed at treating the underlying disease and eliminating factors that are known to cause ectopic beats such as alcohol and caffeine intake. In symptomatic, beta-blockers should be the first line of therapy followed by calcium channel blockers and class IC agents such as flecainide and propafenone. Class III agents such as sotalol and amiodarone should be avoided because of pro-arrhythmia risks.

JUNCTIONAL PREMATURE COMPLEXES

A junctional premature complex (JPC) refers to a premature beat originating from the AV junction area, which includes the AV node, the peri-nodal area, and the His bundle. After impulse formation, propagation occurs both in the ante-

grade direction down the His bundles and in the retrograde direction up to the atria. The result is near simultaneous atrial and ventricular depolarization with a surface P wave buried in the QRS complex (see Fig. 10–3B). At times, retrograde atrial activation precedes ventricular activation, resulting in a PR interval as long as 90 ms. This action is more common when the impulse originates from a peri-nodal site. When the impulse originates from the His bundle itself, retrograde atrial activation always follows ventricular depolarization, resulting in a retrograde P wave that follows the QRS complex. On some occasions, the impulse fails to propagate in the antegrade direction, resulting in a retrograde P wave that mimics an APC. When a JPC fails to conduct in the retrograde direction, the result is a QRS complex without a P wave. Finally, the impulse might not conduct in either direction but may affect the conduction of subsequent impulses (concealed JPCs), resulting in AV block. In such instances, the diagnosis is based on the presence of manifest JPC in a patient with otherwise normal QRS duration and evidence of intermittent AV block. The mechanism of JPC is believed to be abnormal automaticity, although triggered activity may also be a potential mechanism. They can occur in both normal and abnormal hearts. JPCs are more common in the setting of digitalis toxicity, high-catecholamine states, hypokalemia, and MI.

Most patients with JPCs are asymptomatic. When symptoms occur, skipped beats and palpitations are the most common complaints. More severe symptoms such as dizziness, near syncope, and syncope might occur if the patient has AV block caused by concealed JPCs. Management of JPCs should be focused on correcting the underlying problems. In symptomatic patients with no underlying cause, beta-blockers are often helpful in suppressing JPCs. Classes I and III antiarrhythmic drugs should only be used in patients with symptoms refractory to beta-blocker therapy. In patients with AV block secondary to concealed JPCs, therapy should be aimed at suppressing the junctional beats rather than implanting a pacemaker.

VENTRICULAR PREMATURE COMPLEXES

A ventricular premature complex (VPC) refers to a premature depolarization originating from the ventricles. The impulse often does not conduct to the atria and thus does not reset the sinus node. The result is a wide QRS complex with a compensatory pause (see Fig. 10–3C). When retrograde conduction occurs and the sinus node is reset, a noncompensatory pause will be inscribed. A VPC that occurs very early and fails to affect both the next ventricular depolarization and sinus node activity is referred to as interpolated VPC. With an interpolated VPC, the RR interval surrounding the VPC is equal to the sinus RR interval. A supraventricular premature beat may conduct with aberrancy, resulting in a wide QRS complex similar to a VPC. Criteria in favor of a ventricular origin include (1) the absence of a preceding P wave, (2) AV dissociation, (3) marked left axis deviation, (4) a QRS interval longer than 160 ms, (5) certain configurational characteristics such as Rsr' in lead V1, QS or rS in lead V6, and concordance (upright or downward QRSs in all precordial leads), and, finally, (6) the presence of a full compensatory pause. VPCs occur in patients with normal and abnormal hearts. The underlying mechanisms include reentry, abnormal automaticity, and triggered activity.

When associated with symptoms, patients with VPCs often complain of *skipped* beats and palpitations. The presence of frequent VPCs such as in a bigeminal rhythm (VPCs alternating with sinus beats) can significantly lower the effective heart rate, resulting in a low cardiac output state. In such instances, symptoms might include dizziness, near syncope, and syncope. In addition to the presence of symptoms, VPCs can have an impact on prognosis and risk of sudden death. Although VPCs have no prognostic significance in patients with normal hearts, their presence in patients with heart disease is often associated with poor outcome. In patients with a history of MI, the presence of VPCs increases mortality. Suppression of VPCs with antiarrhythmic drugs, however, has not been shown to reduce mortality. In the Cardiac Arrhythmia Suppression Trial (CAST), randomization of patients with a history of MI, ventricular arrhythmias, and documented arrhythmia suppression with flecainide or encainide showed increased mortality. The largest trial that assessed the effect of amiodarone on the risk of arrhythmic death among MI survivors with frequent VPCs was the Canadian Amiodarone Myocardial Infraction Arrhythmia Trial (CAMIAT). The consensus from this trial was that, unlike other anti-arrhythmic drugs, amiodarone was not associated with excess risk of death. At present, the first drug of choice for the treatment of symptomatic VPCs should be a beta-blocker. If beta-blocker therapy fails, amiodarone or catheter ablation should be considered. With catheter ablation, the VPC site of origin is identified, and radiofrequency energy is applied to eliminate the ectopy. Both amiodarone therapy and catheter ablation

should only be considered in patients who continue to have symptomatic VPCs despite beta-blocker therapy. In the asymptomatic patient, no drug therapy is needed.

II. Bradyarrhythmias

Bradyarrhythmias are usually the result of either *sinus node dysfunction* or *atrioventricular block*.

SINUS NODE DYSFUNCTION

Sinus node dysfunction may be exhibited as sinus bradycardia, sinus pauses or arrest, or sinoatrial exit block. Patients with sinus node disease may have lightheadedness, dizziness, near syncope, or syncope, or may not have any symptoms at all.

Sinus bradycardia indicates, by definition, a sinus rate less than 60 beats/min (Fig. 10–4A). The diagnosis of sinus node disease requires that secondary causes be excluded. Increases in vagal tone are frequently seen in young healthy athletes and are a common cause of sinus node slowing. Increased vagal tone also occurs during carotid sinus massage, Valsalva maneuvers, vomiting, increased intracranial pressure, and vasovagal syncope. Other causes of sinus bradycardia include drugs (digitalis, beta-blockers, calcium channel blockers, and some anti-arrhythmic agents such as sotalol and amiodarone), hyperkalemia, hypothyroidism, and hypothermia. Sinus bradycardia also occurs in the setting of many organic heart diseases, including coronary artery disease, cardiomyopathy, and myocarditis.

Sinus pause is the result of transient failure of impulse formation in the sinus node. When this inactivity is prolonged, it is called *sinus arrest*. Both conditions are visualized on the ECG as a flat line with no P waves. Depending on the duration of sinus node inactivity, the pause may be terminated by a junctional or ventricular escape beat. Sinus pause or arrest should be differentiated from (1) nonconducted atrial premature beats and (2) sinoatrial exit block (see later discussion). A nonconducted APC usually shows as a small deformity on the T wave (see Fig. 10–4B). Causes of sinus pauses and sinus arrest are similar to those of sinus bradycardia.

Sinoatrial exit block is the result of abnormal transmission between the sinus node and the atrium. Several types of sinoatrial conduction block exist (see later discussion). Because sinoatrial electrograms are not routinely available, only second-degree sinoatrial block might be diagnosed from the surface ECG. Second-degree (Type II) sinoatrial exit block is usually inferred by the presence of a pause equal to a multiple of the basic PP interval (see Fig. 10–4C). In some instances, the Wenckebach phenomenon (second-degree [Type I]) is observed, resulting in progressive shortening of the PP interval before seeing the absence of a P wave (see Fig. 10–4D). Patients with sinoatrial exit block often have other arrhythmias, including atrial fibrillation, atrial tachycardia (tachycardia-bradycardia syndrome) (see Fig. 10–4E), sinus bradycardia, and AV block.

ATRIOVENTRICULAR BLOCK

The sinus impulse has to traverse the atrium, the AV node, and the His-Purkinje system before reaching the ventricles.

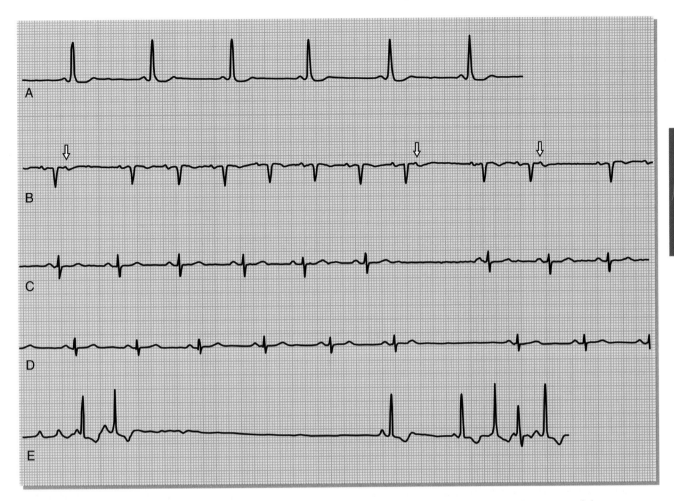

Figure 10–4 Sinus node disturbances. *A,* Sinus bradycardia at a rate of 49 beats/min in a patient receiving metoprolol. *B,* Nonconducted APCs. Note the small deformity on the T wave *(arrows)* caused by the APCs. The following pause is caused by resetting of the sinus node. *C,* Sinoatrial exit (second-degree type II) block. Note that the pause is equal to a multiple of the basic PP interval (twice). *D,* Sinoatrial exit (Wenckebach) block. Note the progressive shortening of the PP interval before seeing the absence of a P wave. *E,* Sick sinus syndrome. Coarse AF was followed by a prolonged spontaneous period of asystole before restoration of sinus rhythm *(tachy-brady* syndrome).

This interval is reflected on the ECG as the PR interval. Conduction delay or block can occur at any level, resulting in various types of AV block. AV block is classified into (1) first-degree AV block, (2) second-degree AV block (types I and II), and (3) third-degree AV block.

First-degree AV block occurs when enough prolongation in AV conduction occurs, resulting in a PR interval greater than 200 ms (Fig. 10–5A). Despite the prolonged PR interval, each P wave is followed by a QRS interval. In patients with first-degree AV block and a narrow QRS complex, the site of block is usually in the AV node. In the setting of a wide QRS complex, the site of block can be at any level but remains most commonly at the level of the AV node. A PR interval longer than 290 ms is almost always associated with AV nodal disease.

Second-degree AV block is associated with intermittent failure of the P wave to be conducted to the ventricles. The ratio of P waves to QRS complexes may vary in the same patient. Two types of second-degree AV block have been classified: *type I,* also called Mobitz 1 or Wenckebach phenomenon, and *type II,* or Mobitz II. *Type I* second-degree AV block is characterized by (1) progressive lengthening of the PR interval until a P wave is blocked, (2) progressive shortening of the RR interval until a P wave is blocked, and (3) the RR interval surrounding the blocked P wave is shorter than two PP intervals (see Fig. 10–5B). In the presence of narrow QRS complex, the site of AV block is in the AV node. In patients with a wide QRS complex, the site of AV block can be infranodal in up to 25% of instances. *Type II* AV block is characterized by intermittent blocked P waves with no change in the PR interval (see Fig. 10–5C). The sinus cycle length is usually constant with the RR interval surrounding the nonconducted P wave equal to twice the sinus cycle length. In the presence of a wide QRS complex, the site of AV block is usually infranodal. In the setting of a narrow QRS complex, the site of block is usually in the His bundle above the bifurcation but may occasionally be in the AV node. In 2:1 AV block (see Fig. 10–5D), the site of block is unknown. Findings that favor infranodal block include (1) a history of near syncope or syncope, (2) a QRS duration above 120 ms, (3) the presence of type II second-degree AV block or third-degree AV block during continuous ECG

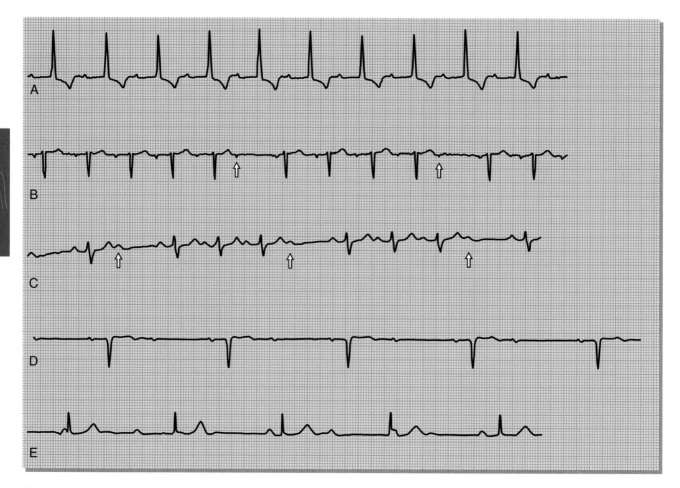

Figure 10–5 Heart block. *A,* First-degree atrioventricular (AV) block; the PR interval is prolonged (>200 ms). *B,* Second-degree AV block, type 1 (Wenckebach). Progressive PR prolongation preceding a nonconducted P wave *(arrows)* occurs. *C,* Second-degree AV block, type II. Nonconducted P waves are seen *(arrows)* in the absence of progressive PR prolongation. *D,* 2:1 AV block in which every other P wave is conducted. *E,* Third-degree (complete) AV block with AV dissociation and a narrow-complex (AV nodal) escape rhythm.

monitoring, (4) improved AV conduction with carotid sinus massage, and (5) worsening AV conduction with atropine and exercise. Identifying the site of block is important in the asymptomatic patient with 2:1 AV block because infranodal block is associated with worse prognosis and mandates the implantation of a pacemaker.

Third-degree AV block or complete AV block is defined by the presence of atrioventricular dissociation *and* an atrial rate that is faster than the ventricular rate. By definition, the sinus P waves are not conducted and the QRS complexes are from a subsidiary pacemaker, which usually has a slower rate. The RR and PP intervals are usually constant but bear no relation to each other. The PR interval will vary as the Ps are independent of the QRSs (see Fig. 10–5E).

III. Tachyarrhythmias

Tachyarrhythmias are divided into *supraventricular, ventricular,* and *preexcited tachycardias.* During supraventricular tachycardia (SVT), the ventricles are depolarized via the normal His-Purkinje system, with or without aberrancy, resulting in a narrow or wide complex tachycardia. During

VT, the impulse originates from the ventricle and depolarizes the ventricles in an asynchronized fashion, resulting in a wide QRS complex. With preexcited tachycardias, some or all ventricular activation is caused by antegrade conduction down an accessory pathway, resulting in a wide complex tachycardia. A summary of the most common tachyarrhythmias follows.

ATRIAL TACHYARRHYTHMIAS

Atrial tachycardia results from an ectopic atrial focus discharging at a rate faster than the sinus rate. The rate is usually 100 to 250 beats/min, and the P wave morphology is different than the sinus P wave (Fig. 10–6A) unless the tachycardia focus site is close to the sinus node. The PR interval is usually normal or longer than the PR interval during sinus rhythm. The rhythm is usually regular, though episodes of AV block may result in some irregularities. Most commonly, AV conduction is 1:1; however, variable AV block might be seen. When atrial tachycardia occurs with AV block, digoxin toxicity is suggested. Atrial tachycardias are more likely to occur in patients with concomitant heart disease, including coronary artery disease, valvular disease, cardiomyopathies,

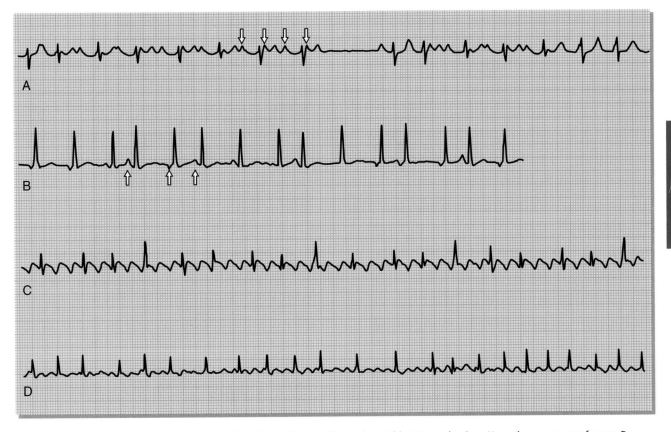

Figure 10–6 Atrial tachyarrhythmias. *A,* Atrial tachycardia with 2:1 and variable AV conduction. Note the presence of more P waves *(arrows)* than QRS complexes. *B,* Multifocal atrial tachycardia demonstrating an irregularly irregular rhythm at a rate of approximately 110 beats/min, with at least three different P wave morphologies *(arrows)* and without a dominant underlying rhythm. *C,* Atrial flutter. Flutter waves are seen as the discrete undulations of the baseline *(saw-tooth pattern)*. The conduction rate is variable. *D,* Atrial fibrillation. The rhythm is irregularly irregular without evidence of organized atrial electrical activity.

cor pulmonale, and congenital heart disease. The mechanism of atrial tachycardia can be automaticity, reentry, or triggered activity. In a young patient, automaticity is the most likely mechanism, and, as the age increases, reentry becomes more common. Triggered activity has been suggested, but its role remains poorly defined. In patients with cardiac surgery resulting in atrial scars, reentry around the existing scar can result in atrial tachycardia, called *incisional tachycardia.* The ECG manifestation of the latter is similar to focal atrial tachycardia, except that the P wave duration is usually longer. The P wave morphology and axis are determined by the exit site. Vagal maneuvers usually do not terminate atrial tachycardias but can result in transient AV block, thus unmasking the P waves. When the arrhythmia is not a result of digoxin toxicity, β-blockers and calcium channel blockers are the mainstays of therapy, with class I or class III anti-arrhythmic agents reserved for refractory patients. Catheter ablation can eliminate this arrhythmia in 75% to 90% of patients. When atrial tachycardia is the result of digoxin therapy, withholding the agent should be the first step, followed by the administration of digoxin-specific antibodies if the patient is symptomatic.

Multifocal atrial tachycardia (MAT) is an irregular rhythm defined by the presence of three or more P wave morphologies and a rate greater than 100 beats/min (see Fig. 10–6B). It occurs most commonly in patients with underlying lung

disease; is also seen in the setting of an acute MI, hypokalemia, or hypomagnesemia; and may be a precursor of atrial fibrillation. Aminophylline use may also be a contributing factor. Treatment is directed at the underlying disease. Rate control of this arrhythmia may be difficult, although verapamil is frequently effective.

Atrial flutter (AFL) is a reentrant tachycardia localized to the right atrium with passive activation of the left atrium. The reentrant circuit is limited anteriorly by the tricuspid valve and posteriorly by the cristae terminalis and the eustachian ridge. The direction of impulse propagation around the tricuspid annulus determines the P wave morphology. If propagation is in the counterclockwise direction, the impulse propagates up the septum and down the lateral wall, resulting in a negative P wave in the inferior leads with a typical saw-tooth pattern (see Fig. 10–6C), called *typical AFL.* If propagation is in the clockwise direction, the P wave is upright in the inferior leads, and the tachycardia is called *atypical AFL.* The atrial rate during AFL is usually around 250 to 350 beats/min, with an average rate of 300 beats/min. The ventricular rate depends on the conduction down the AV node. Usually, conduction is 2:1, resulting in a ventricular rate of approximately 150 beats/min. In young patients with enhanced AV nodal conduction, the ventricular rate can be as high as the atrial rate, reaching 300 beats/min. Similarly, in the presence of an accessory pathway, the ventricular rate can be very rapid, resulting in hemodynamic compromise and ventricular fibrillation.

AFL may occur in patients with or without structural heart disease and may be precipitated by thyrotoxicosis, pericarditis, and alcohol ingestion. When AFL is associated with hemodynamic compromise or angina, immediate cardioversion should be performed. Relatively low-energy shocks are frequently effective because of the stable nature of the circuit. When the patient is hemodynamically stable, the focus should be on rate control to reduce the risk of tachycardia-induced cardiomyopathy and anticoagulation to reduce the risk of stroke. If patients remain symptomatic despite rate control, rhythm control either pharmacologically or with catheter ablation should be attempted. When class IA anti-arrhythmic agents are used to convert AFL to sinus rhythm, the ventricular rate must first be controlled with digoxin, β-blockers, or calcium channel blockers. Class IA agents may slow the flutter rate and augment AV nodal conduction, resulting in 1:1 conduction with very rapid ventricular rates. Radiofrequency catheter ablation of the reentrant flutter circuit is quite effective, resulting in the restoration of sinus rhythm in 90% to 95% of patients.

Atrial fibrillation (AF) is the most common sustained supraventricular tachyarrhythmia. According to *Moe's hypothesis,* AF is maintained by having a critical number of wavelets circulating in the atria. These wavelets may shrink, undergo decremental conduction, collide with another wavelet or a boundary and be mutually annihilated, or may encounter functional and/or anatomic obstacles and create new wavelets by wave breaks, a mechanism referred to as *vortex shedding.* Other mechanisms such as rapidly firing foci leading to *fibrillatory conduction,* and the presence of a *mother rotor* defined as a stable, high-frequency rotating pattern that drives AF, have recently emerged. Technologic advances using optical mapping and frequency analysis have provided evidence for such alternative theories. During AF, multiple reentrant loops continuously circulating in both atria result in ineffective atrial contraction. In addition, the AV node is bombarded at rates greater than 400 beats/min. Because of the conductive properties, many of the impulses are blocked at the AV node. The resultant ventricular rhythm is irregularly irregular at rates between 120 and 170 beats/min. At rapid ventricular rates, the rhythm may appear to be regular, although careful measurements will disclose the irregularity. A truly regular ventricular rate in the setting of AF suggests the development of a junctional or ventricular rhythm, both of which may be a reflection of digoxin toxicity. AF may be paroxysmal or chronic and may be the only arrhythmia present or be part of a more generalized rhythm disturbance (sick sinus syndrome). The surface ECG demonstrates an irregular ventricular pattern and the absence of organized atrial activity; that is, no P waves are present (see Fig. 10–6D). Physical examination of a patient in AF reveals variation in the intensity of S_1, an irregular cardiac rhythm, and absence of *a* waves in the jugular venous pulsations. At the very short RR intervals that occur intermittently during rapid heart rates, the minimal diastolic filling time and subsequent low stroke volume fail to produce a palpable pulse. A discrepancy may therefore exist between the auscultated heart rate and the palpable pulse rate, with the auscultated rate being a more accurate reflection of the true ventricular rate.

A clear association of AF with age exists, and a sharp increase in incidence is noted after the seventh decade of life. AF may occur without any identifiable cardiac abnormality but is common in the setting of underlying cardiac disease, including valvular heart disease (especially rheumatic), heart failure, and ischemic cardiac disease. The most frequent predisposing cardiovascular condition for the development of AF is hypertension. AF may also be precipitated by pericarditis, thyrotoxicosis, pulmonary emboli, pneumonia, and acute alcohol ingestion and occurs postoperatively in approximately one third of patients who undergo cardiac surgery. AF is frequently asymptomatic or associated with only minor symptoms, such as palpitations. In patients with obstructive coronary artery disease, the rapid heart rate associated with the onset of AF may precipitate ischemia. In patients with aortic or mitral stenosis and in other patients who are dependent on the atrial contribution to cardiac output (e.g., patients with left ventricular hypertrophy or with a dilated or hypertrophic cardiomyopathy), the loss of effective atrial contraction with the onset of AF may result in significant hemodynamic compromise. In addition, in patients with bypass tracts (see later discussion), AF may result in extremely rapid ventricular rates with subsequent hemodynamic collapse.

The treatment of AF is threefold: (1) prevention of thromboembolic complications, (2) rate control, and (3) restoration and maintenance of sinus rhythm.

Because of the ineffective mechanical function of the atria during fibrillation, stasis of blood may occur, especially in the atrial appendages, and result in thrombus formation and subsequent thromboembolic events. In the absence of anticoagulation therapy, AF is associated with a 5%- to 6%-per-year risk of embolic stroke. This risk is increased in the setting of rheumatic valvular disease (>10%). Other clinical factors that increase the risk of stroke in patients with AF include prior stroke, diabetes, hypertension, heart failure, left atrial enlargement, and increasing age. No difference in stroke rate occurs between paroxysmal and chronic AF. Restoration of normal sinus rhythm has not been shown to reduce the risk of stroke. In fact, in the Atrial Fibrillation Follow-up Investigation of Rhythm Management (AFFIRM) trial, a trend toward a higher incidence of stroke in patients randomized to rhythm control was found when compared with rate control, albeit not statistically significant. This trend was most likely caused by the decreased use of warfarin in the rhythm control group. Therefore, any patient with paroxysmal, persistent, or permanent AF who does not have a contraindication to anticoagulation should be treated with warfarin therapy with a target international normalized ratio between 2.0 and 3.0.

Rate control in AF is important for several reasons. It has been shown to improve symptoms and quality of life. Symptoms and hemodynamic compromise are increased at faster ventricular rates, and the tachycardic response may induce ischemia in patients with coronary artery disease. In addition, the poorly controlled heart rate may result in the development of progressive ventricular dysfunction. The heart rate can usually be controlled with digoxin, β-blockers, or calcium channel blockers. In rare instances, the ventricular rate cannot be controlled by pharmacologic means, and catheter ablation of the AV node and permanent pacemaker implantation are necessary for adequate heart rate control.

Occasionally, patients exhibit AF and a relatively slow ventricular rate in the absence of rate-lowering medications. This circumstance usually reflects significant underlying conduction system disease that also often involves the sinus node.

Rhythm control has several advantages, including (1) abolition of symptoms, (2) halting atrial enlargement (an independent predictor of stroke), and (3) improvement of left ventricular function and exercise capacity. The main disadvantage is subjecting patients to a drug therapy and/or procedure that might be associated with complications. As stated before, rhythm control has not been shown to reduce the risk of stroke or to have an impact on mortality when compared with rate control. Therefore, rhythm control should be attempted in patients who are symptomatic despite rate control and in those who have left ventricular dysfunction. When AF is associated with hemodynamic compromise, electrical cardioversion (with 100 to 360 joules) is the treatment of choice. In hemodynamically stable patients with less than 48 hours of AF, the risk of thromboembolism is low, and pharmacologic or electrical cardioversion can be attempted without the need for 3 weeks of anticoagulation (see later discussion). Patients with more than 48 hours of AF, or in whom the duration of the arrhythmia is unknown, are at increased risk of having atrial thrombi and should be treated with anticoagulation for at least 3 weeks before an attempt at cardioversion. An alternative approach is to perform a transesophageal echocardiogram; if atrial thrombi are not present, cardioversion can be safely performed. Anticoagulation should be continued for at least 4 weeks after successful cardioversion because effective atrial contraction may be slow to return. The options for maintaining rhythm control include (1) pharmacologic therapy, (2) catheter ablation, and (3) surgical Maze procedure. The class IA (quinidine, procainamide, and disopyramide), class IC (propafenone and flecainide), and class III (sotalol and amiodarone) agents are effective in restoring sinus rhythm and for long-term maintenance therapy. However, the benefits of such therapy must be weighed against the risks of toxicity with these agents, and the probability of maintaining sinus rhythm must be taken into account. The preferred choice of drug therapy for the maintenance of sinus rhythm in patients with paroxysmal and persistent AF, based on the most recent American College of Cardiology/American Heart Association guidelines, is provided in Figure 10–7. Radiofrequency ablation of the ostia of the pulmonary veins or electrical isolation of the pulmonary veins from the left atrium is a procedure that should be reserved to symptomatic patients who have failed drug therapy. Ablation therapy frequently abolishes the arrhythmia, improving symptoms and, at times, left ventricular function in patients with baseline congestive heart failure. The surgical maze procedure involves making surgical lesions in the atria that interrupt reentrant circuits and may restore sinus rhythm in more than 90% of patients. This procedure is usually performed in conjunction with mitral valve surgery.

ATRIOVENTRICULAR NODAL (JUNCTIONAL) RHYTHM DISTURBANCES

AV nodal reentrant tachycardia (AVNRT) is the most common type of paroxysmal SVT and is characterized by the sudden onset and termination of a regular narrow QRS complex tachycardia at rates of 150 to 250 beats/min

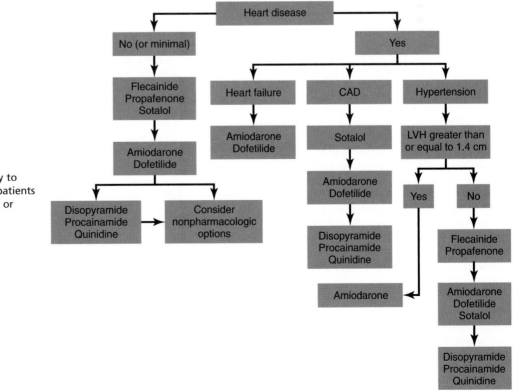

Figure 10–7 Drug therapy to maintain sinus rhythm in patients with recurrent paroxysmal or persistent AF.

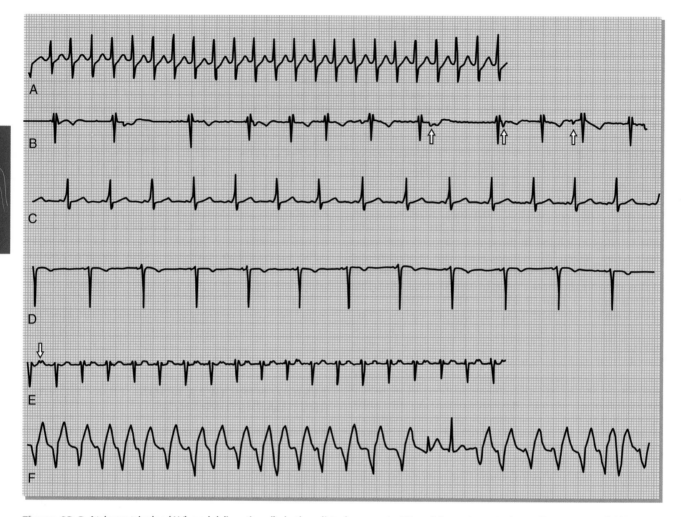

Figure 10–8 Atrioventricular (AV) nodal (junctional) rhythm disturbances. *A,* AV nodal reentrant tachycardia at a rate of 185 beats/min. The retrograde P waves are hidden in the QRS complexes. *B,* Automatic junctional tachycardia. Note the presence of AV dissociation during tachycardia. The P waves *(arrows)* are dissociated form the QRS complexes. *C,* Normal sinus rhythm in a patient with Wolff-Parkinson-White (WPW) syndrome. Note the short PR interval (<120 ms), the *slurring* of the initial portion of the QRS (delta wave), and the wide QRS complex. *D,* Normal sinus rhythm in a patient with Lown-Ganong-Levine (LGL) pattern. Note the short PR interval without the presence of a delta wave or wide QRS complex. *E,* Orthodromic AV reentrant tachycardia at a rate of 146 beats/min in a patient with WPW syndrome. The retrograde P waves are clearly seen altering the normal T wave contour *(arrow). F,* Atrial fibrillation in a patient with WPW syndrome. Note the rapid and irregular ventricular response with widening of the QRS secondary to preexcitation.

(Fig. 10–8A). A wide QRS complex may occur if aberrant conduction occurs in the His-Purkinje system. These rhythms may occur at any age, are somewhat more common in women than men, may occur in the absence of organic heart disease, may be short lived or sustained, and may produce palpitations, chest pain, dyspnea, and presyncope. The substrate for this tachycardia is dual AV node pathways with different effective refractory period (ERP), a fast pathway with a longer ERP and a slow pathway with a shorter ERP. Whether these pathways are exclusively intranodal or not remains controversial, but catheter ablation studies of these pathways have revealed distinct atrial insertion sites, with the fast pathway inserting anteriorly near the His bundle and the slow pathway posteriorly near the coronary sinus ostium.

At least two types of AVNRT have been identified. In the usual form (typical), the impulse propagates antegrade down the slow pathway and retrograde up the fast pathway. Because retrograde conduction is over the fast pathway, atrial and ventricular depolarizations are almost simultaneous, resulting in a P wave buried in the QRS complex, or appearing at its terminal portion, resulting in pseudo S wave in the inferior leads and a pseudo R' in lead V1 (see Fig. 10–8A). In the unusual form of AVNRT, antegrade conduction is over the fast pathway, and retrograde conduction is over the slow pathway, resulting in a P wave after the QRS complex with a long RP interval. AVNRT is usually initiated with premature stimuli and terminated by premature beats, vagal maneuvers, adenosine, or other cardiac medications known to cause block in the AV node. Vagal maneuvers (e.g., carotid sinus massage, Valsalva maneuver, coughing) may terminate an episode by causing a transient AV nodal blockade. Adenosine (6 to 12 mg intravenously) terminates episodes in more than 95% of patients and is the treatment of choice if vagal maneuvers fail. In rare instances, direct current cardioversion is necessary. Intravenous β-blockers, digoxin, or calcium channel blockers are also an extremely effective acute therapy, and their oral formulations are effective chronically. Classes IC and III anti-arrhythmic agents are useful in resistant patients. In rare instances, direct current cardioversion is necessary. Radiofrequency catheter ablation of one limb of the reentrant circuit (slow pathway) can cure AVNRT in more than 90% of patients, with a low risk of inducing complete heart block (<2%) that might require the placement of a permanent pacemaker.

Automatic junctional tachycardia (AJT) is characterized as a rapid irregular SVT with episodes of AV dissociation (see Fig. 10–8B). The rate ranges between 110 and 250 beats/min, and the QRS interval is usually narrow but may be wide secondary to bundle branch block. AJT was first described in infants and children but has also been reported in adults in which the prognosis is more benign. Abnormal automaticity is believed to be the mechanism responsible for AJT. This tachycardia is usually sensitive to catecholamines but can sometimes be terminated with carotid sinus massage and adenosine. Beta-blockers, calcium channel blockers, and classes IC and III anti-arrhythmic drugs should be the first line of therapy. When drug therapy fails, radiofrequency can result in cure; however, it is associated with a significant risk of AV block (20%), requiring the implantation of a permanent pacemaker. AJT must be differentiated from the more common nonparoxysmal junctional tachycardia. The latter is regular, has a slower rate (70 to 120 beats/min) and occurs in the setting of digitalis toxicity, inferior MI, metabolic derangements, chronic lung disease, or after cardiac surgery. The mechanism of nonparoxysmal junctional tachycardia is believed to be triggered activity secondary to DADs. Digoxin toxicity must always be excluded as a cause. Specific therapy for nonparoxysmal junctional tachycardia is usually not necessary.

WOLFF-PARKINSON-WHITE SYNDROME AND ATRIOVENTRICULAR RECIPROCATING ARRHYTHMIAS

Normally, the AV node is the only pathway that allows the wave of depolarization to conduct from the atria to the ventricles. However, anomalous bands of tissue (accessory pathways or bypass tracts) may exist and form an additional conduction pathway. The conductive properties of these bypass tracts differ from those of the AV node in that they do not produce the decremental conduction property of normal conduction tissue. In other words, they do not conduct slower at rapid rates. Conduction via the bypass tracts may be unidirectional or bidirectional. These properties provide the substrate for macro-reentrant arrhythmias (see previous discussion) using the bypass tract as one limb of the reentrant circuit and the AV node as the other. Other less frequent pathways have been reported such as AV nodal bypass tract, a direct communication between the atria and the His-Purkinje system, nodoventricular fibers connecting the AV node to the ventricular myocardium, and fasciculoventricular connections from the His-Purkinje system to the ventricles. The majority of patients with bypass tracts have otherwise anatomically normal hearts, although the incidence of right-sided accessory pathways is increased in

patients with Ebstein's anomaly of the tricuspid valve. Similarly, an association with left-sided accessory pathways and mitral valve prolapse and hypertrophic cardiomyopathy has been noted.

During *normal sinus rhythm,* when the AV bypass tract conducts in an antegrade fashion, the ventricular muscle will be activated by the atrial impulse sooner than would be expected if the impulse reached the ventricles only by way of the normal AV conduction. This activity is referred to as *preexcitation.* The result is a short PR interval (<120 ms) and a wide QRS complex with *slurring* of the initial portion of the QRS, referred to also as a *delta wave.* The QRS is wide because it is a fusion complex created by ventricular activation through two separate pathways, the AV node and the accessory pathway (see Fig. 10–8C). The extent of preexcitation is determined by the conductive properties of the pathway and the AV node in addition to the accessory pathway location. Wolff-Parkinson-White (WPW) syndrome refers to the presence of preexcitation and a history of paroxysmal tachycardia. When preexcitation is present alone without paroxysmal tachycardia, the patient is referred to as having WPW pattern. Occasionally, the accessory pathway conducts only in the retrograde direction or from the ventricle to the atrium without any antegrade conduction and thus ventricular preexcitation. This circumstance is referred to as a *concealed* accessory pathway because its presence is not evident on the surface ECG when the patient is in normal sinus rhythm. As stated before, some accessory pathways connect the atria to the His-Purkinje system. The result is a short PR interval because the atrial impulse will be bypassing the AV node, but a normal QRS complex is seen because the ventricles are activated via the normal His-Purkinje system (see Fig. 10–8D). This circumstance is referred to as Lown-Ganong-Levine (LGL) pattern; when it is associated with a history of tachycardias, it is referred to as the LGL syndrome.

The most common *arrhythmia* in WPW syndrome is *orthodromic* AV reentrant tachycardia (AVRT) in which the AV node is used as the antegrade limb of the circuit and the bypass tract as the retrograde limb. This circumstance results in a narrow-complex QRS tachycardia on the surface ECG (see Fig. 10–8E), unless aberrant conduction is present. A retrograde P wave may be noted, usually with a short RP interval. Less commonly, *antidromic* AVRT may occur that uses the accessory pathway as the antegrade limb and the AV node as the retrograde limb. This circumstance results in complete preexcitation of the ventricles with a wide, bizarre QRS complex on the ECG. Because the AV node is an intrinsic component of both forms of AVRT, transient blockade of the AV node by vagal maneuvers or medications will interrupt the circuit and terminate the tachyarrhythmia. The incidence of *atrial tachyarrhythmias,* such as AF or AFL, is increased in patients with bypass tracts. When these arrhythmias occur, AV nodal–blocking drugs are contraindicated; in this setting, digoxin, β-blockers, or calcium channel blockers may result in slowing of conduction through the AV node with resultant preferential excitation of the ventricles through the accessory AV connection. Extremely rapid ventricular rates are possible and may precipitate hemodynamic collapse and sudden death (see Fig. 10–8F).

In a patient with a delta wave noted on the ECG but without any symptoms, no specific therapy is required.

In patients with frequent episodes of AVRT, chronic pharmacologic therapy with drugs that prolong the refractory period of the accessory pathway (class IA, IC, or III antiarrhythmic agents) is effective. Drugs that slow conduction in the AV node (digoxin, β-blockers, or calcium channel blockers) should be avoided in patients with WPW because they may enhance conduction down the accessory pathway and increase the ventricular rate during AF and AFL. Intravenous procainamide is the drug of choice for acutely controlling the rate of AF or AFL in patients with bypass tracts. Electrical cardioversion should be considered early in these patients. Radiofrequency catheter ablation of the accessory pathway has become the therapy of choice for symptomatic patients and has a success rate in excess of 95%.

VENTRICULAR RHYTHM DISTURBANCES

VT is defined as three or more consecutive ventricular depolarizations occurring at a rate greater than 100 beats/min. The resulting QRS complexes on the surface ECG are aberrant, as described earlier for VPCs, and may be monomorphic or polymorphic (Fig. 10–9A). Evidence of independent atrial activity may be present (AV dissociation); however, when retrograde conduction to the atria is present, AV dissociation is not seen. Occasionally, a normal sinus depolarization may be conducted to the ventricles before the pathologic ventricular depolarization occurs and results in a normal-appearing QRS complex, called a *capture* beat. If the atrial depolarization reaches the ventricles simultaneously with the spontaneous ventricular depolarization, a *fusion* complex will result. These abnormalities are pathognomonic for VT. VT that lasts for more than 30 seconds or requires termination because of hemodynamic instability is considered *sustained;* VT that lasts less than 30 seconds and is hemodynamically stable is considered *nonsustained.*

When a wide-complex tachycardia occurs, determining whether it is VT or SVT with aberrancy is important because the therapeutic and prognostic implications differ significantly. When an SVT is associated with a narrow-complex

QRS, the diagnosis is straightforward. However, when an SVT occurs in the setting of a preexisting bundle branch block or conducts aberrantly as a result of rate-related block in the His-Purkinje system, the resulting QRS complex is wide and may be difficult to distinguish from VT. Several features may be helpful in making this distinction. The presence of AV dissociation, capture beats, or fusion complexes is diagnostic of VT. However, the absence of these findings is not helpful because they are present in less than 50% of instances. A wide-complex tachycardia occurring in the presence of ischemia or in a patient with known ischemic heart disease is VT in more than 90% of instances. The heart rate, blood pressure, and presence or absence of symptoms do not differentiate these arrhythmias, whereas intermittent cannon *a* waves in the jugular venous pulsations suggest VT. If an abnormal QRS complex is present when the patient is in normal sinus rhythm and the QRS complex during the tachycardia is identical to this, the rhythm is likely SVT. Adenosine may be useful in determining the cause; with SVT, adenosine-induced blockade of the AV node will terminate the tachycardia in the majority of instances, given that 90% of SVT involve the AV node (60% AVNRT, 30% AVRT). In the remainder of patients, adenosine-induced AV block will unmask the atrial activity and thus help make the diagnosis. In rare instances, adenosine may terminate a VT when the tachycardia originates from the right ventricular outflow tract. Verapamil should never be used as a diagnostic test because it may precipitate ventricular fibrillation if the initial rhythm is VT. Table 10–1 lists the features that may help differentiate these arrhythmias from one another.

VT occurs most frequently in patients with underlying heart disease, including acute ischemia, prior infarction with scar formation, congestive cardiomyopathy, right ventricular dysplasia, and hypertrophic heart disease. The mechanism is usually reentry in the ventricular myocardium, although it may also arise in a diseased portion of the conduction system (e.g., bundle branch reentry). Metabolic abnormalities, such as hyperkalemia and hypoxia, and medications, such as

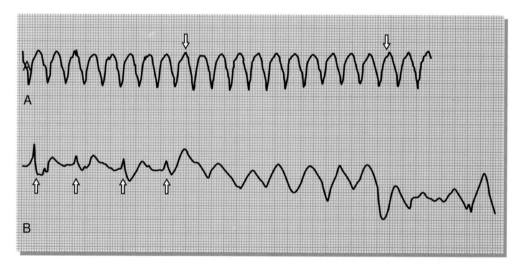

Figure 10–9 Ventricular rhythm disturbances. *A,* Monomorphic ventricular tachycardia at a rate of 200 beats/min. The QRS complex is wide, and P waves are seen to occasionally alter the QRS morphology *(arrows),* reflecting AV dissociation. *B,* Ventricular fibrillation. An *agonal* rhythm is initially present *(arrows)* but deteriorates into ventricular fibrillation. The baseline is irregular without evidence of organized ventricular electrical activity.

Table 10–1	**Features That May Differentiate Ventricular Tachycardia from Supraventricular Tachycardia with Aberrancy**

Helpful Features	**Implications**
Positive QRS concordance	Diagnostic of VT
Presence of AV dissociation, capture beats, or fusion beats	Diagnostic of VT
Atypical RBBB (monophasic R, QR, RS, or triphasic QRS in V1; R to S ratio <1, QS or QR, monophasic R in V6)	Suggests VT
Atypical LBBB (R >30 ms or R to S [nadir or notch] >60 ms in V1 or V2; R to S ratio <1, QS or QR I V6)	Suggests VT
Shift of axis from baseline	Suggests VT
History of CAD	Suggests VT
QRS during tachycardia identical to QRS during sinus rhythm	Suggests SVT
Termination with adenosine	Suggests SVT

AV = atrioventricular; CAD = coronary artery disease; LBBB = left bundle branch block; RBBB = right bundle branch block; SVT = supraventricular tachycardia; VT = ventricular tachycardia.

digoxin and antiarrhythmic agents, may also precipitate VT, likely as a result of triggered activity. On the other hand, VT can occur in the absence of structural heart disease. This type of VT accounts for only 6% of all clinical VTs and is called idiopathic VT. Idiopathic VT is best classified according to its site of origin. Right ventricular outflow tract VT (RVOT-VT) is the most common type of idiopathic VT originating from the right ventricular outflow tract with left bundle branch block–inferior axis morphology. The mechanism of this tachycardia is believed to be triggered activity. This tachycardia occurs in otherwise healthy individuals, is very sensitive to catecholamines, and terminates with adenosine, thus the term *adenosine-sensitive VT*. The other type of idiopathic VT originates from the septum near the apex of the left ventricle resulting in right bundle branch block–superior axis morphology. The mechanism of idiopathic left VT has been shown to be reentry with involvement of the distal His-Purkinje system. Idiopathic left VT is known to be verapamil sensitive, thus the term *verapamil-sensitive VT*.

Nonsustained VT requires no treatment unless the patient is symptomatic. In most instances, nonsustained VT is associated with left ventricular dysfunction, which independently, if moderate to severe, is an indication for the implantation of an implantable cardioverter-defibrillator (ICD). When patients are symptomatic, the choice of medical therapy is dictated by the presence or absence of structural heart disease. In patients with normal left ventricular function, beta-blockers, calcium channel blockers,

and class IC and class III agents should be used, in that order. In patients with left ventricular dysfunction, beta-blockers followed by amiodarone are usually the drugs of choice. An important point to note is that, although this arrhythmia is often a marker for increased cardiac mortality in some patients with structural or ischemic heart disease, suppression of this arrhythmia with pharmacologic treatment has not been shown to decrease mortality in most settings. Patients with sustained VT that is associated with hemodynamic compromise, angina, or heart failure should undergo synchronized cardioversion. When stable, sustained VT should be managed with intravenous drug therapy such as amiodarone or lidocaine. If left ventricular function is normal, procainamide and sotalol may also be used. If drug therapy fails, synchronized cardioversion should be performed. Following the acute treatment, most patients receive an ICD unless a reversible cause has been identified (e.g., ischemia, metabolic abnormalities, drug toxicity). Ventricular tachyarrhythmias that occur in the setting of acute MI respond to treatment of the ischemia and do not necessarily require prolonged anti-arrhythmic therapy. In the rare instances of idiopathic VT, catheter ablation may provide a permanent cure, with a success rate of 90%. Catheter ablation is also used as an adjunctive therapy in patients with ICDs who have recurrent or incessant VT. With improvements in interventional techniques, localization of the abnormal ventricular foci and subsequent radiofrequency ablation may be curative in many forms of VT, including those associated with previous MI.

Ventricular flutter (VFL) is a form of monomorphic VT occurring at a rate of 280 to 300 beats/min and is a hemodynamically unstable rhythm. *Ventricular fibrillation* (VF) is a disorganized, chaotic, ventricular rhythm that results in ineffective ventricular contraction, rapid hemodynamic collapse, and death if not immediately terminated (see Fig. 10–9B). VF is recognized on ECG by coarse undulations of the baseline without identifiable QRS complexes, ST segments, or T waves. It may occur in the setting of ischemia, metabolic abnormalities, and drug toxicity, or it may degenerate from VT, either spontaneously or after attempted cardioversion. Treatment with immediate nonsynchronized direct current shock at 360 joules (or equivalent biphasic) is required in all instances. Several shocks may be required for termination of this arrhythmia, and concurrent treatment of precipitating causes is essential. Once the rhythm has been successfully terminated, an intravenous anti-arrhythmic agent such as amiodarone or lidocaine should be started to prevent recurrences. If VF is the result of an acute reversible cause, no chronic therapy is required. However, if VF occurs as a result of fixed underlying cardiac disease, implantation of an ICD is indicated.

Approach to the Patient with Suspected Arrhythmias
HISTORY

Many, if not most, arrhythmias occur intermittently, and patients are often asymptomatic at the time of evaluation. Therefore, with the suggestion of an arrhythmic problem, the necessity and urgency for further evaluation must frequently be determined by the history alone. Palpitations, syncope, presyncope, dizziness, chest pain, and symptoms of heart failure are the most common complaints of patients with arrhythmic disorders. Palpitations give a sensation of a rapid or irregular heart beat. Characterizing the pattern (regular or irregular, intermittent or continuous) and rate of palpitations by having patients tap their fingers on a table to the rhythm of the palpitations may help determine their cause. For instance, occasional *skipped beats* are likely the result of premature atrial or ventricular beats, whereas periods of rapid, irregular heartbeats may be reflective of paroxysmal AF. The perception of palpitations does not invariably correlate with arrhythmias; some patients have tachyarrhythmias without palpitations, whereas other patients have palpitations without tachyarrhythmias. Correlation between the symptoms and an arrhythmia can be confirmed only by simultaneously recording the ECG and documenting the symptoms. Syncope is the sudden, transient loss of consciousness. Obtaining a complete history of the events immediately preceding and after a syncopal episode will suggest the diagnosis in the majority of patients for whom a diagnosis is eventually determined. Chest pain may be a manifestation of palpitations or may represent arrhythmia-induced cardiac ischemia. Similarly, cardiac arrhythmias may also precipitate or exacerbate congestive heart failure. A prior history of cardiac disease is important to elicit. Patients with palpitations or syncope and a history of cardiomyopathy or prior MI frequently have ventricular tachyarrhythmias, whereas patients with valvular heart disease or hypertension frequently develop AF. A family history of cardiac disease (e.g., dilated or hypertrophic cardiomyopathy, bypass tracts, sudden cardiac death, LTQS) is important to note.

PHYSICAL EXAMINATION

In addition to noting the pulse rate and rhythm, a thorough examination is useful for identifying evidence of underlying cardiac disease. When patients are examined during an arrhythmic episode, several clues to the nature of the arrhythmia may be present. Evidence of AV dissociation suggests a ventricular arrhythmia and includes variable intensity of S_1 (because of variations in the PR interval), intermittent cannon *a* waves in the jugular venous pulsation, and a cacophony of sounds (as a result of atrial systole occurring during various parts of the cardiac cycle, generating intermittent S_3 and S_4). The S_2 may become widely or paradoxically split if a bundle branch block develops during an arrhythmia. Nonetheless, these findings are not diagnostic of

a ventricular source of the arrhythmia because bundle branch blocks and, rarely, AV dissociation may occur during supraventricular tachyarrhythmias as well.

USEFUL TESTS

Electrocardiogram

The *ECG* taken during the arrhythmia is usually diagnostic. If P waves are not obvious, moving the arm leads to a parasternal position (Lewis leads) or using an esophageal electrode (placed 40 cm into the esophagus by means of a nasogastric tube) may help discern atrial activity. In patients who exhibit a hemodynamically stable supraventricular tachyarrhythmia, carotid sinus massage or pharmacologic therapy with adenosine or verapamil may slow or block conduction in the AV node, resulting in either tachycardia termination or the identification of the underlying rhythm. Carotid sinus massage is performed with the patient in the supine position by applying light pressure for 5 to 10 seconds over the carotid impulse at the angle of the jaw. A successful test should result in slowing of the ventricular rate (Fig. 10–10). If no effect is noted, massage can be performed over the contralateral carotid impulse. This test should not be performed if carotid bruits are present. Unfortunately, many patients are examined after the arrhythmia has resolved. Nonetheless, clues may be present on the resting ECG. A delta wave is diagnostic of WPW syndrome, which is associated with AV reentrant arrhythmias and AF. Evidence of prior MI raises the suspicion of ventricular tachyarrhythmias.

Recording Devices

Because of the intermittent nature of arrhythmias, prolonged *recording devices* are more effective than a single ECG in electrocardiographically capturing an arrhythmia. Ambulatory ECG (Holter) monitors continuously record the rhythm and are useful in patients who have frequent episodes of presumed arrhythmic symptoms. Patient-activated event monitors, or loop recorders, can be worn for weeks at a time and continuously monitor the patient's heart rhythm. If symptoms occur, the patient activates the device, which then permanently records the rhythm for several minutes before and after the event and transmits the recorded rhythm by telephone to a central monitoring facility. This type of monitor is useful if the patient has infrequent symptoms. For patients with very infrequent symptoms, an implantable event monitor can be placed under the skin of the chest wall and can remain in place for

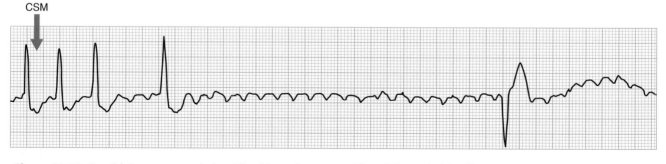

Figure 10–10 Carotid sinus massage during AFL with resultant unmasking of the underlying flutter waves.

up to a year. All of these devices are useful in diagnosing arrhythmias, determining the relationship (if any) of the patient's symptoms to an arrhythmia, monitoring the efficacy of anti-arrhythmic therapy, and evaluating artificial pacemaker function. If a patient's symptoms are exertion related, formal exercise testing may be useful.

Head-Up Tilt-Table Testing

In patients with suggested neurocardiogenic syncope, *head-up tilt-table* testing may reproduce their symptoms. This procedure is performed by strapping a patient to the tilt table, then tilting the table 60 to 80 degrees vertically for 15 to 60 minutes. The presumed mechanism of tilt-induced syncope involves a postural decrease in ventricular filling, resulting in increased sympathetic activity and ventricular contraction. This increased contraction is believed to result in the activation of cardiac mechanoreceptors (C-fibers), leading to reflex increase in vagal tone and withdrawal of peripheral sympathetic tone. The result is bradycardia-induced low cardiac output and hypotension. The sensitivity of the test in detecting neurocardiogenic syncope can be up to 85% depending on the tilt protocol used, with a relatively low false-positive rate (<15%). The administration of intravenous isoproterenol or sublingual nitroglycerin increases the diagnostic yield of the test while decreasing its specificity.

Electrophysiologic Study

Invasive electrophysiologic (EP) studies are performed by recording the electrical activity of the heart through catheters strategically positioned in the right atrial and ventricular chambers. This test may be useful in a group of patients in whom conduction disorders of the sinus or AV node are suggested. The results may help determine the mechanism of heart block and the need for permanent pacemaker implantation. More commonly, EP studies are used to evaluate patients with documented tachyarrhythmias or with syncope for which a tachyarrhythmia is suggested as the cause. Both supraventricular and ventricular tachyarrhythmias may be reproduced by programmed electrical stimulation. If a tachyarrhythmia is induced, the application of radiofrequency energy at the arrhythmia site of origin or targeting a critical component of the arrhythmia circuit often leads to tachycardia termination.

Syncope

Syncope is defined as sudden, transient loss of consciousness and may be the result of a variety of cardiac and noncardiac conditions (Table 10–2). Presyncope is a feeling of impending syncope without true loss of consciousness. Cardiovascular causes are responsible for the vast majority of syncope episodes and produce loss of consciousness by means of a drop in blood pressure, with resultant bilateral cortical or brainstem hypoperfusion. Cerebrovascular disease is an uncommon cause of syncope, unless bilateral carotid artery disease or vertebrobasilar disease is present.

The most important aspect of the approach to the patient with syncope is obtaining a thorough history, both from the patient and from any witnesses to the episode. The conditions during which a syncopal episode occurs may suggest the cause. For instance, syncope that occurs on arising from a lying or sitting position suggests orthostasis. Exercise-induced syncope suggests obstructive cardiac disease, such as aortic or mitral valve stenosis or hypertrophic cardiomyopathy. Syncope during straining, coughing, or micturition is the result of Valsalva-induced decrease in venous return. A history of palpitations preceding the event suggests an arrhythmic cause. Syncope that occurs during emotional stress suggests a vasovagal episode. Certain features may suggest a noncardiac cause, including incontinence or tonic-clonic movements, which suggest seizure. Patients who suffer a cardiac syncopal episode usually regain consciousness rapidly (<5 min). Longer episodes of unresponsiveness suggest a noncardiac cause. Review of the patient's medications is important and may suggest drug-induced hypotension or arrhythmias as the cause of a syncopal episode.

The physical examination of a patient with syncope should include evaluation of orthostatic changes in the heart rate and blood pressure, a thorough cardiac examination to exclude significant murmurs, a neurologic examination, and carotid sinus massage when the history suggests carotid sinus sensitivity as the diagnosis. A 12-lead ECG should be obtained and may be diagnostic of the cause of syncope (e.g., complete heart block) or reveal abnormalities that warrant further evaluation (e.g., prior myocardial infarction, conduction system disease, nonsustained VT, a delta wave of WPW syndrome).

Further cardiac testing is useful in select patients. An echocardiogram is helpful in patients in whom structural heart disease or an arrhythmic cause is suspected. A 24-hour Holter monitor or an event monitor may be helpful in evaluating for possible arrhythmias. In patients with recurrent syncope without evidence of a structural or arrhythmic cause and in patients in whom the history suggests vasovagal or neurocardiogenic syncope, tilt-table testing may be useful (see earlier discussion). In patients in whom the history, ECG, or Holter monitoring suggest a tachyarrhythmia or bradyarrhythmia as the cause of syncope, EP testing is indicated (see earlier discussion). However, in patients with a normal resting ECG and no structural heart disease, the diagnostic yield of EP testing is so low that it is rarely useful. Figure 10–11 offers a diagnostic approach to the patient with syncope. In spite all of these diagnostic modalities, in more than 30% of all patients with syncope, the cause remains unknown. Fortunately, these patients can be reassured of a good prognosis.

Sudden Cardiac Death

Sudden cardiac death (SCD) is commonly defined as a natural, unexpected death occurring within 1 hour of the onset of symptoms. Sudden death may be the result of a variety of cardiac and noncardiac diseases (Table 10–3), although cardiac causes are by far the most common. SCD accounts for an estimated 300,000 deaths per year—over 50% of all deaths from cardiac causes—and is the leading cause of death among men ages 20 to 60. Ventricular tachyarrhythmias (VT and VF) occurring in the setting of ischemic heart disease account for the mechanism of death in the vast majority of these patients. Polymorphic VT occurring in the setting of LTQS (see later discussion), short

Table 10–2 Causes of Syncope

Cause	Features
Peripheral Vascular or Circulatory	
Vasovagal syncope (neurally mediated)	Prodrome of pallor, yawning, nausea, diaphoresis; precipitated by stress or pain; occurs when patient is upright, aborted by recumbency; fall in blood pressure with or without a decrease in heart rate
Micturition syncope	Syncope with urination (probably vagal)
Post-tussive syncope	Syncope after paroxysm of coughing
Hypersensitive carotid sinus syndrome	Vasodepressor and/or cardio-inhibitory responses with light carotid sinus massage (see text)
Drugs	Orthostasis
	Occurs with antihypertensive drugs, tricyclic antidepressants, phenothiazines
Volume depletion	Orthostasis
	Occurs with hemorrhage, excessive vomiting or diarrhea, Addison's disease
Autonomic dysfunction	Orthostasis
	Occurs in diabetes, alcoholism, Parkinson's disease, deconditioning after a prolonged illness
Central Nervous System	
Cerebrovascular	Transient ischemic attacks and strokes are unusual causes of syncope; associated neurologic abnormalities are usually present
Seizures	Warning aura sometimes present, jerking of extremities, tongue biting, urinary incontinence, postictal confusion
Metabolic	
Hypoglycemia	Confusion, tachycardia, jitteriness before syncope; patient may be taking insulin
Cardiac	
Obstructive	Syncope is often exertional; physical findings consistent with aortic stenosis, hypertrophic obstructive cardiomyopathy, cardiac tamponade, atrial myxoma, prosthetic valve malfunction, Eisenmenger syndrome, tetralogy of Fallot, primary pulmonary hypertension, pulmonic stenosis, massive pulmonary embolism
Arrhythmias	Syncope may be sudden and occurs in any position; episodes of dizziness or palpitations; may be a history of heart disease; brady- or tachyarrhythmias may be responsible—check for hypersensitive carotid sinus

QT syndrome (see later discussion), Brugada syndrome (see later discussion), and hypertrophic cardiomyopathy are also common causes of SCD, particularly in young patients. VT in the absence of underlying heart disease and rapid conduction of AF or AFL over an accessory bypass tract precipitating VT-VF account for other tachyarrhythmic causes of SCD. Bradyarrhythmias and pulseless electrical activity, a condition during which the electrical activity of the heart continues in the absence of mechanical contraction, account for only a small proportion of SCD.

Ischemic heart disease is present in at least 80% of patients who die suddenly of a cardiac cause, and as many as 75% of these patients have a prior history of a MI. In the remainder, SCD is their first manifestation of ischemic heart disease. Nonetheless, only 20% of patients resuscitated from an episode of SCD have evidence of having had an acute transmural MI at the time of the event. This circumstance is of prognostic importance—survivors of SCD that occurred in the setting of an acute MI have a recurrence rate of less than 5% in the following year compared with a 30% recurrence rate in survivors in whom SCD occurred in the absence of an acute infarction.

The only effective treatment of an acute episode of SCD is immediate circulatory support with cardiopulmonary resuscitation (CPR) and establishment of an effective cardiac rhythm with electrical defibrillation. Once a stable rhythm has been restored, intravenous anti-arrhythmic therapy, usually with amiodarone, should be instituted for the first 24 hours while determination of the precipitating cause is made. That VT-VF was the mechanism of SCD cannot be assumed, unless these rhythms were documented at the time of arrest. A thorough search for other possible causes is mandatory. In SCD survivors, a full cardiac evaluation should be performed to define cardiac function, identify the presence of reversible heart disease, and assess the risk of recurrent arrhythmias. Echocardiography can identify possible structural cardiac causes of SCD (e.g., aortic stenosis, hypertrophic cardiomyopathy) and allows assessment of left ventricular function. This identification is important prognostically—patients with depressed ventricular function have a higher likelihood of recurrent SCD, a poorer response to anti-arrhythmic drug therapy, and a higher mortality rate than do those with normal ventricular function. Ambulatory ECG monitoring and stress testing are useful in

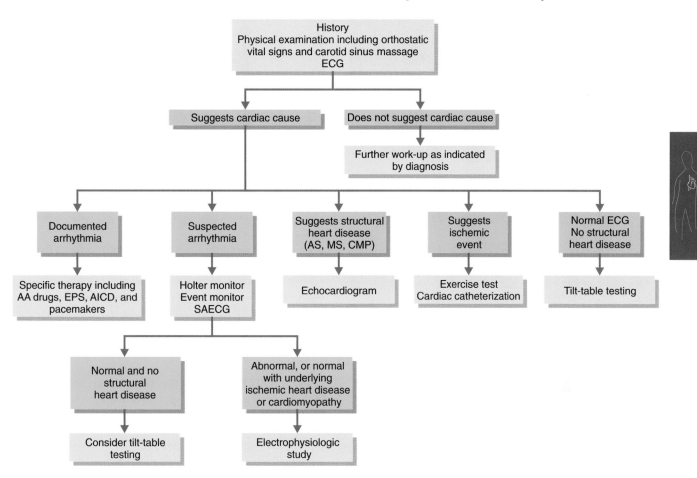

Figure 10–11 Diagnostic approach to the patient with syncope. AA = anti-arrhythmic; AICD = automatic implantable cardioverter-defibrillator; AS = aortic stenosis; CMP = cardiomyopathy; ECG = electrocardiogram; EPS = electrophysiologic study; MS = mitral stenosis; SAECG = signal-averaged ECG.

documenting the frequency and severity of recurrent ventricular arrhythmias and in assessing for residual ischemia.

Patients in whom acute MI precipitates SCD do not require anti-arrhythmic therapy. Cardiac catheterization and revascularization should be performed if possible. In SCD survivors in whom the event occurred in the absence of an acute MI, and in patients with recurrent ventricular tachyarrhythmias, the implantation of an ICD has been the mainstay of treatment. Trials during the 1990s suggested that sotalol and amiodarone are effective anti-arrhythmic drugs in the treatment of patients with SCD or recurrent VT. Several secondary prevention trials including the Antiarrhythmics Versus Implantable Defibrillators (AVID) trial significantly changed the therapeutic approach to SCD survivors. This study was a randomized trial of anti-arrhythmic therapy (primarily amiodarone) versus ICD implantation in patients with depressed ventricular function who had survived an episode of life-threatening ventricular tachyarrhythmia, and it demonstrated a mortality benefit with ICD therapy.

Perhaps the most effective method of treating SCD is by identifying patients at highest risk and instituting therapy aimed at preventing its occurrence. In the patient who has had MI, several factors have been shown to be associated with an increased risk of SCD (Table 10–4). The occurrence of frequent complex ventricular ectopy in patients after an acute MI is associated with a near tripling of the risk of subsequent SCD; however, attempts at suppression of these arrhythmias with anti-arrhythmic agents have resulted in an increased mortality. Several studies have, however, demonstrated a decrease in overall mortality, as well as in SCD, in patients treated with beta-blocking agents after a MI. Therefore these agents should be instituted in these patients unless a contraindication to their use exists. Patients who have had MI with moderate left ventricular dysfunction, nonsustained VT on ambulatory ECG monitoring, and inducible monomorphic VT during EP testing have been shown to have an improved survival with ICD implantation (according to the Multicenter Unsustained Tachycardia Trial [MUSTT] and Multicenter Automatic Defibrillator Implantation Trial [MADIT]). Recently, the MADIT-II and Sudden Cardiac Death in Heart Failure Trial (SCD-HeFT) demonstrated improved survival with ICD therapy regardless of the presence of spontaneous or inducible ventricular arrhythmias. The MADIT-II trial was designed to evaluate the effect of prophylactic ICD therapy on survival in patients with prior MI and left ventricular ejection fraction ≤30%. The trial was stopped in November 2001 because ICD therapy was shown to save lives. The SCD-HeFT trial compared ICD therapy with amiodarone and placebo in patients with ischemic or nonischemic dilated cardiomyopathy with a left

Table 10–3	**Causes of Sudden Cardiac Death**

Noncardiac

Central nervous system hemorrhage
Massive pulmonary embolus
Drug overdose
Hypoxia secondary to lung disease
Aortic dissection or rupture

Cardiac

Ventricular fibrillation
Myocardial ischemia/injury
Long QT syndrome
Short QT syndrome
Brugada syndrome
Arrhythmogenic right ventricular dysplasia
Ventricular tachycardia
Bradyarrhythmias, sick sinus syndrome
Aortic stenosis
Tetralogy of Fallot
Pericardial tamponade
Cardiac tumors
Complications of infective endocarditis
Hypertrophic cardiomyopathy (arrhythmia or obstruction)
Myocardial ischemia
Atherosclerosis
Prinzmetal's angina
Kawasaki's arteritis

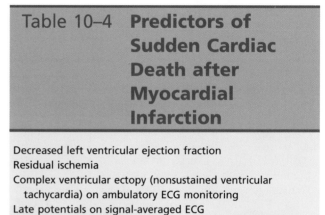

Table 10–4	**Predictors of Sudden Cardiac Death after Myocardial Infarction**

Decreased left ventricular ejection fraction
Residual ischemia
Complex ventricular ectopy (nonsustained ventricular tachycardia) on ambulatory ECG monitoring
Late potentials on signal-averaged ECG
Decreased heart rate variability
Prolonged QT on ECG
Induction of sustained monomorphic ventricular tachycardia with programmed electrical stimulation

ECG = electrocardiogram.

ventricular ejection fraction ≤35%, New York Heart Association (NYHA) Functional Classification II–III, and no history or suspicion of sustained VT or VF. Similar to the MADIT-II, ICD therapy was shown to improve all-cause mortality in this patient population. As a result of these multicenter trials, patients with moderate to severe left ventricular dysfunction should be referred for an ICD implant for primary prevention of SCD.

Management Of Cardiac Arrhythmias

When initiating treatment of an arrhythmia, several clinical factors should be considered, including the nature of the specific arrhythmia, the setting in which the arrhythmia occurred, the consequences of the arrhythmia, and the potential risks of therapy. Certain arrhythmias (e.g., VT) can cause hemodynamic instability or SCD and warrant aggressive treatment to prevent recurrences. Other arrhythmias are hemodynamically stable but produce intolerable symptoms (e.g., palpitations, dizziness) and should be similarly suppressed. Certain arrhythmias may not be a problem acutely but warrant treatment to prevent long-term complications (e.g., stroke prevention in AF). The situation in which an arrhythmia occurs may dictate the need for therapy. For example, VF occurring in the setting of an acute MI is

unlikely to recur if the underlying ischemic process is treated and warrants no specific therapy for the arrhythmia itself. Conversely, VF occurring in the absence of acute ischemia is likely to recur and requires aggressive therapy. Arrhythmias that are tolerated well and require no therapy in patients with structurally normal hearts may not be tolerated at all in patients with depressed left ventricular systolic function or valvular heart disease and may require aggressive therapy in these settings. Some arrhythmias are secondary to an underlying disease process. Metabolic abnormalities (e.g., hypokalemia, hypomagnesemia, hypoxia, hyperthyroidism) and acute illness (e.g., congestive heart failure, sepsis, anemia) may precipitate arrhythmias, as may emotional upset, certain foods or beverages (e.g., caffeine-containing products, alcohol), and both prescription (e.g., digoxin, theophylline, anti-arrhythmic agents) and nonprescription (e.g., decongestants, certain antibiotics, cocaine) drugs. Although treatment of arrhythmias associated with these factors may be warranted acutely, long-term therapy is not required, provided that the inciting factor is removed or controlled.

Asymptomatic arrhythmias are difficult clinical problems. Ventricular premature contractions and nonsustained VT may be markers of underlying heart disease and, although benign themselves, may progress to more malignant arrhythmias. Treatment with anti-arrhythmic medications in these instances has not been shown to decrease mortality, and, in fact, some agents are associated with increased mortality because of their pro-arrhythmic side effects. The presence of symptoms is clearly important in deciding whether or not to treat an arrhythmia. In patients who are asymptomatic, the risks of the arrhythmia must be compared with the risks of therapy before instituting an anti-arrhythmic agent.

Pharmacologic Therapy

Anti-arrhythmic medications work by interfering with various aspects of myocardial depolarization or repolarization and can be classified based on their particular mechanism of action. The most frequently used classification system is the Vaughn Williams classification, which categorizes these drugs based on their in vitro EP effects on normal Purkinje fibers (Table 10–5). This classification is a helpful construct; however, several limitations to its interpretation and use exist. First, whether the in vivo effects of a drug in a specific class are the same as those seen in vitro is unclear. Second, a given drug may have properties of more than one class. Third, drugs in the same class may differ somewhat in their modes of action, side effect profile, and clinical effectiveness for treating a given arrhythmia. Nonetheless, the classification remains a useful communication tool.

Several general points are worth noting in the management with anti-arrhythmic agents. Many drugs are given as a standard dose, whereas others are titrated, depending on clinical effect. Therapeutic blood levels of many drugs have been established; however, the absolute concentration of the agent in the patient's blood is a much less useful guide to therapy than is the clinical effectiveness of the drug and the presence or absence of side effects. The therapeutic-to-toxic ratio of most anti-arrhythmic agents is small such that, at therapeutically effective doses, toxic side effects are common. Knowledge of the metabolism of these agents is important. Either the kidney or the liver metabolizes most anti-arrhythmic drugs (Table 10–6), and doses must be decreased in patients with renal or hepatic dysfunction to avoid toxicity. Many of these agents have negative inotropic effects, and, even at nontoxic levels, noncardiac side effects are common. These drugs frequently interact with other medications and may interfere with nonpharmacologic modes of therapy. For example, quinidine and amiodarone increase the serum digoxin level and augment the anticoagulant effect of warfarin. Flecainide and propafenone increase the amount of energy required for an artificial pacemaker to pace the heart effectively (pacing threshold), whereas amiodarone increases the amount of energy required to defibrillate the heart effectively (defibrillation threshold). For this reason, artificial pacemakers and ICDs need to be checked after instituting anti-arrhythmic agents.

Table 10–6 and Table 10–7 summarize the important characteristics of the most commonly used anti-arrhythmic agents. An in-depth discussion of each agent is beyond the scope of this chapter; however, several points warrant specific mention.

Class IA anti-arrhythmic agents block sodium channels to a moderate degree and are useful for the long-term oral treatment of both supraventricular and ventricular arrhythmias. Procainamide is also available in an intravenous preparation and is useful for the acute management of these arrhythmias. These agents prolong the conduction time and the ERP of most cardiac tissues, including accessory pathways, and may be effective therapy for patients with AVNRT or AVRT. Because these agents slow the spontaneous sinoatrial rate and can enhance conduction through the AV node through vagolytic effects, they can induce more rapid ventricular rates in patients with AF and AFL. Therefore, care must be taken to ensure that the ventricular rate is controlled with a β-blocker, calcium channel blocker, or digoxin before instituting a type IA agent in patients with atrial arrhythmias. As a result of its α-adrenergic blocking effects, quinidine may cause significant hypotension and may also produce syncope in 0.5% to 2% of patients as a result of QT prolongation and subsequent polymorphic VT. This pro-arrhythmic effect may also be seen with the other agents in this class. Between 60% and 70% of patients who receive procainamide develop antinuclear antibodies (specifically antihistone antibodies), whereas a clinical lupus–like syndrome occurs in only 20% to 30%; this rate is reversible on stopping the drug. Disopyramide has significant negative inotropic effects and should be used with extreme caution (if at all) in patients with left ventricular dysfunction.

Class IB agents are weak sodium-channel blockers. They are useful for treating ventricular tachyarrhythmias, but, because they have minimal effects on the sinus or AV nodes, they are not effective for supraventricular arrhythmias. Lidocaine is the most clinically useful drug in this class and is the initial intravenous drug of choice in patients with ventricular tachyarrhythmias. Lidocaine appears particularly effective in ischemia-related arrhythmias; however, its prophylactic use during an acute infarction is not indicated and may increase mortality. Phenytoin is a potent anti-epileptic that also has class IB anti-arrhythmic properties. It is

Table 10–5	**The Vaughn Williams Classification of Anti-arrhythmic Drugs**	
Class	**Physiologic Effect***	**Examples**
I	Blocks sodium channels; predominantly reduces the maximum velocity of the upstroke of the action potential (phase 0)	—
IA	Intermediate potency blockade	Quinidine, procainamide, disopyramide
IB	Least potent blockade	Lidocaine, tocainide, mexiletine, phenytoin
IC	Most potent blockade	Flecainide, propafenone, moricizine
II	β-Adrenergic-receptor blockade	Propranolol, metoprolol, atenolol
III	Potassium-channel blockade: predominantly prolongs action potential duration	Amiodarone, sotalol, bretylium, ibutilide, dofetilide
IV	Calcium channel blockade	Verapamil, diltiazem

*Several agents have physiologic effects characteristic of more than one class.

Table 10–6 Select Characteristics of Anti-arrhythmic Drugs

Drug	Effect on Surface ECG	Effect on LV Function	Important Drug Interactions	Effect on Pacing and Defibrillation Thresholds	Major Route of Elimination
Quinidine	Prolongs QRS and QT	Negative inotropic effect	Increases digoxin level and warfarin effect Cimetidine increases quinidine level Phenobarbital, phenytoin, and rifampin decrease quinidine level	Increases PT and DT at high doses	Liver and kidney
Procainamide	Prolongs PR, QRS, and QT	Negative inotrope	Cimetidine, alcohol, and amiodarone increase procainamide level	Increases PT at high doses	Liver and kidney
Disopyramide	Prolongs QRS and QT	Negative inotrope	Phenobarbital, phenytoin, and rifampin all decrease disopyramide level	Increases PT at high doses	Liver and kidney
Lidocaine	Shortens QT	None	Propranolol, metoprolol, and cimetidine all increase lidocaine level	Increases DT	Liver
Mexiletine	Shortens QT	None	Increases theophylline level Phenobarbital, phenytoin, and rifampin all decrease mexiletine level	Variable effects	Liver
Flecainide	Prolongs PR and QRS	Negative inotrope	Increases digoxin level	Increases PT; variable effect on DT	Liver and kidney
Propafenone	Prolongs PR and QRS	Negative inotrope	Increases digoxin, theophylline, and cyclosporine levels; increases warfarin effect Phenobarbital, phenytoin, and rifampin decrease propafenone level Cimetidine and quinidine increase propafenone level	Increases PT; variable effect on DT	Liver
Moricizine	Prolongs PR and QRS	Negative inotrope	Decreases theophylline level Cimetidine increases moricizine level	—	Liver
Amiodarone	Prolongs PR and QT; slows sinus rate	None	Increases digoxin and cyclosporine levels; increases warfarin effect	Increases DT	Liver
Sotalol	Prolongs PR and QT; slows sinus rate	Negative inotrope	Additive effects with other β-blockers	Decreases DT	Kidney
Bretylium	Prolongs PR and QT	None	—	—	Kidney
Ibutilide	Prolongs PR and QT	None	—	Decreases DT	Liver
Dofetilide	Prolongs QT	None	Verapamil, diltiazem, cimetidine, and ketoconazole all increase dofetilide level	Decreases DT	Liver and kidney

DT = defibrillation threshold; ECG = electrocardiogram; LV = left ventricle; PT = pacing threshold.
PR, QRS, and QT refer to their respective intervals on the surface ECG.

Table 10–7 Common Side Effects of Select Anti-arrhythmic Drugs

Drug	Major Side Effects
Quinidine	Nausea, diarrhea, abdominal cramping Cinchonism: decreased hearing, tinnitus, blurred vision, delirium Rash, thrombocytopenia, hemolytic anemia Hypotension, torsades de pointes, quinidine syncope
Procainamide	Drug-induced lupus syndrome Nausea, vomiting Rash, fever, hypotension, psychosis, agranulocytosis Torsades de pointes
Disopyramide	Anticholinergic: dry mouth, blurred vision, constipation, urinary retention, closed-angle glaucoma Hypotension, worsening heart failure
Lidocaine	CNS: dizziness, peri-oral numbness, paresthesias, altered consciousness, coma, seizures
Mexiletine	Nausea, vomiting CNS: dizziness, tremor, paresthesias, ataxia, confusion
Flecainide	CNS: blurred vision, headache, ataxia Congestive heart failure, ventricular pro-arrhythmia
Propafenone	Nausea, vomiting, constipation, metallic taste to food Dizziness, headache, exacerbation of asthma, ventricular pro-arrhythmia
Moricizine	Nausea, dizziness, headache
β-Blockers	Bronchospasm, bradycardia, fatigue, depression, impotence Congestive heart failure
Calcium channel blockers	Congestive heart failure, bradycardia, heart block, constipation
Amiodarone	Agranulocytosis, pulmonary fibrosis, hepatopathy, hyper- or hypothyroidism, corneal micro-deposits, bluish discoloration of the skin, nausea, constipation, bradycardia Hypotension with intravenous administration
Sotalol	Same as β-blockers, torsades de pointes
Bretylium	Orthostatic hypotension Transient hypertension, tachycardia, and worsening of arrhythmia (initial catecholamine release)
Ibutilide	Torsades de pointes
Dofetilide	Torsades de pointes, headache, dizziness, diarrhea

CNS = central nervous system.

particularly effective in treating atrial and ventricular arrhythmias caused by digoxin toxicity. These agents have relatively little effect on hemodynamics, and clinically important pro-arrhythmia is rare.

Class IC agents are potent blockers of sodium channels. They are effective therapy for both ventricular and supraventricular arrhythmias; however, the use of flecainide and moricizine to treat asymptomatic ventricular arrhythmias after MI has been proved to increase mortality, especially in patients with left ventricular dysfunction. Flecainide remains an effective and relatively safe therapy for supraventricular arrhythmias (especially paroxysmal AF) in patients with structurally normal hearts. Propafenone is similar to flecainide but with β-blocking effects and therefore may exacerbate bradycardia, heart block, heart failure, and bronchospasm. Both drugs can convert AF to AFL (class IC AFL), which usually conducts at faster rates. Therefore, similar to class IA agents, class IC agents should only be used after the initiation of an AV-nodal agent (beta-blockers, calcium channel blockers, digoxin) when treating patients with atrial arrhythmias.

The β-blockers and nondihydropyridine calcium channel blockers constitute class II and class IV anti-arrhythmic agents, respectively. The anti-arrhythmic effectiveness of these drugs relates mainly to their ability to slow the rate of the sinus node and decrease conduction through the AV node. They are effective for controlling the rate of AF and AFL, although they are not effective for converting these arrhythmias to normal sinus rhythm. Intravenous administration of these agents may acutely terminate some supraventricular tachyarrhythmias, especially reentrant rhythms that use the AV node as one limb of the reentrant circuit (i.e., AVNRT, AVRT). By virtue of their ability to slow conduction in the AV node selectively, these agents may facilitate conduction down a bypass tract and are contraindicated in patients with WPW syndrome and atrial tachyarrhythmias. These agents also have a negative inotropic effect and thus must be used with caution in patients with left ventricular dysfunction or overt heart failure.

Class III anti-arrhythmic drugs prolong the action potential duration. Amiodarone is mainly a class III agent but has physiologic effects of all four classes. It is an effective therapy for a wide range of both supraventricular and ventricular arrhythmias and is safe to use in patients with left ventricular dysfunction. Amiodarone is the drug of choice for the treatment of AF in patients with heart failure and may decrease arrhythmic death after MI and in patients with nonischemic cardiomyopathy. It is more effective than other antiarrhythmic agents in preventing recurrences of VT or VF and is the drug of choice for treating these arrhythmias in the setting of cardiac arrest. In addition, amiodarone may be administered intravenously for the acute treatment of refractory ventricular tachyarrhythmias. Its use has been somewhat limited by the fear of significant side effects; however, with maintenance doses under 300 mg/day, adverse effects are less common. The most serious side effect is pulmonary fibrosis, which shows as an interstitial pattern on chest radiographs and a restrictive pattern on pulmonary function tests. Excess sinus bradycardia and AV block are also serious cardiovascular adverse effects, particularly when combined with classes II and IV agents. Thyroid function abnormalities are relatively common, however, they are rarely a cause for drug discontinuation. Patients receiving amiodarone therapy should have liver and thyroid function tests performed at least twice a year and a yearly chest radiograph and pulmonary function tests. A more comprehensive list of the potential side effects is available in Table 10–7. Sotalol has both class III and β-blocking effects. It is particularly effective for treating ventricular tachyarrhythmias, but it is also effective for a large number of supraventricular arrhythmias, including AF. Ibutilide is a parenteral class III agent that is effective for the acute termination of AF and AFL of recent onset (<90 days), and it enhances the success of electrical cardioversion of this arrhythmia. Dofetilide is a pure class III agent that is effective for treating atrial arrhythmias; it is especially effective for the termination and prevention of AF and AFL. Dofetilide has no demonstrable negative inotropic effect, is more effective than sotalol is for the acute conversion of AF, and is not associated with the risk of pulmonary and hepatic toxicity that is seen with amiodarone. All of these agents at initiation are routinely monitored for prolongation of the QT intervals and are potentially associated with an increased risk of torsades de pointes. The incidence of this arrhythmia is quite low in patients given amiodarone but is as high as 2% and 5% in patients with impaired ventricular function who are given dofetilide or ibutilide, respectively. Bretylium causes an initial release of norepinephrine from nerve terminals and may result in transient hypertension and aggravation of arrhythmias. It subsequently prevents norepinephrine release and thus prevents arrhythmia recurrence. Bretylium is administered intravenously and is indicated for treating life-threatening ventricular tachyarrhythmias when other agents have failed.

Several other anti-arrhythmic agents that do not fit into the Vaughn Williams classification are worthy of mention. Adenosine is an endogenous nucleoside that, when given intravenously in pharmacologic doses, results in profound, albeit transient, slowing of AV conduction, and sinus node discharge rate. Flushing, chest pain, and dyspnea commonly occur after adenosine injection but are short lived because of the short half-life of this agent (approximately 6 seconds). The main use of adenosine is in the treatment of SVT; it terminates more than 95% of AVNRTs and AVRTs. During rapid atrial tachyarrhythmias, transient adenosine-induced heart block may help unmask the underlying rhythm. Theophylline blocks the effects of adenosine, and dipyridamole potentiates its effects. Atropine blocks the effects of the vagus nerve on the heart and results in an increased sinus rate and increased conduction through the AV node. It is indicated for the treatment of symptomatic bradycardia. Digoxin enhances vagal tone and results in a slowing of the sinus node rate and slowed conduction through the AV node. It is useful for controlling the ventricular response to a SVT when combined with a beta-blocker or a calcium channel blocker.

Nonpharmacologic Therapy of Bradyarrhythmias

CARDIAC PACEMAKERS

Artificial cardiac pacemakers are devices that deliver a small electrical impulse to a localized region of the heart, causing the affected myocytes to depolarize to the threshold potential, thus initiating an action potential that then spreads to the remainder of the heart. These devices can be used temporarily to treat a transient bradyarrhythmia resulting from a reversible cause, or they can be implanted permanently to treat irreversible disorders of impulse formation or conduction that result in recurrent or persistent bradyarrhythmias. Temporary pacemakers can deliver the electrical impulse indirectly through the chest wall (transcutaneous pacing), or they can be placed intravenously into the right side of the heart to deliver the impulse locally (transvenous pacing). Transcutaneous pacing requires higher energy to *capture* the heart electrically and therefore can be somewhat uncomfortable. In addition, some patients, especially obese individuals, cannot be effectively paced transcutaneously. Nonetheless, this type of pacemaker can be an effective mode of pacing in most patients, may help stabilize a patient who has an unstable bradyarrhythmia until a transvenous or permanent pacemaker can be inserted, and is useful to have as prophylaxis for acutely ill patients who are at high risk of developing significant bradyarrhythmias. Permanent pacemakers are usually inserted intravenously. The pulse generator is buried in a *pocket* created in the pectoral region of the chest wall, and the leads pass from the generator through the cephalic, axillary, or subclavian vein and into the right atrium and/or ventricle where they are anchored in place. Indications for permanent pacemaker insertion are listed in Table 10–8.

Current pacemakers allow for the tailoring of the pacemaker function to the specific needs of the patient. A code has been developed that describes these various functions. The first letter reflects the cardiac chamber being paced (V = ventricle; A = atrium; D = dual chamber/atrium and ventricle). The second letter reflects the chamber in which electrical activity is being sensed (V = ventricle; A = atrium; D = dual chamber/atrium and ventricle; O = none). The third letter reflects the response mode of the pacemaker. If the pacemaker senses the patient's own native beat, it may respond by being inhibited (I), being triggered to fire at the same time as the native beat (T), or being triggered to fire after a sensed atrial event but inhibited by a sensed ventricular event (D). Newer pacemakers are also capable of sensing a patient's activity level (through temperature, vibration, or respiratory sensors) and changing their paced rate in response to a sensed increase in metabolic need. This mode is termed a *rate-responsive* mode and is indicated by an *R* after the first three letters. Examples of common pacing modes are listed in Table 10–9.

The choice of pacing mode depends on the needs of the individual patient. Dual-chamber pacing maintains AV synchrony, which is an advantage because the timing of atrial contraction is important for maximizing cardiac output. Therefore, AV synchronous pacing is useful for patients with left ventricular dysfunction in whom loss of AV synchrony may result in the precipitation of heart failure. For patients who have structurally normal hearts or who have a pacemaker implanted for only occasional symptomatic bradyarrhythmias, maintaining AV synchrony is not as important, and a single ventricular pacing electrode is sufficient. In patients with chronic AF, AV synchrony is not possible, and a single ventricular pacing electrode is also adequate.

Safeguards have been programmed into the pacemakers that limit the upper pacing rate, thus preventing rapid ventricular pacing in response to a supraventricular tachyarrhythmia. Newer pacemakers can detect the onset of an atrial tachyarrhythmia and switch to an appropriate pacing mode (mode switching). Pacemaker malfunction may be demonstrated as failure of a pacemaker impulse to depolarize the heart (failure to capture), abnormalities of sensing (oversensing or undersensing), or pacing at an abnormal rate. Many pacemakers decrease their pacing rate or change their pacing mode as the battery life is depleted.

Table 10–8 Indications for Pacemaker Insertion

Pacing is definitely indicated.	Acquired third-degree AVB with or without symptoms*
	Congenital third-degree AVB with symptoms
	Mobitz I (Wenckebach) second-degree AVB with symptomatic bradycardia
	Mobitz II second-degree AVB with or without symptomatic bradycardia
	Sinus bradycardia (heart rate <40 beats/min) with symptoms
	Alternating bundle branch block
Pacing is probably indicated.	Congenital AVB with moderate bradycardia
	Bifascicular block (RBBB + LAFB or RBBB + LPFB) with a history of syncope after ruling our other causes
	Incidental finding of significant His-Purkinje disease during invasive cardiac electrophysiologic evaluation
	Transient third-degree AVB or Mobitz II second-degree heart block after an AMI
	Neurocardiogenic syncope with a positive tilt-table test
Pacing is not indicated.	Asymptomatic sinus bradycardia
	Asymptomatic sinus node dysfunction
	Bradycardia during sleep
	First-degree AVB
	Asymptomatic Mobitz I (Wenckebach) second-degree AVB
	Transient asymptomatic pause during atrial fibrillation
	Asymptomatic >3-sec pause with CSM
	Recurrent syncope of undetermined cause

*Symptoms include syncope, dizziness, confusion, congestive heart failure, and decreased exercise tolerance.
AMI = acute myocardial infarction; AVB = atrioventricular block; CSM = carotid sinus massage; LAFB = left anterior fascicular block; LBBB = left bundle branch block; LPFB = left posterior fascicular block; RBBB = right bundle branch block.

Table 10–9   Common Pacemaker Modes

Pacemaker Type	Code	Chamber Paced	Chamber Sensed	Mode
Ventricular asynchronous	VOO	V	None	Continuous ventricular pacing regardless of the presence of intrinsic QRS complexes
Ventricular demand	VVI	V	V	Ventricular pacing inhibited by spontaneous QRS complexes
Atrial demand	AAI	A	A	Atrial pacing inhibited by spontaneous P waves
Atrial synchronous, ventricular inhibited	VDD	V	AV	Ventricular pacing follows a sensed P wave after a preset AV delay; ventricular pacing inhibited by spontaneous QRS complexes; no atrial pacing
AV sequential	DVI	AV	V	Ventricular pacing follows atrial pacing after a preset AV delay; ventricular and atrial pacing inhibited by spontaneous QRS; no P wave sensing
Optimal sequential	DDD	AV	AV	Ventricular pacing follows sensed P waves or atrial pacing after a preset AV delay; ventricular pacing inhibited by spontaneous QRS complexes; atrial pacing inhibited by spontaneous P waves
Rate responsive	VVIR	V	V	Same as VVI or DDD, but pacing rate increases with physiologic demand
	DDDR	AV	AV	

A = atrial; AV = atrioventricular; V = ventricular.

Nonpharmacologic Therapy Of Tachyarrhythmias

DIRECT CURRENT CARDIOVERSION AND DEFIBRILLATION

Direct current cardioversion and electrical defibrillation are effective methods for treating atrial or ventricular tachyarrhythmias and are the methods of choice for terminating hemodynamically unstable tachyarrhythmias, as well as stable tachyarrhythmias that are refractory to pharmacologic therapy. Cardioversion refers to the synchronized application of an electrical shock to the heart in an attempt to terminate a tachyarrhythmia. Synchronization of the shock to the QRS complex is a critical feature because the inadvertent administration of an electrical shock during ventricular repolarization (i.e., during the T wave) may precipitate VF. Defibrillation refers to the asynchronous delivery of an electrical shock to terminate VF. Synchronization in this setting is not possible because no organized ventricular activity (QRS) occurs during VF.

Small, although real, risks are inherent with electrical cardioversion. For this reason, several factors need to be addressed before elective procedures. Hyperkalemia should be excluded, as should a supratherapeutic digoxin level; cardioversion in the setting of digoxin toxicity may precipitate refractory ventricular arrhythmias. Adequate sedation is important and can usually be accomplished by the intravenous administration of benzodiazepines (e.g., midazolam) or short-acting anesthetic agents (e.g., propofol). Aspiration of gastric contents can occur because patients are unable to protect their airways during this type of sedation; therefore, patients should have fasted for at least 6 hours before the procedure. Minor cutaneous burns at the site

of application of the electrical current are common, especially if multiple shocks are delivered. Even with appropriate synchronization, electrical cardioversion may precipitate VF, in which case immediate defibrillation is required. In patients with AF, systemic embolization of atrial thrombus may occur after conversion to normal sinus rhythm. Therefore, patients who are undergoing elective cardioversion of AF must be adequately anticoagulated with warfarin for at least 3 weeks before and 4 weeks after electrical cardioversion.

The electrical shock is delivered through paddles applied to the patient's chest. These shocks can be arranged either with both paddles placed on the anterior chest (one paddle at the upper sternal border and the other at the cardiac apex) or with one paddle anteriorly located over the right upper sternal border and the other posteriorly over the left interscapular region. Lubrication with electrolyte gel or the use of electrolyte pads improves contact and decreases burns. AFL can frequently be converted to normal sinus rhythm with low-energy shocks (<50 joules), whereas AF frequently requires higher energy (100 to 360 joules). VT can be cardioverted with low-energy shocks (10 to 50 joules), but VF should always be defibrillated with high-energy shocks (200 to 360 joules). If the initial shock is not successful, the energy should be titrated up and several paddle positions tried before accepting failure. Traditional defibrillators deliver monophasic electrical impulses, whereas newer devices deliver biphasic impulses. These biphasic defibrillators require significantly reduced energy for successful arrhythmia termination and are more effective than monophasic systems. Many tachyarrhythmias recur after initially successful cardioversion. Administering an antiarrhythmic agent may help maintain sinus rhythm in these patients.

RADIOFREQUENCY CATHETER ABLATION AND AUTOMATIC IMPLANTABLE CARDIOVERTER-DEFIBRILLATORS

Because of the frequent recurrence of tachyarrhythmias despite pharmacologic therapy and the risk of pro-arrhythmia with most anti-arrhythmic agents, several nonpharmacologic approaches to the chronic management of tachyarrhythmias have been developed. Radiofrequency catheter ablation involves the application of alternating current electrical energy in the radiofrequency range to a strategically chosen area of the endocardium. An arrhythmogenic focus or the pathway by which the arrhythmia is perpetuated can be identified (mapped), and a radiofrequency-induced lesion can be created at that site, thereby eliminating (i.e., ablating) the arrhythmia. Ablation is effective in eliminating AFL and supraventricular tachyarrhythmias caused by accessory pathways (e.g., WPW syndrome) and dual pathways in the AV node such as AVNRT. The success rate of this procedure in curing these arrhythmias is greater than 95%. In addition, radiofrequency ablation is effective in treating AF, although the success rate is less with this arrhythmia. Ablation is associated with a relatively low risk of complications that include tamponade, stroke, and inadvertent complete AV block in up to 2% of patients, depending on the site of ablation. In patients with AF or AFL that is refractory to pharmacologic rate control, production of iatrogenic complete heart block by ablation of the AV node and subsequent placement of a permanent ventricular pacemaker offers a definitive method of controlling the ventricular rate. Catheter ablation of VT is more difficult than it is for SVT but can be effective in select patients. Patients with monomorphic VT in the absence of structural heart disease (e.g., RVOT-VT, idiopathic left VT, bundle branch reentry VT) are good candidates, and success can be expected in approximately 90% of these instances. Patients with VT related to prior MI are difficult to treat with ablation, and such therapy should be attempted only if these patients have incessant or recurrent VT despite anti-arrhythmic therapy.

ICD therapy is the anti-tachycardic equivalent of a pacemaker and is used for treating ventricular tachyarrhythmias. Similar to the pacemaker, the ICD has a generator that is buried in the pectoral region and is connected to an electrode that is placed transvenously and anchored to the endocardium. The device monitors heart rate and identifies a tachyarrhythmia as any rhythm that is faster than the rate programmed into the device. Most ICDs have several possible therapeutic responses to a sensed tachyarrhythmic event. Pacing the ventricle at a faster rate (anti-tachycardia pacing) may successfully terminate a relatively slow VT. If this level is not successful, the device may then deliver a 20- to 36-joule electrical discharge, which may be repeated several times at escalating energy levels in an attempt to terminate the tachyarrhythmia. Fast VT and VF are usually treated with high-energy shock, although painless anti-tachycardia pacing has been used with some success in treating fast VT. Most of the current devices also have pacemaker capabilities in the event of a bradyarrhythmia.

The indications for the implantation of an ICD are continuously changing as trials demonstrate their effectiveness (or lack of effectiveness) in specific situations. ICDs have been shown to decrease mortality compared with anti-arrhythmic therapy in survivors of VF or hemodynamically unstable VT. They also offer a mortality benefit in patients with ischemic and nonischemic cardiomyopathy who have a left ventricular ejection fraction less than 35%. Anti-arrhythmic therapy is often necessary after ICD implantation to decrease the frequency of ventricular tachyarrhythmic events or to control the rate of SVTs that might lead to inappropriate shocks. Given the effectiveness of radiofrequency ablation and ICDs, surgical therapy of tachyarrhythmias is rarely necessary. Surgery is occasionally used after failed ablation in patients with accessory bypass tracts and those with recurrent or incessant VT that failed medical therapy and ablation. In addition, in patients with refractory VT in the setting of a ventricular aneurysm, surgical aneurysmectomy may eliminate the arrhythmia, with a success rate of approximately 70%, and improve pharmacologic control of the arrhythmia in an additional 20% of patients.

Clinical Syndromes

LONG QT SYNDROME

LTQS refers to specific congenital and acquired abnormalities of repolarization that result in prolongation of the QT interval on the surface ECG (Table 10–10). This circumstance is defined as a QTc greater than 440 ms (QTc equals the QT interval divided by the square root of the RR interval). Acquired forms are the result of various drugs or metabolic abnormalities. At least four separate genetic mutations account for the congenital forms of this disorder and do so by alterations in potassium or sodium channels. Congenital

Table 10–10	Conditions Associated with Prolongation of the QT Interval	
Condition	**Examples**
Congenital	Romano-Ward syndrome (without deafness) Jervell and Lange-Nielsen syndrome (with deafness)
Acquired	Class IA and class III anti-arrhythmic agents
Drugs	Tricyclic antidepressants Phenothiazines Antibiotics (macrolides, pentamidine, trimethoprim-sulfamethoxazole) Terfenadine (especially when combined with macrolides or anti-fungal agents)
Metabolic	Hypokalemia Hypocalcemia Hypomagnesemia
Other	Liquid protein diets

forms may be associated with deafness (Jervell and Lange-Nielsen syndrome) or occur in isolation (Romano-Ward syndrome). The significance of the LTQS is its association with the development of a specific type of VT called *torsades de pointes*. This arrhythmia occurs in the setting of a prolonged QT interval, is usually initiated when a VPC occurs during the susceptible period of repolarization (i.e., at the peak of the T wave), and is characterized by a wide-complex tachyarrhythmia with QRS complexes of varying axis and morphology that appear to rotate around the isoelectric baseline. Frequently, these episodes are self-limited, although syncope and sudden death may occur.

The treatment of torsades de pointes differs from that of other forms of VT. Many anti-arrhythmic agents will prolong the QT interval and exacerbate the arrhythmia. Intravenous magnesium (2 to 3 g) is effective in terminating this arrhythmia even in the presence of normal serum magnesium levels. Treatment with isoproterenol or temporary transvenous pacing at rates of 100 to 120 beats/min can effectively help prevent the arrhythmia, presumably through tachycardia-induced shortening of the QT interval. Removing the inciting agent is of paramount importance in acquired cases. Chronic treatment in patients with the congenital syndromes is with β-blocker therapy at the highest doses tolerated. Chronic pacemaker and/or ICD implantation is indicated in patients with recurrent arrhythmia despite β-blocker therapy. Screening family members of these patients is also important to identify those at risk for this arrhythmia.

SHORT QT SYNDROME

Short QT syndrome is a new clinical entity that is associated with a high incidence SCD and/or AF. The diagnosis is made when a patient exhibits syncope and a corrected QT interval less than 320 ms. Missense mutations in *KCNH2 (HERG)* linked to a gain-of-function of the rapidly activating delayed-rectifier current $I(Kr)$ have been identified in the first two reported families with familial SCD. In addition, two more gain-of-function mutations in the *KCNJ2* gene encoding the strong inwardly rectifying channel protein *Kir2.1* and in the *KCNQ1* gene encoding the α-subunit of the *KvLQT1 (I[Ks])* channel confirmed a genetically heterogeneous disease. The treatment of choice for patients with syncope or SCD is the implantation of an ICD. In the asymptomatic patient, the treatment remains unclear.

BRUGADA SYNDROME

Brugada syndrome is characterized by the presence of a ST-segment elevation in V1–V3 that is unrelated to ischemia, structural heart disease, or electrolyte abnormalities. This syndrome has been linked to mutations in *SCN5A*, the gene encoding for the α-subunit of the sodium channel. Brugada syndrome is a familial disease with an autosomal-dominant mode of transmission with incomplete penetrance and an incidence between 5 and 66 per 10,000 persons. Unfortunately, syncope and SCD caused by rapid polymorphic VT are often the first symptoms in patients with this disease. Unlike ischemia-induced polymorphic VT, the arrhythmia in patients with Brugada syndrome often occur during sleep. Elevated parasympathetic activity and sodium channel blockers such as procainamide and flecainide exacerbate the occurrence of ventricular arrhythmias in patients with Brugada syndrome. On the other hand, high catecholamine states, Isuprel, and potassium I_{to} blockers such as quinidine are effective in suppressing ventricular arrhythmias in patients with this syndrome. Similar to other clinical syndromes associated with SCD, ICD implantation is the preferred therapy in patients with Brugada syndrome and a history of near-syncope, syncope, or SCD. In the asymptomatic patient, the performance of a diagnostic EP study for further risk stratification has been suggested. In patients with inducible sustained ventricular arrhythmias, the implantation of an ICD has been shown to improve long-term outcome. In the asymptomatic patient with a negative EP study, close follow-up is usually sufficient.

Prospectus for the Future

- Identification of specific populations of patients with paroxysmal AF who benefit from pulmonary vein isolation and ablation for maintenance of sinus rhythm
- Evaluation of atrial pacing as a modality to prevent recurrences of AF
- Further clarification of which patient populations benefit from implantation of a cardioverter-defibrillator
- Programming of cardioverter-defibrillators to provide therapy before arrhythmia onset by identifying electrical characteristics that may predict impending arrhythmias (long RR intervals, R-on-T phenomenon, T wave alternans, etc.)
- Progress on the development of genetically engineered biologic pacemakers as alternatives to mechanical pacemakers

References

American College of Cardiology/American Heart Association Task Force on Practice Guidelines: ACC/AHA/NASPE 2002 guideline update for implantation of cardiac pacemakers and antiarrhythmia devices: Summary article. Circulation 106:2145–2161, 2002.

American College of Cardiology/American Heart Association Task Force on Practice Guidelines and the European Society of Cardiology Committee for Practice Guidelines and Policy Conferences: ACC/AHA/ESC guidelines for the management of patients with atrial fibrillation: Executive summary. J Am Coll Cardiol 38:1231–1265, 2001.

Bardy GH, Lee KL, Mark DB, et al: Amiodarone or an implantable cardioverter-defibrillator for congestive heart failure. N Engl J Med 352(3):225–237, 2005.

Wyse DG, Waldo AL, DiMarco JP, et al: The Atrial Fibrillation Follow-up Investigation of Rhythm Management (AFFIRM) investigators: A comparison of rate control and rhythm control in patients with atrial fibrillation. N Engl J Med 347:1825–1833, 2002.

Pericardial and Myocardial Disease

Christopher J. McGann

Saurabh Gupta

Ivor J. Benjamin

Pericardial Disease

ACUTE PERICARDITIS

The pericardium is a protective sac around the heart composed of two distinct layers: The *parietal* pericardium is the fibrous outer layer, and the inner layer, abutting the myocardial surface, is the *visceral* pericardium. These two layers are separated by 5 to 15 mL of clear fluid, produced by the visceral pericardium, which acts as a lubricant between the heart and surrounding structures.

Acute pericarditis results from inflammation of the visceral and parietal pericardium, and, in most instances, its cause is unknown. Viral infection is the most common cause and is believed to account for many of the idiopathic cases. Though less common, pericarditis caused by bacterial infection or tuberculosis can result in life-threatening complications. Inflammation of the pericardium following myocardial infarction (Dressler's syndrome) is a less common clinical diagnosis in the current era of revascularization treatments using thrombolytic drugs and coronary angioplasty. A comprehensive list of conditions that can involve the pericardium is shown in Table 11–1.

The classic clinical presentation of pericarditis is chest pain. Chest pain from myocardial ischemia or pulmonary embolism may mimic pericarditis, and their differentiation can be challenging. Symptoms of pericarditis are typically abrupt in onset, sharp, and positional, with relief after sitting upright and leaning forward. On physical examination, the presence of a pericardial rub indicates contact between two inflamed layers of the pericardium. Pericardial rubs have a characteristic high-pitched, leathery quality, with three components that correspond to movement of the heart during the cardiac cycle (ventricular systole, early ventricular diastole, and atrial contraction). Given that friction rubs may be intermittent and variable in intensity, with only one or two components audible, detection may require serial cardiac examinations. However, the absence of an audible rub does not exclude the diagnosis of pericarditis.

Electrocardiographic (ECG) changes are common and evolve over time. During the acute phase, diffuse ST-segment elevation and PR depression are the classic findings and result from superficial inflammation of the heart. This ECG pattern can be confused with the injury current of transmural ischemia in acute myocardial infarction. However, more EGC leads are involved in pericarditis, and the presence of reciprocal ST-segment depression in ischemia can help differentiate the two entities. Most of the ECG abnormalities resolve over several days to weeks, but T-wave abnormalities may persist much longer. Laboratory testing directed at excluding specific causes of pericarditis may include tuberculin skin testing, evaluation of thyroid and renal function, antinuclear antibody, complement levels, rheumatoid factor, and human immunodeficiency virus (HIV) serologic testing. An elevated erythrocyte sedimentation rate, C-reactive protein, or white blood cell count suggests active inflammation but remains nonspecific for the causal agent. Viral serologic studies have been insensitive and generally do not alter the therapeutic decision. Cardiac enzymes may be elevated if concomitant involvement of the myocardium exists. Chest x-ray and echocardiographic findings are normal in most cases of acute pericarditis unless complicated by a pericardial effusion.

The treatment of acute pericarditis is directed at managing the underlying cause and providing pain relief. For most patients, nonsteroidal anti-inflammatory drugs (NSAIDs) are effective for relieving the chest discomfort and resolving the pericardial inflammation. Oral colchicines (either alone or in combination with NSAIDs) can be an effective alternative. Therapy with glucocorticoids should be reserved for pericarditis that is secondary to neoplasm or unresponsive to combination therapy because some studies suggest that the early use of glucocorticoids may increase the risk of recurrence. Though most cases are self limited and resolve without sequelae, recurrent episodes of pericarditis are not uncommon. In addition, complicated cases of pericarditis can result in cardiac tamponade, pericardial constriction,

Table 11–1   Categories of Pericardial Disease and Select Specific Causes

Idiopathic*

Infectious

Viral* (echovirus, coxsackievirus, adenovirus, cytomegalovirus, hepatitus B, infectious mononucleosis, HIV/AIDs)

Bacterial* (Pneumococcus, Staphylococcus, Streptococcus, Mycoplasma, Lyme disease, *Hemophilus influenzae, Neisseria meningitidis*)

Mycobacteria* (Pneumococcus, Staphylococcus, *Streptococcus avium-intracellulare*)

Fungal (histoplasmosis, coccidioidomycosis)

Protozoal

Immune Inflammatory

Connective tissue disease* (systemic lupus erythematosus, rheumatoid arthritis, scleroderma, mixed)

Arteritis (polyarteritis nodosa, temporal arteritis)

Early postmyocardial infarction

Late postmyocardial infarction (Dressler's syndrome),* late postcardiotomy or thoracotomy,* late posttrauma*

Drug Induced* (e.g., procainamide, hydralazine, isoniazid, cyclosporine)

Neoplastic disease

Primary: mesothelioma, fibrosarcoma, lipoma, etc.

Secondary:* breast and lung carcinomas, lymphomas, leukemias

Radiation Induced*

Early postcardiac surgery

Device and procedure related

Coronary angioplasty, implantable defibrillators, pacemakers

Trauma

Blunt and penetrating* post-cardiopulmonary resuscitation*

Congenital

Cysts, congenital absence

Miscellaneous

Chronic renal failure, dialysis related

Hypothyroidism

Amyloidosis

Aortic dissection

*Causes that exhibit as acute pericarditis.
AIDS = acquired immunodeficiency syndrome;
HIV = human immunodeficiency virus.

and myocardial injury when the process evolves into a myopericarditis.

PERICARDIAL EFFUSION

Pericardial effusion refers to an abnormal accumulation of fluid within the pericardial space. Although symptoms may depend on the underlying disease process (e.g. tuberculosis, rheumatoid arthritis, hypothyroidism), a hemodynamically insignificant pericardial effusion is generally asymptomatic from a cardiovascular perspective. If the pericardial effusion is large, it may result in chest pressure or symptoms related to compression of adjacent structures. For instance, cough, hoarseness, dyspnea, or dysphagia can be initial signs if the effusion impinges on the phrenic nerve, recurrent laryngeal nerve, lungs, or esophagus, respectively.

The hemodynamic consequences of a pericardial effusion are associated with the rate of fluid accumulation rather than the size of the effusion. If fluid accumulates slowly, the pericardial space can accommodate up to 2 L of fluid without a significant increase in pericardial pressure, whereas a rapidly accumulating effusion such as in hemopericardium caused by trauma may result in cardiac tamponade (see later discussion) with the collection of as little as 100 to 200 mL of fluid.

The physical examination in a patient with a small pericardial effusion is often normal. If the effusion is large, the apical impulse may be difficult to palpate, and the heart sounds are muffled. On chest radiographic examination, the cardiac silhouette may be enlarged without pulmonary vascular congestion. When a large volume of pericardial fluid is present, the voltage of the QRS complexes on ECG may be diminished. In addition, the amplitude of the QRS complexes may vary from beat to beat (QRS alternans), an abnormality thought to be secondary to changes in the electrical axis by the heart's *swinging* within the pericardial sac. Echocardiography is a sensitive test to detect pericardial effusion and provides an accurate assessment of its size, location, and hemodynamic significance. Computed tomography (CT) and magnetic resonance imaging (MRI) are emerging techniques being used to determine the cause through enhanced tissue characterization and evaluation of surrounding structures. Unsuspected cases of pericardial effusion are discovered incidentally when these imaging studies are ordered for other indications.

Drainage of the pericardial fluid by percutaneous fine needle aspiration (peri-cardiocentesis) can be performed for diagnostic and therapeutic reasons. In general, *diagnostic pericardiocentesis* is usually of low yield and should be reserved for patients with persistent (>2 wk) pericardial effusions or suspected purulent or tuberculous pericarditis. Pericardiocentesis is usually performed in the cardiac catheterization laboratory under fluoroscopic or echocardiographic guidance. Laboratory analysis of the fluid is important to determine whether the effusion is transudative or exudative, with an accompanying examination and culture for microorganisms. In addition, cytologic examination is performed to rule out malignancy, and triglycerides are measured for evidence of a chylous effusion, which can result from thoracic duct injury. When tuberculosis is suggested, elevated levels of adenosine deaminase are detected in the fluid and support the diagnosis. A tissue sample of the pericardium can be obtained by surgical excision when the diagnosis remains unclear after fluid analysis. Tissue examination is especially important for effusion resulting from a chronic infectious process because pericardial fluid alone identifies the organism in a minority of patients. *Therapeutic pericardiocentesis* is performed to remove excess fluid in patients with effusions resulting in significant symptoms or evidence of hemodynamic compromise. However, for patients with recurrent or loculated effusions, pericardiotomy (pericardial window) may provide an efficient means of drainage.

The treatment for asymptomatic pericardial effusions is directed at the underlying illness, and, in turn, the prognosis depends on the underlying disease. Pericardial effusion caused by neoplastic invasion has a guarded outlook, whereas those caused by treatable infections, connective tissue diseases, or hypothyroidism often resolve with appropriate medical therapy. Some effusions respond to a short course of NSAIDs or colchicines, particularly when associated with suggested viral pericarditis.

CARDIAC TAMPONADE

Cardiac tamponade occurs when accumulation of fluid in the pericardial space exerts pressure on the heart. Initially, cardiac tamponade leads to increased intracardiac filling pressures and elevated venous pressure. With equalization of the intrapericardial and diastolic filling pressures of the heart, ventricular filling is reduced, and stroke volume declines. Adrenergic activation leads to an increase in heart rate, myocardial contractility, and systemic vascular resistance. Eventually, however, these compensatory mechanisms are unable to maintain normal cardiac output, and systemic arterial pressure falls.

The hemodynamic consequences of a pericardial effusion are largely dependent on the rate at which the fluid accumulates. In addition, the restraining characteristics of the pericardium (i.e., normal pericardium is relatively compliant) and the state of intravascular volume can influence the amount of pericardial fluid that is required to induce tamponade. For instance, when hypovolemia is present, compressive effusions result in tamponade more quickly than is seen in euvolemic or hypervolemic states. Patient complaints in cardiac tamponade are attributable to reduced cardiac output. When tamponade develops slowly, symptoms typically include dyspnea, fatigue, and lightheadedness. In contrast, patients with acute tamponade are often critically ill, with symptoms and signs of cardiogenic shock.

On physical examination, patients appear anxious and pale, with tachypnea and diaphoresis. Tachycardia is a compensatory sign and helps maintain cardiac output. Pulsus paradoxus (fall in the systolic blood pressure of more than 10 mm Hg with inspiration) is a characteristic finding in patients with cardiac tamponade. Under normal conditions, the filling of the right ventricle increases with inspiration when intrathoracic pressure is lowered, which results in distention of the right ventricle with minimal impingement on left ventricular inflow. With cardiac tamponade, the compressive effects of the pericardial fluid limit expansion of the right ventricle. As a result, the interventricular septum bulges into the left ventricular cavity to accommodate the increased volume of blood in the right ventricle. This action further

impedes left ventricular filling, leading to a reduction in stroke volume and a fall in systolic pressure. Pulsus paradoxus is not specific for cardiac tamponade, however, and may occur with other disease states such as chronic obstructive pulmonary disease, asthma, severe congestive heart failure, pulmonary embolism, and, in some instance, with constrictive pericarditis. The jugular veins are distended because of elevated right ventricular heart pressures. The x descent is typically prominent, whereas the y descent is absent. The lung fields are clear. The cardiac examination usually reveals quiet heart sounds, though a friction rub may be audible.

If the effusion is large, the chest x-ray examination may reveal an enlarged cardiac silhouette with a globular configuration. The ECG may show reduced voltage or electrical alternans. Echocardiography is the gold standard for noninvasive assessment. The right atrium and right ventricle are thin-walled low-pressure chambers and are most susceptible to the effects of increased intrapericardial pressures. As a result, collapse of these chambers is seen when intrapericardial pressure exceeds right-sided filling pressures. In addition, characteristic interventricular septal motion varies with respiration as do left ventricular filling and output, and the inferior vena cava is typically distended. Despite the usefulness of echocardiography, right-sided heart catheterization may be necessary to document the hemodynamic importance of a pericardial effusion. Typical findings of tamponade include elevation and equalization of atrial and ventricular diastolic pressures. If the intrapericardial pressure is measured simultaneously, it is elevated and equal to the atrial and ventricular filling pressures.

Cardiac tamponade is a medical emergency and requires immediate treatment. Temporizing measures include intravenous hydration. Vasopressors may be necessary to stabilize the patient while definite plans for pericardiocentesis are made. If the effusion is large and circumferential, pericardiocentesis can quickly restore hemodynamic stability. If the effusion is loculated or recurrent, surgical drainage with the formation of a pericardial window may be necessary.

CONSTRICTIVE PERICARDITIS

Constrictive pericarditis develops from permanent scarring of the pericardium in response to various inflammatory conditions. It is characterized by a thickened, fibrotic (or calcified) pericardium that restricts diastolic filling of the heart. The disease process is often diffuse and symmetric and results in elevated and equalized diastolic pressures in all four cardiac chambers. However, in contrast to tamponade, in which ventricular filling is impaired throughout diastole, early diastolic filling in constrictive pericarditis is not impaired. This circumstance leads to rapid early filling of the ventricle secondary to elevated atrial pressure, followed by an abrupt rise and plateau (*square-root sign*) in ventricular pressure during middle and late diastole as the ventricular volume reaches the limit set by the nondistensible pericardium (Fig. 11–1). The causes of pericardial constriction are similar to those that result in pericarditis and include infection, radiation exposure, connective tissue disorders, and uremia. In addition, the condition can occur in the months to years following cardiac surgery. Before the advent of effective antituberculous treatment, mycobacterium

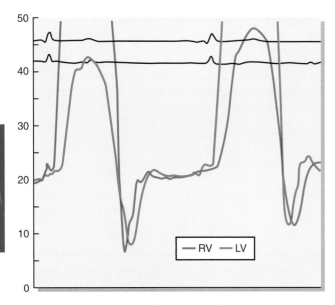

Figure 11–1 Pressure recordings in a patient with constrictive pericarditis: simultaneous right ventricular and left ventricular pressure tracings with equalization of diastolic pressure, as well as *dip and plateau* morphology.

tuberculosis was the most common cause. However, as with pericarditis, most instances of pericardial constriction have no discernable cause and are therefore termed *idiopathic.*

Patients with mild to moderate constriction complain of abdominal pain and exhibit lower extremity swelling from hepatic congestion and peripheral edema. As the process becomes more severe, fatigue and dyspnea result from diminished cardiac output, and pulmonary congestion may cause cough, paroxysmal nocturnal dyspnea (PND), and orthopnea. On physical examination, the jugular veins are distended and paradoxically rise with inspiration (Kussmaul's sign), which occurs because negative intrathoracic pressure is not transmitted to the pericardium in constrictive physiology. As a result, increased venous return cannot be accommodated by the right atrium and right ventricle, and the jugular veins become more distended. Elevation in central venous pressure is accompanied by prominent x and y descents. The y descent, which is absent or diminished in tamponade, is prominent and abbreviated because of a rapid rise in pressure in mid diastole. Pulsus paradoxus is not typically present in constrictive pericarditis because inspiration does not result in an increase in right ventricular filling. Other findings include signs of right ventricular heart failure, such as hepatomegaly, ascites, and peripheral edema. On cardiac examination, an early diastolic sound (pericardial knock) may be heard at the left sternal border, just after the aortic component of S$_2$, and corresponds to cessation of early, rapid diastolic filling.

Chest x-ray examination may reveal pericardial calcification and pleural effusions. QRS voltage may be diminished on ECG with nonspecific ST- and T-wave abnormalities. Although most patients maintain sinus rhythm, some develop atrial ectopy or atrial fibrillation. On echocardiographic examination, the pericardium may appear thickened and immobile. Ventricular septal wall motion abnormalities

and dilation of the inferior vena cava are also common. Doppler echocardiography demonstrates abnormal flow velocities in the pulmonary and hepatic veins and an abnormal pattern of ventricular diastolic filling. CT and MRI are now increasingly used to measure pericardial thickness. As with echocardiography, MRI can be useful to detect the hemodynamic consequences of constrictive pericarditis.

In most patients, right-sided heart catheterization is necessary to establish a diagnosis. Typical findings include elevation and equalization of atrial and ventricular diastolic pressures. Elevation in central venous pressure is accompanied by prominent x and y descents. The y descent, which is absent or diminished in tamponade, is prominent because of rapid emptying of the atrium in early diastole but abbreviated because of the rapid rise in right ventricular pressure in mid diastole. Both the right and left ventricular diastolic pressures show an early diastolic fall in pressure followed by a rapid rise and plateau during mid and late diastole, *square root sign,* as additional filling is impaired by the noncompliant pericardium. As opposed to restrictive cardiomyopathy, the left and right ventricular diastolic pressure tracings are nearly superimposable and do not change with volume loading or exercise. In difficult cases in which the differentiation from restrictive cardiomyopathy is uncertain, a pericardial or myocardial biopsy may be helpful.

Constrictive pericarditis is a progressive disease. Patients with mild constrictive pericarditis may be successfully treated with salt restriction and diuretics. Sinus tachycardia is a compensatory mechanism, therefore the use of drugs that slow heart rate (beta-blockers or calcium channel blockers) warrants caution. In most symptomatic patients, surgical removal of the pericardium (pericardiectomy) is the treatment of choice. Patients with constrictive pericarditis secondary to radiation exposure have relatively worse long-term prognosis. Pericardial disease that results in constriction disqualifies an athlete from all competitive sports.

EFFUSIVE CONSTRICTIVE PERICARDITIS

Effusive constrictive pericarditis refers to a clinical hemodynamic syndrome in which constriction of the heart by the visceral pericardium occurs in the presence of tense effusion in the free pericardial space. It may represent an intermediate stage in the development of constrictive pericarditis. The causes of effusive constrictive pericarditis are the same as those for constriction. However, effusive constrictive pericarditis appears more frequent in radiation-induced pericarditis and relatively less frequent in postsurgical cases. The clinical features resemble those of both tamponade and constriction, with signs of right ventricular heart failure most common.

Though echocardiography, MRI, and CT are useful noninvasive tests, the diagnosis is generally made after successful pericardiocentesis. After fluid drainage and intrapericardial pressure fall to zero, intracardiac pressures remain elevated, with associated constrictive physiology. Ventricular pressure tracing show a typical *square root sign,* whereas the atrial and jugular venous pressure pulses show a prominent y descent. As a result, pericardiocentesis fails to relieve the patient's symptoms. Surgical management by excision of the visceral and parietal pericardium is usually effective.

Diseases of the Myocardium

Cardiomyopathy is a general term that refers to primary disease of the heart muscle. Myocardial injury from coronary artery disease and hypertension is responsible for the vast majority of heart disease. In this section, we will discuss myocardial diseases of nonischemic and nonhypertensive origins, which account for approximately 5% to 10% of patients in the United States with heart failure.

DILATED CARDIOMYOPATHY

Dilated cardiomyopathy (DCM) is characterized by cardiac enlargement and impaired systolic function of one or both ventricles. DCM represents an end-stage process resulting from many specific cardiomyopathies listed in Table 11–2. Idiopathic dilated cardiomyopathy (IDCM) refers to primary myocardial disease in the absence of coronary occlusive, valvular, or systemic disease. Histologic examination of

Table 11–2 Specific Cardiomyopathies

Disorder	Description
Dilated cardiomyopathy	Dilation and impaired contraction of the left or both ventricles. Caused by familial—genetic, viral, immune, alcoholic—toxic, or unknown factors or is associated with recognized cardiovascular disease.
Hypertrophic cardiomyopathy	Left and/or right ventricular hypertrophy, often asymmetric, which usually involves the interventricular septum. Mutations in sarcoplasmic proteins cause the disease in many patients.
Restrictive cardiomyopathy	Restricted filling and reduced diastolic size of either or both ventricles with normal or near-normal systolic function. Is idiopathic or associated with other disease (e.g., amyloidosis, endomyocardial disease).
Arrhythmogenic right ventricular cardiomyopathy	Progressive fibrofatty replacement of the right and, to some degree, left ventricular myocardium. Familial disease is common.
Unclassified cardiomyopathy	Diseases that do not fit readily into any category. Examples include systolic dysfunction with minimal dilation, mitochondrial disease, and fibroelastosis.
Ischemic cardiomyopathy	Arteries as dilated cardiomyopathy with depressed ventricular function not explained by the extent of coronary artery obstructions or ischemic damage.
Valvular cardiomyopathy	Arises as ventricular dysfunction that is out of proportion to the abnormal loading conditions produced by the valvular stenosis and/or regurgitation.
Hypertensive cardiomyopathy	Arises with left ventricular hypertrophy with features of cardiac failure related to systolic or diastolic dysfunction.
Inflammatory cardiomyopathy	Cardiac dysfunction as a consequence of myocarditis.
Metabolic cardiomyopathy	Includes a wide variety of causes, including endocrine abnormalities, glycogen storage disease, deficiencies (such as hypokalemia), and nutritional disorders.
General systemic disease	Includes connective tissue disorders and infiltrative diseases such as sarcoidosis and leukemia.
Muscular dystrophies	Includes Duchenne, Becker-type, and myotonic dystrophies.
Neuromuscular disorders	Includes Friedreich's ataxia, Noonan syndrome, and lentiginosis.
Sensitivity and toxic reactions	Includes reactions to alcohol, catecholamines, anthracyclines, irradiation, and others.
Peripartal cardiomyopathy	First shows in the peripartum period but it is probably a heterogenous group.

Derived from Richardson P, McKenna W, Bristow M, et al: Report of the 1995 World Health Organization/International Society and Federation of Cardiology Task Force on the Definition and Classification of Cardiomyopathies. Circulation 93:841, 1996.
Copyright 1996 American Heart Association. Copyright 2005 Elsevier, Inc.

the heart muscle reveals nonspecific changes of hypertrophy and fibrosis in most patients with this condition. A genetic predisposition to DCM is found in certain families, although these cases may still be classified as idiopathic if no clear genetic link can be identified. Many familial forms of DCM are associated with mutations in genes encoding for the cytoskeletal (e.g., desmin), nuclear membrane, (e.g., lamin C), or contractile proteins (e.g., myosin, troponin-T).

DCM is more common in men than it is in women and usually occurs in middle age. A large number of patients may remain clinically asymptomatic for prolonged periods until severe ventricular systolic dysfunction develops. The clinical features are related to decreased cardiac output. Early symptoms include fatigue, weakness, and dyspnea. As disease progresses with increasing volume overload, orthopnea, PND, and ankle swelling are common complaints. Simultaneous right and left ventricular heart failure occurs if the disease involves both ventricles; however, right ventricular heart failure more commonly arises secondary to left ventricular systolic dysfunction in most patients.

On physical examination, tachycardia is often present, with a narrow pulse pressure. With advanced disease, patients may have significant respiratory distress and tachypnea at rest. Jugular venous distention is usually present and reveals prominent V waves if tricuspid regurgitation is present. Crackles may be present over the lung fields but are absent in patients with chronic heart failure and elevated pulmonary wedge pressure. Breath sounds are diminished over regions with pleural effusions. The cardiac apex is diffuse and may be laterally displaced. Murmurs of mitral and tricuspid regurgitation are frequently heard because of dilation of the mitral or tricuspid annulus from ventricular enlargement. Gallops are common on auscultation, with prominent S_3 in patients with decompensated heart failure. In some patients, the clinical features of right ventricular heart failure may predominate with hepatomegaly, ascites, and peripheral edema.

Initial laboratory evaluation should focus on identifying potential reversible causes of DCM. These assessments include serum electrolytes, thyroid studies, iron studies (to exclude hemochromatosis), and HIV serologic tests. In patients with a strong family history, a referral for genetic testing should be considered. B type natriuretic peptide (BNP) levels may be obtained in patients whose diagnosis is unclear and may require serial follow-up. Cardiomegaly is seen on chest x-ray examination, and evidence of pulmonary venous congestion and pleural effusions is present in advanced cases. The ECG may show nonspecific ST- and T-wave abnormalities and a pseudomyocardial infarct pattern, despite the absence of an infarction. Echocardiography plays an important role and provides a comprehensive evaluation of ventricular size, function, and associated valvular abnormalities. In addition, the presence of atrial or ventricular thrombus can be identified on echocardiography. An aggressive work-up for secondary causes of DCM should be pursued before a patient is diagnosed with idiopathic DCM. Radionuclide imaging or coronary angiography should be performed to exclude ischemic heart disease. In some patients, a myocardial biopsy is performed to evaluate for infiltrative causes or storage diseases (e.g. amyloidosis, sarcoidosis, hemochromatosis).

Management of patients with idiopathic disease follows standard heart failure guidelines. In patients with clinical evidence of fluid overload, initial intravenous diuretic therapy with a loop diuretic such as furosemide is often needed. Oral diuretics may be subsequently titrated to achieve a euvolemic state and the optimal control of symptoms. Therapeutic approaches involve targeting the effects of the renin-aldosterone and the adrenergic systems, both of which are activated in patients with DCM and produce adverse effects that lead to harmful negative remodeling of the left ventricular cavity. Beta-adrenergic blockers (specifically with carvedilol and long-acting preparations of metoprolol) can result in significant improvement in survival and symptoms. However, these drugs should be initiated with caution in patients with fluid overload to avoid decompensation caused by negative chronotropic and inotropic effects. Angiotensin-converting enzyme (ACE) inhibitors or angiotensin-receptor blockers are also standard therapies, with proved survival benefit. In addition, aldosterone-receptor blockade with spironolactone or eplerenone may provide additional benefits. These patients should be monitored closely for development of life-threatening hyperkalemia. Digoxin may have a role in treating patients who are still symptomatic despite these therapies or in patients with concomitant atrial fibrillation who are either intolerant to beta-blockers or need further control of ventricular rate. Digoxin should either be avoided in patients with renal dysfunction or titrated to maintain serum levels between 0.5 and 0.8 ng/mL because high serum levels can slightly increase mortality. The addition of fixed-dose isosorbide dinitrate plus hydralazine to standard therapy for heart failure is efficacious and can increase the survival among patients with advanced heart failure.

Patients with significantly diminished exercise capacity and suboptimal response to maximal medical management should be considered for orthoptic cardiac transplantation. Left ventricular assist devices (LVAD), as a bridge to transplantation, represent alternate therapy for patients with advanced heart failure. Patients with left ventricular ejection fraction of less than 35% despite maximal medical management are candidates for an implanted cardioverter-defibrillator (ICD) for primary prevention of sudden cardiac death. With current interventions, the overall prognosis of DCM remains poor, with an annual mortality rate of approximately 12%.

HYPERTROPHIC CARDIOMYOPATHY

Hypertrophic cardiomyopathy (HCM) is a disorder characterized by left ventricular hypertrophy with normal or small left ventricular cavity size in the absence of an apparent cause (e.g. hypertension, aortic stenosis). It is a relatively common form of genetic heart disease (0.2%; 1:500 in the general population) and results from over 400 specific mutations on at least 12 genes coding for cardiomyocyte contractile proteins. Both familial and sporadic forms occur with known mutations that affect sarcomeric proteins, myosin heavy chains, myosin light chains, tropomyosin, troponins, and myosin-binding C protein. The familial forms account for nearly one half of the patients and are transmitted in an autosomal-dominant pattern, with phenotypic expression of the disease varying markedly within and between families. Despite the wide variety of genetic abnormalities, all forms are associated with a common phenotype that includes cardiomyocyte dysfunction, myofibril disarray, cardiomyocyte hypertrophy, and interstitial fibrosis.

HCM may be *obstructive* or *nonobstructive*, depending on whether a pressure gradient that impedes left ventricular outflow can be detected. Diastolic dysfunction frequently occurs in patients with HCM, even in the absence of a significant outflow tract gradient, and may be independent of the degree of left ventricular hypertrophy. Myocardial hypertrophy increases wall stiffness and impairs ventricular relaxation, which results in elevated left ventricular end-diastolic and pulmonary venous pressures. The obstructive form is found in 25% of patients and is typically identified by a markedly thickened, asymmetric ventricular septum and systolic anterior motion (SAM) of the mitral valve, resulting in dynamic obstruction to left ventricular outflow. Alternatively, the hypertrophied myocardium may cause a mid-cavitary gradient with apposition of the walls during systole. Previous names for this syndrome included hypertrophic obstructive cardiomyopathy (HOCM), asymmetric septal hypertrophy (ASH), and idiopathic hypertrophic subaortic stenosis (IHSS).

Symptomatic HCM occurs in adolescents and young adults between the ages of 20 and 40 years. It is the most common cause of unexpected sudden death in young, competitive athletes. Nonetheless, one third of adults will have symptomatic HCM after the age of 60 years. The most frequent symptom is dyspnea on exertion (present in approximately 90% of patients) because exercise-induced augmentation of cardiac output is associated with diastolic dysfunction and elevation in left ventricular filling pressures. Ischemic chest pain can occur in the absence of epicardial coronary artery disease and is caused by increased oxygen demand by the hypertrophied ventricle and elevated wall tension that reduce blood flow to the subendocardium. Patients may complain of syncope or near syncope resulting from outflow tract obstruction and an inability to increase cardiac output during exertion. In other persons, sudden death caused by ventricular arrhythmia is the initial manifestation of the disease. The risk of sudden death is increased in individuals with a history of syncope, a family history of sudden death, or significant ventricular arrhythmias on ambulatory ECG monitoring or electrophysiologic study.

On cardiovascular examination, a precordial apical impulse, which is forceful, diffuse, and displaced laterally, is prominent in patients with HCM. In obstructive HCM, the initial carotid upstroke is brisk and is followed by a mid-systolic dip corresponding to the development of left ventricular tract outflow obstruction. The carotid impulse rises again in late systole of the cardiac cycle (pulsus bisferiens). Even without severe obstruction, the carotid upstroke remains rapid and brisk, an important distinguishing feature of HCM but not of aortic valve stenosis. On auscultation, S_1 is normal, whereas S_2 may be normal or paradoxically split in obstructive HCM. Decreased compliance of the left ventricle during atrial contraction may lead to an audible S_4 gallop. A harsh crescendo-decrescendo systolic murmur, best heard along the left sternal border, radiates to the base of the heart. The murmur typically increases in intensity with physiologic or pharmacologic maneuvers that reduce left ventricular volume or increase contractility, such as standing, Valsalva maneuvers, or after administering nitro-

glycerin or catecholamine. Conversely, the intensity of the murmur decreases with maneuvers that increase left ventricular volume or decrease contractility, as with squatting, handgrip, volume loading, or administration of beta-blockers. In addition to the outflow tract murmur, patients may have an apical holosystolic murmur of mitral regurgitation that results from displacement of the anterior mitral leaflet during systole.

The ECG in HCM typically shows increased QRS voltage secondary to left ventricular hypertrophy and may lead to the diagnosis in young patients with abnormalities on a screening ECG. Prominent, abnormal Q waves are frequently present in the inferior and lateral leads and reflect depolarization of the hypertrophied septum. A pseudo-infarct pattern with poor R-wave progression in the precordial leads is also seen in some patients. Echocardiography allows assessment of left ventricular function, the degree and location of the hypertrophy, and the severity of the SAM of the mitral leaflets. Doppler techniques can be used to estimate the severity and location of left ventricular outflow tract obstruction and to monitor changes in the gradient during provocative maneuvers or after specific treatment. Echocardiography is also useful for screening family members of patients diagnosed with HCM. Cardiac catheterization is indicated if the echocardiogram is inadequate in defining the severity of obstruction or if evaluation for coronary artery disease is indicated.

Management of HCM is aimed at improving diastolic dysfunction and minimizing left ventricular outflow obstruction. Both beta-blockers and calcium channel blockers have been used extensively in this disease and have been shown to improve symptoms. The beneficial effects of these medications are primarily related to decreasing heart rate, which prolongs diastole and allows for increased ventricular filling. In addition, the negative inotropic effect mitigates the hypercontractile state and relieves the severity of left ventricular outflow tract obstruction. Because vasodilation can aggravate a dynamic outflow obstruction in some patients, caution is recommended with use of calcium channel blockers. Disopyramide has also been used in HCM to improve symptoms and relieve outflow tract obstruction. Disopyramide decreases the inotropic state but can increase atrioventricular conduction if atrial fibrillation develops. As a result, if used, disopyramide is often combined with a beta-blocking agent. In a recent series, two thirds of patients with obstructed HCM treated with disopyramide experienced improvement in symptoms, with approximately 50% reduction in subaortic gradient over 3 years. Based on these findings, disopyramide should be considered before proceeding to surgical myectomy or alternate invasive strategies (discussed later).

If refractory symptoms develop from left ventricular outflow obstruction, the insertion of a dual-chamber pacemaker may help relieve the obstruction and symptoms. Because asynchronous ventricular contraction with pacing decreases inward motion of the interventricular septal wall, an increase in left ventricular outflow dimension and reduction in outflow obstruction are seen in some patients. Surgical myectomy, a procedure that resects the basal anterior septum, is considered the gold standard for the treatment of patients with symptomatic HCM who are refractory to medical therapy (Fig. 11–2). A successful operation can

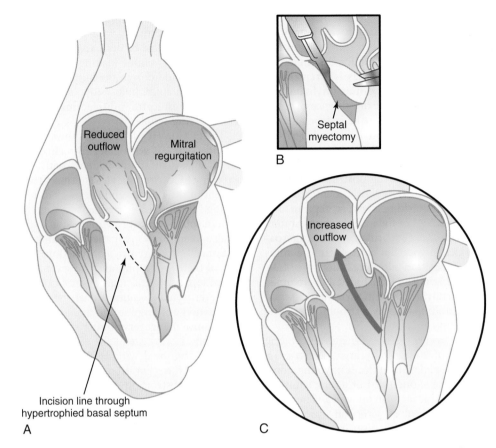

Figure 11–2 Schematic diagram of a patient undergoing surgical septal myectomy. (From Nishimura RA, Holmes DR Jr: Clinical practice: Hypertrophic obstructive cardiomyopathy. N Engl J Med 350:1320–1327, 2004.)

markedly attenuate the gradient and produce marked improvement in symptoms. Many patients are restored to near-normal exercise capacity, and nearly 90% are free of symptoms of dyspnea, angina, and exertional syncope postoperatively. Long-term follow-up studies after septal myectomy show lasting improvements in symptoms and exercise capacity without recurrence of outflow tract obstruction.

Alcohol-induced septal ablation, performed in the cardiac catheterization laboratory, is an alternative and more recent treatment for HCM. The procedure involves using myocardial perfusion echocardiography and cineangiography to localize a septal perforator artery perfusing the proximal septum. Alcohol is then selectively injected into this artery, the occlusion of which produces a controlled myocardial infarction. The subsequent thinning and remodeling of the basal anterior septal region have been shown to improve functional capacity and decrease the left ventricular outflow gradient. Complete heart block requiring permanent pacing is a known complication, although this adverse outcome is becoming less frequent with increased experience and improved technique.

Atrial fibrillation is often poorly tolerated hemodynamically because patients with HCM are especially dependent on atrial contraction to fill a stiff, noncompliant ventricle. Thus, restoration of sinus rhythm for patients with atrial fibrillation is critical to avoid the adverse outcomes associated with rapid ventricular rate. Prompt cardioversion is indicated, and long-term therapy for rhythm control may be needed.

The clinical course of patients with HCM is unpredictable. In general, clinical deterioration occurs slowly, with the incidence of symptomatic cases increasing with advancing age. Sudden death can occur at any time, even in an asymptomatic individual, and is the leading cause of death in this population. Ventricular tachycardia or fibrillation is the primary mechanism of sudden death. The most prominent characteristics of patients at high risk for experiencing sudden death include the following: (1) prior cardiac arrest or sustained ventricular tachycardia, (2) a history of a first-degree relative who has experienced sudden cardiac death, (3) left ventricular hypertrophy with a wall thickness greater than 30 mm, (4) syncope, if exertional and repetitive or in a young patient if no other cause is documented, and (5) nonsustained ventricular tachycardia on ECG monitoring if frequent, repetitive, and prolonged. High-risk patients, in general, receive treatment with amiodarone or an ICD. The efficacy of beta-blockers and calcium channel blockers in preventing sudden death has not been established. Endocarditis prophylaxis is indicated in all patients with HCM.

Athletes with a probable or unequivocal clinical diagnosis of HCM should be excluded from most competitive sports. This recommendation is independent of age, gender, phenotypic appearance, symptoms, or degree of outflow obstruction. In addition, the recommendation to avoid vigorous exercise remains, despite treatment with the medical or surgical therapies described previously.

The clinical significance and natural history of genotype-positive, phenotype-negative individuals remain unresolved.

Systematic follow-up (every 12 to 18 mo) of this subgroup is strongly recommended, particularly if a family history of HCM and sudden cardiac death exists. Routine testing includes serial two-dimensional echocardiography, 12-lead ECG, and ambulatory Holter (ECG) monitor. Exercise stress testing and imaging with cardiac magnetic resonance (CMR) are also recommended but at less frequent intervals.

RESTRICTIVE CARDIOMYOPATHIES

Restrictive cardiomyopathy is a less common form of cardiomyopathy in the Western world. The condition is characterized by impaired ventricular filling with normal or decreased diastolic volume of either or both ventricles. Systolic function usually remains normal, at least early in the disease, and wall thickness may be normal or increased, depending on the underlying cause. Increased myocardial stiffness of the myocardium causes left ventricular pressure to rise significantly with only small changes in volume. Known causes include infiltrative, noninfiltrative, or inherited storage disorders (Table 11–3).

Amyloidosis is the most common cause of restrictive cardiomyopathy. Although any type of amyloidosis may affect the heart muscle, cardiac involvement is more common in primary amyloidosis. This form of amyloidosis is caused by plasma cell production of immunoglobulin light chains, as seen in multiple myeloma. Secondary amyloidosis is caused by the deposition of protein other than immunoglobulin and is familial, senile, or the result of a chronic inflammatory process. Restrictive cardiomyopathy results from replacement of normal myocardial contractile elements by infiltrative interstitial deposits.

Hemochromatosis is the most common storage disease in adults and can lead to a restrictive cardiomyopathy caused by iron overload in the heart. Although conditions such as amyloidosis and sarcoidosis are seen infiltrating the interstitium around myocytes, storage diseases are characterized by intracellular accumulation. Iron deposited in the perinuclear area of cardiac myocytes disrupts cellular architecture and myocardial function, resulting in cell death and replacement fibrosis. Classic hereditary hemachromatosis is an autosomal-recessive disorder caused by mutations in the gene that regulates iron absorption. Symptomatic organ involvement generally begins in midlife, often with nonspecific symptoms such as unexplained fatigue or joint pain. Liver disease usually predominates, but restrictive cardiomyopathy may also develop. Nongenetic causes of hemochromatosis include iron overload from hemolytic anemia and blood transfusions.

The diagnosis of restrictive cardiomyopathy should be considered in patients with predominantly right ventricular heart failure without evidence of either cardiomegaly or systolic dysfunction. Patients may show symptoms and signs of right or left ventricular failure, although findings of right ventricular heart failure are more common. Distinguishing restrictive cardiomyopathy from constrictive pericarditis is important (Table 11–4), the latter of which can also exhibit *restrictive physiology* but may be cured surgically. Treatment for restrictive cardiomyopathies is generally focused on alleviating the symptoms of heart failure. Diuretics should be used judiciously to treat venous congestion in the pulmonary and systemic circulation because excess diuresis may decrease ventricular filling pressures, leading to reduced

Table 11–3	Classification of Types of Restrictive Cardiomyopathy According to Cause

Myocardial

Noninfiltrative

Idiopathic cardiomyopathy*
Familial cardiomyopathy
Hypertrophic cardiomyopathy
Scleroderma
Pseudoxanthoma elasticum
Diabetic cardiomyopathy

Infiltrative

Amyloidosis*
Sarcoidosis*
Gaucher's disease
Hurler's disease
Fatty infiltration

Storage diseases

Hemochromatosis
Fabry's disease
Glycogen storage disease

Endomyocardial

Endomyocardial fibrosis*
Hypereosinophilic syndrome
Carcinoid heart disease
Metastatic cancers
Radiation*
Toxic effects of anthracycline*
Drugs causing fibrous endocarditis (serotonin, methysergide, ergotamine, mercurial agents, busulfan)

*This condition is more likely than the others to be encountered in clinical practice.
Kushwaha SS, Fallon JT, Fuster V: Medical progress: Restrictive cardiomyopathy. N Engl J Med 336(4):267–276, 1997.

cardiac output and hypoperfusion. Digoxin can be arrhythmogenic in patients with amyloidosis and should be avoided. Atrial fibrillation may worsen existing diastolic dysfunction, and a rapid ventricular response may further compromise cardiac function. Therefore, maintaining sinus rhythm is important. In patients with advanced conduction system disease, a permanent pacemaker may be indicated.

Limited success has been reported with the use of chemotherapeutic agents for treating restrictive cardiomyopathies. In the case of amyloidosis, when associated with heart failure, the median survival is less than 1 year, with most deaths occurring suddenly. Experience with

Table 11–4   Differentiation between Restrictive Cardiomyopathy and Constrictive Pericarditis

Type of Evaluation	Restrictive Cardiomyopathy	Constrictive Pericarditis
Physical examination	Kussmaul's sign present Apical impulse may be prominent S₃ may be present, rarely S₄ Regurgitant murmurs common	Kussmaul's sign usually present Apical impulse usually not palpable Pericardial knock may be present
Electrocardiography	Low voltage (especially in amyloidosis), pseudo-infarction, left-axis deviation, atrial fibrillation, conduction disturbances common Increased wall thickness (especially thickened interatrial septum in amyloidosis)	Regurgitant murmurs uncommon Low voltage
Echocardiography	Decreased RV and LV velocities with inspiration	Normal wall thickness Pericardial thickening may be seen Prominent early diastolic filling with abrupt displacement of interventricular septum
Doppler studies	Inspiratory augmentation of hepatic-vein diastolic flow reversal Mitral and tricuspid regurgitation common	Increased RV systolic velocity and decreased LV systolic velocity with inspiration Expiratory augmentation of hepatic-vein diastolic flow reversal
Cardiac catheterization	LVEDP often >5 mm Hg greater than RVEDP but may be identical	RVEDP and LVED usually equal RV systolic pressure <50 mm Hg RVEDP greater than one third of RV systolic pressure
Endomyocardial biopsy	May reveal specific cause of restrictive	May be normal or show nonspecific myocyte hypertrophy or myocardial fibrosis
CT/MRI	Pericardium usually normal	Pericardium may be thickened

CT = computer tomography; LV = left ventricular; LVEDP = left ventricular end-diastolic pressure; MRI = magnetic resonance imaging; RV = right ventricular; RVEDP = right ventricular end-diastolic pressure.

treatment for hemachromatosis is more encouraging. With early diagnosis, phlebotomy and iron chelation therapy with desferoxamine may improve cardiac function before cell injury becomes irreversible. Deaths from hemachromatosis usually result from cirrhosis and liver carcinoma rather than cardiac disease. In cardiac sarcoidosis, malignant ventricular arrhythmias are a frequent mode of presentation and may require treatment with an ICD. Endomyocardial fibrosis and eosinophilic cardiomyopathy can respond to medical therapy with corticosteroids, whereas cytotoxic drugs are effective during the early phase of Löffler's endocarditis.

ALCOHOLIC CARDIOMYOPATHY

In the United States, long-term heavy alcohol consumption is a major cause of nonischemic DCM. In general, alcoholic patients who consume more than 90 g of alcohol a day (approximately seven to eight standard drinks per day) for more than 5 years are at risk for developing asymptomatic alcoholic cardiomyopathy. With longer periods of alcohol use, cardiomyopathy may progress and result in signs and symptoms of heart failure.

Alcoholic cardiomyopathy is characterized by an increase in myocardial mass, dilation of the ventricles, and wall thinning. Changes in ventricular function depend on the stage: Asymptomatic alcoholic cardiomyopathy is associated with diastolic dysfunction, whereas systolic dysfunction is a common finding in symptomatic patients. The pathophysiologic factors of this disorder are complex. Three major proposed mechanisms are (1) direct toxic effect of alcohol on myocytes, (2) nutritional effects (most commonly thiamine deficiency), and (3) toxic effects of additives in alcoholic beverages (cobalt-induced cardiomyopathy in Canada several years ago).

Women appear to be more sensitive than men to the cardiotoxic effects of alcohol and require a lower total lifetime dose of ethanol to develop the disease. Despite the fact that the mean lifetime dose of alcohol in female alcoholics is lower than the dose in male alcoholics, cardiomyopathy and myopathy appear to be equally common.

The findings on physical examination are similar to those seen in DCM but vary with the involvement of one or both ventricles and the degree of myocardial dysfunction. Because of the adrenergic effects of alcohol use, the incidence of supraventricular tachyarrhythmia is increased.

Abstinence along with medical therapy for heart failure may lead to sustained improvements in ventricular function and prognosis. Patients with alcoholic cardiomyopathy have a similar outcome as patients with IDCM. Alcoholism without abstinence is a strong predictor of early cardiac death. Therefore an aggressive approach to achieve alcohol cessation is needed in these patients (see Chapter 133).

ARRHYTHMOGENIC RIGHT VENTRICULAR CARDIOMYOPATHY

Arrhythmogenic right ventricular cardiomyopathy or dysplasia (ARVC, ARVD) is characterized by fibrofatty replacement of the right ventricular myocardium. It is an autosomal-dominant familial disorder with male predominance. ARVC is a major cause of sudden death in young adults and athletes, particularly in the northeastern region of Italy, and is less commonly seen in the United States by comparison. ARVC is characterized by a broad phenotypic spectrum, with loss of myocytes during early development in the right ventricular myocardium with fatty or fibrofatty replacement. Right ventricular aneurysm formation and segmental wall motion abnormalities are other criteria. ARVC is frequently associated with myocarditis.

The clinical diagnosis is challenging. Patients may complain of palpitations or syncope often associated with reentrant arrhythmias. The diagnosis may be established by a familial history, ventricular tachyarrhythmia, particularly ventricular tachycardia of right ventricular origin elicited by exercise-induced catecholamine release. Classic ECG findings include T-wave inversion in precordial leads V1 through V3 and epsilon waves. Echocardiography may identify right ventricular dilatation, segmental wall motion abnormalities, or aneurysm formation. However, imaging criteria for ARVC are better evaluated by CMR because of superior imaging of right ventricular structure and function and tissue characterization used to identify myocardial fatty infiltration.

Anti-arrhythmic therapy with beta-blockers or amiodarone is used to help control arrhythmias, and in patients at high risk for sudden death, ICD therapy may provide protection from life-threatening ventricular arrhythmias. Athletes with probable or definite diagnosis of ARVC should be excluded from most competitive sports.

MYOCARDITIS

Myocarditis is a self-limited but, occasionally, life-threatening inflammatory condition that affects humans of all ages. *Viral myocarditis* refers to inflammation during active replication of virus in the myocardium or the subsequent autoimmune phase of the disease. *Postviral myocarditis* has also been used to describe specifically the autoimmune phase. When neither a direct causal relationship nor a specific cause can be established, the term *lymphocytic myocarditis* has gained more widespread acceptance to reflect this predominant histologic feature in affected patients.

In the United States, an estimated 25% of the 750,000 persons with heart failure have DCM, accounting for 50% of the patients requiring cardiac transplantation. Although DCM has multiple causes, viral infection plays s a key role in its pathogenesis and accounts for 21% of DCM on mean follow-up of 33 months. In military recruits and adults younger than 40 years of age, epidemiologic studies have estimated viral myocarditis as an etiologic factor in 20% of cases of sudden death. Histologic evidence of myocarditis is routinely seen in 1% to 9% of postmortem examinations.

Viral infection accounts for the majority of cases of myocarditis in industrialized societies. Enteroviruses such as Coxsackie B viruses are nonenveloped RNA viruses in the picornavirus family. The coxsackievirus B group, in particular subtypes B3 and B4, and adenovirus lead the list of human pathogens. Coxsackieviruses are distinguished from other types of picornaviruses based on their pathogenesis in susceptible hosts and antigenic classifications. These main classes are coxsackievirus group A (A1 to A22, A24) and the coxsackievirus group B (B1 to B6). Group A coxsackieviruses after inoculation in suckling mice produce myositis and generalized paralysis. Group B coxsackieviruses produce distinctive focal muscle lesions, necrosis of interscapular fat pads, cerebral lesions, and spastic paralysis. Improvements in molecular detection have implicated other viruses, such as hepatitis C viruses, and human cytomegalovirus (CMV), alone or in combination with cardiotropic agents such as the HIV.

HIV has emerged as a major etiologic agent in viral-induced CDM. In patients who are HIV positive, cardiac decompensation with lymphocytic interstitial myocarditis is a frequent complication, with an estimated prevalence between 8% and 50% or more. The precise mechanism of HIV-induced cardiac disease has been debated, but the available evidence suggests that the HIV exhibits cardiotropism. Among patients with active acquired immunodeficiency syndrome (AIDS) myocarditis and other viral, protozoa, and bacteria infections are commonly seen, suggesting that these co-morbid conditions and autoimmunity might be contributing factors to HIV-induced myocarditis.

Nonviral infectious agents can also cause myocarditis. In Central and South America, infection with the protozoa *Trypanosoma cruzi* (Chagas' disease) is the major cause of myocarditis. This parasitic infection is largely immune mediated for which treatment with antiprotozoal therapy with nifurtimox or benzimidazole is beneficial. Similarly, diphtheritic myocarditis has been reported in 22% of patients, with a case-fatality rate of 3%. Combination therapy with diphtheria antitoxin and antibiotics are usually effective. Bacterial infections, toxoplasmosis, or infection with the tick-borne spirochete, *Borrelia burgdorferi* (Lyme disease), are also known to result in myocarditis. Though no clear cause for peripartum cardiomyopathy has been discovered, lymphocytic infiltration has been found in up to 50% of myocardial biopsy specimens, raising the possibility of an autoimmune process or enhanced susceptibility to viral myocarditis. Finally, numerous noninfectious causes of myocarditis are well documented and include pharmacologic agents, drugs, systemic inflammatory disorders, and granulomatous diseases.

The clinical features of inflammatory myocarditis vary widely. Viral myocarditis may be indicated when patients are examined after a recent febrile illness followed by onset of cardiac symptoms such as dyspnea, fatigue, chest pain, or palpitations from arrhythmias. Others may exhibit conduction system abnormalities, acute congestive heart failure, or an embolic event from intracardiac thrombi. After the initial insult, several days may be required for any cardiac symptoms to appear. On physical examination, the patient is often tachycardic. In severe cases, typical signs of congestive heart failure are elevated jugular veins, pulmonary rales, peripheral edema, hepatomegaly, and a S_3 gallop on cardiac examination. A friction rub may be audible if pericardial inflammation is present.

Elevated cardiac enzymes and rising viral titers support the diagnosis. Though no pathognomonic findings of myocarditis are found on an ECG, sinus tachycardia and nonspecific ST- and T-wave abnormalities are common. With pericardial involvement, ECG findings typical for acute pericarditis are seen, including diffuse ST-segment elevation. Electrophysiologic complications may include arrhythmias, conduction defects, or heart block; sudden death caused by ventricular fibrillation has also been reported. Echocardiography is used to confirm the severity of systolic ventricular dysfunction and, in some instances, affords qualitative changes in image texture heterogeneity brightness, which is indicative of myocarditis. However, MRI has become a powerful diagnostic tool, with high sensitivity and specificity in the noninvasive assessment of suspected viral myocarditis caused by advances in myocardial tissue characterization.

The use of transvenous endomyocardial biopsy, first introduced in 1962, facilitates the diagnosis and treatment of myocarditis in antemortem samples. Although reliance on histomorphologic abnormalities on light microscopy has been heavy, termed the *Dallas criteria,* many pathologists and clinicians have now abandoned these arbitrary clinicopathologic classifications owing to wide intra- and interobserver variability. The histomorphologic abnormalities that support such a classification in DCM include interstitial fibrosis, myocyte degeneration, and increased *reparative* fibrosis of the extracellular matrix. A faster diagnosis of myocarditis is now possible by applying the polymerase chain reaction (PCR) to detect specific viral genomes in the myocardium. When biopsy is guided by imaging techniques such as MRI, increased sensitivity and specificity of this diagnostic tool have been reported in a limited number of studies.

Based on the available literature, the indications for endomyocardial biopsy are (1) to establish the diagnosis of suggested myocarditis in a patient with new onset heart failure, (2) to consider alternative diagnoses (e.g., giant cell myocarditis) in patients who are unresponsive to conventional therapy for heart failure, (3) to monitor response after immunosuppression therapy if clinically indicated (e.g., disease recurrence or progression), and (4) to decide about placement of a permanent pacemaker when an inflammatory process is the cause. Both the sensitivity and the specificity of the endomyocardial biopsy are reduced when viral infection is focal, remote, or subclinical.

In the pediatric population, a viral cause is a common diagnosis for new onset of heart failure and/or cardiogenic shock. In adults, viral myocarditis will exhibit more insidiously and, without a high index of clinical suspicion, can be misdiagnosed as heart failure secondary to ischemic heart disease, diabetes, hypertension, or valvular heart disease. For new-onset heart failure of less than 3 months duration, idiopathic giant cell myocarditis (IGCM) should be considered in patients who do not respond to conventional therapy for heart failure. The diagnosis requires endomyocardial biopsy with histologic evidence for diffuse inflammatory lymphocytic infiltrate and myocyte necrosis interspersed with eosinophils and multinucleated giant cells. Immunosuppression therapy has been used for IGCM, but no published studies have established benefit.

New insights about the molecular mechanisms related to the different phases of disease from viral infection to cardiac remodeling suggest the need to re-evaluate existing practices for the diagnosis and treatment of viral myocarditis. Early disease can escape clinical recognition because viral replication may be entirely asymptomatic and go unnoticed without myocardial sequelae. Complete recovery with an excellent prognosis can be expected in most cases of uncomplicated myocarditis. The development of myocarditis in neonates, often from nursery outbreak or from infected mothers, can progress into multisystemic disease involving the liver and central nervous system. Clinical signs such as feeding difficulty, lethargy, and fever are preceded by either cardiac or respiratory distress syndrome, or both. The initial infection with myocardial involvement sets the stage for the multiple phases of myocarditis with increased risk of re-infection and autoimmune reactivation of the disease. The older patient typically seeks medical attention for management of congestive heart failure and, perhaps, CDM. In patients with DCM, the risk factors for sudden death are a positive signal-averaged ECG, low heart rate variability index, inducible ventricular tachycardia or fibrillation, nonsustained ventricular tachycardia, and left ventricular dysfunction.

To date, no effective therapy for viral myocarditis has been established. Clinical trials of immunosuppressive therapy have failed to show clinical efficacy. Empiric trials in which specific antiviral agents are administered based on genomic diagnosis lack long-term follow-up of clinical outcomes. The treatment of heart failure resulting from myocarditis follows well-established clinical therapy and encompasses diuretics, α-adrenergic blockers, ACE inhibitors, and aldosterone antagonists.

Patients with probable or definite evidence of myocarditis should be withdrawn from all competitive sports and undergo a convalescent period for at least 6 months following the onset of clinical manifestations. Athletes may return to training and competition after this period if cardiac size and function return to normal, clinically relevant arrhythmias are absent, and serum markers of inflammation and heart failure have normalized.

Prospectus for the Future

Genetically engineered animal models have emerged as powerful tools for molecular and genetic studies of human diseases. Susceptible populations at high risk such as children and young adults might benefit from an effective vaccination program. Emerging technologies such as proteomics and genomics might lend important insights into the pathogenesis of human viral myocarditis. Molecular aids using PCR and other serologic methods are likely to speed diagnosis with greater accuracy and specificity. In parallel, medical providers must be alert to epidemiologic shifts in the prevalence of cardiotropic agents such as hepatitis C that can contribute to new cases of viral myocarditis worldwide. Most importantly, future efforts are needed to forge consensus for the treatment of inflammatory phases and prevention of viral sequelae. Lastly, the global effort in basic and clinical research on AIDS is anticipated to yield spin-offs in pathogenesis, vaccine development, and other unforeseen benefits for the treatment and prevention of viral-mediated diseases in humans.

References

American College of Cardiology/American Heart Association Task Force on Practice Guidelines (Writing Committee): ACC/AHA 2005 guideline update for the diagnosis and management of chronic heart failure in the adult—summary article. Circulation 112(12):1825–1852, 2005.

American College of Cardiology/European Society of Cardiology: Clinical expert consensus document on hypertrophic cardiomyopathy. J Am Coll Cardiol 42:1687–1713, 2003.

Kadish A, Dyer A, Daubert JP, et al: Prophylactic defibrillator implantation in patients with non-ischemic dilated cardiomyopathy. New Engl J Med 350:2151–2158, 2004.

Maron BJ, Ackerman MJ, Nishimura RA, et al: Task Force 4: HCM and other cardiomyopathies, mitral valve prolapse, myocarditis, and Marfan syndrome. J Am Coll Cardiol 45:1340–1345, 2005.

Chapter 12

Other Cardiac Topics

David A. Bull

Ivor J. Benjamin

Cardiac Tumors

Primary cardiac tumors are extremely rare, with a prevalence of less than 0.3% in most pathologic series (Table 12–1). Myxoma is the most common primary tumor of the heart and is usually benign. These tumors are frequently isolated lesions, arising most often in the left atrium in the region of the fossa ovalis. Less commonly, myxomas may be detected in the right atrium, in the right or left ventricle, or in multiple sites within the heart. A familial pattern of myxomas can occur and is transmitted in an autosomal-dominant manner. In these patients, multiple cardiac myxomas may be present in association with a constellation of extracardiac abnormalities, including pigmented nevi, cutaneous myxomas, breast fibroadenomas, and pituitary and adrenal gland disease. In addition, patients with familial myxoma may have recurrence of the tumor or tumors after surgical excision. Whether sporadic or familial, less than 10% of myxomas are malignant.

Symptoms associated with myxoma are usually related to embolization of tumor fragments and obstruction of the mitral valve. In addition, patients may exhibit a constellation of nonspecific symptoms and laboratory abnormalities, including fever, malaise, weight loss, anemia, and elevated erythrocyte sedimentation rate. The diagnosis is usually made with echocardiography; the transesophageal approach is the most sensitive method for detecting small left atrial tumors. Considering the propensity for embolization, most myxomas are surgically removed when diagnosed. Because tumors may recur, follow-up echocardiograms should be performed.

Other less common benign tumors include papillary fibroelastomas, fibromas, and rhabdomyomas. Fibroelastomas are pedunculated tumors with frondlike attachments that usually arise from the surface of the mitral and aortic valve leaflets. These tumors do not result in valve dysfunction but may be a source of systemic embolization. Fibromas most often arise within the interventricular septum and may be associated with arrhythmias or conduction disturbances. Rhabdomyomas are the most common cardiac tumors found in children and are often associated with tuberous sclerosis.

Cardiac lipomas may occur throughout the heart and pericardium. Pericardial lipomas can be quite large, whereas intramyocardial lipomas are small and often encapsulated. Surgical excision is the treatment of choice. Lipomatous hypertrophy of the interatrial septum should be considered in the differential of atrial masses. This lesion is a consequence of nonencapsulated adipose tissue hyperplasia and, although occasionally found incidentally at autopsy, may be associated with supraventricular arrhythmias, conduction disturbances, and, in rare cases, sudden cardiac death.

Approximately one fourth of all primary cardiac tumors are malignant, and most are sarcomas. These tumors grow rapidly and often result in chamber obliteration and obstruction of blood flow. If there is involvement of the pericardium, then a hemorrhagic effusion with pericardial tamponade may develop. The prognosis in affected individuals is poor; surgical excision is possible in rare cases. Irradiation and chemotherapy may provide palliative relief.

In contrast with primary cardiac tumors, metastatic disease involving the heart is common, occurring in up to one in five patients dying with malignancy. The most common tumors to metastasize to the heart are carcinomas of the lung, breast, and kidney; melanoma and lymphoma may also have cardiac involvement. Metastasis to the pericardium is common and often complicated by a hemorrhagic effusion and pericardial tamponade. Infiltration of the myocardium may result in conduction disturbances and arrhythmias. Intracavitary masses are unusual but may result from local tumor invasion or direct extension of the malignancy through the venous system (i.e., renal cell carcinoma may metastasize to the heart through the inferior vena cava). Treatment is directed at the underlying malignancy. If pericardial tamponade is present, then immediate drainage will help stabilize the patient. A pericardotomy is often necessary to prevent reaccumulation of fluid within the pericardial sac. Surgical excision of an obstructing tumor mass is usually palliative.

Table 12–1	**Examples of Tumors of the Heart and Pericardium**

Primary

Benign

Myxoma
Lipoma
Papillary fibroelastoma
Rhabdomyoma
Fibroma

Malignant

Angiosarcoma
Rhabdomyosarcoma
Mesothelioma
Fibrosarcoma

Metastatic

Melanoma
Lung
Breast
Lymphoma
Renal cell

Table 12–2	**Cardiac Lesions From Nonpenetrating Trauma**

Pericardium

Hematoma
Hemopericardium
Rupture
Pericarditis
Constriction (late complication)

Myocardium

Contusion
Intracavitary thrombus
Aneurysms and pseudoaneurysms
Rupture (e.g., free wall, septum)
Acute rupture (e.g., atrium, ventricle, septa)

Valves

Rupture (e.g., leaflets, chordae, papillary muscle)

Coronary Arteries

Laceration

Great Vessels

Aortic rupture

From Schick EC: Nonpenetrating cardiac trauma. Cardiol Clin 13:241–247, 1995.

Traumatic Heart Disease

NONPENETRATING CARDIAC INJURIES

Blunt cardiac trauma accounts for approximately 10% of all traumatic heart disease (Table 12–2). Motion-related injuries secondary to abrupt body deceleration (motor vehicle accidents) and chest wall compression (e.g., steering wheel impact, athletic blow, cardiac resuscitative maneuvers) are the most common causes of blunt injury to the heart. Changes in the myocardium range from small ecchymotic areas in the subepicardium to transmural injury with myocardial hemorrhage and necrosis. Pericarditis is present in most patients and may be complicated by a tear or rupture of the pericardium or cardiac tamponade. Less common complications include rupture of a papillary muscle or chordae tendineae and coronary artery laceration.

Patients most often experience precordial pain that is similar to that associated with myocardial infarction. However, musculoskeletal pain secondary to chest wall injury may confuse the clinical presentation. Congestive heart failure is unusual unless myocardial injury has been extensive or valve dysfunction has occurred. Life-threatening ventricular arrhythmias may occur with severe trauma and are a frequent cause of death in such patients. The electrocardiogram most often demonstrates nonspecific repolarization abnormalities or ST-segment and T-wave changes consistent with acute pericarditis. If myocardial injury is extensive, then localized ST-segment elevation and pathologic Q waves may be present. Elevation of the myocar-

dial component of the creatine kinase muscle band (CK-MB) is supportive of a diagnosis of cardiac contusion but is of limited diagnostic use in patients with massive chest wall trauma because the CK-MB fraction may be elevated as a result of severe skeletal muscle injury. Newer markers of myocardial injury, such as troponins T and I, may be more specific for establishing a diagnosis of myocardial contusion. Echocardiography is a useful, noninvasive tool to assess for wall motion abnormalities, valve dysfunction, and the presence of hemodynamically significant pericardial effusion.

Treatment of patients with cardiac contusion is similar to that for myocardial infarction, with initial observation and monitoring, followed by a gradual increase in physical activity. Anticoagulants and thrombolytic agents are contraindicated given the risk of hemorrhage into the myocardium and pericardial sac. Most patients who survive the initial injury will have partial or complete recovery of myocardial function. However, patients should be monitored for late complications that include aneurysm formation, free-wall or papillary muscle rupture, and significant arrhythmias.

GREAT VESSEL INJURY

Rupture of the aorta is one of the most common cardiovascular injuries resulting from blunt chest wall trauma. In over

90% of the cases, rupture occurs in the descending thoracic aorta just distal to the origin of the subclavian artery. Most individuals die immediately of exsanguination. However, up to 20% of patients may survive the initial injury if the blood is confined within the aortic adventitia and surrounding mediastinal tissues (pseudoaneurysm). Characteristic symptoms and findings on presentation include chest and interscapular back pain, increased arterial pressure and pulse amplitude in the upper extremities, decreased pressure and pulse amplitude in the lower extremities, and mediastinal widening on the chest radiograph. Previously, aortography had been the standard for diagnosing blunt aortic injury. Aortography, however, is a relatively invasive, time-consuming procedure with the potential for additional morbidity in this critically ill group of patients. Although conventional chest computed tomographic (CT) scanning could not match the diagnostic accuracy of aortography, helical thin-cut CT angiography has emerged as a superior alternative to aortography for diagnosing blunt aortic injury. Helical CT scanning is an ideal diagnostic method for aortic injury because of its relatively low cost compared with aortography, its nearly universal availability in emergency departments, and its lack of operator dependence. In addition, at most trauma centers, CT scanning is already an integral part of the diagnosis and management of serious blunt injury, with patients typically undergoing simultaneous CT scanning of other areas of the body to evaluate potential injuries.

The overall diagnostic accuracy for helical CT scanning in the setting of blunt aortic injury exceeds 99%, with the positive- and negative-predictive values for helical CT scanning meeting or exceeding the same values for aortography. Patients without direct helical CT scan evidence of blunt aortic injury require no further evaluation. Aortography should be reserved for indeterminate helical CT scans. Such a strategy helps substantially reduce the morbidity and cost of unnecessary aortograms for blunt aortic injury.

The force from rapid deceleration necessary to tear the aorta often leads to injuries of other organs. Associated injuries may be present in more than 90% of patients with aortic transection, and 24% of these patients require a major surgical procedure before aortic repair. The extremely high death rate of acute blunt rupture of the thoracic aorta has led surgeons in the past to repair the tear as quickly as possible. This form of management, however, has resulted in high rates of death and complications, often because of associated injuries in other organs. Patients with traumatic rupture of the aorta fall into two broad categories: (1) Approximately 5% are hemodynamically unstable or deteriorate within 6 hours of admission. These patients require emergent surgical correction because mortality without intervention exceeds 90%. (2) The other 95% of patients are hemodynamically stable at the time of presentation, allowing time for a work-up and staging of any intervention. Mortality in this group is as low as 25% and is rarely the result of free rupture if the blood pressure is controlled. In the past decade, the philosophy of managing traumatic rupture of the aorta in this subgroup of patients has changed to emphasizing blood pressure control and assessing the need for emergent repair against the risks of operation. Recent prospective studies have demonstrated the value of initial antihypertensive therapy to allow delayed repair of blunt aortic injury in patients with severe co-existent injuries to

other organ systems. In a substantial number of cases, associated injuries or co-morbidities make the risks of immediate surgical repair prohibitive. The current indications for considering delayed aortic repair include trauma to the central nervous system, contaminated wounds, respiratory insufficiency from lung contusion or other causes, body surface burns, blunt cardiac injury, tears of solid organs that will undergo nonoperative management, and retroperitoneal hematoma, as well as patients 50 years or older and those with medical co-morbidities. Patients with significant neurologic, pulmonary, or cardiac injuries have better outcomes if their confounding pathologic condition can be ameliorated before thoracotomy.

PENETRATING CARDIAC INJURIES

Penetrating cardiac injuries are frequently the result of physical violence secondary to bullet and knife wounds. Similar wounds may result from the inward displacement of bone fragments or fractured ribs secondary to blunt chest wall injury. Iatrogenic injuries may occur during placement of central venous catheters and wires.

With traumatic perforations, the right ventricle is the most frequently involved chamber, considering its anterior location in the chest, and is often associated with pericardial laceration. Symptoms are related to the size of the wound and the nature of the concomitant pericardial injury. If the pericardium remains open, then extravasated blood drains freely into the mediastinum and pleural cavity, and symptoms are related to the resulting hemothorax. If the pericardial sac limits blood loss, then pericardial tamponade results. In this situation, treatment includes emergent pericardiocentesis, followed by emergent surgical closure of the wound. Small penetrating wounds to the ventricles that are not associated with extensive cardiac damage have the highest rate of survival. Late complications include chronic pericarditis, arrhythmias, aneurysm formation, and ventricular septal defects.

Cardiac Surgery

CORONARY ARTERY BYPASS GRAFTING

Despite the effectiveness of current medical therapy for the treatment of coronary artery disease, many patients may require revascularization. Coronary artery bypass grafting (CABG) is an effective means of reducing or eliminating symptoms of angina pectoris. In addition, previous studies have shown that CABG may improve survival in certain subgroups of patients, including patients with angina refractory to medical therapy, patients with greater than 50% stenosis of the left main coronary artery, and patients with severe three-vessel coronary artery disease associated with left ventricular dysfunction. In addition, patients with two-vessel coronary artery disease in which a severe stenosis (>75%) is present in the proximal left anterior descending artery appear to benefit from CABG even if left ventricular function is normal.

Standard CABG is performed through a median sternotomy incision with cardiopulmonary bypass and cardioplegic arrest. Operative mortality is 1% or less in stable patients with normal left ventricular function; the incidences of peri-operative myocardial infarction and stroke range from 1% to 4%. An increase in adverse events is associated with advancing age, sex, short stature, diabetes, unstable angina or recent myocardial infarction, and severely reduced left ventricular function. Overall survival at 10 years is approximately 80%, with recurrent or progressive angina occurring in approximately 50% of patients.

Long-term success of surgery is dependent on the type of conduit used during surgery (saphenous vein grafts versus internal mammary artery) and the progression of atherosclerotic disease in the native and graft vessels. The internal mammary artery is particularly resistant to atherosclerotic disease and has a patency rate of approximately 90% at 10 years. In comparison, venous grafts are subject to closure both during the immediate postoperative period (usually secondary to technical factors) and months to years after surgery, secondary to intimal hyperplasia and progression of atherosclerosis. As a result, only 50% of venous grafts are patent 7 to 10 years after CABG. The major predictor of the subsequent development of atherosclerotic disease in the surgically placed bypass grafts is the ability of patients to control their risk factors for the development of atherosclerotic disease generally after surgery, particularly cigarette smoking, hypertension, diabetes, hypercholesterolemia, and obesity. Aggressive lowering of low-density lipoprotein levels after CABG, as well as the administration of a daily aspirin, have been shown to reduce the incidence of venous graft occlusion. Most cases of recurrent angina can be managed successfully with medication (see Chapter 9). In many cases, percutaneous revascularization of a native vessel or graft will provide symptomatic relief and is the initial procedure of choice in this setting. In patients with refractory symptoms not amenable to percutaneous revascularization, repeat CABG is an option; however, in this setting, repeat CABG is associated with increased peri-operative mortality and less satisfactory long-term control of angina.

MINIMALLY INVASIVE CARDIAC SURGERY

Minimally invasive approaches for cardiac surgery can be broadly grouped into two categories: (1) those approaches that avoid the performance of a sternotomy, and (2) those approaches that avoid the use of cardiopulmonary bypass. Over the last 15 years, progressive experience incorporating these approaches has led to the application of minimally invasive techniques to select patients undergoing cardiac surgery. Many of the approaches have significant limitations, however, and the development of minimally invasive techniques for the performance of cardiac surgery continues to evolve.

In highly select patients, minimally invasive direct coronary artery bypass (MIDCAB) can be performed through a limited thoracotomy, sparing the patient the peri-operative morbidity associated with a median sternotomy. This technique also avoids the use of cardiopulmonary bypass. The most common approach is through a small left anterior thoracotomy incision and allows for the harvesting of the left internal mammary artery under direct visualization. Therefore, this technique is most suitable for patients with proximal disease in the distribution of the left anterior descending coronary artery, although other coronary arteries can be bypassed using different thoracotomy approaches.

The major limitation to this approach has been the lower patency rates in the left internal mammary grafts placed using this technique and a higher incidence of recurrent ischemia compared with conventional CABG. The MIDCAB procedure therefore is only applicable to highly select patients with disease in the distribution of the left anterior descending coronary artery and significant co-morbidities, which preclude the performance of a median sternotomy and use of cardiopulmonary bypass.

The initial experience with the MIDCAB approach and the subsequent demonstration of its limitations prompted the development of port-access cardiac surgery. This technique incorporates the MIDCAB approach of a limited lateral thoracotomy, thereby avoiding a median sternotomy but uses cardiopulmonary bypass to facilitate performance of intracardiac procedures, including mitral valve repair or replacement, as well as the potential for access to other coronary artery distributions beyond the left anterior descending coronary artery for CABG. The port-access approach uses an endo-aortic balloon via cannulas placed in the femoral vessels for cardiopulmonary bypass. A few centers have successfully used the port-access platform for performance of select cardiac surgical procedures, particularly mitral valve repair or replacement. The widespread adoption of this platform has been limited by persistent difficulties with access to all areas of the heart for coronary revascularization and the potentially catastrophic complication of aortic dissection in a small number of patients.

The limitations encountered with both the MIDCAB and port-access platforms have spurred the development of performing coronary bypass surgery through a median sternotomy but without cardiopulmonary bypass (e.g., off-pump coronary artery bypass [OPCAB]), allowing for surgery on the beating heart. The advantage of OPCAB over other platforms for minimally invasive coronary surgery is that complete revascularization can be performed and both internal mammary arteries can be harvested. Compared with conventional CABG, OPCAB is associated with decreased blood loss, decreased need for transfusion, decreased myocardial enzyme release up to 24 hours after surgery, decreased renal dysfunction, and, typically, decreased number of grafts placed per patient. Also compared with conventional CABG, however, OPCAB is not associated with a decreased length of hospital stay, a decreased mortality rate, or improved long-term neurologic function. Although the OPCAB platform has become the most widely adopted approach for minimally invasive cardiac surgery, major questions remain regarding the intermediate and long-term patencies of the bypass grafts placed using this technique and whether the decreased number of grafts placed per patient compromises the long-term cardiac outcomes of patients undergoing this procedure, compared with conventional CABG. Large-scale prospective clinical trials need to be conducted to answer these questions definitively.

VALVULAR SURGERY

Surgical repair or replacement of a diseased valve is dependent on multiple factors, including the type and severity of the valve lesion, the presence of symptoms, and the functional status of the left and in some cases the right ventricle (see Chapter 8). In most adults, the diseased valve is usually replaced with a prosthesis, although some forms of valve disease, such as mitral valve regurgitation or mitral stenosis without significant valvular or chordal calcification, may be amenable to repair. Because prosthetic heart valves are associated with a number of complications, including thrombosis, endocarditis, and hemolysis, the decision to proceed with valve surgery should only be made after the risks of valve replacement are weighed against the potential benefits of symptom relief and improved survival.

Valve surgery is performed in a manner similar to CABG, with most cases requiring a median sternotomy, cardiopulmonary bypass, and cardioplegic arrest. Minimally invasive surgery through a modified sternotomy or thoracotomy incision may be possible in select patients with isolated aortic or mitral valve disease. Operative mortality for all techniques ranges from 1% to 8% for most patients with preserved left ventricular function and good exercise capacity. The risk of surgery increases further with advancing age, depressed left ventricular ejection fraction, presence of severe coronary artery disease, and replacement of multiple valves. Symptomatic patients usually have significant clinical improvement after valve surgery; however, long-term survival is strongly dependent on the patient's preoperative functional status and ventricular function.

CARDIAC TRANSPLANTATION

Over the last two decades, cardiac transplantation has become a life-saving treatment choice in patients with end-stage congestive heart failure. With advances in surgical techniques and immunosuppressive therapy, 1- and 5-year survival rates are approximately 90% and 75%, respectively. These rates are far superior to the 1-year survival rate in patients with advanced heart failure, which can be as low as 50%. Unfortunately, many patients suitable for cardiac transplantation die before surgery as a result of the limited number of donor hearts available each year. The development and widespread application of left ventricular assist devices has allowed many of these patients who would otherwise die awaiting transplantation to survive until a donor heart becomes available. In many cardiac transplant centers today, more than one half of the patients undergoing cardiac transplantation have previously undergone placement of a left ventricular assist device.

The major indications for cardiac transplantation are to prolong survival and improve the quality of life. Determining which patients are suitable for cardiac transplantation can be difficult because many patients may have clinical and hemodynamic improvement with intensification of medical therapy. In general, functional capacity as assessed by exercise stress testing with measurement of maximal oxygen consumption at peak exercise is the best predictor of which patients should be selected for cardiac transplantation. Those individuals with severely impaired exercise capacity (e.g., peak oxygen consumption less than 10 to 12 mL/min/kg, with the lower limit of normal 20 mL/min/kg) are most likely to experience a survival benefit from transplantation. Exclusion criteria include irreversible pulmonary vascular hypertension, malignancy, active infection, diabetes mellitus with end-organ damage, and advanced liver or kidney disease. Although advanced age is associated with higher surgical and 1-year mortality rates, an age limit for cardiac transplantation is no longer strictly enforced at most centers, with patients instead being listed for transplantation based on an overall assessment of their physiologic status and potential for long-term survival after transplantation.

The procedure is performed through a median sternotomy incision. The posterior walls of the left and right atria with their venous connections are left in place and used to suture to the donor heart. The aorta and pulmonary artery are directly anastomosed to the recipient's great vessels. Immunosuppressive therapy is begun immediately after surgery and continued throughout the patient's life. Although new immunosuppressive agents are available, most regimens still include combinations of cyclosporine, azathioprine, and prednisone. Frequent complications during the first year include infection and rejection of the donor heart. In addition, hyperlipidemia and hypertension are common medical problems that may require treatment.

The major long-term complication is the development of coronary vasculopathy in the transplanted heart. In contrast to coronary artery atherosclerosis, which tends to be a focal process affecting primarily the proximal vessels, this disease is characterized by diffuse myointimal proliferation involving primarily the medial and distal segments of the coronary arteries. Although the cause of this disease is not entirely known, coronary vasculopathy is thought to be secondary to an immune-mediated response directed against the donor vessels. Monitoring for this complication can be difficult because angina is not provoked in the denervated heart and standard exercise stress testing has a low sensitivity for detecting this disease. Coronary angiography is performed after transplantation and yearly thereafter to monitor for significant narrowing of the coronary arteries. Unfortunately, the diffuse nature of the vasculopathy makes coronary angiography less accurate for the detection of this disease. Intracoronary ultrasound, with measurements of the intimal layer and coronary artery lumen size, is a new technique that appears to be more sensitive than coronary angiography for the detection of this complication. Treatment options are limited, but aggressive management of hypercholesterolemia and the use of calcium channel blockers, specifically diltiazem, have been associated with a slowing of disease progression and a higher survival rate. Retransplantation is reserved for patients with severe, three-vessel coronary artery disease with reduced left ventricular function and symptoms of congestive heart failure.

NONCARDIAC SURGERY IN THE PATIENT WITH CARDIOVASCULAR DISEASE

Noncardiac surgery in patients with known cardiovascular disease may be associated with an increased risk of death or cardiac complications, such as myocardial infarction, congestive heart failure, and arrhythmias. To determine an individual patient's risk for a procedure, the consulting physician must have knowledge of the type and severity of the patient's cardiac disease, his or her co-morbid risk factors, and the type and urgency of surgery. In general, the preoperative evaluation and management of patients with cardiovascular disease are similar to those in the nonoperative setting, with additional noninvasive and invasive testing targeted toward those at-risk patients in whom the results would affect treatment or outcome.

Usually, estimation of a patient's peri-operative risk can be determined by a careful clinical evaluation, including a

Table 12–3 Clinical Predictors of Increased Perioperative Cardiovascular Risk (Myocardial Infarction, Congestive Heart Failure, Death)

Major

Unstable coronary syndromes
Recent myocardial infarction (e.g., >1 wk and ≤1 mo)
Unstable or severe angina (Canadian Cardiovascular Society angina class III or IV)
Decompensated heart failure
Significant arrhythmias
High-grade atrioventricular block
Symptomatic ventricular arrhythmias
Supraventricular arrhythmias with uncontrolled ventricular response
Severe valvular disease

Intermediate

Mild angina (Canadian Cardiovascular Society angina class I or II)
Prior myocardial infarction
Compensated or prior congestive heart failure
Diabetes mellitus

Minor

Advanced age
Abnormal electrocardiogram (e.g., left ventricular hypertrophy, left bundle branch block)
Rhythm other than sinus
Low functional capacity (i.e., unable to climb one flight of stairs with a bag of groceries)
History of a stroke
Uncontrolled systemic hypertension

Table 12–4 Cardiac Risk Stratification for Noncardiac Surgical Procedures

High (reported cardiac risk >5%)

Emergent major operations, particularly in the older adult population
Major vascular surgery, aortic aneurysm repair
Peripheral vascular surgery
Prolonged procedures associated with large fluid shifts or blood loss or both

Intermediate (reported cardiac risk <5%)

Carotid endarterectomy
Head and neck
Intraperitoneal and intrathoracic
Orthopedic
Prostate

Low (reported cardiac risk <1%)

Endoscopic procedures
Cataract extraction
Breast biopsy

From Eagle KA, Brundage BH, Chaitman BR, et al: Guidelines for perioperative cardiovascular evaluation for noncardiac surgery: Report of the ACC/AHA Task Force on Practice Guidelines. J Am Coll Cardiol 27:910–948, 1996.

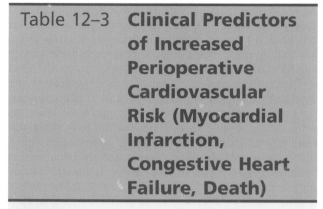

history, physical examination, and review of the electrocardiogram. Patients at highest risk for a peri-operative cardiac event are those with a recent myocardial infarction (defined as more than 7 days but less than 1 month earlier), unstable or severe angina, decompensated congestive heart failure, significant arrhythmias, or severe valvular disease (Table 12–3). Predictors of moderate or intermediate cardiac risk include a history of stable angina, compensated heart failure, prior myocardial infarction, or diabetes mellitus. Advanced age, an abnormal electrocardiogram, low-functional capacity, and poorly controlled hypertension are associated with cardiovascular disease but are not independent predictors of a peri-operative cardiac event.

Risks associated with the type of surgery are highest in patients undergoing major emergency procedures, especially when performed in the older adult population (Table 12–4). Cardiac complications are also common after vascular surgery, considering that the prevalence of underlying coronary artery disease is high in this patient population. In addition, any surgery associated with large volume shifts or blood loss may place increased demands on an already diseased heart. Procedures associated with the lowest risk in the patient with cardiac disease are cataract extraction and endoscopy.

Once the clinical evaluation is complete and the type of surgery is known, the need for additional testing and treatment can be determined. If emergency surgery is contemplated, then little in the way of cardiac assessment can be performed, and recommendations may be directed at peri-operative medical management and surveillance. If surgery is not urgent, then additional evaluation is based on the clinical assessments of the risk and type of surgery. Patients with major risk factors for cardiac complications should have surgery delayed until the cardiac condition is treated and stabilized. Patients with intermediate predictors of cardiac risk scheduled for high-risk surgery should undergo noninvasive testing, such as exercise or pharmacologic stress testing or echocardiography. The results of these tests will help determine future management, such as cardiac catheterization or intensification of medical therapy. Those patients scheduled for low- or intermediate-risk surgery, especially if the patient has good exercise capacity, should proceed with surgery with appropriate medical management and postoperative surveillance. Noncardiac surgery is generally safe for patients with minor or no clinical risk factors for cardiac complications, although some patients with poor functional capacity scheduled for high-risk operations may benefit from additional cardiac evaluation.

Disease-Specific Approaches

CORONARY ARTERY DISEASE AND MYOCARDIAL INFARCTION

Approximately 70% of postoperative myocardial infarctions occur within the first 6 days, with the peak incidence between 24 and 72 hours. Mortality associated with noncardiac surgery has been reported as high as 30% to 40%, especially if associated with congestive heart failure or significant arrhythmias. Multiple stresses associated with surgery can provoke ischemia. Physiologic tachycardia and hypertension secondary to volume shifts, anemia, infection, and the stress of wound healing increase myocardial oxygen demand and may provoke ischemia. In addition, increased platelet reactivity during the postoperative period may increase the risk of coronary thrombosis and subsequent infarction.

Despite the high mortality associated with peri-operative myocardial infarction, few studies have examined the effects of anti-ischemic therapy on the prevention of this complication. Several small, uncontrolled trials have suggested that β-blockers may reduce intra-operative ischemia. More recently, the use of atenolol before and after surgery was associated with a reduction in myocardial infarction and cardiac death, especially during the first 6 to 12 months after surgery. Although the data are limited, the use of a peri-operative β-blocker should be considered in all patients with suggested or known coronary artery disease unless a specific contraindication to its use is present. The data available on the usefulness of calcium channel blockers and nitrates are even more limited, but this approach may be appropriate for the treatment of symptomatic coronary disease in individuals who are not candidates for revascularization. Coronary angiography and revascularization should be reserved for individuals in whom this treatment would otherwise result in significant improvement in symptoms or long-term survival. In rare cases, revascularization may be indicated in high-risk patients undergoing major noncardiac surgery.

All patients with suggested or known cardiac disease should have routine electrocardiograms the first 3 days after surgery to monitor for ischemia. When the electrocardiogram is inconclusive, measurement of troponin levels may be helpful to document an ischemic event. Treatment of a myocardial infarction in this setting is similar to that for the nonsurgical patient (see Chapter 9), although the use of anticoagulants and thrombolytic agents may be contraindicated in the immediate postoperative period. Special attention should be paid to correcting abnormalities that may provoke additional ischemia (e.g., hypoxia, anemia).

CONGESTIVE HEART FAILURE

Several studies have shown that decompensated heart failure is associated with increased peri-operative cardiac compli-

cations. In these patients, surgery should be postponed until appropriate treatment is instituted and symptoms have been stabilized. If planned surgery is associated with large blood loss or fluid shifts, then a pulmonary artery catheter may be helpful in managing the patient.

During the postoperative period, congestive heart failure most commonly occurs during the first 24 to 48 hours when fluid administered during surgery is mobilized from the extravascular space. However, heart failure may also result from myocardial ischemia and new arrhythmias. Initial management includes identification and treatment of the underlying cause. In addition, intravenous diuretics usually provide rapid relief of pulmonary congestion. If heart failure is complicated by hypotension or poor urine output, then insertion of a pulmonary artery catheter may be helpful to guide additional therapy (see Chapter 6).

VALVULAR HEART DISEASE

Aortic and mitral stenosis are associated with the greatest risk for complications after noncardiac surgery. Patients with symptomatic, severe aortic stenosis should have valve replacement before noncardiac surgery. In patients with mild-to-moderate mitral stenosis, careful attention to volume status and heart rate control are necessary to optimize left ventricular filling and to avoid pulmonary congestion. Patients with severe mitral stenosis should be considered for percutaneous valvuloplasty or mitral valve replacement before high-risk surgery. In patients with valve disease or prosthetic heart valves, prophylactic antibiotics are recommended when appropriate.

ARRHYTHMIAS AND CONDUCTION DEFECTS

Patients with symptomatic, high-grade conduction disturbances, such as third-degree atrioventricular (AV) block, have an increased peri-operative risk of cardiac complications and should have a temporary pacemaker inserted before surgery. Patients with first-degree AV block, Mobitz type I AV block, or bifascicular block (right bundle branch block and left anterior fascicular block) do not require prophylactic pacemaker insertion.

Atrial arrhythmias, such as atrial fibrillation, are common after surgery and are usually not associated with significant complications if the ventricular rate is well controlled. Ventricular premature beats and nonsustained ventricular tachycardia are also common after noncardiac surgery and do not require specific therapy unless associated with myocardial ischemia or heart failure. In most instances, treatment of the underlying cause (e.g., hypoxia, metabolic abnormalities, ischemia, volume overload) will result in significant improvement or resolution of the rhythm disturbance without specific anti-arrhythmic therapy.

CARDIAC DISEASE IN PREGNANCY

Pregnancy is associated with dramatic changes in the cardiovascular system that may result in significant hemodynamic stress to the patient with underlying heart disease. During a normal pregnancy, plasma volume increases an average of 50%, beginning in the first trimester and peaking between the 20th and 24th weeks of pregnancy. This change is accompanied by an increase in stroke volume, heart rate, and, accordingly, cardiac output. In addition, a concomitant fall in systemic vascular resistance and mean arterial pressure occurs because of the effects of gestational hormones on the vasculature and the creation of a low-resistance circulation in the pregnant uterus and placenta. During labor, uterine contractions result in a transient increase of up to 500 mL of blood in the central circulation, resulting in further increases in stroke volume and cardiac output. After delivery, intravascular volume and cardiac output increase further as compression of the inferior vena cava by the gravid uterus is relieved and extravascular fluid is mobilized. Symptoms and signs that may mimic cardiac disease often accompany these hemodynamic changes and include fatigue, reduced exercise tolerance, lower extremity edema, distention of the neck veins, S_3 gallop, and new systolic murmurs. Differentiating symptoms produced by cardiac disease versus those attributable to a normal pregnancy can be difficult. Under such circumstances, echocardiography can be a safe and helpful noninvasive test to assess cardiac structure and function in the pregnant patient.

Many pregnant patients with known cardiac disease can complete a normal pregnancy and delivery without significant harm to the mother or fetus. However, certain cardiac conditions, including irreversible pulmonary hypertension, cardiomyopathy associated with severe heart failure, and Marfan syndrome with a dilated aortic root, are associated with a high risk for cardiovascular complications and death. Under these circumstances, patients should be advised against having children. If pregnancy should occur, then a first-trimester therapeutic abortion should be strongly recommended.

Specific Cardiac Conditions
MITRAL STENOSIS

Mitral stenosis secondary to rheumatic heart disease frequently occurs in young women of childbearing age. The physiologic increases in heart rate and cardiac output during pregnancy result in a significant increase in the gradient across the mitral valve and a rise in left atrial and pulmonary venous pressures. Congestive heart failure may develop as the pregnancy progresses through the second and third trimesters or may occur more acutely with the onset of atrial fibrillation. The management of the patient with mitral stenosis depends on her pre-pregnant functional capacity and the severity of the valve obstruction. In general, patients with severely symptomatic mitral valve stenosis should have percutaneous or surgical correction of the valve before conception. Women with minimal symptoms (New York Heart Association functional classes I to II) usually tolerate pregnancy and vaginal delivery well even if moderate-to-severe stenosis is present. Management includes salt restriction, diuretic therapy, and aggressive treatment of pulmonary infections. Patients who develop atrial fibrillation with a rapid ventricular response should be treated with AV nodal blocking agents and cardioversion if possible. Patients who develop refractory heart failure during pregnancy should be considered for mitral balloon valvuloplasty because surgical

commissurotomy or valve replacement may be associated with fetal demise.

AORTIC STENOSIS

Aortic stenosis in a pregnant woman is usually congenital in origin. Patients with significant outflow obstruction may develop angina or heart failure during the later portion of the pregnancy as cardiac output increases. Supportive therapy includes bedrest and prevention of hypovolemia. If these measures fail to control symptoms and the fetus is not near term, then balloon valvuloplasty or aortic valve surgery should be considered to reduce the risk of maternal death.

MARFAN SYNDROME

Pregnant women with Marfan syndrome are at an increased risk of aortic dissection and rupture, especially during the third trimester and first postpartum month. Patients with an aortic root diameter greater than 40 mm are at greatest risk for this complication and should strongly consider therapeutic abortion during the first trimester. Women with an aortic root diameter less than 40 mm should have serial echocardiograms to monitor the size of the aortic root during pregnancy. In addition, restriction in physical activity and treatment with a β-blocker may help prevent further dilation of the aorta.

CONGENITAL HEART DISEASE

Survival to reproductive age is common in patients with corrected congenital defects. The risk of pregnancy in these patients is related to the completeness of the repair and the mother's functional capacity. Uncomplicated atrial or ventricular septal defects not associated with symptoms or pulmonary hypertension are usually well tolerated during pregnancy. Intracardiac shunts associated with pulmonary vascular hypertension are associated with a high maternal mortality during pregnancy, as a result of an increase in right-to-left shunting and worsening oxygen desaturation of the blood. In these women, pregnancy is contraindicated. If pregnancy should occur, then a therapeutic abortion during the first trimester should be recommended. Women with uncorrected tetralogy of Fallot should undergo palliative or definitive repair before conception to improve maternal and fetal outcomes with pregnancy. Women with residual obstruction of the right ventricular outflow tract remain at high risk for right ventricular heart failure during pregnancy.

PROSTHETIC HEART VALVES

Most patients with a normal-functioning prosthetic valve tolerate pregnancy without complications. However, in patients with mechanical valves, special attention to the choice and dose of anticoagulant therapy is necessary to avoid thromboembolic complications in the mother and teratogenic effects in the fetus. Women should start subcutaneous heparin before conception to avoid the potential teratogenic effects of warfarin during the first several months of critical fetal organ development. This therapy can be continued throughout pregnancy, or, alternatively, warfarin can be reinstituted late in the second trimester or during the third trimester. Heparin therapy, although reducing the risk of teratogenicity associated with warfarin use, is associated with a high risk of maternal bleeding complications. Low–molecular-weight heparin may be an acceptable alternative; however, no firm data are available to support these recommendations. At the time of delivery, anticoagulation therapy is interrupted to avoid bleeding complications. Antibiotic prophylaxis is generally not recommended at the time of delivery.

HEART DISEASE ARISING DURING PREGNANCY

Cardiovascular disease can develop during pregnancy and may pose a significant risk to the mother and/or fetus. Hypertension is not an uncommon problem during pregnancy and is defined as a consistent increase in blood pressure of 30/15 mm Hg or as an absolute blood pressure greater than 140/90 mm Hg. The three major forms of hypertension that may develop during pregnancy include chronic hypertension, gestational hypertension, and toxemia. Toxemia is a form of hypertension that develops during the second half of pregnancy and is associated with proteinuria, edema, and, in severe forms, seizures. This problem is primarily managed by the obstetrician and is not discussed in this text. Gestational hypertension is an elevation in blood pressure that occurs late in the pregnancy, during delivery, or in the first postpartum days. This disease entity is not associated with proteinuria or edema and resolves within 2 weeks of delivery. Chronic hypertension is presumed to be present if an elevation in blood pressure is detected before the 20th week of pregnancy. No matter what the cause, fetal mortality correlates with the severity of the hypertension and begins to rise when the diastolic pressure exceeds 75 mm Hg during the second trimester and 85 mm Hg during the third trimester. Initial treatments include a reduction in physical activity and salt restriction. If the blood pressure remains greater than 150/90 mm Hg, then antihypertensive treatment should be instituted. Agents that have been safely used in pregnancy include hydralazine, α-methyldopa, clonidine, β-blockers, and labetalol. Diuretics should be used with caution because of the increased risk of placental hypoperfusion.

Peripartum cardiomyopathy (PCM) is a form of dilated cardiomyopathy that may begin during the last trimester of pregnancy or within the first 6 months after delivery in a woman without prior heart disease or other definable causes for cardiac dysfunction. The true incidence of the disease is unknown, but estimates conclude that one woman in 3000 to 4000 pregnancies is affected. Although the cause of PCM is unknown, myocardial injury is thought to be immunologically mediated. Women usually exhibit symptoms and signs of congestive heart failure. Echocardiography is useful to assess chamber size and degree of ventricular dysfunction. The outcome with PCM is variable, with death or progressive heart failure occurring in approximately one third of affected women. The prognosis is particularly poor if symptoms develop before delivery. Despite this risk, many patients will have complete recovery of ventricular function, although recurrence is possible, especially with subsequent pregnancies. Treatment is similar to that for congestive heart failure (see Chapter 6) and usually includes vasodilators, such as hydralazine, digoxin, and diuretics. Angiotensin-converting enzyme inhibitors have been associated with increased fetal wastage in pregnant animals and should be avoided. A thorough evaluation of cardiac function should be performed before subsequent pregnancies. If a woman decides to proceed with another pregnancy, then she should be monitored regularly for signs of cardiac decompensation.

Approximately 50% of aortic dissections that occur in women younger than the age of 40 years are associated with pregnancy. Although the cause of aortic dissection during pregnancy is unknown, it has been postulated that hemodynamic and hormonal changes associated with pregnancy may weaken the aortic wall. The highest incidence of dissection is during the third trimester, although it may occur at any time during the pregnancy and during the early postpartum period. The presenting symptoms and diagnostic work-up are similar to those for the nonpregnant patient (see Chapter 13). Transesophageal echocardiography is highly sensitive and specific for the detection of aortic dissection and offers the advantage of not exposing the fetus to ionizing radiation. Management includes aggressive blood pressure control and β-blocker therapy to reduce shear forces of the ejected blood. Recommendations for corrective surgery are similar to those for the nonpregnant patient and are discussed in Chapter 13.

Prospectus for the Future

CABG remains an important but less commonly used mode for revascularization of symptomatic coronary artery disease. Prospective studies are needed to evaluate the efficacy, health outcomes, and cost benefits for combined approaches of CABG and percutaneous coronary angioplasty (PTCA) with drug-eluting stents. Percutaneous and minimally invasive surgical options will gain greater widespread application in the management of heart disease. With the limited donor pool for cardiac transplantation, advanced heart failure will be managed with resynchronization therapy, left ventricular assist devices, and stem- and cell-based therapies.

References

Butany J, Nair V, Naseemuddin A, et al: Cardiac tumours: Diagnosis and management. Lancet Oncol 6(4):219–228, 2005.

Elkayam U, Bitar F: Valvular heart disease and pregnancy. Part I: Native valves. J Am Coll Cardiol 46(2):223–230, 2005.

Elkayam U, Bitar F: Valvular heart disease and pregnancy. Part II: Prosthetic valves. J Am Coll Cardiol 46(3):403–410, 2005.

Froehlich JB, Karavite D, Russman PL, et al: ACC/AHA preoperative assessment guidelines reduce resource utilization before aortic surgery. J Vasc Surg 36(4):758–763, 2002.

Gray DT, Veenstra DL: Comparative economic analyses of minimally invasive direct coronary artery bypass surgery. J Thorac Cardiovasc Surg 125(3):618–624, 2003.

Vascular Diseases and Hypertension

Wanpen Vongpatanasin

Ronald G. Victor

Diseases of the systemic and pulmonary vasculature are among the most common clinical problems encountered in internal medicine. Yet these important diseases are not often given the emphasis they deserve; they fall between the cracks of traditional medical subspecialties. Early clinical recognition is important because in many cases effective therapy can prevent or at least delay needless suffering and death. This chapter reviews the causes, clinical manifestations, diagnostic evaluations, and therapeutic approaches to the major forms of systemic and pulmonary vascular diseases, as well as arterial hypertension. New qualifying examinations are now available in both vascular medicine and hypertension, highlighting the increasing need for expertise in these fields.

Systemic Vascular Disease

PERIPHERAL ARTERIAL DISEASE

Peripheral arterial disease (PAD) refers to atherosclerotic vascular disease of mainly the lower extremities. Similar to other atherosclerotic vascular diseases, PAD is more prevalent in men than it is in women, particularly before the age of menopause. The prevalence increases with age, ranging from 2% to 6% for adults under the age of 60 years to 20% to 30% for those over the age of 70 years. As with coronary atherosclerosis, the major reversible risk factors are cigarette smoking, diabetes mellitus, hyperlipidemia, and hypertension. Only 30% to 50% of patients with PAD become symptomatic. The classic syndrome of intermittent claudication refers to ischemic muscle pain or weakness that is brought on by exertion and promptly relieved by rest. Claudication is associated with a significant 10-year risk of morbidity and mortality. Approximately 25% of patients will develop worsening claudication, 5% will require amputation, 10% to 20% will require revascularization (e.g., surgery, angioplasty), and 30% will die of a cardiovascular event (e.g., heart attack, stroke) as a result of concomitant coronary or cerebrovas-

cular atherosclerosis. To minimize the progression of PAD and avoid complications, risk factor modification is absolutely essential. This modification includes tight control of blood pressure (BP), plasma lipids, and blood glucose. Complete cessation of tobacco use is a must.

The diagnosis of PAD begins with a careful history and physical examination and is confirmed with noninvasive laboratory testing. Ischemic pain occurs in the leg muscles supplied by arterial segments that are distal to the site of stenosis. Thus, calf claudication is the hallmark of femoral-popliteal disease, whereas discomfort in the thigh, hip, buttock associated with impotence indicates aortoiliac disease (Leriche's syndrome). Depending on the severity of the stenosis, the pain is experienced at a predictable walking distance and is promptly relieved by rest. Claudication must be differentiated from the pseudoclaudication of lumbar degenerative spinal canal stenosis. In the latter condition, walking can also aggravate leg pain, but it is not relieved simply by the cessation of exercise. Rather, assuming positions that minimize lumbar extension such as stooping forward or sitting alleviates the pain. The characteristic physical findings of PAD are absent or diminished pulses distal to the stenosis, bruits over the diseased artery, hair loss, thin shiny skin, and muscle atrophy. Severe ischemia causes pallor, cyanosis, decreased skin temperature, ulceration, and gangrene.

Noninvasive techniques are quite good. The *ankle-brachial index* (ABI) is the ratio of the highest systolic BP measured from either the dorsalis pedis or posterior tibialis artery to the highest systolic BP obtained from the brachial artery using a Doppler stethoscope. The normal ABI range is 0.9 to 1.3. An ABI of less than 0.9 indicates PAD. This simple noninvasive test has a sensitivity and specificity of 95% and 99%, respectively. In some patients with diabetes mellitus or renal failure, the media of the affected leg vessels become so heavily calcified that they resist compression except during very high levels of cuff inflation. The result is a falsely elevated ankle BP and an artificially normal or supernormal ABI (Table 13–1)

Table 13–1	Interpretation of Ankle-Brachial Index
Ankle-Brachial Index	**Interpretation**
0.90–1.30	Normal
0.70–0.89	Mild PAD
0.40–069	Moderate PAD
<0.40	Severe PAD
>1.30	Noncompressible vessels

PAD = peripheral arterial disease.

Duplex ultrasonography is an important adjunct to the ABI, with a similar sensitivity and specificity. This test is particularly useful to diagnose PAD in patients with noncompressible vessels from medial wall calcification. The Doppler velocity waveform remains abnormal, despite a spuriously normal or elevated ABI. Magnetic resonance (MR) angiography and computed tomographic (CT) angiography are newer techniques that now permit excellent visualization of vascular stenosis and identification of runoff vessels. With these noninvasive imaging modalities, spatial resolution is comparable with that of traditional invasive angiography. Catheter-based angiography, the gold standard, now is reserved for patients undergoing revascularization.

The medical management of patients with PAD includes lifestyle and risk factor modification, as well as antiplatelet therapy. Smoking cessation reduces the risk of limb loss, myocardial infarction, and death. Lipid-lowering therapy with a statin hydroxymethylglutaryl–coenzyme A (HMG CoA) reductase inhibitor should be initiated and intensified if low-density lipoprotein (LDL) cholesterol is greater than 100 mg/dL. Hypertension should be treated with appropriate medication, which should be intensified until BP is less than 140/90 mm Hg. The target BP is even lower (<130/80 mm Hg) in PAD patients with diabetes or chronic kidney disease or patients who have had a prior cardiovascular event or who have left ventricular hypertrophy (LVH) visualized by electrocardiography (ECG) or echocardiography. In contrast to traditional teaching, β-adrenergic blockers do not reduce walking capacity or worsen intermittent claudication in patients with PAD. Aspirin reduces the risk of myocardial infarction, death, and stroke. However, clopidogrel has proven to be more effective than aspirin in this setting. Each patient needs an exercise prescription because exercise training improves walking capacity and quality of life. Pentoxifylline is a methylxanthine derivative that may improve maximal walking distance, but the data are inconclusive. Better data is available with cilostazol, a phosphodiesterase III inhibitor, whereas sildenafil is a phosphodiesterase V inhibitor. In several studies of patients with symptomatic PAD, cilostazol consistently improved walking capacity and quality of life. It is one of the most effective agents for intermittent claudication. However, cilostazol must be avoided in patients with congestive heart failure because its use increases mortality.

Revascularization (percutaneous or surgical) is indicated for patients with severe claudication that is resistant to medical therapy, limb-threatening ischemia, or vasculogenic impotence. Percutaneous revascularization offers a comparable patency rate with less morbidity and mortality than does surgery in patients with short focal stenoses in large arteries such as the distal aorta or iliac arteries (Fig. 13–1). Surgical revascularization is more suitable for longer areas of stenosis or obstructive lesions distal to the origin of the iliac arteries.

Acute limb ischemia constitutes a vascular emergency. Sudden occlusion of a peripheral artery is caused by either arterial embolism or thrombosis in situ. Arterial emboli usually originate in the cardiac chambers in the setting of pre-existing cardiac disease such as myocardial infarction (e.g., left ventricular mural thrombus), congestive heart failure, or atrial arrhythmias (e.g., left atrial thrombus in a patient with atrial fibrillation). Thrombosis in situ usually occurs in arteries with a pre-existing severe stenosis in the setting of long-standing PAD with or without previous vascular surgery. Patients with arterial embolism usually experience sudden onset of symptoms without a history of claudication, whereas those with thrombosis in situ typically have a history of claudication that has previously been stable and then suddenly assumes a crescendo pattern over a period of days. In either case, the physical examination reveals a cold, cyanotic (bluish) extremity with absent pulses distal to the site of arterial occlusion and diminished motor and/or sensory function. A hand-held Doppler device is used to assess signals at different arterial segments and confirms the diagnosis of acute vascular occlusion. Anticoagulation should be initiated immediately with intravenous heparin titrated to maintain the activated partial thromboplastin time equal to 2.0 to 2.5 times control. Patients with embolic occlusion generally require surgical thromboembolectomy, whereas those with thrombosis in situ should be treated with catheter-directed infusion of plasminogen activator. After revascularization, patients with acute arterial embolism should undergo transesophageal echocardiography to determine the potential cardiac source. Patients with thrombosis in situ may need additional revascularization procedures to improve perfusion distal to severely diseased arteries. Patients with irreversible tissue necrosis, regardless of the cause, should be treated with emergent amputation rather than revascularization to reduce the risk of kidney failure (myoglobinemia), sepsis, and multi-organ failure.

AORTIC ANEURYSM

Abdominal aortic aneurysm is a common vascular disease in older adults, affecting 4% to 8% of men and 0.5% to 1.5% of women over the age of 65 years. Thoracic aortic aneurysm is much less prevalent (0.4% to 0.5%). Besides age, the major risk factors for abdominal aortic aneurysms are cigarette smoking, hypertension, and a family history of aortic aneurysms. Atherosclerosis is responsible for most cases of abdominal aortic aneurysm, but other causes include cystic medial necrosis (Marfan syndrome, Ehlers-Danlos syndrome), vasculitis with connective tissue disease (Takayasu's

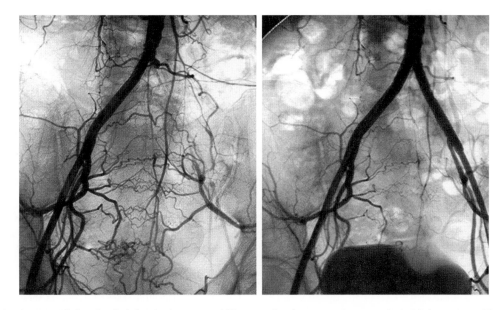

Figure 13–1 Angiogram of the distal abdominal aorta and iliac arteries demonstrates an occluded left common iliac artery with extensive collateral circulation from the contralateral internal iliac artery *(left)*, which resolved after successful stent implantation *(right)*. (Images courtesy of Bart Domatch, MD, Radiology Department, University of Texas Southwestern Medical Center, Dallas, Texas.)

arteritis, giant-cell arteritis), chronic infection (syphilitic aortitis), and trauma. Abdominal aortic aneurysms gradually grow in size over time at an average rate of 1 to 4 mm per year. The risk of rupture is low until the diameter reaches 5 cm, and then it increases exponentially. The risk of aortic rupture is 1% per year for aneurysms between 3.5 and 4.9 cm in diameter and 5% per year for aneurysms larger than 5 cm.

Most patients with aortic aneurysms are asymptomatic, but some develop vascular complications such as aneurysm expansion with compression of adjacent structures. Occasionally, mural thrombi form within the aneurysm embolize, causing acute occlusion of distal arterial segments. Patients with iliac aneurysm may develop hydronephrosis or recurrent urinary tract infection from ureteral compression. Others develop neurologic symptoms from compression of sciatic or femoral nerves. The classic physical finding is a pulsatile nontender mass below the umbilicus (distal to the origin of the renal arteries). In thin patients, normal aortic pulsations are often palpable but above the umbilicus. Hypotension and acute abdominal pain should prompt consideration of aneurysm rupture, which requires emergent operative repair. Duplex ultrasonography is an accurate and reliable diagnostic tool for abdominal aortic and iliac aneurysms. Routine screening for abdominal aortic aneurysm with ultrasonography is recommended for all men between the ages of 65 and 75 years. Such screening has a proven mortality benefit. CT and MR angiography allow visualization of the thoracic and abdominal aorta, as well as the iliac arteries and its branches (Fig. 13–2). Medical treatment for aortic aneurysm includes smoking cessation, tight BP control, and cholesterol reduction. β-Adrenergic blockade reduces the rate of aortic root enlargement in patients with Marfan syndrome but has not proven beneficial in patients with abdominal aortic aneurysm from other causes. Patients with large aneurysms or rapid aneurysm

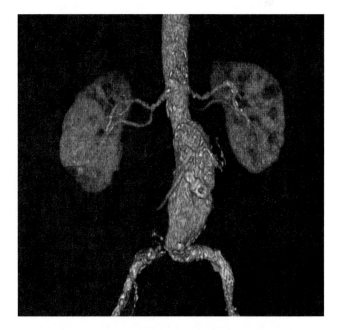

Figure 13–2 CT angiogram of the distal abdominal aorta shows abdominal aortic aneurysm with the largest diameter of 6.2 cm and severe stenosis at the origin of the right common iliac artery. (Image courtesy of Bart Domatch, MD, Radiology Department, University of Texas Southwestern Medical Center, Dallas, Texas.)

expansion regardless of the size should undergo aneurysm repair (Table 13–2). Elective abdominal aortic aneurysm repair carries a peri-operative mortality rate of 2% to 6%. Furthermore, a large randomized study failed to demonstrate any benefit of surgery in patients with aneurysms 4.0 to 5.5 cm in diameter. For these reasons, patients with small aortic aneurysms should be treated medically with close

Table 13–2	**Indications for Surgical Treatment of Arterial Aneurysms**

Symptoms from expansion of aneurysm or compression of adjacent structure

Rupture of aneurysm

Rapid aortic aneurysm expansion of ≥1 cm per year

Large aneurysm
   Ascending aorta >4.5 cm for patients with Marfan
      syndrome and >5.0 cm for all others
   Aortic arch >5.5 cm
   Descending thoracic aorta >5.0 cm
   Abdominal aorta >5.5 cm
   Iliac aneurysm >3 cm

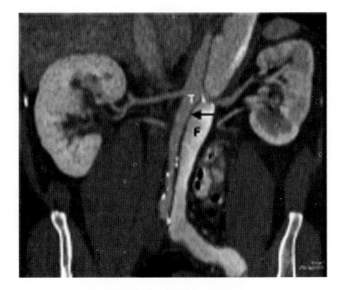

Figure 13–3 CT angiogram of the aorta shows type B aortic dissection. The intimal flap *(arrow)* separates the true lumen *(T)* from the false lumen *(F)* and compromises blood flow to the right kidney causing renal atrophy and cortical thinning. (Image courtesy of Bart Domatch, MD, Radiology Department, University of Texas Southwestern Medical Center, Dallas, Texas.)

monitoring of aneurysm size with periodic imaging studies every 6 to 12 months (see Table 13–2).

Percutaneous endovascular graft placement is an alternative method to open surgical intervention for the repair of abdominal aortic aneurysm. An early mortality benefit can be realized with percutaneous rather than with surgical repair (1% to 2% versus 2% to 5%). However, after the first postoperative year, percutaneous repair is associated with a higher number of both repeat interventions and late complications.

Aortic Dissection

In aortic dissection, the intimal layer is torn from the aortic wall leading to the formation of a false lumen in parallel with the true lumen. Risk factors include hypertension, cocaine use, trauma, hereditary connective tissue disease (e.g., Marfan syndrome, Ehlers-Danlos syndrome), vasculitis (e.g., Takayasu's arteritis, giant-cell arteritis), Behçet's disease, bicuspid aortic valve, and aortic coarctation. Aortic dissection can be classified as types A and B (Stanford system). Type A dissection involves the ascending aorta, whereas type B dissection involves the distal aorta. The DeBakey system subdivides aortic dissection into three subtypes—types I, II, and III. Type 1 dissection involves the entire aorta, whereas type II involves only the ascending aorta, and type III involves only the descending aorta. Aortic dissection involving the ascending aorta carries a high mortality rate of 1% to 2% per hour during the first 24 to 48 hours. Patients usually develop acute onset of severe chest or back pain. Abdominal pain, syncope, and stroke are common. Retrograde propagation of the dissection can cause pericardial tamponade or coronary artery dissection with acute myocardial infarction. Dissection involving the aortic valve causes acute severe aortic insufficiency with acute pulmonary edema. The dissection plane may propagate in an antegrade direction to compromise flow in the carotid and subclavian arteries, producing a stroke or acute upper limb ischemia.

Patients with distal (type B) aortic dissection exhibit acute onset of back pain or chest pain often accompanied by lower extremity ischemia and ischemic neuropathy. The physical findings include pulse deficits, neurologic deficits, or a diastolic murmur of aortic regurgitation. However, acute aortic regurgitation into an unprepared ventricle produces only a short, soft diastolic murmur that is often missed. The widened pulse pressure and associated physical findings of chronic aortic regurgitation are absent, and the clinical picture is that of an acutely ill patient with tachypnea, tachycardia, and a narrow pulse pressure. Hypotension, jugular venous distention, and pulsus paradoxus should prompt the diagnosis of pericardial tamponade. Transesophageal echocardiography, MR angiography, or CT angiography confirm the diagnosis by demonstrating an intimal flap that separates the true lumen from the false lumen (Fig. 13–3). Type A aortic dissection is uniformly fatal without emergent surgical repair. With surgery, mortality is reduced to 10% at 24 hours and 20% at 30 days. Patients with type B aortic dissection should be treated medically because 1-year survival is higher with medical therapy than it is with surgery (75% versus 50%). However, surgery is indicated if type B dissection compromises blood flow to the legs, kidneys, or other viscera. Tight control of BP is essential because aortic aneurysm develops in 30% to 50% of patients with type B aortic dissection studied for 4 years.

Penetrating Aortic Ulcers and Intramural Hematoma

Penetrating aortic ulcers and intramural hematomas exhibit chest pain that is indistinguishable from that of aortic dissection. In contrast to aortic dissection, however, the pathologic condition is localized. No identifiable intimal flap and thus no branch vessel occlusion are produced. Disruption of the internal elastic lamina produces aortic ulcers that erode

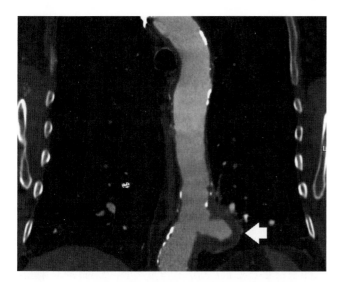

Figure 13–4 CT angiogram of the descending thoracic aorta shows a large penetrating aortic ulcer above the diaphragm *(arrow)*. (Image courtesy of Bart Domatch, MD, Radiology Department, University of Texas Southwestern Medical Center, Dallas, Texas.)

into the medial wall and protrude into the surrounding structures. Rupture of the vasa vasorum causes formation of localized hematoma underneath the adventitia with resultant asymmetric thickening of the aortic wall. Patients with either condition typically are older than those with aortic dissection, have a larger aortic size, and have a higher prevalence of abdominal aortic aneurysm. Aortic rupture is the major complication of both penetrating ulcers and intramural hematomas, particularly with those aneurysms located in the ascending aorta. The diagnosis is made with invasive angiography, CT angiography, or MR angiography (Fig. 13–4). Surgical intervention should be considered for ulcers and hematomas of the ascending aorta, deeply penetrating ulcers, or severely bulging hematomas, irrespective of their location. Ulcers and hematomas of the descending aortic may be managed successfully with β-adrenergic blockade and tight control of BP.

Other Arterial Diseases

Buerger's disease is a nonatherosclerotic disease of the arteries, veins, and nerves of the arms and legs affecting mostly young men before the age of 45 years. The cause is unknown, but all patients have a history of heavy tobacco addiction. The presenting symptom is claudication of the feet, legs, hands, or arms. Multiple-limb involvement and superficial thrombophlebitis are common. The C-reactive protein and Westergren sedimentation rate typically are normal, and a search for serologic markers for connective tissue disease (e.g., antinuclear antibody or rheumatoid factor, antiphospholipid antibody) is negative. The diagnosis is usually based on the typical clinical presentation. If the presentation is atypical, then biopsy may be needed to make the diagnosis. The histologic hallmark is inflammatory intramural thrombi within the arteries and veins with sparing of internal elastic lamina and other arterial wall structures. The most effective treatment for Buerger's disease is complete tobacco absti-

nence. The prostacyclin analog iloprost constitutes adjunctive therapy to reduce limb ischemia and improve wound healing.

Raynaud's phenomenon is a vasospastic disease of the small arteries of mainly the fingers and toes. Primary (idiopathic) Raynaud's phenomenon occurs in the absence of underlying disorders. Secondary Raynaud's phenomenon occurs in association with connective tissue diseases (e.g., scleroderma, polymyositis, rheumatoid arthritis, systemic lupus erythematosus), as well as with repeated mild physical trauma (e.g., use of jack hammers), certain drugs (e.g., antineoplastic chemotherapeutic agents, interferon, monamine-reuptake inhibitors such as tricyclic antidepressants, serotonin agonists), and Buerger's disease. Patients usually complain of recurrent episodes of digital ischemia, with a characteristic white-blue-red color sequence. Pallor is followed by cyanosis if ischemia is prolonged and then by erythema (reactive hyperemia) when the episode resolves. Episodes are precipitated by cold temperature or emotional stress. Physical examination can be entirely normal between attacks with normal radial, ulnar, and pedal pulses. Some patients may have digital ulcers or thickening of fat pad (sclerodactyly). Patients should be instructed to avoid cold temperatures and dress warmly. Calcium channel blockers (CCBs) reduce the frequency and severity of vasospastic episodes.

Giant-cell arteritis is an immune-mediated vasculitis predominantly involving medium-sized and large arteries such as the subclavian artery, axillary artery, and aorta of the older adult with a strong male predominance. Approximately 40% of patients with giant-cell arteritis also have polymyalgia rheumatica, a syndrome characterized by severe stiffness and pain originating in the muscles of the shoulders and pelvic girdle. Patients may exhibit headache from temporal arteritis, jaw claudication from ischemia of the masseter muscles, or visual loss from involvement of ophthalmic artery. Chest pain suggests the co-existence of aortic aneurysm or dissection. Physical findings include low-grade fever, scalp tenderness in the temporal area, pale and edematous fundi, or a diastolic murmur of aortic regurgitation. BP difference of more than 15 mm Hg between arms suggests subclavian artery stenosis. Laboratory findings include significantly elevated C-reactive protein and Westergren sedimentation rate plus anemia. The diagnosis is confirmed by histologic examination of the arterial tissue (frequently from temporal artery biopsy), showing infiltration of lymphocytes and macrophages (i.e., giant cells) in all layers of the vascular wall. High-dose corticosteroids are highly effective. To minimize complications from long-term corticosteroid administration, the steroid dose should be tapered to find the lowest dose needed to suppress symptoms, which often wane. Every attempt should be made to discontinue corticosteroids over time.

Takayasu's arteritis is an idiopathic granulomatous vasculitis of the aorta, its main branches, and the pulmonary artery. This condition is particularly common in young women of Asian descent, but it also occurs in Occidental women and men. The inflammatory process in the vascular wall can lead to stenosis and/or aneurysm formation. Hypertension, as a result of renal artery stenosis or aortic coarctation, is the most common manifestation and is present in as many as 80% of affected individuals. Because the vascular involvement is so widespread, patients may have symptoms and signs of coronary ischemia, congestive heart failure, stroke, vertebrobasilar insufficiency, or intermittent claudication. Physical findings include bruits over the subclavian arteries or aorta, as well as diminished brachial pulses and thus a low brachial artery BP. The diagnosis is based primarily on this clinical presentation. First-line treatment is with corticosteroids. Other immunosuppressive agents such as methotrexate or cyclophosphamide are often added to prevent disease progression and relapse. Immunosuppressive therapy does not cause regression of pre-existing vascular stenoses or aneurysms. For this reason, percutaneous or surgical revascularization is usually required.

Arteriovenous (AV) fistulas are abnormal vascular communications that shunt blood flow from the arterial system directly into the venous system, bypassing the capillary beds that normally ensure optimal tissue perfusion and nutrient exchange. AV fistulas may be congenital, as in AV malformation (AVM), or acquired. The main causes of acquired AV fistula are penetrating trauma (e.g., gunshot, knife wound) and surgically created shunts for hemodialysis access. Patients may exhibit a pulsatile mass, symptoms related to compression of an adjacent organ, or bleeding from spontaneous rupture of an AVM. Systolic and diastolic bruits or thrills may be detectable over the fistula or AVM. An AVM in skeletal muscle may lead to bone malformation or a pathologic fracture, whereas AVM in the brain may result in neurologic deficits or seizures. High-output heart failure is another complication from a large AVM or fistula. MR angiography, CT angiography, or conventional angiography confirms the diagnosis. Depending on the size and location of the AVM, treatment options include surgical resection, transcatheter embolization, or pulse laser irradiation. Patients with acquired AV fistulas from trauma usually need surgical closure.

Pulmonary Vascular Disease

Pulmonary hypertension is characterized by elevated mean pulmonary pressure of greater than 25 mm Hg at rest or greater than 30 mm Hg during exercise. The many causes of pulmonary hypertension are summarized in Table 13–3.

Patients with pulmonary hypertension not only have an elevated pulmonary arterial pressure but also a low cardiac output, causing symptoms of exertional dyspnea, fatigue, and syncope. Pulmonary capillary wedge pressure is usually normal except in patients with pulmonary venous hypertension and congenital heart disease.

PULMONARY ARTERIAL HYPERTENSION

Pulmonary arterial hypertension (PAH) is caused by a combination of pulmonary vasoconstriction, endothelial cell and/or smooth muscle proliferation, intimal fibrosis, and thrombosis in the pulmonary capillaries and arterioles. PAH is either idiopathic (primary pulmonary hypertension [PPH]) or secondary to connective tissue disease, congenital heart disease, portal hypertension, or human immunodeficiency viral (HIV) infection, as well as anorexigenic drugs or toxins. Connective tissue diseases, particularly scleroderma, are the most common secondary causes of PAH.

Table 13–3 Classification of Pulmonary Hypertension
Pulmonary Arterial Hypertension (PAH)
Primary pulmonary hypertension (PPH) or idiopathic pulmonary hypertension (IPAH):
Sporadic
Familial
PPH associated with:
Connective tissue disease
Congenital heart disease
Portal hypertension
Human immunodeficiency viral infection
Drugs and toxins: Anorexigens, cocaine
Pulmonary Venous Hypertension
Left ventricular heart failure
Left ventricular valvular heart disease
Pulmonary Hypertension Associated with Chronic Respiratory Disease or Hypoxemia
Chronic obstructive pulmonary disease
Obstructive sleep apnea
Pulmonary Hypertension Associated with Chronic Venous Thromboembolism

Patients with mild PAH can be asymptomatic, but patients with more advanced disease complain of dyspnea, chest pain, syncope, or presyncope. Physical findings include a left parasternal lift, loud pulmonary component of the second heart sound, murmur of tricuspid or pulmonic regurgitation, hepatomegaly, peripheral edema, or ascites. Associated ECG abnormalities indicate right ventricular hypertrophy, right atrial enlargement, or right axis deviation. Echocardiography provides important information about the severity of the pulmonary hypertension (i.e., estimated pulmonary artery pressure, right ventricular dimensions and function) and its potential causes (e.g., left ventricular failure, valvular lesions, congenital heart disease with left-to-right shunts). Pulmonary function tests, ventilation-perfusion (V/Q) lung scans, polysomnography or overnight oximetry, autoantibody tests, HIV serology, and liver-function tests also should be performed to determine other potential causes. Right ventricular catheterization should be performed in all patients with suggested PAH. Under basal conditions in the catheterization laboratory, an elevated mean pulmonary artery pressure exceeding 25 mm Hg, a pulmonary capillary wedge pressure exceeding 15 mm Hg, and a pulmonary vascular resistance exceeding 3 units confirm the diagnosis. Acute vasodilator drug challenge should be performed during right ventricular catheterization to guide appropriate treatment.

Without treatment, the prognosis of PAH is poor with a median survival of less than 3 years. Patients with severe symptoms should be treated with prostacyclin or epoprostenol (an intravenous prostacyclin analog) because of their proven efficacy to improve exercise capacity, quality of life, and survival. A newer prostacyclin analog, treprostinil, can be delivered subcutaneously and is also effective in reducing symptoms and improving exercise capacity. Bosentan, an oral nonselective endothelin-receptor blocker, is approved for use in patients with moderate or severe PAH. Oral CCBs are indicated for the small subset of patients with mild-to-moderate symptoms who demonstrate significant reduction in pulmonary pressure with acute CCB challenge. Supplemental home oxygen is indicated for all patients with hypoxemia. Higher elevations exacerbate hypodemia, and relocation to sea level improves symptoms. Oral anticoagulation is recommended for all patients with PAH. Diuretics should be prescribed for patients with peripheral edema or hepatic congestion. Lung transplantation is recommended only for patients in whom severe symptoms occur despite intensive medical therapy.

Venous Thromboembolic Disease

Venous thromboembolism (VTE) encompasses both deep vein thrombosis (DVT) and pulmonary embolism (PE). Among the adult United States population, the overall combined annual incidence is as high as 1 new case per 1000 persons. The incidence of VTE is higher in men than it is in women and higher in African Americans and whites than it is in Asians and Hispanics. Over 150 years ago, Dr. Rudolf Virchow recognized three predisposing factors: (1) endothelial damage, (2) venous stasis, and (3) hypercoagulation (Virchow's triad). Endothelial damage is common with surgery or trauma, venous stasis is common with prolonged bed rest or immobilization (leg cast), and hypercoagulation is common with cancer. Trousseau's syndrome consists of migratory thrombophlebitis with noninfectious vegetations on the heart valves (marantic endocarditis) typically in the setting of mucin-secreting adenocarcinoma. Dr. Trousseau, a pathologist, diagnosed his own pancreatic carcinoma on the basis of the association that now bears his name. Hypercoagulable states include hereditary diseases such as deficiencies in antithrombin III, protein C, or protein S; mutation in factor V gene (factor V Leiden) or factor II gene (prothrombin G20210A); as well as hyperhomocysteinemia. However, a thorough search for identifiable risk factors will come up negative in 25% to 50% of patients with VTE.

DEEP VEIN THROMBOSIS

Most DVT starts in the calf veins. Without treatment, 15% to 30% of these clots propagate to the proximal calf veins. The risk of a subsequent PE is much higher with proximal DVT than those confined to the distal calf vessels (40% to 50% versus 5% to 10%, respectively). Involvement of the upper extremities is much less common, but subclavian and/or axillary vein thrombosis also can lead to PE in as many as 30% of affected individuals. The same risk factors that cause lower-extremity DVT also cause upper-extremity DVT. In addition, other specific causes of upper-extremity DVT include traumatic damage of the vessel intima from heavy exertion such as rowing, wrestling, or weight lifting (Paget-Schroetter syndrome), from extrinsic compression at the level of thoracic inlet (thoracic outlet obstruction), or from insertion of central venous catheters or pacemakers. Pain and/or swelling are the major complaints from patients with DVT; however, a large number of patients with DVT are asymptomatic, particularly if the DVT is restricted to the calf. Patients with upper-extremity DVT can develop the superior vena caval syndrome of facial swelling, blurred vision, and dyspnea. Thoracic outlet obstruction can compress the brachial plexus leading to unilateral arm pain associated with hand weakness. Physical examination frequently reveals tenderness, erythema, warmth, and swelling below the site of thrombosis. Pain with dorsiflexion of the foot (Homan's sign) may be present, but the low sensitivity and the low specificity limit its usefulness in the diagnosis of lower-extremity DVT. A palpable tender cord, dilated superficial veins, and low-grade fever occur in some patients. Upper-extremity DVT can cause brachial plexus tenderness in the supraclavicular fossa and atrophic hand muscles. For patients with probable thoracic outlet obstruction, several provocative tests should be performed. Adson's test is positive if the radial pulses weaken during inspiration and during extension of the arm of the affected side while rotating the head to the same side. Wright's test is positive if the radial pulses become weaker and painful symptoms are reproduced while abducting the shoulder of the affected side with the humerus externally rotated.

The laboratory diagnosis of DVT includes measurement of D-dimers, which are fibrin degradation products. D-dimer elevation is a highly sensitive indicator of DVT that can be performed rapidly in the emergency department. In a patient in whom the index of probability is low, a negative D-dimer test effectively excludes the diagnosis of DVT. However, the test is not specific and can be elevated in many other conditions frequently encountered in hospitalized patients (e.g., inflammation, recent surgery, malignancy). Duplex ultrasonography can be used to demonstrate the presence of a blood clot and/or noncompressibility of the affected veins proximal to the site of occlusion. Duplex ultrasonography has greater sensitivity in detecting proximal DVT (90% to 100%) than distal DVT (40% to 90%) of the lower extremities. With upper-extremity DVT, acoustic shadowing of the clavicle may obscure detection of thrombosis in subclavian vein segments. MR angiography is particularly helpful in making the diagnosis of upper extremity DVT and pelvic vein thrombosis. Contrast venography is the conventional gold standard test, but it is invasive and technically difficult in patients with edematous extremities. Therefore, invasive venography should be reserved for patients in whom the clinical suggestion is high, despite negative or inconclusive results from noninvasive imaging.

Patients with proximal lower-extremity DVT and those with upper-extremity DVT should be treated initially with intravenous unfractionated heparin (UFH) or subcutaneous fixed-dose low–molecular-weight heparin (LMWH) to prevent thrombus propagation and to maintain the patency of venous collaterals. Intravenous UFH should be given as a bolus, followed by continuous infusion to maintain an activated partial thromboplastin time of at least 1.5 times the control value. LMWH has a longer half-life than UFH and can be given once or twice daily with similar efficacy. After initiation of either form of heparin, oral anticoagulation with warfarin should be initiated and titrated until the international normalized ratio (INR) reaches a value between 2 and 3. When DVT is confined to the calf, the risk of PE is low and the risk-to-benefit ratio of anticoagulation remains controversial.

When upper-extremity DVT occurs in young patients who are otherwise healthy, two invasive approaches to thrombus removal should be considered: (1) infusion of a fibrinolytic drug through a catheter inserted directly into the affected vein, or (2) mechanical fragmentation of the thrombus via catheter-based technology. The purpose of these invasive procedures is to prevent or minimize the post-thrombotic syndrome, which includes chronic arm pain, swelling, hyperpigmentation, and ulceration from residual venous obstruction.

Catheter-based placement of a filter in the inferior vena cava should be considered for patients with proximal DVT who either have an absolute contraindication to anticoagulation or develop recurrent PE despite an adequate trial of anticoagulation. Vena cava filters are effective in reducing the incidence of PE, but they increase the risk of recurrent DVT. Some proximal or distal migration of the filter occurs in up to 50% of cases; however, clinically evident filter embolization is limited to case reports.

PULMONARY EMBOLISM

PE occurs when a thrombus dislodges from the deep veins of the upper or lower extremities. Pulmonary vascular resistance and pulmonary arterial pressure increase from two mechanisms: (1) anatomic reduction in cross-sectional area of the pulmonary vascular bed, and (2) functional hypoxia-induced pulmonary vasoconstriction. The pressure overload on the right ventricle can lead to dilation, hypokinesis, and tricuspid regurgitation. When severe, elevated right ventricular end-diastolic pressure can compress the right coronary artery, causing subendocardial ischemia. In acute PE, areas of lung tissue are ventilated but under perfused. This V/Q mismatch and the resultant redistribution of pulmonary blood flow from obstructed pulmonary artery to other lung regions with lower V/Q ratios cause arterial hypoxemia. In patients with a patent foramen ovale, hypoxemia worsens when the sudden elevation in right atrial pressure causes right-to-left shunting across the foramen.

The classic symptoms of acute PE are the sudden onset of dyspnea and pleuritic chest pain. Additional symptoms include anginal chest pain from right ventricular ischemia, hemoptysis from pulmonary infarction, and syncope or pre-syncope from massive PE with acute right ventricular failure (cor pulmonale). The most common physical findings are tachypnea and tachycardia. Additional physical findings include a right ventricular lift, inspiratory crackles, a loud pulmonary component of the second sound, expiratory wheezing, and a pleural rub. Symptoms and signs of proximal DVT are present in 10% to 20% of patients. Arterial blood gas analysis often reveals hypoxemia, respiratory alkalosis, and a high alveolar–to–arterial oxygen tension gradient. However, normal arterial blood gases values do not exclude the diagnosis. The most common finding with ECG analysis is sinus tachycardia. Atrial fibrillation, premature

atrial contraction, and supraventricular tachycardia are less common. Other ECG changes suggest acute right ventricular strain. These include the S1-Q3-T3 pattern, a new right bundle branch block or right-axis deviation, and P-wave pulmonale. However, these findings are present in only 30% of patients with even massive PE. Common but nonspecific abnormalities with chest radiographic studies include atelectasis, pleural effusion, and pulmonary infiltrates. Less common but more specific radiographic findings include Hampton's hump (i.e., wedge-shaped infiltrate in the peripheral lung field), which is indicative of pulmonary infarction and Westermark's sign (decreased vascularity). The plasma D-dimer test is elevated in most patients with PE as a result of activation of the endogenous fibrinolytic system, which is not sufficient to dissolve the clot. Commercially available D-dimer assays have a high sensitivity and negative predictive value but low specificity. Therefore, a normal D-dimer test effectively excludes the diagnosis of PE in patients in whom the clinical suggestion is low. On the other hand, elevated venous blood levels of cardiac troponin I and troponin T and other markers of myocardial injury indicate right ventricular dysfunction and a poor prognosis.

In patients with suggested PE, a completely normal V/Q scan effectively excludes the diagnosis without further testing. However, less than 10% of V/Q scans are interpreted as definitively normal. In patients in whom a moderate or high level of clinical probability of PE exists, a high-probability V/Q scan has a diagnostic accuracy of 90% to 100%; however, a low or intermediate probability scan is no more helpful than a coin flip. More recently, spiral CT angiography has become the imaging modality of choice in patients with acute PE because of its excellent visualization of the pulmonary artery (Fig. 13–5). The resolution of 1 mm or less rivals that of conventional invasive angiography. The speed of the newer generation scanners allows acquisition of all images within a single breath hold, avoiding respiratory motion artifacts. According to a recent meta-analysis, the overall negative predictive value of CT angiography exceeds 99%. A negative CT excludes the diagnosis of PE and eliminates the need for further diagnostic testing. The CT

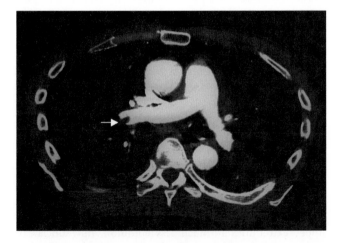

Figure 13–5 Spiral chest CT angiogram shows a large thrombus in the right main pulmonary artery *(arrow)*. (Image provided by Michael Landay, MD, Department of Radiology, University of Texas Southwestern Medical Center, Dallas, Texas.)

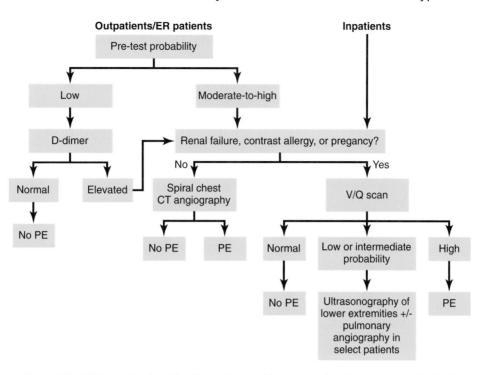

Figure 13–6 Diagnostic algorithm for patients with suggested pulmonary embolism (PE).

scan also permits detection of other pathologic conditions involving the lung parenchyma, pleura, and mediastinal structures. Such pathologic findings may mimic PE and constitute alternative causes of chest pain and dyspnea. CT angiography is not yet available at all centers. The requirement for intravenous injection of iodinated contrast material restricts applicability to nonpregnant patients and to those without a history of kidney disease or an allergic reaction to contrast dye. Figure 13–6 presents an algorithm for the work-up of PE based on current evidence. Echocardiography is not helpful in making or excluding the diagnosis, but it is helpful in determining right ventricular size and function, which is frequently abnormal in patients with hemodynamically significant PE. Invasive pulmonary angiography should be reserved for patients in whom noninvasive testing is inconclusive.

Treatment of acute PE includes immediate anticoagulation with intravenous UFH. Thrombolytic therapy with recombinant tissue plasminogen activator (rt-PA) is reserved for patients with hypotension and severe hypoxemia from massive PE. Patients with right ventricular dysfunction also should be treated with rt-PA and intravenous heparin because of greater improvement in right ventricular function than treatment with heparin alone. After initiation of heparin, warfarin should be administered. The heparin infusion needs to be continued for at least the first 5 days of warfarin therapy. Warfarin's antithrombotic action depends on a substantial reduction in the circulating blood level of factor II, which has a long half-life of more than 48 hours. After 5 days (at least two half-lives), the heparin infusion can be discontinued once the warfarin dose is adjusted to maintain a therapeutic INR of 2 to 3.

The time necessary to continue anticoagulation after an acute PE or DVT episode depends on the presence or absence of reversible risk factors for recurrent VTE. Patients with a history of trauma or surgery generally have a low rate of recurrent VTE; therefore, warfarin can be discontinued after 3 to 6 months of administration. Patients with cancer and VTE should be treated continuously with long-term subcutaneous fixed-dose LMWH because of its greater efficacy than warfarin in preventing recurrent thromboembolism in this setting. Patients with idiopathic VTE are at higher risk for recurrent episodes if anticoagulation is discontinued 1 or more years after treatment. Therefore, this patient group should be treated with warfarin indefinitely unless contraindicated. However, in patients with idiopathic VTE who are at high risk of bleeding, duration of anticoagulation may be shortened to 3 to 6 months.

VENOUS THROMBOEMBOLISM PROPHYLAXIS

Patients who are at high risk for VTE should receive prophylaxis with subcutaneous UFH or LMWH. Patients at high risk include those who are hospitalized with acute medical illness—particularly congestive heart failure, acute respiratory illness, acute inflammatory diseases—and those who are expected to be immobilized for 3 days or longer. In particular, elective or urgent or emergent surgery is an important indication for VTE prophylaxis. Subcutaneous UFH is equally effective to LMWH in preventing symptomatic DVT in patients undergoing general surgery, gynecologic surgery, or neurosurgery. However, LMWH has several advantages over UFH, including ease of administration (once a day versus three times a day), lower incidence of heparin-induced thrombocytopenia, and lower risk of osteoporosis. Hip surgery or total knee replacement is an indication for LMWH rather than UFH because of its superior efficacy in preventing DVT. Mechanical prophylaxis with intermittent pneumatic compression provides additional protection from VTE and should be administered in all surgical patients whenever possible.

Many newer anticoagulants, such as inhibitor of factor X (e.g., fondaparinux, idraparinux) and oral thrombin inhibitor ximelagatran, have been introduced for clinical use in many countries. The role of these agents in the prevention and treatment of VTE is being investigated in large clinical trials.

Arterial Hypertension

Affecting one quarter of the adult population (60 million in the United States and 1 billion people worldwide), arterial hypertension is the leading cause of death in the world, the most common cause for an outpatient visit to a physician, and the most easily recognized treatable risk factor for stroke, myocardial infarction, heart failure, peripheral vascular disease, aortic dissection, atrial fibrillation, and end-stage kidney disease. Despite this knowledge and unequivocal scientific proof that treating hypertension with medication dramatically reduces its attendant morbidity and mortality, hypertension remains untreated or undertreated in the majority of affected individuals in all countries, including those with the most advanced systems of medical care (Fig. 13–7). Thus, hypertension remains one of the world's great public health problems. The asymptomatic nature of the condition impedes early detection, which requires regular BP measurement. Because most cases of hypertension cannot be cured, BP control requires life-long treatment with prescription medications, which are costly and may cause more symptoms than the underlying disease

process. Effective hypertension management requires continuity of care by a regular and knowledgeable medical provider, as well as sustained active participation by an educated patient. This section reviews the most important principles in the early detection and effective treatment of hypertension.

INITIAL EVALUATION FOR HYPERTENSION

The initial evaluation for hypertension needs to accomplish three goals: (1) staging of BP, (2) assessing the patient's overall cardiovascular risk, and (3) detecting clues of secondary hypertension. The initial clinical data needed to accomplish these goals are obtained through a thorough history and physical examination, routine blood tests, a spot (preferably first morning) urine specimen, and a resting 12-lead ECG. In some patients, ambulatory BP monitoring and an echocardiogram provide helpful additional data about the time-integral burden of BP on the cardiovascular system.

GOAL 1: ACCURATE ASSESSMENT OF BLOOD PRESSURE

Across populations, the risks of heart disease and stroke increase continuously and logarithmically with increasing levels of systolic and diastolic BPs at or above 115/75 mm Hg (Fig. 13–8). Thus, the dichotomous separation of *normal* from *high* BP is artificial. BP is currently staged as normal, prehypertension, or hypertension based on the average of two or more readings taken at two or more office visits. When a patient's average systolic and diastolic pressures fall into different stages, the higher stage applies (Table 13–4).

Prehypertension is a newly added designation of BPs in the 120 to 139 mm Hg systolic, 80 to 89 mm Hg diastolic ranges. Prehypertensive individuals are twice as likely to progress to hypertension as are those with lower values.

BP normally varies dramatically throughout a 24-hour period. To minimize variability in readings, BP should be measured at least twice after 5 minutes of rest with the

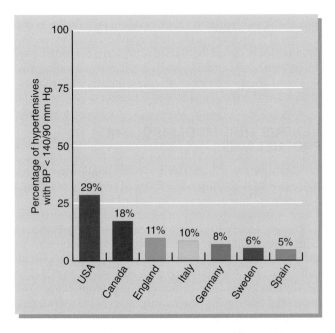

Figure 13–7 Hypertension control rates in North America and Europe. (Wolf-Maier K, Cooper RS, Kramer H, et al: Hypertension treatment and control in five European countries, Canada, and the United States. Hypertension 43:10–17, 2004.)

Table 13–4	**Staging of Office Blood Pressure***	
Blood Pressure Stage	**Systolic Blood Pressure (mm Hg)**	**Diastolic Blood Pressure (mm Hg)**
Normal	<120	<80
Prehypertension	120–139	80–89
Stage 1 hypertension	140–159	90–99
Stage 2 hypertension	≥160	≥100

*Calculation of seated blood pressure is based on the mean of two or more readings on two separate office visits. From Chobanian A, et al: The Seventh Report of the Joint National Committee on the Prevention, Evaluation, and Treatment of High Blood Pressure: The JNC 7 Report. JAMA 289:2560–2572, 2003.

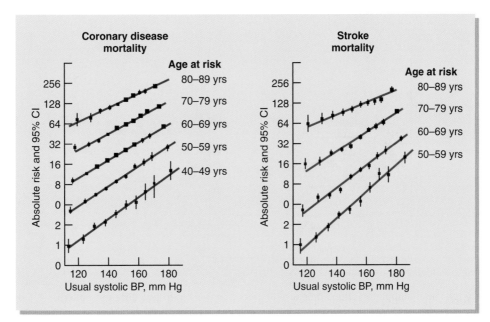

Figure 13–8 Absolute risk of coronary artery disease and stroke mortality by usual systolic blood pressure (BP) levels. (Prospective studies collaboration age-specific relevance of usual BP to vascular mortality: A meta-analysis of individual data for one million adults in 61 prospective studies. Lancet 360:1903–1913, 2002.)

patient seated, the back supported, and the arm bare and at heart level. The most common mistake in measuring BP is using a standard-issue cuff that is too small for a large arm, producing spuriously elevated readings. Most overweight adults will require a large adult cuff. Tobacco and caffeine should be avoided for at least 30 minutes. To avoid underestimation of systolic pressure in older adults who may have an *auscultatory gap* as a result of arteriosclerosis, radial artery palpation should be performed to estimate systolic pressure; then the cuff should be inflated to a value 20 mm Hg higher than the level that obliterates the radial pulse and deflated at a rate of 3 to 5 mm Hg per second. BP should be measured in both arms and after 5 minutes of standing, the latter to exclude a significant postural fall in BP, particularly in older persons and in those with diabetes or other conditions (e.g., Parkinson's disease) that predispose the patient to autonomic insufficiency.

Because of the anxiety of going to the physician, BPs often are higher in the physician's office than when measured at home or during normal daily life outside the home. Self-monitoring of BP outside of the physician's office actively engages a patient in his or her own health care and provides a better estimate of a person's usual BP for medical decision making. Many **electronic home monitors** are available, but only a handful of models have been rigorously validated against mercury sphygmomanometry and can be recommended.

Ambulatory monitoring provides automated measurements of BP over a 24-hour period while patients are engaged in their usual activities, including sleep (Fig. 13–9). With ambulatory monitoring, current recommendations for *upper limits of normal* are a mean daytime BP of 135/85 mm Hg, mean nighttime BP of 120/70 mm Hg, and a mean 24-hour BP of 130/80 mm Hg. However, an *optimal* mean daytime ambulatory BP is less than 130/80 mm Hg. To

avoid undertreating hypertension, these lower treatment thresholds must be used when incorporating ambulatory monitoring in medical decision making. With self-monitoring of BP at home, an average value of 130/80 mm Hg should be considered the upper limit of normal; BP should be lower in the patient's own home than with daily activities outside the home.

Up to one third of patients with elevated office BPs have normal home or ambulatory BPs. If the 24-hour BP profile is completely normal and no target organ damage has occurred despite consistently elevated office readings, then the patient has *office only,* or *white coat,* hypertension, presumably the result of a transient adrenergic response to the measurement of BP in the physician's office (see Fig. 13–9). In other patients, office readings underestimate ambulatory BPs, presumably because of sympathetic overactivity in daily life owing to job or home stress, tobacco abuse, or other adrenergic stimulation that dissipates when coming to the office (Fig. 13–10). Such documentation prevents underdiagnosing and undertreating this *masked hypertension,* which is present in up to 10% of patients and increases cardiovascular risk.

GOAL 2: CARDIOVASCULAR RISK STRATIFICATION

The great majority of patients with BPs in the prehypertensive or hypertensive range will have one or more additional modifiable risk factors for atherosclerosis (e.g., hypercholesterolemia, cigarette smoking, diabetes). Many patients already have evidence of target organ involvement at the time of the initial office evaluation for newly diagnosed hypertension. In addition to hypertensive stage, the other two components to cardiovascular risk are (1) co-morbidity, and (2) target organ damage (Table 13–5).

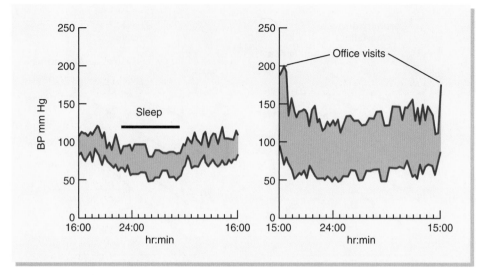

Figure 13–9 Twenty-four hour ambulatory blood pressure (BP) monitor tracings in two different patients. *A,* Optimal blood pressure (BP) in a healthy 37-year-old woman. The normal variability in BP, the nocturnal dip in BP during sleep, and the sharp increase in BP on awakening are noted. *B,* Pronounced white-coat effect in an 80-year-old woman referred for evaluation of medically refractory hypertension. Documentation of the white-coat effect prevented overtreatment of the patient's isolated systolic hypertension. (*A,* Courtesy of Meryem Tuncel, MD, Hypertension Division, Department of Internal Medicine, University of Texas Southwestern Medical Center, Dallas, Texas. *B,* Tracing provided by Wanpen Vongpatanasin, MD, Hypertension Division, Department of Internal Medicine, University of Texas Southwestern Medical Center, Dallas, Texas.)

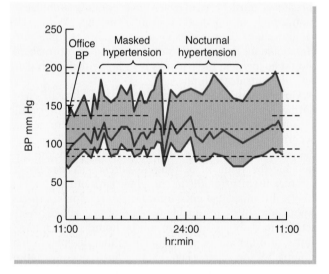

Figure 13–10 Twenty-four hour ambulatory blood pressure (BP) monitor tracing shows both masked hypertension and nocturnal hypertension in a 55-year-old man with stage 3 chronic kidney disease. Treatment with three different antihypertensive medications in this patient produced an office BP of 125/75 mm Hg, which seems to be at goal. However, progressive hypertensive heart disease and deterioration of renal function suggested masked hypertension. Ambulatory monitoring revealed that the patient's treated BP was much higher out of the office, documenting both masked hypertension (ambulatory BP of 175/95 mm Hg and sustained nocturnal hypertension (BP of 175/90 mm Hg). Additional medication was added. (Tracing provided by Ronald G. Victor, MD, Hypertension Division, Department of Internal Medicine, University of Texas Southwestern Medical Center, Dallas, Texas.)

The current United States treatment guidelines recommend a usual BP of 140/90 mm Hg as the threshold for initiating a lifetime of antihypertensive medication in most patients and a lower threshold of 130/80 mm Hg for high-risk patients, including those with diabetes or chronic kidney disease. Based on evidence that has come to light after the publication of the set of practice guidelines in 2003, the definition of *high-risk* patients has been expanded to include those with any of the following four conditions: (1) clinically evident cardiovascular disease (coronary disease, stroke), (2) chronic kidney disease (estimated glomerular filtration rate [GFR] <60 m/min/1.73 m^2 or estimated urinary albumin excretion >300 mg/24 hr), (3) diabetes mellitus, or (4) LVH confirmed by ECG or echocardiography.

GOAL 3: IDENTIFICATION OF SECONDARY (IDENTIFIABLE) CAUSES OF HYPERTENSION

A thorough search for secondary causes is not cost effective in most patients with hypertension, but it becomes critically important in two circumstances: (1) when a compelling cause is found on the initial evaluation, or (2) when the hypertensive process is so severe that it either is refractory to intensive multiple-drug therapy or requires hospitalization. Table 13–6 summarizes the major causes of secondary hypertension that should be suggested on the basis of a good history, physical, and routine laboratory tests.

Renal Parenchymal Hypertension

Chronic kidney disease is the most common cause of secondary hypertension. Hypertension is present in more than 85% of patients with chronic kidney disease and is a major factor causing their increased cardiovascular morbidity and

Table 13–5 Components of Cardiovascular Risk Stratification in Patients with Hypertension or Prehypertension

Indications for BP <130/80 mmHg	Other CVD Risk Factors
Diabetes mellitus	Age
Chronic kidney disease	Older than 55 years of age for men
GFR <60 mL/min/1.73 m²	Older than 65 years of age for women
Urine albumin: Cr ≧30 mg/g	Family history of premature CVD
Prior cardiovascular event	Men under 55 years of age
Angina pectoris	Women under 65 years of age
Myocardial infarction	Tobacco use
Coronary revascularization	LDL cholesterol >130 mg/dL
Congestive heart failure	Physical inactivity
Stroke or TIA	Metabolic syndrome
Left ventricular hypertrophy	Waist circumference
	Men: >40 inches
	Women: >35 inches
	Serum triglycerides ≧150 mg/dL
	HDL cholesterol
	Men: <40 mg/dL
	Women: <50 mg/dL
	Fasting glucose ≧110 mg/dL
	Blood pressure ≧130/85 mmHg

BP = blood pressure; CVD = cardiovascular disease; GFR = glomerular filtration rate; Cr = serum creatinine; TIA = transient ischemic attack; LDL = low-density lipoprotein; HDL = high-density lipoprotein.
Executive Summary of the Third Report of the National Cholesterol Education Program (NCEP) Expert Panel on Detection, Evaluation, and Treatment of High Cholesterol in Adults (Adult Treatment Panel III). JAMA 285:2486–2497, 2001.

mortality. The mechanisms causing the hypertension include an expanded plasma volume and peripheral vasoconstriction, with the latter caused by both activation of vasoconstrictor pathways (renin-angiotensin and sympathetic nervous systems) and inhibition of vasodilator pathways (nitric oxide). Renal insufficiency should be considered when proteinuria is found by dipstick or when the serum creatinine level is greater than 1.2 mg/dL in women with hypertension or greater than 1.4 mg/dL in men with hypertension.

Renovascular Hypertension

Unilateral or bilateral renal artery stenosis is present in less than 2% of patients with hypertension in a general medical practice but up to 30% in patients with medically refractory hypertension. The main causes of renal artery stenosis are atherosclerosis (85% of patients), typically in older adults with other clinical manifestations of systemic atherosclerosis and fibromuscular dysplasia (15% of patients), typically in women between the ages of 15 and 50 years. Unilateral renal artery stenosis leads to underperfusion of the juxtaglomerular cells, thereby producing renin-dependent hypertension even though the contralateral kidney is able to maintain normal blood volume. In contrast, bilateral renal artery stenosis (or unilateral stenosis with a solitary kidney) constitutes a potentially reversible cause of progressive renal failure and volume-dependent hypertension. The following clinical clues increase the suggestion of renovascular hypertension: any hospitalization for urgent or emergent hypertension; recurrent *flash* pulmonary edema; recent worsening of long-standing, previously well-controlled hypertension; severe hypertension in a young adult or in an adult after 50 years of age; precipitously and progressively worsening of renal function in response to angiotensin-converting enzyme (ACE) inhibition or angiotensin II-receptor blockade (ARB); unilateral small kidney by any radiographic study; extensive peripheral arteriosclerosis; or a flank bruit. The diagnosis is confirmed by noninvasive testing with MR or spiral computed tomographic (CT) angiography (Fig. 13–11). Renal artery angioplasty often cures fibromuscular dysplasia. Atherosclerotic renal artery stenosis should be treated with intensive medical management of atherosclerotic risk factors (hypertension, lipids, smoking cessation). Revascularization should be considered for the following indications: (1) medically refractory hypertension, (2) progressive renal failure on medical therapy, and (3) bilateral renal artery stenosis or stenosis of a solitary functioning kidney.

Primary Aldosteronism

The most common causes of primary aldosteronism are (1) a unilateral aldosterone-producing adenoma and (2) bilateral adrenal hyperplasia. Because aldosterone is the principal ligand for the mineralocorticoid receptor in the distal nephron, excessive aldosterone production causes excessive renal Na⁻-K⁻ exchange, often resulting in hypokalemia. The diagnosis should always be suggested when hypertension is accompanied by either unprovoked hypokalemia (serum K⁺

Table 13–6 Guide to Evaluation of Secondary Hypertension

Probable Diagnosis	Clinical Clues	Diagnostic Testing
Renal parenchymal hypertension	Estimated GFR <60 mL/min/1.73 m^2 Urine albumin:creatinine ≧30 mg/g	Renal ultrasound
Renovascular disease	New elevation in serum creatinine, significant elevation in serum creatinine with initiation of ACEI or ARBs, refractory hypertension, flash pulmonary edema, abdominal bruit	MR or CT angiography, invasive angiogram
Coarctation of the aorta	Arm pulses >leg pulses, arm BP >leg BP, chest bruits, rib notching on chest radiograph	MR imaging, aortogram
Primary aldosteronism	Hypokalemia, refractory hypertension	Plasma renin and aldosterone, 24-hr urine potassium, 24-hr urine aldosterone and potassium after-salt loading, adrenal CT scan, adrenal vein sampling
Cushing's syndrome	Truncal obesity, wide and blanching purple striae, muscle weakness	Plasma cortisol, urine cortisol after dexamethasone, adrenal CT scan
Pheochromocytoma	Spells of paroxysmal hypertension, palpitations, perspiration, pallor, pain in the head Diabetes	Plasma metanephrine and normetanephrine, 24-hr urine catechols, adrenal CT scan
Obstructive sleep apnea	Loud snoring, daytime somnolence, obesity, large neck	Sleep study

ACEI = angiotensin-converting enzyme inhibitor; ARBs = angiotensin-receptor blockers; BP = blood pressure; CT = computed tomography; GFR = glomerular filtration rate; MR = magnetic resonance.
Modified from Kaplan NM: Clinical Hypertension, 8th ed. Philadelphia, Williams & Wilkins, 2002.

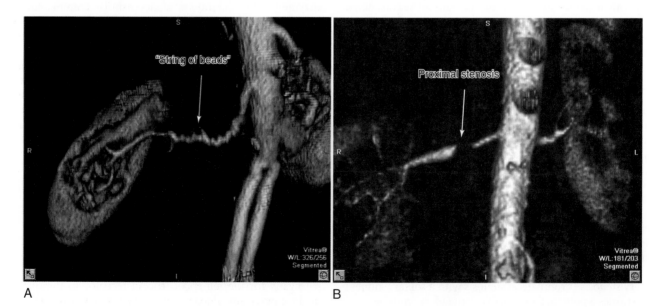

A   B

Figure 13–11 Computed tomography (CT) angiogram with three-dimensional reconstruction. *A,* Classic *string-of-beads* lesion of fibromuscular dysplasia. *B,* Severe proximal atherosclerotic stenosis of the right renal artery. (Images courtesy of Bart Domatch, MD, Radiology Department, University of Texas Southwestern Medical Center, Dallas, Texas.)

<3.5 mmol/L in the absence of diuretic therapy) or a tendency to develop excessive hypokalemia during diuretic therapy (serum K^+ <3.0 mmol/L). However, more than one third of patients do not have hypokalemia on initial presentation, and the diagnosis should be considered in any patient with refractory hypertension. The diagnosis is confirmed by the demonstration of nonsuppressible hyperaldosteronism during salt loading, followed by adrenal vein sampling to distinguish between a unilateral adenoma and bilateral hyperplasia. Laparoscopic adrenalectomy is the treatment of choice for unilateral aldosterone-producing adenoma, whereas pharmacologic mineralocorticoid-receptor blockade with eplerenone is the treatment for bilateral adrenal hyperplasia.

Mendelian Forms of Hypertension

Nine very rare forms of severe early-onset hypertension are inherited as Mendelian traits. In each case, the hypertension is mineralocorticoid induced and involves excessive activation of the epithelial sodium channel *(ENaC),* the final common pathway for reabsorption of sodium from the distal nephron. The resultant salt-dependent hypertension can be caused by both gain-of-function mutations of *ENaC* (Liddle's syndrome) or the mineralocorticoid receptor (i.e., a rare form of pregnancy-induced hypertension) and by increased production or decreased clearance of mineralocorticoids. These include aldosterone (glucocorticoid-remediable aldosteronism), deoxycorticosterone (17-hydroxylase deficiency), and cortisol (syndrome of apparent mineralocorticoid excess).

Pheochromocytoma

Pheochromocytomas are rare catecholamine-producing tumors of the adrenal (or sometimes extra-adrenal) chromaffin cells. The diagnosis should be suggested when hypertension is accompanied by paroxysms of headaches, palpitations, pallor, or diaphoresis. In some patients, pheochromocytoma is misdiagnosed as panic disorder. A family history of early-onset hypertension may suggest pheochromocytoma as part of the multiple endocrine neoplasia syndromes. If the diagnosis is missed, then outpouring of catecholamines from the tumor can cause an unsuspected hypertensive crisis during unrelated radiologic or surgical procedures; the peri-operative mortality rate exceeds 80% in such patients.

Laboratory confirmation of pheochromocytoma is made by demonstrating elevated levels of serum or urine catecholamines or their metabolites (vanillylmandelic acid or metanephrines). These are typically large tumors that can usually be localized by CT or MR imaging, although nuclear scanning with specific isotopes that localize to chromaffin tissue is occasionally needed to identify smaller tumors.

Treatment of these tumors is surgical resection. Patients must receive adequate α-blockade (phentolamine), β-blockade, and volume expansion before surgery to prevent the hemodynamic swings that can occur during manual manipulation of the tumor peri-operatively. For unresectable tumors, chronic therapy with the α-adrenergic blocker phenoxybenzamine is usually effective.

The differential diagnosis includes other causes of neurogenic hypertension such as sympathomimetic agents (cocaine, methamphetamine), baroreflex failure, and obstructive sleep apnea. A history of surgery and radiation therapy for head-and-neck tumors suggests the possibility of baroreceptor damage. Loud snoring, obesity, and somnolence suggest obstructive sleep apnea. Weight loss, continuous positive airway pressure, and corrective surgery improve BP control in some patients with sleep apnea.

Other causes of secondary hypertension include hypothyroidism, hyperthyroidism coarctation of the aorta, and immunosuppressive drugs, especially cyclosporine and tacrolimus.

TREATMENT OF HYPERTENSION

Prescription medication is the cornerstone of treating hypertension. Lifestyle modification should be used as an adjunct but not as an alternative to life-saving BP medication. Most dietary sodium comes from processed foods, and daily salt consumption can be reduced from 10 to 6 g by teaching patients to read food labels (6 g of NaCl = 2.4 g of Na^{-+} = 100 mmol of Na$^+$. The **Dietary Approaches to Stop Hypertension** (DASH), which is rich in fresh fruits and vegetables (for high potassium content) and low-fat dairy products, has been shown to lower BP in feeding trials. Other lifestyle modifications that can lower BP include weight loss in overweight patients with hypertension, regular aerobic exercise, smoking cessation, and moderation in alcohol intake.

Currently, 92 prescription medications and many fixed-dose combinations are marketed for the treatment of hypertension in the United States (see Table 13–4).

WHICH DRUGS FOR WHICH PATIENTS?
Patients with Uncomplicated Hypertension

Choosing the best drugs to treat hypertension in a given patient comes down to two considerations: (1) effectively lowering BP and preventing hypertensive complications with minimal side effects and cost, and (2) concomitant treatment of co-morbid cardiovascular diseases (e.g., angina, heart failure). The seventh report of the United States Joint National Committee (JNC 7) recommends a thiazide-type diuretic as cost-effective first-line therapy for most patients with hypertension. It also recommends initiating therapy with two drugs—one being a thiazide—for stage 2 hypertension. In contrast, the European Society of Hypertension makes no specific drug class recommendation, arguing that the most effective drugs are those that the patient will tolerate and take. The British Hypertension Society advocates a treatment strategy that is based on the patient's age and ethnicity. It recommends initiating therapy with an ACE inhibitor or ARB or a β-blocker (*A or B* drug) for young white patients (under 55 years of age) who often have high-renin hypertension but a CCB or diuretic (*C or D* drug) for older and black patients who often have low-renin hypertension (Tables 13–7 and 13–8).

A growing body of evidence from clinical trials emphasizes the overriding importance of lowering BP with combinations of drugs rather than belaboring the choice of a single, best agent to begin therapy. Primary hypertension is multifactorial, and typically several medications (usually

Table 13–7   Oral Antihypertensive Agents

Drug	Dose Range, Total mg/day (doses per day)	Drug	Dose Range, Total mg/day (doses per day)
Diuretics		**Angiotensin-Converting Enzyme Inhibitors**	
Thiazide Diuretics		Benazepril	10–80 (1–2)
		Captopril	25–150 (2)
HCTZ	6.25–50 (1)	Enalapril	2.5–40 (2)
Chlorthalidone	6.25–50 (1)	Fosinopril	10–80 (1–2)
Indapamide	1.25–5 (1)	Lisinopril	5–80 (1–2)
Metolazone	2.5–5 (1)	Moexipril	7.5–30 (1)
		Perindopril	4–16 (1)
Loop Diuretics		Quinapril	5–80 (1–2)
		Ramipril	2.5–20 (1)
Furosemide	20–160 (2)	Trandolapril	1–8 (1)
Torsemide	2.5–20 (1–2)		
Bumetanide	0.5–2 (2)	**Angiotensin-Receptor Blockers**	
Ethacrynic acid	25–100 (2)	Candesartan	8–32 (1)
		Eprosartan	400–800 (1–2)
Potassium-sparing		Irbesartan	150–300 (1)
		Losartan	25–100 (2)
Amiloride	5–20 (1)	Olmesartin	5–40 (1)
Triamterene	25–100 (1)	Telmisartan	20–80 (1)
Spironolactone	12.5–400 (1–2)	Valsartan	80–320 (1–2)
Eplerenone	25–100 (1–2)		
		α-Blockers	
β-Blockers		Doxazosin	1–16 (1)
Acebutolol	200–800 (2)	Prazosin	1–40 (2–3)
Atenolol	25–100 (1)	Terazosin	1–20 (1)
Betaxolol	5–20 (1)	Phenoxybenzamine	20–120 (2) for pheochromocytoma
Bisoprolol	2.5–20 (1)		
Carteolol	2.5–10 (1)	**Central Sympatholytics**	
Metoprolol	50–450 (2)	Clonidine	0.2–1.2 (2–3)
Metoprolol XL	50–200 (1–2)	Clonidine patch	0.1–0.6 (weekly)
Nadolol	20–320 (1)	Guanabenz	2–32 (2)
Penbutolol	10–80 (1)	Guanfacine	1–3 (1) (q hs)
Pindolol	10–60 (2)	Methyldopa	250–1000 (2)
Propranolol	40–180 (2)	Reserpine	0.05–0.25 (1)
Propranolol LA	60–180 (1–2)		
Timolol	20–60 (2)	**Direct Vasodilators**	
		Hydralazine	10–200 (2)
β/α-Blockers		Minoxidil	2.5–100 (1)
Labetalol	200–2400 (2)		
Carvedilol	6.25–50 (2)	**Fixed-Dose Combinations**	
		Amiloride/HCTZ	5/50 (1)
Calcium Channel Blockers		Amlodipine/benazepril	2.5–5/10–20 (1)
Dihydropyridines		Atenolol/Chlorthalidone	50–100/25 (1)
		Benazepril/HCTZ	5–20/6.25–25 (1)
Amlodipine	2.5–10 (1)	Bisoprolol/HCTZ	2.5–10/6.25 (1)
Felodipine	2.5–20 (1–2)	Candesartan/HCTZ	16–32/12.5–25 (1)
Isradipine CR	2.5–20 (2)	Enalapril/HCTZ	5–10/25 (1–2)
Nicardipine SR	30–120 (2)	Eprosartan/HCTZ	600/12.5–25 (1)
Nifedipine XL	30–120 (1)	Fosinopril/HCTZ	10–20/12.5 (1)
Nisoldipine	10–40 (1–2)	Irbesartan/HCTZ	15–30/12.5–25 (1)
		Losartan/HCTZ	50–100/12.5–25 (1)
Nondihydropyridines		Olmesartan/HCTZ	20–40/12.5 (1)
		Spironolactone/HCTZ	25/25 ($^1/_2$–1)
Diltiazem CD	120–540 (1)	Telmisartan/HCTZ	40–80/12.5–25 (1)
Verapamil HS	120–480 (1)	Trandolapril/verapamil	2–4/180–240 (1)
		Triamterene/HCTZ	37.5/25 ($^1/_2$–1)
		Valsartan/HCTZ	80–160/12.5–25 (1)

The major contraindications and side effects of these drugs are summarized in Table 13–8.

Table 13–8 Major Contraindications and Side Effects of Antihypertensive Drugs

Drug Class	Major Contraindications	Side Effects
Diuretics		
Thiazides	Gout	Insulin resistance, new onset type 2 diabetes (especially in combination with β-blockers) Hypokalemia, hyponatremia Hypertriglyceridemia Hyperuricemia, precipitation of gout Erectile dysfunction (more than other drug classes) Potentiate nondepolarizing muscle relaxants Photosensitive dermatitis
Loop diuretics	Hepatic coma	Interstitial nephritis Hypokalemia Potentiate succinylcholine Potentiate aminoglycoside ototoxicity
Potassium-sparing diuretics	Serum K >5.5 mEq/L GFR <30 mg/mL/1.73 m^2	Fatal hyperkalemia if used with salt substitutes, ACE inhibitors, ARBs, high-potassium foods, NSAIDs
β-Blockers	Heart block Asthma Depression Cocaine and/or methamphetamine abuse	Insulin resistance, new onset type 2 diabetes (especially in combination with thiazides) Heart block, acute decompensated CHF Bronchospasm Depression, nightmares, fatigue Cold extremities, claudication (β2 effect) Stevens-Johnson syndrome Agranulocytosis
ACE Inhibitors	Pregnancy Bilateral renal artery stenosis Hyperkalemia	Cough Hyperkalemia Angioedema Leukopenia Fetal toxicity Cholestatic jaundice (rare fulminant hepatic necrosis if the drug is not discontinued)
ARBs	Pregnancy Bilateral renal artery stenosis Hyperkalemia	Hyperkalemia Angioedema (very rare) Fetal toxicity
Dihydropyridine CCBs	As monotherapy in chronic kidney disease with proteinuria	Headaches Flushing Ankle edema CHF Gingival hyperplasia Esophageal reflux
Nondihydropyridine CCBs	Heart block Systolic heart failure	Bradycardia, AV block (especially with verapamil) Constipation (often severe with verapamil) Worsening of systolic function, CHF Gingival edema and/or hypertrophy Increase cyclosporine blood levels Esophageal reflux

Continued

Table 13–8 Major Contraindications and Side Effects of Antihypertensive Drugs—cont'd

Drug Class	Major Contraindications	Side Effects
α-Blockers	Monotherapy for hypertension Orthostatic hypotension Systolic heart failure Left ventricular dysfunction	Orthostatic hypotension Drug tolerance (in the absence of diuretic therapy) Ankle edema CHF First-dose effect (acute hypotension) Potentiate hypotension with PDE-5 inhibitors (e.g., sildenafil)
Central sympatholytics	Orthostatic hypotension	Depression, dry mouth, lethargy Erectile dysfunction (dose dependent) Rebound hypertension with clonidine withdrawal Coombs' positive hemolytic anemia and elevated LFTs with α-methyldopa
Direct vasodilators	Orthostatic hypotension	Reflex tachycardia Fluid retention Hirsutism, pericardial effusion with minoxidil Lupus with hydralazine

ACE = angiotensin-converting enzyme; ARBs = angiotensin-receptor blockers; AV = arteriovenous; CCBs = calcium channel blockers; CHF = congestive heart failure; GFR = glomerular fiiltration rate; LFTs= liver function tests; MI = myocardial infarction; NSAIDs = nonsteroidal anti-infllammatory drugs; PDE-5= phosphodiesterase type 5.

three or more) with different mechanisms of action (see Table 13–4) are required simultaneously to reach currently recommended BP levels (<140/90 mm Hg for most patients, <130/80 mm Hg for high-risk patients). In most patients with hypertension, low-dose combination drug therapy is the only way to control BP adequately and to minimize side effects. With many classes of antihypertensive medication, the dose-response relationship for BP is rather flat. Most of the BP lowering occurs at the lower end of the dose range. However, many of the side effects are steeply dose-dependent, becoming problematic mainly at the high end of the clinical class range. Thus, low-dose combinations achieve therapeutic synergy and minimize side effects. Fixed-dose combinations reduce pill burden and cost. Additional ways to facilitate patient adherence include: (1) titrating medical therapy based on home readings, which engages the patient's active participation; (2) teaching the patient to know his or her goal BP values, and (3) prescribing long-acting preparations with once-daily dosing.

Along with antihypertensive medication and lifestyle modification, additional cardiovascular risk reduction with low-dose aspirin (81 mg per day) and lipid-lowering medication should be strongly considered as an integral part of most antihypertensive regimens. In patients who are treated for hypertension, low-dose aspirin has been shown to reduce the risk of myocardial infarction by 36% without increasing the risk of intracerebral hemorrhage. Recent data document a sizeable cardiovascular benefit of adding 10 mg of the HMG CoA reductase inhibitor atorvastatin to antihypertensive therapy in patients over 60 years of age with moderate

hypertension and an average LDL cholesterol of only 130 mg/dL.

Hypertension in African Americans

Hypertension disproportionately affects African Americans. The explanation is unknown, but the dominant importance of environmental factors is indicated by a significant geographic variation in hypertension prevalence among African-origin and European-origin populations. Hypertension is rare in Africans living in Africa and is more prevalent in several European countries than it is in the United States. As monotherapy, an ACE inhibitor or ARB or a β-blocker generally yields a smaller decrease in BP in an African American than it does in a white person with hypertension and thus affords less protection against stroke. However, when high doses of an ACE inhibitor or ARB are used in combination with a diuretic, antihypertensive efficacy is amplified and ethnic differences seem to disappear. When used as part of an appropriate multidrug regimen, an ACE inhibitor–based treatment can achieve excellent control of hypertension in African-American patients with hypertensive nephrosclerosis, and it slows the deterioration in renal function.

Hypertensive Nephrosclerosis

Hypertension is the second most common cause of chronic kidney disease, accounting for over 25% of cases. Hypertensive nephrosclerosis is the result of persistently uncontrolled hypertension, causing chronic glomerular ischemia. Typically, proteinuria is mild (<0.5 g/24 hr). Nondiabetic chronic kidney disease is a compelling indication for ACE inhibitor–based or ARB-based antihypertensive therapy. ACE inhibitors cause greater dilation of the efferent renal arterioles, thereby minimizing intraglomerular hypertension. In contrast, arterial vasodilators such as dihydropyridine CCBs, when used without an ACE inhibitor or ARB, preferentially dilate the afferent arteriole and impair renal autoregulation. Glomerular hypertension can result if systemic BP is not sufficiently lowered. The ACE inhibitor should be withdrawn only if the rise in serum creatinine exceeds 30% of the baseline value or the serum K⁻ increases to greater than 5.6 mmol/L.

Hypertensive Patients with Diabetes

Compared with its 25% prevalence in the general adult population, hypertension is present in 75% of patients with diabetes and is a major factor contributing to excessive risk of myocardial infarction, stroke, heart failure, microvascular complications, and diabetic nephropathy progressing to end-stage renal disease. To reduce these risks, BPs should be lowered to less than 130/80 mm Hg. The cardiovascular benefits of tight BP control in patients with diabetes cannot be overemphasized because they exceed and are additive to those of tight glucose control. To achieve such stringent BP goals typically requires three to five drugs. An ACE inhibitor or ARB should be the drug of first choice for the hypertensive patient with diabetes because of mounting evidence that these agents provide special reno-protective effects. However, an ACE inhibitor or ARB alone rarely achieves the stringent BP goals in patients with diabetic nephropathy. A loop diuretic is usually needed to shrink the expanded plasma volume. A dihydropyridine CCB is usually needed for antihypertensive synergy. The dihydropyridine CCB should not be started until antihypertensive therapy has been initiated with an ACE inhibitor or ARB. A β-blocker should be added

if the patient has coronary disease, which is prevalent in diabetes or heart failure. The α,β-blocker carvedilol has a better metabolic profile than standard β-blockers.

Hypertensive Patients with Coronary Artery Disease

To lower myocardial oxygen demands in patients with coronary disease, the antihypertensive regimen should reduce BP without causing reflex tachycardia. For this reason, a β-blocker is often prescribed in conjunction with a dihydropyridine CCB. β-Blockers are indicated for patients with hypertension who have sustained a myocardial infarction and for most patients with chronic heart failure. ACE inhibitors are indicated for almost all patients with left ventricular systolic dysfunction and may be considered for patients after myocardial infarction even in the absence of ventricular dysfunction. In patients with very high cardiovascular risk profiles but without known left ventricular dysfunction, the ACE inhibitor ramipril (10 mg/day) reduces cardiovascular events, an effect that may or may not be beyond what can be explained by BP reduction alone. In patients with stable coronary artery disease, a cardioprotective effect of ACE inhibition has also been demonstrated in patients with moderate cardiovascular risk profiles but not in those with lower risk profiles.

Isolated Systolic Hypertension in Older Adults

In developed countries, systolic pressure rises progressively with age; if individuals live long enough, then almost all (>90%) develop hypertension. Diastolic pressure rises until the age of 50 years and decreases thereafter, producing a progressive rise in pulse pressure (i.e., systolic pressure minus diastolic pressure) (Fig. 13–12).

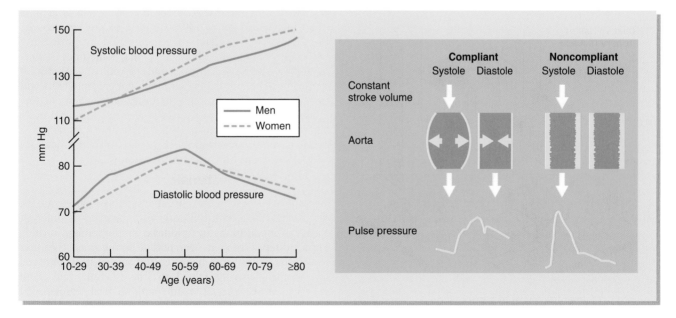

Figure 13–12 Age-dependent changes in systolic and diastolic blood pressure (BP) in the United States *(left panel).* Schematic diagram explains the relation between aortic compliance and pulse pressure *(right panel).* *(Left panel,* From Burt V, Whelton P, Rocella EJ, et al: Prevalence of hypertension in the U.S. adult population: Results from the Third National Health and Nutrition Examination Survey, 1988–1991. Hypertension 25:305–313, 1995. *Right panel,* From Dr. Stanley Franklin University of California at Irvine. Used with permission.)

Different hemodynamic faults underlie hypertension in young and old persons. Patients who develop hypertension before 50 years of age typically have *combined systolic and diastolic hypertension*: systolic pressure greater than 140 mm Hg *and* diastolic pressure greater than 90 mm Hg. The main hemodynamic fault is vasoconstriction at the level of the resistance arterioles. In contrast, the majority of patients who develop hypertension after 50 years of age have *isolated systolic hypertension*: systolic pressure greater than 140 mm Hg but diastolic pressure less than 90 mm Hg (often less than 80 mm Hg). In isolated systolic hypertension, the primary hemodynamic fault is decreased distensibility of the large conduit arteries (see Fig. 13–12). Collagen replaces elastin in the elastic lamina of the aorta, an age-dependent process that is accelerated by atherosclerosis and hypertension. The cardiovascular risk associated with isolated systolic hypertension is related to pulsatility, the repetitive pounding of the blood vessels with each cardiac cycle and a more rapid return of the arterial pulse wave from the periphery, both begetting more systolic hypertension. In the United States and Europe, the majority of uncontrolled hypertension occurs in older patients with isolated systolic hypertension. A BP of 160/60 mm Hg (pulse pressure of 100 mm Hg) carries twice the risk of fatal coronary heart disease as 140/110 mm Hg (pulse pressure of 30 mm Hg) (Fig. 13–13)!

In older persons with isolated systolic hypertension, lowering systolic pressure from higher than 160 to lower than 150 mm Hg reduces the risks of stroke, myocardial infarction, and overall cardiovascular mortality; it also reduces heart failure admissions and slows the progression of dementia. Trial data do not yet exist in older persons to determine whether the treatment of isolated elevations in systolic pressure between 140 and 160 mm Hg is beneficial; however, in the absence of such data, most authorities recommend treatment to prevent progression of systolic hypertension. No studies have specifically tested for a mortality benefit of treating systolic hypertension in patients above 80 years of age; however, post-hoc analyses strongly suggest a large reduction in strokes and heart failure admissions.

Based on data from several large randomized trials, low-dose thiazide diuretics and dihydropyridine CCBs are the drugs of choice for isolated systolic hypertension. For many older patients with hypertension, especially those with diabetes, the addition of an ACE inhibitor or ARB will be necessary to achieve recommended BP goals. To prevent the development of orthostatic hypotension, medication should be titrated to standing BP.

Blood Pressure Lowering for Secondary Prevention of Stroke

Most neurologists do not recommend BP reduction during an acute stroke. After the acute phase, BP should be lowered with a thiazide diuretic, adding an ACE inhibitor or additional drugs as needed to achieve BP goals.

Hypertensive Disorders of Women

Oral contraceptives cause a small increase in BP in most women but rarely cause a large increase into the hypertensive range. If hypertension develops, oral contraceptive therapy should be discontinued in favor of other methods of contraception. Oral estrogen replacement therapy seems to cause a small increase in BP. In contrast, transdermal estrogen (which bypasses first-pass hepatic metabolism) seems to cause a small but consistent decrease in BP.

Hypertension, the most common nonobstetric complication of pregnancy, is present in 10% of all pregnancies. Of these women, one third are caused by chronic hypertension and two thirds are due to preeclampsia, which is defined as an increase in BP to 140/90 mm Hg or greater after the twentieth week of gestation accompanied by proteinuria (>300 mg/24 hr) and pathologic edema, sometimes accompanied by seizures (eclampsia) and the multisystem HELLP syndrome of hemolysis (H), elevated liver enzymes (EL), and low platelets (LP). Although the cause remains an enigma, preeclampsia is the most common cause of maternal mortality and perinatal mortality. α-Methyldopa remains the drug of choice for chronic hypertension in pregnancy, and hydralazine (plus bed rest) for preeclampsia.

Resistant Hypertension

Defined as persistence of usual BP above 140/90 mm Hg despite treatment with full doses of three or more different classes of medications in rational combination and including a diuretic, *resistant hypertension* is the most common reason for referral to a hypertension specialist. In practice, the problem usually falls into one of four categories: (1) pseudoresistance, (2) inadequate medical regimen, (3) nonadherence or ingestion of pressor substances, or (4) secondary hypertension. Pseudoresistant hypertension is caused by *white-coat aggravation,* a white-coat effect superimposed on chronic hypertension that is well-controlled with medication outside the physician's office. The most common cause of apparent drug resistance is the absence of

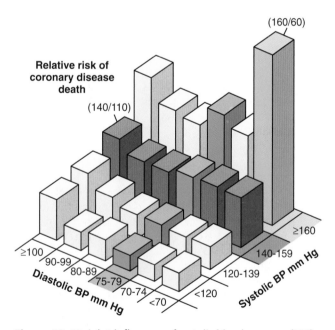

Figure 13–13 Joint influences of systolic blood pressure (SBP) and diastolic BP on coronary heart disease (CHD) risk in the Multiple Risk Factor Intervention Trial. (Neaton JD, Wentworth D: Serum cholesterol, blood pressure, cigarette smoking, and death from coronary heart disease: Overall findings and differences by age for 316,099 white men. Arch Intern Med 152:56–64, 1992.)

appropriate diuretic therapy. Significant impairment in renal function can be present with serum creatinine in the 1.2 to 1.4 mg/dL range or even lower, particularly in older patients with little muscle mass. To avoid this pitfall, calculation of GFR by equations based on serum creatinine, age, and weight and measurement of the urinary albumin-to-creatinine ratio from a spot-urine specimen should be an essential part of the routine evaluation of every patient with hypertension. Other common shortcomings of the medical regimen include reliance on monotherapy and inadequate dosing. Several common causes of resistant hypertension are related to the patient's behavior: medication nonadherence, recidivism with lifestyle modification (e.g., obesity, a high-salt diet, excessive alcohol intake), or habitual use of pressor substances such as sympathomimetics (e.g., tobacco, cocaine, methamphetamine, phenylephrine-containing cold or herbal remedies) or nonsteroidal anti-inflammatory drugs (NSAIDs), with the latter causing renal sodium retention. Once these behavioral factors have been excluded, the search should begin for secondary hypertension. The most common unrecognized factors are chronic kidney disease and primary aldosteronism.

Acute Severe Hypertension

Of all the patients in the emergency department, 25% have an elevated BP. *Hypertensive emergencies* are acute, often severe elevations in BP that are accompanied by acute or rapidly progressive target organ dysfunction such as myocardial or cerebral ischemia or infarction, pulmonary edema, or renal failure. *Hypertensive urgencies* are severe elevations in BP without severe symptoms and without evidence of acute or progressive target organ dysfunction. Thus the key distinction and approach to the patient depends on the state of the patient and the assessment of target organ damage, not simply the absolute level of BP. The full-blown clinical picture of a hypertensive emergency is a critically ill patient with a BP greater than 220/140 mm Hg, headaches, confusion, blurred vision, nausea and vomiting, seizures, heart failure, oliguria, and grade III or IV hypertensive retinopathy (Fig. 13–14). Hypertensive emergencies require immediate admission in an intensive care unit (ICU) for intravenous therapy and continuous BP monitoring, whereas hypertensive urgencies can often be managed with oral medications and appropriate outpatient follow-up in 24 to 72 hours. The most common hypertensive cardiac emergencies include acute aortic dissection, hypertension after coronary artery bypass graft surgery, acute myocardial infarction, and unstable angina. Other hypertensive emergencies include eclampsia, head trauma, severe body burns, postoperative bleeding from vascular suture lines, and epistaxis that cannot be controlled with anterior and posterior nasal packing. Neurologic emergencies, which include acute ischemic stroke, hemorrhagic stroke, subarachnoid hemorrhage, and hypertensive encephalopathy, can be difficult to distinguish from one another. Hypertensive encephalopathy is characterized by severe hypertensive retinopathy (i.e., retinal hemorrhages and exudates, with or without papilledema) and a posterior leukoencephalopathy affecting mainly the white matter of the parieto-occipital regions as seen on cerebral MR imaging or CT scanning. A new focal neurologic deficit suggests a stroke-in-evolution, which demands a much more conservative approach to correcting the elevated BP.

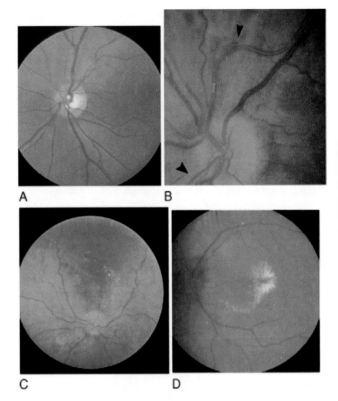

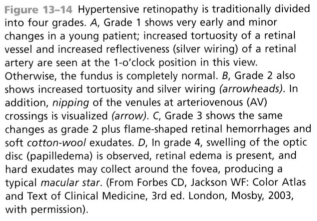

Figure 13–14 Hypertensive retinopathy is traditionally divided into four grades. *A*, Grade 1 shows very early and minor changes in a young patient; increased tortuosity of a retinal vessel and increased reflectiveness (silver wiring) of a retinal artery are seen at the 1-o'clock position in this view. Otherwise, the fundus is completely normal. *B*, Grade 2 also shows increased tortuosity and silver wiring *(arrowheads)*. In addition, *nipping* of the venules at arteriovenous (AV) crossings is visualized *(arrow)*. *C*, Grade 3 shows the same changes as grade 2 plus flame-shaped retinal hemorrhages and soft *cotton-wool* exudates. *D*, In grade 4, swelling of the optic disc (papilledema) is observed, retinal edema is present, and hard exudates may collect around the fovea, producing a typical *macular star*. (From Forbes CD, Jackson WF: Color Atlas and Text of Clinical Medicine, 3rd ed. London, Mosby, 2003, with permission).

In most other hypertensive emergencies, the goal of parenteral therapy is to achieve a controlled and gradual lowering of BP. A good rule of thumb is to lower the initially elevated arterial pressure by 10% in the first hour and by an additional 15% over the next 3 to 12 hours to a BP of no less than 160/110 mm Hg. BP can be reduced further over the next 48 hours. Unnecessarily rapid correction of the elevated BP to completely normal values places the patient at high risk for worsening cerebral, cardiac, and renal ischemia. In chronic hypertension, cerebral autoregulation is reset to higher-than-normal BPs. This compensatory adjustment prevents tissue overperfusion (i.e., increased intracranial pressure) at very high BPs, but it also predisposes the patient to tissue underperfusion (i.e., cerebral ischemia) when an elevated BP is lowered too quickly. In patients with coronary disease, overly rapid or excessive reduction in diastolic BP in

Table 13–9   Parenteral Agents for Management of Hypertensive Emergencies

Agent	Dose	Onset of Action	Precautions
Parenteral Vasodilators			
Sodium nitroprusside	0.25–10 mcg/kg/min IV infusion	Immediate	Thiocyanate toxicity with prolonged use
Nitroglycerin	5–100 mcg/min IV infusion	2–5 min	Headache, tachycardia, tolerance
Nicardipine	5–15 mg/hr IV infusion	1–5 min	Protracted hypotension after prolonged use
Fenoldopam mesylate	0.1–0.3 mcg/kg/min IV infusion	1–5 min	Headache, tachycardia, increased intraocular pressure
Hydralazine	5–10 mg as IV bolus or 10–40 mg IM; repeat every 4–6 hr	10 min IV 20 min IM	Unpredictable and excessive falls in blood pressure; tachycardia; angina exacerbation
Enalaprilat	0.625–1.25 mg every 6 hr IV bolus	15–60 min	Unpredictable and excessive falls in blood pressure; acute renal failure in patients with bilateral renal artery stenosis
Parenteral Adrenergic Inhibitors			
Labetalol	20–80 mg as slow IV injection every 10 min, or 0.5–2.0 mg/min IV as infusion	5–10 min	Bronchospasm, heart block, orthostatic hypotension
Metoprolol	5 mg IV every 10 min for three doses	5–10 min	Bronchospasm, heart block, heart failure, exacerbation of cocaine-induced myocardial ischemia
Esmolol	500 mcg/kg IV over 3 min; then 25–100 mg/kg/min as IV infusion	1–5 min	Bronchospasm, heart block, heart failure
Phentolamine	5–10 mg IV bolus every 5–15 min	1–2 min	Tachycardia, orthostatic hypotension

IM = intramuscular; IV = intravenous.

the ICU can precipitate an acute myocardial ischemia or infarction. Secondary causes of hypertension should be considered in every patient admitted to the ICU with hypertensive crisis.

Parenteral agents for the treatment of hypertensive emergency are summarized in Table 13–9. Sodium nitroprusside, a nitric oxide donor, is the most popular agent because it can be titrated rapidly to control BP. Intravenous nitroglycerin, another nitric oxide donor, is indicated mainly for hypertension in the setting of acute coronary syndrome or decompensated heart failure. Nicardipine is a parenteral dihydropyridine CCB that is particularly useful in the postoperative cardiac patient and patients with renal failure to avoid the thiocyanate toxicity with nitroprusside. Fenoldopam is a selective dopamine-1 receptor agonist that causes both systemic and renal vasodilation, as well as increased glomerular filtration, natriuresis, and diuresis. Intravenous labetalol is an effective treatment of a hypertensive crisis particularly in the setting of myocardial ischemia with preserved ventricular function.

Most patients in the emergency department with hypertensive urgencies are either nonadherent with their medical regimen or are being treated with an inadequate regimen. To expedite the necessary changes in medications, outpatient follow-up should be arranged within 72 hours. To manage the patient during the short-interim period, effective oral medication includes labetalol, clonidine, or captopril, which is a short-acting ACE inhibitor.

BPs greater than 160/110 mm Hg are a common incidental finding among patients in emergency departments and other acute care settings for urgent medical or surgical care of symptoms that are unrelated to BP (e.g., musculoskeletal pain, orthopedic injury). In these settings, the elevated BP is more often the first indication of chronic hypertension than a simple physiologic stress reaction, providing an important opportunity to initiate primary care referral for formal evaluation and treatment of chronic hypertension. Home and ambulatory BP monitoring are indicated to determine whether the patient's BP normalizes completely once the acute illness has resolved.

PROGNOSIS

One of the most important prognostic factors in hypertension is ECG or echocardiographic LVH, with the latter already present in as many as 25% of patients with newly diagnosed hypertension. LVH predisposes the patient to heart failure, atrial fibrillation, and sudden cardiac death. For these reasons, BP should be lowered to below 130/80 mm Hg in hypertensive patients with LVH.

Because of their relatively short duration (typically <5 years), randomized trials underestimate the life-time protection against premature disability and death afforded by several decades of antihypertensive therapy in clinical practice. In the Framingham Heart Study, treating hypertension for 20 years in middle-aged adults reduced total cardiovascular mortality by 60%, which is considerably greater than the results of most randomized trials despite the less intense treatment guidelines when therapy was initiated in the 1950s through the 1970s.

Prospectus for the Future

1. Further delineation of genetic causes of hypertension and application of this research to the treatment of hypertension, including development of antihypertensive drugs that target the various signaling pathways in hypertension and the development of gene therapy for the control of hypertension
2. Improvement of endovascular techniques (stent grafts) for the treatment of aortic aneurysms, aortic dissection, and peripheral vascular diseases
3. Evaluation of drug-eluting stents for the prevention of restenosis after percutaneous revascularization of infra-inguinal vascular disease
4. Further evaluation of gene therapy with vascular growth factors to stimulate angiogenesis in patients with vascular disease
5. Improvements in noninvasive imaging techniques of the vasculature, including three-dimensional reconstruction using CT angiography, MR angiography, and duplex ultrasonography

References

Agodoa LY, Appel L, Bakris GL et al: African American Study of Kidney Disease and Hypertension (AASK) Study Group. Effect of ramipril vs amlodipine on renal outcomes in hypertensive nephrosclerosis: A randomized controlled trial. JAMA 285:2719–2728, 2001.

American Heart Association Proceedings: Atherosclerotic Vascular Disease Conference. Circulation 109:2595–2650, 2004.

Aneurysm Detection and Management Veterans Affairs Cooperative Study Group: Immediate repair compared with surveillance of small abdominal aortic aneurysms. N Engl J Med 346:1437–1444, 2002.

Chobanian A, Bakris G, Black H, et al: The seventh report of the Joint National Committee on Prevention, Detection, Evaluation, and Treatment of High Blood Pressure. The JNC 7 report. JAMA 289:2560–2572, 2003. (The latest United States consensus guidelines).

Dalhof B, Sever PS, Poulter NR et al., for the ASCOT investigators: Prevention of cardiovascular events with antihypertensive regimen of amlodipine adding perindopril as required versus atenolol adding bendroflumethiazide as required, in the Anglo-Scandinavian Cardiac Outcomes Trial-Blood Pressure Lowering Arm (ASCOT-BPLA): A multicentre randomised controlled trial. Lancet 366:895–906, 2005.

Fleming C, Whitlock EP, Beil TL: Screening for abdominal aortic aneurysm: A best-evidence systematic review for the U.S. Preventive Services Task Force. Ann Intern Med 142:203–211, 2005.

Goldhaber SZ: Prevention of recurrent idiopathic venous thromboembolism. Circulation 110:IV-20–IV-24, 2004.

Goldhaber SZ, Elliott CG: Acute pulmonary embolism: Part I: Epidemiology, pathophysiology, and diagnosis. Circulation 108:2726–2729, 2003.

Julius S, Kjeldsen SE, Weber M, et al., for the Value Group: Outcomes in hypertensive patients at high cardiovascular risk treated with regiments based on valsartan or amlodipine: The VALUE randomised trial. Lancet 363, 2022–2031, 2004.

Sever PS, Dalhof B, Poulter NR et al., for the ASCOT investigators: Prevention of coronary and stroke events with atorvastatin in hypertension patients who have average or lower-than-average cholesterol concentrations, in the Anglo-Scandinavian Cardiac Outcomes Trial-Lipid Lowering Arm (ASCOT-LLA): A multicentre randomized controlled trial. Lancet 361:1149–1158, 2003.

The ALLHAT Officers and Coordinators for the ALLHAT Collaborative Research Group: The major outcomes in high risk hypertensive patients randomized to angiotensin-converting enzyme inhibitor or calcium channel blocker vs. diuretic: The antihypertensive and lipid-lowering treatment to prevent heart attack trial (ALLHAT). JAMA 288:2981–2997, 2002.

Section IV

Pulmonary and Critical Care Medicine

Cecil
Andreoli and Carpenter's
Essentials of Medicine

The Lung in Health and Disease

Jesse Roman

Kenneth L. Brigham

The lung is a complex organ with an extensive array of airways and vessels arranged to efficiently transfer the gases necessary for sustaining life. This organ has an immense capacity for gas exchange and, therefore it is not a limiting factor in exercise tolerance in healthy individuals. However, gas exchange becomes compromised in lung disease, rendering the host unable to function properly. The most dramatic consequence of acute and chronic abnormalities in lung function is systemic hypoxemia, leading to tissue hypoxia. Thus, the sequelae of lung dysfunction involve detrimental effects to other organs.

Lung disorders are common and range from well-known conditions such as asthma and chronic obstructive pulmonary disease (COPD) to rarely encountered disorders such as lymphangioleiomyomatosis. This section discusses the diagnosis, evaluation, and treatment of disorders that develop in direct response to lung injury, as well as disorders that develop indirectly through injuries to other organs. This chapter begins with a brief discussion of how the basic structural-functional relationships of the lung are established during lung development, followed by a description of the classification of pulmonary disorders discussed in the chapters in this section.

Lung Development

The lung begins to develop during the first trimester of pregnancy through complex and overlapping processes that transform the embryonic lung bud into a functioning organ with an extensive airway network, two complete circulatory systems, and millions of alveoli responsible for the transfer of gases to and from the body. Lung development can be described in five consecutive stages: *embryonic, pseudoglandular, canalicular or vascular, saccular,* and *alveolar postnatal* (Table 14–1). During the embryonic stage, the rudimentary lung emerges from the foregut as a single epithelial bud surrounded by mesenchymal tissue and occurs between 26 days

and 6 weeks of gestation. This stage is followed by the pseudoglandular stage (between 6 and 16 weeks of gestation) during which repeated monochotomous and dichotomous branching forms rudimentary airways—a process termed *branching morphogenesis* (Fig. 14–1). Coinciding with airway formation, new bronchial arteries arise from the aorta. The canalicular stage is next (between 16 and 28 weeks of gestation) and is characterized by the formation of the acinus, the differentiation of the acinar epithelium, and the development of the distal pulmonary circulation. Through the process of *vasculogenesis,* capillary networks derived from endothelial cell precursors are formed, extend from and around the distal air spaces, and connect with the developing pulmonary arteries and veins. By the end of this stage, the thickness of the alveolar-capillary membrane is similar to that of the adult. During the saccular or prenatal alveolar stage (between 26 and 36 weeks of gestation), vascularized crests emerging from the parenchyma divide the terminal airway structures termed *saccules.* Thinning of the interstitium continues bringing capillaries from adjacent alveolar structures into close apposition, leading to a double capillary network. Near birth, capillaries from opposing networks fuse to form a single network, and capillary volume increases with continuing lung growth and expansion. After birth, the lung continues to grow through the first few years of childhood with the creation of more alveoli through the septation of the air sacs. By age 2 years the lung contains double arterial supplies and venous drainage systems, a complex airway system designed to generate progressive decreases in resistance to airflow as the air travels distally, and a vast alveolar network that efficiently transfers gases to and from the blood.

The processes that drive lung development are tightly controlled, but mishaps do happen, leading to congenital lung disorders such as cystic adenomatoid malformation of the lung, lung hypoplasia or agenesis, bullous changes in the lung parenchyma, and abnormalities in the vasculature including aberrant connections between systemic vessels and

Table 14–1	Stages of Lung Development	
Stage	**Period**	**Comments**
Embryonic	26 days–6 wk	Embryonic lung bud emerges from the foregut.
Pseudoglandular	6–16 wk	Airway tree is formed through a process of monochotomous and dichotomous branching accompanied by growth.
Canalicular	16–28 wk	Angiogenesis and vasculogenesis occur to form the developing vascular network.
Saccular	28–36 wk	Alveoli begin to form through thinning of the mesenchyme and apposition of vascular structures with the air spaces and maturation.
Alveolar (postnatal)	Birth-2 yr	Further development of alveoli and maturation occurs.

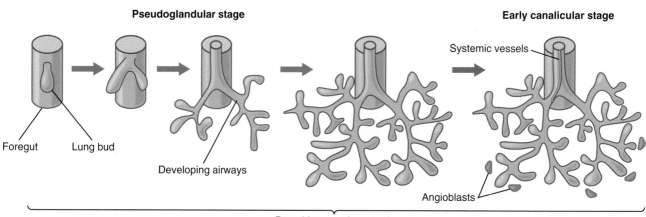

Figure 14–1 Lung branching morphogenesis. Branching morphogenesis occurs during the pseudoglandular stage of lung development and is the process by which the embryonic lung develops the primitive airway system through monochotomous and dichotomous branching.

lung compartments (e.g., lung sequestration) and congenital absence of one or both pulmonary arteries. However, these conditions are rare when compared with the number of infants born annually with abnormal lung function as a result of prematurity. In premature infants the lung is underdeveloped, producing insufficient quantities of surfactant, a surface-active substance produced by specific alveolar epithelial cells that helps decrease surface tension, thereby preventing alveolar collapse. To sustain life while allowing maturation, mechanical ventilation and oxygen supplementation are required but may promote the development of bronchopulmonary dysplasia. In children without congenital abnormalities, lung disorders are relatively rare except for those caused by infection and accidents.

Pulmonary Disease

Pulmonary disorders in the adult are some of the most common clinical entities confronted by physicians. At least four of the top ten causes of death by medical illnesses in the United States are related to pulmonary dysfunction in one way or another: cancer (of which lung cancer is the most common), COPD, pneumonia, and sepsis. COPDs such as emphysema and chronic bronchitis are the fourth leading cause of death and the second leading cause of disability in this country. At a time when a decrease in the age-adjusted death by other common disorders such as coronary artery disease and stroke is occurring, death by COPD continues to increase and is projected to become the third leading cause of death in this country by the year 2020. Over 16 million Americans are estimated to have COPD, but since COPD takes years to develop and the incidence of cigarette smoking (the most common etiologic factor for COPD) is staggering (in 2005, more than 44.5 million Americans were daily smokers), the true disease burden of COPD is much greater.

Asthma is also a common illness, affecting 6% to 8% of the population in the United States. Between the decades of 1960 and 1990, the prevalence, hospitalization rate, and mortality related to asthma increased dramatically. Sleep-disordered breathing is estimated to affect 7 to 18 million people in the United States, with 1.8 to 4 million of these having severe sleep apnea. More rare diseases such as interstitial lung diseases are being increasingly recognized, and their true incidence seems to have been underestimated. For example, idiopathic pulmonary fibrosis, the most common of the idiopathic interstitial pneumonias, affects 85,000 to 100,000 Americans annually. Another interstitial lung disease, sarcoidosis, affects approximately 45,000 Americans each year. Acute respiratory conditions are also common. Viral upper respiratory infections account for 40% of all acute respiratory conditions. Pneumonia occurs in 6 million people per year and is one of the top leading causes of death in the United States.

These conditions affect individuals of all ages, races, and sex. However, a disproportionate increase in the incidence, morbidity, and mortality related to lung diseases exists in minority populations. This finding is true for COPD, asthma, and certain interstitial lung disorders, among others. Although these differences point to genetic differences among these populations, they also point to differences in culture, socioeconomic status, exposure to pollutants (e.g., inner city living), and access to health care.

This section reviews the epidemiologic factors, pathophysiologic conditions, clinical presentation, evaluation, and management of the most common lung diseases. Lung diseases are often classified on the basis of the affected anatomic areas of the lung (e.g., interstitial lung diseases, pleural diseases, airways diseases) and/or the physiologic abnormalities detected by pulmonary function testing (e.g., obstructive lung diseases, restrictive lung diseases). In general, classification schemes based exclusively on physiologic factors are inaccurate because distinctly different disorders with different causes, consequences, and responses to therapy show similar physiologic abnormalities (Fig. 14–2).

The *obstructive lung diseases* share a common physiologic characterization of airflow limitation, as determined by pulmonary function testing (referred to as an *obstructive pattern*). Obstructive lung diseases include emphysema, chronic bronchitis, asthma, and bronchiectasis, among others. The *interstitial lung diseases* are less common disorders, but are more difficult to subclassify because this category includes over 120 distinct entities, some that are inherited and most without an obvious cause. In general, a restrictive physiologic condition that is due to decreased lung compliance and small lung volumes characterizes these disorders, and this characterization is the reason they are often referred to as restrictive lung disorders (e.g., idiopathic pulmonary fibrosis). However, not all interstitial lung diseases exhibit a restrictive pattern on pulmonary function testing. They can even have airflow limitation as a result of small airway involvement (e.g., sarcoidosis, bronchiolitis obliterans). The *pulmonary vascular diseases* make up a rare group of disorders in which involvement of the pulmonary vasculature causes increased intraluminal pressure or pulmonary hypertension. These range from disorders caused by obstruction to blood flow as a result of blood clots (e.g., pulmonary embolus) to disorders characterized by tissue remodeling and obliteration or compression of the vascular structures by connective tissue (e.g., primary pulmonary hypertension). The *disorders of respiratory control* include conditions in which extrapulmonary abnormalities are responsible for dysfunction of the respiratory system, causing abnormal ventilation. These include disorders of

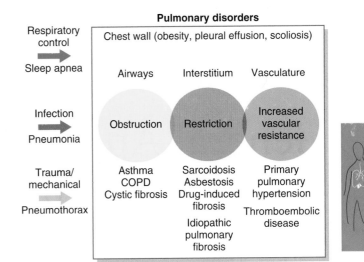

Figure 14–2 Lung diseases. Lung diseases are caused by abnormalities in the lung structure (e.g., airways, interstitium, vasculature), the chest wall, or external forces (e.g., infection). Disorders affecting the lung structure cause physiologic derangements (e.g., obstruction to airflow, restricted lung volumes, pulmonary hypertension, and hypoxia), but these derangements are not necessarily specific to any particular lung disease caused by the extensive overlap among the mechanisms responsible for their manifestation.

sleep such as obstructive sleep apnea. These also include disorders of the neuromuscular system in which ventilatory abnormalities are due to poor excursion of the respiratory muscles as observed in myasthenia gravis and polymyositis. *Disorders of the pleura, chest wall, and mediastinum* are classified as such because they affect these specific structures. However, more often than not, these abnormalities extend into adjacent pulmonary structures in which case they might cause lung atelectasis (as seen in asbestos-related pleural fibrosis), vascular or lung airway occlusion (as seen in fibrosing mediastinitis), and restrictive physiologic disorders (as seen in severe scoliosis and morbid obesity). Infectious agents, of which viral and bacterial infections are the most frequent, cause conditions that include *infectious diseases of the lung*. *Neoplastic disorders* of the lung include both benign (e.g., hamartomas) and malignant (e.g., lung carcinoma) disorders, which can affect the lung parenchyma or its surrounding pleura (e.g., mesothelioma). This section also discusses illnesses requiring critical care such as acute lung injury and sepsis, which are often triggered by injuries to the lung and are frequently managed by pulmonologists and critical care specialists.

References

Burri PH: Development and growth of the lung. In Fishman AP (editor-in-chief): Fishman's Pulmonary Diseases and Disorders. New York, McGraw-Hill, 1998, pp 91–105.

King TE: Clinical advances in the diagnosis and therapy of the interstitial lung diseases. Am J Respir Crit Care Med. 172:268–279, Aug 1, 2005. Epub May 5, 2005.

Mannino DM: Epidemiology and global impact of chronic obstructive pulmonary disease. Semin Respir Crit Care Med 26:204–210, 2005.

Von Hertzen L, Haahtela: Signs of reversing trends in prevalence of asthma. Allergy, 60:283–292, 2005.

Chapter 15

General Approach to Patients with Respiratory Disorders

Bonnie S. Slovis

Jesse Roman

Kenneth L. Brigham

History

As with any patient, a detailed history is necessary to assess effectively a patient who may have pulmonary disease. Patients with lung disorders often complain of one or more of the following symptoms: dyspnea or shortness of breath, fatigue, exercise intolerance, chest tightness, cough, sputum production, and chest pain, among others. Although individually these symptoms are not specific, the presence of certain symptoms coinciding in the same individual may point to a specific diagnosis.

Important to note, common symptoms of respiratory disease, such as dyspnea and cough, are frequently seen in diseases of other organ systems. For example, dyspnea is also a cardinal symptom of heart disease, and cough may be caused by gastroesophageal reflux or chronic sinusitis. An organized approach to the patient, starting with a careful history and a detailed physical examination, will focus further investigation to determine the cause of the symptom.

Common Presenting Complaints

Dyspnea (shortness of breath) is a common complaint of patients with pulmonary disease. Timing and acuity of onset, exacerbating and alleviating factors, and degree of functional impairment are key elements of the history. Associated symptoms such as cough, hemoptysis, chest pain, wheezing, orthopnea, and paroxysmal nocturnal dyspnea, as well as environmental triggers, should be elicited and are helpful in developing a differential diagnosis. If dyspnea is recent, of sudden onset, and accompanied by chest pain, then diseases such as pneumothorax, pulmonary embolism, and pulmonary edema should come to mind. If the dyspnea is long standing and is slowly progressive, then chronic conditions such as chronic obstructive pulmonary disease (COPD), pulmonary fibrosis, and neuromuscular disorders

are in the differential diagnosis. The progression of chronic dyspnea may be insidious. Asking specific questions to quantify changes in functional status over time is important. Dyspnea may occur during exertion or at rest and may be episodic or continuous. Episodic dyspnea associated with exertion suggests parenchymal lung disease or cardiac dysfunction. Dyspnea that is seasonal or triggered by environmental exposure suggests diseases such as asthma or hypersensitivity pneumonitis. Positional dyspnea can occur in patients with severe obstructive lung disease, diaphragmatic paralysis, or neuromuscular weakness.

Orthopnea is defined as dyspnea that occurs in the supine position. This condition may occur as a result of a decrease in vital capacity caused by abdominal contents exerting force against the diaphragm. *Paroxysmal nocturnal dyspnea* is dyspnea that occurs one to several hours after lying down and is associated with congestive heart failure. Increased venous return to the heart causes this condition, resulting in mild interstitial edema. Asthma can also be associated with nocturnal dyspnea and is thought to be due to decreased vital capacity, decreased body temperature, decreased production of endogenous agents with bronchodilator functions, and increased exposure to allergens present in beddings. Exercise-induced asthma causes dyspnea out of proportion to the degree of exertion, with dyspnea often being most severe in the 15 to 30 minutes after the cessation of exercise.

Wheezing, although associated with asthma, has many causes. The absence of wheezing does not rule out asthma in any setting, and the presence of wheezing does not establish the diagnosis. Other conditions that cause wheezing are congestive heart failure; endobronchial obstruction by tumor, foreign body, or mucus; vocal cord abnormalities; and acute bronchitis.

Cough is a frustrating symptom for both the patient and the physician. The three most common causes of chronic cough are postnasal drip, asthma, and gastroesophageal reflux disease. Cough may be mild and infrequent, or it may be severe enough to induce emesis or syncope. Cough may be dry or may produce sputum or blood (*hemoptysis*). The symptom may begin months after initiation of a drug (e.g., angiotensin-converting enzyme inhibitors) leading to a dry, hacking cough. *Bordetella pertussis* infection (whooping cough) and viral lower respiratory infections can produce a cough that may last for 3 months or longer. Patients with asthma often have a cough. On occasion, cough is their only symptom, a condition sometimes referred to as *cough-variant asthma.* Nocturnal cough should raise the suggestion of asthma, heart failure, or gastroesophageal reflux disease.

More than occasional production of *sputum* is abnormal and should be characterized by quantity, color, presence or absence of blood, and timing. The physician should ask the patient to estimate the frequency and volume of sputum produced in 24 hours, as well as any diurnal variation. *Chronic bronchitis* is defined as a persistent cough resulting in sputum production for more than 3 months in each of the last 3 years. Patients with asthma often have a productive cough resulting from excess mucus production. Colored sputum does not always signify a bacterial infection because the concentration of cellular debris, predominantly white cells present in any inflammatory process, influences sputum color. Patients with difficult-to-control asthma who report brown plugs or casts of the small bronchi in their sputum may have *allergic bronchopulmonary aspergillosis.*

Hemoptysis is a frightening symptom. The volume of blood may be scant or large enough to cause asphyxiation or exsanguination. The most common cause of hemoptysis in the United States is bronchitis, whereas the most common cause worldwide is pulmonary tuberculosis. Most cases of hemoptysis are small in volume and self limited and resolve with the treatment of the underlying process. Massive hemoptysis, defined as more than 500 mL of blood in 24 hours, is rare and considered a medical emergency when it occurs. Causes of massive hemoptysis include lung cancer, lung cavities containing mycetomas, cavitary tuberculosis, pulmonary hemorrhage syndromes, pulmonary arteriovenous malformations, and bronchiectasis. The physician should distinguish among hemoptysis, epistaxis, and hematemesis. Because many patients have trouble identifying the source of the bleeding, a careful upper airway physical examination is essential.

Chest pain attributable to the lungs usually results from pleural disease, pulmonary vascular disease, or musculoskeletal pain precipitated by coughing because no pain receptors exist in the lung parenchyma. Lung cancer, for example, does not cause pain until it invades the pleura, chest wall, vertebral bodies, or mediastinal structures. Disease or inflammation of the pleura causes pleuritic chest pain characterized as a sharp or stabbing pain with deep inspiration. Pain caused by pulmonary emboli, infection, pneumothorax, and collagen vascular disease is also usually pleuritic. Pulmonary hypertension may produce dull anterior chest pain unrelated to respiration caused by right ventricular strain and demand ischemia. Other examples of noncardiac causes of chest pain include esophageal disease, herpetic neuralgia, musculoskeletal pain, and trauma. Older patients or those with a history of chronic systemic steroid use may have thoracic pain resulting from vertebral compression or rib fractures. Adequate analgesia, including narcotics, is essential in the treatment of chest pain in patients with underlying lung disease to prevent the reduction in vital capacity caused by splinting of the chest in reaction to the pain. Musculoskeletal chest pain should be a diagnosis of exclusion after serious causes have been ruled out. This pain is usually reproducible with movement or palpation over the affected area.

An accurate history of tobacco use, as well as other *toxic* and *environmental exposures,* is essential in patients with respiratory complaints. Tobacco smoke is the most prevalent environmental toxin causing lung disease. Patients may be anxious about other inhaled toxins or irritants and yet may continue to smoke without concern. Asking about tobacco use and attempting to motivate patients to quit smoking is the physician's duty. The risk of lung disease from smoking is directly related to individual genetic susceptibility and the total pack–years of exposure, and it is inversely related to the age at onset of smoking and, in the case of lung cancer, the interval since smoking cessation.

A history of exposure to other inhaled toxins, irritants, or allergens should be elicited. A careful occupational history often uncovers exposure to inorganic dust or fibers such as asbestos, silica, or coal dust. Organic dusts may cause hypersensitivity pneumonitis and other interstitial lung diseases. Solvents and corrosive gases are also causes of pulmonary disease. The presence of household pets should be documented. Cats are the most allergenic for asthma, and birds may cause hypersensitivity or fungal lung disease. A travel history is important in evaluating infectious causes of pulmonary disease. For example, histoplasmosis is common in the Ohio and Mississippi River valleys, and coccidioidomycosis is found in the desert Southwest. Travel to developing countries increases the risk of exposure to tuberculosis. A family history is important in assessing the risk of genetic lung diseases such as cystic fibrosis and α_1-antitrypsin deficiency, as well as the susceptibility to asthma, emphysema, or lung cancer.

Physical Examination

The physical examination should be complete with emphasis on areas highlighted by the history. The first steps in the physical examination of the patient with pulmonary disease are observation and inspection, which must be done when the patient's chest is bare (Table 15–1). The physician should start by evaluating the general appearance of the patient. In particular, attention should be given to the presence or absence of respiratory distress. This observation will not only help in diagnosis, but it will point to the urgency of the case.

Body habitus is important because morbid obesity in a patient with exercise intolerance and sleepiness might point to a diagnosis of sleep-disordered breathing, whereas dyspnea in a thin middle-aged man with pursed lips might suggest emphysema. Race and sex should also be noted because certain conditions are more frequently encountered in specific populations. For example, sarcoidosis is most common in African Americans in the Southeast, whereas lymphangioleiomyomatosis is a rare disorder that essentially affects young women of childbearing age.

The physician should watch the patient breathe and note the effort required for breathing. Increased respiratory rate, use of accessory muscles of respiration, pursed-lip breath-

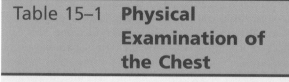

Table 15–1   Physical Examination of the Chest

Inspection

Observation for anxiety, distress, malnutrition, somnolence
Chest wall shape, deformity
Respiratory rate, depth, pattern
Paradoxic respiratory motion of chest and abdomen
Retractions
Use of accessory muscles
Pursed-lip breathing
Cyanosis

Palpation

Tracheal deviation
Chest expansion
Vocal fremitus
Lymphadenopathy
Subcutaneous emphysema

Percussion

Normal, dull, or hyperresonant

Auscultation

Breath sounds: normal vesicular over periphery and bronchial
  centrally
Pleural rub
Added sounds: wheezes, crackles
Stridor

---

be kept in place while the patient takes several deep inspirations. The physician's thumbs should separate slightly and the hands should move symmetrically apart during the patient's inspiration.

Fremitus is a faint vibration felt best with the edge of the hand against the patient's chest wall while the patient speaks. Fremitus is increased in areas with underlying lung consolidation, and it is decreased over a pleural effusion. Next, the patient's chest should be percussed. The level of the diaphragms on each side should be noted. The percussion note should be compared on the two sides starting at the apex and moving down, including the posterior, anterior, and lateral aspects. A pleural effusion, consolidation, mass, or an elevated diaphragm can cause dullness to percussion; a pneumothorax or hyperinflation can cause hyperresonance.

Auscultation of the lungs is performed to evaluate the quality of the breath sounds and to detect the presence of extra (adventitious) sounds not heard in normal lungs. Normal breath sounds have two qualities, vesicular and bronchial. Bronchial breath sounds are heard over the central airways and are louder and coarser than vesicular breath sounds, which are heard at the periphery and base of the lungs. Bronchovesicular sounds are a combination of the two and are heard over medium-sized airways. Bronchial sounds have a longer inhaled component, whereas vesicular sounds have a much longer expiratory component and are much softer. Bronchial breath sounds and bronchovesicular breath sounds at the periphery of the lungs are abnormal and may be caused by underlying consolidation. In the presence of consolidation, increased transmission of vocal sounds, called *whispered pectoriloquy,* occurs; *egophony,* in which the spoken letter *e* sounds like an *a* over the area of consolidation is heard and sometimes compared with the bleating of a goat.

Abnormal or extra pulmonary sounds are crackles, wheezes, and rubs. *Crackles* can be coarse rattles or fine, *Velcro-like* sounds. Mucus in the airways or the opening of large- and medium-sized airways often causes coarse crackles. Fine crackles, produced with inspiration by the opening of collapsed alveoli, are most common at the bases and are heard in pulmonary edema and interstitial fibrosis, as well as in healthy older patients during deep inspiration. *Wheezing* is a higher pitched sound and, when heard locally, suggests large airway obstruction. The wheezing of patients with asthma or congestive heart failure is lower in pitch and heard diffusely over all lung fields. Localized wheezing can be heard in conditions such as pulmonary embolism, obstruction of a bronchus by a tumor, and foreign body aspiration. A *rub* is a pleural sound caused by inflamed pleural surfaces rubbing together. A rub has been described as the sound of pieces of leather rubbing against each other. Rubs are often evanescent and depend on the amount of fluid in the pleural space. Often, pleuritic chest pain and a rub develop after large-volume thoracentesis. A crunching sound timed with the cardiac cycle, called *Hamman's crunch,* is heard in patients with a pneumomediastinum. The complete absence of breath sounds on one side should cause the examiner to think of pneumothorax, hydrothorax, or hemothorax; obstruction of a main stem bronchus; or surgical or congenital absence of the lung. The physical findings associated with various pulmonary disorders are outlined in Table 15–2.

---

ing, and paradoxic abdominal movement all indicate increased work of breathing. The patient's inability to speak in full sentences indicates severe airway obstruction or neuromuscular weakness. The physician should listen for cough during the history and physical examination and should note the strength of the cough because this may signal respiratory muscle weakness or severe obstructive lung disease. The patient's rib cage should expand symmetrically with inspiration. The shape of the thoracic cage should also be noted. Increased anteroposterior diameter is observed in those with obstructive lung disease. Severe kyphoscoliosis, pectus excavatum, ankylosing spondylitis, and morbid obesity can produce restrictive ventilatory disease as a consequence of distortion and restriction of the volume of the thoracic cavity.

Palpation of the chest is performed by first palpating the accessory muscles of respiration in the patient's neck—the scalene and sternocleidomastoid muscles. Hypertrophy and contraction indicate increased respiratory effort. The trachea should be palpated and should lie in the midline of the neck. Deviation of the trachea may suggest lung collapse or a mass. Neck masses should be noted. The physician should place both hands on the lower half of the patient's posterior thorax with thumbs touching and fingers spread; the hands should

Table 15–2 Physical Findings in Common Pulmonary Disorders

Disorder	Mediastinal Displacement	Chest Wall Movement	Vocal Fremitus	Percussion Note	Breath Sounds	Added Sounds	Voice Sounds
Pleural effusion	Heart displaced to opposite side	Reduced over affected area	Absent or markedly decreased	Dull	Absent over fluid; bronchial breath at upper border	Absent; pleural rub may be found above effusion	Absent over effusion; increased with egophony at upper border
Consolidation	None	Reduced over affected area	Increased or normal	Dull	Bronchial	Crackles	Increased with egobronchophony and whispered pectoriloquy
Pneumothorax	Tracheal deviation to opposite side if under tension	Decreased over affected area	Absent	Resonant	Absent or decreased	Absent	Absent
Atelectasis	Ipsilateral shift	Decreased over affected area	Variable	Dull	Absent or diminished	Crackles may be heard	Absent
Bronchospasm	None	Decreased symmetrically	Normal or decreased	Normal or decreased	Bronchovesicular	Wheezing	Normal or decreased
Interstitial fibrosis	None	Decreased symmetrically	Normal or increased	Normal	Bronchovesicular	End-inspiratory crackles unaffected by cough or posture	Normal

Evaluation

The clinician should be able to develop a differential diagnosis based on a detailed history and a thorough physical examination. This preliminary differential diagnosis is the basis on which a battery of tests is ordered, recognizing that these tests might unveil disorders not considered in the initial assessment. The objective of this extended evaluation is twofold: (1) to confirm a diagnosis or discard other disorders, and (2) to assess the severity of the lung derangement. In general, patients with a suggested lung disorder should undergo pulmonary function testing. *Spirometry* evaluates airflows and helps distinguish between an obstructive pattern characteristic of COPD, asthma, and related disorders, as well as a restrictive pattern observed in fibrosing lung disease. Spirometry will also provide information regarding the severity of the physiologic derangement. *Lung volume measurements* are helpful in assessing hyperinflation or confirming a restrictive process. Measuring diffusion capacity for carbon monoxide (D_LCO) will provide information about alterations in gas-exchanging capability. Further assessment of gas exchange can be obtained through the determination of *arterial blood gas* levels. A *6-minute walk test* will evaluate oxygenation during exertion; through this test, patients are often found to require supplemental oxygen for the first time. Other more specialized tests (e.g., bronchoprovocation, cardiopulmonary stress testing, polysomnography) might be required, depending on the circumstances.

Imaging studies of the chest are extremely useful in evaluating lung structure. The *chest radiograph* will provide information about the lung parenchyma and pleura, the cardiac silhouette, mediastinal structures, and even body habitus. Frequently, examining old chest radiographic images is useful to assess progression of disease. *Computed tomography* will provide more accurate information about the pulmonary and mediastinal structures, and it is essential in the assessment of interstitial lung disease and lung masses, among other disorders. Together with *ventilation/perfusion scanning* and *pulmonary angiography,* the computed tomogram is one of the many tools available to evaluate the lung vasculature. *Magnetic resonance imaging, positron-emission tomography,* and related tests are becoming more frequently used in the evaluation of patients with lung masses and other lung disorders. Standard blood tests such as the *blood counts* and *blood chemistry* point to specific disorders or may provide information about the severity of a lung disorder (e.g., polycythemia in chronic hypoxemia, leukocytosis in lung infection). Some specialized tests should be reserved when specific diagnoses such as *serologic conditions* (e.g., rheumatoid factor, antinuclear antibodies) are suggested in patients who may have connective tissue–related lung disease or *hypersensitivity profile* when the diagnosis of hypersensitivity pneumonitis is being entertained.

Together with the history and physical examination, these tests are useful at narrowing a diagnosis to establish a specific plan of treatment. This plan can often be created in a single visit. However, patients will frequently require several visits to a clinician. These follow-up visits serve to assess progression of disease, patient compliance with therapy, and response to management. If these noninvasive tests do not allow for diagnosing the problem, then more invasive tests might be necessary. *Fiberoptic or rigid bronchoscopy* allows for direct visualization of the airways and for obtaining valuable clinical samples for study. *Transthoracic percutaneous needle aspiration* is useful in evaluating peripheral lung lesions. Ultimately, surgery might be required to obtain tissue through *open or video-assisted thoracoscopic-guided lung biopsy.*

References

Fishman AP (Editor-in-chief): Fishman's Pulmonary Diseases and Disorders, 3rd ed. New York: McGraw-Hill, 1998, pp 361–393.

Murray JF: History and Physical Examination. In Murray JF, Nadel JA (eds): Textbook of Respiratory Medicine. 2nd Ed. Philadelphia: WB Saunders, 1994, pp 563–584.

Snider GL, Gale ME: Section III. Approach to the Clinical and Radiographic Evaluation of Patients with Common Pulmonary Syndromes. In Baum GL, Crapo JD, Celli BR, Karlinsky JB (eds): Textbook of Pulmonary Diseases. Philadelphia: Lippincott-Raven, 1998, pp 283–310.

Evaluating Lung Structure and Function

Bonnie S. Slovis

Jesse Roman

Kenneth L. Brigham

The primary function of the lung is the efficient transfer of oxygen into the blood and the removal of carbon dioxide. Gas exchange requires adequate cardiac output, alveolar ventilation, alveolar-capillary surface area, and regional matching of blood flow to ventilation. These processes require a normal lung structure and function, which can be assessed together or individually in a noninvasive fashion through pulmonary function testing and imaging studies. The interpretation of these studies requires a good understanding of the anatomy and physiology of the lung. This chapter discusses the anatomy and physiology of the lung in broad strokes, followed by a more detailed discussion of the tests available to evaluate lung structure and function.

Anatomy and Physiology of the Lung

The primary function of the lungs is gas exchange. The entire cardiac output goes through the lungs, where oxygen is absorbed and carbon dioxide is removed from the blood. Gas exchange requires adequate cardiac output, alveolar ventilation, alveolar-capillary surface area, and regional matching of blood flow to ventilation. In the normal lung, alveolar-capillary surface can double from 50 to $100\,m^2$ by recruiting closed capillaries and alveoli. Lung disease can affect ventilation, pulmonary blood flow, or alveolar-capillary surface area and usually reduces the ability of the lung to match pulmonary blood flow with ventilation. These changes compromise the ability of the lung to meet the body's demand for gas exchange.

AIRWAY

Inspired air travels through the nose and pharynx, where it is heated, humidified, and filtered of particles greater than $10\,\mu m$ in diameter, and where soluble gases are removed.

Entrance to the trachea is through the larynx, which is open during ventilation and closed and covered by the epiglottis during swallowing and Valsalva maneuvers.

The trachea, which is 10 to 12 mm in diameter, is held open by anterior, U-shaped, incomplete, cartilage rings. The trachea divides into the two main stem bronchi at the level of the sternomanubrial junction. The right main stem bronchus takes off at a less acute angle than the left and therefore foreign bodies are more commonly aspirated into the right lung. The large airways are supported by circumferential cartilage rings and continue to branch, with the cartilage disappearing in the smaller airways. These bronchial branches are conducting airways and do not participate in gas exchange. The airways become respiratory bronchioles at approximately the eighteenth branch and contain increasing numbers of alveolar sacs. They continue to branch, becoming alveolar ducts, which ultimately terminate in alveoli (Fig. 16–1). Gas exchange takes place in the branches from the respiratory bronchioles to the alveoli, called the *respiratory zone*. The total cross-sectional area of the airways increases rapidly after the tenth branch, and resistance to air flow decreases. Airflow is laminar proximal to the respiratory zone, where turbulent flow begins and diffusion becomes the dominant mechanism of gas movement. The alveolar lining cells are predominantly flat, *type I pneumocytes,* which rest on a very thin basement membrane and allow rapid diffusion of gases to and from the adjacent capillary blood. *Type II pneumocytes,* approximately 5% of the alveolar lining cells, are round and secrete surfactant, a complex lipoprotein that coats the alveolar surface and decreases surface tension, thus stabilizing alveoli against collapse at low volumes. Type II pneumocytes are capable of regeneration and repair and are also the precursors of type I cells after injury.

BLOOD VESSELS

The lungs have a dual circulation. The bronchial circulation originates from the aorta and, under systemic pressure, sup-

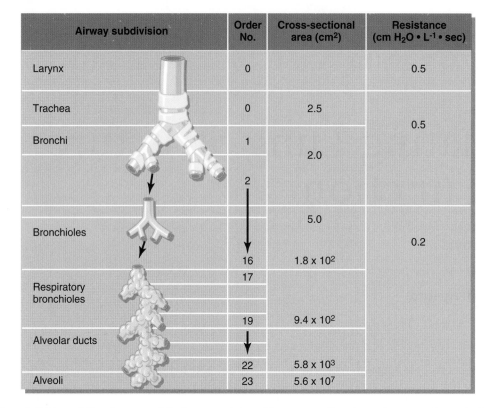

Airway subdivision	Order No.	Cross-sectional area (cm²)	Resistance (cm H$_2$O · L^{-1} · sec)
Larynx	0		0.5
Trachea	0	2.5	0.5
Bronchi	1	2.0	
	2		
Bronchioles		5.0	0.2
	16	1.8×10^2	
Respiratory bronchioles	17		
	19	9.4×10^2	
Alveolar ducts			
	22	5.8×10^3	
Alveoli	23	5.6×10^7	

Figure 16–1 The subdivision of the airways and their nomenclature. The cross-sectional area increases dramatically toward the peripheral, small airways. (Adapted from Weibel ER: Morphometry of the Human Lung. Berlin, Springer, 1963.)

plies nutrient flow to lung structures proximal to the alveoli. One third of the venous outflow from the bronchial circulation returns through the bronchial veins to the right side of the heart, similar to other organs perfused by systemic blood. The remainder of the bronchial circulation drains into the pulmonary veins, which then empty into the left atrium and form part of the normal anatomic right-to-left shunt.

The pulmonary circulation is a low-resistance circuit that receives the entire output of the right cardiac ventricle. Pulmonary arterial pressure and pulmonary vascular resistance are approximately one tenth those of the systemic circulation. Pulmonary arteries and arterioles are thin walled and have much less smooth muscle than systemic arteries. They accompany the bronchial tree to supply bronchopulmonary segments. At the level of the alveolar ducts, the pulmonary arterioles terminate in a meshwork of capillaries, which form a sheet of blood surrounding the alveoli and create the large surface area necessary for gas exchange. Blood returns to the heart through pulmonary veins that course between lung lobules, coalesce into four main pulmonary veins, and empty into the left atrium.

VENTILATION

Ventilation is the movement of air in and out of the lungs. The volume of air in the lungs is determined by the balance between the outward elastic force of the thoracic cage and the inward elastic recoil of the lungs. During inspiration, active contraction of the respiratory muscles increases intrathoracic volume and creates sub-atmospheric pressure in the pleural space and alveoli. Air enters the lung down the pressure gradient between atmospheric and intrathoracic pressures. Exhalation is passive in normal lungs and begins when inspiratory muscles relax. Intrinsic elastic recoil passively returns the lungs to their resting volume, when alveolar pressure and ambient pressure are equal. With active contraction of expiratory muscles, alveolar pressure can be increased above ambient pressure, emptying additional volume from the lung. In disease states such as emphysema when the elastic recoil of the lung is greatly diminished, active contraction of the expiratory muscles is required to empty enough air from the lungs to permit ventilation.

The primary respiratory muscle is the diaphragm. The so-called accessory muscles of respiration—the intercostal, sternocleidomastoid, scalene, and abdominal muscles—normally contribute little. The diaphragm is dome shaped at rest, curving into the thoracic cavity. It flattens during contraction, increasing the thoracic volume and distending the abdominal wall. If the lungs are hyperinflated because of trapped gas from emphysema or asthma (obstructive lung diseases [OLDs]), then the diaphragm is flat or inverted at end expiration and its contraction will not produce an appreciable change in thoracic volume. In this situation the scalene and sternocleidomastoid accessory muscles of respiration contract and elevate the anterior chest wall. Although this action increases intrathoracic volume, the increase is much less than that produced by the normal diaphragm, the effects of which on air movement are also much reduced. In addition to recruitment of accessory muscles during inspiration, OLD requires contraction of the abdominal muscles

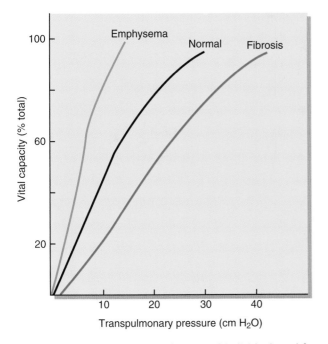

Figure 16–2 Compliance curves for normal individuals and for patients with emphysema and pulmonary fibrosis. An elevation in the transpulmonary pressure required to achieve a given lung volume increases the work of breathing.

during expiration to exert pressure on the flattened diaphragm, which in turn increases intrathoracic pressure to force exhalation.

Respiratory muscles must overcome both elastic and resistive forces. The opposing elastic forces of the chest wall (outward force) and lungs (inward force) determine the resting lung volume at the end of passive expiration, called the *functional residual capacity* (FRC). The FRC should be less than 50% of the total lung capacity (TLC), which is the total amount of air that the lung can contain. Elasticity is usually measured as its inverse function, compliance. Compliance is the change in lung volume produced by a given change in transpulmonary pressure. In normal lungs at FRC, it takes approximately 1 cm of water (H_2O) pressure to inflate the lungs 200 mL. Compliance would then be 200 mL/cm H_2O, decreasing as lung volume increases toward TLC. Compliance is decreased in diseases such as pulmonary fibrosis or pulmonary edema, which restrict lung volume expansion. Compliance is increased in emphysema because of the loss of elastic recoil (Fig. 16–2). When compliance is decreased, the work of breathing is increased, because of the increased pressure required to inflate the lungs. In diseases such as emphysema in which compliance is increased, the work of breathing is also increased during inspiration as a result of the loss of mechanical advantage from hyperinflation and flattened diaphragms, and during expiration because decreased lung elastic recoil requires active muscle contraction to empty the lungs in preparation for the next inspiration. In patients with severe obstructive or restrictive lung disease, the work of breathing may be a major contributor to the resting metabolic rate. In extreme circumstances, this increase in energy expenditure can result in weight loss

known as pulmonary cachexia. With normal lungs, the work of breathing uses only 4% to 5% of the total calories burned, but in severe lung disease up to 30% of the total body oxygen consumption can be consumed by the work of breathing. Under these extreme circumstances, minute ventilation may decrease and partial pressure of carbon dioxide in arterial blood ($PaCO_2$) may increase as a homeostatic response of the body to decreasing the energy cost of breathing.

Airway resistance is inversely related to the total cross-sectional area of the airways. Normal resistance is in the range of 1 to 2 cm H_2O/L/sec. Although the peripheral airways are narrow, their total cross-sectional area is large; consequently, resistance to air flow at that level of the tracheobronchial tree is low. Airway resistance decreases as lung volume increases because of an increase in airway diameter resulting from tethering of airway walls to lung tissue. Causes of increased airway resistance include airway obstruction by an intrinsic mass or a mucous plug, airway smooth muscle contraction (bronchospasm), and the dynamic compression of a forced exhalation.

Not all air entering the lungs is in contact with gas-exchanging units. The portion of an inhaled breath that fills the respiratory zone is the alveolar volume (V_A), and the portion remaining in the conducting airways is the dead space volume (V_D). At end expiration, the V_D contains exhaled alveolar gas that has equilibrated with pulmonary capillary blood; thus, the amount of fresh air reaching the alveoli on the next breath is the V_A minus the V_D. The sum of V_A and V_D ventilation with quiet breathing is the tidal volume (V_T). The proportion of the V_T that is V_D varies with the V_T. Although V_D increases slightly with larger inspirations because of traction on the bronchi, the increase is less than the increase in V_A. Slow, deep breathing results in greater V_A and therefore greater gas exchange than rapid shallow breathing at the same volume of air per minute or minute ventilation. V_D in the seated position with quiet respiration is approximately 1 mL per pound of ideal body weight.

The distribution of ventilation in the lungs is unequal, with greater ventilation in the base and less at the apex in the upright position. The same inequality is true for lung perfusion. This matching of ventilation and perfusion optimizes gas exchange.

CONTROL OF VENTILATION

Ventilation is the primary short-term homeostatic mechanism for maintaining normal blood pH, the strongest factor controlling ventilation. Normal blood pH is accomplished through the elimination or retention of carbon dioxide. The $PaCO_2$ in blood is inversely proportional to the minute ventilation. Hypoxia is the second strongest drive to ventilation. Maintaining pH and adequate oxygenation is accomplished through the respiratory control system, which consists of neurologic respiratory control centers, respiratory effectors, and respiratory sensors.

Respiratory Control Centers

Neuronal control of autonomic respiration resides in the brainstem, primarily the medullary reticular formation. The medulla receives input from the pons, which may modify or fine tune the rhythm of breathing. Voluntary ventilation originates in the cerebral cortex and can override autonomic ventilatory control.

Respiratory Effectors

The muscles of respiration include the diaphragm and accessory muscles, as previously discussed. For effective ventilation, these muscles must be coordinated by the respiratory control center through the phrenic, intercostal, cranial, and cervical nerves.

Respiratory Sensors

Two types of respiratory receptors are present: chemoreceptors and mechanoreceptors. Central and peripheral chemoreceptors detect changes in pH, $PaCO_2$, and partial pressure of oxygen in arterial blood (PaO_2). Central chemoreceptors located in the medulla respond rapidly to changes in hydrogen ion concentration and $PaCO_2$ by stimulating or inhibiting ventilation to maintain blood pH within the normal range. The peripheral chemoreceptors also respond to hydrogen ion concentration and $PaCO_2$ but are most sensitive to changes in PaO_2. In contrast to the linear response of ventilation to $PaCO_2$, the response to changes in PaO_2 is minimal until the PaO_2 drops below 60 mm Hg. A steep relationship develops below this threshold between the PaO_2 and ventilation (Fig. 16–3). The PaO_2 versus ventilation curve is a mirror image of the oxygen dissociation curve for hemoglobin. Mechanoreceptors in the chest wall and airways modulate rate and depth of breathing in response to stretch. *J receptors* located in juxtacapillary regions in the lung periphery stimulate ventilation in response to pulmonary vascular engorgement. In addition, airway irritant receptors respond to physical and chemical stimuli.

PERFUSION

The pulmonary vascular bed receives the entire output of the right ventricle. Because the pulmonary circulation is a low-pressure system, it is affected by gravity, with the greatest blood flow going to the dependent portions of the lungs. The hydrostatic pressure increases from the top to the bottom of the lungs. Alveolar pressure, assuming open airways, is relatively constant throughout the lung. The relationship between alveolar and pulmonary vascular pressures is the mechanism that largely determines blood flow in the normal lung.

In 1964, West devised a model of blood flow within the lungs that divides the lung into three zones, determined by the relationship between pulmonary vascular and alveolar pressures (Fig. 16–4). *Zone 1* is defined as an area of the lungs in which alveolar pressure exceeds pulmonary artery pressure, thus inhibiting perfusion. Zone 1 conditions tend to occur in the most superior portions of the lungs in situations such as shock, in which pulmonary artery pressure falls below alveolar pressure, or with positive pressure ventilation, in which the alveolar pressure rises above pulmonary artery pressure. This ventilated but unperfused area of the lung is called alveolar or physiologic dead space and, depending on size, can significantly increase the minute ventilation required to remove carbon dioxide from the blood. *Zone 2* conditions exist when pulmonary arterial pressure is higher than alveolar pressure but alveolar pressure is higher than pulmonary venous pressure. In zone 2, the hydrostatic pres-

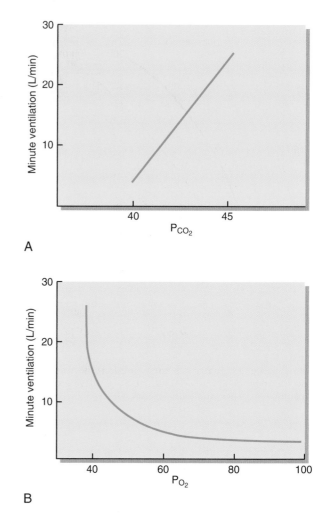

A

B

Figure 16–3 A rising PCO_2 leads to a linear increase in minute ventilation (*A*). The ventilatory response to hypoxemia (*B*) is less sensitive and is clinically relevant only when the PO_2 has dropped significantly.

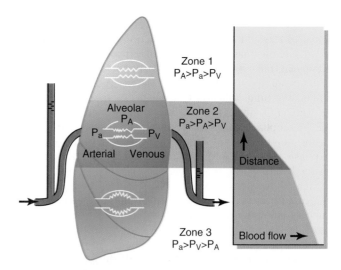

Figure 16–4 Zonal model of blood flow in the lung. Because of the inter-relationship of vascular and alveolar pressures, the lung base receives the most flow (*see text for explanation*). (From West JB, Dollery CT, Naimark A: Distribution of blood flow in isolated lung: Relation to vascular and alveolar pressures. J Appl Physiol 19:713–724, 1964.)

sure driving blood flow is the difference between pulmonary artery pressure and alveolar pressure. In *zone 3*, pulmonary venous pressure exceeds alveolar pressure and blood flow is determined by the arterial-venous pressure difference.

In states of increased oxygen demand, cardiac output rises and pulmonary vascular resistance actually falls through recruitment of previously unperfused vessels, increasing the total vascular cross-sectional area. This response allows blood flow to increase dramatically with relatively small increases in pulmonary artery pressure. The relationship between lung volume and pulmonary vascular resistance is U-shaped. At low volumes, vascular resistance decreases with increasing volume because of tethering of vessels to lung tissue; however, at high lung volumes, resistance rises again, with compression of capillaries by increasing alveolar volume.

Alveolar hypoxia causes local constriction of arterioles that supply the hypoxic area (hypoxic pulmonary vasoconstriction), which decreases blood flow to areas of low ventilation and thus helps maintain ventilation-perfusion (V/Q) matching in a heterogeneously ventilated lung. In the instance of generalized alveolar hypoxia, such as at altitude, global vasoconstriction results in pulmonary hypertension. Acidosis and increased sympathetic tone also cause lesser degrees of vasoconstriction, whereas mediators produced in the pulmonary vascular bed (e.g., nitric oxide, prostacyclin) can cause local vasodilation.

GAS TRANSFER

Oxygen and carbon dioxide are easily dissolved in plasma. Other atmospheric gases are much less soluble and are not significantly exchanged across the alveolar-capillary interface. The solubility of oxygen and carbon dioxide allows complete equilibration between alveolar and plasma concentrations during each respiratory cycle. The majority of oxygen contained in the blood is bound to hemoglobin, with a small fraction dissolved measured as the PaO_2. Each molecule of hemoglobin is capable of carrying four molecules of oxygen. Under normal conditions at a PaO_2 of 150 mm Hg, hemoglobin is completely saturated and further increases in PaO_2 have little effect on the oxygen content of blood. The oxygen-hemoglobin dissociation curve is a graph of the relationship between PaO_2 and hemoglobin saturation. Its shape reflects the cooperative binding of oxygen to hemoglobin (Fig. 16–5). Decreased blood pH, increased temperature, increased 2, 3-diphosphoglycerate, and increased $PaCO_2$ all act to decrease the affinity of hemoglobin for oxygen, which facilitates unloading of oxygen into tissues. Carbon monoxide binds hemoglobin with 240 times greater affinity than does oxygen at the same sites and also induces cooperative binding. Binding of hemoglobin by carbon monoxide decreases the oxygen content of blood by decreasing the amount of oxygen bound to hemoglobin, but it has no effect on PaO_2. Binding of hemoglobin simultaneously decreases the off-loading of oxygen into tissues by increasing the affinity of hemoglobin for oxygen.

Carbon dioxide is also bound to hemoglobin, but it does not exhibit cooperative binding; thus, the shape of the carbon dioxide dissociation curve is more linear than that of oxygen and is determined by the mass effect of PaO_2. In the lung, oxygen displaces carbon dioxide from hemoglobin, and

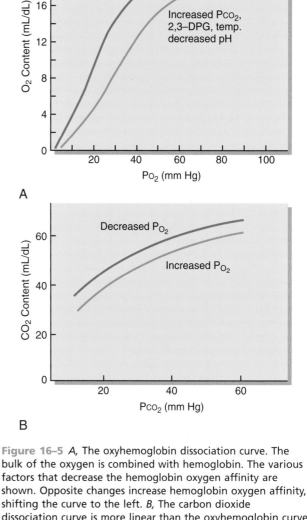

A

B

Figure 16–5 *A,* The oxyhemoglobin dissociation curve. The bulk of the oxygen is combined with hemoglobin. The various factors that decrease the hemoglobin oxygen affinity are shown. Opposite changes increase hemoglobin oxygen affinity, shifting the curve to the left. *B,* The carbon dioxide dissociation curve is more linear than the oxyhemoglobin curve throughout the physiologic range. Increased PaO_2 shifts the curve to the right, which decreases carbon dioxide content for any given $PaCO_2$ and thus facilitates carbon dioxide off-loading in the lungs. The shift to the left at a lower PaO_2 facilitates carbon dioxide on-loading at the tissues. DPG = diphosphoglycerate.

the release of oxygen allows on-loading of carbon dioxide in tissues.

ABNORMALITIES OF PULMONARY GAS EXCHANGE

PaO_2 and $PaCO_2$ are determined by the degree of equilibration between the alveolar gas and capillary blood. The degree of equilibration depends on four main factors: (1) matching of ventilation with perfusion, (2) ventilation, (3) shunt, and (4) diffusion.

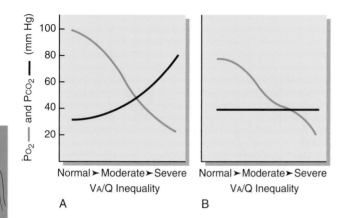

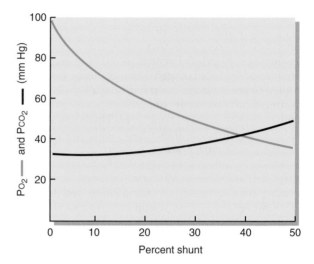

Figure 16–6 *A,* The effect of increasing ventilation/perfusion (V/Q) inequality on PaO_2 and $PaCO_2$ when cardiac output and minute ventilation are held constant. *B,* The gas tensions change when ventilation is allowed to increase. Increased ventilation can maintain a normal $PaCO_2$ but can only partially correct the hypoxemia. (Adapted from Dantzker DR: Gas exchange abnormalities. In Montenegro H [ed]: Chronic Obstructive Pulmonary Disease. New York, Churchill Livingstone, 1984, pp 141–160.)

Figure 16–7 The effect of increasing shunt on the arterial PaO_2 and $PaCO_2$. The minute ventilation has been held constant in this example. Under usual circumstances, the hypoxemia would lead to increased minute ventilation and a fall in the $PaCO_2$ as the shunt increases. (From Dantzker DR: Gas exchange abnormalities. In Montenegro H [ed]: Chronic Obstructive Pulmonary Disease. New York, Churchill Livingstone, 1984, pp 141–160.)

Ventilation/Perfusion Inequality (Mismatch)

The lung is composed of units with varying ratios of V/Q. In normal lungs, the range of ratios is narrow, from about 0.5 to 3.0. As lung disease develops, the range widens; consequently, V/Q is matched in fewer lung units. This mismatch without compensation will cause the PaO_2 to fall and the $PaCO_2$ to rise. In patients with normal respiratory drive and ventilatory capacity, the increasing $PaCO_2$ triggers an increase in minute ventilation, which maintains $PaCO_2$ and pH levels within normal range but has very little effect on PaO_2. When the ability to increase minute ventilation is exceeded, both hypoxemia and hypercarbia result (Fig. 16–6). Inequality is the primary cause of abnormal gas exchange in diseased lungs.

Hypoventilation

Hypoventilation is defined as ventilation inadequate to keep $PaCO_2$ from increasing above normal. In this situation, hypoxia may occur when increased carbon dioxide in alveoli displaces sufficient oxygen. $PaCO_2$ is directly proportional to minute ventilation. The alveolar gas equation describes the reciprocal relationship between $PaCO_2$ and PaO_2 as follows:

$$PaO_2 = [(P_B - P_{H_2O}) \times FIO_2] - [PaCO_2 \div R]$$

where P_B is atmospheric pressure, P_{H_2O} is the partial pressure of water vapor, FIO_2 is the fractional concentration of inspired oxygen, and R is the respiratory exchange ratio. As minute ventilation falls, the $PaCO_2$ rises and the PaO_2 falls. Administering supplemental oxygen (i.e., increased FIO_2) can reverse hypoventilation-induced hypoxia in patients who are breathing room air.

Shunt

Shunt is the portion of the blood that goes from the right side of the heart to the left without an opportunity for exchange of oxygen and carbon dioxide. Anatomic shunt occurs across intracardiac septal defects, via pulmonary arteriovenous malformations, and from the very small percentage of venous return from cardiac and bronchial circulations that empties directly into the left atrium. Physiologic shunt occurs when pulmonary capillary blood traverses unventilated lung units and is actually one extreme of mismatch. Shunt is the most potent source of hypoxemia because the oxygen content of shunted blood cannot be affected by increases in the FIO_2. At values less than 50% of the cardiac output, shunt has very little effect on $PaCO_2$ (Fig. 16–7).

The fraction of blood shunted can be calculated only when the FIO_2 is 100%, as calculated by the following formula:

$$Qs \div Qt = [Cc'O_2 - CaO_2] \div [Cc'O_2 - CvO_2]$$

where Qs = shunted blood flow, Qt = total blood flow, $C'O_2$ = end pulmonary capillary oxygen content, and CvO_2 = mixed venous oxygen content.

Diffusion Impairment

With normal cardiopulmonary function, blood spends an average of 0.75 seconds in the pulmonary capillaries at rest. During vigorous exercise, this time may be decreased to 0.25 seconds. Because it takes only 0.25 seconds for blood and alveolar oxygen to equilibrate across the thin alveolar-capillary membrane, no fall in the end-capillary oxygen concentration occurs even under these conditions. Increased diffusing distance resulting from a thickening of the alveolar-capillary membrane requires more time for oxygen to equilibrate between alveolar gas and capillary blood, resulting in a decrease in PaO_2 first with exercise and in extreme cases at rest. Hypoxemia is rarely caused solely by diffusion

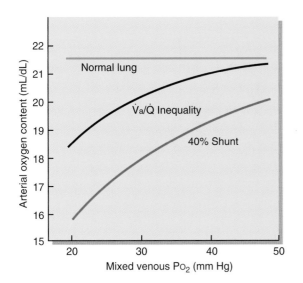

Figure 16–8 The effect of altering mixed venous $P\bar{v}O_2$ on the arterial oxygen content under three assumed conditions: a normal lung, severe ventilation/perfusion (V/Q) inequality, and the presence of a 40% shunt. For each situation, the patient is breathing 50% oxygen and the $P\bar{v}O_2$ or mixed veous PO_2 is altered, keeping all other variables constant. (From Dantzker DR: Gas exchange in the adult respiratory distress syndrome. Clin Chest Med 3:57–67, 1982.)

impairment. The abnormalities in carbon monoxide diffusing capacity measured during pulmonary function testing reflect mismatching far more often than diffusion impairment.

NONPULMONARY CAUSES OF HYPOXEMIA

The PaO_2 can be affected by the partial pressure of mixed systemic venous blood (PvO_2) entering the pulmonary circulation. PvO_2 is decreased when the demand for oxygen in the tissues outstrips the supply. Inadequate cardiac output, low hemoglobin concentration, or low hemoglobin oxygen saturation all result in low PvO_2. The effect of decreased PvO_2 on PaO_2 is usually only clinically significant in patients with underlying lung disease producing V/Q mismatch or shunt (Fig. 16–8). Hypoxia caused by a combination of heart and lung disease should be understood and managed according to the contribution of each.

GROWTH AND AGING OF THE NORMAL LUNG

The lung grows by alveolar multiplication up to 8 years of age, after which it continues to grow by increasing alveolar diameter until about the age of 20 years. Thereafter both total alveolar surface area and elastic recoil decrease progressively with age. By 80 years of age, the alveolar surface area is reduced by about 30%. Loss of elastic recoil increases FRC. In aging, small airways and alveoli in the lower lung zones tend to collapse during expiration, increasing V/Q mismatch and contributing to the progressive increase in the difference of the alveolar-arterial oxygen found in the normal lung with age.

Evaluation of Lung Function

A careful history and physical examination will unveil important information about lung function. However, accurate measurements of lung function require pulmonary function testing in an accredited laboratory. A series of invasive and noninvasive tests are available to evaluate ventilatory function, gas exchange, and gas distribution, among other functions. These tests are useful in pointing toward a particular diagnosis. However, a definitive diagnosis cannot be derived from them; the clinician must put together the clinical presentation, imaging studies, and results of pulmonary function tests to reach a diagnosis to develop an appropriate plan of treatment.

Pulmonary function tests are indicated to (1) assess the presence, type, and severity of respiratory impairment in patients with unexplained respiratory symptoms or signs; (2) monitor the course of a known disease and its modification by therapy; (3) screen or monitor patients at risk of developing lung disease (e.g., smokers, high-risk populations, patients on drugs with known pulmonary toxicity); and (4) provide the preoperative assessment of patients with possible or existing lung disease.

Routine pulmonary function testing evaluates four areas of lung function: *airflow, lung volumes, gas exchange,* and *lung mechanics.* Accurate interpretation of these tests requires appropriate reference standards. Variables that affect the standard values include age, height, sex, race, and hemoglobin concentration. The standard deviation of these variables and the day-to-day and test-to-test variations must be considered when interpreting a given set of pulmonary function tests.

SPIROMETRY

Airflow can be estimated by spirometry, a test that allows the plotting of the volume exhaled during a forced expiration against time of exhalation. The patient breathes into an apparatus that measures inspiratory and expiratory flow rates with changing lung volumes. Airflow is measured during a forced vital capacity (FVC) maneuver. Several components are derived from this maneuver:

- FVC is the maximal amount of air that can be exhaled after a maximal inspiration.
- Forced expiratory volume in 1 second (FEV_1) is that portion of the FVC exhaled in the first second.
- FEV_1/FVC ratio (FEV_1/FVC%) is the FEV_1 divided by the FVC expressed as a percentage.
- Forced expiratory flow (FEF 25% to 75%) is the average expiratory flow from the point at which 25% of the FVC has been exhaled to the point at which 75% has been exhaled.

The values measured or derived are compared with normal values predicted on the basis of age, sex, height, and race. Abnormal values are defined as being in the fifth percentile (i.e., the mean predicted value −1.64 × the standard error of the estimate).

Spirometry can unveil abnormalities that are classified into two patterns: *obstructive* and *restrictive*. Obstructive impairments are defined by a low FEV_1 and a low

Table 16–1	Determining Severity of Impairment	
Percent Predicted (FEV$_1$ or TLC or D$_L$CO)	**Severity (Obstruction or Restriction or Diffusion)**
>80	Normal
>70–80	Minimal
60–70	Mild
50–60	Moderate
<50	Severe

FEV$_1$ = forced expiratory volume in 1 second; TLC = total lung capacity; D$_L$CO = diffusing capacity for carbon monoxide.

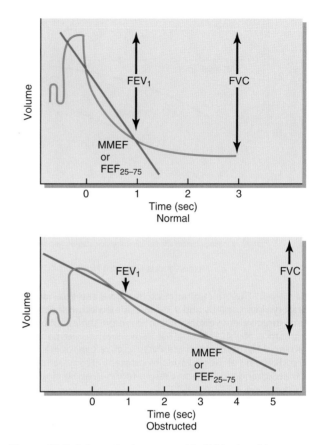

Figure 16–9 Spirometry in a normal individual and in a patient with OLD. FEV$_1$ represents the forced expired volume in 1 second, and FVC represents the forced vital capacity. The slope of the line connecting the points at 25% and 75% of the FVC represents the forced expired flow (FEF at 25% to 75%) or maximum mid-expiratory flow (MMEF). The FEF at 25% to 75% is less reproducible and less specific than the FEV$_1$.

FEV$_1$/FVC%, indicating an impairment of expiratory flow. The severity of the impairment is determined by the FEV$_1$ (Table 16–1). However, in early obstructive impairments, the FEF of 25% to 75% may be the first value to become abnormal. Diseases characterized by an obstructive pattern with spirometry are asthma, chronic bronchitis, emphysema, bronchiectasis, cystic fibrosis, and central airway lesions, among others. Increased airway resistance (e.g., asthma) and/or decreased elastic recoil (e.g., emphysema) cause airflow obstruction in these disorders (**Web Fig. 16–1**). Spirometry will not distinguish between these processes. A restrictive pattern is characterized by loss of lung volume, which is highlighted by a proportional decrease in both the FEV$_1$ and FVC, thereby leading to a preserved FEV$_1$/FVC% (Fig. 16–9). A restrictive pattern is best evaluated by measuring lung volumes (see next section on "Lung Volumes").

Obstructive or restrictive patterns generated by spirometry can be readily assessed by a volume-time curve (**Web Fig. 16–2**). However, the same measurements generated during the FVC maneuver can be depicted in a flow-volume loop (Fig. 16–10 and **Web Fig. 16–3**) (see also Fig. 16–9). As previously described, the patient first inspires to TLC during the FVC maneuver, followed by forced exhalation to residual volume (RV). The patient must sufficiently contract the chest wall muscles to overcome the outward elastic recoil of the chest wall to ensure that expiratory flow is not inhibited. Once this threshold effort is made, maximal airflow at any given volume is dependent only on the driving pressure (i.e., lung elasticity) and airway resistance and is independent of effort. For the flow-volume loop, the flow rate is plotted on the vertical axis and the volume is plotted on the horizontal axis. Expiratory flow is positive and inspiratory flow is negative. In this fashion, flows at specific lung volumes are depicted.

Examination of the pattern of the flow-volume loop is useful because obstructive and restrictive impairments show characteristic loops that can be readily recognized. Early

obstructive impairments result in a distal concavity of the expiratory curve, whereas more severe obstructive impairments that cause hyperinflation and air trapping shift the curve to the left. In restrictive impairments, the curve is shifted to the right (smaller lung volumes).

In addition to depicting an obstructive or restrictive pattern, the flow-volume loop can assist in evaluating the type of central airway obstruction. A fixed obstruction results in equal attenuation of higher expiratory and inspiratory flows so that the loop becomes flattened (see Fig. 16–10). This pattern can be seen in patients with fibrotic tracheal stenosis. Variable extrathoracic central airway obstruction results in a somewhat normal-appearing expiratory curve but a significantly flattened inspiratory curve. This pattern can be observed in patients with laryngeal narrowing from laryngospasm, edema, tumors, or vocal cord paralysis. Obstruction to airflow within the thorax (intrathoracic variable airflow obstruction) shows an attenuation of the expiratory curve but a more normal inspiratory curve. This pattern may be observed in those with tracheomalacia or tracheal tumors and is difficult to distinguish from those observed in patients with chronic obstructive pulmonary disease (COPD) and other OLDs.

To evaluate airway hyper-reactivity, spirometry can be performed before and 10 minutes after administration of an

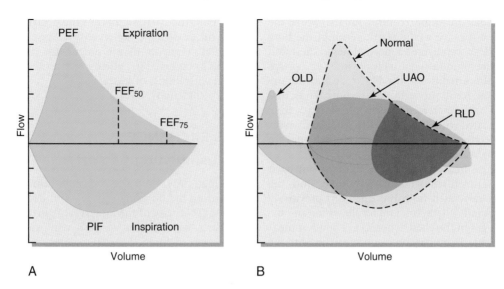

Figure 16–10 *A,* The maximum expired flow and volume curve in a normal individual. The peak expiratory flow (PEF) and forced expiratory flows at 50% and 75% of the exhaled vital capacity (FEF at 50% and 75%) are indicated. PIF = peak inspiratory flow. *B,* In obstructive lung disease (OLD), hyperinflation pushes the position of the curve to the left, and characteristic scalloping on expiration develops. In restrictive lung disease (RLD), lung volumes are reduced, but flow for any point in volume is normal. The flow-volume curve displays different patterns with various forms of upper airway obstruction (UAO), with reduction in respiratory flow if the obstruction is outside the thoracic cavity and, in addition, in expiratory flow if the obstruction is caused by a fixed deformity.

inhaled beta-agonist. In general, a significant response is considered to be an improvement in FEV_1 or FVC of at least 12% to 15%. However, this test alone should not be used to prescribe chronic bronchodilator therapy. In addition, the test is not specific and the absence of a response does not totally discard airways hyper-reactivity; a bronchoprovocation test is more accurate at defining this problem.

LUNG VOLUMES

The lung volume measurements can be divided into four lung volumes and four capacities. Each capacity is the sum of two or more volumes (Fig. 16–11):

- T_V is the amount of air inhaled or exhaled during normal breathing.
- RV is the amount of air remaining in the lungs after a maximal expiration.
- Inspiratory reserve volume (IRV) is the amount of air that can be exhaled maximally from FRC.
- TLC is the amount of gas in the lungs after a maximal inspiration.
- Vital capacity (VC) is the maximal amount of air that can be exhaled after maximal inspiration; if VC is exhaled with maximal effort, then it is classified as FVC.
- FRC is the volume in the lungs at end-expiration of a normal tidal breath.
- Inspiratory capacity (IC) is the maximal amount of air that can be inhaled from FRC.

Because the RV cannot be measured, the TLV cannot be estimated in this way. Rather, FRC is measured by either gas dilution or plethysmography, and this value is then used with

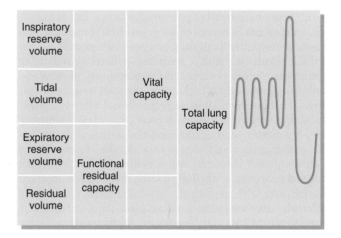

Figure 16–11 Lung volumes and capacities. Although spirometry can measure vital capacity (VC) and its subdivisions, calculation of residual volume (RV) requires measurement of functional residual capacity (FRC) by body plethysmography, helium dilution technique, or nitrogen washout.

the values determined by spirometry to derive the RV and related volumes and capacities using one or more of the following equations:

$$TLC = VC + RV = IC + FRC = IRV + T_V + ERV + RV$$
$$VC = IC + ERV = IRV + T_V + ERV$$
$$FRC = ERV + RV$$
$$IC = IRV + T_V$$

The FRC is the lung volume at which the elastic recoil of the lung inward equals the elastic recoil of the lung outward. No energy is required to hold FRC; although the inspiratory component of tidal breathing requires muscle work, the expiratory phase is passive as the elastic recoil of the lung restores to the FRC. Because most abnormalities in chest wall elastic recoil are uncommon and usually obvious (e.g., severe scoliosis), most abnormalities in the FRC reflect an abnormality in the elastic recoil properties of the lung. Thus, diseases associated with increased elastic recoil (e.g., lung fibrosis) are associated with decreased FRC, whereas diseases associated with decreased elastic recoil (e.g., emphysema) are associated with increased FRC.

The FRC is measured by either a gas dilution (nitrogen or helium) or a plethysmographic technique, and the TLC and RV are calculated from the equations previously described. Importantly, plethysmography allows for an estimation of all the gas in the chest, whereas gas dilution measures only the gas in spaces that communicate freely with the airways. Thus, under certain conditions, FRC measured by the gas dilution technique may underestimate the FRC because of poor distribution of the gas. This can be observed in noncommunicating bullae and in the setting of bronchospasm or mucous plugging.

Restrictive impairments are defined as a low TLC and a low FRC, and their severity is based on the percentage predicted for a particular patient based on age, sex, height, and race. Restrictive disorders can occur in three circumstances: lung disorders, disorders of the chest wall, and neuromuscular disease. Lung disorders with interstitial infiltration typically show restriction caused by increased elastic recoil such as observed in idiopathic pulmonary fibrosis and sarcoidosis. Lung edema as a result of congestive heart failure can also cause a restrictive pattern. Chest wall abnormalities may exhibit themselves with a restrictive pattern by restricting lung expansion as observed in kyphoscoliosis, obesity, and ankylosing spondylitis. Included in the chest wall abnormalities are the pleural diseases (e.g., pleural effusion, pneumothorax), space-occupying lesions (e.g., pleural tumors), and conditions causing increased abdominal girth such as pregnancy, ascites, and large intra-abdominal tumors. Some neuromuscular disorders cause restriction by preventing normal excursion of the lung during breathing as observed in patients with myasthenia gravis, amyotrophic lateral sclerosis, diaphragmatic paralysis, and the Guillain-Barré syndrome. Patients may also restrict lung excursion during inspiration as a result of pain or somnolence (e.g., drug overdose). Similarly, lung resection during lobectomy or pneumonectomy will cause a restrictive defect.

In summary, spirometry and lung volume measurements can identify lung disorders characterized by obstruction and restriction. In obstructive disorders, spirometry shows decreased FEV_1 and decreased $FEV_1/FVC\%$. When obstruction is significant, lung volumes may be increased (increased TLC and RV) as a result of hyperinflation and air trapping. The severity of the obstructive defect is estimated on the basis of the FEV_1. In restrictive disorders, the FEV_1 may be decreased, but the $FEV_1/FVC\%$ will be preserved. However, the TLC, FRC, and RV will be decreased. The severity of the restrictive defect is based on the TLC.

PEAK EXPIRATORY FLOW RATE

The peak expiratory flow rate (PEFR) can be measured with a hand-held device that can be used at the bedside. The lower the PEFR, the more significant the obstruction. The device is useful to evaluate the severity of an obstructive impairment at home or in the emergency department. Severe attacks as observed in patients with asthma are usually associated with PEFRs of less than 120 to 200 L/min (normal is 500 to 600 L/min).

GAS EXCHANGE

Diffusing Lung Capacity

Information about gas exchange can be obtained by measuring the diffusing capacity and PaO_2 and $PaCO_2$. The diffusing capacity of the lung is estimated by measuring the diffusing capacity for carbon monoxide (D_LCO). This maneuver requires the measurement of exhaled carbon monoxide after inhalation of a known concentration of this gas. Carbon monoxide diffuses freely and has a high affinity for hemoglobin. The rate of transfer of carbon monoxide into the blood (mL/min per mm Hg concentration gradient) can be calculated after measuring the amount of carbon monoxide remaining in the exhaled gas.

The D_LCO is often decreased in interstitial lung disease and is a good marker of poor gas exchange. However, this measurement provides only an overall assessment of gas exchange and depends on many factors including access of the gas to the gas exchanging area, surface area of the lung, the physical properties of the gas (e.g., carbon monoxide), perfusion of the ventilated areas, hemoglobin concentration, and thickness of the alveolar-capillary membrane. Alterations in any of these variables can affect the D_LCO measurement. Therefore, an abnormal D_LCO does not always signify defects in gas transfer as a result of derangements in the alveolar-capillary membrane. Rather, an abnormal measurement could be related to decreased surface area (e.g., pneumonectomy), poor perfusion (e.g., pulmonary embolism), or poor access of the gas to the alveoli (e.g., acute bronchospasm, mucous plugging). A prolonged circulatory transit time (e.g., mild congestive heart failure) and polycythemia may be associated with a mildly increased D_LCO.

The D_LCO is often affected early in interstitial lung disease related to toxic drugs and related disorders and is therefore an important component of the evaluation of patients with interstitial lung disease. In emphysema, destruction of the vasculature within the alveolar septa also leads to decreased D_LCO (**Web Fig. 16–4**). However, in diseases where isolated involvement of the airways (e.g., asthma) develops, the D_LCO is typically not affected.

Arterial Blood Gases

The measurement of PaO_2 and $PaCO_2$ provides information about the adequacy of oxygenation and ventilation. This requires arterial blood sampling through arterial puncture or indwelling cannula (Table 16–2). Oxygenation can also be measured through noninvasive devices including the pulse oximeter, which measures hemoglobin oxygen saturation, and through transcutaneous devices that measure PaO_2 and $PaCO_2$. These devices are particularly useful for measuring oxygenation during exertion in the office setting. Often, alterations in oxygenation are not detected at rest, but they are unveiled during exertion. The 6-minute walk test is a standardized test in which the patient walks for 6 minutes

Table 16–2	**Normal Values for Arterial Blood Gases**

Po_2: 104 − (0.27 × age)

Pco_2: 36–44

pH: 7.35–7.45

Alveolar-arterial O_2 difference = 2.5 + 0.21 × age

Po_2 = partial pressure of oxygen; Pco_2 = partial pressure of carbon dioxide; O_2 = oxygen.

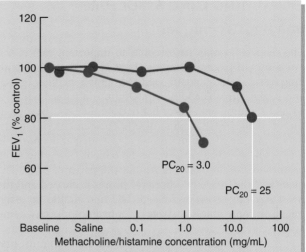

Figure 16–12 Bronchoprovocation challenge. Patients are exposed to increasing concentrations of an inhaled challenge (e.g., methacholine, histamine) followed by evaluation of FEV_1 (percent control). The FEV_1 falls at lower concentrations of the challenge drug in a patient with asthma (*blue circles*) when compared with an individual without asthma (*red circles*).

while the oxygen hemoglobin saturation is measured. A decrease in the oxygen hemoglobin saturation is abnormal and suggests impaired gas exchange capabilities.

A flow diagram depicting how these pulmonary function tests can be used to evaluate patients with obstructive and restrictive disorders is depicted in **Web Fig. 16–5**.

Specialized Studies

CARDIOPULMONARY EXERCISE TESTING

During cardiopulmonary exercise testing, the cardiac rhythm, ventilation, oxygen uptake, carbon dioxide output, and arterial blood gases are measured. Exercise requires adequate ventilation, diffusion, and oxygen uptake by hemoglobin, distribution of cardiac output, and uptake and use of oxygen by tissue. Thus, any abnormalities interfering with one or more of these steps can cause exercise limitation. Similar to other pulmonary function tests, this cardiopulmonary test does not provide a diagnosis; however, monitoring the variables previously described provides the clinician the information to determine whether dyspnea is related to an intrinsic lung abnormality, a cardiac process, or deconditioning.

BRONCHIAL BRONCHOPROVOCATION TESTING

Some OLDs might be associated with hyper-reactive airways such as in the patient with asthma in whom identifying this abnormality is sometimes important for establishing a diagnosis. However, patients with asthma are occasionally asymptomatic and show little physiologic abnormalities at the time of evaluation. If the patient's history, physical examination, or prebronchodilator and postbronchodilator testing cannot identify hyperreactive airways, then a bronchoprovocation (challenge) test might be useful. This test is also useful in the evaluation of certain allergens that might be causing airway symptoms in patients by recreating the challenge in a safe environment.

The test requires the inhalation of bronchoconstrictors such as methacholine and histamine, or stimulation with hypertonic or hypotonic solutions, exercise, or cold and dry air hyperventilation. When drugs are used, they are administered in incremental doses until 20% or more fall in FEV_1 from baseline is noted. Patients with asthma demonstrate this fall in FEV_1 at doses considerably smaller than normal individuals (Fig. 16–12).

SLEEP STUDIES

Sleep disordered breathing is the term used to define abnormal lung function that is triggered during sleep. During the transition between wakefulness and sleep, input from the behavioral control system decreases, the hypoxic drive to breathing is reduced, and the ventilatory response to $PaCO_2$ is diminished. These changes are most dramatic during rapid eye movement (REM) sleep and are heightened in sleep disordered breathing, which causes abnormal respiratory function, hypoxemia, and fragmented sleep.

Sleep disordered breathing is best assessed with overnight polysomnography. Continuous recordings of electrocardiographic and electroencephalographic tracings are made while the patient sleeps. In addition, airflow, oxygen saturation, and respiratory, eye, chin, and limb muscle movements are monitored and recorded. This test serves to identify patients with obstructive sleep apnea during which a cessation of airflow occurs, despite the presence of breathing movements. In central sleep apnea, cessation of airflow follows cessation of breathing movements. These disorders can be associated with nocturnal oxygen hemoglobin desaturation and cardiac arrhythmias. The test can also help evaluate for other sleep disturbances including insomnias, narcolepsy, and parasomnias.

EVALUATING LUNG STRUCTURE

Imaging Techniques

The *chest radiograph* has become an important tool in the evaluation of patients who may have or are diagnosed with lung disease. The standard chest radiograph includes frontal and lateral films. The ideal frontal film is obtained with the patient standing with his or her back to the x-ray beam and the chest against the film cassette (posteroanterior film). Sometimes, an ideal film cannot be obtained and a portable film is taken, which usually has the patient facing the x-ray beam and the film cassette behind the patient's back. The quality of the image in a portable film is decreased and the heart size can be overestimated. The film should be taken on inspiration unless a suggested pneumothorax is being assessed.

When reading a chest radiograph, the clinician must first assess the quality of the film. Importantly, the clinician must assess proper positioning of the patient during the filming and distinguish between a standard posteroanterior film and a portable film to interpret the image appropriately. A posteroanterior film usually shows careful centralization of the body (as observed when the heads of the clavicles are equidistant to the spinous process) and an absence of scapular densities within the lung field. Often, a gastric bulb can be detected, indicating that the film was obtained while the patient was upright. In a properly penetrated film, the lower thoracic vertebral interspaces and the left lower lobe should be barely visible through the cardiac silhouette. If these interspaces are not easily seen, then the film is over penetrated. After proper positioning is assessed, the clinician should proceed with examination of the film by evaluating the lungs and pulmonary vasculature, the bony thorax, the heart and great vessels, the diaphragms and pleura, the mediastinum, the soft tissues, and the sub-diaphragmatic areas. The chest radiograph can eliminate some structural abnormalities from consideration and can demonstrate abnormalities such as infiltrates, interstitial disease, vascular disease, masses, pleural effusions and thickening, cavitary lung disease, cardiac enlargement, and some airway diseases. The plain radiograph in combination with the history and physical examination are often sufficient to diagnose chest disease. In many circumstances, however, additional imaging techniques are necessary to define the disease process more clearly.

Computed tomographic (CT) imaging has many applications in pulmonary medicine and, because it avoids the superimposition of shadows, it provides information that cannot be obtained through regular chest radiography. The CT image is created by measuring the attenuation coefficients of a 1-cm thick axial beam in many projections, and a computerized algorithm reconstructs a cross-sectional image. Sequential CT imaging at intervals of a few seconds during contrast administration is called a *dynamic computed tomogram*. Progressive opacification of a structure in question implies that it is a vessel or an extremely vascularized lesion. Important uses of CT imaging are to:

- Evaluate pulmonary nodules and masses
- Distinguish pleural thickening from pleural fluid
- Estimate the size of the heart and the presence of pericardial fluid or thickening

- Identify discriminate patterns of involvement in interstitial lung disease
- Detect and define cavities
- Identify intracavitary processes such as mycetomas or fluid
- Quantify the extent and distribution of emphysema
- Detect and measure mediastinal adenopathy and masses
- Evaluate proximal clots in pulmonary arteries.

Increased attention has been given to the *spiral CT* scan because of its usefulness as a screening technique in patients with suggested acute pulmonary embolus, and this test has become the test of choice in this setting at many institutions. Certain patterns of calcification of pulmonary nodules, such as eggshell or popcorn calcification, can rule out malignancy and the need for invasive diagnostic procedures.

High-resolution CT (HRCT) is a variant of CT that uses thin collimation (1- to 2-mm slice), a special reconstruction algorithm that sharpens soft-tissue interfaces, and image reconstruction, among others, to provide a superior visualization of the pulmonary parenchyma, including secondary lobule and interlobular septa. HRCT is very useful in the evaluation of patients who may have interstitial lung disease and bronchiectasis.

Magnetic resonance imaging (MRI) is a tomographic imaging technique based on nuclei of a target element, usually hydrogen, aligning as a result of a strong magnetic field. In response to stimulation by a radiofrequency signal, a radio signal with the same frequency is emitted. Differing images can be obtained by varying the times between stimulations and the time after maximum signal. Fat produces the strongest signal, whereas air and air-containing lung, bone, and flowing blood produce little to no signal. MRI may differentiate tumor from normal tissues, pneumonia, or atelectasis.

Pulmonary angiography is used to evaluate the pulmonary vasculature after the administration of intravascular dye followed by imaging of the lungs via x-ray studies. This procedure is considered the gold standard for evaluating patients who may have acute pulmonary embolism. Risk factors are mainly related to bleeding, allergic reactions to the dye, and transient pulmonary hypertension.

Positron-emission tomographic (PET) imaging can aid in the diagnosis and staging of lung cancer. It detects metabolically active masses greater than 1 cm in diameter and enlarged mediastinal nodes with considerable sensitivity. However, it does not distinguish between inflammation and malignancy, an important issue in areas with endemic fungal lung disease.

Bronchoscopy

Fiberoptic bronchoscopy is commonly performed by pulmonologists under sedation. The bronchoscope can be introduced nasally, orally, or through an artificial airway or tracheostomy. This procedure allows for direct visualization of the airways and photography. Bronchial washing allows for harvesting fluid from the more proximal airways, whereas bronchoalveolar lavage allows for suctioning fluid from the distal air spaces, which could be submitted for study (e.g., cytology, cell counts, culture, special stains). Bronchial brushings allow for scraping of the bronchial mucosa.

Bronchial tissue can be obtained through bronchial biopsies, whereas transbronchial biopsies are performed with forceps that allow sampling of the distal airways and lung parenchyma. Transthoracic needle aspiration can be performed through the bronchoscope to assess submucosal or extrabronchial areas.

Bronchoscopy is most often used to evaluate the airways and to examine for infection. However, it can be used to retrieve foreign bodies, to suction secretions to re-expand an atelectatic lung, to perform neodymium–yttrium-aluminum-garnet (YAG) laser therapy of endobronchial lesions, to assist with difficult endotracheal intubations, or to guide the placement of catheters for brachytherapy of lung cancer. It is a safe procedure with major complications (e.g., significant bleeding, pneumothorax, respiratory failure) occurring in 0.1% to 1.7% of patients and mortality in 0.01% to 0.1% of patients. Transbronchial biopsies increase the rate of complications.

Thoracic surgeons or pulmonologists with extensive training (invasive pulmonologists) usually perform *rigid bronchoscopy* under general anesthesia in the surgical department. It is the preferred procedure when evaluating or treating massive hemoptysis, for laser ablation of large intraluminal lesions, for removal of foreign bodies, and for placing airway stents and dilating tracheobronchial strictures.

Other

Percutaneous transthoracic needle aspiration and biopsy of lung lesions can be performed under fluoroscopic, sono-graphic, or CT guidance. It is performed mainly for the cytologic diagnosis of malignancy. The diagnostic yield for malignancy is 82% to 97%, and it is 73% to 94% for benign disease. *Mediastinoscopy* is a procedure by which an instrument is inserted in the mediastinum anteriorly and passed posteriorly to the sternum and anteriorly to the trachea to visualize and sample lymph nodes in that area and in the subcarinal area. It is often used for staging in lung cancer. *Open-lung biopsy* is usually indicated when less invasive procedures fail to provide a diagnosis, when the patient is not responding to empiric therapy, and when the clinician believes that histologic findings are likely to affect management. Recently, the use of *video-assisted thoraco-scopic-guided lung biopsy* has diminished the morbidity inherent with the procedure while allowing for adequate sampling of tissue.

References

Grippi MA, Metzger LF, Sacks AV, et al (Eds-in-Chief): Fishman's Pulmonary Diseases and Disorders. New York, McGraw-Hill, 1998, pp 533–574.

Miller WT: Radiographic evaluation of the chest. In Fishman AP (Ed-in-Chief): Fishman's Pulmonary Diseases and Disorders. New York, McGraw-Hill, 1998, pp 433–486.

Rubin LJ: Primary pulmonary hypertension. N Engl J Med, 336:111–117, 1997.

West JB: Pulmonary Pathology: The Essentials, 5th ed. Baltimore, Williams & Wilkins, 1998.

West JB: Respiratory Physiology: The Essentials, 5th ed. Baltimore, Williams & Wilkins, 1995.

West JB, Wagner PD: Pulmonary gas exchange. Am J Respir Crit Care Med, 157:S82–S87, 1988.

Obstructive Lung Diseases

Jesse Roman

Kenneth L. Brigham

The obstructive lung diseases are a group of disorders that cause dyspnea and are characterized by airflow limitation on pulmonary function testing (*obstructive pattern*). These disorders are very common and include *emphysema, chronic bronchitis, bronchiolitis, asthma, cystic fibrosis,* and *bronchiectasis,* among others. Some of these disorders co-exist in the same patient; are induced by the same etiologic factors (e.g., tobacco exposure); cannot be distinguished from each other by physical examination, physiologic testing, or imaging studies; and their treatments are similarly based on the current understanding of the pathophysiologic features of each. Such disorders (e.g., emphysema, chronic bronchitis, chronic bronchiolitis) have been classified together in the clinical term *chronic obstructive pulmonary disease* (COPD). In general, COPD is characterized by irreversible or poorly reversible airflow limitation, and this definition serves to distinguish this group of disorders from asthma, a chronic inflammatory disease of the airways characterized by airway hyperactivity and reversible airflow limitation (Fig. 17–1).

The flow of air through the bronchial tree is directly proportional to the driving pressure and is inversely proportional to the resistance. In obstructive lung disease, alterations in one or both of these processes might be involved. For example, in emphysema, airflow limitation is mainly caused by decreased elastic recoil resulting in decreased driving pressure. In asthma, airflow limitation is due to bronchoconstriction that causes increased airway resistance. Airway obstruction to flow causes characteristic changes in lung volumes. The residual volume and functional residual capacity are increased, whereas the total lung capacity remains normal or increased. Vital capacity is reduced by the increase in residual volume. Several factors contribute to the increase in functional residual capacity and residual volume in obstructive lung disease. Decreased lung elastic recoil increases the functional residual capacity because of reduced opposition to the outward force exerted by the chest wall. Loss of airway tone and decreased tethering by surrounding lung in COPD, as well as bronchoconstriction and mucous plugging in acute asthma, allow airways to collapse at higher lung volumes and trap excessive air. Finally, under demands for increased minute ventilation, the increased resistance to airflow may not allow the lungs to empty completely during the time available for expiration.

The three major consequences of these changes in lung volume are as follows: (1) Breathing at higher lung volumes requires a higher change in pressure for the same change in lung volume, and this requirement increases the work of breathing. (2) Larger lung volumes place the inspiratory muscles at a mechanical disadvantage. The diaphragm is flattened, thereby decreasing its ability to change intrathoracic volume, and all the inspiratory muscle fibers are shortened, decreasing the tension they are able to exert to effect changes in lung volume. (3) Larger lung volumes occur, during which the tethering of the narrowed and collapsing airways by the surrounding lung parenchyma tend to retain airway patency and reduce airway resistance and air trapping; this consequence is beneficial. These three physiologic derangements explain many of the clinical features of obstructive lung diseases (Table 17–1).

Although the consequences to lung function are similar in the obstructive lung diseases, their pathogenesis and prognosis are different. Therefore, a careful evaluation is needed to reach a definitive diagnosis that will guide targeted therapy.

Chronic Obstructive Pulmonary Disease

COPD is a term that includes a group of pulmonary disorders that cause dyspnea and that are characterized by structural changes in the lung that lead to progressive irreversible or fixed airflow limitation. This term encompasses emphysema, chronic bronchitis, and chronic bronchiolitis, as well as pulmonary disorders that have common clinical, radiographic, and physiologic manifestations and, more importantly, often co-exist in the same patient. The term excludes other causes of airflow obstruction such as cystic fibrosis, bronchiectasis, which may also cause irreversible airflow obstruction, and asthma.

COPD is one of the most common disorders seen by physicians, and it is the fourth leading cause of death in the United States. Prevalence rates for COPD are higher in men than in women and are correlated with increasing age, lower socioeconomic status, and smoking. Hispanics appear to be more affected than whites, who are more affected than African Americans. COPD accounts for 10% bed occupancy in most hospitals around the country, and approximately 500,000 patients with COPD are discharged from the hospital each year.

Cigarette smoking is the most common cause of COPD (over 90%); however, other factors such as air pollution, occupational exposures to dust and fumes, and infections contribute to the occurrence, severity, and progression of the disease. Although cigarette smoking is the most common cause, it is important to note that only 20% of smokers develop clinically significant COPD. This finding suggests that COPD results from a susceptibility to environmental factors (e.g., tobacco) as a result of a genetic predisposition. A genetic predisposition is also implied by the documentation of familial clusters of COPD.

Several longitudinal studies have defined patterns of age-related decline in lung function and have documented the concept of susceptibility to COPD. These studies show that most adult nonsmoking men exhibit a decline in forced expiratory volume in 1 second (FEV_1) of 35 to 40 mL per year. This rate is increased to 45 to 60 mL per year in the majority of cigarette smokers. However, the susceptible smoker may demonstrate losses of 70 to 120 mL per year (Fig. 17–2). This information allows the physician to project the rate of decrease of lung function in patients with COPD and assess the effects of therapeutic interventions.

The only genetic disorder thus far linked to COPD is α_1-antitrypsin deficiency, which accounts for less than 1% of all

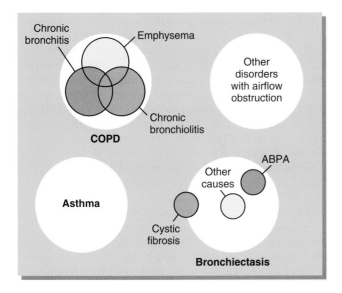

Figure 17–1 Classification of obstructive lung diseases.

Table 17–1 Features of Obstructive Lung Diseases

Disorder	Clinical Features	Laboratory Findings
Chronic obstructive lung disease	Chronic progressive dyspnea	Decreased expiratory flow rates, hypoxia and hypercapnia in end-stage disease
Emphysema	Little or no sputum, end-stage cachexia	Hyperinflation, increased compliance, low D_LCo, rarely α_1-antitrypsin deficiency
Chronic bronchitis	Sputum, history of smoking, industrial exposure	Nonspecific; rarely occurs in isolation without varying degrees of emphysema
Asthma	Episodic dyspnea, cough, wheezing, with or without environmental triggers	Airway hyper-reactivity, response to bronchodilators
Bronchiectasis	Usually large volume of sputum	Chest radiograph: dilated bronchi, thick-walled, tram track shadows, obstruction with or without restriction on pulmonary function tests
Immotile cilia syndrome	Situs inversus, dextrocardia, sinusitis, infertility	Abnormal dynein in ciliated cells
Hypogammaglobulinemia		Decrease in one or more immunoglobulins
Cystic fibrosis	Sinusitis, bronchiectasis, meconium ileus, malabsorption, infertility	Increased sweat chloride, mutation in CFTR chloride channel, elevated fecal fat, abnormal nasal mucosal potential difference

CFTR = CF transmembrane conductance regulator; D_LCo = diffusion capacity for carbon monoxide.

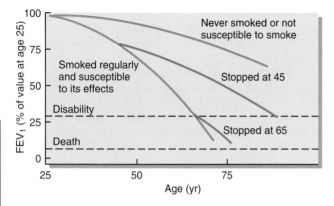

Figure 17–2 Pattern of decline in forced expiratory volume in 1 second (FEV$_1$) with risks of morbidity and mortality from respiration disease in a susceptible smoker in comparison with a normal patient or a nonsusceptible smoker. Although cessation of smoking does not replenish the lung function already lost in a susceptible smoker, it decreases the rate of further decline. (Data from Fletcher C, Peto R: The natural history of chronic airflow obstruction. BMJ 1:1645–1648, 1977.)

cases. The deficient enzyme, α_1-antitrypsin, is produced primarily in the liver from which it travels to the lung where it deactivates elastases released by inflammatory cells that are capable of degrading connective tissue matrices. In doing so, α_1-antitrypsin prevents the uncontrolled degradation of elastin in the lung parenchyma and protects against the development of emphysema. Patients who develop emphysema at a young age (<40 years) should be evaluated for this condition whether or not they smoke.

Emphysema

Emphysema is an entity included within the general term COPD. It is defined in pathologic terms as permanent enlargement of air spaces as a result of destruction of the lung parenchyma in the absence of significant fibrosis. These changes result in an abnormal acinus with limited capabilities for gas exchange. Based on thin gross lung sections, emphysema can be classified into *centriacinar* and *panacinar*. In centriacinar emphysema, the proximal part of the acinus (the respiratory bronchiole) is affected, which represents the most common histologic feature observed in emphysema related to smoking, whereas panacinar emphysema is typically seen in α_1-antitrypsin deficiency.

The discovery of the association between α_1-antitrypsin and emphysema in the 1960s led to the hypothesis that emphysema is caused by an imbalance in protease-antiprotease systems favoring the former and leading to uncontrolled destruction of the lung connective tissue. In particular, elastin was believed to be the main target of lung proteases because the absence of α_1-antitrypsin prevents elastase inactivation. Excessive destruction of elastin fibers that is due to the absence of inhibitory proteases leads to decreased elastic recoil and explains many of the clinical manifestations of emphysema. Although excess elastase that is due to chronic lung inflammation might overwhelm even normal levels of α_1-antitrypsin, other protease-antiprotease systems might contribute to the development of this condi-

tion (i.e., the *protease-antiprotease hypothesis*). Currently, increased interest exists in the potential role of matrix metalloproteinases in the lung and how disturbances in their expression and activation in cigarette smokers might lead to emphysema.

Because elastases, matrix metalloproteinases, and other proteases can be delivered to the lung by neutrophils, macrophages, and other immune cells, *inflammation* is also considered a key process in the development of emphysema. Many studies have documented an increase in the expression and protein levels of pro-inflammatory cytokines in emphysema leading to the idea that the persistent delivery of pro-inflammatory molecules to the lung stimulates immune cell recruitment with subsequent delivery of proteases that destroy lung tissue. Inflammation also results in mucosal edema and increased mucus production, both of which narrow the airway. Persistent or recurrent inflammation can destroy structural elements of the bronchial walls and can result in the fixed bronchial dilation and distortion found in bronchiectasis. *Oxidant stress* also contributes by causing lipid peroxidation, activation of proteases, and expression of pro-inflammatory cytokines, among other effects (**Web Fig. 17–1**). *Neurogenic stimuli* are also considered important in the pathogenesis of obstructive airway disease. The conducting airways are surrounded by smooth muscle, which contains adrenergic and cholinergic receptors. Stimulation of β_2-adrenergic receptors by circulating catecholamines dilates airways, whereas stimulation of airway irritant receptors constricts airways through a cholinergic mechanism via the vagus nerve. The irritant bronchoconstricting pathways are normally present to protect against inhalation of noxious agents, but in pathologic states, these pathways may contribute to airway hyper-reactivity. A host of endogenous chemical mediators such as proteases, growth factors, and cytokines can affect airway tone.

Clearly, the mechanisms that lead to emphysema are complex and multifactorial, and more studies are required to elucidate its pathogenesis. Because tobacco is the most common offender leading to emphysema, many studies, not surprisingly, document the ability of tobacco smoke to activate these pathways.

CLINICAL MANIFESTATIONS

In general, emphysema caused by chronic cigarette smoking is not observed in patients before 40 years of age. If it is, then consideration should be given to genetic disorders such as α_1-antitrypsin deficiency. Emphysema related to chronic tobacco exposure is exhibited by slowly progressive dyspnea that is first noted during exertion but that progresses over years until it is evident at rest. Affected individuals might complain of exercise intolerance and fatigue, and the disease eventually leads to weight loss, depression, and/or anxiety as a result of increased work of breathing. Chronic cough can be present, and it could be productive or dry depending on the degree of airway involvement (e.g., chronic bronchitis).

During the early stages of emphysema, the physical examination may be normal. A normal examination and the absence of symptoms often delay diagnosis. Inspection of the thorax and palpation may fail to reveal findings. As the disease progresses, the lungs might be hyper-resonant to percussion, and auscultation may show few rhonchi, wheezes, or faint crackles. During the late stages of emphysema, patients show evidence of increased work of breathing as highlighted by the use of accessory muscles and pursed lips, and weight loss. Despite their respiratory insufficiency, these patients are able to work to sustain relatively normal oxygen levels in blood until very late in the disease, leading to the classic clinical presentation of the "pink puffer." However, hypoxemia may occur during exercise and sleep.

As the disease progresses the lung volumes increase (hyperinflation) and the diaphragms flatten, which renders the inspiratory excursions inefficient. Tidal volume decreases and respiratory rate increases in an effort to decrease work of breathing. In advanced disease, the cardio-vascular system becomes affected as a result of a loss of vasculature in destroyed alveolar walls. With limited area for blood flow, pulmonary pressures rise (i.e., pulmonary vascular hypertension), leading to right ventricular strain. This development, together with the constriction of the pulmonary vessels as a result of hypoxemia, can accelerate the development of right ventricular failure, which is referred to as *cor pulmonale* in the setting of lung disease. Heart gallop, distended neck veins, hepatojugular reflux, and leg edema characterize cor pulmonale.

EVALUATION

Airway narrowing, which increases resistance to airflow, or a loss of elastic recoil of the lung, which decreases driving pressure, can decrease airflow in the lungs. Both of these physiologic abnormalities are often present in COPD. They can be detected by pulmonary function tests, which are essential for the diagnosis of obstructive pulmonary disease, for assessing its severity, and for evaluating response to therapy. Emphysema is characterized by airflow obstruction as defined by a reduced maximum expiratory flow mainly the result of a loss of elastic driving pressures but also by increased resistance to flow in the small airways. *Spirometry,* which reveals decreased FEV_1, best detects this characterization. The decrease in FEV_1 predominates when compared with that of the forced vital capacity (FVC) leading to reduction of the FEV_1/FVC %; a reduced FEV_1 and FEV_1/FVC% is pathognomonic of airflow limitation.

Although some degree of reversibility can be detected with bronchodilators and hyper-reactivity can be unveiled by bronchoprovocation challenge, the obstructive defect is not entirely reversible in emphysema. This characteristic and the progressive nature of the obstruction represent key features that help distinguish this entity (and COPD in general) from asthma. The severity of disease and prognosis can be estimated by the FEV_1; an FEV_1 around 1 L (usually 50% of predicted levels) suggests severe obstruction and, in the case of COPD, predicts a mean survival of 50% at 5 years.

Lung volumes should be measured because the limitation to expired airflow and decreased elastic recoil lead to lung hyperinflation, evidenced by increased residual volumes, functional residual capacity, and, ultimately, total lung capacity. Increased lung volume leads to flattening of the diaphragm, which causes shortening of its muscle fibers, reducing contractile efficiency.

Destruction of alveoli decreases the surface area for gas exchange. This loss of surface area, coupled with bronchial obstruction and altered distribution of ventilated air, result in ventilation/perfusion (V/Q) inequality or mismatch, which may cause hypoxemia. Hyperinflation of the lungs increases zone 1 conditions, in which alveolar pressure exceeds pulmonary arterial pressure, a process that stops perfusion and creates a physiologic dead space. Hypercarbia, but not hypoxemia, can be avoided by hyperventilation, even with substantial V/Q mismatching. However, eventually, the metabolic costs of breathing become excessive and respiratory muscles fatigue. Over time, chemoreceptors *reset*, allowing the level of partial pressure of carbon dioxide in arterial blood ($PaCO_2$) to rise, which increases the efficiency of ventilation by eliminating a higher concentration of carbon dioxide per breath, lowering the metabolic cost. Significant individual variation is observed in the degree of mechanical impairment and in the magnitude of increase in $PaCO_2$. Derangements in gas exchange can be detected by performing arterial blood gases. They can also be detected by showing a decrease in lung *diffusion capacity for carbon monoxide* (D_LCO) or by evaluating hemoglobin oxygen desaturation during exertion.

Chest radiographs might fail to reveal abnormalities during the early stages of emphysema, but in later stages, radiographic studies show hyperinflation, hyperlucency, flattening of the diaphragms, and bullous changes in lung parenchyma. Pleural abnormalities, lymphadenopathy, and mediastinal widening are not characteristic of emphysema and should point to other diagnoses such as lung cancer. *Computed tomography* (CT) is more sensitive than plain radiographs because CT allows for a more detailed evaluation of the lung parenchyma and surrounding structures. The *electrocardiogram* might show evidence of right ventricular strain. Blood tests might reveal erythrocytosis in the setting of chronic hypoxemia, whereas increased white blood cell counts might suggest infection.

MANAGEMENT

Because a cure for emphysema does not exist, the best approach to this condition resides in its prevention. The majority of cases of emphysema in the United States are due to cigarette smoking. Thus, a major emphasis has been placed on the development of educational programs that emphasize smoking prevention and promote smoking cessation. Currently, available smoking cessation strategies are effective in only 30% of patients and, for the most part, are not long lasting without strong commitment demonstrated by the patient. Nicotine replacement with gum or transdermal patches, bupropion, behavior modification, and long-term physician and group support increase the success of cessation attempts. Most patients who are successful at smoking cessation have had at least one prior failed attempt; this finding should encourage physicians to continue to counsel patients against smoking at every opportunity.

Once emphysema is established, therapy is directed at avoiding complications (e.g., infection), relieving airflow obstruction by increasing the caliber of the airways, and diminishing the effects of inadequate oxygenation. Drugs that are used to diminish airway obstruction include bronchodilators, anti-inflammatory drugs, and mucolytics. Sympathomimetic agents (β_2-adrenoreceptor agonists) are the most potent bronchodilators, although the anticholinergic drug ipratropium bromide may be superior in the management of COPD. In practice, a combination of the two agents and/or the use of long-acting agents are preferable to improve compliance. Albuterol is the most commonly used β-agonist; its bronchodilator effect is rapid in onset and is relatively short lived. The long-acting β-agonists salmeterol and salbutamol can be administered twice daily and are effective for maintenance therapy. Tiotropium is a long-acting anticholinergic that has been found to improve symptoms in patients with COPD. Combinations of these agents (e.g., albuterol, ipratropium bromide) are available commercially.

Bronchodilator drugs can be delivered either by a metered-dose inhaler (MDI) or nebulizer. The MDI offers advantages of portability and ease of administration and convenience. When used correctly with a spacer, MDIs are as effective as nebulizers in delivering the drug. Nebulization has no advantage over the use of MDIs in the long-term management of obstructive lung disease except in patients unable to use an MDI properly.

Methylxanthine medications, such as theophylline, are weak systemic sympathomimetic agents with a narrow therapeutic window; they are not first-line drugs in the treatment of obstructive lung disease, although long-acting derivatives with improved safety profiles have been recently developed. Theophylline preparations have some anti-inflammatory activity and may provide additional bronchodilation in patients with COPD who do not respond adequately to inhaled β-agonists. When these preparations are used, blood concentrations should be maintained in the lower end of the therapeutic range (between 8 and 12 mcg/mL). Toxicity is common at concentrations higher than 20 mcg/mL. The metabolism of theophylline is decreased by many commonly used drugs (e.g., erythromycin), and toxic serum concentrations of theophylline can be reached quickly when these other drugs are administered unless the theophylline dose is adjusted appropriately. Toxic effects of theophylline may be observed in the gastrointestinal, cardiac, and neurologic systems. Severe theophylline toxicity could be fatal and may require treatment with charcoal hemoperfusion.

Until the mid-1990s, the use of anti-inflammatory agents for the treatment of stable (not acute) airway obstruction was uncommon mainly because of limited data indicating a role for these agents in improving symptoms and prolonging survival. However, current data suggest that the chronic use of inhaled corticosteroids improves symptoms, decreases exacerbations, and may improve survival. For this reason, inhaled long-acting corticosteroids (e.g., fluticasone propionate, budesonide) are indicated in the treatment of emphysema. These agents can be found combined with long-acting β-agonists. Systemic use of corticosteroids is indicated during acute exacerbations, and intravenous corticosteroids have been proved useful in the acute setting. Intravenous corticosteroids have also proved effective for the management of acute exacerbations of most obstructive lung diseases including cases of asthma (Fig. 17–3). The use of other agents with anti-inflammatory capabilities such as leukotriene inhibitors is not indicated at the present time.

Chronic oxygen supplementation is now commonly used in patients with advanced emphysema and related obstructive lung disorders because oxygen is the only intervention

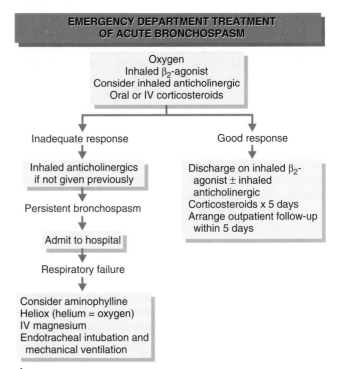

EMERGENCY DEPARTMENT TREATMENT OF ACUTE BRONCHOSPASM

Oxygen
Inhaled β₂-agonist
Consider inhaled anticholinergic
Oral or IV corticosteroids

Inadequate response

Inhaled anticholinergics if not given previously

Persistent bronchospasm

Admit to hospital

Respiratory failure

Consider aminophylline
Heliox (helium = oxygen)
IV magnesium
Endotracheal intubation and mechanical ventilation

Good response

Discharge on inhaled β₂-agonist ± inhaled anticholinergic
Corticosteroids x 5 days
Arrange outpatient follow-up within 5 days

A

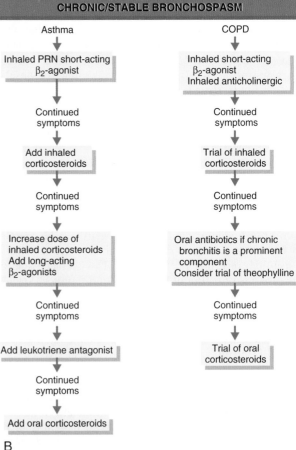

OUTPATIENT TREATMENT OF CHRONIC/STABLE BRONCHOSPASM

Asthma

Inhaled PRN short-acting β₂-agonist

Continued symptoms

Add inhaled corticosteroids

Continued symptoms

Increase dose of inhaled corticosteroids
Add long-acting β₂-agonists

Continued symptoms

Add leukotriene antagonist

Continued symptoms

Add oral corticosteroids

COPD

Inhaled short-acting β₂-agonist
Inhaled anticholinergic

Continued symptoms

Trial of inhaled corticosteroids

Continued symptoms

Oral antibiotics if chronic bronchitis is a prominent component
Consider trial of theophylline

Continued symptoms

Trial of oral corticosteroids

B

Figure 17–3 Algorithms for the treatment of bronchospasm in the emergency department (*A*) and in outpatients with stable disease (*B*).

that has been shown to improve survival in patients with COPD. Oxygen supplementation is recommended once the partial pressure of oxygen in arterial blood (PaO_2) drops below 55 mm Hg or the hemoglobin oxygen saturation decreases to 88%. Oxygen supplementation might be needed at earlier stages if end-organ damage as a result of hypoxemia is documented (e.g., congestive heart failure, mental deterioration, pulmonary hypertension).

Oxygen therapy is frequently necessary in acute exacerbations of obstructive lung disease. In patients who hypoventilate chronically and therefore have an elevated $PaCO_2$, elevating the inspired oxygen content may acutely worsen hypercarbia by decreasing ventilatory drive. Nonetheless, arterial oxygen must be maintained in a range compatible with life even at the expense of precipitating respiratory failure requiring mechanical ventilation.

Exacerbations of airway obstruction may result from viral or bacterial infection. The most common bacterial pathogens in COPD are *Streptococcus pneumoniae*, *Haemophilus influenzae*, and *Moraxella catarrhalis*. Management of acute exacerbations should include empiric antibiotics. Immunization with influenza vaccines directed at specific epidemic strains is the single most effective intervention for reducing morbidity and mortality from obstructive lung disease. Pneumococcal vaccination is recommended in older patients and in those with underlying lung disease.

Multiple airway clearance techniques exist to aid clearing of airway secretions, but their effectiveness in the management of emphysema and other obstructive lung diseases is questioned. If needed, then chest physiotherapy and postural drainage might be useful in patients with co-existing chronic bronchitis and increased sputum production. However, the use of mucolytics (e.g., Mucomyst) is questionable in view of the fact that they might irritate the airways.

Patients with pulmonary disease of sufficient severity to compromise normal activities of daily living commonly demonstrate improved quality of life and less subjective dyspnea when enrolled in a comprehensive, high-quality *pulmonary rehabilitation program*. Pulmonary rehabilitation has not been shown to improve objective measures of pulmonary function, to affect the rate of decline in lung function, or to improve survival. However, it has been shown to improve the quality of life in motivated patients. An important part of pulmonary rehabilitation is nutritional assessment and careful attention to maintaining adequate nutrition. Malnutrition and cachexia are common in later stages of obstructive lung disease and result in decreased respiratory muscle strength and compromised immune function.

In certain patients with advanced disease, surgical interventions might prove beneficial. Of these, bullectomy, lung volume reduction surgery (LVRS), and lung transplantation are all potentially effective surgical options for select patients. Resection of nonfunctional areas of lung (e.g., bullectomy) may allow for compressed functional areas to expand and might improve symptoms, airflows, and oxygenation by improving V/Q matching in a subgroup of patients. A similar benefit may be seen after LVRS. The best candidates for LVRS are those with predominantly upper lobe disease, without an asthmatic or a bronchitic component, and without other major co-morbidities. However, in general, a high surgical mortality risk exists in patients with an FEV_1 or D_LCO of less than 20% predicted.

Single or bilateral lung transplantation is an option for patients with end-stage airflow obstruction. In general, the average survival after lung transplantation is 4 to 5 years. Chronic rejection, viral infections, transplant-associated lymphoproliferative disease, and late occurrence of obliterative bronchiolitis remain significant problems of lung transplantation, but the procedure can clearly improve the quality of life and can extend productive life in properly selected patients. Guidelines for the management of COPD in general have been recently revised by the Gold Initiative for COPD and are referred to as the ***GOLD Guidelines***.

Chronic Bronchitis

Chronic bronchitis often coincides with emphysema in the patient with COPD, and it is defined as a persistent cough resulting in sputum production for more than 3 months in each of the past 2 years. Cigarette smoking is the major cause, although exposure to pollutants may also play a role. Pathologic findings are goblet-cell hyperplasia, mucous plugging, and fibrosis.

Many of the inflammatory mechanisms involved in the development of emphysema are considered important in the pathogenesis of chronic bronchitis. However, in contrast to emphysema, chronic bronchitis is primarily a disease of the airways and not the lung parenchyma. Therefore, the main clinical findings are related to airflow limitation that is a result of airway resistance; it is not due to decreased driving force unless emphysema co-exists.

The clinical presentation of patients with chronic bronchitis is similar to that described for patients with emphysema, but a predominant symptom is sputum production. Recurrent bacterial airway infections might also be present. As with other patients with COPD, the evaluation of patients with chronic bronchitis should include pulmonary function tests and a chest radiograph in addition to standard laboratory testing.

The treatment includes the use of inhaled bronchodilators and corticosteroids as described for emphysema. If significant sputum production and retention are considered to cause recurrent exacerbations as a result of airway infection, then chest physiotherapy to promote expectoration is recommended. In selected patients, continuous antibiotic therapy with alternating courses of different agents (rotating antibiotics) may improve outcomes by diminishing exacerbations, hospitalization or visits to the emergency department, and improve symptoms.

Chronic Bronchiolitis

Chronic bronchiolitis is a disease associated with inflammation, fibrosis, and distortion of the small airways (membranous and respiratory bronchioles) that result in airflow limitation that is due to increased airway resistance. These changes can be accompanied by airway muscle hyperplasia. Chronic bronchiolitis often co-exists with other pathologic conditions in patients with COPD, and cigarette smoking is the major cause. In general, the clinical presentation and evaluation of this disorder are similar to those described for

COPD. However, a significant number of cases of bronchiolitis are related to acute viral infections (e.g., paramyxoviruses). Bronchiolitis can also be seen after chronic exposure to occupation-related mineral dusts such as silica and asbestos. This disorder should not be confused with obliterative bronchiolitis typically seen in chronic rejection after lung transplantation.

Bronchiectasis

Bronchiectasis is an abnormal dilation of the bronchi that results from inflammation and permanent destructive changes in the elastic and muscular layers of the bronchial walls. Bronchiectasis may be localized to a certain bronchus or may be diffuse. This disorder is usually caused by recurrent or chronic severe infections such as necrotizing pneumonias (e.g., *Staphylococcus aureus* pneumonia), tuberculosis, or infection with atypical mycobacteria (e.g., *mycobacterium avium-intracellulare*). Viral (e.g., *measles*) and fungal (e.g., *histoplasmosis* and *coccidioidomycosis*) infections and even anatomic obstruction may cause bronchiectasis as well. *Allergic bronchopulmonary aspergillosis* is a condition associated with hypersensitivity to aspergillus fungi that is usually exhibited as severe intractable asthma, central bronchiectasis, high levels of immunoglobulin E (IgE), and precipitins for aspergillus species.

Bronchiectasis is more frequent in middle-aged to older individuals, but it occurs in younger patients when associated with congenital defects like *cystic fibrosis* or *immotile cilia syndrome* (Kartagener's syndrome), a rare inherited abnormality of the ciliary microtubules that impairs airway clearance and is associated with recurrent infections. The classic triad of this syndrome includes sinusitis, *situs inversus,* and infertility. Other congenital syndromes associated with bronchiectasis include α_1-antitrypsin deficiency and immunodeficiency states related to hypogammaglobulinemia.

Similar to individuals with chronic bronchitis, patients with bronchiectasis may exhibit chronic cough and foul-smelling sputum, shortness of breath, abnormal chest sounds, and fatigue. Blood-streaked sputum is common, but massive hemoptysis rarely occurs. Clubbing may be exhibited in up to 40% of patients. Pulmonary function tests may show varying degrees of obstruction. Chest radiographs may be normal or may show increased interstitial markings. The classic finding is parallel lines in peripheral lung fields described as *tram tracks,* which represent thickened bronchial walls that do not taper from proximal to distal sites. High-resolution CT is more sensitive for the detection of dilated airways.

Cystic Fibrosis

Cystic fibrosis is an autosomal recessive genetic disorder that affects approximately 30,000 children and adults in the United States. This disorder affects many organs, and it is the most common lethal genetic disorder in the white population, with a carrier frequency of 1 in 25, affecting 1 in 3500 live births. About 1000 new patients with cystic fibrosis are diagnosed each year. Cystic fibrosis results from a mutation in a single gene that encodes the cystic fibrosis transmembrane conductance regulator (CFTR), which is a cyclic adenosine monophosphate–regulated chloride channel present on the apical surface of epithelial cells (**Web Fig. 17–2**). The most common mutation is the ΔF508 mutation, which is a loss of the codon for phenylalanine at the 508 position of the protein. However, more than 800 mutations have been identified to date. This defect results in defective chloride transport and increased sodium reabsorption in airway and ductal epithelia, creating abnormally thick and viscous secretions in the respiratory, hepatobiliary, gastrointestinal, and reproductive tracks. The thick secretions cause luminal obstruction and destruction of exocrine ducts.

In patients with cystic fibrosis, the airways become colonized initially with *Staphylococcus aureus* or *Haemophilus influenza,* followed by *Pseudomonas aeruginosa.* Persistent inflammation and infection cause bronchial wall destruction and bronchiectasis. Mucous plugging of small airways causes postobstructive cystic dilations and parenchymal destruction. Progressive airflow obstruction ensues, and most patients die of respiratory failure.

Table 17–2	**Organ Involvement in Cystic Fibrosis**

Pulmonary

Cough and sputum production
Recurrent pneumonias
Bronchial hyperreactivity
Hemoptysis
Pneumothorax
Significant digital clubbing
Cor pulmonale

Upper Respiratory Tract

Nasal polyps
Chronic sinusitis

Gastrointestinal

Meconium ileus in the neonate
Distal intestinal obstruction
Rectal prolapse
Hernias
Exocrine pancreatic dysfunction causing steatorrhea, malnutrition, and vitamin deficiency
Acute pancreatitis (rare)
Diabetes mellitus
Cirrhosis and portal hypertension
Salivary gland inflammation
Cholelithiasis

Genitourinary

Azoospermia
Decreased fertility rate in women
Nephrolithiasis

Patients with cystic fibrosis may exhibit salty-tasting skin, persistent coughing with and without sputum production, wheezing, shortness of breath, poor appetite or failure to thrive, and greasy bulky stools. Although the predominant symptoms are related to the respiratory system, patients may be infertile and/or diagnosed with diabetes and osteoporosis (Table 17–2). The diagnosis of cystic fibrosis should be considered in any patient with unexplained chronic sinus disease, bronchiectasis, or malabsorption. Pulmonary function tests may show varying degrees of obstruction, but progressive airway obstruction is common. Chest imaging studies may be normal or may show bronchiectasis.

The diagnosis of cystic fibrosis is made by measuring the concentration of chloride in sweat (*sweat test*). The diagnosis is considered definitive if the clinical picture is consistent with cystic fibrosis and if the chloride concentration performed in a certified laboratory is greater than 60 mEq/L on at least two occasions. Genotyping confirms the diagnosis.

Although most patients are diagnosed in childhood, some patients remain without a diagnosis until adulthood. Nearly 40% of the population with cystic fibrosis is estimated to be older than 18 years of age. Before 1940, infants with cystic fibrosis rarely lived to their first birthday. Currently, the median survival for a person with cystic fibrosis is in the third decade of life.

The treatment of cystic fibrosis relies on aggressive airway hygiene, nutritional support including pancreatic enzyme replacement, antibiotics, bronchodilators, and aerosolized recombinant human DNase, which decrease sputum viscosity. Inhaled tobramycin provided twice daily every other month slows the rate of decline in pulmonary function. As is the case for other obstructive lung diseases, the ultimate therapy for patients with cystic fibrosis with end-stage lung disease is lung transplantation; bilateral lung transplantation is preferred in this condition.

Asthma

Asthma is a chronic pulmonary disorder characterized by airway inflammation, airway hyper-reactivity, and reversible airflow obstruction. The incidence of asthma is highest in children, but it affects all ages, and it occurs worldwide with a preponderance of incidences in developed industrialized countries. Up to 7% of the United States population is estimated to have asthma. Despite a better understanding of its causes and pathophysiologic features and the development of new drugs with bronchodilator activity, the prevalence of asthma in the United States increased 75% between 1960 and 1994. During this period, physician visits for asthma doubled, hospitalizations increased dramatically, and mortality increased by 40% in the 1980s. By 1995, close to 15 million people in the United States were affected with asthma, causing over 5500 deaths each year.

The cause of asthma remains unknown, but it is likely to be a polygenic disease influenced by environmental factors. Several genetic abnormalities have been detected in asthma including variations in the β-adrenergic receptor leading to diminished responsiveness to β-agonists. Atopy is strongly linked to asthma. Exposure to indoor allergens like dust mites, cockroaches, furry pets, and fungi are significant risk factors, as are outdoor pollution and other irritants. Of note, obesity has been linked to a higher incidence of asthma, a disturbing observation in view of the increasing prevalence of obesity. Certain infectious agents and other conditions can cause acute bronchospasm even in patients without the diagnosis of asthma. Such is the case for viral infections, gastroesophageal reflux disease, and exposure to gases or fumes.

Airway inflammation is considered the major pathogenetic mechanism responsible for asthma. Patients with asthma have higher numbers of activated inflammatory cells within the airway wall, and the epithelium is infiltrated with eosinophils, mast cells, macrophages, and T lymphocytes, which produce multiple soluble mediators (e.g., cytokines, leukotrienes, bradykinins). An imbalance in pro-inflammatory versus inhibitory cytokines may be a fundamental part of the pathogenesis of asthma. In addition, a disruption of the continuity of the ciliated columnar epithelium occurs, as well as increased vascularity and edema.

Asthma is also associated with *airway wall remodeling*, which is characterized by hyperplasia and hypertrophy of smooth muscle cells, edema, inflammatory infiltration, and increased deposition of connective tissue components such as types I and III collagens. The latter not only leads to a thickening of the subepithelial lamina reticularis, but an expansion of the entire airway wall also occurs. Whether inflammation leads to remodeling or these processes represent two independent manifestations of the disease is unknown. Nevertheless, airway inflammation and remodeling together may functionally dissociate the airway from the lung parenchyma, thereby preventing the *stenting* of the airways during exhalation. Over time, airway wall remodeling leads to irreversible airflow limitation, which worsens the disease by rendering bronchodilator drugs less efficient; airway wall remodeling also makes it more difficult to distinguish this disease from COPD in which airflow obstruction is irreversible.

CLINICAL MANIFESTATIONS

The classic triad of symptoms is persistent wheeze, chronic episodic dyspnea, and chronic cough. Although wheezing is not a pathognomic feature of asthma, in the setting of a compatible clinical picture, asthma is the most common diagnosis. Asthma can develop at any age as episodic cough, shortness of breath, and chest tightness. Often these symptoms worsen at night or during the early hours of the morning. Physical examination may be normal or may show evidence of wheezing. Other associated symptoms are sputum production and chest pain or tightness. If hemoptysis is present, then Churg-Strauss vasculitis, allergic bronchopulmonary aspergillosis, or bronchiectasis should be suggested. Patients may exhibit only one or a combination of the foregoing symptoms. In the case of severe airflow limitation, the clinician may find that the patient has difficulty talking, is using accessory muscles of inspiration, shows *pulsus paradoxus,* is diaphoretic, and has mental status changes ranging from agitation to somnolence. In patients with these findings, treatment should be immediate and aggressive.

EVALUATION

A diagnosis of asthma requires documentation of hyperactivity and reversible airway obstruction to flow. The history

Table 17–3 **Diagnostic Studies in Asthma**

Routine pulmonary function test Special pulmonary function test	Decreased FEV_1; hyperinflation; improvement with bronchodilator
Methacholine or cold-air challenge	Indicates the presence of nonspecific bronchial hyper-reactivity; bronchoconstriction occurs at lower doses in asthma
Challenge with specific agents: occupational, drugs	Occasionally performed
Chest radiograph Skin tests	Fleeting infiltrates and central bronchiectasis in ABPA Demonstrate atopy; little value except prick test to *Aspergillus fumigatus* positive in ABPA
Blood tests	Eosinophils and IgE are usually increased in atopy; levels may be very high in ABPA; *Aspergillus precipitins* increased in many but not all patients with ABPA

ABPA = allergic bronchopulmonary aspergillosis; FEV_1 = forced expiratory volume in 1 second; IgE = immunoglobulin E.

might be sufficient to assess this because most patients complain of repeated but reversible episodes of wheezing. Airflow limitation is easily detected by spirometry when present. However, because asthma is episodic, patients might exhibit symptoms at a time when this cannot be documented. Depending on the circumstances, it might be necessary to formally test for airway hyperactivity via bronchoprovocation challenge (Table 17–3). The patient is given an airway application of a stimulant with bronchoconstrictor activity; histamine, methacholine, and cold air are among the most commonly used stimulants. Exercise can also be used to trigger an attack. Although most patients with or without asthma may develop some degree of airflow limitation during bronchoprovocation testing, the diagnosis depends on the dose of the stimulus needed to elicit an effect; those with asthma develop airflow limitation at much lower doses than patients without.

Lung volume measurements may show hyperinflation during active disease, but D_LCO is typically normal because asthma is an airways disease and does not cause destruction of the acinus. Decreased D_LCO may be due to artifacts created by the measurement, which is highly sensitive to distribution of the gas (as is the case in mucous plugging). In this setting, the D_LCO value normalizes when corrected for gas volume distribution. During acute exacerbations of asthma, arterial blood gases are useful to determine gas-exchange status. A chest radiograph should be obtained if a concern for pulmonary infection exists. Blood tests might reveal eosinophilia and increased levels of IgE. Skin tests might be useful to identify household and other antigens that may precipitate asthma attacks in a particular patient (see Table 17–3).

MANAGEMENT

The management of asthma requires education and cooperation on the part of the patient. Simple, inexpensive peak expiratory flow meters can be used at home to monitor airflow obstruction. A diary should be maintained, and a clear plan should be in place for using the peak flow information to intervene early in exacerbations and to alter long-term therapy for optimal control of symptoms. The cornerstone of maintenance therapy in all but mild intermittent asthma is scheduled administration of inhaled corticosteroids. Long- and short-acting bronchodilators are added for additional symptomatic control as needed. Leukotriene inhibitors have been shown to be effective adjuncts in maintenance therapy, but they do not replace corticosteroids. Theophylline preparations may have additional beneficial effects in some patients, but the narrow therapeutic window and modest efficacy of these preparations limit their value.

Acute severe asthma, or status asthmaticus, is an attack of severe bronchospasm that is unresponsive to routine therapy. Such attacks may be sudden (*hyperacute asthma*) and may be rapidly fatal, often before medical care can be obtained. In most cases, however, patients have a history of progressive dyspnea over hours to days, with increasing bronchodilator use. Patients with severe exacerbations may have difficulty talking; they may use accessory muscles of inspiration and show *pulsus paradoxus,* orthopnea, and/or diaphoresis, or have mental status changes ranging from agitation to somnolence. In patients with these findings, treatment should be immediate and aggressive, with continuous monitoring of blood oxygen saturation by pulse oximetry, often supplemented by arterial blood gas analysis to evaluate hypercarbia. A rising $PaCO_2$ in a patient with asthma is an ominous sign and may portend a medical emergency. These patients require continuous direct observation and monitoring, and many require mechanical ventilation. Peak expiratory flow rates should be frequently measured to assess response to therapy. **Guidelines for the diagnosis and management of asthma** have been devised by the National Asthma Education and Prevention Program Expert Panel and were updated in 2002.

Prospectus for the Future

The chronic obstructive lung diseases are among the most common disorders encountered by pulmonologists. However, despite the development of new drugs with bronchodilator and anti-inflammatory activity, the increasing incidence of disorders such as asthma and COPD and their consequences have not been significantly curtailed. Recently, alterations in the expression and activation of proteases of the matrix metalloproteinase family have been linked to the development of emphysema. Consequently, agents capable of modulating the activity of these proteases are being tested in preclinical studies for their ability to prevent experimental emphysema. Because tobacco is the most common etiologic factor related to irreversible obstructive lung disease, newer strategies to facilitate smoking cessation are needed, and further studies designed to elucidate the mechanisms that control habit formation should be encouraged. In asthma, a new understanding about the interplay between inflammation and airway remodeling has sparked interest in elucidation of the mechanisms that mediate tissue remodeling, but effective strategies specifically targeting this process remain unavailable. Remodeling of the lung connective tissue is not unique to asthma and emphysema; it is also an important component of bronchiectasis and other obstructive lung diseases, as well as in interstitial lung disorders. However, agents capable of effectively modulating lung tissue remodeling have not been identified. In the meantime, new information about the genetics involved in the control of airway inflammation and tissue destruction is emerging, and it is not difficult to envision a day when this new information will allow for the early detection of susceptibility to obstructive lung disease that will be the basis for personalized therapy.

References

American Thoracic Society: Standards for the diagnosis of care of patients with chronic obstructive pulmonary disease. Am J Respir Crit Care Med 152:S77–S121, 1995.

Barnes PJ: Inhaled glucocorticoids for asthma. N Engl J Med 332:868–875, 1995.

Cote CG, Celli BR: New treatment strategies for COPD: Pairing the new with the tried and true. Postgrad Med 117:27–34, 2005.

Drazen JM, Israel E, O'Byrne PM: Treatment of asthma with drugs modifying the leukotriene pathway. N Engl J Med, 340:197–206, 1999.

Mannino DM: COPD: Epidemiology, prevalence, morbidity and mortality, and disease heterogeneity. Chest 121:121S–126S, 2002.

Nelson HS: Beta-adrenergic bronchodilators. N Engl J Med 333:499–506, 1995.

Niederman MS: Introduction: Mechanisms and management of COPD: We can do better—it's time for a re-evaluation. Chest, 113:233S–283S, 1998.

Ramsey BW: Management of pulmonary disease in patients with cystic fibrosis. N Engl J Med 335:179–188, 1996.

Shapiro SD. Evolving concepts in the pathogenesis of chronic obstructive pulmonary disease. Clin in Chest Med, 21:621–632, 2000.

Wagner PD, Pauwels RA: National Asthma Education and Prevention Program: Highlights of the Expert Panel Report II: Guidelines for the Diagnosis and Management of Asthma (NIH Publication No. 97-4051). Bethesda, MD: National Heart, Lung and Blood Institute, 1997.

Chapter 18

Interstitial Lung Diseases

Jesse Roman

Kenneth L. Brigham

The interstitial lung diseases (ILDs) comprise a group of over 120 distinct entities that are characterized by diffuse chronic lung injury and inflammation that frequently progress to irreversible fibrosis. A major difficulty in assessing these disorders is that they share common clinical, radiographic, and physiologic manifestations. The classification of an ILD has changed over the years as new information about their pathogenesis has emerged. This text uses a classification that divides ILDs into the following categories: *idiopathic interstitial pneumonitides, granulomatous disorders, connective tissue–related ILDs, drug-induced ILDs, pulmonary vasculitic disorders,* and *distinct entities of unknown origin that exhibit well-defined syndromes such as sarcoidosis, eosinophilic granuloma, and lymphangioleiomyomatosis.*

In general, ILDs are characterized by four manifestations that together are referred to as the *ILD syndrome:* (1) respiratory symptoms such as dyspnea and cough, (2) bilateral infiltrates visualized on chest radiographic films, (3) physiologic abnormalities with lung restriction being the most frequently encountered, and (4) histologic abnormalities showing fibrosis and inflammation. The early identification of this syndrome in patients will suggest ILD and will often avoid misdiagnosis and inappropriate tests.

Respiratory symptoms in patients with ILD are usually subacute or chronic with some patients diagnosed weeks, months, or even years after the symptoms arise. Fatigue, fever, and weight loss are not infrequent. During the early stages of disease, symptoms are exhibited during exertion with few or no indications of disease during rest. This presentation often leads to delays in seeking medical assistance because patients often ascribe these symptoms to increasing age, poor conditioning, or other diseases (e.g., cardiac illness). Some patients are identified during routine evaluation, whereas others require extensive evaluation to reach a diagnosis.

A thorough history is helpful in narrowing the diagnosis. Age, for example, is an important diagnostic factor because some patients with ILD are typically examined after age 50 (e.g., idiopathic pulmonary fibrosis [IPF]), whereas others are seen at a younger age (e.g., sarcoidosis, eosinophilic granuloma). Sex is also an important consideration because some

rare forms of ILDs develop almost exclusively in women; such is the case of lymphangioleiomyomatosis, which is almost always seen in young women of childbearing age. Some racial groups experience a disproportionate higher incidence of certain ILDs; such is the case for sarcoidosis in the southeast United States where it is most common in patients of African-American descent.

An attempt should be made to elicit a history of connective tissue disease (e.g., lupus, rheumatoid arthritis, scleroderma) because these often involve the lung interstitium. Environmental and occupational histories are also important, particularly because they can reveal exposure to agents that promote lung fibrosis such as asbestos or beryllium. Other medical illnesses can mimic ILD such as congestive heart failure, and yet other seemingly innocuous disorders can worsen it (e.g., chronic aspiration of gastric contents). A list of pharmacologic agents used should be elicited because certain drugs are linked to the development of ILDs (e.g., amiodarone, bleomycin).

The physical examination may reveal an otherwise healthy individual with few physiologic abnormalities detectable only during exertion (e.g., oxygen desaturation during exercise). Patients with ILD show evidence of decreased chest expansion during inspection. Palpation and percussion rarely reveal changes, but auscultation shows Velcro crackles at the bases of both lungs. Other manifestations may include clubbing of the fingers. Skin rashes, arthritis and joint deformities, Raynaud's phenomenon, and dysphagia may point to a connective tissue–related ILD such as *dermatomyositis* or *polymyositis, progressive systemic sclerosis,* or *mixed connective tissue disorder.* Evidence of right ventricular heart failure with jugular vein distention, a cardiac gallop, loud P2 sound, and leg edema suggests pulmonary hypertension; right ventricular heart failure is usually the result of chronic hypoxemia and often related to end-stage lung disease.

A chest radiograph can narrow the possible diagnosis based on the distribution of the reticulonodular changes. For example, sarcoidosis, lymphangioleiomyomatosis, hypersensitivity pneumonitis, eosinophilic granuloma, and ankylosing spondylitis most often affect the upper- and mid-level

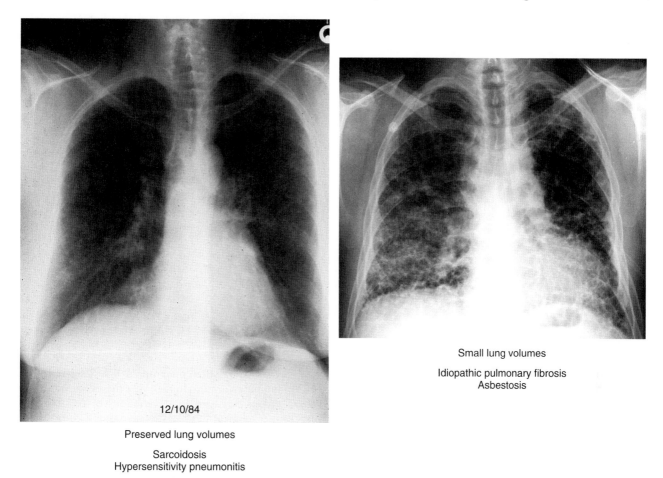

Small lung volumes

Idiopathic pulmonary fibrosis
Asbestosis

12/10/84

Preserved lung volumes

Sarcoidosis
Hypersensitivity pneumonitis

Figure 18–1 Radiographic manifestations of interstitial lung diseases (ILDs). Left image shows well-preserved lung volumes with bilateral interstitial reticulonodular infiltrates as seen in diseases similar to sarcoidosis and hypersensitivity pneumonitis. Right image shows reduced lung volumes with bilateral basilar infiltrates as seen in idiopathic pulmonary fibrosis (IPF).

lung fields, whereas IPF, asbestosis, and many connective tissue–related ILDs typically involve the lower-level lung fields. Some of these conditions exhibit more proximal airway involvement such as that seen in sarcoidosis, whereas involvement of the lung periphery as seen in IPF characterizes others. Some patients with ILDs exhibit cystic changes (e.g., lymphangioleiomyomatosis, eosinophilic granuloma), whereas others show cavitation as that seen in Wegener's granulomatosis and sarcoidosis. A careful examination of other chest structures is important, such as the pleural surfaces and the mediastinum. Sarcoidosis, for example, typically exhibits hilar and mediastinal lymphadenopathies. Pleural effusions may accompany connective tissue–related ILDs. These patterns are best analyzed through the use of high-resolution computed tomography (HRCT) of the chest, a test considered essential in the evaluation of patients suggested as having ILD.

Pulmonary function tests typically reveal a restrictive pattern characterized by proportionately decreased air flows with preserved forced expiratory volume in 1 second–percent of forced vital capacity (FEV_1/FVC%) ratio (no obstruction to airflow) and decreased lung volumes as highlighted by decreased total lung capacity and functional residual capacity. The diffusion capacity for carbon dioxide (D_LCO) of the lung is often decreased, and desaturation of

hemoglobin for oxygen occurs during exertion. During the advanced stages of disease, the partial pressure of oxygen in arterial blood (PaO_2) decreases at rest.

Although the physiologic abnormalities described represent the classic manifestations of ILDs, an obstructive pattern that resembles chronic obstructive pulmonary disease (COPD) characterizes other IDLs. In this setting, the imaging studies show preservation of lung volume (Fig. 18–1). This presentation is in contrast with what is considered to be the *classic* manifestations of ILD: bilateral infiltrates and reduced lung volumes on imaging studies coupled with physiologic restriction. These manifestations can cause confusion and lead to delays in diagnosis. However, careful consideration of the histologic changes seen in these entities provides a useful explanation. Histologically, ILD affects the interstitium of the lung, the space located between the basement membrane of the vascular structures within the distal airspaces and the basement membranes of the epithelial cells that line the alveoli (Fig. 18–2). This space also extends proximally toward the alveolar ducts and respiratory bronchioles. Normally, the interstitium of the lung contains a few fibroblasts and connective tissue components within a very thin wall that allows for the efficient diffusion of gases. In ILD, however, this space expands with the accumulation of fibroblasts and the deposition of an aberrant matrix that

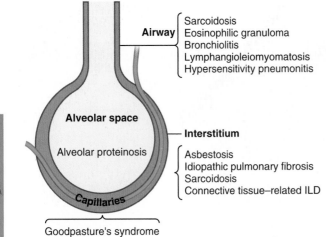

Figure 18–2 Interstitial lung diseases (ILDs) affect the interstitium of the lung at different locations. Depending on the site of disease activity, its consequences may vary. Specifically, diseases that affect the interstitium that surrounds the distal part of the alveoli lead to physiologic restrictions with reduced lung volumes. In contrast, diseases that preferentially affect the interstitium located near the more proximal parts of the acinus near the distal bronchioles may exhibit predominantly with well-preserved lung volumes and physiologic obstruction.

increases the distance between the alveolar space and vascular structures, thereby delaying and sometimes preventing gas exchange. This thickened interstitium accounts for the poor oxygenation and increased lung stiffness exhibited as decreased compliance, small lung volumes, and increased work of breathing. These findings account for the clinical manifestations seen in disorders like *IPF* and *asbestosis*. In ILDs characterized by the involvement of the more proximal interstitial spaces extending into the respiratory bronchioles, a narrowing of these small airways occurs, leading to an obstruction to airflow that resembles the physiologic abnormalities seen in COPD. These ILDs are distinguishable from other ILDs because, in addition to their obstructive physiologic characteristics (and as a consequence of it), the radiograph does not show small lung volume. Rather, lung volumes are preserved and may even appear hyperinflated. ILDs that may develop such derangements include *sarcoidosis, lymphangioleiomyomatosis, eosinophilic granuloma, bronchiolitis obliterans and organizing pneumonia (BOOP)*, and *hypersensitivity pneumonitis*.

Although the clinical manifestations, imaging studies, and physiologic characteristics might point to a specific entity, histologic manifestations are frequently required to confirm a diagnosis. However, histologic findings may not always be diagnostic because the lung displays a limited number of patterns of repair after injury that often lead to nonspecific pathologic changes. For example, granulomatous inflammation is characteristic of sarcoidosis, but granulomas can also be seen in infectious disorders (e.g., tuberculosis), berylliosis, Wegener's granulomatosis, and hypersensitivity pneumonitis. A pattern of usual interstitial

pneumonitis is typical of IPF, but it can also be seen in ILDs related to connective tissue disorders, among others. Thus the diagnosis of ILD is based on the clinical, radiographic, and histologic manifestations that individually are nonspecific but together point to a specific diagnosis. The summary of the typical manifestations of several ILDs is included in Table 18–1.

In general, the management of ILD is dependent on the specific entity causing the interstitial process. If environmental or occupational hazards or drugs are identified as culprits, then evasion of the injuring agents is necessary. However, in most cases a cause cannot be identified. If so, a trial with immunosuppressants might be warranted because many of these conditions are related to lung inflammation. Oxygen supplementation and pulmonary rehabilitation might be useful in select patients with more advanced disease. In progressive fibrosing ILD in which no effective therapies are available, lung transplantation should be considered.

Idiopathic Interstitial Pneumonias

The idiopathic interstitial pneumonias (IIPs) are a group of ILDs of unknown origins. In the 1970s these conditions were generally considered different variations of *IPF*. However, the distinct clinical presentations, natural courses, and responses to treatment observed in these patients led to their reclassification into a group of idiopathic interstitial disorders based on the following histologic patterns: *usual interstitial pneumonitis (UIP), nonspecific interstitial pneumonitis (NSIP), acute interstitial pneumonitis (AIP)*, and *desquamative interstitial pneumonitis (DIP)*.

Of the IIPs, IPF, also known as cryptogenic fibrosing alveolitis, is the most common affecting 85,000 to 100,000 individuals in the United States. Although initially thought to be a relatively rare disease, IPF is now considered to be one of the most common ILDs with prevalence in some populations of 29 cases per 100,000; the prevalence is much higher in patients over the age of 70. In most patients with IPF, the disease is sporadic; however, IPF has been found in members of certain families (termed *familial IPF*), indicating that genetic alterations might predispose patients to this illness. The disease is idiopathic, but gamma herpesviruses have been detected in the lungs of a large proportion of patients with IPF, and an animal model resembling this condition has been reported. Many environmental, occupational, and infectious agents can cause lung fibrosis including asbestos, silica, and tuberculosis. Therefore, distinguishing IPF from these other lung disorders is important because of the implications for prognosis and therapy.

IPF is characterized by progressive fibrosis of the lungs resulting in nonproductive cough and shortness of breath that worsens with exertion and, ultimately, causes hypoxemic respiratory failure. A typical patient with IPF is between 50 and 70 years of age, and the symptoms frequently develop 1 to 2 years before a diagnosis is confirmed. Physical examination often reveals crackles in the bases of both lungs, indicating the predominant site of scarring. With increased connective tissue deposition, the lung becomes stiff as evidenced by decreased compliance. Pulmonary function tests

Table 18–1 Manifestations of Interstitial Lung Disease

Disease	Physical Examination	Radiographs	Laboratory Findings	Histologic Findings
Pneumoconioses Coal worker's pneumoconiosis Asbestosis Silica-induced ILD Beryllium exposure	Variable findings Normal Crackles Clubbing	Diffuse reticulonodular infiltrates Large nodules Eggshell calcification of hilar nodes Pleural plaques	Nonspecific except beryllium: lymphocyte transformation test Obstructive and/or restrictive PFTs	Fibrosis Coal: anthracotic pigment Silicas: inflammation, bi-refringent crystals, alveolar proteinosis Asbestos: mesothelioma
Hypersensitivity pneumonitis	Fever Cough Crackles	Waxing and waning reticulonodular infiltrates Fibrosis	Serum precipitins to specific proteins Obstructive and/or restrictive PFTs	Obliterative bronchiolitis without granulomas Desquamative interstitial pneumonitis and diffuse alveolar damage Diffuse or patchy, intra-alveolar
IPF DIP and/or RB-ILD UIP AIP NSIP	Variable findings Normal Crackles Clubbing	Normal to end-stage honeycombing Abnormalities usually diffuse	Nonspecific Restrictive PFTs	Macrophages Patchy, fibroblasts, fibrosis Uniform, fibroblasts, no fibrosis Patchy or diffuse, prominent interstitial inflammation, fibrosis
Collagen vascular	Collagen vascular disease Crackles Pleural rub	Pleural effusions Diffuse interstitial infiltrates Nodular infiltrates Occasional cavities	Serologic findings for specific disease Occasionally obstructive, usually restrictive PFTs	Interstitial inflammation Vasculitis Bronchiolar obstruction Organizing pneumonia Fibrosis
Drug-induced ILD	Fever Crackles Pleural rub	Fibrosis Migratory infiltrates Diffuse interstitial infiltrates Pulmonary edema	Restrictive PFTs Anti-RNP antibodies	Alveolar macrophages with lamellar bodies in amiodarone Interstitial inflammation Fibrosis Eosinophilic infiltration
Sarcoidosis	Fever Malaise Weight loss Erythema nodosum Lupus pernio and skin plaques Salivary and lacrimal gland enlargement	Reticulonodular infiltrates Nodules Hilar adenopathy Mediastinal adenopathy Fibrosis	Lymphocytic bronchoalveolar lavage T8 > T4 subsets Obstructive and/or restrictive PFTs Elevated transaminases with liver involvement Occasional hypercalcemia	Noncaseating granuloma with giant cells and negative acid-fast bacilli and fungal stains Fibrosis

Continued

Table 18–1 Manifestations of Interstitial Lung Disease—cont'd

Disease	Physical Examination	Radiographs	Laboratory Findings	Histologic Findings
	Iritis, uveitis, chorioretinitis; keratoconjunctivitis Cranial nerve palsies Arthritis Occasional rales or wheezes			
Radiation exposure	Crackles Fever	Focal interstitial infiltrates corresponding to radiation port Occasional diffuse infiltrates Fibrosis	None	*Acute:* endothelial and alveolar lining cell damage *Chronic:* fibrosis
Eosinophilic granuloma	None to cough Dyspnea Chest pain Fatigue Weight loss Occasional fever	Spontaneous pneumothorax Nodules Reticulonodular infiltrates Middle and upper lobe predominance Honeycombing Sparing of costophrenic angle Cysts and nodules on HRCT	Normal lung volumes with decreased D_LCo	OKT-6 (CD1) and S-100 positive immunostaining Few eosinophils Peri-bronchiolar inflammation Macrophages filling lumen of bronchioles and intraluminal fibrosis
Lymphangioleiomyomatosis	Dyspnea Cough Chest pain Decreased breath sounds or rales Hemoptysis Ascites	Spontaneous pneumothorax Pleural effusions Reticulonodular infiltrate Miliary pattern Honeycombing Hyperinflation Diffuse, small, thin-walled cysts on HRCT	Obstructive and/or restrictive PFTs Chylous pleural effusions Chylous ascites	HMB-45 positive immunostaining Atypical smooth muscle cell proliferation around bronchovascular bundles
BOOP	Fever Chills Malaise Fatigue Cough Dyspnea on exertion Weight loss	Peripheral patchy infiltrates, occasionally migratory CT scan: patchy consolidation, ground glass opacities, small nodules	Restrictive and occasionally obstructive PFTs in smokers	Patchy peri-bronchiolar distribution Foamy macrophages in alveolar spaces Intraluminal buds of granulation tissue

AIP = acute interstitial pneumonia; BOOP = bronchiolitis obliterans and organizing pneumonia; CT = computed tomography; DIP/RB-ILD = desquamative interstitial pneumonia/respiratory bronchiolitis with interstitial lung disease; HRCT = high-resolution computed tomography; IPF = idiopathic pulmonary fibrosis; NSIP = nonspecific interstitial pneumonia; PFTs = pulmonary function tests; RNP = anti-ribonucleoprotein antibodies; UIP = usual interstitial.

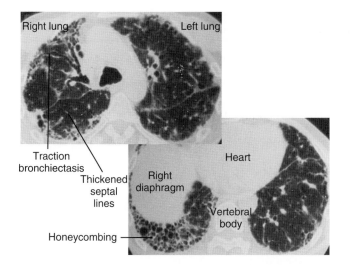

Right lung

Left lung

Traction
bronchiectasis

Thickened
septal
lines

Heart

Right
diaphragm

Vertebral
body

Honeycombing

Figure 18–3 Computer tomography (CT) of the chest in a patient with idiopathic pulmonary fibrosis (IPF).

show decreased lung volumes consistent with a restrictive process. Poor oxygenation in IPF often requires long-term oxygen supplementation. The chest radiograph shows infiltrates that are most predominant at the bases and periphery of the lungs. HRCT allows for better visualization of the lung and is very useful in evaluating the extent of disease. It delineates the areas of fibrosis and provides information about other structures in the chest. The classic HRCT findings of IPF are bilateral reticulonodular infiltrates with peripheral distribution and the presence of honeycombing and traction bronchiectasis in the absence of ground glass opacification, lymphadenopathy, and pleural disease (Fig. 18–3). In the setting of a typical clinical presentation and classic HRCT findings, a lung biopsy may not be necessary. Unfortunately, a lung biopsy is required for confirmation in many patients.

The histologic patterns of IPF shows areas of scar tissue interspersed with normal alveolar structures. An interesting pathologic feature is the presence of *fibroblastic foci*, which are areas in which fibroblasts accumulate and are believed to be the site of disease activity. This overall pattern of tissue organization is UIP, which can accompany other disorders (e.g., connective tissue–related ILD); thus, the diagnosis of IPF depends on a clinical, radiographic, and histologic picture that includes the syndrome of ILD in the absence of an obvious cause and a histologic manifestation consistent with UIP.

Currently, no known effective treatments are available for IPF. Because inflammation is considered to be an important factor, corticosteroids and other immunosuppressants (e.g., azathioprine, cyclosphosphamide) have been used, but it is now recognized that these drugs do little to stop the progression of the disease and could be harmful. Consequently, several other drugs, including interferon, pirfenidone, and n-acetylcysteine, among others, are being tested in clinical trials.

The second most common IIP is *NSIP.* As the term suggests, this condition exhibits a histologic picture that is nonspecific and characterized by diffuse interstitial inflammation. It is often associated with other conditions

such as connective tissue disorders (e.g., systemic lupus erythematosus, rheumatoid arthritis, polymyositis) or hypersensitivity pneumonitis. The association with these disorders is so strong that histologic confirmation of NSIP should prompt a search for these conditions. As in IPF, patients with NSIP exhibit slowly progressive dyspnea and bilateral interstitial infiltrates. Ground glass opacification is often noted by HRCT. NSIP is more responsive to immunosuppressants than is IPF, and a 3-month trial period with these agents should be considered. However, occasionally, NSIP is associated with significant fibrosis (*fibrosing NSIP*), and lung transplantation should be considered in these patients, if possible.

DIP is usually seen in young individuals and is associated with a history of cigarette smoking. Patients exhibit a progressive shortness of breath and bilateral infiltrates on chest radiograph. The HRCT pattern is nonspecific, and a biopsy may be required for diagnosis. Tissue histologic findings show the accumulation of activated macrophages in the alveolar spaces. Treatment relies on immunosuppressant therapy and the avoidance of tobacco exposure. DIP is often confused with (and is considered by some experts to be identical to) *respiratory bronchiolitis ILD (RB-ILD)*, which has a similar clinical presentation and is associated with tobacco exposure.

AIP is another IIP that is not commonly seen. Its presentation differs from other IIPs in that it is more acute with dyspnea progressing from days to a few weeks, invariably leading to respiratory failure. The histologic pattern shows diffuse interstitial fibrosis. Although a trial with immunosuppressants is recommended, this condition is often fatal, independent of treatment.

BOOP is often considered within the group of IIPs because it mimics these disorders clinically. Patients with BOOP exhibit subacute or chronic dyspnea first noted on exertion and sometimes triggered after an acute illness like an upper respiratory viral infection. Connective tissue disorders, inhaled irritants, and drugs (e.g., methotrexate) can cause BOOP. Histologically, BOOP is characterized by distal airway and interstitial inflammation and obliteration of distal airspaces with fibroblasts and fibrosis. Similar to NSIP and DIP, this condition is likely to respond to immunosuppressant therapy.

Granulomatous Disorders

Of the ILDs characterized by granulomatous lung inflammation, *sarcoidosis* is the most common. Sarcoidosis is a multisystem illness with a prevalence of 1 to 40 cases per 100,000 worldwide. In Northern Europe, a higher incidence of sarcoidosis occurs among Scandinavian, German, and Irish individuals. In the United States, the prevalence rates of sarcoidosis are 10.9 per 100,000 for whites and 35.5 per 100,000 for African Americans with women being more frequently affected. Sarcoidosis occurs most often in young individuals between 10 and 40 years of age with women being affected more often than men.

Sarcoidosis is characterized by the formation in tissues of noncaseating granulomas that organize in an inner core of epithelioid cells, monocytes, lymphocytes, and macrophages surrounded by fibroblasts and connective tissue. These gran-

Table 18–2 Clinical Manifestations of Sarcoidosis

Organ Systems

Pulmonary	Dyspnea, cough, wheezing, hemoptysis, laryngeal, endobronchial lesions
Dermatologic	Erythema nodosum, papules, plaques
Ocular	Uveitis, chorioretinitis, keratoconjunctivitis, lacrimal gland enlargement, optic neuritis
Neurologic	Cranial nerve palsy, headache, diabetes insipidus, mass lesions, seizures, meningitis, encephalitis
Rheumatologic	Arthralgias, arthropathy, myopathy
Gastrointestinal	Elevated transaminases, abdominal pain, jaundice
Cardiologic	Arrhythmias, conduction abnormalities, congestive heart failure
Hematologic	Lymphadenopathy (especially hilar), hypersplenism
Endocrine	Hypercalcemia, hypercalciuria, epididymitis, parotitis
Renal	Renal failure, renal calculi

Syndromes

Löfgren's syndrome	Fever, arthralgias, bilateral hilar adenopathy, erythema nodosum
Heerfordt's syndrome (uveoparotid fever)	Fever, swelling of parotid gland and uveal tracts, cranial nerve VII palsy

ulomas involve the airways and/or lung parenchyma in over 90% of patients. The upper respiratory system, lymph nodes, skin, and eyes may be involved. Other organs that may also be affected include the liver, bone marrow, spleen, musculoskeletal system, heart, salivary glands, and nervous system (Table 18–2). The cause of these lesions is unknown, but inhaled antigens have been suggested, ranging from bacterial products to environmental exposures. To date, neither genetic factors nor specific triggers have been firmly established.

Sarcoidosis is associated with abnormal immune function as evidenced by cutaneous anergy and as exhibited in lung by increased CD4+ lymphocytes and increased concentrations of pro-inflammatory cytokines such as interleukin-1β, interferon-γ, and tumor necrosis factor-α (TNF-α). These derangements can be detected in the bronchoalveolar lavage fluid and are consistent with an imbalance in the production of Th1 versus Th2 cytokines, favoring the production of the former and promoting persistent inflammation.

In about one half of patients, the disease is detected on routine chest radiograph before the development of symptoms. The range and severity of symptoms associated with sarcoidosis vary greatly, depending on the organs involved. In some cases, the first symptoms are often vague and may include low-grade fever, weight loss, or joint pain. Shortness of breath, dry cough, and chest pain occur in one third to one half of patients. Skin manifestations include erythema nodosum, plaques, nodules, and lupus pernio. Ocular symptoms are also common. Patients may also develop well-described syndromes such as *uveoparotid fever*, also known as Heerfordt's syndrome, which exhibits the triad of uveitis, parotitis, and facial nerve palsy. *Löfgren's syndrome* includes erythema nodosum, plaques, arthralgias, and hilar adenopathy. Both syndromes are associated with better outcomes when compared with other clinical presentations of sarcoidosis.

In 90% of patients, the chest radiograph shows abnormalities that include bilateral hilar adenopathy (**Web Fig. 18–1**), infiltrates, and fibrosis. The radiographic changes

Table 18–3 Radiographic Staging of Sarcoidosis

Stage	Radiographic Findings
0	Normal radiograph
1	Adenopathy without parenchymal abnormality
2A	Adenopathy and parenchymal disease
2B	Parenchymal disease without adenopathy Fibrosis and honeycombing
3	Fibrosis and honeycombing

characteristic of sarcoidosis have been classified in stages 0 through 3 (Table 18–3), but little data are available to indicate that these represent chronologic stages of the disease. Pulmonary function tests may be normal or show physiologic abnormalities consistent with obstruction, restriction, or a combination of both. Liver involvement may cause mild elevation of transaminases, and cirrhosis has been reported although it is rare. Hypercalcemia and hypercalciuria may be detected and are due to increased intestinal absorption and increased conversion of vitamin D to its active form in sarcoid granulomas.

The diagnosis of sarcoidosis is dependent on a typical clinical, radiographic, and histologic picture. Tissues show noncaseating granulomas, but because sarcoidosis is nonspecific, careful attention should be given to rule out infectious causes such as mycobacterial infection through stains and cultures of clinical samples. Necrotizing granulomas have been reported in sarcoidosis, but this finding should

Table 18–4	Indications for Use of Corticosteroids in Sarcoidosis
Disorder	**Treatment**
Iridocyclitis	Corticosteroid eye drops Local subconjunctival deposit of cortisone
Posterior uveitis	Oral prednisone
Pulmonary involvement	Steroids rarely recommended for stage 1; usually used if infiltrate remains static or worsens over 3-month period or if the patient is symptomatic
Upper airway obstruction	Rare indication for intravenous steroids
Lupus pernio	Oral prednisone shrinks the disfiguring lesions
Hypercalcemia	Responds well to corticosteroids
Cardiac involvement	Corticosteroids usually recommended if patient has arrhythmias or conduction disturbances
Central nervous system involvement	Response is best in patients with acute symptoms
Lacrimal and salivary gland involvement	Corticosteroids recommended for disordered function, *not* gland swelling
Bone cysts	Corticosteroids recommended if symptomatic

prompt an intense search for infectious causes. In contrast to most ILDs in which tissue diagnosis requires open-lung biopsy, the granulomas in sarcoidosis can be identified in skin lesions or in mediastinal or peripheral lymph nodes. A transbronchial lung biopsy is positive in 50% to 60% of patients with normal parenchyma and close to 90% of patients with parenchymal abnormalities detected by chest radiograph. Once the diagnosis is made, all patients should have an ophthalmologic evaluation, as well as a 24-hour collection of urine to evaluate for hypercalciuria. Electrocardiographic (ECG) examination is also important because sarcoid can involve the heart and cause arrhythmias as a result of the disruption of the conducting system by granulomatous infiltration.

The course of sarcoidosis varies among individuals. Race seems to play a role. For example, African Americans (especially women) tend to be affected more acutely and with more severity than whites who tend to develop asymptomatic and chronic disease. An exception to this statement occurs in young, fair-skinned Scandinavian white women who exhibit acute uveitis, fever, so-called *sarcoid arthritis,* and myopathy. In these patients, corticosteroid therapy is a mainstay of acute therapy, particularly when uveitis is present.

Although corticosteroid use has remained the mainstay of treatment, the long-term beneficial effects have not been confirmed. The evaluation of the effectiveness of this treatment is limited by the fact that roughly one third of patients with sarcoidosis have a spontaneous remission within 3 years of onset. One third of patients remains stable and one third shows a progression of disease with about 10% developing severe lung fibrosis. Therefore, treatment with corticosteroids should be withheld until evidence of organ dysfunction or evidence of progression is determined through pulmonary function testing or imaging studies. Patients with radiographic changes consistent with stage 2A and higher (with parenchymal infiltrates) have lower rates of spontaneous remission. Special indications for the use of corticosteroids in sarcoidosis include involvement of the heart, eyes, and central nervous system, among others (Table 18–4). Methotrexate, plaquenil, topical steroids, anti–TNF-α agents, and thalidomide have been tested with varying results in small studies.

Interstitial Lung Diseases Related to Connective Tissue Disorders

Many connective tissue disorders can cause lung inflammation that is indistinguishable from other ILDs (Table 18–5). *Systemic lupus erythematosus, rheumatoid arthritis, mixed connective tissue disorder, progressive systemic sclerosis (scleroderma), polymyositis or dermatomyositis,* and *Sjögren's syndrome,* among others, are examples. Although not normal, an ILD related to connective tissue disorders can develop before other symptoms typical of connective tissue disorders (e.g., arthritis), making the diagnosis even more difficult. Clinical manifestations are nonspecific and include dyspnea, cough, fever, weight loss, and general malaise.

In patients with a suggested connective tissue disorder–related ILD, a thorough history and physical exami-

Table 18–5	**Pulmonary Involvement in Connective Tissue Disorders**				
Syndrome	**RA**	**Lupus**	**SS**	**PM/DM**	**Sjögren's Syndrome**
Pleurisy effusion	+ (5–40%)	+ (30–40%)			
Necrobiotic nodules	+				
Fibrosis	+ (20–60%)	+ (3%)	+ (15–90%)	+ (10–40%)	+ (33%)
Bronchiolitis	+	+			+
Pulmonary arthropathy	+	+	+	+	
Atelectasis		+			
Pulmonary edema		+			
Pneumonitis, hemorrhage		+			
Diaphragm dysfunction		+			
Aspiration			+	+ (14%)	
Secondary carcinoma			+		

DM = Dermatomyositis; PM = Polymyositis; RA = Rheumatoid arthritis; SS = Sjögren's syndrome.

nation can elicit related abnormalities such as arthritis and hand deformities, rashes, esophageal dysmotility, Raynaud's syndrome, and skin changes. Lung examination might reveal bi-basilar crackles, and pulmonary function tests will often show a restrictive pattern with decreased lung-diffusion capacity. Chest imaging studies are often useful because they show the pattern of distribution of the infiltrates (e.g., *ankylosing spondylitis* is associated with bilateral fibrocavitary lesions in the lung apices), and they provide information about adjacent thoracic structures (e.g., pleural effusions are more commonly seen in rheumatoid arthritis and systemic lupus erythematosus). Pulmonary hypertension can occur in these patients, especially with scleroderma and systemic lupus erythematosus. Pneumonitis can be seen in systemic lupus erythematosus, Sjögren's syndrome, polymyositis, and dermatomyositis.

Bronchoscopy, with bronchoalveolar lavage and transbronchial biopsy, is often used to rule out infectious causes, and tissue biopsy findings may be nonspecific. Currently, many of these disorders are recognized as showing histologic patterns consistent with those of IIPs with NSIP being the most common, but UIP and BOOP are also frequently found. A thorough history and physical examination are necessary to distinguish these entities from one another because imaging studies and histologic patterns might not discriminate. As with other ILDs, immunosuppressants are

the mainstay of treatment and, in general, these disorders are more responsive to this therapy than is IPF. Supportive care and treatment of the underlying disease are important.

Drug-Induced Lung Disorders

Drug-induced ILDs comprise a group of disorders in which the cause of the ILD can be ascribed to a reaction to a drug (Table 18–6). Frequently, an association between ILD and any particular drug use is elusive because the symptoms might not necessarily coincide with the time of drug use or because the patient might not relate his or her symptoms to the use of the drug, especially when taking multiple medications. Of the drugs typically known to cause ILDs, the anti-arrhythmic drug *amiodarone* is one of the most recognizable. Amiodarone can cause acute or chronic alveolar and interstitial disease exhibited as cough or dyspnea on exertion. Acute toxicity is rare, and chronic toxicity is more common in patients taking 400 mg/day or more. Physical examination might show bi-basilar crackles, and pulmonary function testing might show a restrictive pattern. A decreased diffusion lung capacity is often detected early and is considered a good test for the follow-up of patients on this drug. Chest imaging studies might show unilateral or bilat-

Table 18–6   Common Drug-Induced Lung Diseases

Drug	Dose Relation	Manifestation
Chemotherapeutic		
Bleomycin	Acute or chronic, >450 U increased risk	Pneumonitis, fibrosis, BOOP
Busulfan	Chronic	Fibrosis, alveolar proteinosis
Cyclophosphamide	Chronic	Fibrosis, BOOP
Cytosine arabinoside	Acute	Pulmonary edema, ARDS
Methotrexate	Acute or chronic	Hypersensitivity pneumonitis, resolves with discontinuation, BOOP
Mitomycin C	Acute or delayed	Pneumonitis, ARDS, BOOP, hemolytic uremic syndrome
Antimicrobial		
Nitrofurantoin	Acute or chronic	Acute pneumonitis, fibrosis
Sulfasalazine	Acute or chronic	Pulmonary infiltrate with eosinophilia, BOOP
Cardiovascular		
Amiodarone	Acute or chronic, >400 mg/day	Pneumonitis, fibrosis
Flecainide	Acute	ARDS, LIP
Tocainide	Weeks or months	Pneumonitis
Procainamide	Subacute or chronic	Drug-induced systemic lupus erythematosus, pleural effusions, infiltrates
Anti-inflammatory		
Aspirin	Acute	Pulmonary edema, bronchospasm
Illicit		
Opiates	Acute	Pulmonary edema
Cocaine	Acute	Pulmonary edema, diffuse alveolar damage, pulmonary hemorrhage, BOOP
Talc (in intravenous and inhaled illicit drugs)	Acute or chronic	Granulomatous interstitial fibrosis, granulomatous pulmonary artery occlusion, particulate embolization
Tocolytics		
Terbutaline, albuterol, ritodrine	Acute	Pulmonary edema

ARDS = acute respiratory distress syndrome; BOOP = bronchiolitis obliterans and organizing pneumonia; LIP = lymphoid interstitial pneumonia.

eral infiltrates that are nonspecific. Analyses of cells obtained by bronchoalveolar lavage or biopsy typically show *foamy* macrophages.

The antineoplastic drug, *bleomycin*, causes dose-related cytotoxicity, which occurs in most patients who receive a cumulative dose of more than 450 U. The risk of bleomycin toxicity is increased in patients receiving radiation therapy, and high-inspired oxygen concentrations can precipitate lung toxicity in patients previously treated with this drug. *Methotrexate* is thought to produce a type of hypersensitivity pneumonitis and has been associated with the development of pulmonary fibrosis. *Nitrofurantoin* can produce hypersensitivity pneumonitis that may progress to fibrosis. Other drugs (e.g., *procainamide*) can cause drug-induced

lupus syndrome with pleural effusions and interstitial and alveolar infiltrates.

Pulmonary Vasculitis and Diffuse Alveolar Hemorrhage

Diffuse alveolar hemorrhage syndromes are characterized by the abrupt onset of cough, fever, and dyspnea. Hemoptysis is common but not universal. Anemia and the presence of hemorrhagic fluid in the airways visualized with bronchoscopy support the diagnosis. The chest radiograph commonly shows patchy infiltrates or diffuse alveolar infiltrates.

The presence of azotemia may point to a pulmonary-renal syndrome. Some lung disorders characterized by diffuse alveolar hemorrhage are associated with the production of antineutrophil cytoplasmic antibodies (ANCA) directed against neutrophil cytoplasmic antigens and detectable in peripheral blood. ANCAs were first described in patients with pauci-immune glomerulonephritis.

Repeated episodes of diffuse alveolar hemorrhage can result in irreversible interstitial fibrosis, particularly in middle-aged patients with Wegener's granulomatosis. The mortality rates from diffuse alveolar hemorrhage related to ANCA-positive vasculitis range between 25% and 50%.

The most common histologic pattern seen on lung biopsy obtained from patients with diffuse alveolar hemorrhage is pulmonary capillaritis, which is characterized by neutrophilic infiltration of the alveolar septa. This sequentially leads to necrosis, loss of capillary structural integrity, and pouring of red blood cells into the interstitium and alveolar spaces. Other histologic findings may include bland pulmonary hemorrhage and diffuse alveolar damage.

ANCAs are associated with several specific disorders including *Wegener's granulomatosis, microscopic polyangiitis, Churg-Strauss syndrome, pauci-immune glomerulonephritis without evidence of extrarenal disease,* and certain drug-induced vasculitis syndromes. In these conditions, ANCAs consistently have specificities for either proteinase-3 or myeloperoxidase.

Wegener's granulomatosis is a systemic necrotizing granulomatous vasculitis that often involves the small- and medium-sized vessels of the upper airway, the lower respiratory track, and the kidney. The most frequent manifestations of this illness are pulmonary, as highlighted by cough, chest pain, hemoptysis, and dyspnea. Other manifestations include upper airway involvement of the tracheobronchial tree, kidneys, musculoskeletal system, eyes, heart, nervous system, and constitutional symptoms such as fever and weight loss.

The diagnosis of Wegener's granulomatosis is suggested from the clinical and laboratory findings and from the presence of circulating ANCAs that are usually directed against proteinase-3 (C-ANCA). The sensitivity of positive C-ANCA for Wegener's granulomatosis is 90% to 95%, but it is not specific. Chest imaging may show bilateral disease, and infiltrates tend to evolve over the course of the illness. Lung nodules are common and may cavitate. Effusions and adenopathy are not common. Sinus films or computed tomographic (CT) scans serve to diagnose upper airway involvement.

Tissue biopsy at a site of active disease is generally needed to confirm Wegener's granulomatosis. The presence of granulomatous inflammation is common, but actual vasculitis is seen in close to 35% of patients. Usually, a renal biopsy is preferred because it is easier to perform and more often diagnostic. In the absence of renal involvement, a lung biopsy should be considered. The typical histopathologic findings are vasculitis and granulomatous inflammation. Special stains and cultures should be performed to exclude the presence of infections that can produce similar findings.

Microscopic polyangiitis is a form of systemic necrotizing small-vessel vasculitis that most often affects venules, capillaries, arterioles, and small arteries without clinical or pathologic evidence of necrotizing granulomatous inflammation. The absence or paucity of immunoglobulin localization in vessel walls distinguishes microscopic polyangiitis from immune complex-mediated small-vessel vasculitis such as *Henoch-Schönlein purpura* and *cryoglobulinemic vasculitis.* This rare condition has a prevalence of 1 to 3 cases per 100,000, but it is the most common cause of pulmonary-renal syndrome. The signs and symptoms of microscopic polyangiitis are similar to those of Wegener's granulomatosis.

The treatment of Wegener's granulomatosis and microscopic polyangiitis is similar. Combination therapy with corticosteroids and cyclosphosphamide is the standard of care. Other drugs used in maintenance include methotrexate, trimethopin-sulfamethaxazole, and azathioprine.

Allergic granulomatosis or *Churg-Strauss syndrome* is a multisystemic disorder characterized by vasculitis and necrotizing granulomatous inflammation that involves the lungs, nervous system, and skin. Other organs are less commonly involved. It is usually accompanied by eosinophilia and elevated immunoglobulin E, suggesting an immediate hypersensitivity reaction. Patients with this condition may develop allergic rhinitis or asthma. The vasculitis might be associated with skin nodules and purpura. Most patients respond well to corticosteroids, but other immunosuppressants similar to cyclosphosphamide may be required in patients with refractory disorders.

In addition, other well-known causes of alveolar capillaritis may occur, including the systemic vasculitides, collagen vascular disorders, anti-glomerular membrane antibody syndrome (*Goodpasture's syndrome*), and *Henoch-Schönlein purpura.* Goodpasture's syndrome causes diffuse alveolar hemorrhage associated with glomerulonephritis caused by antiglomerular basement membrane antibodies to the α3 chain of type IV collagen that is also found in the lung basement membrane. The treatment of Goodpasture's syndrome is plasmapheresis and immunosuppression. The disease is fatal if left untreated.

Idiopathic pulmonary hemorrhage or *hemosiderosis* is a diagnosis of exclusion. Patients with this syndrome have recurrent diffuse alveolar hemorrhage without associated renal or systemic disease. Histologically, the lung shows hemorrhage and hemosiderin accumulation without inflammation. Treatment includes supportive care, immunosuppression, and occasionally plasmapheresis, but response to therapy is varied. This syndrome is most common in children, who have a worse prognosis than adults.

Environmental and Occupational Interstitial Lung Diseases

Several environmental and occupational exposures may cause ILDs. These include the *pneumoconioses, drug-induced ILD,* and *hypersensitivity pneumonitis.* Pneumoconiosis and hypersensitivity pneumonitis are discussed in this text. The most common pneumoconioses result from inhalation of asbestos, coal, dust, silica, or beryllium. Hypersensitivity pneumonitis is caused by the inhalation of organic dusts.

PNEUMOCONIOSIS

Silicosis is a chronic fibrotic lung disease caused by exposure to crystalline-free silica. Certain occupations that have a higher propensity for exposure to silica include mining, stone cutting, carving, polishing, foundry work, and abrasive clearing (sandblasting). Exposure is usually chronic (over 5 years), but more acute cases are described especially if exposure is heavy. Manifestation of silica-induced ILD can be *simple nodular silicosis,* which is usually asymptomatic unless the patient is also exposed to tobacco, and *progressive massive fibrosis* (PMF), which is characterized by extensive bilateral apical fibrosis. Hilar node enlargement may be seen accompanied by *eggshell* nodal calcification. Pulmonary function tests in simple nodular silicosis may be normal or show a mixed obstructive or restrictive pattern, whereas PMF is typically associated with severe restriction and hypoxemia.

Coal worker's pneumoconiosis is an uncommon cause of pulmonary fibrosis in workers exposed to coal dust and graphite. Usually, the patients are exposed while working in underground mines. Most patients show chronic cough, which is usually productive because the bronchitis is related to coal exposure or to tobacco. The chest radiograph shows diffuse small rounded opacities.

Asbestosis is due to chronic exposure to asbestos, which is a silicate used for insulation, friction-bearing surfaces, and to strengthen materials. Typically, asbestos exposure may lead to pleural disease characterized by pleural plaques, effusion, and fibrosis, but it does not necessarily affect the lung parenchyma. If it does, then it is called asbestosis and is associated with interstitial lung fibrosis. Asbestosis is characterized by a gradual onset of dyspnea after 20 to 30 years of exposure. The clinical presentation, pulmonary function tests, and imaging studies are similar to those found in restrictive lung diseases like IPF. However, the detection of significant pleural disease is useful in distinguishing this

illness from other ILDs. The diagnosis is made from the history and demonstration of pleural plaques. In uncertain cases, the demonstration of asbestos in tissue specimens may be necessary. A higher incidence of malignancy in the presence of asbestosis, including lung carcinoma and mesothelioma, is found particularly in patients who smoke. No specific treatment exists. *Berylliosis* results from exposure to beryllium, a rare metal useful in modern, high technology industries. Exposure to be beryllium can lead to an acute chemical bronchitis and pneumonitis or chronic beryllium disease. Chronic beryllium disease is characterized by a multisystemic granulomatosis that is sometimes difficult to distinguish from sarcoidosis. The diagnosis is made by history of exposure, histologic examination, and laboratory confirmation through a lymphocyte transformation test that is available at specialized centers. Corticosteroids may be useful in the treatment of berylliosis.

HYPERSENSITIVITY PNEUMONITIS

Hypersensitivity pneumonitis (also termed *extrinsic allergic alveolitis*) is a disease mediated by an exaggerated immune reaction to repeated inhalation of and sensitization to organic dusts in susceptible people (Table 18–7). The disease may develop after an acute reaction (acute form) elicited after intense exposure to the antigen and followed 4 to 6 hours later by cough, dyspnea, fever, chills, and malaise that last for up to 24 hours. Subacute manifestations differ only in the severity of the symptoms and have a more insidious course. Chronic hypersensitivity pneumonitis results in progressive fibrosis and restrictive lung disease that are difficult to distinguish clinically from IPF.

Diffuse crackles are a common physical finding. Chest radiographic findings are variable and nonspecific; however, in general, hypersensitivity pneumonitis is characterized by

Table 18–7 Hypersensitivity Pneumonitis

Antigen	Source	Disease Examples
Thermophilic bacteria	Moldy hay, sugar cane, compost	Farmer's lung, bagassosis, mushroom worker's disease
Other bacteria	Contaminated water, wood dust, fertilizer, paprika dust	Humidifier, detergent worker's disease, and familial hypersensitivity pneumonitis
Fungi	Moldy cork, contaminated wood dust, barley, maple logs	Suberosis, sequoiosis, and maple bark strippers, malt worker's disease, and paprika splitter's lung
Animal protein	Bird droppings, animal urine, bovine and porcine pituitary powder	Pigeon breeder's lung, duck fever, turkey handler's disease, pituitary snuff taker's disease, laboratory worker's hypersensitivity pneumonitis
Chemically altered human proteins (albumin and others)	Toluene diisocyanate Trimellitic anhydride Diphenylmethane diisocyanate	Hypersensitivity pneumonitis
Phthalic anhydride	Heated epoxy resin	Epoxy resin lung

infiltrates in the mid- and upper-lung fields. In chronic hypersensitivity pneumonitis, lower lobe disease may predominate.

In the appropriate setting, a presumptive diagnosis of hypersensitivity pneumonitis can be made on clinical grounds. Most patients with hypersensitivity pneumonitis have precipitating antibodies to the offending agent, but serum precipitins also develop in up to 50% of asymptomatic patients with the same exposure. On occasion, environmental or laboratory challenge with the probable antigen may be repeated in specialized settings. Effective treatment requires eliminating exposure to the offending antigen. Systemic corticosteroids can relieve symptoms in the acute phase, but their efficacy in chronic forms of the disease is less clear.

Specific Entities

EOSINOPHILIC GRANULOMA

Eosinophilic granuloma is a disease of young- to middle-aged adults. Nearly all cases occur in white men who smoke, in whom it is more common than it is in Asians and African Americans. The patients exhibit dyspnea on exertion or cough. The chest radiograph typically shows micronodular and macronodular lesions and cysts that predominate in the mid- and upper-lung zones. Pulmonary function tests show an obstructive pattern. Specific diagnosis can be made with open lung biopsy and special stains. Electron microscopy may reveal X bodies (Birbeck granules). In the right clinical setting and with a typical HRCT, a biopsy might not be needed for diagnosis. The development of *diabetes insipidus* as a result of involvement of the central nervous system is a poor sign. Cystic lesions in flat bones (e.g., skull, ribs, pelvis) occur in the minority of patients and suggest presence of a systemic illness termed *histiocytosis X*. Treatment includes avoidance of tobacco use; corticosteroids have been used with variable response.

LYMPHANGIOLEIOMYOMATOSIS

Lymphangioleiomyomatosis is a rare disorder that occurs in women of childbearing age. The disease is characterized by extensive hamartomatous smooth muscle infiltration of the lungs. Dyspnea, pneumothorax, chylous pleural effusions, and hemoptysis are common clinical presentations. The chest radiograph shows an interstitial pattern with mid- and upper-lung predominance, multiple cystic lesions, and preserved lung volumes. Pulmonary function tests may show a mixed obstructive and restrictive pattern. In the right clinical setting, the diagnosis can be made with HRCT. However, lung biopsy might be necessary to demonstrate interstitial infiltration of smooth muscle involving the alveolar walls, lobular septa, venules, small airways, and pleura. Hormonal manipulation with progesterone or oophorectomy might be useful.

EOSINOPHILIC LUNG DISEASE

The pulmonary infiltrate with peripheral blood eosinophilia (PIE) syndrome is characterized by lung infiltrates on chest radiograph and peripheral blood eosinophilia. The cause of both disorders is unknown, but the presence of eosinophilia

and occasional bronchospasm suggest that acute hypersensitivity mechanisms are involved. Although not included in this classification, the hypereosinophilic syndrome is sometimes associated with pulmonary involvement. Other disorders associated with eosinophilia that are included in the differential diagnosis of PIE syndromes include tuberculosis, brucellosis, fungal infections, tumors, and sarcoidosis.

Simple pulmonary eosinophilia (Löeffler's syndrome) is characterized by transient migratory infiltrates that last less than 1 month. In some cases, no symptoms are present, but dyspnea and dry cough may occur. Pathologic examination of tissues reveals interstitial and intra-alveolar accumulation of eosinophil, macrophages, and edema. The syndrome might be idiopathic or caused by parasitic infections (e.g., *Ascaris* sp., *Strongyloides* sp.) or drugs (e.g., penicillin). Treatment requires removal of the offending agent or treatment of the parasitic infection. In idiopathic cases, corticosteroids may be used.

In the absence of asthma, *prolonged pulmonary eosinophilia* is an idiopathic disease predominantly of middle-aged women. Also termed *chronic eosinophilic pneumonia*, this illness is characterized by productive cough, dyspnea, malaise, weight loss, night sweats, and fever associated with progressive peripheral lung infiltrations that, on chest radiography, look like "the photographic negative of pulmonary edema." Lung histologic examination shows mixed inflammatory infiltrates with many eosinophils. However, in the right clinical setting, confirmation of eosinophilia in the bronchoalveolar lavage might be sufficient. Spontaneous remissions have been reported, but respiratory failure can also develop. Typically, treatment with corticosteroids is rapidly effective. Prolonged therapy is recommended because relapses are common. If the patient has asthma, then pulmonary infiltrates and severe intractable symptoms may suggest a diagnosis of *allergic bronchopulmonary aspergillosis*, a hypersensitivity reaction to *Aspergillus* sp. that is quite responsive to corticosteroids.

Tropical pulmonary eosinophilia represents a form of filariasis and is characterized by PIE syndrome, new onset of asthma, and fever. The diagnosis should be considered especially in travelers to the Far East. *Acute eosinophilic pneumonia* is characterized by rapid onset accompanied by fever and can be confused with PIE syndromes related to infectious causes. The patient is usually a young healthy individual with bilateral diffuse interstitial infiltrates. Treatment with corticosteroids is usually effective.

PULMONARY ALVEOLAR PROTEINOSIS

Pulmonary alveolar proteinosis is a disorder in which the alveoli fill with protein and phospholipid material similar to surfactant. The cause of this condition is unknown, but it is thought to be due to an unknown inhaled insult, perhaps an infection. Alveolar macrophages help clear surfactant in abnormal lungs. However, in pulmonary alveolar proteinosis, it appears that macrophage function is inhibited. Although patients may remain stable for years, some progress to fibrosis. Bilateral whole-lung lavage may help patients with profound hypoxemia, and it dramatically improves oxygenation. More recently, administration of granulocyte-macrophage colony-stimulating factor (GM-CSF) has been shown to effect remission of the disorder.

Prospectus for the Future

Sensitive and specific noninvasive methods are needed for the early identification of ILDs when attempts at preventing progression of lung fibrosis are likely to be more effective. IPF, the most common of the IIPs, is almost invariably fatal, and current treatment strategies are ineffective. Several clinical trials are examining the effectiveness of novel drugs in its treatment, including interferon-γ, anti–TNF-α agents, endothelin receptor antagonists, and antioxidants. The National Institutes of Health have established the *Idiopathic Pulmonary Fibrosis Clinical Research Network* to accelerate discovery. However, much confusion about this disease remains in the community, and educational strategies will be needed to accelerate diagnosis. Sarcoidosis is another enigmatic disease that, when progressive, is largely unresponsive to current treatment strategies. Small studies suggest agents capable of immunomodulation might be useful, but further work is needed in this arena. The advent of new technology able to evaluate genetic abnormalities related to disease has unveiled gene polymorphisms associated with IPF and sarcoidosis, among other ILDs. However, the true role of these abnormalities in causing the disease remains unclear, and the ability to exploit this information for early detection of disease is still limited. Interesting research is ongoing related to less common ILDs such as lymphangioleiomyomatosis, which affects women of childbearing age, and is focusing on the intracellular pathways that lead to cellular dysfunction in these disorders. Further work in this area and in the detection of the environmental hazards responsible for ILD is desperately needed. Until new and effective treatment strategies are generated, lung transplantation represents the only hope for an increasing number of patients with fibrosing ILDs. Therefore, efforts to extend life in lung transplant recipients are under way, particularly those targeting chronic rejection and bronchiolitis obliterans, the main cause of death in this population.

References

Gross TJ, Hunninghake GW: Idiopathic pulmonary fibrosis. N Engl J Med 345:517–525, 2001.

King TE: Clinical advances in the diagnosis and therapy of the interstitial lung diseases. Am J Respir Crit Care Med 172:268–279, 2005.

Pipavath S, Godwin JD: Imaging of interstitial lung disease. Clin Chest Med 25:455–465, 2004.

Schwarz MI, King TE, Raghu G: Approach to the evaluation and diagnosis of interstitial lung disease. In Schwarz MI, King TE, (eds): Interstitial Lung Disease, Hamilton, BC Decker, 2003, pp 1–53.

Chapter **19**

Pulmonary Vascular Disease

Jesse Roman

Kenneth L. Brigham

Pulmonary vascular diseases make up a heterogenous group of disorders with multiple causes that affect the pulmonary vasculature. Pulmonary vascular disorders can be caused by conditions that directly affect the pulmonary vessels as in primary pulmonary hypertension (PPH), or by disorders outside of the lung as in thromboembolic disease. Secondary causes of pulmonary hypertension are presented in Table 19–1. The main complication of these disorders is the development of pulmonary hypertension, which is defined as a mean pulmonary artery pressure over 25 mm Hg at rest or over 30 mm Hg with exercise. Pulmonary hypertension is caused by the loss of a cross-sectional area of the vascular bed, which increases vascular resistance. The loss of a cross-sectional area may be the result of mechanical occlusion, loss of vessels, vascular remodeling, or inflammation. Clinical manifestations of the disease may not be exhibited until late in the course of the disease. This delayed onset is due to the fact that the pulmonary vasculature is a high-flow, low-resistance, highly compliant system that can accept the entire output of the right ventricle with only slight increases in pressure even when one half of the pulmonary vasculature is removed.

Pulmonary Thromboembolic Disease

Pulmonary thromboembolic disease is a relatively common entity with an incidence ranging from 400,000 to 650,000 patients per year in the United States. Pulmonary thromboembolic disease is usually a complication of venous thrombosis. The deep veins of the femoral and popliteal systems of the lower extremities are most often affected, but right atrial, right ventricular, and upper-extremity thrombosis can also embolize to the lung. In view of this, predisposing factors for pulmonary embolism are the same as those for venous thrombosis and include venous stasis, hypercoagulability, and endothelial injury. Congenital or acquired procoagulant disorders (e.g. activated protein C deficiency) are also considered predisposing factors.

Once a clot dislodges from the lower extremity circulation, it travels to the pulmonary circulation where it can obstruct a branch of the pulmonary artery. The affected lung segment develops an increased ventilation/perfusion (V/Q) ratio. This development increases overall dead space ventilation, which leads to an inefficient excretion of partial pressure of carbon dioxide in arterial blood ($PaCO_2$). In addition, blood flow is shifted from the obstructed site to other areas, which may include areas of low V/Q ratios, thereby leading to shunting and hypoxemia. Pulmonary infarction of the area distal to the occlusion is rare because of the redundancy of the pulmonary circulation, which includes the bronchial arteries.

CLINICAL PRESENTATION

The classic presentation of acute pulmonary embolism includes acute shortness of breath accompanied by chest pain, hemoptysis, severe hypoxemia, and circulatory collapse as a result of shock. However, more often than not, the presentation is subtle and the diagnosis might be difficult to make without a high level of suspicion, particularly in young individuals with otherwise healthy lungs. Mildly increased dyspnea on exertion and atypical chest pain might be the only symptoms on initial presentation. Therefore, a careful history is paramount when evaluating patients for thromboembolic disease, especially those at high risk for this disorder as a result of stasis, malignancy, and previous history of venous thrombosis, as well as other risk factors. The physical examination might reveal abnormalities in lung auscultation ranging from isolated crackles to diffuse wheezing. Pleural effusions might be underlying areas of dullness to percussion during the physical examination. Edema of the extremities, especially if the edema is asymmetric, might point to venous thrombosis. In deep-vein thrombosis, dorsiflexion of the foot may cause calf pain as a result of stretching the calf muscles and deep veins (Homan's sign).

EVALUATION

In severe cases, determining the level of arterial blood gas may show acidemia, hypoxemia, and hypercapnia, but subtle changes such as mild alkalosis might be the only abnormalities. A normal $PaCO_2$ in a patient with tachypnea and

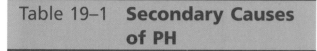

Table 19–1   Secondary Causes of PH

Cardiac Disease

- Valvular disease
- Left ventricular failure
- Intracardiac shunt

Pulmonary Disease

- Interstitial lung disease
- Chronic obstructive pulmonary disease
- Alveolar hypoventilation
- Hypoxia-induced

Collagen Vascular Disease

- Progressive systemic sclerosis
- Systemic lupus erythematosus
- Rheumatoid arthritis

Drug-Induced

- Chemotherapy-induced
- Crack cocaine
- Anorexic agents
- L-tryptophan
- Toxic old syndrome

Pulmonary Thromboembolic Disease

Other

- Human immunodeficiency viral infection
- Portal hypertension
- Schistosomiasis

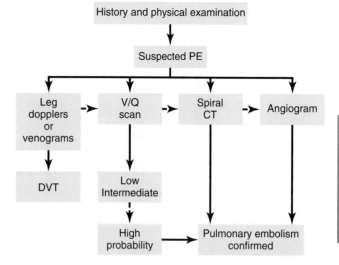

Figure 19–1 Tests commonly used in the evaluation of patients who may have pulmonary embolism. Doppler ultrasounds or venograms of the leg are useful to evaluate deep-vein thrombosis. Ventilation/perfusion (V/Q) scans are most useful when they are normal or show lesions highly suggestive of intravascular clot. Unfortunately, this finding is not the case in many patients requiring further investigation. Spiral computed tomography (CT) has a high sensitivity and specificity, and it allows for the evaluation of thoracic structures in addition to assessing the vasculature. Angiography is considered the gold standard, but it is often not needed if other noninvasive tests are used alone or in combination.

presumably hyperventilation suggests dead space and, in the appropriate setting, might point to the diagnosis. However, a normal alveolar-arterial oxygen-tension gradient (A-aDo$_2$) is not sensitive enough to exclude acute pulmonary embolism. An elevated level of lactic dehydrogenase (LDH) might be the result of tissue infarction, but this test is also insensitive and nonspecific. Some have advocated the use of plasma D-dimer levels in patients who might have pulmonary thromboembolism, but these are not specific either because they are elevated in patients with several unrelated medical conditions such as congestive heart failure, chronic illness, and connective tissue disorders. The main usefulness of plasma D-dimer levels is its negative predictive value.

The electrocardiogram may show atrial tachyarrhythmias or evidence of right heart strain as evidenced by a new right bundle branch block, right ventricular strain pattern, and the S$_I$Q$_{II}$T$_{III}$ pattern that mimics inferior myocardial infarction. The chest radiograph is often normal but may show atelectasis, isolated infiltrates, or a small pleural effusion. Oligemia (Westermark sign), an abrupt cutoff of pulmonary vessels or enlarged central pulmonary arteries (Fleischer sign), and pleural-based area of increased opacity (Hampton

hump) might also be noted. Independent of these findings, chest radiographs are not sensitive enough to diagnose pulmonary embolism. Three diagnostic methods are used for the diagnosis of pulmonary embolism: the V/Q scan, chest computed tomographic (CT) imaging, and pulmonary arteriography (Fig. 19–1). Nuclear tests based on radiolabeled fibrinogen are considered too insensitive and nonspecific.

The V/Q scan compares lung ventilation by radiolabeled tracer gas with lung perfusion by radiolabeled micro-occlusive particles. The usefulness of the V/Q scan depends greatly on the pre-test probability of the disease, which, in turn, is dependent on the expertise of the clinician and his or her level of certainty. A *high-probability* V/Q scan is characterized by a lobar or multilobar perfusion defects that coincide with areas of normal or relatively normal ventilation and is over 90% accurate in diagnosing pulmonary embolism. A *normal* V/Q scan shows no perfusion or ventilation defects and can exclude pulmonary embolism in essentially all cases. However, the test is less reliable when interpreted as *low, intermediate,* or *indeterminate* probability. Under such circumstances, pulmonary embolism is likely between 4% and 66% of patients (Table 19–2) and further testing is necessary to rule in or rule out accurately the diagnosis of pulmonary embolism.

Recently, spiral CT angiography has been found to provide a noninvasive and sensitive way to evaluate for pulmonary emboli (**Web Fig. 19–1**). Pulmonary arteriography is the gold standard and should be considered in patients

Table 19–2	Pulmonary Embolism Likelihood Using Clinical Suggestion and Ventilation/Perfusion Scan			
Scan Result	**Clinical Probability**			
	80–100%	**20–79%**	**0–19%**	**All**
High	96	88	56	87
Intermediate	66	28	16	30
Low	40	16	4	14
Normal	0	6	2	4
All scans	68	30	9	28

Data from PIOPED Study. JAMA, 263:2753–2759, 1990.

without contraindications to the procedure when other tests are inconclusive and a high suggestion of pulmonary embolism exists. Although complication rates related to this procedure are low, the complications are significant if developed, ranging from pulmonary hypertension and sudden death to idiosyncratic hypersensitivity reactions to dye. For this reason, many clinicians rely on a combination of interventions to arrive to the diagnosis particularly when pulmonary tests are combined with tests that evaluate the deep veins of the lower extremities such as venography and Doppler ultrasound.

MANAGEMENT

Pulmonary embolism is treated with supportive measures directed at sustaining organ function (e.g., fluid replacement for hypotension, mechanical ventilation for respiratory failure). To date, the only mechanical way to dislodge reliably a pulmonary artery clot is with surgical thromboembolectomy, a procedure with high mortality that requires a high level of expertise. Consequently, medical treatments are preferred and these are directed to prevent further clotting or to dissolve an existing clot. Anticoagulation with regular–

or low–molecular-weight heparin is recommended in patients without major contraindications to anticoagulation (e.g., upper gastrointestinal bleeding, hemorrhagic stroke). Their administration through subcutaneous injection appears to be as efficient as intravascular administration. The use of thrombolytic medications (e.g., streptokinase, urokinase) is usually reserved for patients with increased risk of mortality as a result of circulatory collapse caused by obstruction to the flow in large or multiple pulmonary vessels. However, recent data suggest that thrombolytic medications may improve outcomes when provided to patients without circulatory collapse but who show signs of new right ventricular strain on echocardiogram.

Primary Pulmonary Hypertension

PPH is an uncommon disorder that is progressive and usually fatal without treatment. The median survival after the diagnosis of the disease is approximately 3 years. Variables associated with poor survival include heart failure, Raynaud's phenomenon, elevated right atrial pressure, significantly elevated mean pulmonary arterial pressure, and decreased cardiac index. The peak incidence of PPH is between the ages of 20 and 45 years, and it affects women more frequently than men. In general, the cause of PPH is unknown; however, it has been associated with the use of anorexic drugs. Exogenous factors like human immunodeficiency viral (HIV) infection, cocaine use, and oral contraceptives have also been implicated.

The histologic characteristics of PPH are changes in both the arterial and venous systems. The arteries are more commonly affected, showing medial hypertrophy, plexogenic changes, and thrombosis. Plexogenic pulmonary arteriopathy represents the classic finding in PPH and it consists of medial hypertrophy, intimal proliferation and fibroelastosis, and necrotizing arteritis.

Treatment options for patients with PPH can improve survival and include drugs with vasodilator activity such as calcium channel blockers and prostacyclin. Because of the potential adverse effects of calcium channel blockers (decreased preload leading to acute hypotension), continuous intravenous prostacyclin is considered the most effective medical treatment. Often, this treatment option is used to bridge patients to lung transplantation. Other interventions include supplemental oxygen, anticoagulation, and judicious use of diuretic medications. Heart-lung, double-lung, or single-lung transplantations have been performed in these patients with some success, but the overall 5-year survival rate in all patients undergoing lung transplantation is only 50%. Recently, a group of new drugs with vasodilatory activities (and potential antiproliferative effects) have been shown to be effective in reducing pulmonary arterial pressure. Among these, endothelin-receptor antagonists and sildenafil have been tested and appear to be effective.

Prospectus for the Future

The mechanisms responsible for the development of PPH continue to elude scientists. However, the management of this condition will change dramatically in the next few years with the availability of selective inhibitors of cyclic guanosine monophosphate (cGMP)–specific phosphodiesterase type 5 (e.g., sildenafil) and endothelin-receptor antagonists (e.g., bosentan). These oral medications promote vasodilation and may even affect vascular remodeling, although the latter remains speculative. Independent of their mechanisms of action, these drugs are relatively safe and allow for ambulatory treatment of pulmonary hypertension. Some advocate the use of these drugs in secondary hypertension as well, but large prospective and well-controlled clinical trials are needed to assess their effectiveness in this arena. On the other hand, less new information is available about pulmonary thromboembolic disease. Although new inhibitors of the coagulation cascade are currently under investigation (e.g., antithrombin agents, inhaled heparin), understanding the mechanisms that lead to this illness has not dramatically changed over the last decade. Studies are needed in the area of genetic predisposition for thromboembolic disease, as well as in vascular dysfunction leading to thrombus formation.

References

Bull TM: New and future therapies in pulmonary arterial hypertension. Semin Respir Crit Care Med 26:429–436, 2005.

Fedullo PF, Auger WR, Channick RN, et al: Chronic thromboembolic pulmonary hypertension. Clin Chest Med 22:561–581, 2001.

Rubin LJ, Badesch DB: Evaluation and management of the patient with pulmonary arterial hypertension. Ann Intern Med 143:282–292, 2005.

Ramzi DW, Leeper KV: DVT and pulmonary embolism: Part I. Diagnosis. Am Fam Physician 69:2829–2836, 2004.

Ramzi DW, Leeper KV: DVT and pulmonary embolism: Part II. Treatment and prevention. Am Fam Physician 69:2841–2848, 2004.

Chapter 20

Disorders of Respiratory Control

Jesse Roman

Kenneth L. Brigham

During the transition between wakefulness and sleep, input from the behavioral control system decreases, the hypoxic drive to breathing is reduced, and the ventilatory response to partial pressure of carbon dioxide in arterial blood ($PaCO_2$) is diminished. These changes are most dramatic during rapid eye movement (REM) sleep. Sleep-disordered breathing refers to a diverse group of conditions in which these physiologic variations are heightened, resulting in abnormal respiratory function and fragmented sleep.

Of the sleep-related disorders, sleep apnea has received the most attention. *Apnea* is defined as the complete cessation of airflow for 10 or more seconds. *Hypopnea* is a significant decrease in airflow. Occasional episodes of apnea and hypopnea are expected during normal sleep, and their frequency increases with age. However, in patients with sleep apnea, the frequency and duration of the episodes are increased, leading to sleep fragmentation, as well as to hypoxemia and hypercapnia. Upper airway obstruction (i.e., obstructive sleep apnea) or decreased central respiratory drive (i.e., central sleep apnea) may be the cause of sleep apnea. In some patients, both disorders are present.

Some studies suggest that the prevalence of sleep-disordered breathing may be as high as 9% in women and 24% in men, but prevalence levels depend on the definition used. Sleep-disordered breathing is usually defined as a respiratory disturbance index or frequency of abnormal respiratory events that number five episodes per hour of sleep. Higher prevalence estimates occur in the older adult population with some studies showing over 80% prevalence in older patients. Children are also affected, although less frequently (~2%).

Obstructive Sleep Apnea

Obstructive sleep apnea is the most common of the sleep apnea syndromes and is considered to affect close to 6% of middle-aged and older men and is less common in women. In these patients, the upper airway relaxation that occurs during sleep is such that complete occlusion of the airway results and, consequently, cessation of airflow occurs. After variable periods of airway occlusion, the patient arouses, reestablishes muscle tone, and opens the airway. This vicious cycle is repeated many times during the night, resulting in recurring episodes of hypoxemia and hypercapnia. During airway occlusion, an increased sympathetic tone also occurs, producing vasoconstriction and hypertension. Episodes of hypoxemia can be associated with bradycardia and cardiac arrhythmias. These events are believed to be linked mechanistically to the increased incidence of stroke and coronary artery disease in patients with obstructive sleep apnea.

Clinical Manifestations

Obstructive sleep apnea should be suggested when patients complain of morning headaches, recurrent awakenings, and daytime somnolence that affects daytime activities including driving. Complaints of snoring and gasping episodes may be elicited from sleeping partners. Difficulties in maintaining sleep as a result of frequent awakenings may lead to mood effects and decreased quality of life. Recent weight gain, sedatives and sleeping pills, or alcohol intake may heighten these symptoms.

The primary risk factors for obstructive sleep apnea are obesity (although variable) and abnormal upper airway anatomy caused by macroglossia, long soft palate and uvula, enlarged tonsils, or micrognathia. Increased neck diameter (over 17 cm in men and over 16 cm in women) may also be noted. A narrow oropharynx as a result of a small pharyngeal opening or redundant soft tissue is often observed. Patients may be hypertensive and, in extreme cases, may show right-sided ventricular heart failure, which results as a consequence of prolonged episodes of hypoxemia and pulmonary vasoconstriction leading to pulmonary hypertension.

Evaluation

Chest radiographic images and pulmonary function testing are usually not helpful in the evaluation of patients with sleep apnea. In some cases, obstructive sleep apnea is associated with the obesity-hypoventilation syndrome, which is characterized by significant obesity associated with chronic hypoventilation and hypoxemia (*pickwickian syndrome*). In such cases, arterial blood gases show hypoxemia and hypercapnia, and blood cell counts might suggest polycythemia. Although rare, hypothyroidism, acromegaly, and amyloidosis can cause or enhance obstructive sleep apnea, and these conditions should be ruled out.

A formal diagnosis requires overnight polysomnography during which continual recordings of electrocardiographic and electroencephalographic tracings are made while the patient sleeps. In addition, airflow, oxygen saturation, and respiratory, eye, chin, and limb muscle movements are monitored and recorded. Obstructive sleep apnea is diagnosed in sleeping patients (confirmed by the electroencephalographic tracings) who develop cessation of airflow despite repeated muscular efforts to breathe (**Web Fig. 20–1**). These episodes may be accompanied by transient hypoxemia and cardiac arrhythmias. A score is derived from these data that defines clinically significant sleep apnea.

Polysomnography will distinguish obstructive sleep apnea from central sleep apnea, during which cessation of airflow is associated with halted respiratory movements. Polysomnography is also important to rule out other sleep disturbances such as insomnia, narcolepsy, and parasomnias, as well as restless leg syndrome.

The treatment of sleep apnea includes behavioral and medical approaches. When associated with obesity, weight loss should be enthusiastically encouraged. Avoidance of sedatives and alcohol is also important. Airway obstruction can be prevented with the use of continuous positive airway pressure (CPAP) provided through a tightly fitted mask. CPAP maintains positive airway pressure throughout expiration, thereby preventing collapse of the upper airway. The amount of pressure needed can be titrated, and oxygen can be added to further prevent hypoxemic episodes. CPAP is effective in most patients, but compliance with this technique is variable. Surgical removal of obstructing tonsils, adenoids, and polyps, or uvulopalatopharyngoplasty may be useful in patients with specific anatomic abnormalities. A permanent tracheostomy may be necessary in severe cases when other approaches fail. However, in general, the surgical approach to this disorder is limited to select patients usually after CPAP has failed.

Other Disorders Related to Respiratory Control

Central sleep apnea is a rare disorder. It predominates in men and is generally associated with normal body habitus. Patients may complain of daytime sleepiness and insomnia with frequent awakenings. This disorder is due to apnea or hypopnea, resulting from decreased central respiratory drive and may be a consequence of central nervous system injury (i.e., central apnea may be the result of a structural abnormality of the brainstem) or idiopathic. Affected individuals may hypoventilate even while awake, although they are capable of normal voluntary breaths. During sleep, frequent apnea is common.

In patients with obstructive lung disease, increased work of breathing eventually makes it difficult to maintain sufficient ventilation to maintain normal levels of $PaCO_2$. When ventilatory capacity declines, hypoventilation causes $PaCO_2$ to increase; the kidneys respond by retaining bicarbonate to keep arterial blood pH at normal levels. These patients appear to have normal ventilatory drive, but they lack the ability to increase minute ventilation to meet increased metabolic demand. This characteristic is observed in certain patients with chronic bronchitis who exhibit the classic description of the "blue bloater."

Lower brainstem and upper pontine lesions may cause *central hyperventilation.* However, this disorder rarely occurs in the absence of other physiologic or chemical abnormalities. Hepatic cirrhosis and extreme anxiety are all causes of central hyperventilation. Pregnancy can also cause hyperventilation and is thought to be caused by elevated levels of progesterone and other hormones that increase central actions. *Apneustic breathing* consists of sustained inspiratory pauses, resulting from damage to the midpons, most commonly caused by basilar artery infarction. *Biot's respiration* or *ataxic breathing* is a haphazardly random pattern of sleep and is characterized by shallow breaths; a disruption of the respiratory rhythm generator in the medulla causes this sign.

The regular cycling of crescendo-decrescendo tidal volumes, separated by apneic or hypopneic pauses, characterizes *Cheyne-Stokes respiration.* Patients with this disorder usually have generalized central nervous system disease or congestive heart failure. Heart failure prolongs circulatory times, causing a delay between changes in blood gases at the tissue level, and delays the arrival of those changes at the brainstem chemoreceptors. This delay sets up a cycle of gradual increase to hyperventilation, followed by gradually decreasing ventilation to apnea and then a repetition of the cycle.

Prospectus for the Future

With over 5% of the population in the United States suffering from sleep-disordered breathing and with the recognition that these disorders may contribute to systemic illnesses such as hypertension and cardiovascular disorders, interest in early diagnosis and treatment of disorders of respiratory control is growing. In view of the high incidence and potential health consequences of sleep-disordered breathing, physicians must be on the lookout for this condition. The increased incidence of obstructive sleep apnea parallels that of obesity in the United States, a public health problem that has been associated with asthma and increased risk of death. Sleep medicine is an emerging clinical and research area that will continue to receive great attention in the coming decade.

References

Abad VC, Guilleminault C: Neurological perspective on obstructive and nonobstructive sleep apnea. Semin Neurol 24:261–269, 2004.

Caples SM, Gami AS, Somers VK: Obstructive sleep apnea. Ann Intern Med 142:187–197, 2005.

Parish JM, Somers VK: Obstructive sleep apnea and cardiovascular disease. Mayo Clin Proc 79:1036–1046, 2004.

Stephen GA, Eichling PS, Quan SF: Treatment of sleep disordered breathing and obstructive sleep apnea. Minerva Med 95:323–336, 2004.

Chapter 21

Disorders of the Pleura, Chest Wall, and Mediastinum

Jesse Roman

Kenneth L. Brigham

Pleural Disease

The *pleura* is a continuous, thin, connective-tissue membrane that lines the internal thoracic cavity and mediastinum (parietal pleura) and the external surface of the lung (visceral pleura). Mesothelial cells, which are supplied by a vascular network derived from the systemic and lymphatic circulations, line the pleural membranes. Sensory nerve endings supply the parietal pleura but not the visceral pleura. The pleural membranes form a closed space that normally contains a film of a few milliliters of serous fluid. However, in certain systemic illnesses or diseases of the thorax, this space is violated by the accumulation of air (pneumothorax), fluid (effusion), or blood (hemothorax), as well as the formation of tumors (e.g., mesothelioma) or traumatic disruption.

The elastic recoil of the lung exerts an inward force, and the chest wall exerts an outward force, which results in a net pressure in the pleural space that is slightly less than atmospheric pressure when those forces are in balance (i.e., when the lung is at functional residual capacity). Under these conditions, fluid is normally transferred by a hydrostatic gradient from the parietal and visceral surfaces into the pleural space. The normal fluid turnover is approximately 10 to 20 mL/day.

Visceral pleural vessels are supplied from the pulmonary circulation, and parietal pleural vessels are part of the systemic circulation. Therefore, elevated pulmonary venous pressure increases the entry of fluid into the pleural space, and increased systemic venous pressure decreases absorption from the space. Pleural inflammation increases the permeability of pleural vessels and causes excessive fluid to enter the space for a given driving force. In addition, protein concentration in the fluid increases and creates an increased oncotic force that favors fluid accumulation. Hypoalbuminemia decreases intravascular oncotic pressure and favors sequestration of fluid in extravascular spaces that include the pleural space. Central lymphatic obstruction or obstruction of the channels at the pleural surface by tumor or exudates decreases pleural fluid absorption. Thus, normal fluid turnover in the pleural space can be disturbed when the dynamics are altered by increased hydrostatic pressure as observed with congestive heart failure, decreased blood oncotic pressure (e.g., low albumin states), increased permeability as observed with inflammatory processes of the pleura, increased negative pleural pressure as caused by atelectasis, or impaired lymphatic drainage as observed after trauma or neoplastic infiltration.

Patients with abnormalities of the pleura can be asymptomatic or exhibit dyspnea and/or pleuritic chest pain; this pain sharply increases in intensity during inspiration or coughing and may be referred to the ipsilateral shoulder and substernal area. Fever may be present, depending on the origin of the problem. Physical examination may reveal splinting, limited hemithorax excursion, and friction rub. Decreased breath sounds, egophony, and dullness to percussion are expected in pleural effusion, atelectasis, consolidation, or lung mass. These lesions can be further distinguished by evaluating for tactile fremitus, which is elevated in atelectasis, consolidation, and mass but diminished in pleural effusion.

A chest radiographic image may show a number of findings including a homogenous density with meniscus formation at the lateral chest wall, blunted costophrenic angle, and thickened fissure lines. When the volume of fluid in the pleural space exceeds 250 mL, the costophrenic angle is blunted. A mediastinal shift toward the abnormal hemithorax suggests atelectasis, whereas an ipsilateral shift suggests a massive pleural effusion. Lateral decubitus images may confirm suggested subpulmonic effusions and assess freemoving fluid. Ultrasound is useful to localize an effusion. However, a chest computed tomographic (CT) image allows for evaluation of the pleural space and adjacent structures that might be involved and could point to a specific diagnosis.

Pleural Effusion

Benign or malignant illnesses may cause pleural effusions. The most common cause is congestive heart failure. Parapneumonic effusions are also common and rarely evolve into

Table 21–1   Pleural Effusions

Transudates		Exudates	
Congestive heart failure	Infection	Systemic lupus erythematosus	Trauma
Hypoalbuminemia	Empyema	Rheumatoid arthritis	Hemothorax
Nephrotic syndrome Malnutrition	Para-pneumonic Malignancy	Intra-abdominal pathologic abnormalities	Chylothorax Ruptured esophagus
Cirrhosis	Primary lung cancer	Pancreatitis	Miscellaneous
Intraabdominal fluid	Lymphoma	Subphrenic abscess	Myxedema
Ascites	Metastatic cancer	Complications of abdominal surgery	Uremia
Peritoneal dialysis	Pulmonary embolism and infarction Collagen vascular disease	Meigs' syndrome Urinothorax	Asbestosis Lymphedema Drug-induced lupus Dressler's syndrome

From Light RW, Macgregor MI, Luchsinger PC, et al: Pleural effusions: The diagnostic separation of transudates and exudates. Ann Intern Med 77:507–513, 1972.

Table 21–2   Differentiation of Exudative and Transudative Pleural Effusions

	Exudate	Transudate
Protein	>3 g/dL	<3 g/dL
Pleural and serum protein	>0.5	<0.5
LDH	Two thirds upper limit of normal	Two thirds upper limit of normal
Pleural and serum LDH	>0.6	<0.6

LDH = lactate dehydrogenase.
Adapted from Light RW, Macgregor MI, Luchsinger PC, et al: Pleural effusions: The diagnostic separation of transudates and exudates. Ann Intern Med 77:507–513, 1972.

empyema. Malignancy may cause an effusion as a result of a primary tumor or metastatic lesions involving the pleura, which promotes infection through obstructive pneumonitis, or as a result of an obstruction in the lymphatic system.

When the cause for a pleural effusion is not evident, obtaining pleural fluid for examination is necessary. The objective is to determine the pathophysiologic mechanism that is causing the pleural fluid to accumulate. Osmotic and hydrostatic forces are responsible for the development of a *transudate,* as observed in cirrhosis, congestive heart failure, and low-protein states. Transudate develops in approximately one third of the patients and typically requires no further invasive studies (Table 21–1). Altered vascular permeability, as observed in inflammation, infection, or neoplasm, causes an exudate to develop. In some conditions

(e.g., thromboembolic disease), pleural fluid is a transudate or an exudate. To distinguish an exudate from a transudate, one of three criteria must be fulfilled: (1) pleural fluid/serum protein ratio is >0.5, (2) pleural fluid/serum lactate dehydrogenase (LDH) is >0.6, and (3) pleural fluid LDH is >200 (Table 21–2). When all three criteria are met, the sensitivity, specificity, and predictive value exceed 98% for an exudative effusion.

If an exudate is identified, then determining whether it is a *complicated* or an *uncomplicated* effusion is important (**Web Fig. 21–1**). A complicated effusion usually refers to fluid accumulation as a result of infection as observed in empyema. In this setting, evacuation of the effusion is necessary, and this evacuation can be attained with the insertion of a thoracostomy tube. A pH level of <7.2 usually identifies a complicated effusion; however, this finding is not specific because malignancy, rheumatoid arthritis, and trauma with esophageal disruption can also be associated with reduced pH levels.

After the previously discussed examination is completed and the laboratory findings are recorded, additional laboratory studies are obtained, selectively depending on the clinical presentation of the disorder. Microbiologic and cytologic studies are useful to evaluate for infection and malignancy. Frank pus defines an empyema, and organisms by Gram's stain procedure or in culture medium define a pleural space infection. Cytologic examination for malignant cells is positive in 60% of malignant effusions on first thoracentesis, and sensitivity rises to 80% if three separate samples are obtained. Blood in the effusion suggests malignancy, trauma, tuberculosis, collagen vascular disease, or thromboembolism. Lymphocytosis suggests chronicity but may also be related to tuberculosis or lymphoproliferative disorders. Eosinophils are found with blood or air in the pleural space. Glucose levels are decreased (<20 mg/dL) with infection and rheumatoid disease. An elevated amylase level may be observed with pancreatitis. Triglyceride levels over 110 mg/dL are characteristic of chylothorax. Elevated levels of adenosine deaminase are useful to diagnose tuberculous pleuritis.

If necessary, a biopsy of the pleura may be performed *blindly* through a *Cope's* or *Abrams' needle* or under direct visualization with video-assisted thoracoscopy. Pleural biopsies are positive for acid-fast bacilli in more than 50% of patients with tuberculous effusions, whereas fluid culture is positive in only 25% of those tested. Blind pleural biopsies can occasionally diagnose malignancy when pleural fluid is negative. However, visually directed biopsies have the highest yield.

Transudative effusions are typically small and rarely require drainage to improve symptoms. In contrast, exudative effusions as a result of infection need drainage to avoid sepsis but also to prevent the development of loculation, cutaneous fistulas (e.g., *empyema necessitatis*), lung abscess, and bronchopleural fistula. Fibrothorax may also develop, which will impair lung function caused by encasement of the underlying lung. The injection of fibrinolytic agents into the pleural space may prevent the occurrence of fibrothorax. Once established, however, treatment of a fibrothorax may require thoracotomy and decortication, an extensive surgical procedure with a high rate of complications. The recurrence of malignant pleural effusions may improve with chemical pleurodesis with talc or tetracycline derivatives, but effectiveness is variable, achieving a complete response in little more than 50% of patients. The life expectancy of patients with malignant pleural effusions resulting from lung cancer is a few months.

Pneumothorax

Pneumothorax is the accumulation of air in the pleural space. When the volume of air is significant, it causes dyspnea and pleurisy. Physical examination may show decreased breath sounds, hyperresonance, limited lateral excursion, and tracheal shift to the opposite side. Management usually requires insertion of a thoracostomy tube and suction.

Pneumothorax may occur spontaneously, typically in young, tall, thin men, presumably as a result of the rupture of congenital apical blebs. For a small pneumothorax, observation alone might be indicated; however, larger pneumothoracic accumulations require aspiration, small-bore tube insertion, or placement of a large-bore thoracostomy tube with suction, followed by water-seal drainage. *Complicated pneumothoraces* occur as a result of underlying lung disease as observed in emphysema, cystic fibrosis, granulomatous inflammation, necrotizing pneumonias, pulmonary fibrosis, and lung abscess. *Pneumocystis carinii* infection can also lead to pneumothorax because the development of thin-walled, cystlike lesions or pneumatoceles can be associated with pneumothorax. Other causes of pneumothorax include barotrauma in the setting of mechanical ventilation. Traumatic pneumothorax may occur as a result of penetrating or blunt trauma and is usually managed by tube thoracostomy. *Catamenial pneumothorax* refers to a pneumothorax that develops at the time of menstruation in women between the ages of 30 and 40 years and with a history of pelvic endometriosis. Extrauterine endometriosis in the lung is believed to be the cause of catamenial pneumothorax, but this suggestion cannot be confirmed in all patients.

A *tension pneumothorax* is the accumulation of air in the pleural space, creating positive pressure. Because tension pneumothorax can cause hemodynamic compromise, this medical emergency requires immediate decompression. All patients with pneumothorax who are receiving mechanical ventilation require a chest tube because of the risk of developing a tension pneumothorax. Occasionally, needle drainage can be performed without reaccumulation; in other situations, small-bore catheters are placed percutaneously. In patients with recurrent pneumothoraces as a result of emphysema or subpleural blebs, pleurodesis via mechanical or chemical abrasion of the pleura with or without thoracoscopy or thoracotomy with oversewing of the blebs is required.

Malignant Mesothelioma

Malignant mesothelioma typically occurs in individuals over age 55 years, particularly in men who have been exposed to asbestos in the distant past. The patient may exhibit dyspnea, chest pain, and weight loss; chest-imaging studies show pleural effusion and mass. Diagnosis requires a pleural biopsy. Chemotherapy and radiation are common treatment options, but the overall prognosis is poor with a mean survival of 1 to 2 years, independent of treatment.

Mediastinal Diseases

The mediastinum includes the central portion of the thorax posterior to the sternum, medial to the medial surface of the lungs, anterior to the chest wall, and bounded inferiorly by the diaphragm and superiorly by the thoracic inlet. For clinical purposes, this space is divided into three compartments: anterior, middle, and posterior (Fig. 21–1).

MEDIASTINITIS

Acute mediastinitis is a rapidly progressive inflammatory process that occurs as a result of trauma and necrotic tumor

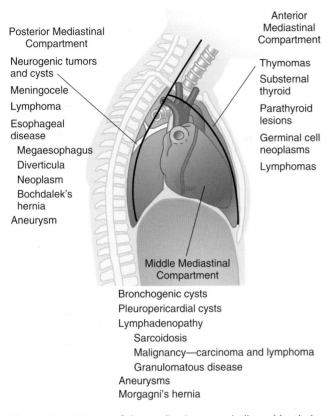

Posterior Mediastinal Compartment

Neurogenic tumors and cysts

Meningocele

Lymphoma

Esophageal disease

  Megaesophagus

  Diverticula

  Neoplasm

  Bochdalek's hernia

Aneurysm

Anterior Mediastinal Compartment

Thymomas

Substernal thyroid

Parathyroid lesions

Germinal cell neoplasms

Lymphomas

Middle Mediastinal Compartment

Bronchogenic cysts

Pleuropericardial cysts

Lymphadenopathy

  Sarcoidosis

  Malignancy—carcinoma and lymphoma

  Granulomatous disease

Aneurysms

Morgagni's hernia

Figure 21–1 Masses of the mediastinum are indicated by their anatomic locations.

or iatrogenically during invasive procedures such as esophageal endoscopy. The infection leads to fever, sepsis, pain, and subcutaneous emphysema. Chest imaging studies may show widening of the mediastinum, pneumothorax, or hydrothorax. Treatment requires antibiotics, pleural drainage, and mediastinal evacuation. *Chronic mediastinitis* (also termed *fibrosing mediastinitis*) is a slow, progressive illness that could be idiopathic or caused by granulomatous infections such as tuberculosis and histoplasmosis. Other causes include neoplasm, radiotherapy, and rarely drugs (e.g., methysergide). The condition is usually indolent, and patients remain asymptomatic until vascular or neurologic structures are affected. Superior vena cava syndrome may be a complication. Diagnosis and treatment often require surgical exploration. In some cases, fibrosis progresses inexorably to occlude vital structures with a fatal outcome.

MEDIASTINAL MASSES

Both benign and malignant masses can develop in the mediastinum. The major causes are neurogenic neoplasms, thymomas, congenital cysts, lymphomas, and germ-cell tumors. Mediastinoscopy can be used to evaluate some of these lesions. The treatment depends on the type of tumor. For example, thymic cancer tumors are best treated by resection, followed by radiation and/or chemotherapy. Lymphoma tumors are treated with chemotherapy and radiation. Neurogenic tumors of the posterior mediastinum require surgical resection.

Chest Wall Disease

Adequate ventilation depends on the efficient movement of the chest wall and diaphragm in response to neural stimulation. Thus, any disease that restricts the motion of the chest wall, distorts its symmetry, or interferes with neuromuscular function may produce hypoventilation. In these diseases, the total lung and vital capacities are decreased, but the residual volume is usually normal or even increased. Hypoventilation produces hypercapnia and progressive atelectasis. The decrease in vital capacity leads to ventilation/perfusion inequality, resulting in hypoxemia.

VERTEBRAL DISEASE

Disorders of the chest wall may limit ventilatory movements and are associated with lung restriction and hypoventilation. *Scoliosis* is an abnormal lateral curvature and decreased mobility of the vertebral column. *Kyphosis* is extreme flexion of the thoracic supine. Usually, these deformities co-exist, and the resulting restriction of the thoracic cavity volume may cause respiratory failure. Surgical correction of the deformity in adults does not improve respiratory function or the incidence of complications.

OBESITY

Obesity causes a decrease in the expiratory reserve volume, decreased ventilation of basilar portions the lungs, and hypoxemia as a result of ventilation/perfusion inequality. The abnormalities are magnified when the patient is in the supine position and are frequently accompanied by disorders of ventilatory control and upper airway obstruction. When obesity is associated with hypoventilation, it is termed the obesity-hypoventilation syndrome (*pickwickian syndrome*). The most important consequence of this and related conditions associated with chronic hypoventilation is pulmonary hypertension.

DIAPHRAGMATIC PARALYSIS

Unilateral diaphragmatic paralysis in the absence of other diseases may be asymptomatic. Most patients retain 75% of normal vital capacity, despite the functional loss of a hemidiaphragm. Encroachment of abdominal contents on the thoracic cavity causes symptoms to worsen when the patient is in the supine position. Causes of diaphragmatic paralysis include injury of the phrenic nerve by tumor invasion or compression, viral neuropathy, systemic lupus erythematosus, or other neuropathic diseases. Surgical injury could be a cause, and difficulties in weaning from mechanical ventilation after thoracic surgery should prompt an evaluation of diaphragmatic function. The diagnosis of diaphragmatic paralysis is made by fluoroscopic observation of the diaphragm during the sniff maneuver in which the affected diaphragm moves paradoxically. Definitive diagnosis is made from nerve conduction studies.

Bilateral diaphragmatic paralysis causes significant dyspnea and orthopnea. Paradoxic inward motion of the abdominal wall during inspiration is a classic finding. Maximal inspiratory force is significantly decreased. Chest radiographic images show decreased lung volumes and can

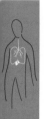

be mistaken for pulmonary interstitial lung disease because of crowding of the parenchyma and vasculature at the bases. Bilateral diaphragmatic paralysis is rarely idiopathic and is usually a manifestation of an acute or a chronic generalized neuromuscular disease such as *Guillain-Barré syndrome,* muscular dystrophy, amyotrophic lateral sclerosis, or post-polio syndrome, a diagnosis that is frequently overlooked.

Bilateral diaphragmatic paralysis is usually irreversible, shifting the focus to the management of progressive respiratory failure. Decisions to use supplemental oxygen, non-invasive positive pressure ventilation, or tracheostomy with long-term mechanical ventilation depend on the medical condition, the prognosis, and the patient's preference.

References

Colice GL, Curtis A, Deslauriers J, et al: A new classification of parapneumonic effusions and empyema. Chest 108:299–301, 1995.

Light RW: Useful tests on the pleural fluid in the management of patients with pleural effusions. Curr Opin Pulm Med 5:245–249, 1999.

Yusen, RD: Medical and surgical treatment of parapneumonic effusions: An evidence-based guideline. Chest 118:1158–1171, 2000.

Chapter 22

Infectious Diseases of the Lung

Jesse Roman

Kenneth L. Brigham

Pulmonary infections are common, with pneumonia occurring in over 6 million people annually; pneumonia represents one of the top 10 causes of death in the United States. Pulmonary infection can be due to several organisms including viruses, bacteria, and fungi. Patients usually exhibit respiratory symptoms including productive cough, dyspnea, chest pain, and occasionally hemoptysis. Other less specific symptoms include fever, general malaise, muscle aches, and weight loss. The presentation may be acute (days to weeks), as observed with bacterial pneumonia, or subacute or chronic (weeks to years), as observed with tuberculosis. Patients with certain underlying conditions (e.g., human immunodeficiency viral [HIV] infection) may be predisposed to specific illnesses, and knowledge of the specific impairment in host defense mechanisms may help determine the cause of the infection.

Diagnosis and therapy will depend on clinical, imaging, and laboratory data. Of these, the chest radiograph plays an important role. A parenchymal opacity is observed in the patient with pneumonia (**Web Fig. 22–1**); however, noninfectious disorders that mimic pneumonia exist, and no radiographic finding is entirely specific for infection. A para-pneumonic effusion may also be present (**Web Fig. 22–2**).

Community-Acquired Pneumonia

A good understanding of the epidemiology of infectious organisms at a particular location and the efficiency of the patient's host defense mechanisms will help guide therapy when evaluating the patient with pneumonia. Table 22–1 describes the most common types of infections in community-acquired and nosocomial pneumonias.

Streptococcus pneumoniae is a gram-positive, diplococcal bacterium that accounts for up to 26% of all pneumonias and 60% to 75% of those acquired in the community. When encapsulated, *S. pneumoniae* is a pathogenic organism (e.g., serotype III) and carries a high mortality rate. Affected patients are usually the older adult, immunocompromised patients, and those who abuse alcohol. The rates of pneumococcal pneumonia are 19/100,000 but are increased in patients with acquired immunodeficiency syndrome (AIDS) (2000/100,000). Patients may have an antecedent upper respiratory tract infection, followed by the sudden onset of fever, shaking chills, dyspnea, and pleurisy. Cough productive of purulent, rust-colored sputum is common. Imaging studies show alveolar consolidation.

The sputum Gram's stain is positive in only 45% of bacteremic cases. Therefore, isolation of the organism from a usually sterile site, such as blood, pleural fluid, or cerebrospinal fluid, confirms the diagnosis. In clinical practice, the diagnosis is presumptive. Invasive diagnostic procedures are seldom indicated when appropriate empirical therapy has been instituted. Penicillin G and erythromycin were once the antibiotic medications of choice. However, a rapid increase in the prevalence of *Streptococcus* sp. resistant to penicillin, erythromycin, and trimethoprim-sulfamethoxazole has occurred. Thus the second- and third-generation cephalosporins, the newer macrolides (e.g., azithromycin, ad clarithromycin), and quinolones (e.g., Levaquin, Tequin) are the treatments of choice. The majority of patients become afebrile in 5 days after starting antibiotherapy, but radiographic clearing make take up to 14 days and even longer in the older adult.

Mycoplasma pneumoniae is a slow-growing, facultative anaerobic organism that accounts for 25% to 60% of all atypical pneumonias. *M. pneumoniae* is common in patients between the ages of 5 and 35 years who may initially exhibit upper respiratory tract symptoms, pharyngitis, and bullous myringitis. Dry cough, fever, gastrointestinal symptoms, headache, and myalgias are common. The chest radiograph may show fine interstitial reticulonodular infiltrates that progress to air-space consolidation. Pleural effusions may be observed, but hilar enlargement is rare.

The diagnosis is difficult and based on clinical and epidemiologic features. Acute and convalescent serologic findings are required to confirm the diagnosis but are not helpful during the acute illness. Cold agglutinins are nonspecific, and cultures take up to 2 to 3 weeks to grow. Newer techniques are more rapid and sensitive, including enzyme-linked immunosorbent assay (ELISA) and DNA probes

Table 22–1	Organisms Causing Pulmonary Infections	
Pathogen	**Community Acquired**	**Nosocomial**
Bacterial	**70–80%**	**90%**
Streptococcus pneumoniae	60–75%	3–9%
Hemophilus influenza	4–5%	
Legionella sp.	2–5%	Up to 25%
Staphylococcus aureus	1–5%	10–20%
Gram-negative bacilli	Rare	50%
Atypical	**10–20%**	**Rare**
Mycoplasma pneumoniae	5–18%	—
Chlamydia psittaci	2–3%	—
Coxiella burnetii	1%	—
Virus	**10–20%**	**Rare**
Influenza	—	8%
Hantavirus	—	Rare

Adapted from: Modai J. Empiric therapy of severe infections in adults. Am J Med 88:12S–17S, 1990.

coupled with hybridization techniques. Macrolide medications are recommended for treatment.

Nosocomial Pneumonia

Nosocomial pneumonia is pneumonia that occurs after 72 hours of hospitalization and is the second most common cause of hospital-acquired infection. Nosocomial pneumonia is associated with significant morbidity and mortality; pneumonia is the most common cause of mortality from nosocomial infections. Mechanical ventilation is the most potent risk factor for developing nosocomial pneumonia, and the disorder is termed *ventilator-induced pneumonia* (VAP). The most common bacterial pathogens responsible for VAP are *S. pneumoniae, Hemophilus influenza,* and *Moraxella catarrhalis,* especially when the infection occurs in the first 4 days after intubation. Later, VAP is caused by *Pseudomonas aeruginosa, Acinetobacter* sp., *Enterobacter* sp., and *Staphylococcus aureus.* The incidence of nosocomial pneumonia is 10% for patients in the general surgical setting, 20% for patients in medical intensive care units, and 70% in the setting of acute respiratory distress syndrome.

Many nosocomial pneumonias are polymicrobial and include gram-negative bacilli, anaerobes, and *Staphylococcus* sp. Gram-negative bacilli include *P. aeruginosa* and methicillin-resistant staphylococci. *Legionella* sp. are also recognized as important pathogens responsible for outbreaks of nosocomial pulmonary infections.

The pathogenesis of nosocomial pneumonia is based on colonization of the oropharynx and stomach with virulent pathogens and the subsequent aspiration of these organisms into the lower respiratory tract. Gastric colonization by gram-negative organisms is enhanced by neutralization of

gastric acidity. Other risk factors include co-existing illness, impaired nutritional status, invasive therapeutic interventions, smoking history, advanced age, nursing home residence, and mechanical ventilation. Clinical criteria for diagnosis are relatively poor, and radiographic findings are nonspecific, usually showing multilobar infiltrates and effusions. Multiple-cavitating nodular infiltrates are suggestive of staphylococcus septic emboli. The diagnosis of nosocomial pneumonia could be enhanced by quantitative cultures of secretions obtained by bronchoscopic lavage or sterile protective specimen endobronchial brushing.

Treatment is dependent on combined chemotherapy with g-lactam antipseudomonal penicillin or cephalosporin, together with an aminoglycoside or a quinolone. Vancomycin is added if methicillin-resistant *Staphylococcus* sp. is suspected. Clindamycin and related drugs are useful if aspiration pneumonia is strongly suggested.

Mycobacterium Tuberculosis Infection

Infection with *Mycobacterium tuberculosis,* an aerobic, nonmotile, acid-fast rod with niacin production, causes tuberculosis. In 1997 the World Health Organization Global Surveillance and Monitoring Project estimated 8 million new cases per year of tuberculosis, including 3.5 million cases of infectious pulmonary disease. In addition, 16.2 million cases of the disease existed. An estimated 1.87 million individuals die of tuberculosis each year, and the global case fatality rate was 23%, with 50% in some African countries with high HIV rates. In the United States, tuberculosis increased at an alarming rate in the early 1990s as a result of the surge of HIV infection, drug abuse, inner city poverty, and homelessness.

The infection is acquired through the inhalation of droplets of bacilli that are engulfed by alveolar macrophages in which intracellular growth occurs, followed by the release of bacilli from dead cells. Confinement of infection depends on specific cellular immunity, requiring coordination between T lymphocytes and macrophages. Histologically, tissues infected with *M. tuberculosis* show caseating or necrotizing granulomas (Fig. 22–1). This host defense mechanism is impaired in those with HIV, leading to poor development of granulomas.

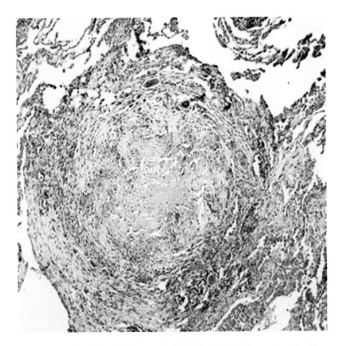

Figure 22–1 Necrotizing granuloma in lung infected with *M. tuberculosis.*

Patients exhibit insidious symptoms that progress over weeks to months. Fever, weight loss, night sweats, and productive cough are often observed. Chest radiographs may show patchy infiltrates with cavitation in the apical and posterior segments of the upper lobes. Bronchogenic spread occurs through aspiration of infected material to the lower lobes. A military pattern may be observed in a chest radiograph image and indicates hematogenous dissemination. Atypical presentations may be encountered in the older adult and in the patient with an immunosuppressed system.

The diagnosis of *M. tuberculosis* infection is dependent on a positive tuberculin test, which does not indicate active disease but only exposure or previous infection. Patients are at high risk for developing active tuberculosis early after tuberculin conversion, and thus the reason for recommending prophylaxis, particularly within 2 years after conversion (Table 22–2). Prophylaxis is also recommended in patients with a history of inadequately treated tuberculosis and positive tuberculin reactors less than 35 years of age. Patients with an immunocompromised system and with radiographic evidence of old inactive tuberculosis should be treated for a year. Prophylaxis can be achieved by administering isoniazid 300 mg daily for 6 to 12 months.

Treatment of patients suspected of having active disease includes at least four drugs: isoniazid, 5 mg/kg/day; rifampin, 10 mg/kg/day; ethambutol, 5 to 25 mg/kg/day; pyrazinamide, 15 to 30 mg/kg/day, and should be considered before a formal diagnosis is made (e.g., exposure to tuberculosis, pulmonary symptoms, cavitary disease on imaging studies). If diagnosis is confirmed, then the drugs are continued for 2 months, barring adverse reactions to the drug therapy. After 2 months, the regimen can be tailored, depending on drug-sensitivity studies and continued for another 4 months with at least two active drugs. Identifying the bacilli or growing it from clinical samples in cultured medium (e.g., sputum, bronchoalveolar lavage fluid, tissue) can confirm the diagnosis of tuberculosis.

Rates of drug-resistant tuberculosis are increased in certain populations (e.g., Hispanics, Southeast Asians).

Table 22–2	**Prophylaxis Against Tuberculosis in Adults**	
PPD	**Prophylaxis Indicated Regardless of Age**	**Prophylaxis Indicated If < 35 Years Old**
5 mm	Close contacts recently diagnosed with TB HIV positive or HIV risk factors Fibrotic changes on chest radiograph	
10 mm	Diabetes mellitus Immunosuppression Hematologic malignancy Injection drug use Renal failure Malnutrition	PPD increased over 10 mm within 2 years Native of high-prevalence country High-risk ethnic minorities Residents and staff of long-term care facilities
15 mm	PPD increased over 15 mm within 2 years	No risk factors

HIV = human immunodeficiency virus; PPD = purified protein derivative of tuberculin; TB = tuberculosis.

Resistance is detected in 9% of patients who have not received previous therapy and of 22.8% in those with prior treatment. In patients with drug-resistant tuberculosis, treatment should include at least three drugs that have not been administered before and to which the organism is susceptible *in vitro.* Treatment should continue for at least 18 to 24 months. Direct observation of therapy may be required to ensure compliance.

Pneumocystis Carinii Pneumonia

Pneumocystis carinii is an opportunistic fungus that occurred mainly in malnourished premature infants, as well as adults with hematologic malignancy undergoing chemotherapy in the pre-AIDS era. However, its incidence rose significantly in the late 1980s and 1990s as a result of the increase number of patients with AIDS with low CD4+ lymphocyte counts (<250). Patients may complain of nonproductive cough, fever, dyspnea, and weight loss. The symptoms are slowly progressive over weeks in the patient infected with HIV. Oral candidiasis, increased serum lactic dehydrogenase (LDH), increased Aa-oxygen gradient, and a decreased CD4+ count are independent predictors of HIV-related *P. carinii* pneumonia.

Chest radiographic images may show diffuse, bilateral interstitial infiltrates, but they may be clear in up to 15% of patients (**Web Fig. 22–3**). Other findings include isolated infiltrates, cavitary lesions, nodular masses, pneumothorax, and a military pattern. Hilar and mediastinal adenopathy are rare. Identifying the organism in sputum, which is effective in 60% to 85% of patients, will help obtain a diagnosis. Bronchoscopy with bronchoalveolar lavage can increase the yield (86%), especially if a transbronchial biopsy is included (98% to 100%).

Prophylaxis can be provided by oral trimethoprim-sulfamethoxazole or aerosolized pentamidine. When pneumonia is present, the therapy of choice is trimethoprim-sulfamethoxazole; however, significant adverse effects, including leukopenia, nausea, vomiting, and elevation of liver transaminases, are associated with this therapy. Intravenous pentamidine is a reasonable alternative to trimethoprim-sulfamethoxazole; this therapy could be complicated by hypoglycemia. Less toxic drug regimens are available (e.g., trimethoprim and dapsone, clindamycin and primaquine) but are recommended only after failure of other medications. Corticosteroids should be considered in patients with severe disease as demonstrated by significant hypoxemia (e.g., partial pressure of oxygen in arterial blood [PaO$_2$] <70 mm Hg). Corticosteroids are expected to decrease the likelihood of progression to respiratory failure.

Prospectus for the Future

Lung infection continues to represent a source of high morbidity and mortality rates, both in the community and in hospitals. A significant portion of this infection affects the extremes of age—children and older adults. Although industry continues to search for new antibiotics with higher safety and effectiveness profiles, the judicious use of agents currently available will help prevent or delay drug resistance while newer agents are being developed. Continued efforts are needed to reinforce vaccination against infectious agents including influenza. HIV infection and tuberculosis continue to have important negative consequences in the United States, but none is as dramatic as those witnessed in Africa and other underdeveloped countries. In addition to continued efforts toward the development of antiviral medications and effective vaccines, concerted international efforts will be necessary to reduce the relentless drive of these illnesses by improving education, enhancing the economy of underdeveloped countries, and reducing poverty. Most importantly, promoting sustained vigilance by relevant government agencies is the priority of future international efforts.

References

Enarson DA, Murray JF: Global Epidemiology of Tuberculosis. In Rom WN, Gray SM (eds): Tuberculosis. Boston: Little Brown, 1996, pp. 57–75.

Markewitz BA, Mayer J, Sud PR, et al: Treatment of hospital-acquired pneumonia. Semin Respir Infect 15:248–257, 2000.

Segreti J, House HR, Siegel RE: Principles of antibiotic treatment of community-acquired pneumonia in the outpatient setting, Am J Med 118:S1S–S8S, 2005.

Essentials in Critical Care Medicine

Jesse Roman

Kenneth L. Brigham

Critical care medicine has evolved dramatically over the past decades, thanks to the development of new technologies but also because of information from clinical trials that have established standards for the management of patients in the critical care setting. Since the epidemic of poliomyelitis in the 1950s, intensive care units have clearly proved to be beneficial in treating acute reversible disorders. However, because of the innovative nature of the technology used and the need for close monitoring and intensive management, the delivery of critical care medicine is expensive, accounting for up to 30% of total hospital costs.

Patients in intensive care units (ICUs) are a heterogenous population treated for diverse conditions ranging from septic shock and respiratory failure to diabetic ketoacidosis and upper gastrointestinal bleeding. This chapter discusses a few of the most common conditions encountered in the ICU setting that are often managed by pulmonologists. These topics include acute respiratory failure and mechanical ventilation, acute lung injury, and shock.

Acute Respiratory Failure and Mechanical Ventilation

Acute respiratory failure results when the lung can no longer accomplish adequate gas exchange, a condition that is fatal if left untreated. Hypoxemic respiratory failure refers to respiratory failure associated with failure to oxygenate, whereas hypercarbic respiratory failure is the failure to ventilate. These disorders are manifested by alterations in arterial partial pressure of oxygen (PaO_2) and carbon dioxide ($PaCO_2$), respectively. The values of PaO_2 and $PaCO_2$ that define respiratory failure are somewhat arbitrary, but respiratory compromise is evident when the PaO_2 is less than 60 mm Hg while the patient breathes room air or the $PaCO_2$ is over 45 mm Hg.

Respiratory failure is common in patients with chronic lung disease who develop an exacerbation of their lung condition from infection, pulmonary embolism, congestive heart failure, or related processes. However, respiratory failure can also develop in otherwise healthy individuals as a result of severe trauma, heavy sedation, neurologic dysfunction, or a variety of other processes. The management of respiratory failure depends on the clinical presentation. Patients with respiratory failure while awake, cooperative, and hemodynamically stable may tolerate aggressive respiratory therapy without intubation and mechanical ventilation, as long as gas exchange and overall status are continually monitored. This setting often described patients with chronic obstructive pulmonary disease (COPD) who can sometimes tolerate a $PaCO_2$ level as high as 85 mm Hg. In contrast, patients in respiratory failure with evidence of severe respiratory distress (e.g., respiratory rate >30 breaths/min), mental deterioration (e.g., impaired judgment, confusion, hallucinations, somnolence) or hemodynamic instability (e.g., bradydysrhythmias or tachydysrhythmias, hypotension) usually require intubation and mechanical ventilation. In the latter circumstances, waiting for arterial blood gas determinations is not necessary and could dangerously delay therapy. Although arterial blood gas evaluation is crucial when determining the need for mechanical ventilation in the patient with respiratory failure, the patient's clinical status will ultimately dictate the course of action.

Although intubation and mechanical ventilation are usually the preferred options in respiratory failure that is considered reversible and noninvasive, positive- and negative-pressure ventilation have proved useful in select patients with COPD and other disorders. Noninvasive positive pressure is provided through a tightly fitted mask connected to a respirator. However, frequently, noninvasive ventilation is insufficient to deliver the pressure needed to address the ventilatory demands of the patient.

Once a decision to intubate is made, an experienced operator should expeditiously perform intubation. Complications of intubation are usually related to prolonged hypoxemia as a result of delays in the procedure, but they also include vomiting and aspiration of gastric contents, trauma to the vocal cords, bleeding, pneumothorax, cardiac arrhythmias, and cardiac arrest. Once inserted, the tube should be secured and its position assessed by examining for breath sounds, followed by chest radiography for confirmation. Direct visualization through a bronchoscope is rarely needed. A ventilator should be available before the procedure is begun so that mechanical ventilation can start as soon as the endotracheal tube is secured.

Mechanical Ventilation

Initial ventilator settings may vary, but typically they include a ventilator mode of assist control, fraction of inspired oxygen (FiO_2) of 1.0 (or 100%), respiratory rate set at 10 to 12 breaths per minute, and tidal volume of 400 to 600 mL. The adequacy of the ventilator settings needs to be determined with repeated arterial blood gas levels and the clinical evaluation of the patient. Persistent cyanosis, pallor, diaphoresis, and restlessness may suggest that the tube is misplaced or that the ventilator settings are insufficient to ventilate the patient appropriately. Positive-end expiratory pressure (PEEP) might be required in patients with refractory hypoxemia. PEEP prevents the premature collapse of the alveoli during expiration and improves ventilation/perfusion matching, leading to improve oxygenation. Once the settings are adjusted to maintain relatively normal levels of arterial blood gases (pH between 7.3 and 7.45, PaO_2 >60 mm Hg, PCO_2 between 30 and 45 mm Hg), attention should be given to developing a *maintenance* plan that will secure adequate oxygenation and ventilation until the cause of the respiratory failure is treated and the failure is reversed. This plan should include assessment of the need for sedation, appropriate strategy of mechanical ventilation, supportive measures to achieve hemodynamic stability, nutritional assessment, and therapies targeting the initial injurious process that triggered the respiratory failure (e.g., pneumonia, pulmonary embolism, asthma, shock). Most patients will require sedation to diminish discomfort and to decrease the work of breathing, but it should be administered carefully because sedation is often accompanied by a decrease in blood pressure.

The most common type of ventilation currently used is positive-pressure ventilation, which can be delivered through volume-cycled or pressure-controlled ventilators. Volume-cycled ventilators cyclically deliver a predetermined volume that is set on the machine. In this setting the amount of inspiratory pressure depends on lung compliance. Thus, in the patient with highly compliant lungs (e.g., emphysema), the predetermined lung volume that will be delivered should cause a relatively small increase in inspiratory pressure. In contrast, in the patient with low compliant lungs (e.g., lung fibrosis or edema), inspiratory pressures will be higher during the delivery of an equal volume. When using a pressure-controlled ventilator, the clinician sets the inspiratory pressure for a prescribed time. In this setting, the tidal volume may vary because it will depend directly on the inspiratory pressure provided and the compliance of the lung. Thus, in the volume-cycled ventilators, tidal volume remains constant despite variations in pressure, whereas in pressure-controlled ventilators, inspiratory pressure remains constant; however, the tidal volume may not. Pressure-controlled ventilation is most often used when the clinician is concerned about limiting the pressure delivered by the ventilator.

When using a positive-pressure, volume-cycled ventilator, several modes are available. In the 1980s, the most popular mode of ventilation was intermittent mandatory ventilation (IMV). IMV allows the clinician to set the tidal volume and the lowest needed respiratory rate considered necessary. A *ventilated* or *supported* breath is triggered by negative pressure generated by a spontaneous effort to breathe (usually 1 to 2 cm of water) that opens a valve through which the predetermined tidal volume is delivered. The respiratory rate of the patient may vary, but the rate of *supported breaths* will not. Although this mode can adequately ventilate patients, it is often associated with asynchrony characterized by a dissociation of spontaneous breaths and supported breaths. In addition, if the patient's spontaneous respiratory rate is higher than the set rate, then the spontaneous breaths would not be supported. These two processes lead to increased work of breathing. To decrease asynchrony, synchronized intermittent mandatory ventilation (SIMV) was developed, which allows for the synchronization of spontaneous breaths with the supported breaths. Unfortunately, increased work of breathing during the unsupported breaths remains in this mode.

In view of this brief history, the current preferred mode of ventilation is assisted-control (AC) ventilation (also called controlled mechanical ventilation [CMV]). In AC ventilation the clinician sets the tidal volume and the lowest allowed respiratory rate; however, each spontaneous breath is supported. In other words, the entire tidal volume is delivered with each breath, independent of the set ventilator rate. AC ventilation is considered a more physiologic ventilatory mode and is associated with decreased work of breathing when compared with other volume-cycled or pressure-controlled ventilatory modes.

Another mode of ventilation is pressure-support ventilation. This mode is delivered by a pressure-controlled ventilator and, as previously mentioned, requires the clinician to set the inspiratory pressure. A ventilated breath is triggered by a spontaneous breath, which is detected by a change in flow. The latter triggers the delivery of air, but the volume delivered depends on the set pressure and the compliance of the lung. In this setting the clinician has to adjust the inspiratory pressure to deliver the appropriate tidal volume. Nevertheless, in practice, differences between this mode and AC ventilation are minimal in the hands of an experienced clinician.

Weaning from Mechanical Ventilation

The complications of endotracheal intubation and mechanical ventilation are many; barotrauma and pneumonia are the most significant. Therefore, the patient who is mechanically ventilated must be treated aggressively and monitored carefully. Weaning from mechanical ventilation should be considered when the original insult that caused respiratory failure has cleared, especially if the patient is awake and cooperative and shows no signs of respiratory or hemodynamic instability. Weaning is usually not attempted if

Table 23-1	Conventional Weaning Parameters	
Parameters	**Weanable Values**	**Normal Ranges**
NIF (cm of water)	<–20	<–50
VC (mL/kg)	>10	>65–75
V_T (mL/kg)	<5	>5–7
RR (breaths/min)	<32	12–20
V_E (L/min)	>10	>10

NIF = negative inspiratory force; RR = respiratory rate; VC = vital capacity; V_E = minute ventilation; V_T = tidal volume.

requirements for oxygen supplementation remain high (FiO_2 >0.5). Conventional parameters that determine whether weaning is possible include negative inspiratory force, vital capacity, tidal volume, respiratory rate, and minute ventilation (Table 23–1). Unfortunately, the strength of these parameters lies in the ability to predict failure to wean rather than in the ability to predict successful spontaneous breathing. A better way to assess weaning capability is to engage the patient in a short *weaning trial* during which support from the ventilator is diminished. This trial can be achieved by allowing the patient to breathe oxygen for 1 hour through a T tube without providing supporting pressure. Another strategy is to decrease the pressure generated by the ventilator during a trial of continuous positive airway pressure (CPAP). The patient is monitored for any signs of distress or hemodynamic instability, and arterial blood gas levels are measured to determine the effectiveness of spontaneous ventilation. If the patient tolerates the trial, then extubation may be indicated, depending on the patient's clinical status and his or her underlying condition. In general, only 10% to 15% of patients who are extubated on the basis of the results of these trials require reintubation.

If the patient fails the weaning trial, then attempts should be made to identify the factors responsible for the failure to wean. Frequently, all obvious contributory factors are identified and corrected, but the patient requires a more prolonged weaning trial before extubation. Two weaning strategies are recommended in this setting. The first is to engage the patient in spontaneous ventilation trials through a T tube for 1 hour once or twice each day with total ventilatory support between trials, usually via AC ventilation. The length of the T-tube trials can be progressively increased until the patient no longer requires mechanical support. The other strategy is dependent on the use of pressure support ventilation. The ventilator is set to deliver a low respiratory rate (usually at 6 breaths/min or lower) during the SIMV mode, and the inspiratory pressure is progressively decreased until the patient can breathe spontaneously without ventilatory support. Both strategies seem to be equally effective, although weaning via pressure support ventilation might be preferred in patients with chronic lung disease who have been mechanically ventilated for prolonged periods.

Acute Lung Injury

Acute diffuse lung injury in its most severe form is called acute respiratory distress syndrome (ARDS). Acute lung injury is characterized by increased permeability of the alveolar-capillary membrane leading to flooding of the alveolar spaces with proteinaceous material, and ARDS is defined by clinical measures of the severity of lung dysfunction (e.g., PaO_2/FiO_2). This process is triggered by direct injury to the lung as observed in aspiration pneumonia, smoke inhalation, and a near-drowning event, or systemic injury such as trauma, surgery, sepsis, burns, long-bone fractures, pancreatitis, uremia, transfusion therapy, shock, drug intoxication, or cardiopulmonary bypass. Approximately 150,000 cases of ARDS are reported each year in the United States, and aspiration pneumonia and sepsis are the most common associated conditions. The morbidity rate associated with ARDS is high and approximately 40% to 50% of patients die.

ARDS is the pulmonary manifestation of a systemic disorder that appears to trigger a dysregulated inflammatory response to injury. Uncontrolled inflammation causes injury to the pulmonary vascular endothelium and epithelium, which results in increased permeability of both physiologic barriers, allowing the extravasation of proteinaceous edema fluid from the intravascular space and its accumulation into the lung interstitium and alveolar spaces. This condition is often referred to as noncardiogenic pulmonary edema. In the lung, these processes cause refractory hypoxemia and decreased lung compliance, thereby increasing the work of breathing. Failure of other organs is frequent; consequently, multiorgan failure is common, especially in the setting of sepsis.

Histologically, ARDS is characterized by diffuse alveolar damage with hyaline membranes. The damage is further exaggerated by reductions in the quantity and quality of the synthesized surfactant leading to atelectasis. After a few days, the tissue shows hyperplasia of type II pneumocytes and deposition of connective tissue matrices resulting in fibrosis. These events can be worsened by mechanical ventilation via positive pressure, hyperdistention, and hyperoxia.

A diagnosis of ARDS should be considered in patients with a predisposing condition (e.g., sepsis), bilateral pulmonary infiltrates, and refractory hypoxemia (i.e., usually a PaO_2/FiO_2 of 200 mm Hg or less), in the absence of significant cardiac dysfunction. Currently, the treatment of ARDS relies on supportive measures directed at eradicating the injurious agent, sustaining the cardiovascular system, providing nutrition, and avoiding such complications as infection and barotrauma. Recently, a ventilatory management strategy designed to deliver low-tidal volumes (~6 mL/kg body weight) has proved beneficial, resulting in increased survival. Corticosteroids, surfactant replacement, and extracorporeal oxygenation have not proved beneficial and are not recommended. Oxygenation can be improved by PEEP and prone ventilation, but these interventions do not appear to affect the natural course of the disease. Nitric oxide added to the inspired gas has been tested with variable effects on oxygenation, and its true role in the management of ARDS remains undefined.

Shock

Shock is defined as systemic organ hypoperfusion, usually associated with hypotension, that leads to cell injury and death. Four classifications are provided: (1) cardiogenic shock (i.e., decreased cardiac output as a result of dysfunction), (2) hypovolemic shock (i.e., decreased intravascular volume), (3) septic or redistributive shock (i.e., decreased systemic vascular resistance) or (4) obstructive shock (i.e., decreased cardiac output as a result of obstruction to flow). (Anaphylactic shock caused by an allergic reaction to a drug or a related insult is not discussed in this text.)

When encountering a patient in shock, the strategy is to gain vascular access quickly and to replace volume aggressively while making a careful assessment of the situation. This strategy is particularly appropriate when shock is thought to be the result of hypovolemia or sepsis. In the case of cardiogenic shock, strategies designed to improve cardiac function should be implemented, including inotropes or, in severe unresponsive cases, cardiac bypass or cardiac-assist devices. In the case of severe hypovolemia, administration of saline is usually sufficient, but colloid administration (e.g., albumin, blood) may also be required. With sepsis, fluid replacement, antibiotic therapy, and drainage of any infected space are paramount. In select patients in whom severe sepsis is diagnosed early, intravascular administration of a recombinant version of activated protein C (drotrecogin alfa [activated]) has been shown to improve survival. Obstructive shock is the result of obstruction to blood flow, as observed in massive pulmonary embolism or *saddle embolus* lodged at the bifurcation of the right and left pulmonary arteries. In this setting, relieving the obstruction mechanically or through other methods (e.g., thrombolysis) or supporting the patient's circulation until the obstruction subsides is important.

In the management of shock, monitoring blood pressure and organ perfusion is of utmost importance. A central venous line will facilitate the delivery of fluids, and an arterial line will allow for accurate monitoring of blood pressure. In cases where aggressive fluid replacement is not effective and the exact cause of shock remains unknown, the placement of a pulmonary artery catheter (Swan-Ganz) may be useful. This catheter allows for the direct assessment of pressures in the right atrium, right ventricle, pulmonary artery, and pulmonary capillary wedge pressure, and it allows for the assessment of the cardiac output. These values can then be used in equations that allow for calculating derived parameters such as cardiac index, systemic and pulmonary vascular resistance, and oxygen content. Information generated by the use of this catheter and the equations needed to calculate derived parameters are described in Tables 23–2 and 23–3. These values are useful in distinguishing the different types of shock (Table 23–4). Concerns have been raised about the true usefulness and benefit-risk ratio associated with this procedure. Significant expertise is required for the insertion of these catheters and for the adequate interpretation of the data generated.

Table 23–2	**Useful Resting Hemodynamic Parameters (PA Catheter)**
Parameters	**Normal Ranges**
Right atrial pressure or CVP	0–5 mm Hg
Right ventricular pressure (systolic/diastolic)	25/0–5 mm Hg
Pulmonary artery pressure (systolic/diastolic)	25/8–12 mm Hg
Pulmonary capillary wedge pressure	8–12 mm Hg
Cardiac output	3.5–7.0 L/min
Cardiac index	2.5–4.5 L/min/m²
Oxygen consumption	200–250 mL/min
Arteriovenous oxygen content	3.5–5.5 mL/100 mL
Mixed venous oxygen content	18 mL/100 mL
Mixed venous oxygen saturation	75%
Stroke volume	70–130 mL/beat
Stroke volume index	40–50 mL/beat/m²
Left ventricular stroke work index	45–60 g/beat/m²
Systemic vascular resistance	800–1200 dyne/sec/cm⁻⁵
Pulmonary vascular resistance	150–250 dyne/sec/cm⁻⁵

CVP = central venous pressure; PA = pulmonary artery.

Systemic Inflammatory Response Syndrome

The systemic inflammatory response syndrome (SIRS) is a constellation of clinical signs and symptoms triggered by the host response to diverse insults. The most common cause of SIRS is infection, which is called *sepsis*. However, not infrequently, SIRS can be triggered by noninfectious disorders such as pancreatitis and drug intoxication. The diagnosis of SIRS requires at least two of the following criteria: (1) temperature higher than 38°C or less than 36°C; (2) tachycardia greater than 90 beats/min; (3) tachypnea greater than 20 breaths/min, or (4) $PaCO_2$ less than 32 mm Hg; and (5) white blood cell count greater than 12,000/mcl or less than 4000 mcl. This systemic response may result in dysfunction of many organs, including the lung, liver, kidneys, heart, and

Table 23–3 Equations to Calculate Derived Parameters

$$CO = \frac{VA}{(CaO_2 - CvO_2)}$$

$$CI = \frac{CO}{BSA(m^2)}$$

$$(CxO_2) = \% \text{ Saturation} \times Hgb (g/dL) \times 1.39 + (PxO_2 \times 0.003)$$
$$DO_2 (mL/min/m^2) = CI \times CaO_2$$

$$SV = \frac{CO}{HR(beats/min)}$$

$$SVI = \frac{SV}{BSA}$$

$$LVSWI = \frac{1.36 \times (MAP - PCWP) \times SI}{100}$$

$$MAP = \frac{(2 \times diastolic) + systolic}{3}$$
$$= \frac{diastolic + systolic - diastolic}{3}$$
$$= \frac{diastolic + pulse \; pressure}{3}$$

$$SVR = \frac{MAP - CVP}{CO} \times 80$$

$$PVR = \frac{Mean \; PA \; pressure - PCWP}{CO} \times 80$$

BSA = body surface area; CaO2 = arterial oxygen content; CI = cardiac index; CO = cardiac output; CVP = central venous pressure; CxO2 = oxygen content; DO2 = oxygen delivery; HR = heart rate; LVSWI = left ventricular stroke work index; MAP = mean arterial pressure; PA = pulmonary artery; PCWP = pulmonary capillary wedge pressure; PVR = pulmonary vascular resistance; PxO2 = partial pressue of oxygen; SV = stroke volume; SVR = systemic vascular resistance.

central nervous system, which is referred to as multiple-organ dysfunction syndrome or multiple-organ system failure. The prognosis worsens as more organs become involved with mortality ranging from 30% in less severe cases to over 90% with five or more failing organs.

Noxious Gases, Fumes, and Smoke Inhalation

The inhalation of certain gases and fumes may cause asphyxia or cellular and metabolic injury (Table 23–5). Carbon monoxide poisoning is a common and frequently unsuspected cause of inhalational injury and results in tissue hypoxia by competitively displacing oxygen from hemoglobin. Affinity of carbon monoxide for hemoglobin is approximately 250 times greater than that of oxygen. The correlation between carbon monoxide levels and symptoms is weak, but generally patients with levels greater than 30% are symptomatic. Symptoms may range from confusion or fatigue to nausea, headache, and profound coma. The diagnosis is based on clinical grounds and supported by laboratory data. Carbon monoxide intoxication might occur in closed automobiles and exposure to kerosene heaters or charcoal fires in closed spaces. In suggested cases, arterial blood gas levels should be obtained with measured, noncalculated, hemoglobin-oxygen saturation. A carbon monoxide level should be measured in patients with a measured systemic arterial oxygen saturation (SaO_2), lower than the calculated SaO_2 obtained from the arterial oxygen tension. Treatment includes 100% inspired oxygen. Hyperbaric oxygen might be useful, but the clinical use of this therapy is unclear.

Inhalation of caustic substances such as ammonia, chlorine, and hydrogen fluoride causes acute symptoms of eye and upper airway inflammation. Pain, lacrimation, rhinorrhea, and upper airway symptoms usually prompt the individual to flee the environment. Inhalation of nitrogen dioxide (silo filler's disease) occurs in farmers who work in silos where fermentation of grain produces large quantities of the gas. Most patients recover without sequelae, but a small minority of patients may develop bronchiolitis obliterans with organizing pneumonia (BOOP).

Table 23–4 Hemodynamic Variables in the Four Types of Shock

Type of Shock	Pulmonary Capillary Wedge Pressure	Cardiac Index	Systemic Vascular Resistance Index
Hypovolemic	Low	Low	High
Cardiogenic	Low	Low	High
Extracardiac obstructive	Normal or low (high in tamponade)	Low	High
Distributive	Normal or low	High (rarely low)	Low

Adapted from Parrillo JE, Ayres SM (eds): Major Issues in Critical Care Medicine. Baltimore: Williams & Wilkins, 1984.

Table 23–5 Toxic Gases and Fumes

Injuries	Agents	Occupational Exposures
Simple asphyxia	Carbon dioxide	Mining, foundries
	Nitrogen	Mining, diving
	Methane	Mining
Cellular hypoxia and oxygen transport	Carbon monoxide	Mining, combustion in closed spaces
		Smoke inhalation
	Cyanide	Petroleum refining
	Hydrogen sulfide	
Direct tissue injury	Ammonia	Fertilizer, cleaning agents
	Chlorine	Bleaches, swimming pools
	Nitrogen dioxide	Farming, fertilizer, combustion in closed spaces
	Phosgene	Welding, paint removal
	Cadmium, mercury	Welding

Metal fume fever causes influenza-like symptoms as a result of the inhalation of metal oxides generated by welding. Inhalation of platinum, formalin, and isocyanates may precipitate asthma. Pneumonitis can be induced by high-intensity inhalation of cadmium and mercury vapors.

Smoke inhalation may cause direct thermal injury that is usually confined to the upper airways, but it may also produce injury to the lower airways if exposure to sufficient steam occurs as a result of the high thermal content of water. Laryngeal edema, airway inflammation, and mucus can lead to airway obstruction, which requires intubation. Anoxia occurs from consumption of oxygen by fire, as well as from cytotoxic injury from gases such as carbon monoxide, cyanide, and oxidants liberated during combustion. Cyanide poisoning uncouples oxygen from energy production and requires prompt treatment with 100% oxygen and sodium thiosulfate. The combustion of natural and synthetic polymers often produces aldehydes, acetaldehyde, and acrolein, which have a high irritant potential. The treatment of patients with inhalation injuries is supportive with close attention to the airway. Oxygen should be provided, and continuous monitoring of cardiac and hemodynamic status is necessary. Sometimes intubation and mechanical ventilation are needed to overcome airway obstruction and the development of respiratory failure.

Prospectus for the Future

The administration of critical care medicine units and the delivery of care in those units are changing at a rapid pace with the standardization of care through the development of critical care pathways. Over the past few years, studies unveiling the value of early assessment and aggressive treatment of shock through *goal-directed therapy*, the understanding that tight glucose control enhances survival in severely ill patients, and the development of new drugs for the treatment of shock have radically altered the way critical care medicine is practiced. Further, the use of low-volume ventilation in patients with ARDS, the development of new strategies designed to accelerate weaning from mechanical ventilation, and the development of methods for the early detection of ventilator-associated pneumonia promise to improve the outcomes in patients with respiratory failure as well. Although more information about critical care illnesses is generated each year, the main obstacle to improving the outcomes in the critical care setting is the limited use of these relatively new strategies in critical care units inside and outside academic institutions. Of note, compliance with proved new therapies is being fostered, among other mechanisms, through the so-called leap-frog initiative that promotes 24-hour coverage of critical care units by trained experts, the use of electronic records, and other strategies. Well-randomized, controlled studies designed to test new drugs and other strategies in the critical care setting are under way and are likely to change further the way we deliver medicine to the critically ill patient in the near future.

References

Calandra T, Cohen J: International sepsis forum definition of infection in the ICU consensus conference. Crit Care Med 33:1538–1548, 2005.

Cohen J, Brun-Buisson C, Torres A, et al: Diagnosis of infection in sepsis: An evidence-based review. Crit Care Med 32:S466–S494, 2004.

Hill NS. Noninvasive ventilation for chronic obstructive pulmonary disease. Respir Care 49:87–89, 2004.

Sehti JM, Siegel MD: Mechanical ventilation in chronic obstructive pulmonary disease. Clin Chest Med 21:799–818, 2000.

Rello J, Paiva JA, Baraibar J, et al: International conference for the development of consensus on the diagnosis and treatment of ventilator-associated pneumonia. Chest 120:955–970, 2001.

Ware LB, Matthay MA: The acute respiratory distress syndrome. N Engl J Med 342:1334–1349, 2000.

Neoplastic Disorders of the Lung

Jesse Roman

Kenneth L. Brigham

Lung Cancer

Lung cancer is the leading cause of cancer death in both men and women in the United States, and an estimated 1 million people die worldwide of lung cancer each year. Despite recent advances in the understanding of the biology of lung cancer and the introduction of new chemotherapeutic agents for its treatment, the 5-year survival rate for patients with lung cancer is less than 15%. A major reason for this poor rate of survival relates to the fact that most patients with lung cancer are diagnosed during the advanced stages of the disease when surgical resection is less likely to be curative.

Smoking is the leading cause of lung cancer, a cause-effect relationship that was recognized as early as the 1940s. The risk of lung cancer is proportionate to cigarette pack–years smoked (packs per day × years smoked) with a peak incidence in the sixth and seventh decades. Ex-smokers show a persistent risk of lung cancer throughout life. Passive smoking is thought to be the cause of lung cancer in a significant percent of nonsmokers who develop the disease. Nonsmokers who live with smokers have over a 30% increased risk of developing lung cancer. Other risk factors for lung cancer include environmental hazards such as asbestos exposure. Tobacco smoking is an important co-factor of lung cancer in the setting of asbestos exposure. Radon increases the risk of lung cancer; and this risk is most common in miners. Radon exposure in the home is less significant, but in view of the increased risk, home radon testing is recommended.

The exact mechanisms by which these factors promote lung cancer remain unclear, but they are likely to cause genetic abnormalities that, when unopposed, promote the oncogenic transformation of lung epithelial cells. Because of the redundant repair mechanisms available to the lung, many individual genetic *hits* appear necessary. These *hits* affect the expression of proto-oncogenes, suppressor genes, and growth factors. Proto-oncogenes, similar to members of the *ras* family (e.g., *k-ras*) control cell cycling, growth, and differentiation. Mutations in *ras* genes have been detected in over 50% of squamous cell cancers and in 68% of adenocarcinoma cells. Other proto-oncogenes implicated in the pathogenesis of lung cancer are *c-erb, rb, p53, c-myc,* and *c-src.* Mutations in tumor suppressor genes (e.g., p21) might also promote the development of lung cancer. Growth factors, such as gastrin-releasing peptide, insulin-like growth factor, and epidermal growth factor, promote tumor-cell proliferation through the activation of protein kinase pathways (e.g., protein kinase B, mammalian target of rapamycin [mTOR]) that stimulate cellular proliferation.

The majority of bronchogenic carcinomas are one of the following two major types: (1) *small-cell* carcinoma (SCLC) and (2) *non–small-cell* carcinoma (NSCLC). NSCLCs are the most common and include squamous cell carcinoma (30%), adenocarcinoma (32%), and large-cell carcinoma (10%), whereas SCLCs account for less than 20% of all bronchogenic carcinomas.

CLINICAL PRESENTATION

Patients may complain of mild cough, dyspnea, increased sputum production, hemoptysis, chest pain, and weight loss. Localized pleuritic chest pain suggests chest wall invasion. Shoulder pain might indicate bone metastasis or the involvement of the brachial plexus. Hoarseness is caused by involvement (or compression) of the left recurrent laryngeal nerve and suggests mediastinal or hilar involvement. A pleural effusion is observed in 9% of patients and can be related to direct tumor involvement of the pleura or obstruction of lymph flow from the mediastinal nodes. The presence of a malignant pleural effusion precludes resection. The superior vena cava is involved in less than 5% of patients; despite its implications, its involvement does not represent an emergency. Dysphagia suggests esophageal involvement.

The physical examination may be normal or may reveal changes in the lung examination, such as crackles (e.g., post-obstructive pneumonia); inspiratory wheeze, suggestive of airway obstruction; or dullness to percussion as a result of underlying pleural effusion. Lymph node enlargement in the neck or axillary areas is suggestive of metastatic disease. The most common sites of metastases are the lymph nodes, liver, brain, adrenal glands, kidneys, and lungs.

NON–SMALL-CELL CARCINOMAS

Most cases of lung cancer are due to NSCLCs. Of these, *adenocarcinomas* and *squamous cell carcinomas* are the most common. A central airway lesion that may be accompanied by postobstructive pneumonitis is the usual presentation of squamous cell carcinoma. These tumors may be cavitating tumors with thick walls. Because of their slow rate of growth, these tumors have the lowest propensity for metastasis. Pathologically, squamous cell carcinomas can be distinguished from other NSCLCs by the presence of keratinization, pearl formation, and intercellular bridging.

In contrast to squamous cell carcinomas, adenocarcinomas are most often found in the periphery of the lung. This tumor is frequently associated with malignant pleural effusions and has a high propensity to distant metastasis. Pathologically, the tumor cells stain positive for carcinoembryonic antigen, mucin, and surfactant apoprotein. This tumor responds poorly to therapy and carries a very poor prognosis. Alveolar or bronchoalveolar cell carcinoma represents a subset of adenocarcinomas and is the most common form of lung cancer found in nonsmokers and young patients. It can develop as a lung infiltrate or as a solitary nodule and can be accompanied by bronchorrhea.

Large-cell carcinoma also frequently develops as a peripheral lesion and may be associated with pneumonitis and hilar adenopathy. Two subtypes can exist: giant cell, an anaplastic tumor that has a median survival for patients of less than 1 year; and clear cell, a tumor that resembles renal cell carcinoma and has fewer malignant features.

SMALL-CELL LUNG CARCINOMA

Most SCLCs are found in the central or proximal locations in the lung. These tumors metastasize rapidly, and most patients (over 70%) have metastatic disease at the time of presentation. Tumor cells show neuroendocrine cell features and are often associated with paraneoplastic syndromes. Although a few SCLCs can be resected if no evidence of metastasis is found, the SCLCs for the majority of patients have progressed beyond the time when resection is feasible; chemotherapy is necessary. SCLC is an aggressive lung tumor and, without treatment, the median survival of patients with this cancer is less than 5 months. The overall survival at 5 years is 5% to 10%.

MANAGEMENT

The management of lung cancer includes strategies targeting prevention, early detection, and treatment. Of these, the most effective approach is prevention. Because tobacco abuse is the main causal agent known to promote the development of lung cancer, strategies designed to prevent people from smoking or to promote smoking cessation should be encouraged. The use of beta-carotene, retinol, or N-acetylcysteine for prevention should be discouraged because they remain untested and could potentially increase the risk for lung cancer.

Early detection in high-risk populations is important because essentially all patients with advanced lung cancer die from this disease. This fact has prompted an increased interest in lung cancer screening. Unfortunately, randomized trials of screening with chest radiographic studies or sputum cytologic testing have not demonstrated a decrease in lung cancer mortality. Tantalizing data have emerged about the use of chest computed tomography (CT) for screening; however, additional studies are needed to demonstrate the value of this strategy.

Once a lung cancer is diagnosed, staging is necessary to determine the best course of action. Chest CT is useful to delineate the location of the tumor and to examine for mediastinal nodes or extension into the pleura (**Web Fig. 24–1**). However, it has limited use in distinguishing benign versus malignant nodules in the mediastinum. In patients with enlarged mediastinal nodes, mediastinoscopy is indicated to determine whether resection is feasible. Recently, positron-emission tomography (PET) has proved useful for evaluating extent of disease because it can provide information about metastases to distant organs. Any symptoms pointing to involvement of nonpulmonary sites (e.g., head CT, bone scan) should be evaluated. In addition to mediastinoscopy, on occasion, other invasive techniques might be required for staging.

The treatment of lung carcinoma depends on the staging. Endobronchial malignancies can be treated with brachytherapy, cryotherapy, laser therapy, and related modalities to relieve obstruction. In clinical stage I (IA and IB) lung cancer, complete surgical resection of the tumor is recommended in cases without contraindications to surgery. If tumor is present in the margins of the surgical specimen, then local treatment (e.g., radiation) or re-resection might be considered. To avoid this problem, most experts recommend lobar or greater resection because sublobar (i.e., wedge or bronchopulmonary segment resection) leads to higher rates of recurrence. In stage II (with N1 lymph node metastasis), postoperative radiation might improve local recurrence, but it is unlikely to affect overall survival. For patients with stage IIIA lung cancer, the optimal treatment is unclear. Surgical resection followed by adjuvant radiotherapy and/or chemotherapy are considerations, but more studies are required. In stage IIIB, surgery may be indicated for T4N0M0 tumors (Table 24–1). However, combined chemotherapy and radiotherapy is preferable. In stage IV, chemotherapy is the recommended strategy because it improves survival and provides palliation for symptoms.

Special Circumstances
SOLITARY PULMONARY NODULE

A solitary pulmonary nodule is a spheric lesion in the lung that is less than 3 cm in diameter. Depending on the population, up to 50% clinically encountered solitary pulmonary nodules are malignant. Benign nodules are related to infectious granulomas (e.g., histoplasmosis), noninfectious granulomas, hamartomas, and other benign tumors.

When confronted with a patient with a solitary pulmonary nodule, determining the likelihood of its malignancy is critically important because early resection of

Table 24–1	**Paraneoplastic Syndromes Associated with Bronchogenic Carcinoma**	
Syndrome	**Cell Type**	**Mechanism**
Hypertrophic pulmonary osteoarthropathy and clubbing	All except small cell	Unknown
Hyponatremia	Small cell most common; may be any type	SIADH, ectopic antidiuretic hormone production by tumor
Hypercalcemia	Usually squamous cell	Bone metastases, osteoclast-activating factor, parathyroid hormone–like hormone, prostaglandins
Cushing's syndrome	Usually small cell	Ectopic ACTH production
Eaton-Lambert myasthenic syndrome	Usually small cell	Voltage-sensitive calcium channel antibodies in >75%; affects presynaptic neuronal calcium channel activity
Other neuromyopathic disorders	Small cell most common; may be any type	Antineuronal nuclear antibodies, also known as anti-Hu; others unknown
Thrombophlebitis	All types	Unknown

ACTH = Adrenocorticotropic hormone; *SIADH* = syndrome of inappropriate secretion of antidiuretic hormone.

malignant nodules are usually curative, whereas resection of benign nodules exposes the patient to an unnecessary risk of surgery. Advanced age and significant smoking history increase the likelihood of malignancy. Imaging studies should be compared with previous studies if available because the presence of a solitary nodule without changes in size for over 2 years dramatically reduces the likelihood of it being malignant. The characteristics of the nodule are also important. Nodules with smooth edges and calcification are usually benign, whereas nodules with irregular edges and without calcification are more likely to be malignant. Central calcification is more consistent with benign lesions as opposed to extrinsic calcification. A chest CT is recommended when evaluating a nodule to better define its contour, to evaluate for occult calcification, and to examine other thoracic structures (e.g., mediastinal nodes).

In general, patients with nodules that are suggestive of malignancy should undergo thoracotomy for surgical resection unless the patient is reluctant or contraindications for anesthesia or surgery exist. In the latter setting, a transthoracic needle-aspiration biopsy should be considered for diagnosis, recognizing that a negative biopsy does not entirely rule out the possibility of malignancy. Depending on the clinical picture and the estimated probability of malignancy (based on risk assessment), observation for a period of up to 2 years might be warranted, especially in patients where the suggestion of malignancy is low. More recently,

PET scanning has enhanced the accuracy in diagnosing solitary nodules. In general, malignant nodules are positive by PET scanning, but this test is not specific and false-positive results can be obtained in infectious lesions, whereas false-negative results can be obtained in nodules smaller than 1 cm and in bronchoalveolar carcinomas, among others.

PARANEOPLASTIC SYNDROMES

Paraneoplastic syndromes are usually neurologic syndromes that are rare and are elicited by a patient's immune response to tumors of the lung, ovaries, breast, and lymphatic system (Table 24–2). Neurologic symptoms develop over weeks and may include difficulties in walking or swallowing, loss of muscle tone, loss of fine-motor coordination, slurred speech, memory loss, vision problems, dementia, sleep disturbances, seizures, and vertigo. Neurologic paraneoplastic syndromes include stiff-person syndrome, encephalomyelitis, cerebellar degeneration, neuromyotonia, and sensory neuropathy. Neuromuscular junction disorders can occur, as observed in the Lambert-Eaton myasthenic syndrome and in myasthenia gravis. Myopathies are observed and can exhibit symptoms reminiscent of polymyositis. Retinopathies, certain visual-loss syndromes, hyponatremia, hypercalcemia, and Cushing's syndrome can also be manifestations of a paraneoplastic syndrome.

Table 24–2   International Staging System for Lung Cancer (1997 Revision)

Primary Tumor (T)

T1—Tumor >3 cm diameter without invasion more proximal than lobar bronchus
T2—Tumor >3 cm diameter *or* tumor of any size with any of the following characteristics:
    Invasion of visceral pleura
    Atelectasis of less than entire lung
    Proximal extent at least 2 cm from carina
T3—Tumor of any size with any of the following characteristics:
    Invasion of chest wall
    Involvement of diaphragm, mediastinal pleura, or pericardium
    Atelectasis involving entire lung
    Proximal extent within 2 cm of carina
T4—Tumor of any size with any of the following:
    Invasion of mediastinum
    Invasion of heart or great vessels
    Invasion of trachea or esophagus
    Invasion of vertebral body or carina
    Presence of malignant pleural or pericardial effusion
    Satellite tumor nodule(s) within same lobe as primary tumor

Nodal Involvement (N)

N0—No regional node involvement
N1—Metastasis to ipsilateral hilar and/or ipsilateral peribronchial nodes
N2—Metastasis to ipsilateral mediastinal and/or subcarinal nodes
N3—Metastasis to contralateral mediastinal or hilar nodes *or* ipsilateral or contralateral scalene or supraclavicular nodes

Metastasis (M)

M0—Distant metastasis absent
M1—Distant metastasis present (includes metastatic tumor nodules in a different lobe from the primary tumor)

Stage Groupings of TNM Subsets

Stage IA	T1 N0 M0	Stage IIIA	T3 N1 M0
Stage IB	T2 N0 M0		T1–3 N2 M0
Stage IIA	T1 N1 M0	Stage IIIB	Any T N3 M0
Stage IIB	T2 N1 M0		T4 Any N M0
	T3 N0 M0	Stage IV	Any T Any N M1

Adapted from Mountain CF: Revisions in the international system for staging lung cancer. Chest 111:1710, 1997.

Evaluation of Surgery for the Patient With Lung Cancer

The presurgical evaluation of patients with lung cancer involves staging of the tumor (see Table 24–2), the determination of surgical resectability, and the evaluation of lung function to determine whether the patient is a good candidate for surgery. Staging of a tumor begins with a careful history and physical examination, followed by a CT scan of the chest. Mediastinoscopy is often needed to evaluate mediastinal nodes. Other tests (e.g., PET scans, CT scans of the head) are necessary if specific symptoms or findings from the physical examination or laboratory results are suggestive of extrapulmonary involvement. Once it is determined that surgery is the most appropriate approach based on staging, evaluation of the patient's general status and ability to tolerate the procedure is necessary. Cardiac evaluation is often necessary in older patients who smoke. Because lung cancer is more common in smokers, many patients have chronic lung disease (e.g., chronic obstructive pulmonary disease [COPD]), and lung-function testing will be necessary. Patients with lung disease are rarely good candidates for pneumonectomy. Those with severe lung dysfunction, as evidenced by a very low level of forced expiratory volume in 1 second (FEV_1) (usually below 1.5 L), and/or those who need oxygen supplementation are not good candidates for lobectomy. Sometimes, a ventilation/perfusion (V/Q) scan is required to evaluate perfusion to the site of the lung cancer to avoid resection in cases where the procedure might cause massive pulmonary hypertension and circulatory collapse.

Prospectus for the Future

Lung cancer is the number one cause of cancer death in both women and men in the United States, with tobacco exposure representing the main predisposing factor. Despite the use of aggressive chemotherapy, the 5-year survival rate in the setting of NSCLC, the most common lung cancer in America, is less than 15%. However, many clinical studies are testing the effectiveness of new agents that target intracellular signaling responsible for cell-cycle control in tumor cells, including inhibitors of cyclooxygenase-2 and mammalian target of rapamycin pathways. In a significant number of patients with cancer, abnormalities in the activity of regulatory kinases are suggested and drugs targeting these kinases are under active investigation. In addition, new information is available suggesting that screening with sophisticated imaging techniques (e.g., CT scanning) is beneficial, but its cost effectiveness is still in question. Further work is needed in the biologic study of lung cancer through the development of more relevant animal models and through the rapid translation of information generated experimentally to the clinical arena.

References

Hensing TA: Clinical evaluation and staging of patients who have lung cancer. Hematol Oncol Clin North Am 19:219–235, 2004.

Horiike A, Saijo N: Small cell lung cancer: Current therapy and novel agents. Oncology 19:47–52, 2005.

Isobe T, Herbst RS, Onn A: Current management of advanced non-small cell lung cancer: Targeted therapy. Semin Oncol 32:315–328, 2005.

Lee YC, Light RW: Management of malignant pleural mesothelioma: A critical review. Curr Opin Pulm Med 6:267–274, 2000.

Mazzone PJ, Arroliga AC: Lung cancer: Preoperative pulmonary evaluation of the lung resection candidate. Am J Med 578–583, 2005.

Mulshine JL, Sullivan DC: Clinical practice: Lung cancer screening. N Engl J Med 352:2714–2720, 1005.

Section V

Renal Disease

Cecil

Andreoli and Carpenter's
Essentials of Medicine

Elements of Renal Structure and Function

Robert L. Safirstein

Elements of Renal Structure

GROSS ANATOMY

The human kidneys are a pair of bean-shaped organs situated in the retroperitoneal space, positioned on either side of the vertebral column at the level of the lower thoracic and upper lumbar vertebrae. The right kidney is slightly lower than the left kidney because of the location of the liver. Each adult kidney weighs approximately 120 to 170 g and measures approximately $12 \times 6 \times 3$ cm. A coronal section of the kidney shows two distinct regions (Fig. 25–1A). The pale outer region, or cortex, is approximately 1 cm in thickness. The dark inner region is the medulla and contains 6 to 15 (average 8) conical structures called pyramids. The base of each pyramid is situated at the corticomedullary junction, and the apex extends into the hilum of the kidney as the papilla. The medulla is subdivided further into an outer zone containing the outer and inner stripes of the outer medulla and an inner zone containing the papilla. This distinction, which is apparent grossly, is important because of the specific tubular and vascular components distinct to each region, all of which are important in the function of the kidney to be described in subsequent sections.

The concave medial aspect of the kidney is the site of the renal hilum through which pass the branches of the renal artery and vein, lymphatics, nerves, and the expanding upper region of the ureter, called the renal pelvis. The renal pelvis communicates with a flattened space within the kidney, called the renal sinus, in which the renal pelvis branches into major and minor calyces to collect the urine emerging through the merged collecting ducts within the renal pyramids.

RENAL BLOOD SUPPLY

Blood is delivered to each kidney from a main renal artery branching from the aorta at the level of the first lumbar vertebra (see Fig. 25–1B). The renal artery enters the hilum and usually divides into two main segmental branches, which are further subdivided into several lobar arteries supplying the upper, middle, and lower regions of the kidney. These vessels branch further as they enter the renal parenchyma and create interlobar arteries that course toward the renal cortex along the lateral margin of the medullary pyramids. At the corticomedullary junction, these smaller arteries provide perpendicular branches that continue in an archlike manner, appropriately named the arcuate arteries. Interlobular arteries arise from the arcuate arteries and branch radially within the cortex. The glomerular capillaries receive blood through afferent arterioles that originate from these terminal interlobular arteries. The efferent arteriole leaves the glomerular capillary bed and supplies a network of vessels that surround the tubular structures. The efferent arterioles of the juxtamedullary glomeruli form hairpin loops called vasa recta that extend deep into the medulla.

INNERVATION OF THE KIDNEY

Kidneys are richly innervated by the autonomic nervous system. Sympathetic nerve endings are present in all segments of renal vasculature, tubules, and the juxtaglomerular apparatus. Stimulation of the renal sympathetic nerves enhances the release of renin from the juxtaglomerular cells, thereby increasing angiotensin and aldosterone production.

NEPHRON

The basic structural and functional unit of the kidney is the nephron (Fig. 25–2). Each human kidney contains approximately 1 million nephrons, and each nephron is composed of two major components: (1) a filtering element that consists of an enclosed capillary network (the renal corpuscle) and (2) its attached tubule. Most of the components of the renal corpuscle are contained within the glomerulus, which consists of Bowman's capsule, which, in turn, encloses the glomerular tuft. The tubule components that emerge from Bowman's capsule include in succession the proximal tubule, a convoluted and straight portion, the loop of Henle

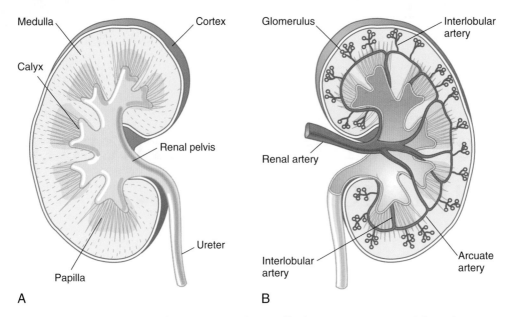

Figure 25–1 Basic renal structure. *A,* Urinary collecting structures. *B,* Arterial supply.

(composed of the straight portion of the proximal tubule, the thin descending limb, thin ascending limbs of long-looped nephrons, and the medullary thick ascending limb [MTAL]), the distal tubule, which includes the cortical segment of the thick ascending limb that courses close to its glomerular pole and includes the macula densa, the post-macula densa segment, and the convoluted portion of the distal tubule. The collecting duct system follows and is comprised first of the connecting segment followed by the collecting ducts, which have both cortical segments and outer and inner medullary segments.

Nephrons are mainly classified based on whether they possess a short or a long loop of Henle. The short-looped nephrons usually originate from the superficial and midcortical regions, and their loops of Henle bend within the outer medulla. By contrast, the long-looped nephrons originate from the juxtamedullary (corticomedullary) region, and their loops of Henle extend into the inner medulla. A minority of these juxtamedullary nephrons have loops that penetrate deeply in the inner medulla to reach the papilla before turning upward.

RENAL CORPUSCLE (GLOMERULUS)

The glomerulus (Fig. 25–3) is a unique network of capillaries suspended between the afferent and efferent arterioles enclosed within an epithelial structure (Bowman's capsule). The capillaries are arranged into lobular structures called glomerular tufts and are lined by a thin layer of endothelial cells. The core of the glomerulus consists of the mesangial, which consists of mesangial cells and a surrounding mesangial matrix. Other components of the glomerulus include the glomerular basement membrane and visceral and parietal epithelial cells. The afferent and efferent arterioles enter and leave the glomerulus at the vascular pole, and Bowman's capsule continues as the proximal tubule at the urinary pole. The efferent arteriole splits into another capillary network

that surrounds the adjacent tubules to form the peritubular capillary network. The renal corpuscle thus consists of the parietal epithelium of Bowman's capsule, a visceral epithelium surrounding the glomerular tuft, endothelial cells lining the capillaries, the glomerular basement membrane, and the intraglomerular mesangial cells within a mesangial matrix.

Epithelial Cells

The visceral epithelial cells, or podocytes, are highly specialized pericytes with a complex cytoarchitecture and prominent surface features best exemplified by interdigitating projections onto the surface of the glomerular endothelium, called foot processes. Between these projections are slit diaphragms. Injury to the podocytes leads to proteinuria, and disturbances of podocyte architecture result in the retraction, or effacement, of these foot processes and proteinuria. These changes are characteristic of all progressive renal disease syndromes. Considering that hereditary forms of nephrotic syndrome are associated with mutations in genes whose products are localized to these cells, the podocyte appears to be a primary target of many of the acquired diseases of the kidney in which proteinuria is prominent.

Endothelial Cells

A thin layer of fenestrated endothelial cells lines the glomerular capillary lumen. These fenestrae are larger than most in the body and are responsible, in part, for the high ultrafiltration coefficient of the human glomerulus. A cell coat that is rich in polyanionic glycoproteins covers the endothelial surface and accounts for the lower permeability of negatively charged proteins, such as albumen, of the glomerular filtration barrier. As is the case elsewhere in the body, these endothelial cells regulate coagulation, inflammation, and vasomotor tone. They express surface antigens of the class 2 histocompatibility complex, express adhesion

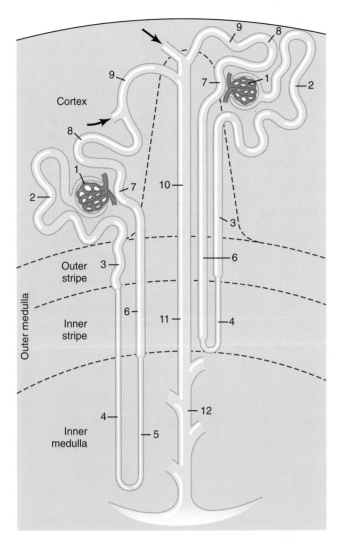

Figure 25–2 Organization of two nephrons. Each nephron consists of a glomerulus *(1)*, proximal convoluted tubule *(2)*, proximal straight tubule *(3)*, thin descending limb of the loop of Henle *(4)*, thin ascending limb *(5)*, thick ascending limb *(6)*, macula densa *(7)*, distal convoluted tubule *(8)*, and connecting tubule *(9)*. Several nephrons coalesce to empty into a collecting duct *(10)*, the outer medullary collecting duct *(11)*, and the inner medullary collecting duct *(12)*. The deeper glomerulus gives rise to nephrons along with loop of Henle, which descend to the papillary tip, whereas the more superficial glomerulus has a loop of Henle that bends at the junction between the inner and outer medulla. (Modified from Briggs JP, Kriz W, Schnermann JB: Overview of kidney function and structure. In Primer on Kidney Diseases, 4th ed. Philadelphia: WB Saunders, 2005.)

molecules for leukocytes, bind factors IXa and Xa, release and bind von Willebrand factor, and synthesize and release endothelin-1 and nitric oxide.

Glomerular Basement Membrane

The glomerular basement membrane is a layer of hydrated gel composed of glycoproteins that contain interwoven collagen fibers (type IV and type V collagen). Heparinases that digest heparin-rich glycoproteins lead to dramatic increases

in the permeability of the basement membrane to anionic proteins, indicating that the basement membrane is an important determinant of the glomerular protein filtration barrier. These components are made by both podocytes and endothelial cells. The lack of type IV collagen as a result of mutation of the collagen type IV α5 subunit gene on the X chromosome leads to Alport's syndrome.

Mesangium

Glomerular capillaries course along a structure called the mesangium and is composed of mesangial cells embedded in a mesangial matrix (see Fig. 25–3). Mesangial cells have structural characteristics of smooth muscle cells and contain actin, myosin, and α-actin. The cells are attached through cytoplasmic projections that tether them to the basement membrane through microfibrils that associate with fibronectin, the most abundant protein of the mesangial matrix. This arrangement affects the contractile force of the mesangial cells. A minority of the mesangial cells also participate in the phagocytosis of macromolecules, including immune complexes. These cells possess receptors for growth factors, such as platelet-derived growth factor (PDGF), constrictor peptides, such as endothelin and arginine vasopressin, and cytokines. The cells can also produce extracellular matrix when stimulated by these factors and may participate in the abnormal matrix production in many forms of glomerular disease.

Juxtaglomerular Apparatus

Tightly adherent to every glomerulus at a site between the entrance and exit of the arterioles is a plaque of distal tubule cells called the macula densa. These specialized cells, together with the intervening matrix of the mesangium and the specialized granular cells of the contacting arterioles, form the juxtaglomerular apparatus. Under conditions of varying salt delivery, this region regulates glomerular filtration, whereby the flow of sodium chloride (NaCl) past this region is kept constant by a process termed tubuloglomerular feedback. The structure is also the site of renin formation, which is also sensitive to salt concentration. These cells are richly innervated by sympathetic neurons.

TUBULE

The glomerular corpuscle funnels ultrafiltrate into the renal tubules. The proximal tubule begins at the urinary pole of the glomerulus and consists of two segments. The initial segment, the proximal convoluted tubule, is located in the cortex. The second segment, the straight portion of the proximal tubule, is located in the medullary ray and enters the medulla to form part of the loop of Henle. The thin descending limb of the loop of Henle forms a hairpin turn in the medulla and returns toward the cortex, forming the distal tubule. The distal tubule consists of two segments: (1) the thick ascending limb of the loop of Henle and (2) the distal convoluted tubule. The distal tubule leads to the connecting segment, which marks the transition between the distal tubule and the collecting segment. The collecting segment comprises the cortical collecting duct (CCD) and the outer and inner medullary collecting ducts. These segments of the collecting duct differ not only in regional distribution, but also in the mix of cells found within each segment, the

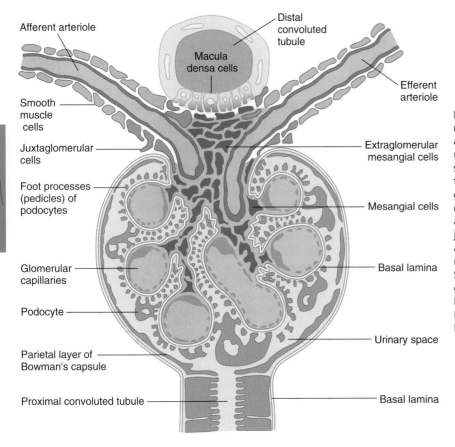

Afferent arteriole

Distal convoluted tubule

Macula densa cells

Efferent arteriole

Smooth muscle cells

Juxtaglomerular cells

Extraglomerular mesangial cells

Foot processes (pedicles) of podocytes

Mesangial cells

Glomerular capillaries

Basal lamina

Podocyte

Parietal layer of Bowman's capsule

Urinary space

Proximal convoluted tubule

Basal lamina

Figure 25–3 Schematic diagram of a renal glomerulus and the structures associated at the vascular pole *(top)* and urinary pole *(bottom)* (not drawn to scale). Mesangial cells are associated with the capillary endothelium and the glomerular basement membrane. The macula densa cells of the distal tubule are shown intimately associated with the juxtaglomerular cells of the afferent arteriole and the extraglomerular mesangial cells. (Modified from Kriz W, Sakai T: Morphological aspects of glomerular function. In Davison AM [ed]: Nephrology: Proceedings of the Tenth International Congress of Nephrology. London: Baillière-Tindall, 1987, p. 3.)

distribution of transporters specific to each segment, and responsiveness to hormones that regulate transport. The collecting ducts terminate as the papillary collecting ducts, or the ducts of Bellini, which empty into the renal pelvis at the tips of the renal papillae.

Elements Of Renal Physiology

The main functions of the kidney are to maintain and regulate body fluid composition (including its red blood cell mass), excrete waste products of metabolism and xenobiotics, and regulate calcium and phosphate balance (Table 25–1). Although filtration, reabsorption, and secretion are fundamental to the regulation of body fluid composition, less obvious is how its capacity to synthesize, metabolize, and secrete hormones and lipids contributes to the kidney's regulation of electrolyte metabolism and blood pressure. The first step in this complex process is the formation of an ultrafiltrate of plasma at the glomerulus. This fluid, which is free of cellular elements and most of the plasma proteins, flows through the various tubular segments, where it is modified by the processes of reabsorption and secretion to restore the fluid and ionic composition of the body perturbed by metabolism and diet. How each of the structures of the nephron contributes to the achievement of this balance

in which intake matches output is outlined in the following sections.

RENAL BLOOD FLOW

Approximately one fifth of the cardiac output perfuses the kidneys and represents the highest blood flow rate by weight of any organ in the body. The glomerulus filters approximately one fourth of the blood reaching the kidney per minute. Blood cells and protein are excluded from the filtration barrier, and this blood passes to the peritubular capillary network where its high oncotic pressure helps return the fluid that is reabsorbed from the filtrate to the blood. The medulla, which receives its blood from the postglomerular blood through the specialized capillaries of the vasa recta, receives only 15% of the renal blood flow (RBF). The normal kidney possesses the ability to autoregulate RBF, during which it is held constant over a wide range of arterial pressures. When arterial pressure increases, the operation of the system increases resistance in the afferent arteriole and reduces resistance in the efferent arteriole, whereas a fall in arterial pressure results in the opposite changes in afferent and efferent resistance. Both the inherent reaction of the arterioles to changes in perfusion pressure and the operation of the tubuloglomerular feedback system participate in these autoregulatory adjustments under normal physiologic conditions. In the diseased kidney, however, this process is severely restricted.

Table 25–1 Renal Homeostatic Functions

Function	Mechanism	Affected Elements
Waste excretion	Glomerular filtration	Urea, creatinine
	Tubular secretion	Urate, lactate, drugs (diuretics)
	Tubular catabolism	Pituitary hormones, insulin
Electrolyte balance	Tubular NaCl absorption	Volume status, osmolar balance
	Tubular K^+ secretion	K^+ concentration
	Tubular H^+ secretion	Acid-base balance
	Tubular water absorption	Osmolar balance
	Tubular Ca^+, Phos, Mg^+ transport	Ca^+, Phos, Mg^+ homeostasis
Hormonal regulation	Erythropoietin production	Red blood cell mass
	Vitamin D activation	Ca^+ homeostasis
Blood pressure regulation	Altered Na^+ excretion	Extracellular volume
	Renin production	Vascular resistance
Glucose homeostasis	Gluconeogenesis	Glucose supply (maintained) in prolonged starvation

Ca^+ = calcium; H^+ = hydrogen ion; K^+ = potassium; Mg^+ = magnesium; Na^+ = sodium; NaCl = sodium chloride; Phos = phosphate.

GLOMERULAR FILTRATION RATE

An ultrafiltrate of the blood is formed in the glomerulus driven by Starling forces as in other capillary beds. The glomerular circulation is ideally suited for high rates of filtration as the high ultrafiltration pressure generated by the afferent and efferent arterioles, the unusually high hydraulic permeability of the filtration barrier, and the tortuous course of the capillaries in the glomerular stalk, which increases the surface area available for filtration, all contribute to the large volume of fluids entering the tubule compartment. Normal glomerular filtration rate (GFR), which depends on body size, age, diet, and physiologic state, is typically given as 100 mL/min for women and 120 mL/min for men. Normal pregnancy raises GFR. Although the most accurate means by which GFR is measured is the clearance of inulin, this method is labor intensive and thus not clinically useful for screening purposes. Instead, serum creatinine and endogenous creatinine clearance are used most frequently to estimate changes in GFR. Multiple changes in glomerular function can cause reductions in GFR, the hallmark of renal disease. These changes include reductions in the numbers of nephrons, as occur in chronic renal disease, reduction in glomeruli perfusion from circulatory collapse or specific elevation in the resistance in the afferent arteriole, or obstruction to the flow of urine by urinary bladder outflow obstruction. Reductions in blood flow, without reduced hydrostatic pressure, as occur in severe heart failure, also reduce GFR by reducing effective net ultrafiltration pressure. Renal disease, whether primary or secondary, impairs the generation of filtrate by different combinations of these mechanisms and will be highlighted by other contributors in subsequent chapters.

TUBULAR FUNCTION

The glomerular filtrate is modified as it courses down the nephron to become the urine. Net absorption of the filtrate and its constituents best characterized as sodium (Na^+), chloride (Cl^-), water, bicarbonate (HCO_3^-), glucose, amino acids, phosphates, calcium (Ca^+), magnesium (Mg^+), uric acid, and others, whereas hydrogen ions (H^+), ammonium ions (NH_4^+), and a large number of organic acids and bases are added to the filtrate. Urea and potassium (K^+) undergo both processes, and the net result depends primarily on the underlying physiologic state and diet. One of the most striking characteristics of the renal tubule is its cellular heterogeneity, and these differences underlie their unique transport characteristics. The transport proteins that are unique to each segment and the responsiveness to drugs that inhibit transport best exemplify this heterogeneity. Each segment's role in modifying the final urine will be discussed separately.

PROXIMAL TUBULE

The proximal tubule reclaims at least 60% of the filtered load of Na^+, Cl^-, water, urea, K^+, and fully 90% of the filtered HCO_3^-. These high rates of absorption are achieved without detectable differences in osmotic gradients between blood and filtrate. Almost all of the filtered glucose and amino acids are reclaimed from the filtrate during passage along the proximal tubule. Phosphates are reabsorbed at this site, and the activity of this transport route is significantly affected by parathyroid hormone (PTH). The primary mechanisms of transport of these solutes across the proximal tubule is linked to NA^+ by coupling primary active transport via the sodium-potassium adenosine triphosphatase (Na^+,K^+-

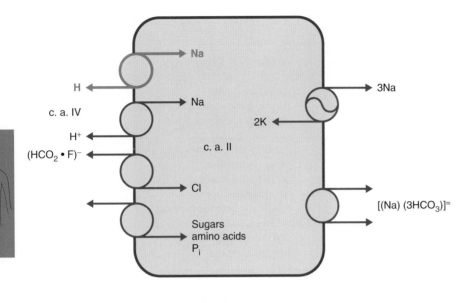

Figure 25–4 The major transport processes of the proximal tubular cells. (See text for explanation.)

ATPase) at the basolateral membrane, with secondary active transport mechanisms primarily distributed in the luminal brush border membranes of the proximal tubule (Fig. 25–4). The structural feature of the proximal tubule that enables large transepithelial mass flow is the large brush border of the luminal membrane, which enlarges membrane area greatly. This polarity of the renal epithelium is basic to achieving vectorial transport throughout the nephron.

The other structural attribute that defines a transporting epithelium is the presence of highly specialized regions where cells are joined, called junctional complexes. These complexes are found at the apical surface and not only bind the cells together and maintain polarity, but also establish a potential space by which solute and water may pass via a paracellular transport route. The electrical classification of the proximal tubule as a *leaky epithelium* is determined by the specific characteristics of the constituents of the junctional complex. Water movement through these channels and the differing selectivity for solutes establish the solvent drag effect in which significant movement of salt and water may be accomplished. Protein constituents of the junctional complex may be defective and lead to transport defects such as the congenital hypercalciuria noted in the syndrome of hypomagnesemic hypercalciuria in which a mutation of paracellin seems to be responsible for the urinary Ca^+ and Mg^+ loss.

The reabsorption of HCO_3^- in the proximal tubule perhaps best illustrates the exquisite efficiency of the structural-functional relationships illustrated in Figure 25–4. Protons are secreted into the lumen via the operation of the Na^+-H^+ exchanger (NHE) located in the brush border. The transporter is regulated by cyclic adenosine monophosphate (cAMP) whose action depends on specific structural associations with the NHE-related factor (NHERF) and the cytoskeleton (**Web Fig. 25–1**). The potential energy stored in the Na^+ gradient established by the operation of the Na^+,K^+-ATPase drives this exchange. The HCO_3^- thus generated is extruded across the basolateral membrane accompanied by Na^+ via the Na^+-HCO_3^- co-transporter. The efficient operation of the system is facilitated by two isozymes of carbonic

anhydrase, one at the luminal membrane to dehydrate the carbonic acid formed by H^+ excretion into the lumen and another intracellularly to form HCO_3^- from the hydroxyl ions formed by H^+ exit from the cell. When the operation of the NHE is coupled to a formate-Cl^- exchanger present on the apical membrane of the proximal tubule, the net result is NaCl reabsorption. Thus, the polarity of these transport processes and their coupling achieves efficient proton secretion and NaCl and $Na^+HCO_3^-$ reabsorption at low expenditure of energy.

In the straight portion of the proximal tubule, organic acids such as uric acid and drugs such as penicillin are secreted. Most diuretics are also secreted in this nephron segment and inhibit luminal solute transport at sites downstream in the nephron. Furthermore, ammonia synthesis, an important step in renal acid excretion, also occurs in the proximal tubule.

The physical forces surrounding the tubule also govern solute and water reabsorption in proximal tubules. For example, a high peritubular capillary hydrostatic pressure, as occurs in volume by fusion, impairs water and Na^+ reabsorption from the proximal tubule. By contrast, a high colloid oncotic pressure in the peritubular capillary favors the absorption of water and electrolytes from the proximal tubule. The primary determinant of these physical forces is the filtration fraction or the portion of the glomerular plasma that is filtered; the amount is low in volume expansion and high in heart failure.

LOOP OF HENLE

The loop of Henle begins at the corticomedullary junction as the thin descending limb and then makes a hairpin turn and continues as the thin ascending limb. The structure becomes the MTAL at the level of the outer medulla and ends in the macula densa at the level of the glomerulus from which it originated. Each segment of the loop has a different permeability for NaCl and water such that approximately 15% of the volume of the isosmotic ultrafiltrate is absorbed, and approximately 25% of the NaCl is absorbed. Passive

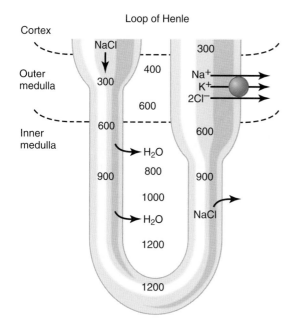

Loop of Henle

Cortex

Outer
medulla

Inner
medulla

NaCl

300

400

600

600

900

800

1000

1200

1200

300

Na⁺
K⁺
2Cl⁻

600

900

NaCl

H_2O

H_2O

Figure 25–5 The loop of Henle is responsible for additional absorption of filtrate. Water is absorbed in the solute-impermeable descending limb. The concentrated medullary interstitium, established by solute transport at the water-impermeable ascending limb, drives water absorption from the descending limb. The hyperosmolar interstitium also provides the driving force for urinary concentration at the collecting duct. The relative osmolarity of the tubular fluid and interstitium is demonstrated by the numerals.

water absorption in the thin descending limb and salt absorption in the thin ascending limb of the loop occur as a result of the selective permeability of these segments. This differential absorption converts the isotonic fluid entering from the proximal tubule into a dilute fluid delivered to the distal tubule (Fig. 25–5).

A major participant in both diluting the tubule fluid and generating high medullary interstitial solute concentration is the MTAL (Fig. 25–6). The MTAL absorbs NaCl by an active, energy-dependent process. Specifically, luminal transport involves a Na⁺-K⁺-2Cl⁻ co-transporter (NKCC2). Cl⁻ exit from the cell is through a Cl⁻ channel whose activity is augmented by raising intracellular Cl⁻ concentration. K⁺ entering the cell through the co-transporter is recycled at the luminal membrane via a K⁺ channel and supports several functions. It maintains co-transporter activity, enables K⁺ secretion, and generates a positive transcellular potential that drives Na⁺, Ca⁺, and Mg⁺ absorption through the cation-selective paracellular pathway. This cation selectivity is determined by the specific paracellular protein paracellin. Genetic defects in each of these proteins have been found in patients with phenotypes typical of Bartter's syndrome (see Chapter 27). Because this segment is impermeable to water, the luminal fluid leaving the thick ascending limb is made hypotonic with regard to plasma by active salt absorption, a critical step in urinary dilution. The addition of NaCl to the medullary interstitium is the primary step that allows a multiplicative process to build and maintain the interstitial

hypertonicity necessary to absorb water from thin descending limbs and from collecting ducts during antidiuresis. Furosemide is a potent inhibitor of the co-transporter. Antidiuretic hormone (ADH) increases thick ascending limb NaCl transport by raising cAMP within the cell, whereas prostaglandin inhibits ADH-induced increased intracellular cAMP content and NaCl transport. A newly recognized regulatory role occurs through the activation of the Ca⁺-sensing receptor (CaSR; **Web Fig. 25–2**), which inhibits NaCl transport by reducing K⁺ recycling and reduces the concentration of urine. This latter function is important to prevent urinary stone formation in periods of high Ca⁺ intake.

The hairpin arrangement and countercurrent flow of the loop help maintain high interstitial osmolality in comparison with the isotonic nature of the cortex. A similar organization of the vasa recta allows the NaCl absorbed from the loop of Henle and urea absorbed from the papillary collecting duct to be trapped within the interstitium and increases interstitial osmolality further. The integrity of these anatomic relationships is essential to the concentrating ability of the kidney.

A significant portion of Ca⁺ reabsorption occurs within the loop of Henle. Ca⁺ absorption in the medullary portion of the thick ascending limb varies with the magnitude of the positive luminal transepithelial voltage generated by active salt absorption and occurs through the Ca⁺-selective paracellular pathway. The thick ascending limb of the loop of Henle is also the major site of Mg⁺ reabsorption and most probably occurs by a similar mechanism.

DISTAL NEPHRON

The distal nephron may be divided into three segments: (1) the distal convoluted tubule (DCT), the connecting tubule (CNT), which is a transitional epithelial, and (3) the collecting duct. The collecting duct in the cortex consists of both intercalated cells and principal cells, whereas those in the medulla are exclusively composed of principal cells.

The DCT (Fig. 25–7) is a water-impermeable segment of the nephron that continues the dilution of luminal fluid initiated by the thick ascending limb. NA⁺ absorption in the distal convoluted tubule occurs primarily by a thiazide diuretic–sensitive, Cl⁻-coupled co-transporter similar to the one found in the thick ascending limb but which does not depend on K⁺. Genetic defects in the NaCl co-transporter are responsible for Gitelman's syndrome (discussed in Chapter 27). This segment is important also in the regulation of Ca⁺ balance because PTH and vitamin D increase Ca⁺ transport here. Luminal Ca⁺ uptake proceeds through channels in the luminal membrane driven by the large electrochemical gradient for Ca⁺ entry. Ca⁺ exit, which is active, proceeds predominantly via a Na⁺-Ca⁺ exchanger and to a minor degree via a Ca⁺-ATPase. The exit step is the major site by which PTH regulation occurs. Na⁺ transport in this segment is not affected by ADH or aldosterone. Inhibition of the NaCl co-transporter, by thiazides for example, augments Ca⁺ reabsorption by increasing Ca⁺ entry and promoting Ca⁺ exit as a consequence of reduced NaCl entry.

The collecting duct begins with the connecting tubule, which possesses a mixture of distal tubule and CCD transport characteristics. The functional aspects of the collecting duct epithelium are crucial to achieving salt and water

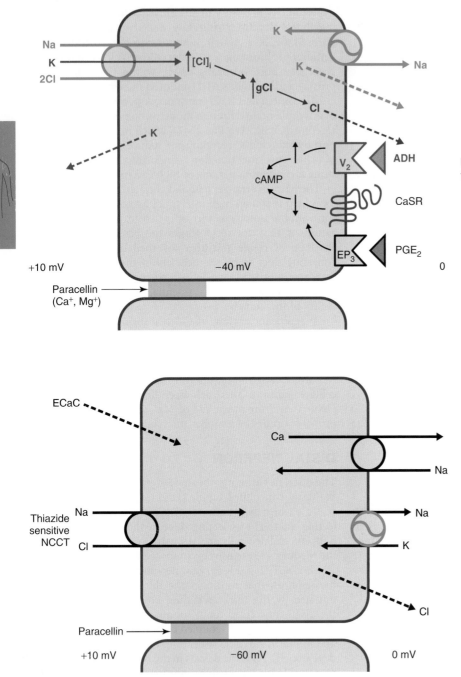

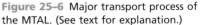

Figure 25–6 Major transport process of the MTAL. (See text for explanation.)

Figure 25–7 Major transport processes of DCT. (See text.)

homeostasis (Fig. 25–8). In states of volume depletion and maximal aldosterone production, the urine can be rendered virtually free of Na^+. The first or cortical regions of the collecting duct are lined by a mixture of principal cells and intercalated cells (Fig. 25–9). The number of the intercalated cells decreases as the collecting descend into the medulla so that they are absent in collecting ducts below the first portion of the inner medulla. Transepithelial Na^+ reabsorption is accomplished by the operation of the epithelial-Na^+ channel (ENaC; see **Web Fig. 25–3**) at the luminal membrane and the basolateral Na^+,K^+-ATPase. Aldosterone increases the rate of Na^+ transport in this segment, as does ADH, whereas prostaglandins and the natriuretic peptides reduce it. Aldosterone also hyperpolarizes the basolateral mem-

brane, provoking net K^+ secretion through K^+ channels in each membrane.

The intercalated cells do not participate in Na^+ reabsorption or K^+ secretion but instead participate in acid-base homeostasis. Two types of intercalated cells exist. The first type secretes acid, whereas the second type secretes base, depending on the polarity of the transport proteins. The A-type cell (see Fig. 25–9) reclaims the last amount of filtered HCO_3^- and achieves final titration of urinary buffers, including ammonia, by proton secretion. Evidence has been found for the existence of both an H^+ and an H^+,K^+-ATPase. Basolateral HCO_3^- exit is accomplished in exchange for Cl^- through an anion exchanger, and the Cl^- that enters the cell is extruded through a Cl^- channel. Reversal of this polarity

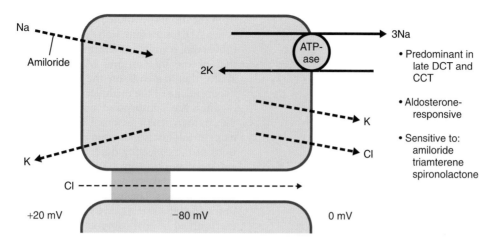

Figure 25–8 Major transport processes of the CCD. (See text.)

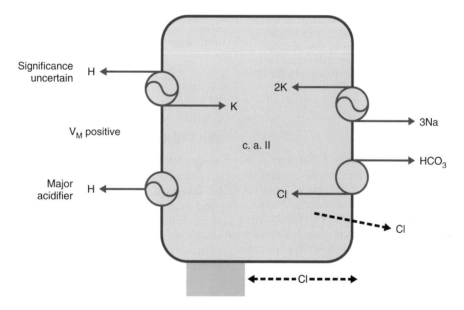

Figure 25–9 Major transport processes of the A-type intercalated cell of the outer medullary collecting duct. (See text for information.)

of the proton pumps and anion exchanger leads to HCO_3^- secretion in the B-type intercalated cell, but these cells disappear at the inner stripe of the outer medulla. Aldosterone stimulates urinary acidification principally by promoting Na^+ reabsorption and increasing luminal electronegativity. Increased Na^+ delivery to these sites, as occurs during volume expansion and diuretic use, stimulates proton excretion by stimulating Na^+ transport at this site as well.

The epithelial cells of the inner medullary collecting duct (IMCD) (Fig. 25–10) are taller and have less mitochondria than those of the outer medullary collecting duct (OMCD). Additionally, a richly featured lateral intercellular space is found that probably facilitates the transfer of fluid and urea that is provoked by ADH here. This site demonstrates the presence of inhibitory cyclic guanosine monophosphate (cGMP)-responsive ENaC proteins that are activated by natriuretic peptides, such as atrial natriuretic peptide (ANP).

This area is the site for the operation of the *escape phenomenon,* where atrial stretch caused by volume expansion leads to the release of ANP and suppression of collecting duct Na^+ transport and natriuresis. Another key regulator is nitric oxide, which also inhibits ENaC via a cGMP pathway. Failure of these systems to operate during congestive heart failure is an important determinant of edema production and suggests that the area would be a fruitful therapeutic target.

POTASSIUM SECRETION ALONG THE DISTAL NEPHRON

K^+ secretion, which may begin in the thin descending limb of the loop of Henle, is significant along the collecting ducts because the K^+ that appears in the urine is mostly a result of secretion by these segments. Many factors influence K^+ secretion and can be classified as apical and peritubular factors.

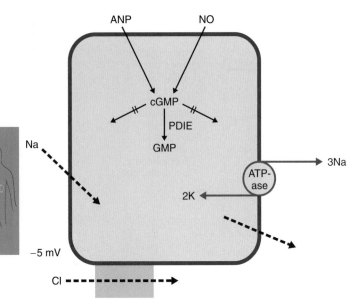

Figure 25–10 The IMCD cell and the effect of intracellular cGMP elevation in its inhibition. The failure of this inhibitory system to repress salt transport during congesting heart failure suggests that this area is an important therapeutic site for its treatment.

The principal apical factor determining K^+ secretion is tubule flow rate, which reduces the luminal K^+ concentration and stimulates the diffusion of intracellular K^+ down its concentration gradient into the tubular lumen. Volume expansion with NaCl also raises Na^+ delivery to the collecting ducts that stimulates Na^+ reabsorption and increases luminal electronegativity. Increased luminal weak acids and decreased Cl^- concentration increase K^+ secretion, whereas intraluminal acidity inhibits K^+ secretion. Studies show that the latter effect is caused by a decrease in luminal membrane K^+ conductance. Inhibitors of K^+ secretion are either inhibitors of Na^+ channels, such as triamterene and amiloride, which depolarize the luminal membrane potential, or inhibitors of the K^+ channel itself, such as barium. The peritubular factors that affect K^+ transport are K^+, H^+, HCO_3^-, and hormones. Increased K^+ concentration in the plasma increases K^+ secretion directly and by provoking aldosterone secretion. This stimulation by aldosterone is inhibited by spironolactone. Distal K^+ secretion is decreased by metabolic acidosis and increased by metabolic alkalosis.

WATER REABSORPTION ALONG THE DISTAL NEPHRON

The ability of the distal nephron to alter its ability to reabsorb water and urea in response to reduced water intake is in striking contrast to the relative invariability of water reabsorption in the proximal nephron. This task is accomplished by changing its permeability characteristics for water and urea along the nephron in response to ADH. The cells of the distal nephron are minimally permeable to water and urea in the absence of ADH and, in this circumstance, can deliver the hypotonic (50 to 100 mOsm/kg of water) fluid issuing

from the distal convoluted tubule unchanged into the urine. When ADH is present, water passes across the collecting duct tubule wall readily, and the luminal fluid tonicity approaches that of the interstitium. Maximal urinary concentrating ability thus depends on the availability of ADH plus the hypertonicity of the medullary generated from thick ascending limb NaCl absorption and trapping of salt and urea via the countercurrent system. Urea plays a special role because its permeability is increased only in the most terminal portions of the collecting duct, thus establishing a large gradient for deposition in the deep papilla as continued water reabsorption takes place at sites proximal to these terminal-collecting ducts. The urea moving into the interstitium deep in the medulla is trapped by the countercurrent system and exerts an additional osmotic force to draw water out of the collecting ducts and thin descending limbs that extend to these regions. Prostaglandins impair distal water reabsorption through several mechanisms, including blockade of ADH action in the collecting duct, as well as increasing medullary blood flow. Thus nonsteroidal anti-inflammatory drugs, by blocking prostaglandins, may impair renal free-water excretion.

Other Renal Homeostatic Functions

WASTE EXCRETION

The kidney is responsible for eliminating nitrogenous products of protein catabolism, which is accomplished primarily by filtration at the glomerulus. Because homeostatic requirements necessitate the maintenance of low concentrations of these compounds, large volumes of ultrafiltrate formation are necessary for excretion of the absolute quantity of material. The normal daily GFR of 180 L makes such mass elimination possible.

Tubule secretion, especially at the straight portion of the proximal tubule, is another route by which toxins are cleared from the blood. Organic acids (e.g., hippurates, urate, lactate), organic bases (e.g., morphine), and many xenobiotics are excreted in this manner. The secretory process is the major route of elimination for substances that are protein bound. A large number of drugs, including antibiotics and diuretics, are excreted through this mechanism.

REGULATION OF BLOOD PRESSURE

The kidney plays a major role in the genesis of hypertension, as confirmed by genetic disorders of salt transport. Perhaps most important among these roles is the gain in function mutation discovered in patients with Liddle's syndrome, in which the ENaC is activated. These patients have severe hypertension and die of early-onset cardiovascular and cerebrovascular disease. Increasing evidence suggests that essential hypertension may represent a primary defect in Na^+ excretion by the kidney, which leads to expanded intravascular volume and hypertension. Overproduction of renin, made by the granular cells of the juxtaglomerular apparatus, as occurs in some forms of renovascular disease, causes severe hypertension as well.

RENAL HORMONAL REGULATION

The kidney contributes to the metabolic degradation of a significant number of peptide hormones, including most pituitary hormones, glucagon, and insulin, by tubular cells. Decreased renal catabolism of insulin in patients with diabetes and renal insufficiency may cause hypoglycemic episodes.

The kidney is also the major site of erythropoietin production. This hormone is a highly glycosylated, 39,000-Da protein. Erythropoietin is produced in the renal cortex, but the cell has not been identified with certainty. Erythropoietin stimulates red blood cell production by its effect on the bone marrow. Erythropoietin production increases in states of decreased tissue oxygen delivery. This increase of production may occur as a result of chronic hypoxemia, as seen in persons living at high altitudes or in patients with lung disease, or as a result of decreased oxygen-carrying capacity of blood, as seen in individuals with anemia.

The kidney contributes to Ca^+ homeostasis not only by directly regulating the excretion of Ca^+, phosphate, and acid, but also by affecting hormonal production. Vitamin D requires two enzymatic hydroxylations to become a potent hormone that regulates intestinal Ca^+ absorption. After hydroxylation in the liver at the 25 position of the molecule, renal proximal tubular cells add a second hydroxyl ion at the 1 or 24 position. This hydroxylation step is controlled and stimulated by PTH and low phosphate. As noted previously, the juxtaglomerular cells produce and secrete renin. Renin promotes the formation of angiotensin II, a potent vasoconstrictor that is a stimulus to aldosterone secretion. Aldosterone stimulates renal Na^+ absorption and excretion of K^+ and H^+.

GLUCOSE HOMEOSTASIS

The kidney participates in regulating plasma glucose by its ability to synthesize glucose via the gluconeogenetic pathway. The kidney uses lactate, pyruvate, and amino acids for gluconeogenesis. This function becomes important in prolonged starvation states, during which the kidney contributes up to 40% of plasma glucose. Absence of this gluconeogenetic pathway in patients with severe renal dysfunction may contribute to hypoglycemia in persons with diabetes.

Prospectus for the Future

The role of podocyte injury in renal disease progression will be elucidated further.

The detailed three-dimensional molecular structure of the major salt and water transporters will reveal not only the mechanism by which they accomplish transfer of molecules across biologic membranes, but also how they interact with regulatory proteins—how disease-causing mutations work. Such detailed information will help in the design of newer therapeutic agents for such disorders.

More detailed understanding of the operation of the tubuloglomerular feedback system will have important therapeutic implications for the treatment of acute and chronic renal disease.

Molecular biology and molecular genetics will continue to provide information about the pathophysiologic mechanisms of human renal disease.

References

Ellison DH: Divalent cation transport by the distal nephron: Insights from Bartter's and Gitelman's syndromes. Am J Physiol 279:F616–F625, 2000.

Schrier RW, Gottschalk CW (eds): Diseases of the Kidney, Biochemical, Structural, and Functional Correlations in the Kidney, vol 1. Boston, Little Brown and Co, 1997, pp 3–201.

Approach to the Patient with Renal Disease

Michelle W. Krause

Sudhir V. Shah

Assessment of the Patient with Kidney Disease

HISTORY AND PHYSICAL EXAMINATION

It is estimated that kidney disease affects approximately 10 percent of the adult population in the United States and worldwide. Particularly disturbing is the recognition related to inadequate physician awareness of chronic kidney disease and limited utility of databases for identification of these patients. The recognition that both acute and chronic forms of kidney disease are very common should prompt physicians to pay particular attention to the detection of kidney disease. Individuals with kidney disease may exhibit either few or vague symptoms such as fatigue, malaise, or anorexia, especially with insidious chronic kidney disease or more intensely in acute renal failure with hypertension, edema, changes in urine production, hematuria, or dark-colored (*cola-colored*) urine. A history of diabetes and hypertension along with duration and other concomitant organ complications such as retinopathy or neuropathy are important in determining the association to the cause of kidney disease. Similarly, a history of recurrent urinary tract infections with reflux nephropathy, chronic obstruction with recurrent renal calculi, or a family history of kidney disease in Alport's syndrome is helpful in determining the cause of kidney disease. Other pertinent historical information required when assessing kidney disease includes inquiry into other systemic disorders that affect kidney function such as arthralgias and skin rash in autoimmune diseases, fever and pharyngitis in postinfectious glomerulonephritis, and medications—including prescription drugs, over-the-counter medications, illicit drugs, and herbs—in acute and chronic interstitial nephritis. One of the most important factors in determining whether kidney disease is acute or chronic in nature is to review previous medical records to obtain a baseline assessment of kidney function.

The physical examination may show signs of systemic illness that is responsible for the patient's kidney disease. A careful examination of the retina may suggest the presence of diabetes, hypertension, bacterial endocarditis, and cholesterol emboli (**Web Fig. 26–1**). In addition, examination of skin for the presence of edema, rash, and purpura and joint examination for signs of arthritis are important (**Web Fig. 26–2**). A rectal examination in men or a pelvic examination in women is crucial to exclude a process that might cause urinary obstruction.

RENAL FUNCTION TESTS

An approximate assessment of glomerular filtration rate (GFR) is most easily obtained by measuring the concentration of creatinine and urea nitrogen in the serum. Creatinine is a metabolite of creatine, a major muscle constituent. In a specific individual, the daily rate of production of creatinine is constant and is determined by the mass of skeletal muscle. Glomerular filtration eliminates nearly all creatinine, and the concentration of creatinine in the serum has been used as a marker of renal function. The normal range for serum creatinine concentration is 0.8 to 1.3 mg/dL in men and 0.6 to 1.1 mg/dL in women. The serum creatinine value is lower in women because of less muscle mass, which leads to a lower rate of creatinine production. However, a value in this range does not necessarily imply normal renal function. For example, in a patient whose creatinine increases from 0.6 to 1.2 mg/dL, a 50% decrease in GFR has occurred, despite creatinine remaining in the normal range. Certain drugs such as cimetidine, trimethoprim, triamterene, and amiloride may interfere with creatinine excretion and cause a false elevation in the serum creatinine value.

The blood urea nitrogen (BUN) concentration is often used in conjunction with the serum creatinine concentration as a measure of renal function. Urea is the major end-product of protein metabolism, and its production reflects both the dietary intake of protein and the protein catabolic rate. Glomerular filtration excretes urea, but a significant amount of urea is reabsorbed along the tubule, particularly in sodium-avid states such as volume depletion. Consequently, the BUN value may vary in relation to the extracellular fluid volume, whereas the serum creatinine

Table 26–1 Factors Affecting Blood Urea Nitrogen Level Independent of Renal Function

Disproportionate Increase in Blood Urea Nitrogen

Volume depletion
Gastrointestinal hemorrhage
Corticosteroid or cytotoxic agents
High-protein diet
Obstructive uropathy
Sepsis
Catabolic states tissue breakdown

Disproportionate Decrease in Blood Urea Nitrogen

Low-protein diet
Liver disease

Table 26–2 Calculation of the Creatinine Clearance

24-Hour Urine Collection

$$C_{cr} = U_{cr} \times V/P_{cr}$$

where C_{cr} = clearance of creatinine (mL/min)
U_{cr} = urine creatinine (mg/dL)
V = volume of urine (mL/min) (for 24-hr volume: divide by 1440)
P_{cr} = plasma creatinine (mg/dL)

Cockroft-Gault Formula

C_{cr} = (140 – age in years) × (lean body weight in kg)
Scr = serum creatinine in mg/dL × 72
For women, multiply final value by 0.85

Modification of Diet in Renal Disease Formula

GFR = 186 × (Cr)$^{-1.154}$ × age$^{-0.203}$ × 1.212 (if African American) × 0.742 (if woman)
Normal range: 95–105 mL/min/1.75 m^2

concentration is less dependent on volume status. The usual ratio of urea nitrogen to creatinine concentration in the serum is 10:1. This ratio is increased in a large number of clinical settings (Table 26–1).

Based on the limitations of creatinine and BUN alone in estimating kidney function, the National Kidney Foundation (NKF) and the Kidney Disease Outcomes Quality Initiative (K/DOQI) developed clinical practice guidelines that recommend measuring the creatinine clearance (C_{cr}) to estimate the GFR (see **website www.kdoqi.org**). The C_{cr} may be measured by 24-hour urine collection or mathematically by the Cockroft-Gault formula or Modification of Diet in Renal Disease (MDRD) formula (Table 26–2). Two major errors limit the accuracy of C_{cr} in 24-hour urine collections: (1) increasing creatinine secretion and (2) incomplete urine collection. Approximately 10% of creatinine is secreted by proximal tubular cells into the urine in individuals with normal kidney function, and this percentage may be increased in individuals with kidney disease, thus leading to an overestimation of the true GFR. Therefore, the NKF K/DOQI clinical practice guidelines recommend using mathematical equations rather than 24-hour urine collections for C_{cr} to estimate the GFR.

Recently, cystatin C has been described as a valid marker in estimating kidney function. Cystatin C is a cysteine protease that is produced by all nucleated cells, released into the bloodstream, and then completely filtered by the glomerulus. Cystatin C is not affected by conditions that alter muscle mass such as sex, age, and chronic diseases (e.g., cancer, liver disease), and it may be more reliable than creatinine is in estimating the GFR. The widespread use of cystatin C, however, has not been uniformly adopted, and its future use in assessing kidney function is not clear.

Tests that examine the ability of the kidney to maintain salt and water balance, as well as acid-base homeostasis, are used to evaluate renal tubular function. The water deprivation test can assess the maximal urinary concentrating ability. In the patient with polyuria who may have a defect in urinary concentrating ability, the administration of 5 units of aqueous vasopressin, once the urinary osmolality reaches a steady state, distinguishes patients with either central or nephrogenic diabetes insipidus. Patients with central diabetes insipidus develop a doubling of the urinary osmolality with aqueous vasopressin. In contrast, individuals with nephrogenic diabetes insipidus do not respond with further increase in urinary concentration.

The fractional excretion of various solutes in the urine provides useful information about the tubular handling of a solute relative to its GFR. The fractional excretion of sodium (Fe_{Na}) is the fraction of sodium filtered at the glomerulus that is ultimately excreted in the urine (Table 26–3). Determination of the Fe_{Na} is most useful in the differential diagnosis of acute oliguric renal failure. Notably, the Fe_{Na} can be calculated on a spot specimen because the volume terms in the numerator and denominator cancel each other. A value for Fe_{Na} less than 1% suggests prerenal failure, such as volume depletion, whereas a value greater than 1% is consistent with parenchymal renal disease, such as acute tubular necrosis or interstitial nephritis. The Fe_{Na} may, however, be less than 1% in patients with acute glomerular disease or radiocontrast-induced acute renal failure. In patients with persistent vomiting, volume depletion may be associated with high Fe_{Na} because of metabolic alkalosis leading to increased urinary sodium. However, the urinary chloride concentration is typically low and is an accurate index of volume depletion.

Table 26–3 Calculation of the Fractional Excretion of Sodium

Fractional Excretion of Sodium (Fe_{Na}) = Fraction of Sodium Filtered at the Glomerulus that Is Ultimately Excreted in the Urine

Fe_{Na} = clearance of sodium/clearance of creatinine
Fe_{Na} = $U_{Na}/P_{Na}(P_{cr}/U_{cr})$
where P_{Na} = plasma sodium (mEq/L)
P_{cr} = plasma creatinine (mg/dL)
U_{Na} = urine sodium (mEq/L)
U_{cr} = urine creatinine (mg/dL)

Acidification of the urine is an important tubular function that can be assessed by the measurement of the urine pH. In the presence of systemic acidosis (arterial pH <7.3), the urine pH should be less than 5.3. Failure to acidify urine in the presence of systemic acidosis suggests distal renal tubular acidosis.

A normal individual excretes less than 150 mg/day of protein. The glomerular basement membrane serves as an effective barrier to the passage of high–molecular-weight proteins such as albumin, and the renal tubules have the capacity to reabsorb the small amount of protein that is filtered. An increase in proteinuria may occur as a transient phenomenon in individuals with febrile illnesses or after vigorous exercise. Postural or orthostatic proteinuria is a benign condition that is confirmed by the absence of proteinuria in overnight urine collection while the patient is supine. Persistent proteinuria almost always indicates renal disease. Proteinuria may be quantified with either a 24-hour urine collection or a random urine protein-to-urine creatinine ratio (U pro/Cr). For example, a random U pro/Cr ratio of 1.0 correlates to 1.0 g proteinuria. Because of the limitations of 24-hour urine collections previously discussed, the NKF K/DOQI clinical practice guidelines recommend that a U pro/Cr ratio assessment be performed for quantifying proteinuria. Individuals who excrete more than 3.5 g of protein have, with rare exceptions, glomerular disease. Less than 3.5 g of urinary protein can be found in patients with glomerular and tubular diseases. For individuals without overt proteinuria on urinalysis but with conditions that are associated with kidney disease such as diabetes mellitus, early identification of underlying kidney damage can be assessed by measuring microalbuminuria. Microalbuminuria is defined as the excretion of 30 to 300 mg/24 hr of albumin and is associated with progression of renal disease and with higher cardiovascular morbidity and mortality in patients with diabetes mellitus and hypertension.

URINALYSIS

Urinalysis is a simple, noninvasive, and inexpensive means of detecting renal disease. A clean-catch voided urine speci-

men should be examined promptly using both chemical and microscopic means. Normal urine color ranges from almost colorless to deep yellow, depending on the concentration of the urochrome pigment. Abnormal urine colors may be a sign of disease or may indicate the presence of an infection, pigment, drug, or dye. The presence of red blood cells or myoglobin often results in red or smoke-colored urine. Cloudiness of the urine may occur when a high concentration of white blood cells is present (pyuria) or when amorphous phosphates precipitate in alkaline urine.

A chemical assessment of the urine is performed with the *dipstick,* a plastic strip impregnated with various reagents that detect the pH, protein, hemoglobin, glucose, ketones, leukocyte esterase, and nitrite in the urine. These assays are semiquantitative and are graded on the basis of color changes in the various reagent strips. The dipstick method for detecting urinary protein is sensitive for albumin but does not detect immunoglobulins or tubular proteins (Tamm-Horsfall mucoprotein). The disadvantage of the dipstick method is its failure to detect immunoglobulin light chains or Bence Jones proteins secreted in multiple myeloma. The urine sulfosalicylic acid test is an alternate test that detects all urinary proteins by a process of precipitation. Highly concentrated urine may show trace to 1+ protein (10 to 30 mg/dL) in a normal individual. The finding of blood in the urine is abnormal and generally indicates the presence of intact red blood cells. Blood detected by a dipstick that cannot be accounted for by red blood cells in the urine sediment is the result of either hemoglobin or myoglobin often in association with rhabdomyolysis. Leukocyte esterase and nitrites are usually positive in the presence of infection. A negative test, however, does not rule out infection.

Microscopic examination of the urine sediment is used to detect cellular elements, casts, crystals, and micro-organisms (Table 26–4) (**Web Fig. 26–3**). *Microscopic hematuria* is defined as more than two red blood cells per high-power field on a centrifuged urine specimen. Red cells of glomerular origin tend to be dysmorphic, whereas nonglomerular red cells are uniform in size and shape. *Pyuria* is defined as the presence of more than four white blood cells per high-power field. The presence of pyuria suggests urinary tract infection or inflammation. Sterile pyuria (negative culture in the presence of pyuria) suggests the diagnosis of prostatitis, chronic urethritis, renal tuberculosis, renal stones, papillary necrosis, or interstitial nephritis. A more specific test for interstitial nephritis involves documenting eosinophiluria by Wright's stain or Hansel's stain. Renal tubular epithelial cells are large, with prominent nuclei, and are often seen in acute tubular necrosis, glomerulonephritis, or pyelonephritis. Epithelial cells in the urinary sediment may derive from any site along the urinary tract from the renal pelvis to the urethra. Renal tubular cells that contain absorbed lipids are termed *oval fat bodies.* Free fat droplets in the urine are usually observed in association with heavy proteinuria.

Urinary casts are cylindric structures derived from the intratubular precipitation of Tamm-Horsfall protein. The presence of red or white blood cells in the casts provides presumptive evidence of inflammatory parenchymal renal disease. *Red blood cell casts* most frequently indicate the presence of a proliferative glomerular lesion but may also be seen in patients with acute interstitial nephritis. *Renal tubular cell casts* in a patient with acute renal failure help confirm the diagnosis of acute tubular necrosis. The pres-

Table 26–4	**Microscopic Examination of the Urine**

Finding	Associations
Casts	
Red blood cells	Glomerulonephritis, vasculitis
White blood cells	Interstitial nephritis, pyelonephritis
Epithelial cells	Acute tubular necrosis, interstitial nephritis, glomerulonephritis
Granular	Renal parenchymal disease (nonspecific)
Waxy, broad	Advanced renal failure
Hyaline	Normal finding in concentrated urine
Fatty	Heavy proteinuria
Cells	
Red blood cells	Urinary tract infection, urinary tract inflammation
White blood cells	Urinary tract infection, urinary tract inflammation
Eosinophils	Acute interstitial nephritis, atheroembolic disease
(Squamous) epithelial cells	Contaminants
Crystals	
Uric acid	Acid urine, acute uric acid nephropathy, hyperuricosuria
Calcium phosphate	Alkaline urine
Calcium oxalate	Acid urine, hyperoxaluria, ethylene glycol poisoning
Cystine	Cystinuria
Sulfur	Sulfa-containing antibiotics

ence of *leukocyte casts* in a patient with urinary tract infection indicates a diagnosis of pyelonephritis rather than a lower urinary tract infection. Leukocyte casts may also be observed in patients with interstitial nephritis and, less commonly, in those with glomerulonephritis.

In the absence of specific symptoms, crystals of calcium oxalate (envelope shaped) and uric acid (rhomboid shaped) identified in acidic urine are of little clinical significance. The presence of cystine crystals (benzene-ring shaped) in the urine indicates the rare disease cystinuria. Triple phosphate crystals (coffin-lid shaped) may be identified in alkaline urine. Presence of bacteria in an unspun urine specimen is significant and provides presumptive evidence for a urinary tract infection.

Major Renal Syndromes

A patient with renal disease may be classified into separate clinical syndromes based on type and manifestation of renal injury as described in Table 26–5.

Acute nephritic syndrome is a clinical syndrome characterized by the relatively abrupt onset of kidney dysfunction accompanied by the presence of red blood cell casts and dysmorphic erythrocytes in the urine sediment, as well as varying degrees of proteinuria, which are highly suggestive of glomerular origin. Sodium avidity in the acute nephritic syndrome is considerably greater than what would be expected from decreased GFR. Plasma albumin is generally normal; consequently, a significant fraction of the retained sodium remains intravascularly and may explain the presence of hypertension, plasma volume dilution, circulatory overload, and congestive heart failure. Although acute post-streptococcal glomerulonephritis is the prototype for the acute nephritic syndrome, other infections may also lead to this syndrome. Acute nephritic syndrome may also be caused by primary glomerular diseases, such as mesangioproliferative glomerulonephritis, and multisystem diseases that include systemic lupus erythematosus, Henoch-Schönlein purpura, and essential mixed cryoglobulinemia (see **Web Fig. 28–26** in Chapter 28, "Glomerular Diseases").

Nephrotic syndrome is characterized by increased glomerular permeability exhibited by proteinuria in excess of 3.5 g/day/1.73 m² body surface area. A variable tendency exists toward edema, hypoalbuminemia, and hyperlipidemia. Patients with the nephrotic syndrome, in addition to proteinuria, may demonstrate oval fat bodies, coarse granular casts, and occasional cellular elements, but the lack of *active* sediment with dysmorphic red blood cells and red blood cell casts is characteristic. The differential diagnosis includes glomerular diseases such as minimal change disease, membranous nephropathy, focal segmental glomerulosclerosis (FSGS), diabetic nephropathy, and amyloidosis. In patients with a mixed clinical picture (nephrotic/nephritic syndrome), membrane-proliferative nephritis, systemic lupus erythematosus, postinfectious glomerulonephritis,

Table 26–5 **Major Renal Syndromes**

Syndrome	Definition	Example
Acute nephritic syndrome	Abrupt onset of renal insufficiency accompanied by hematuria that is glomerular or tubular in origin	Poststreptococcal glomerulonephritis
Nephrotic syndrome	Increased glomerular permeability manifested by massive proteinuria (>3.5 g/day/1.73 m^2), edema, and hypoalbuminuria	
With *bland* urine sediment (pure nephrotic)	Oval fat bodies, coarse granular casts	Minimal change disease
Asymptomatic urinary abnormalities	Isolated proteinuria (<2.0 g/day/1.73 m^2) or hematuria (with or without proteinuria)	Immunoglobulin A nephropathy
Tubulointerstitial nephropathy	Renal insufficiency associated with non–nephrotic-range proteinuria and functional tubular defects	Sarcoidosis
Acute renal failure	An abrupt decline in renal function sufficient to result in retention of nitrogenous waste (e.g., blood urea nitrogen and creatinine)	Acute tubular necrosis
Rapidly progressive renal failure	Rapid deterioration of renal function over a period of weeks to months	Rapidly progressive glomerulonephritis
Tubular defects	Isolated or multiple tubular transport defects	Renal tubular acidosis

and mixed essential cryoglobulinemia are the most likely diagnostic considerations.

The term *rapidly progressive renal failure* is applied to patients who have more than a 50% loss in kidney function over weeks to months. This condition is in contrast to patients with *acute renal failure,* who have an abrupt decline in renal function over several days, and to patients with *chronic renal failure,* who have a decline in renal function over months to years. The differential diagnosis of a patient who presents with rapidly progressive renal failure is shown in Table 26–6. One of the important but uncommon causes of rapidly progressive renal failure is rapidly progressive glomerulonephritis. This condition is a clinical syndrome that is typically associated with extensive glomerular crescent formation (**Web Fig. 26–4**) as the principal histologic finding on renal biopsy. Dysmorphic erythrocytes, red blood cell casts, and moderate proteinuria are characteristic in rapidly progressive glomerulonephritis.

Acute renal failure is a syndrome that can be broadly defined as an abrupt decline in renal function sufficient to result in kidney impairment over days to a few weeks. Acute renal failure can result from a decrease in renal blood flow (prerenal azotemia), intrinsic parenchymal disease (intrarenal azotemia), or obstruction to urine flow (postre-

Table 26–6 **Causes of Rapidly Progressive Renal Failure**

Obstructive uropathy
Malignant hypertension
Rapidly progressive glomerulonephritis
Thrombotic thrombocytopenic purpura, hemolytic uremic syndrome
Atheromatous embolic disease
Bilateral renal artery stenosis
Scleroderma crisis
Multiple myeloma

nal azotemia). The general approach for evaluating acute renal failure is detailed in Chapter 32.

Tubulointerstitial nephropathy represents a group of clinical disorders that principally affect the renal tubules and interstitium, with relative sparing of the glomeruli and renal vasculature. In the majority of patients, the disease can possibly be classified into acute interstitial nephritis or chronic interstitial nephropathy based on the rate of progression of renal dysfunction. Chronic tubulointerstitial nephropathy is characterized by renal insufficiency, non–nephrotic-range proteinuria, and tubular damage disproportionately severe relative to the degree of kidney impairment. Thus, patients with chronic tubulointerstitial disease often have modest degrees of sodium wasting, hyperkalemia, and a normal anion gap metabolic acidosis even when renal dysfunction is modest. Acute interstitial nephritis, often caused by a medication, is characterized by the sudden onset of clinical signs of renal dysfunction associated with a prominent inflammatory cell infiltrate within the renal interstitium and is often important in the differential diagnosis of patients with acute renal failure.

Imaging of the Urinary Tract

One of the most common imaging studies of the urinary tract is the renal ultrasound. Renal ultrasonography is a noninvasive method of obtaining an anatomic image of the kidney and the collecting system. This technique is particularly useful for determining kidney size, for detecting renal masses, cysts, and dilation of the collecting system, and for identifying hydronephrosis. The absence of hydronephrosis on a sonogram does not rule out obstructive uropathy, particularly in the presence of acute obstruction, volume depletion, or retroperitoneal fibrosis. In a patient with advanced renal failure, the presence of bilaterally small kidneys typically less than 8 cm implies a chronic, irreversible process, whereas the presence of normal-size kidneys of 11 to 13 cm indicates acute renal failure or chronic renal failure caused by diseases such as diabetes, amyloidosis, or multiple myeloma. Duplex ultrasonography, in which B-mode ultrasonography has been combined with pulsed Doppler imaging, may be useful in detecting disease of the major renal arteries or veins. Ultrasound can easily identify simple cysts. However, complex cysts or solid lesions require further investigation by computed tomography or magnetic resonance imaging. Discrepancy in kidney size by more than 2.0 cm may suggest ischemic damage to the kidney such as renovascular disease, reflux nephropathy with scarring of the kidney, or congenital abnormalities. Ultrasonography is routinely used to guide kidney biopsy, to introduce nephrostomy tubes, or to drain fluid collection around the kidney.

Intravenous pyelography (IVP) involves the intravenous administration of iodinated radiographic contrast medium that is excreted through the kidney by glomerular filtration. The contrast medium concentrates in the renal tubules and produces a nephrogram image within the first few minutes after injection. As the medium passes into the collecting system, the calyces, renal pelvis, ureters, and bladder are visualized. The use of IVP over ultrasonography is required when a more detailed imaging study of anatomic structures is required or when evaluating obstruction and acute nephrolithiasis. The disadvantage of IVP is the requirement for radiocontrast, which can induce nephrotoxicity, particularly in patients with renal insufficiency as defined by an estimated GFR of less than 60 mL/min/1.73 m^2, volume depletion, diabetes, or congestive heart failure.

Retrograde pyelography is performed by injecting radiocontrast material directly into the ureters at the time of cystoscopy. This technique is useful in defining obstructing lesions within the ureter or renal pelvis, particularly in the setting of a nonvisualizing kidney on IVP. Ureteric stones can be removed during this procedure using a special basket.

Computed tomography of the kidney is usually done by instilling a contrast medium, except when investigating renal calculi or hemorrhage. Computed tomography is most helpful in evaluating renal masses, complex cysts, and perinephric and vascular pathologic conditions such as renal-vein thrombosis. In select cases, computed tomography is used to guide kidney biopsy or fluid collection, such as that from a peri-nephric abscess. As in other imaging studies of the urinary tract, computed tomography often uses radiocontrast agents and is contraindicated in individuals with impaired kidney function.

Magnetic resonance imaging uses high magnetic fields and radiofrequencies to construct images. Magnetic resonance imaging is most helpful in delineating complex renal masses, staging renal tumors and detecting invasion of renal veins, and diagnosing renovascular disease; it is also used as an alternative to computed tomography in patients with kidney failure to avoid using radiocontrast agents, as gadolinum is non-nephrotoxic. Technical improvement in magnetic resonance angiography has enhanced the detection of renal artery stenosis and may grade the severity of the disease. Magnetic resonance imaging should be avoided in patients with implanted ferromagnetic devices such as pacemakers.

Radionuclide imaging provides important noninvasive information about kidneys. The test involves the intravenous administration of radiolabeled compounds, after which images are taken with a gamma camera. Pregnancy is the only contraindication for the renal radionuclide imaging. The uses of renal radionuclide imaging are listed in the Table 26–7.

Renal arteriography involves the direct injection of radiographic contrast medium into the aorta and renal arteries and is used to assess renal vasculature. It is particularly useful in evaluating patients with suggested renal artery stenosis or thrombosis and those with a renal mass. Patients with unexplained hematuria or with a suggested vascular malformation should have a renal arteriogram. Individuals with polyarteritis nodosa may require selective renal arteriogra-

Table 26–7	**Common Uses of Radionuclide Renal Imaging**

Renal perfusion
Renovascular hypertension
GFR estimation
Pyelonephritis, renal abscess
Interstitial nephritis
Renal cortical scarring
Obstruction
Renal pseudotumor

GFR = glomerular filtration rate.

Table 26–8 Indications for Kidney Biopsy

Nephrotic syndrome

Persistent proteinuria, particularly with abnormal sediment or abnormal renal function

Hematuria associated with abnormal urine sediment or proteinuria

Unexplained hematuria after exclusion of lower urinary tract causes

Systemic disorders with kidney involvement (e.g., systemic lupus erythematosus, Henoch-Schönlein purpura)

Acute renal failure with atypical features or failure to recover renal function in 8 weeks

Rapidly progressive renal failure

Renal allograft dysfunction

phy to detect microaneurysms. Renal vein catheterization is used to confirm the diagnosis of renal vein thrombosis or to obtain blood samples from the renal vein. Although computed tomography or magnetic resonance imaging is used to confirm the diagnosis of renal vein thrombosis, renal venography may be required when the diagnosis is in doubt or when the initial diagnostic suspicion is high.

Renal Biopsy

Most renal biopsies are performed when a glomerular lesion is suggested and less commonly in patients with unexplained acute renal failure. Table 26–8 lists the indications for kidney biopsy. The percutaneous biopsy is the most commonly used technique and is a relatively safe procedure. Potential complications of a closed renal biopsy include hematuria, renal hematoma, vascular laceration with the development of arteriovenous fistula, and the inadvertent biopsy of liver, spleen, or bowel. Percutaneous kidney biopsy is contraindicated in solitary or ectopic kidneys (except kidney transplants), horseshoe kidney, uncontrolled bleeding disorders, uncontrolled hypertension, renal infection, renal neoplasm, and uncooperative patients.

Prospectus for the Future

The early identification of kidney disease needs to be determined well before changes in serum parameters that are elevated after significant kidney impairment has occurred. The use of urinary biomarkers is emerging as diagnostic tools that will help identify individuals at risk for kidney disease and will allow for the development of novel therapeutic interventions that prevent the development of kidney failure or limit progressive loss of kidney function.

Additionally, genetic analysis of individuals with kidney disease may allow for directed therapeutic regimens that decrease the risk of progressive kidney disease and the ultimate need for dialysis therapies or renal transplantation in the future.

References

National Kidney Foundation: K/DOQI clinical practice guidelines for chronic kidney disease: Evaluation, classification, and stratification. Am J Kidney Dis 39:S1–S62, 2002.

Stevens LA, Fares G, Fleming J, et al: Low rates of testing and diagnostic codes usage in a commericial clinical laboratory: Evidence for lack of physician awareness of chronic kidney disease. J Am Soc Nephrol 16:2439–2448, 2005.

Chapter 27

Fluid and Electrolyte Disorders

Thomas E. Andreoli

Robert L. Safirstein

The content of fluid and electrolytes in the cells and fluid compartments of the body are remarkably constant under normal conditions despite a widely varying intake. This constancy is maintained by fluid and solute shifts across the cells of the body and by the capacity of the kidney to adjust the urinary excretion of water, electrolytes, and solutes to match intake and the needs of the body. In health, the solute content of body water is maintained between 285 and 295 mOsm/kg of water. Tight regulation of body water and solute concentrations is made possible by the remarkable ability of the kidney to regulate urine volume from 500 mL to 24 L per 24-hour period. The ability of the kidney to carry out its functions is intrinsically tied to the thirst-neurohypophyseal-renal axis.

Volume Disorders

Water constitutes approximately 60% of total-body weight in humans (Fig. 27–1). Total-body water is inversely proportional to the amount of body fat, which varies with age, gender, and nutritional status. Approximately two thirds of the total-body water are in the intracellular compartment. Three fourths of the extracellular water are in the interstitial space, and one fourth is in the plasma. Potassium and magnesium constitute the major cations of the intracellular space, whereas sodium is the major cation of the extracellular space. Phosphate and protein are the major anions of the intracellular space, whereas chloride and bicarbonate are the major anions of extracellular space. The cell membrane represents the barrier between the intracellular and extracellular fluid compartments. Because membranes are relatively permeable to water, the osmotic gradient determines the movement of fluid across the cell membrane. Thus, except for transient changes, the intracellular and extracellular fluid compartments are in *osmotic equilibrium*. The transfer of fluid between the vascular and interstitial compartments occurs across the capillary wall and is governed by the balance between hydrostatic pressure gradients and plasma oncotic pressure gradients, as related in the *Starling equation*:

$$J_V = (K_f \times [\Delta P - \sigma \Delta \Pi])$$

Where J_V is the rate of fluid transfer between vascular and interstitial compartments, K_f is the water permeability, ΔP is the difference between capillary and interstitial hydrostatic pressure, $\Delta \Pi$ equals the difference between capillary and interstitial oncotic pressure, and σ is the reflection coefficient (albumin = 1). Thus, an increase in the driving force for fluid movement into the interstitial compartment may result from a decrease in the colloid oncotic pressure of plasma, as may occur in hypoalbuminemia, and/or an increase in the capillary hydrostatic pressure, as occurs in congestive heart failure.

NORMAL VOLUME HOMEOSTASIS

The kidney plays a crucial role in regulating the constancy of extracellular fluid (ECF) volume. The response to a reduction in ECF volume consists of hemodynamic responses that adjust cardiac output and peripheral vascular resistance to maintain blood pressure, as well as primary renal responses that adjust external sodium and water balance. Together, this response has been termed the *integrated volume response* (Fig. 27–2). Hemodynamic alterations occur within minutes of a perceived volume reduction and are characterized by tachycardia, increased peripheral resistance from arterial vasoconstriction, and decreased venous capacitance from venoconstriction. Renal conservation of salt and water lags behind by 12 to 24 hours and involves the release of various hormones (see Fig. 27–2). Stimulation of the extrarenal baroreceptors also results in the release of antidiuretic hormone (ADH), which promotes water retention in the kidney. Vasoconstrictive factors, such as endothelins produced and released by vascular endothelial cells, also play a role in modulating systemic hemodynamics. Elevation of the efferent arteriolar resistance increases the filtration fraction, increases peritubular protein concentration, and increases sodium and water reabsorption in proximal tubules. Vasodilator prostaglandins, such as prostaglandin E_2, modulate these vasoconstrictive influences and maintain the glomerular filtration rate (GFR) by enhancing the renal blood flow in states associated with ECF volume depletion. This action is the reason that nonsteroidal anti-inflammatory drugs are so deleterious during volume depletion.

In response to volume expansion, the renal excretion of salt and water is increased because of the suppression of the aforementioned pathways. The release of atrial natriuretic peptide is a major factor promoting natriuresis in volume-expanded states. Atrial natriuretic peptide is released from the atrial myocytes in response to atrial stretch associated with volume expansion. This peptide release promotes natriuresis by increasing GFR and inhibiting collecting duct sodium reabsorption.

ABNORMAL VOLUME REGULATION

The integrated volume response depends on afferent mechanisms that sense changes in the *effective circulating volume* (ECV). ECV is difficult to define because it is not a measurable and distinct body fluid compartment. ECV relates to the *fullness* and tension within the arterial tree. Because only 15% of total blood volume is in the arterial compartment, arterial blood volume can be decreased in relation to the holding capacity of the arterial tree. In most circumstances, ECV correlates with the total ECF volume, except in certain disorders in which ECV is decreased in the presence of an increased total ECF volume (Table 27–1). In these disorders, the ECV is decreased as a result of either decreased cardiac output or arterial vasodilation, which decreases fullness and tension in the arterial circulation.

Because the afferent sensors respond to ECV rather than to the total ECF volume, in disease states such as congestive heart failure and hepatic cirrhosis, during which ECV is low, continued activation of the *integrated volume response* occurs and thus promotes further salt and water retention.

VOLUME DEPLETION

Disorders of extracellular volume result from alterations in sodium balance. The causes of true volume depletion—that is, decreased ECV and total ECF volume—are listed in Table 27–2. Extra renal losses are the most common clinical causes of volume depletion, and when they occur with normal renal function, the urine is highly concentrated, salt poor, and acidic. When volume depletion occurs from renal losses, the

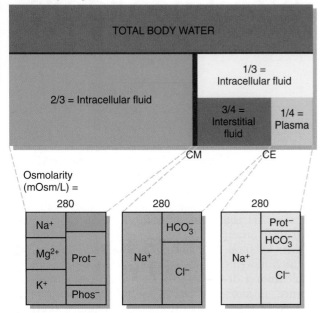

Figure 27–1 Composition of body fluid compartments. The compartments are anatomically defined by the cell membrane *(CM)* and capillary endothelium *(CE)*. The osmolar concentration among compartments is equivalent despite wide variation in cation and anion composition.

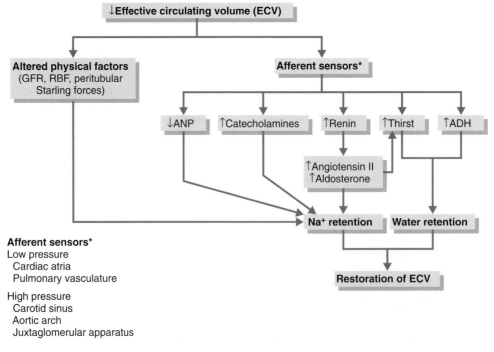

Figure 27–2 Volume repletion reaction. ADH = antidiuretic hormone; ANP = atriopeptin; GFR = glomerular filtration rate; RBF = renal blood flow.

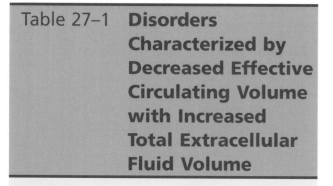

Table 27–1	**Disorders Characterized by Decreased Effective Circulating Volume with Increased Total Extracellular Fluid Volume**

Congestive heart failure
Liver disease
Sepsis
Nephrotic syndrome (minority)
Pregnancy
Anaphylaxis

Table 27–2	**Causes of Volume Depletion**

Gastrointestinal losses
  Upper: bleeding, nasogastric suction, vomiting
  Lower: bleeding, diarrhea, enteric or pancreatic fistula,
    tube drainage

Renal losses
  Salt and water: diuretics, osmotic diuresis, post-obstructive
    diuresis, acute tubular necrosis (recovery phase),
    salt-losing nephropathy, adrenal insufficiency, renal
    tubular acidosis
  Water: diabetes insipidus

Skin and respiratory losses
  Sweat, burns, insensible losses

Sequestration without external fluid loss
  Intestinal obstruction, peritonitis, pancreatitis,
    rhabdomyolysis

Table 27–3	**Causes of Volume Excess**

**Primary Renal Sodium Retention
(Increased Effective Circulating Volume)**

Oliguric acute renal failure
Acute glomerulonephritis
Severe chronic renal failure
Nephritic; nephrotic syndrome
Primary hyperaldosteronism
Cushing's syndrome
Early stages of severe liver disease
Conn's syndrome
Gordon's syndrome
Liddle's syndrome

**Secondary Renal Sodium Retention
(Decreased Effective Circulating Volume)**

Heart failure
Later stages of severe liver disease
Nephrotic syndrome (minimal change disease)
Pregnancy

urine is inappropriately dilute and sometimes rich in salt. The syndrome of nephrogenic diabetes insipidus is one such cause, and in congenital forms of the syndrome, loss-of-function mutations occur in the V2 vasopressin receptor (X-linked), as well as autosomal-dominant and -recessive forms cause by inactivating mutations of the collecting duct water channel aquaporin-2. The clinical findings in states of true volume depletion are secondary to an underfilling of the arterial tree and to the renal and hemodynamic responses to this underfilling. Mild volume depletion may be associated with orthostatic dizziness and tachycardia. As the intracellular compartment becomes further depleted, recumbent tachycardia becomes evident, and urine output diminishes.

Patients with severe volume depletion may exhibit vasoconstriction, hypotension, mental obtundation, cool extremities, and negligible urine output. Many of these clinical features can be explained based on effects of vasoconstrictor hormones, such as catecholamine and angiotensin II, that are released in response to hypovolemia.

Significant volume depletion can occur in the absence of classic clinical findings. States of volume depletion in patients receiving cardiovascular drugs and excess renal sodium loss from intrinsic renal disease or diuretics are examples of clinical circumstances in which an assessment of the state of hydration may be difficult. An appropriate clinical history is always mandatory, particularly prior knowledge of the patient's body weight. If doubt exists about the state of hydration, particularly in critically ill patients, measurement of the pulmonary capillary wedge pressure by means of right-sided heart catheterization permits assessment of the intravascular volume status.

The absolute quantity and the rate of fluid replacement depend on the severity of volume depletion, which is estimated by the clinical presentation. If fluid repletion is to involve parenteral infusions, the distribution of the infused fluid should be considered. Nearly all of the volume of solutions containing 0.9% sodium chloride and colloid are retained in the extracellular space and are the preferred parenteral solutions for the treatment of hypovolemia. By contrast, only one third of infused 5% glucose in water (D_5W) remains in the extracellular compartment.

VOLUME EXCESS

Volume expansion occurs when salt and water intake exceeds renal and extrarenal losses. The causes are listed in Table 27–3. The underlying disturbance common to these disorders is sodium and water retention by the kidney. The

Table 27–4   Characteristics of Commonly Used Diuretics

Agent	Site	Primary Effect	Secondary Effect
Carbonic anhydrase inhibitors (acetazolamide)	Proximal tubule	Blocking of ↓ Na$^+$-H$^+$ exchange	K$^+$, HCO$_3^-$ loss
Loop diuretics (furosemide, bumetanide, ethacrynic acid)	Thick ascending limb of loop of Henle	↓ Na$^+$/K$^+$/2Cl$^-$ transport	K$^+$ loss ↑ H$^+$ secretion ↑ Ca^{2+} excretion
Thiazide Diuretics			
Thiazides	Distal convoluted tubule	↓ NaCl co-transport	↓ K$^+$ loss ↓ H$^+$ secretion ↓ Ca^{2+} excretion
Metolazone	Distal tubule, proximal tubule	↓ NaCl reabsorption	—
Aldosterone antagonists (spironolactone)	Cortical collecting duct	↓ Na$^+$ reabsorption	↓ K$^+$ loss ↓ H$^+$ secretion
Primary sodium-channel blockers (triamterene, amiloride)	Cortical collecting duct	↓ Na$^+$ reabsorption	↓ K$^+$ loss ↓ H$^+$ secretion

Ca^{2+} = calcium; Cl$^-$ = chloride; H$^+$ = hydrogen; HCO$_3^-$ = bicarbonate; K$^+$ = potassium; Na$^+$ = sodium; NaCl = sodium chloride.

sodium and water retention may be primary, resulting in increased ECV, or secondary, in response to a decreased ECV. The net result of renal sodium and water retention is an alteration of Starling forces that leads to increased capillary hydrostatic pressure and favors fluid shifts from the intravascular to interstitial space. Most patients with nephrotic syndrome have an increased ECV resulting from primary renal sodium retention. In advanced liver disease, the ECV is decreased because of arterial underfilling from vasodilation that results in secondary renal sodium retention. However, in early liver disease, the volume excess may result from primary renal sodium retention. Severe hypoalbuminemia associated with liver disease, nephrotic syndrome, or severe malnutrition may overwhelm the local capillary homeostatic mechanisms and may lead to edema formation.

The mainstay in treating volume excess is dietary sodium restriction in combination with diuretics (Table 27–4). Diuretics enhance natriuresis by inhibiting the reabsorption of sodium at various sites along the nephron. The cardinal example of a proximal tubular diuretic is acetazolamide, a *carbonic anhydrase inhibitor,* which blocks proximal reabsorption of sodium bicarbonate. Consequently, prolonged use of acetazolamide may lead to hyperchloremic acidosis. Metolazone, a member of the thiazide class of diuretics, in addition to blocking sodium reabsorption in the distal tubule, exerts its natriuretic effect in the proximal tubule. Because the proximal tubule is the major site for phosphate reabsorption, profound phosphaturia may accompany the use of metolazone. *Loop diuretics* such as furosemide and bumetanide inhibit the sodium, chloride, and potassium cotransporter of the thick ascending limb of the loop of Henle. *Thiazide diuretics* inhibit the sodium and chloride cotransporter of the distal tubule. The loop diuretics promote calcium excretion, and the thiazide diuretics decrease calcium excretion. Thus, the former are useful in managing hypercalcemia, whereas the latter are useful in preventing calcium stone formation. Spironolactone, an *aldosterone antagonist,* decreases sodium reabsorption in the cortical collecting duct. Primary *sodium channel blockers* such as amiloride also block sodium reabsorption in the cortical collecting duct by an aldosterone-independent mechanism. The last two groups of diuretics do not cause hypokalemia, which is a common complication associated with the use of other diuretics. In states of severe sodium retention and edema formation, such as severe congestive heart failure and nephrotic syndrome, a combination of diuretics working at different sites in the nephron may be more effective than the use of a single class of diuretics. Moreover, using potassium-sparing diuretics in combination with a potassium-wasting diuretic can minimize potassium and magnesium deficits. In patients with cirrhosis and ascites, abdominal paracentesis with concomitant intravenous infusion of some colloid has been used as a good therapeutic alternative to diuretics.

Osmolality Disorders

Body fluid osmolality, the ratio of solute to water in all fluid compartments, is maintained within an extremely narrow range. Because water moves freely across most cell membranes, changes in the ECF osmolality cause reciprocal changes in the intracellular volume. The ECF osmolality can be approximated by calculating the serum osmolality based on the major solutes in that compartment:

$$\text{Calculated osmolality} = (2 \times \text{sodium}) + (\text{glucose} \div 18) + (\text{BUN} \div 2.8)$$

Where the glucose and blood urea nitrogen (BUN) concentrations are expressed as milligrams per deciliter and the serum sodium concentration is expressed as milliequivalents per liter.

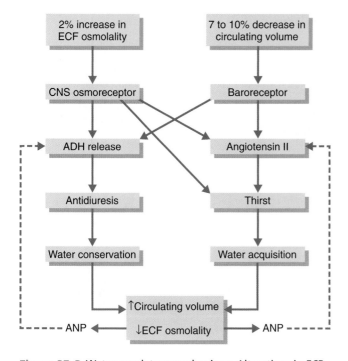

Figure 27–3 Water regulatory mechanisms. Alterations in ECF osmolality or volume stimulate *(solid lines)* thirst and release of ADH. The net result is a positive water balance. Counter-regulation is provided by the inhibitory effects *(dashed lines)* of atriopeptin (ANP). CNS = central nervous system; ECF = extracellular fluid.

Measured osmolality usually equals the calculated osmolality. However, in the presence of osmotically active substances, such as ethanol, methanol, or ethylene glycol, the measured osmolality is higher than the calculated osmolality. Under these circumstances, the *osmolar gap* (measured minus calculated osmolality) provides a clue to the presence of toxins and gives an estimated concentration of these solutes. Alterations in the plasma sodium concentration almost always reflect changes in water balance. Because sodium is the major cation in the ECF, disorders of osmolality are generally reflected by an abnormal sodium concentration in the ECF.

Regulation of osmolality involves changes in renal water excretion, and the sodium excretion is not affected by osmoregulatory factors unless concomitant ECV depletion exists. ECF osmolality is regulated by dual pathways in the *water repletion reaction* (Fig. 27–3). Osmoreceptor cells in the central nervous system that are located in the wall of the third ventricle sense minor changes in the osmolality of blood in the internal carotid circulation. Neuronal signals from osmoreceptors stimulate the release of ADH from the posterior pituitary gland and simultaneously stimulate the sensation of thirst. ADH causes renal water conservation by increasing water permeability and water reabsorption in the collecting ducts. Thirst leads to an increase in water intake. When the ECF volume is reduced by approximately 10%, water retention is activated as a means of replenishing ECF volume irrespective of osmolality. In this case, baroreceptors in the venous and arterial circulation stimulate ADH release through neuronal pathways. This *nonosmotic* stimulation of

ADH release occurs independently of osmoreceptor function. Water repletion activates mechanisms that counter-regulate water conservation. Suppression of thirst and inhibition of ADH release lead to decreased water intake and increased renal water excretion.

Hyponatremia

PATHOPHYSIOLOGIC FACTORS

A diagnostic approach to hyponatremia is outlined in Figure 27–4. The causes of hyponatremia show an association with normal, high, or low total-body sodium content. In some hyponatremic disorders, the serum osmolality is elevated; thus, the intracellular water content is not increased, and no risk of brain edema exists. Hyperglycemia and the use of hypertonic mannitol may result in hyponatremia because of water shift from the intracellular to extracellular space. Hyponatremia associated with normal serum osmolality may be seen in patients with extreme hyperlipidemia and hyperproteinemia, resulting from methodologic errors in techniques to measure serum electrolyte concentration. The increasing use of ion-selective electrodes for these measurements is making these causes of *pseudohyponatremia* uncommon. Hyponatremia may also be seen in patients who undergo transurethral resection of the prostate or hysteroscopic examination because of the absorption of large amounts of hypo-osmolar glycine or sorbitol irrigating solutions.

Most hyponatremic disorders are associated with hypo-osmolality. In principle, hypo-osmolality can result from an increase in water intake and/or a decrease in renal water excretion. Under normal circumstances, the kidneys can excrete 16 to 20 L of water free of solutes, or *free water,* per day. Water excretion may be impaired secondary to a reduced GFR, reduced ECV, impaired sodium-chloride reabsorption in the renal diluting segments of the distal nephron, failure to suppress ADH secretion in response to hypotonicity (syndrome of inappropriate secretion of ADH [SIADH]). Finally, there is a rare congenital syndrome, the nephrogenic syndrome of inappropriate antidiuresis (NSIAD), which is caused by a gain in function mutation of the V2 vasopressin receptor, such that the latter is activated even in the absense of vasopressin.

Because of the large capacity of normal kidneys to excrete free water, even in patients with *primary polydipsia,* the hyponatremia is caused by both large water intake and impaired water excretion. Hyponatremia may also occur with modestly increased water intake in the presence of impaired GFR or decreased solute intake. In patients with decreased GFR, renal water excretion is impaired because of decreased delivery of filtrate to the distal nephron. Patients with chronic starvation or beer potomania have deficient oral intake of solutes. Because renal water excretion depends on osmolar intake, these patients may develop hyponatremia at a modestly increased level of water intake.

More commonly, hyponatremia occurs as a result of the inability to dilute urine maximally because of reduction in the rate of salt absorption by the diluting segment, sustained nonosmotic release of ADH, or a combination of these two factors. In the disorders associated with decreased ECV, nonosmotic ADH release occurs and promotes water

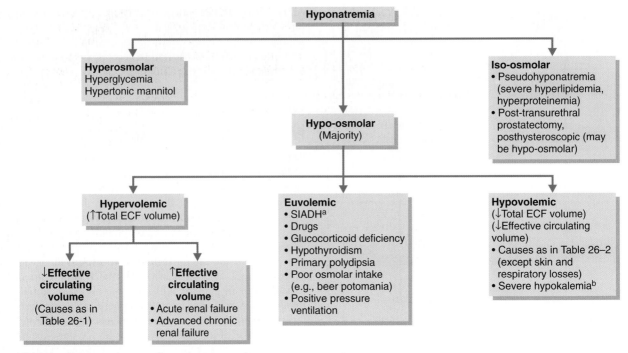

aSIADH patients may have modest volume expansion.
bSeen in patients with hypokalemia due to diuretic use and may be due to Na+ entry into the cells to replace K+ loss.

Figure 27–4 Diagnostic approach to hyponatremia. ECF = extracellular fluid; SIADH = syndrome of inappropriate secretion of ADH.

retention by the kidney. In addition, these patients have enhanced proximal sodium-chloride reabsorption with diminished distal delivery. These disorders may be associated with signs of either volume expansion or volume depletion.

SIADH is the prototype of the primary release of ADH or ADH-like substances. It occurs most often in association with pathologic processes of the central nervous system or pulmonary system. Many medications can enhance the release of ADH or can potentiate its effect (Table 27–5). The circulating ADH allows excessive water absorption in the collecting duct with a modest expansion of the ECF volume. With the increase in volume, renal perfusion is increased, and the kidney subsequently decreases sodium reabsorption in an attempt to reestablish euvolemia. Two infants have recently been described with apparent SIADH in which the serum vasopressin levels are suppressed. Evaluation revealed gain of function mutations of the V2 vasopressin receptor in these patients.

DIAGNOSIS AND TREATMENT

The signs and symptoms of hyponatremia are related to brain cell swelling caused by an increase in the brain water content resulting from water shift from a hypo-osmolar extracellular environment. Hence, hyponatremic disorders should be considered in any patient who has acute mental status changes. An assessment of the volume status by physical examination is the most important initial step in the diagnostic approach to patients with hyponatremia. The most difficult differential diagnosis among hyponatremic disorders involves the distinction between patients who have reduced ECV and those who have SIADH. In both instances,

the urine osmolality may be inappropriately concentrated relative to the serum osmolality. In reduced ECV, the urine sodium concentration is negligible, whereas it is usually higher than 30 mEq/L in patients with SIADH. High BUN and serum uric acid levels also suggest reduced ECV. When hyponatremia is associated with a low BUN and uric acid level, SIADH is the most likely diagnosis.

Baseline data should include body weight, serum electrolytes, serum osmolality, urine electrolytes, and urine osmolality; frequent measurement of serum and urine electrolytes, intake, and urine output should be performed during the treatment of hyponatremia. As a general rule, the administration of sodium solutions with a tonicity greater than that of urine raises serum sodium concentrations. The treatment should depend on the underlying clinical disease and volume status of the patient. Sodium and water intake should be restricted in the volume-expanded patient. In patients with decreased ECV and true hypovolemia, secondary to extrarenal losses, treatment should include isotonic sodium chloride.

In patients with SIADH, restriction of water intake is the mainstay of therapy. However, this is difficult to achieve because patients are invariably thirsty, particularly in the southern regions of the United States. Demethylchlorotetracycline and lithium, while proposed, are not generally acceptable. Hypertonic saline, particularly in patients with SIADH, will produce a profound natriuresis and hyponatremia will develop rapidly. The most rational approach to therapy is the use of furosemide in combination with normal saline. Furosemide forces the excretion of a urine which is $1/2$ normal saline, while the administration of normal saline helps correct the hyponatremia.

Table 27–5	**Causes of Syndrome of Inappropriate Secretion of Antidiuretic Hormone**

Central Nervous System Disorders

Trauma
Infection
Tumors
Porphyria

Pulmonary Disorders

Tuberculosis
Pneumonia
Positive pressure ventilation

Neoplasia

Carcinoma: bronchogenic, pancreatic, ureteral, prostatic, bladder
Lymphoma and leukemia
Thymoma and mesothelioma

Drugs

Increased ADH release
  Chlorpropamide
  Clofibrate
  Carbamazepine
  Vincristine
Potentiated ADH action
  Chlorpropamide
  Cyclophosphamide
  Nonsteroidal anti-inflammatory agents

ADH = antidiuretic hormone.
Modified from Andreoli TE: Disorders of fluid volume, electrolyte, and acid-base balance. In Wyngaarden JB, Smith LH Jr, Bennett JC (eds): Cecil Textbook of Medicine, 19th ed. Philadelphia: WB Saunders, 1992, p 509.

When hyponatremia occurs acutely (<48 hours), cerebral edema can ensue. The typical signs and symptoms include headache, nausea, vomiting, weakness, incoordination with falls, delirium, and seizures. Patients in whom hyponatremia develops over days to weeks may exhibit more subtle neurologic signs and symptoms.

The rate of correction of serum sodium depends on the symptoms and duration of hyponatremia. The correction of serum sodium with acute hyponatremia may be achieved rapidly (up to 2.5 mEq/L/hr) until central nervous system symptoms and seizures subside. Even under these circumstances, an absolute change of serum sodium of more than 20 mEq/L/day should be avoided. In patients with chronic hyponatremia (>48 hours), the serum sodium concentration should be corrected at a rate of 0.5 mEq/L/hour until it reaches 120 mEq/L. Patients with asymptomatic hyponatremia (acute or chronic) do not need aggressive therapy. This caution is necessary because of the occurrence of central pontine myelinolysis with too rapid correction.

Hypervolemic hypotonic hyponatremia secondary to cirrhosis, congestive heart failure, or renal failure should be treated not only by measures directed at the underlying disease, but also with loop diuretics to help promote the excretion of hypotonic urine. Water restriction should be maintained at less than 1 L/24-hour period. For patients with chronic SIADH that is not responsive to treatment of the underlying cause, free-water restriction alone is often sufficient. In resistant cases and in patients with neurologic symptoms, a combination of furosemide and normal or high dietary sodium intake is necessary. Demeclocycline, by blocking the effect of ADH on the renal collecting duct, can be useful in select cases at doses of 900 to 1200 mg/24-hour period.

Hypernatremia

PATHOPHYSIOLOGIC FACTORS

In most instances, hypernatremia is caused by excess water loss, rather than by sodium gain. Hypertonicity of the plasma is a powerful stimulus for thirst. Patients who are unable to sense thirst owing to diseases of the brain or patients who are physically unable to obtain water may develop hypernatremia. Most patients with hypernatremia, however, exhibit a primary defect in urinary concentrating ability along with insufficient administration of free water (Fig. 27–5).

Water can be lost in the urine, in excess of electrolytes, in conditions characterized by the presence of large quantities of osmotically active solutes in the filtrate. This type of *osmotic diuresis* can occur in patients with hyperglycemia, after the infusion of mannitol, or in patients who are excreting excessive amounts of amino acids or urea. The last situation occurs in patients receiving high-protein tube feedings or total parenteral nutrition.

Diabetes insipidus is a disorder in which the collecting tubule is impermeable to water. Patients may have a central defect in the release of ADH or a defect in renal responsiveness to the hormone (nephrogenic).

In hypernatremia caused by osmotic diuresis, urine osmolality may be higher than serum osmolality because of the presence of solutes such as glucose, mannitol, or urea in the urine.

TREATMENT

Hypernatremia that is associated with hypovolemia implies a sodium deficit in addition to the water deficit and requires isotonic saline infusion. In other patients, hypotonic intravenous solutions (D_5W, half-normal saline, or quarter-normal saline) should be administered to correct hypernatremia. The water content of these fluids varies according to the electrolyte concentration. For example, 1 L of D_5W essentially equals 1 L of free water, because glucose is eventually metabolized. However, 1 L of half-normal saline or quarter-normal saline contains 500 or 750 mL, respectively, of free water. In addition, if other solutes, such as potassium or magnesium, are added to the intravenous fluids, their contribution to the tonicity of the administered

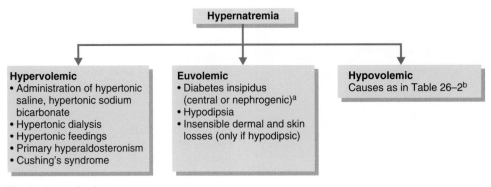

aMay be hypovolemic.
bUnder "sequestration," only rhabdomyolysis may cause hypernatremia due to shift of water from extracellular to intracellular space.

Figure 27–5 Diagnostic approach to hypernatremia.

fluid should be taken into account. Administration of solutions that are hypotonic relative to the urine corrects hypernatremia.

The serum sodium concentration can be used as a guide to the replacement of free water by the following formula:

$$\text{Water deficit} = 0.6 \times \text{body weight (kg)} \times (1 - [140/\text{Na}^+])$$

Where Na^+ = plasma sodium, and body weight (kg) = estimated body weight when hydrated.

The treatment of patients with central diabetes insipidus is discussed in Chapter 64.

As is the case in patients with hyponatremia, the rate of correction of hypernatremia is important. In chronic hypernatremia (>36 to 48 hours), the brain generates compounds that raise the intracellular osmolality and thereby minimize cell shrinkage. This process is metabolically driven and is slow to return to normal. Thus, rapid correction of plasma osmolality may lead to a shift of water to the relatively hypertonic intracellular compartment and may result in brain edema. As a general rule, hypernatremia should be corrected over 48 hours at a rate not exceeding 0.5 mEq/L/hr, or 12 mEq/L/day.

Disturbances in Potassium Balance

The human body contains approximately 3500 mEq of potassium. With a normal concentration of 3.5 to 5.0 mEq/L, the ECF contains approximately 70 mEq of potassium, or only 2% of total-body stores. In response to a dietary potassium load, rapid removal of potassium from the extracellular space is necessary to prevent life-threatening hyperkalemia. For example, in the absence of a homeostatic mechanism, if a person ingests 50 mEq of dietary potassium in a single meal (the average daily American diet contains 100 to 120 mEq of potassium per day), the serum potassium might rise to 7 mEq/L (assuming an extracellular volume of 14 L with a baseline serum potassium of 4 mEq/L). Thus, the initial adaptation to a potassium load is the rapid redistribution of potassium from the extracellular space to the intra-

cellular space. Various hormones, including insulin, aldosterone, and catecholamines, cause movement of potassium into cells. The acid-base status of the patient is another determinant of the serum potassium concentration, as potassium moves across cell membranes driven by pH gradients between the cell and the ECF compartments. The greatest effect on the serum potassium concentration is associated with metabolic acidosis involving mineral acids. The cellular permeability to the anions of the mineral acids is low; consequently, the basolateral membrane is hyperpolarized, provoking potassium movement into the blood. By contrast, metabolic acidosis caused by organic acids, such as lactic acid and keto acids, does not cause hyperkalemia. The anions of these acids are relatively permeable and accompany hydrogen into the cell. This situation diminishes the electrochemical gradient favoring potassium efflux.

Although these mechanisms affect the distribution of potassium between the fluid compartments, other mechanisms are necessary to maintain overall potassium balance. People ingest approximately 100 mEq of potassium daily, the bulk of which is eliminated by the kidneys. Increased potassium excretion results from enhanced distal nephron potassium secretion by the principal cells of the connecting tubule and collecting duct into the tubular lumen down an electrochemical gradient. Factors that enhance this gradient promote potassium secretion. These factors include the rate of distal tubular flow, the distal delivery of sodium, the presence of poorly reabsorbable anions in the tubular fluid, and stimulation by aldosterone.

The ratio of extracellular to intracellular potassium establishes the resting membrane potential of the cell. Hence hyperkalemia or hypokalemia is associated with alteration of the resting membrane potential, which accounts for most of the symptoms and findings in these disorders.

DIAGNOSTIC APPROACH

A careful history with emphasis on the patient's diet and use of medications and laxatives should be obtained. Spurious hyperkalemia and hypokalemia must be excluded. In addition to serum electrolytes and magnesium, urine electrolytes and urine osmolality should be obtained. The next step

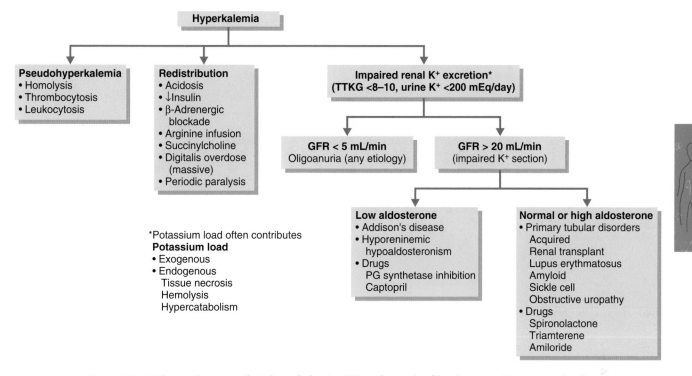

Figure 27–6 Diagnostic approach to hyperkalemia. GFR = glomerular filtration rate; PG = prostaglandin.

should be to determine whether abnormal renal potassium handling is involved in the genesis of the disorder. This state may be determined by measuring the 24-hour urine potassium excretion. In extrarenal hyperkalemia, renal potassium excretion should be more than 200 mEq/day, and if hypokalemia is caused by extrarenal losses, the renal potassium excretion should be less than 20 mEq/day.

HYPERKALEMIA

The ratio of intracellular to extracellular potassium concentration is the major determinant of the resting potential of the cell membrane. As the extracellular potassium concentration increases, the cell membrane is partially depolarized, the sodium permeability is diminished, and the ability to generate action potentials is decreased. In muscle tissue, this change accounts for muscle weakness and paralysis. In the heart, hyperkalemia exhibits as changes in the electrocardiogram. These changes include peaked T waves, decreased amplitude or the absence of P waves, wide QRS complexes, sinus bradycardia, and conduction defects.

A pathophysiologic approach to the causes of hyperkalemia is outlined in Figure 27–6. Vigorous phlebotomy techniques can result in lysis of red blood cells, a process that releases intracellular potassium into the serum sample. Thrombocytosis ($>1 \times 10^6/\mu L$) and leukocytosis ($>60,000/\mu L$) may also be associated with *spurious hyperkalemia*. These disorders can be diagnosed rapidly by determining the plasma and serum concentrations of potassium. True hyperkalemia is present if these values differ by less than or equal to 0.2 mEq/L.

Chronic renal insufficiency does not cause hyperkalemia unless it is advanced, with a GFR ranging from less than 10 to 15 mL/min. Thus, hyperkalemia in chronic renal insufficiency is usually caused by a distal nephron defect in potassium secretion rather than by the impaired GFR, as shown in Figure 27–6. Failure to increase plasma aldosterone by the administration of corticotropin or furosemide confirms the diagnosis of *hyporeninemic hypoaldosteronism*. Prostaglandin deficiency may play a role in the pathogenesis of this disorder. Determination of the urine potassium in response to a single dose of an oral mineralocorticoid (such as 9α-fludrocortisone) may help differentiate hypoaldosteronism from aldosterone resistance. In aldosterone resistance, no increase in urine potassium excretion occurs in response to the mineralocorticoid.

Treatment of hyperkalemia depends on the urgency of clinical findings. When electrocardiogram changes consistent with hyperkalemia are present, the most rapid method of reversing the effects of hyperkalemia is to reestablish the normal membrane potential. Calcium antagonizes the membrane effects of hyperkalemia and can provide rapid protection of the cardiac conduction system. This protection, however, is short lived and must be accompanied by other therapies to decrease the extracellular potassium concentration. The distribution of potassium into the intracellular compartment by administration of sodium bicarbonate, β_2-adrenergic agonists, or insulin rapidly decreases the serum concentration of potassium. The ultimate goal of the treatment is the net removal of potassium from the body. Exchange resins, such as sodium polystyrene sulfonate, can enhance potassium excretion from the gastrointestinal tract. Attempts can be made to enhance renal excretion by improving the distal delivery of sodium with sodium bicarbonate and administration of loop diuretics. Finally, dialysis can be used to remove excess extracellular potassium. For long-

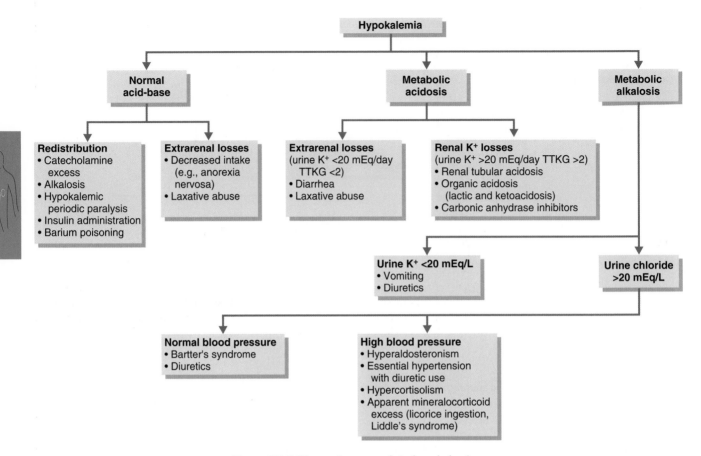

Figure 27–7 Diagnostic approach to hypokalemia.

term management of patients with an aldosterone deficiency, an oral preparation of a mineralocorticoid can be used. Discontinuing any offending drug that may contribute to the patient's hyperkalemia is mandatory.

HYPOKALEMIA

Because potassium is the most abundant intracellular cation, its deficiency results in a wide variety of defects. For example, rhabdomyolysis and adynamic ileus have been associated with hypokalemia. Chronic hypokalemia stimulates thirst and may cause nephrogenic diabetes insipidus. However, the most prominent abnormalities relate to the cardiovascular system. Typically, hypokalemia is associated with flattening of the T waves and development of U waves. The most urgent abnormality is an association with arrhythmias, particularly in patients receiving digitalis. Hypokalemia, through stimulation of renal ammonia synthesis, may worsen hepatic encephalopathy in patients with hepatic cirrhosis.

A diagnostic approach to hypokalemia is outlined in Figure 27–7. As in hyperkalemia, spurious hypokalemia can also occur with leukocytosis (>60,000 cells/μL), resulting from active uptake of potassium by white blood cells from the serum. True hypokalemia is caused by redistribution, extrarenal potassium loss, poor intake, or renal potassium losses. Because only 2% of total-body potassium is distributed in the extracellular compartment, serum potassium

measurements may not accurately reflect the total-body stores. In fact, hypokalemia can occur in the presence of normal total-body potassium stores. This state occurs when potassium shifts from the extracellular space to the intracellular space. Excess circulating catecholamines, insulin administration, and alkalosis are the major causes of redistribution of potassium from the extracellular space to the intracellular space. Redistribution hypokalemia is particularly important in the clinical setting of myocardial infarction and exacerbation of chronic obstructive pulmonary disease. These patients are especially prone to arrhythmias, because excess catecholamines (in response to stress or inhaled β_2-agonists) cause potassium shifts in the setting of total-body potassium depletion from frequent diuretic usage.

In patients with hypokalemia, the acid-base status, the presence or absence of hypertension, and measurement of urinary chloride and potassium are helpful in narrowing the diagnostic possibilities. In patients with diuretic abuse (usually patients with eating disorders), the urine sodium and chloride concentrations are high in the presence of metabolic alkalosis, a profile similar to that of *Bartter's syndrome*, which is a rare genetic defect usually seen in adolescents with other neurologic abnormalities and caused by reduced activity of the sodium, potassium, and chloride (NKCC2) co-transporters in the thick ascending limb (see below). In this setting, a urine screen for diuretics may be necessary to make the diagnosis. In comparison, patients with surreptitious vomiting have a low urinary chloride concentration. Patients who abuse laxatives have low urine sodium and chloride concentrations, with metabolic acidosis or normal acid-base status. Glycyrrhizic acid, the active ingredient in licorice, blocks 11β-dehydrogenase, an enzyme that inactivates glucocorticoids, and its inhibition results in unregulated activation of the mineralocorticoid receptors in the distal nephron.

Determination of serum magnesium should always be performed in a patient with hypokalemia. Hypokalemia that is associated with hypomagnesemia is resistant to therapy unless concomitant magnesium deficiency is corrected.

Given the factors that determine transmembrane potassium shifts, the net potassium deficit may be difficult to calculate. An estimate for a 70-kg man based on the serum concentration is a 100- to 200-mEq deficit in total-body potassium when the serum concentration decreases from 4 to 3 mEq/L. At less than 3 mEq/L, every 1-mEq/L decrease in the serum concentration of potassium reflects an additional 200- to 400-mEq deficit in total-body potassium. Hypokalemia should be treated with oral potassium supplementation. Intravenous potassium administration should only be used in urgent situations, such as in patients with arrhythmias or digitalis toxicity, and intolerance to oral formulations in patients with adynamic ileus. The rate of intravenous potassium administration generally should not exceed 10 mEq/hour; only under electrocardiographic monitoring, the potassium administration rate can be increased up to 20 mEq/hour. Hypokalemia associated with long-term diuretic therapy may be treated with the addition of a potassium-sparing diuretic.

Bartter's and Gitelman's Syndromes

A major advance in the study of inherited disorders of salt wasting syndromes has been the demonstration that Bartter's and Gitelman's syndromes result from mutation of specific ion transport proteins expressed by cells of the distal nephron. The dysfunction of the thiazide-sensitive sodium-chloride co-transporter (NCCT) in Gitelman's syndrome, and the bumetanide-sensitive sodium-potassium-chloride (NKCC2) co-transporter in Bartter's syndrome cause salt wasting, extracellular volume depletion, secondary hyperaldosteronism, and hypokalemia.

The various characteristics of the five different Bartter's syndromes and the Gitelman's syndromes are shown in Tables 27–6 and 27–7. Stated briefly, Bartter's syndrome is a genetically heterogeneous disease. Based on molecular genetic studies, 5 different subtypes of Bartter's syndromes can be distinguished. Type I, or neonatal Bartter's syndrome, is caused by loss of function mutations in the sodium-potassium-chloride co-transporter NKCC2. NKCC2 is encoded by the *SCL12A1* gene on chromosome 15. This sodium-potassium-chloride co-transporter is expressed in the apical cell membranes of the thick ascending limb of the loop of Henle (TAL), and normally accounts for approximately 30% of total reabsorption of sodium filtered by the glomerulus. Patients with this syndrome present early in life with a severe systemic disorder characterized by marked sodium and potassium wasting, polyhydramnios, and significant hypercalciuria and nephrocalcinosis. Prostaglandin synthesis and excretion are significantly increased and may account for much of the systemic symptoms.

Bartter's syndrome type II is due to loss of function mutation of the *KCNJ1* gene on chromosome 11, encoding the inward rectifier voltage-dependent potassium channel ROMK. The potassium channel ROMK is localized in the apical membrane of TAL, but is also expressed in the cortical collecting duct. In the TAL, the potassium flow through this channel into the renal tubule is necessary for NKCC2 activity, which needs adequate luminal potassium supply. In the CCD, this channel is also involved in the excretion of dietary potassium. In this syndrome, an aberrant ROMK channel leads to malfunction of the NKCC2 co-transporter and results in salt wasting, high tubular flow, and distal potassium wasting. Bartter's syndrome type III is caused by

Table 27–6	**Various Bartter's Syndromes**				
	Type 1	**Type 2**	**Type 3**	**Type 4**	**Type 5**
Gene name	*SLC12A1*	*KCNJ1*	*CLCNKB*	*BSND*	*CASR*
Protein name	NKCC2	ROMK	CLCNKB	Barttin	CaR
Major symptoms	Polyuria, hypocalcemia	As for type 1	Variable	As for type 1	—
Seizures	Dehydration	—	Mild to severe	+ Deafness	—
Urine Ca++	↑	↑	↑	↑	↑
Urine Mg++	↓	↓	↓	↓	↓
Nephrocalcinosis	+++	+++	±	—	+++

Ca++ = calcium; Mg++ = magnesium.

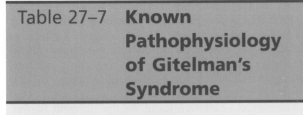

Table 27–7   Known Pathophysiology of Gitelman's Syndrome

Loss of functional mutation: NCCT
NaCl wasting
Secondary hyperaldosteronism: K wasting
Cellular hyperpolarization 2° decreased Cl⁻ entry
  ↑ apical ECaC entry
  ↑ basolateral Na/Ca exchange
  net effect: hypocalciuria
Mg wasting: uncertain mechanism

loss of function mutations of the *CLCNKB* gene on chromosome 1 encoding a chloride channel protein CLC-Kb. This protein is expressed in the basolateral cell membranes of the TAL and is responsible for the reabsorption of sodium chloride in the TAL.

The renal salt wasting in Bartter's type III syndrome is less severe than types I and II. Recently Bartter's syndrome type IV was found to be caused by loss of function mutation of the *BSND* gene (Bartter's Syndrome and Sensori-Neural Deafness) on chromosome 1p31. The BSND gene encodes "barttin," a protein expressed in the basolateral membrane of the TAL. Barttin is the β-subunit of the ClC-Kb chloride channel, and it is necessary for ClCKb delivery to the plasma membrane, and in the cochlea co-localizes with chloride channels ClCKa and ClCKb. These patients present also with sodium, potassium wasting, and impaired cochlear function and deafness. Recently, the presence of hypokalemic alkalosis due to Bartter's syndrome type V was found in patients with autosomal dominant hypocalcemia. In this disease, hypocalcemia was related to gain of function mutation of the calcium-sensing receptor (CaSR). The CaSR is heavily expressed at the basolateral membrane of the TAL, where it is thought to play an important inhibitory role in regulating the transcellular transport of sodium, chloride, and calcium. Activation of the basolateral CaSR in the TAL reduces apical K⁺ channel activity, which induces a Bartter-like syndrome. Genetic activation of the CaSR by these mutations is also expected to increase urinary calcium excretion by inhibiting the generation of the lumen positive potential difference that drives paracellular calcium transport in the TAL.

To date, Gitelman's syndrome appears to be molecularly homogeneous. Although a loss of function mutation of the *SLC12A3* gene in chromosome 16q13 has been identified as one of the causes, recent genetic characterization of Gordon's syndrome, a disease with clinical features opposite to Gitelman's syndrome, suggests the possibility that similar mirror-image mutations and possibly more than one, might account for Gitelman's syndrome. The *SLC12A3* gene encodes the renal thiazide-sensitive sodium-chloride co-transporter NCCT. NCCT is responsible for the sodium reabsorption in the distal tubule, which accounts for approximately 7% of the total filtered sodium. Although Gitelman's syndrome is a milder disorder than Bartter's syndrome,

patients do report significant morbidity related to muscular symptoms, fatigue, and increased risk for cardiac arrhythmias in patients having a prolonged QT interval. Although plasma renin activity is increased, renal prostaglandin excretion is not elevated, another feature that distinguishes Gitelman's syndrome from Bartter's syndrome.

A major phenotypic difference between Bartter's and Gitelman's syndromes involves urinary calcium excretion. The hypercalciuria of Bartter's syndrome is believed to result largely from dysfunction of thick ascending limb cells. Calcium absorption which is passive and paracellular is driven by lumen positive transepithelial voltage, that is generated by NKCC2 co-transport and luminal K⁺ recycling. When NKCC2 co-transport is reduced or blocked by loop diuretics or genetic abnormality, the lumen positivity declines, and calcium reabsorption declines. What is not entirely clear is why the loss of luminal positivity does not lead to increased magnesium excretion. In addition to this mechanism, increased distal delivery of NaCl, as a result of dysfunction of the thick ascending limb raises intracellular chloride concentration which in turns inhibits apical calcium channel of distal convoluted tubule (DCT) cells, further contributing to calcium retention and nephrolithiasis. In contrast to patients with Bartter's syndrome, patients with Gitelman's syndrome invariably demonstrate hypocalciuria.

The hypocalciuria of Gitelman's syndrome resembles the clinical beneficial effects of DCT diuretics (thiazides and others) to reduce urinary calcium excretion. The mechanisms of hypocalciuria in Gitelman's syndrome are well established. First, mild contraction of the ECF volume increases calcium reabsorption along the proximal tubule. Second, reduction in NaCl entry to DCT cells stimulates transepithelial calcium transport. When apical Na and Cl entry into DCT cells is inhibited, because of either diuretic treatment or genetic disease, the intracellular chloride concentration declines. Lower intracellular Cl activity hyperpolarizes the cell, and activates calcium entry via distinctive apical calcium channels ECaC and CaT2, expressed in the DCT cells. Because calcium movement from lumen to cell must be balanced, the increased calcium entry to DCT cells stimulates calcium efflux via the basolateral Na⁺/Ca⁺ exchanger and the Ca-ATPase. Therefore, the resultant effect is the development of hypocalciuria.

Although the pathogenesis of calcium disorders in Bartter's and Gitelman's syndromes is relatively clear, the pathogenesis of magnesium disorders associated with these syndromes is rather confusing. Gitelman's syndrome is associated with severe hypomagnesemia whereas Bartter's syndrome is not. This is surprising because more magnesium is reabsorbed along the loop of Henle than along the distal tubule, and because DCT diuretics induce less magnesium wasting than loop diuretics when given acutely. Recent molecular genetic studies of families affected with a rare autosomal recessive disease termed Renal Hypomagnesemia with Hypercalciuria and Nephrocalcinosis, led to the discovery of several mutations of a human gene Paracellin-1(*PCLN-1*). The protein encoded by this gene is a tight junction protein predominantly localized in both the TAL and the distal convoluted tubule. Mutations of *PCLN-1* cause massive renal magnesium wasting with hypomagnesemia and hypercalciuria resulting in nephrocalcinosis and renal failure.

Therefore, current studies suggest that *PCLN-1* alone, or in partnership with other constituents, forms an intercellular pore permitting paracellular passage of Mg^{2+} and Ca^{2+} down their electrochemical gradients. This conclusion is supported by the location of *PCLN-1* in tight junctions of TAL and DCT, the phenotype of patients with mutations in this gene, and the prior physiologic studies implicating the paracellular pathway of the TAL in Mg^{2+} homeostasis. To date, the mechanisms by which magnesium wasting occurs in patients with Gitelman's syndrome remain unknown.

Disturbances in Acid-Base Balance

Most metabolic processes occurring in the body result in the production of acid. The largest source of endogenous acid production is from the complete catabolism and oxidation of glucose and fatty acids ultimately to carbon dioxide and water. Pulmonary ventilation excretes the volatile acid produced by such cellular respiration, approximately 22,000 mEq of hydrogen daily, as carbon dioxide. Cellular metabolism of sulfur-containing amino acids, the oxidation of phosphoproteins and phospholipids, nucleoprotein degradation, and the incomplete combustion of carbohydrates and fatty acids result in the formation of nonvolatile acids. These processes produce approximately 1 mEq/kg body weight of hydrogen daily. Nonvolatile acid excretion is effected through the kidney. The primary factors regulating alteration in the rate of minute ventilation are changes in cerebrospinal fluid and arterial blood pH.

The normal concentration of hydrogen in arterial blood is 40 mEq/L, equal to a pH of 7.40. This concentration is maintained relatively constant despite variations in the endogenous and exogenous acid inputs. Circulating and intracellular buffers acutely neutralize an acid load. The capacity of these buffering systems is limited, however, and would be quickly depleted by normal endogenous acid production. Mechanisms for excreting acid must therefore be effective to regenerate these buffers to maintain acid-base homeostasis.

RENAL HYDROGEN ION EXCRETION

The kidney contributes to acid-base homeostasis by the reclamation of 4500 mEq of bicarbonate filtered at the glomerulus daily and by the generation of new bicarbonate. This renal bicarbonate generation is given by the equation for net acid excretion (NAE):

$$E_{NAE} = E_{NH_4^+} + E_{TA} - E_{HCO_3^-}$$

Where $E_{NH_4^+} + E_{TA}$ is the rate of ammonium and titratable acid excretion, respectively, and $E_{HCO_3^{-1}}$ is the rate of bicarbonate excretion. Although not difficult, measurement of NAE is not routinely done, and thus analysis of acid base disorders has relied on indirect but more readily available measurements.

The principal process of renal bicarbonate generation is accomplished by urinary acidification and ammonia generation. Ammonia is generated from glutamine and secreted into the tubule fluid by the proximal tubule epithelium.

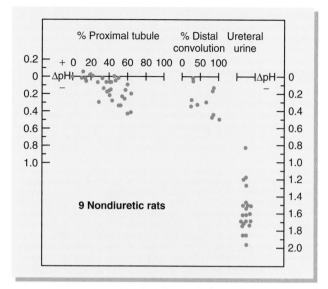

Figure 27–8 pH changes along the rat nephron.

Acidification is accomplished by proton secretion by distinct transporters uniquely distributed along the nephron. These transporters were highlighted in Chapter 25, and here we will discuss how they modify the tubular fluid pH. The acidification profile of tubular fluid is shown in Figure 27–8. Tubule fluid pH falls slightly along the proximal tubule by the operation of the sodium-hydrogen exchanger type 3 (NHE3) located at the luminal membrane. This proton secretion is linked to bicarbonate reabsorption, and nearly 90% of the filtered load of bicarbonate is reabsorbed from the tubule fluid during its course along the proximal tubule. The proximal tubule is a high-capacity bicarbonate reabsorption system whose rate results from the presence of carbonic anhydrase in the luminal membrane. Carbonic anhydrase in the luminal membrane rapidly catalyzes the dehydration of carbonic acid to carbon dioxide and water and thus restricts the fall in tubule fluid pH along the proximal tubule and prevents the development of too steep a pH gradient into which sodium-hydrogen exchange takes place. The distal tubule, on the other hand, lacks a luminal carbonic anhydrase and has a limited capacity to reabsorb bicarbonate. However, given that the bicarbonate concentration reaching these sites is low and the principal buffers in the tubule fluid along these sites are ammonia and phosphate ions, the continued operation of the distal proton pumps lowers the prevailing urinary pH to sometimes a thousand-fold below the pH of the initial filtrate. Along these sites, however, the full operation of the kidney in acid-base homeostasis is observed as the urinary buffers are titrated by secreted protons from pumps distributed along the distal nephron and excreted into the urine.

The rate of bicarbonate generation is not fixed and responds to changes in volume and electrolyte status, hormones, and acid-base parameters. Proximal bicarbonate reabsorption is increased during volume depletion, by elevation in the partial pressure of carbon dioxide (P_{CO_2}), as seen in chronic respiratory acidosis, and by hypokalemia. Conversely, volume expansion or the reduction of the P_{CO_2}

lowers the proximal tubular reabsorptive rate for bicarbonate. Aldosterone and ambient P_{CO_2} affect the rate of distal nephron hydrogen ion secretion.

ASSESSMENT OF ACID-BASE STATUS

A systematic approach to assessing acid-base status consists of several steps, as summarized in Table 27–8. The initial step is to obtain arterial and venous blood samples to measure blood pH and P_{CO_2}, as well as serum electrolytes to

Table 27–8	Systemic Approach to the Analysis of Acid-Base Disorders

Assess the accuracy of the acid-base parameters using the Henderson equation ($H^+ = 24 \times [PaCO_2/HCO_3^-]$) or the Henderson-Hasselbalch equation ($pH = 6.1 + \log[HCO_3^-/0.03 \times PaCO_2]$).

Obtain a good history and perform a complete physical examination, looking for clues to a particular acid-base disturbance.

Calculate the serum anion gap: $Na^+ - (HCO_3^- + Cl^-)$.

Identify the primary acid-base disturbance and assess whether a simple or mixed acid-base disturbance is present.

Examine serum electrolytes and ancillary laboratory data.

Measure urine pH and urine electrolytes, urine urea nitrogen, and glucose to calculate the urine anion gap ($Na^+ + K^+ - Cl^-$) or urine osmolal gap (measured osmolality $- [2(Na^+ + K^+) + [urea nitrogen/2.8] + [glucose/18]]$).[a]

[a]Measurement of urine Na^+ and Cl^- and urine pH should be obtained when metabolic alkalosis is present. Measurement of urine electrolytes, urine glucose, and urine pH should be obtained when an element of normal anion gap metabolic acidosis is present.
Cl^- = chloride; H^+ = hydrogen; HCO_3^- = bicarbonate; K^+ = potassium; Na^+ = sodium; $PaCO_2$ = partial pressure of carbon dioxide in arterial blood.

determine the nature of the acid-base disturbance. Validation of the internal consistency of the calculated and measured bicarbonate should be carried out. Based on the pH, P_{CO_2}, and serum bicarbonate, a minimum diagnosis should be established. Next, a measurement of the compensatory response and the anion gap should be performed. If the compensation of a primary acid-base defect is inappropriate, then a mixed acid-base disorder is considered (Table 27–9). The anion gap is useful in the diagnostic approach to metabolic acidosis. When an organic acid, such as lactic acid, is added to the ECF compartment, the bicarbonate concentration falls as the acid is buffered. The anion gap increases as the organic base is accumulated. Quantitatively, the increase in anion gap should be equivalent to the decrease in bicarbonate concentration. Thus, by adding the difference between the calculated and normal anion gap to the prevailing bicarbonate concentration, an estimate of the *starting* bicarbonate concentration can be made. An abnormally elevated initial bicarbonate concentration indicates concomitant metabolic alkalosis. After establishing the nature of the acid-base disorder and whether it is complex or simple, examination of the urine pH and urine anion or osmolal gap can also provide useful information.

METABOLIC ACIDOSIS

Metabolic acidosis is characterized by a decrease in the serum bicarbonate concentration. This decrease occurs either by excretion of bicarbonate-containing fluids or by utilization of bicarbonate as a buffer of acids. In the latter instance, the nature of the base may affect the electrolyte composition. Thus, considering metabolic acidosis by means of the anion gap is convenient (Table 27–10).

Metabolic acidoses with a normal anion gap is most commonly caused by extrarenal losses of bicarbonate, as occurs in diarrheal diseases, but may also be caused by abnormally high renal excretion of bicarbonate and by the addition of substances yielding hydrochloric acid, as when arginine hydrochloride is administered.

Table 27–9	Nature of Adaptive Response to Primary Acid-Base Disorders	
Primary Acid-Base Disturbance	**Initiating Mechanism**	**Secondary Physiologic Response**
Metabolic acidosis	↓ plasma HCO_3^-	↓ $PaCO_2$ of 1.0–1.3 mm Hg for each mEq/L fall in plasma HCO_3^- $PaCO_2 = (1.5 \times HCO_3^-) + 8 \pm 2$
Metabolic alkalosis	↑ plasma HCO_3^-	↑ $PaCO_2$ of 0.4–0.7 mm Hg for each mEq/L rise in plasma HCO_3^-
Respiratory acidosis	↑ $PaCO_2$	*Acute:* ↑ plasma HCO_3^- of 1.0 mEq/L for every 10-mm Hg rise in $PaCO_2$ *Chronic:* ↑ plasma HCO_3^- of 3.5 mEq/L for every 100-mm Hg fall in $PaCO_2$
Respiratory alkalosis	↓ $PaCO_2$	*Acute:* ↓ plasma HCO_3^- of 2 mEq/L for every 10-mm Hg fall in $PaCO_2$ *Chronic:* ↓ plasma HCO_3^- of 4–5 mEq/L for every 10-mm Hg fall in $PaCO_2$

Note: Rare cases with $PaCO_2$ values greater than 55 mm Hg have been reported.
HCO_3^- = bicarbonate; $PaCO_2$ = partial pressure of carbon dioxide in arterial blood.

Table 27–10   Causes of Metabolic Acidosis

Normal Anion Gap

Bicarbonate losses
Extrarenal
Small bowel drainage
Diarrhea
Renal
Proximal renal tubular acidosis
Carbonic anhydrase inhibitors
Primary hyperparathyroidism
Failure of bicarbonate regeneration
Distal renal tubular acidosis
Aldosterone deficiency
Addison's disease
Hyporeninemic hypoaldosteronism
Aldosterone insensitivity
Interstitial renal disease
Aldosterone antagonists
Ureteroileostomy (ileal bladder)
Acidifying salts
Ammonium chloride
Lysine or arginine hydrochloride
Diabetes mellitus (recovery phase)

Wide Anion Gap

Reduced excretion of acids
Renal failure
Overproduction of acids
Ketoacidosis
Diabetic
Alcoholic
Starvation
Lactic acidosis
Toxin ingestion
Methanol
Ethylene glycol
Salicylates

Modified from Andreoli TE: Disorders of fluid volume, electrolyte, and acid-base balance. In Wyngaarden JB, Smith LH Jr, Bennett JC (eds): Cecil Textbook of Medicine, 19th ed. Philadelphia: WB Saunders, 1992, p 523.

The urinary anion gap is defined as follows:

Urinary anion gap = (sodium + potassium) − chloride

The equation provides an approximate index of urinary ammonium excretion, as measured by a negative urinary anion gap. Thus, a normal renal response would be a negative urinary anion gap, generally in the range of 30 to 50 mEq/L. In such an instance, the acidosis is probably caused by gastrointestinal losses rather than by a renal lesion.

The causes of acidosis characterized by a wide anion gap are listed in Table 27–10. In severe *renal failure,* inorganic compounds such as phosphates and sulfates are the major contributors to the increased anion gap. Organic com-pounds also accumulate in patients with severe renal failure. *Ketoacidosis* results from accelerated lipolysis and ketogene-sis caused by relative or absolute insulin deficiency. Alcoholic ketoacidosis and starvation ketoacidosis result from the suppression of endogenous insulin secretion caused by inadequate carbohydrate ingestion. In addition, in alcoholic ketoacidosis, insulin resistance contributes to ketone forma-tion. The syndrome of *lactic acidosis* results from impaired cellular respiration. Lactate is produced from the reduction of pyruvate in muscle, red blood cells, and other tissues as a consequence of anaerobic glycolysis. In situations of dimin-ished oxidative metabolism, excess lactic acid is produced. This anaerobic state also favors a shift of keto acids to the reduced form, β-hydroxybutyrate. The nitroprusside reac-tion, which is catalyzed by the keto acids acetoacetate and acetone, is thus nonreactive in the setting of lactic acidosis. Lactic acidosis occurs most commonly in disorders charac-terized by inadequate oxygen delivery to tissues, such as shock, septicemia, and profound hypoxemia. Certain toxins may also sufficiently alter mitochondrial function and estab-lish an effective anaerobic state. Some of these toxins may undergo metabolism into organic acids that can contribute to the generation of acidosis characterized by a large anion gap. Methanol is metabolized by alcohol dehydrogenase to formic acid. Ethylene glycol is metabolized to glycolic and oxalic acids. Salicylates are themselves acidic compounds and can cause acidosis characterized by a wide anion gap.

The treatment of metabolic acidosis depends on the underlying cause and the severity of the manifestations. The rapid administration of parenteral sodium bicarbonate is generally indicated when the pH is less than 7.1 and hemo-dynamic instability is evident. Oral bicarbonate supplemen-tation may be sufficient if the acidosis is caused by gastrointestinal bicarbonate loss or renal tubular acidosis (RTA). Treatment of organic acidosis should be directed at the underlying disorder. If the generation of the organic acid can be interrupted, the organic base pair may be metabo-lized, effectively regenerating bicarbonate. The acidemia of diabetic ketoacidosis, for example, can be effectively treated by administration of insulin, thereby inhibiting further keto-genesis. In lactic acidosis, therapy should be directed toward improving tissue perfusion. In alcoholic and starvation ketoacidosis, administration of dextrose-containing intra-venous fluids corrects the acidosis.

RENAL TUBULAR ACIDOSIS SYNDROMES

Currently, three major renal tubular acidosis syndromes have been identified. These syndromes are discussed later, and their principal characteristics are described in Table 27–11.

Proximal Renal Tubular Acidosis Syndromes

Proximal RTA occurs either alone or as the full Fanconi's syndrome, with glycosuria, aminoaciduria, and phospha-turia. In proximal RTA, the threshold is reduced from 25 mM to approximately 18 to 20 mM (Fig. 27–9). Thus, a single-pulse loss of bicarbonate of approximately 850 to 900 mEq takes place.

Proximal RTA occurs in a significant number of systemic diseases, most notably Wilson's disease, cystinosis, and the gammopathies, especially light-chain disease; it is also seen in renal transplantation. Several molecular defects have been identified that also cause proximal RTA:

- Mutations in the carbonic anhydrase II gene, which reduce its expression. It is transmitted as an autosomal-recessive syndrome characterized by osteopetrosis, cerebral calcification, and mental retardation.
- Mutations in the *SCLC4A4b* gene that codes for the basolateral membrane sodium bicarbonate transporter. This lesion is also an autosomal-recessive disease characterized by glaucoma, cataracts, band keratopathy, and psychomotor retardation.

- Mutations in the *SLC9A3* gene, which encodes the luminal NHE3 transport protein.
- Generalized Fanconi's syndrome, which appears to be the consequence of a deficit in adenosine triphosphate (ATP) production in the proximal tubule, which reduces the activity of the basolateral sodium-potassium adenosine triphosphatase (Na$^+$, K$^+$-ATPase). This reduction is seen in severe phosphate depletion, as well as in hereditary fructose intolerance.

The focus of treatment is to enhance proximal bicarbonate reabsorption by reducing ECF volume. This reduction is achieved most commonly by salt restriction. An attempt to raise serum bicarbonate by oral bicarbonate therapy is counterproductive because it raises extracellular volume, enhances bicarbonaturia, provokes kaliuresis and phosphaturia, and produces hypokalemia and hypophosphatemia. Supplemental potassium to correct the hypokalemia is often necessary.

Hyperkalemic Renal Tubular Acidosis Syndromes

This second major group of RTA is theoretically caused by defects in principal cell function and takes three clinical forms. Pseudohypoaldosteronism I is inherited as an autosomal-recessive disease characterized by hyperkalemia, sodium wasting, and failure to thrive. Serum aldosterone is elevated, and the defect is unresponsive to administration of mineralocorticoids. A truncated form of epithelial sodium channel (ENaC) is found with low activity and massive sodium loss and is treated by large amounts of oral sodium. A second form, termed Gordon's syndrome, is characterized

Table 27–11	**Renal Tubular Acidosis Syndromes**	
Type	**Locus**	**Defect**
Proximal	S$_1$–S$_3$	↓ HCO$_3^-$ threshold
Hyperkalemic	CCD principal cell	↓ V$_M$ (–) leading to ↓ H$^+$ secretion
Gradient limited	OMCD intercalated cells	Three specific defects in H$^+$ secretion

CCD = cortical collecting duct; H$^+$ = hydrogen; HCO$_3^-$ = bicarbonate; OMCD = outer medullary collecting duct; S = Segment; V$_M$ (–) = negative transepithelial voltage in the OMCD.

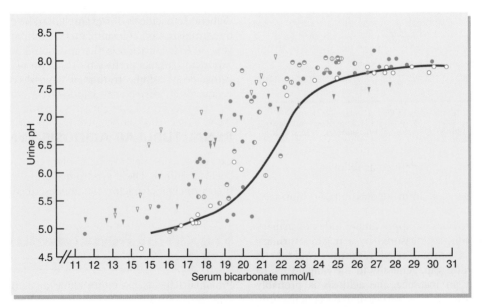

Figure 27–9 Bicarbonate titration curve in proximal RTA. Normal bicarbonate titration is given by the solid line. Note that in patients with proximal RTA, bicarbonate excretion begins to appear in the urine when serum bicarbonate concentration exceeds 16 to 18 mM, whereas in normal individuals, bicarbonate does not appear until serum bicarbonate is above 22 to 24 mM. Below the threshold, patients with proximal RTA can reabsorb filtered bicarbonate nearly completely.

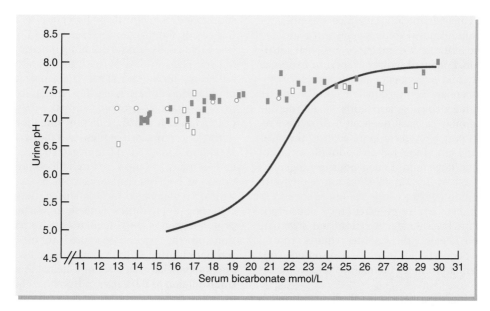

Figure 27–10 Bicarbonate titration curve in gradient-limit RTA. Note the fixed bicarbonate excretion at any level serum bicarbonate. (Compare with Figure 27–9.)

by hyperkalemia and sodium avidity, often accompanied by low renin and mild hypertension. The defect is responsive to loop diuretics and sodium restriction. Indirect assessment of the ability of the collecting duct to generate a steep electrical gradient suggests that an abnormal chloride shunt exists that reduces the negative transepithelial potential generated by sodium reabsorption.

Gordon's syndrome is also responsive to thiazide diuretics, which inhibit the sodium-chloride co-transporter (NCC) in the distal tubule. Recent evidence suggests that this form of hyperkalemic RTA is caused by a loss of function mutation of a newly identified kinase, *WNK-4* (with no lysine), that itself inhibits NCC function. Thus, the activity of the NCC is increased, reducing delivery to the collecting duct, and induces an apparent shunt-induced defect in potassium excretion. Because sodium reabsorption is increased in the distal tubule, hypercalciuria is prominent and nephrocalcinosis occurs.

The third form of hyperkalemic RTA is an acquired disease usually associated with interstitial fibrosis. In this form, serum aldosterone and renin are reduced even in the presence of hyperkalemia. The reason for this defect in aldosterone secretion and responsiveness to administered mineralocorticoids is unknown but suggests defects in principal cell function. The disease responds partially to furosemide and cautious liberalization of salt intake without provoking hypertension.

The third major category of RTA is the so-called gradient-limited form and seems to be caused by a defect in outer medullary collecting duct function. Both principal and intercalated cell transports are defective. This disease is characterized by a fixed defect in bicarbonate excretion without apparent threshold (Fig. 27–10) and a fixed excretion of alkaline urine. Most commonly, the disease is the consequence of an inherited defect in the activity of the hydrogen-ATPase or potassium-hydrogen-ATPase. Acquired damage to

the latter can also occur in autoimmune diseases, most notably Sjögren's syndrome. This damage also occurs in sickle cell disease and primary hyperparathyroidism when these are associated with interstitial kidney damage. Drugs such as amphotericin and lithium may also cause damage. Impaired function of the basolateral band III chloride-bicarbonate exchanger is also thought to explain isolated cases as mutations have been found in the *AEI* gene that codes for it. Multiple mutations in *AEI* gene may also occur and in such cases RTA is associated with ovalocytosis.

In all cases of distal, gradient-limited RTA, hyperchloremic acidosis occurs and is accompanied, because of sodium loss, by secondary hyperaldosteronism, leading to potassium depletion. In children, the syndrome impairs growth, and it may be associated with hypokalemic muscle paralysis, hypercalciuria, and nephrocalcinosis. Therapy consists of bicarbonate replacement, as well as potassium replacement. Particularly in children, large amounts of bicarbonate may be required to ensure normal growth. Distal RTA is also complicated by a low urinary excretion of citrate, which leads to severe nephrocalcinosis.

METABOLIC ALKALOSIS

A gain in base or loss of acid increases the bicarbonate concentration of the ECF. Normally, an elevation of the serum bicarbonate concentration is corrected by excretion of the excess bicarbonate. The maintenance of *metabolic alkalosis* therefore implies a defect in the renal mechanism regulating bicarbonate excretion. This failure to excrete excess bicarbonate occurs by both physiologic responses to volume depletion, especially if hypercapnia and hypokalemia accompany the alkalosis, or by pathophysiologic responses, as occur in autonomous mineralocorticoid excess.

The most common cause of metabolic alkalosis is gastric loss of hydrochloric acid by vomiting or mechanical drainage. Diuretic (thiazide and loop) use is commonly associated with metabolic alkalosis. Volume depletion associated with vomiting and diuretic use enhances proximal bicarbonate reabsorption. Enhanced activity of sodium-hydrogen exchange at this site, and consequent enhanced volume reabsorption, results in enhanced bicarbonate reabsorption (see Chapter 25). Volume depletion also leads to aldosterone secretion, which stimulates distal nephron hydrogen secretion and augments potassium secretion. Repair of the alkalosis under these circumstances requires administration of sodium chloride and potassium. Endogenous or exogenous mineralocorticoid excess (see Fig. 27–7) is unresponsive to volume administration as extracellular volume is expanded. The stimulation of distal hydrogen secretion by aldosterone is sufficient to limit bicarbonate excretion and stimulate potassium secretion. Repair of this disorder requires removal of the excess mineralocorticoid. In all these disorders, concomitant hypokalemia promotes the maintenance of metabolic alkalosis.

Excessive alkali ingestion (e.g., milk-alkali syndrome) is an uncommon cause of metabolic alkalosis and results from impaired renal bicarbonate excretion caused by renal failure in the setting of excess alkali intake. In this instance, both hypercalcemia and vitamin D excess are thought to play roles in damaging the kidney. Removal of alkali often corrects the alkalosis, but renal function remains reduced if nephrocalcinosis is prominent.

The determination of urinary chloride concentrations is helpful in formulating a rational approach to the diagnosis and treatment of metabolic alkalosis. In patients with hypertension since childhood, alkalosis, hypokalemia, and low urinary chloride, consideration should be given to Liddle's syndrome. These features resemble mineralocorticoid excess, but renin and aldosterone levels are suppressed (pseudohypoaldosteronism). The disorder is inherited as an autosomal-recessive disorder with mutations in the ENaC gene that result in deletion of the C-terminal region of the protein. This condition results in reduced degradation and increased density of sodium channels in the luminal membrane of the principal cells of the collecting duct (see Chapter 25). The clinical features are a consequence of the enhanced salt reabsorption, resultant volume expansion, and increased distal nephron potassium and proton secretion.

Patients with high urinary chloride and alkalosis and who are hypertensive require work-up for hypercorticism, which may be autonomous, as in primary aldosteronism and Cushing's disease or secondary to renal artery stenosis. Rarer still are the 11 β-hydroxylase deficiencies, or *apparent mineralocorticoid excess* (AME), in which reduced conversion of glucocorticoids reaching the collecting duct leads to overstimulation of ENaC. Another such syndrome of congenital hypertension and alkalosis is glucocorticoid-remediable aldosteronism (GRA), which is caused by a gene duplication in which the promoter for the 11 β-hydroxylase gene drives the aldosterone synthase gene and leads to adrenocorticotropic hormone–responsive aldosterone synthesis. In each of these instances, hyperactivity of ENaC leads to all clinical features of the syndrome.

Normotensive or hypotensive conditions with alkalosis, hypokalemia, and high urinary chloride consist of two distinct forms: Bartter's syndrome and Gitelman's syndrome. Each syndrome involves distinct abnormalities in segment specific sodium chloride reabsorption, as well as differences in calcium and magnesium excretion. In Bartter's syndrome (see Table 27–6), several disabling mutations in genes affecting the reabsorption of sodium chloride across the thick ascending limb have been characterized, including loss of function mutations in the NKCC2 co-transporter, the *ROMK* channel protein, and the basolateral chloride channel, and a gain in function mutation of the calcium-sensing receptor. Each of these mutations causes salt wasting, including enhanced calcium excretion, volume depletion, and, in many instances, reduced blood pressure. The reduction in ECF volume causes a secondary hyperaldosteronism, which, when coupled with enhanced sodium delivery to the collecting duct, causes potassium wasting and enhanced proton excretion. In Gitelman's syndrome, disabling mutations in the distal convoluted tubule thiazide-sensitive sodium-chloride co-transporter have been described. The phenotypic characteristics of Gitelman's syndrome in contradistinction to Bartter's syndrome are the reduced calcium excretion and hypercalcemia observed, as might be expected from inhibition of the sodium-chloride co-transporter (see Chapter 25). The cause of hypermagnesuria in Gitelman's syndrome is much less certain.

RESPIRATORY ACIDOSIS

Respiratory acidosis occurs with any impairment in the rate of alveolar ventilation. Acute respiratory acidosis occurs with a sudden depression of the medullary respiratory center (narcotic overdose), with paralysis of the respiratory muscles, and with airway obstruction. Chronic respiratory acidosis generally occurs in patients with chronic airway disease (emphysema), with extreme kyphoscoliosis, and with extreme obesity (pickwickian syndrome).

The serum bicarbonate concentration is increased, the magnitude of which depends on the acuity and the severity of the respiratory disorder. The compensatory increase in serum bicarbonate in prolonged hypercapnia (>1 week) is primarily a function of bone buffering as the kidney plays a relatively minor role in the increase. Acute increases in the Pco_2 result in somnolence, confusion, and, ultimately, carbon dioxide narcosis. Asterixis may be present. Because carbon dioxide is a cerebral vasodilator, the blood vessels in the optic fundi are often dilated, engorged, and tortuous. Frank papilledema may be present in patients with severe hypercapnic states.

The only practical therapy of acute respiratory acidosis involves treatment of the underlying disorder and ventilatory support. In patients with chronic hypercapnia who develop an acute increase in the Pco_2, attention should be directed toward identifying the factors that may have aggravated the chronic disorder. Diuretics often exacerbate the increase in serum bicarbonate and result in a mixed disorder of metabolic alkalosis and respiratory acidosis. Under these circumstances, acidification of the serum may be necessary to improve ventilation.

RESPIRATORY ALKALOSIS

Respiratory alkalosis occurs when hyperventilation reduces the arterial Pco_2 and consequently increases the arterial pH. Acute respiratory alkalosis is most commonly a result of pregnancy; it may also occur in damage to the respiratory centers, in acute salicylism, in fever and septic states, in advanced liver disease, and when respiratory rate is increased in pneumonia, pulmonary embolism, and congestive heart failure. The disorder may be produced iatrogenically by injudicious mechanical ventilatory support. Chronic hyperventilation occurs in the acclimatization response to high altitudes cause by reduced ambient partial pressure of oxygen.

Acute hyperventilation is characterized by lightheadedness, paresthesias, circumoral numbness, and tingling of the extremities. Tetany occurs in severe cases. When anxiety provokes hyperventilation, air rebreathing with a paper bag generally terminates the acute attack.

Prospectus for the Future

- Identification of additional gene mutations informative about the renal regulation of water and solute transport

- Design of small molecules to inhibit salt and water transport in specific nephron segments for the treatment of hypertension and edema

References

Andreoli TE: Water: Normal balance, hyponatremia and hypernatremia. Ren Fail 22:711–735, 2000.

Brater DC: Drug-induced electrolyte disorders and use of diuretics. In Kokko JP, Fanner RL (eds): Fluid and Electrolytes, 3rd ed. Philadelphia, WB Saunders, 1996, pp 693–728.

Feldman BJ, Rosenthal MD, Vargas GA, et al: Nephrogenic syndrome of inappropriate antidiuresis. N Engl J Med 352:1884–1890, 2005.

Kokko JP: Fluid and electrolytes. In Goldman L, Bennett JC (eds): Cecil Textbook of Medicine, 21st ed. Philadelphia, WB Saunders, 2000, pp 540–567.

Tannen RL: Dyskalemias. In Massry SG, Glasscock FJ (eds): Textbook of Nephrology, 4th ed. Philadelphia, Lippincott Williams & Wilkins, 2001, pp 295–307.

Chapter 28

Glomerular Diseases

Michelle W. Krause

Patrick D. Walker

Glomerulus

The glomerulus consists of a capillary bed that receives blood from the afferent arteriole and is drained by the efferent arteriole. It contains four different cell types: (1) the visceral epithelial cell (podocyte), (2) the endothelial cell, (3) the mesangial cell, and (4) the parietal epithelial cell (Fig. 28–1). The podocyte and endothelial cells support the glomerular basement membrane (GBM) by means of an extensive trabecular network (**Web Fig. 28–1**). The mesangium provides a skeletal framework for the entire capillary network and, owing to its contractile capability, can control blood flow along the glomerular capillaries in response to a host of mediators. The endothelial cells line the capillary lumen, and the parietal epithelial cells cover the interior of Bowman's capsule.

Clinical Manifestations of Glomerular Disease

Vascularized tissues such as glomeruli respond to injury primarily by acute inflammation, including both humoral and cell-mediated immune mechanisms. The initial manifestations of glomerular disease include urinary abnormalities such as hematuria and proteinuria, as well as nonspecific systemic symptoms such as new-onset hypertension, edema, and malaise.

The glomerular capillaries provide a filtration barrier that prevents the passage of proteins into the urine based on protein size, shape, and electrical charge, resulting in less than 50 mg of protein excreted in the urine per day (**Web Fig. 28–2**). Nephrotic-range proteinuria (>3.5 g/day in adults) represents diffuse glomerular injury with loss of the net negative charge on the capillary wall and/or structural defects in the filtration barrier. The presence of either red blood cell (RBC) casts or dysmorphic RBCs in the urine characterizes glomerular bleeding indicative of a proliferative glomerulonephritis (GN). Occasionally, RBC casts are seen in patients with acute interstitial nephritis. Dysmorphic RBCs are best seen using phase-contrast microscopy and

consist of cells of varying size, shape, and hemoglobin content (**Web Figs. 28–3 and 28–4**).

Renal function at presentation varies in different types of glomerular disease from normal renal function (e.g., minimal change disease) to relentlessly progressive decline (e.g., rapidly progressive glomerulonephritis [RPGN]). Figure 28–2 provides a schematic description of the cardinal mechanisms of glomerular injury.

Approach to the Patient with Glomerular Disease

Glomerular diseases have been classified in numerous ways. Here, these diseases are organized as they relate to the four major glomerular syndromes: (1) acute nephritic syndrome, (2) RPGN, (3) nephrotic syndrome, and (4) asymptomatic urinary abnormalities (Table 28–1). The diagnosis of glomerular diseases is based on pathologic features related to glomerular alterations. Definitions of some of the more commonly used terms are given in Table 28–2.

Acute Nephritic Syndrome

Acute nephritic syndrome is characterized by the abrupt onset of hematuria with RBC casts and/or dysmorphic RBCs, proteinuria (usually non-nephrotic range), and impaired renal function (see **Web Figs. 28–3** and **28–4**). Altered renal function exhibits oliguria, a rise in blood urea nitrogen and creatinine values, and retention of salt and water resulting in hypertension. Acute nephritic syndrome is most commonly caused by proliferative GN, the prototype being poststreptococcal glomerulonephritis (PSGN). Table 28–3 lists the diseases commonly associated with this condition organized by serum complement levels.

PSGN occurs as a postinfectious complication of nephritogenic strains of group A β-hemolytic streptococcal infection. Pharyngitis (strep throat) is followed by PSGN in fewer than 5% of people infected, usually within a 7- to 28-day latent period. Streptococcal pyoderma is less common than

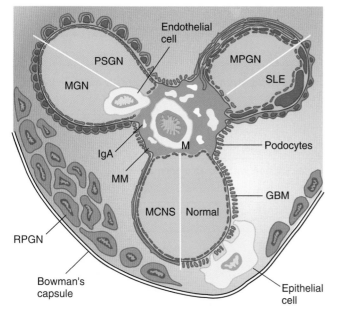

Figure 28–1 Schematic drawing of a glomerulus illustrating the normal features, as well as several diseases. GBM = glomerular basement membrane; IgA = immunoglobulin A deposits in IgA nephropathy; M = mesangial cell; MCNS = minimal change nephrotic syndrome; MN = membranous nephropathy; MM = mesangial matrix; MPGN = membranoproliferative glomerulopathy; PSGN = poststreptococcal glomerulonephritis; RPGN = rapidly progressive glomerulonephritis; SLE = systemic lupus erythematosus.

pharyngitis but leads to PSGN in as many as 50% of infected individuals. PSGN is typically seen in children ages 3 to 12, although it can occur in adults. Both sexes are affected equally. In North America, PSGN occurs frequently in the summer and autumn.

Laboratory findings include RBCs and RBC casts (**Web Figs. 28–5** through **28–10**), white blood cells, and proteinuria on urinalysis; antibodies to streptococcal antigens; a low serum complement (usually returning to normal at 6 to 12 weeks); and abnormal kidney function. Histologically, PSGN is a diffuse proliferative (mesangial and endothelial cells) (**Web Fig. 28–11**) and exudative (neutrophils and monocytes) GN (Fig. 28–3) with coarsely granular capillary loop deposits of immunoglobulin G (IgG) and C3 (see Fig. 28–3) and subepithelial electron-dense humplike deposits (**Web Figs. 28–12 and 28–13**) by electron microscopy.

The differential diagnosis includes other hypocomplementemic causes of the acute nephritic syndrome (Table 28–4), including other postinfectious GNs (e.g., bacterial endocarditis, shunt nephritis), systemic lupus erythematosus (SLE), and membranoproliferative GN (MPGN). Because the diagnosis of PSGN is most often straightforward, a renal biopsy is indicated only if the disease follows an atypical course in children. Most adults with acute nephritic syndrome require a kidney biopsy to establish the diagnosis.

No specific therapy for PSGN has been developed, although antibiotics should be administered if continued streptococcal infection is present. Salt restriction and, in some cases, diuretics and antihypertensive agents may be required to manage hypertension, edema, and congestive heart failure from sodium retention and oliguria. Complete recovery occurs in at least 90% to 95% of all patients. Less than 5% of patients have oliguria for more than 7 to 9 days, and the prognosis in these patients is less favorable. Proteinuria and/or hematuria may continue for 1 to 2 years in some

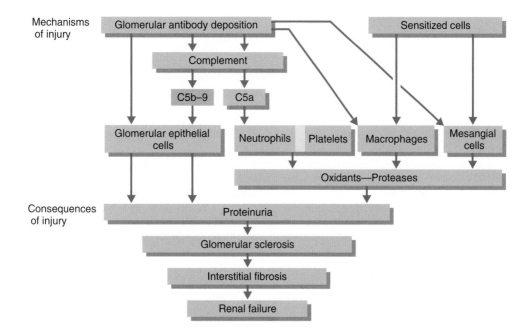

Figure 28–2 Mechanisms of glomerular injury. (From Shah SV: Mechanisms of glomerular injury. Semin Nephrol 11:320–331, 1991.)

Table 28–1   Characteristics of Glomerular Syndromes

Syndrome	Features
Acute nephritic syndrome	Glomerular hematuria (RBC casts and/or dysmorphic RBCs) temporally associated with acute renal failure
Rapidly progressive glomerulonephritis	Glomerular hematuria (RBC casts and/or dysmorphic RBCs) with renal failure developing over weeks to months and diffuse glomerular crescent formation
Nephrotic syndrome	Massive proteinuria (>3.5 g/day/1.73 m^2) with variable edema, hypoalbuminemia, hyperlipidemia, and hyperlipiduria
With "bland" sediment	"Pure" nephrotic syndrome
With "active" sediment	"Mixed" nephrotic/nephritic syndrome
Asymptomatic urinary abnormalities	Isolated proteinuria (usually <2.0 g/day/1.73 m^2) or hematuria (with or without proteinuria)

RBC = red blood cell.

Table 28–2   Pathologic Features of Glomerular Disease

Type of Disease	Feature
Focal	Some (but not all) glomeruli contain the lesion.
Diffuse (global)	Most glomeruli ($>75\%$) contain the lesion.
Segmental	Only a part of the glomerulus is affected by the lesion (most focal lesions are also segmental, e.g., focal segmental glomerulosclerosis).
Proliferation	An increase in cell number resulting from hyperplasia of one or more of the resident glomerular cells with or without inflammatory cell infiltration.
Membrane alterations	Capillary wall thickening caused by deposition of immune deposits or alterations in basement membrane.
Crescent formation	Epithelial cell proliferation and mononuclear cell infiltration in Bowman's space.

patients. Progression to chronic renal failure, although uncommon, is much more likely to occur in adults compared with children.

Nonstreptococcal postinfectious GN may occur after other bacterial infections (e.g., staphylococcal, pneumococcal), viral infections (e.g., mumps, hepatitis B, varicella, coxsackievirus infection, infectious mononucleosis), protozoal infections (e.g., malaria, toxoplasmosis), and a host of others (e.g., schistosomiasis, syphilis). The clinical and histologic manifestations may vary somewhat, depending on the infecting agent. Still, most infections have features similar to those of PSGN and an equally good prognosis if the underlying infection is eradicated.

GN associated with infective endocarditis usually exhibits as a mild form of the acute nephritic syndrome with hematuria and/or proteinuria and a mild decrease in renal function. Endocarditis is now more common in patients with prosthetic valves and in those engaging in intravenous drug abuse rather than patients with rheumatic heart disease. *Staphylococcus aureus* is the most common organism, although a variety of gram-positive and gram-negative organisms may be involved. In patients with infected ventriculoatrial shunts (shunt nephritis), the most common organism is *Staphylococcus epidermitis*. Shunt nephritis usually shows itself as hematuria and proteinuria, with nephrotic-range proteinuria in approximately one fourth of

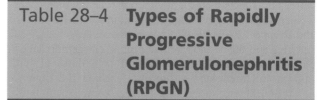

Table 28–3	Differential Diagnosis of Acute Nephritic Syndrome	
Low Serum Complement Level	**Normal Serum Complement Level**	

Low Serum Complement Level	Normal Serum Complement Level
Acute postinfectious glomerulonephritis	Immunoglobulin A nephropathy
Membranoproliferative glomerulonephritis	Idiopathic rapidly progressive glomerulonephritis
Systemic lupus erythematosus	Antiglomerular basement membrane disease
Subacute bacterial endocarditis	Polyarteritis nodosa
Visceral abscess "shunt" nephritis	Wegener's granulomatosis
Cryoglobulinemia	Henoch-Schönlein purpura
	Goodpasture's syndrome

Table 28–4 Types of Rapidly Progressive Glomerulonephritis (RPGN)

Antiglomerular Basement Membrane Antibody-Mediated RPGN (Linear Immunofluorescent Pattern)
Idiopathic antiglomerular basement membrane antibody-mediated RPGN
Goodpasture's syndrome
Associated with other primary glomerular diseases
Membranous nephropathy
Immune Complex–Mediated RPGN (Granular Immunofluorescent Pattern)
Idiopathic immune complex-mediated RPGN
Associated with other primary glomerular diseases
Membranoproliferative glomerulopathy (type II > type I)
Immunoglobulin A nephropathy
Associated with secondary glomerular diseases
Postinfectious glomerulonephritides
Systemic lupus erythematosus
Mixed essential cryoglobulinemia
Henoch-Schönlein purpura
Non–Immune-Mediated RPGN (Negative Immunofluorescent Pattern)
Idiopathic pauci-immune RPGN (ANCA associated)
Vasculitides, including Wegener's granulomatosis and microscopic polyarteritis

ANCA = antineutrophil cytoplasmic antibodies.

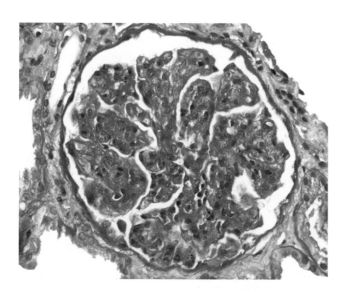

Figure 28–3 Glomerulus showing diffuse proliferation and inflammatory cell infiltration.

the patients. Light microscopy shows a focal proliferative GN. Elimination of infection with appropriate antibiotic therapy is almost always associated with a return of renal function to normal.

GN associated with abscess has been reported in patients with brain, pulmonary, hepatic, retroperitoneal, and other types of abscesses. The presentation is similar to shunt nephritis, and successful antibiotic therapy usually results in normalization of renal function.

SLE, Henoch-Schönlein purpura, and essential mixed cryoglobulinemia (EMC) may present as acute nephritic syndrome but are discussed later in this chapter.

Rapidly Progressive Glomerulonephritis

RPGN is a syndrome characterized by glomerular hematuria (RBC casts and/or dysmorphic RBCs) and renal failure developing over weeks to months associated with diffuse glomerular epithelial cell proliferation in Bowman's space leading to crescent formation evident on renal biopsy (Fig. 28–4). Classification is complicated by the fact that RPGN can occur with immune deposits (either anti-GBM or immune-complex type) or without immune deposits. In addition, RPGN can be an idiopathic primary glomerular disease, or it can be superimposed on other glomerular diseases. The classification scheme used here is based on the immunofluorescence information obtained from renal biopsy (see Table 28–4).

Anti-GBM GN, characterized by linear capillary loop staining with IgG and C3 (Fig. 28–5) and extensive crescent formation, accounts for 10% to 20% of all cases of RPGN. Approximately two thirds of these patients have Goodpasture's syndrome (RPGN associated with pulmonary hemorrhage). The pathogenesis of anti-GBM GN appears to be linked to the development of autoimmunity to the noncollagenous domain of the α3 chain of type IV collagen. Anti-GBM GN occurs in two peaks, the first in the third and fourth decades and the second in the sixth and seventh decades. Goodpasture's syndrome is more common in the young and affects men slightly more frequently than it does women, usually exhibiting RPGN along with hemoptysis and dyspnea. A strong association exists between cigarette smoking and the development of pulmonary hemorrhage in patients with anti-GBM GN. Laboratory findings, in addition to impaired kidney function, include the presence of anti-GBM antibodies and normal complement levels. Therapy consists of high-dose oral prednisone, cytotoxic agents such as cyclophosphamide, and plasma exchange. A high index of suspicion resulting in earlier diagnosis and vigorous treatment has increased survival to more than 50%, as compared with 10% to 15% survival 20 years ago.

Immune-complex RPGN is almost always associated with another underlying disease, and the correct diagnosis can usually be made by seeking the other clinical and laboratory features of these conditions (see Table 28–4). Approximately 30% of all cases of RPGN are of this type (granular deposits of immunoglobulins and complement).

Pauci-immune RPGN is found in approximately 50% of patients with crescentic GN and is seen in association with small-vessel vasculitides such as microscopic polyangiitis or Wegener's granulomatosis (**Web Fig. 28–14**). An idiopathic form is also thought to represent a vasculitis limited to glomeruli. Antineutrophil cytoplasmic antibodies (ANCA) are found in 80% to 85% of patients with pauci-immune GN and is thought to be pathogenic in the endothelial cell injury. Two forms of ANCA antibodies have been developed: myeloperoxidase ANCA, termed MPO-ANCA; and proteinase 3-ANCA, termed PR3-ANCA. Both antibodies are studied using enzyme-linked immunoabsorbent assays (ELISAs). MPO-ANCA is generally in a perinuclear pattern (p-ANCA), while PR3-ANCA is generally cytoplasmic in distribution (c-ANCA) based on immunofluorescent studies (**Web Fig. 28–15**). The majority of MPO-ANCA antibodies are also p-ANCA positive, whereas PR3-ANCA antibodies are predominately c-ANCA positive. Cytotoxic agents and corticosteroids have been successful in the initial treatment of pauci-immune RPGN. Approximately 20% to 30% of individuals will experience a relapse of the disease, and maintenance therapy with azathioprine or mycophenolate mofetil has been suggested, although the duration of treatment has not been resolved.

Nephrotic Syndrome

Nephrotic syndrome is characterized by the presence of proteinuria, hypoalbuminemia, edema, hyperlipiduria, and hyperlipidemia. However, the finding of proteinuria of more than $3.5 \, g/24 \, hr/1.73 \, m^2$, so-called nephrotic-range proteinuria, is sufficient for the designation of nephrotic syndrome. Table 28–5 includes the renal lesions commonly associated with the nephrotic syndrome. These lesions are divided into

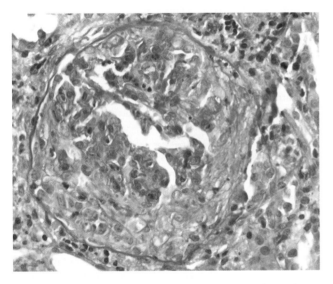

Figure 28–4 Glomerulus demonstrating crescent formation.

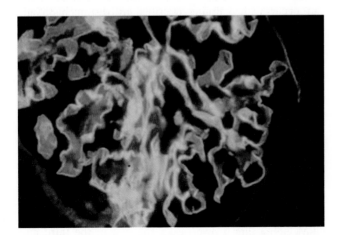

Figure 28–5 Immunofluorescence demonstrating a linear pattern of immunoglobulin G.

Table 28–5	**Glomerulopathies Associated with Nephrotic Syndrome**

Nephrotic-Range Proteinuria with "Bland" Urine Sediment (Pure Nephrotic)
Primary glomerular disease
Minimal change nephrotic syndrome (nil lesion, lipoid nephrosis)
Membranous nephropathy
Focal segmental glomerulosclerosis
Secondary glomerular disease
Diabetic nephropathy (Kimmelstiel-Wilson glomerulosclerosis)
Amyloidosis
Nephrotic-Range Proteinuria with "Active" Urine Sediment ("Mixed" Nephrotic/Nephritic)
Primary glomerular disease
Membranoproliferative glomerulopathy, types I, II, and III
Secondary glomerular disease
Membranoproliferative glomerulopathy
Systemic lupus erythematosus
Henoch-Schönlein purpura
Mixed essential cryoglobulinemia

diseases with "active" versus "bland" urine sediment (i.e., with or without RBC casts) (see **Web Figs. 28–3**, **28–4**, and **28–5**). Each of these entities may occur as a primary renal lesion or secondary to a systemic disease.

Nephrotic Syndrome with "Bland" Urine Sediment

MINIMAL CHANGE NEPHROTIC SYNDROME (NIL DISEASE)

Minimal change nephrotic syndrome (MCNS) is also known as nil lesion or lipoid nephrosis; 85% to 90% of all children with nephrotic syndrome have MCNS. The condition usually exhibits the sudden onset of the nephrotic syndrome in children ages 2 to 8 years, with a male-to-female ratio of 2 : 1. In adults, MCNS accounts for 15% to 20% of patients with idiopathic nephrotic syndrome, with a more equal male-to-female ratio. As children approach the teenage years and early adulthood, the incidence of MCNS as a cause of nephrotic syndrome diminishes. In adults, the association of MCNS with nonsteroidal anti-inflammatory agents (see Chapter 29) and Hodgkin's disease must be kept in mind.

Laboratory features of MCNS usually include those of nephrotic syndrome, with bland urinary sediment, normal renal function, and normal complement levels. Histologically, light microscopy is normal (hence the term *nil disease*), no immunoglobulin or complement deposition is seen, and effacement of the foot processes is observed (**Web Figs. 28–16, 28–17**).

MCNS is extremely responsive (90% to 95%) to corticosteroids. In children, prednisone at 60 mg/m^2/day (up to a maximum of 80 mg/day) for 4 to 6 weeks and then 40 mg/m^2/day every other day for 4 to 6 weeks is recommended. The time to clinical response may be slower in adults compared with children, and adults should not be considered steroid resistant until they fail to respond to 16 weeks of treatment. Following remission, as many as 75% of patients have one or more relapses. The first relapse is treated similarly to the initial episode. Patients who have three or more relapses, or those who become corticosteroid dependent, are generally treated with an 8-week course of an alkylating agent, chlorambucil (0.1 to 0.2 mg/kg/day), or cyclophosphamide (2.0 mg/kg/day). Recent studies indicate that cyclosporine therapy is of value in select patients and may induce remissions more often in corticosteroid-dependent patients and less often in corticosteroid-resistant patients. Approximately three fourths of individuals are disease free at 10 years, with a 10-year survival rate of 95%.

FOCAL SEGMENTAL GLOMERULOSCLEROSIS

Focal segmental glomerulosclerosis (FSGS) accounts for 10% to 15% of nephrotic syndrome in children and is now the most common cause of nephrotic syndrome in adults (Table 28–6). Although heavy proteinuria and edema are usually present at onset, some patients have asymptomatic proteinuria and hematuria. Hypertension, impaired kidney function, and microscopic hematuria are commonly found at the time of diagnosis. Serum complement levels are normal. Recently, a glomerular permeability factor present

Table 28–6	**Features of Focal Segmental Glomerulosclerosis**

Etiology
  Primary
    Idiopathic
  Secondary
    Hypertension
    Obesity
    Sickle cell disease
    Heroin
    Acquired immunodeficiency syndrome (AIDS)
    Reflux nephropathy
    Medications

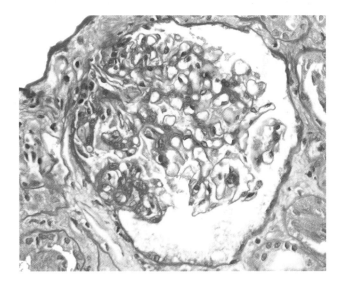

Figure 28–6 Glomerulus demonstrating a focus of sclerosis and hyalinosis.

in the blood has been implicated in the proteinuria in some patients with FSGS. FSGS is classified into distinct histologic variants based on the location of sclerosis on light microscopy on renal biopsy. The most common sclerotic lesion is located in the perihilar area of the glomerulus (Fig. 28–6) with glomerular tip variant (**Web Fig. 28–18**), collapsing glomerulopathy (**Web Fig. 28–19**), cellular variant, and those not otherwise specified occurring less frequently. Heroin users and patients with acquired immune deficiency syndrome may develop the nephrotic syndrome associated with the histologic lesion of collapsing glomerulopathy. Collapsing glomerulopathy has an African-American predominance and is typically associated with massive proteinuria and advanced kidney failure at the time of diagnosis. These patients typically follow a more rapid downhill course, often with progression to end-stage renal failure in less than 1 year.

Approximately one third of patients respond to corticosteroid therapy with a lasting remission and good long-term

Table 28–7	**Features of Membranous Nephropathy**

Nephrotic-range proteinuria with "bland" urinary sediment
Glomerular basement membrane thickening with "spike" formation, granular deposits of IgG and complement, and subepithelial electron-dense deposits
Etiology
  Idiopathic
  Secondary
    Infections: hepatitis B, syphilis
    Neoplasms: carcinomas of the lung, stomach, and breast
    Drugs: gold, D-penicillamine, captopril
    Collagen vascular diseases: systemic lupus erythematosus, mixed connective tissue disease

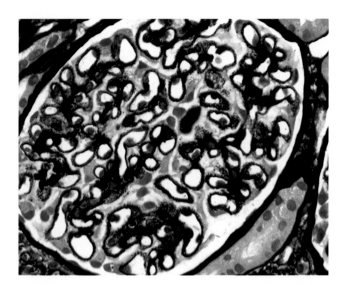

Figure 28–7 Membranous glomerulopathy showing "spikes" on capillary loops.

renal function. However, most patients, particularly those with persistent nephrotic syndrome, progress to chronic renal failure (50% to 55% by 10 years). Approximately 10% to 15% of patients follow a long-term course with relapses and remissions and late onset of renal failure. Secondary causes of FSGS are generally resistant to immunosuppressive treatment, and control of hypertension and reduction in proteinuria with angiotensin blockade is recommended. Recurrence of FSGS in transplants occurs in 40% to 50% of patients.

MEMBRANOUS NEPHROPATHY

Membranous nephropathy (MN) accounts for 25% to 30% of nephrotic syndrome in adults, with peak occurrence in the fourth and fifth decades. MN is primary in 80% to 85% of patients. In patients older than 60 years, MN is an indicator of an underlying malignancy in 10% to 15% of cases. Other secondary causes include SLE and hepatitis, with hepatitis B much more commonly associated with MN than is hepatitis C (Table 28–7). Microscopic hematuria without RBC casts is present in approximately 50% of the patients. Light microscopy reveals thickening of capillary loops with basement membrane "spike" formation on silver stain (Fig. 28–7). Cellular proliferation is absent. Immunofluorescence studies are generally positive for IgG and C3 in a granular pattern within the loops (**Web Fig. 28–20**). Electron microscopy shows subepithelial electron-dense deposits with basement membrane extensions adjacent to the deposits with complete effacement of foot processes (**Web Fig. 28–21**).

The *rule of thirds* applies to MN, with spontaneous remission in up to one third of patients, another third continuing to have proteinuria but stable renal function, and a third progressing to end-stage renal failure at 5 to 10 years. This prevalence has remained unchanged over the last 3 decades in spite of earlier recognition, better control of hypertension, and use of proteinuria-decreasing agents. Treatment of MN is controversial. Meta-analysis of multiple large prospective studies indicates that no justification exists for the use of corticosteroids alone as primary therapy. In addition, sponta-

neous partial or complete remission in up to 40% of patients does not justify the routine use of cytotoxic therapy for all patients with MN. Cytotoxic therapy should therefore be offered to patients who are at high risk of progression based on clinical factors such as age, male gender, renal function, persistence of nephrotic syndrome, or histologic presence of tubulointerstitial damage. In these patients, either chlorambucil or cyclophosphamide along with oral steroids is currently recommended. Some evidence from a recent meta-analysis suggests the beneficial effects from cytotoxic agents in progressive idiopathic MN.

DIABETIC NEPHROPATHY

Diabetic nephropathy is the single most important cause of end-stage renal disease (ESRD) in the United States, accounting for approximately 40% of all patients with ESRD, and is rising exponentially. The cumulative incidence of nephropathy is 30% to 50% in type 1 diabetes and approximately 20% in type 2 diabetes, although certain populations of patients with type 2 diabetes (e.g., Pima Indians) have a higher incidence of nephropathy. More than one half of patients with ESRD secondary to diabetes have type 2 diabetes.

Diabetic nephropathy is a clinical syndrome characterized by persistent albuminuria (>300 mg/24 hr), a relentless decline in GFR, and hypertension. Nephropathy is rare during the first 5 years of diabetes, increasing to a peak at 15 to 20 years after the onset of disease. Microalbuminuria (30–300 mg/day) strongly predicts the development of diabetic nephropathy and is associated with increased cardiovascular mortality. After the onset of microalbuminuria, macroalbuminuria or overt nephropathy (>300 mg/day) almost inevitably develops during the next 5 years associated with a significant risk for the development or worsening of hypertension and progressive decline in renal function. Fifty percent of patients have ESRD 7 to 10 years after the onset of proteinuria. The rate at which patients with proteinuria progress is highly variable, but if nephropathy is untreated,

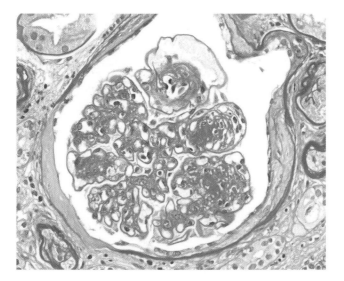

Figure 28–8 Glomerulus with diffuse mesangial matrix increase and aneurysmal dilation of capillary loops typical of diabetic nephropathy.

the GFR decreases by 1 mL/min/month. A high percentage of patients with type 2 diabetes (in contrast to type 1 diabetes) have modest proteinuria and hypertension when initially examined, indicating that other diseases may be responsible for the renal damage. Diabetic retinopathy is found in more than 90% of patients with type 1 diabetes, whereas nearly one third of patients with type 2 diabetes and diabetic nephropathy have no evidence of retinopathy. Regardless, the absence of retinopathy and/or renal insufficiency without proteinuria, the presence of RBC casts, and/or the low levels of complement should lead to a search for other causes of renal disease.

The Kimmelstiel-Wilson nodule described as the classic diabetic glomerular lesion is found in only 15% to 20% of patients with diabetic nephropathy. The more common lesion is that of diffuse glomerulosclerosis, with a uniform increase in mesangial matrix (Fig. 28–8). Hyaline arteriolosclerosis involving both afferent and efferent arterioles, as well as tubulointerstitial atrophy and fibrosis, accompanies both the nodular and the diffuse forms of diabetic glomerulosclerosis.

Although no cure for diabetic nephropathy exists, treatment interventions include vigorous control of blood sugar, antihypertensive treatment with angiotensin blockade to a goal blood pressure of less than 130/80 mm Hg, and restriction of dietary proteins to slow the progressive loss of the GFR. Angiotensin II receptor blockers in diabetic nephropathy have shown a significant decrease in the progressive loss of kidney function above and beyond that expected by antihypertensive effects alone and should be used in all patients, unless significant side effects such as angioedema, uncontrollable hyperkalemia, or acute renal failure preclude their use.

DYSPROTEINEMIAS AND AMYLOIDOSIS

Multiple myeloma (see Chapter 50), the most common dysproteinemia, is associated with light chain cast nephropathy (LCCN), previously called myeloma kidney, monoclonal immunoglobulin deposition disease (MIDD), and amyloidosis. LCCN and light chain deposition disease (LCDD) occur together 10% to 15% of the time, whereas amyloidosis usually occurs alone. As many 50% of patients with multiple myeloma have renal insufficiency at presentation.

Patients with LCCN usually exhibit proteinuria and renal insufficiency and may rapidly progress to ESRD despite stable paraprotein production and excretion. LCCN is characterized by large, often fractured distal tubular casts surrounded by multinucleated giant cells. The casts are composed primarily of light chains and Tamm-Horsfall protein.

MIDD includes LCDD, mixed light and heavy chain disease, and heavy chain disease. MIDD is a monoclonal gammopathy characterized by deposition of immunoglobulins in the kidney and other vital organs (liver, heart, and peripheral nerves). Monoclonal light chains predominate, with LCDD accounting for 85% to 90% of all cases of MIDD. Proteinuria is present in 85% to 90% at presentation. Most patients also exhibit renal insufficiency, and rapid progression to renal failure is the usual course. MIDD is secondary to myeloma in 50% to 60% of cases, with the other 40% to 50% having either normal bone marrow or slight plasmacytosis and minimal or no paraproteinemia. The characteristic light microscopic finding is nodular glomerulosclerosis similar to diabetic nodular sclerosis. LCDD is confirmed by linear deposits of monoclonal light chains ($\kappa : \lambda$ in a ratio of 4:1) along glomerular and tubular basement membranes.

Systemic amyloidosis is classified into four types according to the chemical composition of fibrillar deposits, which correspond to clinical patterns, termed *primary, secondary, hereditary,* and *dialysis-associated amyloidosis.* The most common form in the United States is primary amyloidosis, which is derived from light chains. Secondary amyloidosis, which develops after chronic inflammatory or infectious disease, is composed of AA proteins (see Chapter 89). Several autosomal-dominant hereditary forms have been found, of which the most well known is familial amyloidotic polyneuropathy with amyloid derived from transthyretin. The fourth form occurs in patients with chronic hemodialysis, and the amyloid fibril is a β_2-microglobulin. Up to 80% of patients with amyloidosis or AA forms of amyloidosis have renal involvement. Nephrotic syndrome is the initial feature in 80% to 85% of patients with secondary amyloidosis and in approximately 15% to 20% of patients with primary amyloidosis and is rare in familial amyloidosis. Renal insufficiency is present in 40% to 50% at diagnosis. The median survival period is approximately 2 years, with cardiac failure the most common cause of death.

No reliable biochemical tests exist for diagnosis, and definitive diagnosis must be made by tissue biopsy. Fine-needle aspirate of abdominal fat is often positive for amyloid in patients with primary or secondary amyloidosis but only rarely in patients with dialysis-associated amyloidosis. However, a kidney biopsy is commonly needed to make a definitive diagnosis and to rule out other diseases. By light microscopy, amyloid is Congo-red positive and apple-green bi-refringent, and it is fibrillar by electron microscopy (Fig. 28–9). No specific treatment for amyloidosis has been developed. In patients with primary amyloidosis and multiple myeloma, treatment of the myeloma may slow the

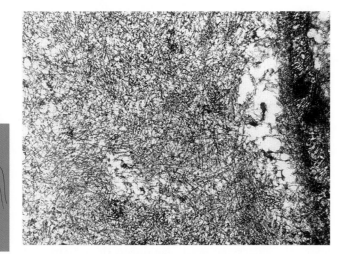

Figure 28–9 Electron micrograph demonstrating the nonbranching fibrils characteristic of amyloidosis.

Table 28–8	Features of Membranopro-liferative Glomerulopathy

Nephrotic-range proteinuria with "active" urinary sediment
Idiopathic
Type I: Mesangial hypercellularity and capillary loop "splitting"
Type II: Mesangial hypercellularity with glomerular basement membrane "dense deposits"
Type III: Morphologic variants
Type I changes plus subepithelial deposits
Changes intermediate between type I and type II
Associated with other diseases (secondary)
Hepatitis C and B
Systemic lupus erythematosus
Mixed essential cryoglobulinemia
Sickle cell disease
Partial lipodystrophy (type II)

progression of amyloidosis. Treatment of AA amyloid is also focused on correction of the underlying inflammatory disease. Colchicine is used in patients with amyloidosis secondary to familial Mediterranean fever.

Nephrotic Syndrome with "Active" Urine Sediment

Patients usually exhibit the manifestations of the nephrotic syndrome and are found to have microscopic hematuria with dysmorphic red cells with or without RBC casts. Occasionally, the primary presenting complaints are related to the acute nephritic syndrome, and the patient is found to have nephrotic-range proteinuria. A variety of glomerular diseases must be considered, including MPGN, lupus nephritis, Henoch-Schönlein purpura, and essential mixed cryoglobulinemia.

MEMBRANOPROLIFERATIVE GLOMERULONEPHRITIS

MPGN may be idiopathic or associated with a significant number of other diseases (Table 28–8). Idiopathic MPGN is a disease of young persons, with most cases diagnosed in those between the ages of 5 and 30 years. Overall, MPGN accounts for 10% to 15% of all cases of idiopathic nephrotic syndrome. The clinical manifestations are variable, with approximately 50% having nephrotic syndrome, 25% to 30% with asymptomatic proteinuria, and 15% to 20% with acute nephritic syndrome. Concurrent hematuria and proteinuria are almost always present. Serum C3 levels are depressed in more than 70% of patients at disease onset and in almost all patients at some point in their disease (see Table 28–3). The presence of C3 nephritic factor is most likely an associated event rather than a cause of MPGN, and its presence does not appear to alter the prognosis.

MPGN is characterized by capillary loop thickening with basement membrane duplication and mesangial hypercellularity, often with lobular accentuation. Several subtypes exist. Type I MPGN has subendothelial deposits with double-contoured basement membranes (**Web Fig. 28–22**). Complement components with or without immunoglobulins are found in a granular pattern along capillary loops alone or with mesangial involvement (**Web Fig. 28–23**). Type II MPGN (dense deposit disease) shows sweeping replacement of whole segments of the GBM by highly electron-dense material, causing a marked widening of the GBM. Immunofluorescence reveals linear C3 deposition in the capillary loops sometimes associated with mesangial "ring" deposits.

MPGN is a slow but progressive disease, with approximately 50% to 60% of patients in chronic renal failure at the end of 10 years. Poor prognostic indicators include the presence of nephrotic syndrome, hypertension, azotemia, tubulointerstitial disease, and/or crescents at the time of diagnosis. Spontaneous remission of proteinuria rarely occurs but does not usually affect the long-term outcome. No therapeutic regimen that is considered effective in treating MPGN currently exists. Type II MPGN recurs in virtually 100% of renal transplants, but recurrence is far less common in type I MPGN (approximately 25%). Recurrence rarely alters long-term outcome, though this may change as graft survival increases.

ESSENTIAL MIXED CRYOGLOBULINEMIA

Mixed cryoglobulins are composed of monoclonal IgM rheumatoid factor and polyclonal IgG and produce EMC. EMC occurs usually in middle age, affecting women slightly more than it does men, and presents as purpura, fever, Raynaud's phenomenon, arthralgias, and weakness. Renal manifestations are seen in 40% to 50% of patients and vary from proteinuria and/or hematuria to the acute nephritic syndrome. Many patients are hypocomplementemic, with a decrease in early complement components such as C4 and normal levels of C3 (see Table 28–3). Thus, the presence of

Table 28–9	**Histologic Classification of Lupus Nephritis**
Class I	Minimal mesangial lupus nephritis
Class II	Mesangial proliferative lupus nephritis
Class III	Focal lupus nephritis involving <50% of glomeruli
Class IV	Diffuse segmental lupus nephritis involving >50% of glomeruli
Class V	Membranous lupus nephritis
Class VI	Advanced sclerosing glomerulonephritis

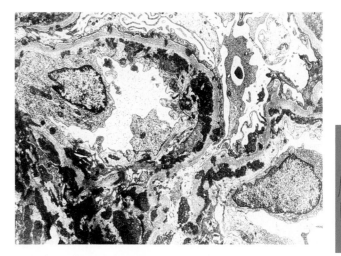

Figure 28–10 Electron micrograph from a patient with SLE with massive subendothelial deposits, a few subepithelial deposits, and mesangial deposits.

palpable purpura in a patient with proteinuria and hematuria, with high titers of rheumatoid factor with or without low levels of C4, is highly suggestive of EMC. MPGN with intraluminal hyaline thrombi is characteristic of EMC. IgG, IgM, and C3 are usually present in subendothelial areas, the mesangium, and the thrombi (**Web Fig. 28–24**).

Approximately 50% of patients with EMC have chronic hepatitis C. Antihepatitis C viral antibody, hepatitis C viral core antigens, and hepatitis C RNA can be found in the cryoglobulins and in the renal deposits. Treatment of the hepatitis C with antiviral therapy can also positively affect the glomerular lesions. The overall survival rate in patients with renal manifestations is approximately 75%. However, patients with renal insufficiency or acute nephritic syndrome usually progress to ESRD. Plasmapheresis to decrease the circulating cryoprecipitates and use of cytotoxic agents may improve the prognosis of patients with severe renal disease. Nonetheless, relapses are common after stopping treatment.

SYSTEMIC LUPUS ERYTHEMATOSUS GLOMERULONEPHRITIS

SLE is primarily a disease of young women, although it may occur in both sexes at any age (see Chapter 80). SLE accounts for 5% to 10% of patients with nephrotic syndrome, and it can be the presenting manifestation of a patient with SLE without any other systemic manifestations. Lupus nephritis is in the differential of hypocomplementemic glomerulonephritis exhibiting as any of the glomerular disease syndromes (see Table 28–3). Diagnosis rests on serologic evidence of antinuclear antibody production in the presence of inflammation of multiple organs. Clinical evidence of renal disease is present in as many as 85% to 90% of patients with SLE, varying from minimal changes to crescentic glomerulonephritis. Virtually all patients are found to have renal injury if a kidney biopsy is performed. The nephrotic syndrome with an active sediment is most common, and 10% to 15% of patients also have impaired kidney function. Serum complement levels are usually low during periods of active renal disease. A small number of patients have RPGN.

The clinical presentation and the severity of renal disease correlate with the underlying histopathologic condition, best classified using the new classification of lupus nephritis in 2003 from the International Society of Nephrology and the Renal Pathology Society (Table 28–9). Essentially, these categories can be grouped as proliferative (types II, III, and IV) or membranous (type V) glomerulopathies, with greater proliferation associated with a poorer prognosis. Multiple immunoglobulins and various components of complement are almost invariably present within the glomeruli and may involve all levels of the GBM, as well as the mesangium (Fig. 28–10). Some studies have suggested that the presence and amount of subendothelial deposits seen by electron microscopy are good predictors of progression.

Treatment strategies are aimed at disease severity based on histologic classification. In general, patients with class I and II disease do not need treatment directed at the renal lesions. Patients with class III glomerular lesions are managed with the lowest possible dose of corticosteroids and observed carefully for the development of more diffuse renal disease. Several long-range studies of patients with diffuse segmental proliferative GN (class IV) have suggested that the addition of cytotoxic drugs to a regimen of prednisone may offer better long-term preservation of renal function. The outlook for patients even with class IV lupus nephritis has improved enormously over the last 25 years, with renal survival now as high as 85% to 90% at 10 years.

Patients with SLE tolerate dialysis about as well as do patients with non-SLE renal failure. Indeed, for reasons that are not yet understood, patients with SLE who are placed on chronic dialysis often note dramatic amelioration of other manifestations of SLE. Renal transplantation is also well tolerated, with recurrence of SLE GN being relatively rare.

HENOCH-SCHÖNLEIN PURPURA

Henoch-Schönlein purpura (HSP) is seen most often in children (boys more than girls) and is characterized by purpuric lesions on the buttocks and legs, episodic abdominal pain, arthralgias, fever, malaise, and proteinuria (often nephrotic range) with hematuria and RBC casts. Serum C3 levels are not decreased.

The glomeruli show varying degrees of mesangial hypercellularity, with the prognosis declining as the proliferation increases. Uncommonly, exuberant crescent formation

Table 28–10	Asymptomatic Urinary Abnormalities

Isolated Proteinuria

Proteinuria without hematuria
Postural proteinuria

Isolated Hematuria (with or without Proteinuria)

Immunoglobulin A nephropathy (Berger's disease)
Hereditary nephritis
Alport's syndrome
Thin basement membrane disease
Benign recurrent hematuria

occurs associated with a rapid progression to renal failure. IgA and C3 staining of the mesangium are prominent, with numerous mesangial electron-dense deposits seen by electron microscopy. Both lesional skin and nonlesional skin show IgA and C3 in dermal capillaries, with linear IgA at the dermal-epidermal junction in 15% to 20% of cases.

HSP tends toward a benign, self-limited course of remission and relapse, usually disappearing after a few months to years. More than one half of the patients recover completely from their renal injury, but approximately 10% progress to ESRD. Persistent nephrotic syndrome, acute nephritic syndrome at onset, and older age suggest a poorer prognosis. An association has been found in adults of HSP with underlying lung or gastrointestinal malignancies. Therapy is unproved for the renal manifestations of HSP, although patients with extensive crescent formation should be managed aggressively. Recurrence is uncommon in renal transplants.

ASYMPTOMATIC URINARY ABNORMALITIES

A variety of renal lesions may exhibit as either isolated proteinuria or hematuria, with or without proteinuria (Table 28–10). Isolated proteinuria without hematuria is usually an incidental finding in a patient who is asymptomatic. These patients generally excrete less than 2 g of protein per day with and without cellular elements in the urine and have normal renal function. Approximately 60% of these patients have postural, or orthostatic, proteinuria, with an absence of proteinuria while lying flat and a return of proteinuria on standing. The long-term outcome of isolated proteinuria (postural or nonpostural) is excellent, with the majority of patients showing steady decline in protein excretion. However, in some patients, this condition represents an early manifestation of a more serious glomerular disease such as MGN, IgA nephropathy (IgAN), focal glomerulosclerosis, diabetic nephropathy, or amyloidosis. Finally, notably, mild proteinuria may accompany a febrile illness, exercise, congestive heart failure, or infectious diseases.

Asymptomatic hematuria is the primary presenting manifestation of a significant number of specific glomerular diseases, including IgAN, hereditary nephritis, thin basement membrane syndrome, and benign recurrent hematuria. Hematuria may also represent the fortuitous early discovery of another glomerular disease such as SLE or postinfectious GN.

IgA Nephropathy (Berger's Disease)

IgAN, characterized by mesangial IgA deposits (**Web Fig. 28–25**), accounts for 40% to 50% of patients with asymptomatic hematuria and is the most common cause of primary glomerular disease worldwide. IgAN is usually uncovered during a routine examination of the urine, revealing asymptomatic hematuria. The symptomatic patient usually exhibits gross hematuria after a viral illness, with men affected two to three times more frequently compared with women and whites much more commonly affected compared with African Americans. Most patients are between the ages of 15 and 35. Microscopic hematuria usually remains after the gross hematuria resolves. Mild proteinuria of less than 1 g/day is common, but nephrotic-range proteinuria may be seen in 10% to 15% of patients. Serum complement is normal.

Light microscopic changes (see **Web Fig. 28–26**) vary from normal glomeruli (grade I), through mesangial hypercellularity (grade II), to a mixed group of abnormalities, including segmental sclerosis, crescent formation, tubular atrophy, and interstitial fibrosis (grade III). Mesangial deposits of IgA are diagnostic of this disease (**Web Fig. 28–26**).

Progressive renal insufficiency develops in 40% to 50% of patients after 20 years. Some individuals have a more rapid progression, with renal failure in less than 5 years. Poor prognostic indicators include nephrotic-range proteinuria, hypertension, and the higher-grade renal biopsy changes. Immunosuppressive therapy has been advocated for progressive IgA nephropathy or patients with the nephrotic syndrome, but no curative therapy is currently available. Mesangial IgA deposits recur frequently in renal transplants but with minimal long-term effects on function.

Hereditary Nephritis (Alport's Syndrome)

Hereditary nephritis usually shows in childhood with microscopic hematuria, with or without intermittent gross hematuria. Mild proteinuria is often present, but nephrotic syndrome is rare. Sensorineural deafness begins to occur after age 15 in approximately 50% of the patients. Family history may show any of a large number of different patterns, although 80% of pedigrees show some X-linkage, and over one half of these results from a mutation of COL4A5, the gene located at Xq22 that codes for the α5 chain of type IV collagen. Boys are usually more affected than are girls and often develop renal failure by age 30.

No effective treatment is currently available. Studies have shown that the GBM in patients with Alport's syndrome does not react with anti-GBM antibody, implying a lack of certain GBM antigens. Therefore, although Alport's syndrome does not recur in renal transplants, allografts may develop anti-GBM GN, owing to the presence of GBM antigens for which the recipient lacks immune "tolerance."

Thin Basement Membrane Disease

Thin basement membrane disease is an autosomal dominant basement membrane glomerulopathy, with some cases resulting from mutation of the COL4A4 gene at the 2q35q37 location. The disease usually exhibits as microscopic hematuria without proteinuria in an otherwise asymptomatic young adult. Light microscopy and immunofluorescence examinations are normal, whereas ultrastructural examination demonstrates the markedly thinned GBM. Prognosis is excellent, although a few kindreds with progressive renal failure have been reported.

Benign Recurrent Hematuria

The majority of these patients are young adults found to have microscopic hematuria on routine examination or display gross hematuria associated with a febrile illness, exercise, or immunization. The common causes of hematuria are depicted in Table 28–11. Hypercalciuria is a common cause of macroscopic and microscopic hematuria in children. Recent studies indicate that adults have similar consequences from hypercalciuria and/or hyperuricosuria. Benign recurrent hematuria is diagnosed in patients with asymptomatic hematuria when the other possibilities are excluded. Renal biopsy is essentially normal. Overall, the prognosis is excellent, with as many as 50% in complete remission at 5 years and only a few with declining renal function.

Table 28–11	**Common Causes of Hematuria by Age and Sex**
Age 0–20 yr	
Glomerulonephritis	
Urinary tract infection	
Congenital urinary tract anomalies	
Age 20–40 yr	
Urinary tract infection (females > males)	
Calculi	
Bladder cancer	
Age 40–60 yr	
Urinary tract infection (females > males)	
Bladder cancer	
Calculi	
Age ≥ 60 yr (men)	
Benign prostatic hypertrophy	
Bladder cancer	
Urinary tract infection	
Age ≥ 60 yr (women)	
Urinary tract infection	
Bladder cancer	

From Koenig KG, Bolton WK: Clinical evaluation and management of hematuria and proteinuria. In Neilson EG, Couser WG (eds): Immunologic Renal Diseases. Philadelphia: Lippincott-Raven, 1997, p 809.

Prospectus for the Future

The most common cause of glomerular disease and progressive kidney disease is diabetic nephropathy. A strong effort is underway to detect patients at risk for diabetic nephropathy using genetic and other urinary biomarkers through proteomics. By early identification of individuals at risk for kidney failure, novel treatment strategies may be developed that would prevent the progressive loss of kidney function and end-stage renal disease.

Additionally, better understanding of the mechanisms of glomerular injury in the various forms of glomerulonephritis has paved the way for development of disease-specific therapy, rather than systemic immunosuppression, to limit the extensive side effects and result in higher remission and cure rates for the disease.

References

Glassock RJ: Glomerular diseases. In Massry SG, Glassock RJ (eds): Massry and Glassock's Textbook of Nephrology. Philadelphia: Lippincott, Williams & Wilkins, 2001, pp 649–744.

Lewis EJ, Hunsicker LG, Clarke WR, et al. Renoprotective effect of the angiotensin-receptor antagonist irbesartan in patients with nephropathy due to type 2 diabetes. NEJM 345(12):851–860, 2001.

Madaio MP, Harrington JT. The diagnosis of glomerular diseases: Acute glomerulonephritis and the nephrotic syndrome. Arch Intern Med 161(1):25–34, 2001.

Neilson EG, Couser WG (eds): Immunologic Renal Diseases, 2nd ed. Philadelphia: Lippincott, Williams & Wilkins, 2001.

Weening JJ, D'Agati VD, Schwartz MM, et al. The classification of glomerulonephritis in systemic lupus erythematosus revisited. Kidney Intern 65:521–530, 2004.

Major Nonglomerular Disorders

Jayant Kumar

Patrick D. Walker

Tubulointerstitial Nephropathy

Tubulointerstitial nephropathy encompasses a group of clinical disorders that affect principally the renal tubules and interstitium, with relative sparing of the glomeruli and renal vasculature. Glomerular and vascular diseases in their chronic phase can affect the interstitial compartment. Most cases of tubulointerstitial nephropathy can be classified into two types based on morphologic changes and the rate of decline in the renal function. Acute interstitial nephritis causes a rapid (days to weeks) decline in renal function and is characterized histologically by an acute inflammatory infiltrate. Chronic interstitial nephropathy causes a slowly progressive (years) decline in renal function and is characterized histologically by predominantly interstitial scarring and fibrosis, with a variable but less impressive amount of monocytic infiltration.

Acute Interstitial Nephritis

Acute interstitial nephritis (AIN) is a clinicopathologic syndrome that is characterized by an acute rise in serum creatinine with fever, rash, eosinophilia, eosinphiluria, and histologically by interstitial edema with cellular infiltrates. AIN is an important cause of acute renal failure (ARF) and may account for 10% to 20% of all cases of ARF.

ETIOLOGY

The most common causes of AIN are listed in Table 29–1. The best-documented cases of AIN have resulted from complications of therapy with a wide variety of drugs, especially antibiotics and nonsteroidal anti-inflammatory drugs. Certain infectious agents such as leptospirosis, legionnaires' disease, and mononucleosis appear to have a particular tendency to cause AIN.

Acute pyelonephritis can be classified histologically as a form of AIN. In contrast to the allergic form of AIN, acute pyelonephritis is associated with direct bacterial invasion of the renal medulla. The clinical manifestations are predominantly those of infection, fever, chills, and flank pain. Acute pyelonephritis only rarely causes ARF.

Severe glomerulonephritis, although sometimes accompanied by an interstitial inflammatory infiltrate, is generally excluded from classifications of AIN. In some patients, such as those with systemic lupus erythematosus (SLE), interstitial inflammation may be out of proportion to the degree of glomerular injury, and interstitial nephritis is the predominant finding.

CLINICAL FEATURES

The major clinical manifestation of AIN is the development of acute renal insufficiency. Many patients develop a systemic manifestation of hypersensitivity reaction with some combination of fever, skin rash, peripheral eosinophilia, and eosinophiluria. The absence of any or all of these features is common and therefore does not preclude the diagnosis of AIN. Hypertension and edema, important features of acute glomerulonephritis, are uncommon in AIN.

Urine analysis provides important clues. Hematuria (sometimes macroscopic), sterile pyuria, and leukocyte casts are common findings in AIN. Eosinophiluria (seen by Hansel's staining) is highly suggestive of AIN but is not often observed. Mild to moderate proteinuria (usually <1 g/day) is present in the majority of patients. Electrolyte abnormalities associated with AIN include hyperkalemia, renal tubular acidosis (RTA), and renal sodium wasting. Definitive diagnosis of AIN can be made only by renal biopsy, which may be indicated if the diagnosis of ARF is uncertain (**Web Fig. 29–1**). A gallium scan can be helpful to differentiate AIN from acute tubular necrosis (ATN). In AIN caused by intense inflammatory infiltrate, kidneys will light up, whereas in ATN, they do not. However, false-negative results can be seen, and a negative scan does not rule out AIN.

Discontinuing use of the offending drug is the primary treatment of drug-induced AIN. In situations in which antibiotics are used to treat underlying infection, another

Table 29–1 Causes of Acute Interstitial Nephritis

Drugs

Antimicrobial drugs
Penicillins (especially methicillin)
Rifampin
Sulfonamides
Ciprofloxacin
Cephalosporins
Nonsteroidal anti-inflammatory drugs
Allopurinol
Sulfonamide diuretics

Systemic Infections

Legionnaires' disease
Leptospirosis
Streptococcal infections
Cytomegalovirus infection
Infectious mononucleosis

Primary Renal Infections

Acute bacterial pyelonephritis

Immune Disorders

Acute allograft rejection
Systemic lupus erythematosus
Sjögren's syndrome

Table 29–2 Clinical Findings That Suggest Chronic Tubulointerstitial Disease

Hyperchloremic metabolic acidosis (out of proportion to the degree of renal insufficiency)
Hyperkalemia (out of proportion to the degree of renal insufficiency)
Reduced maximal urinary concentrating ability (polyuria, nocturia)
Partial or complete Fanconi's syndrome
Phosphaturia
Bicarbonaturia
Aminoaciduria
Uricosuria
Glycosuria
Urinalysis
May be normal but may contain cellular elements; absence of RBC casts
Modest proteinuria (<2.0 g/day); absence of nephrotic-range proteinuria

RBC = red blood cell.

appropriate drug can be substituted. In most cases, this approach usually results in restoration of renal function within several weeks. A short course of high-dose corticosteroids (e.g., prednisone 1 mg/kg/day for 1 to 2 weeks) may accelerate recovery, but the added risk in patients with underlying infections must be weighed against possible benefits.

Chronic Tubulointerstitial Nephropathy

Chronic tubulointerstitial nephropathy is a clinicopathologic entity characterized clinically by slowly progressive renal insufficiency, non–nephrotic-range proteinuria, and functional tubular defects. Pathologically, chronic tubulointerstitial nephropathy is characterized by interstitial fibrosis with atrophy and loss of renal tubules (**Web Fig. 29–2**). Chronic interstitial nephropathy is an important cause of chronic renal failure and appears to be responsible for 15% to 30% of all cases of end-stage renal disease (ESRD).

DIAGNOSIS AND CLINICAL FEATURES

Chronic tubulointerstitial nephropathy is characterized by an interstitial mononuclear cell infiltrate along with fibrosis

and tubular atrophy. These tubular defects (similar to acidosis) are disproportionately severe in relation to the degree of renal failure (Table 29–2). Most patients with chronic interstitial nephropathy have little or no clinical evidence of active renal inflammation. The urinalysis may show modest pyuria and minimal hematuria and in some cases shows white blood cell and granular casts. Proteinuria levels are usually less than 1 g/day.

Certain causes of chronic interstitial nephritis tend to damage a specific segment of the nephron and thereby alter only the tubular functions that are normally ascribed to that segment. Conditions such as multiple myeloma or heavy metal toxicity, which affect primarily proximal tubule structures, may exhibit proximal RTA, glycosuria, aminoaciduria, and uricosuria. Distal RTA, salt wasting, and hyperkalemia are seen in patients with isolated distal tubular damage, as may occur with chronic obstruction or amyloidosis. Alternatively, patients with analgesic nephropathy, sickle cell disease, or polycystic kidney disease (PKD) may reveal polyuria that is caused by a urinary concentrating defect secondary to medullary involvement.

SPECIFIC CAUSES OF CHRONIC TUBULOINTERSTITIAL NEPHROPATHY
(TABLE 29–3)

Urinary Tract Obstruction

Urinary tract obstruction is the most important cause of chronic tubulointerstitial nephropathy and is discussed later in this chapter.

Table 29–3 Conditions Associated with Chronic Tubulointerstitial Nephropathy

Urinary Tract Obstruction Drugs

Analgesics, NSAIDs
Nitrosourea
Cisplatin
Cyclosporine
Tacrolimus
Lithium

Vascular Diseases

Nephrosclerosis
Atheroembolic disease

Heavy Metals

Lead
Cadmium

Metabolic Disorders

Hyperuricemia, hyperuricosuria
Hypercalcemia, hypercalciuria
Hyperoxaluria
Potassium depletion
Cystinosis

Hereditary Diseases

Medullary cystic disease
Hereditary nephritis
Polycystic kidney disease
Sickle hemoglobinopathies

Malignancies and Granulomatous Diseases

Multiple myeloma
Sarcoidosis
Tuberculosis
Wegener's granulomatosis

Immunologic Diseases

Systemic lupus erythematosus
Sjögren's syndrome
Cryoglobulinemia
Goodpasture's syndrome
Vasculitis
Amyloidosis
Renal allograft rejection

Other Diseases

Balkan nephropathy
Radiation nephritis
Chinese herb nephropathy

NSAID = nonsteroidal anti-inflammatory drug.

Chronic Pyelonephritis and Reflux Nephropathy

The term *chronic pyelonephritis* is reserved specifically for radiologic findings that demonstrate deformities of the pelvis and calyces that are typically most pronounced in the upper and lower poles. Experts now generally agree that bacteriuria alone is unlikely to result in chronic renal injury. The lesion of chronic pyelonephritis results from vesicoureteral reflux or urinary tract infection in association with obstruction.

DRUGS

Analgesic Nephropathy

Excessive consumption of certain analgesic agents such as phenacetin or acetaminophen (phenacetin is largely converted to acetaminophen), usually in combination with aspirin, may result in chronic interstitial nephritis. Analgesic nephropathy occurs more frequently in women who have ingested large quantities (cumulative ingestion >3 kg) of antipyretic-analgesic mixtures. Patients frequently do not report taking analgesics. Emotional stress, neuropsychiatric disturbances, and gastrointestinal disturbances are commonly associated with analgesic nephropathy. Anemia is present in most patients and is frequently more severe than can be attributed to the degree of renal insufficiency; this tendency is because of associated gastrointestinal blood loss that is commonly seen in this condition. Sloughing of a necrotic papilla into the urinary tract may be associated with gross hematuria, flank pain (ureteral colic), passage of tissue in the urine, and an abrupt decline in renal function.

A variety of findings on intravenous urography or retrograde pyelography, including calyceal-filling defects resulting from the presence of a sloughed papilla (ring sign), may suggest the diagnosis. Demonstration of papillary necrosis in the absence of other common causes (e.g., diabetes mellitus, urinary tract obstruction, infection, sickle cell disease) suggests analgesic nephropathy. Plain computed tomography (CT) of kidneys is the diagnostic method of choice; it can show papillary calcification and abnormal contour of the renal cortex. Patients with analgesic nephropathy are at increased risk for the development of transitional cell carcinoma of the urinary tract, particularly of the renal pelvis. With cessation of analgesic use, renal function generally stabilizes.

Cytotoxic and Immunosuppressive Agents

Several agents such as cyclosporine, tacrolimus, cisplatin, and nitrosoureas can cause chronic tubulointerstitial nephropathy. Cyclosporine and tacrolimus are calcineurin inhibitors used as antirejection drugs. These agents cause interstitial fibrosis in the kidneys over time and lead to loss of renal function in solid organ transplant recipients.

Hypertensive Nephrosclerosis

The pathologic hallmark of benign nephrosclerosis is an arteriolopathy that is most pronounced in the interlobular and afferent arterioles. Interstitial and glomerular changes appear to result from the subsequent ischemia. Tubular atrophy and interstitial scarring may precede signs of glomerular injury in arteriolar nephrosclerosis.

Radiation Nephritis

Clinically evident renal injury is uncommon with less than 1000 to 2000 cGy but develops in approximately 50% of patients receiving higher doses. In the early stage of radiation nephritis, tubular necrosis, medial and intimal thickening of the small renal arteries, and damage to the glomerular endothelium are present. Later, glomerulosclerosis, collagenous thickening of the small renal arteries, and interstitial fibrosis are prominent. Evidence of renal damage occurs several months to years after renal irradiation.

HEAVY METALS

Lead

Although occupational lead exposure has declined since the 1960s, environmental exposure to lead aerosols has remained relatively high. Lead exposure sometimes occurs as a result of consuming contaminated drinking water (from lead pipes and soldered joints) or from consuming "moonshine" whiskey. Lead accumulates in tubule cells and causes a predominantly proximal tubular injury, which may lead to glycosuria, aminoaciduria, and chronic interstitial disease. The clinical triad of hypertension, gout ("saturnine" gout), and renal insufficiency in a patient suggests the possibility of lead nephropathy. Disodium ethylenediaminetetraacetic acid, a chelator of lead, may be used to test for a lead burden, as well as to treat some cases of lead nephropathy.

Metabolic Abnormalities

Although prolonged hyperuricemia is associated with renal dysfunction, the role of chronic hyperuricemia in producing renal insufficiency is not entirely clear. The classic urate nephropathy is associated with tophaceous gout and is uncommon these days. It is characterized by urate tophi in the renal parenchyma. Association of elevated serum uric acid and renal insufficiency might be the result of decreased secretion of uric acid by proximal tubular cells.

Primary hyperoxaluria, enteric hyperoxaluria, and cystinosis are inherited diseases that may lead to chronic interstitial nephritis and subsequent end-stage renal failure (ESRF). Hypokalemia and hypercalcemia can also cause chronic tubular injury, leading to nephrogenic diabetes insipidus. Chronic hypercalcemia may result in nephrocalcinosis and chronic interstitial nephritis that may be only slowly and incompletely reversible.

Malignancies

Renal involvement is common in patients with multiple myeloma; progressive renal insufficiency is seen in more than two thirds of these patients. The so-called *myeloma kidney* (cast nephropathy) is characterized by laminated refractile tubular casts (surrounded by inflammatory cells and multinucleated giant cells) and by tubular atrophy and interstitial fibrosis. Cast nephropathy leads to rapid onset of renal failure. Furthermore, in 5% to 15% of cases of myeloma, nephrotic syndrome develops as a result of glomerular lesions (amyloidosis and light chain deposition disease).

Immune Disorders

A variety of immune disorders may be associated with both acute and chronic interstitial nephritis, including several types of glomerulonephritis, chronic renal transplant rejection, and SLE. Renal involvement in Sjögren's syndrome is usually in the form of chronic interstitial nephritis. The most common functional abnormalities are distal hypokalemic RTA and urinary concentrating defects. Sarcoidosis can have renal involvement leading to noncaseating granulomas in the interstitium.

CYSTIC DISEASES OF THE KIDNEY

Renal cystic diseases are characterized by epithelium-lined cavities filled with fluid or semisolid debris within the kidneys. Certain clinical settings suggest specific cystic disorders (Table 29–4). An abdominal mass in a neonate or older infant suggests the possibility of either autosomal-dominant polycystic kidney disease (ADPKD) or autosomal-recessive polycystic kidney disease (ARPKD). Renal failure in adolescence suggests ARPKD or medullary cystic disease. The finding of a solitary cyst in a healthy 50-year-old person is suggestive of a simple cyst. A history of renal disease in a family raises the possibility of ADPKD, ARPKD, or medullary cystic disease. Recurrent renal stones can occur in patients with ADPKD or medullary sponge kidney. The onset of hematuria in a patient undergoing chronic hemodialysis may indicate the possibility of acquired cystic disease.

Simple Cysts

Simple renal cysts increase in frequency with age, being present in up to 50% of the population over 50 years of age. Simple cysts are most often asymptomatic and are usually incidental findings during imaging studies. Renal ultrasonography, together with CT, permit accurate differentiation of benign from malignant lesions in most instances.

Polycystic Kidney Disease

The PKDs include ADPKD, usually referred to as adult PKD, and ARPKD, often referred to as infantile or childhood PKD. ARPKD occurs in association with congenital hepatic fibrosis and causes death from renal failure during the first year of life.

Autosomal-Dominant Polycystic Kidney Disease

ADPKD is the most common hereditary renal disease and affects more than 500,000 people in the United States and 4 to 6 million worldwide. The clinical disorder can be caused by at least three different genes. The most common one, *ADPKD1*, is carried on the short arm of chromosome 16, and the *ADPKD2* gene is carried on chromosome 4. The location of the *ADPKD3* gene has not yet been determined. The protein product from the genes is polycystin-1 and polycystin-2, and they occur on the renal tubular epithelium. Polycystin-1 interacts with proteins, lipids, and carbohydrates, eliciting an intracellular phosphorylation pathway. Polycystin-2 acts as a calcium-permeable channel (**Web Fig. 29–3**). Cysts separate from the parent tubules and

Table 29–4 Characteristics of Renal Cystic Disorders

Feature	Simple Cysts	ADPKD	ARPKD	ACKD	MCD	MSK
Inheritance pattern	None	Autosomal dominant	Autosomal recessive	None	Often present, variable pattern	None
Incidence or prevalence	Common, increasing with age	1/200–1/1000	Rare	40% in dialysis patients	Rare	Common
Age at onset	Adulthood	Usually adulthood	Neonatal period, childhood	Late adulthood	Adolescence, early adulthood	Adulthood
Presenting symptoms	Incidental finding	Pain, hematuria, infection, family screening	Abdominal mass, renal failure, failure to thrive	Hematuria	Polyuria, polydipsia, enuresis failure to thrive	Incidental, urinary renal failure to calculi
Hematuria Recurrent infections	Occurs Rare	Common Common	Occurs Occurs	Occurs No	Rare Rare	Common Common
Renal calculi Hypertension	No Rare	Common Common	No Common	No Present from underlying disease	No Rare	Common No
Method of diagnosis	Ultrasonography	Ultrasonography, gene linkage analysis	Ultrasonography	CT scan	None reliable	Excretory urogram
Renal size	Normal	Normal to very large	Large initially	Small to normal, occasionally large	Small	Normal

ACKD = acquired cystic kidney disease; ADPKD = autosomal dominant polycystic kidney disease; ARPKD = autosomal recessive polycystic kidney disease; CT = computed tomography; MCD = medullary cystic disease; MSK = medullary sponge kidney.
From Gabow PA: Cystic diseases of the kidney. In Wyngaarden JB; Smith LH Jr, Bennett JC (eds): Cecil Textbook of Medicine, 19th ed. Philadelphia: WB Saunders, 1992, p 609.

accumulate fluid secreted into them by cyclic adenosine monophosphate (cAMP)-mediated salt secretion. ADPKD leads to cyst formation in less than 1% of tubules, which suggests that, apart from the inherited gene, another genetic event in the form of somatic mutation or a "second hit" is required to cause the disease.

Clinical manifestations of ADPKD rarely occur before the age of 20 to 25 years. Therefore, many affected people of childbearing age pass the genetic trait on to offspring while they are still asymptomatic. Patients are usually seen either for screening because of a family history of the disease or for evaluation of symptoms. Acute abdominal flank pain along with hematuria is the most common clinical manifestation.

Nonspecific and dull lumbar pain is a frequent symptom and usually occurs when the kidneys are sufficiently enlarged to be palpable on examination of the abdomen. Sharp, localized pain may result from cyst rupture or infection or from passage of a renal calculus. Microhematuria is frequently the initial sign of PKD; gross hematuria may also occur.

Hypertension, the most common cardiovascular manifestation of ADPKD, occurs in approximately 60% of patients before the onset of renal insufficiency. Urinary tract infection, pyelonephritis, and cyst infections are common complications. The extra-renal involvement in ADPKD is common and includes hepatic, pancreatic, and splenic cysts; approximately 10% of patients have cerebral aneurysms; and approximately 25% of patients have mitral valve prolapse. Diverticulosis has also been commonly associated with ADPKD.

The natural history of renal functional impairment with ADPKD is variable. The disease progresses to ESRD in almost 50% of patients by age 60 years. The type II disease generates about a decade later in the onset of symptoms and development of renal failure. Some of the conditions associated with poor prognosis in ADPKD include presence of the *ADPKD1* gene, male sex, African-American race, hypertension, clinical presentation at an earlier age, and episodes of gross hematuria.

The diagnosis of PKD is made based on radiographic evidence of multiple cysts distributed throughout the renal parenchyma in association with renal enlargement. The demonstration of the characteristic bilateral renal cystic involvement is best accomplished by renal ultrasound. In adults, CT scan with contrast medium occasionally reveals more cystic involvement than is apparent by ultrasonography. Imaging studies that show only a few cysts require differentiation of early ADPKD from multiple simple cysts **(Web Fig. 29–4)**. Recommendations are based on the age and number of cysts present in one or both kidneys for the diagnosis of ADPKD in individuals with a family history. The presence of extrarenal involvement, particularly hepatic cysts, lends support to the diagnosis of ADPKD. A commercial genetic test is available that identifies PKD-1 versus PKD-2 in approximately 60% of individuals with ADPKD. This test is probably best reserved for patients with nondiagnostic imaging studies.

The treatment for patients with ADPKD is aimed at preventing complications of the disease and preserving renal function. Patients and family members should be educated about the inheritance and manifestations of the disease. Screening of all patients with ADPKD for cerebral aneurysms is not cost effective. However, screening is recommended in patients with a strong family history of aneurysmal hemorrhages and for individuals with certain occupations (e.g., pilots). Therapy for PKD is directed toward control of hypertension and toward prevention and early treatment of urinary tract infections. Cyst infections should be treated with trimethoprim-sulfamethoxazole, chloramphenicol, or ciprofloxacin, which penetrate cyst walls and attain therapeutic levels. ESRD is managed by either dialysis or transplantation. Bilateral nephrectomy may be required before transplantation in patients with large kidneys or those with a history of frequent or persistent urinary tract infections.

Acquired Cystic Kidney Disease

Acquired cystic kidney disease refers to the development of cysts in patients with chronic renal failure or ESRD who are undergoing dialysis. On occasion, carcinomas may complicate this disorder. After 3 to 4 years on dialysis, annual screenings are recommended to rule out malignancy. Although the diagnosis can be established with ultrasonography, CT scan is the diagnostic method of choice in acquired cystic kidney disease.

Medullary Cystic Disorders

Medullary cystic disease is part of a group of congenital tubulointerstitial nephropathies known as juvenile nephronophthisis-medullary cystic disease complex. It occurs as a rare, autosomal-dominant disease, sometimes accompanied by eye deformities. Anemia and prolonged childhood enuresis caused by a urinary concentrating defect are early indications of the renal disease. Other associated clinical features include short stature and failure to thrive. Neither radiography nor renal biopsy has a high rate of success in demonstrating the small medullary cysts because they are only approximately 1 to 2 mm in diameter. Medullary cystic disease regularly results in ESRD during adolescence or early adulthood.

Medullary sponge kidney is a more common, benign disorder that is often detected incidentally on abdominal radiographs. Medullary sponge kidney is relatively common and often exhibits as a result of passage of a renal calculus. Estimates suggest that approximately 10% of patients who have renal stones may also have medullary sponge kidney. Nephrocalcinosis occurs in approximately one half the patients and accounts for identification of asymptomatic patients on routine abdominal radiography. The diagnosis is made on intravenous pyelography (IVP) by the characteristic radial pattern ("bouquet of flowers" or "bunch of grapes") of contrast-filled medullary cysts. Treatment for urinary tract infection and renal calculus formation is indicated. Renal failure is not a feature of this condition.

URINARY TRACT OBSTRUCTION

Obstruction to urine flow may occur at any point from the renal pelvis to the urethral meatus. The several causes of urinary tract obstruction are classified in Table 29–5. Unilateral ureteral obstruction usually causes no detectable change in urinary flow or total renal function. Azotemia or renal failure occurs only if the drainage of both kidneys is significantly compromised. Total urinary tract obstruction is an important cause of ESRD.

A change in urinary habits is often the presenting sign of urinary tract obstruction. Complete obstruction is the most common cause of true anuria. However, polyuria, especially nocturia, is not uncommon in partial obstruction and may occur as a consequence of defective urinary concentration.

Urinary tract obstruction as a cause of renal failure must be sought in any patient who has renal failure of unknown origin, especially in the absence of proteinuria. In addition, total anuria in a setting of ARF or widely varying urine output is highly suggestive of urinary tract obstruction. Renal sonography is the preferred means of diagnosing urinary tract obstruction and depends on identification of hydronephrosis. Dilation of the urinary tract may not be evident within the first 24 hours of obstruction or in some patients who are severely dehydrated. Nuclear scan with administration of furosemide can be useful in this setting. Retrograde examination of the ureters is rarely necessary for making the diagnosis but may be necessary for defining the anatomy of the obstruction before surgical intervention.

Management of urinary tract obstruction is directed toward identifying the site and cause of obstruction and relieving the obstruction, usually through surgical intervention. In urgent situations, a temporary percutaneous nephrostomy can be preformed until definite measures can be taken. Eliminating the obstruction is occasionally associated with a *postobstructive diuresis,* which is caused partially by a solute diuresis from salt and urea retained during obstruction and partially by the renal concentrating defect. Urinary tract infection in an obstructed kidney constitutes a urologic emergency and necessitates prompt relief of the obstruction.

NEPHROLITHIASIS

Nephrolithiasis is a common cause of morbidity in the United States. The peak incidence is in the age group of 20 to 45 years, with a predilection for men (the incidence is five times higher in men than it is in women). The incidence of nephrolithiasis is higher in developed countries, mainly because of high intake of animal protein coupled with a low-fiber diet.

Depending on stone composition, five types of renal calculi are recognized (Table 29–6). Calcium stones are the most common, accounting for 75% of all stones. The majority of these calculi are calcium oxalate stones, which contribute to more than 50% of all diagnosed renal calculi. Calcium phosphate stones require an alkaline pH for their precipitation and therefore are less common, except in patients with RTA, primary hyperparathyroidism, or milk-alkali syndrome.

Patients with nephrolithiasis usually have hematuria (both gross and microscopic) and sudden onset of excruciating colicky pain located in the flank and radiating to the groin on the same side. Nephrolithiasis may sometimes be associated with polyuria, dysuria, vomiting, and ileus. Initial evaluation of the patient with nephrolithiasis should include a history of hematuria or passing a stone, urinary tract infections, family history, and a detailed dietary analysis. Initial screening should include measurements of electrolytes, creatinine, serum calcium, phosphate, and uric acid. Manage-

---

Table 29–5 Causes of Urinary Tract Obstruction

Congenital Urinary Tract Malformation

Meatal stenosis
Ureterocele
Posterior urethral valves

Intraluminal Obstruction

Calculi
Blood clots
Sloughed papillary tissue

Extrinsic Compression

Pelvic tumors
Prostatic hypertrophy
Retroperitoneal fibrosis

Acquired Anomalies

Urethral strictures
Neurogenic bladder
Intratubular precipitates

Table 29–6 Frequency Distribution, Risk Factors, and Radiologic Appearance of Renal Calculi

Type of Stone	Percentage of All Stones	Risk Factors	Radiologic Appearance
Calcium oxalate, calcium phosphate	75	Hypercalciuria (40–50%) Hypocitraturia (20–40%) Hyperuricosuria (15–25%) Hyperoxaluria (<5%) Decreased urine volume (5–10%)	Opaque, round, multiple calculi
Magnesium ammonium phosphate (triple phosphate, struvite)	10–15	Anatomic urologic abnormality Infection with urease-producing organism Hypercalciuria Hyperuricosuria	Opaque, staghorn
Uric acid	10–15	Hyperuricosuria Urine pH < 5.0 Decreased urine volume	Radiolucent
Cystine	1	Hypercystinuria Decreased urine volume	Radiopaque, may be staghorn

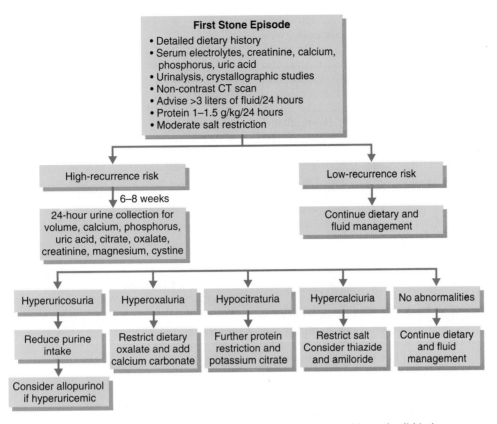

Figure 29–1 Management protocol for patients with idiopathic nephrolithiasis.

ment of patients with nephrolithiasis requires identifying the specific type of stone. Urinalysis is helpful in determining the pH, identifying hematuria, ruling out infection, and, most important, identifying the type of crystals. Uric acid stones are easily identifiable because they are the only radiolucent stones. Cystine stones are less radiopaque and may assume the calyceal shape. Additionally, triple phosphate stones have a staghorn appearance and can be easily identified radiologically. The most reliable method of identifying stones is crystallographic study when the stone is identified through straining of urine.

Forty percent of patients with a first episode of nephrolithiasis have a second episode within 2 to 3 years, and 75% have a recurrence in 7 to 10 years. After 20 years of follow-up, less than 10% of the patients remain stone free. Based on these figures, all patients with a first episode of nephrolithiasis should be advised to consume approximately 3 L of fluid per day to maintain at least 2 L of urinary volume per day. During the night, 8 to 10 ounces should be consumed because this is the period of maximum urinary concentration. Restricting intake of animal protein and reducing daily salt intake are the two dietary modifications that have been shown to lower the risk of recurrent nephrolithiasis. Accordingly, patients should be advised to restrict their intake of protein to 1 to 1.5 g/kg and to use salt in moderation. A comprehensive metabolic work-up may be initiated 6 to 8 weeks after passage of the first stone. This work-up should include two 24-hour urine collections for volume, pH, creatinine, urea, sodium, calcium, phosphate, urate,

oxalate, and citrate excretion, together with serum parathyroid hormone determination (Fig. 29–1).

The majority of renal stones (approximately 90%) are passed spontaneously. The probability of passing a stone depends on the size (especially the width), as well as on its anatomic location. Ureteral stones that are less than 4 mm in width usually pass within a year. Stones that are wider than 8 mm are unlikely to pass. Symptoms of obstruction, pain, and fever may necessitate surgical intervention. Extracorporeal shock wave lithotripsy treatment is more beneficial in patients with renal pelvic or upper ureteral stones. Ureteroscopy with basket retrieval or ultrasonic lithotripsy may be more successful in patients with lower ureteral stones.

Calcium Stones

As mentioned previously, calcium stones can be made up of either calcium oxalate or calcium phosphate. Only a minority of patients with calcium stones have identifiable systemic disease such as hyperparathyroidism, sarcoidosis, hypervitaminosis D, RTA, or gastrointestinal disease responsible for hyperoxaluria. Approximately 50% of patients have hypercalciuria in the absence of any of the diseases described here, along with normal serum calcium and parathyroid hormone levels.

Several risk factors are identified in patients with calcium stones. Hypercalciuria can result from hypercalcemia secondary to primary hyperparathyroidism, sarcoidosis, malignancy, and immobilization; it can sometimes also result from familial hypercalciuric syndromes. RTA, volume overload, and loop diuretics can also increase calcium concentration in the urine. In 90% of patients with hypercalciuria, the condition is idiopathic. In these patients, the presence of hypercalciuric levels of more than 4 mg/kg/24 hr in the absence of the causes described here is usual. Hypercalciuria tends to be familial, with hyperabsorption at the gut, normal or low serum parathyroid hormone levels, increased 1,25-vitamin D levels, and mild hypophosphatemia.

Other risk factors for calcium stones include low urinary volume and increased intake of animal protein. Epidemiologic studies have shown that urine volumes of less than 1100 mL/day are significantly associated with increased risk of calcium stones. Increased intake of animal protein leads to increased acid load that results in increased urinary calcium excretion. The high protein intake also increases urinary calcium excretion by increasing the glomerular filtration rate.

Hyperuricosuria is a risk factor because urate crystals increase the precipitability of calcium oxalate and calcium phosphate. Hypocitraturia is a well-known risk factor for calcium stones, in as much as citrate in urine binds calcium and prevents its precipitation. Normally, citrate is reabsorbed in the proximal tubule, and this reabsorption is enhanced in the presence of acidosis. Accordingly, conditions such as distal RTA, renal failure, severe hypokalemia, chronic diarrheal states, or treatment with acetazolamide can result in hypocitraturia and increased risk for calcium stones. A subset of patients with hypocitraturia have none of the risk factors described here and are said to have idiopathic hypocitraturia.

Oxalate is a by-product of normal metabolism. Increased excretion of oxalates occurs in primary hyperoxaluria as a result of an enzymatic defect. More commonly, hyperoxaluria is a result of increased gastrointestinal absorption in patients with small bowel dysfunction, such as inflammatory bowel disease. Increased gastrointestinal absorption of oxalates can also be seen with intestinal malabsorption syndromes, as well as with diets high in oxalates (found in tea, colas, citrus juices, spinach, and peanuts).

Medical management of patients with calcium stones depends on identifying the metabolic disorder contributing to the stone formation. Reducing dietary sodium and protein intake, consuming a high-fiber diet, and increasing fluid intake can decrease hypercalciuria. Thiazides, by virtue of increasing distal renal tubular calcium reabsorption, can also help in managing hypercalciuria. Reducing the intake of dietary oxalates can help manage hyperoxaluria. Magnesium-containing supplements are also helpful by reducing the gastrointestinal oxalate load by binding intestinal oxalate. Dietary calcium supplements can also help manage enteric hyperoxaluria. Hypocitraturia is effectively treated by controlling the underlying condition as well as by treatment with potassium citrate.

Calcium stones 4 to 7 mm in diameter have a 50% chance of passing spontaneously. Surgical intervention is indicated when a stone is unlikely to pass spontaneously or when serial studies show loss of renal function or increasing hydronephrosis, when infection is present, and when intractable pain is present.

Uric Acid Stones

Uric acid stones are caused by the precipitation of uric acid in the urine. The main risk factors are dehydration, persistently acidic urine, hyperuricosuria resulting from overproduction of uric acid, or increased secretion associated with RTA. Ten percent to 15% of patients have elevated serum uric acid levels, whereas 80% of those forming uric acid stones have no definable abnormality of either serum uric acid or urinary uric acid excretion. More than 75% of patients with recurrent uric acid stones have hyperacidic urine, which accelerates the precipitation of uric acid.

The mainstay of treatment of uric acid stones is to increase volume and alkalinize the urine in an effort to reduce precipitation of uric acid. Alkalinization of urine (with a urinary pH goal of 6.5 to 7) can be achieved during the day with oral sodium bicarbonate. To achieve alkalinization at night when the urine is most acidic, acetazolamide may be used in an evening dose. In a very small number of patients with hyperuricosuria, allopurinol may be indicated. The majority of uric acid stones dissolve with effective urinary alkalinization within a few weeks. Patients in whom such treatment fails can be treated with extracorporeal shock wave lithotripsy.

Magnesium Ammonium Phosphate (Struvite) Stones

Patients with struvite stones usually have a medical history of several urinary tract infections treated with multiple courses of antibiotics. Infection with urease-producing organisms (*Proteus* and *Providencia* species) results in formation of ammonium. Ammonium raises the urine pH, making the urine alkaline, which, in turn, precipitates struvite and apatite. Ammonium phosphate traps calcium and magnesium, which results in magnesium ammonium phosphate stones. Radiologically, triple phosphate stones appear as radiopaque stones, usually filling the collecting system of the involved kidney. Although infection is an important factor in producing triple phosphate stones, a nidus is often responsible for initiation of infection. Forty percent of patients with struvite stones have hypercalciuria, and approximately 15% have hyperuricosuria. Patients with metabolic abnormalities resulting in either hypercalciuria or hyperuricosuria should be managed in the same way as patients with calcium or uric acid stones. Management of patients with triple phosphate stones should focus on treating risk factors and on evaluating for anatomic abnormalities. The goal of treatment is to eradicate infection, which is difficult to achieve. Percutaneous nephrolithotomy is currently the primary surgical intervention of choice.

Cystine Stones

Cystine crystals are hexagonal in shape and, when present in urine, indicate the presence of excess cystine excretion that leads to the formation of cystine stones. The normal solubility of cystine is 240 to 400 mg/L, and patients with cystine stones have an excretion rate of approximately 480 to 3600 mg per 24 hours. Solubility of cystine in the urine can be achieved by maintaining high urine output, as well as by alkalinizing the urine. The goal is to ensure a urine output of 3 to 4 L/day and achieve a urine pH of approximately 7.0. Drugs such as penicillamine or tiopronin can be added to the therapeutic armamentarium in patients who experience failure of fluid management and urine alkalinization. Cystine stones are refractory to extracorporeal shock wave lithotripsy; therefore ultrasonic lithotripsy may be indicated in managing patients in whom medical treatment fails.

Prospectus for the Future

- Attention needs to be focused on evaluating ways of preventing polycystic kidney disease, possibly using EGF-receptor tyrosine kinase inhibitors.
- There are now a variety of sensible strategies for minimizing renal calculi. These include allopurinol for hyperuricemia. A more vexing problem is the individual who has hypercalciuria. At present, the use of thiazide diuretics is helpful, since it minimizes urinary excretion. On the other hand, more rational therapies, particularly identifying the disease in children and using calcium restriction or sodium restriction may be helpful.
- One should definitely avoid combination analgesic use. Obviously, antibiotics and cytotoxic or immunosuppressive agents must be used for certain disorders. The only option is to follow those patients with extreme caution, including renal biopsy when appropriate.

References

Eknoyan G: Tubulointerstitial diseases and toxic nephropathies. In Goldman L, Bennett JC (eds): Cecil Textbook of Medicine, 21st ed. Philadelphia: WB Saunders, 2000, pp 594–600.

Fick GM, Gabow PA: Hereditary and acquired cystic disease of the kidney. Kidney Int 46:951–964, 1994.

Hruska K: Renal calculi (nephrolithiasis). In Goldman L, Bennett JC (eds): Cecil Textbook of Medicine, 21st ed. Philadelphia: WB Saunders, 2000, pp 622–627.

Kelly CJ, Neilson EG: Tubulointerstitial diseases. In Brenner BM (ed): The Kidney, 5th ed. Philadelphia: WB Saunders, 1995, pp 1655–1679.

Wilson, Patricia D: Mechanism of Disease: Polycystic Kidney Disease. NEJM 350:151–164, 2004.

Chapter 30

Vascular Disorders of the Kidney

Muhammad G. Alam

Sameh R. Abul-Ezz

In this chapter, a wide spectrum of diseases is covered that have the common theme of affecting the renal vasculature. These diseases include those that affect larger vessels (e.g., renal artery occlusion) and the more recently recognized ischemic nephropathy, as well as atheroembolic disease, which involves the smaller vessels. Also discussed are malignant hypertension and scleroderma, which have common histologic patterns, and thrombotic microangiopathy.

Renal Artery Occlusion

Renal artery occlusion is an important and potentially reversible cause of kidney failure. A wide spectrum of diseases can lead to renal artery occlusion (Table 30–1). Early recognition and appropriate treatment can prevent permanent loss of kidney function.

Clinical symptoms associated with acute occlusion of primary or secondary branches of the renal artery depend on the presence of collateral circulation. Acute renal infarction is associated with lumbar or flank pain, nausea, vomiting, and fever. Laboratory tests show leukocytosis and increased levels of serum aspartate aminotransferase, lactate dehydrogenase, and alkaline phosphatase. Microscopic hematuria may also be seen. Significant renal dysfunction may be associated with bilateral renal infarction or infarction of a solitary functioning kidney. It is frequently associated with acute onset of hypertension caused by the activation of the renin-angiotensin system.

Radiologic evaluation is necessary to establish the diagnosis of renal vascular occlusive disease. Radionuclide imaging with technetium-labeled diethylenetriamine pentaacetic acid or dimercaptosuccinic acid will show no blood flow to the affected kidney. Enhanced computed tomography or magnetic resonance angiography and duplex Doppler studies have shown improved diagnostic accuracy. However, the diagnosis is more reliably established by renal arteriography.

To avoid irreversible renal damage, prompt localization of the thrombus and restoration of blood flow to the ischemic kidney is critical. Traumatic renal artery thrombosis can lead to irreversible renal damage unless surgical thrombectomy is performed within 4 to 6 hours. In acute atheroembolic disease, early diagnosis and revascularization within hours has the highest success in preserving renal function. In contrast, in chronic ischemic renal disease and in the presence of collateral circulation, the return of renal function may occur even when diagnosis and treatment are delayed. Return of renal function has been documented after surgical treatment even up to 6 weeks after thrombosis. Therapeutic options include anticoagulation, intravenous or intra-arterial thrombolytic therapy, percutaneous angioplasty, clot extraction by a percutaneous catheter, and surgical thrombectomy. In the case of aortic dissection, surgical intervention may become necessary.

Ischemic Renal Disease

Ischemic nephropathy is defined as chronic renal impairment secondary to hemodynamically significant renal artery stenosis and is an important cause of renal insufficiency and end-stage renal disease. Approximately 15% of patients with end-stage renal disease who are older than age 50 years have ischemic renal disease. The prevalence of renal vascular disease is even higher in patients with evidence of coronary, cerebral, or peripheral vascular disease, ranging up to 30% to 40%.

The diagnosis of atherosclerotic ischemic nephropathy should be considered in patients with significant risk factors (Table 30–2). The urinalysis is usually remarkable for few cells and mild to moderate proteinuria. Nephrotic-range proteinuria is unusual. Renal vascular disease is usually progressive in nature. Angiographic progression of renal artery stenosis has been documented in 40% to 50% of patients over a period of 2 to 5 years. With progression,

Table 30–1 Conditions Associated with Renal Artery Occlusion

Abdominal trauma or surgery
Embolism (from heart, paradoxic thromboemboli)
Hypercoagulable states
Dissecting abdominal aortic or renal artery aneurysm
Vasculitis (polyarteritis nodosa, Kawasaki disease, Takayasu's arteritis)
Renal artery stenosis (fibromuscular dysplasia, atherosclerosis)
External compression to renal artery (enlarged lymph node, malignancy)
Postprocedure (percutaneous renal artery intervention)

Table 30–2 Risk Factors Associated with Ischemic Nephropathy

Severe or refractory hypertension
Hypertensive crisis
Asymmetry of kidney size
Presence of renal bruit
Flash pulmonary edema with normal left ventricular function
Age > 50 years
Rise in serum creatinine level with angiotensin-converting enzyme inhibitor use
History of smoking
Presence of atherosclerosis elsewhere (e.g., coronary arteries)

atherosclerotic renal vascular disease can lead to end-stage renal disease.

The diagnosis of ischemic nephropathy depends on the finding of significant renal artery stenosis and proving that these lesions are the cause of renal impairment. Initial selection of diagnostic tests depends on the clinical suspicion. Discrepancy in renal size on ultrasound is an important clue for considering the diagnosis. Duplex Doppler ultrasonography is a good screening test, but it is highly operator dependent, may be technically difficult, and is time consuming. Angiotensin-converting enzyme inhibitor renography is considered a good screening test, but it is not reliable in patients with moderate to advanced renal dysfunction. Computed tomographic angiography and magnetic resonance angiography are effective noninvasive tests to detect the stenosis of renal vessels. The *gold standard* test for the diagnosis of ischemic nephropathy is renal arteriography. However, the risks of arteriography include contrast medium–induced acute renal failure, atheroembolic renal disease, and irreversible loss of renal function. These patients usually have underlying renal insufficiency and are at an increased risk for contrast medium–induced acute renal failure, which may be prevented by hydration, using iso-osmolar contrast, limiting the volume of contrast, or carbon dioxide angiography. The recommended approach is to proceed to renal arteriography in patients with multiple risk factors for ischemic nephropathy. However, in patients with equivocal risk factors, ordering initial noninvasive tests such as duplex Doppler ultrasonography or magnetic resonance angiography before proceeding to angiography is the best approach.

Treatment options for these patients include medical therapy, percutaneous angioplasty, and surgical revascularization. Medical therapy does not reliably prevent disease progression. However, medical therapy with appropriate antihypertensive agents may be the only available option for patients who are unlikely to tolerate invasive procedures. The major goals for surgical revascularization or percutaneous angioplasty with or without stent placement are to preserve kidney function in the presence of progressive kidney disease caused by ischemia or to control blood pressure that is otherwise uncontrolled despite the use of multiple appropriate antihypertensive medications. Either percutaneous angioplasty or surgical revascularization can restore renal function lost as a result of renal artery stenosis. The selection of either procedure will be dependent on individual patients. Percutaneous angioplasty with or without endovascular stent is the treatment of choice in patients at high surgical risks. However, surgical revascularization may be the best option in patients with bilateral high-grade osteal renal artery stenosis that is not amenable to angioplasty or in patients with renal and aortic disease.

Fibromuscular Dysplasia

Fibromuscular dysplasia is a noninflammatory, nonatheromatous vascular disorder that commonly affects renal arteries, although it can affect virtually any artery in the human vascular bed. Fibromuscular dysplasia can involve intimal, medial, or adventitial layers of the artery with medial involvement of the artery being the most frequent lesion. It commonly affects women between the ages of 15 and 50 years. The disease is asymptomatic in most cases and is usually discovered incidentally. Hypertension is common in these patients, and progressive renal failure is less frequent. Duplex ultrasonography, captopril renography, computed tomographic arteriography, and magnetic resonance angiography are commonly used tools for screening and diagnosis. A definitive diagnosis is usually made on renal angiography. Intervention is necessary to treat hypertension or salvage kidney function. When indicated, treatment options include endovascular or surgical revascularization. Percutaneous angioplasty is considered the mainstay of treatment, although its superiority over surgical revascularization is not proved.

Arterioles and Microvasculature

The processes that involve the smaller vessels of the kidney are usually diffuse and involve both kidneys. Most of the diseases of renal arterioles are associated with systemic involvement of other organ systems. Clinically, arteriolar diseases are usually associated with hypertension as a result of the activation of the renin-angiotensin system. Renal insufficiency may be of acute onset but more commonly is progressive over weeks to months.

Atheroembolic Diseases of the Kidney

Atheroembolic renal disease is a progressive disorder exhibiting worsening renal insufficiency as a result of embolic obstruction of small- and medium-size renal blood vessels by atheromatous emboli. It usually occurs in patients with widespread atheromatous disease, either spontaneously or more commonly after surgery, or after procedures such as angiography or percutaneous angioplasty, especially those involving the renal arteries. Atheroembolic disease may also occur after treatment with anticoagulants or thrombolytic therapy, which may interfere with the healing of ulcerated plaques (Table 30–3).

The most common clinical problem is acute, subacute, or chronic renal dysfunction. Labile hypertension may occur secondary to renal ischemia and activation of the renin-angiotensin system. Renal insufficiency may be nonoliguric and is usually progressive. Evidence of cholesterol embolization in the retina, muscles, or skin displayed as livedo reticularis may be helpful in making the diagnosis. Atheroembolic disease may also involve other organs, leading to cerebrovascular disease, acute pancreatitis, ischemic bowel, or peripheral gangrene.

The urinalysis is typically benign with few cells, and proteinuria is usually mild. Eosinophilia, eosinophiluria, leukocytosis, and hypocomplementemia may occur during the active phase of the disease. These findings indicate immunologic activation of the surface of the exposed atheroemboli. Pathologic examination of the kidney shows the presence of cholesterol clefts surrounded by tissue reaction in small- to medium-size renal arteries. No effective treatment for this disorder exists. Avoiding angiographic and surgical procedures in patients with diffuse atherosclerosis may help prevent this disease. Anticoagulants and thrombolytic agents may worsen the atheroembolic process and should be avoided. Steroids and lipid-lowering agents have no proved benefit in this condition. Peritoneal dialysis is preferred in patients who develop end-stage renal disease to avoid heparin use with hemodialysis. The prognosis is generally poor and is dependent on the extent of organ involvement and the degree of embolization.

Table 30–3	**Risk Factors for Atheroembolic Renal Disease**

Angiography or angioplasty (aortic, coronary, renal)
Surgical procedures with manipulation of the aorta and/or renal arteries
Anticoagulation or thrombolytic therapy
Spontaneous in patients with severe atherosclerotic disease

Chronic Hypertensive Nephrosclerosis

Hypertension is the leading cause of chronic kidney disease and the second most common cause of end-stage kidney disease next to diabetes mellitus. Chronic hypertensive nephrosclerosis is described as a slow process of intrarenal vascular sclerosis and ischemic changes associated with chronic hypertension. When advanced, these changes can lead to end-stage renal disease. Risk factors for this disorder include race (African American), marked elevation in blood pressure, and underlying chronic kidney disease. Patients usually have long-standing hypertension (>10 years) and a slowly progressive rise in serum creatinine value.

The diagnosis of chronic hypertensive nephrosclerosis is based on clinical presentation in the setting of long-standing hypertension. Typically, patients have normal urinary sediment, non–nephrotic-range proteinuria, and small kidneys on ultrasound examination. Kidney biopsy is rarely necessary for diagnosis. Progression of kidney failure is related to the degree of blood pressure control. Accelerated hypertension may worsen the rate of progression of kidney disease. The primary goal of therapy is to control the blood pressure. Angiotensin-converting enzyme inhibitors are considered the drug of choice. The outcomes of these patients depend on blood pressure control, compliance with medications, and regular follow-up. In some patients, worsening kidney function occurs despite apparently good blood pressure control. The possibility exists that genetic factors are important in some of these patients. Some evidence suggests that fewer number of nephrons at birth lead to hyperperfusion of each nephron, resulting in glomerular sclerosis.

Malignant Nephrosclerosis

Malignant nephrosclerosis describes renal vascular changes associated with accelerated hypertension leading to renal ischemia and acute renal failure. The rise in arteriolar and capillary pressure leads to disruption of the vascular endothelium, resulting in the characteristic fibrinoid necrosis. The plasma renin-angiotensin system is activated and may contribute to the development of fibrinoid necrosis.

Patients usually exhibit extreme elevations in diastolic blood pressure (>120 mm Hg). Hypertensive encephalopathy often occurs concurrently. Proteinuria and hematuria occur in association with acute renal failure. Renal biopsy shows fibrinoid necrosis of the arterioles and produces a histologic picture similar to microangiopathy seen in hemolytic uremic syndrome (HUS). Characteristic concentric proliferation and thickening of the intima of interlobular arteries produces an *onionskin lesion*. The initial goal of therapy is rapid lowering of the diastolic blood pressure to 100 to 110 mm Hg within 6 hours. Lowering the mean arterial pressure initially by more than 25% is not recommended. More aggressive blood pressure control is unnecessary and may lead to ischemic events as a result of decreased perfusion. More gradual lowering of the diastolic blood pressure to less than 80 mm Hg and systolic blood pressure to less than 130 mm Hg can be achieved over weeks. Renal function commonly deteriorates further during the initial phase of blood pressure control but recovers as the vascular lesions heal and autoregulation of blood flow is reestablished. Most patients with accelerated hypertension will have moderate to severe chronic and acute vascular damage and are at increased risk for coronary, cerebrovascular, and renal disease. Patients who develop renal insufficiency tend to have a low survival rate. Work-up for secondary causes of hypertension is warranted in patients who have malignant hypertension.

Scleroderma

Scleroderma is a progressive connective tissue disorder associated with proliferation of connective tissue, thickening of vascular walls, and vascular lumen narrowing. Approximately 50% of patients may have signs of kidney involvement such as mild proteinuria, abnormal serum creatinine level, and associated systemic hypertension. Scleroderma renal crisis occurs in 10% to 15% of patients and is characterized by acute kidney failure accompanied by an abrupt onset of severe hypertension. A minority of patients with scleroderma renal crisis may have normal blood pressure. Risk factors associated with kidney disease caused by scleroderma include rapidly progressive diffuse skin involvement, cooler months, and race (African American). The typical manifestations associated with kidney involvement include intimal proliferation, medial thickening, increased collagen deposition, and *onionskin* hypertrophy of the small renal arteries. Other findings with renal crisis include microangiopathy, volume overload, visual symptoms, and hypertensive encephalopathy. The renin-angiotensin system is activated and may contribute to the development or worsening of renal crisis. The diagnosis of scleroderma renal crisis requires the presence of other features of scleroderma. In rare instances, renal crisis may be the first presentation of scleroderma. Antinuclear antibody, anticentromere antibody, Scl-70 antibody, and anti-RNP polymerase antibodies may be positive. Therapy should be started before the occurrence of irreversible changes. Blood pressure control is the primary goal to slow progression of kidney failure. Angiotensin-converting enzyme inhibitors are the drugs of choice and lead to improvement of blood pressure control in the majority of patients. With adequate blood pressure control and use of angiotensin-converting enzyme inhibitors, some patients may regain sufficient renal function to discontinue dialysis.

Hemolytic Uremic Syndrome and Thrombotic Thrombocytopenic Purpura

HUS and thrombotic thrombocytopenic purpura (TTP) are characterized by thrombotic microangiopathy and thrombocytopenia. The clinical features of and therapy for these disorders are similar, although some differences exist (Table 30–4). Renal involvement is common in HUS and is characterized by fibrin thrombi in the glomerular capillary loops. The arterioles may also show thrombi with fibrinoid necrosis.

HUS is common in children after nonspecific diarrheal illnesses. Verotoxin-producing *Escherichia coli* (O157:H7) have been associated with hemorrhagic colitis and HUS. HUS may be associated with kidney failure, thrombocytopenia, and microangiopathic hemolytic anemia. Similar features are observed with TTP. However, mental status changes and neurologic symptoms are observed frequently with TTP. Both disorders may be associated with malignancy, oral contraceptives, antineoplastic agents, infections, and autoimmune diseases. The clinical course of kidney

Table 30–4	**Comparison between Hemolytic Uremic Syndrome and Thrombotic Thrombocytopenic Purpura**		
Feature	**Hemolytic Uremic Syndrome**	**Thrombotic Thrombocytopenic Purpura**	
Neurologic manifestations	Rare	Common	
Thrombocytopenia	Moderate	Severe	
Renal failure	Common	Occasionally	
Diarrhea and colitis	Common	Rare	
Multiorgan involvement	Unusual	Common	
Recurrence	Rare	Common	
Mortality	Low	High	

involvement may be acute or rapidly progressive kidney failure. The rate of spontaneous recovery from HUS is high in children, and only supportive therapy may be required. The prognosis in adults by comparison is less favorable, and additional therapy is usually necessary. Plasma exchange is the most effective modality, with a good response in up to 90% of cases; it also has a greater efficacy compared with fresh frozen plasma infusion. Therefore, plasma exchange should be initiated as soon as the diagnosis is made. In patients with TTP, plasma exchange daily for 1 week, then on alternate days until remission is achieved, is recommended as initial therapy. Vincristine is of value in patients who do not respond to plasma exchange. Corticosteroids are usually given in combination with other therapies, and it is difficult to evaluate their efficacy. Splenectomy is reserved for patients with TTP who are resistant to therapy.

Antiphospholipid-Antibody Syndrome and the Kidney

Patients with the antiphospholipid-antibody syndrome may develop venous or arterial thrombosis, thrombocytopenia, and recurrent fetal loss. This disorder may be associated with systemic disorders such as systemic lupus erythematosus or other autoimmune diseases, certain infections, and drugs, or it may occur alone as a primary disease. Antiphospholipid-antibody syndrome may be associated with lupus anticoagulants, anticardiolipin antibodies, and a false-positive result on a Venereal Disease Research Laboratory test.

Kidney involvement is associated with vascular occlusive disease affecting renal blood vessels, ranging from glomerular capillaries to the main renal artery. A finding of glomerular microthrombi similar to those seen in HUS has been reported and is the most characteristic finding. Some patients have mild proteinuria with normal renal function, whereas others develop acute or rapidly progressive kidney failure associated with proteinuria and active urinary sediment. Large renal artery thrombosis with renal infarction may be associated with flank pain, hematuria, and worsening kidney function. Renal vein thrombosis may be asymptomatic or acute and associated with flank pain and acute kidney dysfunction.

Kidney transplantation in patients with antiphospholipid antibodies might be complicated with increased incidence of renal allograft thrombosis and loss. Treatment with anticoagulants may prevent recurrence of thrombosis and loss of the renal allograft. Treatment of antiphospholipid-antibody syndrome is the same regardless of the presence of renal involvement. A patient with thrombotic microangiopathy or thrombosis of a small or larger artery requires anticoagulation to prevent vascular injury. High-intensity anticoagulation with warfarin (international normalized ratio >3) markedly reduces the incidence of new thrombotic events in these patients. Immunosuppressive agents are not successful in the treatment of this syndrome.

Renal Vein Thrombosis

Renal vein thrombosis is a common disorder in a certain group of patients. The incidence of renal vein thrombosis may be as high as 30% in patients with nephrotic syndrome, especially those with membranous nephropathy. However,

Table 30–5	**Conditions That Predispose to Renal Vein Thrombosis**

Hypercoagulable States

Nephrotic syndrome
Oral contraceptives and pregnancy
Protein S or C deficiency
Antiphospholipid-antibody syndrome
Systemic lupus erythematosus
Extracellular fluid depletion
Extrinsic compression of the renal vein
Lymph node enlargement
Tumors
Retroperitoneal fibrosis
Aortic aneurysm

Other Disorders

Renal cell carcinoma
Trauma or surgery
Sickle cell disease
Renal papillary necrosis
Steroid use

renal vein thrombosis can also occur in association with other hypercoagulable states, volume depletion and hemoconcentration, extrinsic compression, renal cell carcinoma, sickle cell disease, papillary necrosis, and sepsis (Table 30–5). In nephrotic syndrome, antithrombin III levels are decreased and protein C and S levels may be altered and contribute to the hypercoagulable state.

Symptoms of renal vein thrombosis depend on whether the occlusion is acute or chronic. Patients with acute renal vein thrombosis may have nausea, vomiting, flank pain, testicular pain, microscopic or gross hematuria, and marked elevation of the plasma lactate dehydrogenase level. A rise in serum creatinine value and increased renal size may also be noted. Patients with chronic renal vein thrombosis, however, may have nonspecific findings such as worsening proteinuria or evidence of renal tubular dysfunction. Renal vein thrombosis of the transplant renal vein commonly produces anuria and acute kidney injury.

The gold standard for the diagnosis of renal vein thrombosis is selective renal venography. Recently, computed tomography, magnetic resonance angiography, and ultrasonography have been useful noninvasive screening tools, but they are less reliable compared with renal venography.

Treatment of established renal vein thrombosis consists of anticoagulation with heparin and then long-term anticoagulation with warfarin. Therapy is usually continued for 1 year or indefinitely in the case of recurrence or persistence of risk factors. Thrombolytic therapy is considered in patients with acute renal vein thrombosis accompanied by acute kidney injury. Rarely, surgical thrombectomy may be required in patients who fail to respond to anticoagulant therapy.

Prospectus for the Future

Cardiovascular disease is the major cause of death in patients with chronic kidney disease. Experts believe that ischemic nephropathy is associated with heart disease and congestive heart failure. The hypothesis that improving blood flow to the affected kidney improves renal survival and patient survival or decreases cardiovascular mortality needs to be tested in a prospective controlled trial.

References

Bidani AK, Griffin KA: Pathophysiology of hypertensive renal damage: Implications for therapy. Hypertension 44:595–601, 2004.

Slovut DP, Olin JW: Current concepts: Fibromuscular dysplasia. New Engl J Med 350(18):1862–71, 2004.

Vasbinder GB, Nelemans PJ, Kessels AG, et al: Accuracy of computed tomographic angiography and magnetic resonance angiography for diagnosing renal artery stenosis. Ann Intern Med 141(9):674–82, 2004.

Chapter 31

Acute Kidney Injury

Didier Portilla
Sudhir V. Shah

Definition and Etiology

Acute renal failure (ARF) is a syndrome that can be broadly defined as an abrupt decrease in glomerular filtration rate (GFR) sufficient to result in retention of nitrogenous waste products (blood urea nitrogen [BUN] and creatinine) and perturbation of extracellular fluid volume and electrolyte and acid-base homeostasis. In the absence of a universally accepted definition of acute renal failure, and in recognition that ARF as previously defined includes a spectrum of clinical conditions, the term *acute kidney injury* (AKI) has been proposed to reflect the entire spectrum of the syndrome. In addition, a consensus conference involving key societies in nephrology and critical care worldwide has recommended the following diagnostic criteria for AKI: an abrupt (within 48 hours) reduction in kidney function currently defined as:

- an absolute increase in serum creatinine of either ≥0.3 mg/dL (≥25 mmol/L), or
- a percentage increase of ≥50%, or
- a reduction in urine output (documented oliguria of <0.5 mL/kg/hr for >6 hours).

These criteria include both an absolute and a percent change in creatinine to accommodate variations related to age, gender, and body mass index. The urine output criteria were included based on the predictive importance of this measure, but with the recognition that urine outputs may not be measured routinely in non-ICU settings. AKI can result from (1) diseases that cause a decrease of renal blood flow (*prerenal azotemia*), (2) diseases that directly involve renal parenchyma (*renal azotemia*), or (3) diseases associated with urinary tract obstruction (*postrenal azotemia*) (Fig. 31–1). Despite technical advances in renal replacement therapy and supportive care over the last few years, the mortality rate of patients with AKI remains high. Several recent studies highlight the clinical importance of AKI. AKI has been shown to be an independent risk factor for morbidity and mortality, and even a modest increase (0.3 mg/dL) in serum creatinine is associated with high in-hospital mortality. In addition, recent studies indicate that AKI is an important contributor to post-hospital discharge mortality and

end-stage kidney disease (ESKD). Estimates are that approximately 15% of patients with AKI will progress to ESKD within 3 years.

The most common intrinsic renal disease that leads to AKI is an entity referred to as *acute tubular necrosis* (ATN), which is a clinical syndrome characterized by an abrupt and sustained decline in GFR occurring within minutes to days in response to an acute ischemic or nephrotoxic insult. The clinical recognition of ATN is largely predicated on exclusion of prerenal and postrenal causes of sudden azotemia, followed by exclusion of other causes of intrinsic AKI (glomerulonephritis, acute interstitial nephritis, and vasculitis). The other defined renal syndromes must be excluded before concluding that ATN is present. Although the name *acute tubular necrosis* is not an entirely valid histologic description of this syndrome, the term is ingrained in clinical medicine and is therefore used in this chapter.

Differential Diagnosis and Diagnostic Evaluation of the Patient

ACUTE AZOTEMIA DURING HOSPITALIZATION

AKI complicates approximately 5% of hospital admissions and up to 30% of admissions to intensive care units. Despite the exhaustive list of conditions that can cause acute azotemia in hospitalized patients, a thorough history and physical examination and simple laboratory tests often suffice for diagnosis. In hospitalized adults, prerenal azotemia is the single most common cause of acute azotemia, and ATN is the most common intrinsic renal disease that leads to AKI. Thus, the most important differential diagnosis is between prerenal azotemia (e.g., volume depletion) and ATN (secondary to ischemia or nephrotoxins). In the elderly male patient, bladder outlet obstruction must also be excluded. In addition, depending on the clinical setting, other diagnoses to be considered are acute interstitial nephritis (secondary to antibiotics), atheromatous emboli (from prior aortic surgery and/or aortogram),

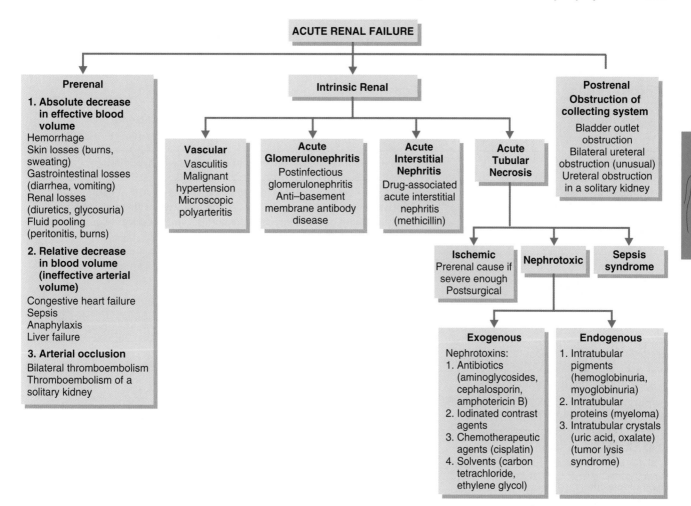

Figure 31–1 Causes of ARF.

APPROACH TO DIAGNOSIS: CHART REVIEW, HISTORY, AND PHYSICAL EXAMINATION

ureteral obstruction (pelvic or colon surgery), or intrarenal obstruction (acute uric acid nephropathy).

Determination of the cause of AKI depends on a systematic approach, as depicted in Table 31–1. The difficulty in arriving at a correct diagnosis in a hospitalized patient is not the failure to identify a possible cause of the AKI; the problem is often just the opposite in that several causes of AKI may be possible. The correct diagnosis depends on a thorough analysis of available data concerning the patient with AKI and on examination of the sequence of deterioration in renal function in relation to chronology of the potential causes of AKI. The correct diagnosis also requires knowledge of the natural history of the different causes of AKI. Some of the important data that should be sought from the patient's chart review are presented in Table 31–2.

Reduced body weight, postural changes in blood pressure and pulse, and decreased jugular venous pulse all suggest a reduction in extracellular fluid volume. Prerenal azotemia

Table 31–1	**Diagnostic Approach to Acute Kidney Injury**

1. Record review (see Table 31–2); special attention to evidence of recent reduction in GFR and sequence of events leading to deterioration of renal function to determine possible causative factors
2. Physical examination, including evaluation of hemodynamic status
3. Urinalysis, including thorough sediment examination
4. Determination of urinary indices
5. Bladder catheterization
6. Fluid diuretic challenge
7. Radiologic studies, particular procedure dictated by clinical setting (e.g., ultrasonography to look for obstruction)
8. Renal biopsy

GFR = glomerular filtration rate.

Table 31–2 Record Review in a Hospitalized Patient Who Develops Acute Kidney Injury

Record Finding	Comments
Prior renal function	Determination of whether the azotemia is acute; patients with prior renal insufficiency particularly susceptible to AKI, secondary to contrast dyes
Presence of infection	Sepsis a possible cause of AKI, even in the absence of hypotension
Nephrotoxic agents	Aminoglycosides (e.g., gentamicin) important cause of ATN in hospitalized patients, typically nonoliguric ATN during first 2 wk of therapy; antibiotics possible cause of acute interstitial nephritis; cytotoxic drugs (e.g., cisplatin) possible cause of AKI
Contrast studies including oral cholecystography, intravenous pyelography, angiography	Important cause of ATN in hospitalized patients; typically causes oliguric ATN within 24–48 hr after study
Episodes of hypotension	Suggestion of prerenal azotemia or ischemic ATN
History of blood transfusions	Incompatible blood transfusion an unusual cause of ATN
Review of chart for history of loss or sequestration of extracellular fluid volume, intake-output, and serial weights	Important clues to the possibility of prerenal azotemia
Type of surgery	Patients who have had cardiac or vascular surgery or with obstructive jaundice particularly susceptible to ATN
Type of anesthesia	Methoxyflurane and the related less toxic enflurane causes of nonoliguric ATN
Amount of blood loss during surgery and whether associated with hypotension	Suggestion of prerenal azotemia or ischemic ATN

ARF = acute renal failure; ATN = acute tubular necrosis.

may also develop in states in which extracellular fluids are expanded (cardiac failure, cirrhosis, and nephrotic syndrome), but the *effective* blood volume is decreased. Thorough abdominal examination may show a distended, tender bladder that indicates lower urinary tract obstruction. When lower urinary tract obstruction is suspected as a cause of acute azotemia, examination of the prostate and a sterile *in-and-out* diagnostic postvoid bladder catheterization should be performed as a part of the physical examination. The urine volume should be recorded and a specimen saved for studies described later.

Additional findings that may be helpful are the occurrence of fever and rash in some patients with acute interstitial nephritis. A history of recent aortic catheterization and the finding of livedo reticularis are diagnostic clues for cholesterol or atheromatous emboli.

Differentiating prerenal azotemia from ATN may be difficult, partly because evaluation of volume status in a critically ill patient is not easy, and any cause of prerenal azotemia, if severe enough, may lead to ATN. Evaluation of the urine volume and urine sediment and of certain urinary indices is particularly helpful in making the correct diagnosis.

URINE VOLUME

The urine volume is often less than 400 mL/day in oliguric ATN. Normal urine output does not exclude the diagnosis of ATN because many patients with ATN have urine outputs as high as 1.5 to 2.0 L/day. This nonoliguric ATN is frequently associated with nephrotoxic antibiotic-induced AKI. In contrast, anuria (no urine output) should suggest a diagnosis other than ATN, the most important being obstruction. Widely varying daily urine outputs also suggest obstruction.

URINE SEDIMENT

In prerenal failure, a moderate number of hyaline and finely granular casts may be seen, but coarsely granular and cellular casts are infrequent. In ATN, the sediment is usually quite characteristic: *dirty* brown granular casts and renal tubular epithelial cells, free and in casts, are the most striking elements and are present in 70% to 80% of patients with ATN (**Web Fig. 31–1A and B**). A benign sediment containing few formed elements should alert the physician to the possibility that obstruction is present. In AKI associated with intratubular oxalate (e.g., methoxyflurane anesthesia) or uric acid deposition (associated with acute hyperuricemia after chemotherapy of neoplastic disease), the sediment contains abundant oxalate or uric acid crystals.

URINARY INDICES

An important series of diagnostic tests relates to an assessment of renal tubular function. The most widely used and convenient tests are measurements of sodium and creatinine simultaneously obtained from plasma and urine serum samples to calculate the fractional excretion of sodium (Fe_{Na}). The rationale for the use of these indices is as follows: The ratio of urine to plasma creatinine (U/P_{Cr}) provides an index of the fraction of filtered water excreted. If the assumption is made that all of the creatinine filtered at the glomerulus is excreted into the urine and that relatively little is added by secretion (an oversimplification but an acceptable one), then any increment in the concentration of creatinine in urine over that in plasma must result from the removal of water.

In prerenal azotemia, owing to the reduction in the amount of glomerular filtrate entering each nephron and to an added stimulus to salt and water retention, U/P_{Cr} typically is considerably greater than it is in ATN, and urinary sodium concentrations characteristically are low (Table 31–3). In contrast, in the ATN variety of AKI, the nephrons excrete a large fraction of their filtered sodium and water, and the

results are a lower U/P_{Cr} and a higher Fe_{Na}. An exception to the rule that low Fe_{Na} indicates prerenal and high Fe_{Na} indicates ATN is the use of a diuretic or the presence of glucosuria that decreases tubular sodium reabsorption and increases Fe_{Na}. Recent studies show that, in the presence of diuretics, the rate of fractional excretion of urea (Fe_{urea}) of less than 35 indicates intact tubular function thus favoring prerenal rather than established ARF as a cause of the azotemia. Because of the adaptive responses, in a patient with advanced chronic kidney disease (CKD), prerenal azotemia may not be associated with a Fe_{Na} of less than 1%. Interpretations of these tests therefore must be made in conjunction with other assessments of the patient because clinically important exceptions to these generalizations exist. For example, certain types of ATN, such as in the case of severe burns, sepsis, and radiographic dye–induced kidney injury, or conditions associated with vascular inflammation, such as acute glomerulonephritis, acute vasculitis, or kidney transplant rejection, may exhibit all of the clinical characteristics of ATN but with a Fe_{Na} of less than 1%.

INDICATIONS FOR OTHER DIAGNOSTIC TESTS AND RENAL BIOPSY

If the diagnosis of prerenal azotemia or ATN is reasonably certain, and if the clinical setting does not require the exclusion of other causes of acute azotemia, then no further diagnostic evaluation is necessary. Further assessment is indicated in the following situations: (1) when the diagnosis is uncertain, especially if the clinical setting suggests other possibilities (obstruction or vascular accident); (2) when clinical findings make the diagnosis of prerenal azotemia or ATN unlikely (anuria); and/or (3) when oliguria persists beyond 4 weeks.

Ultrasonography of the urinary tract is a noninvasive way to determine the presence of dilation of the collecting system that would suggest postrenal AKI. Radionuclide methods are available to assess the presence or absence of renal blood flow, differences in flow to the two kidneys, and excretory (secretory) function. However, these studies have reduced accuracy in quantitating absolute rates of flow. Renal biopsy is useful in cases in which clinical and laboratory assessment suggest diagnoses other than ischemic or nephrotoxic injury that may respond to disease-specific therapy. These conditions include glomerulonephritis, vasculitis, hemolytic uremic syndrome (HUS), thrombotic thrombocytopenic purpura, and allergic interstitial nephritis.

Approach to the Patient with Renal Failure

Azotemia first discovered outside the hospital may be either chronic or acute in origin. Useful points in deciding whether renal failure is acute or chronic are summarized in Table 31–4. Most patients who have advanced azotemia have chronic renal failure. Before a detailed evaluation is carried out, priority should be given to identifying complications of renal failure that may be lethal without prompt treatment. Some of these complications, such as marked fluid overload and pericardial tamponade, may be detected on clinical examination. However, life-threatening complications such

Table 31–3	**Urinary Diagnostic Indices**	
Index	**Prerenal Azotemia**	**Acute Tubular Necrosis**
Urine sodium (U_{Na}) (mEq/L)	<20	>40
Urine creatinine (U_{Cr}) (mg/dL)/P_{Cr} (mg/dL)	>40	<20
Urine osmolarity (U_{OSM}) (mOsm/kg H_2O)	>500	<350
Renal failure index (RFI) RFI = $U_{Na}U_{Cr}/P_{Cr}$	<1	>1
Fractional excretion of filtered sodium (Fe_{Na}) $Fe_{Na} = U_{Na}P_{Cr}/P_{Na}U_{Cr}$ (100)	<1	>1

P_{Cr} = plasma creatinine; P_{Na} = plasma sodium; U_{Cr} = urine creatinine; U_{Na} = urine sodium.

Table 31–4　Useful Features That Suggest Acute or Chronic Kidney Disease

Feature	Acute Kidney Injury	Chronic Kidney Disease
Previous history	Normal renal function	History of elevated blood urea nitrogen or creatinine
Kidney size	Normal	Small, with exception of multiple myeloma, diabetes, amyloid, polycystic kidney disease
Bone film	No evidence of renal osteodystrophy	Possible evidence of renal osteodystrophy
Hemoglobin, hematocrit	Anemia possible, but normal hemoglobin level in a patient with advanced azotemia is presumptive evidence of acute renal failure	Anemia common

as severe hyperkalemia or extreme metabolic acidosis require laboratory evaluation.

Even before the nature of the underlying disease causing azotemia is known, a decision to initiate dialysis has to be made. Dialysis should be instituted promptly in patients with severe hyperkalemia, acidosis, marked fluid overload, or uremic manifestations. Many uremic manifestations are nonspecific. However, a pericardial rub and neurologic manifestations such as asterixis are indications for prompt dialysis.

LABORATORY EVALUATION

In hospitalized adults in whom the diagnoses of prerenal and postrenal azotemia have been excluded, AKI is usually caused by ATN. By contrast, in an outpatient setting in which prerenal and postrenal causes have been excluded, other renal parenchymal diseases cause AKI more often. Examination of the urine for blood and protein and of the urine sediment can give valuable information that often helps narrow considerably the diagnostic possibilities and suggest further appropriate laboratory evaluation.

The presence of 3+ to 4+ protein, 2+ to 3+ blood, and an active sediment with red blood cells (RBCs) and RBC casts is characteristic of proliferative glomerulonephritis. A history of an underlying systemic disease and various laboratory tests such as complement levels, antinuclear factor, and protein electrophoresis may suggest the presence of glomerulonephritis, but a kidney biopsy is required for a definitive diagnosis (reviewed in Chapter 28).

The presence of only a few RBCs in the urine sediment with strongly heme-positive urine or a heme-positive supernatant (with the RBCs removed by centrifugation) most commonly results from myoglobinuria or hemoglobinuria. Patients with rhabdomyolysis have a marked increase in the muscle enzymes such as creatine phosphokinase (CPK). The urine sediment in patients with myoglobinuria may show RBCs, pigmented casts, granular casts, and numerous uric acid crystals.

IMAGING STUDIES

Kidney size gives important clues about whether the kidney failure is acute or chronic and whether obstruction is present. Renal ultrasonography is the initial procedure of choice because it is noninvasive and reliable. The finding of normal-size kidneys in a patient with advanced azotemia generally suggests that the patient has acute rather than chronic kidney disease; however, several important causes of chronic kidney disease, including diabetes mellitus, human immunodeficiency virus nephropathy, multiple myeloma, and amyloidosis, may be associated with normal-size kidneys. The renal ultrasound examination is also helpful in (1) making a diagnosis of polycystic kidney disease, (2) determining whether one or two kidneys are present, and (3) localizing the kidney for renal biopsy.

Normal kidney size in a patient with kidney failure is often an indication for renal biopsy. Before a renal biopsy is carried out, the patient's blood pressure must be controlled, bleeding and coagulation parameters must be checked, and the presence of two kidneys must be confirmed.

CYSTATIN C: A NEW MARKER FOR KIDNEY FUNCTION?

Cystatin C is a nonglycosylated 13 kDa basic cysteine protease that all nucleated cells produce, and inflammatory conditions or muscle mass do not alter the production rate; only thyroid dysfunction has been shown to alter serum levels independent of GFR. Serum cystatin C levels increase before serum creatinine levels in patients with progressive CKD. Recent data also suggests that cystatin C levels increase 1 to 2 days before serum creatinine in patients developing AKI in the setting of radiocontrast nephropathy, kidney transplantation, and AKI in the intensive care unit. Cystatin C is excreted by glomerular filtration and then undergoes essentially complete tubular reabsorption and catabolism, without secretion, so that it is not normally found in urine in significant amounts. Based on these preliminary studies, cystatin C holds a promise as a potential novel diagnostic test to indicate the early development of acute tubular injury.

Clinical Presentation, Complications, and Management of Acute Tubular Necrosis

AKI produces signs and symptoms that reflect loss of the regulatory, excretory, and endocrine functions of the kidney. The loss of excretory ability of the kidney is expressed by a rise in the plasma concentration of specific substances that the kidney normally excretes. The most widely monitored indices are the concentrations of BUN and creatinine in the serum. In patients without other complications, the BUN rises by approximately 10 to 20 mg/dL/day, and the bicarbonate level falls to a steady-state level of 17 to 18 mEq/L. The serum potassium level need not rise appreciably, except in the presence of a hypercatabolic state, gastrointestinal bleeding, or extensive tissue trauma.

Because ATN is inherently a catabolic disorder, patients with ATN generally lose approximately 0.5 lb/day. Providing adequate calories (1800 to 2500 kcal or 35 kcal/kg body weight/day) and approximately 1.0 to 1.4 g/kg body weight of protein per day may minimize further weight loss. The use of hyperalimentation with 50% dextrose and essential amino acids has had little effect on minimizing mortality and morbidity in patients with ATN, except in patients who also have significant burns.

Hyperkalemia is a life-threatening complication of AKI and often necessitates urgent intervention. The electromechanical effects of hyperkalemia on the heart are potentiated by hypocalcemia, acidosis, and hyponatremia. Thus, the electrocardiogram, which measures the summation of these effects, is a better guide to therapy compared with a single potassium determination. The cardiac effects of hyperkalemia are primarily referable to blunting of the magnitude of the action potential in response to a depolarizing stimulus. The sequential electrocardiographic changes observed in hyperkalemia are peaked T waves, prolongation of the PR interval, widening of the QRS complex, and a sine wave pattern, and these changes are mandatory indications for prompt treatment. The most common biochemical abnormality responsible for death in patients with ATN is hyperkalemia.

Moderate acidosis is generally well tolerated and does not need treatment unless used as an adjunct to controlling hyperkalemia or when plasma bicarbonate levels fall to less than 15 mEq/L. Hyperkalemia and acidosis not easily controlled by medical therapy are indications for initiating dialysis.

In most patients, hypocalcemia is asymptomatic and does not require treatment. Phosphate-binding gels may be used in patients with significant hyperphosphatemia. Anemia regularly develops in patients with ATN and does not require treatment unless it is symptomatic or contributes to heart failure.

In a well-managed patient (with use of early dialysis), many of the uremic manifestations outlined in Table 31–5 either do not develop or are minimal. However, infection

Table 31–5 **Major Complications of Acute Kidney Injury**	
Impairment of Fluid and Electrolyte Excretion	
Water	Hyponatremia
Sodium chloride	Volume expansion
	Congestive heart failure
Potassium	Hyperkalemia
	Arrhythmias
Hydrogen	Acidosis
Phosphate	Hyperphosphatemia
	Hypocalcemia
	Metastatic calcifications
Magnesium	Hypermagnesemia
Uric acid	Hyperuricemia
Retention of urea and other solutes	Uremia
	Cardiac: pericarditis
	Neurologic: asterixis, confusion, somnolence, coma, seizures
	Hematologic: anemia, coagulopathy, bleeding diathesis
	Infection
	Gastrointestinal: nausea, vomiting, gastritis, bleeding
	Skin: pruritus
	Glucose intolerance
Synthetic Impairment	
1,25-Dihydroxyvitamin D$_3$	Hypocalcemia
Erythropoietin	Anemia
Impaired drug metabolism and excretion	Drug toxicity, decreased diuretic effectiveness

remains the main cause of death despite vigorous dialysis. Thus, meticulous aseptic care of intravenous catheters and wounds and avoidance of the use of indwelling urinary catheters are important in the management of such patients.

The indications for initiating dialysis are severe hyperkalemia and/or acidosis not easily controlled by medical treatment or fluid overload. In the absence of any of the foregoing conditions, most nephrologists advocate dialysis when the BUN reaches approximately 80 to 100 mg/dL because the goal of modern therapy is to avoid the occurrence of uremic symptoms. Therefore, the patient is dialyzed as frequently as is necessary to keep the BUN at less than 80 mg/dL. When this approach is used, most patients do not develop uremic symptoms, the diet and fluid intake can be liberalized, and the overall management of the patient is easier. Finally, the clinician must review thoroughly the indications for and the doses of all drugs administered to patients with ATN. Monitoring of blood concentrations of drugs is an important adjunct to effective treatment.

Outcome and Prognosis

The oliguric phase of ATN typically lasts for 1 to 2 weeks and is followed by the diuretic phase. Approximately one fourth to one third of the deaths occur in the diuretic phase. This finding is not surprising because, with the availability of dialysis, the most important determinant of the outcome is not the uremia itself but rather the underlying disease that causes the ATN.

As noted previously, infection continues to be the most important cause of death in patients with ATN. In modern acute-care hospitals, the outcome of patients who develop ATN is highly variable, and, depending on the nature of the underlying disease, mortality rates may be in excess of 50%. In patients who survive the acute episode, renal function returns essentially to normal, with the only residual findings being a modest reduction in GFR and an inability to concentrate and acidify urine maximally.

Prevention

The first principle of good management is prophylaxis. This approach requires recognition of the clinical settings in which ATN normally occurs (e.g., in patients undergoing cardiac or aortic surgery) and recognition of patients particularly susceptible to ATN. Useful measures include correcting fluid deficiencies before surgical procedures and keeping patients who are particularly at risk adequately hydrated before radiocontrast studies. Nephrotoxic drugs should be used only when essential and then only with careful monitoring of the patient. Finally, pretreatment with allopurinol before chemotherapy of massive tumors diminishes uric acid excretion.

Pathogenesis of Acute Tubular Necrosis

Although an initial decrease in renal blood flow appears to be a requisite for the development of ischemic ATN, blood flow returns nearly to normal within 24 to 48 hours after the initial insult. Despite adequate renal blood flow, tubular dysfunction persists, and the GFR remains depressed. Despite the common use of the term *acute tubular necrosis,* necrosis of the tubules is seen infrequently in either ischemic or nephrotoxic AKI. In addition, although two kinds of cell death, *apoptosis* and *necrosis,* are recognized, one of the major advances in the medical community's understanding of cell death has been the recognition that the pathways traditionally associated with apoptosis may be critical in the form of cell injury associated with necrosis. Thus, evidence indicates that apoptotic mechanisms, including increased mitochondrial membrane permeability resulting in the release and activation of apoptogenic factors such as endonuclease, are important in renal tubular injury and that certain mediators (increased fatty acids, oxidants, caspases, and ceramide) regulate this process. The pathway that the cell follows depends on both the nature and the severity of insults. Integral to the path that is followed is thought to be the expression of many genes involved in cell cycle regulation, as well as a group of genes that are pro-inflammatory and chemotactic. The cascades that lead to the apoptotic or necrotic mode of cell death probably are activated almost simultaneously and may share some common pathways (see Table 31–3).

Various biochemical changes have been implicated in proximal tubule cell injury in ARF. These changes include mitochondrial dysfunction, adenosine triphosphate (ATP) depletion, phospholipid degradation, elevation in cytosolic free calcium, decrease in sodium (Na^+), potassium (K^+)-ATPase activity, alterations in substrate metabolism, lysosomal changes, and the production of oxygen-free radicals. Which changes are causative and which may simply be by-products of advanced cell injury are not yet clear.

Recent studies provide support for the role of microvascular endothelium and inflammatory cells in the pathophysiology of ischemic AKI. An early elevation on circulating levels of von-Willebrand factor (a marker for endothelial cell injury) is seen, as well as increases in F-actin aggregates in the basolateral aspects of renal microvascular endothelial cells, accompanied by increased leukocyte and perhaps T cell endothelial–adhesive interactions. Leakage of glomerular ultrafiltrate from the tubular lumen into the renal interstitium across the damaged renal tubular cells, obstruction to flow resulting from debris or crystals in the lumen of the tubules, and a decrease in the glomerular capillary ultrafiltration coefficient, have all been proposed to play a pathophysiologic role in sustaining the clinical picture of ATN.

Specific Causes of Acute Renal Failure

EXOGENOUS NEPHROTOXINS

Radiographic Contrast Agents

Contrast media–associated acute kidney injury has been associated with increased mortality, permanent loss of kidney function, kidney failure requiring dialysis, prolonged hospitalization, and increased cost of medical care. Contrast media–associated AKI is fortunately rare in patients who are not at high risk for contrast nephropathy. Risk factors associated with contrast-media nephropathy are listed in Table 31–6. Patients with a combination of advanced chronic kidney disease and diabetes are considered at extremely high risk for developing acute kidney disease.

The exact mechanism by which contrast medium causes acute kidney disease is not well understood. Suggested mechanisms include severe vasoconstriction of renal medullary vessels and direct renal tubular toxicity likely related to release of oxidants.

Although acute kidney disease in this setting is usually defined as an increase in serum creatinine of 0.5 mg/dL or 25% or more from the baseline, an increase in serum creatinine of as little as 0.3 mg/dL is associated with unfavorable outcomes. Most patients develop acute kidney failure within 24 to 96 hours after parenteral administration of contrast media and, in the majority of these patients, kidney function recovers within 7 to 10 days. In a small proportion of patients, kidney function may not recover completely, or the patients may require dialysis. A diagnosis of contrast media–associated AKI is made on the temporal association of exposure to contrast media and kidney injury without any other obvious cause for acute kidney injury. Most patients

Table 31–6	**Major Risk Factors Associated with Contrast Media–Associated Nephropathy**

Chronic kidney disease
Diabetes mellitus
Age > 65
Volume depletion
Study requiring large volume of contrast
High osmolar contrast media
Presence of more than one risk factor

Table 31–7	**Prevention of Contrast Media–Associated Nephropathy**

Identify high-risk patients
Avoid volume depletion
Use adequate saline hydration before and after the procedure
Limit contrast volume
Use iso-osmolar contrast media

have a Fe_{Na} of less than 1. To date, no treatment for contrast media–associated renal failure is available, and therefore prevention is the key (Table 31–7). Hydration with saline has proved beneficial. In high-risk groups, intravenous administration of saline 4 to 12 hours before and 8 to 12 hours after administering contrast media is recommended. Hydration with a solution containing bicarbonate has been shown to decrease the incidence of contrast nephropathy, but until more data are available, normal saline is recommended. Iso-osmolar contrast media has also been shown to have lower incidence of contrast nephropathy. Prophylactic use of N-acetylcysteine has not shown to be of consistent benefit.

Aminoglycosides

One of the most important manifestations of aminoglycoside (e.g., tobramycin, gentamicin, amikacin) nephrotoxicity is AKI, which occurs in approximately 10% of patients receiving these drugs. Maintaining blood levels in the therapeutic range reduces but does not eliminate the risk of nephrotoxicity. AKI is usually mild and nonoliguric and produces a rise in the serum creatinine level after approximately one week of therapy with one of the aminoglycosides. The prognosis for recovery of kidney function after several days is excellent, although some patients may need dialysis support before recovery.

Nonsteroidal Anti-Inflammatory Drugs

Nonsteroidal anti-inflammatory drugs (NSAIDs) have several acute renal effects. NSAIDs are potent inhibitors of prostaglandin synthesis, a property that contributes to their nephrotoxic potential in certain high-risk patients in whom renal vasodilation depends on prostaglandins. The most frequent pattern of injury related to NSAIDs is prerenal azotemia, particularly in patients who either are volume contracted or have a reduced effective circulating volume. Susceptible persons include those with congestive heart failure, cirrhosis, chronic kidney disease, and volume depletion. Hyperchloremic metabolic acidosis, often associated with hyperkalemia, has also been recognized as an effect of the NSAIDs, particularly in persons with preexisting chronic interstitial kidney disease. Hyporeninemic hypoaldosteronism occurs in these persons in states of renal prostaglandin inhibition. Finally, NSAIDs have been associated with the development of acute interstitial nephritis, often associated with renal insufficiency and nephrotic-range proteinuria. This complication appears to be an idiosyncratic reaction to propionic acid derivatives such as ibuprofen, naproxen, and fenoprofen. In contrast to acute interstitial nephritis associated with other drugs, the incidence of hypersensitivity symptoms and eosinophilia is low. Discontinuation of the offending agent usually results in resolution of this disorder.

Cyclooxygenase-2 Inhibitors

Cyclooxygenase-2 (COX-2) inhibitors have recently become a frequently used component of drug therapy in the adult population to treat acute inflammatory states, including arthritis and pain. Results from recent clinical trials have indicated that prostaglandins formed by COX-2 have important roles in renal physiology under certain conditions and that the effects of COX-2 inhibitors on kidney function are similar to those of traditional NSAIDs. Patients who are considered at elevated risk for adverse kidney events, including those with advanced age, kidney or hepatic disease, congestive heart failure, and diuretic or angiotensin-converting enzyme inhibitor therapy, should be monitored with the same caution when receiving therapy with COX-2 inhibitors as they would be while receiving NSAIDs. A total of 15 cases of AKI associated with the use of these drugs have been reported to date: nine with celecoxib and six with rofecoxib. All cases occurred in patients with the risk factors listed previously, and all patients returned to baseline renal function within 3 days to 3 weeks after discontinuation of COX-2 inhibitor therapy.

Cisplatin

Kidney injury is a well-recognized and dose-dependent complication of cisplatin, an antineoplastic agent used in the treatment of several carcinomas. Hypomagnesemia resulting from renal losses of magnesium may be severe and can occur in as many as 50% of patients. Patients should be well hydrated before they receive cisplatin, and simultaneous treatment with other known nephrotoxins should be avoided whenever possible. The usual lesion is that of ATN, but with severe damage or recurrent administration of the drug, chronic interstitial disease may ensue.

ETHYLENE GLYCOL TOXICITY

Ethylene glycol is a colorless, odorless, sweet liquid found in solvents and antifreeze. Ingestion of ethylene glycol, usually in the form of antifreeze, produces a characteristic syndrome of severe high anion gap $\{(Na^+) - [(Cl^-) + (HCO_3^-)]\}$ metabolic acidosis with a large osmolar gap $[(2)(Na^+) + (BUN)/2.8 + (glucose)/18 + (ethanol)/4.7]$. Ethylene glycol is metabolized by alcohol dehydrogenase to glycolic acid, which is believed to be the major contributor to acidosis. The key clinical findings in patients who have ingested ethylene glycol are disorientation and agitation initially, progressing to central nervous system depression, renal failure, metabolic acidosis, respiratory failure, and circulatory insufficiency. Hypocalcemia is a prominent feature attributed to the deposition of calcium oxalate in multiple tissues but may be aggravated by a decreased parathyroid hormone response. The typical urine sediment is calcium oxalate crystals. AKI generally follows after 48 to 72 hours.

Aggressive intervention with intravenous sodium bicarbonate to enhance renal clearance of glycolate through ion trapping, intravenous ethanol or Antizol (fomepizole) to block the metabolism of ethylene glycol, and hemodialysis for removing ethylene glycol and glycolate should be initiated at the time of diagnosis. Regular monitoring of the osmolar gap (corrected for ethanol level if intravenous ethanol is being used during treatment) and anion gap will help guide therapy during hemodialysis.

ANGIOTENSIN-CONVERTING ENZYME INHIBITORS

AKI associated with angiotensin-converting enzyme inhibitors is thought to be hemodynamic in origin, resulting from loss of autoregulation of renal blood flow and GFR, and has been typically reported when these drugs are given to patients with bilateral renal artery stenosis or with moderately advanced azotemia. Allergic acute interstitial nephritis similar to that observed with antibiotic administration has also been reported.

ENDOGENOUS NEPHROTOXINS

Rhabdomyolysis

Since the first description of the causative association between rhabdomyolysis and AKI in persons with crush injuries during World War II, the spectrum of causes of rhabdomyolysis, myoglobinuria, and renal failure has broadened. Rhabdomyolysis is most frequently the result of trauma or other injury, leading to muscle compression, ischemia, excess muscle activity associated with exercise or seizures, metabolic derangements (hypokalemia and hypophosphatemia), drugs, and infections. Cocaine use, neuroleptic malignant syndrome, and the use of hydroxymethylglutaryl coenzyme A reductase inhibitors (statin drugs) in the treatment of hypercholesterolemia also contribute to or cause rhabdomyolysis. Muscle pain and dark brown orthotoluidine-positive urine without RBCs are important diagnostic clues, but the diagnosis must be confirmed by elevations of CPK and myoglobin. Approximately one third of patients with rhabdomyolysis develop ARF, frequently associated with hyperkalemia, hyperuricemia,

hyperphosphatemia, early hypocalcemia, and a reduced ratio of BUN to creatinine because of excessive creatinine release from muscle. Late hypercalcemia is also a typical feature of the disease.

The most important aspect of management will be rapid volume repletion. When patients are encountered in the field, intravenous fluids of normal saline at 200 to 300 mL/hr should be initiated. If urine output increases in 4 to 6 hours, then the solution should be continued to match the urine output until the rhabdomyolysis resolves. However, if the patient continues to be oliguric (urine output < 400 mL/day) the infusion should be discontinued and the patient treated conservatively for AKI. Experience from recent disasters documents that early aggressive hydration and alkalinization (3 ampules of sodium bicarbonate to 1 L of 5% dextrose in water at 250 mL/hr) are capable of preventing myoglobinuric AKI by protecting the kidney from the nephrotoxicity of myoglobin and urate. The metabolic alkalosis induced will help protect the patient from hyperkalemia, which can be a lethal complication of rhabdomyolysis.

Hyperuricemic Acute Kidney Injury

AKI may occur in patients with *high-turnover* malignant diseases (acute lymphoblastic leukemia and poorly differentiated lymphomas) who either spontaneously or, more frequently, after cytotoxic therapy release massive amounts of purine uric acid precursors. This process leads to uric acid precipitation in the renal tubules. During massive cell lysis, phosphate and potassium are also released in large amounts, with resulting hyperphosphatemia and hyperkalemia. The peak uric acid level is often greater than 20 mg/dL, and a ratio of urinary uric acid to creatinine concentrations greater than 1:1 suggests the diagnosis of acute uric acid nephropathy. Prevention of AKI includes establishing a urinary output of 3 L or more per 24 hours, and treatment with allopurinol before cytotoxic therapy is instituted.

Hepatorenal Syndrome

Hepatorenal syndrome is defined as kidney failure in patients with severely compromised liver function in the absence of clinical, laboratory, or anatomic evidence of other known causes of kidney failure. It closely resembles prerenal failure, except it does not respond to conventional volume replacement. In the United States and Europe, most cases of hepatorenal syndrome occur in patients with advanced alcoholic cirrhosis. Hepatorenal syndrome may begin insidiously over a period of weeks to months, or it may appear suddenly and may cause severe azotemia within days. The common precipitating causes are deterioration of liver function, sepsis, use of nephrotoxic antibiotics or NSAIDs, overzealous use of diuretics, diarrhea, and gastrointestinal bleeding. The disorder can, however, occur without any apparent precipitating cause. The hallmark of hepatorenal syndrome is oliguria with urine osmolality two to three times the concentration of plasma, as well as urine that is virtually sodium free, similar to that of patients with prerenal azotemia.

The initial step in management is to search diligently for and to treat correctable causes of azotemia. An important step in the management of these patients is to exclude reversible prerenal azotemia. Because hepatorenal syndrome and prerenal azotemia have similar urinary diagnostic indices, a functional maneuver, such as the administration of volume expanders, must often be used to differentiate between these two entities. Once a diagnosis of hepatorenal syndrome is established, no specific treatment exists, and management is conservative. The prognosis is poor.

Acute Kidney Injury Related to Pregnancy

AKI of pregnancy is presently a rare occurrence in industrialized nations, occurring in approximately 1 in 20,000 deliveries. This decreased incidence is directly related to legalization of abortion in many countries.

AKI associated with infection following an abortion may be precipitated by hypotension, hemorrhage, sepsis, and disseminated intravascular coagulopathy. Although many organisms can be involved, the most serious and common infection associated with AKI is that caused by *Clostridium* species. The clinical picture may be associated with hemolysis as a result of the production of a toxin. Aggressive management with broad-spectrum antibiotics and dialysis support are the mainstays of therapy for this group of patients.

Pyelonephritis, or urinary tract infection, is one of the most common medical complications of pregnancy. Approximately 25% of patients can develop a transient decline in GFR during pyelonephritis. These patients should be treated initially with intravenous antibiotics followed by oral antibiotics for up to 2 weeks of therapy.

In the third trimester, AKI is associated with and secondary to complications of pregnancy to include preeclampsia, postpartum hemorrhage, amniotic fluid embolism, placental abruption, and retained fetal and placental parts. A renal failure pattern resembling ATN is seen in patients suffering from preeclampsia and peripartum hemorrhage. Bilateral cortical necrosis may occur in association with any type of ischemic injury and appears to have a disproportionate incidence in pregnancy as compared with the non-pregnant adult. Abruptio placentae can also cause ATN but is most commonly associated with renal cortical necrosis. The syndrome involving hemolysis, elevated liver enzymes, and low platelets (HELLP syndrome) in association with preeclampsia has been associated with ARF in up to 7.7% of patients.

Postpartum ARF, also known as *postpartum hemolytic uremic syndrome,* is characterized by hypertension and microangiopathic hemolytic anemia and occurs from 1 day to several months after delivery, the most common time frame being from 2 to 5 weeks postpartum. The mainstay of treatment is plasma exchange, with a maternal survival rate of 70% to 80% as compared with the 90% mortality rate that existed before the use of plasma exchange. Elevation of lactate dehydrogenase in HUS versus elevated transaminases in HELLP syndrome may provide help in distinguishing these two syndromes.

Prospectus for the Future

Members representing key societies in nephrology and critical care worldwide have organized a group called Acute Kidney Injury Network (AKIN) to address many of the critical issues facing this field. Consensus conferences and research initiatives as well as establishment of a clinical trials network emerging from such an initiative are likely to provide significant advances in the field in the next decade. It is generally accepted that many of the clinical trials in AKI have failed because of late intervention. There is urgent need to identify biomarkers that indicate early renal injury and/or predict development of renal failure prior to the changes in serum creatinine. There are several groups in the United States and elsewhere critically evaluating biomarkers for this purpose, and other biomarkers which may have prognostic and therapeutic implications. Patients at risk to develop acute kidney injury (AKI) are likely to be identified by specific genetic differences that predispose patients to the development of AKI. For example, patients who develop repeated episodes of rhabdomyolysis-induced AKI have been found to have genetic polymorphisms of carnitine palmitoyltransferase enzymes, a series of mitochondrial enzymes involved in the metabolism of fatty acids. Similarly, it may be possible to detect why, for example, only about 15% of patients develop aminoglycoside nephrotoxicity. Thus, in the future, it may be possible to target specific therapies minimizing potential side effects.

References

Chertow GM, Burdick E, Honour M, et al: Acute kidney injury, mortality, length of stay, and costs in hospitalized patients. J Am Soc Nephrol 11:3365–3370, 2005.

Dangas G, Iakovou I, Nikolsky E, et al: Contrast-induced nephropathy after percutaneous coronary interventions in relation to chronic kidney disease and hemodynamic variables. Am J Cardiol 95(1):13–19, 2005.

Herget-Rosenthal S, Marggraf G, Hüsing J, et al: Early detection of acute renal failure by serum cystatin C. Kidney Int 66:1115–1122, 2004.

Lassnigg A, Schmidlin D, Mouhieddine M, et al: Minimal changes of serum creatinine predict prognosis in patients after cardiothoracic surgery: A prospective cohort study. J Am Soc Nephrol 15:1597–1605, 2004.

Portilla D, Kaushal GP, Basnakian AG, Shah SV: Recent progress in the pathophysiology of acute renal failure. In Runge MS, Patterson C (eds): Principles of Molecular Medicine, 2nd ed. Totawa, N.J.: Humana Press, 2006, pp 643–649.

Schrier RW, Wang W, Poole B, Mitra A: Acute renal failure: Definitions, diagnosis, pathogenesis and therapy. J Clin Invest 114(1):5–14, 2004.

Uchino S, Kellum J, Bellomo R, et al: Acute renal failure in critically ill patients. JAMA 294(7):813–818, 2005.

Chapter 32

Chronic Renal Failure

Jayant Kumar

Sameh R. Abul-Ezz

Chronic kidney disease (CKD) is defined as progressive and irreversible loss of renal function, most often leading to end-stage renal disease (ESRD). The most common causes of CKD are listed in Table 32–1. The spectrum of CKD ranges from proteinuria to elevated creatinine and finally ESRD. In the United States, the prevalence of CKD estimated by population-based studies is approximately 20 million people. The public health impact of this problem is phenomenal. First, many of these 20 million people will progress to ESRD, requiring dialysis or transplant. Second, elevated serum creatinine has been increasingly recognized as an independent risk factor for cardiovascular disease. Thus, identification of elevated creatinine will put the patient at risk not only for renal loss, but also for decreased survival (**Web Fig. 32–1**). CKD has been classified into various stages according to the National Kidney Foundation, starting from proteinuria in stage 1 to ESRD in stage 5 (Table 32–2).

During evaluation, every attempt should be made to arrive at the specific cause of chronic renal failure. Prior laboratory measurement of the serum creatinine concentration will help differentiate between acute renal failure and CKD. Renal biopsy is the most specific tool to reach a definitive diagnosis, which allows treatment of the underlying cause, assessment of the prognosis, and determination of suitability for kidney transplantation. If the biopsy is not performed, diagnosis is made based on present, past, and family histories, serology, examination of the urine sediment, and renal ultrasound. Although most CKDs are associated with a progressive decrease in bilateral kidney size (<8.5 cm in length by ultrasound or computed tomographic [CT] scan), a few systemic diseases are characterized by normal kidney size despite advanced renal failure. These diseases include diabetes mellitus, multiple myeloma, polycystic kidney disease, nephropathy related to human immunodeficiency virus, and amyloidosis.

Adaptation to Nephron Loss

To ensure adequate solute, water, and acid-base balance, the surviving nephrons must adjust by increasing their filtration and excretion rates. Patients with chronic renal failure are vulnerable to edema formation and severe volume overload,

hyperkalemia, hyponatremia, and azotemia. During progressive renal disease, sodium balance is maintained by increasing fractional excretion of sodium by the nephrons. Acid excretion is maintained until the late stages of chronic renal failure, when the glomerular filtration rate (GFR) falls to less than 15 mL/min. Initially, increased tubular ammonia synthesis provides an adequate buffer for hydrogen in the distal nephron. Later, a significant decrease in distal bicarbonate regeneration results in hyperchloremic metabolic acidosis. Further loss of nephron mass leads to the retention of organic ions such as sulfates, which results in an anion gap metabolic acidosis.

Once renal insufficiency is established, the tendency for renal disease is to progress regardless of the initial insult. Glomerular sclerosis ensues, most likely as a result of glomerular hyperfiltration and/or hypertension. Compensatory glomerular hypertrophy is invariably associated with tubular hypertrophy in the remaining nephrons. Tubular hypertrophy is associated with increased energy expenditure, a metabolic event related to generation of reactive oxygen metabolites. Reactive oxygen metabolites have been proposed as a mechanism of tubulointerstitial damage in animal models. In addition, hyperlipidemia is believed to play a role in progressive renal insufficiency through mesangial proliferation and sclerosis. The adaptive mechanism can be beneficial in maintaining fluid, electrolyte, and acid-base balance. However, these short-term adaptation mechanisms become maladaptive in the long term, secondary to activation of the renin-angiotensin-aldosterone pathway and increased transforming growth factor (TGF-[beta]) leading to renal fibrosis.

Interventions that reduce intraglomerular pressure, such as protein restriction and the use of angiotensin-converting enzyme inhibitors or angiotensin-receptor blockers, have been shown to help attenuate progression of renal disease. Figure 32–1 illustrates different pathways through which these maladaptive mechanisms can result in progression of renal insufficiency and ultimately ESRD.

Conservative Management

Conservative management of chronic renal failure should include (1) instituting measures to slow progression, (2) identifying potentially reversible causes of renal failure when unexpected declines in renal function occur, (3) identifying and treating complications of chronic renal failure, and (4) preparing patients emotionally and physically for ESRD and renal replacement therapy (RRT). Methods used to slow progressive kidney disease include optimal control of hypertension, optimal management of diabetes and hyperlipidemia, avoidance of nephrotoxins, cessation of smoking, and, most importantly, use of medications that block the renin-angiotensin-aldosterone pathway.

MANAGEMENT OF HYPERTENSION

Several controlled trials have conclusively confirmed that aggressive management of hypertension attenuates the rate of progression of renal failure, with significant benefits being shown in patients with diabetic nephropathy, as well as in other CKDs. The present recommendation is to target blood pressure to lower than 130/80 mm Hg in patients with hypertension and diabetes or kidney disease. In addition, studies demonstrate the nephroprotective effect of medications that block the production or effect of angiotensin II, above and beyond control of hypertension in patients with diabetic and nondiabetic renal disease. The use of nondihydropyridine calcium channel blockers (e.g., verapamil, diltiazem) has also been shown to be beneficial in slowing the progression of renal disease. To reach optimal blood pressure control, an average of 2.7 antihypertensive medications will be needed per patient, as proved in many large trials. To ensure patient compliance, individualized drug regimens to suit a person's lifestyle become important.

Table 32–1	Percentage Distribution of Incidence of End-Stage Renal Disease by Primary Diagnosis, 1995–1999

Primary Cause	Incidence (%)
Diabetes	42.9
Hypertension; large vessel disease	26.4
Glomerulonephritis (GN)	9.9
Cystic, hereditary, congenital disease	3.1
Interstitial nephritis; pyelonephritis	4.0
Secondary GN; vasculitis	2.4
Miscellaneous conditions	3.8
Cause unknown	7.5

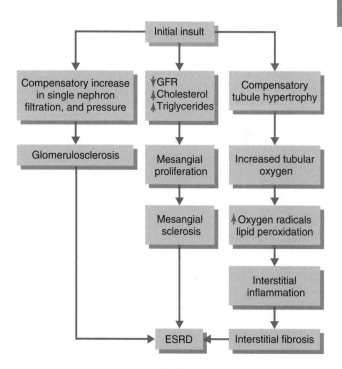

Figure 32–1 Factors responsible for the progression of renal disease. ESRD = end-stage renal disease; GFR = glomerular filtration rate.

Table 32–2	Stages of Chronic Kidney Disease and the U.S. Prevalence Rates			
Stage	**Description**	**GFR[1], mL/min/1.73 m²**	**U.S. Prevalence (1000s)**	**U.S. Prevalence (%)**
1	Kidney damage with normal or increased GFR	≥90	5900	3.3
2	Kidney damage with mildly decreased GFR	60–89	5300	3.0
3	Moderately decreased GFR	30–59	7600	4.3
4	Severely decreased GFR	15–29	400	0.2
5	Kidney failure	<15 or dialysis	300	0.1

[1]As defined by the National Kidney Foundation, 2002.
GFR = glomerular filtration rate.

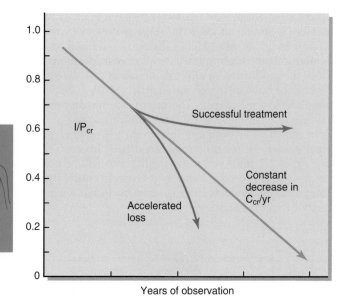

Figure 32–2 Use of the reciprocal of plasma creatinine concentration ($1/P_{Cr}$) to follow the progress of glomerular disease in a patient. (Data from Sullivan LP, Grantham JJ: Physiology of the Kidney, 2nd ed. Philadelphia, Lea & Febiger, 1982.)

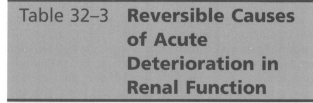

Table 32–3	**Reversible Causes of Acute Deterioration in Renal Function**

Decreased Renal Perfusion

Intravascular volume depletion
Heart failure

Obstruction
Infection

Urinary tract infection
Sepsis

Nephrotoxins

Endogenous: myoglobulin, hemoglobin, uric acid, calcium, phosphorus
Exogenous: contrast media, drugs

Poorly controlled hypertension: malignant or accelerated hypertension

DIET

In the past, dietary protein restriction was advocated to reduce uremic symptoms. More recently, animal and human studies have shown that dietary protein restriction tends to slow the rate of progression of renal insufficiency. The recommended dietary protein intake is 0.60 g/kg/day and, if this is not accepted or tolerated, can be increased to 0.75 g/kg/day with at least 50% of the protein being of high biologic value. At present, advising aggressive dietary management in patients with renal insufficiency, with proper restriction of sodium, potassium, phosphorus, and protein intake, seems prudent. Sodium should be restricted, especially in patients who are hypertensive and edematous. Malnutrition at the initiation of dialysis is a strong predictor of increased mortality. Therefore, a protein-restricted diet must be approached with great surveillance and caution, and all efforts must be made to deliver adequate calories.

MANAGEMENT OF REVERSIBLE CAUSES OF ACUTE DETERIORATION IN RENAL FUNCTION

The rate of decline in GFR for individual patients is log linear. Accordingly, plotting 1/serum creatinine against time usually predicts the rate at which a specific patient will reach ESRD, as shown in Figure 32–2. When such a patient suddenly shows acceleration of kidney failure, the differential diagnosis for such acceleration should be considered, as presented in Table 32–3. Patients with chronic renal impairment are susceptible to factors leading to acute renal failure, and these entities should be investigated aggressively.

AVOIDING TOXIC DRUG EFFECTS

Many drugs that are excreted by the kidney should be avoided or adjusted in patients with renal insufficiency, as shown in Table 32–4. In hospitalized patients, aminoglycosides are one of the most common offenders. By inhibiting vasodilatory prostaglandins, nonsteroidal anti-inflammatory drugs including cyclooxygenase-2 (COX-2) inhibitors can decrease GFR, as well as cause acute interstitial nephritis. Radiocontrast agents can cause acute or acute-on-chronic renal failure in hospitalized patients. Risk factors for contrast-induced acute renal failure include volume depletion and preexisting renal insufficiency. Patients at high risk of contrast-induced acute renal failure should receive intravenous fluid hydration with normal saline or 0.45% saline with 50 mEq of sodium bicarbonate/L 8 to 10 hours before and after the procedure. Iso-osmolar contrast agents are less toxic than high-osmolar agents, and the volume of the contrast should be minimized. Recent studies have also suggested a protective role of N-acetyl-cysteine, 600 mg twice a day, the day before and the day of the contrast exposure, suggesting a role of reactive oxygen species in the injury.

Clinical Manifestations

GENERAL FEATURES OF UREMIC SYNDROME

Patients with renal insufficiency usually become symptomatic when the GFR is less than 10 mL/min. *Uremia* is a syndrome that affects every organ system. Uremic syndrome is likely the consequence of a combination of factors, including retained molecules, deficiencies of important hormones,

Table 32–4 **Drug Dosages in Chronic Renal Failure**

Major Dosage Reduction	Minor or No Reduction	Avoid Usage
Antibiotics		
Aminoglycosides	Erythromycin	NSAIDs
Penicillin	Nafcillin	Nitrofurantoin
Cephalosporins	Clindamycin	Nalidixic acid
Sulfonamides	Chloramphenicol	Tetracycline
Vancomycin	Isoniazid; rifampin	
Quinolones	Amphotericin B	
Fluconazole	Aztreonam/tazobactam	
Acyclovir; ganciclovir	Doxycycline	
Foscarnet		
Imipenem		
Others		
Digoxin	Antihypertensives	Aspirin
Procainamide	Benzodiazepines	Sulfonylureas
H$_2$ antagonists	Quinidine	Lithium carbonate
Meperidine	Lidocaine	Acetazolamide
Codeine	Spironolactone	
Propoxyphene	Triamterene	

NSAIDs = nonsteroidal anti-inflammatory drugs.

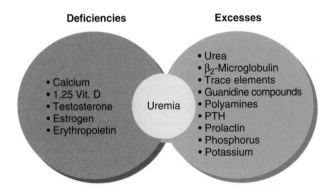

Figure 32–3 Etiologic factors of uremia. PTH = parathyroid hormone.

and metabolic factors, rather than the effect of a single uremic toxin (Fig. 32–3). Urea can cause symptoms of fatigue, nausea, vomiting, and headaches. Its breakdown product (cyanate) can result in carbamylation of lipoproteins and peptides and adverse effects, leading to multiple organ dysfunctions.

Guanidines, by-products of exogenous or endogenous protein metabolism, are increased in renal failure. These by-products can inhibit α_1-hydroxylase activity within the kidney and can lead to deficient calcitriol production and secondary hyperparathyroidism. High parathyroid hormone levels have been implicated in various manifestations of uremia, especially in cardiomyopathy and metastatic calcifications. β_2-Microglobulin accumulation in patients with

renal failure has been associated with neuropathy, carpal tunnel syndrome, and amyloid infiltration of the joints.

SPECIFIC MANIFESTATIONS OF UREMIA

Major manifestations of uremia are shown in Figure 32–4.

Cardiovascular Effects

Mortality from cardiovascular disease in patients with renal failure is 3.5 times that of an age-matched population (**Web Figs. 32–2 and 32–3**). Heart disease accounts for more than 50% of the deaths in patients with uremia. More than 60% of patients who start dialysis have echocardiographic manifestations of left ventricular hypertrophy, dilation, and systolic or diastolic dysfunction. Anemia and hypertension contribute to left ventricular hypertrophy and congestive heart failure. Secondary hyperparathyroidism can lead to metastatic calcification in the myocardium, cardiac valves, and arteries. Accelerated atherogenesis is responsible for the high prevalence of coronary artery disease in this population and the high rate of recurrent coronary artery stenosis after angioplasty. Pericarditis can occur in patients with uremia before they start dialysis, as well as in patients who are already undergoing dialysis, usually related to inadequate dialysis. Initiation of dialysis or intensifying dialysis therapy usually results in the resolution of pericarditis.

Gastrointestinal Disease

Gastrointestinal disturbances are among the earliest and most common signs of the uremic syndrome. Patients with renal failure usually describe a metallic taste and loss of appetite. Later, they experience anorexia, nausea, vomiting,

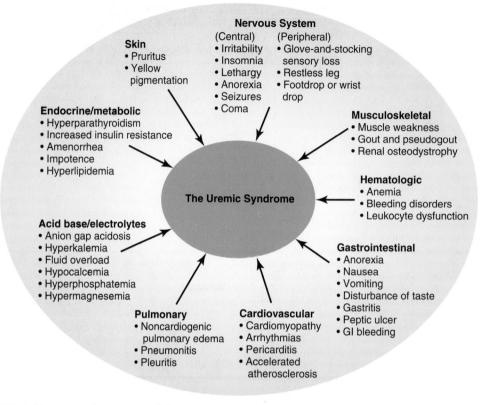

Figure 32–4 Diagrammatic summary of the major manifestations of the uremic syndrome. GI = gastrointestinal.

and weight loss, which should improve after dialysis is initiated. Several pathologic processes can lead to gastrointestinal bleeding, which is caused by gastritis, peptic ulceration, and arterial venous (AV)-malformations, in addition to platelet dysfunction.

Neurologic Manifestations

Central nervous system manifestations are frequent and occur early, often with subtle changes in cognitive function and memory and disturbances in sleep. Lethargy, irritability, frank encephalopathy, asterixis, and seizures are late manifestations of uremia and are usually avoided by early initiation of dialysis. Peripheral neurologic manifestations appear as symmetric sensory neuropathy in a glove-and-stocking distribution. Peripheral motor impairment can result in restless legs and footdrop or wristdrop. Clinically, these patients have decreased distal tendon reflexes and loss of vibratory perception.

Musculoskeletal Manifestations

Alterations in calcium and phosphate homeostasis and renal osteodystrophy are common manifestations of ESRD. Hyperparathyroidism and disturbance of vitamin D metabolism are commonly found. Hypocalcemia and secondary hyperparathyroidism are the results of phosphate retention and the lack of α_1-hydroxylase activity in the failing kidney, with consequent deficiency of the most active form of vitamin D. Over time, the adaptive parathyroid hypertrophy becomes maladaptive and leads to bone disease and tissue calcification. Calcium and phosphate homeostasis in the

setting of renal failure is demonstrated in Figure 32–5. Control of hyperparathyroidism with dietary phosphate restriction, phosphate binders, calcium supplementation, $1,25(OH)_2$-vitamin D, and vitamin D analogs (Zemplar and Hectorol), together with dialysis therapy, is now achievable. Calcimimetics are a novel class of drug that targets calcium-sensing receptors on the parathyroid gland and sensitizes them to the inhibitory effect of serum calcium. This action inhibits parathyroid hyperplasia.

Hematologic Effects

Erythropoietin (EPO), a hormone produced by the kidney that regulates erythrocyte production, becomes progressively deficient as renal mass declines. EPO and iron deficiency are common causes of anemia in CKD. Routine administration of EPO to patients with ESRD results in correction of anemia, improved quality of life, and decreased dependence on blood transfusions. EPO is given typically once a week. A longer-acting preparation, darbapoetin-α, can be given once every 2 weeks. Bleeding disorders, primarily from defects in platelet adherence and aggregation, are common in patients with uremia. Uremic bleeding can be generally controlled with cryoprecipitate, 1-deamino-(8-D-arginine)-vasopressin, conjugated estrogens, and dialysis.

Endocrine Abnormalities

Alterations in thyroid function testing may contribute to difficulty diagnosing thyroid disease in patients with uremia. Common laboratory findings may include an increased triiodothyronine resin uptake, a low triiodothyronine level

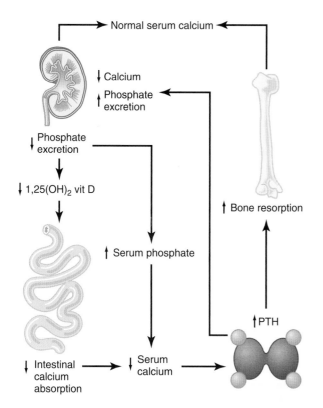

Figure 32–5 Calcium and phosphate homeostasis in the setting of renal failure. The decreased excretion of phosphate initiates the cycle directed at normalization of the serum calcium concentration. PTH = parathyroid hormone.

resulting from the impaired conversion of thyroxine to tri-iodothyronine peripherally, and normal thyroxine levels. Thyroid-stimulating hormone levels are usually normal. On occasion, the use of a thyrotropin-releasing hormone–stimulation test may be needed for a diagnosis of thyroid disorders in uremia. Interestingly, goiter is present in up to one third of patients with chronic renal failure.

A deranged pituitary-gonadal axis can result in sexual dysfunction exhibited by impotence, decreased libido, amenorrhea, sterility, and uterine bleeding. Hyperprolactinemia may be responsible for some of the abnormalities of the pituitary-gonadal axis. Patients have decreased plasma levels of testosterone, estrogen, and progesterone, with normal or increased levels of follicle-stimulating hormone and luteinizing hormones. Pregnancy is uncommon in female patients who have a GFR of less than 30 mL/min.

Immunologic Function

Defects occur in both the humoral and cellular immune systems in patients with ESRD. These patients are generally immunosuppressed and are susceptible to infections.

Metabolic Disorders

As renal function diminishes, many patients with diabetes have a decreased insulin requirement. This change is partly a result of the increased half-life of exogenously administered insulin secondary to decreased insulin clearance, which leads to development of frequent episodes of hypoglycemia in a person with diabetes who was well controlled on a stable

insulin regimen. At the same time, increased peripheral insulin resistance in patients with uremia has been recognized. Insulin resistance occurs secondary to tissue insensitivity to insulin, as well as metabolic acidosis and hyperparathyroidism, which impair insulin release and secretion.

Lipid abnormalities are common findings in the early course of renal failure. They are most consistent with type IV hyperlipoproteinemia, with a marked increase in plasma triglycerides and less of an increase in total cholesterol. The activity of lipoprotein lipase is decreased in uremia, with a reduction in the conversion of very–low-density lipoprotein to low-density lipoprotein and thus hypertriglyceridemia. These abnormalities of lipid metabolism are considered contributors to accelerated atherosclerosis and contribute to mesangial proliferation and progressive renal failure. The treatment of choice is a hydroxymethylglutaryl–coenzyme A (HMG-CoA) reductase inhibitor class of drugs because of their pluripotent effects on inflammation and atherosclerosis.

Dermatologic Manifestations

Uremic hue, a yellowish skin color, is likely the result of retained liposoluble pigments, such as lipochromes and carotenoids. Pruritus is a common complaint of patients with renal failure. Uremic hue usually responds to dialysis, control of hyperparathyroidism, improved calcium and phosphate balance, and, occasionally, ultraviolet rays. Calciphylaxis, which is rare in patients with well-managed renal failure, results from painful skin calcification in patients with a serum calcium × phosphate product that exceeds 70 mg/dL in the presence of severe hyperparathyroidism. Nail findings include the half-and-half nail, characterized by red, pink, or brownish discoloration of the distal nail bed, pale nails, and splinter hemorrhages. Thickening and fibrosis of skin, especially starting in the lower extremities are seen in renal disease. This entity is called nephrogenic fibrosing dermopathy and is differentiated from scleroderma by relative sparing of the face.

Treatment of End-Stage Renal Disease

A plan for a modality of RRT should be discussed with the patient early in the course of renal failure and before the appearance of uremic symptoms. The current criteria for initiating dialysis is a GFR of 15 mL/minute or less. Creatinine clearance overestimates GFR in advanced renal failure because of tubular secretion of creatinine. A more accurate estimation of the GFR can be calculated from the average of the creatinine and urea clearances. Patients with volume overload that is resistant to diuretics, metabolic acidosis, pericarditis, persistent hyperkalemia, intractable gastrointestinal symptoms, or encephalopathy should be started on dialysis even though their creatinine clearance may exceed the previously set criteria. The choice of RRT largely depends on the patient's physical and sociodemographic characteristics. Most patients are started either on hemodialysis or on peritoneal dialysis. Renal transplantation is encouraged because it allows a better quality of life, increased survival rate, and a greater chance for rehabilitation.

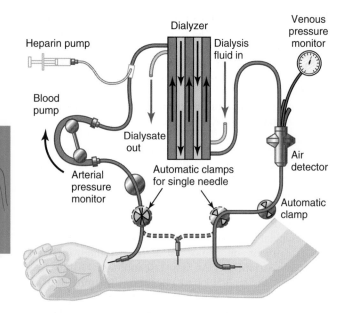

Figure 32–6 Essential components of a dialysis delivery system that, together with the dialyzer, make up an *artificial kidney.* In isolated ultrafiltration, no dialysis fluid is used (bypass mode). Also shown is the apparatus for using a single needle for inflow and outflow of blood from the patient. (From Keshaviah PR: Hemodialysis Monitors and Monitoring. In Maher JF [ed]: Replacement of Renal Function by Dialysis, 3rd ed. Boston: Kluwer Academic Publishers, 1989. Reprinted by permission of Kluwer Academic Publishers.)

HEMODIALYSIS

According to United States Renal Data System 2002 data, approximately 100,000 patients in the United States were initiated on RRT: 92% began hemodialysis, 6% began peritoneal dialysis, and 2% underwent renal transplantation as their first modality of RRT. The point prevalence rate for that year was 308,000 patients on dialysis and 122,000 patients with a functioning transplant (see Web Fig. 32–1). The annual cost to Medicare, which covers most of the patients with ESRD in the United States, was $15 billion in 2002.

This distribution of patients on various modalities differs in other countries. Hemodialysis continues to be the most common modality of RRT for patients in the United States. As illustrated in Figure 32–6, blood is pumped from a temporary or permanent vascular access into tubing that leads to a large number of capillaries bundled together in a dialyzer (**Web Fig. 32–4**). The capillaries are made up of semisynthetic materials that are biocompatible. This membrane is semipermeable and is capable of allowing exchange of small molecules across the concentration gradient by diffusion. Moving in the opposite direction to blood is a dialysate solution that is passing through outside the capillaries, thus allowing countercurrent exchange. This solution contains sodium chloride, bicarbonate, and varying concentrations of potassium. Diffusion through the membrane allows low–molecular-weight substances such as urea, potassium, and organic acids to move across according to the concentration gradient. Removal of fluid is achieved by ultrafiltration, which is achieved by applying transmembrane hydrostatic pressure.

Hemodialysis Modalities

In the setting of ESRD, an average patient undergoing hemodialysis requires 4.0 hours of dialysis three times a week to achieve adequate toxin removal. The typical complications associated with dialysis treatments are hypotension and muscle cramping. Avoiding excessive weight gain between treatments can minimize these complications. This process is called *intermittent dialysis,* as is obvious from the frequency of treatments provided per week. The treatment requires a blood flow of approximately 400 mL/min from the access to the dialysis machine. All the fluid gained between two treatments is removed during a short duration. On average, 3 to 4 kg of fluid removal is performed in 4 hours, which makes patients prone to hypotension.

In the setting of acute renal failure, when patients are in an intensive care unit, a continuous modality of hemodialysis can be used called continuous venovenous hemodialysis (CVVHD). In CVVHD, slower blood flow of 100 mL/min is used 24 hours a day to achieve the fluid removal over an extended period. This modality is well tolerated in patients who are critically ill and who are hemodynamically compromised, but it requires a special machine. A hybrid modality called sustained low-efficiency dialysis (SLED) can also be used, which uses a regular intermittent hemodialysis machine. A blood flow rate of 200 mL/min and longer duration of approximately 8 to 12 hours are prescribed to avoid hypotension. SLED obviates the necessity of buying a new machine for the treating facility and training of the intensive care unit staff to monitor CVVHD. Various dialysis modalities are described in **Web Table 32–1.**

Accesses for Hemodialysis

The catheters used for dialysis are associated with high infection rates. Temporary catheters are placed the way central venous lines are placed and can be used for a short time. They can be inserted into internal jugular, subclavian, or femoral veins. Permanent catheters have a cuff around the outer wall of the tubing and tunnel under the chest wall skin for some distance before entering the internal jugular vein. The cuff causes local fibrosis in the subcutaneous tissue, thus sealing the access of skin flora into the catheter and reducing the infection rates. Permanent accesses such as arteriovenous fistulas or arteriovenous grafts are preferred because they provide high blood flow rates and lead to fewer infections. Fistulas are preferred because they reduce the likelihood of clotting or getting stenosis, which causes access failure (**Web Fig. 32–5**).

PERITONEAL DIALYSIS

Peritoneal dialysis is a type of RRT in which the peritoneal capillaries act as a semipermeable membrane similar to a hemodialysis filter. This technique has several advantages because it allows independence from the long time spent in dialysis units, it does not require stringent dietary restrictions as in hemodialysis, and rehabilitation rates are better than those observed in hemodialysis, with more patients returning to full-time employment. Residual renal function is maintained for a longer period (e.g., 1 to 2 years) while the patient is undergoing peritoneal dialysis, thus improving morbidity and mortality. In continuous ambulatory peritoneal dialysis, dialysate of 2- to 3-L volumes is instilled in the peritoneal cavity for varying amounts of time and exchanged four to six times daily. In continuous cyclic peritoneal dialysis, the patient is connected to a machine referred to as a *cycler* that allows inflow of smaller volumes of dialysate with shorter dwell time through the night. This process allows patients to be actively working during the day. Several modifications in this regimen can be made to fit specific patients to achieve adequate clearance. The rate of removal of various solutes depends on the concentration gradient, surface area, and permeability of the peritoneal membrane to the solute. Smaller molecules move across the peritoneal membrane with ease and are influenced by ultrafiltration rates. Ultrafiltration is achieved through increasing dextrose concentration in the dialysate. The two major drawbacks of peritoneal dialysis are peritonitis and difficulty in achieving adequate clearances in patients with excess body mass. Peritonitis in patients undergoing peritoneal dialysis can be treated with intraperitoneal antibiotics, most often as outpatients. Catheter removal is indicated in some cases of peritonitis, for instance, bacterial peritonitis that is not responding to antibiotics and fungal peritonitis. Additionally, a slow deterioration occurs in the permeability of the membrane, leading to inadequate dialysis, hence the need to change the modality of RRT to hemodialysis.

KIDNEY TRANSPLANTATION

Renal transplantation is the preferred modality of RRT, with hemodialysis or peritoneal dialysis often required before, during, or after transplantation. When cyclosporine became available in 1983, the success rate for renal transplantation from deceased donors improved significantly, with an 85%

to 90% 1-year graft survival rate compared with 65% with azathioprine and steroids. A decrease in the incidence of acute rejection has been seen secondary to the introduction of newer immunosuppressive agents that include rapamycin, mycophenolate mofetil, tacrolimus, and anti-interleukin-2–receptor antibodies (daclizumab and basiliximab). This advance has been associated with some improvement in long-term allograft survival.

Deceased Donor Versus Living Donor Kidney Transplantation

Advantages and disadvantages of deceased versus living, related or unrelated, kidney donor transplantation are listed in Table 32–5. Because the deceased donor organ supply fails to meet the demand, the pressure for living kidney donation has increased. Unrelated donors with a stable and close emotional relationship with the recipient, such as a spouse, are considered to be appropriate. Survival of grafts from these unrelated donors is better than survival of grafts from deceased donors, despite less histocompatibility matching of human leukocyte antigen (HLA). Living or deceased donor kidney transplantation should only be performed with ABO blood group–compatible pairs. The main advantages of a living related donor transplant are less ischemic injury and histocompatibility matching. Figure 32–7 is a representation of the inheritance pattern of HLA within a family. HLA-identical matches consistently demonstrate superior graft survival and reduced chance for rejection than less-matched living or deceased donor renal transplants.

Table 32–5 **Comparison of Donor Sources for Kidney Transplantation**	
Advantages	**Disadvantages**
Living Donor	
Better tissue match with less likelihood of rejection	Small potential risk of operation to donor
Smaller doses of drugs for immunosuppression	Requirement of willing, medically suitable family member or other person
Waiting time for transplant reduced	
Sequelae of long-term dialysis avoided	
Elective surgical procedure	
Better early graft function with shorter hospitalization	
Better short-term and long-term success	
Cadaver Donor	
Availability to any recipient	Tissue match not as similar
Availability of other organs for combined transplants (i.e., kidney-pancreas transplant)	Waiting time variable
	Operation performed urgently
Availability of vascular conduits for complex vascular reconstruction	Early graft function possibly compromised
	Short-term and long-term success not as good as from living donor

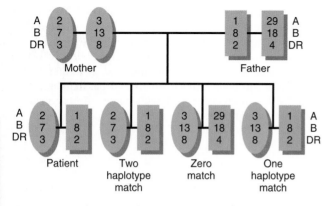

Figure 32–7 Diagrammatic representation of inheritance of human leukocyte antigen (HLA) tissue types in a family with four siblings.

Immunosuppressant Drug Therapy

Prophylaxis against and treatment of graft rejection are at the heart of the success of kidney transplantation. Since the 1960s, the immunosuppressive protocols for renal transplantation have undergone remarkable evolution. All protocols for immunosuppression aim at disruption of the lymphocyte cell cycle. Azathioprine and steroids, with or without antilymphocyte preparations, were the mainstay of clinical immunosuppression in the 1960s and 1970s. Since the introduction of cyclosporine in the early 1980s, the number of drugs capable of suppressing the immune system has increased steadily. These agents, by virtue of their specific mode of action, have succeeded in preventing most patients from having early and irreversible graft rejections without severe toxic effects. The mechanism of action of some of the most commonly used immunosuppressants is illustrated in Figure 32–8.

The hepatic cytochrome P-450 system is essential for cyclosporine, tacrolimus, and rapamycin metabolism. Significant changes in the levels of these drugs may occur when patients start or discontinue taking any of several drugs that can induce or inhibit this system.

Cyclosporine exerts its specific immunosuppressive activity by inhibiting immunocompetent lymphocytes in the G_0 and G_1 phases of the cell cycle. Some of the most important side effects of cyclosporine are listed in Table 32–6, and most respond to an appropriate reduction in the dose. The most significant of these effects is nephrotoxicity, which is usually secondary to decreased glomerular blood flow.

Tacrolimus has a mechanism of action and side effect profile similar to those of cyclosporine but with additional problems of hyperglycemia and an increased tendency toward neurotoxicity.

Mycophenolate mofetil/mycophenolic acid (CellCept/ Myfortic) specifically inhibits T-lymphocyte and B-lymphocyte proliferation by interfering with purine synthesis and thus DNA synthesis. Mycophenolate mofetil has been associated with a 60% to 70% reduction in acute transplant rejection when compared with conventional therapies and thus promotes long-term graft survival.

Rapamycin (sirolimus) is a macrolide antibiotic produced by the fungus *Streptomyces hygroscopicus.* Rapamycin binds to the immunophilins, thus blocking the phosphorylation of *p70(s6)* kinase and the eukaryotic initiation factor-4E-binding protein, *PHAS-I.* This action leads to the dampening of cytokine and growth factor activity on T, B, and nonimmune cells. Rapamycin is used for maintenance immunosuppressive therapy. The major side effects are thrombocytopenia and dyslipidemia (primarily hypertriglyceridemia).

Acute Rejection

T lymphocytes survey the human body and are capable of recognizing foreign antigens when these antigens are presented in association with HLA antigens, especially class II histocompatibility antigens. When the recipient's T-helper cells identify foreign HLA class II antigens presented by dendritic or other antigen-presenting cells in the transplanted kidney, lymphocyte activation results. Activated cytotoxic lymphocytes invade the tubular interstitial region of the transplanted kidney, with resulting tubulitis. Clinically, acute rejection is detected by graft tenderness, rise in serum creatinine levels, oliguria, and, in some instances, fever. Frequent monitoring of renal function has allowed early detection of acute rejection based on rising serum creatinine before any clinical signs or symptoms become apparent. Acute rejection episodes have a negative impact on long-term graft survival. Acute humoral rejection involves the intrarenal arteries and leads to vasculitis, carrying a poor prognosis. This type of rejection is usually resistant to steroids, thus necessitating antilymphocyte therapy.

Post-transplant Infection

Infection is second only to vascular disease as the leading cause of mortality in kidney transplant recipients. In addition to common community-acquired bacterial and viral infections, kidney transplant recipients are also susceptible to numerous viral, fungal, and other opportunistic infections that normally do not cause severe illness in the immunocompetent host. Fortunately, the timetable of these infections is predictable, and an educated guess based on the time of infection after transplantation, together with the specific set of syndromes associated with each infection, can help early recognition and prompt empiric treatment pending confirmatory tests. Figure 32–9 shows the temporal relationship of infections in renal transplantation.

Post-transplant Malignant Disease

Immunosuppression increases the risk of developing malignant disease. Skin cancer (mostly squamous cell) has the highest incidence in transplant recipients as compared with all other types of malignancy. Sun exposure is the most significant risk factor, and skin protection provides excellent primary prevention. With continuous surveillance and aggressive management, metastasis from skin cancers is rare.

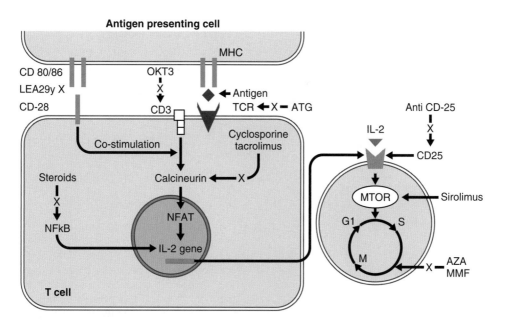

Figure 32–8 Pathways of T-cell activation and site of action of immunosuppressive agents. IL = interleukin.

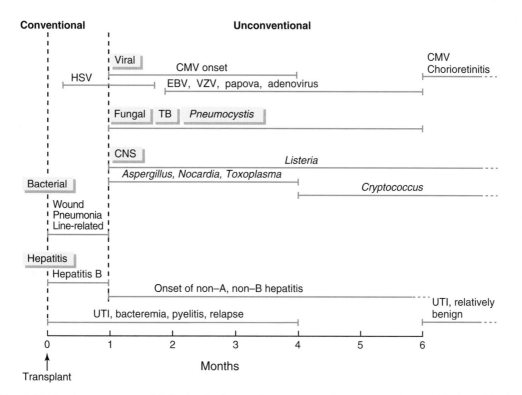

Figure 32–9 Timetable for the occurrence of infection in the renal transplant recipient. Exceptions to this timetable should initiate a search for an unusual hazard. CMV = cytomegalovirus; CNS = central nervous system; EBV = Epstein-Barr virus; HSV = herpes simplex virus; TB = tuberculosis; UTI = urinary tract infection; VZV = varicella-zoster virus. (From Rubin RH, Wolfson JS, Cosimi AB, et al: Infection in the renal transplant recipient. Am J Med 70:405–411, 1981. Copyright 1981 by Excerpta Medica, Inc.)

Table 32-6　Side Effects of Commonly Used Immunosuppressive Drugs

Effect	Corticosteroids	Azathioprine	Cyclosporine	Mycophenolate Mofetil	Tacrolimus	Sirolimus
Renal	Fluid retention		Preglomerular vasoconstriction Striped interstitial fibrosis Hyperkalemia		Preglomerular vasoconstriction Less marked than with cyclosporine Interstitial fibrosis Hyperkalemia Hypomagnesemia	Increased creatinine Peripheral edema
Cardiovascular	Hypertension	—	—	—	—	—
Hematologic	Bone marrow suppression	Macrocytosis	Hemolytic uremic syndrome	Leukopenia Anemia	Hemolytic uremic syndrome	Anemia Leukopenia Thrombocytopenia
Neurologic	Proximal muscle weakness Mood changes Depression	—	Tremor Seizures	—	Headaches Insomnia Paresthesias Pruritus Coarse tremor	Headache Insomnia Tremor
Gastrointestinal	Gastritis	Acute pancreatitis	Cholestasis	Vomiting Diarrhea Abdominal pain CMV invasive gastritis/esophagitis	Nausea Vomiting Diarrhea	Abdominal pain Nausea Vomiting Diarrhea Constipation Dyspepsia
Metabolic	Glucose intolerance Dyslipidemia	—	Dyslipidemia Decreased glucose tolerance	—	Decreased glucose tolerance	Hypercholesterolemia Hyperlipidemia
Dermatologic	Acne Easy bruisability	Alopecia	Hypertrichosis Brittle fingernails	—	Alopecia	Delayed wound healing Rash
Miscellaneous	Osteoporosis Aseptic necrosis Obesity Accelerated cataract formation	—	Gingival hypertrophy	—	—	—

CMV = cytomegalovirus

Transplant recipients are also at high risk of developing non-Hodgkin's lymphoma and Kaposi's sarcoma, a rare occurrence in the immunocompetent host. Cancer surveillance should be an essential part of post-transplant follow-up. Transplant recipients should be educated to recognize and report early changes in bowel habits, respiratory symptoms, hematuria, musculoskeletal symptoms, skin changes, or weight changes.

Prospectus for the Future

In the CKD population, the major challenge will be to slow the progression of kidney disease by identifying novel targets. Serum cystatin-C may be used increasingly as a sensitive marker of kidney function as it correlates better with low GFR. Other efforts include the following:

- The development of an artificial kidney
- Development and transplantation of cultured islet cells with minimized immunosuppression as an acceptable treatment for type 1 diabetes mellitus
- Development of laboratory tests to measure the overall immune-reactivity of solid organ transplant recipients in order to customize treatment protocols without the risk of rejection or opportunistic infections
- Development of new immunosuppressive regimens or therapies to achieve tolerance
- Genetic manipulation of animals to succeed in xenotransplantation

References

Abbate M, Remuzzi G: Progression of renal insufficiency: Mechanisms. In Massry SG, Glassock RJ (eds): Massry and Glassock's Textbook of Nephrology, 4th ed. Philadelphia: Lippincott, Williams & Wilkins, 2001, pp 1210–1217.

American Kidney Foundation: K/DOQI clinical practice guidelines for chronic kidney disease: Evaluation, classification and stratification. Am J Kidney Dis 39(2 suppl 1):S1–S266, 2002.

Halloran PF: Drug therapy: Immunosuppressive drugs for kidney transplantation. N Engl J Med 351(26):2715–2729, 2004.

Luke RG: Chronic renal failure. In Goldman L, Bennett JC (eds): Cecil Textbook of Medicine, 21st ed. Philadelphia: WB Saunders, 2000, pp 571–577.

Rubin RH, Marty FM: Principles of antimicrobial therapy in the transplant patient [Editorial]. Transpl Infect Dis 6(3):97–100, 2004.

Sarnak MJ, Levey AS, Schoolwerth AC et al: Kidney disease as a risk factor for development of cardiovascular disease: A statement from the American Heart Association Councils on Kidney in Cardiovascular Disease, High Blood Pressure Research, Clinical Cardiology, and Epidemiology and Prevention. Circulation 108:2154–2169, 2003.

Section VI

Gastrointestinal Disease

Common Clinical Manifestations of Gastrointestinal Disease

A. Abdominal Pain

Charles M. Bliss, Jr.

M. Michael Wolfe

Abdominal pain is a frequent manifestation of intra-abdominal disease. Abdominal pain is difficult to localize or grade because the sensation of pain is colored by emotional and physical factors. Abdominal pain may be classified as acute or chronic. Acute pain occurs suddenly and suggests serious physiologic alterations. Conversely, chronic pain may be present for several months; although it does not mandate immediate attention, chronic pain may lead to prolonged evaluation. Appropriate evaluation of abdominal pain requires knowledge of pain mechanisms, close attention to history and physical examination findings, and recognition of important accompanying symptoms, as well as awareness of the strengths and weaknesses of the tests that might be used.

Physiology

Abdominal pain results from stimulation of receptors specific for thermal, mechanical, or chemical stimuli. Once these receptors are excited, pain impulses travel through sympathetic fibers. Abdominal pain can be characterized as somatic or visceral. Somatic pain originates from the abdominal wall and parietal peritoneum, whereas visceral pain originates in internal organs and from the visceral peritoneum. Two types of neurons carry pain: A fibers, which have rapid conduction, and C fibers, which have slow conduction. Most visceral neurons are of the C type, and the pain resulting from their stimulation tends to be variable with regard to sensation and localization. In contrast, fibers originating from the parietal peritoneum and abdominal wall are of both the A and the C types, and the pain tends to be sharp and distinctly localized.

Because of this pattern of innervation, abdominal viscera are not sensitive to cutting, tearing, burning, or crushing. However, visceral pain results from stretching of the walls of hollow organs, or of the capsule of solid organs, as well as from inflammation or ischemia.

Causes of Abdominal Pain

Multiple intra-abdominal and extra-abdominal disorders can produce abdominal pain. Distinguishing acute from chronic abdominal pain is helpful. The approach varies with each specific cause, but acute abdominal pain generally demands prompt intervention.

Clinical Features

HISTORY

The differential diagnosis of abdominal pain, whether acute or chronic, requires thorough history taking with regard to pain characteristics, location and radiation, timing, and the presence of any other accompanying symptoms.

Table 33-1   **Key Abdominal Pain Syndromes**

Condition	Type	Location	Radiation
Acute Abdominal Pain			
Appendicitis	Crampy, steady	Periumbilical, RLQ	Back
Cholecystitis	Intermittent, steady	Epigastric, RUQ	Right scapula
Pancreatitis	Steady	Epigastric, periumbilical	Back
Perforation	Sudden, severe	Epigastric	Entire abdomen
Obstruction	Crampy	Periumbilical	Back
Infarction	Severe, diffuse	Periumbilical	Entire abdomen
Chronic Abdominal Pain			
Esophagitis	Burning	Retrosternal	Left arm, back
Peptic ulcer	Gnawing	Epigastric	Back
Dyspepsia	Bloating, dull	Epigastric	None
IBS	Crampy	LLQ, RLQ	None

IBS = irritable bowel syndrome; LLQ = left lower quadrant; RLQ = right lower quadrant; RUQ = right upper quadrant.

Pain location often indicates the organ responsible for the problem. For instance, epigastric pain is usually typical of peptic ulcer or dyspepsia, whereas right upper quadrant pain is more suggestive of cholecystitis and other biliary disorders. Early in the course of illness, pain may be perceived in one location and subsequently be felt in another; this pattern of progression may be suggestive of specific pain syndromes. In acute cases, abdominal pain tends to be sharp and severe. The pain of a perforated viscus is intense, and the pain from a dissecting aneurysm may be described as tearing or crushing. Chronic pain may be less severe; pain from irritable bowel or dyspepsia is constant and dull, and the pain of chronic peptic ulcer is described as gnawing or hunger pain. The pattern of pain relief is helpful for diagnosing some conditions. The physician should also inquire about whether pain is steady or intermittent and whether it occurs at night. For nocturnal pain, a distinction should be made between pain that awakens the patient and pain that is felt when the patient wakes up for other reasons.

Table 33-1 outlines characteristics, location, and radiation of pain for a few common acute and chronic abdominal conditions.

PHYSICAL EXAMINATION

Examination of the abdomen may provide invaluable clues to the diagnosis, but the examination should start with the general appearance of the patient. A patient writhing in bed and unable to find a comfortable position may be suffering from obstruction. In contrast, a patient lying with the lower extremities flexed and avoiding any motion may be suffering from peritonitis. Abdominal distention indicates obstruction or ascites. Visual inspection for peristalsis is helpful for the diagnosis of small bowel obstruction, but this sign is present only in the early stages. Focal areas of disten-

tion may indicate hernias; note should also be made of any scars from previous surgery.

Auscultation should be performed in several areas to evaluate the timber and pattern of bowel sounds, as well as to search for bruits or hums. Absence of bowel sounds suggests ileus, whereas the presence of hyperactive, high-pitched sounds may indicate obstruction. Multiple bruits alert the examiner to the possibility of significant vascular disease, suggesting ischemia.

The abdomen should be palpated gently, starting in an area away from the area of pain. The physician searches for areas of localized tenderness and rebound, as well as for masses and enlarged organs. Percussion is performed to identify size of organs or to determine the presence of ascites. Pain on percussion of the abdomen indicates peritoneal reaction, as does severe rebound tenderness.

A rectal examination is important for identifying a rectal tumor in the case of colon obstruction or tenderness high in the rectum in acute appendicitis. Pelvic examination should be performed in women to rule out pelvic inflammatory disease.

Acute Abdomen

The acute abdomen is a challenging condition in medical practice. The first question to be answered is whether immediate surgery is needed. Therefore, a quick evaluation is necessary to avoid undue delay in intervention for patients who require surgery. Early surgical consultation should be obtained, even in doubtful cases, rather than awaiting confirmation of the diagnosis via laboratory or radiologic studies.

The acute abdomen is caused by sudden inflammation, perforation, obstruction, or infarction of various intra-abdominal organs. However, many extra-abdominal conditions such as pneumonia, myocardial infarction, nephrolithiasis, and metabolic disorders may cause acute abdominal pain.

In some instances, the acute abdomen, in its early stages, may show few findings. The examiner should be aware that patients with benign chronic conditions might come to the emergency department with severe pain that is out of proportion to any physical findings. With the acute abdomen, inquiring about medical history, particularly previous abdominal surgery, is important. Indeed, a patient with sudden crampy pain and abdominal distention may have intestinal obstruction caused by adhesions or an incarcerated hernia. Performing an entire examination of the patient, looking for jaundice, skin lesions, or evidence of chronic liver disease, is also important.

A complete blood cell count with differential, a urinalysis, and measurements of serum amylase, lipase, bilirubin, and electrolytes are necessary components of the laboratory examination. Additional studies may be done but usually do not aid in the rapid decision making required in the evaluation of the acute abdomen. An elevated white blood cell count may indicate inflammatory disease, and extremely high values are quite typical of acute intestinal ischemia. An elevated serum amylase concentration usually indicates acute pancreatitis, although a perforated ulcer or mesenteric thrombosis may also cause hyperamylasemia.

Radiographic examination is an important part of the evaluation of the patient with an acute abdomen. An abdominal film is important in revealing the intra-abdominal gas pattern, and an upright film that includes the diaphragm or left lateral decubitus film may identify intra-abdominal air. Ultrasonography can be helpful in the diagnosis of acute cholecystitis or appendicitis. Computed tomography (CT) scans have become more helpful with technologic improvements in scanners; early CT scans allow prompt diagnosis of sometimes unsuspected abdominal diseases. Examination with a radiopaque medium should be used judiciously, especially if surgery is anticipated. **Web Figures 33–1 through 33–4** are CT images of appendicitis, diverticulitis, pancreatitis, and ulcerative colitis.

Chronic Abdominal Pain

Chronic abdominal pain poses a challenge for the physician to distinguish organic pain resulting from a specific pathologic process from functional pain. The location and characteristics of pain, as already discussed, serve as important guides, as do other accompanying symptoms. The presence of postprandial nausea and vomiting suggests chronic peptic ulcer, disorders of gastric emptying, or outlet obstruction. The documentation of weight loss mandates the search for an organic cause, such as inflammatory bowel disease or celiac disease. If anorexia accompanies weight loss, particularly in elderly patients, cancer must be excluded. If no cancer can be found and all objective tests are normal, the possibility of chronic depression must be entertained.

The most frequent causes of chronic abdominal pain are *functional*. Dyspepsia is characterized by chronic intermittent epigastric discomfort, sometimes accompanied by nausea or bloating. These symptoms are not always relieved by acid suppression and may be the result of an underlying motor disorder. Furthermore, the eradication of *Helicobacter pylori (H. pylori)*, when found in a patient with dyspeptic symptoms, may not necessarily lead to the resolution of symptoms. Controversy thus presently exists regarding the most effective strategy for the treatment of dyspepsia when *H. pylori* are found in the absence of peptic ulcer disease.

Irritable bowel syndrome (IBS) is a common disorder. Estimates are that 15% of Americans suffer from IBS on a regular basis and that 40% to 50% of referrals to gastroenterologists are related to IBS. The syndrome consists of abdominal distention, flatulence, and disordered bowel function. The abdominal pain of IBS tends to be in the left lower quadrant, but it can be located elsewhere or be more generalized. Any patient with weight loss, anemia, nocturnal symptoms, steatorrhea, or onset of symptoms after age 50 should be carefully evaluated for organic disease. The Rome criteria, developed for research studies, may be helpful in the diagnosis of IBS. These criteria include pain associated with change in bowel habits, relieved with defecation or accompanied by distention or bloating. Patients are reassured, counseled, and treated with anticholinergic agents and stool softeners. Alosetron, a serotonin 5 HT_3 antagonist, has been shown to help relieve symptoms in patients with diarrhea-predominant IBS. Tegaserod, a serotonin 5 HT_4 agonist, has been found to be effective in relieving pain and constipation in constipation-predominant IBS and has recently been approved for use in both men and women.

The more challenging clinical problem is the one of functional abdominal pain syndrome. This term describes a condition in which the pain has been present for months or years. The complaints of pain are often not related to eating, defecation, or menses, unlike other causes of chronic pain. The patient is likely to be a woman who has undergone numerous examinations and diagnostic studies with negative findings and, in many cases, surgical operations without any relief. Lengthy or repeated diagnostic work-ups are counterproductive and only convince the patient that one more test is what is needed to determine the source of the pain. The physician must establish that organic disease is not present and must also realize that the pain is real. The patients are not malingerers in spite of the fact that the pain does not fit any familiar pattern. Depression may be the result rather than the cause of the pain.

Chronic abdominal pain is a clinical situation requiring as much tact, diplomacy, and compassion as it does scientific knowledge. An effort should be made to inquire about social factors, including history of physical and sexual abuse, particularly in women. Psychiatric evaluation may be necessary, but the suggestion for such a consultation may be interpreted by the patient as a belief from the physician that the "pain is in my head." A referral to a competent pain management specialist is helpful in a certain number of cases. This approach offers the possibility of providing relief with nerve blocks when the pain is localized or other pain relieving devices. If this approach fails, referral to a psychologist or psychiatrist may be acceptable to the patient.

For a practical approach to chronic abdominal pain, see the algorithm in Figure 33–1.

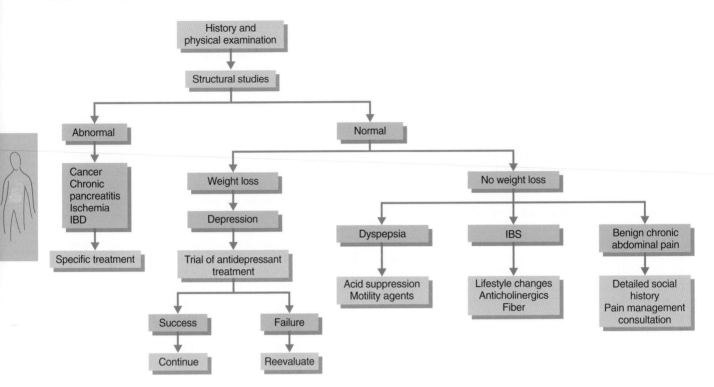

Figure 33–1 Approach to the patient with chronic abdominal pain. IBD = inflammatory bowel disease; IBS = irritable bowel syndrome.

References

Chang L, Ameen VZ, Dukes GE, et al: A dose-ranging, phase II study of the efficacy and safety of alosetron in men with diarrhea-predominant IBS. Am J Gastroenterol 100:115–123, 2005.

Drossman DA: Functional abdominal pain syndrome. Clin Gastroenterol Hepatol 2:353–365, 2004.

Johanson JF, Wald A, Tougas G, et al: Effect of tegaserod in chronic constipation: A randomized, double-blind, controlled trial. Clin Gastroenterol Hepatol 2:796–805, 2004.

Lembo A, Ameen VZ, Drossman DA: Irritable bowel syndrome: Toward an understanding of severity. Clin Gastroenterol Hepatol 3:717–725, 2005.

Ng CS, Watson CJE, Palmer CR, et al: Evaluation of early abdominopelvic computed tomography in patients with acute abdominal pain of unknown cause: Prospective randomized study. BMJ 325:1387–1390, 2002.

B. Gastrointestinal Hemorrhage

Chi-Chuan Tseng

M. Michael Wolfe

Acute Gastrointestinal Hemorrhage

Acute gastrointestinal (GI) bleeding remains a common and major medical problem, despite recent advances in diagnosis and treatment. Bleeding occurs as the result of different diseases, and adequate treatment depends on assessing hemodynamic stability, determining severity of blood lost, and identifying sources of bleeding. Although advancements in intensive medical and surgical care, pharmacologic therapy, and the prompt deployment of endoscopic therapies have significantly decreased the rate of rebleeding, the overall mortality rate from acute bleeding episode has remained essentially unchanged during the last half century and remains approximately 7% to 10% because of an aging population and an increased prevalence of serious concomitant illnesses.

PRESENTATION OF GASTROINTESTINAL BLEEDING

If massive GI bleeding occurs, patients generally exhibit weakness, dizziness, lightheadedness, shortness of breath, postural changes in blood pressure or pulse, cramping abdominal pain, and diarrhea. The characteristics of bleeding may help localize the source of bleeding to the upper or lower GI tract. Patients with acute bleeding commonly exhibit one of the following symptoms.

Hematemesis

The patient usually exhibits vomiting of bright red blood or of material that resembles coffee grounds. After excluding swallowed blood from the nasopharynx or secondary to hemoptysis, the source of bleeding is likely proximal to the ligament of Treitz.

Melena

As little as 50 to 100 mL of blood in the stomach can produce melena. Black, tarry, usually foul-smelling stools are most often a manifestation of upper GI bleeding; however, a small bowel or proximal colonic source of bleeding may, on occasion, lead to melenic stools.

Hematochezia

The passage of bright red blood or maroon stools per rectum frequently indicates a lower GI source of bleeding. However, approximately 10% to 15% of patients with acute severe hematochezia have an upper GI source of bleeding. This group of patients commonly displays signs of hemodynamic instability.

ETIOLOGY OF GASTROINTESTINAL BLEEDING

A major goal during early management of bleeding is to distinguish between upper and lower GI bleeding. In addition to the symptoms and signs stated previously, certain aspects of the history, physical examination, laboratory studies, and age of the patient may assist in localizing the site of bleeding. However, determining the site of bleeding is frequently not possible after initial evaluation. Common sources of acute GI hemorrhage are listed in Table 33–2.

APPROACH TO THE PATIENT WITH ACUTE GASTROINTESTINAL BLEEDING

Assessment of Vital Signs and Resuscitation

The first step in the evaluation and therapy for the patient with acute GI hemorrhage is to determine the severity of blood loss. Vital signs with postural changes should be recorded immediately. If the systolic blood pressure drops more than 10 mm Hg and/or the pulse increases more than 10 beats per minute as the patient changes positions from supine to standing, the patient has likely lost at least 800 mL (15%) of circulating blood volume. Hypotension, tachycardia, tachypnea, and mental status changes in the setting of acute GI hemorrhage suggest at least a 1500-mL (30%) loss of circulating blood volume (Fig. 33–2).

The goal of resuscitation is to restore the normal circulatory volume and to prevent complications from red blood cell loss, such as cardiac, pulmonary, renal, or neurologic consequences. Initially, at least two large-bore intravenous catheters are used to administer isotonic solutions (e.g., lactated Ringer's solution, 0.9% sodium chloride [NaCl]), and blood products, if indicated. If the patient is in shock, central venous access should be established. The amount of blood products to be transfused must be individualized, and in view of a potential risk of blood transfusion, simply transfusing until an arbitrary hematocrit level is achieved is inappropriate. If coagulation studies are abnormal, as commonly observed in cirrhotic patients, fresh frozen plasma and/or platelets may be required to control ongoing hemorrhage.

Initial Evaluation

As the patient is being fluid resuscitated, the following information should be obtained by history and physical examination to determine the source of bleeding:

1. The nature of bleeding: melena, hematemesis, hematochezia, or occult blood. A digital rectal examination is essential for the determination of stool color and the identification of anal fissures or rectal neoplasms.
2. The duration of GI bleeding, which helps dictate the appropriate pace of the evaluation to determine the bleeding source.
3. The presence or absence of abdominal pain; for example, hematochezia caused by diverticula or angiodysplasia is typically painless, but when caused by ischemia, it may be accompanied by abdominal pain.
4. Other associated symptoms, including fever, urgency and/or tenesmus, recent change in bowel habits, and weight loss.
5. Current or recent medication use, particularly nonsteroidal anti-inflammatory drugs (NSAIDs) or aspirin, which may predispose to ulceration or gastritis (see Chapter 36), anticoagulants, and alcohol. Many over-the-counter products may contain aspirin or NSAIDs.
6. Relevant medical and surgical history, including a history of GI bleeding, abdominal surgery (prior abdominal aorta repair should raise suspicion for an aortoenteric fistula), history of radiation therapy (radiation proctitis), history of major organ disease (including cardiopulmonary, hepatic, or renal disease), history of inflammatory bowel diseases, and recent polypectomy (postpolypectomy bleeding).

The physical examination must include an assessment of vital signs, cardiac and pulmonary examination, and abdominal and digital rectal examination. The initial laboratory examination should include complete blood cell count, blood typing, and cross-matching, as well as measurements of serum electrolytes, blood urea nitrogen, creatinine, and coagulation factors. The first hematocrit measurement may not reflect the degree of blood loss, but it will decrease gradually to a stable level over 24 to 48 hours.

The initial disposition of the patient must also be considered. Patients over age 60 years, those with severe blood

Table 33–2 Common Sources of Acute Gastrointestinal Hemorrhage

Source	Associated Clinical Features	Treatments
Upper Gastrointestinal Tract		
Esophagitis	Heartburn, dysphagia, odynophagia	Medication*
		Antireflux surgery or procedures
Esophageal cancer	Progressive dysphagia, weight loss	Chemoradiotherapy, surgery
		Palliative endoscopy procedures
Gastritis, gastric ulcer	Aspirin, NSAID use	Withdraw NSAIDs
Duodenitis, duodenal ulcer	Abdominal pain, dyspepsia	Medication†
	Helicobacter pylori infection	Endoscopic therapy for acute bleeding
Gastric cancer	Early satiety, weight loss, abdominal pain	Surgery, chemotherapy
Esophagogastric varices	History of CLD	Variceal banding, sclerotherapy
	Stigmata of CLD on examination	Vasopressin, octreotide
		TIPS or decompressive surgery
Mallory-Weiss tear	History of retching before hematemesis	Supportive (usually self limited)
		Endoscopic therapy
Lower Gastrointestinal Tract		
Infection	History of exposure, diarrhea, fever	Supportive, antibiotics
Inflammatory bowel diseases	History of colitis, diarrhea, abdominal pain, fever	Steroids, 5-ASA, immunotherapy
		Surgery if unresponsive to medication
Diverticula	Painless hematochezia	Supportive
		Surgery for recurrent disease
Angiodysplasia	Painless hematochezia	Endoscopic therapy
	Often in ascending colon	Supportive
Commonly involves stomach and small bowel as well	Surgery for localized disease	
Colon cancer	Change in bowel habit, anemia, weight loss	Surgery
Colon polyp	Usually asymptomatic	Endoscopic or surgical removal
Ischemic colitis	Typically elderly patients	Supportive (self limited)
	History of vascular disease	
	May produce abdominal pain	
Meckel's diverticulum	Painless hematochezia in young patient	Surgery
	Located at distal ileum	
Hemorrhoids	Rectal bleeding associated with bowel movement	Supportive
		Surgery, banding

*Proton pump inhibitors or histamine$_2$ receptor antagonists.
†Proton pump inhibitors or histamine$_2$ receptor antagonists in the absence of *H. pylori* infection; various combinations of antibiotics, proton pump inhibitors, and bismuth products in the presence of *H. pylori* infection.
CLD = chronic liver disease; NSAIDs = nonsteroidal anti-inflammatory drugs; TIPS = transjugular intrahepatic shunt; 5-ASA = 5-aminosalicylic acid compounds.

loss or with continued bleeding (as reflected by a significant decrease in hematocrit or postural changes in blood pressure or pulse rate), and those with significant co-morbid illness are at the greatest risk of complications of GI hemorrhage and are best managed in an intensive care setting until stabilized.

Identification of the Bleeding Source

In approximately 80% to 90% of cases, acute GI hemorrhage resolves spontaneously without recurrence. Nevertheless, localizing the bleeding source is prudent because proper identification allows for direct treatment in cases in which bleeding does not spontaneously resolve and allows for the identification of the patient at risk for further bleeding. For

example, in the patient with a bleeding duodenal ulcer, various stigmata of hemorrhage may be identified within the ulcer crater during endoscopy. These signs include active bleeding, a pigmented protuberance (artery visible within the ulcer crater), and clot over the ulcer. The patient with a *clean base*, in which no such stigmata are found, has an excellent prognosis for cessation of bleeding. The patient with an actively bleeding ulcer or visible artery without active bleeding is extremely likely (>50% chance) to have continued bleeding. Furthermore, the site of bleeding may be injected with vasoconstrictors or sclerosants or may be cauterized at the time of endoscopy, all of which decrease the need for transfusion, the need for surgery, and length of hospital stay.

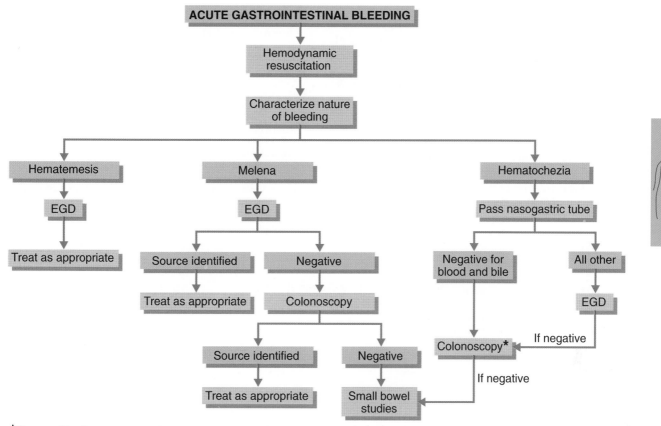

ACUTE GASTROINTESTINAL BLEEDING

*If severe bleeding prevents endoscopic visualization, arteriography may be performed.

Figure 33–2 Approach to the patient with acute gastrointestinal bleeding. EGD = esophagogastroduodenoscopy.

An approach to the patient with acute GI bleeding is outlined in Figure 33–2. Historical points and objective findings often enable localization of the bleeding site to the upper GI tract (proximal to the ligament of Treitz) or to the lower GI tract (distal to that point). For the patient with melena or hematemesis, the upper GI tract should be examined first. Patients with hematochezia more commonly have lower GI bleeding, but when the pace of bleeding is brisk, an upper GI tract lesion may reveal hematochezia. Placement of a nasogastric tube with aspiration of contents is a reasonable first step. The absence of blood does not by itself rule out the presence of an upper GI source because blood from a duodenal bulb ulcer may not flow back into the stomach and allow for sampling by the nasogastric tube. In general, in patients who have acute GI hemorrhage and significant blood loss, an upper endoscopy should be the initial step in the evaluation. Once the lower GI tract has been identified as the source of bleeding, sigmoidoscopy or colonoscopy is the test of choice. In cases of lower GI bleeding in which the pace of bleeding is so brisk as to preclude endoscopic visualization of the colon and rectum, scintigraphic Technetium-99m (^{99m}Tc)-sulfur colloid– or ^{99m}Tc-pertechnetate–labeled erythrocyte scans can localize the bleeding site if the rate of blood loss exceeds 0.5 mL per minute. However, the bleeding site identified by scintigraphic examination may not be accurate, but it will direct visceral arteriographic search while minimizing the dye

used. Barium studies have *no* role in the evaluation of acute GI hemorrhage.

Chronic Gastrointestinal Hemorrhage

Chronic GI hemorrhage may exhibit self-limited, recurrent episodes of melena or hematochezia, usually not with the degree of hemodynamic compromise discussed earlier. Patients may also have no overt evidence of blood loss but may have persistent anemia and consistent occult blood loss.

The evaluation of this condition differs from that of acute GI hemorrhage. Obviously, the pace of the evaluation is less urgent by comparison. Furthermore, the likely causes for this bleeding differ from those of acute GI bleeding. Patients with this condition usually have undergone upper and lower endoscopies at least once, with no bleeding source identified. Therefore, the bleeding either must have an upper GI tract or colonic source that is difficult to identify or that emanates from the small intestine. The small intestine is a difficult area to examine in this regard because of its length and configuration. In general, the small intestine is initially evaluated radiographically. The patient may ingest barium, which is followed through the length of the small intestine. To distend the small bowel and give greater mucosal detail, an enteroclysis tube may be placed with its distal tip near the ligament of Treitz, allowing more forceful administration of barium and air. This type of study has limited diagnostic utility because flat mucosal lesions such as vascular ectasias, a common cause of obscure bleeding, may easily be missed. Endoscopic evaluation may be attempted by push or double-balloon enteroscopy or with newer *capsule endoscopy* (see Chapter 34). For the patient with persistent blood loss, no source of bleeding in the upper GI tract or colon as determined by endoscopy, and negative findings on radiologic studies, the entire small intestine may be examined at laparotomy with endoscopy in the operative suite. In addition, angiographic evaluation of the whole GI tract may reveal the source of chronic blood loss.

References

Barkum A, Bardou M, Marshall JK: Consensus recommendations for managing patients with nonvariceal upper gastrointestinal bleeding. Ann Intern Med 139:843–857, 2003.

Bounds BC, Friedman LS: Lower gastrointestinal bleeding. Gastroenterol Clin of North Am 32:1107–1125, 2003.

Huang CS, Lichtenstein DR: Nonvariceal upper gastrointestinal bleeding. Gastroenterol Clin North Am 32:1053–1078, 2003.

Manning-Dimmitt LL, Dimmitt SG, Wilson GR: Diagnosis of gastrointestinal bleeding in adults. Am Fam Phys 71:1339–1346, 2005.

Marek TA: Gastrointestinal bleeding. Endoscopy 35:891–901, 2003.

Mitchell SH, Schasfer DC, Dubagunta S: A new view of occult and obscure gastrointestinal bleeding. Am Fam Phy 69:875–881, 2004.

Rupp T, Singh S, Waggenspack W: Gastrointestinal hemorrhage: The prehospital recognition, assessment, and management of patients with GI bleed. J Emerg Med Serv 29:80–95, 2004.

C. Malabsorption

Elihu M. Schimmel

The main purpose of the GI tract is the digestion and absorption of major nutrients (fat, carbohydrate, and protein), essential micronutrients (vitamins and trace minerals), water, and electrolytes. Digestion involves both mechanical and enzymatic breakdown of food. Mechanical processes include chewing, gastric churning, and the to-and-fro mixing in the small intestine. Enzymatic hydrolysis is initiated by intraluminal processes requiring gastric, pancreatic, and biliary secretions and is completed at the intestinal brush border. The final products of digestion are absorbed through the intestinal epithelial cells. The regulation of gastric emptying, normal intestinal progression, and adequate intestinal surface area are additional important factors.

Most food components can be absorbed throughout the length of the small intestine but some can be absorbed only at specific areas (e.g., vitamin B_{12} and cholesterol are absorbed only in the terminal ileum). Several molecules undergo an enterohepatic circulation with release into and reabsorption from the intestine, notably the bile acids needed for fat absorption. The primary absorptive function of the colon is the absorption of water and electrolytes; in addition, colonic salvage of much of the carbohydrate from indigestible fiber occurs through bacterial enzymatic activity. This section discusses normal assimilation of the major nutrients and the approach to patients with maldigestion or malabsorption.

Digestion and Absorption of Fat

Dietary fat is composed predominantly of triglycerides (~95%) with long-chain fatty acids (16- and 18-carbon-length molecules). In animal fat, the constituent fatty acids are mostly saturated (e.g., palmitic and stearic), whereas those of vegetable origin are rich in unsaturated fatty acids (i.e., having one or more double bond in the carbon chain, e.g., oleic and linoleic acids). Fats are insoluble (hydrophobic), and digestion begins with emulsification (i.e., fat droplets are dispersed in the aqueous medium of the lumen). Bile salts and pancreatic enzymes are bound to the surface of these globules by colipase, resulting in the release of fatty acids and a monoglyceride. These substances are taken up as mixed micelles with bile salts, allowing these hydrophobic particles to cross the unstirred water layer that overlies the epithelial brush border. Within the cell, the fatty acids are resynthesized into triglycerides and, together with cholesterol and phospholipids, are packaged into chylomicrons and very-low-density lipoproteins (VLDLs) to be exported via lymphatic channels. Bile salts that remain in the lumen are recycled into new micelles and are finally reabsorbed in the terminal ileum with 95% efficiency. Most dietary lipids are absorbed in the jejunum, together with the fat-soluble vitamins (A, D, E, and K). Whereas fat constitutes 40% to 45% of diet calories in developed countries, a goal of 35% or less is set as a dietary recommendation for reduction of risk from cardiac disease and some cancers.

Digestion and Absorption of Carbohydrates

The bulk of dietary carbohydrates consists of starch, a glucose polymer, and the disaccharides sucrose and lactose, but only monosaccharides are absorbed. Salivary and pancreatic amylases release oligosaccharides from starch, and the final hydrolysis to glucose monomers occurs at the brush border, including disaccharide hydrolysis by sucrase and lactase. Glucose and galactose are actively transported in conjunction with sodium, whereas fructose absorption occurs by facilitated diffusion. Approximately one half of dietary energy is ordinarily derived from carbohydrate, with a nutritional goal of 55%, and an increased component of insoluble fiber (i.e., that which is indigestible by mammalian enzymes but variably broken down by colonic bacteria).

Digestion and Absorption of Proteins

Dietary proteins are the major source for amino acids and the only source for the essential amino acids. Digestion starts in the stomach with pepsins secreted by the gastric mucosa, but most of the hydrolysis is accomplished by pancreatic enzymes in the proximal small bowel. The pancreas secretes the proteases trypsin, elastase, chymotrypsin, and carboxypeptidase as inactive proenzymes. Enterokinase (more properly termed *enteropeptidase*) is secreted by the intestinal brush border and splits trypsinogen to its active form, trypsin, which, in turn, converts the other proenzymes to their active forms. The products of luminal brush border peptidase digestion consist of amino acids and oligopep-

tides, which are transported across the epithelial cell. The transfer of most amino acids is sodium dependent and takes place in the proximal small bowel. Dietary need for amino acid nitrogen is met with about 15% of calories from protein.

Mechanisms of Malabsorption

The term *maldigestion* refers to defective hydrolysis of nutrients, whereas *malabsorption* refers to impaired mucosal absorption. In clinical practice, however, malabsorption refers to all aspects of impaired nutrient assimilation. Malabsorption can involve multiple nutrients or be more selective, and the clinical manifestations of malabsorption are thus highly variable. The complete process of absorption consists of a *luminal phase,* in which various nutrients are hydrolyzed and solubilized; a *mucosal phase,* in which further processing takes place at the brush border of the epithelial cell with subsequent transfer into the cell; and a *transport phase,* in which nutrients are moved from the epithelium to the portal venous or lymphatic circulation. Impairment in any of these phases can result in malabsorption (Table 33–3).

Table 33–3　Pathophysiologic Mechanisms in Malabsorption

Luminal Phase	Mucosal Phase	Transport Phase
Reduced nutrient availability	Extensive mucosal loss (resection or infarction)	Vascular conditions (vasculitis; atheroma)
Cofactor deficiency (pernicious anemia; gastric surgery)	Diffuse mucosal disease (celiac sprue)	Lymphatic conditions (lymphangiectasia; irradiation; nodal tumor, cavitation, or infiltrations)
Nutrient consumption (bacterial overgrowth)	Crohn's disease; irradiation; infection; infiltrations; drugs: alcohol, colchicine, neomycin, iron salts	
Impaired fat solubilization	Brush border hydrolase deficiency (lactase deficiency)	
Reduced bile salt synthesis (hepatocellular disease)	Transport defects (Hartnup cystinuria; vitamin B_{12} and folate uptake)	
Impaired bile salt secretion (chronic cholestasis)	Epithelial processing (abetalipoproteinemia)	
Bile salt inactivation (bacterial overgrowth)		
Impaired CCK release (mucosal disease)		
Increased bile salt losses (terminal ileal disease or resection)		
Defective nutrient hydrolysis		
Lipase inactivation (ZE syndrome)		
Enzyme deficiency (pancreatic insufficiency or cancer)		
Improper mixing or rapid transit (resection; bypass; hyperthyroidism)		

Adapted from Riley SA, Marsh MN: Maldigestion and malabsorption. In Feldman M, Scharschmidt BF, Sleisenger MH (eds): Sleisenger and Fordtran's Gastrointestinal and Liver Disease: Pathophysiology/Diagnosis/Management, 6th ed. Philadelphia: WB Saunders, 1998, pp 1501–1522.
CCK = cholecystokinin; ZE = Zollinger-Ellison.

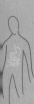

LUMINAL PHASE

Digestion is accomplished for the most part by pancreatic enzymes, particularly lipase, colipase, and trypsin; the gastric digestive enzymes do not play a major role. As a consequence, chronic pancreatitis can result in malabsorption, particularly for fat and protein. Deficiency in bile salts also contributes to fat malabsorption and may be the result of cholestatic liver disorders (impaired secretion of bile), bacterial overgrowth (resulting in luminal bile salt deconjugation), or ileal disease or resection (with loss of effective enterohepatic circulation of the bile acids). The major part of digestion occurs in the duodenum and most proximal jejunum.

MUCOSAL PHASE

Mucosal disease is a common cause of malabsorption and can occur because of diffuse small intestinal disease, such as in celiac sprue or Crohn's disease, or from a decrease of surface area (e.g., after surgical resection for small bowel infarction). Selective defects in an otherwise normal intestine may result in specific entities such as lactase deficiency or abetalipoproteinemia.

TRANSPORT PHASE

After absorption, nutrients leave the cells through venous or lymphatic channels. Consequently, malabsorption may occur after mesenteric venous obstruction, lymphangiectasia, or lymphatic obstruction from malignancy or infiltrative processes (such as Whipple's disease).

Multiple Mechanisms

Occasional disorders can impair the absorptive process at many stages. For example, patients with subtotal gastrectomy often have malabsorption. Resultant defects can be found at all phases: impaired gastric churning, premature emptying, and impaired mixing (in the jejunum) of food with bile and pancreatic enzymes. The last of these defects is a consequence of anatomic changes (gastrojejunostomy bypassing the duodenum) and reduced production of pancreatic enzymes (given that cholecystokinin and secretin release is blunted when gastric contents bypass the duodenum.) Finally, stasis may lead to bacterial overgrowth in the afferent loop, with changes in the bile acids needed for fat absorption. Another example of manifold mechanisms is diabetes mellitus, with delayed gastric emptying, abnormal intestinal motility, bacterial overgrowth, and pancreatic exocrine insufficiency.

Clinical Manifestations of Malabsorption

The clinical manifestations of malabsorption are usually nonspecific. A change in bowel movements—usually diarrhea—and weight loss may occur early. Later, symptoms and signs of nutrient deficiency develop. Muscle wasting and edema result from protein malabsorption. Nutritional anemia, caused by iron and vitamin deficiencies (folate and

B_{12}), contributes to fatigue. Bleeding tendency, such as ecchymosis, may be attributed to prolonged prothrombin time (high international normalized ratio) from vitamin-K deficiency. Bulky, oily stools are the hallmark of steatorrhea resulting from fat malabsorption, whereas bloating (abdominal distention) and soft diarrheal movements occur as a result of carbohydrate malabsorption. Signs associated with malabsorption are presented in Table 33–4.

Clinical Tests for Malabsorption

Blood assays of albumin, carotene, cholesterol, calcium, and folic acid and assessment of the prothrombin time are useful screening studies for malabsorption. These tests are helpful in assessing the severity of malabsorption but are not specific for the differential diagnosis. Many tests are available in the work-up of malabsorption; those that have been most useful clinically are discussed later in this section.

FECAL FAT ANALYSIS

The simplest qualitative method for detecting stool fat is the microscopic examination of a Sudan stain of a drop of stool. Sensitivity is limited, but it is quick and easy, and it correlates well with the quantitative measurement of fecal fat when moderate to severe steatorrhea is present. To quantify fat, stool is collected for 3 consecutive days while the patient is on a diet containing 100 g of fat per day, and the specimen is analyzed for fat content. Normal fat excretion should not exceed 6 g/day. Although the test is cumbersome and nonspecific, it offers an accurate quantification of fecal fat excretion, provided fat consumption is appropriate.

TESTS OF PANCREATIC EXOCRINE FUNCTION

Intubation study of the duodenum with a fluoroscopically placed double-lumen tube may be the best index of pancreatic exocrine function. After stimulation of the pancreas, duodenal contents are aspirated and analyzed for bicarbonate and enzyme output. The test is invasive and time consuming; much experience is needed for its accurate interpretation; and it remains more of a research tool than a useful clinical test. The measurement of pancreatic enzymes in the blood (trypsinogen) or in the stool (chymotrypsin or elastase) is simple and provides helpful laboratory evidence for the diagnosis of moderate to severe pancreatitis. Pancreatic calcifications seen on abdominal films or CT scan indicate the presence of chronic pancreatitis. Abnormal ductal anatomy can be demonstrated by an endoscopic retrograde cholangiopancreatography (ERCP), but this test is invasive and has significant adverse side effects. Magnetic resonance cholangiopancreatography is a less sensitive, but noninvasive, imaging procedure that may supplement the ERCP for diagnostic purposes.

SMALL INTESTINAL BIOPSY

Peroral small intestinal mucosal biopsy is a key diagnostic test for diseases that affect the cellular phase of absorption.

Table 33–4 Signs Associated with Malabsorption Syndromes

Gastrointestinal Signs

Mass	Crohn's disease, lymphoma, tuberculosis, glands
Distention	Intestinal obstruction, gas, ascites, pseudocyst (pancreatic), motility disorder
Steatorrheic stool	Mucosal disease, bacterial overgrowth, pancreatic insufficiency, infective and/or inflammatory, drug induced

Extraintestinal Signs

Skin

Nonspecific	Pigmentation, thinning, inelasticity, reduced subcutaneous fat
Specific	Blisters (dermatitis herpetiformis), erythema nodosum (Crohn's disease), petechiae (vitamin-K deficiency), edema (hypoproteinemia)

Hair

Alopecia	Gluten sensitivity
Loss or thinning	Generalized inanition, hypothyroidism, gluten sensitivity

Eyes

Conjunctivitis, episcleritis	Crohn's disease, Behçet's syndrome
Paleness	Severe anemia

Mouth

Aphthous ulcers	Crohn's disease, gluten sensitivity, Behçet's syndrome
Glossitis	Deficiencies of vitamin B_{12}, iron, folate, niacin
Angular cheilosis	Deficiencies of vitamin B_{12}, iron, folate, B complex
Dental hypoplasia (pitting, dystrophy)	Gluten sensitivity

Hands

Raynaud's phenomenon	Scleroderma
Finger clubbing	Crohn's disease, lymphoma
Koilonychia	Iron deficiency
Leukonychia	Inanition

Musculoskeletal

Mono- and polyarthropathy	Crohn's disease, gluten sensitivity, Whipple's disease, Behçet's syndrome
Back pain (osteomalacia, osteoporosis, sacroiliitis)	Crohn's disease, malnutrition, gluten sensitivity
Muscle weakness (low potassium, magnesium, vitamin D, generalized inanition)	Diffuse mucosal disease, bacterial overgrowth, lymphoma

Nervous system

Peripheral neuropathy (weakness, paresthesias, numbness)	Vitamin-B_{12} deficiency
Cerebral (seizures, dementia, intracerebral calcification, meningitis, pseudotumor, cranial nerve palsies)	Whipple's disease, gluten sensitivity, diffuse lymphoma

From Riley SA, Marsh MN: Maldigestion and malabsorption. In Feldman M, Scharschmidt BF, Sleisenger MH (eds): Sleisenger and Fordtran's Gastrointestinal and Liver Disease: Pathophysiology/Diagnosis/Management, 6th ed. Philadelphia: WB Saunders, 1998, pp 1501–1522.

In some diseases, the histologic features are diagnostic; in others, the findings may be highly suggestive (Table 33–5). Endoscopic duodenal biopsies have largely replaced the more cumbersome jejunal sampling obtained by aspiration biopsy tubes. Several tissue samples should be taken from the distal duodenum to enhance the diagnostic accuracy.

D-XYLOSE TEST

D-Xylose is a 5-carbon monosaccharide that is transported across the intestinal mucosa largely by passive diffusion. In this test, a patient ingests 25 g of D-xylose, and urine is collected for the next 5 hours. Healthy individuals excrete more

Table 33–5 Utility of Small Bowel Biopsy Specimens in Malabsorption

Often Diagnostic

Whipple's disease
Amyloidosis
Eosinophilic enteritis
Lymphangiectasia
Primary intestinal lymphoma
Giardiasis
Abetalipoproteinemia
Agammaglobulinemia
Mastocytosis

Abnormal But Not Diagnostic

Celiac sprue
Systemic sclerosis
Radiation enteritis
Bacterial overgrowth syndrome
Tropical sprue
Crohn's disease

From Trier JS: Diagnostic value of peroral biopsy of the proximal small intestine. N Engl J Med 285:1470, 1971.

than 4.5 g of D-xylose in 5 hours (or ≥20% of the ingested load). The test reflects intestinal transport function and surface area and it serves as an indicator of mucosal absorption. Abnormally low (false-positive) results may occur in the presence of impaired renal excretory function, massive peripheral edema, or ascites. Abnormal results can also be seen in the presence of bacterial overgrowth, but this *pseudomalabsorption* may be corrected after treatment with antibiotics serving as a therapeutic trial.

RADIOGRAPHIC STUDIES

Barium studies of the small bowel in malabsorption are usually nonspecific. Occasionally, however, distinct anatomic changes are seen in jejunal diverticulosis, lymphoma, Crohn's disease, strictures, or enteric fistulas; also, a distinctive barium pattern of thin-walled, dilated loops, suggestive of celiac sprue, may exist.

SCHILLING TEST

Absorption of vitamin B_{12} requires several steps. First, the ingested vitamin binds to salivary R-factor protein; gastric parietal cells secrete intrinsic factor that mixes with the ingested meal. In the duodenum, pancreatic trypsin hydrolyzes the R-factor protein, freeing the vitamin to bind with intrinsic factor. The vitamin B_{12}–intrinsic factor complex is then absorbed by specific receptors found on enterocytes in the distal ileum. Consequently, malabsorption of vitamin B_{12} can occur because of lack of intrinsic factor (e.g., pernicious anemia or gastric resection), pancreatic

insufficiency, bacterial overgrowth, or ileal resection or mucosal disease (i.e., Crohn's disease). The Schilling test quantifies vitamin B_{12} absorption using radiolabeled vitamin B_{12} as a marker. The test may be expanded to several stages to amplify its diagnostic spectrum. In stage 1, after the injection of 1000 μg of unlabeled vitamin B_{12} to saturate hepatic storage, the patient ingests 0.5 μg of radiolabeled vitamin. Urine is then collected for the measurement of radioactivity; reduced radioactivity suggests B_{12} malabsorption. The test is repeated (stage 2) with the addition of oral intrinsic factor to the ingested vitamin B_{12}. If urinary excretion of the radiolabel is corrected, pernicious anemia is diagnosed. If malabsorption is still present, the patient is given a short course of oral antibiotics (stage 3), and the test is repeated; correction of radiolabeled B_{12} excretion establishes bacterial overgrowth. If the test result remains abnormal, oral pancreatic enzymes are given (stage 4), and the test is repeated; correction of the abnormality implies pancreatic deficiency. Finally, if all these interventions fail, ileal disease or the absence of transcobalamin protein is determined by other diagnostic tests. This long outline serves more as an example of an algorithm of clinical analysis; the usual routine in clinical settings is to administer parenteral vitamin B_{12}, whereas the cause is delineated by other modalities.

BREATH TESTS

Breath tests rely on bacterial degradation of luminal compounds, which releases metabolic by-product gases (such as hydrogen, methane, and carbon dioxide [CO_2]) that can be measured in the exhaled breath. In the case of disaccharidase deficiency, a specific disaccharide (such as lactose) that is orally ingested but not properly absorbed in the small intestine is delivered to the colon where bacterial fermentation liberates metabolites; hydrogen gas is the marker assayed in the breath. In the presence of bacterial overgrowth of the small intestine, orally ingested glucose ferments in the proximal small bowel (instead of being absorbed), resulting in increased breath hydrogen; here, the timing of exhaled hydrogen aids in the diagnosis. The measurement of radioactive CO_2 (tested with a nutrient labeled with ^{14}C in the breath) has been used to estimate the malabsorption of fat or bile acids and for measurement of bacterial overgrowth (^{14}C-xylose). The radioactive tests are cumbersome, and their usefulness in clinical practice is limited.

Approach to the Patient with Suspected Malabsorption

A large number of diagnostic tests are available for the workup of malabsorption, necessitating the use of a rational algorithm (Fig. 33–3). The most accurate test for fat malabsorption remains the 72-hour fecal fat analysis; however, the test is difficult to carry out in clinical practice. Surrogate screening for steatorrhea is done with the qualitative stool fat examination (Sudan stain) and serum carotene. If the stool fat content is normal, the patient may still have selective impairment of the absorption of a specific carbohydrate. This latter condition should be suspected if the primary symptoms are cramps, flatulence, and diarrhea. The most common

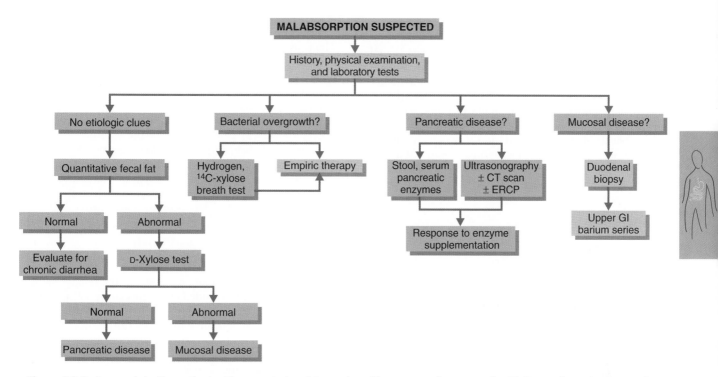

Figure 33–3 Approach to the patient with suspected malabsorption. CT = computed tomography; ERCP = endoscopic retrograde cholangiopancreatography; GI = gastrointestinal. (Adapted from Riley SA, Marsh MN: Maldigestion and malabsorption. In Feldman M, Scharschmidt BF, Sleisenger MH [eds]: Sleisenger and Fordtran's Gastrointestinal and Liver Disease: Pathophysiology/Diagnosis/Management, 6th ed. Philadelphia: WB Saunders, 1998, pp 1501–1522.)

example of carbohydrate malabsorption is lactose intolerance; specific tests include the oral lactose tolerance test, but measurement of breath hydrogen is more sensitive and specific. More generally, an osmotic gap in fecal water suggests a dietary (rather than secretory) cause of the diarrhea related to luminal short-chain fatty acids or carbohydrates. The osmotic gap is calculated by the following formula: plasma osmolality − {2 × (fecal sodium [Na^+] + fecal potassium [K^+])}. The osmotic gap is not calculated by directly measuring stool osmolality because it increases with time in the specimen container. In addition, luminal osmolality is equal to serum osmolality because the colon cannot establish a gradient against the serum concentration of solutes.

When fat malabsorption is demonstrated (>6 g/24 hr, or increased qualitative stool fat and decreased serum carotene), a D-xylose absorption-excretion test should be performed next. A normal D-xylose test makes diffuse mucosal disease unlikely and suggests maldigestion, principally pancreatic enzyme or bile salt deficiency. Clues to chronic pancreatitis include a history of alcohol abuse or previous episodes of pancreatitis; unusual causes of pancreatic malabsorption, such as cystic fibrosis, microlithiasis, or drug toxicity, require specific testing and a detailed history. In the search for maldigestion, serum enzyme tests and abdominal imaging (plain film or, with much greater sensitivity, abdominal CT scan) can be obtained next to identify pancreatic disease. If the urinary D-xylose excretion is abnormal, the breath hydrogen test may be used to diagnose bacterial overgrowth using glucose for the carbohydrate load. When no bacterial overgrowth is present, a mucosal biopsy should be performed (see Table 33–5). Radiologic studies of the small bowel with barium may be helpful on occasion.

When the origin of malabsorption remains unclear, other considerations should include parasitic infection, such as *Giardia lamblia* or ascariasis involvement of the pancreatic duct (more common in undeveloped countries). These diagnoses require a careful stool examination for ova and parasites or fecal antigen studies. Occasionally, therapeutic trials for treatable conditions should be instituted, such as a gluten-free diet for celiac disease, pancreatic enzyme replacement for pancreatic exocrine function, metronidazole for *G. lamblia* infection, or broad-spectrum antibiotics for suspected bacterial overgrowth.

The specific treatment of malabsorption depends on identifying the underlying condition. Parenteral nutrition may have a role in maintaining an adequate nutritional status. Treatment modalities are discussed in the sections devoted to the corresponding diseases.

Specific Disorders

A large number of disorders, some of them listed in Table 33–3, can cause malabsorption. Two of these disorders, celiac sprue and bacterial overgrowth, are discussed in this section as illustrative of the pathophysiologic aspects of malabsorption.

CELIAC SPRUE (ALSO NONTROPICAL SPRUE OR GLUTEN-SENSITIVE ENTEROPATHY)

Celiac disease is characterized by intestinal mucosal injury resulting from immunologic damage from gluten in persons genetically predisposed to this condition. The prevalence of the disease among relatives of patients with celiac sprue is approximately 10%. A strong association of celiac sprue exists with human leukocyte antigen (HLA) class II molecules, particularly HLA-DQ2 and HLA-DQ8. The disease is induced by exposure to storage proteins found in grain plants such as wheat (which contains gliadin), barley, rye, and their products. Oats are implicated not because of gliadin but rather because of contamination with wheat during packaging and transportation. The exposure initiates a cellular immune response that results in mucosal damage, particularly in the proximal intestine. Results of investigations suggest that an enzyme, tissue transglutaminase, may be the autoantigen of celiac sprue.

Clinical Presentation

Celiac disease can exhibit the classic constellation of symptoms and signs of a malabsorption syndrome. Not uncommonly, the manifestation may be atypical, with nonspecific GI symptoms such as bloating, chronic diarrhea (with or without steatorrhea), flatulence, lactose intolerance, or deficiencies of a single micronutrient, as in iron deficiency anemia. Extra-intestinal complaints such as depression, weakness, fatigue, arthralgias, osteoporosis, or osteomalacia may predominate. A significant number of diseases, including dermatitis herpetiformis, type 1 diabetes mellitus, autoimmune thyroid disease, and selective immunoglobulin A (IgA) deficiency, are found in significant association with celiac disease.

Diagnosis

Although celiac disease is a leading consideration in every patient with the malabsorption syndrome, it should be included as well in the differentials of patients with atypical manifestations. Intestinal biopsy is the most valuable test in establishing the diagnosis, and the spectrum of pathologic changes ranges from normal villous architecture with an increase in mucosal lymphocytes and plasma cells (the infiltrative lesion) to partial blunting or total villous flattening. Although abnormal biopsy findings are not specific, they are highly suggestive, particularly because most other conditions that can mimic celiac disease (such as Crohn's disease, gastrinoma, lymphoma, tropical sprue, graft-versus-host disease, or immune deficiency) may be distinguished clinically. A clinical response to a gluten-free diet establishes the diagnosis and precludes the need, in adults, to document healing by repeated biopsies. Serologic blood tests (anti-gliadin, anti-endomysial, and reticulin antibodies) are helpful in screening of patients with atypical symptoms or asymptomatic relatives of patients with celiac sprue.

Treatment

Strict, lifelong adherence to a gluten-free diet is the only treatment for celiac disease. Specific nutritional supplementation should be provided to correct deficiencies, particularly those of iron, vitamins, and calcium. A clinical response may be seen within a few weeks. Patients should be monitored to ensure adequate response and proper adherence to the diet. The long-term prognosis is excellent in patients who adhere to the diet, although a slight increase in the incidence of malignancies may occur, particularly lymphoma.

BACTERIAL OVERGROWTH SYNDROME

The proximal small bowel normally contains fewer than 10^4 bacteria per milliliter of fluid, with no anaerobic *Bacteroides* organisms and few coliforms. Overgrowth of luminal bacteria can result in diarrhea and malabsorption by a significant number of mechanisms: (1) deconjugation of bile salts, which leads to impaired micelle formation and impaired uptake of fat; (2) patchy injury to the enterocytes (small intestinal epithelial cells); (3) direct competition for the use of nutrients (e.g., uptake of vitamin B_{12} by gram-negative bacteria or the fish tapeworm *Diphyllobothrium latum*); and (4) stimulated secretion of water and electrolytes by-products of bacterial metabolism, such as hydroxylated bile acids and short-chain (volatile) organic acids.

Conditions Associated with Bacterial Overgrowth

The most important factors maintaining the relative sterility of the upper gut include (1) gastric acidity, (2) peristalsis, and (3) intestinal immunoglobulins (IgA). Thus, conditions that impair these functions can result in bacterial overgrowth. Impaired peristalsis can be caused by motility disorders (e.g., scleroderma, amyloidosis, diabetes mellitus) or anatomic changes (e.g., surgically created blind loops, obstruction, jejunal diverticulosis). Achlorhydria (resulting from atrophic gastritis or the inhibition of gastric acid secretion), pancreatic insufficiency, and hypogammaglobulinemia are also associated with bacterial overgrowth but uncommonly result in clinical steatorrhea.

Diagnosis

Direct culture of jejunal aspirate is the most definitive diagnostic test, but it is invasive, uncomfortable, and a costly laboratory undertaking. The ^{14}C-xylose breath test is an accurate and sensitive laboratory test, whereas breath hydrogen after an oral challenge with glucose is simpler, although not as sensitive or specific. Empiric therapeutic trial with antibiotics is an acceptable alternative to diagnostic testing.

Treatment

When appropriate, specific therapy, such as surgery for intestinal obstruction, should be provided. More commonly, patients are treated with antibiotics, the most appropriate being those effective against aerobic and anaerobic enteric organisms. Tetracycline, trimethoprim-sulfamethoxazole, or metronidazole (each in combination with a cephalosporin or quinolone) is a suitable agent. A single course of therapy for 7 to 10 days may be therapeutic for months. In other patients, intermittent therapy (1 of every 4 weeks) or even an extended period of continuous therapy may be the most effective management.

Malabsorptive Therapy

Cardiovascular disease and other consequences of obesity have reached epidemic proportions in the United States, and as a result, one approach to the problem has included the deliberate induction of malabsorption (primarily of fats) to reduce lipid levels and the body mass index (BMI). Medication used for this purpose includes bile acid–binding resins, such as cholestyramine and colestipol and, more recently, the lipase inhibitors, orlistsat (Xenical) and ezetimibe (Zetia). Surgical treatment usually consists of gastric partition combined with some degree of small intestinal bypass, which induces significant weight loss by several proposed mechanisms, including malabsorption, improved nutrient deposition, and enhanced satiety.

References

Alaedidni A, Green PH: Narrative Review: Celiac disease: Understanding a complex disease. Ann Intern Med 142:289–298, 2005.

DiBaise JK, Young RJ, Vanderhoof JA: Intestinal rehabilitation and the short bowel syndrome. Am J Gastroenterol 99:1386–1395, 2004.

MacDonald TT, Montelone G: Immunity, inflammation, and allergy in the gut. Science 307:1920–1925, 2005.

Marth T, Raoult D: Whipple's disease. Lancet 361:239–246, 2003.

Pietzak MM, Thomas DW: Childhood malabsorption. Pediatr Rev 24:195–206, 2003.

Romanuglo J, Schiller D, Bailey RJ: Using breath tests wisely in a gastroenterology practice: An evidence-based review of indications and pitfalls in interpretation. Am J Gastroenterol 97:1113–1126, 2002.

Swallow DM: Genetics of lactase persistence and lactose intolerance. Ann Rev Genetics 37:197–219, 2003.

Thompson T: National Institutes of Health consensus statement on celiac disease. Am J Dietetic Assoc 105:194–195, 2005.

D. Diarrhea

Satish K. Singh

Definition

Diarrhea is both a symptom and a sign. As a symptom, diarrhea is most often reported as a decrease in stool consistency and an increase in stool volume; often, patients will also use the term to describe frequency, urgency, and fecal incontinence. As a sign, diarrhea is defined as a stool weight (i.e., water content) that exceeds 200 g in 24 hours. This section discusses the physiologic aspects of intestinal solute and water transport and the pathophysiologic factors and management of diarrheal diseases.

Normal Physiology

Approximately 8 to 9 L of fluid enter the small intestines daily: 1 to 2 L originate from dietary intake, whereas the balance represents normal salivary, gastric, pancreatic, biliary, and intestinal secretions. The small intestine absorbs most of this fluid so that only 1.0 to 1.5 L pass into the colon. In the colon, further water salvage results in a final stool output of only 100 to 200 mL/day.

Different types of specialized epithelial cells line the small and large intestines. However, all epithelial cells possess (1) polarity, in that they have distinct apical (facing the lumen) and basolateral (facing the blood) domains, (2) intercellular *tight* junctions that join their apical poles, and (3) a basolateral Na+-pump (sodium-potassium adenosine triphosphatase [Na+,K+-ATPase]) that maintains an electrochemical gradient. Among different small and large intestinal segments, epithelial cells mediate a range of different transport processes but share in common the fact that ions are moved by transport processes, whereas water moves down passive osmotic gradients. Movement of ions across the epithelium can be either passive, along electrochemical and concentration gradients, or active, against such gradients, requiring energy expenditure. Active ion transport is always transcellular, that is, it occurs *through* cells. Because of their

charge, ions do not readily penetrate lipid bilayers and are moved through the plasma membrane in a regulated fashion via specialized proteins known as *pumps, carriers, and channels.*

Pumps are energy (ATP)-requiring transporters capable of moving ions and solutes against an electrochemical gradient. The most important pump in the intestinal epithelium is Na+, K+ATPase, which removes Na+ from the inside of the cell across the basolateral membrane against electrochemical gradients. With each cycle of the pump, three Na+ ions are exported, and two K+ ions are imported, creating an electronegative, Na+-poor cell interior that ultimately drives transepithelial Na+ and water absorption (Fig. 33–4).

Fluid secretion throughout the gut depends on electrogenic chloride (Cl−) secretion. Active Cl− secretion is predominantly mediated by cells within the crypts that possess tandem pathways for basolateral uptake and apical exit of Cl−. Typically, basolateral Cl−-uptake mechanisms are coupled to the Na+ gradient, thus maintaining intracellular Cl− concentration above electrochemical equilibrium. As a result, increased apical Cl− permeability following activation of an apical Cl−-channel protein causes Cl− to exit the cell into the lumen, resulting in Cl− and water secretion. One Cl− channel, in particular, has been identified as the defective gene product in cystic fibrosis. Known as the *cystic fibrosis transmembrane regulator* (CFTR), it is activated by elevations in intracellular cyclic adenosine monophosphate (cAMP), as well as by several other mediators implicated in secretory diarrhea. The process of active chloride secretion is shown in Figure 33–5.

Although the small bowel and the colon share many basic mechanisms with regard to ion transport, differences exist. As a result, the small intestinal fluid that enters the colon has a plasma-like electrolyte composition, whereas fecal fluid contains twice as much K+ as it does Na+. At no time does either the small or the large intestine maintain standing osmotic gradients.

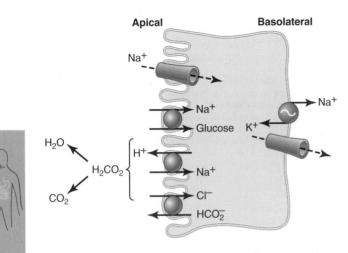

Apical   Basolateral

Figure 33–4 Apical sodium transporters. Sodium moves down its electrochemical gradient across the apical membrane of the epithelial cell. Pathways for apical sodium uptake include (1) channel proteins specific for sodium that can be blocked by amiloride, (2) carriers that couple the movement of sodium to the movement of nutrients such as glucose, and (3) antiport carriers that mediate electroneutral entry of sodium in exchange for intracellular hydrogen ion (i.e., acid). The common exit pathway across the basolateral membrane is the sodium pump. (From Sellin JH: Intestinal electrolyte absorption and secretion. In Feldman M, Scharschmidt BF, Sleisenger MH [eds]: Sleisenger and Fordtran's Gastrointestinal and Liver Disease: Pathophysiology/Diagnosis/Management, 6th ed. Philadelphia: WB Saunders, 1998, pp 1451–1471.)

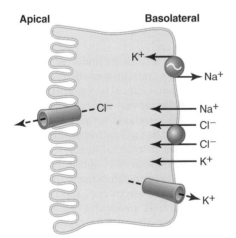

Apical   Basolateral

Figure 33–5 Chloride secretion. Discrete basolateral entry steps and apical exit steps are integral to chloride secretion. A carrier couples the movement of sodium, potassium, and chloride in a 1:1:2 stoichiometry and permits chloride to accumulate in the cell above its electrochemical equilibrium. Chloride exits the cell across the apical membrane by means of a chloride channel. The sodium and potassium that entered with the chloride are recycled by, respectively, the sodium pump and a basolateral potassium channel. (From Selin JH: Intestinal electrolyte absorption and secretion. In Feldman M, Scharschmidt BF, Sleisenger MH [eds]: Sleisenger and Fordtran's Gastrointestinal and Liver Disease: Pathophysiology/Diagnosis/Management, 6th ed. Philadelphia: WB Saunders, 1998, pp 1451–1471.)

Pathophysiologic Factors

A significant number of mechanisms can cause diarrhea, and these mechanisms are listed in Table 33–6. However, most diarrheal states are caused by either inadequate absorption of ions, solutes, and water or by increased secretion of electrolytes that result in water accumulation in the lumen.

SECRETORY DIARRHEA

Secretory diarrhea is caused by abnormal ion transport across the intestinal epithelium, which results in decreased absorption, increased secretion, or both. Secretory diarrheas are typically caused by neurohumoral mediators and/or bacterial toxins that affect intracellular levels of cAMP, cyclic guanosine monophosphate (cGMP), and/or calcium. Elevated levels of these intracellular second messengers, in turn, typically inhibit electroneutral NaCl absorption and induce Cl^- secretion, the net result being increased water accumulation in the gut lumen. A classic example of a secretory diarrhea is cholera. A toxin produced by the bacterium binds to membrane receptors on enterocytes, irreversibly activating a guanine nucleotide–binding protein (G protein) that leads to enhanced cAMP production. The increased intracellular cAMP (1) inhibits apical electroneutral NaCl absorption (mediated by coupled Na^+–hydrogen ion [H^+] and Cl^-–bicarbonate ion [HCO_3^-] exchange) and (2) simultaneously induces Cl^- secretion by activating apical Cl^- channels. These events result in massive diarrhea, intravascular volume loss, and, absent fluid resuscitation, eventual circulatory collapse. The hallmark of toxigenic and hormone-mediated secretory diarrheas is that no associated epithelial injury occurs, leaving intact apical Na^+–coupled nutrient transporters (Na^+-glucose, Na^+-amino acid) that are not inhibited by intracellular second messengers. The persistence of these intact, alternative Na^+–absorption pathways is what can be exploited effectively by glucose and starch-based oral rehydration therapies.

Clinically, secretory diarrheas (1) are high output (often >1 L/day), (2) persist during fasting, and (3) display a minimal (<50 mOsm) stool osmotic gap (i.e., the amount by which stool osmolality exceeds what is accounted for by measured electrolytes, estimated from $2[Na^+] + 2[K^+]$) because salt secretion alone is causing the diarrhea. Some causes of secretory diarrhea are listed in Table 33–7. Although these features are classic for cases of pure secretory diarrhea, a more complex picture can ensue when mixed mechanisms co-exist, for example, in malabsorptive syndromes such as celiac disease. Osmotic forces from malabsorbed fatty acids inhibit fluid absorption from both the small intestine and the colon, whereas bile acids interfere with absorption of water and electrolytes in addition to inducing Cl^- secretion in the colon. Thus, the component of water loss from fat malabsorption may fall substantially during fasting (see discussion of osmotic diarrhea later), an osmotic gap might be present as a result of carbohydrate malabsorption fermentation and organic anion production, and a secretory component may exist as well if, for example, bile acids are substantially malabsorbed.

Table 33–6   Classification of Diarrhea

Type	Mechanism	Examples	Characteristics
Secretory	Increased secretion and/or decreased absorption of Na^+ and Cl^-	Cholera Vasoactive intestinal peptide-secreting tumor Bile salt enteropathy Fatty acid-induced diarrhea	Large-volume, watery diarrhea No gas or pus No solute gap Little or no response to fasting
Osmotic	Nonabsorbable molecules in gut lumen	Lactose intolerance (lactase deficiency) Generalized malabsorption (particularly carbohydrates) Mg^{2+}-containing laxatives	Watery stool; no blood or pus Improves with fasting Stool may contain fat globules or meat fibers and may have an increased solute gap
Inflammatory	Destruction of mucosa Impaired absorption Outpouring of blood, mucus	Ulcerative colitis Shigellosis Amebiasis	Small frequent stools with blood and pus Fever Variable
Decreased absorptive surface	Impaired reabsorption of electrolytes and/or nutrients	Bowel resection Enteric fistula	
Motility disorder	Increased motility with decreased time for absorption of electrolytes and/or nutrients	Hyperthyroidism	Variable
	Decreased motility with bacterial overgrowth	Irritable bowel syndrome Scleroderma Diabetic diarrhea	Malabsorption

Na^+ = sodium; Cl^- = chloride; Mg^{2+} = magnesium.

Table 33–7   Some Causes of Secretory Diarrhea

Infections

Bacterial toxins (enterotoxigenic *Escherichia coli*)

Stimulant Laxatives

Ricinoleic acid (castor oil), senna (Senokot), bisacodyl (Dulcolax)

Bile Acid and Fatty Acid Malabsorption

Intestinal Resection

Neuroendocrine Tumors

Zollinger-Ellison syndrome (gastrin)
Carcinoid syndrome (serotonin, substance P, prostaglandins)
Medullary carcinoma of the thyroid (calcitonin, prostaglandins)
Pancreatic cholera syndrome (vasoactive intestinal peptide)

OSMOTIC DIARRHEA

Water and solute movement is coupled throughout the GI tract, and no standing osmotic gradients are maintained across the mucosa. As a result, osmotic diarrhea is simply caused by excessive levels of poorly absorbed, osmotically active solutes in the lumen. Some causes of osmotic diarrhea are presented in Table 33–8. Osmotic diarrhea has two important clinical features. First, diarrhea stops when patients fast because they are no longer taking in poorly absorbed osmoles or the nutrients that they are malabsorbing. Second, stool analysis reveals an elevated osmotic gap because of the presence in stool of osmotically active and/or nonabsorbed agents.

ABNORMAL INTESTINAL MOTILITY

Altered GI motility can cause diarrhea by two mechanisms:

1. Enhanced motility, resulting in rapid gut transit and decreased contact time between luminal contents and absorptive epithelial cells. Decreased transit time and enhanced propulsive contractions contribute to post-vagotomy, post-gastrectomy, carcinoid, hyperthyroid, and diabetic diarrheas, as well to diarrhea-predominant IBS.
2. Decreased motility, caused by diseases such as scleroderma or diabetes. These diseases promote

Table 33–8 Some Causes of Osmotic Diarrhea

Laxatives Containing Poorly Absorbed Anion

Sodium phosphate (Phospho-Soda)

Laxatives Containing Poorly Absorbed Cation

Magnesium hydroxide (Philip's Milk of Magnesia), magnesium citrate (Citrate of Magnesia)

Disaccharidase Deficiency

Lactose intolerance

Poorly Absorbed Carbohydrate

Lactulose, sorbitol ("sugar-free" gum), mannitol, congenital glucose-galactose or fructose malabsorption

General Malabsorption Syndromes

small intestinal stasis that can result in overgrowth of largely anaerobic bacteria that deconjugate bile acids, causing steatorrhea and diarrhea.

EXUDATIVE DIARRHEA

Inflammatory or infectious conditions that result in damage to the intestinal mucosa can cause diarrhea by a large number of mechanisms. Blood, mucus, and serum proteins are lost, the extent of which depends largely on the degree of injury. However, mucosal damage and attendant inflammation can interfere with absorption, induce secretion, and affect motility, all of which contribute to diarrhea.

Evaluation of Diarrhea

HISTORY AND PHYSICAL EXAMINATION

A thoroughly obtained history will yield valuable clues that guide appropriate and cost-effective investigation of diarrheal diseases. The *duration* of diarrhea is particularly useful because most acute diarrheas are caused by microbial pathogens and typically resolve independent of intervention. Chronic diarrhea, defined as lasting more than 4 weeks, is unlikely to be infectious. The presence of blood is also a useful clue because it suggests inflammation, neoplasm, ischemia, or infection by invasive organisms. Large-volume diarrhea suggests small bowel or proximal colonic disease; in contrast, frequent small stools with associated urgency suggest left-sided colonic and/or rectal disease. All current and recent medications (specifically new medications, antibiotics, and antacids) and alcohol intake should be reviewed. Intake of nutritional supplements should also be reviewed, including sugar substitutes that contain poorly absorbed carbohydrates, fat substitutes, milk products, shell-

fish, and heavy intake of fruits, fruit juices, and caffeine. The social history should include travel, source of drinking water (treated city water or well water), consumption of raw milk in rural populations, exposure to farm animals that may spread *Salmonella* or *Brucella,* and sexual practices. Familial occurrence of celiac disease, inflammatory bowel disease, or multiple endocrine neoplasia syndromes should be considered as well. Physical examination in acute diarrhea is helpful in determining severity of disease and hydration status. Physical findings are less helpful in chronic diarrhea, although certain findings have been associated with specific diseases: oral ulcers and pyoderma gangrenosum with inflammatory bowel disease, dermatitis herpetiformis with celiac disease, and lymphadenopathy with lymphoma.

Further evaluation with appropriate laboratory tests depends largely on the duration and severity of diarrhea and the presence of blood, overt or occult, in the stool.

ACUTE DIARRHEA

Acute diarrhea is defined as lasting less than 4 weeks and is most commonly caused by infectious organisms or toxins. It is usually self limited and, in the absence of blood in the stool, usually remains undiagnosed. If a patient is seen early in the course of illness and has mild diarrhea without systemic symptoms or blood in the stool, expectant management with observation and follow-up is the most appropriate course of action. Otherwise, and certainly in the presence of blood, stool should be evaluated for infectious organisms and antimicrobials initiated when appropriate. If organisms are not identified, sigmoidoscopy should be performed and biopsies obtained. Further investigations should be guided by findings on sigmoidoscopy (e.g., if inflammatory bowel disease is suspected), severity of diarrhea, immunocompetence of the patient, and the presence of systemic toxicity. A general algorithm for the evaluation of acute diarrhea is shown in Figure 33–6.

CHRONIC DIARRHEA

Clinicians have numerous tests at their disposal for investigating a patient with chronic diarrhea, and a rational approach should be exercised in making the most appropriate choices. Duration of diarrhea, evidence of systemic involvement, nutritional deficiencies, and prior work-up should guide the evaluation of the patient. In contrast to acute diarrhea, infectious origin is uncommon with chronic diarrhea. However, certain persistent parasitic infections, such as giardiasis and postviral syndromes that result in persistently disturbed brush border enzyme and transport activities, can produce a chronic malabsorptive diarrheal picture.

Weight loss and evidence of nutritional deficiencies suggest malabsorption caused by a pathologic process in the small intestine or pancreas, the latter associated with a history of excessive alcohol intake and/or chronic pancreatitis. Chronic bloody diarrhea suggests inflammatory bowel disease, particularly ulcerative colitis. Chronic diarrhea with no evidence of nutritional or metabolic derangements suggests lactose intolerance (common); IBS, particularly when associated with abdominal pain (common); microscopic colitis (particularly in elderly women); fecal incontinence; or surreptitious laxative abuse. Colon cancer should always be

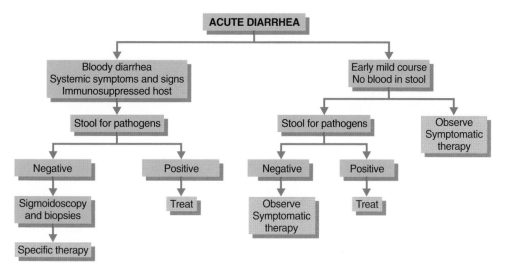

Figure 33–6 Algorithm for the evaluation of the patient with acute diarrhea.

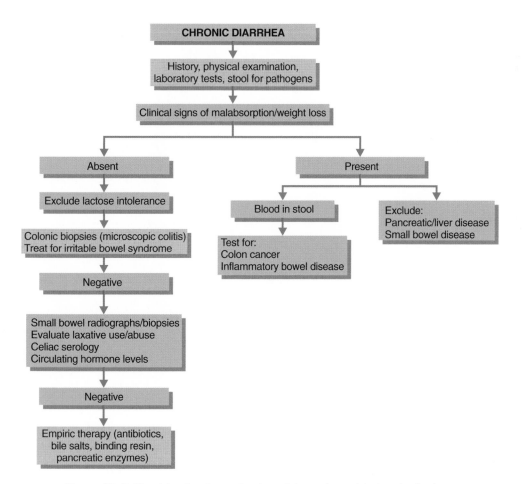

Figure 33–7 Algorithm for the evaluation of the patient with chronic diarrhea.

considered. Large-volume diarrhea in the absence of nutritional deficiencies, with features of a secretory process, usually prompts a search for hormone-producing tumors, although more often than not, they remain occult. Whenever possible, therapy is directed specifically toward the underlying cause. When no specific treatment is available (as in microscopic colitis) or no cause is determined, empiric

therapies (e.g., antibiotics for possible bacterial overgrowth, *G. lamblia* infection, cholestyramine for bile acid malabsorption) and/or agents that decrease motility and secretion in general (e.g., loperamide, diphenoxylate and, in more severe cases, codeine, paregoric, long-acting somatostatin analog) can be tried. A general algorithm for the approach to chronic diarrhea is presented in Figure 33–7.

Prospectus for the Future

When viewed in a long-term perspective, the addition of diagnostic studies such as CT scanning, endoscopy, and most recently capsule endoscopy, have clearly heightened diagnostic accuracy. The hope is that, in the future, even more sophisti-cated diagnostic instruments, including biochemical measurements, will enhance even more the understanding of the complex manifestations of abdominal pain.

References

Afzalpurkar RG, Schiller LR, Little KH, et al: The self-limited nature of chronic idiopathic diarrhea. N Engl J Med 327:1849, 1992.

Eherer AJ, Fordtran JS: Fecal osmotic gap and pH in experimental diarrhea of various causes. Gastroenterology 103:545, 1992.

Field M: Intestinal ion transport and the pathophysiology of diarrhea. J Clin Invest. 111(7):931–943, 2003.

Fine KD, Schiller LR: AGA technical review on the evaluation and management of chronic diarrhea. Gastroenterology 116:1464–1486, 1999.

Mertz HR: Irritable bowel syndrome. N Engl J Med 349:2136–2146, 2003.

Schiller LR, Sellin JH: Diarrhea. In Feldman M, Friedman L, Sleisenger MH (eds): Sleisenger & Fordtran's Gastrointestinal and Liver Disease, 7th ed. Philadelphia: WB Saunders, 2002, pp 131–153.

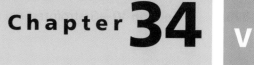

Endoscopic and Imaging Procedures

Brian C. Jacobson

Daniel S. Mishkin

Since Mikulicz first used a prototype esophagoscope to visualize the lumen of the esophagus in 1880, physicians have been attempting to peer into every portion of the gastrointestinal (GI) tract in an attempt to understand disease and to restore their patients to health. No other field in internal medicine is associated with as many imaging modalities as gastroenterology, with its broad focus on the GI tract, pancreas, liver, and biliary tree, including the gallbladder. A wide variety of both invasive and noninvasive imaging procedures is available for evaluating GI signs and symptoms, performing cancer screening, and providing therapeutic interventions. This chapter reviews the various endoscopic and radiographic procedures currently in use, including their indications and basic information regarding their performance.

Gastrointestinal Endoscopy

The once-rigid endoscope has been supplanted by today's flexible instruments. These instruments are composed of long shafts 6 mm to 12 mm in diameter (Fig. 34–1) that house wires for deflecting the endoscope's tip in multiple directions, digital imaging equipment, and an accessory channel for the passage of biopsy forceps or other tools. The distal end contains lenses for both lighting and visualization, and the proximal end includes a series of knobs and buttons used to deflect or *steer* the endoscope's tip, insufflate air into the GI lumen, wash the lens, and suction air or liquid from the GI lumen.

GI endoscopy can be performed in dedicated endoscopy suites or at a patient's bedside in emergency situations. After positioning the patient appropriately and providing sedation, if necessary, the lubricated endoscope is passed through the intended orifice and advanced manually by the endoscopist. Bends and turns in the GI lumen are navigated by deflecting the endoscope tip and by applying torque to the instrument shaft (i.e. rotating the shaft along the long axis of the instrument). Endoscopy is generally safe, with complications that include bleeding (0.3% to 1% after colono-

scopic polypectomy), perforation (0.05% in general, but 0.1% to 0.5% after polypectomy), and sedation-associated hypotension and hypoxia (1% to 5%). Death related to endoscopic procedures is exceedingly rare (0% to 0.01%).

ESOPHAGOGASTRODUODENOSCOPY

Esophagogastroduodenoscopy (EGD), often referred to as *upper endoscopy*, is performed with a *gastroscope* and allows the endoscopist to visualize the esophagus, stomach, and duodenum to its third and sometimes fourth portions (Fig. 34–2). Diagnostic indications for EGD include dysphagia and odynophagia, screening for and surveillance of Barrett's esophagus, screening for esophagogastric varices, upper GI symptoms suggestive of ulcer disease or malignancy, suspected upper GI bleeding, and occasionally investigation of less common entities, such as celiac sprue or protein-losing enteropathy. The therapeutic interventions performed during EGD include the treatment of esophageal varices; dilation of esophageal strictures; rupture of esophageal rings and webs; dilation of the gastroesophageal junction in the setting of achalasia; removal or ablation of neoplastic lesions such as polyps, foci of high-grade dysplasia, or small malignancies; therapy for upper GI bleeding; and the placement of palliative stents for malignant obstruction of the esophagus, pylorus, or duodenum.

ENTEROSCOPY

Examination of the small intestine beyond the ligament of Treitz is not feasible with a standard gastroscope. However, in the setting of obscure GI bleeding (defined as persistent GI blood loss despite a normal EGD and normal colonoscopy), evaluation of the 15 or more feet of small bowel becomes necessary. In addition, small bowel irregularities identified on barium studies may also require direct visualization to enable appropriate therapy. *Push* enteroscopy using a long (>200 cm) endoscope allows the endoscopist to both image and biopsy or cauterize lesions in the

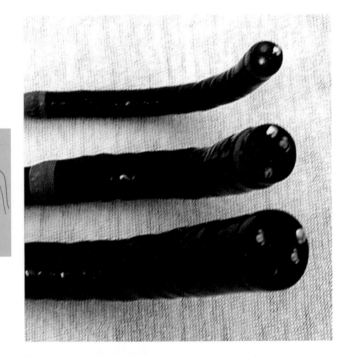

Figure 34–1 Endoscopes used for upper GI endoscopy. Endoscopes of varying sizes are available for use in different situations. The uppermost endoscope (6-mm diameter) can be used for unsedated endoscopy. The middle endoscope (9-mm diameter) is used for standard diagnostic endoscopy. The lowermost endoscope (12-mm diameter) is used for therapeutic endoscopy, such as the placement of enteral stents. (Courtesy Brian C. Jacobson.)

small intestine. Advancing this instrument beyond the first 50 cm of jejunum can be difficult, and, in some cases, intra-operative enteroscopy may be necessary. In this setting, a surgeon will make small incisions in a patient's abdomen and then pleat the small bowel onto the enteroscope while the endoscopist visualizes the luminal surface. Once a lesion is identified, the surgeon may elect to proceed directly to a resection of the affected intestine.

A new technique for providing endoscopic access to the majority of the small bowel can be performed using a double balloon enteroscope. This method uses an endoscope equipped with two balloons spaced several centimeters apart. By inflating and deflating the balloons in sequence, the enteroscope can be advanced through extremely long stretches of small intestine. Combining an anterograde (via the mouth) and retrograde (via the anus) approach, the entire small intestine can be investigated in more than 85% of cases.

VIDEO CAPSULE ENDOSCOPY

The desire to obtain visualization of the GI lumen in the least invasive way has resulted in the development of video capsule endoscopy, the use of pill-size wireless cameras that the patient swallows (**Web Fig. 34–1; Web Video 34–1**). Currently, two capsule endoscopes are available, one for the esophagus and another for the small intestine. Both capsules are 11 × 26 mm, and can transmit images wirelessly to a data recorder as they travel through a patient's GI tract, without the need for sedation. At the end of the study, the data recorder allows for stored images to be uploaded into a computer for viewing while the capsule is ultimately passed in the patient's stool. The small bowel capsule endoscope has become the gold standard for visualizing the small intestine, most commonly for the purpose of investigating obscure GI bleeding (**Web Figs. 34–2 and 34–3; Web Video 34–2**) and suspected inflammatory bowel disease (**Web Figs. 34–4 and 34–5**).

A second capsule endoscope exists specifically for evaluating the esophagus. This capsule is helpful in patients being screened for esophageal varices or individuals with suspected complications of acid-reflux, such as reflux esophagitis or Barrett's esophagus.

SIGMOIDOSCOPY AND COLONOSCOPY

Flexible sigmoidoscopy allows visualization of the rectum, sigmoid colon, and descending colon to the level of the splenic flexure. Enemas are given before the procedure to clear stool from the distal colon. Because sigmoidoscopy is quick (<10 minutes) and not particularly painful, sedation is typically not provided, making it a convenient tool for colorectal cancer screening. Additional indications for sigmoidoscopy include acute and chronic diarrhea and rectal bleeding and for evaluating responses to therapies for colitis.

Colonoscopy allows direct visualization of the entire large bowel and even several centimeters of terminal ileum. Bowel cleansing for colonoscopy requires the ingestion of osmotically active solutions, such as sodium phosphate or polyethylene glycol, coupled with a liquid diet for 24 hours before the procedure. Colonoscopy is more uncomfortable for the patient than sigmoidoscopy is, which requires sedation. Indications for colonoscopy include those for sigmoidoscopy, as well as iron deficiency anemia, frank and occult GI blood loss, and assessing inflammatory bowel disease, including surveillance for dysplasia. Therapeutic interventions possible during colonoscopy include polypectomy, thermal ablation of vascular ectasias, decompression of colonic dilation associated with pseudo-obstruction, and occasionally the endoscopic control of lower GI bleeding.

ENDOSCOPIC RETROGRADE CHOLANGIOPANCREATOGRAPHY

Endoscopic retrograde cholangiopancreatography (ERCP) is a combined endoscopic and radiographic procedure for imaging the biliary and pancreatic ducts. A *duodenoscope* is a specially designed instrument for use during ERCP that includes an imaging lens oriented on the side of the endoscope's tip, allowing a direct view of the ampulla of Vater on the medial wall of the second portion of the duodenum. A tiny finger-like projection called an *elevator* helps the endoscopist guide a catheter into the duct of interest. Contrast is then injected through the catheter, filling the duct, and fluoroscopic images are obtained (Fig. 34–3). ERCP is indicated for evaluating obstructive jaundice with or without suppurative cholangitis, biliary colic with suspected bile duct stones, chronic or recurrent acute pancreatitis, and suspected primary sclerosing cholangitis. Bile duct brushings and even biopsies may be obtained to determine if a biliary stricture is neoplastic. With the use of a special manometry catheter, sphincter of Oddi pressures can also be measured in cases of

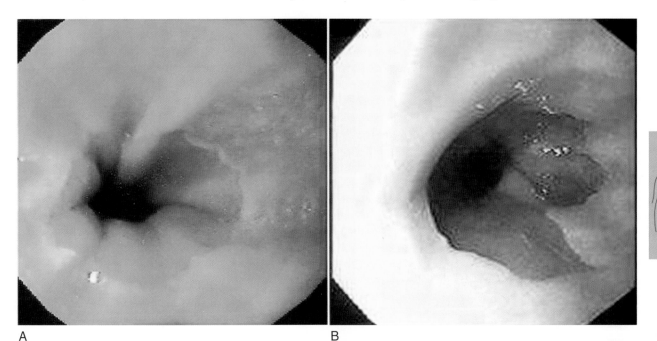

A   B

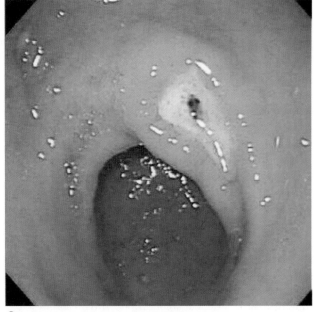

C

Figure 34–2 *A,* Endoscopic view of the distal esophagus. The distal esophagus contains an abrupt transition between its squamous-lined mucosa and the columnar-lined mucosa of the stomach. *B,* Endoscopic view of Barrett's esophagus, in which the squamous epithelium of the distal esophagus is replaced by columnar-lined epithelium. Evident in this view is a tongue of columnar-lined mucosa extending proximally into the esophagus. *C,* Endoscopic view of a gastric ulcer. A yellow-based ulceration with a pigmented spot is visualized on the gastric wall at the transition between the corpus and the antrum. (Courtesy M. Michael Wolfe.)

suspected sphincter of Oddi dysfunction. Therapeutic interventions possible during ERCP include sphincterotomy (an incision through the sphincter of Oddi using a catheter with an electrocautery cutting wire), removal of bile duct stones, and the placement of biliary or pancreatic duct stents to alleviate signs and symptoms of obstruction. ERCP carries a significant (5%) risk of complications, including pancreatitis, postsphincterotomy bleeding, and perforation.

Choledochoscopy and *pancreatoscopy* are techniques in which an endoscope 3 mm or less in diameter is passed through the accessory channel of a duodenoscope and into the bile or pancreatic ducts. The use of this small endoscope permits direct visualization of ductal abnormalities, guides electrohydraulic lithotripsy of large stones, and allows for direct sampling of ductal lesions.

ENDOSCOPIC ULTRASOUND

Endoscopic ultrasound (EUS) or endosonography is performed with an endoscope containing an ultrasound transducer in its tip. Because this transducer can be placed within the GI lumen, high-resolution images of the bowel wall can be obtained, revealing distinct layers that correspond to the mucosa, submucosa, muscularis propria, and serosa (Fig. 34–4). This technique allows the endoscopist to stage tumor depths and determine the layer of origin of subepithelial masses. In addition, EUS can penetrate the luminal wall, providing sonographic images of the mediastinum, pancreas, liver, gallbladder, and mesenteric vessels. Thin EUS probes can be passed through the accessory channel of a duodenoscope and into the biliary and pancreatic ducts to provide

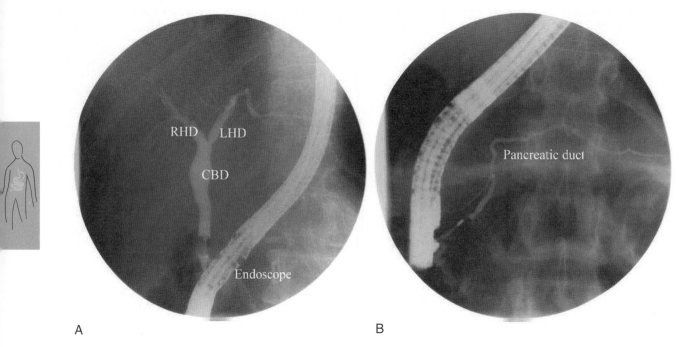

A   B

Figure 34–3 Endoscopic retrograde cholangiopancreatography (ERCP). *A,* Normal cholangiogram. Contrast injected into the biliary tree during ERCP demonstrates the intraductal anatomy of the common bile duct (CBD), right hepatic duct (RHD), left hepatic duct (LHD), and smaller intrahepatic biliary radicals. *B,* Normal pancreatogram. Contrast injected into the pancreatic duct during ERCP defines the intraductal anatomy throughout the length of the pancreas. (Courtesy Brian C. Jacobson.)

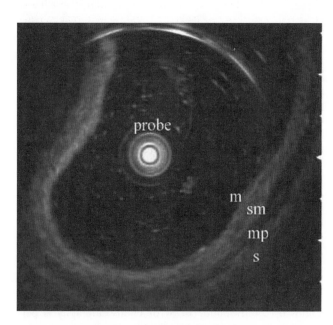

Figure 34–4 Endoscopic ultrasound of the gastrointestinal wall. A 12-MHz ultrasound probe, passed through the accessory channel of an endoscope, demonstrates the normal layers of the rectal wall. The mucosa *(m)* appears as a superficial, hyperechoic *(white)* band and a deeper hypoechoic *(black)* band. The submucosa *(sm)* appears as the next hyperechoic layer. The muscularis propria *(mp)* appears hypoechoic, and the serosa *(s)* appears as the outermost, hyperechoic layer. (Courtesy Brian C. Jacobson.)

sonographic images of small tumors and stones. Fine-needle aspiration (FNA) can be performed under EUS guidance, enhancing the diagnostic capability of EUS. Tissue samples obtained by EUS-guided FNA are analyzed by cytopathologists and can distinguish benign from malignant lesions and metastatic spread of cancer to lymph nodes or the liver. FNA can also be performed to drain cystic lesions, such as pancreatic cystic neoplasms and pseudocysts.

Nonendoscopic Imaging Procedures

PLAIN ABDOMINAL RADIOGRAPHS

Plain abdominal radiographs include upright, supine, and lateral decubitus films obtained with standard x-ray equipment and without the use of contrast agents. Plain abdominal radiographs can reveal evidence of a pneumoperitoneum, dilated bowel loops and air-fluid levels, excessive amounts of stool, or displacement of bowel loops. These findings are indicative of a perforation, obstruction or ileus, constipation or fecal impaction, and volvulus or organ enlargement, respectively (Fig. 34–5). Calcifications, such as those seen in chronic pancreatitis and gallstone disease, may also be visible on these radiographs. Plain films are most useful in the initial evaluation of abdominal pain or nausea and vomiting.

CONTRAST STUDIES

Contrast agents such as barium or the water-soluble diatrizoate (e.g., Gastrograffin) can be administered by mouth or

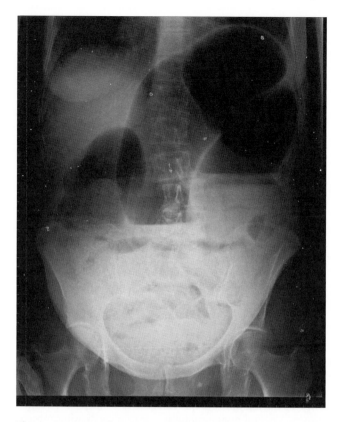

Figure 34–5 Upright plain x-ray image of the abdomen. Air in dilated loops of colon and air-fluid levels can be seen in this patient with a sigmoid volvulus. (Courtesy Brian C. Jacobson.)

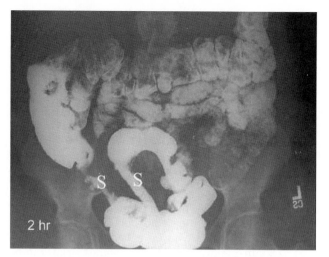

Figure 34–6 Small bowel follow-through. Ingested barium defines the contours of the small and large bowel lumen. A long stricture (S) of the terminal ileum can be seen in this patient with Crohn's disease. (Courtesy Brian C. Jacobson.)

rectum to detect mucosal abnormalities (ulcerations and masses), strictures, herniations, diverticula, and abnormal peristalsis. Contrast agents can be used alone (single contrast) or with the instillation of air or ingestion of gas-forming agents (double contrast). The former method is more useful for detecting obstructing lesions and motility disturbances, whereas the latter method aids in detecting more subtle findings such as small ulcerations or polyps.

A video esophogram entails the filming of a patient's oral cavity and pharynx during the ingestion of contrast materials of various thicknesses and textures. This imaging modality permits careful assessment of a patient's ability to manipulate a food bolus, swallow effectively, and avoid aspiration events. A video esophogram is indicated for evaluating patients with oropharyngeal dysphagia and recurrent aspiration pneumonia. A more generalized barium esophogram focuses attention on the esophagus during the ingestion of a bolus of contrast. This study can detect esophageal rings, webs, strictures, and motility problems that endoscopy might miss. A barium esophogram may be useful for evaluating nonoropharyngeal dysphagia, as well as odynophagia.

An upper GI series includes serial radiographic images as an ingested contrast agent travels through the esophagus, stomach, and duodenum. This study can define gastric abnormalities, such as ulcerations and mucosal thickening. It is indicated in evaluating abdominal pain and suspected gastric outlet obstruction. If radiographic imaging continues as the contrast agent traverses the jejunum and ileum, the study is called a small bowel follow-through (Fig. 34–6).

During this more involved procedure, a radiologist will obtain multiple films, including spot films, or close-up views of regions that appear abnormal. Fluoroscopy can be used to follow a contrast agent during the journey through the small bowel. Attention is paid not only to structural findings, but also to the length of time required for contrast to reach and enter the colon. For more detailed small bowel images, enteroclysis can be performed. This method requires the infusion of concentrated contrast directly into the small bowel through a nasojejunal tube placed under fluoroscopic guidance. Because of its invasive nature, enteroclysis is becoming less common in this era of wireless capsule endoscopy. Indications for a small bowel follow-through include suspected small bowel obstruction or partial obstruction from any cause, suspected small bowel mucosal diseases such as Crohn's disease, and obscure GI blood loss.

Single- and double-contrast barium enemas can detect colonic strictures, diverticula, polyps, and colonic ulcerations, and they can reduce an intussusception. A barium enema may be used in conjunction with flexible sigmoidoscopy to provide screening for colorectal cancer, or it may be used to visualize the proximal colon when colonoscopy cannot be completed for various reasons. In general, the upper GI series and barium enema have been superseded by upper endoscopy and colonoscopy because the endoscopic procedures offer increased sensitivity for detecting mucosal abnormalities, the ability to obtain mucosal biopsies, and the potential for resection of identified lesions.

TRANSABDOMINAL ULTRASOUND

Ultrasonography is often the first imaging study obtained in the evaluation of suspected biliary colic, jaundice, and abnormal liver tests. Its use of sound waves to create an image avoids radiation exposure, and the addition of Doppler techniques permits the assessment of vascular patency. Ultrasound can detect parenchymal abnormalities, such as fatty liver or cirrhosis, focal masses or cysts, ascites, biliary ductal dilation, gallstones, and large vessel thromboses. It may detect thickening of the gut wall and areas of intussusception. Ultrasound is also used to guide needle placement for biopsies or fluid aspiration. Ultrasound cannot penetrate bone or air, preventing its use as a more general diagnostic tool for the GI tract.

COMPUTED TOMOGRAPHY, COMPUTED TOMOGRAPHY ENTEROGRAPHY, AND COMPUTED TOMOGRAPHY COLOGRAPHY

Computed tomography (CT) uses computer-aided reconstruction of multiple radiographic images obtained in a circular or helical course around a patient's vertical axis. Internal organs are visualized based on their inherent tissue densities compared with their surroundings. The GI lumen is usually opacified by having the patient drink an oral contrast agent. In addition, intravenous contrast agents can be administered to highlight regions with increased blood flow, thereby improving detection of pathologic lesions, such as tumors. CT can detect parenchymal lesions, such as tumors, cysts, and abscesses, as well as define the size, shape, and parenchymal characteristics of organs, such as the liver and spleen. Vascular abnormalities, such as perigastric varices or large vessel thromboses, and intra-abdominal fluid, such as ascites, can also be seen with CT. The caliber and contour of the GI tract wall are demonstrated by CT, aiding in the diagnosis of inflammatory lesions, such as colitis, diverticulitis, and appendicitis. CT can also be used to guide needle biopsies of abdominal masses and to place electrodes into tumors for ablative therapies such as radiofrequency ablation. The use of CT to guide placement of drainage catheters has made possible the percutaneous treatment of intra-abdominal abscesses, pseudocysts, and pancreatic necrosis.

CT enteroclysis and *CT enterography* are two emerging techniques developed to provide better images of the small intestine. CT enteroclysis uses a nasojejunal tube to deliver contrast into the small intestine, whereas CT enterography uses an orally ingested intraluminal contrast to highlight the small intestinal mucosa. Early data suggest that these studies are at least equivalent to, if not better than, the current standard small bowel follow-through.

CT can also be used to obtain high-resolution images of the colon. CT colography, or *virtual colonoscopy,* makes use of special image reconstruction software to create accurate visualization of the colonic lumen, provided that the patient has completed a bowel-cleansing regimen identical to that used for colonoscopy. These CT images are 70% to 90% sensitive for detecting polyps or masses within the colon, helping to determine which patients need therapeutic colonoscopy. Virtual colonoscopy is presently being used in some centers to complete colonic visualization in the setting of an incomplete endoscopic colonoscopy.

MAGNETIC RESONANCE IMAGING AND MAGNETIC RESONANCE CHOLANGIOPANCREATOGRAPHY

Similar to CT, magnetic resonance imaging (MRI) provides multiple cross-sectional images of the abdomen and pelvis. These images are created using powerful field magnets to orient small numbers of nuclei within the body in such a way as to produce a measurable magnetic moment. MRI therefore avoids radiation exposure but requires the patient to lie nearly motionless, and often within a small enclosed tube, for prolonged periods. MRI can visualize parenchymal lesions such as masses and cysts and may better characterize abnormalities seen on CT, such as hemangiomas, hepatic focal nodular hyperplasia, and fatty liver. MRI is also helpful in better characterizing perirectal abscesses and fistulas in Crohn's disease. Special rectal MRI probes or coils can provide detailed images of rectal cancer used for tumor staging.

MRI of the biliary and pancreatic ducts (*magnetic resonance cholangiopancreatography,* MRCP) is a noninvasive method that can detect ductal dilation, strictures, stones, pancreatic parenchymal changes in chronic pancreatitis, and congenital ductal abnormalities, such as pancreas divisum. Although MRCP techniques continue to improve, this technique fails to visualize small bile duct stones (<4 mm) and strictures, and it may be inaccurate for diagnosing primary sclerosing cholangitis. *Magnetic resonance angiography* is a magnetic resonance method for visualizing blood vessels and serves as an important noninvasive tool for evaluating patients with suspected mesenteric ischemia.

VISCERAL ANGIOGRAPHY

Angiography is an invasive technique whereby a catheter is introduced into a blood vessel, and intravascular contrast is injected during fluoroscopic imaging to visualize the vessel's lumen. Visceral angiography is used for evaluating mesenteric vessels in the setting of GI bleeding and suspected mesenteric ischemia. For GI bleeding, angiography is sensitive enough to detect 1.0 to 1.5 mL/min of blood loss. Once the site of bleeding has been localized, the radiologist can infuse vasopressin (a vasoconstrictor) or embolize the vessel using tiny coals or gelatin sponges to ensure hemostasis. In the setting of mesenteric ischemia, angiography permits localization of a vascular stenosis or obstruction, followed by possible therapeutic interventions (e.g. balloon angioplasty, stent placement, infusion of vasodilators and thrombolytics). Other indications for angiography include the placement of transjugular intrahepatic portosystemic shunts (TIPS) in cirrhotic patients with intractable variceal bleeding or refractory ascites and chemoembolization of liver tumors.

RADIONUCLIDE IMAGING

Technetium-99m (^{99m}Tc) is currently the major radionuclide used in GI imaging. Its 6-hour half-life and ready availability make it ideal for clinical use. ^{99m}Tc is used to label various substances for use in several imaging techniques. ^{99m}Tc-sulfur colloid scanning and ^{99m}Tc-labeled red blood cell scanning are two distinct methods that can be used to detect active GI bleeding. The latter uses the patient's own blood cells to carry the radionuclide throughout the body. These methods can detect as little as 0.05 to 0.4 mL/min of blood loss. However, localization of the site of bleeding is less accurate with these methods compared with angiography. ^{99m}Tc scans are often performed before angiography to document ongoing bleeding before subjecting a patient to the more invasive, less sensitive study. A ^{99m}Tc-labeled red blood cell scan can also be used to diagnose a hepatic hemangioma with an almost 100% positive predictive value.

Cholescintigraphy using ^{99m}Tc-iminodiacetic acid (IDA) analogs is the most commonly performed liver study in nuclear medicine. The radionuclide is taken up by the liver, excreted into bile, and passes through the biliary tree into the gallbladder and duodenum. Failure to visualize the gallbladder during a hepatobiliary IDA scan may indicate cholecystitis secondary to cystic duct obstruction by a gallstone.

Meckel's diverticulum can be a source of abdominal pain and bleeding, but it can be difficult to visualize with standard endoscopic and radiographic imaging. The agent ^{99m}Tc-pertechnetate has a high affinity for gastric mucosa and is therefore used to demonstrate the presence of this congenital anomaly.

Prospectus for the Future

Through continued technologic advances, improvements in both endoscopic and radiologic image quality and resolution will also continue. In addition, the gastrointestinal lumen will no longer be regarded as a boundary to therapeutic endoscopy. Examples of expected innovations include:

- *The implementation of transgastric endoscopically guided surgical procedures.* With the use of recently introduced instruments, an endoscopist will be able to incise the gastric wall, advance an endoscope into the peritoneal cavity, and then perform surgical procedures such as elective cholecystectomy. A new field of *endosurgery* will develop to accompany these advances and will require training in both surgical principles and gastroenterology.
- *Commercial availability of new endoscopic imaging methods, such as confocal microscopy and fluorescence endoscopy.* Confocal microscopy allows an endoscopist to obtain magnified endoscopic images similar to those seen with a low-power microscope. Fluorescence endoscopy entails the use of special wavelengths of light to excite naturally occurring fluorophores in benign and neoplastic tissue. These fluorophores, such as collagen and nicotinamide adenine dinucleotide plus hydrogen (NADH), then fluoresce in a predictable manner, thereby providing a means of identifying, by endoscopy, otherwise microscopic changes, such as dysplasia without the need for a biopsy.
- *Video capsule endoscopes with advanced diagnostic and possibly therapeutic capabilities.* Through further advances in nanotechnology, video capsule endoscopes will be able to sample gastrointestinal secretions, measure intraluminal pressures, take biopsies, and perhaps even provide focal ablation of lesions using thermal energy or radiofrequency ablation.

References

Byrne MF, Jowell PS: Gastrointestinal imaging: Endoscopic ultrasound. Gastroenterology 122:1631–1648, 2002.

Fleischer D: Capsule imaging. Clin Gastroenterol Hepatol 3:S30–S32, 2005.

Gore RM, Levine MS: Textbook of Gastrointestinal Radiology, 2nd ed. Philadelphia: WB Saunders, 2000.

Thrall JH, Ziessman HA: Nuclear medicine: The requisites, 2nd ed. St. Louis: Mosby, 2000.

Esophageal Disorders

Robert C. Lowe

M. Michael Wolfe

The esophagus appears to be a simple organ with a single function, the transmission of ingested food and fluids to the stomach. This task is achieved, however, by a tightly coordinated pattern of motility, coupled with a protective barrier that prevents gastric secretions from entering the esophagus and pharynx. Derangement of these activities can cause a significant number of distressing symptoms that are among the most common reasons for patients to seek medical care.

Normal Function of the Esophagus

The esophagus is a hollow muscular tube designed to transport ingested materials from the mouth to the stomach in a coordinated fashion. It is composed of both striated muscle (the proximal one third) and smooth muscle (the distal two thirds), bounded by two sphincters that are tonically contracted between swallows. The upper esophageal sphincter (UES) opens to admit a bolus into the esophagus and then closes rapidly to prevent aspiration of material into the trachea. The lower esophageal sphincter (LES) opens at the initiation of a swallow and remains open until the bolus passes into the stomach. It then closes to prevent reflux of ingested material into the esophageal body.

The act of swallowing begins with propulsion of the chewed bolus into the posterior oropharynx by the tongue. During the next phase of swallowing, several actions occur:

- The soft palate elevates to close off the nasopharynx.
- The epiglottis closes over the larynx, sealing off the trachea.
- The larynx is pulled upward to facilitate esophageal opening.
- The UES relaxes.
- The pharyngeal constrictors contract to propel the bolus into the esophagus.

Once the bolus has entered the esophagus, it is propelled downward by a series of coordinated contractions (primary peristalsis). The motility of the esophagus is mediated by local neurotransmitter release from enteric neurons. Contraction of esophageal segments above a bolus is induced by acetylcholine, whereas relaxation of segments below the bolus is mediated by both nitric oxide (NO) and vasoactive intestinal peptide (VIP).

Symptoms of Esophageal Disease

Heartburn (pyrosis) is the most common symptom of esophageal disease, occurring in 44% of Americans at least once a month. Approximately 10% of persons in the United States experience heartburn every day. It is most often described as a burning sensation in the epigastrium that rises into the chest. Patients often move their hand up and down between the xiphoid and sternal angle when describing this symptom. Given that heartburn is a cardinal sign of gastroesophageal reflux, it tends to occur after meals, when a patient is lying supine, or after an increase in intra-abdominal pressure (bending or lifting). Specific types of food, including fatty or spicy foods and chocolate, may also induce heartburn. Symptoms are often relieved temporarily by antacid preparations. Heartburn may be accompanied by regurgitation of bitter or sour fluid into the back of the throat or by excessive saliva production (the so-called *water brash,* which is caused by a vagal reflex induced by the presence of acid in the esophagus).

Dysphagia refers to a sensation of difficulty swallowing; patients report that a food bolus "gets stuck" or "goes down slowly." Although patients may point to their neck or chest when describing where the bolus gets held up, the location to which they point is poorly correlated with the actual level of obstruction. Dysphagia may result from a mechanical obstruction of the esophagus, inflammation of the esophageal mucosa, or an abnormality of motility of the esophagus.

Odynophagia, or pain on swallowing, needs to be differentiated from dysphagia in the patient history because it can be an important clue to the cause of the swallowing disorder. Painful swallowing is most often associated with infectious esophagitis or pill-induced esophageal ulcers but is only rarely present in acid-mediated esophageal disease.

Chest pain may also be a sign of esophageal disease, most often caused by gastroesophageal reflux or esophageal dysmotility. Unfortunately for the clinician, the symptoms of cardiac and esophageal chest pain overlap because of the shared neural pathways mediating pain sensation to these organs. Typical features of angina may occur in reflux-induced chest pain, including radiation to the neck and jaw, relief with nitrates, which modulate esophageal motility, and onset of symptoms with exertion. Chest pain that wakes a patient from sleep, however, is uncommon in true cardiac disease and may suggest an esophageal disorder, as does pain that is relieved with antacids or pain that lasts for several hours without associated symptoms. Esophageal chest pain is often thought to occur in response to esophageal spasm, but most data suggest that gastroesophageal reflux is responsible for the majority of cases.

Gastroesophageal Reflux Disease

Gastroesophageal reflux disease (GERD) is the most common disorder of the esophagus, causing occasional heartburn in nearly one half of the population and daily symptoms in nearly 15% of Americans. GERD is responsible for approximately $10 billion to $12 billion in direct medication costs per year, and acid antisecretory therapies used in the treatment of GERD are among the most commonly prescribed drugs in the United States.

PATHOGENESIS

GERD occurs when the esophageal mucosa is bathed in acid-containing gastric secretions. Under normal conditions, several defensive mechanisms exist to minimize esophageal acid exposure. The most important of these mechanisms is the LES, which remains closed between swallows, separating the gastric and esophageal compartments. In a minority of patients with GERD, the LES is tonically weak, whereas the most common abnormality seen in these patients is an increase in transient LES relaxations (TLESRs). These brief relaxations occur in all persons, but those with GERD have a large number of episodes, allowing excessive acid exposure to the esophagus. The presence of a hiatal hernia contributes to deficient LES function by removing the added constriction of the diaphragmatic crura; thus, hiatal hernia is often noted in patients with GERD. However, reflux and hiatal hernia may occur independently of one another. Other factors contributing to esophageal protection include:

- Esophageal bicarbonate secretion
- Esophageal motility—acid in the esophagus induces contractions (so-called *secondary peristalsis*) to clear the refluxate. Patients with motility disorders cannot empty refluxed acid into the stomach, leading to increased esophageal exposure to acid and symptoms of GERD.
- Saliva—salivary bicarbonate helps neutralize refluxed acid. Patients with sicca syndrome therefore have an increased incidence of GERD symptoms.

These factors are summarized in Figure 35–1.

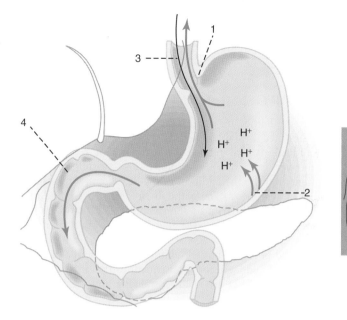

Figure 35–1 Pathogenesis of GERD: *1,* impaired lower esophageal sphincter-low pressures or frequent transient lower esophageal sphincter relaxation; *2,* hypersecretion of acid; *3,* decreased acid clearance resulting from impaired peristalsis or abnormal saliva production; *4,* delayed gastric emptying or duodenogastric reflux of bile salts and pancreatic enzymes.

CLINICAL FEATURES

Heartburn is the cardinal clinical feature of GERD, and, when present, the diagnosis of GERD is made easily. Complaints of bitter regurgitation or water brash add to the diagnostic accuracy, but these features are not always present. In some cases, atypical symptoms dominate in patients with no history of heartburn. The majority of cases of noncardiac chest pain, which can mimic angina, are believed to be caused by GERD. In addition, a significant number of additional symptoms, including chronic cough, asthma, hoarseness, chronic sore throat, and globus sensation, may be the result of occult gastroesophageal reflux (**Web Table 35–1**).

DIAGNOSIS

The diagnosis of GERD is most often made on clinical grounds in patients with typical symptoms. Endoscopy is not a sensitive means of diagnosing GERD, given that only 15% of patients with GERD will have endoscopic evidence of esophagitis; endoscopy is useful, however, in identifying complications of GERD, including esophageal ulcers, strictures, and Barrett's esophagus. A barium upper gastrointestinal series may demonstrate reflux of contrast material, but this, too, is insensitive as a diagnostic test for GERD. If a diagnosis of GERD is in question owing to the presence of atypical symptoms or comorbid illnesses, the appropriate diagnostic test is a 24-hour ambulatory pH study. A nasogastric probe is placed into the stomach, and transducers continuously monitor the pH of the esophagus while the patient participates in his or her usual daily routine. Symptomatic episodes are recorded in a diary and compared with the recorded pH values. Although pH monitoring is the most accurate means of diagnosing GERD, it is not often used because an empiric trial of antisecretory therapy that leads to symptom resolution is considered diagnostic and is often used in place of expensive and invasive pH monitoring.

THERAPY

Many modalities are used in the treatment of GERD; these are outlined in Table 35–1. Therapy begins with lifestyle modifications that reduce the incidence of reflux. These maneuvers are often not completely successful, and most patients require the addition of medical therapy to achieve relief of symptoms. The pathophysiologic process underlying GERD is primarily an abnormality of LES motility, but current therapies directed at augmenting motility are rarely successful. Promotility agents such as metoclopramide have been used in GERD but with limited efficacy and a preponderance of side effects. Consequently, the mainstays of therapy for GERD are acid-neutralizing and antisecretory

therapy, which neutralize or inhibit gastric acid secretion and render the refluxate less irritating to the esophageal mucosa. Magnesium and aluminum-based antacids (Mylanta, Maalox, Rolaids) offer temporary relief of symptoms, but lasting relief is better achieved with histamine receptor antagonists (H_2RAs) and proton pump inhibitors (PPIs). Provided their optimal administration, PPIs are the most effective preparations, controlling GERD symptoms in greater than 85% of patients with daily (before breakfast) or twice-daily (before breakfast and dinner) dosing.

SEQUELAE OF GASTROESOPHAGEAL REFLUX DISEASE

Common complications of GERD include esophagitis, ulceration, and esophageal stricture. Strictures typically produce progressive dysphagia to solids and often require endoscopic dilation to relieve the obstruction followed by intensive antisecretory therapy to prevent recurrence.

BARRETT'S ESOPHAGUS

Barrett's esophagus is a condition in which the squamous mucosa of the esophagus undergoes metaplasia, becoming a columnar-lined epithelium with features of intestinal mucosa (goblet cells, Paneth cells). This *specialized intestinal epithelium* appears to occur as a result of years of acid exposure and is present in 5% to 15% of patients who undergo endoscopy for chronic GERD symptoms (**Web Fig. 35–1**). Barrett's changes may be localized to the area of the gastroesophageal junction or may extend several centimeters proximally. The clinical significance of Barrett's metaplasia lies in its propensity to undergo neoplastic change and develop into adenocarcinoma (**Web Fig. 35–2**). The risk of cancer in Barrett's esophagus is estimated to be 40 to 100 times that of the general population, with a 0.5% risk of developing cancer per patient-year. Neither acid suppression therapy nor fundoplication leads to regression of Barrett's metaplasia. At present, endoscopic surveillance is recommended for all patients with Barrett's esophagus. Endoscopy is performed every 2 years, and biopsies are taken from the area of abnormal mucosa. If the biopsies reveal low-grade dysplasia, then the frequency of endoscopies is increased. If high-grade dysplastic changes are seen and confirmed by a second pathologist, then the risk of subsequent adenocarcinoma is greater than 25%, and surgical resection should be considered.

Dysphagia

Evaluation of a patient complaining of difficulty swallowing begins with the discrimination between oropharyngeal and true esophageal disease. Oropharyngeal dysphagia is a disorder of initiation of swallowing caused by neurologic or muscular disease, including Parkinson's disease, stroke, multiple sclerosis, myasthenia gravis, and amyotrophic lateral sclerosis (ALS). Patients with oropharyngeal dysphagia may complain of an inability to move the bolus to the back of the mouth and may note pooling of food in the cheeks after a swallow. Coughing or sputtering while eating may indicate aspiration of food, and nasal regurgitation is a classic sign of

---

Table 35–1 Treatment of Gastroesophageal Reflux Disease

Simple (Lifestyle) Measures

Elevation of the head of the bed
Avoidance of food or liquids 2–3 hr before bedtime
Avoidance of fatty or spicy foods
Avoidance of cigarettes, alcohol
Weight loss
Liquid antacid (aluminum hydroxide, magnesium hydroxide), 30 mL 30 min after meals and at bedtime, *or* over-the-counter H_2-receptor blockers

Persistent Symptoms

Without Esophagitis

Alginic acid antacids (Gaviscon), 10 mL 30 min after meals and at bedtime
Promotility drugs
Cisapride, 10 mg four times daily (qid)
Metoclopramide, 10 mg qid
H_2-receptor blockers
Cimetidine, 400 mg twice daily (bid)
Ranitidine, 150 mg bid
Famotidine, 20 mg bid
Nizatidine, 150 mg bid

With Esophagitis

H_2-Receptor blockers—regular or double dose depending on severity
H_2-Receptor blocker and promotility agent
Proton pump inhibitor
Omeprazole, 20 mg every morning
Lansoprazole, 30 mg every morning
Antireflux surgery

oropharyngeal dysphagia caused by a lack of coordination of the soft palate, which fails to close off the nasopharynx during swallowing. Treatment of oropharyngeal dysphagia consists of treating the underlying disorder, if possible, along with intensive speech and swallowing therapy that teaches patients techniques for improving their swallowing function.

If a patient is found to truly have esophageal dysphagia, the next step in evaluation is to distinguish between mechanical obstruction of the esophagus and an abnormality of esophageal motility. Patients with motility disorders often describe dysphagia to both solids and liquids, whereas patients with obstruction generally have progressive obstruction *only to solids* until very late in their disease, when the obstruction becomes so narrow as to interfere with the passage of liquids. An important diagnostic feature in patients with dysphagia to solids is whether the dysphagia is intermittent or progressive. Intermittent dysphagia indicates the presence of an esophageal ring or web, whereas progressive symptoms are more likely to be caused by a stricture or mass lesion. A barium swallow is useful in outlining obstructive lesions of the esophagus, although endoscopy will then be necessary for purposes of biopsy and possible dilation; many gastroenterologists choose to evaluate dysphagia with an initial upper endoscopy to avoid numerous diagnostic tests.

If radiologic testing or endoscopic examination fail to demonstrate an obstructing lesion, the motility of the esophagus should be evaluated using esophageal manometry, a procedure in which a nasogastric tube with pressure transducers is placed in the esophagus, and pressures are measured during a specific number of swallows. This procedure permits diagnosis of motility disorders such as achalasia, diffuse esophageal spasm, or other nonspecific motility disorders. An algorithm for the management of patients with dysphagia is presented in Figure 35–2.

Esophageal Motility Disorders

Many patients with esophageal dysmotility have a nonspecific disorder that cannot be definitively characterized; however, three of the more common disorders of esophageal motility are achalasia, diffuse esophageal spasm, and scleroderma. The features of these three diseases are outlined in Table 35–2.

ACHALASIA

Achalasia is a rare disorder of esophageal motility characterized by a tonically contracted LES that fails to relax appropriately during swallows, along with a dilated, aperistaltic esophagus. The disorder is caused by a degeneration of neurons in the myenteric plexus of the esophagus and in the vagal nuclei supplying the esophagus. Patients with achalasia typically have progressive dysphagia and weight loss and commonly experience chest pain and regurgitation of undigested food. Diagnosis is made using esophageal manometry, which reveals a tightly contacted LES that fails to relax with swallowing, along with poor or absent peristalsis in the esophageal body. Endoscopy is indicated to rule out an obstructing lesion of the lower esophagus or gastric cardia, which can mimic achalasia. Barium study in achalasia demonstrates a characteristic pattern shown in Figure 35–3. The widely dilated esophagus that tapers to a narrow *bird's beak* is highly suggestive of achalasia but does not obviate the need for endoscopy and manometric evaluation. Treatment is directed at opening the contracted LES, either by balloon dilation or by surgical myotomy. Botulinum toxin injections are also used to relax the LES, but relief is usually transient and re-treatment is almost always necessary.

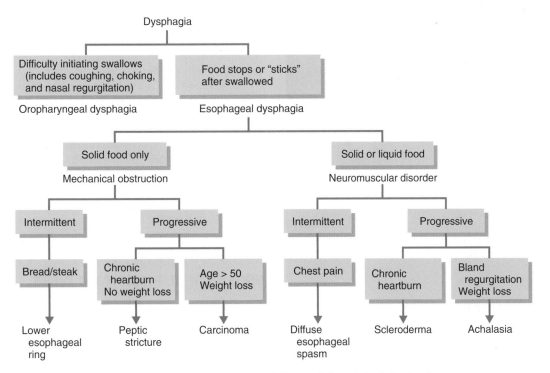

Figure 35–2 Algorithm for the differential diagnosis of dysphagia.

Table 35–2	**Esophageal Motor Disorders**		
	Achalasia	**Scleroderma**	**Diffuse Esophageal Spasm**
Symptoms			
	Dysphagia Regurgitation of nonacidic material	Gastroesophageal reflux disease Dysphagia	Substernal chest pain (angina-like) Dysphagia with pain
Radiographic Appearance			
	Dilated, fluid-filled esophagus Distal *bird beak* stricture	Aperistaltic esophagus Free reflux Peptic stricture	Simultaneous noncoordinated contractions
Manometric Findings			
Lower esophageal sphincter	High resting pressure Incomplete or abnormal relaxation with swallow	Low resting pressure	Normal pressure
Body	Low-amplitude, simultaneous contractions after swallowing	Low-amplitude peristaltic contractions or no peristalsis	Some peristalsis Diffuse and simultaneous nonperistaltic contractions, occasionally high amplitude

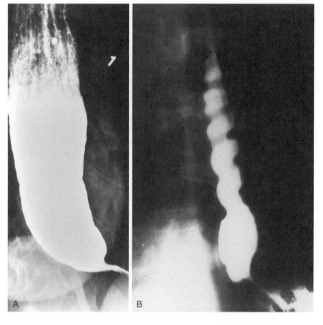

Figure 35–3 Radiologic appearance of achalasia *(A)* and diffuse esophageal spasm *(B)*. In achalasia, the esophageal body is dilated and terminates in a narrowed segment or *bird beak*. The appearance of numerous simultaneous contractions is typical of diffuse esophageal spasm.

DIFFUSE ESOPHAGEAL SPASM

Diffuse esophageal spasm is a motility disorder of the esophagus that usually produces episodes of chest pain and intermittent dysphagia to both solids and liquids. Manometric examination of the esophagus reveals uncoordinated, non-peristaltic contractions of normal or increased amplitude. This disorder is difficult to treat, given that pharmacologic therapy with nitrates and calcium channel blockers often proves minimally effective. Balloon dilation of the esophagus has been associated with relief in a minority of patients, as has surgical myotomy.

SCLERODERMA (PROGRESSIVE SYSTEMIC SCLEROSIS)

Esophageal dysmotility is a cardinal feature of scleroderma, occurring in up to 80% of patients. Scleroderma affects the distal two thirds of the esophagus (i.e., the smooth muscle portion), leading to fibrosis, atrophy, aperistalsis of the distal esophagus, and decreased LES tone. The manometric features of scleroderma include poor peristalsis in the distal esophageal body and a weak LES. As a result of this dysmotility, gastroesophageal reflux is typically present and is often severe; erosive esophagitis and peptic strictures are not uncommon, and patients may exhibit dysphagia caused by the primary dysmotility or to mechanical obstruction associated with stricture. The use of PPIs has significantly decreased the incidence of erosive GERD and its sequelae in patients with scleroderma.

Other Esophageal Disorders
ESOPHAGEAL RINGS AND WEBS

Esophageal rings (also called Schatzki or B rings) are rings of fibrous tissue that occur in the lower esophagus and cause intermittent dysphagia to solids. Classically, patients experience dysphagia when eating a large piece of meat or soft bread (leading to the name *steakhouse syndrome*). Between episodes of dysphagia, patients report normal swallowing and no associated symptoms. On endoscopic examination, rings are visible in the distal esophagus and may be partial or completely circumferential (**Web Fig. 35–3**). Treatment with balloon or bougie dilation is effective in relieving symptoms, though some patients require repeated dilations to remain symptom free. Esophageal webs are similar to rings but tend to occur in the proximal esophagus. An association between esophageal webs and iron deficiency anemia (sideropenic dysphagia) has been described (also known as Plummer-Vinson or Patterson-Kelly syndrome).

ESOPHAGEAL INFECTIONS

Infections of the esophagus occur but are uncommon in patients who are immunocompetent. They are, however, a major source of morbidity in patients with compromised immunity, including organ transplant recipients, patients infected with human immunodeficiency virus (HIV), and patients on chronic steroids. Infectious esophagitis tends to produce both dysphagia and odynophagia, with the latter being the predominant symptom. Candida esophagitis is often associated with oral thrush and tends to produce dysphagia and only mild pain on swallowing. Candida has a characteristic appearance on endoscopic examination and esophageal brushings and biopsies demonstrate fungal hyphae (**Web Fig. 35–4**). Treatment with oral fluconazole is generally effective. Herpes simplex virus (HSV) causes mul-

tiple esophageal ulcers and exhibits clinically with severe odynophagia. Acyclovir is the treatment of choice for herpes esophagitis. Cytomegalovirus (CMV) also causes esophageal ulceration and odynophagia. Endoscopic examination usually demonstrates a single large ulcer in the distal esophagus, and biopsies often detect viral inclusions that confirm the diagnosis. Both ganciclovir and foscarnet are effective treatments for CMV esophagitis. HIV infection is itself associated with esophageal ulceration and odynophagia, although much less commonly in the era of effective anti-retroviral therapy.

PILL ESOPHAGITIS

Several medications can cause esophageal ulceration following prolonged contact with the esophageal mucosa. The most common medications associated with this condition include tetracyclines, potassium preparations, nonsteroidal anti-inflammatory drugs (NSAIDs), iron sulfate, and the bisphosphonate alendronate. Patients report epigastric pain, sometimes radiating to the back, and both dysphagia and odynophagia. Treatment is symptomatic, and topical preparations such as viscous lidocaine may be helpful in relieving discomfort. Prevention of pill esophagitis is accomplished by ensuring that patients drink sufficient fluid (>120 mL) when taking oral medications. Patients should also be counseled to avoid lying down immediately after swallowing pills.

Prospectus for the Future

Our understanding of a significant number of issues regarding GERD, including extra-esophageal manifestations and disease sequelae, will continue to evolve in the future, leading to progress in the treatment options for this common disorder. These issues include:

- The development of effective and safe prokinetic agents that are aimed at treating the pathophysiologic motor abnormalities underlying GERD and the development of new medication aimed at providing prompt and sustained improvement in symptoms associated with GERD, such as episodic heartburn.
- Improvements in the understanding of the precise role and contribution of gastric contents to the development of non-cardiac chest pain and tracheopulmonary symptoms attributed to GERD.

- Improvement in the early detection of Barrett's metaplasia, dysplasia, and early esophageal adenocarcinoma (including chemoprevention) in patients with GERD. These improvements will include a better understanding of the cellular and molecular pathways that underlie metaplastic and neoplastic transformation and tumor progression, which will serve to provide additional targets for selective pharmacologic or immunologic forms of therapy.
- Technologic advances in the performance of both instrument and capsule endoscopic methods, including endoscopic spectrophotometry, for the diagnosis and treatment of Barrett's-associated dysplasia and esophageal adenocarcinoma.
- A better definition of the roles of surgical and endoscopic methods to treat GERD and its complications and the precise role of photodynamic therapy and other novel methods for the ablation of dysplastic and neoplastic mucosa.

References

Baehr PH, McDonald GB: Esophageal infections: Risk factors, presentation, diagnosis, and treatment. Gastroenterology 106:509–532, 1994.

Barrison AF, Jarboe LA, Weinberg BM, et al: Patterns of proton pump inhibitor use in clinical practice. Am J Med 111:469–473, 2001.

Mittal RK, Balaban DH: The esophagogastric junction. NEJM 336:924–932, 1997.

Shaheen N, Ransohoff DF: Gastroesophageal reflux, Barrett esophagus, and esophageal cancer: Scientific review. JAMA 287:1972–1981, 2002.

Shaker R, Castell DO, Schoenfeld PS, Spechler SJ: Nighttime heartburn is an under-appreciated clinical problem that impacts sleep and daytime

function: The results of a Gallup survey conducted on behalf of the American Gastroenterological Association. Am J Gastroenterol 98(7): 1487–1493, 2003.

Spechler SJ: Clinical practice: Barrett's esophagus. NEJM 346:836–842, 2002.

Spechler SJ, Castell DO: Classification of oesophageal motility abnormalities. Gut 49:145–151, 2001.

Vakil N: Review article: New pharmacological agents for the treatment of gastro-oesophageal reflux disease. Aliment Pharmacol Ther 19:1041–1049, 2004.

Chapter 36

Diseases of the Stomach and Duodenum

Jaime A. Oviedo

M. Michael Wolfe

The stomach, a J-shaped dilation of the alimentary tract, acts as a reservoir for recently ingested food and initiates the process of digestion. By storing large quantities of food (1.5 to 2.0 L in the adult), the stomach allows intermittent feeding. Once solid particles have been reduced in size to accommodate the much smaller capacity of the duodenum, the gastric contents are released through the pylorus in a controlled fashion. This chapter focuses on the anatomy and physiology of the stomach and duodenum, as well as on the most common disease processes that may involve these two organs.

Gastroduodenal Anatomy

The stomach is in continuity with the esophagus proximally and the duodenum distally. A circular smooth muscle structure, the *lower esophageal sphincter,* located at the distal end of the esophagus, creates a high-pressure zone that, under normal conditions, prevents gastric contents from refluxing into the esophagus. Similarly, the pyloric sphincter, the most distal portion of the stomach, plays an important role in the trituration of solid food particles and ensures the downstream propulsion of the food bolus, preventing duodenogastric reflux. The stomach is divided into four regions (**Fig. 36–1; Web Video 36–1**). The cardia is a poorly defined transition from the esophagogastric junction to the fundus. The dome-shaped fundus projects upward above the cardia and is the most superior part of the stomach in contact with the left hemidiaphragm and the spleen. The body, or corpus, located immediately below and continuous with the fundus, is the largest part of the stomach and is characterized by the presence of longitudinal folds known as rugae. The antrum extends from the incisura angularis, a fixed sharp indentation that marks the end of the gastric body, to the *pylorus,* or *pyloric channel,* a tubular structure that joins the stomach to the duodenum.

The mucosa, or inner lining of the stomach, is formed by a layer of columnar epithelium. The submucosa, immediately deep to the mucosa, provides a skeleton of dense connective tissue in which lymphocytes, plasma cells, arterioles, venules, lymphatics, and the myenteric plexus are contained. The third tissue layer, the muscularis propria, is a combination of an inner oblique, a middle circular, and an outer longitudinal smooth muscle layer. The serosa, a thin, transparent continuation of the visceral peritoneum, is the final layer of the stomach wall. The autonomic innervation of the stomach stems from both the sympathetic and parasympathetic nervous systems. The anterior and posterior trunks of the vagus nerve provide parasympathetic innervation, whereas the celiac plexus, coursing along the vascular supply of the stomach, provides sympathetic innervation.

The gastric mucosal surface is composed of a single layer of mucus-containing columnar epithelial cells. The surface lining is invaginated by gastric pits, which provide access to the gastric lumen for gastric glands. The gastric glands of different regions of the stomach are lined with different types of specialized cells. The oxyntic or acid-producing region of the stomach is found in the fundus and body, where gastric glands contain characteristic parietal cells, which secrete both acid and intrinsic factor. These glands also contain zymogen-rich chief cells, which synthesize pepsinogen, and enterochromaffin-like endocrine cells, which secrete histamine. Antral glands have different endocrine cells, including gastrin-secreting G cells and somatostatin-secreting D cells.

The duodenum, the most proximal portion of the small intestine, forms a C-shaped loop around the head of the pancreas and is in continuity with the pylorus proximally and the jejunum distally (see Fig. 36–1 and Web Video 36–1). Angular changes in course divide the duodenum into four portions. The first part of the duodenum is the duodenal bulb or cap and is characterized by a smooth, featureless luminal surface. The remainder of the duodenum has characteristic circular folds known as the *plica circularis* or *valvulae conniventes,* which increase the surface area available for digestion. Similar to the stomach, the duodenal wall is formed by mucosa, submucosa, muscularis, and serosa layers. The duodenal mucosa is lined with columnar cells

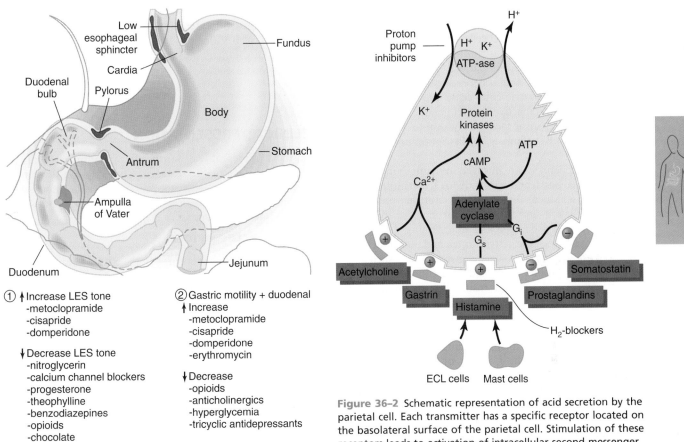

Figure 36–1 Anatomic regions of the stomach and duodenum. Agents that affect LES tone and gastroduodenal motility.

① ↑Increase LES tone
-metoclopramide
-cisapride
-domperidone

↓Decrease LES tone
-nitroglycerin
-calcium channel blockers
-progesterone
-theophylline
-benzodiazepines
-opioids
-chocolate
-coffee
-peppermint

② Gastric motility + duodenal
↑Increase
-metoclopramide
-cisapride
-domperidone
-erythromycin

↓Decrease
-opioids
-anticholinergics
-hyperglycemia
-tricyclic antidepressants

Figure 36–2 Schematic representation of acid secretion by the parietal cell. Each transmitter has a specific receptor located on the basolateral surface of the parietal cell. Stimulation of these receptors leads to activation of intracellular second messenger systems: Gastrin and acetylcholine promote the accumulation of intracellular calcium, whereas histamine causes a stimulatory G protein (G_s) to activate adenylate cyclase, which, in turn, generates cyclic adenosine monophosphate (cAMP). These intracellular messengers then activate protein kinases, which activate the proton pump (the H^+, K^+-ATPase enzyme), located at the apical surface of the parietal cell, to secrete H^+ ion in exchange for K^+ ions. Prostaglandins and somatostatin inhibit parietal cell function by binding to receptors that act through inhibitory G proteins (G_i) to inhibit adenylate cyclase. Long arrows indicate sites of action of various drugs that inhibit acid secretion. ECL = enterochromaffin-like endocrine cells.

forming villi surrounded by crypts of Lieberkühn. The submucosa includes characteristic Brunner's glands that produce bicarbonate-rich secretions involved in acid neutralization. The innervation of the duodenum is also similar to that of the stomach.

Gastroduodenal Mucosal Secretions and Protective Factors

Although hydrochloric acid (HCl) is the primary gastric secretion, the stomach also secretes water, electrolytes (hydrogen [H^+], sodium [Na^+], potassium [K^+], chloride [Cl^-], and bicarbonate [HCO_3]), enzymes (pepsin and gastric lipase), and glycoproteins (intrinsic factors and mucin) to assist in a wide variety of physiologic functions. The digestion of proteins and triglycerides, as well as the complex process of vitamin B_{12} absorption, begins in the gastric lumen. Gastric acid also prevents the development of enteric colonization and systemic infections. The normal human stomach contains approximately 1 billion parietal cells that secrete H^+ ions into the gastric lumen in response to various physiologic stimuli. Parietal cells located in the oxyntic

glands of the fundus and body of the stomach are stimulated to secrete H^+ ions by three different pathways: neurocrine, paracrine, and endocrine (Fig. 36–2). The neurocrine pathway involves the vagal release of acetylcholine, which stimulates H^+ ion generation via a parietal cell muscarinic M_3 receptor. The paracrine pathway is mediated by the release of histamine from mast cells and enterochromaffin-like (ECL) cells in the stomach. Histamine binds to histamine$_2$-specific receptors on parietal cells, activating adenylate cyclase, which, in turn, leads to an increase in adenosine 3′, 5′-cyclic monophosphate (cAMP) levels and subsequent generation of H^+ ions. The secretion of gastrin from antral G cells constitutes the endocrine pathway and stimulates H^+ ion generation both directly on the parietal cell and indirectly by stimulating histamine secretion from ECL cells. The sodium-potassium adenosine triphosphatase (H^+, K^+-ATPase) enzyme, or proton pump, located at the apical surface of the parietal cell, is the final step of acid secretion.

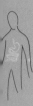

A negative feedback loop governs both gastrin release and acid secretion, preventing postprandial acid hypersecretion. Somatostatin, produced by D cells in the gastric corpus and fundus, inhibits release of gastrin from G cells and may also reduce acid secretion from parietal cells and histamine release from ECL cells. Acid is necessary to convert pepsinogen, secreted from gastric chief cells, into pepsin, a proteolytic enzyme that is inactive at a pH greater than 4. Parietal cells also secrete intrinsic factor, a glycoprotein that binds to ingested vitamin B_{12}, allowing its absorption in the terminal ileum.

Several mechanisms are involved in maintaining the protective mucosal barrier. Mucus and HCO_3 constitute the first line of defense. Mucus forms a stable layer that prevents H^+ ion back-diffusion and lubricates the mucosa, protecting against mechanical damage and maintaining a significant pH gradient between the gastric lumen and the epithelial cell surface. Endogenous epithelial defensive factors, such as cell migration and proliferation, lead to a constant and rapid renewal of the mucosa and ensure the continuity of the epithelium and the integrity of the tight intercellular junctions. Subepithelial defensive factors such as an adequate mucosal blood flow constitute a second line of protection and play a crucial role in maintaining a normal pH environment and thereby the integrity of the gastroduodenal mucosa.

Gastroduodenal Motor Physiology

Based on electrophysiologic and functional characteristics, the stomach can be divided into two functional compartments. The proximal stomach (fundus and proximal third of the body) acts as a reservoir for recently ingested food, whereas the distal stomach grinds, mixes, and sieves food particles. The smooth muscle of the proximal stomach has a characteristic tonic contraction that allows for gastric accommodation, a process by which the fundus relaxes in response to incoming food and fluid, with little increase in intragastric pressure. In contrast, the distal stomach produces high-amplitude contractions originating from the pacemaker region in the midportion of the greater curvature.

Gastroduodenal motor events vary in response to fasting and food intake. During fasting, gastric motility is characterized by a pattern of phasic contractions known as the migrating motor complex (MMC). The MMC clears the stomach and small intestine of undigested food particles, mucus, and sloughed epithelial cells. The MMC begins in the stomach and migrates down the length of the small bowel with a combined duration of 84 to 112 minutes. Following a meal, irregular contractile activity propels the ingested material distally.

Gastric emptying of a mixed solid and liquid meal involves the coordinated actions of the distinct regions of the stomach with feedback from the small intestine. While liquids empty from the stomach at a relatively linear rate, solids are propelled forward by gastric contractions toward the antrum, where particles are triturated by high-amplitude contractions. Once solids have been reduced in size to particles of 1 to 2 mm, they are emptied into the pylorus.

A variety of medications and foods that exert significant effects on gastroduodenal motility are described in Figure 36–1 (see **Web Video 36–1**). Agents that modify the lower esophageal sphincter and esophageal motility are explained in Chapter 35.

Gastritis
CLINICAL PRESENTATION

Gastritis represents a nonspecific inflammation of the mucosal surface of the stomach. Clinically, the three most common causes of gastritis are *Helicobacter pylori*, nonsteroidal anti-inflammatory drugs (NSAIDs), and stress-related mucosal changes.

Helicobacter pylori

Helicobacter pylori are curved, flagellated, gram-negative rods found only in gastric epithelium or in gastric metaplastic epithelium. It is the most common worldwide microbial infection, with an estimated 50% of the world's population being infected. *H. pylori* clearly cause histologic gastritis and are found in 50% to 95% of patients with gastroduodenal ulcers. However, only a minority of patients with *H. pylori* gastritis develop peptic ulcer disease (PUD) or gastric cancer. In the Western world, a clear age-related prevalence of *H. pylori* infection exists in healthy individuals, increasing from 10% in those younger than age 30 to 60% in those older than age 60, and the mode of transmission appears to be via the fecal-oral route. Improvements in sanitation and standards of living have been associated with a decline in the rate of infection. *H. pylori* colonization is more common in individuals in lower socioeconomic strata compared with other groups. In the developing world, infection is far more common, with over 80% of the population being infected by age 20. *H. pylori* infection is typically lifelong, unless antimicrobial treatment is instituted.

H. pylori reside in the mucus layer overlying gastric epithelium and are characterized as noninvasive organisms. Factors important in the organism's ability to colonize the stomach include its motility, production of urease, and bacterial adherence. Ammonia generated from urea by *H. pylori* urease neutralizes acid, creating a more hospitable microclimate in which the bacteria can survive. *H. pylori* also have the ability to bind specifically to gastric-type epithelium, which prevents the organisms from being shed during cell turnover and mucus secretion or gastric motility. Tissue injury is mediated by the production of lipopolysaccharide, leukocyte-activating factors, and *CagA* and *VacA* proteins, which have been associated with cytotoxic effects, inflammation, and cytokine activation. Colonization causes acute and chronic inflammation consisting of neutrophils, plasma cells, T cells, and macrophages accompanied by varying degrees of epithelial cell injury, all of which resolve after treatment.

Although predicting the ultimate outcome of *H. pylori* infection is impossible, the clinical manifestations can be correlated with various distributions of gastric histopathologic states. Antral-predominant *H. pylori* gastritis is associated with duodenal ulcers, whereas corporal and fundic colonizations are more likely to cause atrophic gastritis. Other important factors that may influence the outcomes of the infection include the host response, environmental factors, and age at the time of infection. Virtually all patients with *H. pylori* infection have a chronic superficial gastritis; however, duodenal and gastric ulcers develop in only 20% of infected patients. Patients with *H. pylori* infection and severe atrophic gastritis, corpus-predominant gastritis, or both, along with intestinal metaplasia, are at increased risk for intestinal-type gastric cancer. Finally, the mucosal lymphocytic response to *H. pylori* infection may lead to a monoclonal B-cell proliferation in mucosa-associated lymphoid tissue (MALT). MALT lymphomas, also known as maltomas, are rare, with approximately 1 in 1 million infected patients developing the disease. Complete histologic regression has been demonstrated in 50% to 80% of maltomas following eradication of *H. pylori*. Flat, localized, nonbulky lesions of the distal stomach are associated with greater rates of cure following antibiotic therapy.

Nonsteroidal Anti-inflammatory Drugs

NSAIDs are one of the most widely used classes of drugs. Although generally well tolerated, NSAIDs are associated with a small but significant percentage of adverse gastrointestinal (GI) events. Concepts about NSAID-induced gastroduodenal mucosal injury have evolved from a simple notion of topical injury to theories involving multiple mechanisms with both local and systemic effects. According to the dual-injury hypothesis, NSAIDs have direct toxic effects on the gastroduodenal mucosa and indirect effects through active hepatic metabolites and decreased synthesis of mucosal prostaglandins. Hepatic metabolites are excreted into the bile and subsequently into the duodenum, where they may cause mucosal damage to the stomach by duodenogastric reflux and to the small intestine by antegrade passage through the GI tract. Prostaglandin inhibition, in turn, leads to reduction in epithelial mucus, decreased secretion of HCO_3, impaired mucosal blood flow, reduced epithelial proliferation, and decreased mucosal resistance to injury. The impairment in mucosal resistance facilitates mucosal injury by endogenous factors, including acid, pepsin, and bile salts.

Prostaglandins are derived from arachidonic acid, which originates from cell membrane phospholipids through the action of phospholipase A2. The metabolism of arachidonic acid to prostaglandins and leukotrienes is catalyzed by the cyclooxygenase (COX) pathway and the 5-lipoxygenase (LOX) pathway, respectively (Fig. 36–3) Two related but unique isoforms of COX, designated COX-1 and COX-2, have been demonstrated in mammalian cells. Despite their structural similarities, each is encoded by distinct genes that differ with regard to their distribution and expression in tissues; the COX-1 gene is primarily expressed constitutively, whereas the COX-2 gene is inducible. COX-1 appears to function as a housekeeping enzyme in most tissues, including the gastric mucosa, whereas the expression of COX-2 can be induced by inflammatory stimuli and mitogens in many different types of tissue. Theories have therefore suggested that the anti-inflammatory properties of NSAIDs are mediated through the inhibition of COX-2, whereas adverse effects, such as gastroduodenal ulceration, occur as a result of the effects on COX-1. The discovery of the two COX isoforms led to the development of COX-2–specific inhibitors (e.g., celecoxib, rofecoxib, valdecoxib), drugs that maintain

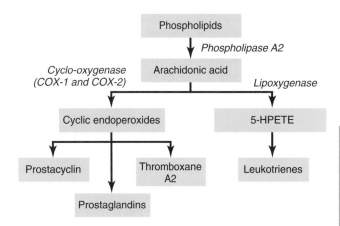

Figure 36–3 Biosynthesis of prostaglandins and leukotrienes via the cyclooxygenase and lipoxygenase pathways.

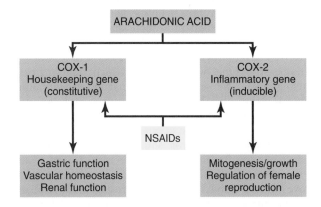

Figure 36–4 Depiction of the two cyclooxygenase (COX) isoenzymes that catalyze the synthesis of tissue prostaglandins from arachidonic acid.

their anti-inflammatory properties while preserving the biosynthesis of protective prostaglandins (Fig 36–4).

The spectrum of NSAID-related mucosal injury includes a combination of subepithelial hemorrhages, erosions, and ulcerations that is often referred to as *NSAID gastropathy*. Erosions are likely to be small and superficial, whereas ulcers tend to be larger (more than 5 mm in diameter) and deeper. Although no area of the stomach is resistant to NSAID-induced mucosal injury, the most frequently and severely affected site is the antrum. Microscopically, a *reactive* pattern of injury can be found that is characterized by mucin depletion and little or no increase in inflammatory cells. Endoscopic studies have shown a prevalence of gastroduodenal ulcers of 10% to 25% in patients with chronic arthritis treated with NSAIDs, which is 5 to 15 times the expected prevalence in an age-matched healthy population.

Stress-Related Gastric Mucosal Damage

During critical illness, events such as shock, hypotension, and catecholamine release are associated with reduced blood flow and mucosal ischemia. When blood flow to the mucosa is inadequate, the normal mucosal protective mechanisms, including epithelial turnover and mucus and HCO_3 secretion, are altered. In addition, mediators such as cytokines and oxygen-free radicals are released. The combination of these events reduces the mucosal resistance to acid back-diffusion, causing erosions that may progress to ulceration and bleeding. Although mucosal damage develops in the majority of critically ill patients, stress ulcers usually remain superficial and do not erode through the stomach wall to cause perforation. The major problem is blood loss, which is occult in most instances. Although occult stress ulcer bleeding occurs in 20% of patients in long-term intensive care units, gross hemorrhage occurs in only 5%.

TREATMENT

Aggressive volume resuscitation, control of sepsis, and adequate oxygenation in critically ill patients are important measures that may reduce the occurrence of low-flow states and subsequent mucosal damage. A wide variety of prophylactic strategies are used to prevent GI bleeding in critically ill patients. Pharmacologic agents used in this setting exert their effects through three main mechanisms: (1) acid neutralization, (2) mucosal protection, and (3) inhibition of gastric acid secretion. Acid neutralization with antacids is effective but requires administration every 1 to 2 hours via a nasogastric tube, which is inconvenient and increases nursing time. The side effects of magnesium-containing antacids include diarrhea, hypermagnesemia, and alkalemia, whereas aluminum-based antacids cause hypophosphatemia, constipation, and metabolic alkalosis, as well as potentially toxic plasma aluminum levels in patients with renal insufficiency. Mucosal protective agents such as sucralfate, an aluminum salt of sucrose sulfate, may improve mucosal blood flow through a prostaglandin-mediated mechanism. Sucralfate is well tolerated at doses of 1 g every 4 to 6 hours. Constipation occurs in 2% to 4% of patients, and aluminum toxicity has occurred in patients with chronic renal failure. Prostaglandin analogs (e.g., misoprostol) exert a protective effect on the gastric mucosa but have not been carefully studied for stress ulcer prophylaxis, and their use in this setting cannot be recommended. Antisecretory agents inhibit gastric acid secretion and are frequently used in the prevention of stress-induced mucosal damage in critically ill patients. Histamine$_2$-receptor antagonists (H$_2$-RAs) (e.g., cimetidine, ranitidine, famotidine, nizatidine), given either as a continuous infusion or by bolus injection, have been shown to reduce the incidence of clinically significant stress bleeding. An increase in intragastric pH to greater than 4.0 has been demonstrated with these agents; however, tolerance occurs rapidly and may limit their clinical efficacy. Although H$_2$-RAs are considered safe, they do possess both class-specific and individual side effect potentials. The most prominent class-specific effect is central nervous system toxicity, which occurs more frequently in elderly patients compared with other age groups. Proton pump inhibitors (PPIs) irreversibly block parietal cell H$^+$, K$^+$-ATPase. These agents (e.g., omeprazole, lansoprazole, rabeprazole, pantoprazole, esomeprazole) are prokinetic agents that are normally activated following systemic absorption and localization to the highly acid milieu of the secretory canaliculus of *activated* parietal cells. Activation occurs following a meal, and because critically ill patients are generally fasting, PPIs administered orally or via nasogastric tube are significantly less active in this setting and are thus not recommended.

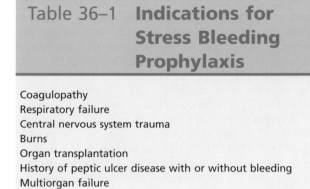

Table 36–1	Indications for Stress Bleeding Prophylaxis

Coagulopathy
Respiratory failure
Central nervous system trauma
Burns
Organ transplantation
History of peptic ulcer disease with or without bleeding
Multiorgan failure
Trauma or major surgery

Pantoprazole, the first intravenous PPI available in the United States, has shown promising results in several small studies and may prove beneficial in stress bleeding prophylaxis. Intravenous preparations of lansoprazole and esomeprazole have recently become available. No published data evaluating the use of the newer intravenous PPIs exist in this setting.

Prophylaxis is recommended in patients with coagulopathy and in patients with respiratory failure requiring mechanical ventilation for more than 48 hours. Other patients in whom stress bleeding prophylaxis is indicated include those with central nervous system trauma, burns, organ transplantation, a history of PUD with or without bleeding, multiorgan failure, trauma, and major surgery (Table 36–1).

OTHER CAUSES OF GASTRITIS

Autoimmune atrophic gastritis exhibits an autosomal-dominant inheritance pattern and is associated with autoantibody formation. Histologically, autoimmune atrophic gastritis is characterized by chronic inflammation, gradual atrophy of glands, and loss of parietal cells. The process is usually confined to the corpus and fundus, where the gastric glands tend to undergo intestinal metaplasia. Loss of parietal cells results in achlorhydria, vitamin B$_{12}$ deficiency, and megaloblastic anemia (pernicious anemia). These patients have an increased risk of carcinoma, especially in Scandinavian countries. No overall increased cancer risk has been documented in American patients, and routine surveillance has not been advocated in the United States.

Lymphocytic gastritis is characterized by a mononuclear infiltration of T cells, usually antral predominant, and is often associated with celiac disease, collagenous-lymphocytic colitis, and Ménétrier's disease. Eosinophilic gastritis is characterized by an eosinophilic infiltration of the stomach, especially the antrum. All layers of the gastric wall may be affected, but selective predominance of eosinophilic infiltrates may be found in the submucosa, muscle layers, or subserosa, making biopsy diagnosis difficult. Clinical manifestations include delayed gastric emptying or manifestations of anemia from chronic blood loss caused by associated mucosal ulceration. Corticosteroids are used to control symptoms.

Ménétrier's disease is a rare disease characterized by giant gastric folds in the fundus and the body of the stomach.

Histologically, increased mucosal thickness, glandular atrophy, and an increase in the size of the gastric pits are characteristic findings. Hypochlorhydria and hypoalbuminemia are commonly seen. In children, Ménétrier's disease is thought to be caused by cytomegalovirus (CMV), whereas overexpression of a tissue growth factor has been implicated in the adult form of the disease.

In addition to *H. pylori*, a variety of infectious pathogens may involve the stomach. Gastric infections are typically seen in patients who are immunocompromised in the settings of human immunodeficiency virus infection, chemotherapy, and organ transplantation. Bacterial infections such as tuberculosis and syphilis rarely involve the stomach. CMV and herpesvirus infection, as well as fungal (e.g., *Candida*, histoplasmosis, mucormycosis, cryptococcosis, aspergillosis), and parasitic infections (e.g., *Cryptosporidium*, *Strongyloides*) are also possible. Other diseases such as sarcoidosis and Crohn's disease may also involve the stomach. The presence of granulomas on histologic specimens along with systemic manifestations of the disease confirm the diagnosis.

The stomach is occasionally involved by acute *graft-versus-host* disease. Gastric erosions or ulcers may be encountered in the investigation of bone marrow transplantation patients with abdominal pain or GI bleeding. Biopsy specimens should be obtained to rule out opportunistic infections (e.g., CMV).

Alcohol, drugs (e.g., cocaine, iron, potassium chloride), and physical agents (nasogastric tubes) are also associated with nonspecific forms of gastritis. Similarly, ischemia as a result of vascular injuries, embolization, vasculitis, and amyloidosis have been described as causes of gastritis.

Peptic Ulcer Disease

Peptic ulcers are a common clinical problem characterized by mucosal defects of the GI mucosa of the stomach or the duodenum. The proteolytic enzyme pepsin and gastric acid were initially identified as the key factors involved in the pathogenesis of ulcers. Thus, the concept of *no acid, no ulcer* has been widely used and accepted for many years. However, in the last 2 decades, the roles of factors other than acid and pepsin in the development of ulcers have been recognized. Men and women are at equal risk of developing PUD, and the overall lifetime risk for both genders is 10%. Peptic ulcers are uncommon in children, but the risk increases with age. Over 70% of all ulcer cases occur in individuals between the ages of 25 and 64 years. However, whereas the incidence of PUD is decreasing in the young age groups, more persons 65 years of age and older are developing ulcers. These trends are likely related to the overall decrease in the prevalence of *H. pylori* infection and the increasing use of NSAIDs by the older population. The most important risk factors for the development of peptic ulcers are infection with *H. pylori* and use of NSAIDs. If neither of these factors is present, an alternative cause must be sought, such as hypersecretory states (e.g., Zollinger-Ellison syndrome [ZES]) or one of the other less common causes of ulcer disease, including Crohn's disease, vascular insufficiency, viral infection, radiation therapy, and cancer chemotherapy. Although a significant number of environmental factors, including stress, personality, occupation, alcohol consumption, and diet, have been linked to the development of ulcers, no convincing evidence suggesting that any of these factors can by itself cause PUD has been found.

PATHOPHYSIOLOGIC FACTORS

By killing ingested bacteria and other micro-organisms, gastric acid prevents the development of enteric colonization and ensures both efficient absorption of nutrients and prevention of systemic infections. Gastric acid is also an important factor in protein hydrolysis and digestion and, under various conditions, may play an etiologic role in inciting gastroduodenal mucosal injury. Postprandial gastric acid secretion is regulated primarily by increases in gastrin expression, which is controlled by a negative feedback loop wherein postprandial gastrin–mediated acid secretion stimulates the release of somatostatin from antral D cells. Somatostatin appears to act via a paracrine mechanism to inhibit further release of gastrin from G cells. Somatostatin produced by D cells in the gastric corpus and fundus may also directly inhibit acid secretion from parietal cells and may suppress histamine release from ECL cells. Although the presence of acid is necessary for ulcers to form, acid secretion is normal in nearly all patients with gastric ulcers and is increased in only one third of patients with duodenal ulcers. Therefore, acid is clearly not the only factor involved in the pathogenesis of peptic ulcers, and the balance between aggressive factors that act to injure the gastroduodenal mucosa and defensive factors that normally protect against corrosive agents is also important. When this delicate balance is disrupted for any reason, an ulcer may ensue.

In addition to the regulation of intragastric acidity, mechanisms involved in maintaining the protective mucosal barrier include mucus and HCO_3 secretion, mucosal blood flow, cell restitution and repair, and changes in local immune factors. The mucosal defensive properties appear to be mediated to a large extent by endogenous prostaglandins, nitric oxide, and trefoil proteins. When the synthesis of any or all is diminished, the ability of the gastroduodenal mucosa to resist injury is reduced, and even normal rates of acid secretion may be sufficient to injure the mucosa. As stated previously, the pathogenesis of peptic ulcer is complex and involves an imbalance between defensive and aggressive factors. Individuals infected with *H. pylori* have been shown to have a diminished number of somatostatin-secreting D cells, which decreases the magnitude of the response to luminal acidification. Thus, in patients with *H. pylori* infection limited to the antrum, the negative inhibition of gastrin release is disrupted, resulting in higher postprandial gastrin levels and hypersecretion of acid. In addition, *H. pylori* penetrate the mucous layer and adhere to surface epithelial cells by attaching to phospholipids and glycoproteins. Once attached, the bacteria synthesize and release phospholipases and proteases that are harmful to the mucous layers and the underlying cells. Interleukin-8 and other cytokines that contribute to mucosal injury are subsequently released from the gastric epithelium. Approximately 65% of *H. pylori* isolates produce a vacuolating toxin. Toxin-producing strains may be more pathogenic than those that do not produce toxins, and their presence correlates with a more intense polymorphonuclear cell infiltration. A cytotoxin-associated gene (*cagA*) has been found to be a marker for strains that make

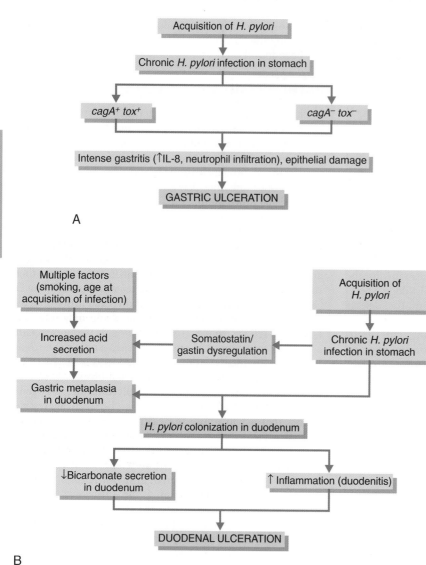

A

B

Figure 36–5 Mechanisms by which *H. pylori* may cause gastric ulcers *(A)* and duodenal ulcers *(B)*. IL-8 = interleukin-8. (From Peek RM, Blaser MJ: Pathophysiology of *Helicobacter pylori*-induced gastritis and peptic ulcer disease. Am J Med 102:200–207, 1997.)

the vacuolating toxin. Patients infected with *cagA*-positive strains are more likely to develop ulcers (Fig. 36–5).

Although a large number of gastroduodenal ulcers are associated with *H. pylori* infection, at least 60% of individuals with complicated ulcers (e.g., hemorrhage, perforation) report the use of NSAIDs, including aspirin. Topical injury caused by NSAIDs certainly contributes significantly to the development of gastroduodenal mucosal injury. However, the systemic effects of these agents appear to play the predominant role, largely through the decreased synthesis of mucosal prostaglandins. NSAID-induced ulceration occurs with all traditional NSAIDs, regardless of enteric coating or delivery as a prodrug formulation. The risk of NSAID-induced ulceration and complications is dose related and increases with age older than 60 years, concurrent corticosteroid use, increasing duration and dose of therapy, anticoagulant therapy, and a history of prior ulcer disease.

ZES, produced by gastrin-secreting tumors, accounts for 0.1% of patients who have PUD and should be considered in patients with ulcers in unusual sites (e.g., distal duodenum, jejunum); multiple, recurrent, or complicated duodenal ulcers; or ulcers associated with chronic diarrhea.

CLINICAL PRESENTATION

Peptic ulcers can exhibit in a variety of forms ranging from asymptomatic iron deficiency anemia to abdominal pain, obstruction, perforation, and hemorrhage. Symptoms may mimic those of other diseases, including cholecystitis, pancreatitis, gastric cancer, and gastroesophageal reflux. Myocardial ischemia or infarction, especially of the inferior wall, can cause abdominal pain that resembles peptic ulcer. Abdominal pain is generally epigastric and is usually described as a dull ache but may be sharp or burning. Less than 20% of patients report the hunger-like pain traditionally associated with both gastric and duodenal ulcers. Similarly, the character of the symptoms and their relation with meals, specifically pain relief after food intake for duodenal ulcer and pain worsening for gastric ulcer, do not always correlate with endoscopic diagnosis and are less useful in predicting ulcer location. Nocturnal pain and pain relief with milk or antacids are common with duodenal ulcers but can also occur with gastric ulcers. NSAID-associated ulcers typically produce painless bleeding. Nausea and vomiting are commonly associated with peptic ulcers, being slightly more common with gastric ulcers. Gastric outlet obstruction may be caused by antropyloric or duodenal ulcers but should be differentiated from malignant obstruction resulting from gastric or pancreatic cancer. Weight loss, although suggestive of malignancy, is frequently reported by patients with peptic ulcers.

DIAGNOSIS

Because the clinical features of gastroduodenal ulcers may overlap with other disorders, and the physical examination is often not helpful in the diagnosis, imaging studies of the GI tract are required to confirm the presence of peptic ulcers. Although contrast radiology (barium upper GI series) can be used, endoscopy is usually preferred because, in addition to characterizing the ulcer, it allows tissue sampling to exclude malignancy, assessment of *H. pylori* infection, and, in cases of acute ulcer hemorrhage, delivery of endoscopic therapy for the control of hemorrhage.

DIAGNOSTIC TESTS FOR *H. PYLORI*

The fact that the eradication of *H. pylori* infection is associated with a significant reduction in ulcer recurrence is now recognized. *H. pylori* testing is thus essential in all patients with PUD. Diagnostic tests for detecting *H. pylori* infection and the indications for their use are summarized in Figure 36–6. Immunoglobulin G serologic testing is the noninvasive test of choice for diagnosing *H. pylori* infection in the untreated patient. However, because the antibodies may persist for several years, serologic analysis is not useful as a means to document cure of the infection. Positive results of antibody testing may thus indicate past exposure but not necessarily current infection with *H. pylori*. Another noninvasive mean of detecting *H. pylori* is the ^{13}C- or ^{14}C-labeled urea breath test. When present, *H. pylori* urease splits the urea, which may be detected as labeled carbon dioxide in the breath of a patient. The urea breath test is more accurate than serologic tests, and although more expensive and less widely available, is the noninvasive test of choice to document successful *H. pylori* eradication after antibiotic therapy. Patients should not receive PPIs for at least 14 days before administration of breath tests to avoid false-negative results. Stool antigen testing is also available and useful in the initial diagnosis of *H. pylori* infection. If endoscopic examination is performed, the diagnosis is made by the rapid urease test or histologic testing. In the rapid urease test, mucosal biopsies are placed in a urea-containing medium with a pH-sensitive indicator that changes color when ammonia is produced from urea by the urease of the organism. The rapid urease test has high sensitivity and specificity equivalent to histologic analysis and is inexpensive. Recent treatment with antibiotics or PPIs may decrease the yield of the test. Histologic analysis is frequently the standard for detecting *H. pylori* infection and can establish the degree, type, and location of inflammation. Gastric biopsy specimens should be taken from both the antrum and the corpus because the bacteria are not uniformly distributed throughout the stomach. The presence of chronic active gastritis is strongly suggestive of *H. pylori* infection, even if bacteria are difficult to identify.

Complications of Peptic Ulcer Disease

BLEEDING

PUD is the leading cause of upper GI bleeding, accounting for approximately 50% of instances and more than 150,000 hospital admissions annually in the United States. Although bleeding ceases spontaneously in 80% of the patients, the mortality of bleeding ulcers is 5% to 10%. Patients with bleeding ulcers exhibit hematemesis, melena, or hematochezia, often without abdominal pain. The major risk factor for bleeding ulcers is NSAID use. Predictors for an adverse outcome include hemodynamic instability at presentation, bright red blood via the rectum and/or through the nasogastric tube, age older than 60 years, ongoing transfusion requirements, and an increasing number of underlying medical illnesses. All patients with upper GI bleeding should undergo early upper endoscopic examination, which allows for both therapeutic intervention and the determination of other predictors for rebleeding. Rebleeding rates are approximately 5% for clean-based ulcers, 10% for ulcers with flat spots, 22% for adherent clots, 43% for nonbleeding visible vessels, and 55% for active oozing or spurting from an ulcer (Fig. 36–7). Patients with large ulcers, greater than 1 to 2 cm in diameter, also have increased rebleeding rates and mortality. Endoscopic therapy with techniques such as multipolar or thermal coagulation or injection with epinephrine clearly improves the outcome in patients with bleeding ulcers by decreasing mortality, length of hospital stay, number of blood transfusions, and need for emergency surgery.

Because most ulcer bleeding recurs within 3 days of initial presentation, patients with active bleeding or stigmata of hemorrhage, such as raised pigmented spots in an ulcer crater or clot, can be discharged within 2 to 3 days if they are stable. Given the excellent prognosis for patients with clean-based ulcers, discharge within 24 hours of presentation or immediately after endoscopic examination appears to be safe. Approximately 20% of patients rebleed after endoscopic therapy, and 50% of these can be successfully re-treated. The remainder may be treated angiographically with either intra-arterial vasopressin or embolization techniques. Surgery is generally reserved for instances in which all other measures have failed. Although endoscopic therapy is the first treatment modality in the management of actively bleeding gastroduodenal ulcers, some evidence also suggests that adjuvant use of acid suppression therapy can reduce recurrent bleeding after initial endoscopic control. A continuous infusion of intravenous omeprazole has been shown to reduce the incidence of recurrent ulcer hemorrhage following endoscopic therapy. Thus, patients with significant upper GI bleeding in whom a peptic ulcer is suggested should be treated with an intravenous PPI using a loading dose (80 mg of pantoprazole) followed by a continuous infusion (8 mg/hr of pantoprazole). If at the time of endoscopic examination no evidence of recent or active bleeding can be found, and once feeding has been initiated, oral administration can be substituted for the parenteral route.

PERFORATION

Perforation, which occurs when a peptic ulcer erodes through the full thickness of the stomach or duodenum, is a

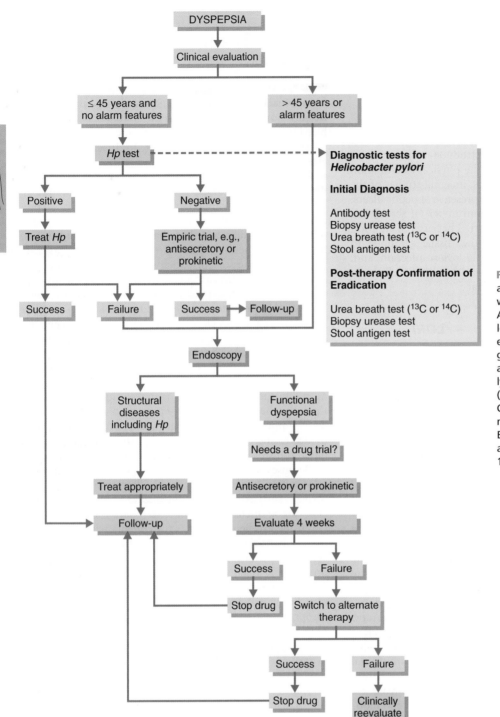

Figure 36–6 Diagnostic approach to patients presenting with uninvestigated dyspepsia. Alarm features include weight loss, vomiting, dysphagia, evidence of anemia, gastrointestinal bleeding, or an abdominal mass or lymphadenopathy. *Hp = H. pylori.* (Modified from American Gastroenterological Association medical position statement: Evaluation of dyspepsia. [No authors listed]. Gastroenterology 114:579–581, 1998.)

far less common complication than bleeding. Ulcer perforation usually leads to peritonitis, which, if untreated, may result in sepsis and death. Patients exhibit sudden onset of severe abdominal pain that typically begins in the epigastrium and radiates throughout the entire abdomen. When peritonitis has occurred, physical examination is remarkable for abdominal pain, guarding, rebound tenderness, and boardlike rigidity. The clinical suggestion of perforation may be confirmed in most cases by the presence of free intra-abdominal air (pneumoperitoneum) with either an upright chest radiograph or upright and supine abdominal radio-

graphs. In less obvious instances, computed tomography (CT) or an upper GI water-soluble contrast study may be helpful. Perforation mandates surgical intervention. A perforated duodenal ulcer is typically repaired with an omental patch, whereas a perforated gastric ulcer necessitates either an omental patch or a resection.

GASTRIC OUTLET OBSTRUCTION

In the era before acid suppression and *H. pylori*, PUD accounted for 60% of the cases of gastric outlet obstruction.

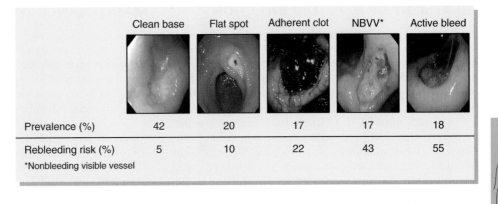

	Clean base	Flat spot	Adherent clot	NBVV*	Active bleed
Prevalence (%)	42	20	17	17	18
Rebleeding risk (%)	5	10	22	43	55

*Nonbleeding visible vessel

Figure 36–7 Endoscopic classification of peptic ulcers with prevalence and risk of rebleeding. (From Laine L, Peterson WL: Medical progress: Bleeding peptic ulcer. N Engl J Med 331:717–727, 1994.)

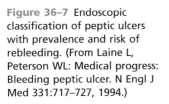

More recently, the incidence of both ulcers and obstruction requiring surgery has declined, and estimates indicate that fewer than 5% of patients with duodenal ulcer and less than 1% to 2% with gastric ulcer develop significant gastric outlet obstruction. Gastric outlet obstruction is typically caused by either pyloric channel or duodenal ulcers and may be seen in the setting of acute ulceration, in which edema, spasm, and inflammation lead to obstruction, or as a consequence of chronic ulceration with scarring and fibrosis. Patients usually exhibit symptoms of early satiety, bloating, nausea, vomiting, and weight loss. Endoscopy is the diagnostic test of choice but is frequently obscured by the presence of retained food residue. Patients in whom gastric outlet obstruction is suggested should undergo gastric decompression and lavage to remove retained gastric contents before endoscopic examination. Malignancy may now account for 50% of instances of gastric outlet obstruction and should be excluded with adequate biopsy and cytology samples. Occasionally, imaging techniques such as barium upper GI series and radionuclide gastric emptying scans can also be used to determine the length of the obstructed area and to evaluate gastric emptying. In addition to the correction of fluid, electrolyte, and pH imbalances resulting from persistent vomiting, patients with gastric outlet obstruction should undergo nasogastric decompression for 3 to 5 days. During that time, acid suppression with an intravenous H_2-RA or PPI should also be instituted. Adequacy of response may be assessed empirically with a trial of refeeding. For patients failing to respond to medical therapy, treatment options include endoscopic balloon dilation and surgery.

Treatment of Peptic Ulcer Disease

HEALING ULCERS BY SUPPRESSING ACID SECRETION

Regardless of the cause, the inhibition of gastric acid secretion continues to be the cornerstone of therapy for PUD. Antacids are effective agents for healing ulcers and may provide some symptom relief. However, because of the need to take these drugs at least four, and up to seven, times every day, and the frequency of associated adverse effects, antacids are now rarely used in the healing of gastroduodenal ulcers.

H_2-RAs reduce acid secretion by competitively and selectively inhibiting the histamine receptor on the parietal cell. H_2-RAs increase intragastric pH and inhibit pepsin activity. In general, H_2-RAs are safe and well tolerated, although the occurrence of adverse effects is slightly increased with cimetidine because of binding to cytochrome P-450 and hence increased risk of drug interactions. H_2-RAs heal 90% to 95% of duodenal ulcers and 88% of gastric ulcers at 8 weeks. Given as a single full dose at bedtime, cimetidine (800 mg), ranitidine and nizatidine (300 mg), and famotidine (40 mg) have comparable efficacies for ulcer healing. The recommended duration of treatment is 4 weeks for duodenal ulcers and 8 weeks for gastric ulcers.

PPIs, the most potent inhibitors of gastric acid secretion available, heal gastroduodenal ulcers more rapidly than H_2-RAs. However, because they are most effective when the parietal cell is stimulated to secrete acid in response to a meal, PPIs should only be taken before a meal and should not be used in conjunction with H_2-RAs or other antisecretory agents. Moreover, because acid secretion must be stimulated for maximum efficacy, PPIs are administered before the first meal of the day. These agents are safe and well tolerated; adverse effects are unusual and include headache, diarrhea, and nausea. Single daily doses of omeprazole (20 mg), pantoprazole (40 mg), rabeprazole (20 mg), lansoprazole (30 mg), or esomeprazole (40 mg) all before breakfast are effective in healing gastroduodenal ulcers. The recommended duration of treatment is again 4 weeks for duodenal ulcers and 8 weeks for gastric ulcers.

HEALING BY ENHANCING MUCOSAL DEFENSE

Sucralfate, a complex salt of sucrose sulfate and aluminum hydroxide, appears to be as effective as H_2-RAs in the treatment of duodenal ulcer disease. The evidence for efficacy in healing of gastric ulcers is less compelling. Sucralfate has little or no effect on acid secretion and acts through several different mucosal protective mechanisms. In the gastroduodenal lumen, sucralfate becomes a gel-like substance that binds to both defective and normal mucosa, acting as a physical barrier to the diffusion of acid, pepsin, and bile acids. The recommended dose is 1 g four times daily, which makes it less convenient than other agents for treating PUD.

Although bismuth compounds and prostaglandin analogs have been shown to provide protective effects on the gastroduodenal mucosa and may have some effect on ulcer healing, these agents are not routinely used in the initial treatment of peptic ulcers.

TREATMENT OF *H. PYLORI* INFECTION

Eradication of *H. pylori* should be attempted in all patients with documented, current or past PUD and evidence of infection. The various niches of *H. pylori* within the gastric mucosa provide a challenge for antimicrobial therapy. Successful therapy requires a combination of drugs that prevents the emergence of resistance and effectively reaches the bacteria. Therapy must be of sufficient duration to ensure that a small population of bacteria does not remain viable. Combinations of two antibiotics, plus either a PPI or ranitidine bismuth citrate, are used to maximize the chance of eradication. Current treatment regimens for *H. pylori* are shown in Table 36–2. Factors such as antibiotic resistance and noncompliance with therapy have been identified as predictors of treatment failure. Metronidazole resistance is most common, and both metronidazole and clarithromycin resistance are increasing in frequency, with rates of 37% and 10%, respectively. Because compliance is essential for treatment success, the current regimens offer simpler dosing than earlier options. A failed initial course of antibiotic therapy suggests antibiotic resistance, and it may be assumed that, if the patient received metronidazole or clarithromycin in the original regimen, resistance to that antibiotic is present. When possible, repeat use of the same antibiotic should be avoided. The recommended duration for repeat treatment courses is 14 days.

Table 36–2	Treatment Regimens for *Helicobacter pylori* Infection

Triple therapy (cure rates 85 to >90%)

BMT triple therapy for 14 days
  Bismuth subsalicylate 524 mg by mouth four times daily
  Metronidazole 250 mg by mouth four times daily
  Tetracycline HCl 500 mg by mouth four times daily + H$_2$-RA
    for additional 4 wk

LAC for 10 or 14 days
  Lansoprazole 30 mg by mouth twice daily
  Amoxicillin 1 g by mouth twice daily
  Clarithromycin 500 mg by mouth twice daily

OAC for 10 or 14 days
  Omeprazole 20 mg by mouth twice daily
  Amoxicillin 1 g by mouth two times daily
  Clarithromycin 500 mg by mouth twice daily

RBC-AC (cure rate >90%)
  Ranitidine bismuth citrate + amoxicillin + clarithromycin

MOC (cure rate >90% in the absence of metronidazole resistance)
  Metronidazole + omeprazole + clarithromycin

H$_2$-RA = histamine$_2$-receptor antagonist; HCl = hydrochloric acid.

MAINTENANCE THERAPY

Before embarking on long-term maintenance therapy for PUD, careful attention must be paid to eliminating the most important risk factors for ulcer recurrence: *H. pylori* infection and NSAID use. Moreover, hypersecretory states, including gastrinoma, should be excluded before considering maintenance therapy in individuals with recurrent ulcers without *H. pylori* infection. Patients with a history of ulcer complications, frequent ulcer recurrence, continued NSAID use, or *H. pylori*-negative ulcers, and in those who fail to clear *H. pylori* infection despite appropriate therapy, should be considered as candidates for maintenance antisecretory therapy. However, even patients who have had a complicated ulcer may not require maintenance therapy, provided *H. pylori* infection is cured. Maintenance regimens include an H$_2$-RA at bedtime at one half the dose required for initial healing or a PPI taken before breakfast.

TREATMENT AND PROPHYLAXIS OF NSAID-INDUCED ULCERATION

The optimal treatment for patients with NSAID-induced gastroduodenal ulcers is the discontinuation of the offending agent. If NSAIDs must be continued, therapy with an antisecretory agent should be instituted. Based on their superior safety profile and their ability to heal gastroduodenal ulcers at an accelerated rate whether or not NSAID use is continued, PPIs are preferred over both H$_2$-RAs and misoprostol in the treatment of NSAID-associated gastroduodenal ulcers.

Because of the significant rate of serious complications associated with NSAIDs and the poor correlation of dyspeptic symptoms (e.g., abdominal pain, distention, nausea, heartburn) with the presence of gastroduodenal mucosal injury, prevention of ulceration has become the principal goal in the management of NSAID-related GI toxicity. Risk factors for NSAID-related injury have been identified and include advanced age (older than 60 years), prior history of PUD or ulcer hemorrhage, concomitant use of anticoagulants or corticosteroids, significant co-morbid conditions, and the use of high NSAID doses (Table 36–3). Two strategies have been used to prevent ulcers: (1) the concomitant use of medications such as misoprostol or PPIs and (2) the development of safer anti-inflammatory agents, such as COX-2–specific inhibitors. Misoprostol, a prostaglandin E$_1$ analog, significantly reduces the development of both gastric and duodenal ulcers in patients using NSAIDs. By augmenting prostaglandin-dependent pathways, misoprostol reduces gastric acid secretion and enhances mucosal defenses. However, misoprostol is associated with significant adverse effects and a high frequency of therapy discontinuation as a result of these effects, especially when administered four times a day. The most frequent symptom is diarrhea, although symptoms such as abdominal pain, nausea, and bloating may also occur. A lower dose of misoprostol (200 mcg three times daily) is nearly as effective as four-times-a-day dosing for preventing duodenal and gastric ulcers, with a slight reduction in the occurrence of adverse effects.

The second strategy to prevent NSAID-induced ulcers involves the co-administration of an antisecretory agent,

Table 36–3 Risk Factors for Development of NSAID-Related Ulcers

Definite

Advanced age
History of ulcer
Concomitant corticosteroid therapy
Concomitant anticoagulation therapy
High doses of NSAIDs
Serious systemic disorders

Possible

Concomitant infection with *Helicobacter pylori*
Cigarette smoking
Consumption of alcohol

NSAIDs = nonsteroidal anti-inflammatory drugs.

usually a PPI, or the substitution of the traditional NSAID with one of the newer COX-2–specific inhibitors.

According to available evidence from clinical trials, PPIs are superior to H_2-RAs in preventing gastroduodenal ulceration, as well as in improving dyspeptic symptoms during continued NSAID use. Similarly, PPIs provide protection against endoscopic NSAID ulcers at a rate at least comparable with that of misoprostol, with fewer associated GI symptoms. However, misoprostol, but not PPIs, has been shown in a prospective analysis to decrease the prevalence of ulcer complications.

COX-2–specific inhibitors (e.g., celecoxib, rofecoxib, valdecoxib) have shown an improved GI safety profile with reduced incidence of ulcers and ulcer complications and at least similar effectiveness when compared with traditional NSAIDs.

However, recent evidence suggesting an increased risk of cardiovascular events, specifically myocardial infarctions and strokes, associated with the use of selective COX-2 inhibitors, has led to significant public concern with subsequent market withdrawal of some of these agents and restricted use of others. These adverse effects are thought to be related, at least in part, to the inhibition of prostacyclin with the resultant unopposed *thrombogenic* effects of thromboxane A_2.

Although the issue is controversial, most current evidence does not suggest that *H. pylori* potentiates the risk of NSAID-induced GI ulcers or clinical events. Therefore, a strategy of *H. pylori* testing and treatment in NSAID users without a history of ulcer disease is not recommended. Conversely, patients with a prior history of ulcers or ulcer complications should be tested and treated for *H. pylori*, if present, before beginning NSAID therapy.

Other new *GI-safe* NSAIDs are now being tested in clinical trials. Nitric oxide–releasing NSAIDs have shown reduced gastroduodenal toxicity when compared with traditional NSAIDs in small endoscopic studies.

SURGERY

Because of the remarkable progress in pharmacologic acid suppression therapy and the recognition that ulcer disease can be cured by eliminating *H. pylori* infection and NSAIDs, surgery now plays a marginal role in treating uncomplicated PUD. Surgical intervention is now mostly reserved for managing the complications of peptic ulcers, especially gastric outlet obstruction and perforation. Some of the different surgical approaches are shown in Figure 36–8.

NONULCER DYSPEPSIA

Dyspepsia, a classic symptom of PUD, is a common clinical problem and may be seen in 25% to 40% of adults. However, only 15% to 25% of patients with dyspepsia are found to have a gastric or duodenal ulcer. The remainder is diagnosed with nonulcer or functional dyspepsia, a condition most likely related to an abnormal perception of events in the stomach caused by afferent visceral hypersensitivity. Recent evidence suggests that approximately 40% of patients with nonulcer dyspepsia (NUD) have impairment in the fundic accommodation response of the stomach. Dyspeptic symptoms may be chronic, recurrent, or of new onset. The diagnostic work-up should focus on excluding other causes of dyspepsia such as gastroparesis and gastric cancer.

MANAGEMENT

Three possible strategies for managing patients with NUD have been formulated (see Fig. 36–6). Immediate endoscopic evaluation is indicated for individuals older than age 45 years or persons exhibiting alarm features *(red flags)* such as weight loss, recurrent vomiting, dysphagia, GI bleeding, anemia, a strong family history of GI cancer, or an abdominal mass. Urgent endoscopic examination is indicated to exclude a serious underlying disease process, particularly gastric and esophageal carcinoma. If a gastric ulcer is found during endoscopic examination, multiple biopsies and cytologic analysis should be obtained to exclude malignancy. Ulcer treatment is subsequently employed, and ulcer healing should be confirmed with a follow-up endoscopic examination because nonhealing ulcers can occasionally be a manifestation of gastric carcinoma. Barium radiography offers poor sensitivity and specificity and is thus no longer recommended in the evaluation of dyspepsia.

The second option when treating patients younger than age 45 with NUD but without alarm features is an empiric trial of antisecretory therapy for 1 to 2 months. Endoscopy is indicated in patients who fail to respond to this regimen. Avoiding the introduction of long-term drug use in this situation is important, particularly because of the considerable benefit of placebo in such individuals.

The third strategy for managing of NUD involves initial noninvasive testing for *H. pylori* followed by antimicrobial therapy in patients with positive tests. This strategy is presumed to heal ulcers if present, eliminate the ulcer diathesis, and save on resources, particularly in patients younger than age 45 years without alarm symptoms. The frequency of *H. pylori* infection in the community should also be taken into account because noninvasive tests show decreased accuracy when the prevalence of *H. pylori* is less than 10%. This

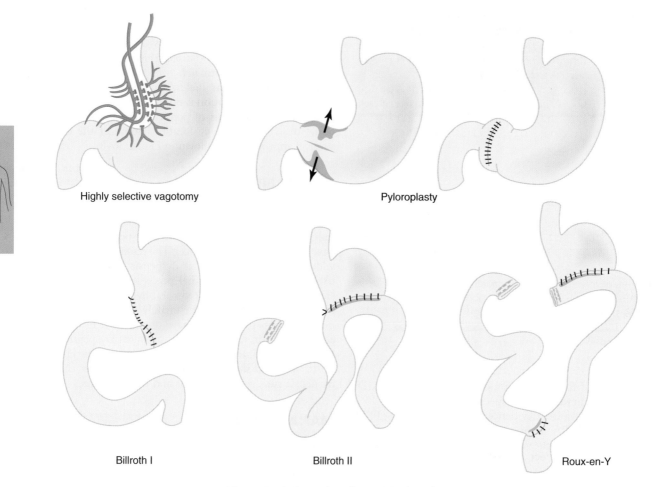

Highly selective vagotomy   Pyloroplasty

Billroth I   Billroth II   Roux-en-Y

Figure 36–8 Operations for peptic ulcer disease.

approach, although advocated by some physicians, has not been proved to be effective in relieving NUD. Moreover, indiscriminate use of antimicrobial therapy may be associated with altering normal intestinal flora, increasing resistance of *H. pylori* and other bacteria that are not a target of therapy, and producing a series of adverse events such as antibiotic-associated and *Clostridium difficile* colitis.

Zollinger-Ellison Syndrome

ZES is characterized by elevated levels of serum gastrin produced by gastrin-secreting tumors that are most often located in the pancreas and duodenum. Hypergastrinemia stimulates hypersecretion of gastric acid and pepsin, which may produce peptic ulcers, duodenojejunitis, esophagitis, and diarrhea. ZES is an uncommon cause of PUD, accounting for less than 1% of the instances. The gastrin-secreting tumor in ZES, referred to as a gastrinoma, is frequently located in the *gastrinoma triangle,* an area encompassed by the second and third portions of the duodenum, the junction of the head and neck of the pancreas, and the cystic duct. Seventy-five percent of all gastrinomas are sporadic; the remaining 25% are part of the type I multiple endocrine

neoplasia (MEN-I) syndrome, an autosomal-dominant condition with a locus on chromosome 11, typically associated with hyperparathyroidism and pituitary tumors. All patients with sporadic gastrinomas without evidence of liver metastases should be surgically explored with the intent of removing local and regional disease. Unfortunately, despite careful diagnostic testing, no tumor is found in at least 10% of diagnosed instances of ZES.

ZES should be anticipated in patients with recurrent PUD in the absence of *H. pylori* infection or NSAID use, as well as in patients with multiple duodenal ulcers, ulcers in unusual locations (distal duodenum or jejunum), and patients with severe or refractory diarrhea or gastroesophageal reflux disease. Although peptic ulcer occurs in more than 90% of patients with ZES, as many as 35% of individuals exhibit only diarrhea. The diagnosis of ZES is made when a fasting gastrin concentration of more than 1000 pg/mL exists in the setting of gastric acid hypersecretion. In equivocal cases (e.g., gastrin <1000 pg/mL), a positive secretin provocative test will confirm the diagnosis. The secretin test is positive (≥200 pg/mL increase over the pre-injection fasting gastrin level) in approximately 90% of patients with ZES and moderately elevated gastrin levels.

Basal acid output is elevated (>15 mmol/hr without previous gastric acid-reducing surgery and >5 mmol/hr with prior surgery) in more than 90% of patients with ZES. Because gastrinomas constitute a relatively uncommon cause of hypergastrinemia, other causes should be considered. The most common causes of hypergastrinemia are antrum-dominant *H. pylori* infection or achlorhydria related to either decreased intraluminal acid in the setting of atrophic gastritis or antisecretory therapy with PPIs. Hypergastrinemia may be related to other causes, including retained gastric antrum (after ulcer surgery), massive small bowel resection, chronic gastric outlet obstruction, and chronic renal failure. Therefore, acid hypersecretion, as documented by gastric acid analysis, is necessary for the diagnosis of ZES.

Once hypergastrinemia has been established and obvious causes have been excluded, efforts should focus on localizing and resecting the gastrin-secreting tumor. The single best imaging test for gastrinoma is somatostatin-receptor scintigraphy (SRS), which is more sensitive than any conventional imaging study, including CT, magnetic resonance imaging (MRI), and ultrasonography, although endoscopic ultrasonography (EUS) is equally sensitive for localizing primary tumors of the pancreas. If liver metastasis is present, a CT- or ultrasound-guided liver biopsy should be performed. In patients without liver metastasis, SRS will localize a possible primary tumor in 60% of patients. If the patient is a surgical candidate and SRS is positive for a primary tumor, no additional localization studies are required. If the SRS is negative for a possible primary tumor, the use of MRI, angiography, or EUS will detect a possible primary tumor in an additional 15% of patients. Multiple pancreatic or duodenal tumors are generally detected in patients with MEN-I syndrome, and although the precise role of surgery in these patients is less certain, some physicians recommend surgery if a lesion greater than 3 cm is identified with preoperative imaging techniques to decrease the possibility of hepatic metastasis. However, successful and long-lasting remission of MEN-I syndrome occurs rarely, if at all.

All patients with ZES, whether sporadic or familial, require antisecretory therapy after the diagnosis is established and during initial evaluation as attempts are made to localize the gastrinoma. Patients with ZES should be treated initially with a PPI using twice the dose normally employed to treat common gastroduodenal ulcers. Intravenous PPIs such as pantoprazole in daily doses ranging from 80 to 240 mg can be used in patients who are unable to take medications by mouth, including those undergoing surgery. The goal of therapy is a basal acid output of less than 10 mmol/hr in the hour preceding the next dose of the drug. Chronic therapy with PPIs uniformly results in continued inhibition of acid secretion, good symptom control, complete healing of any mucosal lesions, and few adverse effects.

Gastroparesis

Gastroparesis is a syndrome characterized by delayed gastric emptying, resulting in impaired transit of food from the stomach to the duodenum in the absence of mechanical obstruction. Symptoms of gastric stasis include early or easy satiety, bloating, nausea, and vomiting. Because eating exacerbates symptoms, patients frequently exhibit anorexia, weight loss, and nutritional deficiencies. A wide range of clinical disorders is associated with impaired gastric emptying (Table 36-4). Diabetes mellitus is the most common cause of gastroparesis, and up to 60% of patients with diabetes complain of symptoms consistent with gastric stasis. Although gastroparesis is typically seen in individuals with long-standing (>10 years) type 1 diabetes who have other complications, such as peripheral and autonomic

Table 36–4	**Causes of Delayed Gastric Emptying**

Mechanical Causes

Peptic ulcer disease, scarred pylorus
Malignancy: gastric cancer, gastric lymphoma, pancreatic cancer
Gastric surgery: vagotomy, gastric resection, roux-en-Y anastomosis
Crohn's disease

Endocrine and Metabolic Causes

Diabetes mellitus
Hypothyroidism
Hypoadrenal states
Electrolyte abnormalities
Chronic renal failure
Medications
Anticholinergics
Opiates
Dopamine agonists
Tricyclic antidepressants

Abnormalities of Gastric Smooth Muscle

Scleroderma
Polymyositis and/or dermatomyositis
Amyloidosis
Pseudo-obstruction
Myotonic dystrophy
Neuropathy
Scleroderma
Amyloidosis
Autonomic neuropathy

Central Nervous System or Psychiatric Disorders

Brainstem tumors
Spinal cord injury
Anorexia nervosa
Stress

Miscellaneous

Idiopathic gastroparesis
Gastroesophageal reflux disease
Nonulcer (functional) dyspepsia
Cancer cachexia or anorexia

neuropathy, nephropathy, and retinopathy, GI complaints are also common within the first decade of diagnosis. Diabetic gastroparesis appears to occur as a result of permanent neuropathy of autonomic and enteric nerves, transitory variations in glycemic control, or a combination of both. Idiopathic gastroparesis is also common and comprises those instances with no clearly identifiable cause. Up to one third of these patients have viral-induced gastroparesis, with viral infiltration of the myenteric plexus in the stomach. Patients who have undergone gastric surgery, especially those having had preoperative gastric outlet obstruction as a complication of PUD, are also commonly affected by gastroparesis. Finally, Parkinson's disease, rheumatologic disorders, hypo- or hyperthyroidism, chronic intestinal pseudo-obstruction, and a variety of paraneoplastic syndromes can also produce gastroparesis.

The diagnostic evaluation of delayed gastric emptying should focus on excluding structural and metabolic abnormalities. Endoscopy is the preferred initial test to rule out mechanical gastric outlet obstruction, and a small bowel follow-through radiograph may be useful to exclude small bowel lesions. Serum electrolytes, blood cell counts, and thyroid studies should also be performed. When these studies are negative, radionuclide scintigraphy (gastric emptying scan) using a mixed solid-liquid meal can quantitate delayed gastric emptying. Assessment of solid emptying is more clinically relevant than liquid emptying. In especially difficult cases, GI manometry and electrogastrography may help in the diagnosis.

Managing gastroparesis begins with identifying and treating potentially correctable causes. Medications that reduce gastric emptying, such as narcotics, anticholinergics, and tricyclic antidepressants, should be avoided. Because liquids empty easier than solids, and because liquid emptying is often preserved in patients with gastroparesis, simple dietary modifications may be helpful in treatment. The diet should be modified to include blenderized foods and liquid supplements. High-fat and fiber-rich foods should be avoided because they inhibit gastric emptying under normal conditions and are less likely to empty. Medical options are limited and involve the use of prokinetic drugs, which are agents that improve transit in the GI tract.

Metoclopramide is a dopamine$_2$-receptor antagonist that also facilitates the release of acetylcholine from cholinergic nerve terminals in the gut, thereby accelerating gastric emptying. The efficacy of metoclopramide is inconsistent, and adverse effects and the development of tolerance complicate long-term therapy. Adverse effects occur in up to 20% of patients and include drowsiness, anxiety, fatigue, insomnia, restlessness, agitation, extrapyramidal effects, galactorrhea, and menstrual irregularities. The typical dosage is 10 mg, 20 to 30 minutes before meals and at bedtime, although doses as high as 80 mg or as low as 20 mg may be used daily. Doses should be reduced for patients with renal failure.

Cisapride, an agent that increases gastric motor activity by facilitating the release of acetylcholine at the myenteric plexus, is no longer routinely available in the United States and other countries because of serious adverse effects, including ventricular tachycardia, ventricular fibrillation, torsades de pointes, and prolongation of the QT interval, which have been reported when cisapride is administered with other drugs that inhibit cytochrome P-450.

Erythromycin is a macrolide antibiotic that stimulates smooth muscle motilin receptors located at all levels of the GI tract. The prokinetic effects of erythromycin are related to its ability to mimic the effect of the GI peptide motilin to stimulate smooth muscle contraction, which accounts for the acceleration of solid and liquid gastric emptying. Erythromycin may dramatically improve gastric emptying in patients with severe diabetic gastroparesis when given acutely at an intravenous dose of 1 to 3 mg/kg every 8 hours. Long-term use of the drug at a dose of 250 to 500 mg orally every 8 hours in patients with gastric stasis is of limited efficacy because of tachyphylaxis and/or side effects.

In patients who are refractory to these measures, surgical placement of a jejunal tube, with or without a venting gastrostomy, may be necessary. Total parenteral nutrition is rarely indicated. Surgical gastrectomy should only be considered in patients with refractory postsurgical gastric stasis. Gastric pacemakers and other prokinetics, specifically new serotonin-receptor agonists, are under investigation and may be options in the future.

Rapid Gastric Emptying

Rapid gastric emptying is a far less common clinical problem than delayed gastric emptying. Dumping syndrome describes the alimentary and systemic manifestations of early delivery of large amounts of osmotically active food to the small intestine. Dumping syndrome is usually seen when the normal reservoir, grinding, and sieving properties of the stomach are disrupted, most commonly following surgery for PUD. The accelerated emptying of hypertonic boluses of nutrient material into the small intestine results in splanchnic vasodilation and release of vasoactive peptides. Early dumping symptoms, occurring approximately 30 minutes after a meal, include epigastric fullness and pain, nausea, vomiting, early satiety, and vasomotor features such as flushing, palpitations, and diaphoresis. Later symptoms, such as diaphoresis, tremulousness, and weakness, occur approximately 2 hours after a meal and may be caused by hypoglycemia from rebound hyperinsulinemia. Treatment of dumping syndrome involves dietary manipulation to decrease the volume and osmotic load emptied into the intestine. Frequent small feedings of meals low in carbohydrates, separation of liquid and solid intake, and avoidance of hypertonic fluids and lactose are usually helpful. When these measures fail, administration of octreotide at a dose of 25 to 50 mcg subcutaneously 30 minutes before meals may be helpful. Octreotide acts by slowing gastric emptying and intestinal transit, as well as by inhibiting the release of insulin. Surgical procedures to slow gastric emptying have limited success.

Gastric Volvulus

Gastric volvulus occurs when the stomach twists on itself. This event may be transient, producing few if any symptoms, or may lead to obstruction or even ischemia and necrosis. *Primary gastric volvulus,* comprising one third of the patients, occurs below the diaphragm when the stabilizing ligaments are too lax as a result of congenital or acquired causes. *Secondary gastric volvulus* occurs above the diaphragm in association with paraesophageal hernias or other diaphragmatic defects. Acute gastric volvulus produces sudden, severe pain of the upper abdomen or chest, persistent retching producing scant vomitus, and the inability to pass a nasogastric tube. This combination of symptoms, also known as Borchardt's triad, should lead to a strong clinical suggestion of acute gastric volvulus. Chronic gastric volvulus may be associated with mild and nonspecific symptoms, such as epigastric discomfort, heartburn, abdominal fullness or bloating, and borborygmi, especially after meals. The diagnosis of gastric volvulus is made by upper GI series demonstrating an abrupt obstruction at the site of the volvulus. Acute gastric volvulus requires emergency surgical evaluation because of the substantial risk of mortality related to gastric ischemia or perforation. Treatment consists of surgical gastropexy and repair of any associated paraesophageal hernia.

Prospectus for the Future

Our understanding of a significant number of issues involving gastroduodenal pathologic mechanisms and therapeutics will continue to evolve in the next few years. Select goals include:

- Development of variations in the structure and delivery of antisecretory therapy, leading to formulations designed to provide increased rapid onset of action and to improve effectiveness in individuals who are unable to take medications by mouth or those with dysmotility and/or malabsorption
- Further clarification of the role of *H. pylori* infection and its eradication in the decline of the incidence of gastric adenocarcinoma and the perceived increase in the incidence of esophageal adenocarcinoma
- Procurement of evidence-based data to aid in managing stress-related mucosal ulcerations in critically ill patients
- Elucidation of the exact nature and strength of the association between COX-2–selective inhibitors and cardiovascular disease and future development of safer NSAIDs
- Further insight into the mechanism governing GI motility and the development of new agents for the treatment of motility disorders

References

Chan FK, Graham DY: Prevention of non-steroidal anti-inflammatory drug gastrointestinal complications—review and recommendations based on risk assessment. Aliment Pharmacol Ther 19(10):1051–1061, 2004.

Cryer B: COX-2-specific inhibitor or proton pump inhibitor plus traditional NSAID: Is either approach sufficient for patients at highest risk of NSAID-induced ulcers? Gastroenterology 127(4):1256–1258, 2004 Oct.

Go MF: Diagnosis and treatment of *Helicobacter pylori*. Curr Treat Options Gastroenterol 8(2):163–174, 2005 Apr.

Goldstein JL, Johanson J, Hawkey C, et al: Comparative healing of gastric ulcers with esomeprazole versus ranitidine in patients taking either continuous COX-2 selective NSAIDs or nonselective NSAIDs. Gastroenterology 126(4 Suppl 2):A-610, 2004.

Laine L: The gastrointestinal effects of nonselective NSAIDs and COX-2-selective inhibitors. Semin Arthritis Rheum 32(3 Suppl 1):25–32, 2002.

Parkman HP, Hasler WL, Fisher RS: American Gastroenterological Association medical position statement: Diagnosis and treatment of gastroparesis. Gastroenterology 127(5):1589–1591, 2004.

Talley NJ: Dyspepsia: Clinical management. Gastroenterology 125(3):1219–1226, 2003.

Chapter **37**

Inflammatory Bowel Disease

Christopher S. Huang

Lawrence J. Saubermann

Francis A. Farraye

Although a significant number of infectious organisms and noninfectious processes (e.g., medications, radiation, ischemia) can result in intestinal inflammation, the term *inflammatory bowel disease* (IBD) generally refers primarily to two idiopathic diseases: ulcerative colitis and Crohn's disease. The diagnosis of IBD is made by incorporating clinical, endoscopic, radiologic, and histologic information. Ulcerative colitis is characterized by inflammatory changes that involve the colonic mucosa in a continuous superficial fashion, generally starting in the rectum and extending proximally. Depending on the extent of the disease, ulcerative colitis can be divided into proctitis (rectum only), proctosigmoiditis, left-sided colitis (extending to the splenic flexure), or pancolitis. This classification is important for both prognostic and therapeutic reasons. Unlike ulcerative colitis, Crohn's disease can involve any segment of the gastrointestinal system, often in a discontinuous fashion. It is characterized by transmural inflammation, which results in significant complications such as abscesses, fistulas, and strictures. Despite the chronic nature of these two diseases, new and emerging targeted anti-inflammatory treatments hold great promise in helping to reduce morbidity and improve the quality of life of individuals with IBD.

Causes

Although the causes for IBD remain unknown at the present time, recent advances in the understanding of the genetic, immunologic, and environmental factors are beginning to decipher the etiologic factors of these complex disorders. Currently, the main theory regarding IBD pathogenesis involves a dysregulation of the normal intestinal immune processes. This dysregulation results in an over-aggressive response, most likely to the individual's own intestinal microbial flora or some other unidentified environmental component.

GENETIC FACTORS

Approximately 10% of patients with IBD have a first-degree relative with the disease, and first-degree relatives of IBD patients have approximately a 10- to 15-fold increased risk of developing IBD, predominantly with the same disease as the proband. Through advances in genomics, a large number of susceptibility loci on multiple chromosomes have been identified in IBD, supporting a polygenic cause to these disorders. In particular, homozygous mutations of the *Nod2/CARD15* gene located on chromosome 16 are associated with a greater than 20-fold increase in susceptibility for Crohn's disease. Defects in the *Nod2* protein appear to result in abnormal intestinal immune responses to bacterial cell wall components. These gene mutations are estimated to account for approximately 15% to 25% of the cases of Crohn's disease and are linked predominantly to terminal ileal involvement. Many other genes are currently under investigation for their potential involvement in IBD.

The human leukocyte antigen (HLA) gene locus on chromosome 6 has long been thought to play an important role in IBD, especially in Crohn's disease, in which monozygotic twins have a concordance rate of approximately 50%, as compared with ulcerative colitis, in which the rate is approximately 10%. Investigations into both diseases have shown associations with specific HLA haplotypes, but no haplotype is definitively linked to either disorder.

Finally, rare genetic associations have been described in association with IBD or IBD-like disease, including Turner's syndrome, Hermansky-Pudlak syndrome, Down syndrome, glycogen storage disease type 1b, and a wide variety of immunodeficiency disorders.

IMMUNOLOGIC FACTORS

In the normal immunologic state of the intestine, recently activated lymphoid tissue is abundant within the mucosal compartment. This state has been described as controlled, or *physiologic,* inflammation, which has likely developed in response to constant encounters with antigenic substances (derived from dietary, host, or foreign sources) that have crossed the epithelial barrier from the luminal environment. Indeed, one of the main functions of the intestinal immune system is to discriminate noxious or harmful substances and organisms from nonharmful ones. As a result, a large and well-maintained network of many different mucosal immune cells exist, including cells involved in reducing immune responses (regulatory cells) and those involved in activating immune responses. In IBD, this homeostatic balance is dysregulated, and scientific data currently indicate an over-activation response rather than a loss of the down-regulatory component. Central to this hypothesis has been the discovery of the *Nod2* protein in particular immune-related intestinal cell types or in the setting of a response to intestinal epithelial cell activation.

ENVIRONMENTAL FACTORS

Although believed to be important, the role of environmental factors in IBD pathogenesis remains poorly understood. Many infectious agents, including *Mycobacteria paratuberculosis* and measles virus, have been implicated in IBD, but none fulfills the criteria of true pathogens. Environmental factors are suspected because the disease is more common in industrialized countries, and the frequency has been increasing in countries that are becoming more industrialized. However, to date, the only environmental factor clearly associated with IBD is tobacco smoking. Smoking seems to be protective against ulcerative colitis, whereas smokers with Crohn's disease have more aggressive disease than do nonsmokers. No dietary triggers have been found to cause IBD, but elemental diets and diversion of the fecal stream can reduce recurrence of inflammation in Crohn's disease.

Epidemiologic Factors

The incidence and prevalence of IBD reflect the genetic and environmental factors that contribute to these disorders. For example, both diseases are common in northern climates, among whites, and particularly in populations with Northern European ancestry, including North Americans, South Africans, and Australians. Individuals of Ashkenazi Jewish descent have also been found to have a two- to eight-fold increased risk for these disorders compared with non-Jews. Although more common in these groups, IBD can occur in any ethnic or racial group from anywhere in the world.

In the United States, over 1 million individuals have IBD, and the overall incidence of new cases of IBD is approximately 3 to 10 new cases per 100,000 people. Over the last several decades, the incidence of ulcerative colitis has remained stable, whereas the incidence of Crohn's disease has gradually increased. The prevalence of IBD is essentially 10-fold higher at between 30 and 100 per 100,000 people. A bimodal age of presentation exists, with an initial peak between the second and fourth decades of life followed by another peak around the sixth decade of life. Both sexes are equally affected.

Clinical Features of Ulcerative Colitis

Ulcerative colitis is characterized by chronic inflammation of the mucosal surface that involves the rectum (proctitis) and extends proximally through the colon in a continuous manner. The extent and severity of the colonic inflammation determine prognosis and presentation (insidious versus acute onset).

The majority of patients initially exhibit diarrhea, abdominal pain, urgency to defecate, rectal bleeding, and the passage of mucus per rectum. Patients occasionally have extraintestinal manifestations (see later discussion) before they develop intestinal symptoms. Approximately 40% to 50% of patients have proctitis or proctosigmoiditis, 30% to 40% have left-sided colitis (disease extending to the splenic flexure), and the remaining 20% to 25% have pancolitis. Of the patients who initially show proctitis or proctosigmoiditis, approximately 15% will develop more extensive disease over time.

The typical clinical course is of chronic intermittent exacerbations, followed by periods of remission. Signs of a worsening clinical course include the development of abdominal pain, dehydration, fever, and tachycardia. Clinical features, including bowel frequency, fever, increased heart rate, and blood in stools, as well as the presence of anemia and an elevated erythrocyte sedimentation rate (ESR), have been used to assess severity of ulcerative colitis.

MAJOR COMPLICATIONS

Toxic Megacolon and/or Perforation

Toxic megacolon is characterized by gross dilation of the large bowel associated with fever, abdominal pain, dehydration, tachycardia, and bloody diarrhea, which may require urgent surgical intervention. Perforation can occur in the setting of toxic megacolon or in patients with active colitis, especially those on corticosteroids.

Anemia

Anemia is caused by significant amounts of bleeding from the involved colon, as well as bone marrow suppression from the inflammatory condition. Massive hemorrhage is uncommon.

Colonic Adenocarcinoma

The risk of colon cancer is increased in patients with ulcerative colitis, the magnitude of which is related to the extent and duration of disease. Colon cancer risk is increased 10- to 20-fold (if disease extends proximal to the sigmoid colon) after 10 years of disease compared with unaffected individuals. Colonoscopy with surveillance biopsies are recommended every 2 years after 8 years of disease in patients with pancolitis and after 12 to 15 years in patients with left-sided colitis, followed by yearly examinations after 20 years of disease. Whenever dysplasia, a precursor to cancer, is found (outside the setting of a colonic polyp), colectomy is recommended. Proctitis is not associated with an increased cancer risk. Patients with IBD and primary sclerosing cholangitis appear to be at particularly increased risk, and yearly surveillance is recommended after the initial diagnosis.

Crohn's Disease

Crohn's disease may involve any portion of the gastrointestinal tract, and it is the site of involvement, as well as the type of inflammation, that defines the clinical presentation. Unlike ulcerative colitis, the inflammation in Crohn's disease is transmural, and the bowel wall can become thickened, fibrotic, and strictured. The mucosal surface may develop *cobblestoning* related to edema with linear ulcerations. Deep fissures can develop and result in microperforations and the formation of fistulous tracts. The disease may be continuous but often has *skip* lesions with intervening segments of normal intestine. The mesentery can become infiltrated with fat, known as *creeping fat.* The disease is often present for months or years before diagnosis, and, in children, growth retardation may be the sole presenting sign.

Distribution of Crohn's disease is divided into three major patterns. The most common is ileocecal, which involves the distal portion of the small intestine (terminal ileum) and the proximal large bowel, and is observed in approximately 40% of patients. Ileocecal Crohn's disease may mimic many other diseases, including acute appendicitis. Common symptoms include right lower quadrant abdominal pain, fever, weight loss, and sometimes a palpable inflammatory mass. Chronic inflammation, which leads to fibrosis and stricture formation, may result in partial or complete intestinal obstruction, as demonstrated by abdominal pain, distention, nausea, and vomiting. Because vitamin B_{12} and bile salts are absorbed in the terminal ileum, ileal Crohn's disease or surgical resection of the terminal ileum may lead to B_{12} deficiency, as well as deficiencies of the fat-soluble vitamins (A, D, E, and K) as a result of bile salt malabsorption.

The second major site of Crohn's disease involves the small intestine, especially the terminal ileal portion, and is seen in approximately 30% of individuals at the time of presentation. Similar complications develop, including fistulas, which may form between different segments of bowel (e.g., enteroenteric, enterocolonic), bowel and skin (enterocutaneous), bowel and bladder (enterovesicular), and bowel and vagina (rectovaginal).

The third site of disease is confined to the colon and is observed in 25% of individuals at the time of presentation. Although the disease often spares the rectum, 30% to 40% of patients may develop disabling perianal involvement with fissures, fistulas, and abscesses. Diarrhea is the major consequence but usually with less bleeding than that seen in ulcerative colitis. Distinguishing Crohn's colitis from ulcerative colitis can be difficult.

The remaining sites of Crohn's disease are rare (5%) and include the esophagus, stomach, and duodenum.

MAJOR COMPLICATIONS

Stenosis (Stricture) of the Small Intestine or Colon

Stenosis may lead to bowel obstruction or stasis with bacterial overgrowth.

Extensive Ileal Mucosal Disease (or Resection)

Extensive ileal mucosal disease may lead to malabsorption of vitamin B_{12} (resulting in a megaloblastic anemia and neurologic side effects if not corrected) and malabsorption of bile salts (resulting in diarrhea induced by unabsorbed bile salts and potential fat soluble vitamin deficiency). Weight loss may result from generalized malabsorption caused by loss of absorptive surfaces.

Fistulas

Transmural inflammation may lead to spontaneous drainage into adjacent bowel loops (enteroenteric fistula), bladder (enterovesical fistula), skin (enterocutaneous fistula), and vagina (rectovaginal), or it may lead to abscess formation around bowel or in other surrounding tissues.

Urinary Calcium Oxalate Stones

Chronic fat malabsorption leads to luminal binding of free fatty acids to calcium, allowing oxalate, which normally is poorly absorbed because it complexes to calcium in the gut lumen, to be absorbed. This increase in oxalate absorption increases the risk of urinary calcium oxalate stone formation. Patients with an ileostomy and/or chronic volume loss from diarrhea are also at increased risk for uric acid stones.

Carcinoma

For colonic Crohn's disease, the risk is equivalent to ulcerative colitis (see previous discussion). The rates of small bowel carcinoma and lymphoma are slightly increased in patients with Crohn's disease.

Massive Hemorrhage

Massive hemorrhage in Crohn's disease is uncommon.

Diagnosis

The diagnosis of IBD is based on a constellation of clinical features, laboratory tests, and endoscopic, radiographic, and histologic findings. Laboratory tests are not specific and usually reflect inflammation (leukocytosis) and/or anemia. Perinuclear antineutrophil cytoplasmic antibody (p-ANCA) is positive in up to 70% of patients with ulcerative colitis but rarely positive in patients with Crohn's disease, whereas anti-*Saccharomyces cerevisiae* antibodies (ASCA) are common in Crohn's disease and are rarely found in ulcerative colitis. However, these serologic tests are not sensitive or specific enough to use in routine clinical practice. Stool examination for ova and parasite identification and testing for *Clostridium difficile* toxin and enteric bacterial pathogens should be performed to exclude infections that can mimic IBD.

Colonoscopy in patients with ulcerative colitis reveals a granular mucosa, decreased vascular markings, decreased mucosal reflection, and superficial ulcerations (Fig. 37–1). In more severe cases, the mucosa is friable, with deeper ulcerations and exudate. Patients with long-standing disease have *pseudopolyps,* which represent islands of normal tissue in

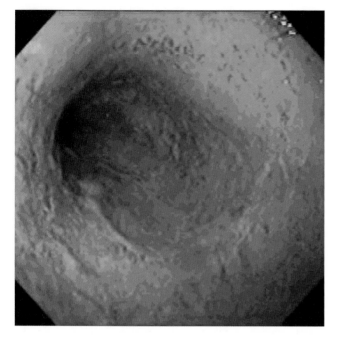

Figure 37–1 Endoscopic image in ulcerative colitis demonstrating diffuse inflammation characterized by erythema, edema, friability, and hemorrhage.

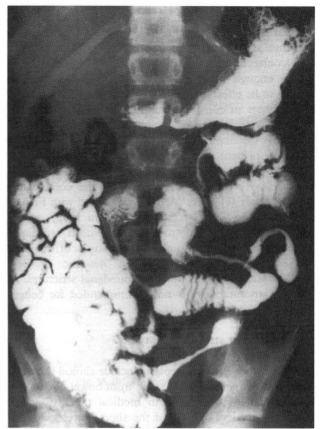

Figure 37–3 Radiograph demonstrating small bowel Crohn's disease with skip areas and a *string* sign.

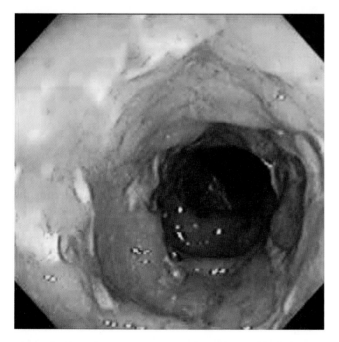

Figure 37–2 Endoscopic image in Crohn's disease demonstrating linear ulcers in areas of otherwise normal mucosa.

regions of previous ulceration. On endoscopic examination in Crohn's disease (Fig. 37–2), the involved mucosa may show aphthoid ulcerations, deep linear or stellate ulcers, edema, erythema, exudate, and friability with intervening areas of normal mucosa (skip lesions).

In Crohn's disease, small bowel radiography has traditionally been the best study with which to investigate the jejunum and ileum, although video capsule endoscopy has recently become increasingly used in this setting. After ingestion of the *PillCam,* over 50,000 total images are obtained over 8 hours (two images per second), transmitted to the data recorder and reviewed by the gastroenterologist. Using this technology, small ulcerations and strictures can be detected (**Web Fig. 37–1**), although patients with known or suspected strictures and/or fistulas should not undergo capsule endoscopy. On small bowel radiography, involved areas have edema and thickening of the bowel wall that lead to bowel loop separation and can also show ulcerations of the mucosa, fistulas, or strictures. A tight, long stricture in the small bowel is commonly called the *string sign* (Fig. 37–3). Linear ulcers with segments of edematous or uninvolved mucosa lead to the characteristic pattern referred to as *cobblestoning.* Computed tomographic scanning can often identify bowel wall thickening with surrounding inflammation, as well as identify intra-abdominal abscesses and fistulas.

Mucosal biopsies in ulcerative colitis reveal crypt architectural distortion, with crypt abscesses and infiltration by plasma cells, neutrophils, lymphocytes, and eosinophils (Fig. 37–4). In Crohn's disease, the inflammation is transmural and more commonly focal. Granulomas are found in 25% to 30% of histologic specimens in Crohn's disease, but not in ulcerative colitis, and can assist in the diagnosis of Crohn's disease in the right clinical setting (Fig. 37–5).

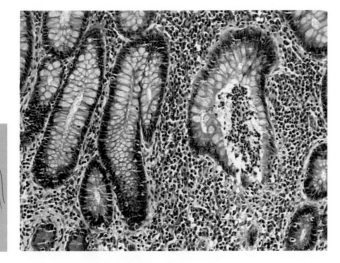

Figure 37–4 Mucosal biopsy demonstrating crypt branching and a crypt abscess characteristic of ulcerative colitis (H & E image). (Courtesy Niall Swan, MD.)

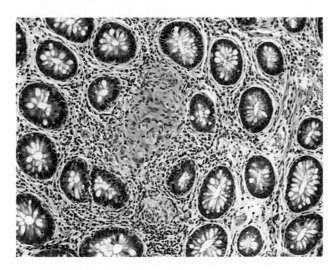

Figure 37–5 Colonic biopsy demonstrating chronic inflammatory infiltrate with a granuloma (H & E image; magnification 10×). (Courtesy Niall Swan, MD.)

Differential Diagnosis

The differential diagnosis of IBD includes infectious colitis, ischemic colitis, radiation enteritis, enterocolitis induced by nonsteroidal anti-inflammatory drugs, diverticulitis, appendicitis, gastrointestinal malignancies, and irritable bowel syndrome. In patients with acute onset of bloody diarrhea, infectious causes that must be excluded include *Salmonella enteritidis, Shigella, Campylobacter jejuni, Escherichia coli* O157, and *Clostridium difficile.* Among the infectious causes, *Yersinia enterocolitica* can mimic Crohn's disease because the pathogen causes ileitis, mesenteric adenitis, fever, diarrhea, and right lower quadrant abdominal pain. *Mycobacterium tuberculosis,* strongyloidiasis, and amebiasis must be excluded in high-risk populations because these infections can mimic IBD, and treatment with corticosteroids can lead to disseminated infection and death.

Table 37–1	**Extraintestinal Manifestations of Inflammatory Bowel Disease**

Skin

Pyoderma gangrenosum
Erythema nodosum

Hepatobiliary

Primary sclerosing cholangitis
Cholelithiasis
Autoimmune hepatitis

Musculoskeletal

Seronegative arthritis
Ankylosing spondylitis
Sacroiliitis

Ocular

Uveitis
Episcleritis

Miscellaneous

Hypercoagulable state
Autoimmune hemolytic anemia
Amyloidosis

Extraintestinal Manifestations

Although both ulcerative colitis and Crohn's disease primarily involve the bowel, they are associated with inflammatory manifestations in other organ systems, reflecting the systemic nature of these disorders (Table 37–1). Most of these manifestations occur frequently when the bowel is involved, and, in some cases, they may become more difficult to treat than the bowel disease itself.

The most common extraintestinal manifestation is arthritis, of which two major types have been identified. The first is a peripheral, large joint, asymmetric, seronegative, oligo-articular, nondeforming arthritis (~20% of patients) that may involve the knees, hips, wrists, elbows, and ankles. This *peripheral arthropathy* usually parallels the course of the large bowel disease *(colitic arthritis)* and usually lasts for only a few weeks. A second arthritis is axial in location, and its activity does not mirror that of the bowel disease. It consists of sacroiliitis and/or ankylosing spondylitis. Ankylosing spondylitis (~5% to 10% of IBD patients) exhibits low back pain and stiffness. Although the HLA genotype B27 is not increased in IBD, up to 75% of individuals with IBD and ankylosing spondylitis are HLA-B27 positive. Sacroiliitis alone (without ankylosing spondylitis) is common in IBD (up to ~80% of patients), but many of these patients are asymptomatic.

Liver complications of IBD include both intrahepatic and biliary tract diseases. Intrahepatic diseases include fatty liver, pericholangitis, chronic active hepatitis, and cirrhosis. Pericholangitis, also known as small-duct sclerosing cholangitis, is the most common of these diseases and usually is asymptomatic, identified only by abnormalities in alkaline phosphatase and γ-glutamyl transpeptidase on laboratory tests and histologically by portal tract inflammation and bile ductule degeneration. Small-duct sclerosing cholangitis may progress to cirrhosis.

Biliary tract disease includes an increased incidence of gallstones and primary sclerosing cholangitis (PSC). PSC is a chronic cholestatic liver disease marked by fibrosis of the intrahepatic and extrahepatic bile ducts, occurring in 1% to 4% of patients with ulcerative colitis and less often in Crohn's disease. Overall, approximately 70% of patients with PSC have ulcerative colitis. Fibrosis leads to strictures of the bile ducts, which, in turn, may lead to recurrent cholangitis (fever, right upper quadrant pain, and jaundice) and progression to cirrhosis. In addition, approximately 10% of patients develop cholangiocarcinoma. Medical or surgical therapy for the IBD does not modify the course of PSC, and most patients will progress to cirrhosis and liver failure over 5 to 10 years unless a liver transplantation is performed.

The two classic dermatologic manifestations of IBD are pyoderma gangrenosum and erythema nodosum. Pyoderma gangrenosum (~5% of patients) exhibits as a discrete ulcer with a necrotic base, usually on the legs. The ulcer may spread and become large and deep, destroying soft tissues. Pyoderma parallels the activity of the IBD in 50% of cases. Treatment is usually with systemic and/or intralesional steroids. Other treatment options include dapsone, cyclosporine, and infliximab. Erythema nodosum (10% of patients, usually with peripheral arthropathy) exhibits raised, tender nodules, usually over the anterior surface of the tibia. It heals without scarring and responds to treatment for the underlying bowel disease.

Ocular manifestations of IBD include uveitis and episcleritis (5%). Uveitis (or iritis) is an inflammatory lesion of the anterior chamber and produces blurred vision, photophobia, headache, and conjunctival injection. Local therapy includes steroids and atropine. Episcleritis is less serious compared with uveitis, producing burning eyes and scleral injection, and is treated with topical steroids.

Other complications of IBD include chronic anemia (common), digital clubbing and hypertrophic osteoarthropathy (uncommon in adults), an increased incidence of thromboembolic disease (uncommon), and amyloidosis (rare).

Differentiation Between Ulcerative Colitis and Crohn's Disease

Generally, the diagnoses of ulcerative colitis and Crohn's disease can be made based on the findings as described in their respective sections presented earlier and those outlined in Table 37–2. As noted, the majority of Crohn's patients have small bowel involvement, skip lesions, and pain, whereas the majority of ulcerative colitis patients have bloody diarrhea with involvement of the rectum and a continuous, superficial spread of the disease. The endoscopic, radiologic, and histologic criteria aid in the phenotypic differentiation of these disease entities. However, occasionally, a diagnosis of *indeterminate* colitis is made as a result of an overlap of findings. For example, colonic Crohn's disease may produce superficial continuous rectal involvement similar to ulcerative proctitis. Similarly, chronic ulcerative colitis can infrequently result in inflammation of the terminal ileum, called *backwash ileitis*. In many indeterminate cases, repeated examination is necessary and/or complications develop that help identify the form of the disease.

Table 37–2 Differentiating Features

	Ulcerative Colitis	Crohn's Disease
Site of involvement	Only involves colon	Any area of the gastrointestinal tract
	Rectum almost always involved	Rectum usually spared
Pattern of involvement	Continuous	Skip lesions
Diarrhea	Bloody	Usually nonbloody
Severe abdominal pain	Rare	Frequent
Perianal disease	No	In 30% of patients
Fistula	No	Yes
Endoscopic findings	Erythematous and friable	Aphthoid and deep ulcers
	Superficial ulceration	Cobblestoning
Radiologic findings	Tubular appearance resulting from loss of haustral folds	String sign of terminal ileum
		RLQ mass, fistulas, abscesses
Histologic features	Mucosa only	Transmural
	Crypt abscesses	Crypt abscesses, granulomas (~30%)
Smoking	Protective	Worsens course
Serology	p-ANCA more common	ASCA more common

ASCA = anti-*Saccharomyces cerevisiae* antibodies; p-ANCA = perinuclear antineutrophil cytoplasmic antibody; RLQ = right lower quadrant.

Treatment (Induction of Remission and Maintenance of Remission)

As part of the initial management of patients with IBD, the clinician must determine the extent and assess the severity of the disease. Patients with mild or moderate disease can be managed as outpatients with close monitoring in association with a gastroenterologist. Patients with severe or fulminant disease, as indicated by abdominal pain, fever, tachycardia, anemia, and leukocytosis, require hospital admission and multidisciplinary team management. Because IBD is a chronic recurrent illness, treatment is centered on controlling the acute attack with induction of remission followed by maintenance of remission. Treatment options for ulcerative colitis and Crohn's disease are reviewed in Table 37–3.

5-AMINOSALICYLIC ACID

The aminosalicylates are given either orally or topically (suppository and enema) and are safe and effective in the treatment of mild to moderate disease, as well as in maintenance of remission. This category includes sulfasalazine (Azulfidine) at a dose of 4 to 6 g/day in divided doses, which consists of 5-aminosalicylic acid (5-ASA) linked to a sulfapyridine moiety and which is activated following the release of the 5-ASA after bacterial lysis in the colon. Side effects, including headache, nausea, and skin reactions, may require discontinuation of sulfasalazine in approximately 30% of patients. Reversible oligospermia may occur with sulfasalazine, and rare serious side effects include pleuropericarditis, pancreatitis, agranulocytosis, interstitial nephritis, and hemolytic anemia. Patients who take sulfasalazine need folic acid supplementation. Newer derivatives of oral 5-ASA compounds, such as mesalamine (Pentasa, 4 g/day in divided doses; Asacol, 2.4 to 4.8 g/day in divided doses), olsalazine (Dipentum, 1 to 2 g/day in divided doses), and balsalazide (Colazal, 6.75 g/day in divided doses), as well as topical forms (Canasa suppositories, 1000 mg as needed daily; or Rowasa enemas, 4 g as needed every night), are being commonly used because of a favorable side effect profile. The majority of patients with sulfasalazine allergy or intolerance can successfully take the newer 5-ASA compounds. The delivery system (pH dependent, slow release) of the orally administered 5-ASA products allows targeting of different areas within the small bowel or colon.

CORTICOSTEROIDS

Corticosteroids may be used topically, orally, or intravenously and are effective for controlling active disease but are not useful for maintaining remission. They are indicated for moderate or severe disease and in patients in whom treatment with 5-ASA fails. The most commonly used agent is prednisone, started in doses between 40 and 60 mg/day. Patients improve rapidly, and the medication is usually tapered down slowly, that is, 5 to 10 mg/week until discontinuation. Patients who do not improve after 1 week of oral treatment or those with more severe disease are best treated in the hospital with intravenous corticosteroids, such as intravenous hydrocortisone, 300 mg/day, or methylprednisolone, which can be given either by continuous infusion or in three divided doses. Corticosteroids have numerous side effects with long-term use. Budesonide (oral Entocort EC, 9 mg daily), a new corticosteroid, which undergoes extensive first-pass hepatic metabolism, is now available for inducing and maintaining remission of ileocolonic Crohn's disease and may offer long-term benefits with decreased corticosteroid side effects.

ANTIBIOTICS

Antibiotics are primarily used in patients with Crohn's disease who have colonic or perianal involvement. Intravenous antibiotics are also part of the initial treatment in patients with severe, toxic, or fulminant colitis. The two commonly used antibiotics are metronidazole (Flagyl) and ciprofloxacin (Cipro). Ciprofloxacin is prescribed at a dosage of 500 mg twice a day. Metronidazole is prescribed at a dosage of 20 mg/kg/day in three divided doses. Patients should be warned of potential side effects, such as a disulfiram (Antabuse) effect and peripheral neuropathy.

IMMUNOMODULATORS

Included in this category are azathioprine (Imuran, 2.0 to 2.5 mg/kg/day) and its active metabolite 6-mercaptopurine (6-MP) (Purinethol, 1.0–1.5 mg/kg/day), as well as methotrexate and cyclosporine. Azathioprine and 6-MP are effective therapies for maintaining remission in both Crohn's disease and ulcerative colitis and are used primarily as steroid-sparing agents. They have a slow onset of action (months) but are generally safe and well tolerated. Other regimens include intramuscular methotrexate for induction (25 mg weekly) and maintenance of remission (15 mg weekly) in active Crohn's disease and intravenous cyclosporine (2.0 to 4.0 mg/kg/day given over 24 hours) as *bridge* treatment for severe steroid-refractory ulcerative colitis. Given the

Table 37–3	**Treatment Options**	
Disease Severity	**Ulcerative Colitis**	**Crohn's Disease**
Mild	Oral and topical 5-ASA compounds	5-ASA compounds Antibiotics Elemental diet
Moderate	Oral and topical 5-ASA compounds Oral steroids Azathioprine, 6-MP	5-ASA compounds Antibiotics Budesonide or oral steroids Azathioprine, 6-MP Methotrexate Infliximab
Severe	Intravenous steroids Cyclosporine Azathioprine, 6-MP Surgery	Intravenous steroids Infliximab Azathioprine, 6-MP Surgery

5-ASA = 5-aminosalicylic acid; 6-MP = 6-mercaptopurine.

potential for both short-term and long-term side effects, as well as the need for close follow-up, patients needing these medications are best managed by gastroenterologists.

BIOLOGIC THERAPY

Biologic therapy involves an important new class of agents that selectively inhibits specific aspects of the immune system. Chimeric monoclonal antibodies (infliximab, or intravenous Remicade, 5 mg/kg) targeted against the pro-inflammatory cytokine, tumor necrosis factor-α, have been shown to be effective in managing moderate to severely active Crohn's disease and also in patients with fistulizing disease. The use of infliximab in the treatment of ulcerative colitis is not yet widely accepted, although recent studies have demonstrated a benefit in patients with moderate to severe disease refractory to conventional medical therapy. Other agents in this biologic therapeutic class that are being developed include fully humanized monoclonal antibodies against tumor necrosis factor-α (adalimumab) and the humanized anti-alpha-4 integrin antibody (natalizumab).

PROBIOTICS

Probiotics are viable nonpathogenic organisms that, after ingestion, may prevent or treat intestinal diseases. Probiotics are being explored as treatment in IBD and may help prevent recurrence after surgery for Crohn's disease and to treat *pouchitis* after ileal pouch-anal anastomosis.

NUTRITIONAL SUPPORT

Nutritional support is an important adjunctive aspect in the management of patients with IBD. However, the role of nutrition as a primary treatment has been limited to patients with small bowel Crohn's disease. These patients may achieve and maintain remission with total parenteral nutrition or elemental diets after prolonged periods (at least 4 weeks). Many patients with Crohn's disease and ulcerative colitis experience weight loss during exacerbations of their illness and need caloric supplements. Vitamins and minerals can be given orally as a multivitamin with folic acid. Vitamin B_{12} should be supplemented parenterally in patients who have extensive ileal disease or an ileal resection. Patients taking corticosteroids require supplemental calcium and vitamin D, and individuals with extensive small bowel involvement can also develop malabsorption of fat-soluble vitamins (A, D, E, and K), iron deficiency, and rarely trace minerals. Lactose-free diets may be necessary, as well as low-fiber diets, in patients with active disease or strictures.

ANTIDIARRHEALS AND BILE SALT RESIN BINDERS

Antidiarrheal agents should be used cautiously during exacerbations of colitis because they can precipitate toxic megacolon. The main role of these medications involves controlling diarrhea in patients who have undergone previous resections. Generally, when less than 100 cm of terminal ileum has been resected, patients can develop a bile salt malabsorptive state during which bile salts enter the colon and result in a secretory diarrhea. Bile salt resin binders such as cholestyramine are an effective treatment in these cases. When patients have undergone one or more extensive resections, the bile salt pool is depleted, and fat malabsorption develops. These patients may require a low-fat diet supplemented with medium-chain triglycerides and antidiarrheal agents, but bile salt resin binders should not be used.

SURGICAL MANAGEMENT

Surgical intervention is indicated for patients with severe disease that does not respond to medical treatment (toxic colitis or megacolon), for those with symptomatic strictures, and for patients with side effects resulting from medical therapy. The other main indication for surgical treatment is the presence of dysplasia or cancer. For patients with ulcerative colitis, regardless of the extent of disease, the entire colon must be removed, and the operation is essentially curative. Approximately 20% to 25% of patients have pancolitis, and one third to one half will require colectomy within 2 to 5 years of diagnosis, depending on the severity of their colitis. In contrast, less than 10% of individuals with mild disease or proctitis will undergo colectomy by 10 years after diagnosis. Historically, the initial operation for ulcerative colitis was a total proctocolectomy and Brooke ileostomy. More recently, the ileal pouch-anal anastomosis has become the operation of choice in most patients. In this operation, the colon is removed, and the small bowel is constructed into a reservoir (ileal pouch) that is anastomosed to the anus, allowing defecation through the anus. A complication of this operation is the development of inflammation of the pouch, called *pouchitis*.

Surgery is not curative in Crohn's disease and is generally avoided, if possible. Nonetheless, 10 years after a diagnosis of Crohn's disease, more than 60% of patients will require surgery. Many surgical procedures in patients with Crohn's disease are performed to manage complications of the disease, including segmental resection, stricturoplasty, fistulectomy, and abscess drainage. Unfortunately, the recurrence rate is high, with 70% of patients having an endoscopic recurrence within 1 year of surgery and 50% having a symptomatic recurrence within 4 years.

Prospectus for the Future

As our understanding of the etiologic and pathophysiologic aspects of inflammatory bowel disease increases, major advancements in diagnosis and treatment are anticipated. These advancements include the following:

- The use of molecular, genetic, and serologic tests to differentiate between subtypes of disease, as well as identify individ-

uals at high risk of developing complications of inflammatory bowel disease
- The increased, and earlier, use of biologic agents in the treatment of inflammatory bowel disease
- Improvements in the detection of dysplasia and prevention of colorectal cancer (including chemoprevention) in patients with chronic colitis

References

Cima RR, Pemberton JH: Medical and surgical management of chronic ulcerative colitis. Arch Surg. 140:300, 2005.

Egan LJ, Sandborn WJ: Advances in the treatment of Crohn's disease. Gastroenterology 126:1574, 2004.

Hanauer SB, Present DH: The state of the art in the management of inflammatory bowel disease. Rev Gastroenterol Disord 3:81, 2003.

Hanauer SB, Sandborn W: Management of Crohn's disease in adults. Am J Gastroenterol 96:635, 2001.

Hanauer SB: Medical therapy for ulcerative colitis 2004. Gastroenterology 126:1582, 2004.

Itzkowitz SH, Present DH: Crohn's and Colitis Foundation of America, Colon Cancer in IBD Study Group: Consensus Conference—colorectal cancer screening and surveillance in inflammatory bowel disease. Inflamm Bowel Dis. 11:314, 2005.

Katz S: Update in medical therapy of ulcerative colitis: Newer concepts and therapies. J Clin Gastroenterol 39:557, 2005.

Kornbluth A, Sachar DB: Ulcerative colitis practice guidelines in adults (update): American College of Gastroenterology, Practice Parameters Committee. Am J Gastroenterol 99:1371, 2004.

Newman B, Siminovitch KA: Recent advances in the genetics of inflammatory bowel disease. Curr Opin Gastroenterol 21:401, 2005.

Oviedo J, Farraye FA: Self-care for the inflammatory bowel disease patient: What can the professional recommend? Semin Gastrointest Dis 12:223, 2001.

Podolsky DK: Inflammatory bowel disease. N Engl J Med 347:417, 2002.

Sandborn WJ, Targan SR: Biologic therapy of inflammatory bowel disease. Gastroenterology 122:1592, 2002.

Siegel CA, Sands BE: Review article: Practical management of inflammatory bowel disease patients taking immunomodulators. Aliment Pharmacol Ther 22:1, 2005.

Van Assche G, Vermeire S, Rutgeerts P: Medical treatment of inflammatory bowel diseases. Curr Opin Gastroenterol. 21:443, 2005.

Chapter 38

Neoplasms of the Gastrointestinal Tract

Paul C. Schroy III

Esophageal Carcinoma

Carcinoma of the esophagus is one of the most lethal of all cancers. The lack of early symptoms and serosal barrier, as well as the rich, bidirectional esophageal lymphatic flow, often results in advanced disease by the time of diagnosis. The American Cancer Society estimates that approximately 14,550 new cases of esophageal cancer and 13,770 esophageal cancer deaths will occur in the United States in 2006. Historically, squamous cell carcinoma (SCC) constituted 95% of all esophageal carcinomas. Since 1980, however, the incidence of adenocarcinoma of the esophagus has rapidly increased, and adenocarcinoma now represents up to 50% of newly diagnosed cases of esophageal carcinoma. The epidemiologic mechanism of SCC differs from that of adenocarcinoma of the esophagus, but the symptoms, treatments, and prognoses are similar.

INCIDENCE AND EPIDEMIOLOGIC FACTORS

The incidence of SCC varies dramatically throughout the world. The highest rates are found in developing countries such as China, Iran, Zimbabwe, and parts of Latin America. SCC is relatively uncommon in the United States, with an annual incidence rate of approximately 5 individuals per 100,000 persons. Esophageal cancer is rare among individuals younger than 40 years of age but thereafter increases in incidence with each subsequent decade. Men are more often affected than women, and African Americans have a fivefold increase in incidence compared with other racial and ethnic groups. The cause of SCC is unknown, but environmental, dietary, and local esophageal factors have been implicated. Heavy alcohol consumption and smoking are the predominant risk factors for SCC in the United States. In developing countries, nutritional deficiencies (e.g., selenium), betel nut chewing, human papillomavirus infection, and consumption of extremely hot drinks (e.g., tea), nitrates, and pickled vegetables, are also important risk factors. Predisposing conditions include lye strictures, radiation injury,

Plummer-Vinson syndrome, achalasia, tylosis, and celiac disease.

Adenocarcinoma of the esophagus is primarily a disease of white men. The primary risk factor for adenocarcinoma is Barrett's esophagus, a condition in which specialized intestinal-type columnar mucosa replaces the normal squamous mucosa in response to chronic gastroesophageal reflux disease. The presumption is that intestinal metaplasia progresses to low-grade dysplasia and then high-grade dysplasia and finally adenocarcinoma. The risk for developing adenocarcinoma in the setting of Barrett's esophagus is approximately 0.5% per year. Long-standing gastroesophageal disease, obesity, and cigarette smoking have also been implicated as potential causative factors. Endoscopic surveillance with biopsy is recommended for Barrett's esophagus but not chronic gastroesophageal reflux disease.

CLINICAL PRESENTATION

Early and curable esophageal carcinoma is frequently asymptomatic and detected serendipitously. The presence of symptoms heralds an advanced and most often incurable stage of disease. Under careful questioning, most patients will have had symptoms for a few months before they sought medical attention. Dysphagia is the most common symptom of esophageal carcinoma, occurring when the esophageal lumen has been compromised by approximately 75% of its normal diameter. Difficulty swallowing solid foods precedes dysphagia to liquids. With complete obstruction, regurgitation, aspiration, and cough or pneumonia may occur. Pulmonary symptoms may also occur if a tracheoesophageal fistula is present. Patients uniformly have weight loss and anorexia. Chest pain, hiccups, or hoarseness indicates involvement of adjacent structures such as the mediastinum, diaphragm, and recurrent laryngeal nerve, respectively. If gastrointestinal bleeding occurs, it is often occult or associated with an iron deficiency anemia. Life-threatening gastrointestinal hemorrhage can occur if the tumor has invaded major vessels. Clubbing of the nails and paraneoplastic syndromes, such as hypercalcemia and Cushing's syndrome, are rarely seen.

DIAGNOSIS

Patients with dysphagia or other suggestive symptoms should be evaluated by upper endoscopy or a double-contrast esophageal barium study. The advantage of endoscopy includes the opportunity to obtain tissue of the cancer, either by biopsy or brush cytologic study. Esophageal carcinoma may appear as a plaque, an ulcer, a stricture, or a mass. Nearly 90% of adenocarcinomas develop in the distal esophagus, whereas 50% of SCCs occur in the middle one third of the esophagus, and the other 50% are evenly distributed in the proximal and distal esophagus. Computed tomographic scanning of the chest and abdomen is performed to detect invasion of local structures and metastases to the lung and liver. Endoscopic ultrasonography (EUS), with its ability to image the esophageal wall as a five-layer structure that correlates with histologic layers, is more accurate than computed tomography is for staging tumor depth, local invasion, and regional node involvement. EUS also permits targeted fine-needle aspiration of suspicious findings.

THERAPY

Stage is the most important prognostic factor for the survival of patients with esophageal cancer and influences the treatment options. Staging is based on the tumor-node-metastasis (TNM) classification system. Only localized tumors confined to the wall of the esophagus are potentially curable by surgery. Overall 5-year survival rates for patients undergoing curative resection, however, are only 5% to 20%. Preoperative chemotherapy with multidrug regimens combined with radiation therapy may reduce local recurrence rates and improve survival. Chemotherapy plus radiation therapy is also recommended for patients with locally unresectable disease, those with medical conditions that preclude surgery, and those who refuse surgery. Patients with metastatic disease should be considered for palliative treatment of dysphagia. Local treatment with endoscopic methods (e.g., malignant stricture dilation), placement of an endoprosthesis (stent), and tumor ablation by laser or photodynamic therapy are often the methods of choice for rapid palliation. More sustained palliation can be achieved using combined chemotherapy and radiation therapy.

Gastric Carcinoma

Gastric carcinoma is one of the leading causes of cancer-related deaths worldwide. For unknown reasons, the incidence of gastric cancer has declined dramatically in the United States since the 1930s. Despite its declining incidence, the American Cancer Society estimates that approximately 22,280 new cases and 11,430 gastric cancer deaths will occur in 2006. Unfortunately, gastric cancer is often advanced at the time of diagnosis; the 5-year survival rate is 5% to 15%.

INCIDENCE AND EPIDEMIOLOGIC FACTORS

More than 90% of gastric cancers are adenocarcinomas. The incidence of gastric cancer varies widely throughout the world. The disease is more common in developing countries than in industrialized nations and shows a predilection for urban and lower socioeconomic groups. Japan, China, South America, and Eastern Europe exhibit the highest rates. The United States has among the lowest incidence rates at less than 10 cases per 100,000 persons. Gastric cancer rarely occurs before age 40; thereafter, the incidence rises steadily, peaking in the seventh decade. Men are afflicted at a rate nearly twice that of women. African Americans, Hispanic Americans, and Native Americans are 1.5 to 2.5 times more likely to develop gastric cancer than whites. Migrants typically acquire the risk of their host countries, suggesting an important role for environmental factors. Low socioeconomic status, improper food storage, and other dietary and local gastric factors are associated with the disease. Dietary factors include deficiencies in fats, protein, and vitamins A and C and excesses in salted meat or fish and nitrates. Predisposing conditions that include atrophic gastritis, postgastrectomy states, achlorhydria, pernicious anemia, adenomatous polyps, and Ménétrier's disease are also associated with an increased incidence. The World Health Organization has classified *Helicobacter pylori* as a carcinogen and epidemiologically linked to gastric adenocarcinoma (Fig. 38–1). However, only a small proportion of patients infected with *H. pylori* develop gastric adenocarcinoma.

Gastric lymphomas account for fewer than 5% of primary gastric malignancies. The stomach is the most common site of extranodal non-Hodgkin's lymphoma, but Hodgkin's lymphoma of the stomach is rare. Gastric mucosa-associated lymphoid tissue (MALT) lymphomas are associated with *H. pylori* infection in 90% of cases and are reported to regress in 60% to 70% of cases after eradication of *H. pylori*. MALT lymphomas can also occur in association with various autoimmune and immunodeficiency syndromes. Most of these lymphomas develop in individuals over the age of 50, and a slight male predominance exists.

CLINICAL PRESENTATION

The location, size, and growth pattern of gastric malignancies may influence the presenting symptoms. Abdominal discomfort is the most frequent symptom; however, early satiety, nausea, and vomiting may occur, especially with gastric outlet

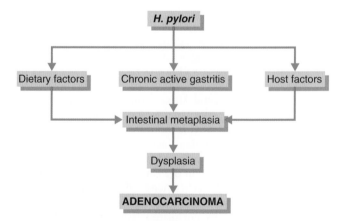

Figure 38–1 Model for the development of gastric adenocarcinoma.

obstruction. Gastrointestinal bleeding may present as iron deficiency anemia, occult bleeding, or frank upper gastrointestinal hemorrhage. Anorexia and weight loss often accompany other symptoms. The signs of metastatic disease, which may be found on physical examination and signify incurability, include a Virchow (left supraclavicular) node, a Blumer shelf (mass in the perirectal pouch found on digital rectal examination), and a Krukenberg tumor (metastasis to the ovaries). A wide variety of paraneoplastic syndromes have been associated with gastric adenocarcinoma and warrant an investigation for a gastrointestinal malignancy. They include Trousseau's syndrome (thrombosis), acanthosis nigricans (pigmented dermal lesions), membranous nephropathy, microangiopathic hemolytic anemia, Leser-Trélat sign (seborrheic keratosis), and dermatomyositis.

DIAGNOSIS

The diagnostic tests for gastric malignancies include double-contrast upper gastrointestinal radiography or endoscopy. Lesions detected on barium study require endoscopic biopsy and cytologic study for histologic evaluation. Gastric carcinomas may appear as ulcers, masses, enlarged gastric folds, or an infiltrative process with a nondistensible stomach wall (linitis plastica). The accuracy of endoscopic ultrasonography is 90% for determining the depth of invasion and 80% for predicting regional node involvement. Computed tomographic scanning of the chest and abdomen may detect metastases in the lung and liver but is otherwise poor for staging. Laparoscopy is increasingly being used for staging and determination of resectability with high accuracy.

THERAPY

The standard treatment of gastric cancer is complete surgical resection with removal of all gross and microscopic disease. The postoperative local-regional recurrence rate remains at 80%. A postoperative combination of chemotherapy plus radiation therapy reduces local recurrence rates and improves survival in patients undergoing curative resection. In the United States, nearly two thirds of patients exhibit advanced disease (stages III to IV), with a survival rate of less than 5%. Chemotherapy is the mainstay of treatment for such patients, but long-term survival is rare. Palliative resection may be performed to prevent obstruction or treat bleeding; radiation therapy and endoscopy may also be of palliative benefit in select patients. Treatment options for gastric lymphomas include some combination of chemotherapy, radiation therapy, and/or surgery, depending on the stage of disease.

Colorectal Polyps and Carcinoma

Carcinoma of the colon and rectum is the third most common cancer and the second most common cause of cancer deaths in American men and women. More than 148,610 new cases and 55,170 colorectal cancer–related deaths will occur in 2006. Screening has been shown to be an effective strategy for reducing both colorectal cancer mor-

tality, through early detection, and incidence, through the identification and removal of premalignant adenomas.

INCIDENCE AND EPIDEMIOLOGIC FACTORS

Worldwide incidence and mortality of colorectal cancer vary considerably. With the notable exception of Japan, industrialized countries are at greatest risk. In the United States, incidence rates have declined slightly over the last decade but remain in excess of 40 cases per 100,000 persons. Approximately 6% of Americans will develop colorectal cancer during their lifetime. Age is an important determinant of risk. Although extremely uncommon in individuals younger than age 35 (except those with rare predisposing genetic syndromes), the incidence of colorectal cancer increases steadily with age, beginning around age 40, with an approximate doubling with each successive decade thereafter to around age 80. Cancer of the colon affects men and women at similar rates, whereas cancer of the rectum is more common in men than it is in women. Colorectal cancer does not appear to have a racial predilection, although African Americans have a slightly increased incidence of stage IV disease. Epidemiologic studies have identified a significant number of modifiable risk factors related to colorectal cancer. Factors associated with an increased risk of the disease include obesity, consumption of red meat and alcohol, and use of tobacco; conversely, factors associated with a decreased risk include physical activity and consumption of certain vegetables and multivitamins with folic acid.

The majority of colorectal cancers are believed to arise from benign adenomatous polyps (adenomas). The epidemiologic factors of colorectal adenomas are similar to those of colorectal cancer. In general, the prevalence of colorectal adenomas in a given country parallels the prevalence of colorectal cancer. Age is an important determinant of prevalence in high-risk countries. In the United States, autopsy studies suggest an overall prevalence of 50%, ranging from approximately 30% at age 50 to 55% at age 80 years. Fortunately, only a minority of adenomas progress to colorectal cancer. The length of time an adenoma takes to develop into an invasive cancer is unknown, but data from multiple observational studies suggest at least 10 years. Insight into the molecular mechanisms responsible for the adenoma-carcinoma sequence suggests that colorectal carcinogenesis is a multistage process (Fig. 38–2) resulting from the accumulation of genetic alterations involving various oncogenes (e.g., K-*ras*), tumor-suppressor genes (e.g., *APC* or *β-catenin, DCC, SMAD4, SMAD2, p53*) and, in some instances, DNA mismatch repair genes (e.g., *hMLH1*).

High-risk groups have been identified and include those with a personal or family history of colorectal cancer or adenomas, various genetic polyposis and nonpolyposis syndromes, and inflammatory bowel disease (Table 38–1). Hereditary nonpolyposis colorectal cancer (HNPCC) and familial adenomatous polyposis (FAP) are well-defined genetic syndromes associated with the highest risk of colorectal cancer. HNPCC (Lynch syndromes) is characterized by inherited mutations in one of the DNA mismatch repair genes (e.g., *hMLH1* or *hMSH2*), early-onset colorectal cancer (average age 44 years) in the absence of polyposis, a predominance (60% to 70%) of tumors proximal to the splenic

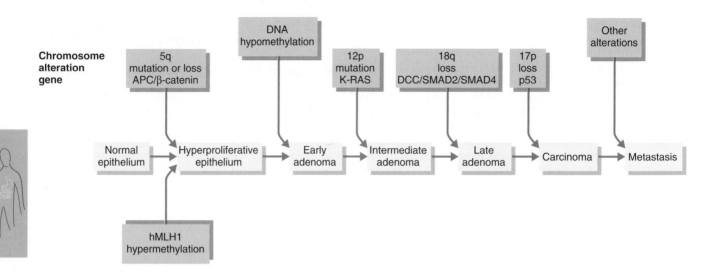

Figure 38–2 A genetic model for colorectal tumorigenesis.

Table 38–1	**Risk Factors for Colorectal Cancer**

Age ≥50
Personal history of adenomatous polyps or colorectal cancer
Familial adenomatous polyposis/Gardner's syndrome
MYH-associated adenomatous polyposis
Hereditary nonpolyposis colon cancer
Ulcerative colitis or Crohn's colitis
First-degree relative with colon cancer or adenomatous
  polyps diagnosed before age 60
Hamartomatous polyposis syndrome (Peutz-Jeghers, juvenile
  polyposis)

HNPCC = hereditary nonpolyposis colorectal cancer;
MYH = *mutY* homologue.

flexure, an excess of both colorectal and extracolonic (e.g., endometrial) cancers, and a estimated lifetime risk of colorectal cancer of 80% to 90%. In contrast, FAP is characterized by inherited mutations in the *APC* gene, the appearance of hundreds of colorectal adenomas during the second or third decade of life, and a risk of colorectal cancer that approaches 100% by the fifth decade if left untreated. FAP is also associated with benign fundic gland polyps in the stomach and duodenal adenomas and adenocarcinomas that have a predilection for the periampullary region. Gardner's syndrome is a variant of FAP in which affected probands also exhibit a variety of extra-intestinal manifestations such as osteomas, desmoids, and other soft-tissue tumors. Congenital hypertrophy of the retinal pigment epithelium is an early benign manifestation of both FAP and Gardner's syndrome. *MYH*-associated adenomatous polyposis syndrome that is indistinguishable from FAP has been described in which mutations of the base excision repair gene, *mutY* homologue *(MYH),* rather than *APC* is causal.

Peutz-Jeghers syndrome is an autosomal dominant condition characterized by hamartomatous polyposis of both the small and large bowel and mucocutaneous pigmentation. Affected individuals are at increased risk of both gastrointestinal (stomach, small bowel, and colon) and extra-intestinal (e.g., genital tract, pancreas, breast) malignancies occurring at a young age. Generalized juvenile polyposis is another inherited hamartomatous polyposis syndrome associated with a small, albeit increased, risk of colorectal cancer.

CLINICAL PRESENTATION

The majority of colorectal neoplasms are asymptomatic until advanced. Gastrointestinal blood loss is the most common symptom and may show as occult bleeding, hematochezia, or unexplained iron deficiency anemia. Other symptoms include abdominal pain from obstruction or invasion, change in bowel habits, and unexplained anorexia or weight loss. A palpable mass may be present in patients with advanced cancers of the cecum.

DIAGNOSIS

All patients with symptoms suggestive of colorectal neoplasia should undergo an evaluation of the colon by colonoscopy. Periodic screening by fecal occult blood testing, flexible sigmoidoscopy, barium enema, or colonoscopy is recommended for asymptomatic, average-risk patients beginning at age 50 years (Table 38–2). Computed tomographic colography *(virtual colonoscopy)* and stool-based DNA testing are two novel screening strategies that show promise but have yet to be endorsed by authoritative groups. Screening recommendations for high-risk patients vary depending on the risk factor (see Table 38–2) but generally rely on colonoscopy performed at a younger age and at more frequent intervals than for those at average risk. Colonoscopic surveillance is recommended for patients with a history of colorectal cancer or adenomas and inflammatory bowel disease. Approximately 50% of colorectal adenomas and cancers are located between the rectum and splenic flexure; however, the prevalence of cancers proximal to the splenic flexure increases with increasing age, especially

Table 38–2 Colorectal Cancer (CRC) Screening and Surveillance Recommendations

Indication	Recommendations

Average risk	Any one of the following beginning at age 50:
	  Annual fecal occult blood testing (FOBT)
	  Flexible sigmoidoscopy every 5 yr
	  Annual FOBT plus flexible sigmoidoscopy every 5 yr
	  Double-contrast barium enema every 5 yr
	  Colonoscopy every 10 yr

One to two first-degree relatives with CRC at any age or one or more adenomas at age <60	Colonoscopy every 5 yr beginning at age 40, or 10 yr younger than earliest diagnosis, whichever comes first
Hereditary nonpolyposis colorectal cancer	Genetic counseling/screening Colonoscopy every 1–2 years beginning at age 25 and then yearly after age 40
Familial adenomatous polyposis and variants	Genetic counseling/testing* Flexible sigmoidoscopy yearly beginning at puberty†
Personal history of CRC	Colonoscopy within 1 yr of curative resection; repeat at 3 yr and then every 5 yr if normal
Personal history of one or more colorectal adenomas	Colonoscopy every 3–5 yr after removal of all index polyps
Inflammatory bowel disease	Colonoscopy every 1–2 yr beginning after 8 yr of pancolitis or after 15 yr if only left-sided disease

*Whenever possible, affected relatives should be tested first because of potential false-negative results.
†Screening recommendation for individuals with positive or indeterminate tests, as well as for those who refuse genetic testing.
From Winawer S, Fletcher R, Rex D, et al: Colorectal cancer screening and surveillance: Clinical guidelines and rationale—update based on new evidence. Gastroenterology 124:544–560, 2003.

among women. Colorectal cancers may arise in sessile (flat) or pedunculated (on a stalk) polyps, or they may appear as a stricture, a fungating mass, or an ulcerated mass. Colonoscopy has greater accuracy than barium enema study in detecting small polyps and early cancers, as well as the ability to remove neoplasms or biopsy lesions at the time of the examination. Lesions detected on barium enema study necessitate colonoscopic evaluation. Computed tomographic scanning of the abdomen and pelvis is used preoperatively to assess the extent of metastatic disease. EUS is used for the preoperative staging of rectal cancer. Carcinoembryonic antigen level is measured preoperatively for a baseline value and, if elevated, monitored to detect tumor recurrence postoperatively.

THERAPY

The rate of survival of patients with colorectal carcinoma is based on the stage of disease (Table 38–3). Unfortunately, 45% of patients first come to medical attention with stage III or IV disease. Surgery alone is curative for early-stage colorectal cancers. Surgery and adjuvant chemotherapy with 5-fluorouracil and leucovorin are recommended for stage III

Table 38–3 Survival Rates and Comparison of Dukes' and Tumor-Node-Metastasis (TNM) Staging in Colorectal Carcinoma

Dukes'	TNM Stage	5-Year Survival Rate
A	I	90%
B	II	75%
C	III	35–60%
D	IV	<10%

colon cancer. For patients with stages II and III rectal cancer, the combination of postoperative radiation and 5-fluorouracil (with or without leucovorin) has been found to significantly reduce the recurrence rate, cancer-related deaths, and overall mortality. For patients with stage IV disease, palliative surgery, chemotherapy, and/or radiation therapy are the mainstays of treatment.

Carcinoid Tumors

The overall incidence of carcinoid tumors in the United States is estimated at 1 to 2 cases per 100,000 people. The most common sites, in descending order of frequency, are the appendix, ileum, rectum, bronchi, stomach, and colon.

Carcinoid tumors arise from neuroendocrine cells and contain a variety of secretory granules containing various hormones and biogenic amines. Serotonin is synthesized from 5-hydroxytryptophan and metabolized in the liver to 5-hydroxyindoleacetic acid, which is biologically inert and secreted in the urine. The release of serotonin (hindgut tumors) and other vasoactive substances into the systemic circulation is thought to cause the carcinoid syndrome. Therefore, carcinoid metastases in the liver or other sites that drain into systemic veins may be associated with the carcinoid syndrome, as may primary carcinoids in the ovary or bronchus. The symptoms include episodic flushing, wheezing, diarrhea, right ventricular valvular heart disease, and, potentially, vasomotor collapse. Localized tumors may produce gross or occult bleeding, obstructive symptoms, or abdominal pain, depending on their location.

Most carcinoids are indolent; however, the malignant potential is variable and appears to be related to the site and, often, the size of the primary tumor. Carcinoids arising in the ileum and those greater than or equal to 2 cm in size have the greatest malignant potential. Surgical resection is the only curative treatment for carcinoid tumors. Somatostatin analogs are highly effective in managing the symptoms of carcinoid syndrome.

Prospectus for the Future

Further elucidation of the clinical and molecular epidemiologic mechanisms of gastrointestinal neoplasms will improve risk stratification and enable clinicians to tailor their use of screening and surveillance strategies, chemopreventive agents, and therapeutic options.

Progress in our understanding of the cellular and molecular pathways that underlie neoplastic transformation and tumor progression will provide additional targets for selective pharmacologic or immunologic therapies.

Technologic advances will facilitate the endoscopic diagnosis and treatment of premalignant and malignant diseases of the gastrointestinal tract.

References

Dicken BJ, Bigam DL, Cass C, et al: Gastric adenocarcinoma: Review and considerations for future directions. Ann Surg 241:27–39, 2005.

Houghton J, Wang TC: *Helicobacter pylori* infection and gastric cancer: A new paradigm for inflammation-associated epithelial cancers. Gastroenterology 128:1567–1578, 2005.

Pignone M, Rich M, Teutsch SM, et al: Screening for colorectal cancer in adults at average risk: A summary of the evidence for the U.S. Preventive Services Task Force. Ann Intern Med 137:132–141, 2002.

Pignone M, Saha S, Hoeger T, Mandelblatt J: Cost-effectiveness analyses of colorectal cancer screening: A systematic review for the U.S. Preventive Services Task Force. Ann Intern Med 137:96–104, 2002.

Shaheen N: Advances in Barrett esophagus and esophageal adenocarcinoma. Gastroenterology 128:1554–1566, 2005.

Winawer S, Fletcher R, Rex D, et al: Colorectal cancer screening and surveillance: Clinical guidelines and rationale—update based on new evidence. Gastroenterology 124:544–560, 2003.

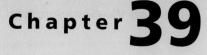

Diseases of the Pancreas

David R. Lichtenstein

Anatomy and Physiology

The pancreas is an organ located in the retroperitoneum (Fig. 39–1) that weighs between 70 and 120 g and is approximately 12 to 20 cm in length. The head of the pancreas is nestled in the C loop of the duodenum, and the tail extends obliquely posterior to the stomach toward the hilum of the spleen. The pancreas consists of the pancreatic acinus and islet cells. The acinar cells comprise more than 95%, and the islets approximately 1% to 2%, of the pancreatic mass. Hormones that the islets produce include insulin, glucagon, somatostatin, and pancreatic polypeptide. The functional exocrine unit of the pancreas is the *pancreatic acinus,* which is composed of both acinar and ductal epithelial cells. Acinar cells synthesize proteolytic digestive enzymes, which are packaged separately in the Golgi region into condensing vacuoles, and transported in an inactive form referred to as zymogens to the apical portions of the cell, where they are discharged into the central ductule of the acinus by exocytosis. The ductules coalesce to form larger ducts, which empty into the duodenum at the ampulla of Vater. Inactive enzymes secreted into the duodenum are converted to an active form by enterokinase secreted from small bowel enterocytes. Trypsinogen, converted to active trypsin in the duodenum by enterokinase, is the trigger enzyme that subsequently converts the other zymogens to active enzymes (Fig. 39–2). Enzymes secreted in an active form include lipase, amylase, and ribonuclease. The *ductal cells* secrete primarily water and electrolytes, which decrease the viscosity of the protein-rich acinar secretions and alkalinize gastric contents emptied into the duodenum to levels at which the pancreatic enzymes become catalytically active (pH ranges from >3.5 to 4).

Normal Pancreas Development

At approximately 4 weeks of gestation, the dorsal pancreas forms as an evagination from the duodenum, and shortly thereafter, the ventral pancreas forms from the hepatic diverticulum. Rotation of the duodenum places the two pancreatic buds in close proximity at 7 to 8 weeks of gestation, at which time their main ducts begin to fuse. If fusion is incomplete, the duct of Wirsung drains only the ventral pancreas through the major ampulla, and the duct of Santorini drains the bulk of the pancreas (dorsal pancreas) through the relatively small accessory ampulla. This common anomaly termed *pancreas divisum* is present in 5% to 10% of the general population and may be associated with acute and chronic pancreatitis. Theories suggest that pancreatitis may result from relative outflow obstruction of the main dorsal duct through the small accessory ampulla. Endoscopic papillotomy or surgical sphincteroplasty are two therapeutic maneuvers that may reduce the incidence of recurrent pancreatitis by increasing drainage through the accessory papilla.

Acute Pancreatitis

Acute pancreatitis is best defined as an acute inflammatory process of the pancreas that may also involve peripancreatic tissues and remote organ systems. The overall incidence is 1 in 4000 for the general population. Gallstones account for 45%, alcohol 35%, miscellaneous causes 10%, and idiopathic causes 10% to 20% of acute pancreatitis cases (Table 39–1). Most patients recover and will have restoration of normal pancreatic function and gland architecture.

CAUSES AND PATHOGENESIS

Most investigators currently believe that acute pancreatitis evolves in multiple stages. The first stage is characterized by changes that occur within pancreatic acinar cells, where the intracellular trafficking of digestive enzyme zymogens such as trypsinogen and lysosomal hydrolases such as cathepsin B is altered. As a result, the two types of enzymes become co-localized within intracellular vacuoles, and cathepsin B catalyzes the activation of trypsinogen. Subsequently, trypsin activates the other digestive zymogens, leading to acinar cell injury. The next stage of pancreatitis involves the initiation of

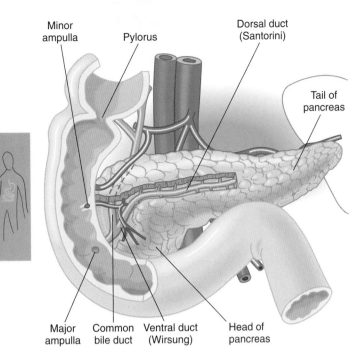

Figure 39–1 Normal anatomy of the pancreas.

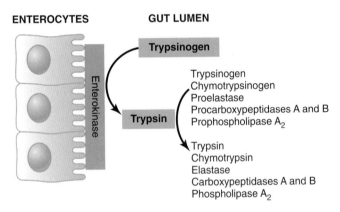

Figure 39–2 Mechanism of proenzyme activation in the intestinal lumen. (Adapted from Solomon TE: Exocrine pancreas: Pancreatitis. In The Undergraduate Teaching Project in Gastroenterology and Liver Disease, Unit 24. Bethesda, Md.: American Gastroenterological Association, 1984.)

an intrapancreatic inflammatory response, which is triggered by the generation, within pancreatic cells, of various pro-inflammatory factors, including chemokines and cytokines. These pancreas-derived chemokines and cytokines cause activation and chemo-attraction of inflammatory cells to the pancreas, and this event, along with increased endothelial permeability, results in an intrapancreatic inflammatory reaction. With further progression of the disease, a third stage evolves during which the pancreatic parenchymal cell injury may worsen and a systemic inflammatory response syndrome (SIRS) may be triggered.

CLINICAL MANIFESTATIONS

Abdominal pain is virtually always present and may be severe and refractory to analgesics. Pain often radiates to the back

and is usually worse when supine. Ileus occurs when the inflammatory process extends into the small intestinal and colonic mesentery or when a chemical peritonitis occurs. Other manifestations include nausea, vomiting, and fever caused by the significant inflammatory process and release of cytokines (Fig. 39–3).

In acute pancreatitis, a wide variety of toxic materials, including pancreatic enzymes, vasoactive materials (e.g., kinins), and other toxic substances (e.g., elastase, phospholipase A_2), are liberated by the pancreas and extravasate along fascial planes in the retroperitoneal space, lesser sac, and the peritoneal cavity. These materials cause chemical irritation and contribute to third-space losses of protein-rich fluid, hypovolemia, and hypotension. These toxic materials may also reach the systemic circulation by lymphatic and venous pathways and contribute to subcutaneous fat necrosis and end organ damage, including shock, renal failure, and respiratory insufficiency (atelectasis, effusions, and acute respiratory distress syndrome [ARDS]). Grey Turner's sign (ecchymosis of the flank) or Cullen's sign (ecchymosis in the periumbilical region) may be seen in association with hemorrhagic pancreatitis.

Metabolic problems are common in severe disease and include hypocalcemia, hyperglycemia, and acidosis. Hypocalcemia is most commonly caused by concomitant hypoalbuminemia. Other mechanisms may include complexing of calcium to released free fatty acids, protease-induced degradation of circulating parathyroid hormone (PTH), and failure of PTH to release calcium from bone. Local spread of inflammation leads to effects on contiguous organs that include gastritis and duodenitis, splenic-vein thrombosis, colonic necrosis, and external compression of the common bile duct, leading to biliary obstruction. Trypsin can activate plasminogen to plasmin and induce clot lysis. On the other hand, trypsin can activate prothrombin and thrombin and produce thrombosis, leading to disseminated intravascular coagulation. *Extrapancreatic fluid collections* occur when fluid extravasates from the pancreas or surrounding leaky tissues. They are located in or near the pancreas and lack a wall of granulation or fibrous tissue. Acute fluid collections occur more commonly with severe pancreatitis. Most of these lesions regress spontaneously and almost all remain sterile. The older term *phlegmon* was used in the past to describe inflammatory collections, but it is too ambiguous and imprecise for current use, given that it does not differentiate acute fluid collections from areas of pancreatic necrosis nor infected from noninfected collections.

A *pancreatic abscess* is a circumscribed intra-abdominal collection of pus, usually in proximity to the pancreas, which contains little or no pancreatic necrosis. *Pancreatic pseudocysts* are defined as encapsulated nonepithelial-lined collections of pancreatic juice formed a minimum of 4 weeks after the onset of acute pancreatitis and located in or adjacent to the pancreas. They occur in the setting of acute or chronic pancreatitis in up to 25% of patients. Treatment of symptomatic pancreatic pseudocysts and abscesses requires radiographic, endoscopic, or surgical drainage. Asymptomatic pseudocysts should be followed. *Pancreatic fistula* occurs as a result of duct disruption and is treated with total parenteral nutrition, endoscopic stenting, and octreotide. Surgical intervention may be needed if this conservative approach is unsuccessful.

Table 39–1   Causes of Acute Pancreatitis

Obstructive Causes

Gallstones
Tumors: ampullary or pancreatic tumors
Parasites: ascaris or *Clonorchis*
Developmental anomalies: pancreas divisum, choledochocele, annular pancreas
Periampullary duodenal diverticula
Hypertensive sphincter of Oddi
Afferent duodenal loop obstruction

Toxins

Ethyl alcohol
Methyl alcohol
Scorpion venom: excessive cholinergic stimulation causes salivation, sweating, dyspnea, and cardiac arrhythmias. Seen mostly in the West Indies
Organophosphorus insecticides

Drugs

Definite association (documented with rechallenges): Azathioprine/6-MP, valproic acid, estrogens, tetracycline, metronidazole, nitrofurantoin, pentamidine, furosemide, sulfonamides, methyldopa, cytarabine, cimetidine, ranitidine, sulindac, dideoxycytidine
Probable association: thiazides, ethacrynic acid, phenformin, procainamide, chlorthalidone, L-asparaginase

Metabolic Causes

Hypertriglyceridemia, hypercalcemia, end-stage renal disease

Trauma

Accidental: blunt trauma to the abdomen (car accident, bicycle)
Iatrogenic: postoperative, endoscopic retrograde cholangiopancreatography, endoscopic sphincterotomy, sphincter of Oddi manometry

Infectious

Parasitic: ascariasis, clonorchiasis
Viral: mumps, rubella, hepatitis A, hepatitis B, non-A and non-B hepatitis, coxsackievirus B, echo, adenovirus, cytomegalovirus, varicella, Epstein-Barr, human immunodeficiency virus
Bacterial: mycoplasma, *Campylobacter jejuni,* tuberculosis, Legionella, Leptospirosis

Vascular

Ischemia: hypoperfusion (such as postcardiac surgery) or atherosclerotic emboli
Vasculitis: systemic lupus erythematous, polyarteritis nodosa, malignant hypertension

Idiopathic

10% to 30% of patients with pancreatitis. Up to 60% of these patients have occult gallstone disease (biliary microlithiasis or gallbladder sludge). Other less common causes include sphincter of Oddi dysfunction, mutations in the cystic fibrosis transmembrane regulator.

Miscellaneous

Penetrating peptic ulcer
Crohn's disease of the duodenum
Pregnancy associated
Pediatric association: Reye's syndrome, cystic fibrosis

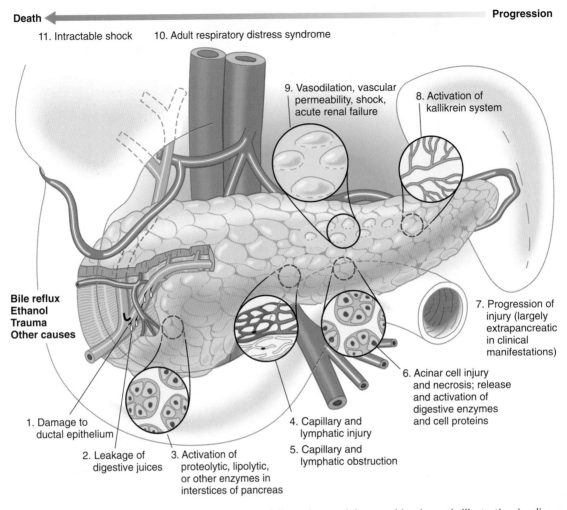

Death ← **Progression**

11. Intractable shock   10. Adult respiratory distress syndrome

9. Vasodilation, vascular permeability, shock, acute renal failure

8. Activation of kallikrein system

Bile reflux
Ethanol
Trauma
Other causes

7. Progression of injury (largely extrapancreatic in clinical manifestations)

6. Acinar cell injury and necrosis; release and activation of digestive enzymes and cell proteins

1. Damage to ductal epithelium

2. Leakage of digestive juices

3. Activation of proteolytic, lipolytic, or other enzymes in interstices of pancreas

4. Capillary and lymphatic injury

5. Capillary and lymphatic obstruction

Figure 39–3 The pathophysiology of acute pancreatitis is not fully understood, but, as this schematic illustration implies, a cascade of events seems likely, beginning with the release of toxic substances into the parenchyma and ending with shock and death. Damage to the ductal epithelium or acinar cell injury may result from bile reflux, increased intraductal pressure, alcohol, or trauma. (Adapted from Grendell JH: The pancreas. In Smith LH Jr, Thier SO [eds]: Pathophysiology: The Biological Principles of Disease, 2nd ed. Philadelphia: WB Saunders, 1985, p 1228.)

DIAGNOSIS

The diagnosis of acute pancreatitis is based on the presence of abdominal pain and is supported by elevations in serum amylase and lipase in excess of three times the upper limit of normal. Elevated serum pancreatic enzymes may occur in a wide variety of other conditions, including bowel perforation, intestinal obstruction, mesenteric ischemia, tubo-ovarian disease, and renal failure. Serum lipase is slightly more specific and remains normal in some conditions associated with an elevation of serum amylase, including macroamylasemia, parotitis, and tubo-ovarian disease. The serum amylase level usually rises rapidly, as does the serum lipase level, and may remain elevated for 3 to 5 days. Serum lipase remains elevated longer than amylase and thus may be helpful if patients seek medical attention several days following symptom onset. Repeated measurements of pancreatic enzymes have little value in assessing clinical progress, and the magnitude of serum amylase or lipase elevation does not correlate with the severity of pancreatitis. Macroamylase and macrolipase can occasionally cause iso-

lated nonpathologic elevations of these enzymes, a situation whereby the measurement of urinary clearance is useful.

Pancreatic imaging with computed tomographic (CT) scanning can be used to confirm a diagnosis of pancreatitis (pancreatic enlargement, peripancreatic inflammatory changes, and extrapancreatic fluid collections). Selective CT scanning may also be useful in evaluating complications and assessing severity of disease (see later discussion), although a normal CT scan is present in 15% to 30% of mild cases. Acute gallstone pancreatitis should be suspected in patients with gallstones on ultrasonography (US) or elevated liver tests, in particular an aspartate aminotransferase level elevated greater than threefold.

SEVERITY OF DISEASE

Supportive therapy alone will be effective in treating 75% of all patients with acute pancreatitis. Twenty-five percent of patients, however, will suffer a complication, with one third of them succumbing to complications, yielding an overall mortality rate of 5% to 10%. Early deaths within the first 2

Table 39–2	**Signs Used to Assess Severity of Acute Pancreatitis**

At Time of Admission or Diagnosis

Age >55 yr
White blood cell count >16,000/mm³
Blood glucose >200 mg/dL
LDH > 2 × normal
ALT > 6 × normal

During Initial 48 hr

Decrease in hematocrit >10%
Serum calcium <8 mg/dL
Increase in blood urea nitrogen >5 mg/dL
Arterial Po₂ <60 mm Hg
Base deficit >4 mEq/L
Estimated fluid sequestration >600 mL

ALT = alanine aminotransferase; LDH = lactate dehydrogenase;
Po₂ = partial pressure of oxygen.
Data from Ranson JH, Rifkind KM, Turner JW: Prognostic signs and
nonoperative peritoneal lavage in acute pancreatitis. Surg Gynecol Obstet
43:209–219, 1976. By permission of Surgery, Gynecology and Obstetrics.

weeks are the result of multisystem organ failure caused by the release of inflammatory mediators and cytokines. Late deaths result from local or systemic infection. The risks of infection and death correlate with disease severity and the presence and extent of pancreatic necrosis. Therefore, a combination of clinical scoring and CT grade provides the most precise prognostic information.

Patients should be stratified into mild or severe levels of illness based on well-established clinical criteria such as Ranson's criteria (Table 39–2) or Acute Physiologic and Chronic Health Evaluation (APACHE II) scores. With increasing scores, the likelihood of a complicated, prolonged, and fatal outcome increases. Mortality is approximately 1% when fewer than three Ranson's signs exist, 10% to 20% when three to five signs exist, and over 50% when six Ranson's signs exist. Similarly, an APACHE-II score greater than 8 has been shown to predict severe pancreatitis. Conversely, a fatal outcome is unlikely with an APACHE-II score less than 8. The distinction between interstitial and necrotizing acute pancreatitis has important prognostic implications (Fig. 39–4). *Interstitial pancreatitis* is characterized by an intact microcirculation and uniform enhancement of the gland on contrast-enhanced CT scanning. Approximately 20% to 30% of patients with acute pancreatitis have necrotizing pancreatitis. *Necrotizing pancreatitis* is characterized by disruption of the pancreatic microcirculation so that large areas do not enhance on CT. The presence of pancreatic necrosis predicts a worse severity of pancreatitis, particularly infection in the necrotic pancreatic tissue, also termed infected necrosis. Infected necrosis develops in 30% to 50% of patients with acute necrotizing pancreatitis but rarely in those with interstitial disease (<1%). The mortality rate for infected necrosis approaches 30% with infected necrosis,

accounting for more than 80% of deaths from acute pancreatitis. Selective gut decontamination or systemic antibiotic prophylaxis is recommended in the setting of necrotizing pancreatitis to reduce the incidence of pancreatic infection. Because clinical and laboratory findings are often similar in patients with either sterile or infected necrosis, the diagnosis of infected necrosis is made by percutaneous CT-guided needle aspiration (Gram stain and culture), which is safe and accurate. Patients with infected necrosis require surgical débridement, whereas patients with sterile necrosis can be followed with supportive therapy, reserving surgical débridement for persistent end organ failure.

TREATMENT

In addition to supportive care, the goals of medical therapy include limiting systemic complications and preventing pancreatic infection once necrosis takes place. No specific treatments have proved effective in lowering morbidity and mortality, including agents that put the pancreas to rest (e.g., somatostatin, calcitonin, glucagon, nasogastric suction, H₂-receptor blockers) and enzyme inhibitors (e.g., aprotinin, gabexate mesilate). All patients should receive close supportive care, including effective analgesia, fluid resuscitation, and nutritional support if oral nutrition is anticipated to be withheld for more than 7 to 10 days. To meet metabolic demands and rest the pancreas, nutrition can be provided by total parenteral nutrition through central venous access or preferably as enteral feeding through a jejunal naso-enteric feeding tube. Systemic complications are best managed in an intensive care unit with aggressive fluid administration and hemodynamic monitoring. Emergency endoscopic retrograde cholangiopancreatography (ERCP) (**Web Video 39–1**) for removing impacted gallstones or establishing biliary drainage is indicated for patients with evidence of biliary sepsis. This procedure should be followed by elective cholecystectomy.

Chronic Pancreatitis

Chronic pancreatitis is defined as an inflammatory disease of the pancreas characterized by irreversible morphologic changes that typically cause pain and or permanent loss of function. Chronic pancreatitis can be classified into non-obstructive and obstructive types (Table 39–3). The most common nonobstructive cause is chronic alcoholism (70%). Alcohol can cause episodes of acute pancreatitis, but at the time of the initial attack, structural and functional abnormalities often exist indicative of underlying chronic pancreatitis. Because most alcoholics do not develop pancreatitis, the presumption is that other unidentified genetic, dietary, or environmental influences exist. If alcoholism is excluded, most patients with chronic pancreatitis in the United States have no demonstrable cause, termed idiopathic (20%). Gallstone pancreatitis, the major cause of acute pancreatitis, almost never leads to chronic pancreatitis. Calcific pancreatitis of the tropics is a major cause of chronic pancreatitis worldwide. Other miscellaneous causes (10%) include trauma, pancreas divisum, cystic fibrosis, hereditary pancreatitis, and metabolic disturbances such as hypercalcemia and hypertriglyceridemia.

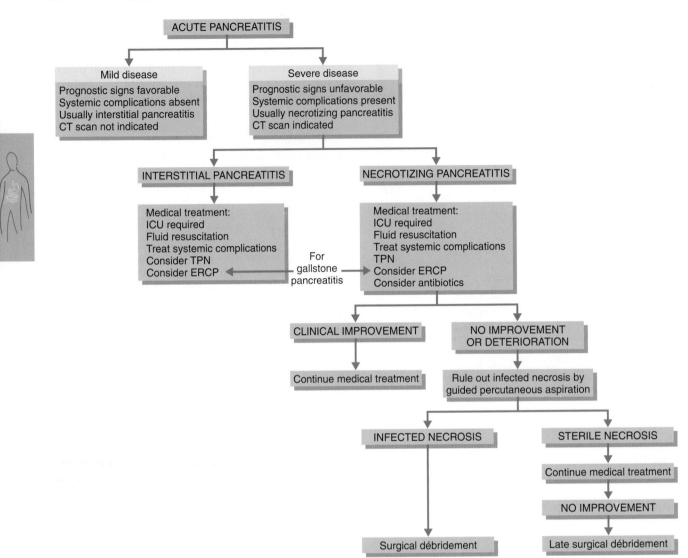

Figure 39–4 Therapeutic algorithm for evaluating acute pancreatitis. CT = computed tomography; ERCP = endoscopic retrograde cholangiopancreatography; ICU = intensive care unit; TPN = total parenteral nutrition. (From Banks PA: Acute and chronic pancreatitis. In Feldman M, Scharschmidt BF, Sleisenger MH [eds]: Sleisenger and Fordtran's Gastrointestinal and Liver Disease: Pathophysiology/Diagnosis/Management, 6th ed. Philadelphia: WB Saunders, 1998, p 833.)

PATHOGENESIS

Alcoholic pancreatitis is the result of abnormal secretion and necrosis-fibrosis of the gland. The *abnormal secretion theory* notes that chronic alcohol ingestion induces hypersecretion of protein from the acinar cell, increased secretion of ionized calcium, concomitant defects in ductal bicarbonate (HCO_3^-) secretion decreasing the solubility of secretory proteins (GP2), and reduced secretion of lithostathine (formerly called pancreatic stone protein), a low-molecular-weight, non-enzymatic protein that inhibits lattice formation by binding to growth sites of calcium carbonate crystals. These secretory defects favor the formation of calcium-protein complexes and ultimately lead to intraductal protein precipitates that obstruct ductules. Progressive blockage of both small ducts and the main pancreatic duct leads to further structural deterioration of ducts, acinar tissue, and eventually islets of Langerhans. The *necrosis fibrosis theory* suggests that alcohol may also have specific cytotoxic effects on acinar cells that act independently to cause tissue damage, possibly even acute pancreatitis. The acute attacks of pancreatitis lead to necrosis of the parenchyma and disruption of the ductal system. After the necrosis subsides and healing occurs, fibrosis of the main duct occurs, which obstructs the gland and leads to large duct disease.

Hereditary pancreatitis results from a mutation of a gene on chromosome 7q that encodes for an abnormal cationic trypsinogen, which cannot be inactivated by intracellular protective proteins. Normally active trypsin is degraded by cleavage of Arg at position 117. In hereditary pancreatitis, Arg is mutated to His, preventing cleavage and resulting in accumulation of active trypsin.

CLINICAL MANIFESTATIONS

Although several different clinical patterns can be seen, most patients with chronic pancreatitis experience pain that can

Table 39–3 Causes of Chronic Pancreatitis

Nonobstructive

Alcohol
Idiopathic: 10–20% of total cases
Tropical, nutritional
Inherited:
  Cystic fibrosis
  Hereditary
Traumatic
Metabolic:
  Hypertriglyceridemia
  Hypercalcemia

Obstructive

Benign obstruction:
  Sphincter of Oddi dysfunction or papillary stenosis
  Pancreas divisum with obstruction of accessory ampulla
    (See Acute Pancreatitis)
Neoplastic obstruction: tumors of the ampulla or ductal
  system

be episodic or continuous. Pain may be accompanied by steatorrhea with symptoms of diarrhea and weight loss. On occasion, patients exhibit exocrine or endocrine insufficiency in the absence of pain. Other patients are asymptomatic and found to have chronic pancreatitis incidentally on imaging.

The pain of chronic pancreatitis is poorly understood. Possible causes include inflammation of the pancreas, increased intrapancreatic pressure, neural inflammation, or extrapancreatic causes, such as stenosis of the common bile duct and duodenum. Evidence in favor of pressure as a cause of pancreatic pain includes reports of pain relief following endoscopic or surgical decompression of a dilated main pancreatic duct. Steatorrhea does not occur until the output of lipase is decreased to less than 10% of normal. Diabetes mellitus is a late complication of chronic pancreatitis, becoming apparent only after 80% to 90% of the gland is severely damaged. The complications of chronic pancreatitis include the development of pseudocysts, pancreatic fistulas, biliary obstruction, pancreatic cancer, small bowel bacterial overgrowth, and gastric varices secondary to splenic-vein thrombosis.

DIAGNOSIS

Because direct biopsy of the pancreas is considered too risky, the diagnosis of chronic pancreatitis is typically based on tests of pancreatic structure and function. Marked structural changes usually, but not always, correlate with severe functional impairment, as determined by pancreatic function tests. In early chronic pancreatitis, however, mild abnormalities of pancreatic function can precede any morphologic changes seen on imaging. Moreover, tests of pancreatic structure may remain normal even with advanced deterioration of pancreatic function and with severe structural deterioration. Laboratory evaluation, such as amylase and lipase, are frequently normal in the setting of well-established chronic pancreatitis, and serum pancreatic enzymes thus neither confirm nor exclude the diagnosis.

TESTS OF FUNCTION

The *secretin stimulation test* is considered the gold standard functional test for diagnosing chronic pancreatitis. The observation that HCO_3^- production is impaired early in chronic pancreatitis has led to the rationale for use of this test to diagnose chronic pancreatitis in the early stages of disease (sensitivity of 95%). This test involves the oral placement of a catheter into the duodenum for aspiration of pancreatic juice before and after stimulation with intravenous secretin. This quantitative measure of pancreatic secretion and enzyme activity is primarily performed in patients with chronic abdominal pain in whom the diagnosis of chronic pancreatitis is suspected and in whom results of imaging studies are negative or equivocal. The secretin test is not widely given because the study is labor intensive and is uncomfortable for patients.

Several less invasive tests have been developed, but they are all less accurate compared with the secretin test, especially in the diagnosis of early chronic pancreatitis. The *72-hour fecal fat* determination is often regarded as the *gold standard* to document steatorrhea (fecal fat >7 g/24 hours); however, the test is not specific for pancreatic exocrine insufficiency. The test also lacks sensitivity because steatorrhea will not occur in chronic pancreatitis until pancreatic lipase output falls to less than 5% to 10% of normal. The *serum trypsinogen* level correlates with functioning acinar parenchyma. A low level (<10 ng/mL) is highly specific for exocrine pancreatic insufficiency. The sensitivity is 80% to 90% in patients with advanced chronic pancreatitis with steatorrhea but only 10% to 20% of those without steatorrhea. *Fecal chymotrypsin* or *elastase* levels may be used as a simple stool test of pancreatic function, but neither is commonly employed in the United States.

TESTS OF STRUCTURE

Findings that suggest chronic pancreatitis include ductal abnormalities (dilation, stones, duct irregularity), parenchymal abnormalities (calcification, inhomogeneity, atrophy), gland contour changes, and pseudocysts. Imaging studies may be normal in the early stages of disease. *Plain film radiography* of the abdomen for detecting pancreatic calcifications can be seen in 20% to 50% of individuals with alcohol-induced chronic pancreatitis. The test should be the first diagnostic test performed when pancreatitis is suspected because it is both simple and inexpensive. Calcifications not detected on plain films can be detected more readily by CT scanning (Fig. 39–5).

ERCP (**Web Video 39–2**) and *endoscopic ultrasonography* (EUS) are the most sensitive imaging studies to evaluate for structural abnormalities of the pancreatic parenchyma and ductular system. The major limitation of ERCP is the development of procedure-related acute pancreatitis in up to 5% of patients. As a result, ERCP should be reserved for patients

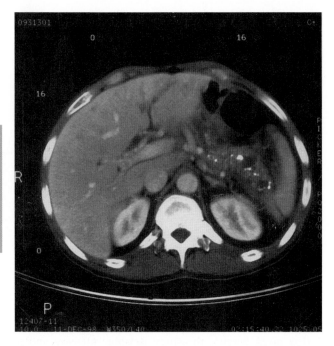

Figure 39–5 Computed tomography scan of a patient with calcifications and small pseudocysts in the pancreas consistent with chronic pancreatitis.

in whom the diagnosis cannot be established or for evaluating symptomatic complications (stones, strictures) associated with chronic pancreatitis. EUS appears to be promising, with early findings that may be more sensitive compared with any other tests of structure or function. Magnetic resonance cholangiopancreatography (MRCP) is a noninvasive diagnostic imaging modality that provides visualization of the pancreatic and biliary systems with images similar to those seen by ERCP but without the risk of precipitating acute pancreatitis.

TREATMENT

Pancreatic enzyme preparations are effective at treating malabsorption and are clinically indicated if patients suffering from chronic pancreatitis lose more than 10% of their body weight, excrete more than 15 g/day of fat with their stool, or suffer from dyspepsia. Four types of pancreatic enzyme preparations are currently available. Most commercial preparations consist of pancreatin, which is the shock-frozen powdered extract of porcine pancreas containing lipase, amylase, trypsin, and chymotrypsin. Enzyme supplements are not absorbed from the gastrointestinal tract, but rather are inactivated by enteral bacterial flora or digestive secretions and fecally eliminated. Administration of acid-stable, encapsulated microspheres or microtablets filled with pancreatic enzymes has greatly increased the efficacy of enzyme supplementation in chronic pancreatitis. Patients with documented exocrine insufficiency should eat three main meals a day and three snacks in between. In general, 25,000 to 50,000 IU of lipase should be ingested simultaneously along with a main meal and 25,000 IU of lipase with snacks; it should not be taken either before or after the

meals. When gastric hyperacidity is present, proton pump inhibitors or H_2-antagonists should be used to delay enzyme inactivation. In cases of progressive maldigestion and steatorrhea, supplementing lipid-soluble vitamins parenterally may be necessary. In cases of severe exocrine insufficiency, one third of the daily caloric intake can be met by administering median-chain triglycerides (MCT), which do not require lipolysis by lipase for absorption. Although clinically effective, patients usually do not like MCT fat because of poor palatability. Symptom improvement, not laboratory tests, demonstrates the efficacy of enzyme supplementation. If these methods do not provide improvement, the next step is to decrease dietary fat intake to less than 50 g/day and to substitute MCTs, which do not require hydrolysis before absorption, for some dietary fat. Other factors may accentuate steatorrhea, including concomitant small bowel bacterial overgrowth, which can occur in up to 25% of patients with chronic pancreatitis. Bacterial overgrowth may be caused by hypomotility of the gut secondary to inflammatory diseases of the head of the pancreas or to chronic use of narcotic analgesics.

The greatest challenge in treating chronic pancreatitis is controlling abdominal pain. Pain is said to improve over time but may take years and is not uniform. Methods of pain relief initially include abstinence from alcohol, analgesics, and pancreatic enzyme supplements. Supplemental pancreatic enzymes are given to decrease cholecystokinin-mediated pancreatic secretion, an approach that alleviates pain in some patients with chronic pancreatitis. Therapy is initiated with large doses of pancrelipases (nonenteric-coated) pancreatic enzyme preparations because, in theory, the enteric-coated preparations release their enzymes further down the intestine away from the stimulatory cholecystokinin (CCK) enterocytes. Nerve blocks (celiac plexus block and splanchnicectomy) yield equivocal results. Endoscopic decompression of pancreatic duct obstruction secondary to strictures or stones may result in pain relief. Surgical ductal drainage, usually with lateral pancreaticojejunostomy (Puestow procedure), may effectively decrease pain in approximately 80% of patients. This procedure is safe and has an operative mortality rate of less than 5%; however, only 50% of patients are free of pain at 5-year follow-up. Patients with nonobstructed, nondilated ductal systems may require pancreatic resection.

Carcinoma of the Pancreas

Carcinoma of the pancreas is the fourth leading cause of cancer in adults, with approximately 28,000 new cases and 25,000 deaths annually. The prognosis is grim; less than 20% of all patients are alive beyond the first year of disease, and only 1% to 3% are alive beyond the fifth year. Carcinoma of the pancreas accounts for approximately 5% of cancer deaths in the United States. More than 90% of these tumors are adenocarcinomas and arise from the ductal cells.

CAUSES AND PATHOGENESIS

Contributing factors include age, gender (male risk ratio 1.4:1), carcinogens, cigarette smoking, hereditary pancreatitis, chronic pancreatitis, and possibly a high-fat diet. Occupational exposure to beta naphthylamine and benzidine are clear risk factors; however, these substances are not thought to be causative agents for the vast majority of patients. Patients with long-standing diabetes may also be at a slight increased risk. Neither alcohol nor coffee consumption appears to be a risk factor.

CLINICAL MANIFESTATIONS

The clinical manifestations of pancreatic carcinoma may be nonspecific and are often insidious. The tumor has usually reached an advanced stage by the time of diagnosis. Common presenting signs and symptoms of pancreatic cancer include jaundice, weight loss, and abdominal pain. The pain is usually constant, with radiation to the back. Because most cancers begin in the pancreatic head, patients may exhibit obstructive jaundice or a large, palpable gallbladder (Courvoisier's sign). Painless jaundice is the most common presentation in patients with a potentially resectable and curable lesion. Anorexia, nausea, and vomiting may also occur, along with emotional disturbances, such as depression. Other, less common presenting symptoms include signs of migratory thrombophlebitis (Trousseau's sign), acute pancreatitis, diabetes, paraneoplastic syndromes (Cushing's syndrome), hypercalcemia, gastrointestinal bleeding, splenic-vein thrombosis, and a palpable abdominal mass.

DIAGNOSIS AND STAGING

Diagnosis of pancreatic cancer is frequently suggested by the presence of a pancreatic mass on imaging studies. Evidence of a dilated pancreatic duct, hepatic metastases, invasion of vessels, or a dilated common bile duct in the setting of biliary obstruction may also be found. The appearance on imaging may be impossible to distinguish from benign causes of pancreatic masses such as focal pancreatitis. CT and magnetic resonance imaging (MRI) are the best initial studies to define a mass and assess for liver metastasis or vascular invasion.

ERCP should be considered if pancreatic cancer is suspected but a mass not found on other imaging studies. ERCP will show a main pancreatic duct stricture in at least 97% of such cases (Fig. 39–6).

The use of tumor markers to diagnose carcinoma of the pancreas has yielded disappointing results. The tumor marker CA 19-9 has a sensitivity of 80% to 90% and a specificity of 85% to 95% in diagnosing pancreatic cancer in patients exhibiting signs and symptoms suggestive of pancreatic cancer. EUS when compared with other imaging studies (spiral CT, MRI, and angiography) is the most accurate diagnostic and staging technique, providing information of tumor location, vascular invasion, and lymph node involvement. The major determinant of both operative resectability and long-term survival is the presence of vascular invasion (superior mesenteric artery or vein, portal vein) or metastatic disease. Unfortunately, only 10% to 20% of carcinomas in the head of the pancreas and essentially no cancers of the body and tail are resectable for cure. If evaluation is conclusive that a pancreatic tumor is not resectable, the first objective is to confirm the cell type, which can be done accurately by CT- or EUS-guided biopsy. When nonoperative staging suggests a resectable tumor, some centers prefer a staging laparoscopy before attempted curative resection.

TREATMENT

Surgery for resectable carcinoma of the head of the pancreas usually involves a Whipple's operation. If resection cannot be done at the time of laparotomy, biliary diversion should be done to relieve jaundice, and gastrojejunostomy is performed if duodenal invasion is present to relieve duodenal obstruction. Surgery offers the only chance for cure. The rate of operative mortality is less than 5%. Attempts at radiation and chemotherapy have met with little success and only modest improvements in patient survival. For patients with inoperable lesions, palliative interventions to alleviate jaundice, pain, and intestinal obstruction often become the focus of therapy.

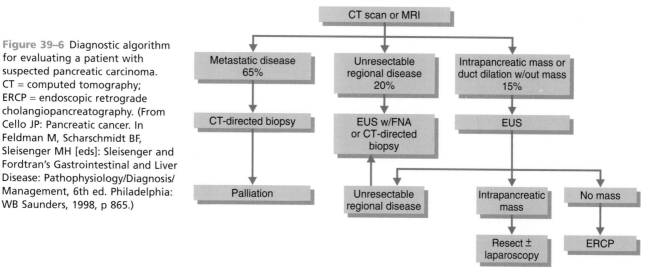

Figure 39–6 Diagnostic algorithm for evaluating a patient with suspected pancreatic carcinoma. CT = computed tomography; ERCP = endoscopic retrograde cholangiopancreatography. (From Cello JP: Pancreatic cancer. In Feldman M, Scharschmidt BF, Sleisenger MH [eds]: Sleisenger and Fordtran's Gastrointestinal and Liver Disease: Pathophysiology/Diagnosis/Management, 6th ed. Philadelphia: WB Saunders, 1998, p 865.)

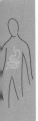

Prospectus for the Future

Our understanding of the pathophysiologic mechanisms responsible for pancreatitis and pancreatic malignancy will continue to evolve. This improved understanding will lead to early diagnosis and improved treatment options.

- Improvements in our understanding of the genetic predisposition for developing pancreatitis will lead to the identification of at-risk individuals and ultimately treatment options to prevent pancreatic injury.
- Elucidation of inciting factors and subsequent inflammatory mediators responsible for the local and systemic injuries seen in acute pancreatitis will offer early treatment options to reduce tissue injury and thereby reduce the severity of the disease process.

- Technologic advances in the endoscopic and minimally invasive surgical treatment of pancreatic necrosis will facilitate care and reduce morbidity and mortality.
- New modalities to evaluate tissue characteristics in early chronic pancreatitis will provide a gold standard for diagnosis and thereby allow for early detection and more appropriate treatment when pain is the presenting symptom.
- Further characterization of the early biologic changes that precede the development of symptomatic pancreatic malignancy will result in prevention, early detection, and new non-surgical modalities for treatment.

References

American Gastroenterological Association: Medical position statement: Epidemiology, diagnosis, and treatment of pancreatic ductal adenocarcinoma. Gastroenterology 117:1463–1484, 1999.

Avgerinos C, Delis S, Rizos S, Dervenis C: Nutritional support in acute pancreatitis. Dig Dis Sci 21:214–219, 2003.

Chowdhury RS, Forsmark CE: Review article: Pancreatic function testing. Aliment Pharmacol Ther 17:733–750, 2003.

Draganov P, Forsmark CE: "Idiopathic" pancreatitis. Gastroenterology 128:756–763, 2005.

Ellis I, Lerch MM, Whitcomb DC: Consensus Committees of the European Registry of Hereditary Pancreatic Diseases, Midwest Multi-Center Pancreatic Study Group, International Association of Pancreatology. Genetic testing for hereditary pancreatitis: Guidelines for indications, counseling, consent and privacy issues. Pancreatology 1:405–415, 2001.

Etemad B, Whitcomb DC: Chronic pancreatitis: Diagnosis, classification, and new genetic developments. Gastroenterology 120:682–707, 2001.

Layer P, Keller J: Lipase supplementation therapy: Standards, alternatives, and perspectives. Pancreas 26:1–7, 2003.

Lockhart AC, Rothenberg ML, Berlin JD: Treatment for pancreatic cancer: Current therapy and continued progress. Gastroenterology 128:1642–1654, 2005.

Rosch T, Daniel S, Scholz M, et al: Endoscopic treatment of chronic pancreatitis: A multicenter study of 1000 patients with long-term follow-up. Endoscopy 34:765–771, 2002.

Schneider G, Siveke JT, Eckel F, Schmid RM: Pancreatic cancer: Basic and clinical aspects. Gastroenterology 128:1606–1625, 2005.

Tenner S: Initial management of acute pancreatitis: Critical issues during the first 72 hours. Am J Gastroenterol 99:2489–2494, 2004.

Vege SS, Baron TH: Management of pancreatic necrosis in severe acute pancreatitis. Clin Gastroenterol Hepatol 3:192–196, 2005.

Warshaw AL, Banks, PA, Fernandez-Del Castillo C: AGA technical review: Treatment of pain in chronic pancreatitis. Gastroenterology 115:765–776, 1998.

Werner J, Hartwig W, Uhl W, et al: Useful markers for predicting severity and monitoring progression of acute pancreatitis. Pancreatology 3:115–127, 2003.

Wray CJ, Ahmad SA, Matthews JB, Lowy AM: Surgery for pancreatic cancer: Recent controversies and current practice. Gastroenterology 128:1626–1641, 2005.

Section VII

Diseases of the Liver and Biliary System

Laboratory Tests in Liver Disease

Gary A. Abrams

Michael B. Fallon

The liver, the largest internal organ in the body, plays a central role in many essential physiologic processes, including glucose homeostasis, plasma protein synthesis, lipid and lipoprotein synthesis, bile acid synthesis and secretion, and vitamin storage (B_{12}, A, D, E, and K). In addition, the liver is vital in biotransformation, detoxification, and excretion of a vast array of endogenous and exogenous compounds. The clinical manifestations of liver disease are varied and can be quite subtle. Clues to the existence, severity, and origin of liver disease may be obtained from a thorough history and physical examination, as well as by routine laboratory screening tests.

Laboratory Tests of Liver Function and Disease

Understanding the utility of different types of laboratory tests of the liver is extremely important in characterizing the underlying liver disease. Unlike tests used to assess function of other organ systems (e.g., arterial blood gas, creatinine clearance), many so-called liver function tests do not directly measure hepatic function and may not accurately reflect the cause or severity of the liver disease process. Specific diagnostic tests such as serologic tests for viral, autoimmune, and inherited liver disease are covered in other chapters.

Tests of Hepatic Function

The great variety of functions that the liver performs has made it difficult to devise a simple, inexpensive, reproducible, and noninvasive test that accurately reflects hepatic capacity for all functions. Instead, currently available tests of liver function are indirect, static measurements of serum levels of compounds that are synthesized, metabolized, and/or excreted by the liver. The liver has a large reserve capacity, and therefore results of *function* tests may remain relatively normal until liver dysfunction is severe.

The most widely available and useful liver function tests are outlined in Table 40–1. The serum albumin level and prothrombin time both reflect the hepatic capacity for protein synthesis. The prothrombin time, which responds rapidly to altered hepatic function because of the short serum half-lives of factors II and VII (hours), is useful as frequently as daily as a marker of hepatic function. However, co-existent vitamin K deficiency must be excluded and/or treated before using the prothrombin time as a measure of hepatic function. In contrast, the serum half-life of albumin is 14 to 20 days, and serum levels fall with prolonged liver dysfunction or in acute liver impairment. Malnutrition and renal or gastrointestinal losses merit consideration in the setting of significant hypoalbuminemia, especially if the prothrombin time is relatively well preserved.

Quantitative tests of liver function, including indocyanine green clearance, galactose elimination capacity, aminopyrine breath test, antipyrine clearance, monoethylglycinexylidide, and caffeine clearance may be superior to conventional biochemical tests in predicting prognosis. However, the clinical utility of these tests has not been established, and they are limited primarily to research centers.

Screening Tests of Hepatobiliary Disease

Screening tests of hepatobiliary disease (Table 40–2) may be divided into two categories, (1) tests of biliary obstruction and/or cholestasis and (2) tests of hepatocellular damage, based on the mechanisms responsible for the abnormal test. However, none of the tests is specific for either category, and the overall pattern and the relative magnitude of abnormalities in these two categories of tests often provide diagnostic clues to the type of liver disease present.

The *serum bilirubin* level reflects a balance between bilirubin production and its conjugation and excretion into bile by the liver. The differential diagnosis for hyperbilirubine-

Table 40–1   Clinical Tests of Hepatic Function

	Property Examined	**Causes of Abnormal Results**
Tests of Hepatic Function (Normal Values)		
Serum albumin (3.5–5.5 mg/dL)	Protein synthetic capacity (over days to weeks)	Decreased synthetic capacity Protein malnutrition Increased protein loss (nephrotic syndrome, protein-losing enteropathy) Increased extracellular fluid volume
Prothrombin time (10.5–13.0 sec)	Protein synthetic capacity (hours to days)	Decreased synthetic capacity (especially factors II and III) Vitamin-K deficiency Consumptive coagulopathy
Screening Test of Hepatobiliary Disease		
Tests of biliary obstruction or impaired bile flow		
Serum bilirubin (0.2–1.0 mg/dL) (3.4–17.1 mol/L)	Extraction of bilirubin from blood; conjugation and excretion into bile	Hemolysis Diffuse liver disease Cholestasis Extrahepatic bile duct obstruction Congenital disorders of bilirubin metabolism
Serum alkaline phosphatase (also 5′-nucleotidase and γ-glutamyl transpeptidase) (56–176 U/L)	Increased enzyme synthesis and release	Bile duct obstruction Cholestasis Infiltrative liver disease (neoplasms, granulomas) Bone destruction/remodeling Pregnancy
Tests of hepatocellular damage		
Aspartate aminotransferase (AST) (10–30 U/L)	Release of intracellular enzyme	Hepatocellular necrosis Cardiac or skeletal muscle necrosis
Alanine aminotransferase (ALT) (5–30 U/L)	Release of intracellular enzyme	Same as AST; however, more specific for liver cell damage

mia (see Chapter 41) requires consideration of an extensive list of disorders in which bilirubin production (hematologic disorders), hepatic metabolism (congenital abnormalities of bilirubin, liver disease), or excretion (biliary obstruction) is altered. Hence, an elevated serum bilirubin determination is not specific for any cause of liver disease. However, such an abnormality, especially in association with predominant elevations in other tests of biliary obstruction, should prompt an evaluation for potentially treatable biliary abnormalities. Recognizing that serum bilirubin levels may not return promptly to normal after relief of biliary obstruction or improvement in liver disease is important because some bilirubin binds covalently to albumin and is removed from the circulation only as albumin is catabolized.

Serum alkaline phosphatase activity reflects a group of isoenzymes derived from liver, bone, intestine, and placenta. Serum levels are elevated in association with a variety of conditions, including cholestasis, partial or complete bile duct obstruction, bone regeneration, pregnancy, and neoplastic, infiltrative, and granulomatous liver diseases. An isolated elevated alkaline phosphatase level may be the only clue to partial obstruction of the common bile duct, to obstruction of ducts in a single lobe or segment of liver, or to neoplastic or granulomatous hepatic disease. In cholestasis, serum alkaline phosphatase levels rise as a result of retention of bile acids in the liver, which solubilize alkaline phosphatase off the hepatocyte plasma membrane, as well as stimulate its synthesis. 5′-Nucleotidase and γ-glutamyl transpeptidase, other hepatocyte plasma membrane enzymes, are similarly released into the circulation during bile duct obstruction or cholestasis and are used to confirm that an elevated alkaline phosphatase level is caused by hepatobiliary disease. An isolated elevated serum alkaline phosphatase with normal 5′-nucleotidase and γ-glutamyl transpeptidase enzymes warrants further testing of alkaline phosphatase isoenzymes to confirm the elevated enzyme is from the liver.

Aspartate (aspartate aminotransferase [AST] or serum glutamic-oxaloacetic transaminase [SGOT]) and *alanine* (alanine aminotransferase [ALT] or serum glutamic-pyruvic transaminase [SGPT]) *aminotransferases* are intracellular amino-transferring enzymes present in large quantities in hepatocytes. After injury or death of liver cells, these

Table 40–2 Abnormal Liver Function Test Patterns and Diagnostic Approach

Hepatocellular Liver Injury	Cholestatic Liver Injury
Predominant increase in AST and ALT ± bilirubin	Predominant increase in alkaline phosphataseγ ± bilirubin
Common causes:	Common causes:
Drug	Drug
Viral	Primary biliary cirrhosis (PBC)
Steatohepatitis	Primary sclerosing cholangitis (PSC)
Autoimmune hepatitis	Autoimmune cholangitis
Metabolic	Sarcoidosis
Initial evaluation	Infiltrative or neoplastic disease
Check drug list	Initial evaluation
Viral serologies (HAV IgM, HBsAg, HBc IgM, HCV Ab), autoimmune hepatitis (antinuclear antibody, smooth muscle antibody)	Check drug list
	PBC (antimitochondrial antibody)
Wilson's (disease) (serum ceruloplasmin), hemochromatosis (iron, total iron-binding capacity, ferritin)	PSC (endoscopic retrograde cholangiopancreatography), autoimmune cholangitis (antinuclear antibody)
Fatty liver (abdominal ultrasound)	Sarcoidosis (angiotensin-converting enzyme level)
Consider liver biopsy (specific indications noted in later chapters)	Infiltrative or neoplastic disease (abdominal ultrasound, CT scan)
	Consider liver biopsy (specific indications noted in later chapters)

ALT = alanine aminotransferase; AST = aspartate aminotransferase; CT = computed tomography; γ = γ-glutamyl transpeptidase; HAV IgM = hepatitis A virus immunoglobulin M; HBc IgM = hepatitis B core immunoglobulin M; HBsAg = hepatitis B surface antigen; HCV Ab = hepatitis C antibody.

enzymes are released into the circulation. In general, the serum aminotransferases are sensitive (albeit nonspecific) tests of liver damage, and the height of the serum aminotransferase activity level reflects the severity of hepatic necrosis, with important exceptions. For instance, both enzymes require pyridoxal 5′-phosphate as a co-factor, and the relatively low serum aminotransferase values seen in patients with severe alcoholic hepatitis (usually 300 U/L) may reflect deficiency of this co-factor. Although aminotransferase levels are increased in a wide array of liver diseases, high levels (15 times the upper limit of normal) generally indicate acute hepatocellular necrosis from viral or toxic causes or, less frequently, indicate acute bile duct obstruction or hepatic ischemia. Patients who have isolated asymptomatic elevations of AST and ALT may have non-alcoholic fatty liver disease (caused by obesity, insulin resistance and diabetes, or hyperlipidemia), alcohol-induced liver disease, or hepatocellular disease, such as hemochromatosis or chronic viral hepatitis. These patients should be screened for treatable diseases. Some patients may require liver biopsy.

Individual liver function tests frequently do not indicate the nature of the underlying liver disease. However, the overall *pattern* of liver test abnormalities and the relative magnitude of abnormalities in individual tests often provide significant insight into whether the nature of the liver disease is primarily hepatocellular or cholestatic. Table 40–2 outlines common patterns of liver test abnormalities and a diagnostic evaluation. Isolated elevation in indirect bilirubin and, rarely, total bilirubin levels greater than 5 mg/dL will occur in hemolysis or Gilbert's syndrome. Bile duct obstruction rarely increases AST and ALT above 500 U/L or alkaline phosphatase above four to five times higher than the upper limits of normal. Ischemic hepatitis often produces ALT and AST levels above 1000 mg/dL, with rapid resolution after fluid resuscitation, excluding other causes of acute hepatocellular necrosis.

Common liver function test patterns in patients with cirrhosis include mildly elevated enzymes (AST and ALT) and elevated bilirubin (primarily conjugated) and alkaline phosphatase associated with thrombocytopenia and prolonged prothrombin time. Specific causes of cirrhosis influence the liver function abnormalities observed (see Chapter 44).

Liver Biopsy

Biopsy and histologic examination of liver tissue are frequently valuable in the differential diagnosis, staging, and consideration of treatment of diffuse or localized parenchymal diseases (e.g., cirrhosis, hepatitis, hemochromatosis, tumors) or hepatomegaly. Liver biopsies can be performed either by a percutaneous or by a transjugular approach. Tissue from a biopsy represents 1/50,000 of total liver tissue, and sampling variability has been noted. Although generally safe, serious complications such as bleeding (1 per 1000) and death (1 per 10,000) may occur. Absolute contraindications include uncooperative patient, prothrombin time greater than 3 to 5 seconds, platelets under 50,000/mm³, nonsteroidal anti-inflammatory drug use in previous 7 to 10 days, and suspected echinococcal cysts in the liver.

Prospectus for the Future

In a significant number of liver disorders that exhibit abnormal liver tests (e.g., hepatitis C, nonalcoholic fatty liver disease), an important diagnostic consideration is the degree of hepatic fibrosis. In general, liver biopsy has been the gold standard for staging disease based on the amount of fibrosis found. Recently, a large number of panels of serum markers have been used to predict the degree of hepatic fibrosis noninvasively, particularly in hepatitis C infection. The use of such tests to predict hepatic fibrosis is likely to increase both in viral and in nonviral liver disease in the near future and may eventually replace liver biopsy as the primary means of assessing degree of hepatic fibrosis.

Another area of active investigation in liver disease is the use of genetic testing to predict susceptibility to drug-induced hepatotoxicity and to predict therapeutic response to specific therapies for liver disease. These pharmacogenomic techniques have the potential to detect genetic markers that may guide the use of drug therapies for liver disease and prevent drug-induced liver disease.

References

Green RM, Flamm S: AGA technical review on the evaluation of liver chemistries. Gastroenterology 123:1367–1384, 2002.

Berk PD: Approach to the patient with jaundice or abnormal liver tests. In Goldman L, Ausiello D (eds): Cecil Textbook of Medicine, 22nd ed. Philadelphia: WB Saunders, 2004, pp 897–906.

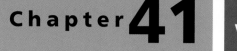

Jaundice

Joseph R. Bloomer
Michael B. Fallon

Jaundice (icterus) connotes the yellow pigmentation of skin, sclerae, and mucous membranes that is caused by hyperbilirubinemia. Jaundice is often a sign of liver disease, and it also occurs in hematologic disorders. Normal serum bilirubin levels range from 0.5 to 1.0 mg/dL, and jaundice becomes clinically evident at levels higher than 2.5 to 3.0 mg/dL.

Bilirubin Metabolism

The normal rate of bilirubin production is approximately 4 mg/kg body weight daily (Fig. 41–1). Approximately 80% originates from the breakdown of heme in senescent red blood cells; most of the remainder comes from ineffective erythropoiesis and catabolism of hepatic hemoproteins such as the cytochromes P-450. The heme ring is cleaved by the enzyme microsomal heme oxygenase to form biliverdin, which is then converted to bilirubin by the enzyme biliverdin reductase. Unconjugated bilirubin is released into the plasma, where it is tightly bound to albumin and transported to the liver. Because unconjugated bilirubin is insoluble in water, it cannot be excreted in urine or bile. However, it will dissolve in lipid-rich environments and thus traverses the blood-brain barrier and placenta.

The three phases of hepatic bilirubin metabolism are (1) uptake, (2) conjugation, and (3) excretion into the bile, the last step being rate-limiting. After dissociating from albumin in the space of Disse, unconjugated bilirubin is transported across the liver cell plasma membrane and attaches to intracellular binding proteins (ligandin). It is then conjugated with glucuronic acid by the enzyme UDP glucuronyltransferase to form bilirubin monoglucuronide and diglucuronide, which are water soluble. Conjugated bilirubin is excreted into bile by active transport across the canalicular membrane by a multispecific canalicular transporter. When biliary excretion of conjugated bilirubin is impaired, the pigment regurgitates from hepatocytes into plasma, causing an increase in the plasma level. Because conjugated bilirubin is water soluble and less tightly bound to albumin than is unconjugated bilirubin, it is readily filtered by the glomerulus and appears in the urine, giving it a dark color (choluria).

Once in bile, bilirubin enters the intestine, where bacteria convert it to colorless tetrapyrroles (urobilinogens) that are excreted in feces. Up to 20% of urobilinogen is reabsorbed and undergoes enterohepatic circulation or excretion in urine.

Laboratory Measurement of Bilirubin

The *van den Bergh reaction,* which is the most commonly used test for detecting bilirubin in biologic fluids, combines bilirubin with diazotized sulfanilic acid to form a colored compound. The direct-reacting fraction is roughly equivalent to conjugated bilirubin and the indirect-reacting fraction (total minus direct fraction) to unconjugated bilirubin. This characteristic provides a means for classifying jaundice into two categories, unconjugated hyperbilirubinemia and conjugated hyperbilirubinemia.

Unconjugated Hyperbilirubinemia

Mechanisms that cause unconjugated hyperbilirubinemia are (1) overproduction, (2) impaired hepatic uptake, and (3) decreased conjugation of bilirubin. These disorders are not usually associated with significant hepatic disease.

OVERPRODUCTION

Overproduction of bilirubin results from hemolysis. Jaundice is characteristically mild, and serum bilirubin levels rarely exceed 5 mg/dL in the absence of co-existent hepatic disease. Ineffective erythropoiesis, which may be significantly increased in megaloblastic anemias, also leads to mild jaundice. Hemolysis can be investigated by examining the peripheral blood smear (and in some cases the bone marrow smear) and measuring the reticulocyte count, haptoglobin, lactate dehydrogenase (LDH), erythrocyte fragility, and Coombs' test.

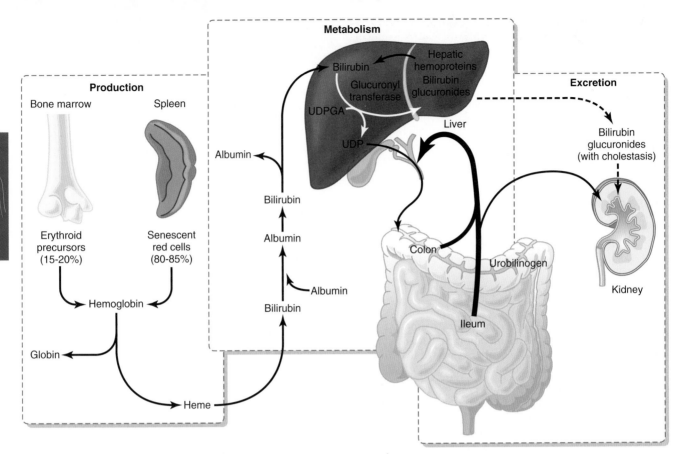

Figure 41–1 Bilirubin production, metabolism, and excretion (see text for detailed description). UDP = uridine diphosphate; UDPGA = uridine diphosphate glucuronic acid.

IMPAIRED HEPATIC UPTAKE

Impaired hepatic uptake causes jaundice that occurs after administering certain drugs, such as rifampin (competition for bilirubin uptake) and those involved in treating Gilbert's syndrome. Gilbert's syndrome is a benign disorder that affects up to 7% of the population with male predominance. It commonly exhibits during the second or third decade of life as mild unconjugated hyperbilirubinemia that is exacerbated by fasting or is noted on routine laboratory testing. Most patients have a bilirubin level that is less than 3 mg/dL. The genetic defect is usually a homozygous abnormality in the TATAA element of the promoter region of the UDP-glucuronyltransferase gene. The diagnosis is strongly suggested by unconjugated hyperbilirubinemia in which normal hepatic enzymes exist and overt hemolysis is absent. Liver biopsy is generally not indicated. Therapy is not usually given, but the bilirubin level does decrease significantly with phenobarbital administration.

IMPAIRED CONJUGATION

Crigler-Najjar syndrome occurs as a result of impaired conjugation of bilirubin that is caused by genetically determined decrease or absence of UDP glucuronyl transferase activity. Conjugation may also be impaired by mild, acquired defects

of UDP glucuronyltransferase induced by drugs such as chloramphenicol.

Neonatal Jaundice

Neonatal jaundice is caused by a combination of mechanisms that result in unconjugated hyperbilirubinemia. In neonates, hepatic bilirubin metabolism is incompletely developed, and bilirubin production is also increased. The major defect is in bilirubin conjugation, which may cause mild to moderate unconjugated hyperbilirubinemia between the second and fifth days of life. Severe unconjugated hyperbilirubinemia in the neonate is usually caused by a combination of hemolysis secondary to blood group incompatibility and defective conjugation. The severe hyperbilirubinemia is associated with a risk of neurologic damage *(kernicterus)*. Phototherapy is the treatment of choice.

Conjugated Hyperbilirubinemia

Conjugated hyperbilirubinemia is generally associated with impaired formation or excretion of *all* components of bile, a situation termed *cholestasis.* The two major mechanisms of conjugated hyperbilirubinemia are (1) a defect in the excretion of bilirubin from hepatocytes into bile (intrahepatic cholestasis) or (2) a mechanical obstruction to the flow of bile through the bile ducts.

IMPAIRED HEPATIC EXCRETION (INTRAHEPATIC CHOLESTASIS)

Intrahepatic cholestasis can result from a wide range of conditions, including those that impair canalicular transport (e.g., drugs) and those that cause destruction of the small intrahepatic bile ducts (e.g., primary biliary cirrhosis).

Primary biliary cirrhosis is a chronic, progressive liver disease that occurs primarily in women and is characterized by the destruction and subsequent disappearance of small lobular bile ducts. The gradual decrease in the number of bile ducts leads to progressive cholestasis, portal inflammation, fibrosis, and eventually cirrhosis. Drug-induced cholestasis may be caused by a wide array of drugs, including phenothiazines, oral contraceptives, and methyltestosterone. Postoperative jaundice typically occurs 1 to 10 days after surgery and has an incidence of 15% after heart surgery and 1% after elective abdominal surgery. It is multifactorial in origin. In hepatocellular disease, all three steps of hepatic bilirubin metabolism are impaired. Excretion, the rate-limiting step, is usually the most affected, leading to predominantly conjugated hyperbilirubinemia. Jaundice may be profound in acute hepatitis (see Chapter 42) without adverse prognostic implications. In contrast, in chronic liver disease, persistent jaundice usually implies irreversible decrease in hepatic function and a poor prognosis.

EXTRAHEPATIC BILIARY OBSTRUCTION

Complete or partial obstruction of the extrahepatic bile ducts may result from a variety of causes that can obstruct the biliary system at any level, from its outlet in the duodenum to the intrahepatic ducts. The list of potential causes is long and includes impaction of gallstones, carcinoma of the head of the pancreas, tumors of the bile ducts, bile duct strictures, and chronic pancreatitis with bile duct compression (Table 41–1).

Clinical Approach to Jaundice

Because the differential diagnosis of jaundice is broad, a thorough history and physical examination and judicious use of laboratory and imaging studies are needed to define its cause. Jaundice appears as yellowing of the skin and sclera. Other conditions may cause yellowing or darkening of the skin (e.g., carotinemia, Addison's disease, quinacrine ingestion), but scleral and mucosal discolorations are absent in these conditions. The most important initial step is to define whether the jaundice is predominately caused by an elevation of unconjugated or of conjugated bilirubin. If jaundice is primarily the result of unconjugated bilirubin, evaluation for hemolysis is appropriate. In patients with elevated conjugated bilirubin, the clinical challenge lies in distinguishing whether biliary obstruction or impaired hepatic excretion is the cause (see Chapter 40).

Table 41–1 Classification of Jaundice

Predominantly Unconjugated Hyperbilirubinemia

Overproduction

Hemolysis (e.g., spherocytosis, sickle-cell disease, hemolysis of the newborn, autoimmune disorders)
Ineffective erythropoiesis (e.g., megaloblastic anemias)

Decreased hepatic uptake

Gilbert's syndrome
Drugs (e.g., rifampin, radiographic contrast agents)
Neonatal jaundice

Decreased conjugation

Gilbert's syndrome
Crigler-Najjar syndrome types I and II
Neonatal jaundice
Hepatocellular disease
Drug inhibition (e.g., chloramphenicol)

Predominantly Conjugated Hyperbilirubinemia

Impaired hepatic excretion

Familial disorders (Dubin-Johnson syndrome, Rotor's syndrome, benign recurrent cholestasis, cholestasis of pregnancy)
Hepatocellular disease
Hepatitis (viral and drug induced)
Drug-induced cholestasis
Primary biliary cirrhosis
Primary sclerosing cholangitis
Autoimmune cholangiopathy
Vanishing bile duct syndrome
Sepsis
Postoperative complications

Extrahepatic biliary obstruction

Gallstones
Tumors of the head of the pancreas (adenocarcinoma, mucinous duct ectasia)
Tumors of bile ducts (cholangiocarcinoma)
Gallbladder cancer
Tumors of the ampulla of Vater (adenoma, adenocarcinoma)
Tumors of the duodenum (adenocarcinoma, lymphoma)
Hemobilia (blood in the biliary tree)
Biliary strictures (postcholecystectomy, postliver transplantation, primary sclerosing cholangitis)
Congenital disorders (biliary atresia)
Metastasis to the hepatic hilum
Primary bile duct lymphoma
Cholangiopathy of acquired immunodeficiency syndrome
Choledocal cysts
Infectious cholangiopathy (Clonorchis sinensis, Ascaris lumbricoides, Fasciola hepatica)
Chronic pancreatitis (fibrosis of the head of the pancreas)

In cholestatic jaundice caused by biliary obstruction or impaired hepatic excretion, the alkaline phosphatase level is typically increased more than three times normal, whereas serum transaminases are usually elevated less than 5-fold to 10-fold (see Chapter 39). Patients with cholestasis also may develop pruritus and malabsorption of fat and fat-soluble vitamins (A, D, E, and K). Recurrent abdominal pain and nausea (gallstones) and epigastric pain radiating to the back with weight loss and gallbladder distention (carcinoma of the pancreatic head) suggest the presence of specific causes of biliary obstruction. In complete biliary obstruction, conjugated hyperbilirubinemia is prominent and usually peaks around 30 mg/dL in the absence of renal failure. Eosinophilia may accompany drug-induced jaundice. Inquiry about the use of drugs known to cause cholestasis, serologic testing for antimitochondrial antibody for primary biliary cirrhosis, and endoscopic retrograde cholangiopancreatography or magnetic resonance cholangiopancreatography to evaluate primary sclerosing cholangitis may be helpful.

In jaundice produced by hepatocellular disease resulting from a variety of causes (see Chapters 42 and 44), serum transaminases are characteristically elevated more than 10-fold, and alkaline phosphatase levels are less than three times normal. Evidence of hepatocellular damage and disease is also frequently present and includes a prolonged prothrombin time, hypoalbuminemia, and clinical features of hepatic dysfunction (i.e., palmar erythema, spider angiomata, gynecomastia, ascites). An inquiry about the use of drugs known to cause hepatocellular injury, alcohol, risk factors for viral hepatitis, and pre-existing liver disease, along with serologic testing for hepatitis (see Chapter 42), may be useful.

A diagnostic approach to jaundice is outlined in Figure 41–2. If extrahepatic obstruction is suspected, noninvasive studies such as ultrasound or computed tomography should be used to determine whether bile ducts are dilated. If dilated ducts are found on noninvasive imaging, then direct cholan-

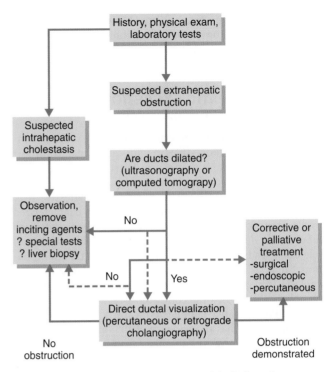

Figure 41–2 Approach to the patient with cholestatic jaundice. The algorithm demonstrates the systematic consideration of the available diagnostic options.

giography (either endoscopic or radiologic) will provide the most reliable approach to management and potential treatment of cholestatic jaundice. If intrahepatic cholestasis is suggested clinically and extrahepatic obstruction is excluded by noninvasive means and/or by direct cholangiography, then liver biopsy will sometimes be useful in determining the cause of cholestasis.

Prospectus for the Future

Important issue regarding both the diagnosis of and therapy for jaundice remain. A fundamental diagnostic issue is distinguishing obstructive jaundice form intrahepatic disease. Over the last 5 to 10 years, both magnetic resonance cholangiopancreatography and endoscopic ultrasound technology have greatly improved. Increasing experience with these modalities and continuing technical advances are likely to reduce dramatically or eliminate endoscopic retrograde cholangiopancreatography as a common diagnostic modality. Furthermore, the use of endoscopic ultrasound–based techniques to enhance

capabilities in therapeutic endoscopic retrograde cholangiopancreatography is likely to expand.

Another rapidly advancing area involves understanding the molecular mechanisms and regulation of bile secretion both under normal conditions and in the setting of specific causes of jaundice. These insights, as well as new information regarding the genetic predisposition to drug-induced cholestasis, will likely lead to novel therapeutic options to diminish the adverse effects of jaundice, as well as provide a means to decrease the incidence of drug-induced cholestatic liver disease.

References

Akobeng A: Neonatal jaundice. Clin Evid 12:501–507, 2004.

Berk PD: Approach to the patient with jaundice or abnormal liver tests. In Goldman L, Ausiello D (eds): Cecil Textbook of Medicine, 22nd ed. Philadelphia: WB Saunders, 2004, pp 897–905.

Bloomer JR, Risheg H: Bilirubin and porphyrin metabolism. In Maddrey WC, Feldman M (eds): Atlas of the Liver, 3rd ed. Philadelphia: Current Medicine 1–17, 2003.

Trauner M, Wagner M, Fickert P, Zollner G: Molecular regulation of hepatobiliary transport systems: Clinical implications for understanding and treating cholestasis. J Clin Gastroenterol 39(4 Suppl 2):S111–S124, 2005.

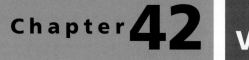

Acute and Chronic Hepatitis

Aasim M. Sheikh

Michael B. Fallon

The term *hepatitis* denotes inflammation of the liver. It is applied to a broad category of clinicopathologic conditions that result from the damage produced by viral, toxic, metabolic, pharmacologic, or immune-mediated attack on the liver. The common pathologic features of hepatitis are hepatocellular necrosis, which may be focal or extensive, and inflammatory cell infiltration of the liver, which may predominate in the portal areas or may extend into the parenchyma.

Acute hepatitis implies a condition lasting less than 6 months, culminating either in complete resolution of the liver damage with return to normal liver function and structure or a rapid progression of the acute injury toward extensive necrosis and a fatal outcome. Physical examination is usually unremarkable but may show enlarged, tender liver and icteric mucous membranes. Laboratory evidence of hepatocellular damage in the form of elevated aminotransferase (aspartate aminotransferase [AST] and alanine aminotransferase [ALT]) levels are the hallmark and may show elevations 20- to 100-fold normal values. Independent of the cause of hepatitis and the level of biochemical abnormality, the clinical course may range from subclinical to severe hepatocellular dysfunction, with evidence of impairment of coagulation, marked jaundice, and disturbance of neurologic function (see Chapter 43).

Chronic hepatitis is defined as a sustained inflammatory process in the liver reflected by liver function test abnormalities lasting longer than 6 months and is often difficult to differentiate from acute hepatitis on clinical or histologic criteria alone. Patients are typically asymptomatic and generally have lower aminotransferase abnormalities as compared with those with acute hepatitis. Histologically, a diagnosis of chronic hepatitis requires the presence of inflammatory cells in the biopsy but also typically has evidence of significant fibrous deposition, disruption of hepatic lobular architecture, and possibly progression toward cirrhosis.

Acute Hepatitis

The causes of acute hepatitis include viral hepatitis (hepatitis A through E), drugs (prescription, nonprescription, and illicit), alcohol, toxins, autoimmune hepatitis, and Wilson's disease. The mechanisms whereby these agents produce hepatic damage include direct toxin-induced necrosis (e.g., acetaminophen, *Amanita phalloides* toxin) and host immune-mediated damage (e.g., viral hepatitis). Massive hepatic necrosis is the dominant process in cases of *Amanita* poisoning, and the clinical course is more aptly described as fulminant hepatic failure (see Chapter 43) than as acute hepatitis. Such a course is less common but well recognized with all other the causative agents. **Web Figure 42–1** is an algorithm detailing diagnostic approach to acute hepatitis.

Acute Viral Hepatitis
ETIOLOGY

Five hepatotropic viruses cause acute viral hepatitis (Table 42–1). Hepatitis viruses A (HAV), B (HBV), C (HCV), D (HDV), and E (HEV) have all been characterized at the molecular level. All are RNA viruses except HBV, which is an enveloped DNA virus. HAV is the most common cause of acute viral hepatitis in the United States, followed by HBV. HBV has been extensively characterized. The complete HBV virion (Dane particle) consists of several components that elicit distinct antibody responses from the host (Fig. 42–1). Clinically relevant is the surface envelope (hepatitis B surface antigen [HBsAg]), a core of partially double-stranded circular DNA (HBV DNA) to which is attached a DNA polymerase, and a nucleocapsid (hepatitis B core antigen [HBcAg] and hepatitis B early antigen [HBeAg]) that encloses the DNA and the polymerase. HCV is the most prevalent hepatitis virus worldwide but is an infrequent cause of symptomatic acute hepatitis. It accounts for most

Table 42–1   **Characteristics of Common Causative Agents of Acute Viral Hepatitis**

	Hepatitis A	Hepatitis B	Hepatitis C	Hepatitis D	Hepatitis E
Causative agent	28-nm RNA virus	42-nm DNA virus; core and surface components	30-nm enveloped/ RNA virus	36-nm hybrid particle with HBsAg coat	30–32-nm nonenveloped RNA virus
Transmission	Fecal-oral; water-borne or food-borne	Parenteral inoculation or equivalent; direct contact	Similar to HBV but poor sexual or vertical transmission	Similar to HBV	Similar to HAV
Incubation period Period of infectivity	2–6 wk 2–3 wk in late incubation and early clinical phase	4 wk–6 mo During HBsAg positivity (occasionally only with anti-HBc positivity)	5–10 wk During HCV RNA positivity	Similar to HBV During HDV RNA or anti-HDV positivity	2–9 wk Similar to HAV
Massive hepatic necrosis	Rare	Uncommon	Rare	Yes	Yes
Carrier state	No	Yes	No	Yes	No
Chronic hepatitis	No	Yes	Yes	Yes	No
Prophylaxis	Hygiene, immune serum globulin, vaccine	Hygiene, hepatitis B immune globulin, vaccine	Hygiene	Hygiene, HBV vaccine	Hygiene, sanitation

HAV = hepatitis A virus; HBc = hepatitis B core; HBsAg = hepatitis B surface antigen; HBV = hepatitis B virus; HCV = hepatitis C virus; HDV = hepatitis D virus.

cases of acute hepatitis previously designated non-A, non-B. Cytomegalovirus and Epstein-Barr virus only occasionally cause acute hepatitis. HDV is an incomplete RNA virus that requires HBsAg for transmission from cell to cell; thus it causes hepatitis only in patients with hepatitis B, both acute (HDV co-infection) and chronic (HDV superinfection). Seven to 10% of presumed acute viral hepatitis has as yet unidentified cause or causes.

TRANSMISSION

The modes of transmission of the hepatitis viruses are noted in Table 42–1.

HAV and HEV are both excreted in the feces before onset of symptoms and are transmitted by the fecal-oral route (Fig. 42–2). They are thus implicated in most instances of waterborne and food-transmitted infection and in epidemics of viral hepatitis. HEV is linked to outbreaks in East Asia, Central Africa, the Middle East, and Mexico. It has a high rate of attack in young adults in these endemic areas and can lead to fulminant hepatitis, particularly in pregnant women.

HBV and HCV are both transmitted parenterally. HBV is present in virtually all body fluids and excreta of carriers. Transmission occurs most commonly through blood and

blood products, contaminated needles, and sexual contact. High-risk transmission groups include the following: sexual partners of acutely and chronically infected persons, with male homosexuals being at particularly high risk, intravenous drug abusers, infants of infected mothers (*vertical transmission*), and health professionals. Patients with increased exposure to blood or blood products and/or with impaired immunity (e.g., patients undergoing dialysis, patients with leukemia, hemophilia, or trisomy 21 syndrome) are also highly susceptible to HBV.

HCV was the main cause of posttransfusion hepatitis prior to 1992. It is presently the most common cause of hepatitis in intravenous drug users, and it accounts for a substantial number of cases of sporadic, community-acquired hepatitis. The risk of vertical and sexual transmission of hepatitis C is much lower than that for hepatitis B.

CLINICAL AND LABORATORY MANIFESTATIONS

Acute viral hepatitis typically begins with a prodromal phase lasting several days and characterized by constitutional and gastrointestinal symptoms including malaise, fatigue, anorexia, nausea, vomiting, myalgia, and headache. A mild fever may be present. Symptoms suggestive of *flu* may be

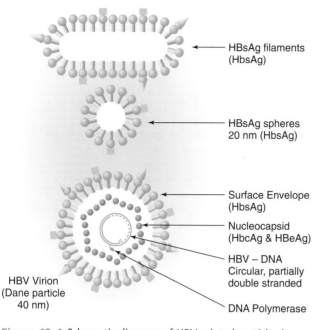

Figure 42–1 Schematic diagram of HBV-related particles in serum and the associated antigens *(in parentheses)*. The spheres and filaments consist of only hepatitis B surface glycoproteins (HBsAg). They are 20 nm in diameter and are 10,000-fold greater in concentration than the complete virion (Dane particle: 40 nm diameter).

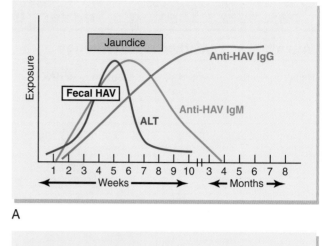

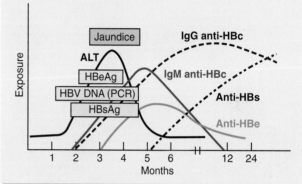

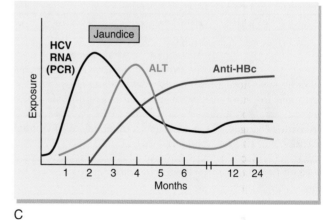

Figure 42–2 Sequence of clinical and laboratory findings in *(A)* a patient with acute HAV infection, *(B)* a patient with HBV infection, and (C) a patient with HCV infection. ALT = alanine transaminase; HBc = hepatitis B core; HBe = hepatitis B early; HBeAg = hepatitis B early antigen; HBs = hepatitis B surface; HBsAg = hepatitis B surface antigen; IgG = immunoglobulin G; PCR = polymerase chain reaction.

prominent. Arthritis and urticaria resembling serum sickness, attributed to immune complex deposition, may be present in 5% to 10% of cases of acute hepatitis B and C. Taste and smell alteration may occur. Jaundice soon appears with bilirubinuria and acholic (pale) stools often accompanied by an improvement in the patient's sense of well being. The liver is usually tender and enlarged; splenomegaly is found in approximately one fifth of patients. Notably, large proportions of all patients with acute viral hepatitis are asymptomatic or have symptoms without jaundice *(anicteric hepatitis)*. In such instances, medical attention is often not sought.

Aminotransferases (ALT and AST) are released from the acutely damaged hepatocytes, and serum levels rise often to greater than 20-fold normal and as high as 100-fold normal. An elevated serum bilirubin (>2.5 to 3.0 mg/dL) results in jaundice and defines *icteric hepatitis*. Values higher than 20 mg/dL are uncommon and approximately correlate with the severity of disease. Elevations in serum alkaline phosphatase are usually limited to three times normal levels, except in cases of cholestatic hepatitis. A complete blood cell count most commonly shows mild leukopenia with atypical lymphocytes. Anemia and thrombocytopenia may also be present. The icteric phase of acute viral hepatitis may last days to weeks, followed by gradual resolution of symptoms and laboratory values.

SERODIAGNOSIS

The ability to detect the presence of viral nucleic acids in hepatitis B, C, and D and antigen or antibodies to

components of hepatitis A through E has fostered progress in the epidemiology of viral hepatitis. These viral markers are used in the diagnosis of acute viral hepatitis (see Figure 42–2; Tables 42–2 and 42–3). An etiologic diagnosis is of great importance in planning preventive and public health measures pertinent to the close contacts of infected

Table 42–2 **Serologic Markers of Viral Hepatitis**

Agent	Marker	Definition	Significance
Hepatitis A virus (HAV)	Anti-HAV IgM type IgG type	Antibody to HAV — —	— Current or recent infection or convalescence Current or previous infection; conferring immunity
Hepatitis B virus (HBV)	HBsAg HBeAg HBV DNA Anti-HBe Anti-HBc (IgM or IgG) Anti-HBs	HBV surface antigen HBe antigen; a component of the HBV core Infectious viral genomic material Antibody to HBe antigen Antibody to HBV core antigen Antibody to HBV surface antigen	Positive in most cases of acute or chronic infection Transiently positive in acute hepatitis B May persist in chronic infection Reflection of presence of viral replication, whole Dane particles in serum, and high infectivity Serum level reflects degree of viral replication; predicts response to therapy Transiently positive in convalescence Persistently present in some chronic cases Usually a reflection of low infectivity Positive in all acute and chronic cases Reliable marker of infection, past or current IgM anti-HBc a reflection of active viral replication and acute infection Not protective Positive in late convalescence in most acute cases Confers immunity
Hepatitis C virus (HCV)	Anti-HCV HCV RNA	Antibodies to a group of recombinant HCV peptides Infectious viral genomic material	Positive on average 12 wk after exposure; not protective Persistent in acute, chronic, or past infection Reflects ongoing infection, level inversely linked to treatment response
Hepatitis D virus (HDV)	Anti-HDV (IgM or IgG) HDV antigen HDV RNA	Antibody to HDV antigen Viral peptide Infectious viral genomic material	Acute or chronic infection seen with + HBsAg; not protective IgM and IgG clear in resolving infection IgG persists in chronic infection Persists in chronic infection Most reliable test for acute or chronic infection
Hepatitis E virus (HEV)	Anti-HEV (IgM or IgG)	Antibody to HEV antigen	Acute or chronic infection IgM may persist up to 6 months

IgG = immunoglobulin G; IgM = immunoglobulin M.

patients and in evaluating prognosis. Epstein-Barr virus and cytomegalovirus hepatitis may also be diagnosed by the appearance of specific antibodies of the immunoglobulin (Ig) M class. In acute hepatitis B, HBsAg and HBeAg are present in serum. Both are usually cleared within 3 months, but HBsAg may persist in some patients with uncomplicated cases for 6 months to 1 year. Clearance of HBsAg is followed after a variable *window* period by emergence of anti-HBs, which confers long-term immunity. Anti-HBc and anti-HBe appear in the acute phase of the illness, but neither provides immunity. Uncommonly, during the serologic window period, anti-HBc IgM, a marker of active viral replication suggesting recent infection may be the only evidence of HBV infection. HDV infection superimposed on HBV infection is most reliably detected by polymerase chain reaction (PCR) test for HDV RNA. Other possible tests include HDV antigen and anti-HDV (IgM and IgG antibodies). Acute hepatitis C can be detected using a sensitive PCR assay for HCV RNA within 2 weeks of exposure. Serum antibodies to HCV develop within 12 weeks of exposure or within 4 to 5 weeks after biochemical abnormalities are discovered. At onset of symptoms, 30% of patients will be missed if checked by serum enzyme immunoassay (EIA) for HCV antibody alone. Commercial EIAs for hepatitis E to detect both IgM and IgG class antibodies are also available but may lack general sensitivity and specificity. The HEV IgM antibody is present for up to 6 months after exposure.

Table 42–3　Interpretation of Serologic Markers and Serum DNA in Hepatitis B

	HBsAg	HBeAg	Anti-HBc IgM	Anti HBc IgG	Anti-HBs	Anti-HBe	HBV DNA§
Acute hepatitis	+	+/−	+				+
Acute hepatitis— window period			+				
Recovery from acute hepatitis			+	+	+	+/−	
Chronic hepatitis	+	+					+
Chronic hepatitis (precore mutant)	+					+	+
Inactive Carrier	+					+/−	
Vaccinated					+		

HBsAg = hepatitis B surface antigen; HBeAg = hepatitis Be antigen; anti-HBc-IgM = hepatitis B core antibody (IgM type); anti-HBc-IgG = hepatitis B core antibody (IgG type); anti-HBs = hepatitis B surface antibody; anti-HBe = hepatitis Be antibody; HBV DNA = hepatitis B viral DNA; § = HBV DNA >10^5 copies/mL.

COMPLICATIONS

Cholestatic Hepatitis

In some patients, most commonly during HAV infection, a self-limited period of cholestatic jaundice may supervene that is characterized by marked conjugated hyperbilirubinemia, elevation of alkaline phosphatase, and pruritus. Investigation may be required to differentiate this condition from mechanical obstruction of the biliary tree (see Chapter 44).

Fulminant Hepatitis

Massive hepatic necrosis occurs in less than 1% of patients with acute viral hepatitis and leads to a devastating and often fatal condition called *fulminant hepatic failure*. This condition is discussed in detail in Chapter 43.

Chronic Hepatitis

Hepatitis A does not progress to chronic liver disease, although occasionally it has a relapsing course. Persistence of aminotransferase elevation and viral antigens or nucleic acids beyond 6 months in patients with hepatitis B and C suggests evolution to chronic hepatitis, although slowly resolving acute hepatitis may occasionally lead to such test abnormalities for up to 12 months, with eventual complete resolution. Chronic hepatitis is considered in detail later in this chapter.

Rare Complications

Acute viral hepatitis may be followed by *aplastic anemia*, which affects mostly male patients and results in a mortality of greater than 80%. Pancreatitis, myocarditis, pericarditis, pleural effusion, and neurologic complications, including Guillain-Barré syndrome, aseptic meningitis, and encephalitis, have also been reported. Cryoglobulinemia and glomerulonephritis are associated with hepatitis B and C, and polyarteritis nodosa with hepatitis B.

MANAGEMENT

All cases of acute hepatitis A, B, and E, unless complicated by fulminant hepatitis, are self-limited (see Table 42–2). The treatment thus is largely supportive and includes rest, maintenance of hydration, and adequate dietary intake. Most patients show a preference for a low-fat, high-carbohydrate diet. Alcohol should be avoided. Vitamin supplementation is of no proven value, although vitamin K may be indicated if prolonged cholestasis occurs. Nausea can be treated with small doses of metoclopramide and hydroxyzine. Hospitalization is indicated for patients with severe nausea and vomiting or those with evidence of deteriorating liver function, such as hepatic encephalopathy or prolongation of the prothrombin time. In general, hepatitis A and E may be regarded as noninfectious after 3 weeks, whereas hepatitis B is potentially infectious to sexual contacts throughout its course, although the risk is low once HBsAg has cleared.

PREVENTION

Both feces and blood from patients with hepatitis A and E contain virus during the prodromal and early icteric phases of the disease (see Fig. 42–2). Raw shellfish concentrate the HAV from sewage pollution and may serve as vector of the disease. General hygienic measures should include hand washing by contacts and careful handling, disposal, and sterilization of excreta and contaminated clothing and utensils. Close contacts of patients with hepatitis A should receive anti-HAV serum immunoglobulin as soon as possible after exposure. HAV vaccination is appropriate for children and travelers to endemic areas, individuals with immunodeficiency or chronic liver disease, and those with high-risk behaviors or occupations. Vaccine for HEV is in development.

　Hepatitis B is rarely transmitted by body fluids other than blood. However, it is highly infectious, and strict adherence to universal precautions is mandatory. Efforts at preventing hepatitis B have involved the use of Ig enriched in anti-HBs (HBIG) and recombinant HBV vaccines. Postexposure prophylaxis with HBIG after blood or mucosal exposure (e.g., needlestick, eye splash, sexual contacts of patients with acute hepatitis B, neonates born to mothers with acute or chronic infection) should be given within 7 days along with HBV vaccine. Preventive vaccination is currently recommended for high-risk groups and individuals (health care professionals, patients undergoing dialysis, patients with advanced liver disease or hemophilia, residents and staff of custodial care institutions, sexually active homosexual men) and is advocated universally for children.

No accepted prevention strategies are available for HCV. Serum Ig is not useful for postexposure prophylaxis. The advent of widespread blood product screening for anti-HCV has made posttransfusion hepatitis a rarity.

Alcoholic Fatty Liver and Hepatitis

Alcohol abuse is a major cause of liver disease in the Western world. Three major pathologic lesions resulting from alcohol abuse are (1) fatty liver, (2) alcoholic hepatitis, and (3) cirrhosis. These lesions are not mutually distinct, and all may be present in the same patient. The first two lesions are potentially reversible and may sometimes be confused clinically with viral hepatitis or gallbladder or biliary tract disease. Alcoholic cirrhosis is discussed in Chapter 44.

MECHANISM OF INJURY

Mechanisms of liver injury caused by alcohol are complex. Ethanol and its metabolites, acetaldehyde and nicotinamide adenine dinucleotide phosphate (NADP), are directly hepatotoxic and cause a large number of metabolic derangements. Induction of cytochrome P-450 (CYP2E1) and cytokine pathways, particularly tumor-necrosis factor-α (TNF-α), are also critical in initiating and perpetuating hepatic injury and producing the lesions of alcoholic hepatitis.

Hepatotoxic effects from alcohol vary considerably among individuals. Nevertheless, consumption by men of 40 to 80 g of ethanol per day (one beer or one mixed drink = 10 g of ethanol) for 10 to 15 years carries a substantial risk of the development of alcoholic liver disease, whereas women appear to have a lower threshold of injury. Malnutrition and presence of other forms of chronic liver disease may potentiate the toxic effects of alcohol on the liver, and genetic factors may contribute to individual susceptibility.

CLINICAL AND PATHOLOGIC FEATURES

Alcoholic fatty liver may exhibit as incidentally discovered tender hepatomegaly. Some patients consult a physician because of pain in their right upper quadrant. Jaundice is rare. Aminotransferases are mildly elevated (less than five times normal). Liver biopsy shows diffuse or centrilobular fat occupying most of the hepatocyte.

Alcoholic hepatitis, a severe and prognostically ominous lesion, is characterized by the following histologic triad: (1) Mallory bodies (intracellular eosinophilic aggregates of cytokeratins), usually seen near or around the cell nuclei of

hepatocytes; (2) infiltration by polymorphonuclear leukocytes; and (3) a network of interlobular connective tissue surrounding hepatocytes and central veins *(pericellular, perivenular, and perisinusoidal fibrosis)*. Patients with this histologic lesion may be asymptomatic or extremely ill with hepatic failure. Anorexia, nausea, vomiting, weight loss, and abdominal pain are common symptoms. Hepatomegaly is present in 80% of patients with alcoholic hepatitis, and splenomegaly is often present. Fever is common, but bacterial infection should always be excluded, because patients with alcoholic liver disease are prone to develop pneumonia, as well as infection of the urinary tract and the peritoneal cavity, when ascites is present. Jaundice is commonly present and may be pronounced, with cholestatic features that require differentiation from biliary tract disease (see Chapter 41). Cutaneous signs of chronic liver disease may be found, including spider angiomas, palmar erythema, and gynecomastia. Parotid enlargement, testicular atrophy, and loss of body hair may be prominent (see Chapter 44). Ascites and encephalopathy may be present and indicate severe disease. The white blood cell count may be strikingly elevated, whereas aminotransferase levels are only modestly increased (range 200 to 400 U/L), which is an important differentiating feature from other forms of acute hepatitis in which aminotransferases are significantly increased (invariably in the thousands). The ratio of AST to ALT nearly always exceeds 2:1, in contrast to viral hepatitis, in which the aminotransferase levels are usually increased in parallel. Prolonged prothrombin time, hypoalbuminemia, and hyperglobulinemia may be found.

DIAGNOSIS

A history of excessive prolonged alcohol intake is often difficult to obtain from patients with alcoholic liver disease. However, historical, clinical, and biochemical features of alcoholic hepatitis are often sufficient to establish the diagnosis. Many patients suspected or found to imbibe alcohol excessively may have causes other than alcohol for their liver disease (e.g., chronic viral hepatitis). Thus, when other causes of liver disease are suggested and the patient's alcohol intake is uncertain, appropriate serologic testing and a liver biopsy may be needed to establish a diagnosis.

COMPLICATIONS AND PROGNOSIS

Alcoholic fatty liver completely resolves with cessation of alcohol intake. Alcoholic hepatitis can also resolve, but more commonly it progresses either to cirrhosis, which may already be present at the time of initial presentation, or to hepatic failure and death. The development of encephalopathy, ascites, deteriorating renal function *(hepatorenal syndrome)*, and gastrointestinal bleeding from varices often complicates alcoholic hepatitis (see Chapter 44). Patients with hepatic discriminant factor (DF) equaling 32 {DF = 4.6 × (prothrombin time [in seconds] − control [in seconds]) + total bilirubin (mg/dL)} have high risk of mortality.

TREATMENT

The cornerstone of treatment of acute alcoholic hepatitis is meticulous supportive care. A high-calorie diet with vitamin (particularly thiamine) supplementation is instituted and may require administration by nasogastric tube in patients with severe anorexia nervosa. Protein should be included, but it may need to be restricted in patients with encephalopathy (see Chapter 44). In the absence of infection, gastrointestinal bleeding, or renal failure, specific patients with alcoholic hepatitis with DF of 32 and hepatic encephalopathy may benefit from corticosteroids. Pentoxifylline (an oral TNF-α antagonist) has in a single randomized trial shown benefit in severe alcoholic hepatitis by diminishing the risk of renal failure.

Drug-Induced and Toxin-Induced Hepatitis

A broad spectrum of hepatic disease may result from a variety of therapeutic drugs or toxins (Table 42–4). The pathophysiologic mechanisms whereby these hepatic lesions are produced are complex. At one end of the spectrum is a predictable, dose-dependent, direct toxic effect on hepatocytes that leads to frank centrilobular hepatocellular necrosis, typical of acetaminophen and carbon tetrachloride toxicity. Other reactions are generally not predictable and usually occur for unknown reasons in susceptible persons (*idiosyncratic drug reaction*). In some instances, genetically determined differences in pathways of hepatic drug metabolism may result in metabolites with greater toxic potential. Classic examples include viral hepatitis-like reactions (halothane and isoniazid), cholestatic hepatitis (chlorpromazine), granulomatous hepatitis (allopurinol), chronic hepatitis (methyldopa), and pure cholestasis without inflammation or hepatocellular necrosis (estrogens and androgens). Immune-mediated hepatic damage may contribute in some cases, possibly when the drugs or their metabolites act as a hapten on the surface of hepatocytes. A few important classes of drugs that cause hepatitis are discussed here.

ANALGESICS

Acetaminophen is metabolized by the hepatic cytochrome P-450 system to a potentially toxic metabolite that is subsequently rendered harmless through conjugation with glutathione. When massive doses are taken (>10 to 15 g), the formation of excess toxic metabolites depletes the available glutathione and produces necrosis. Acetaminophen overdose, commonly taken in a suicide attempt, leads to nausea and vomiting within a few hours. These symptoms subside and are followed in 24 to 48 hours by clinical and laboratory evidence of hepatocellular necrosis (raised aminotransferase levels) and hepatic dysfunction (prolonged prothrombin time and hepatic encephalopathy). Similar findings may occur with therapeutic doses of acetaminophen in patients with chronic alcoholism or malnutrition. Extensive liver necrosis may lead to fulminant hepatic failure and death. In a patient with nonstaggered overdose, a serum acetaminophen level should be drawn 4 to 24 hours after ingestion. If plotted on a treatment nomogram of plasma drug concentration against time, it can predict the severity of outcome and need for therapy. Treatment with *N*-acetylcysteine given orally (140-mg/kg bolus followed by 70 mg/kg × 17

Table 42–4	Classification of Drug-Induced Liver Disease
Category	**Examples**
Predictable hepatotoxins with zonal necrosis	Acetaminophen Carbon tetrachloride
Nonspecific hepatitis	Aspirin Oxacillin Herbs (chaparral, germander)
Viral hepatitis-like reactions	Halothane Isoniazid Phenytoin
Cholestasis	Estrogens Erythromycin Amoxicillin/clavulanic acid
Noninflammatory	17α-Substituted steroids
Inflammatory	Chlorpromazine Antithyroid agents
Fatty liver: large droplet	Ethanol Corticosteroids
Fatty liver: small droplet	Amiodarone Allopurinol
Chronic hepatitis	Methyldopa Nitrofurantoin
Tumors	Estrogens Vinyl chloride
Vascular lesions	6-Thioguanine Anabolic steroids Herbs (senna, comfrey)
Fibrosis	Methotrexate
Granulomas	Allopurinol Sulfonamides

doses), thought to promote hepatic glutathione synthesis, may be life saving.

Nonsteroidal anti-inflammatory drugs (NSAIDs) as a class are a leading cause of drug-induced liver disease. *Salicylates* cause dose-dependent hepatocellular injury that is usually clinically mild and easily reversible. *Diclofenac*, one of the most commonly prescribed NSAIDs worldwide, has been linked to asymptomatic elevation of aminotransferases, acute hepatitis, and to fulminant hepatic failure. *Sulindac* is considered as the most likely NSAID to produce hepatic injury and causes a damage spectrum ranging from hepatocellular to mixed to pure cholestatic injury. Whether the newer cyclo-oxygenase-2–selective NSAIDs have a lower risk of hepatotoxicity is uncertain.

ANTIBIOTICS AND ANTIVIRALS

Isoniazid, as a single-drug prophylaxis against tuberculosis, commonly produces raised serum aminotransferase levels in 20% of patients. This effect appears to be transient and self-limiting in most patients. However, a 1% incidence exists of clinical hepatitis, which progresses to fatal hepatic necrosis in 10% of affected patients. Individual and age-related differences in hepatic acetylation of potentially toxic isoniazid metabolites may be important in this injury. Thus the incidence of severe hepatic damage increases with age such that significant elevation of aminotransferase levels in persons who are older than 35 years of age is an indication for discontinuing the drug.

OTHER ANTIBIOTICS AND ANTIVIRAL AGENTS

Amoxicillin-clavulanic acid suspension is a leading cause of antibiotic-related cholestatic jaundice. Men appear to be more susceptible than women. Erythromycin is an established agent causing cholestatic injury. Trimethoprim-sulfamethoxazole characteristically causes cholestatic or mixed injury. A large number of agents used to treat human immunodeficiency virus infection have been linked with hepatic injury of various forms. Important among these agents are nevirapine, ritonavir, and indinavir.

ANESTHETICS AND ANTICONVULSANTS

Halothane

Historically, the anesthetic agent halothane caused an uncommon acute viral hepatitis-like reaction several days after exposure in susceptible persons. Hepatic injury was caused in part by an allergic response to hepatic neo-antigens produced by halothane metabolism, and the severity of this reaction increased with repeated exposure. Newer, commonly used halogenated anesthetic agents (e.g., isoflurane, enflurane) are hepatotoxic in a much smaller number of patients, though cross-sensitivity does exist.

Anticonvulsants

Phenytoin and carbamazepine have been implicated in an *anti-epileptic hypersensitivity* syndrome, characterized by a triad of rash, fever, and hepatocellular injury that may lead to fulminant hepatic failure. Lymphadenopathy and a mononucleosis-like picture with atypical lymphocytes may be present. Renal and pulmonary involvement may also occur.

HERBS

Herbal supplements are taken throughout the world, and approximately $5 billion per year are spent in the United States alone on herbal agents. Incorrectly considered to be safe because they are *natural,* many herbs are hepatotoxic.

Senecio, Heliotropium, Crotalaria, and comfrey contain pyrrolizidine alkaloids that cause hepatic veno-occlusive disease. Hepatotoxicity ranging from mild hepatitis to massive necrosis and fulminant hepatic failure has been associated with the use of chaparral, germander, pennyroyal oil, mistletoe, valerian root, comfrey, and Ma huang. Milk thistle, often taken by patients with chronic hepatitis and cirrhosis, has not been associated with hepatotoxicity, but its benefit is undefined because of a lack of controlled studies.

Chronic Hepatitis

Chronic hepatitis is defined as a hepatic inflammatory process that fails to resolve after 6 months and in those with acute viral hepatitis persistence of serum viral antigens and nucleic acids beyond a similar period.

ETIOLOGY

Acute viral hepatitis can ultimately lead to chronic hepatitis, with the notable exceptions of HAV and HEV. Nonalcoholic steatohepatitis (NASH) is now considered the most frequent cause of chronic hepatitis in the United States and Western Europe. Several drugs may produce chronic hepatitis, the best recognized being methyldopa. In contrast to acute hepatitis, an etiologic agent is sometimes difficult to identify in cases of chronic hepatitis. The pathogenesis of these idiopathic forms may represent quiescent autoimmune disease, undetected past drug-induced injury or NASH, antibody-negative viral infections, or misdiagnosed cholestatic liver injury (e.g., primary biliary cirrhosis, primary sclerosing cholangitis).

CLASSIFICATION

Current classification of chronic hepatitis is based on the *etiologic agent* responsible for disease, the *grade* of injury (determined by the numbers and location of inflammatory cells), and the *stage* of disease on liver biopsy (determined by the degree, location, and distortion of normal architecture by fibrosis). This classification allows integration of knowledge of the natural history of specific causes with histologic features of hepatic damage to assess the severity and prognosis of the process. Thus, in general, biochemical and serologic studies along with liver biopsy are used in the diagnosis and management of chronic hepatitis.

Chronic Viral Hepatitis

Chronic hepatitis B follows acute hepatitis B in 5% to 10% of adults in the United States. HBV infection without evidence of any liver damage may persist, resulting in asymptomatic or *healthy* hepatitis B carriers. In Asia and Africa, many such carriers appear to have acquired the virus from infected mothers during infancy (vertical transmission). Patients who are HBsAg and Anti-HBe positive and have high serum HBV DNA (>5 million copies/mL) coupled with increased serum aminotransferases are in a high replicative phase (see Table 42–3). In contrast, patients in a low replicative phase are HBsAg and anti-HBe positive, have low serum

HBV DNA (<5 million copies/mL), and near normal or normal aminotransferases. Such patients can go into high replicative phase and exhibit acute on chronic hepatitis B. A subgroup of patients with chronic hepatitis B may be HBeAg negative but still be in a high replicative phase, as evidenced by high HBV DNA levels in serum. These patients have a (precore or core) mutant form of hepatitis B. Patients infected with HBV in high replicative phase are at highest risk of developing cirrhosis and hepatocellular carcinoma. Such patients and those who have already progressed to early cirrhosis are the primary targets of anti-HBV therapy. Current drugs approved as single agents for treating hepatitis B include injectable interferon-α (pegylated and non-pegylated) and oral nucleoside or nucleotide analogues (e.g., lamivudine, adefovir, entecavir). All of these drugs lead to suppression of serum viral DNA to a variable amount, as well as seroconversion from HBeAg to anti-HBe in 10% to 30% of patients. Resistance to the oral agents with prolonged use is a major concern and is highest for lamivudine among the current agents. Interferon, on the other hand, has numerous side effects and may not be well tolerated.

Chronic hepatitis C develops in up to 75% of individuals acutely exposed to HCV and is estimated to affect 1.8% of the US population. Over 20% of these patients may develop cirrhosis in approximately 30 years. Hepatitis C has six major genotypes of which, in the United States, genotype 1 is the most common, followed by genotypes 2 and 3. Genotype has no impact on course of illness but is the most important determinant of successful outcome of treatment. Chronic hepatitis C is currently treated with a combination of pegylated interferon injections and oral ribavirin. Durable suppression of viral activity occurs in as many as 80% of all patients infected with genotype 2 or 3 when treated for 6 months and in 50% of those infected with genotype 1 when treated for 11 months. Both interferon and ribavirin, however, have numerous side effects, which contraindicates their use in 50% or more of patients currently infected with HCV. Out of the remaining 50%, therapy is usually advised for patients with favorable genotypes or those who demonstrate moderate to high fibrosis on liver biopsies. Successful treatment of chronic hepatitis B and C may lead to a decrease in hepatic inflammation and fibrosis and to a reduced risk of progression to cirrhosis and the development of hepatocellular carcinoma.

Autoimmune Hepatitis

Autoimmune liver disease has several forms; however, the typical disease occurs in young women and is characterized by significant hepatic inflammation with a preponderance of plasma cells and fibrosis. The presence of hypergammaglobulinemia, as well as antinuclear or anti-smooth muscle antibodies, represents the classic or type 1 variant. Type 2 autoimmune hepatitis is characterized by anti–liver-kidney microsomal antibodies and also occurs commonly in girls and young women. Type 3 is now considered clinically indistinguishable from type 1 and is identified by the presence of autoantibodies to soluble liver antigen or liver-pancreas antigen. Extrahepatic manifestations that include amenorrhea, rashes, acne, vasculitis, thyroiditis, and Sjögren's syndrome are common. Evidence of hepatic failure and the presence of chronic disease on biopsy at the time of diagnosis are frequent. Treatment with corticosteroids, often in combination with azathioprine for steroid sparing, is efficacious in a majority of patients and, in many instances, prolongs survival.

Nonalcoholic Fatty Liver Disease

Nonalcoholic fatty liver disease (NAFLD), a term that encompasses steatosis (fatty liver), NASH, and cirrhosis secondary to NASH, has become increasingly recognized as the most common reason for abnormal liver function tests among adults in the United States and Western Europe. Though NAFLD most commonly occurs in persons who are overweight, have diabetes, and have hyperlipidemia, it can also occur in persons of normal weight. Estimates indicate that approximately 30 million Americans have NAFLD, and of these, 8.6 million have NASH, with nearly 20% having signs of advanced disease (i.e., bridging fibrosis, cirrhosis) on histologic examination. Histologic criteria for NASH include macrovesicular fatty infiltration (mainly triglyceride); inflammation, including polymorphonuclear leukocytes; and hepatocyte injury (ballooning degeneration or necrotic hepatocytes), with or without fibrosis. The pathogenesis is still under investigation, but insulin resistance plays an essential role leading to lipolysis and hyperinsulinemia, upregulation of cytochrome P-450 pathways, and impaired mitochondrial and peroxisomal fatty acid oxidation. This state leads to excessive oxidative stress, cytokine induction, and inflammation. Clinical trials are investigating the efficacy of weight reduction, exercise, vitamin E (as an antioxidant); lipid-lowering agents, particularly gemfibrozil; and drugs that improve insulin resistance (e.g., metformin).

Genetic and Metabolic Hepatitis

Wilson's disease and α₁-antitrypsin deficiency generally occur before the age of 35 years, and a family history of liver disease may be present. Wilson's disease occurs caused by mutation in the *WD* gene and is autosomal recessive. A resultant accumulation of copper in various tissues occurs, including liver, brain, and the corneas, with neuropsychiatric signs and symptoms and liver disease ranging from steatosis to chronic hepatitis to fulminant liver failure. Diagnostic evaluation for Wilson's disease includes low serum ceruloplasmin and high urinary and hepatic copper levels. Therapy is indefinite and includes copper chelation with d-penicillamine or trientine and diminishing copper absorption with zinc supplementation. A low serum α₁-antitrypsin level and diastase-positive staining of hepatocellular inclusions on liver biopsy suggest α₁-antitrypsin deficiency. A homozygous phenotype (protease inhibitor phenotype Z [PiZZ]) supports the diagnosis, and no specific medical therapy exists apart from liver transplantation.

Prospectus for the Future

A better understanding of the molecular genetics and replication cycles of hepatitis B and C, as well as the role of cell-mediated and humoral immunity (or lack there of) in various forms of chronic viral and nonviral hepatitis, has lead to an expansion of therapeutic options for patients with these diseases. Therapeutic vaccines designed to boost humoral immunity against specific HCV and HBV epitopes are currently in clinical trials. Numerous antiviral agents that target specific enzymes involved in hepatitis C replication are in various stages of development, including ongoing clinical trials. At least five new drugs targeting hepatitis B replication are on the horizon.

The next step is to assess, in combination, the numerous anti-HBV drugs, both old and new, to enhance their efficacy while diminishing the risk of viral resistance. Increasing experience with the use of newer immunosuppressive agents with novel mechanisms of action used in solid organ transplantation opens avenues of studying these agents in patients with autoimmune hepatitis. Finally, recognition of the central role of TNF-α in the pathogenesis of alcoholic hepatitis has led to investigation of a significant number of TNF-α antagonists, currently in use for rheumatologic and autoimmune diseases, in this disorder.

References

Angulo P: Nonalcoholic fatty liver disease. N Engl J Med 346:1221, 2002.

Czaja AJ, Freese DK: Diagnosis and treatment of autoimmune hepatitis. Hepatology 36:479, 2002.

Lee WM: Medical progress: Drug-induced hepatotoxicity. N Engl J Med 349:474, 2003.

Levitsky J, Mailliard ME: Diagnosis and therapy of alcoholic liver disease. Semin Liver Dis 24:233, 2004.

Lindsay KL, Hoofnagle JH: Acute viral hepatitis. In Goldman L, Ausiello D (eds): Cecil Textbook of Medicine. Philadelphia, WB Saunders, 2004, pp 911–917.

Fulminant Hepatic Failure

Brendan M. McGuire

Michael B. Fallon

Fulminant hepatic failure (FHF) is defined as the onset of encephalopathy occurring within 8 weeks of the onset of jaundice in a patient with hepatic injury and no prior history of liver disease. *Late-onset hepatic failure* is recognized as the development of encephalopathy in patients between 8 and 24 weeks after the onset of jaundice. The pathogenesis of FHF involves severe widespread hepatic necrosis, commonly resulting from acute viral infection with hepatitis A, B, C, D, or E viruses (see Chapter 42). It may also result from exposure to hepatotoxins such as acetaminophen, isoniazid, halothane, valproic acid, or mushroom toxins (e.g., those of *Amanita phalloides*). Reye's syndrome (a disease predominantly of children) and acute fatty liver of pregnancy, both of which are characterized by microvesicular fatty infiltration and little hepatocellular necrosis, often resemble FHF. Other rare causes of FHF include Wilson's disease, hepatic ischemia, autoimmune hepatitis, and malignancy. In a significant number of patients with FHF, no cause is found, although a viral infection is usually presumed to be responsible (**Web Figs. 43–1 and 43–2**).

Diagnosis

The diagnosis of FHF is based on the combination of hepatic encephalopathy and liver failure. It is characterized biochemically by significantly elevated serum bilirubin and transaminase levels and marked prolongation of the prothrombin time.

Treatment

Treatment of FHF remains supportive because the underlying cause of liver failure is rarely treatable. However, most processes that result in widespread liver cell necrosis and FHF are transient events, and liver cell regeneration with recovery of liver function often occurs if patients do not die from the complications of liver failure in the interim. Meticulous supportive treatment in an intensive care unit setting has been shown to improve survival. Patients with FHF should be treated in centers with experience with this disease and with a liver transplantation program. Numerous complications result from FHF, and thorough identification and treatment of each are essential (Table 43–1).

Hepatic encephalopathy is often the first and most dramatic sign of liver failure. The pathogenesis of hepatic encephalopathy remains unclear. Hepatic encephalopathy that accompanies FHF differs from that associated with chronic liver disease in two important aspects: (1) it often responds to therapy only when liver function improves, and (2) it is frequently associated with two other potentially treatable causes of coma—hypoglycemia and cerebral edema. Therapy for hepatic encephalopathy in FHF differs slightly from the principles outlined in Chapter 44. Lactulose may be given orally, per nasogastric tube, or rectally, but the oral route should not be used if the patient is at risk for aspiration. Lactulose should be discontinued if no improvement is noted after several doses are administered. Intubation is often necessary to protect the airway from aspiration and to allow ventilation in patients with advanced encephalopathy.

Cerebral edema, the pathogenesis of which is unknown, is a common complication and the leading cause of death in FHF. Clinically, differentiating FHF from hepatic encephalopathy is difficult, and computed tomography of the head is often unreliable. Therefore measuring intracranial pressure is important. The goal is to maintain an intracranial pressure of less than 20 mm Hg. Management includes control of agitation, head elevation of 20 to 30 degrees, hyperventilation, administration of mannitol, treatment of barbiturate-induced coma, and urgent liver transplantation.

Hypoglycemia is a common complication of liver failure resulting from impaired hepatic gluconeogenesis and insulin degradation. All patients should receive 10% glucose intravenous infusions with frequent monitoring of blood glucose levels. Other metabolic abnormalities commonly occur, including hyponatremia, hypokalemia, respiratory alkalosis, and metabolic acidosis. Thus frequent monitoring of blood electrolytes and pH is indicated.

Table 43–1	Management of Selected Problems in Fulminant Hepatic Failure	
Complications	**Pathogenesis**	**Management**
Hepatic encephalopathy	Liver failure	Search for treatable causes (e.g., hypoglycemia, drugs used for sedation, sepsis, gastrointestinal bleeding, electrolyte imbalance, decreased P_{O_2}, increased P_{CO_2}, lactulose)
Cerebral edema	Unknown	Elevate head of bed 20–30 degrees; hyperventilate (P_{CO_2} 25–30 mm Hg); mannitol, 0.5–1.0 g/kg intravenous bolus over 5 min; pentobarbital infusion; urgent liver transplantation
Coagulopathy and gastrointestinal hemorrhage	Decreased synthesis of clotting factors Gastric erosions	Vitamin K; fresh-frozen plasma if actively bleeding and for prevention of bleeding; gastric acid suppression
Hypoglycemia	Decreased gluconeogenesis Insulin degradation	Intravenous 10% dextrose, monitor every 2 hr; 30–50% dextrose may be needed
Agitation	May be caused by: Encephalopathy Intracranial pressure Hypoxemia	Search for treatable causes (e.g., P_{O_2}, skin ulcers, lacerations, abscesses); soft restraints; if severely agitated and a concern for injury, consider sedation along with mechanical ventilation to protect airway
Infection	Liver failure and invasive monitoring	Surveillance cultures and low threshold for empirical antibiotics

P_{CO_2} = partial pressure of carbon dioxide; P_{O_2} = partial pressure of oxygen.

Bleeding occurs frequently and is commonly caused by gastric erosions and impaired synthesis of clotting factors. All patients should receive vitamin K and prophylactic gastric acid suppression. Fresh-frozen plasma should be used if clinically significant bleeding occurs or if major procedures, including intracranial pressure monitoring and central line placement, are performed.

Infection is one of the leading causes of death in FHF. As many as 80% of patients with FHF develop infection (80% bacterial, 20% fungal). Patients are at higher risk of infection as a result of impaired immunity resulting from liver failure and of the need for invasive monitoring. Severe infection may occur without fever or leukocytosis. Therefore frequent cultures and a low threshold for beginning antibiotics are required.

Hepatic Transplantation

Hepatic transplantation (see Chapter 44) has been performed with success in patients with FHF and is the treatment of choice for patients who appear unlikely to recover spontaneously. Because of the urgent need for transplantation, potential candidates should be transferred to transplant centers before significant complications develop (e.g., coma, cerebral edema, hemorrhage, infection). Transplantation is usually indicated in patients with severe encephalopathy or coagulopathy.

Prognosis

The cause of FHF and the degree of hepatic encephalopathy are important in determining prognosis. Patients with FHF from acetaminophen overdose or viral hepatitis A or B have a better survival rate than do patients with Wilson's disease or without a known cause. The short-term survival rate for patients with FHF in coma is 20% without liver transplantation. The 1-year survival rate of patients with FHF after liver transplantation is 80% to 90%. Patients who survive without a transplant also have excellent prognosis because liver tissue usually regenerates normally, regardless of the cause of FHF.

Prospectus for the Future

The development of effective therapy for FHF has been an ongoing focus of clinical and basic investigators for many years. Recently, a significant number of advances suggest the potential for improved treatments. Specifically, basic insights into the mechanisms of hepatocyte cell death and regeneration have defined specific pathways that may be manipulated to decrease hepatocyte loss and improve hepatocyte regeneration in response to acute injury. Such therapies are effective in animal models and are likely to be explored in humans. In addition, ongoing clinical trials with the use of hypothermia in FHF suggest that cooling may decrease cerebral injury and improve overall survival. Multicenter trials will be needed to confirm the efficacy of such an approach.

References

Polson J, Lee WM: AASLD position paper: The management of acute liver failure. Hepatology 41:1179–1197, 2005.

Vaquero J, Chung C, Cahill ME, Blei AT: Pathogenesis of hepatic encephalopathy in acute liver failure. Semin Liver Dis 23:259–269, 2003.

Chapter 44

Cirrhosis of the Liver and Its Complications

Miguel R. Arguedas

Michael B. Fallon

irrhosis is the irreversible end result to a variety of inflammatory, toxic, metabolic, and congestive insults to the liver. These insults lead to the deposition of interconnecting bands of fibrous tissue that surround *nodules* consisting of foci of regenerating hepatocytes. These regenerative nodules may be small (<3 mm; *micronodular cirrhosis*), a typical feature of alcoholic cirrhosis, or large (>3 mm; *macronodular cirrhosis*), more commonly seen as a sequela to chronic active hepatitis. The disruption of the normal hepatic lobular architecture distorts the vascular bed and contributes to portal hypertension and intrahepatic shunting. Normal hepatocyte function is disturbed by the resulting inadequacy of blood flow and ongoing inflammatory, toxic, and/or metabolic damage to hepatocytes. In addition, disturbances in cellular regulation and differentiation during hepatocytes regeneration may lead to the development of hepatocellular carcinoma. Therefore the clinical features of cirrhosis and its complications arise from portal hypertension, hepatocellular dysfunction, and hepatocellular carcinoma (Table 44–1). These disturbances are associated with significant morbidity and mortality, with more than 25,000 deaths occurring annually in the United States as a result of chronic liver disease.

Specific Causes

Alcohol consumption, hepatitis C virus infection, and nonalcoholic fatty liver disease are the most common causes of cirrhosis in Western industrialized nations, whereas hepatitis B is a major cause in the Far East and in developing countries. Cryptogenic cirrhosis remains a diagnosis of exclusion. Chronic active hepatitis, nonalcoholic fatty liver disease, and α_1-antitrypsin deficiency are discussed in Chapter 42. Hemochromatosis and Wilson's disease are covered in Chapter 62. Common and uncommon conditions that may lead to cirrhosis are listed in Table 44–2.

Diagnosis of Cirrhosis

Patients with cirrhosis may often be asymptomatic, and the diagnosis is incidentally established at the time of physical examination, laboratory testing, or radiologic testing for unrelated purposes. Alternatively, patients may exhibit specific complications of cirrhosis such as variceal bleeding, ascites, spontaneous bacterial peritonitis, and hepatic encephalopathy.

For the diagnosis of cirrhosis, liver biopsy has been considered the gold standard. In the majority of cases, though, the diagnosis can be made reliably by a combination of clinical, laboratory, and radiologic findings.

CLINICAL FEATURES

Symptoms are often unspecific and include fatigue, malaise, weight gain, anorexia, nausea, increased abdominal girth, and/or abdominal discomfort. Physical findings include jaundice, spider angiomata, palmar erythema, nail changes (Terry's nails exhibit proximal nail plate discoloration, and Muehrcke's lines exhibit white horizontal lines), gynecomastia, caput medusae, abnormal liver span or consistency, splenomegaly, ascites, lower extremity edema, and testicular atrophy (see Table 44–1).

LABORATORY FEATURES

Hepatocellular dysfunction leads to impaired protein synthesis (hypoalbuminemia and prolongation of prothrombin time), hyperbilirubinemia, low blood urea nitrogen levels, and elevated serum ammonia levels. *Portal hypertension* is responsible for thrombocytopenia and leucopenia resulting from splenic sequestration (hypersplenism).

Table 44–1	**Signs and Symptoms and Pathogenesis of Cirrhosis**
Signs and Symptoms	**Pathogenesis**
Constitutional	
Fatigue, anorexia, malaise, weight loss	Liver dysfunction
Cutaneous	
Spider telangiectasias, palmar erythema	Altered estrogen and androgen metabolism
Jaundice	Altered vascular physiologic factors
	Decreased bilirubin excretion
Endocrine	
Gynecomastia, testicular atrophy, decreased libido	Altered estrogen and androgen metabolism
Gastrointestinal	
Abdominal pain	Hepatomegaly, hepatocellular carcinoma
Abdominal swelling	Ascites
Gastrointestinal bleeding	Variceal hemorrhage
Hematologic	
Anemia, leukopenia, thrombocytopenia	Hypersplenism
Ecchymosis	Decreased synthesis of coagulation factors
Neurologic	
Altered sleep pattern, somnolence, confusion, asterixis	Hepatic encephalopathy

Table 44–2	**Causes of Cirrhosis**

Alcohol
Nonalcoholic steatohepatitis
Hepatitis B and C viruses
Drugs and toxins
Autoimmune hepatitis
Biliary cirrhosis
Primary biliary cirrhosis
Secondary biliary cirrhosis
Bile duct strictures
Sclerosing cholangitis
Biliary atresia
Tumors of the bile ducts
Cystic fibrosis
Chronic hepatic congestion
Budd-Chiari syndrome
Chronic right heart failure
Constrictive pericarditis
Genetically determined metabolic diseases
Hemochromatosis
Wilson's disease
α_1-Antitrypsin deficiency
Galactosemia
Cryptogenic

RADIOLOGIC FEATURES

Current radiologic modalities (ultrasound, computed tomography, and magnetic resonance imaging) are not sensitive or specific enough to replace liver biopsy completely in the diagnosis of cirrhosis. However, when imaging findings supportive of the diagnosis or cirrhosis (relative enlargement of the left hepatic and caudate lobes as a result of right lobe atrophy, surface nodularity, features of portal hypertension including ascites, intra-abdominal varices, and splenomegaly) are found in the presence of clinical and laboratory features of cirrhosis, biopsy is not routinely performed. Liver biopsy is frequently considered if a clinical suspicion of cirrhosis exists but imaging is normal or when the cause of liver disease is in doubt.

Major Complications of Cirrhosis

The major sequelae of cirrhosis are as follows:

1. As a consequence, predominantly of *hepatocellular dysfunction:*
   a. Jaundice
   b. Coagulopathy
   c. Hypoalbuminemia
2. As a consequence, predominantly of *portal hypertension:*
   a. Variceal hemorrhage
   b. Ascites
   c. Spontaneous bacterial peritonitis
   d. Hepatorenal syndrome
   e. Hepatic encephalopathy
   f. Hepatopulmonary syndrome
3. Hepatocellular carcinoma

The pathophysiologic interrelationships among these complications are shown diagrammatically in Figure 44–1.

HEPATOCELLULAR DYSFUNCTION

Cirrhosis results in impaired synthesis of proteins by hepatocytes, which leads to disturbances in the conjugation and excretion of bilirubin, hypoalbuminemia, and deficient production of coagulation factors and to diminished capacity for hepatic detoxification (see Chapters 40 and 43).

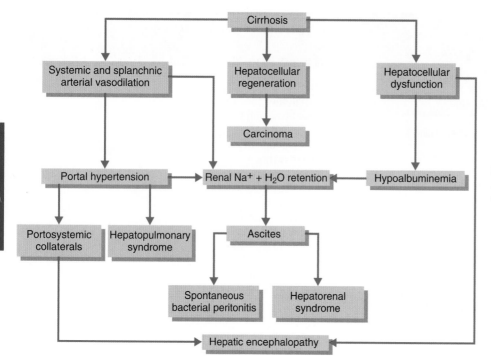

Figure 44–1 Inter-relationships among the complications of cirrhosis.

PORTAL HYPERTENSION

The normal portal pressure gradient is less than 5 mm Hg. In cirrhosis, the distortion of hepatic architecture by fibrous tissue and regenerative nodules, as well as a dynamic component caused by an increase in intrahepatic vascular tone, leads to increased resistance to portal venous flow, resulting in increased portal venous pressure. The portal pressure gradient can be measured using a transvenous approach and is reflected by the value of the wedged hepatic vein pressure minus the free hepatic vein pressure.

Although cirrhosis is the most important cause of portal hypertension, any process leading to increased resistance to portal blood flow into (presinusoidal) or through (sinusoidal) the liver or to hepatic venous outflow from the liver (postsinusoidal) may result in portal hypertension (Table 44–3). In addition, cirrhosis is associated with increased cardiac output, which leads to greater splanchnic blood flow, further aggravating portal hypertension.

In an attempt to decompress the portal system, venous collateral vessels between the portal and systemic circulations develop. Collateral vessels may form at several sites, the most important clinically being those connecting the portal vein to the azygos vein via dilated, tortuous veins (varices) in the submucosa of the gastric fundus and esophagus.

Variceal Hemorrhage

Gastroesophageal varices may develop when the portal pressure gradient exceeds 10 mm Hg, and the risk of variceal rupture leading to hemorrhage occurs when the gradient is greater than 12 mm Hg. Hemorrhage develops in 10% to 30% of patients every year, and each episode of variceal hemorrhage is associated with a mortality rate as high as 50%. Bleeding occurs most commonly from large varices in the esophagus when high tension in the walls of these vessels leads to rupture. Bleeding may produce hematemesis, melena, and/or hematochezia, which typically leads to hemodynamic compromise (see Chapter 33) further aggravated by impaired hepatic synthesis of coagulation factors (from hepatocellular dysfunction) and thrombocytopenia (from hypersplenism).

The management of gastroesophageal varices includes the treatment of acute variceal hemorrhage, the prevention of rebleeding (secondary prophylaxis), and the prevention of the initial episode of bleeding (primary prophylaxis) (Fig. 44–2). In the setting of variceal hemorrhage, the first

Table 44–3 Causes of Portal Hypertension

Increased Resistance to Flow

Presinusoidal
Portal or splenic vein occlusion (thrombosis, tumor)
Schistosomiasis
Congenital hepatic fibrosis
Sarcoidosis
Sinusoidal
Cirrhosis (all causes)
Alcoholic hepatitis
Postsinusoidal
Veno-occlusive disease
Budd-Chiari syndrome
Constrictive pericarditis

Increased Portal Blood Flow

Splenomegaly not caused by liver disease
Arterioportal fistula

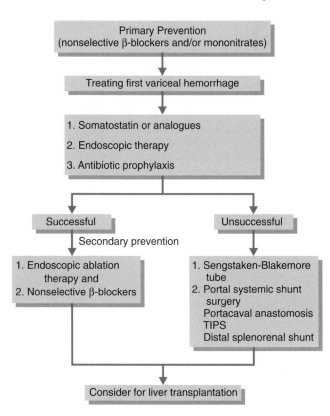

Figure 44–2 Prevention and treatment of variceal bleeding. TIPS = transjugular intrahepatic portosystemic shunt.

Table 44–4 **Causes of Ascites**	
Serum Ascites-Albumin Gradient	
High: >1.1 g/dL	**Low: <1.1 g/dL**
Cirrhosis	Peritoneal carcinomatosis
Chronic hepatic congestion	Peritoneal tuberculosis
Right ventricular heart failure	Pancreatic and biliary disease
Budd-Chiari syndrome	Nephrotic syndrome
Constrictive pericarditis	
Nephrotic syndrome	
Massive liver metastases	
Myxedema	
Mixed ascites	

therapeutic intervention consists of hemodynamic resuscitation with colloids such as blood and/or fresh-frozen plasma and airway protection and ventilatory support, if necessary. Current pharmacologic therapy consists of somatostatin or its synthetic analogues (i.e., octreotide), which are best instituted before endoscopic examination. Endoscopic therapy includes band ligation and/or sclerotherapy (**Web Video 44–1**). Prospective studies have demonstrated that band ligation is the preferred modality given the lower incidence of adverse effects and complications. Balloon tamponade (Sengstaken-Blakemore tube, Linton tube, or Minnesota tube) is a temporary measure reserved for patients in whom endoscopic therapy has failed. These patients may need to undergo portal decompression either surgically or by transjugular intrahepatic portosystemic shunt placement. After an initial episode of variceal bleeding, secondary prophylaxis with nonselective β-blockers alone or in combination with long-acting nitrates and/or variceal obliteration through repeated courses of band ligation would be appropriate.

Endoscopic screening has been recommended to identify patients at high risk for variceal bleeding (i.e., those with large varices) so that primary prophylaxis can be instituted. Several studies suggest that certain clinical features (e.g., thrombocytopenia, ascites, telangiectasias) may help predict patients who are likely to have large varices, but given the poor predictive values of these features, endoscopic screening should be performed in all patients newly diagnosed with cirrhosis. Nonselective β-blockers (propranolol and nadolol) are the agents of choice for primary prophylaxis because they reduce portal blood flow and vascular resistance and hence

portal pressure. In patients with contraindications or intolerance to β-blockers, variceal obliteration through endoscopic band ligation is the best alternative.

Ascites

Ascites is the accumulation of excess fluid in the peritoneal cavity. Although cirrhosis is the most common cause of ascites, this condition may have numerous other causes (Table 44–4). The serum ascites-albumin gradient has replaced the exudative-transudative classification of ascites. An elevated serum ascites-albumin gradient (>1.1 g/dL, serum albumin concentration–ascites albumin concentration) signifies the presence of portal hypertension. Ascites becomes clinically detectable with fluid accumulation greater than 500 mL. Shifting dullness to percussion is the most sensitive clinical sign of ascites, but ultrasonography more readily detects small fluid volumes (250 mL).

The precise sequence of events leading to the development of cirrhotic ascites remains debated. However, both excess renal sodium and water retention resulting from portal hypertension and splanchnic vasodilation resulting in overflow of fluid into the peritoneum (*overflow theory*) and decreased effective circulating blood volume resulting from systemic arterial vasodilation leading to activation of neurohumoral systems and sodium and water retention (*underflow theory*) play a role.

Treatment of ascites consists initially of sodium restriction, preferably to less than 2 g/day. Restricted fluid intake may be necessary if hyponatremia (<125 mEq/L) is present. The administration of spironolactone, an aldosterone antagonist, supplemented with a loop diuretic (e.g., furosemide) is effective in approximately 90% of patients. Diuresis should be monitored closely because aggressive diuretic therapy may result in electrolyte disturbances (i.e., hyponatremia, hypokalemia) and hypovolemia, leading to impaired renal function and potentially precipitating hepatic encephalopathy. *Refractory ascites* occurs in approximately 10% of patients with cirrhosis and is defined as persistent tense ascites despite maximal diuretic therapy (spironolactone, 400 mg/day, and furosemide, 160 mg/day) or the development of azotemia or electrolyte disturbances at submaximal doses of diuretics. Treatment in these patients includes repeated large-volume paracentesis, transjugular intrahepatic portosystemic shunt placement, liver transplantation, and, in some centers, peritoneovenous (LeVeen or Denver) shunts.

Spontaneous Bacterial Peritonitis

Infection of ascitic fluid, usually with *Enterobacteriaceae* or *Pneumococcus,* may occur in patients with cirrhosis. Fever, abdominal pain, and tenderness may be present, or the infection may be clinically silent or may be demonstrated by the development of hepatic encephalopathy and/or renal insufficiency. Therefore diagnostic paracentesis should be considered in any patient with cirrhotic ascites who clinically deteriorates. The diagnosis is strongly suggested if the ascitic fluid polymorphonuclear leukocyte count is greater than 250/L, and if the diagnosis is confirmed by culture, preferably inoculated into blood culture bottles at the time of paracentesis. Treatment with a third-generation cephalosporin for 5 days is usual. The administration of intravenous albumin has been shown to decrease the incidence of renal dysfunction and improves short-term survival. Given the high rates of recurrence, long-term antibiotic prophylaxis is indicated in patients with a prior episode of spontaneous bacterial peritonitis, whereas short-term prophylaxis should be considered in patients with cirrhosis and ascites who are hospitalized with upper gastrointestinal bleeding.

Hepatorenal Syndrome

Serious liver disease from any cause may be complicated by a form of functional renal failure, termed the *hepatorenal syndrome,* which almost invariably occurs in the presence of significant hepatic synthetic dysfunction and ascites. This syndrome occurs in approximately 4% of patients with decompensated cirrhosis, and some prospective series have determined that the probability of developing this syndrome in patients admitted to the hospital for the treatment of ascites may be as high as 30% to 40% at 2 years. Typically, the kidneys are histologically normal, with the capacity of regaining normal function in the event of recovery of liver function such as following liver transplantation. Severe cortical vasoconstriction has been demonstrated angiographically, and it reverses when these kidneys have been transplanted into patients who do not have cirrhosis. The renal dysfunction is characterized by a declining glomerular filtration rate, oliguria, low urine sodium (<10 mEq/L), normal urinary sediment, and azotemia, often with a disproportionately high ratio of blood urea nitrogen to creatinine. Two types of hepatorenal syndrome have been described. Type I is characterized by rapidly progressive renal failure that occurs within 2 weeks and is associated with a dismal prognosis. In type II, renal dysfunction occurs more slowly and is associated with a better prognosis. The decline in renal function often follows one of three events in a patient with cirrhosis and ascites: infection, over-diuresis, or large-volume paracentesis.

Hepatorenal syndrome is usually progressive and fatal, with a mortality of 95%. It should be diagnosed only after plasma volume depletion (a common cause of reversible, prerenal azotemia in patients with cirrhosis, particularly in patients receiving diuretics) and other forms of acute renal injury have been excluded.

Octreotide in combination with midodrine (α-adrenergic agonist), vasopressin analogues (ornipressin),

and transjugular intrahepatic portosystemic shunts have been reported to stabilize or even improve renal function, but liver transplantation has currently become the accepted treatment for hepatorenal syndrome.

Hepatic Encephalopathy

Hepatic encephalopathy is a complex neuropsychiatric syndrome that may complicate severe or advanced liver disease and/or extensive portosystemic collateral formation *(shunting).* Two major forms of hepatic encephalopathy are recognized: acute and chronic.

Acute hepatic encephalopathy usually occurs in the setting of fulminant hepatic failure. Cerebral edema plays an important role in this setting, and progression to coma is common and mortality is extremely high (see Chapter 43). *Chronic hepatic encephalopathy* usually occurs in the setting of cirrhosis and is often reversible. It commonly produces disturbances in the sleep-wake cycle, subtle neurologic dysfunction, and behavioral changes.

The pathogenesis of hepatic encephalopathy in the setting of cirrhosis is thought to involve the inadequate hepatic removal of predominantly nitrogenous compounds or other toxins ingested or formed in the gastrointestinal tract. Ammonia, derived from both amino acid deamination and bacterial hydrolysis of nitrogenous compounds in the gut, has been implicated in the pathogenesis of hepatic encephalopathy, but venous ammonia blood levels correlate poorly with the presence or degree of encephalopathy. Other potential contributors to hepatic encephalopathy have been investigated, including γ-aminobutyric acid, mercaptans, short-chain fatty acids, benzodiazepine-like compounds, imbalance between plasma branched-chain and aromatic amino acids, altered cerebral metabolism (disturbed sodium-potassium adenosine triphosphatase [Na^+-K^+ ATPase] activity), zinc deficiency, and deposition of manganese in the basal ganglia.

The clinical features of hepatic encephalopathy include disturbances of higher neurologic function (e.g., intellectual and personality disorders, dementia, inability to copy simple diagrams *[constructional apraxia],* disturbance of consciousness), disturbances of neuromuscular function (e.g., asterixis, hyperreflexia, myoclonus), and rarely a Parkinson-like syndrome and progressive paraplegia. One of the earliest manifestations is the alteration of the normal sleep-wake cycle. Hepatic encephalopathy is usually divided into stages according to its severity (Table 44–5). Hypoglycemia, subdural hematoma, meningitis, and drug overdose should be considered in the differential diagnosis of hepatic encephalopathy.

Treatment of hepatic encephalopathy is based on identifying and addressing precipitating factors (Table 44–6), short-term restricting of dietary protein, reducing and eliminating substrates for the generation of nitrogenous compounds, and preventing ammonia absorption from the bowel. Gastrointestinal bleeding and increased protein intake may provide increased substrate for the bacterial or metabolic formation of nitrogenous compounds that induce encephalopathy. Patients prone to develop hepatic encephalopathy have increased sensitivity to drugs that depress the central nervous system, and the use of these drugs should be avoided in these patients. Protein restriction may be considered in patients with severe encephalopathy,

Table 44–5	**Stages of Hepatic Encephalopathy**
Stage*	**Clinical Manifestations**
I	Apathy
	Restlessness
	Reversal of sleep rhythm
	Slowed intellect
	Impaired computational ability
	Impaired handwriting
II	Lethargy
	Drowsiness
	Disorientation
	Asterixis
III	Stupor (arousable)
	Hyperactive reflexes, extensor plantar responses
IV	Coma (response to painful stimuli only)

*Stage 0 encephalopathy is used to describe subclinical impairment of intellectual function.

Table 44–6	**Hepatic Encephalopathy: Precipitating Factors**

Gastrointestinal bleeding
Increased dietary protein
Constipation
Infection
CNS-depressant drugs (benzodiazepines, opiates, tricyclic antidepressants)
Deterioration in hepatic function
Hypokalemia: most often induced by diuretics
Azotemia: most often induced by diuretics
Alkalosis: most often induced by diuretics
Hypovolemia: most often induced by diuretics

CNS = central nervous system.

but long-term restriction is associated with worsening malnutrition. Treatment with formulas rich in branched-chain amino acids has shown no benefit in improving encephalopathy or mortality. Reduction and elimination of nitrogenous compound substrates can be achieved by administering enemas and using antibiotics that reduce colonic bacteria (i.e., neomycin, metronidazole, rifaximin). Nonabsorbable disaccharides (i.e., lactulose) are fermented to organic acids by colonic bacteria, lowering stool pH and trapping ammonia in the colon, and thereby preventing absorption.

Hepatopulmonary Syndrome

Hepatopulmonary syndrome occurs in 10% to 15% of patients with cirrhosis and is characterized by gas exchange abnormalities (increased alveolar-arterial gradient and hypoxemia) as a result of intrapulmonary vascular dilation. The vascular dilation leads to impaired oxygen transfer from alveoli to the central stream of red blood cells within capillaries, resulting in *functional* intrapulmonary right-to-left shunt that improves with 100% oxygen. Intrapulmonary shunting can be demonstrated through contrast echocardiography. In this modality, agitated saline, which creates microbubbles, is injected into a peripheral vein while performing two-dimensional echocardiography. Delayed visualization (after the third heartbeat following injection) of microbubbles in the left cardiac chambers indicates intrapulmonary vasodilatation, whereas early visualization occurs with intracardiac shunting. Clinical features range from subclinical abnormalities in gas exchange to profound hypoxemia causing significant dyspnea. No proven medical therapy exists, but using supplemental oxygen may alleviate symptoms. The treatment of choice is liver transplantation, which often leads to complete reversal of the syndrome.

HEPATOCELLULAR CARCINOMA

Hepatocellular carcinoma (HCC) accounts for less than 2.5% of all malignancies in the United States. Recent epidemiologic studies, though, have demonstrated a 71% relative increase in the age-adjusted incidence rate of this malignancy over the last 20 years. In other areas of the world, including sub-Saharan Africa, China, Japan, and Southeast Asia, HCC is one of the most frequent malignancies and is an important cause of mortality, particularly in middle-age men. HCC often arises in a cirrhotic liver and is closely associated with chronic viral hepatitis. Hepatitis B virus DNA has been shown to integrate in the host cell genome, where it may disrupt tumor suppressor genes and/or activate oncogenes. In areas of high prevalence, vaccination to prevent infection with hepatitis B virus has reduced the incidence of this disease. The exact pathophysiologic mechanisms leading to tumorigenesis in patients with other causes of cirrhosis (such as hemochromatosis, alcohol, hepatitis C viral infection) remain poorly understood. Risk factors for development of HCC, as well as its clinical manifestations, are listed in Table 44–7. Currently used imaging techniques for detecting HCC and the most common appearance of the tumor are listed in Table 44–8. A tissue specimen may be necessary to confirm the diagnosis of HCC in some cases but may not be needed if characteristic clinical and radiologic features are present and especially when accompanied by a rise in serum α-fetoprotein levels. Diagnosis of small, treatable tumors is possible with intensive screening programs that employ imaging studies and serum α-fetoprotein levels, although the long-term outcomes and cost effectiveness of these strategies remain unclear. Patients with well-compensated cirrhosis may undergo surgical resection or liver transplantation, whereas, in patients with advanced cirrhosis, liver transplantation should be considered. Nonsurgical options include percutaneous ethanol injection, arterial chemoembolization, and radiofrequency ablation. In patients with widespread, multifocal disease and in those with vascular invasion, the prognosis is poor, with median survival from the time of diagnosis of less than 6 months.

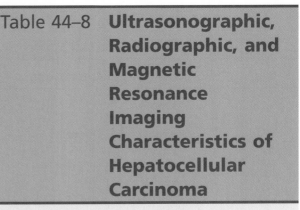

Table 44–7   Hepatocellular Carcinoma

Incidence

From 1–7 per 100,000 to >100 per 100,000 in high-risk areas

Sex

4:1–8:1 male preponderance

Associations

Chronic hepatitis B infection
Chronic hepatitis C infection
Hemochromatosis (with cirrhosis)
Cirrhosis (alcoholic, cryptogenic)
Aflatoxin ingestion
Thorotrast
α_1-Antitrypsin deficiency
Androgen administration

Common Clinical Presentations

Abdominal pain
Abdominal mass
Weight loss
Deterioration of liver function

Unusual Manifestations

Bloody ascites
Tumor emboli (lung)
Jaundice
Hepatic or portal vein obstruction
Metabolic effects
Erythrocytosis
Hypercalcemia
Hypercholesterolemia
Hypoglycemia
Gynecomastia
Feminization
Acquired porphyria

Clinical and Laboratory Findings

Hepatic bruit or friction rub
Serum α-fetoprotein >400 level ng/mL

Table 44–8   Ultrasonographic, Radiographic, and Magnetic Resonance Imaging Characteristics of Hepatocellular Carcinoma

Ultrasonography

Mass lesion with varying echogenicities but usually hypoechoic

Dynamic Computed Tomography

Arterial phase: tumor enhances quickly
Venous phase: quick de-enhancement of the tumor relative to the parenchyma

Magnetic Resonance Imaging

T1-weighted images: hypointense
T2-weighted images: hyperintense
After gadolinium administration, the tumor increases in intensity

HEPATIC TRANSPLANTATION

Liver transplantation is a highly successful procedure in patients with progressive, advanced, and otherwise untreatable liver disease. Advances in surgical techniques and supportive care, the use of cyclosporine and tacrolimus for immunosuppression, and careful selection of patients have all contributed to the excellent results of liver transplantation. From 70% to 80% of patients undergoing liver transplantation survive at least 3 years, usually with good quality of life. The most common indication for liver transplantation in the United States is chronic liver disease resulting from hepatitis C virus infection. Other liver diseases for which transplantation is commonly performed include cirrhosis from alcoholic liver disease, nonalcoholic fatty liver disease, autoimmune hepatitis, primary biliary cirrhosis, and primary sclerosing cholangitis. Patients with hepatitis B are candidates for liver transplantation if they can be given hepatitis B immunoglobulin or nucleoside analogues (i.e., lamivudine) to help prevent recurrence. Excellent results have also been obtained in selected patients with fulminant hepatic failure (see Chapter 43). Liver transplantation for malignant hepatobiliary disease has been less successful because of recurrent disease in the transplanted liver.

The timing of liver transplantation presents a particular challenge given the insufficient availability of donor organs. Liver-assist devices for temporary support until an organ becomes available are currently being evaluated. Recently, the United Network for Organ Sharing has accepted the Model for End-Stage Liver Disease (MELD) system for determining organ allocation. The MELD system consists of a prognostic model that predicts mortality according to selected clinical and laboratory variables, therefore prioritizing organ availability to patients with more advanced disease in whom predicted mortality is high.

VASCULAR DISEASE OF THE LIVER

Disorders of the hepatic vasculature are uncommon and include portal-vein thrombosis, hepatic-vein thrombosis (Budd-Chiari syndrome), and veno-occlusive disease. Affected patients usually have portal hypertension with or without associated liver dysfunction and may mimic the presentation of cirrhosis.

Portal Vein Thrombosis

Thrombosis of the portal vein may develop after abdominal trauma, umbilical vein infection and neonatal sepsis, intra-abdominal inflammatory diseases (e.g., pancreatitis), hypercoagulable states, or in association with cirrhosis. In most cases, however, particularly in children, the cause is unknown. The disease produces the manifestations of portal hypertension (see Chapter 44); however, liver histology is usually normal. The diagnosis is established by angiography, but noninvasive imaging modalities such as Doppler ultrasonography, computerized tomography, and magnetic resonance imaging may reveal thrombus, collateral circulation near the porta hepatis, and/or splenomegaly. In long-standing portal-vein thrombosis, tortuous venous channels develop within the organized clot, leading to *cavernous transformation.*

In acute portal-vein thrombosis, thrombolysis may be attempted. Long-term anticoagulation may be used in chronic thrombosis, especially when associated with hypercoagulable states. Concern exists, though, that anticoagulation may precipitate hemorrhage from varices that arise as a consequence of portal hypertension. If variceal hemorrhage occurs, it is best managed with endoscopic obliteration. Prophylaxis with β-blockers to prevent variceal bleeding may decrease portal pressure and potentially propagate thrombus and is generally not recommended. If endoscopic treatment fails, surgical management with portosystemic shunting may be attempted, but this approach is often difficult because of the absence of suitable patent vessels.

Budd-Chiari Syndrome

The occlusion of the major hepatic veins and/or the inferior vena cava, especially in the intrahepatic and suprahepatic segments, cause Budd-Chiari syndrome. The majority of cases are caused by hematologic disease (e.g., polycythemia vera, paroxysmal nocturnal hemoglobinuria, essential thrombocytosis and other myeloproliferative disorders), pregnancy, oral contraceptive use, tumors (especially hepatocellular carcinoma), hypercoagulable states (e.g., factor V Leiden mutation, protein C & S deficiency), abdominal trauma, and congenital webs of the vena cava. Approximately 20% of cases are idiopathic, but many of these patients may have early, subclinical myeloproliferative disease or genetic mutations associated with a hypercoagulable state.

The presentation of Budd-Chiari syndrome can be acute, which may be associated with fulminant liver failure, or it may exhibit as a subacute or chronic illness. Acute disease produces right upper quadrant abdominal pain, hepatomegaly, ascites, and jaundice, whereas the subacute or chronic form produces primarily portal hypertension. Elevation of serum bilirubin and transaminase levels may be mild, but liver function is often poor, with profound hypoalbuminemia and coagulopathy. The diagnosis can be established noninvasively with Doppler ultrasonography, which may show decreased or absent hepatic vein blood flow, and computed tomography, which shows delayed or absent contrast filling of the hepatic veins and hypertrophy of the caudate lobe. Magnetic resonance angiography may also demonstrate the previously mentioned findings. Hepatic venography is especially useful in cases in which the results of the noninvasive modalities are inconclusive. Venography often shows an inability to catheterize and visualize the hepatic veins; the characteristic *spider-web* pattern of collateral vessels may also be demonstrated, and the inferior vena cava may appear compressed, owing to hepatomegaly or an enlarged caudate lobe. On liver biopsy, centrilobular congestion, hemorrhage, and necrosis are seen with cirrhosis developing in patients with chronic obstruction.

Treatment should be individualized and is dependent on the mode and severity of presentation and the potential cause of the disease. Supportive therapy to relieve ascites and edema (e.g., dietary sodium restriction, diuretics) and chronic anticoagulation may be considered in patients with chronic Budd-Chiari syndrome in whom methods to decompress congestion are not feasible. Thrombolysis followed by anticoagulation is most useful in patients with acute forms. In selected patients (e.g., those with venous webs or strictures and/or single-vessel thrombosis) angioplasty with or without stent placement may be used. Decompressive modalities are most useful before the development of cirrhosis and include transjugular intrahepatic portacaval and side-to-side portacaval shunts. In patients with cirrhosis, liver transplantation is often considered the best option.

Veno-occlusive Disease

Veno-occlusive disease, also called sinusoidal obstruction syndrome, is characterized by jaundice, painful hepatomegaly, and fluid retention that most often occurs after cytoreductive therapy and before bone marrow transplantation but may also follow exposure to other drugs and herbal preparations (e.g., azathioprine, pyrrolizidine alkaloids). Endothelial cell injury leads to obstruction at the level of the hepatic venules and the sinusoids.

The diagnosis is clinically suspected when weight gain, epigastric–right upper quadrant abdominal pain, and jaundice develops within the first 3 to 4 weeks following bone marrow transplant. Laboratory abnormalities include hyperbilirubinemia, elevated transaminases, and in severe cases, profound synthetic dysfunction. Clinical manifestations may be rapidly progressive and may lead to multi-organ dysfunction and death in 20% to 25% of patients. Doppler abdominal ultrasonography may reveal ascites, reversal of portal vein flow, and an elevated hepatic artery resistance index. Liver biopsy is diagnostic and is usually obtained using the transjugular approach. The advantages of this approach compared with the percutaneous route include measurement of the hepatic venous pressure gradient (typically elevated in veno-occlusive disease) and a lower incidence of bleeding.

Mild forms of the disease may favorably respond only to supportive therapy. In moderate to severe disease, treatment has been attempted with tissue plasminogen activator and heparin, defibrotide, antithrombin III, prostaglandin E1, and glutamine plus vitamin E, although their efficacy has not been clearly established.

Prospectus for the Future

For many years, cirrhosis has been viewed as an irreversible fibrotic reaction to chronic liver injury. However, as the mechanisms of hepatic fibrosis have been explored and treatments for chronic liver have been implemented, cirrhosis has been increasingly seen as an imbalance of multiple factors that regulate the generation and degradation of collagen. Among the consequences of the increased understanding of hepatic fibrogenesis is the potential for development of specific agents that influence collagen production and those that may prevent and even diminish hepatic fibrosis. A significant number of antifibrotic agents have been successfully used in animal models of liver injury, and these agents are likely to enter clinical use in the near future.

Another key issue in the therapy of complications of cirrhosis is defining the effectiveness of medical treatment of esophageal varices. Noncardioselective β-adrenergic blockers decrease the risk of variceal bleeding. This effect is established to occur in the subgroup of patients who have a significant reduction in portal pressure measured by hepatic venous pressure recordings. Currently, direct measurement of hepatic venous pressures is not routinely used to assess efficacy of noncardioselective β-adrenergic blockers in lowering portal pressure. The development of noninvasive means to measure portal pressures or targeted measurement of hepatic venous pressure recordings in patients treated with noncardioselective β-adrenergic blockers are likely to help guide treatment of esophageal varices.

References

Arguedas MR: The critically ill liver patient: The variceal bleeder. Semin Gastrointest Dis 14:34–38, 2003.

Cardenas A, Gines P: Management of complications of cirrhosis in patients awaiting liver transplantation. J Hepatol 42:S124–S133, 2005.

De Franchis R, Dell'Era A, Iannuzzi F: Diagnosis and treatment of portal hypertension. Dig Liver Dis 36(12):787–798, 2004 Dec.

Marrero JA: Screening tests for hepatocellular carcinoma. Clin Liver Dis 9:235–251, 2005.

Menon KV, Shah V, Kamath PS: The Budd-Chiari syndrome. N Engl J Med 350:578–585, 2004.

Wadleigh M, Ho V, Momtaz P, Richardson P: Hepatic veno-occlusive disease: Pathogenesis, diagnosis, and treatment. Curr Opin Hematol 10:451–462, 2003.

Webster GJ, Burroughs AK, Riordan SM: Portal vein thrombosis—new insights into aetiology and management. Aliment Pharmacol Ther 21:1–9, 2005.

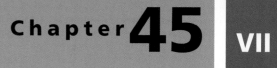

Disorders of the Gallbladder and Biliary Tract

Shyam Varadarajulu

Rudolf Garcia-Gallont

Michael B. Fallon

The main role of the biliary tract and gallbladder is to transport bile into the intestines, which, in turn, is essential for digesting fat. Diseases of the gallbladder and the biliary tract are among the most common afflictions of humankind. This chapter examines the most common gallbladder and biliary tract disorders, focusing on cholelithiasis. The reader is referred to Chapter 41 for a detailed discussion of bilirubin metabolism and the diagnostic approach to jaundice and to Chapter 34 for a review of the various imaging techniques used to study the biliary tract.

Normal Biliary Anatomy and Physiology

Figure 45–1 outlines the normal anatomy of the liver and biliary tract. The liver produces 500 to 1500 mL of bile per day. Bile passes through the canaliculi to the hepatic bile ducts and then into the common hepatic duct. Tonic contraction of the sphincter of Oddi, located in the region of the ampulla of Vater, during fasting diverts approximately one half of the bile through the cystic duct into the gallbladder where it is stored and concentrated. Cholecystokinin, released after food is ingested, causes the sphincter of Oddi to contract and then to relax, allowing delivery of a timed bolus of bile, rich in bile acids, into the intestine. Bile acids, detergent molecules possessing both fat-soluble and water-soluble moieties, convey phospholipids and cholesterol from the liver to the intestine where cholesterol undergoes fecal excretion (see Chapter 41, Fig. 41–1). In the intestinal lumen, bile acids solubilize dietary fat and promote its digestion and absorption. Bile acids are, for the most part, efficiently reabsorbed by the small intestinal mucosa, particularly in the terminal ileum, and are recycled to the liver for re-excretion, a process termed *enterohepatic circulation*.

Gallstones (Cholelithiasis)

In studies performed in the United States, Europe, and South America, approximately 10% to 15% of adults have gallstones. In the United States, gallstone disease leads to over 500,000 cholecystectomies annually, with estimated costs of $4.5 billion per year. Gallstones are of two types: (1) cholesterol (75%) and (2) pigmented (black or brown) (25%), the latter being composed of calcium bilirubinate and other calcium salts. The risk factors for cholelithiasis are shown in Table 45–1.

PATHOGENESIS OF CHOLELITHIASIS

The three main factors that lead to cholesterol gallstone formation are (1) cholesterol supersaturation of bile, (2) nucleation, and (3) gallbladder hypomotility. The liver is the most important organ in regulating total body cholesterol stores. Once secreted, cholesterol, which is insoluble in water, is solubilized in bile by forming mixed micelles with bile acids and phospholipids. In most individuals, many of whom do not develop stones, more cholesterol is in bile than can be maintained in stable solution (supersaturated bile). As bile becomes more supersaturated, aggregation of microscopic cholesterol molecules into coalescent vesicles that crystallize (nucleation) takes place. Gradual deposition of additional layers of cholesterol leads to the appearance of macroscopic stones. Factors that influence nucleation include bile transit time, gallbladder contraction, bile composition (concentration of cholesterol, phospholipids, and bile salts), and presence of bacteria, mucin, and glycoproteins, which act as a nidus to initiate cholesterol crystal formation. The interplay between *pro-* and *antinucleating* factors in the gallbladder may determine whether cholesterol gallstones will form from supersaturated bile. Gallbladder sludge is a supercon-

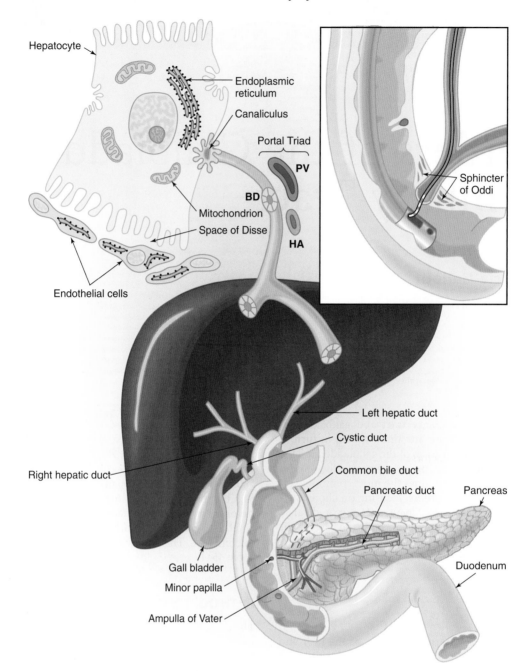

Figure 45–1 Normal anatomy and histology of the liver and biliary tract. Materials destined for metabolism or excretion by the liver (such as unconjugated bilirubin) enter the sinusoidal bed and cross the endothelial barrier and the space of Disse. Unconjugated bilirubin is taken up by the hepatocyte, conjugated with glucuronide to become water-soluble, and excreted into bile across the canalicular membrane of the hepatocyte. The canaliculi empty into bile ductules *(BD)*, which, in turn, lead to the interlobular (small), septal (medium), and large intrahepatic bile ducts and finally to the main branches of the common bile duct *(CHD)*. The portal areas, or *portal triads,* are composed mainly of portal vein *(PV)*, hepatic artery *(HA)*, and BD branches *(left side, magnification)*. Tonic contraction of the sphincter of Oddi, located in the region of the ampulla of Vater, during fasting diverts approximately one half of the bile through the cystic duct into the gallbladder where it is stored and concentrated to be released later during meal times. Diseases at any level of the biliary tree can lead to cholestasis and obstructive jaundice; for example, primary sclerosing cholangitis is caused by inflammatory obstruction of the interlobular bile ducts, whereas stones, cancer of the ampulla of Vater, or pancreatitis can cause distal obstruction of the common bile duct. Investigation of the bile duct is best accomplished using a side-viewing endoscope to insert a catheter into the ampulla of Vater, with injection of contrast to obtain an endoscopic retrograde cholangiogram *(right side, photo insert)*. If pathology is detected (e.g., cholangitis, stricture, stone), therapeutic maneuvers such as stone removal, stenting, or sphincterotomy to enlarge the distal opening of the common bile duct can be performed.

Table 45–1	**Risk Factors for Cholelithiasis**

Primary

Age
Obesity
Female sex
Rapid weight loss
Race (e.g., Native American)

Secondary

Use of oral contraceptives
Pregnancy
Diabetes mellitus
Use of insulin
Low socioeconomic status
Sedentary lifestyle
Total parenteral nutrition
Hemolysis
Biliary parasites (e.g., *Clonorchis sinensis*)

Table 45–2	**Differential Diagnosis of Cholelithiasis**

Peptic ulcer disease
Gastroesophageal reflux disease
Nonulcer dyspepsia
Irritable bowel syndrome
Sphincter of Oddi dysfunction
Hepatitis and perihepatitis (Fitz-Hugh–Curtis syndrome)
Hepatic abscess
Nephrolithiasis
Pyelonephritis
Perinephric abscess
Pneumonia
Pulmonary infarction
Pulmonary embolism
Angina pectoris
Pancreatitis
Ruptured ectopic pregnancy
Appendicitis

centrated mixture of bile acids, bilirubin, cholesterol, mucus, and proteins that exhibits various degrees of fluidity and is prone to precipitate into semisolid or solid form.

The pathophysiologic factors of pigment stones is less well understood compared with gallstone formation; however, increased production of bilirubin conjugates (hemolytic states), increased biliary calcium (Ca^{2+}) and bicarbonate (HCO_3^-, cirrhosis, and bacterial deconjugation of bilirubin to a less soluble form are all associated with pigment stone formation.

Many of the recognized predisposing factors for cholelithiasis and gallbladder sludge can be understood in terms of the pathophysiologic scheme outlined previously:

1. Biliary cholesterol saturation is increased by estrogens, multiparity, oral contraceptives, obesity, rapid weight loss, and terminal ileal disease, which decreases the bile acid pool.
2. Nucleation is enhanced by biliary parasites, recurrent bacterial infection of the biliary tract, and antibiotics such as ceftriaxone, which has a proclivity to concentrate and crystallize with calcium in the biliary tree. Total parenteral nutrition and blood transfusions also promote bile pigment accumulation and *gelfaction* of sludge.
3. Bile stasis is caused by gallbladder hypomotility (resulting from pregnancy, somatostatin, or fasting), bile duct strictures, choledochal cysts, biliary parasites, and total parenteral nutrition.

CLINICAL MANIFESTATIONS OF GALLSTONES

Most individuals with gallstones remain asymptomatic (50% to 60%), approximately one third develop biliary colic or chronic cholecystitis, and 15% develop acute complications.

The natural history of gallstone disease is outlined in Figure 45–2. Obstruction of the biliary tract at any level by stones or sludge is the underlying cause of all manifestations of gallstone disease. Obstruction by gallstones can occur at the level of the cystic duct, common hepatic duct, common bile duct, and ampulla of Vater (see Fig. 45–1). Symptoms arise from contraction of the gallbladder during transient obstruction of the cystic duct by gallstones, whereas persistent obstruction of the cystic duct leads to superimposed inflammation or infection of the gallbladder (i.e., acute cholecystitis). Obstruction of the distal common bile duct may result in abdominal pain, cholangitis (infection of the biliary tract), or pancreatitis (resulting from pancreatic duct obstruction). Common conditions to consider in the differential diagnosis of gallstone disease are listed in Table 45–2.

Asymptomatic Gallstones

Asymptomatic patients should be followed expectantly. Prophylactic cholecystectomy is considered in groups at increased risk for developing complications: (1) patients with diabetes who have a greater morbidity and mortality from acute cholecystitis; (2) persons with a calcified (porcelain) gallbladder or large gallbladder polyps, which are associated with an increased risk of carcinoma of the gallbladder; (3) persons with sickle cell anemia, in whom hepatic crises may be difficult to differentiate from acute cholecystitis; (4) children with gallstones, because they frequently develop symptomatic disease; and (5) Native Americans who are predisposed to developing gallbladder cancer in the setting of gallstones.

Biliary Colic

The term *chronic cholecystitis* has been used to denote recurrent and *nonacute* symptoms caused by the presence of gallstones over a period of days to several years. A better term for this condition is *biliary* colic because the presence of

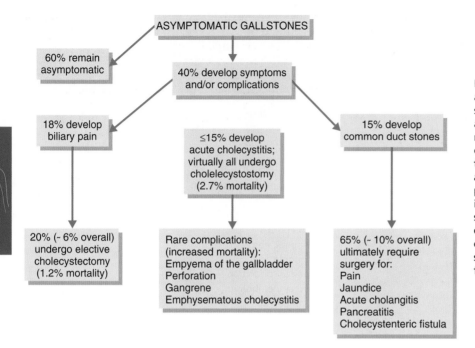

Figure 45–2 Natural history of asymptomatic gallstones. The clinical syndromes associated with gallstones are shown here, and the numbers represent the approximate percentage of adults who develop one or more of these symptoms or complications over a 15- to 20-year period. Over this period, approximately 30% of individuals with gallstones undergo surgery. (The risk of developing complications of gallstones varies considerably among series. The figures shown here represent those derived from more recent studies.)

symptoms correlates poorly with pathologic findings in the gallbladder wall. Biliary colic is typically a steady ache in the epigastrium or right upper quadrant, of sudden onset, reaching a plateau of intensity over a few minutes, which subsides gradually over 30 minutes to several hours. Referred pain may be felt at the tip of the scapula or right shoulder. Nausea and vomiting may occur, whereas fever and a palpable mass (signs of acute cholecystitis) are not evident. Other symptoms such as dyspepsia, fatty food intolerance, bloating and flatulence, heartburn, and belching may occur in patients with gallstones; however, these symptoms are nonspecific and frequently occur in individuals with normal gallbladders.

Gallstones can be best demonstrated by transabdominal ultrasonography (sensitivity and specificity >95%), which has become the initial test to evaluate cholelithiasis. Ultrasound accuracy drops to 20% for visualization of stones within the common bile duct. This limitation of transabdominal ultrasound has been overcome by endoscopic ultrasound (**Web Video 45–1** shows gallstones on endoscopic ultrasonography) and magnetic resonance cholangiopancreatography (MRCP), both of which have an accuracy of 90% to 95% for detecting cholelithiasis and common bile duct stones. Oral cholecystography is no longer used for the routine evaluation of gallstones.

Laparoscopic cholecystectomy has replaced open cholecystectomy as the treatment of choice for recurrent biliary pain. Open cholecystectomy is generally reserved for selected high-risk patients (e.g., those with prior abdominal surgery with adhesions, obesity, or cirrhosis). Laparoscopic cholecystectomy may be accompanied by intraoperative endoscopic retrograde cholangiopancreatography (ERCP) (see Chapter 34 and Fig. 45–1) or transoperative radiologic examination of the common bile duct if concomitant choledocholithiasis is suspected. Factors that may predict the presence of choledocholithiasis include jaundice, pancreatitis, abnormal liver tests, and bile duct dilation.

Cholecystectomy relieves symptoms of biliary pain in virtually all patients with gallstone disease and prevents development of future complications. Dissolution of cholesterol gallstones by orally administered chenodeoxycholic acid or ursodeoxycholic acid is successful in highly selected patients but is slow and costly and requires lifelong administration. Alternative methods to eliminate gallstones, including contact dissolution and fragmentation of stones, are used rarely.

Acute Cholecystitis

Acute cholecystitis refers to distention, edema, ischemia, inflammation, and secondary infection of the gallbladder, generally resulting from obstruction of the cystic duct by gallstones or less commonly by cancer or sludge. The clinical hallmark of acute cholecystitis is the acute onset of upper abdominal pain that lasts for several hours. The pain gradually increases in severity and typically localizes to the epigastrium and/or right hypochondrium with radiation to the right lumbar, scapular, and shoulder area. Nausea and vomiting, anorexia, and low-grade fever are common. Unlike biliary pain, the pain of acute cholecystitis does not subside spontaneously. The findings on physical examination in patients with acute cholecystitis may include inspiratory arrest on palpation of the right upper quadrant (*Murphy's sign),* fever, and less commonly mild jaundice or a palpable gallbladder.

Complications of acute cholecystitis include emphysematous cholecystitis (in people with diabetes, older adults, and individuals who are immunosuppressed), empyema, gangrene, and perforation of the gallbladder. Gallbladder perforation may be *free* into the peritoneum or through a cholecystenteric fistula with gallstone migration and bowel obstruction (gallstone ileus). *Mirizzi syndrome* is the occurrence of profound jaundice resulting from extrinsic compression of the common hepatic duct by an impacted stone in the cystic duct at the gallbladder neck.

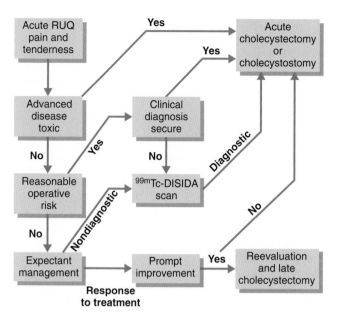

Figure 45–3 Scheme for managing patients with right upper quadrant pain and tenderness who are thought to have acute cholecystitis. This scheme is based on a policy of early operation (conventional or laparoscopic) for appropriate patients and use of cholecystostomy (operative or percutaneous) for patients who are poor operative risks.

The diagnostic modalities employed for acute cholecystitis are similar to those for biliary pain. An ultrasound examination that shows the presence of gallstones, along with pericholecystic fluid, gallbladder wall thickening, and localized tenderness over the gallbladder (*ultrasonographic Murphy's sign*), provides strong supportive evidence for acute cholecystitis. Radionuclide scanning after intravenous administration of technetium-99m (^{99m}Tc)-diisopropyl iminodiacetic acid or hepatobiliary iminodiacetic acid (HIDA) scan is the most accurate test to confirm the clinical impression of acute cholecystitis. If the gallbladder fills with the isotope, acute cholecystitis is highly unlikely, whereas if contrast enters the bile duct and duodenum, but the gallbladder is not visualized, the clinical diagnosis of acute cholecystitis is strongly supported.

Because of the high risk of recurrent acute cholecystitis, most patients need to undergo cholecystectomy, often performed within the first 24 to 48 hours after presentation or, less often, 4 to 8 weeks after an acute episode (Fig. 45–3). Cholecystostomy may be performed on patients with a high operative risk. Antibiotics are generally used when fever or leukocytosis are present. Expectant management is reserved for patients with uncomplicated disease who are not good operative candidates or those in whom the diagnosis is not clear.

Acalculous Cholecystitis

Acalculous cholecystitis accounts for 5% of cases of acute cholecystitis and carries a higher morbidity and mortality than does acute calculous cholecystitis. It is classically associated with the triad of prolonged fasting, immobility, and

hemodynamic instability such as occurs in critically ill patients, especially if they have required total parenteral nutrition or blood transfusions. Gallbladder ischemia and sludge may be important in the pathogenesis. Acalculous cholecystitis is also seen in patients with the acquired immunodeficiency syndrome, in whom it is usually caused by infectious agents such as cytomegalovirus or cryptosporidia. Ultrasonographic features include absence of gallstones, thickened gallbladder wall, and a positive Murphy's sign. As in acute cholecystitis, the gallbladder is not visualized on HIDA scan. Management includes antibiotics and cholecystectomy. If the patient is seriously ill, the gallbladder can be drained percutaneously to relieve the obstruction (cholecystostomy).

Choledocholithiasis and Acute Cholangitis

In the United States, most stones in the common bile duct (choledocholithiasis) originate from the gallbladder, occurring in up to 15% of persons with cholelithiasis. Less commonly, stones may form de novo in the biliary tree. Common bile duct stones may be asymptomatic (30% to 40%), or they may produce biliary colic, jaundice, cholangitis, or pancreatitis.

Acute (suppurative) cholangitis is defined as life-threatening infection and inflammation of the biliary tract as the result of choledocholithiasis. The classic clinical manifestations of acute cholangitis are abdominal pain, jaundice, and fever (*Charcot's triad*). Clinical findings may be absent in elderly or immunosuppressed patients. Cholangitis is a medical-surgical emergency that can lead rapidly to sepsis, shock, and death. Diagnosis is based on a compatible clinical and laboratory picture (abnormal liver function tests and leukocytosis) and radiologic or endoscopic evidence of common bile duct stones.

Treatment of acute cholangitis includes administration of broad-spectrum antibiotics and prompt removal of stones, typically with ERCP (see Fig. 45–1) and endoscopic sphincterotomy. Cholecystectomy is subsequently performed when the patient has stabilized.

Gallstone Pancreatitis

Considering that gallstone pancreatitis recurs in 25% of patients, a cholecystectomy should be performed once the patient has recovered clinically from an attack of pancreatitis. If the patient remains jaundiced during an attack of presumed gallstone pancreatitis, suggestive of a stone in the bile duct, an ERCP is performed so that stones can be extracted by sphincterotomy.

Primary Sclerosing Cholangitis

Primary sclerosing cholangitis is an idiopathic condition of nonmalignant, nonbacterial, chronic inflammatory fibrosis and obliteration of the intrahepatic and extrahepatic bile ducts. It most commonly occurs in young men (two thirds are younger than 45 years of age), often in association with ulcerative colitis (70% of patients with primary sclerosing cholangitis have ulcerative colitis). The clinical spectrum of primary sclerosing cholangitis is broad, ranging from asymptomatic patients with abnormal liver enzymes (typically an elevated alkaline phosphatase) to recurring episodes of fever, chills, abdominal pain, and jaundice. The diagnosis of primary sclerosing cholangitis is made by ERCP or MRCP, which shows characteristic changes (*beading*) of the bile ducts. No proven therapy exists for primary sclerosing cholangitis, although ursodeoxycholic acid and methotrexate are being used in some centers. Other forms of therapy include prophylactic antibiotics for prevention of recurrent bacterial cholangitis, treatment of pruritus, and repletion of fat-soluble vitamin. Endoscopic dilation of a *dominant* biliary stricture during ERCP is an effective treatment of cholestasis in selected patients. Most patients with advanced primary sclerosing cholangitis eventually progress to end-stage liver disease, and evaluation for liver transplantation is appropriate in advanced disease. One third of patients with primary sclerosing cholangitis will develop cholangiocarcinoma; therefore thorough clinical, laboratory (liver function tests and cancer markers such as CA19-9), and radiologic follow-up is warranted.

Other Disorders of the Biliary Tree

BILIARY STRICTURES

Benign biliary strictures usually result from surgical injury or chronic pancreatitis. Biliary strictures resulting from surgical injury may cause symptoms days to years later. Early diagnosis is important because strictures that partially obstruct are clinically asymptomatic and may cause secondary biliary cirrhosis. Biliary stricture should be suspected in any patient with a history of surgery of the right upper quadrant or chronic pancreatitis (typically caused by alcohol) who has a persistently elevated serum alkaline phosphatase and γ-glutamyl transpeptidase. Endoscopic balloon catheter dilation and/or stenting or surgical repair is useful in selected patients.

OTHER NONMALIGNANT CAUSES OF BILIARY OBSTRUCTION

Structural abnormalities such as choledochal cysts, Caroli's disease (congenital saccular intrahepatic bile duct dilation), and duodenal diverticula may also cause bile duct obstruction, often with secondary choledocholithiasis resulting from bile stasis. Hemobilia, with intermittent bile duct obstruction by blood clots, may be caused by hepatic injury, neoplasms, or hepatic artery aneurysms. Biliary parasites should always be considered as a cause of biliary strictures in the appropriate epidemiologic setting. *Ascaris lumbricoides* is a common cause of cholangitis and jaundice

in South America, Africa, and the Indian subcontinent. *Clonorchis sinensis* is the etiologic agent of oriental cholangiohepatitis in Korea and Southeast Asia and in immigrants to the United States. The liver fluke *Fasciola hepatica* is a leading cause of biliary strictures and cholangitis worldwide, most commonly in the Bolivian Andes.

BILIARY NEOPLASMS

Biliary neoplasms such as gallbladder cancer, cancer of the ampulla of Vater, and cholangiocarcinoma are uncommon in the United States, but gallbladder cancer is common in other parts of the world, such as Chile and Southeast Asia. Risk factors for developing these cancers include primary sclerosing cholangitis, chronic ulcerative colitis, choledochal cysts, gallstones, *C. sinensis* infection, hepatolithiasis, and α_1-antitrypsin deficiency. Cholangiocarcinoma and cancer of the ampulla of Vater usually exhibit as unremitting painless jaundice, although necrosis and sloughing of the tumor may cause intermittent biliary obstruction and the appearance of occult fecal blood. If cholangiocarcinoma is present at the bifurcation of the extrahepatic bile duct (50% of cases), the condition is known as *Klatskin's tumor*. Carcinoma of the gallbladder often produces advanced disseminated disease with weight loss, jaundice, pruritus, and large right upper quadrant mass. Symptoms of gallbladder cancer also may resemble those of acute or chronic cholecystitis, particularly when the tumor is small. Although early stage tumors can be treated surgically, most cases are diagnosed at an advanced stage and hence incurable.

GALLBLADDER POLYPS

Gallbladder polyps are outgrowths of the gallbladder mucosal wall. The majority of these lesions are not neoplastic but are hyperplastic or represent lipid deposits (cholesterolosis). Patients who have gallbladder polyps and concomitant gallstones should undergo cholecystectomy regardless of the polyp size or the presence of symptoms because gallstones are a risk factor for gallbladder cancer in patients with gallbladder polyps. Cholecystectomy should also be recommended for patients who have biliary colic or pancreatitis. Patients with gallbladder polyps greater than 1 cm in size should undergo cholecystectomy because of their malignant potential. Polyps less than 1 cm in size should be monitored with periodic imaging.

SPHINCTER OF ODDI DYSFUNCTION

Sphincter of Oddi dysfunction is a benign motility disorder leading to noncalculous obstruction to the flow of bile or pancreatic juice at the level of the pancreatobiliary junction. Patients typically have unexplained abdominal pain (biliary-type pain), with or without elevations of the liver tests. In a selected group of patients, endoscopic or surgical sphincterotomy is of value.

Prospectus for the Future

Imaging of the biliary tract is a critical component of diagnosis and treatment of biliary disorders. Magnetic resonance cholangiopancreatography and endoscopic ultrasound are increasingly used to define which patients require more invasive evaluation and treatment by ERCP. These modalities may also provide important additional information not obtainable by ERCP. As technology improves, these alternate techniques are likely to become the mainstay of diagnosis for biliary disorders, allowing ERCP to be targeted to patients who require specific diagnostic and therapeutic interventions.

A second area of focus in biliary tract disorders is the accurate diagnosis of cholangiocarcinoma, particularly in the setting of primary sclerosing cholangitis. A significant number of novel genetic and immunologic approaches for analysis of bile and biliary epithelium have recently been exploited. These markers may provide a means for significantly enhancing the sensitivity and specificity of detecting cholangiocarcinoma.

References

MacFaul GR, Chapman RW: Sclerosing cholangitis. Curr Opin Gastroenterol 21(3):348–353, 2005.

Browning JD, Horton JD: Gallstone disease and its complications. Semin Gastrointest Dis 14(4):165–177, 2003.

Chattopadhyay D, Lochan R, Balupuri S, et al. Outcome of gallbladder polypoidal lesions detected by transabdominal ultrasound scanning: A nine-year experience. World J Gastroenterol 11(14):2171–2173, 2005.

Section VIII

Hematologic Disease

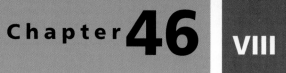

Hematopoiesis and Hematopoietic Failure

Eunice S. Wang

Nancy Berliner

*H*ematopoiesis is the process that determines the formation and development of the wide variety of cellular elements of the blood. The constituents of peripheral blood arise by a complex and carefully regulated process of ontogeny. The pluripotent hematopoietic stem cell both maintains itself by self-renewal and undergoes multilineage differentiation to generate the appropriate numbers and types of cells within the circulating blood compartment (Table 46–1). The hematopoietic system is unique in that it is constantly undergoing this full cycle of maturation by which a primitive cell develops into a variety of highly specialized end-stage cells, all of which have different life spans and are present in different quantities. The bone marrow must have the capacity to produce cells to compensate for the normal rapid turnover of hematopoietic cells that results from senescence, utilization, and migration into tissue spaces. Furthermore, it must have a reserve capacity to produce additional cells in response to unusual demands that arise from bleeding, infection, or other stresses. Understanding of the repeated cycle of cellular ontogeny and self-renewal that meets these challenges provides important insights into normal and pathologic mechanisms in hematology.

Hematopoietic Tissues

Hematopoiesis commences in the embryonic yolk sac, in which early erythroblasts in blood islands form the first hemoglobinized cells. After 6 weeks of gestation, the fetal liver begins producing primitive lymphocytoid cells, megakaryocytes, and erythroblasts, and the spleen becomes a secondary site of erythropoiesis. Hematopoiesis then shifts to its definitive long-term site in the *bone marrow*, the principal site for lifelong hematopoiesis in the normal host. Early in life, all fetal bones contain this regenerative bone marrow, but the marrow becomes progressively replaced by fat with age. In adults, active marrow resides only in the axial skeleton (sternum, vertebrae, pelvis, and ribs) and in the proximal ends of the femur and humerus. Consequently, bone

marrow samples, needed for many hematologic diagnoses, are usually obtained from the iliac crest or sternum. Under pathologic conditions that stress the capacity of the marrow space, as seen in diseases associated with marrow fibrosis (myeloproliferative diseases) or in severe inherited hemolytic anemia (thalassemia major), extramedullary hematopoiesis may be reestablished in sites of fetal hematopoiesis, especially the spleen.

Stem Cell Theory of Hematopoiesis

All mature hematopoietic cells are hypothesized to originate from a small population of *pluripotent stem cells.* Comprising less than 1% of all cells in the bone marrow, these cells bear no distinctive morphologic markings and are best defined by their unique functional properties. Stem cells have two distinctive characteristics. First, they are highly resilient and productive, capable of continuously replenishing huge numbers of granulocytes, lymphocytes, and erythrocytes throughout life. The demand for a continuous fluctuating supply of blood cells requires a hematopoietic system capable of producing large numbers of selected cells in a short time. For example, overwhelming infection by invading microorganisms triggers the release of neutrophils, whereas hypoxia or acute blood loss leads to increased red blood cell production. Second, stem cells represent a self-renewing cell population that is able to maintain its numbers while also providing a continued supply of progenitor cells of multiple different lineages.

In spite of their vast proliferative potential, under normal conditions, most stem cells are quiescent, and few cells undergo expansion or differentiation at any one time. However, their ability to proliferate is striking. Studies with lethally irradiated mice have demonstrated the ability of a few transplanted cells (termed *colony-forming unit–spleen* cells [CFU-S]) to regenerate multilineage hematopoiesis.

The signals regulating the differentiation of pluripotent stem cells into committed progenitors are unknown. Data suggest that the first step toward lineage commitment is a *stochastic* (chance) event; subsequent stages of maturation are hypothesized to occur under the influence of growth factors, or cytokines (Table 46–2). Cytokines act on different cells through specific cytokine receptors. Activation of these receptors induces signal-transduction pathways that lead to changes in gene transcription and eventual cell proliferation and differentiation. These growth factors have also been shown to act as survival factors for the developing hematopoietic cells by preventing *apoptosis* (programmed cell death). This process occurs in the cellular milieu of the bone marrow, and the well-recognized fact is that hematopoiesis also depends in part on the nonhematopoietic cells (fibroblasts, endothelial cells, osteoblasts, and fat cells) that make up the bone marrow microenvironment. Stem cell biology is also regulated by hematopoietic cytokines produced locally and by cell surface ligand interactions between stem cells and the surrounding parenchyma.

Hematopoietic Differentiation Pathway

Traditionally, hematopoiesis has been hypothesized to proceed along a tightly regulated hierarchy (Fig. 46–1) governed by effects of intrinsic transcription factors and cytokines in the bone marrow microenvironment. As more primitive cells mature under the influence of specific regulatory cytokines, they undergo several cell divisions and become *progenitor cells* committed to one lineage. They also

Table 46–1	Normal Values for Peripheral Blood Cells	
Cell Type and Size	**Mean**	**Range**
Hemoglobin	Women: 14.0 g/dL Men: 15.5 g/dL	Women: 12–16 g/dL Men: 13.5–17.5 g/dL
Hematocrit	Women: 41% Men: 47%	Women: 36–46% Men: 41–53%
Reticulocyte Count	1% 60,000/mcL	0.5–1.5% 35,000–85,000/mcL
Mean corpuscular volum	80–100	
Platelet count	250,000/mcL	150,000–400,000/mcL
Total white count	7400/mcL	4500–11,000/mcL
Neutrophils	4400/mcL (40–60%)	1800–7700/mcL
Lymphocytes	2500/mcL (20–40%)	1000–4800/mcL
Monocytes	300/mcL (<5%)	

Table 46–2	Cytokines and Their Activities	
Abbreviation	**Name**	**Effects on Hematopoiesis**
EPO	Erythropoietin	Stimulation of proliferation and maturation of erythroid progenitors; produced by the kidney in response to anemia and hypoxia; important clinically for treatment of anemia associated with low EPO levels (renal failure, anemia of chronic disease)
G-CSF	Granulocyte colony-stimulating factor	Stimulation of proliferation and maturation of granulocytes; more broad-based effect, because also increases release of *stem cells* in peripheral blood; clinically important for treatment of neutropenia and mobilization of stem cells for transplant
GM-CSF	Granulocyte-monocyte colony-stimulating factor	Proliferation of granulocyte and monocyte precursors; role unclear in steady-state hematopoiesis, because knockout has no hematopoietic phenotype
TPO	Thrombopoietin	Proliferation of megakaryocytes; results disappointing in clinical studies
M-CSF	Monocyte colony-stimulating factor	Proliferation of monocytes
IL-2	Interleukin-2	Proliferation of T cells
IL-3	Interleukin-3 (multi-CSF)	Proliferation of granulocytes, monocytes; broad-based effects, appearing to increase the proliferation of *stem cells;* not in use clinically
IL-4	Interleukin-4	Proliferation of B cells
IL-5	Interleukin-5	Proliferation of T cells, B cells; proliferation and differentiation of eosinophils
IL-11	Interleukin-11	Proliferation of megakaryocytes; undergoing clinical testing
LIF	Leukemia inhibitory factor	Proliferation of stem cells and megakaryocytes
SCF	Stem cell factor (kit ligand)	Proliferation of progenitor cells; broad-based effects on multiple lineages

CSF = colony-stimulating factor.

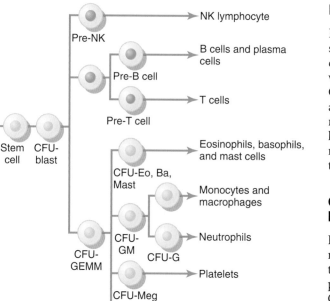

Figure 46–1 Schema of the development of the cells of the bone marrow. Ba = basophil; BFU = blast-forming unit; CFU = colony-forming unit; E = erythroid; Eo = eosinophil; G = granulocyte; GEMM = granulocyte-erythrocyte-macrophage-megakaryocyte; GM = granulocyte macrophage; Meg = megakaryocyte; NK = natural killer.

lose their self-renewal capacity. Morphologically, these cells are transformed from nonspecific blastlike cells into cells that can be identified by their color, shape, and granular and nuclear content. Functionally, they acquire distinguishing cell surface receptors and responses to specific signals. Maturing *granulocytes* and *erythroid cells* undergo several more cell divisions in the bone marrow, whereas *lymphocytes* travel to the thymus and lymph nodes for further development. *Megakaryocytes* cease cellular division but continue with nuclear replication. Eventually, these cells are released from the marrow as fully functional *erythrocytes, mast cells, granulocytes, monocytes, eosinophils, macrophages*, and *platelets*.

PLURIPOTENT STEM CELLS

The pluripotent stem cell is morphologically indistinguishable and is best identified by its expression of the cell differentiation antigen, CD34, and by its ability to form pluripotent colonies in vitro. Under the influence of interleukins (ILs)-1, -3, -6, fms-like tyrosine kinase 3 (flt 3), and a specific stem cell factor (*c-kit* ligand, or steel factor), this cell matures into either a myeloid-lineage stem cell (CFU–granulocyte-erythrocyte-macrophage-megakaryocyte [CFU-GEMM]) or a lymphoid-lineage stem cell. In the presence of granulocyte-macrophage colony–stimulating factor (GM-CSF) and IL-3, the myeloid stem cell will further differentiate into daughter cells of its named lineages (see Fig. 46–1). The lymphopoietic stem cell, in contrast, will become either a pre-B cell or a prothymocyte (pre-T cell) and will leave the marrow for further maturation.

ERYTHROID LINEAGE

Primitive erythroid precursors arising from the myeloid stem cell are called *burst-forming unit–erythroid* cells. These cells then differentiate into CFU-erythroid (CFU-E) cells, which are the committed progenitor cells of erythrocytes. CFU-E cells express receptors for erythropoietin (EPO), an 18-kd molecule produced by renal interstitial cells in response to low oxygenation states or anemia. EPO upregulates proliferation of CFU-E cells and promotes their maturation into proerythroblasts and reticulocytes, which begin to synthesize hemoglobin.

GRANULOCYTE AND MONOCYTE LINEAGES

Human GM-CSF acts early in the hematopoietic pathway to regulate maturation of the CFU-GEMM stem cell. Differentiation of this myeloid precursor into specific committed progenitors occurs under the direction of granulocyte-CSF (G-CSF) and monocyte-CSF. CFU-granulocyte cells undergo sequential transformation into easily recognizable myeloblasts, myelocytes, and eventually early polymorphonuclear neutrophils with their characteristic polysegmented nuclei. CFU-monocyte cells, in contrast, retain a single nucleus as they mature from monoblasts to promonocytes to monocytes and sometimes macrophages.

OTHER LINEAGES

Eosinophils and basophils develop from CFU-GEMM cells under the influence of IL-5 and IL-3–IL-4, respectively. The acquisition of their specific granular contents helps in distinguishing their precursors from those of early monocytes.

The development of platelets is morphologically distinct from the other lineages. CFU-GEMM cells differentiate into CFU-megakaryocyte cells, so named because these cells cease cell division early but not nuclear replication. Megakaryocytes are the only cells in the body with the capacity to double their DNA content (termed endomitosis). Over the course of several cell cycles, the maturing megakaryocyte eventually acquires several times the nuclear content of other cells in preparation for its eventual dissolution into platelets with a fraction of the cytoplasm of other hematopoietic cells. Two growth factors, *thrombopoietin* and *IL-11*, have been shown in both animal and human studies to increase platelet counts, most likely by promoting megakaryocyte development.

STEM CELL PLASTICITY

Provocative recent data has challenged the conventional paradigm of hierarchical hematopoietic stem differentiation. Experts have proposed that hematopoietic stem cells can not only differentiate back into more immature progenitors, but can also cross lineages and transdifferentiate into non-lymphohematopoietic cells such as myocytes, hepatocytes, gastrointestinal epithelial cells and neurons. Whether this *plasticity* of hematopoietic stem cells is truly an intrinsic property of adult stem cells or is caused by contaminating cells of other populations, fusion of hematopoietic cells with other tissue cells, or artifacts introduced by ex vivo stem cell isolation techniques remains controversial. Nevertheless, the suggestion that adult hematopoietic stem cells may be a dynamic renewable resource for tissue repair and regeneration holds great future promise.

Growth Factors in Clinical Use

The discovery of the factors that influence normal hematopoiesis has led to important applications to the treatment of patients with defects in hematopoietic cell production. The discovery that committed hematopoietic cells of each lineage can be stimulated to proliferate and differentiate in the presence of specific cytokines has been of great clinical utility. Advances in DNA technology have led to the synthesis and purification of recombinant human (rh) proteins with similar biologic activity in vivo. The administration of these products to patients has allowed the successful manipulation of the numbers of mature cells in the peripheral blood. For example, exogenous EPO is now considered a mainstay in the management of anemia caused by renal failure, chemotherapy, and marrow failure syndromes. The administration of rhIL-11 to patients with cancer following chemotherapy has been associated with a decreased incidence of thrombocytopenia. The use of rhG-CSF in patients with febrile neutropenia after chemotherapy or radiation therapy has been shown to reduce hospital stays and to shorten the period of high infection risk. Cytokines also have a role in mobilizing peripheral stem cells for collection before and after stem cell transplantation in patients with delayed stem cell engraftment.

Hematopoietic Stem Cell Transplantation

An increasing understanding of hematopoietic stem cell biology has fostered the development of techniques of manipulating stem cells for therapeutic purposes. The fact that the antitumor effects of most chemotherapeutic drugs and radiation therapy are dose-dependent and that both cause a major dose-limiting toxicity of myelosuppression has long been known. Hematopoietic stem cell transplantation permits the administration of intense myeloablative doses of chemotherapy and total body radiation intended to eradicate malignant cells followed by the infusion of stem cells (either from a donor or from the same patient) to replete the ablated marrow. Although historically used in the treatment of primary stem cell disorders such as leukemia, the therapeutic potential of transplantation is now being employed for patients with nonmalignant hematologic malignancies (e.g., aplastic anemia, sickle cell anemia, congenital immunodeficiencies), solid tumors (e.g., renal cell carcinoma, melanoma), and nonmalignant autoimmune diseases (e.g., amyloidosis, systemic lupus). In general, younger patients (<50 years of age) are considered the best candidates for this intensive therapy, although this too is changing in the setting of newer supportive modalities. Several modes of stem cell transplantation have been developed. In *autologous* transplantation, the patient's bone marrow or peripheral blood stem cells are collected during remission following high-dose

chemotherapy and/or rhG-CSF administration. These cells are cryopreserved, thawed, and reinfused. Such an approach incurs a higher risk of relapse as a result of reinfusion of a stem cell product that may remain contaminated with tumor. *Allogeneic* stem cell transplantation is a procedure whereby abnormally functioning hematopoietic bone marrow is eradicated and is replaced with normal bone marrow or stem cells from a compatible source, either a related or an unrelated donor. High-dose chemotherapy with or without total body radiation is administered to destroy the patient's bone marrow, followed by the infusion of new stem cells that engraft and restore normal hematopoiesis. Treatment-related morbidity is significant, with a procedure-related mortality of 10% to 30%; however, improvements in supportive care and immunomodulatory therapy designed to suppress *graft-versus-host disease* (GVHD), an autoimmune phenomenon in which intact lymphocytes in the transplanted marrow attack the host tissues, are continuing to improve outcome. Donor and patient are tested for compatibility of human leukocyte antigen (HLA) and major histocompatibility complex (MHC) proteins expressed on all cells. Three major HLA class I antigens (A, B, and C) and three MHC class II antigens (DP, DQ, and DR) have been developed. The six HLA gene loci are tightly linked on chromosome 6 and are almost always inherited on a single cluster of genes, or *haplotype*. Therefore all children are a *half-match* (haploidentical) to each of their parents, and full siblings have a 25% probability of being HLA identical to one another. HLA-matched nonrelated transplants have higher rates of GVHD than do transplants from HLA-matched related donors as a result of other minor HLA incompatibilities. Patients who receive HLA-mismatched stem cells risk acute GVHD, marrow rejection, and fatal marrow aplasia. Morbidity and mortality associated with non-HLA compatible transplants (less than five of six or all six HLA loci matched) can be prohibitive. *Syngeneic* transplantation occurs when the patient receives marrow from a twin. In these cases, the patient and donor are ideally matched, producing excellent long-term outcomes, although lack of immune response against the primary disease (*graft-versus-leukemia effect*, described later) may increase the rate of relapse.

Historically, stem cell transplants have employed allogeneic bone marrow–derived hematopoietic stem cells aspirated from the posterior iliac crest of the donor and intravenously infused into the patient following myeloablation and immunosuppressive therapy. The process of engraftment or reconstitution of normal hematopoietic function takes several weeks. Patients often require almost daily platelet and red blood cell transfusions and are hospitalized during this period of prolonged neutropenia to minimize life-threatening bacterial, viral, and fungal infections. Other complications include severe mucositis, hemorrhagic cystitis, GVHD, relapsed disease, and graft failure.

New technologies in stem cell transplantation have been stimulated by the discovery that high-dose rhG-CSF treatment results in the mobilization of large numbers of CD34+ hematopoietic progenitor and stem cells from bone marrow sites into circulating blood. In most studies, healthy donors treated with high-dose rhG-CSF had over a 10- to 15-fold transient increase in the concentration of circulating CD34+ cells over baseline levels. These mobilized hematopoietic cells can then be collected via apheresis procedures and employed in place of bone marrow cells for transplantation. When compared with marrow-derived stem cells, peripheral blood stem cells engraft more rapidly, producing improved recovery of neutrophils, erythrocytes, and platelets following myeloablation. Patients receiving allogeneic hematopoietic peripheral blood stem cell transplants for primary hematologic disorders have decreased neutrophil recovery time, transfusion requirements, and length of hospital days with rates of acute GVHD and long-term survival similar to those of marrow transplanted patients. Because peripheral blood stem cell collections often contain three- to fourfold more CD34+ stem cells and 10-fold more lymphoid cells than do harvested marrow grafts, higher rates of chronic GVHD may exist. The discovery of umbilical cord blood as another rich source of CD34+ cells have led to successful cord blood stem cell transplants, with some studies reporting similar long-term outcomes to conventional marrow or peripheral blood transplantation. Although cord transplants provide yet another therapeutic option for patients without other HLA-matched donors, the relatively low numbers of CD34+ cells found in harvested umbilical cords have so far limited this procedure to pediatric patients and smaller-size adults.

Increasing evidence indicates that the excellent response of some patients to hematopoietic stem cell transplantation is partly related to the active suppression of the disease by the newly transplanted graft, referred to as the *graft-versus-leukemia effect*. Studies have documented the compelling observation that infusion of donor lymphocytes can restore remission in patients with evidence of relapse after allogeneic transplantation for chronic myelogenous leukemia (CML). Conversely, procedures that minimize the reactivity between donor and host increase disease relapse. For example, the rate of relapse in patients who receive syngeneic (identical twin) transplants and in patients who receive T-cell–depleted marrow in an attempt to reduce GVHD is increased.

The observation of the effectiveness of donor lymphocyte infusions in controlling CML has led to the conclusion that the immunologic effects of transplanted allogeneic cells may be as important as (or more important than) cytoreduction for the cure of some hematologic malignancies. To further exploit these effects, non-myeloablative transplants are now performed, whereby patients receive conditioning and immunosuppressive regimens in doses sufficient to permit donor stem cell engraftment without aggressive cytoreduction. These *mini-transplants* result in chimeric marrows (part patient, part donor) without significant periods of cytopenias or hematopoietic compromise, although the majority of responding patients convert to a fully donor-derived marrow over time. Although still experimental, these procedures are increasingly being used in patients who are otherwise ineligible for traditional myeloablative transplantation regimens because of age (>50 years of age) and/or other co-morbidities or patients who are suffering from nonmalignant autoimmune disorders.

Disorders of Hematopoiesis

Diseases of the hematopoietic stem cell disrupt the normal regulated pattern of stem cell development and can result in underproduction of mature progeny (*aplastic anemia*), over-production of mature progeny (*myeloproliferative disease*), or failed differentiation with production of too many immature forms (*myelodysplasia* and *acute leukemia*). Myeloproliferative, myelodysplastic, and leukemic disorders are discussed in Chapter 47.

Hematopoietic Failure: Aplastic Anemia
ETIOLOGY AND PATHOGENESIS

Hematopoietic stem cell failure leads to *aplastic anemia (AA)*, a rare disorder characterized by pancytopenia (decreased production of all blood cell lineages) with a markedly hypocellular bone marrow. This disease was first described by Paul Erhlich in 1888, who noted that autopsy bone marrow specimens from a young woman who died of severe anemia and neutropenia were extremely hypoplastic. More recent studies demonstrate that patients with severe AA possess only a fraction of normal pluripotent stem cell numbers despite normal functional marrow stromal cells and normal or even elevated levels of stimulatory cytokines.

AA is an uncommon disease. The incidence ranges from 1 to 5 cases per million in the general population, predominantly in young adults (20 to 25 years of age) and older adults (60 to 65 years of age). Interestingly, the incidence is threefold higher in developing countries (Thailand and China) compared with industrialized western nations (Europe and Israel), a fact that is not explained by differences in drug or radiation exposure. A small proportion of AA cases occur in the context of a congenital bone marrow failure disorder, such as Fanconi's anemia, Schwachmann-Diamond syndrome, and dyskeratosis congenita. The most common congenital AA, Fanconi's anemia, is an autosomal-recessive disorder arising from mutations in genes encoding DNA repair proteins. Patients with autosomal-dominant dyskeratosis congenita have mutations in genes for telomerase complexes, predisposing to premature aging and enhanced marrow failure. The known causes of acquired AA are numerous (Table 46–3) and range from known myeloablative radiation exposure to common viruses and medications. Prior bone marrow toxicity from drugs, chemicals (benzene, cyclic hydrocarbons found in petroleum products, rubber glue, insecticides, chemical dyes), or radiation predisposes a patient to AA because these agents directly injure proliferating and differentiating hematopoietic stem cells by inducing DNA damage. In contrast, therapies such as cytotoxic chemotherapy (especially with alkylating agents) and radiation target all rapidly cycling cells and often induce reversible bone marrow aplasia. Despite these many causes of acquired AA, the majority of AA cases are idiopathic.

Accumulating data point to autoreactive host lymphocytes as the most likely culprits in destroying normal hematopoiesis in AA. Bone marrow stromal cells and cytokine levels in patients with AA are normal. The fact that AA also occurs in diseases of immune dysregulation and after viral infections further suggests an immune-mediated mechanism for the disease. One hypothesis is that antigens presented to the immune system by viruses or drugs trigger cytotoxic T-cell responses that then persist to destroy normal stem cells. In rare instances, 1 in 100,000 patients will develop a severe AA as an idiosyncratic drug reaction.

Table 46–3	**Causes of Acquired Aplastic Anemia**

Drugs (dose-related): chemotherapeutic agents, antibiotics (chloramphenicol, trimethoprim-sulfamethoxazole)
Idiosyncratic (many unproven): chloramphenicol, quinacrine, nonsteroidal anti-inflammatory drugs, anticonvulsants, gold, sulfonamides, cimetidine, penicillamine
Toxins: benzene and other hydrocarbons, insecticides
Viral infection: hepatitis, Epstein-Barr virus, human immunodeficiency virus
Immune disease: graft-versus-host disease in immunodeficiency, hypogammaglobulinemia
Paroxysmal nocturnal hemoglobinuria (PNH)
Radiation
Pregnancy

Table 46–4	**Differential Diagnosis of Pancytopenia**

I. Primary Bone Marrow Disorders

Aplastic anemia (AA)
Congenital aplastic anemia syndromes
Fanconi's anemia
Schwachmann-Diamond syndrome
Dyskeratosis congenital
Acquired aplastic anemia
Hypocellular myelodysplastic (MDS) syndrome
Myelofibrosis (MF)
Paroxysmal nocturnal hemoglobinuria
Acute leukemias (acute lymphocytic leukemia [ALL], acute myeloid leukemia [AML])
Hairy cell leukemia

II. Systemic Diseases with Secondary Bone Marrow Effects

Metastatic solid tumor to marrow
Autoimmune disorders (systemic lupus, Sjögren's syndrome)
Nutritional deficiencies (vitamin B12, folate, alcoholism)
Infections (overwhelming sepsis from any cause, viruses, brucellosis, ehrlichiosis, [mycobacteria])
Storage diseases (Gaucher's disease, Niemann-Pick disease)
Anatomic (hypersplenism)

Whether these individuals unknowingly possess a certain genetic predisposition to sensitivity to exposures (such as nonsteroidal anti-inflammatory drugs, sulfonamides, or the Epstein-Barr virus) commonly found in the general population is unknown.

CLINICAL FEATURES

The clinical onset of AA can be insidious or abrupt. Patients often complain of symptoms related to their cytopenias: weakness, fatigue, dyspnea, or palpitations resulting from anemia; gingival bleeding, epistaxis, petechiae, or purpura caused by low platelet counts; or recurrent bacterial infections caused by low or nonfunctioning neutrophils. Physical examination is often normal except in patients with congenital AA who may have various abnormalities.

LABORATORY STUDIES

The differential diagnosis of pancytopenia is broad and is divided into primary bone marrow disorders (such as AA, hypocellular myelodysplastic syndrome (MDS), acute leukemia, and paroxysmal nocturnal hemoglobinuria and systemic diseases with bone marrow involvement (Table 46–4). Diagnostic confirmation of AA requires bone marrow biopsy to confirm hypocellularity and to rule out other marrow processes. Normal bone marrow cellularity ranges from 30% to 50% up to age 70 and is under 20% above age 70 (**Web Fig. 46–1A**). In contrast, bone marrow cellularity in patients with AA usually ranges from 5% to 15% cellularity with increased fat accumulation and few, if any, hematopoietic cells (primarily plasma cells and lymphocytes) (**see Web Fig. 46–1B**). In AA, hematopoietic progenitor and precursor cells are morphologically normal but number less than 1% of normal levels and have been shown to be markedly dysfunctional with a decreased ability to form differentiated progenitor cell colonies in vitro. Evidence of increased blasts, dysplastic hematopoietic cells (such as pseudo-Pelger-Huët abnormalities or micromegakaryocytes) (see Chapter 47), or clonal cytogenetically abnormal cells in the peripheral blood

or marrow are diagnostic of acute leukemia or MDS and not AA, even in the setting of a hypocellular marrow. In young patients, a diagnosis of Fanconi's anemia is made by demonstrating enhanced sensitivity of cultured cells to mitomycin or diepoxybutane induced chromosomal damage. Although patients with AA typically have a low reticulocyte count (from low red blood cell production) with a paucity of blood cells (**Web Fig. 46–2A**) and macrocytic red cells (**see Web Fig. 46–2B**) on the peripheral smear, patients with other primary marrow disorders may also exhibit similar findings.

TREATMENT

Treatment for AA is based on the severity of disease. Patients with mild cytopenias can be monitored expectantly. However, patients with severe AA based on peripheral blood cells counts (see diagnosis of severe AA in Table 46–5) have a poor median survival rate without treatment, ranging from 2 to 6 months. Because most of these patients die of overwhelming infections, supportive care with broad-spectrum antibiotics, antifungal, and antiviral agents is warranted in patients with advanced neutropenia. Red blood cell and platelet transfusions are helpful in patients who are profoundly symptomatic (with care given to patients eligible for transplantation).

Current therapeutic approaches to AA are focused on either replacing the defective stem cells via stem cell transplantation or controlling an overactive immune response. All young patients with severe AA and an HLA-compatible bone

Table 46–5	**Diagnosis of Severe Aplastic Anemia**

Anemia with corrected reticulocyte counts <1%
Peripheral blood: at least two of the following:
  Neutrophil count <500/μL (0.5 × 10⁹/L) (if neutrophil count
    <200/μL, defined as very severe aplastic anemia)
  Platelet count <20,000/μL (20 × 10⁹/L)
Anemia with corrected reticulocyte counts <1%
Bone marrow: Cellularity <25%; often <5–10%

marrow donor should be considered for allogeneic bone marrow transplantation. This procedure (see Chapter 47) aims to restore normal stem cell function and offers the best chance of definitive cure of the disease. Although long-term survival is excellent in patients younger than 30 years of age transplanted from a sibling donor (75% to 90%), morbidity from the transplant itself and the management of long-term transplant related complications are continuing problems. Outcomes of patients older than 40 years or in patients without an HLA-matched related donor are poor.

The presumed immune mechanisms for drug-induced aplasia have provided the impetus for immunosuppressive approaches to the treatment of AA in older patients, in patients who are unable to find a compatible stem cell donor, and those who are otherwise ineligible for stem cell transplantation. Treatment with a combination of antithymocyte globulin (ATG) and cyclosporine (a specific T-cell inhibitor) allows for restoration of marrow function (i.e., independence from red blood cell or platelet transfusions) in 70% to 80% of patients, with a 5-year survival rate in responders of 90%. Side effects of ATG and ALG include anaphylaxis and serum sickness as a result of the horse or rabbit antigens in the antisera, which are generally self-limited. Patients often relapse and recur with this disease and may warrant retreatment with repeat ATG, newer immunosuppressive agents (such as mycophenolate mofetil), androgens, and experimental agents. Treatment with traditional chemotherapies such as cyclophosphamide has usually proven too toxic. Because endogenous cytokine production is usually high in patients with AA, the routine use of growth factors such as rhG-CSF, EPO, or stem cell factor is generally ineffective; however, in patients who are refractory, long-term administration of combination cytokines appears to have some effects in sustaining blood cell counts. Patients who survive the initial treatment of aplasia, however, remain at increased risk for the emergence of other primary hematologic disorders, such as myelodysplasia, leukemia, and paroxysmal nocturnal hemoglobinuria (PNH). The relationship of such clonal disorders to the pathogenesis of the original aplastic anemia is controversial. For example, some studies demonstrating PNH clones in patients with AA at the time of diagnosis have suggested significant overlap in these disease entities.

Prospectus for the Future

The field of stem cell biology is rapidly changing. Elucidation of normal stem cell differentiation pathways is providing important insights into the pathophysiologic factors of stem cell disorders such as AML and MDS. These observations are also furthering our understanding of the complex interplay among AA, MDS, and PNH. Finally, understanding of stem cell plasticity may open promising new avenues for stem cell therapies of a wide array of nonhematologic disease.

References

Brodsky RA, Jones RJ: Aplastic anemia. Lancet 365(9471):1647–1656, 2005.

Dorshkind K: Multi-lineage development from adult bone marrow cells. Nature Imm 3(4):311–313, 2002.

Korbling M, Estrov Z: Adult stem cells for tissue repair—a new therapeutic concept? N Eng J Med 349:570–582, 2003.

Jaffe ES, Harris NL, Stein H, Vardiman JW: WHO Classification: Pathology and Genetics of Tumours of Haematopoietic and Lymphoid Tissues. Lyon, France, IARC Press, 2001.

Young NS: Acquired aplastic anemia. Annals of Int Med 136(7):534–546, 2002.

Zhu J, Emerson SG: Hematopoietic cytokines, transcription factors and lineage commitment. Oncogene 21: 3295–3313, 2002.

VIII

Chapter 47

Clonal Disorders of the Hematopoietic Stem Cell

Eunice S. Wang

Nancy Berliner

Malignant transformation involves combined defects in cellular maturation and differentiation. The multistep theory of oncogenesis suggests that these defects are often separable and may contribute to a stepwise progression from a normal to a fully transformed cell. The continuous cycling of hematopoietic cells provides a milieu for the development of clonal genetic abnormalities that support this model. Clonal defects of the hematopoietic stem cell give rise to an array of preleukemic and leukemic disorders. Primary defects of maturation give rise to the *myelodysplastic* disorders, whereas loss of normal control of proliferation results in *myeloproliferative* disease. All of these disorders are preleukemic, with a variable but definite rate of transformation to acute leukemia.

Myelodysplastic Syndrome

ETIOLOGY AND PATHOGENESIS

The myelodysplastic syndromes are a heterogeneous group of blood disorders characterized by ineffective and disordered hematopoiesis in one or more of the major myeloid cell lines. Patients have one or more cytopenias despite the presence of normal or increased numbers of hematopoietic cells in the bone marrow. Disordered maturation is accompanied by increased intramedullary *apoptosis* (programmed cell death), which contributes to the decreased release of mature cells into the periphery.

Primary myelodysplastic syndrome (MDS) is predominantly a disease of elderly persons and occurs in approximately 1 in 500 patients between the ages of 60 and 75 years. Most cases are idiopathic and carry an overall risk of transformation to acute myelogenous or myeloid leukemia (AML) of approximately 25%. Persons with prior exposure to radiation, chemotherapy, and organic chemicals (benzene) are at increased risk of MDS. Secondary MDS, which arises following chemotherapy (alkylating agents, anthracyclines), ionizing radiation, radiolabeled antibody therapy, and bone marrow transplantation for other cancers, may occur at any age and comprises 10% to 15% of all diagnosed MDS cases. Therapy-related MDS, which usually arises more than 6 months following completion of myelotoxic therapy, is associated with a poor prognosis of cytogenetic abnormalities and evolves rapidly into AML. As therapies for primary cancers improve with prolonged survival, the incidence of secondary myelodysplasia is likely to rise.

CLINICAL FEATURES

Most patients with MDS are referred for evaluation of an incidental finding of peripheral cytopenias. Symptomatic patients usually exhibit findings related to the secondary effects of cytopenias: bleeding and bruising caused by thrombocytopenia, infection caused by leukopenia, or fatigue and dyspnea related to anemia. Physical examination is usually unremarkable, although 25% or more patients may have splenomegaly. In some patients with MDS, development of skin lesions with fever (acute febrile neutrophilic dermatosis, or Sweet's syndrome) may herald the transformation of MDS into acute leukemia.

LABORATORY STUDIES

In addition to cytopenias, the peripheral blood smear may show characteristic morphologic abnormalities. Erythroid cells are usually macrocytic, often with basophilic stippling. Neutrophils are often hypogranular and hypolobulated, with a characteristic bilobed nuclear morphology termed *pseudo-Pelger-Huët abnormality.* Pelger-Huët anomaly should be anticipated when automated differential cell counts report unusually large numbers of bands.

The bone marrow in MDS is usually normocellular or hypercellular, although 10% of patients may have a hypocellular marrow. Dysplastic changes usually occur in all three cell lines. Erythroid cells appear megaloblastic, with multinucleated cells or asynchronous nuclear-cytoplasmic development. Extremely small *micromegakaryocytes* and agranular megakaryocytes may also be present. The myeloid series shows poor maturation with a *left shift* to earlier hypogranulated myeloid forms. Although elevated numbers of myeloid blasts are common, increasing blasts are indicative of progression toward acute leukemia. Electron microscopy of the marrow shows cellular changes (prominent nuclear chromatin, cytoplasmic vacuoles, and blebs) characteristic of increased apoptosis (**Web Figure 47–1**).

In general, the diagnosis of MDS in adults is largely one of exclusion, given that marrow dysplasia may arise from numerous other causes. In the absence of clonal cytogenetic abnormalities, MDS should never be diagnosed in acute disease states, during chronic hospitalization, or within 6 months of known myelotoxic therapy (radiation, chemotherapy). Causes such as vitamin-B_{12} or folate deficiency, alcohol use, and human immunodeficiency virus infection should be considered. A patient with possible MDS and a hypocellular bone marrow must be distinguished from aplastic anemia (see Chapter 46). Cytogenetic analysis of the bone marrow confirms clonal chromosomal abnormalities in one third to one half of all patients and is diagnostic of MDS in these patients. The identification of characteristic gene deletions (5q-) and translocations diagnostic of MDS and AML subtypes, respectively, underline the likelihood of similar mechanisms of clonal myeloid stem cell injury.

In the past, MDS has been classified according to the French-American-British (FAB) group into five subtypes based on dysplastic marrow morphology and percentage of blasts: refractory anemia, refractory anemia with ringed sideroblasts, refractory anemia with excess blasts, refractory anemia with excess blasts in transformation, and chronic myelomonocytic leukemia (CMML) (Table 47–1). AML was defined as the presence of more than 30% blasts. More recently, the World Health Organization (WHO) has updated the classification criteria to incorporate FAB criteria with new bone marrow and genetic findings (Table 47–2). Because patients with blast counts exceeding 20% fared as poorly as did those with more than 30% blasts, the WHO redefined the criteria for AML as the presence of greater than 20% blasts in the marrow or blood. The five FAB subtypes of MDS were expanded to eight subtypes, with recognition of multilineage dysplasia as an important feature (i.e., refractory cytopenia with multilineage dysplasia, refractory cytopenia with multilineage dysplasia and ringed sideroblasts) and the reclassification of CMML as myelo-

proliferative-myelodysplastic syndrome. The presence of an isolated 5q- cytogenetic abnormality in myelodysplastic marrow was established as a distinct clinical syndrome characterized by anemia with normal to increased platelet count and overall slow progression to leukemia. Most importantly, certain subtypes of AML were redefined *independent of number of marrow blasts*. Identification of classical karyotypic abnormalities in a dysplastic bone marrow, specifically t(8;21), inv(16), and t(15;17), alone are now sufficient to classify these disorders as AML. Moreover, evidence of marrow dysplasia following prior chemotherapy, radiation, or other myeloablative therapy is now considered therapy-related AML (t-AML) rather than MDS because these disorders progress swiftly to acute leukemia.

PROGNOSIS AND TREATMENT

The disease course of MDS varies widely. Some patients may live normal life spans, but most die prematurely of cytopenia-related complications and/or marrow failure. Median survival in MDS is usually less than 2 years. Fifteen to 20% of patients with MDS die of AML. As in AML (see later discussion), the natural history and treatment of some MDS subtypes is correlated with specific cytogenetic abnormalities, and hence careful molecular studies of the marrow should be performed at initial evaluation. For example, MDS associated with an isolated deletion in the long arm of chromosome 5 (termed the *5q- syndrome*) has a well-characterized clinical course. Patients are predominantly older women with a refractory macrocytic anemia, normal or elevated platelet counts, and an overall better clinical prognosis. These patients often live for several years with intermittent red blood cell transfusions and have a low risk of eventual leukemic transformation. In contrast, MDS associated with deletion of the short arm of chromosome 7 (7p-) or complex cytogenetic abnormalities such as monosomy 7 or trisomy 8 often have poor clinical outcomes. In general, patients with refractory anemia and excess blasts or refractory cytopenias with multilineage dysplasia fare poorly. However, this classification correlates only approximately with overall survival (see Table 47–1). In 1998 the International MDS Risk Analysis Workshop developed an International Prognostic Scoring System (IPSS) to better predict clinical outcomes. The IPSS divides patients with MDS into

Table 47–1 French-American-British (FAB) Classification of Myelodysplastic Disorders

Subtype	Blood Findings	Bone Marrow Findings	Evolution to AML (%)	Median Survival (mo)
Refractory anemia (RA)	Blasts <1%	Blasts <5%	16	50
RA with ringed sideroblasts (RARS)	Blasts <1%	Blasts <5%	15	65
RA with excess blasts (RAEB)	Blasts <1%	Blasts 5–20%	48	15
RA with excess blasts in transformation (RAEB-T)	Blasts <1%	Blasts 20–30%	62	9
Chronic myelomonocytic leukemia (CMML)	Monocytes >1 × 10^9/L	Any number of blasts	29	23

Table 47–2 World Health Organization Classification of Myelodysplastic Syndromes

Refractory Anemia (RA)

Blood: Anemia, no or rare blasts
BM: Erythroid dysplasia only, <5% blasts, and <15% ringed
   sideroblasts

Refractory Anemia with Ringed Sideroblasts (RARS)

Blood: Anemia, no blasts
BM: ≥15% ringed sideroblasts, erythroid dysplasia only,
   <5% blasts

Refractory Cytopenia with Multilineage Dysplasia (RCMD)

Blood: Cytopenias (bicytopenia or pancytopenia), no or rare
   blasts, <1 × 10^9/L monocytes
BM: Dysplasia in ≥10% of the cells of two or more myeloid
   cell lines, <5% blasts, no Auer rods, <15% ringed sideroblasts

Refractory Cytopenia with Multilineage Dysplasia and Ringed Sideroblasts (RCMD-RS)

Blood: Cytopenias (two or more), no/rare blasts, no Auer
   rods, and <1 × 10^9/L monocytes
BM: Dysplasia in ≥10% of the cells of two or more myeloid
   cell lines, <5% blasts, ≥15% ringed sideroblasts, no Auer rods

Refractory Anemia with Excess Blasts-1 (RAEB-1)

Blood: Cytopenias, <5% blasts, no Auer rods, and <1 × 10^9/L
   monocytes
BM: Unilineage or multilineage dysplasia, 5–9% blasts, and
   no Auer rods

Refractory Anemia with Excess Blasts-2 (RAEB-2)

Blood: Cytopenias, 5–19% blasts, Auer rods ± <1 × 10^9/L
   monocytes
BM: Unilineage or multilineage dysplasia, 10–19% blasts,
   ± Auer rods

Myelodysplastic Syndrome–Unclassified (MDS-U)

Blood: Cytopenias, no or rare blasts, no Auer rods
BM: Unilineage dysplasia in one myeloid line, <5% blasts,
   and no Auer rods

MDS Associated with Isolated del(5q)

Blood: Anemia, usually normal or increased platelet count,
   and <5% blasts
BM: Normal to increased megakaryocytes with hypolobulated
   nuclei, <5% blasts, isolated cytogenetic abnormality of
   deletion 5q, and no Auer rods

BM = bone marrow.

three prognostic categories based on cytogenetic abnormalities, cytopenias, advanced age, and percentage of bone marrow blasts (Table 47–3) and has been correlated with time to leukemia transformation and overall survival.

Treatment options for MDS are unfortunately limited and are in large part dictated by the patient's age, performance status, quality of life, severity of disease, and prognostic category as defined by the IPSS and cytogenetics. The majority of patients with MDS are elderly individuals who may not tolerate or desire aggressive intervention without hope of cure; therefore most patients with MDS who are considered low risk for disease transformation are best managed supportively with chronic red blood cell and platelet transfusions. One complication of chronic transfusion therapy is iron overload caused by the delivery of between 200 and 250 mg of iron with each unit of transfused red blood cells. Excess iron is stored in macrophages and eventually accumulates in the hepatic parenchyma, myocardium, skin, and the pancreas, leading to secondary hemochromatosis or transfusional iron overload. Clinical symptoms include liver dysfunction, heart failure, hyperpigmentation, or diabetes mellitus. To prevent complications, patients who develop marked elevations in transferrin saturation and serum ferritin levels should undergo iron chelation therapy with deferoxamine (given daily over several hours by subcutaneous or intravenous infusion) or the new oral chelator Exjade. Chronic administration of recombinant growth factors (such as erythropoietin [EPO], granulocyte colony–stimulating factor, and granulocyte-macrophage colony–stimulating factor) alone or in combination have been shown to reduce transfusion needs in some patients, particularly those with low endogenous serum EPO levels. These treatments are palliative and do not affect overall survival.

Patients with high-risk MDS (defined as MDS with cytogenetic abnormalities predisposing to leukemia transformation and/or high levels of circulating blasts based in IPSS Int-2 or higher scores) are candidates for aggressive AML-based chemotherapy (see later discussion in this chapter). Standard chemotherapeutic regimens for MDS or MDS-related AML, however, often result in low remission rates and short disease-free intervals with a high relapse rate in the first 12 to 18 months and no significant prolongation of survival, even in patients who achieve remission. As in other hematologic stem cell disorders, the only curative therapy for MDS is allogeneic stem cell transplantation (see Chapter 46), ideally performed at complete remission. All patients younger than 40 years of age with MDS and human leukocyte antigen (HLA)-matched sibling donors should be offered transplantation at diagnosis. Long-term disease-free survival rates for such patients with low risk disease are over 50%. High transplant-related mortality and relapse rates associated with mismatched or unrelated donor transplants or in older patients with MDS have largely reserved these types of transplantation until development of high-risk disease.

Patients with MDS who are ineligible or unwilling to undergo induction chemotherapy or stem cell transplantation may benefit from a host of therapeutic agents targeting the biologic mechanisms of their disease. Young patients with low-risk MDS and a specific HLA (HLA-DR15) haplotype have demonstrated a 30% to 50% improvement in counts following T-cell immunosuppressive therapy with antithymocyte globulin or cyclosporine A, supporting an

Table 47-3	**International Prognostic Scoring System (IPSS) for Myelodysplastic Disorders**				
Score	**Blasts**	**Karyotype**	**Cytopenias***	**Overall Score**	**Median Survival (yr)**
0	<5%	Normal, Y–, 5q–, 20q–	0–1 cytopenias	0	5.7
0.5	5–10%	All other abnormalities	2–3 cytopenias	0.5–1.0	3.5
1.0		Abnormal 7, >3 abnormalities		1.5–2.0	1.2
1.5	11–20%			2.5 or higher	0.4
2.0	21–30%				

*Cytopenias defined as hemoglobin <10 g/dL; neutrophils <1500/μL; platelets <100,000/μL.

autoimmune cause of marrow suppression. Newer immunomodulatory agents such as thalidomide and its derivative lenalidomide have been shown to exert antigrowth effects on both MDS cells and the marrow microenvironment and have induced responses in up to a third of MDS patients. Patients with MDS characterized by the 5q- aberration are especially sensitive to lenalidomide therapy, with complete and durable response rates up to 66% and disappearance of the abnormal cytogenetic clone in the marrow. In older patients with MDS, treatment with DNA methyltransferase inhibitors such as decitabine or 5-azacytidine may reverse the abnormal hypermethylation and gene silencing contributing to leukemia transformation. In one study, outpatient administration of 5-azacytidine significantly delayed time to leukemia transformation in two thirds of older patients with transfusion-dependent MDS and resulted in notable improvements in quality of life as compared with patients treated with supportive care alone. Although not curative, these and other promising biologic therapies under study have the potential to alter the natural history of MDS and prolong overall survival.

Chronic Myeloproliferative Disorders

ETIOLOGY AND PATHOGENESIS

The chronic myeloproliferative diseases (MPD) are clonal stem cell disorders characterized by leukocytosis, thrombocytosis, erythrocytosis, splenomegaly, and bone marrow hypercellularity. The hallmark of MPD is the failure of a transformed multipotent stem cell to respond to normal feedback mechanisms regulating hematopoietic cell mass. Stem cells from patients with MPD demonstrate clonal colony growth in vitro when these cells are grown in the presence of serum without the addition of exogenous cytokines, and this technique has been used as a diagnostic test for MPD. The MPD were originally divided based on the predominant hyperproliferative cell type into polycythemia vera (PV), essential thrombocytosis (ET), chronic idiopathic myelofibrosis (IMF; also known as agnogenic myeloid metaplasia), and chronic myelogenous leukemia (CML). Hypereosinophilic syndrome (HES) and CML have recently been added to MPD (Table 47–4). Complications of MPD arise from the overproduction of one or more lineages in the blood, and all can be associated with clonal evolution to

Table 47-4	**World Health Organization Classification of Chronic Myeloproliferative Diseases**

Chronic myelogenous leukemia (Philadelphia chromosome, t[9;22] [q34;q11], *bcr-abl* positive)
Chronic neutrophilic leukemia
Chronic eosinophilic leukemia (and the hypereosinophilic syndrome)
Polycythemia vera
Chronic idiopathic myelofibrosis (with extramedullary hematopoiesis)
Essential thrombocythemia
Chronic myeloproliferative disease, unclassifiable

abl = Abelson leukemia; *bcr* = breakpoint cluster region.

acute leukemia, although, with the exception of CML, this is an infrequent and late complication. In the majority of patients with MPD, the pathogenesis of disease is now attributed to dysfunctional kinases. In CML, the Philadelphia chromosome abnormality results in a breakpoint cluster region–Abelson leukemia (*bcr-abl*) fusion protein with constitutive kinase activity, whereas in PV, IMF, and ET, a mutation involving the substitution of a valine for phenylalanine at position 617 (V617) in the Janus kinase 2 (JAK2) has been identified in the majority of patients and may account for the abnormal growth properties that characterize these stem cell disorders.

POLYCYTHEMIA VERA

Etiology and Pathogenesis

PV, literally meaning *increased red blood cells in the blood*, is a syndrome of increased red blood cell mass in the peripheral blood resulting from a clonal multipotent hematopoietic stem cell defect. When patients are first diagnosed with

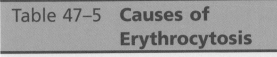

Table 47–5 Causes of Erythrocytosis

I. Relative or spurious erythrocytosis (normal red cell mass)
   A. Hemoconcentration secondary to dehydration (diarrhea, diaphoresis, diuretics, water deprivation, emesis, ethanol, hypertension, pre-eclampsia, pheochromocytoma, carbon monoxide intoxication)

II. True or absolute erythrocytosis
   A. Polycythemia vera
   B. Primary congenital polycythemia
   C. Secondary erythrocytosis caused by:
      1. Congenital causes (e.g., activating mutation of erythropoietin receptor)
      2. Hypoxia caused by carbon monoxide poisoning, high oxygen–affinity hemoglobin, high-altitude residence, chronic pulmonary disease, hypoventilation syndromes such as sleep apnea, right to left cardiac shunt, neurologic defects involving the respiratory center
      3. Nonhypoxic causes with pathologic erythropoietin production
         a. Renal disease (cysts, hydronephrosis, renal artery stenosis, focal glomerulonephritis, renal transplantation)
         b. Tumors (renal cell cancer, hepatocellular carcinoma, cerebellar hemangioblastoma, uterine fibromyoma, adrenal tumors, meningioma, pheochromocytoma)
      4. Drug-associated causes
         a. Androgen therapy
         b. Exogenous erythropoietin growth factor therapy

Adapted from Hoffman R, Benz EJ, Shattil SJ, et al (eds): Hematology: Basic Principles and Practice, 2nd ed. New York, Churchill Livingstone, 1995.

Table 47–6 WHO Criteria for the Diagnosis of Polycythemia Vera

A-Criteria

1. Elevated red cell mass (>25% above mean normal predicted value or hemoglobin >18.5 in men, 16.5 in women, or >99th percentile of reference rage for age, sex, altitude of residence)
2. No cause of secondary erythrocytosis, including absence of familial erythrocytosis and no elevation of erythropoietin caused by hypoxia (arterial pH ≤92%), high-oxygen–affinity hemoglobin, truncated erythropoietin receptor, or inappropriate erythropoietin production by tumor
3. Palpable splenomegaly
4. Clonal genetic abnormality other than the Philadelphia chromosome or *bcr-abl* fusion gene in marrow cells
5. Endogenous erythroid colony formation in vitro

B-Criteria

1. Thrombocytosis (>400 × 10⁹/L)
2. Leukocytosis (>12 × 10⁹/L)
3. Bone marrow biopsy showing panmyelosis with prominent erythroid and megakaryocytic proliferation
4. Low serum erythropoietin levels

Note: Diagnosis of PV requires the presence of the first two A-criteria along with either any one other A-criterion or two B-criteria.
abl = Abelson leukemia; *bcr* = breakpoint cluster region

---

an elevated hemoglobin per unit volume *(erythrocytosis)*, initial evaluation should focus on whether this increase reflects an enhanced red cell mass (i.e., *absolute erythrocytosis or polycythemia*) or a normal red cell mass in the presence of a decreased plasma volume (i.e., *relative erythrocytosis* caused by dehydration or other causes). The latter condition is not true polycythemia (Table 47–5). Polycythemia or absolute erythrocytosis is defined as *an absolute increase in red cell mass caused by increased red blood cell production.* Under normal conditions, the body's ability to increase red blood cell production in states of hypoxemia, anemia, hemolysis, and acute blood loss ensures continuous oxygen delivery to tissues. In response to physiologic stimuli, pluripotent stem cell precursors are activated by EPO to differentiate into erythroid progenitor cells and eventually hemoglobin-carrying erythrocytes. When numbers of mature red blood cells are adequate, a negative feedback mechanism suppresses further EPO production, and the serum hemoglobin level remains normal.

PV is a primary clonal stem cell disorder of unknown origin that is characterized by predominant erythrocytosis associated with other hematopoietic abnormalities.

Although one half of all patients have concurrent leukocytosis and/or thrombocytosis, erythrocytosis is the hallmark and cause of the most serious clinical complications of this disease. Diagnosis of PV was formerly one of *exclusion* based on an elevated red cell mass, splenomegaly, thrombocytosis, leukocytosis, lack of hypoxemia and other secondary causes of polycythemia, and elevated leukocyte alkaline phosphatase and serum B12 levels. More recent information on the disease pathophysiology has led to new diagnostic criteria (Table 47–6). Identification of an abnormal marrow clone, low serum EPO levels, and EPO-independent erythroid colony growth are now helpful in establishing a diagnosis of primary PV. Recent data has demonstrated the presence of an activating mutation in the JAK2 bound to the EPO receptor in the majority of patients with PV.

Clinical Features and Laboratory Studies

PV occurs in 1 to 3 in 100,000 people, with a median age at onset of 65 years. Early recognition and treatment of PV are important because untreated patients with PV suffer significant morbidity and mortality from thromboembolic disease in the cerebral, coronary, and mesenteric circulations. Twenty percent of patients show symptoms of arterial and venous thrombosis, and thrombosis remains the most common cause of death. Typically, patients complain of headache, visual problems, mental clouding, and pruritus after bathing. Occlusive vascular events such as stroke, transient ischemic attacks, myocardial ischemia, and digital pain, paresthesias, or gangrene are common. In addition, pulmonary, deep-venous, hepatic, and portal-venous thromboses may occur. Paradoxically, patients are also predisposed to hemorrhagic events, which are presumably caused by abnormal platelet function, and such patients may exhibit gastrointestinal bleeding. Physical examination often shows retinal-vein occlusion, ruddy cyanosis, and splenomegaly.

Peripheral blood often appears microcytic, with or without iron deficiency. Bone marrow examination shows a hypercellular marrow. Cytogenetic features at the time of diagnosis are usually normal; the development of clonal cytogenetic abnormalities heralds transformation in the later stages of disease. The incidence of the JAK2 (V617) mutation in patients with PV ranges from 65% to 97% in various studies.

Treatment

Without treatment, one half of all patients with PV die of thrombotic complications within 18 months of diagnosis. With therapy, PV is a chronic, progressive disease. The risk of transformation to myelofibrosis and myeloid leukemia is 5% to 20% over 20 years. Patients with advanced age, prior history of thrombosis, and high hematocrit values are at high risk of subsequent vascular events. Therefore intermittent phlebotomy is the mainstay of treatment and usually results in iron-deficiency anemia, which further reduces the rate of red blood cell production. Cytoreductive therapy is indicated for patients with intolerant or failing phlebotomy, with a prior history of or risk factors for thrombosis, or with symptomatic splenomegaly. Low-dose chemotherapeutic agents (such as chlorambucil, busulfan) and radioactive phosphorus (^{32}P) used in the past to treat leukocytosis and thrombocytosis have been associated with increased toxicity and risk of secondary AML. Current therapies include hydroxyurea (a low-dose cytotoxic agent that does not appear to increase leukemic risk), interferon-α (used in young patients and women during pregnancy), and anagrelide (a megakaryotoxic agent used for treating refractory thrombocytosis). Goals of therapy are hematocrit values less than 45% in men and less than 42% in women. As with all myeloproliferative disorders, initiation of cytoreductive therapy may precipitate hyperuricemia (resulting in secondary gout and uric acid stones), warranting treatment with allopurinol. Low-dose aspirin and treatment of asymptomatic thrombocytosis has been demonstrated to decrease thromboembolic events in patients with PV and is especially important in older patients with significant cardiac risk factors. In younger patients, nonsteroidal anti-inflammatory drugs and antiplatelet agents should be used judiciously because of the risk of gastrointestinal hemorrhage. With effective therapy, the long-term survival of these patients is excellent.

ESSENTIAL THROMBOCYTHEMIA

Etiology, Pathogenesis, and Laboratory Studies

ET (also known as *primary thrombocythemia*) is a pluripotent stem cell disorder resulting in elevated levels of platelets and white blood cells. Platelet function and length of survival remain normal. Because elevated platelet counts (termed *thrombocytosis*) can occur secondary to other underlying causes (including bacterial infections, sepsis, iron deficiency, autoimmune diseases, and other malignant diseases), these other causes must be excluded before a diagnosis of ET is considered. In general, diagnosis requires a platelet count exceeding $600,000 \times 10^9$/L with normal red blood cell mass, normal iron studies, and bone marrow examination showing predominant proliferation involving the megakaryocytic lineage with increased mature megakaryocytes and few, if any, dysplastic or micromegakaryocytes. Marrow immunohistochemical and cytogenetic studies to exclude diagnoses of myelodysplasia, myelofibrosis, or the Philadelphia chromosome diagnostic of CML are essential. Although no genetic or biologic marker that is 100% specific for ET has been found, new data demonstrating the presence of the JAK2 V617 mutation in over one half of samples of patients with ET have suggested reclassifying this disease into either V617F-positive or V617F-negative subtypes (Table 47–7). Unlike other MPD, bone marrow cells from patients with ET frequently do not show factor-independent colony growth, and the precise cause of this disease (and relationship with JAK2 mutational status) is under intense investigation.

Table 47–7 Proposed Diagnostic Criteria for Essential Thrombocythemia (ET)

Positive Criteria

A1: Sustained platelet count ≥600×10^9/L

A2: Bone marrow biopsy specimen showing proliferation mainly of the megakaryocytic lineage with increased numbers of enlarged, mature megakaryocytes

A3: Acquired Janus kinase 2 (JAK2) mutation*

Criteria for Exclusion

B1: No evidence of polycythemia vera (PV) (see Table 47–6)

B2: No evidence of chronic myelogenous leukemia (CML)
No Philadelphia chromosome and no *bcr-abl* fusion gene

B3: No evidence of chronic idiopathic myelofibrosis (IMF)
No collagen fibrosis and minimal or absent reticulin fibrosis

B4: No evidence of myelodysplastic syndrome (MDS)
No del(5q) or other cytogenetic abnormalities suggestive of MDS
No significant granulocytic dysplasia and few if any micromegakaryocytes

B5: No evidence of reactive thrombocytosis caused by:
Underlying inflammation or infection
Underlying neoplasm
Prior splenectomy

WHO criteria for ET require A1 + A2 + all B criteria (independent of JAK2 mutation status).
*New proposed criteria for ET distinguishes A1 + A3 + B3–B6 criteria (JAK2 mutation positive ET).
abl = Abelson leukemia; *bcr* = breakpoint cluster region.

Clinical Features and Treatment

ET is an uncommon disorder with an increasing number of cases found in patients who are asymptomatic on routine laboratory testing. Although the median age at onset is 60 to 65 years, 10% to 25% of patients are younger than 40 years of age. Up to two thirds of patients are symptomatic. Vasomotor symptoms include headache, dizziness, visual changes, and *erythromelalgia* (burning pain and erythema of feet and hands). Serious arterial thrombotic complications such as transient ischemic attacks, strokes, seizures, angina, and myocardial infarcts may occur. Patients may rarely have purpuric skin lesions or hematomas. The risk of gastrointestinal bleeding is less than 5%.

In general, patients with this disorder have long-term survival rates similar to those of age-matched control patients. The risk of leukemic transformation is extremely low (3% to 4%) in comparison with other MPD. However, morbidity from recurrent hemorrhagic and thrombotic complications is high and cannot be reliably predicted from the platelet count or platelet function abnormalities. Because treatment requires lifelong administration for disease control, assessment of risk factors and prior history of clinical signs and symptoms dictate therapeutic choices. All patients benefit from aggressive management of cardiovascular risk factors (such as smoking, hypertension, obesity, and hypercholesterolemia). Low-dose enteric aspirin may be used in all patients to relieve neurologic symptoms and carries a minimal risk of bleeding. Although young and/or pregnant patients are often not treated until they become symptomatic, older patients (>60 years) or those with a prior history of thrombosis or long disease duration may benefit from the addition of platelet-lowering agents. Hydroxyurea, a nonspecific myelosuppressive agent, is the most common first-line agent and is generally well tolerated with low long-term leukemogenic risks. Anagrelide (an oral antiplatelet agent that inhibits platelet aggregation and megakaryocyte maturation) is also used, primarily as a second-line agent after hydroxyurea failure resulting from associated acute side effects (fluid retention, palpitations), hemorrhage (with concomitant aspirin use), and risk of myelofibrotic transformation. Both of these agents are known teratogens and therefore cannot be used in the significant fraction of patients with ET who are young women of childbearing age. Because patients with ET have a high incidence of fetal wastage, interferon-α (a cytokine that alters the biologic mechanisms of the malignant clone but does not cross the placenta) in addition to heparin or aspirin has been recommended to improve pregnancy outcomes in these patients.

CHRONIC IDIOPATHIC MYELOFIBROSIS

Etiology, Pathogenesis, and Laboratory Studies

Chronic IMF (also known as *agnogenic myeloid metaplasia*) is a clonal stem cell disorder characterized by abnormal excessive marrow fibrosis leading to marrow failure. An abnormal myeloid precursor is believed to give rise to dysplastic megakaryocytes that produce increased levels of fibroblast growth factors. These cytokines act on normal fibroblasts and other stromal cells, a process that stimulates excessive proliferation and collagen deposition. Over time,

---

Table 47–8 Causes of Bone Marrow Fibrosis

I. Neoplastic causes
  a. Chronic myeloproliferative disorders: chronic idiopathic myelofibrosis (MF), chronic myelogenous leukemia (CML), polycythemia vera (PV)
  b. Acute megakaryoblastic leukemia (FAB-M₇)
  c. Myelodysplasia with myelofibrosis
  d. Hairy cell leukemia
  e. Acute lymphoblastic leukemia
  f. Multiple myeloma
  g. Metastatic carcinoma
  h. Systemic mastocytosis

II. Non-neoplastic causes
  a. Granulomatous diseases: mycobacterial infections, fungal infections, sarcoidosis
  b. Paget's disease of bone
  c. Hypo- or hyperparathyroidism
  d. Renal osteodystrophy
  e. Osteoporosis
  f. Vitamin D deficiency
  g. Autoimmune diseases: systemic lupus erythematosus (SLE), systemic sclerosis

FAB-M₇ = French-American-British acute myeloid leukemia classification subtype 7.

---

increasing fibrosis of the bone marrow leads to premature release of multipotent hematopoietic precursors into the periphery. These cells then migrate and reestablish themselves in other sites, thereby shifting hematopoiesis out of the bone marrow and into other tissues, especially the spleen and liver. This process is termed *extramedullary hematopoiesis*.

Early in the disease, patients may be asymptomatic with incidental findings of abnormal blood counts on routine laboratory tests. Although low blood counts may be present, overall platelet and red blood cell numbers at onset may be increased or normal depending on the degree of compensatory extramedullary hematopoiesis. Review of the peripheral blood will commonly reveal leukoerythroblastic changes characterized by teardrop-shape erythrocytes, giant platelets, and nonleukemic immature myeloid, erythroid, and leukocyte cells (**Web Figure 47–2**). Diagnosis of IMF is made by demonstration of bone marrow fibrosis with normal red blood cell mass, lack of Philadelphia chromosome (diagnostic of CML), splenomegaly, anemia, and evidence of extramedullary hematopoiesis. Other underlying causes of bone marrow fibrosis, both neoplastic and non-neoplastic, should also be excluded (Table 47–8).

Clinical Features and Treatment

IMF is a rare chronic disease of elderly persons with an annual incidence of 0.5 cases per 100,000. Although many patients are asymptomatic at diagnosis, over time, most will complain of progressive fatigue and dyspnea related to anemia or early satiety and left upper quadrant pain associated with splenomegaly and splenic infarction. More than one half of these patients develop massive hepatosplenomegaly. In more advanced disease, patients may have constitutional symptoms such as fever, weight loss, and night sweats. As bone marrow failure evolves, complications of neutropenia and thrombocytopenia develop. Bleeding from occult disseminated intravascular coagulation is a risk. Extramedullary hematopoiesis in the peritoneal and pleural cavities, as well as in the central nervous system (CNS) and spinal cord, may also cause symptoms.

Median length of survival is poor, ranging from 2 to 5 years. The most commonly accepted adverse prognostic factors at onset include a hemoglobin less than 10 g/dL, leukocyte count under 4000/mcL or over 30,000/mcL, a high percentage of circulating blasts, and the presence of constitutional symptoms. Other clinical factors of note are age greater than 60 years, thrombocytopenia, massive hepatosplenomegaly, and cytogenetic abnormalities. Over time, the disease may progress from a chronic phase to an accelerated phase, with acute leukemic transformation in 8% to 10% of patients. Treatment for IMF-related AML is usually ineffective. Other causes of nonleukemic death include heart failure, infection, intracranial hemorrhage, and pulmonary embolism.

At present, no medical therapy has been shown to prolong overall survival or retard disease progression significantly in IMF. Young patients with HLA-matched sibling donors may be considered for potentially curative experimental allogeneic stem cell transplantation at academic medical centers. All patients with symptomatic anemia benefit from palliative transfusions and administration of recombinant erythropoietin, androgens (danazol), or low-dose thalidomide to maintain red blood cell levels. Symptoms caused by excess thrombocytosis and leukocytosis or progressive extramedullary hematopoiesis may be managed with hydroxyurea (as a first-line agent), interferon-α (in younger patients), or low-dose chemotherapeutic agents such as busulfan, interferon-α, or mephalan (with long-term leukemogenic potential). Splenectomy is offered to patients with symptomatic splenomegaly, refractory thrombocytopenia, hypermetabolic symptoms, and portal hypertension but may be associated with significant operative morbidity and mortality. Patients who not surgical candidates may benefit from palliative splenic irradiation or from new biologic agents under development that target the abnormal marrow microenvironment.

CHRONIC MYELOID LEUKEMIA

Etiology and Pathogenesis

CML is one of the MPD characterized by a predominant increase in the granulocytic cell line associated with concurrent erythroid and platelet hyperplasia. It is unique among the MPD in its characteristic natural history, including an inevitable transformation to acute leukemia. CML was the first hematologic malignant disease shown to be associated with a specific chromosomal abnormality. More than 95% of patients with CML have a clonal expansion of a stem cell that has acquired the Philadelphia chromosome, a balanced translocation between chromosomes 9 and 22 (t[9;22] [q34 : q11]). This translocation fuses the *abl* virus gene on chromosome 9 to the *bcr* gene on chromosome 22 and generates a novel *bcr-abl* oncogene. The gene product, the *bcr-abl* protein, is a constitutively active cytoplasmic tyrosine

kinase that has been found to induce leukemia in hematopoietic stem cells. The expression of the *bcr-abl* fusion protein activates multiple downstream signal transduction pathways to permit proliferation independent of cytokine and stromal regulation and render cells resistant to chemotherapy and normal programmed cell death *(apoptosis)*. A subset of patients with CML but lacking a detectable Philadelphia chromosome have subsequently been found to possess detectable *bcr-abl* fusion products by reverse transcriptase–polymerase chain reaction (RT-PCR), indicating a subchromosomal translocation resulting in the same pathologic gene product. The diagnosis of CML is made via detection of the Philadelphia chromosome using karyotype, PCR, or fluorescent in situ hybridization (FISH) analysis. Identification of the Philadelphia chromosome has allowed for easier diagnosis and monitoring of disease. Exquisitely sensitive and quantitative RT-PCR procedures not only allow for detection of up to a single *bcr-abl*–positive cell in 10^5 to 10^6 peripheral cells, but also permit measurement of disease status in both peripheral blood and marrow samples. Responses to treatment regimes in CML are now defined as hematologic (restoration of normal peripheral blood cell counts), cytogenetic (loss of the Philadelphia chromosome by normal karyotypic or FISH analysis), and molecular (loss of detection of the *bcr-abl* gene by RT-PCR) remissions.

Clinical Features and Laboratory Studies

CML is the most common type of the MPD, accounting for 15% to 20% of all leukemias and occurring in 1 in 100,000 people. The median age of onset is 53 years, but patients of any age may be affected. Up to 40% of patients are initially asymptomatic. Other patients exhibit fatigue, lethargy, shortness of breath, weight loss, easy bruising, and early satiety. Physical examination usually shows splenomegaly. Laboratory values are significant for a markedly elevated white blood cell count (median 170×10^9/L), with low leukocyte alkaline phosphatase levels, high uric acid and lactate dehydrogenase levels, and thrombocytosis. Review of the peripheral smear in chronic-phase CML demonstrates a full complement of myeloid cells in all stages of granulocytic development, including immature myeloblasts (usually numbering less than 5%), myelocytes, metamyelocytes, basophils, eosinophils, bands, and neutrophils. In contrast, the peripheral blood smear in reactive granulocytic hyperplastic states (termed *leukemoid reaction*) caused by acute infection or sepsis, consists predominantly of mature neutrophils and bands with few myelocytes, basophils, or eosinophils. The bone marrow in CML is densely hypercellular, with an overwhelming predominance of myeloid cells at all developmental stages and reticulin fibrosis (**Web Figure 47–3**). Detection of the Philadelphia chromosome by conventional or molecular tests will confirm the diagnosis of CML.

The natural history of CML is characterized by a *chronic phase* that evolves into an acute blast crisis. Patients are typically diagnosed during the chronic phase, an indolent stage lasting 3 to 5 years. Peripheral white blood cell counts are elevated with eosinophilia and basophilia (<20%) but few blasts (<5%). With control of peripheral blood cell counts, patients are essentially asymptomatic during this period. Eventually, the disease enters an *accelerated phase* characterized by fever, weight loss, worsening splenomegaly, and bone pain related to rapid marrow cell turnover. Despite therapy, the white blood cell count rises with increased numbers of circulating blasts (between 10% and 19%). The presence of increased peripheral blood basophils (≥20%) results in histamine production, with symptoms of pruritus, diarrhea, and flushing. During accelerated phase, patients may also develop increasing splenomegaly, persistent thrombocytopenia, or thrombocytosis and leukocytosis, with new clonal cytogenetic abnormalities in marrow cells. The last phase of CML, termed *blast crisis,* marks an evolution to acute leukemia, in which marrow is replaced by 20% or more blasts, with accompanying loss of normal mature cellular elements in the marrow and periphery and extramedullary blast proliferation. Death occurs in a few weeks to months. Two thirds of patients develop AML, whereas the rest develop acute lymphoid leukemia, a finding confirming that the initial neoplastic cell is an early stem cell capable of multilineage differentiation.

Treatment

Historically, oral chemotherapeutic agents such as hydroxyurea and busulfan were used to reduce myeloid cell numbers in patients during the chronic phase of CML. Although these drugs decreased the rate of acute disease complications, they did not alter long-term prognosis or prevent progression to blast crises. Treatment with interferon-α results in hematologic remissions in 60% to 80% of patients with chronic-phase CML and was the first agent to induce cytogenetic responses in 20% to 30% of these patients. Achievement of cytogenetic remissions using interferon-α was associated with prolonged survival, with higher response rates obtained by combining chemotherapy with interferon. Although the majority of patients treated with interferon-α still possessed cells with detectable *bcr-abl* translocation by PCR and remained at risk of disease relapse, many remained in hematologic and cytogenetic remission for several years. The mechanism by which the disease is controlled with interferon despite detectable *bcr-abl*–positive cells remains unknown. Unfortunately, patients with accelerated and/or blast crisis CML did poorly with interferon, and high-dose chemotherapy regimens in these patients induced only transient responses, with durations of less than 6 months.

The development of imatinib mesylate (Gleevec, formerly known as STI-571) for the treatment of CML has been heralded as the first successful targeted therapy for cancer. Gleevec is a rationally designed competitive inhibitor of the *bcr-abl* platelet-derived growth factor and *c-kit* tyrosine receptor kinases. Preclinical studies demonstrated that Gleevec potently inhibited the growth of *bcr-abl*–expressing CML cell lines and progenitor cells in vitro and prolonged survival in animal tumor models. Initial early clinical trials of this orally active tyrosine kinase inhibitor were begun in 1998 in CML patients who had failed interferon-α. Not only was the drug well tolerated with manageable side effects, but also 96% of patients receiving a dose greater than 300 mg/day for 4 weeks achieved hematologic remissions, with 33% obtaining cytogenetic remissions after 8 weeks. These striking results have been confirmed in multiple trials, and Gleevec was subsequently shown to be superior to interferon-α and cytarabine in inducing remissions in untreated patients who were newly diagnosed with chronic-phase CML. In these patients, Gleevec not only induced high

rates of cytogenetic and hematologic remissions, but also appeared to delay progression of disease to accelerated and blast phases. High-dose Gleevec has also been demonstrated to be effective in inducing transient hematologic and cytogenetic remissions in some patients with accelerated and blast CML.

Although Gleevec therapy is now standard of care for treatment of CML, with more than 80% of newly diagnosed patients in chronic phase CML achieving complete cytogenetic responses (CCR) on therapy, this agent does not cure the disease. Similar to interferon treatment, the majority of patients achieving CCR on Gleevec still demonstrate persistence of *bcr-abl*–positive leukemic CML stem cells by sensitive molecular testing. Therefore lifelong Gleevec therapy is required to control disease. Moreover, resistance to Gleevec therapy has already been documented, particularly in patients with more advanced stages of CML when *bcr-abl*–expressing cells acquire additional cytogenetic abnormalities and mutations in the *bcr-abl*–receptor kinase domain. Therefore even patients with excellent control of chronic-phase CML on Gleevec therapy remain at risk of eventual disease progression and therapy failure. Studies examining the effects of high-dose Gleevec and newer more potent *bcr-abl* kinase inhibitors on Gleevec-resistant CML are currently under investigation.

Complete eradication of all cells that contain detectable levels of the *bcr-abl* translocation occurs only after allogeneic stem cell transplantation. Given the lack of long-term data with Gleevec, young patients with an HLA-matched donor should still be offered potentially curative allogeneic bone marrow transplantation as definitive therapy at the time of diagnosis of chronic-phase CML. Up to 50% to 75% of such patients can achieve long-term survival following transplant, with an improved outcome (for reasons that are not clear) in patients undergoing the procedure within a year of diagnosis. Increasing evidence indicates that the excellent response of patients with CML to stem cell transplantation is partly related to the active suppression of the disease by the newly transplanted graft, referred to as the *graft-versus-leukemia effect* (GVLE). After allogeneic bone marrow transplantation for CML, RT-PCR reveals that most patients continue to have detectable *bcr-abl* transcripts, especially within the first 6 months after the transplantation procedure. However, detection of *bcr-abl* in this setting is not predictive of imminent hematologic or cytogenetic relapse. Eventually, many patients become *bcr-abl* negative, although low levels of *bcr-abl* transcripts have been shown to persist in some patients in long-term remission. That this characteristic is related to GVLE is supported by several observations. Patients with *graft-versus-host disease* (an autoimmune phenomenon in which intact lymphocytes in the transplanted marrow attack the host tissues) have a decreased rate of relapsed CML. Studies have also resulted in the compelling observation that infusion of donor lymphocytes can restore remission in patients with evidence of relapse after allogeneic transplantation for CML. Conversely, procedures that minimize the reactivity between donor and host increase disease relapse. For example, the rate of relapse in patients who receive syngeneic (identical twin) transplants and in patients who receive T cell–depleted marrow in an attempt to reduce graft-versus-host disease is increased. Because this approach reduces the allogeneic reactivity of the donated stem cells, these patients have a relapse rate of up to 60%, heralded by increasing levels of PCR positivity before hematologic and cytogenetic relapse.

Given the excellent control of CML that Gleevec achieves, the optimal role and timing of allogeneic stem cell transplantation for patients with CML remain unclear. Recently published guidelines suggest that the risks and benefits of allogeneic stem cell transplantation versus Gleevec therapy should be discussed in all patients with chronic-phase CML at the time of diagnosis, with emphasis on patient age, performance status, donor availability, and personal preference; if transplantation is declined, then patients should be reassessed after 3, 6, and 12 months of Gleevec therapy to determine appropriate therapeutic response. Patients who fail to achieve hematologic (after 3 months) or major cytogenetic responses (after 6 to 12 months) should be reconsidered for transplantation, Gleevec dose escalation, interferon-α treatment with cytarabine, or clinical trials with newer biologic agents. Patients in whom RT-PCR demonstrates a three-log or greater reduction in the level of *bcr-abl* transcripts at 1 year have an excellent prognosis, with less than 5% molecular progression and no evolution to accelerated phase or blast crisis at 4 years. Transplantation remains the only curative therapeutic option for advanced-stage CML. Patients with accelerated-phase CML may be treated with high-dose Gleevec while awaiting allogeneic transplantation (if feasible) or experimental therapies, whereas those in blast-phase CML should undergo induction chemotherapy based on acute leukemia regimens followed by transplantation or clinical trials.

Overall, the advances in the management of CML have been impressive. The median length of survival in CML has risen dramatically from a few months to years in the first half of the 20th century, to 6 years for interferon-treated patients, to more than 10 years in patients who undergo allogeneic transplantation. The impact of Gleevec (and newer *bcr-abl* kinase inhibitors presently in development) is likely to prolong survival of patients with CML even more dramatically in the years to come.

ACUTE LEUKEMIAS

Etiology and Pathogenesis

The *acute leukemias* are clonal hematopoietic malignant diseases that arise from the malignant transformation of an early hematopoietic stem cell. Leukemias occur in 8 to 10 in 100,000 people (in comparison with 42 in 100,000 for prostate cancer and 62 in 100,000 for breast cancer). Acute leukemias are classified by cell lineage into AML and *acute lymphoblastic leukemia* (ALL) based on morphology, cytogenetics, cell surface and cytoplasmic markers, and molecular studies. Ninety percent of adult leukemia is AML (with 10% being ALL), whereas 90% of childhood leukemia is ALL (with 10% being AML). The distinction between AML and ALL is crucial diagnostically, therapeutically, and prognostically. AML can be distinguished from ALL by cell morphology and by the presence of *Auer rods*, formed by the aggregation of myeloid granules (**Web Figure 47–4**). Further immunophenotyping of blast cells using cell surface antigens, cytochemistry, and immunohistochemistry confirms cells as being of either myeloid or lymphoid origin (Table 47–9). Morphologic subgroups of both ALL and AML were originally defined by the FAB group and, more recently, revised by the WHO, incorporating newer biologic information (Table 47–10).

Table 47–9   Laboratory Aids to Distinguish Between Acute Myeloblastic Leukemia (AML) and Acute Lymphoblastic Leukemia (ALL)

	AML	ALL
Morphology of leukemic blasts	Granules in cytoplasm; Auer rods* may be present	Agranular, basophilic cytoplasm
	Multiple nucleoli	Regular, folded nucleus with one prominent nucleolus
	FAB (see Table 47–2) subclassification M_1–M_7	FAB subclassification, L_1–L_3
Histochemistry	Myeloperoxidase-positive	Myeloperoxidase-negative; PAS-positive
Cytoplasmic markers	—	Terminal deoxynucleotidyl transferase (Tdt)—positive
Surface markers (% of cases)	—	B-cell markers (5%)
		T-cell markers (15–20%): CD 2, 3, or 5
		CALLA (50–65%): CD 10
Cytogenetic and oncogenetic abnormalities	M_3: t(15;17) Abnormal retinoic acid receptor gene	L3: t(8;14) abnormal *c-myc*
	M_5: t(9;11)	Some ALL: Ph¹ *bcr-abl* fusion gene

*Auer rods are a linear coalescence of cytoplasmic granules that stain pink with Wright's stain.
CALLA = common acute lymphoblastic leukemia antigen; FAB = French-American-British classification system; PAS = periodic acid-Schiff.

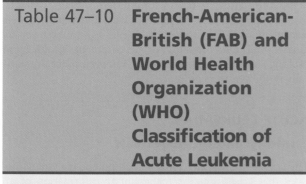

Table 47–10 French-American-British (FAB) and World Health Organization (WHO) Classification of Acute Leukemia

FAB Classification of Acute Myeloid Leukemia

M_0—Acute myelocytic leukemia with minimal differentiation
M_1—Acute myelocytic leukemia without maturation
M_2—Acute myelocytic leukemia with maturation (predominantly myeloblasts and promyelocytes)
M_3—Acute promyelocytic leukemia
M_4—Acute myelomonocytic leukemia
M_5—Acute monocytic leukemia
M_6—Erythroleukemia
M_7—Megakaryocytic leukemia

FAB Classification of Acute Lymphoblastic Leukemia

L_1—Predominantly *small* cells (twice the size of normal lymphocyte), homogeneous population; childhood variant
L_2—Larger than L_1, more heterogenous population; adult variant
L_3—*Burkitt-like* large cells, vacuolated abundant cytoplasm

WHO Classification of Acute Leukemia

I. Acute myeloid leukemia (AML)
  a. AML with recurrent genetic abnormalities
    AML with t(8;21)(q22;q22); (AML [CBFα/ETO])
    AML with abnormal bone marrow eosinophils inv(16)
      (p13;q22) or t(16;16) (p13;q22); (CBFβ/MYH11)
    Acute promyelocytic leukemia (AML with t(15;17)
      (q22;q12) (PML/RARα) and variants
    AML with 11q23 (MLL) abnormalities
  b. AML with multilineage dysplasia
  c. AML and MDS, therapy related
    Alkylating agent related
    Topoisomerase II inhibitor related
  d. AML not otherwise defined
    AML minimally differentiated
    AML without maturation
    AML with maturation
    Acute myelomonocytic leukemia
    Acute monoblastic and monocytic leukemia
    Acute erythroid leukemia
    Acute megakaryoblastic leukemia
    Acute basophilic leukemia
    Acute panmyelosis with myelofibrosis
    Myeloid sarcoma
  e. Acute leukemia of ambiguous lineage
    Undifferentiated acute leukemia
    Bilineal acute leukemia
    Biphenotypic acute leukemia
II. Acute lymphocytic leukemia
  a. Precursor B lymphoblastic leukemia/lymphoblastic lymphoma
  b. Precursor T lymphoblastic leukemia/lymphoblastic lymphoma

CBFα = core binding factor α; CBFb = core binding factor β; ETO = "eight twenty-one"; MDS = primary myelodysplastic syndrome; MLL = mixed lineage leukemia; MYH11 = myosin heavy chain gene; PML = promyelocytic leukemia; RARα = retinoic acid α-receptor.

The pathogenesis of acute leukemia is under intense investigation. Many patients with acute leukemia have detectable characteristic clonal chromosomal abnormalities; however, the role of all but a few of these aberrations in malignant transformation is unknown. In general, unregulated proliferation of immature cells that are incapable of further differentiation *(blasts)* results in marrow replacement and hematopoietic failure. Known risk factors for leukemia are high-dose radiation exposure and occupational exposure to benzene. Patients with secondary AML after exposure to prior chemotherapy have usually received alkylating agents (such as chlorambucil, melphalan, and nitrogen mustard) or topoisomerase II inhibitors (epipodophyllotoxins). An increased incidence of leukemia is also found in patients with chromosomal instability disorders such as Bloom's syndrome, Fanconi's anemia, Down syndrome, and ataxia telangiectasia.

Clinical Features

Patients exhibit clinical evidence of bone marrow failure (similar to other hematopoietic disorders). Complications of disease include anemia, infection, and bleeding from peripheral cytopenias. In addition, proliferating blasts infiltrating the bone marrow may cause bone pain. Blasts also invade other organs and lead to peripheral, mediastinal, and abdominal lymphadenopathy, hepatosplenomegaly, skin infiltration, and meningeal involvement.

Treatment

Therapy of acute leukemias is divided into several stages. *Induction therapy* is directed at reducing the number of leukemic blasts to an undetectable level and restoring normal hematopoiesis *(complete remission)*. At complete remission, however, significant subclinical disease persists, requiring further therapy. Subsequent *consolidation therapy* involves continuing chemotherapy with the same agents to induce elimination of further leukemic cells. With development of a wider range of effective agents, *intensification therapy* has been introduced, involving the use of high-dose therapy with different *non–cross-reactive* drugs, to eliminate cells with potential primary resistance to the induction regimen. *Maintenance therapy* employs low-dose intermittent chemotherapy given over a prolonged period to prevent subsequent disease relapse. The goal of therapy is to induce remission (defined as the presence of less than 5% blasts in the bone marrow and recovery of normal peripheral blood counts).

Adverse clinical prognostic factors for AML and ALL are similar despite widely different treatment approaches. In general, age exceeding 35 years, secondary leukemia or prolonged preleukemic states, high initial leukocyte count, unfavorable cytogenetic abnormalities, and prolonged time to achieve response to initial treatment are associated with poorer outcomes (Tables 47–11 and 47–12).

ACUTE LYMPHOBLASTIC LEUKEMIA

Classification

ALL is a neoplasm of immature lymphoblasts expressing markers of B- or T-cell lineage. The prior FAB classification system divided ALL into three subtypes (L_1, L_2, and L_3) based

Table 47–11 Prognostic Factors in Acute Lymphoblastic Leukemia (ALL)

Factor	Favorable	Unfavorable
Age	2–10 years	Below 2 years or above 10 years
WBC count at diagnosis	Less than 30,000	Greater than 50,000
Phenotype	Precursor B	Precursor T
Chromosome number	Hyperdiploidy	Pseudo/hypodiploidy, near tetraploidy
Chromosome abnormality	t(12;21)	c-Myc alterations (t[8;14], t[2;8], t[8;22])
		MLL alterations (11q23)
		Philadelphia chromosome t(9;22)
CNS disease at diagnosis	No	Yes
Sex	Women	Men
Ethnicity	Caucasian	African American, Hispanic
Time to remission	Short (<7–14 days)	Prolonged time to remission or failure to achieve remission

CNS = central nervous system; MLL = mixed lineage leukemia; WBC = white blood cell.

Table 47–12 Prognostic Factors in Acute Myeloid Leukemia

Clinical

Age >60 years (median for AML = 65 yr of age)
Therapy related or with antecedent hematologic disorder (MDS)
Poor performance status
White blood cell count >20,000–30,000/mm³
Presence of extramedullary disease sites

Biologic

Karyotype: favorable, intermediate, poor (see below)
Immunophenotype: biphenotypic
Abnormal fms-like tyrosine kinase 3 caused by mutation or internal tandem duplication
Multidrug resistance protein expression

Cytogenetic

Abnormality: CR rate, 5-year survival rate

Favorable Prognosis

inv(16), t(16;16), del(16q), t(8;21), t(15;17), 70–95%, 50–85%

Intermediate Prognosis

Normal karyotype, trisomy 8 only, t(9;11), 50–80%, 30–45%

Other Abnormalities not Listed

Poor prognosis:
  5/del(5q), 7/del(7q), inv(3q), t(3;3), 30–50%, 5–15%
  t(6;9), 11q23, t(9;22), complex (≥3 abnormalities)

AML = acute myeloid leukemia; CR = complete remission.

on the morphology of malignant cells. L_1 cells are small, uniform lymphoblasts with indistinct nucleoli and make up 25% to 30% of cases. L_2 cells are larger, more pleomorphic, and occur commonly in adults (65%), whereas the L_3 subtype with large basophilic cells and vacuoles is the most infrequent type, occurring in 2% to 3% of patients. More recently, the WHO system has defined only two subtypes of ALL (precursor B and precursor T ALL) based on the lineage of specific cell surface antigens found on these cells during normal maturation (see Table 47–10). The former ALL-L_3 subtype representing a mature B-cell neoplasm has been reclassified as Burkitt's lymphoma or Burkitt's leukemia.

Clinical Features

ALL is predominantly a pediatric malignancy, with 75% cases occurring in children younger than 6 years of age. Progress in the understanding and treatment of this disease in the 1990s has led to cure rates of up to 80% in children with ALL but only 20% to 40% of adult patients with ALL. These poorer outcomes in adults likely reflect differences in the biologic mechanisms of disease in these different age groups, as well as the inability of older patients to tolerate the intensive chemotherapy and/or transplantation procedures required to achieve long-term responses. In addition, up to 50% of ALL in older adults demonstrate the Philadelphia chromosome abnormality, t(9;22), which has been associated with chemoresistant disease and increased risk of central nervous system disease, as compared with only 20% of pediatric patients with ALL (see Table 47–11).

Treatment

Treatment of ALL is lengthy and involves multiple chemotherapy agents given over a period of 2 to 3 years. Induction chemotherapy typically includes vincristine, corticosteroids, and L-asparaginase, with the addition of an anthracycline, cytarabine, and/or cyclophosphamide in adult patients. Given the propensity of ALL cells to reside in the CNS and testes (so called *sanctuaries* for leukemia cells because standard systemic chemotherapy does not penetrate into these sites), patients should undergo lumbar puncture at time of ALL diagnosis, with routine administration of intrathecal methotrexate and/or whole brain irradiation as an adjunct to systemic induction and consolidation chemotherapy. Complete remission rates are 97% to 99% in children and 75% to 90% in adults. After normal hematopoiesis returns, patients then undergo consolidation and intensification therapy with multiple drugs to eradicate disease. For unknown reasons, ALL tends to relapse several months to years after initial remission. Studies have shown that the frequency of relapse is reduced by maintenance chemotherapy given for up to 2 to 3 years after initial remission achievement. Such prolonged treatment may eliminate slow-growing leukemic clones, prevent further transformation, and/or destroy occult disease in other (particularly CNS) sites.

In ALL, as in AML, the worse the prognosis is, the earlier transplantation should be offered. Studies have shown that patients with Philadelphia chromosome positive (Ph+) ALL, high white blood cell counts, or prolonged time to first remission benefit from bone marrow transplantation in first remission. Early transplantation has achieved 5-year survival rates of 40% to 44%, in comparison with 20% with other therapies. Unfortunately, outcomes for high-risk patients with ALL without an available HLA-matched donor treated with either standard therapy or autologous stem cell transplantation are poor, and no significant benefit has been seen with autologous transplantation over maintenance therapy for ALL. Disadvantages of autologous transplantation for any acute leukemia include higher rates of relapse caused by the lack of GVLE and possible marrow graft contamination with residual leukemia cells despite various marrow purging techniques. Instead, such patients should be considered for HLA-matched unrelated donor allogeneic transplantation or experimental therapies.

Treatment of Ph+ ALL with single-agent, high-dose Gleevec, the specific tyrosine kinase inhibitor of the *bcr-abl* fusion protein used in CML, results in only transient clinical responses. Early studies combining Gleevec with standard induction and consolidation chemotherapy for Ph+ ALL appears to improve outcome versus chemotherapy alone, and further studies investigating the merits of Gleevec with autologous and allogeneic stem cell transplantation for patients with Ph+ ALL are ongoing.

Most ALL relapses occur within 2 years of initial treatment, with leukemic cells recurring in the bone marrow, CNS, or testes. Although relapsed disease responds to local irradiation and further chemotherapy, the duration of second remissions is usually less than 6 months, with an overall 3-year survival rate of less than 10% with chemotherapy alone. All patients whose disease has relapsed and for whom appropriate donors are found should be considered for allogeneic stem cell transplantation or experimental treatments. Again, autologous stem cell transplantation for refractory or relapsed ALL is not routinely recommended because ALL blasts appear to be more chemoresistant with higher failure rates after treatment.

ACUTE MYELOID LEUKEMIA

Classification

AML occurs primarily in older adults, with a median age at diagnosis of 65 years. The original FAB classification of AML divided the disease into eight subtypes (M_0 to M_7) based on morphologic criteria and stage of cellular differentiation (myeloblastic, monocytic, erythroleukemic, megakaryoblastic). In contrast to ALL, some of these FAB subsets correlate with specific clinical syndromes that help determine treatment approaches, as well as prognosis. The most common FAB subtype of AML in adults is AML-M_2. Patients with AML-M_3 (acute promyelocytic leukemia) often exhibit spontaneous bleeding from disseminated intravascular coagulation. Patients with AML-M_4 or -M_5 disease (monocytic leukemias) have high levels of circulating white blood cells and may have swollen gums as a result of infiltration with blasts. Patients with megakaryoblastic leukemia (AML-M_7) have significant marrow fibrosis and usually exhibit organomegaly and pancytopenia similar to those seen in patients with myelofibrosis and myeloid metaplasia. The WHO has recently modified the classification of AML to incorporate new findings. In particular, the number of marrow blasts required for AML diagnosis was decreased from 30% in the FAB system to 20% in the WHO classification, reflecting data that patients with 20% to 30% blasts fared similarly to those with more than 30% blasts. Most importantly, as mentioned previously, certain subtypes of AML were redefined *independent of number of marrow blasts.* Identification of classical karyotypic abnormalities in a dysplastic bone marrow, specifically t(8;21), inv(16), and t(15;17), alone are now sufficient to classify these disorders as AML. Marrow dysplasia following prior chemotherapy, radiation, or other myeloablative therapy is now considered t-AML rather than MDS, given that these disorders proceed swiftly into leukemia (see Table 47–10).

Laboratory Studies

Laboratory evaluation of patients with AML typically show white blood cell counts ranging from neutropenic levels ($1 \times 10^9/L$) to extreme leukocytosis ($200 \times 10^9/L$). Severe thrombocytopenia, normocytic anemia, and circulating peripheral blasts are also common. Bone marrow aspirate and biopsy show a profusion of myeloblasts numbering 20% to 100% with depressed production of normal mature cells. Identification of cytogenetic abnormalities unique to AML subtypes, such as t(15;17) found in acute promyelocytic leukemia and inv(16) found in AML with abnormal bone marrow eosinophils, are crucial for diagnosis, therapy, and prognosis, thereby rendering karyotypic analysis an essential part of any suspected AML diagnosis.

Clinical Features

Newly diagnosed patients with AML may exhibit unique acute emergencies requiring immediate stabilization. *Leukostasis* (also called *hyperleukocytosis syndrome*) caused by high levels of circulating blasts (>80,000 to 100,000) leads to diffuse pulmonary infiltrates and acute respiratory distress. Blast cells may also injure surrounding vasculature, causing life-threatening CNS bleeding. In addition, high cell numbers result in the release of cellular breakdown products, hypokalemia, acidosis, and hyperuricemia that often induce renal failure. Treatment of these complications should be instituted as soon as possible with leukopheresis, hydroxyurea, and induction chemotherapy to reduce circulating cell numbers, along with hydration and urine alkalinization to reduce urine crystallization and dialysis, if indicated. Red blood cell transfusions are contraindicated in patients with high numbers of circulating blast cells because of the risk of further increases in blood viscosity. CNS complications such as intracranial bleeding, cranial nerve invasion, and leukemic meningitis are treated with emergency irradiation of the CNS.

Treatment

Treatment of AML differs from that of ALL in many ways. Therapy for AML involves induction chemotherapy with consolidation chemotherapy administered over 4 to 6 months. Unlike in ALL, maintenance chemotherapy has no established role in prolonging remissions in AML. Routine CNS prophylaxis is also not necessary in AML. Standard induction chemotherapeutic regimens employing cytosine arabinoside (cytarabine) with high-dose anthracycline (daunorubicin or idarubicin) leads to complete remissions in 60% to 80% of younger adults with de novo AML. Lower remission rates are achieved in older adults (>65 years of age), those with antecedent hematologic diseases before AML, or t-AML. After achieving complete remission, depending on their prognostic category (discussed later), age, and performance status, patients may be offered further intensive consolidation chemotherapy or allogeneic or autologous stem cell transplantation. Patients whose disease fails to respond to initial induction therapy have a poor overall prognosis and, if desired, may be re-treated with non–cross-reactive chemotherapy drugs such as epidophyllotoxins (higher-dose cytosine arabinoside–containing regimens).

AML is a biologically heterogeneous neoplasm with widely divergent clinical outcomes. Long-term cure rates (defined as length of survival >5 years) range from 5% to 60% with chemotherapy alone. AML prognosis can be predicted to some degree based on age, cytogenetic abnormalities, disease presentation, prior hematologic disease, or secondary AML (see Table 47–12). Cytogenetics are the most robust prognostic indicator and consist of three categories: favorable, intermediate, and poor. AML subtypes associated with t(8;21), inv(16) or del(16q), t(8;21), or t(15;17) (see discussion of acute promyelocytic leukemia later) aberrations are unusually responsive to induction followed by two to four cycles of high-dose cytosine arabinoside containing consolidation chemotherapy with long-term 5-year survival rates of 55% to 60%. AML subtypes associated with poor prognosis include those with deletions in chromosome 5 or 7, 11q23 aberrations, inv(3q), t(3;3), t(6;9), t(9;22) (the Philadelphia chromosome), or the presence of three or more karyotypic abnormalities. The use of chemotherapy alone in these disease subtypes is less likely to induce remission; if remission is achieved, these patients are at high risk of AML relapse for which chemotherapy alone is rarely successful. Overall survival rates are 5% to 15%. The remaining patients with AML have intermediate risk cytogenetics (defined as normal karyotype, trisomy 8, t(9;11), or other cytogenetic abnormalities not included in the other groups) and demonstrate a 30% to 45% long-term survival rate with standard therapy. Recent evidence has demonstrated that up to one third of all patients with AML also show constitutive activation of the fms-like tyrosine kinase 3 (flt-3) receptor as a result of point mutations or internal tandem duplications (not seen on routine karyotypic testing), which predicts for poor therapeutic response independent of conventional cytogenetics.

Allogeneic transplantation offers the only hope for long-term cure in many patients with AML, particularly those with poor prognosis de novo and relapsed AML whose overall cure rates with chemotherapy alone are less than 20%. Eligible patients with poorer prognoses are recommended for early transplantation, whereas those with favorable disease features may benefit from further chemotherapy before transplantation, or they may undergo bone marrow transplantation only after relapse has occurred. For patients younger than 60 years of age, allogeneic bone marrow transplantation for AML offers an overall long-term cure rate of 40% to 60%, with a procedure-related mortality rate of 10% to 25%. Results are improved when patients undergo bone marrow transplantation after initial induction chemotherapy (in the first remission), rather than after disease relapse (the second remission). However, chemotherapeutic regimens are also more effective in the first remission than they are after transplantation, and the cure rate from transplantation performed during second remissions is still 25%. Decisions about the best time to perform bone marrow transplantation in patients are probably best guided by cytogenetic and clinical data (see Table 47–12). Patients with AML who are ineligible for allogeneic transplants because of advanced age or lack of compatible HLA donors may be offered autologous bone marrow or stem cell transplantation. Marrow or peripheral stem cells are harvested from patients and are purged in vitro to remove neoplastic cells before their reinfusion into patients after myeloablative high-dose chemotherapy with or without radiation. Up to 10% patients die as a result of lack of marrow engraftment and other complications. Whether autologous transplantation improves outcomes when compared with chemotherapy alone is still under debate. However, the long-term survival rates following autologous transplants range from 20% to 40% and are at least equivalent if not better compared with chemotherapy with cytarabine therapy alone. Autologous stem cell transplantation remains an option for patients with poor risk or relapsed AML without compatible HLA donors.

Elderly patients with major co-morbidities and/or secondary leukemia after prior diseases may not tolerate any aggressive chemotherapeutic regimens, with or without stem cell procedures. Infectious complications remain the major cause of morbidity and mortality during intensive chemotherapy regimens. Prophylactic use of growth factor support, antibiotics, and antifungals remains of questionable efficacy. Given the low remission rates (30% to 50%) and high mortality associated with induction therapy, offering supportive therapy or hospice may be more appropriate in some cases. Older patients whose disease relapses after remission achievement may also be treated with gemtuzumab ozogamicin (Mylotarg) an anti-CD33 antibody chemically linked to a cytotoxic agent calicheamicin. This agent binds to CD33-expressing malignant (as well as normal) hematopoietic cells and induces cell death. Complete remission rates are low (15%), with side effects including prolonged pancytopenia with infectious risks and veno-occlusive liver disease. Experimental therapies for AML such as non-myeloablative stem cell transplantation (see

Chapter 46) have resulted in promising long-term remissions in some older individuals and should be pursued based on the patient's overall health status and availability of an appropriate HLA-matched donor.

ACUTE PROMYELOCYTIC LEUKEMIA WITH t(15;17)

Acute promyelocytic leukemia (APL) with t(15;17) comprises 10% to 15% of adult AML, with an increased incidence in younger patients (median age 40 years). APL differs from other acute leukemias because of its unique disease biologic mechanism. APL blasts consist of morphologically distinctive immature promyelocytic cells containing large granules and the characteristic Auer rods of AML. APL cells possess a unique chromosomal translocation, t(15;17), which results in a unique fusion protein (a combination of promyelocytic leukemia protein and retinoic acid α-receptor [PML-RARα]). This protein, a combination of a nuclear transactivation protein, PML, with a retinoic acid receptor on chromosome 17, results in arrested promyelocytic differentiation and enhanced proliferation.

Clinically, patients with APL often exhibit life-threatening bleeding caused by disseminated intravascular coagulation and procoagulant factors released from APL granules. In the past, treatment consisted of low-dose heparin and supportive platelet transfusions alone and resulted in high mortality and morbidity rates. Currently, the centerpiece of APL treatment is *all-trans-retinoic acid* (ATRA), a biologic agent shown to overcome growth arrest and permit differentiation of immature APL blast cells into mature neutrophils. Although ATRA alone induces clinical remissions in up to 90% of patients, high relapse rates observed after monotherapy has led to the standard practice of combining ATRA and anthracycline chemotherapy in induction regimens. Patients initiated on ATRA therapy must be closely observed for development of *retinoic acid syndrome*, acute cardiopulmonary distress caused by pulmonary effusions and infiltrates in the setting of high levels of circulating leukocytes with leukostasis. This serositis-like syndrome is attributed to adhesion of differentiated neoplastic cells to the pulmonary vasculature and carries a 5% to 10% mortality rate. Holding ATRA with initiation of corticosteroids and aggressive diuresis is usually effective. Over two thirds of patients with APL treated with standard ATRA-based induction, consolidation, and maintenance chemotherapy achieve long-term remission. Relapsed patients may be treated with low-dose arsenic trioxide, which also induces incomplete differentiation of APL, with complete remission rates in over 90% of cases. Autologous and/or allogeneic stem cell transplantation may also be considered in the relapsed setting.

Prospectus for the Future

The molecular understanding of the pathogenesis of MDS, MPD, and acute leukemia is progressing rapidly and is having a critical impact on the development of novel therapeutic approaches that promise to transform our clinical approach to these diseases in the coming years.

Myelodysplasia: In MDS, the recent approvals for the use of 5-azacytidine and lenalidomide represent the first innovative therapy for this disease in decades. The trials of 5-azacytidine were prompted by the recognition that epigenetic modifications of the clonal cell population was particularly appropriate for the treatment of MDS, in which epigenetic abnormalities affecting cell growth and apoptosis have been identified as central to the pathogenesis of the disease. Similar approaches promise to widen the therapeutic armamentarium for treating MDS in the future. Furthermore, the particular specificity of lenalidomide for successful treatment of the 5q- syndrome suggests that analysis of its mechanism of action may lay the groundwork for future targeted therapies.

Myeloproliferative disease: The importance of the spectacular success of Gleevec as targeted therapy of CML cannot be overstated. As the first successful therapy based on an understanding of pathogenesis, Gleevec has become emblematic of the translation of our understanding of disease pathogenesis into tangible clinical care innovations. Second-generation tyrosine kinase inhibitors with activity against Gleevec-resistant CML are rapidly coming on line, and we foresee a time when transplant will rarely be the therapy of choice for CML. Similarly, the discovery of the JAK 2 mutations in non-CML myeloproliferative diseases opens new avenues for targeted intervention in these diseases of which previous therapy has been largely supportive. JAK 2 kinase inhibitors are already under development and will be a major focus of research in the coming years.

Acute leukemia: Once again, molecular understanding of the pathogenesis of acute leukemia has led to important therapeutic advances in the treatment of disease. The discovery of the link between the retinoic acid receptor and the origins of APL has provided important insight into the unique sensitivity of this disease to ATRA. Similar approaches may soon provide therapeutic entry points into the treatment of other acute leukemias associated with pathognomonic chromosomal translocations.

References

Barosi G, Hoffman R: Idiopathic myelofibrosis. Semin Hematol 42:248–258, 2005.

Baxter EJ, Scott LM, Campbell PJ, et al: Acquired mutation of the tyrosine kinase JAK2 in human myeloproliferative disorders. Lancet 365:1054–1061, 2005.

Bowen D, Culligan D, Jowitt S, et al: UK MDS Guidelines Group: Guidelines for the diagnosis and therapy of adult myelodysplastic syndromes. Br J Haematol 120:187–200, 2003.

Byrd J, Mrozek K, Dodge R, et al: Pretreatment cytogenetic abnormalities are predictive of induction success, cumulative incidence of relapse, and overall survival in adult patients with de novo acute myeloid leukemia. Blood 100:4325–4336, 2002.

Cappellini MD: Iron-chelating therapy with the new oral agent ICL670 (Exjade). Best Pract Res Clin Haematol 18:289–298, 2005.

Deininger MWN, Goldman JM, Melo JV: The molecular biology of chronic myeloid leukemia. Blood 96(10):3343–3356, 2000.

Harrison CN, Campbell PJ, Buck G, et al: Hydroxyurea compared with anagrelide in high-risk essential thrombocythemia. N Engl J Med 353:33–45, 2005.

Hoew RB, Porwit-MacDonald A, Wanat R, et al: The WHO classification of MDS does make a difference. Blood 103:3265–3270, 2004.

Jaffe ES, Harris NL, Stein H, Vardiman JW (eds): WHO Classification: Pathology and Genetics of Tumours of the Haematopoietic and Lymphoid Tissues. Lyon, France, IARC Press, 2001.

Landolfi R, Marchioli R, Kutti J, et al: Efficacy and safety of low-dose aspirin in polycythemia vera. N Eng J Med 350:114–124, 2004.

Lowenberg B, Downing JR, Burnett A: Acute myeloid leukemia. NEJM 341(14):1051–1062, 1999.

O'Brien SG, Deininger MW: Imatinib in patients with newly diagnosed chronic phase CML. Semin Hematol 40:26–30, 2003.

Radich JP: Philadelphia chromosome positive acute lymphocytic leukemia. Hematol Oncol Clin North Am 15:21–36, 2001.

Sanz MA, Tallman M, Lo-Coco F: Practice points, consensus, and controversial issues in the management of patients with newly diagnosed acute promyelocytic leukemia. Oncologist 10:806–814, 2005.

Tallman M, Gilliland DG, Rowe JM: Drug therapy for acute myeloid leukemia. Blood 106:1154–1163, 2005.

Chapter 48

Disorders of Red Blood Cells

Michal G. Rose

Nancy Berliner

Normal Red Blood Cell Structure and Function

The red blood cells (RBCs) deliver oxygen to all the tissues in the body and carry carbon dioxide back to the lungs for excretion. The erythrocyte is uniquely adapted to these functions. The RBC has a biconcave disc shape that maximizes the membrane surface area for gas exchange, and it has a cytoskeleton and membrane structure that allows it to deform sufficiently to pass through the microvasculature. Passage through capillaries that have a diameter that may be one fourth the resting diameter of the erythrocyte is made possible by interactions between proteins in the membrane (band 3 and glycophorin) and underlying cytoplasmic proteins that make up the erythrocyte cytoskeleton (spectrin, ankyrin, and protein 4.1).

The mature red cell contains no nucleus and is dependent throughout its lifespan on proteins synthesized before extrusion of the nucleus and release from the bone marrow into the peripheral circulation. Approximately 98% of the cytoplasmic protein of the mature erythrocyte is hemoglobin. The remainder is mainly enzymatic proteins, such as those required for anaerobic metabolism and the hexose monophosphate shunt.

As discussed in the text that follows, defects in any of the intrinsic structural features of the erythrocyte can result in hemolytic anemia. Abnormalities of the membrane or cytoskeletal proteins are the causes of alterations in erythrocyte shape and flexibility. Inborn defects in the enzymatic pathways for glucose metabolism decrease the resistance to oxidant stress, and inherited abnormalities of hemoglobin structure and synthesis lead to polymerization of abnormal hemoglobin (sickle cell disease) or to the precipitation of unbalanced hemoglobin chains (thalassemia). All of these changes result in decreased red cell survival.

Oxygen is transported by hemoglobin, a tetramer composed of two α chains and two β-like (β, γ, or δ) chains. In fetal life, the main hemoglobin is fetal hemoglobin (HbF [α_2, γ_2]); the switch from HbF to adult hemoglobin (HbA [$\alpha_2\beta_2$]) occurs in the perinatal period. By 4 to 6 months of age, the level of HbF falls to about 1% of total hemoglobin. HbA$_2$ ($\alpha_2\gamma_2$) is a minor adult hemoglobin, comprising approximately 1% of HbA (Table 48–1).

Clinical Approach to Anemia

Anemia, the reduction in red cell mass, is an important sign of disease. It may reflect decreased production of erythrocytes, either because of primary hematologic disease or in response to systemic illness. Alternatively, anemia may reflect increased cellular turnover from hemolysis. This, in turn, may occur as a result of intrinsic abnormalities of the red cell—primary immune red cell destruction or as a part of a systemic vascular process. The investigation of anemia is a critical component of the evaluation of the patient and commonly provides important insight into systemic illness. Figure 48–1 provides an overview of the differential diagnosis of anemia.

CLINICAL PRESENTATION

The symptoms of anemia usually reflect the rapidity with which the reduction in erythrocyte mass has occurred. Patients with acute hemorrhage or massive hemolysis may exhibit symptoms of hypovolemic shock. However, most patients develop anemia more slowly and may have few symptoms. Usual complaints are fatigue, decreased exercise tolerance, dyspnea, and palpitations. In patients with coronary artery disease, anemia may precipitate worsening symptoms of chest pain. On physical examination, the major sign of anemia is pallor. Patients may be tachycardic and will often have audible flow murmurs. Patients with hemolysis will often exhibit jaundice and splenomegaly.

LABORATORY EVALUATION

The key components of the laboratory evaluation of anemia are the reticulocyte count, peripheral blood smear, erythrocyte indices, nutritional studies, and bone marrow aspirate and biopsy.

The *reticulocyte count* allows the critical distinction between anemia arising from a primary failure of red cell production and anemia resulting from increased red cell destruction. Erythrocytes newly released from the marrow still contain small amounts of RNA; these are termed *reticulocytes* and can be detected by staining the peripheral blood smear with methylene blue or other supravital stains. In response to the stress of anemia, erythropoietin (EPO) production increases and promotes the production and release of increased numbers of reticulocytes. The number of reticulocytes in the peripheral blood therefore reflects the response of the bone marrow to anemia. The reticulocyte count can be expressed either as a percentage of the total red cell number or as an absolute number. In patients without anemia, a normal reticulocyte count is 1% with an absolute count of 50,000/mcL. When anemia is caused by decreased RBC survival, appropriate marrow response results in a reticulocyte count of over 2%, with an absolute reticulocyte count of over 100,000/mcL. When the reticulocyte count is not elevated, a search should begin for a cause for the failure of red cell production. Reticulocyte counts that are expressed as a percentage of total RBCs must be corrected for anemia because decreasing the number of circulating cells will increase the reticulocyte percentage without any increase in release from the marrow. The corrected reticulocyte count is calculated by multiplying the reticulocyte count by the ratio of the patient's hematocrit to a normal hematocrit. The advantage of the absolute reticulocyte count is that this correction is not necessary. The absolute reticulocyte count is becoming increasingly available and will probably supersede the standard reticulocyte count.

Evaluation of the *peripheral blood smear* may provide important clues as to the causes of anemia. Red cell morphologic examination is especially critical in the evaluation of anemia associated with reticulocytosis, wherein an examination of the smear is essential to distinguish between immune hemolysis (which results in spherocytes) and microangiopathic hemolysis (which causes schistocytes or erythrocyte fragmentation). Changes associated with other causes of anemia include sickle and target cells that are characteristic of hemoglobinopathies, teardrop cells and nucleated red cells associated with myelofibrosis and marrow infiltration, intra-

Table 48–1	Structure and Distribution of Human Hemoglobins (Hb)	
Name of Hemoglobin	**Distribution**	**Structure**
A	95%–98% of adult Hb	$\alpha_2\beta_2$
A$_2$	1.5%–3.5% of Adult Hb	$\alpha_2\delta_2$
F	Fetal, 0.5%–1.0% of adult Hb	$\alpha_2\gamma_2$
Gower 1	Embryonic	$\zeta_2\varepsilon_2$
Gower 2	Embryonic	$\alpha_2\varepsilon_2$
Portland	Embryonic	$\zeta_2\gamma_2$

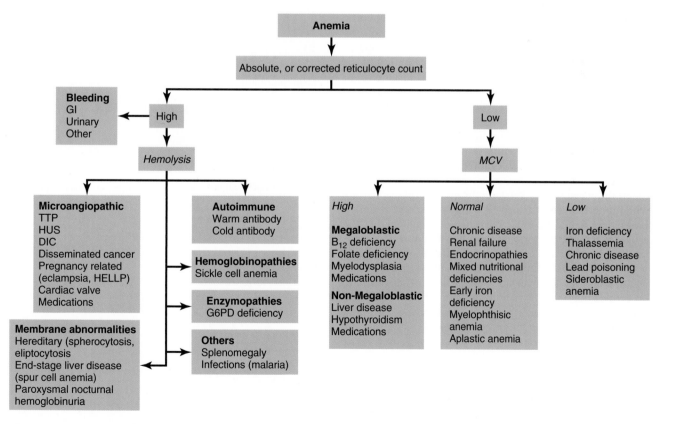

Figure 48–1 Overview of the differential diagnosis of anemia. G6PD = glucose-6-phosphate dehydrogenase; TTP = thrombotic thrombocytopenic purpura; HUS = hemolytic uremic syndrome; DIC = disseminated intravascular coagulation; HELLP = hemolysis, elevated liver enzymes, and low platelet count.

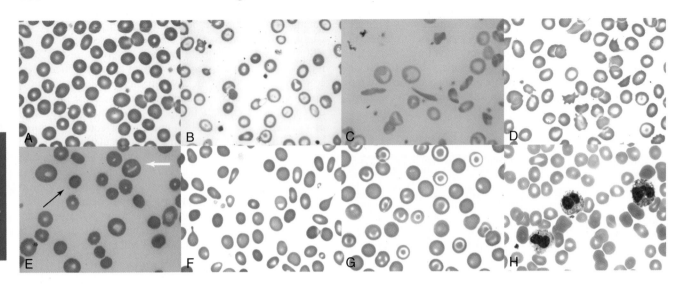

Figure 48–2 Peripheral blood smears in patients with anemia.

corpuscular parasites in malaria and babesiosis, and pencil-shaped deformities associated with severe iron deficiency. In addition, examination of myeloid cells and platelets may also be helpful. Hypersegmented neutrophils and large platelets support the diagnosis of megaloblastic anemia, and the presence of immature blast forms may be diagnostic of leukemia. Figure 48–2 visualizes some common peripheral blood smear findings in patients with anemia.

The *mean corpuscular volume* (MCV) is an extremely helpful tool in the diagnosis of hypoproliferative anemias. In patients with anemia and a low reticulocyte count, the size of the red cells is used to characterize the anemia as microcytic (MCV <80), normocytic (MCV 80 to 100), or macrocytic (MCV >100). The differential diagnosis of hypoproliferative anemia based on red cell size is described in the section that follows.

In patients with anemia and an elevated reticulocyte count, the vigorous production of new erythroid cells suggests that marrow function is normal and responding appropriately to the stress of the anemia. Bone marrow examination in this situation is rarely indicated because the marrow will simply show erythroid hyperplasia, usually without revealing any primary marrow pathologic anomaly. Evaluation should be focused on determining whether the cause for red cell consumption is either bleeding or hemolysis. In contrast, bone marrow examination is often required for the evaluation of hypoproliferative anemia. In patients in whom common abnormalities such as iron deficiency have been ruled out, marrow aspiration and biopsy are indicated to search for abnormalities such as marrow infiltration, marrow involvement with granulomatous disease, marrow aplasia, or myelodysplasia.

Evaluation of Hypoproliferative Anemia

EVALUATION OF MICROCYTIC ANEMIA

The differential diagnosis of microcytic anemia is outlined in Table 48–2. Microcytosis and hypochromia are the hall-

Table 48–2	**Differential Diagnosis of Anemia with Low Reticulocyte Count**

Microcytic Anemia (MCV < 80)

Iron deficiency
Thalassemia minor
Anemia of chronic disease
Sideroblastic anemia
Lead poisoning

Macrocytic Anemia (MCV > 100)

Megaloblastic anemias

Folate deficiency
Vitamin B$_{12}$ deficiency
Drug-induced megaloblastic anemia
Myelodysplasia

Non-megaloblastic macrocytosis

Liver disease
Hypothyroidism
Reticulocytosis

Normocytic Anemia (MCV 80–100)

Early iron deficiency
Aplastic anemia
Myelophthisic disorders
Endocrinopathies
Anemia of chronic disease
Anemia of renal failure
Mixed nutritional deficiency

MCV = mean corpuscular volume.

marks of anemias caused by defects in hemoglobin synthesis, which can reflect either failure of heme synthesis or abnormalities in globin production. The leading cause of microcytic anemia is iron deficiency, in which lack of heme synthesis results from the absence of iron to incorporate into the porphyrin ring. (Iron deficiency is discussed in detail in the section that follows.) Up to 30% of patients with anemia of chronic disease have microcytosis. Lead poisoning blocks incorporation of iron into heme, also resulting in a microcytic anemia. Sideroblastic anemias arise from failure to synthesize the porphyrin ring, usually as a result of inhibition of the heme synthetic pathway enzymes. Congenital sideroblastic anemia may respond to pyridoxine, a co-factor for several of the heme synthetic pathway enzymes. A more common cause of acquired sideroblastic anemia is alcohol abuse; ethanol inhibits most of the enzymes in the heme synthetic pathway. Failure of globin synthesis occurs in thalassemic syndromes, as described in detail in this chapter's section titled "Hemoglobinopathies." All of these disorders lead to decreased mean corpuscular hemoglobin concentration, causing hypochromia and a decrease in red cell size (low MCV).

Iron Deficiency Anemia

Iron deficiency is the leading cause of anemia worldwide. Although the presentation of classic iron deficiency anemia is linked with a microcytic anemia, early iron deficiency is associated with a normocytic anemia. Consequently, iron deficiency should be considered in all patients with anemia, and iron indices should be a part of the evaluation of any patient with hypoproductive anemia, regardless of the MCV.

Iron is acquired in the diet from either heme (found in meat) or nonheme (derived from vegetables such as spinach) sources. Iron from heme is better absorbed than nonheme iron. Iron absorption is increased in iron deficiency and in patients with ineffective erythropoiesis. Iron is absorbed from the proximal small intestine bound to transferrin, which mediates its uptake into red cell precursors via the transferrin receptor. The iron is released and incorporated into heme. Iron outside of hemoglobin-producing cells is stored in ferritin. Men and women have 50 mg/kg and 40 mg/kg of total iron, respectively. Between 60% and 75% of total iron is found in hemoglobin. A small amount (2 mg/kg) is found in heme and nonheme enzymes, and 5 mg/kg are found in myoglobin. The remainder is stored in ferritin, which resides primarily in liver, bone marrow, spleen, and muscle. The capacity for excreting iron is very limited, and iron overload occurs in patients with excessive absorption from the gastrointestinal tract (as a result of ineffective erythropoiesis or congenital hemochromatosis) or from chronic transfusions. Iron overload leads to increased iron deposition in these tissues and secondary deposition in endocrine organs, resulting in liver dysfunction, diabetes, and other endocrine abnormalities.

The most frequent cause of iron deficiency is occult blood loss. All men and postmenopausal women who are found to be iron deficient should have an evaluation for a source of gastrointestinal blood loss, regardless of the detection of occult blood. In premenopausal women, iron deficiency is most frequently secondary to loss of iron with menstruation (about 15 mg/mo) and during pregnancy (about 900 mg per pregnancy). Dietary deficiency of iron is most commonly seen in young children whose growth outstrips their intake of iron and in babies who drink mostly milk at the expense of an intake of iron-containing foods.

Laboratory Evaluation. As previously stated, early iron deficiency does not exhibit the hallmark microcytosis and hypochromia that characterizes classic iron deficiency. Evaluation of the blood smear in advanced iron deficiency often demonstrates hypochromic RBCs, target cells, and *pencil-shaped* elongated cells. Early iron deficiency is frequently associated with reactive thrombocytosis.

The mainstay of the diagnosis of iron deficiency is the peripheral blood iron indices. These include iron and total iron-binding capacity (TIBC) and ferritin. The transferrin saturation is the ratio of serum iron to transferrin concentration (TIBC), and is normally at least 20%. Iron deficiency results in a decrease in serum iron and an increase in iron-binding capacity, leading to a decrease in this ratio to less than 10%. Chronic inflammatory conditions (e.g., infection, inflammation, malignancy) often decrease both iron and TIBC, but the transferrin saturation usually remains above 20%.

The ferritin level is a reflection of total body iron stores. The liver synthesizes ferritin in proportion to total body iron, and a level of less than 12 ng/mL strongly supports a diagnosis of iron deficiency. Unfortunately, ferritin is an acute phase reactant, and levels rise in the setting of fever, inflammatory disease, infection, or other stresses. However, ferritin levels in response to stress should not rise above 50 to 100 ng/mL; therefore ferritin levels over 100 ng/mL usually rule out iron deficiency.

If the indirect measurement of iron indices does not definitively confirm or refute a diagnosis of iron deficiency, then a bone marrow examination can be performed to provide a direct assessment of marrow iron stores. Presence of iron in the marrow excludes iron deficiency anemia because marrow iron stores will be depleted before any fall in red cell production resulting from iron deficiency; conversely, complete absence of marrow iron confirms the diagnosis of iron deficiency.

Treatment. Oral iron supplementation, with administration of ferrous sulfate or ferrous gluconate two to three times daily, is the treatment for iron deficiency. Patients may complain of diarrhea or constipation and should be treated symptomatically. Reduction of the dose and gradual reinstitution of full doses may allow oral therapy to be continued. Iron should be administered for several months after resolution of anemia to allow for the reconstitution of iron stores.

In patients with malabsorption, a complete inability to tolerate oral iron, or iron demands that out strip replacement with oral supplements, parenteral iron may be administered. The parenteral administration of iron, especially iron dextran, has been associated with anaphylaxis. However, newer preparations such as sodium ferric gluconate and iron sucrose are significantly safer. As previously stated, all male patients and postmenopausal women with iron deficiency require evaluation for a source of gastrointestinal bleeding.

EVALUATION OF MACROCYTIC ANEMIA

Two categories of hypoproductive macrocytic anemias exist—megaloblastic anemia and non-megaloblastic macrocyctic anemia. Megaloblastic anemia arises from a failure of DNA synthesis and results in asynchronous maturation of the nucleus and cytoplasm of all rapidly dividing cells. Non-megaloblastic macrocytic anemias usually reflect membrane abnormalities resulting from abnormalities in cholesterol metabolism and are most commonly found in patients with advanced liver disease or severe hypothyroidism. Reticulocytosis greater than 10% will also cause an elevated MCV on automated blood counts because reticulocytes are larger than mature RBCs.

Megaloblastic Anemia

Megaloblastic anemia results from a block to synthesis of critical nucleotide precursors of DNA, which leads to a cell-cycle arrest in S phase. Cytoplasmic maturation occurs, but maturation of the nucleus is arrested. Cells take on a bizarre appearance, with large immature nuclei surrounded by mature-appearing cytoplasm. Interference with DNA synthesis affects all rapidly dividing cells, and therefore patients with megaloblastic syndromes often have pancytopenia and gastrointestinal symptoms such as diarrhea and/or malabsorption. In women, megaloblastic changes of the cervical mucosa occur and may cause alarmingly abnormal Papanicolaou smears. The most common causes of megaloblastic anemia are deficiencies of vitamin B_{12} or folate, medications that inhibit DNA synthesis or that block folate metabolism, and myelodysplasia.

Vitamin B_{12} (Cobalamin) Deficiency. Cobalamin (Cbl) is absorbed from animal protein in the diet. The process of Cbl absorption and metabolism is complex because Cbl is always bound to other proteins. In the stomach, protein-bound vitamins are released by digestion with pepsin and are bound to transcobalamin I. Transcobalamins I and III, termed *R binders* because of their rapid electrophoretic mobility, are found in all secretions, in plasma, and within the secondary granules of neutrophils. Although presumed to be involved with the storage of Cbl, their function is unknown, and isolated congenital deficiency of R binders is clinically silent. Within the proximal duodenum, pancreatic proteases digest Cbl away from the R binder proteins, and Cbl becomes bound to intrinsic factor (IF). IF is secreted by the parietal cells of the stomach and mediates absorption of Cbl via IF-specific receptors in the distal ileum. Within the ileal mucosal cell, the IF-Cbl complex is again digested, and Cbl is released into the plasma bound to transcobalamin II (TCII), the carrier protein that mediates cellular uptake of Cbl by TCII-specific receptors.

Within the cell, Cbl is a co-factor for two intracellular enzymes, methylmalonyl-coenzyme A (CoA) mutase, and homocysteine-methionine methyltransferase (Fig. 48–3). Methylmalonyl-CoA mutase is a mitochondrial enzyme that functions in the citric-acid cycle to convert methylmalonyl-CoA to succinyl-CoA. The cytoplasmic enzyme homocysteine-methionine methyltransferase is necessary for the transfer of methyl groups from *N*-methyltetrahydrofolate to homocysteine to form methionine. Demethylated tetrahydrofolate is necessary as a carbon donor in the conversion of deoxyuridine to deoxythymidine. Absence of Cbl results in a *trapping* of tetrahydrofolate in its methylated form and blocks the synthesis of thymidine 5′-triphosphate for incorporation into DNA. The megaloblastic changes induced by Cbl deficiency are mediated through this functional folate deficiency,

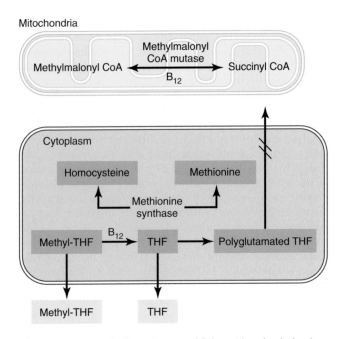

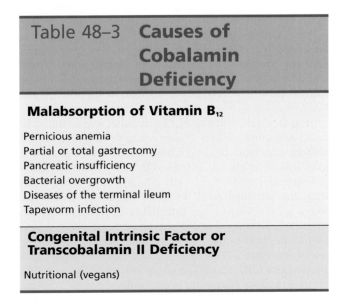

Figure 48–3 Metabolic pathways of folic acid and cobalamin. THF = tetrahydrofolate.

Table 48–3	**Causes of Cobalamin Deficiency**
Malabsorption of Vitamin B_{12}	
Pernicious anemia	
Partial or total gastrectomy	
Pancreatic insufficiency	
Bacterial overgrowth	
Diseases of the terminal ileum	
Tapeworm infection	
Congenital Intrinsic Factor or Transcobalamin II Deficiency	
Nutritional (vegans)	

which explains the similarity in the hematologic abnormalities induced by Cbl and folate deficiency.

Causes of Cobalamin Deficiency. The most common cause of Cbl deficiency is pernicious anemia, an autoimmune disease associated with gastric parietal cell atrophy, defective gastric acid secretion, and absence of IF. Antiparietal cell and anti-IF antibodies are frequently found in patients with pernicious anemia, and it is also associated with other autoimmune diseases such as Graves' disease, Addison's disease, and hypoparathyroidism. Many other lesions in the gastrointestinal tract can interfere with the absorption of Cbl (Table 48–3). Gastrectomy causes loss of parietal cell function and IF secretion. Pancreatic insufficiency interferes with the digestion of the R binder–Cbl complex, hindering the binding of Cbl to IF and ileal absorption. Resection of the terminal ileum prevents vitamin B_{12} absorption, as do

Table 48–4   Causes of Folate Deficiency

Dietary Insufficiency

Increased folate requirements

Pregnancy
Lactation
Hemolysis
Exfoliative dermatitis
Malignancy

Malabsorption

Sprue
Crohn's disease
Short bowel syndrome

Antifolate medications

Methotrexate
Sulfa drugs

---

diseases that affect ileal mucosal function, such as Crohn's disease, sprue, intestinal tuberculosis, and lymphoma. Because the body stores of Cbl are large and daily loss of Cbl is low, the stores of Cbl are adequate for 3 to 4 years if intake stops abruptly; signs of Cbl deficiency do not develop until defective absorption has occurred for several years. Nutritional Cbl deficiency is rare and is only seen in individuals who have been on strict vegan diets, excluding all animal products for many years. Infants born to vegan mothers who are breast-fed are also at risk of developing Cbl deficiency.

Folate Deficiency. Folate is widely present in food—in leafy vegetables, fruits, and animal protein. However, because prolonged cooking destroys it, fresh fruits and vegetables are the most reliable source of folate. Consequently, nutritional folate deficiency is very common in malnourished individuals who eat very little fresh fruits and vegetables. Folate deficiency can also be caused by increased demand, as occurs with pregnancy, hemolysis, and exfoliative dermatitis and by increased losses, which occur with dialysis (Table 48–4). Folate is absorbed in the proximal small intestine, and malabsorption of folate can also lead to folate deficiency.

Other Causes of Megaloblastic Anemia. Drugs and toxins are common causes of megaloblastic anemia. Some drugs, such as methotrexate and sulfa drugs, act as direct folate antagonists and mimic folate deficiency. Purine and pyrimidine analog chemotherapeutic agents (e.g., azathioprine, 5-fluorouracil) are direct DNA-synthesis inhibitors. Antiviral agents cause megaloblastic changes by unclear mechanisms. Alcohol interferes with folate metabolism, increasing the affect of frequent concomitant folate deficiency. Myelodysplasia commonly appears as a macrocytic anemia, with megaloblastic changes primarily in the erythroid series (see the text that follows).

Clinical Manifestations of Megaloblastic Anemia. The development of megaloblastic anemia is usually very gradual, allowing adequate time for concomitant plasma expansion to prevent hypovolemia. Consequently, patients are frequently severely anemic at presentation. They may have yellowish skin as a result of a combination of pallor and jaundice. Some patients have glossitis and cheilosis. With severe anemia, patients usually have a MCV above 110, although concomitant iron deficiency, caused by megaloblastic changes in the intestinal tract, may decrease the macrocytosis. Patients frequently have pancytopenia.

A peripheral smear demonstrates large, oval cells (macro-ovalocytes), hypersegmented neutrophils, and large platelets. The bone marrow is hypercellular, with megaloblastic changes and abnormally large precursors. In addition, evidence for significantly ineffective hematopoiesis is exhibited with elevated bilirubin and lactate dehydrogenase as a result of intramedullary destruction of erythrocytes.

Cbl deficiency is associated with neurologic abnormalities that are not seen with other causes of megaloblastic anemia. The neurologic signs may range widely from a subtle loss of vibratory sensation and position sense caused by demyelination of the dorsal columns to frank dementia and neuropsychiatric disease. The neurologic changes may be present without anemia, especially if a patient with Cbl deficiency is treated with folate, which will correct the hematologic manifestations of megaloblastic anemia but does not treat the neurologic abnormalities. The neurologic manifestations of Cbl deficiency are thought to be secondary to loss of function of the mitochondrial enzyme methylmalonyl-CoA mutase. One proposed explanation is that the failure to metabolize odd-chain fatty acids, which results in their improper incorporation into myelin, causes neurologic dysfunction. This explains why these findings are uniquely seen in patients with Cbl deficiency and are not seen in those with the megaloblastic anemias caused by abnormalities in the folate pathway.

Measuring levels of Cbl and folate in the peripheral blood confirms the diagnosis of megaloblastic anemia. Because megaloblastic changes in the gut mucosa can cause concomitant malabsorption of folate in the presence of Cbl deficiency, and vice versa, both levels should be measured in the patient with megaloblastic hematopoiesis. RBC folate levels better reflect the body folate stores and should be measured when a deficiency is clinically suggested but the serum folate levels are normal. Homocysteine levels are elevated in Cbl and folate deficiency, and methylmalonic acid levels are elevated in Cbl deficiency. These levels can be measured when Cbl deficiency is suggested, but serum Cbl levels are in the low-normal range.

In the setting of Cbl deficiency, a Schilling test may help establish the cause of the deficiency. Radioactive Cbl is given orally with a large parenteral dose of unlabeled Cbl. The absorption of orally administered Cbl is then measured by determining the excretion of radioactivity into the urine. Cbl bound to IF and labeled with a different isotope can be given simultaneously. Selective absorption of IF-bound Cbl supports a diagnosis of pernicious anemia. If neither isotope is absorbed, then the test may be repeated after a course of antibiotics to treat potential bacterial overgrowth or after administering pancreatic enzymes to rule out pancreatic insufficiency. The use of the Schilling test has decreased with the availability of assays for antiparietal cell antibodies and anti-IF antibodies, particularly because the necessity of an adequate urine collection makes it frequently unreliable.

Treatment of Megaloblastic Anemia. Patients with megaloblastic anemia frequently exhibit an extremely low level of hematocrits. Consequently, if the diagnosis is probable, then treatment should be initiated as soon as the folate and Cbl levels have been drawn. Patients with Cbl deficiency should initially receive daily parenteral therapy with 100 mcg intravenously for 7 days. Alternatively, therapy can be given subcutaneously 1 mg daily. Chronic therapy should be 1 mg intramuscularly monthly. Some patients with nutritional Cbl deficiency can receive oral replacement therapy. Oral therapy with high-dose crystalline vitamin B_{12} may overcome blocks to normal Cbl absorption, and oral therapy may be an option in patients who refuse parenteral supplementation. Therapy with Cbl should be accompanied by folate therapy because often concomitant secondary folate deficiency develops.

Patients with folate deficiency can receive replacement with 1 to 5 mg/day of oral folate. As previously noted, it is critical to be certain that patients are not Cbl deficient, because replacement of folate will correct the hematologic parameters in patients with Cbl deficiency, but it will not improve the neurologic sequelae.

After treating megaloblastic anemia, a very rapid response usually occurs. Reticulocytosis is seen as early as 2 days after therapy and peaks within 7 to 10 days. Despite rapid resolution of neutropenia, hypersegmentation of neutrophils may persist for several days. During this period, rapid cellular proliferation and turnover occur, which may precipitate hypokalemia, hyperuricemia, or hypophosphatemia. Patients should also be monitored for the development of iron deficiency in the face of increased demand with the rapid cellular proliferation in response to replacement. Anemia and other cytopenias should respond completely within 1 to 2 months, but the neurologic manifestations of Cbl deficiency improve slowly and may be irreversible.

EVALUATION OF NORMOCYTIC ANEMIA

The differential diagnosis of a normocytic hypoproductive anemia is extensive. Most nutritional anemias that cause microcytosis or macrocytosis begin as a normocytic anemia. Combined nutritional deficiencies may also cause normalization of the MCV. The measurement of EPO levels may be helpful in the diagnosis of normocytic anemia. In addition to helping in the diagnosis of anemia resulting from renal failure, many of the anemias associated with chronic inflammation and endocrinopathies exhibit a depressed EPO level. However, interpretation of EPO levels may be difficult in patients with mild anemia because the levels do not usually rise above the normal range until the hematocrit is depressed below 30%. Even below a hematocrit level of 30% the EPO level will often be in the normal range, but such levels are inappropriately low in the setting of anemia. An elevated EPO level suggests inadequate marrow response to anemia and increases the likelihood of myelophthisis or primary bone marrow failure. In patients for whom the diagnosis is not clear upon routine nutritional and endocrine studies, a bone marrow examination is indicated to rule out primary marrow pathologic conditions.

Anemia of Chronic Disease

The anemia of chronic disease occurs in patients with chronic inflammatory, infectious, malignant, and autoimmune diseases. It is caused by absolute or relative EPO deficiency, direct inhibition of erythropoiesis, poor iron incorporation into developing erythrocytes, and/or shortened erythrocyte survival. Patients have low-serum iron levels, but, in contrast to the iron indices in iron deficiency, the iron-binding capacity is also reduced, and the transferrin saturation is usually greater than 10%. Ferritin levels are usually elevated, both as an acute phase reactant and as a reflection of decreased iron incorporation.

The mainstay of treatment of the anemia of chronic renal failure is EPO replacement. The anemia of chronic disease will resolve if the underlying chronic condition is treated. In the absence of primary treatment, anemia will often respond to therapy with EPO. EPO levels may be helpful in predicting which patients are likely to respond. Therapy with EPO may be successful in patients with levels below 150 units, although it is most successful if the level is below 50 units. Responses to EPO replacement are most dramatic in patients with certain malignancies, especially multiple myeloma, in those with rheumatoid arthritis, and in the anemia associated with human immunodeficiency viral (HIV) infection.

Treatment of other causes of normocytic anemia is dictated by the primary causes of the disorder. The evaluation and treatment of primary marrow failure syndromes and hematologic malignancy are discussed in Chapters 46 and 47, respectively.

Evaluation of Anemia With Reticulocytosis

An elevated reticulocyte count in the setting of anemia signals a compensatory response of a normal marrow to premature loss of erythrocytes. Hemolysis is the premature destruction of RBCs in the reticuloendothelial system (extrinsic hemolysis) or in blood vessels (intrinsic hemolysis). The only other condition that causes anemia with reticulocytosis is acute bleeding. The differential diagnosis of hemolytic anemia is outlined in Table 48–5.

Although examination of the peripheral blood smear is frequently helpful in characterizing any anemia, it is absolutely critical in the evaluation of patients with hemolytic anemia. As previously noted, the morphologic examination of the erythrocytes is helpful in distinguishing immune hemolysis from micro-angiopathic hemolytic anemia. In addition, other red cell morphologic abnormalities are characteristic for specific diseases such as sickle cell disease (sickled cells), enzyme defects (*bite* cells), or erythrocyte membrane abnormalities (spherocytes and elliptocytes).

IMMUNE HEMOLYTIC ANEMIA

Immune-mediated hemolysis results from the coating of the erythrocyte membrane with antibodies and/or complement. It may be mediated by immunoglobulin G (IgG) antibodies (*warm* antibody) or by immunoglobulin M (IgM) antibodies (*cold* antibody). The designation *warm* and *cold* denotes the temperature at which maximal antibody binding takes place, and the clinical syndromes caused by the two types of antibodies are distinct.

The diagnosis of hemolytic anemia is based on the direct and indirect antiglobulin (Coombs' test). To perform a direct

Table 48–5 Differential Diagnosis of Hemolytic Anemia

Immune Hemolytic Anemia

Immunoglobulin G (warm antibody)–mediated hemolysis
Immunoglobulin M (cold antibody)–mediated hemolysis

Other Causes of Hemolysis from Causes Extrinsic to the Erythrocyte

Micro-angiopathic hemolysis

Disseminated intravascular coagulation
Thrombotic thrombocytopenic purpura
Pre-eclampsia, eclampsia, HELLP
Drugs (mitomycin, cyclosporine)
Valvular hemolysis

Splenomegaly

Infection

Hemolytic Anemia Caused by Disorders of the Erythrocyte Membrane

Inherited membrane abnormalities

Hereditary spherocytosis
Hereditary elliptocytosis
Hereditary pyropoikilocytosis

Acquired membrane abnormalities

Paroxysmal nocturnal hemoglobinuria
Spur cell anemia

Hemolysis Caused by Erythrocyte Enzymopathies

Glucose-6-phosphate dehydrogenase deficiency
Other enzyme deficiencies

Hemoglobinopathies

Sickle cell disease
Other sickle syndromes
Thalassemia

HELLP = hemolysis, elevated liver enzymes, and low-platelet count in association with preeclampsia.

Coombs' test, patient erythrocytes are mixed with rabbit antisera directed against either human IgG or human complement. The cells are then monitored for agglutination, the presence of which confirms the presence of antibody and or/complement on the patient's red cells. The indirect Coombs' test is performed by mixing patient serum with ABO-compatible erythrocytes and then combining this mixture with rabbit antisera against IgG; the Coombs' test allows for the evaluation of antibody in the patient's serum.

IgG-Mediated (Warm) Immune Hemolysis

Classic autoimmune hemolytic anemia (AIHA) is caused by IgG antibody directed against erythrocyte antigens. Warm-type hemolysis may be primary (idiopathic) or associated with autoimmune disease, lymphoproliferative disorders, or drugs. Patients exhibit acute anemia, jaundice, and an elevated reticulocyte count. Some patients have splenomegaly. Laboratory analysis confirms the presence of IgG on the erythrocyte membrane, as demonstrated by a positive Coombs' test; some patients will also be associated with complement. The occasional patient will not have reticulocytosis; in such patients the antibody destroys reticulocytes and mature erythrocytes.

The mainstay of therapy for AIHA is corticosteroids. Patients are usually treated with 1 to 2 mg/kg of prednisone, and responding patients are tapered very slowly over several months. Patients who fail to respond to prednisone can be treated with other immunosuppressive agents, such as cyclophosphamide, azathioprine, or chlorambucil. The occasional patient will respond to IV immunoglobulin. Splenectomy may be effective in some patients who are steroid refractory or steroid resistant; however, evidence suggests that patients who do not respond and who have ongoing hemolysis after splenectomy are at high risk for secondary thromboembolic events.

Warm antibodies mediate *drug-induced hemolysis*. Several mechanisms exist through which drugs may induce AIHA (Table 48–6). Penicillin produces hemolysis by binding to erythrocytes and acting as a hapten; the antibody is directed against the drug, and hemolysis occurs only in the presence of the drug. Type 2 hemolysis is caused by the formation of an antibody-drug complex that binds to the erythrocyte membrane and activates complement. Drugs associated with this type of hemolysis include quinidine, quinine, and rifampin. Still other drugs, including methyldopa and procainamide, cause hemolysis by inducing the production of *true* anti-erythrocyte antibodies directed against Rh and other RBC antigens. Antibody may persist in the absence of the drug, but not all patients with a positive Coombs' test will have evidence of hemolysis.

IgM-Mediated (Cold) Hemolytic Anemia

Cold-type immune hemolysis is usually postinfectious. The most common associated illnesses are *Mycoplasma pneumoniae* and Epstein-Barr virus (EBV). IgM antibodies are produced that are directed against the RBC antigen I (*Mycoplasma*) or i (EBV). The antibodies bind at lower temperatures, usually in the distal circulation, and bind complement. During the return to the central circulation, the IgM falls off the red cell, leaving complement bound. The Coombs' test is negative for IgG or IgM but positive for complement. Hemolysis is self-limited, is rarely severe, and resolves with supportive therapy. In cases of severe hemolysis requiring transfusion, blood should be administered through a blood warmer to minimize further hemolysis.

Cold agglutinin disease is a chronic IgM antibody–mediated hemolysis usually seen in association with lymphoproliferative disease. In addition, cold agglutinin disease is usually associated with chronic low-grade hemolysis, although occasionally it may be severe. Patients respond poorly to steroids and splenectomy. Acute severe IgM-

Table 48–6 Drug-Induced Autoimmune Hemolytic Anemia

Type	Mechanism	Drugs Implicated	Direct Coombs-Positive Hemolytic Anemia	Indirect Coombs-Positive Hemolytic Anemia
1	Hapten-mediated	Penicillin Cephalothin (and others)	IgG + Complement +/–	+ Only in the presence of drug
2	Immune complex–mediated	Quinine Quinidine Phenacetin Rifampin Isoniazid Tetracycline Chlorpromazine (and others)	IgG – Complement +	+ Only in the presence of drug
3	*True* anti-RBC antibody	Methyldopa Levodopa Procainamide Ibuprofen Interferon-α (and others)	IgG + Complement –	

RBC = red blood cell.

mediated hemolysis may respond to plasmapheresis. Supportive therapy includes avoidance of exposure to the cold. In the setting of lymphoproliferative disease, patients may respond to immunotherapy with rituximab (anti-CD20 antibody).

HEMOLYSIS FROM CAUSES EXTRINSIC TO THE ERYTHROCYTE

Microangiopathic Hemolysis

Microangiopathic hemolytic anemia (MAHA) is caused by traumatic destruction of RBCs as they pass through small vessels. The leading causes of MAHA include disseminated intravascular coagulation (DIC) and thrombotic thrombocytopenic purpura/hemolytic uremic syndrome (TTP/HUS) (see Table 48–5 and Fig. 48–1). Other causes include pregnancy-related syndromes such as preeclampsia, eclampsia, and the HELLP syndrome (hemolysis, elevated liver enzymes, and low platelets in association with preeclampsia); drugs; and metastatic cancers. A similar hemolytic picture can be seen in traumatic hemolysis on a damaged cardiac valve.

Finding schistocytes (fragmented erythrocytes) on the peripheral blood smear confirms the diagnosis of MAHA. The presence of a normal prothrombin time and partial thromboplastin time supports a diagnosis of TTP/HUS over that of DIC. Treatment is described in Chapter 52.

Infection

Hemolysis can be caused by direct infection of RBCs by parasites, as seen in malaria, babesiosis, and bartonellosis. Severe, overwhelming hemolysis can be seen in clostridial sepsis, in which bacterial toxins directly damages the membrane.

Table 48–7 Congenital Red Blood Cell Membrane Abnormalities

Name of Condition	Abnormal Membrane	
	Proteins	Inheritance
Spherocytosis	Spectrin, ankyrin, band 3, protein 4.2	Autosomal dominant Recessive (rare)
Elliptocytosis	Spectrin, protein 4.1	Autosomal dominant Recessive (rare)
Pyropoikilocytosis	Spectrin	Recessive
Stomatocytosis	Sodium channel permeability defect	Autosomal dominant

HEMOLYTIC ANEMIAS CAUSED BY DISORDERS OF THE ERYTHROCYTE MEMBRANE

Inherited Membrane Abnormalities

Hereditary spherocytosis (HS) is caused by heterogeneous congenital abnormalities in proteins of the erythrocyte cytoskeleton (Table 48–7). The majority of patients with HS have dominantly inherited mutations in spectrin or ankyrin. HS is characterized by hemolytic anemia, splenomegaly, and the presence of prominent spherocytes in the peripheral blood. Spherocytes are the result of *conditioning* of the erythrocytes in the spleen, whereby reticuloendothelial cells remove portions of the abnormal membrane that are the result of the disordered cytoskeleton. Spherocytes reflect membrane loss that decreases the membrane-to-cytoplasm ratio. Because a high membrane-to-cytoplasm ratio is responsible for the flexible, biconcave shape of the normal erythrocyte, the erythrocyte loses its biconcave morphologic characteristics and assumes a spherocytic shape with loss of membrane. Spherocytes are less flexible and may be destroyed in the microvasculature. The laboratory finding characteristic of HS is increased osmotic fragility, caused by the loss of distensibility associated with a decrease in surface membrane. HS is usually a mild disorder with well-compensated hemolysis. Patients typically have exacerbations during infections or when given marrow-suppressing medication. Patients with significant hemolysis should receive folate supplementation. Many patients require cholecystectomy for pigment stones. Severe, symptomatic anemia is treated with splenectomy.

Hereditary elliptocytosis (HE) is typically caused by dominantly inherited mutations affecting the interaction between membrane proteins and underlying cytoplasmic proteins (see Table 48–7). The most common abnormalities affect the interactions with spectrin and protein 4.1, which causes the RBCs to assume an elliptical shape. As in HS, patients usually have mild hemolysis and splenomegaly. *Hereditary pyropoikilocytosis* (HPP) is a rare recessive disorder that is frequently caused by the inheritance of two different membrane disorders (e.g., one allele for HS and one for HE). Patients have much more severe hemolysis with microspherocytes and elliptocytes on the smear. As with HS, treatment for symptomatic anemia in HE and HPP is splenectomy (see Table 48–7).

Acquired Membrane Abnormalities

Paroxysmal Nocturnal Hemoglobinuria. Paroxysmal nocturnal hemoglobinuria (PNH) is an acquired clonal disease that is associated with an abnormality of complement regulation. Normal erythrocytes are protected from complement-mediated cell lysis by the presence of membrane proteins, including delay-accelerating factor (DAF) and membrane inhibitor of reactive lysis (MIRL). Both of these proteins are members of a family of proteins that are anchored to the membrane by a glycosylphosphatidylinositol (GPI) anchor. Patients with PNH have clonal mutations in phosphatydilinositolglycan A (PIG-A), the enzyme required for the synthesis of GPI. These mutations arise in the hematopoietic stem cell, and all hematopoietic cells lack GPI-anchored proteins. Absence of GPI-anchored proteins from erythrocytes renders these erythrocytes susceptible to complement-mediated lysis. Traditional tests for PNH are functional assays based on the increased susceptibility of erythrocytes to lysis by acidic serum (Ham's test) or hypotonic medium (sucrose lysis test). Now that the underlying molecular abnormality in PNH has been defined, diagnosis can be made by flow cytometric documentation of the absence of DAF or MIRL on the surface of RBCs or leukocytes.

PNH is characterized by episodic acute intravascular hemolysis with a release of free hemoglobin that results in the hemoglobinuria for which the disease is named. The disease is considered to be part of the spectrum of myelo-proliferative diseases; it is a clonal stem cell disorder associated with thrombotic risk and with a risk of developing leukemia and/or myelofibrosis. Patients are susceptible to thrombotic complications typical of those seen in myeloproliferative disorders, including Budd-Chiari syndrome, portal vein thrombosis, and cerebrovascular thrombosis. PNH also has an association with aplastic anemia; patients may develop aplasia, and patients with aplastic anemia who respond to immunosuppressive therapy frequently recover with PNH-like clones. Treatment is largely supportive. However, young patients should be considered for allogeneic stem-cell transplantation.

Spur Cell Anemia. Spur cells (acanthocytes) are cells with abnormal morphologic membrane found in patients with advanced liver disease, severe malnutrition, malabsorption, and asplenia. The membrane acquires protrusions as a result of abnormal lipids present in the membrane. The changes may be associated with mild hemolysis, although in patients with advanced liver disease, separating hemolysis from hypersplenism is difficult. Similar changes may be observed in patients with abetalipoproteinemia.

HEMOLYTIC ANEMIAS CAUSED BY DISORDERS OF ERYTHROCYTE ENZYMES

Glucose-6 Phosphate Dehydrogenase Deficiency

Glucose-6-phosphate dehydrogenase (G6PD) is a critical enzyme in the hexose monophosphate shunt pathway, which is required to maintain intracellular stores of reduced glutathione to protect erythrocytes from membrane oxidation and hemoglobin oxidation (Fig. 48–4). The gene for G6PD resides on the X chromosome, and nearly all with the disorder are male patients. However, an occasional heterozygous female patient with skewed lyonization will appear deficient. Most G6PD mutations are found in African and Mediterranean populations and are thought to have been selected because they confer resistance to malaria. The African form

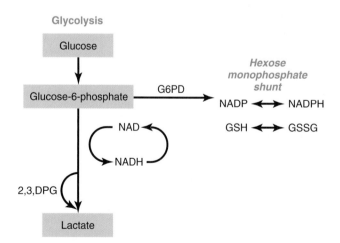

Figure 48–4 Metabolism of the red blood cell (RBC). G6PD = glucose-6-phosphate dehydrogenase; GSH = reduced glutathione; GSSG = reduced and oxidized glutathione; NAD = nicotinamide adenine dinucleotide; NADH = reduced form of NAD; NADP = nicotinamide adenine dinucleotide phosphate; NADPH = reduced form of NADP.

of G6PD deficiency is relatively mild, whereas the Mediterranean form is severe.

Absence of G6PD renders erythrocytes sensitive to oxidative stress. In the setting of infection, acidosis, or oxidant drugs, hemoglobin may precipitate within the cells, causing hemolysis. Many drugs are associated with hemolysis in the setting of G6PD deficiency, including sulfonamides, antimalarials, dapsone, aspirin, and phenacetin. Diagnosis should be suggested in male patients of African-American or Mediterranean extraction who have evidence of hemolysis in the setting of acute infection or recent exposure to oxidant drugs. Patients with the more severe form of the Mediterranean variant of G6PD deficiency may develop hemolysis on exposure to fava beans (favism). Cells with precipitated hemoglobin contain Heinz bodies that can be visualized with crystal violet staining of the peripheral blood smear. These inclusions are removed in the spleen, resulting in the finding of *bite cells* in the blood smear. Diagnosis can be confirmed with measurement of G6PD levels in the peripheral blood. However, reticulocytes and young RBCs in patients with G6PD deficiency have a higher enzyme level; consequently, if the diagnosis is probable, then the patients with a normal G6PD level should be retested at a time removed from the acute episode. The mainstay of preventing hemolysis in these patients is the avoidance of oxidative stress, especially by drugs implicated in causing hemolysis. Splenectomy is recommended only for patients with severe episodic or chronic hemolysis.

Other Enzyme Deficiencies

Deficiencies have been reported involving nearly all of the enzymes of the glycolytic pathway as rare causes of hemolytic anemia. The most common of these is pyruvate kinase deficiency. Autosomal genes encode these enzymes, and the pattern of inheritance is therefore autosomal recessive.

HEMOGLOBINOPATHIES

Hemoglobinopathies are mutations that result in the synthesis of abnormal hemoglobins. The most common of these are the sickle syndromes and the thalassemias, which, like G6PD deficiency, arose in areas of the world in which malaria is endemic.

Sickle Cell Disease

Sickle cell disease is the most common of the sickle syndromes and arises from a point mutation that results in a glutamic acid–to–valine substitution in the sixth amino acid of the β-globin gene. It has arisen as an independent mutation in diverse populations in Africa, India, the Mediterranean, and the Middle East. The substitution of a hydrophobic for a hydrophilic residue renders the deoxygenated sickle hemoglobin (HbS) less soluble and susceptible to polymerization and precipitation. The rate of precipitation of HbS is exquisitely sensitive to the intracorpuscular concentration of deoxygenated hemoglobin. Sickling is therefore increased in settings in which that concentration is increased either by changes in cellular hydration (dehydration) or by changes in the oxygen dissociation curve (e.g., hypoxia, acidosis, high altitude).

Acute Manifestations of Sickle Cell Disease. Most of the acute complications of sickle cell disease are related to vaso-occlusion (Table 48–8). Painful crises, caused by ischemic

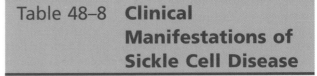

Table 48–8	**Clinical Manifestations of Sickle Cell Disease**

Acute Manifestations

Vaso-occlusive crisis
  Painful crisis
  Acute chest syndrome
  Priapism
Cerebrovascular events
  Thrombotic stroke
  Hemorrhagic stroke
Aplastic crisis
Splenic sequestration
Osteomyelitis

Chronic Manifestations

Chronic renal disease
  Isosthenuria
  Chronic renal failure
Chronic pulmonary disease
Sickle hepatopathy
Proliferative retinopathy
Avascular necrosis
Skin ulcers

pain in organs with occlusions of the microvasculature, can occur anywhere with pain most common in the extremities, chest, abdomen, and back. Painful crises are commonly precipitated by infections, dehydration, rapid changes in temperature, and pregnancy. However, no obvious precipitating cause is often found for an acute painful crisis. Vaso-occlusion in the pulmonary circulation can be a particularly ominous complication of sickle cell disease, resulting in *acute chest syndrome.* The acute chest syndrome is characterized by chest pain, hypoxemia, and chest infiltrates. The roles of infection, infarction, and in situ thrombosis in the acute chest syndrome are indistinguishable, but all patients should receive antibiotics for presumed pneumonia. Because hypoxemia predisposes to further sickling and increasing respiratory compromise, the acute chest syndrome is life threatening and is an indication for emergent exchange transfusion.

Neurologic events are a major cause of morbidity in patients with sickle cell disease. Acute large vessel occlusions occur in children, with a recurrence rate of 70% if untreated; such strokes are an indication for long-term exchange transfusion, which has been shown to decrease the rate of repeated occlusions. For reasons that are poorly understood, such large vessel occlusions rarely occur in adults. Adults may suffer hemorrhagic strokes as a result of aneurysmal dilation of proliferative vessels that form in response to repeated micro-occlusions in the cerebral vessels.

Any toxic or infectious insult that transiently suppresses bone marrow activity may cause an *aplastic crisis.* The shortened survival of the RBC in sickle cell disease renders the patients highly dependent on vigorous ongoing marrow activity, and short intervals of decreased reticulocyte formation can cause profound decreases in hemoglobin and hematocrit. Most dramatic are infections associated with parvovirus B19, which directly infects erythroid precursors. Supportive care is usually all that is required. However, some patients may go on to develop bone marrow necrosis, with a leukoerythroblastic picture; this development may be further complicated by bone marrow embolization to the lungs.

Certain vascular beds are especially prone to complications of sickle cell disease. The renal medulla is highly susceptible to damage by vaso-occlusion because high tonicity and low oxygen tension both significantly increase the concentration of HbS. All patients with sickle cell disease develop defects in urinary concentration ability, and by adulthood they are uniformly isosthenuric. Acute episodes of hematuria secondary to papillary necrosis are common.

The spleen is also a site in which recurrent sickling uniformly occurs. By adulthood, all patients have become functionally asplenic from repeated infarctions of the microvasculature. This contributing factor increases the susceptibility of patients with sickle cell disease to infections with encapsulated organisms. Acute infection remains a significant cause of death in patients with sickle cell disease. For unclear reasons, patients with sickle cell disease are particularly prone to osteomyelitis, with an unusually high incidence of *Salmonella* as the responsible organism.

Chronic Manifestations of Sickle Cell Disease. Sickle cell disease used to be a disease of childhood. As more patients with sickle cell disease survive to adulthood, it has become clear that repeated episodes of vaso-occlusion lead to damage to nearly every end-organ (see Table 48–8). Renal failure and pulmonary failure are leading causes of death in adult patients with sickle cell disease. Other long-term complications include chronic skin ulcers, retinopathy, and liver dysfunction. In addition, most patients require cholecystectomy for pigment stones.

Treatment of Sickle Cell Disease. Treatment of sickle cell disease remains largely supportive. Painful crises are treated with fluid, oxygen supplementation, and analgesics. Patients with any indication of infection should receive antibiotics. Patients with symptomatic anemia should be transfused. Exchange transfusion is indicated for chest syndrome, stroke, bone marrow necrosis, and priapism. More controversial indications for exchange transfusion include intractable pain and slow response to other supportive measures. The goal of exchange transfusion is to achieve a level of 30% to 40% HbS. As previously noted, patients who have sustained a thrombotic large vessel stroke should be chronically exchange transfused.

Recent studies have demonstrated that treatment with hydroxyurea, an agent that increases the concentration of HbF in patients with sickle cell disease, reduces the incidence of vaso-occlusive crises. The efficacy of hydroxyurea in patients with recurrent crises has been demonstrated in a randomized study, and follow-up studies have revealed a survival advantage for patients treated with hydroxyurea. The effect is attributed to the formation of hemoglobin tetramers containing one B^S chain and one γ chain ($\alpha_2\beta^s\gamma$), which do not undergo polymerization. More recently, studies have suggested that response is also related to decreases in leukocyte count and changes in endothelial adherence properties.

Other Sickle Syndromes

Hemoglobin C. Hemoglobin C (HbC) is caused by another substitution, glutamic acid to lysine, in the sixth position of the β-globin chain. Homozygous HbC causes very mild sickle symptoms and is usually nearly clinically silent. Hemoglobin S-C (HbSC) are compound heterozygotes for HbS and HBC. Patients with HbSC are more symptomatic, although the clinical manifestations are milder than those patients with homozygous HbS (HbSS). The patients have a higher hematocrit level, and the higher viscosity increases the degree of retinopathy. They do not sustain splenic infarctions; unlike patients with HbSS, they usually have splenomegaly. Consequently, they occasionally have episodes of acute splenomegaly associated with profound decrease in hemoglobin and hematocrit (splenic sequestration crisis). Although such crises can also occur in children with HbSS, functional asplenia prevents this complication in adults with HbSS.

Sickle Cell β-Thalassemia. Patients who are double heterozygotes for HbS and β-thalassemia have a spectrum of disease dependent on the level of β globin that they produce. Sickle cell β^+-thalassemia is a milder disease than HbSS, probably because of the decreased intracorpuscular concentration of HbS. Patients with sickle cell β^0-thalassemia (see discussion that follows) produce no normal β chains and have essentially the same phenotype as patients with HbSS.

Thalassemia

The thalassemic syndromes (Table 48–9) are a heterogeneous group of disorders associated with decreased or absent synthesis of either α- or β-globin chains. Severe thalassemic syndromes are associated with severe hemolytic anemia and are diagnosed in early childhood. However, mild forms of thalassemia minor frequently cause mild microcytic anemia with little or no evidence of hemolysis. These syndromes are often confused with iron deficiency because of the decreased MCV.

β-Thalassemia. Over 100 mutations have been described that lead to β-thalassemia, in which mutations decrease or eliminate expression from the β-globin locus. The decreased expression of β globin can be caused by structural mutations in the coding region of the gene, resulting in nonsense mutations, truncated messenger RNA (mRNA), and no expression of intact globin from the affected allele (β^0-thalassemia). However, a large number of mutations that result in decreased transcription or translation or altered splicing of the β-globin mRNA may result in reduction but not elimination of globin-chain expression from the affected allele (β^+-thalassemia).

Defective globin-chain synthesis in β-thalassemia causes both decreased normal hemoglobin production and the production of a relative excess of α chains. The decrease in normal hemoglobin synthesis results in a hypochromic anemia, and the excess α chains form insoluble α-chain complexes and cause hemolysis. In mild thalassemic syndromes, the excess α chains are insufficient to cause significant hemolysis, and the primary finding is a microcytic anemia. In severe forms of thalassemia, hemolysis occurs both in the periphery and in the marrow, with intense secondary expansion of the marrow production of red cells. The expansion of the marrow space causes severe skeletal abnormalities, and the ineffective erythropoiesis also provides a powerful stimulus to iron absorption from the intestine.

The clinical spectrum of β-thalassemia reflects the heterogeneity of the molecular lesions causing the disease (see Table 48–9). β-Thalassemia major results from homozygous β^0-thalassemia, leading to severe hemolytic anemia; such patients are diagnosed in infancy and are transfusion-

Table 48–9	Thalassemic Syndromes	
Disorder	**Genotypic Abnormality**	**Clinical Phenotype**
β-Thalassemia		
Thalassemia major (Cooley's anemia)	Homozygous $β^0$-thalassemia	Severe hemolysis, ineffective erythropoiesis, transfusion dependency, iron overload
Thalassemia intermedia	Compound heterozygous $β^0$- and $β^+$-thalassemia	Moderate hemolysis, severe anemia, but not transfusion dependent; main life-threatening complication is iron overload
Thalassemia minor	Heterozygous $β^0$- or $β^+$-thalassemia	Microcytosis, mild anemia
α-Thalassemia		
Silent carrier	α–/αα	Normal complete blood count
α-Thalassemia trait	αα/– – (α-thalassemia 1) OR α–/α– (α-thalassemia 2)	Mild microcytic anemia
Hemoglobin H	α–/– –	Microcytic anemia and mild hemolysis; not transfusion dependent
Hydrops fetalis	– –/– –	Severe anemia, intrauterine anasarca from congestive heart failure; death in utero or at birth

dependent from birth. β-Thalassemia intermedia patients also have two β-thalassemia alleles, but at least one of them is a mild $β^+$ mutation. These patients have severe chronic hemolytic anemia but do not require transfusions. Because of ineffective erythropoiesis, these patients chronically hyperabsorb iron and may develop iron overload in the absence of transfusions. β-Thalassemia minor is usually due to heterozygous β-thalassemia, although it may reflect the inheritance of two mild thalassemic mutations. These are the patients in whom iron deficiency is often misdiagnosed. Iron studies will show normal-to-increased iron with a normal iron saturation. Documenting a compensatory increase in HbA_2 and HbF will confirm the diagnosis.

α-Thalassemia. α-Thalassemia is nearly always caused by mutations that delete one or more of the α-chain loci on chromosome 16. Four α-chain loci exist with two nearly identical copies of the α-globin gene on each chromosome. The spectrum of α-thalassemia therefore reflects whether the patient lacks one, two, three, or all four α-globin genes (see Table 48–9). In general, the clinical manifestations of α-thalassemia are milder than those of β-thalassemia for two reasons. First, the presence of four α-chain genes allows for adequate α-chain synthesis unless three or four loci are deleted. Second, β-chain tetramers are more soluble than their α-chain counterparts and do not cause hemolysis. Patients with the loss of a single α-chain gene are silent carriers and have a normal hematocrit and MCV. Patients with the deletion of two α chains, either on the same chromosome (– –/αα; α-thal 1) or on different chromosomes (α-/α-; α-thal 2), are microcytic and mildly anemic. Patients who inherit one α-thal 1 allele and one α-thal 2 allele (– –/α-) have hemoglobin H disease. Hemoglobin H is the product of excess β-chain production, specifically $β_4$; it causes mild hemolytic anemia and minimal or no intramedullary erythrocyte destruction. Inheritance of the homozygous α-thal 2 allele results in no functional α-chain loci and is incompatible with life. The fetus is unable to make any functional hemoglobin beyond embryonic development because HbF also requires α chains. Free γ chains form tetramers, termed *hemoglobin Barts*. Hemoglobin Barts have an extremely high oxygen affinity, and failure to release oxygen in peripheral tissues results in severe congestive heart failure and anasarca, a clinical picture termed *hydrops fetalis*. Affected fetuses are stillborn or die soon after birth.

Prospectus for the Future

Anemia is increasingly recognized as a marker of increased morbidity and mortality in adults with a wide range of medical conditions, including renal failure, malignancy, cardiac disease, inflammatory conditions, and other chronic diseases. Studies are on going to evaluate the affect of treating anemia on patients' outcome and quality of life. Furthermore, advances in our pathophysiologic understanding of anemia of chronic disease are contributing to our knowledge of iron metabolism and the role cytokines play in hematopoiesis. These developments are paving the way for the development of new therapies for patients with anemia and/or iron overload. Ongoing progress in prenatal diagnosis and stem cell transplantation will contribute to our ability to prevent and treat the thalassemic syndromes and other hemoglobinopathies.

References

Bain BJ: Diagnosis from the blood smear. N Engl J Med 353:498–507, 2005.
Marks PW, Glader B: Approach to anemia in the adult and child. In Hoffman R, Benz EJ, Shatill SJ, et al. (eds): Hematology: Basic Principles and Practice, 4th ed. New York, Churchill Livingstone, 2005, pp 455–464.

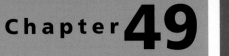

Clinical Disorders of Neutrophils

Michal G. Rose

Nancy Berliner

Leukocytes provide the main defense against bacterial infection. Monocytes and granulocytes are phagocytic cells that can kill ingested bacteria through the generation of reactive intermediates. Monocytes also release inflammatory mediators that increase the activity of lymphocytes. Lymphocyte function is discussed in Chapter 50.

Normal Granulocyte Development, Structure, and Function

NEUTROPHILS

Neutrophils (*polymorphonuclear leukocytes*) are the predominant white blood cell in the peripheral blood. They are morphologically recognizable by their characteristic segmented nucleus. They also contain various cytoplasmic granules that give them a characteristic appearance and are functionally important (Fig. 49–1).

Neutrophil killing of bacteria requires chemotaxis, phagocytosis, and intracellular killing (Fig. 49–2). *Chemotaxis* is the ordered movement of the cell toward an attracting stimulus, such as bacterial formyl peptides or complement fragments (C3b and C5a). Neutrophils adhere to endothelial cells by interaction of neutrophil surface glycoproteins (CD11b/CD18) with endothelial adhesion molecules (intracellular adhesion molecule-1 and endothelial leukocyte adhesion molecule-1), a process termed *margination*. In response to a chemotactic stimulus, these adherent neutrophils move toward the target along the endothelial surface. The syndrome of leukocyte-adhesion deficiency underscores the importance of neutrophil adhesion as the first step in bacterial killing. This rare congenital disease is caused by the absence of surface expression of the CD11b/CD18 complex on neutrophils. Neutrophils fail to adhere to endothelium, are unable to undergo chemotaxis, and do not phagocytose or kill bacteria. Patients have severe, life-threatening bacterial infections despite high levels of circulating neutrophils.

Phagocytosis requires recognition of target bacteria or debris by the neutrophil. Targets are *opsonized* by the surface binding of immunoglobulin or complement factor C3b. The neutrophil has surface receptors for C3b and the Fc portion of immunoglobulin G, which allows recognition and binding to the opsonized target. The target then becomes engulfed in a phagocytic vacuole, which fuses with neutrophil granules inside the cell.

Intracellular killing occurs by both oxygen-dependent and oxygen-independent mechanisms. Contents of the primary granules, including cathepsin G, defensins, and lysozyme, act to break down the bacterial cell wall and kill the target organism. The major mechanism of bacterial killing, however, is through the *respiratory burst*. Stimulation of the neutrophil activates a membrane-bound oxidase complex, which generates superoxide through the transfer of an electron from reduced nicotinamide-adenine dinucleotide phosphate (NADPH). The interaction of superoxide with water generates hydroxyl ions. In addition, myeloperoxidase catalyzes the formation of hypochlorite ion from hydrogen peroxide and chloride. The NADPH oxidase is a multisubunit enzyme. Absence or decreased activity of any one subunit impairs bacterial killing and results in chronic granulomatous disease, another congenital illness in which patients are predisposed to life-threatening bacterial infections.

The granules that give neutrophils their characteristic appearance have important functions in the process of neutrophil-mediated activation and killing. *Primary granules* arise early in myeloid differentiation and are found in both neutrophils and monocytes. They contain a large number of proteins, including myeloperoxidase, acid hydrolases, and neutral proteases. These granules fuse with the phagocytic vacuole and aid in the digestion of ingested bacteria. *Secondary granules* arise later in the differentiation pathway and give the neutrophil its characteristic granular appearance. These granules contain lactoferrin, transcobalamin, and the matrix-modifying enzymes collagenase and gelatinase. On neutrophil stimulation, these granules are released into the extracellular space. Lactoferrin and transcobalamin act as

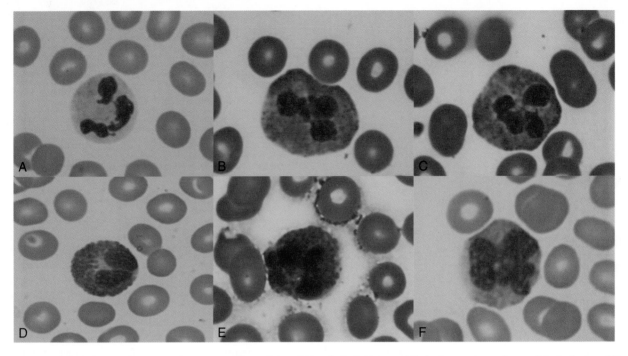

Figure 49–1 Normal granulocytes and monocytes in peripheral blood. *A–C,* Neutrophils (polymorphonuclear cells). *D,* Eosinophils. *E,* Basophils. *F,* Monocytes. (Courtesy of Robert J. Homer, MD, PhD).

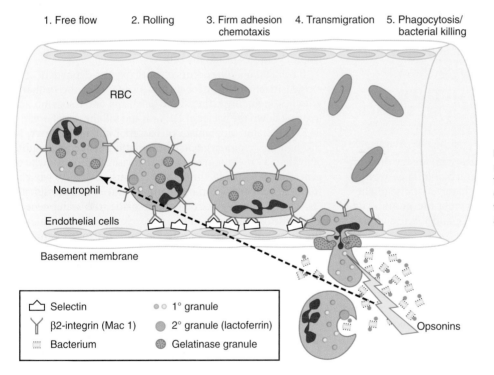

Figure 49–2 Sequence of neutrophil activation that shows the process of rolling, engagement with the vessel wall, attachment, diapedesis, and phagocytosis.

antibacterial proteins by sequestering iron and vitamin B_{12} away from bacteria, and collagenase and gelatinase break down connective tissues at the site of inflammation. Abnormalities in neutrophil granules have been described in rare clinical syndromes. Absence of myeloperoxidase produces surprisingly mild symptoms and may be associated with defects in control of fungal infection. Secondary granule deficiency is extremely rare and is associated with a slight increase in the risk of bacterial infections.

EOSINOPHILS AND BASOPHILS

Eosinophils and basophils arise from myeloid precursors in the bone marrow. They transit rapidly from the marrow to the blood and into the peripheral tissues, where they play a role in allergic and inflammatory reactions. Like neutrophils, they have secondary granules that give them their characteristic appearance and are also functionally important. Both cell types are present in small numbers under normal

Table 49–1	**Differential Diagnosis of Eosinophilia**

Reactive

Infection

Especially parasites; more rarely mycobacteria

Allergic Diseases

Drugs asthma, allergic rhinitis, atopy, urticaria

Pulmonary Diseases

Churg-Strauss, Loeffler's pneumonia, pulmonary infiltrates with eosinophilia (PIE)

Drug Reactions

Usually disappears when drug discontinued

Malignancy

Paraneoplastic, angioimmunoblastic T-cell lymphoma, Hodgkin's Dx

Connective Tissue Diseases

Rheumatoid arthritis, eosinophilic fasciitis, vasculitis

Primary Hypereosinophilic Syndrome

>6 months of eosinophils >1500, with no other apparent cause

conditions. Elevated levels of basophils may be seen in myeloproliferative syndromes.

Although eosinophils are capable of phagocytosis, most of the activity of these cells is mediated through the release of their granules. Their numbers are elevated in parasitic and helminthic infections, in which these cells are thought to play a role in the allergic response to those organisms. Numbers of these cells are also elevated in allergic reactions and in collagen vascular diseases, again linking their function to immunomodulation. *Hypereosinophilic syndromes*, in which extremely high levels of eosinophils can be seen, are rare, and they can be associated with damage to the lung, peripheral nervous system, and endocardial tissues. The differential diagnosis of eosinophilia is outlined in Table 49–1.

MONOCYTES

Monocytes arise from a common myeloid precursor with granulocytes, under the influence of granulocyte-macrophage colony-stimulating factor (GM-CSF) and macrophage colony-stimulating factor (M-CSF). Most circulating monocytes are marginated along the walls of vessels. They migrate from the vessels into tissues, where they develop into macrophages. The monocyte-macrophage lineage has many diverse functions. These phagocytic cells perform chemo-taxis, phagocytosis, and intracellular killing in much the same manner as neutrophils. They are especially important in the killing of mycobacteria, fungi, and protozoal species.

In addition to their role in killing of infectious organisms, monocytes have important interaction with other components of the immune system. They are antigen-presenting cells for T lymphocytes, they are capable of cellular cytotoxicity, and they secrete certain cytokines. The macrophages that process antigens and *present* them to T lymphocytes take on different forms in different tissues. They include the Langerhans cells of the skin, the interdigitating cells of the thymus, and the dendritic cells in the lymph nodes. Antigen-presenting cells are nonphagocytic, and the process by which they internalize antigen is not fully understood. Protein antigens are partially digested and expressed on the cell surface in association with human leukocyte or Ia antigens. This feature permits interaction with and activation of helper T cells. Other macrophages, such as Kupffer cells of the liver and alveolar macrophages of the lung, play an important role in removing particulate and cellular debris and senescent erythrocytes from circulation.

Monocytes also have a role in tumor cell cytotoxicity. They are capable of both antibody-dependent and antibody-independent cytotoxicity against tumor cells. The cytotoxicity is increased by tumor necrosis factor, interleukin-1, and interferon, all of which are also secreted by monocytes. Monocytes secrete a large number of proteins. These include immunomodulatory proteins (tumor necrosis factor, interleukin-1, and interferon), cytokines (G-CSF and GM-CSF), coagulation proteins, cell adhesion proteins, and proteases.

Determinants of Peripheral Neutrophil Number

Most granulocyte precursors are in the bone marrow, where maturation occurs over 6 to 10 days. Marrow precursors represent 20% of the granulocyte mass, and the storage pool represents 75% of the granulocyte mass. Therefore peripheral neutrophils comprise only 5% of the total granulocyte mass. Furthermore, neutrophils circulate in transit between the marrow and peripheral tissues. Of the circulating neutrophils, more than one half are adherent to the vascular endothelium. Again, this process is termed *margination*. The half-life of a neutrophil in the circulation is short, usually only 6 to 12 hours; the neutrophil may then migrate into tissues, where it survives another 1 to 4 days. Therefore the peripheral neutrophil count represents a sampling of less than 5% of the total granulocyte pool and is taken during a period of less than 5% of the total neutrophil lifespan. The peripheral white cell count is therefore a poor reflection of granulocyte kinetics. Abnormalities in neutrophil number can occur rapidly and may reflect either a change in marrow granulocyte production or a shift among various cellular compartments. An elevated peripheral white cell count may result from increased marrow production, or it may reflect mobilization of neutrophils from the marginated pool or release from the marrow storage pool. Similarly, a low granulocyte count may reflect decreased marrow production, increased margination and/or sequestration in the spleen, or increased destruction of peripheral cells.

The *total peripheral white cell count* represents the sum of lymphocytes and granulocytes. The significance of an elevated or depressed leukocyte count therefore depends on the nature of the cellular elements that are increased or decreased. *Leukocytosis* is a nonspecific term that may denote an increase in either lymphocytes (*lymphocytosis*) or neutrophils (*granulocytosis*). In rare cases, increases may reflect excessive numbers of monocytes or eosinophils. Leukocytosis related to an elevation in the neutrophil count is referred to as neutrophil leukocytosis, or *neutrophilia*. Extreme elevation of the white blood cell count to more than 50,000/mcL with the premature release of early myeloid precursors is termed a *leukemoid reaction;* this reaction may be associated with inflammatory reactions and infections, but it requires consideration of a diagnosis of myeloproliferative disease, especially chronic myelogenous leukemia. Evaluation of the peripheral blood smear may reveal characteristic changes that provide clues to the underlying disorder. A *leukoerythroblastic* smear shows the presence of immature granulocytes, teardrop-shaped erythrocytes, nucleated erythrocytes, and increased platelets. Such changes are reflective of marrow infiltration (*myelophthisis*) by fibrous tissue, granulomas, or neoplasm. As with leukocytosis, *leukopenia* may reflect either lymphopenia or *neutropenia*. Neutropenia is defined as an absolute neutrophil count of less than 1500/mcL.

Evaluation of Leukocytosis (Neutrophilia)

Leukocytosis is usually secondary to other processes, and it rarely indicates a primary hematologic disorder (Table 49–2). However, patients with persistent elevation of the neutrophil count, especially in association with elevation of the hematocrit and/or platelet count, should be evaluated to rule out a primary myeloproliferative disorder. A leukocyte alkaline phosphatase determination is helpful in ruling out chronic myelogenous leukemia because it tends to be low in this condition and normal or high in other myeloproliferative disorders and in leukemoid reactions.

Neutrophilia related to acute infection, stress, or acute steroid administration primarily reflects demargination and is usually transient. Persistent neutrophilia usually reflects chronic bone marrow stimulation. Nevertheless, bone marrow aspirate and biopsy are rarely indicated in the workup of neutrophilia. The exception is in those patients who demonstrate leukoerythroblastic changes, in which a bone marrow examination and culture may be indicated to rule out tuberculosis or fungal infection, marrow infiltration with tumor, or marrow fibrosis. Cytogenetic studies should also be performed to help eliminate the diagnosis of chronic myelogenous leukemia.

Evaluation of Leukopenia (Neutropenia)

DIFFERENTIAL DIAGNOSIS OF NEUTROPENIA

Neutropenia can reflect decreased production, increased sequestration, or peripheral destruction of neutrophils (Table 49–3). Patients should first be evaluated for

Table 49–2	**Differential Diagnosis of Neutrophilia**
Primary Hematologic Disease	
Congenital	
Myeloproliferative disorders	
Secondary to Other Disease Processes	
Infection	
Acute	
Chronic	
Acute stress	
Drugs	
Steroids	
Lithium	
Cytokine stimulation (e.g., G-CSF)	
Chronic inflammation	
Malignancy	
Myelophthisis	
Marrow hyperstimulation	
Chronic hemolysis, immune thrombocytopenia	
Recovery from marrow suppression	
Postsplenectomy	
Smoking	

G-CSF = granulocyte colony-simulating factor.

Table 49–3	**Differential Diagnosis of Neutropenia**
Decreased Production of Neutrophils	
Congenital and/or constitutional	
Constitutional neutropenia	
Benign chronic neutropenia	
Kostmann's syndrome	
Benign cyclic neutropenia	
Postinfectious	
Nutritional deficiency (B_{12}, folate)	
Drug-induced	
Primary marrow failure	
Aplastic anemia	
Myelodysplasia	
Acute leukemia	
Increased Peripheral Destruction	
Overwhelming infection	
Immune destruction	
Drug-related	
Associated with collagen vascular disease	
Isoimmune (in newborn)	
Hypersplenism and/or sequestration	

splenomegaly to rule out the possibility of sequestration. In patients who are completely asymptomatic and in whom previous studies are unavailable, the possibility of *constitutional* or *cyclic neutropenia* should be entertained and can be evaluated by serial peripheral blood counts. The normal neutrophil count varies among ethnic groups and is lower in African Americans (*constitutional neutropenia*) than it is in Caucasians. *Cyclic neutropenia* is a relatively benign disorder, in which cyclical changes occur in all hematopoietic cell lines but are most dramatic in the neutrophil lineage. At the nadir of the neutrophil counts, patients may have infections, but the disease is often clinically silent. In contrast, patients with congenital agranulocytosis (*Kostmann's syndrome*) exhibit profound neutropenia and infections in the perinatal period. Until G-CSF became available, most patients with Kostmann's syndrome died in early childhood, but the availability of cytokine therapy has prolonged survival. However, Kostmann's syndrome is also associated with a significantly increased incidence of the development of acute leukemia, a complication that has become apparent as patients survive longer. Acute myelogenous leukemia in these patients is associated with truncation mutations in the G-CSF receptor. These are acquired somatic mutations that may contribute to the pathogenesis of leukemia but do not contribute to the congenital neutropenia. Recent studies have confirmed that Kostmann's syndrome is associated with inherited mutations in the neutrophil elastase gene, although the mechanism by which this gives rise to neutropenia is unknown. Curiously, cyclic neutropenia has been shown to be also linked to mutations in the neutrophil elastase gene, although how different mutations in the same gene can give rise to two such completely different phenotypes is completely unexplained.

Neutropenia may occur during or after viral, bacterial, or mycobacterial infections. *Postviral neutropenia* is especially common in children and probably reflects both increased neutrophil consumption and a viral suppression of marrow neutrophil production. Neutropenia may be seen as a complication of *overwhelming sepsis* and is associated with a poor prognosis.

Drug-induced neutropenia may reflect either dose-dependent marrow suppression or an idiosyncratic immune response. The former is one of the most common complications of chemotherapeutic drugs and is also common with antibiotics such as trimethoprim-sulfamethoxazole. Chloramphenicol causes dose-dependent marrow suppression, although its more ominous complication is the rare idiosyncratic reaction that gives rise to marrow aplasia. Immune-mediated agranulocytosis is a rare complication that can occur with almost any drug. Most drug-induced neutropenias respond rapidly to discontinuation of the offending agent. The administration of G-CSF speeds recovery.

Autoimmune neutropenia may be seen in association with systemic autoimmune disease or as a feature of lymphoproliferative disease. Neutropenia is a common accompaniment to systemic lupus. Although not usually clinically severe, neutropenia is often a marker of disease activity. Neutropenia in rheumatoid arthritis is seen in association with splenomegaly (Felty's syndrome).

LABORATORY EVALUATION OF NEUTROPENIA

Unless the diagnosis of benign or cyclic neutropenia is likely, the evaluation of the patient with neutropenia should include stopping all potentially offending drugs and performing serologic studies to rule out collagen vascular disease. Unlike in patients with leukocytosis, bone marrow examination is indicated early in the evaluation and is frequently diagnostic. Neutropenia more often reflects primary hematologic disease, and bone marrow examination enables one to diagnose marrow failure syndromes, leukemia, and myelodysplasia. In the absence of bone marrow failure, other causes of neutropenia also may give a characteristic bone marrow picture. Drug-induced neutropenia produces a characteristic *maturation arrest* of the myeloid series. Rather than an actual inhibition of neutrophil maturation, this feature reflects the immune destruction of myeloid precursors that leaves only the earliest cells behind. All patients should have cytogenetic studies performed to aid in the diagnosis of myelodysplasia.

MANAGEMENT OF NEUTROPENIA

The therapeutic approach to patients with neutropenia depends on the degree of depression of the neutrophil count. Neutrophil counts between 1000 and 1500/mcL are not usually associated with any significant impairment in the host response to bacterial infection and require no intervention beyond what is demanded for diagnosis and indicated therapy of the underlying cause. Patients with neutrophil counts between 500 and 1000/mcL should be alerted to their slightly increased risk of infection, although serious problems are rarely encountered in patients with functional neutrophils and counts higher than 500/mcL. Patients with neutrophil counts lower than 500/mcL are at significant risk of infection. Such patients must be instructed to notify the physician at the first signs of infection and/or fever, and they must be managed aggressively with intravenous antibiotics regardless of the documentation of a source or infecting organism. Patients with a significantly depressed neutrophil count may exhibit few signs of infection because much of the inflammatory response at the site of infection is generated by the neutrophils themselves. In patients with severe immune-mediated neutropenia, steroids and intravenous immunoglobulin may be helpful in elevating the neutrophil count and in preventing infectious complications. G-CSF may increase the peripheral white count and may help resolve infections in neutropenia induced by drugs, including chemotherapy. It has also been efficacious in some patients with immune neutropenia, as well as in patients with myelodysplasia.

Prospectus for the Future

The delineation of the molecular basis of severe congenital neutropenia and cyclic hematopoiesis has raised important questions about the mechanisms governing the determination of neutrophil mass. The discovery that severe congenital neutropenia and cyclic neutropenia are both linked to mutations in gene encoding, the granule protein neutrophil elastase has raised many questions regarding the link between granule proteins and neutrophil kinetics. A pathophysiologic understanding of these diseases should provide important insights into the regulatory pathways governing the regulation of neutrophil number. Other studies aimed at elucidating the molecular basis for myeloid differentiation are establishing the importance of transcription factor function in neutrophil maturation and are providing insights into the pathogenesis of leukemia and myelodysplasia. Such insights may delineate pathways with entry points for therapeutic intervention in myeloid malignancy.

References

Baehner R: Normal phagocyte structure and function. In Hoffman R, Benz EJ, Shattil SJ, (eds): Hematology: Basic Principles and Practice, 4th ed. New York, Churchill Livingstone, 2005, pp 737–762.

Dinauer MC, Coates TD: Disorders of phagocyte function and number. In Hoffman R, Benz EJ, Shattil SJ, (eds): Hematology: Basic Principles and Practice, 4th ed. New York, Churchill Livingstone, 2005, pp 787–830.

Rose MG, Berliner N: T-cell suppressor disorders. Oncologist 9:247–258, 2004.

Berliner N, Horwitz M, Loughran TP Jr: Congenital and acquired neutropenia. Hematology (American Society of Hematology Education Program) 63–79, 2004.

Disorders of Lymphocytes

Jill Lacy

Stuart Seropian

The central cell of the immune system is the lymphocyte. Lymphocytes mediate the adaptive immune response, providing specificity to the immune system by responding to specific pathogens and conferring long-lasting immunity to reinfection. Lymphocytes are derived from pluripotent hematopoietic stem cells that reside in the bone marrow and give rise to all of the cellular elements of the blood. Two major functional classes of lymphocytes have been developed: (1) B lymphocytes, or B cells, and (2) T lymphocytes, or T cells, which are distinguished by their site of development, antigenic receptors, and function. The major disorders of lymphocytes include (1) neoplastic transformation of specific subsets of lymphocytes resulting in an array of lymphomas or leukemias, (2) congenital and acquired defects in lymphocyte development or function with resultant immunodeficiency syndromes, and (3) physiologic responses to infection or antigenic stimulation that may lead to lymphadenopathy, lymphocytosis, or lymphocytopenia.

Cells of the Immune System: Lymphocyte Development, Function, and Localization

B CELLS

B cells are characterized by the presence of cell surface immunoglobulin (or antibody). Their major function is to mount a humoral immune response to antigens by producing antigen-specific antibody. B cells develop in the bone marrow in a series of highly coordinated steps that involve sequential rearrangement of the heavy- and light-chain immunoglobulin genes and expression of B-cell–specific cell surface proteins (Fig. 50–1). Rearrangement of the immunoglobulin genes results in the generation of a huge repertoire of B cells that are each characterized by an immunoglobulin molecule with unique antigenic specificity. Mature B cells migrate from the bone marrow to lymphoid tissue throughout the body and are readily identified by the presence of cell surface immunoglobulin and antigens that are B-cell–specific, including CD19, CD20, and CD21. In response to antigen binding to cell surface immunoglobulin, mature B cells are activated to proliferate and undergo differentiation into end-stage plasma cells, which lose most of their B-cell surface markers and produce large quantities of soluble antibodies. Neoplastic disorders of B cells arise from B cells at different stages of development, and thus B-cell lymphomas can be highly varied in their morphologic mechanisms and cell surface expression of B-cell antigens, or immunophenotype.

T CELLS

T cells perform an array of functions in the immune response, including those that are classically regarded as cellular immune responses. T-cell precursors migrate from the bone marrow to the thymus, where they differentiate into mature T-cell subsets and undergo selection to eliminate autoreactive T cells that respond to self-peptides. In the thymus, T-cell precursors undergo a coordinated process of differentiation that involves rearrangement and expression of the T-cell receptor (TCR) genes and acquisition of cell surface proteins that are unique to T cells, including CD3, CD4, and CD8. As T cells mature in the thymus, they ultimately lose either the CD4 or CD8 protein, and thus mature T cells are composed of two major groups: CD4+ and CD8+ cells. After T-cell maturation and selection in the thymus, mature CD4 and CD8 T cells leave the thymus and migrate to lymph nodes, spleen, and other sites in the peripheral immune system. Mature T cells constitute approximately 80% of peripheral blood lymphocytes, 40% of lymph node cells, and 25% of splenic lymphoid cells.

Mature CD4 and CD8 T-cell subsets mediate distinct immune functions. CD8+ cells kill virus-infected or foreign cells and suppress immune functions; thus CD8 cells are designated cytotoxic T cells. CD4+ cells activate other immune response cells such as B cells and macrophages by producing cytokines and direct cell contact; thus CD4 cells

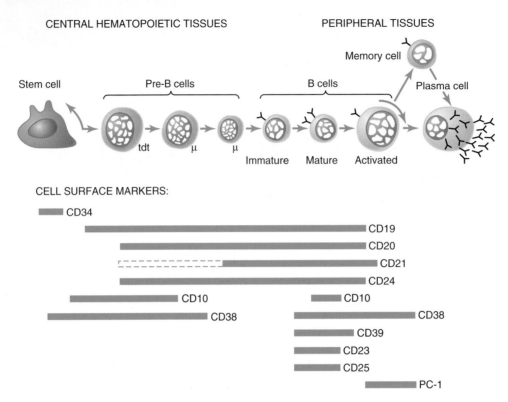

CENTRAL HEMATOPOIETIC TISSUES   PERIPHERAL TISSUES

Figure 50–1 The maturation of B lymphocytes. *Top,* The changes in immunoglobulin production and maturation. *Bottom,* The appearance and disappearance of surface markers. (Adapted from Ferrarini M, Grossi CE, Cooper MD: Cellular and molecular biology of lymphoid cells. In Handin RI, Lux SE, Stossel TP [eds]: Blood Principles and Practice of Hematology. Philadelphia, JB Lippincott, 1995, p 643.)

are considered helper T cells. Similar to B cells, T cells express unique TCR molecules that recognize specific peptide antigens. In contrast to B cells, T cells only respond to peptides that are processed intracellularly and bound to (or presented by) specialized cell surface antigen–presenting proteins, designated major histocompatibility complex (MHC) molecules. Furthermore, CD4 and CD8 T cells are MHC-class restricted in their response to peptide-MHC complexes. CD4 cells recognize antigenic peptide fragments only when they are presented by MHC class II molecules, and CD8 cells recognize antigenic peptide fragments only when they are presented by MHC class I molecules. Antigenic peptides complexed with MHC class I and class II molecules originate from different sources. MHC class I molecules generally produce intracellular or endogenous antigens that are processed in the cytosol and traffic through the endoplasmic reticulum. MHC class II molecules generally produce antigens derived from extracellular sources taken up via endocytosis and processed in intracellular vesicles. Binding of the TCR by a specific peptide-MHC complex triggers activation signals that lead to the expression of gene products that mediate the wide diversity of helper functions in CD4[+] cells or cytotoxic effector functions in CD8[+] cells.

LYMPHOID SYSTEM

Lymphocytes localize to the peripheral lymphoid tissue, which is the site of antigen-lymphocyte interaction and lymphocyte activation. The peripheral lymphoid tissue is composed of lymph nodes, the spleen, and mucosal lymphoid tissue. Lymphocytes circulate continuously through these tissues via the vascular and lymphatic systems.

The lymph nodes are highly organized lymphoid tissues that are sites of convergence of the lymphatic drainage system that carries antigens from draining lymph to the nodes, where they are trapped. A lymph node consists of an outer cortex and an inner medulla (Fig. 50–2). The cortex is organized into lymphoid follicles composed predominantly of B cells; some of the follicles contain central areas or germinal centers, where activated B cells are undergoing proliferation after encountering a specific antigen, surrounded by a mantle zone. The T cells are distributed more diffusely in paracortical areas surrounding the follicles. The spleen traps antigens from blood rather than from the lymphatic system and is the site of disposal of senescent red cells. The lymphocytes in the spleen reside in the areas described as the white pulp, which surround the arterioles entering the organ. As in lymph nodes, the B and T cells are segregated into a periarteriolar lymphoid sheath that is composed of T cells and flanking follicles composed of B cells. The mucosa-associated lymphoid tissues (MALTs) collect antigen from epithelial surfaces and include the gut-associated lymphoid tissue (tonsils, adenoids, appendix, and Peyer's patches of the small intestine), as well as more diffusely organized aggregates of lymphocytes at other mucosal sites.

Lymphocytes circulate in the peripheral blood and comprise 20% to 40% of peripheral blood leukocytes in adults (the proportion is higher in newborns and children). Eighty to 90% of peripheral blood lymphocytes are T cells, and the remainder is largely B cells. The majority of peripheral blood

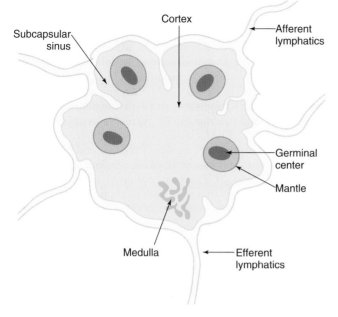

Subcapsular sinus · Cortex · Afferent lymphatics · Germinal center · Mantle · Medulla · Efferent lymphatics

Figure 50–2 The structure of the normal lymph node. The cortical area contains the follicles, which consist of a germinal center and a mantle zone. The medulla contains a complex of channels that lead to the efferent lymphatics.

lymphocytes are mature, resting lymphocytes that morphologically are small, with scant cytoplasm and inconspicuous nucleoli. A small percentage of peripheral blood lymphoid cells represent a third category of lymphoid cells that are referred to as natural killer (NK) cells. These cells do not bear the characteristic cell surface molecules of B or T cells, and their immunoglobulin or TCR genes have not undergone rearrangement. Morphologically, these cells are large, with abundant cytoplasm containing azurophilic granules, and thus they are often called large granular lymphocytes. Functionally, they are part of the innate immune system, responding nonspecifically to a wide range of pathogens without requiring prior antigenic exposure.

Neoplasia of Lymphoid Origin

Malignant transformation of lymphocytes can lead to a diverse array of neoplasia of lymphoid origin, including tumors that arise from T cells or B cells and tumors that represent different stages of lymphocyte development. Lymphoid malignancies usually involve lymphoid tissues, but they can arise in or spread to any site. The major clinical groupings of lymphoid malignancies include non-Hodgkin's lymphomas (NHLs), Hodgkin's disease (HD), lymphoid leukemias, and plasma cell dyscrasias.

The most common clinical presentation of a lymphoid malignancy in adults is painless enlargement of lymph nodes, or lymphadenopathy. Many causes of lymphadenopathy exist, in addition to lymphoid malignancies (Table 50–1). Thus taking a thorough history and performing a careful physical examination is important before performing a lymph node biopsy. The investigation of lymphadenopathy can be organized according to the location of the enlarged nodes

Table 50–1	**Causes of Lymphadenopathy**

Infectious Diseases

Viral: infectious mononucleosis syndromes (cytomegalovirus, Epstein-Barr virus), acquired immunodeficiency syndrome, rubella, herpes simplex, infectious hepatitis
Bacterial: localized infection with regional adenopathy (streptococci, staphylococci), cat-scratch disease, brucellosis, tularemia, listeriosis, bubonic plague (*Yersinia pestis*), chancroid *(Haemophilus ducreyi)*
Fungal: coccidioidomycosis, histoplasmosis
Chlamydial: lymphogranuloma venereum, trachoma
Mycobacterial: scrofula, tuberculosis, leprosy
Protozoan: toxoplasmosis, trypanosomiasis
Spirochetal: Lyme disease, syphilis, leptospirosis

Immunologic Diseases

Rheumatoid arthritis
Systemic lupus erythematosus
Mixed connective tissue disease
Sjögren's syndrome
Dermatomyositis
Serum sickness
Drug reactions: phenytoin, hydralazine, allopurinol

Malignant Diseases

Lymphomas
Metastatic solid tumors to lymph nodes: melanoma, lung, breast, head and neck, gastrointestinal tract, Kaposi's sarcoma, unknown primary tumor, renal, prostate

Atypical Lymphoid Proliferations

Giant follicular lymph node hyperplasia
Transformation of germinal centers
Castleman's disease

Miscellaneous Diseases and Diseases of Unknown Cause

Dermatopathic lymphadenitis
Sarcoidosis
Amyloidosis
Mucocutaneous lymph node syndrome
Multifocal Langerhans cell (eosinophilic) granulomatosis
Lipid storage diseases: Gaucher's and Niemann-Pick diseases

(localized or generalized) and the presence of clinical symptoms. Cervical lymphadenopathy is most often caused by infections of the upper respiratory tract, including infectious mononucleosis syndromes and other viral syndromes, as well as bacterial pharyngitis. Unilateral axillary, inguinal, or femoral adenopathy may be caused by skin infections involving the extremity, including cat-scratch fever. Generalized lymphadenopathy may be caused by systemic infections, such as human immunodeficiency virus (HIV) or cytomegalovirus infection, drug reactions, autoimmune diseases, one of the systemic lymphadenopathy syndromes, or lymphoma. If the cause of persistent lymphadenopathy is not apparent after a thorough evaluation, an excisional lymph node biopsy should be undertaken. An enlarged supraclavicular lymph node is highly suggestive of malignancy and should always be sampled.

The accurate diagnosis of lymphoma requires excisional biopsy of a lymph node or generous biopsy of involved lymph tissue. Fine-needle aspiration or needle biopsy is rarely sufficient for diagnosing malignant lymphoma. Analysis of the pathologic specimen should include routine histologic examination and immunophenotyping. Immuno-phenotyping involves the characterization of the immuno-logic cell surface antigens that are expressed on the malignant lymphocyte by means of a panel of monoclonal antibodies. Immunophenotyping permits a determination of cell of origin (B cell, T cell, NK cell, or nonlymphoid cell) and the pattern of cell surface antigens. In the case of B-cell NHLs, immunophenotyping can also reveal whether the process is monoclonal in origin (i.e., neoplastic) by deter-mining whether the surface immunoglobulin is restricted to either κ or λ light chains. Immunophenotyping has become an essential aspect of the diagnosis and classification of lym-phomas and can be accomplished by flow cytometric analy-sis or by immunohistochemical studies on tissue specimens. In some cases, cytogenetic analysis or molecular studies for immunoglobulin or TCR gene rearrangement may be required to determine the pathologic subtype of lymphoma or to establish a monoclonal (i.e., malignant) process. If a lymph node biopsy is nondiagnostic and unexplained lymph node enlargement persists, the biopsy should be repeated.

Non-Hodgkin's Lymphomas

The NHLs comprise a heterogeneous group of lymphoid malignancies that differ with respect to their histologic appearance, cell of origin and immunophenotype, molecu-lar biologic factors, clinical features, prognosis, and outcome with therapy. In view of the heterogeneity of NHLs, classifi-cation systems have been devised to identify specific patho-logic subtypes that correlate with distinct clinical entities. These systems have evolved steadily over the last 50 years, as correlations between histopathologic and biologic behavior emerged. Until recently, the most widely used classification system in North America was the Working Formulation (WF). The WF classified NHLs based on the architecture of the node (the presence of follicles vs. diffuse infiltrate) and the morphologic features of the malignant lymphocyte (small cell vs. large cell, with cleaved or noncleaved nucleus) and organized the pathologic subtypes into low, intermediate, or high grade based on their natural history and clinical behav-ior. In general, the low-grade histologies were associated with an indolent course and relatively long survival but were incurable, whereas the intermediate- and high-grade his-tologies were biologically aggressive (i.e., short natural history if left untreated) but were potentially curable with appropriate treatment. With the advent of immunopheno-typing and molecular characterization of lymphomas, the fact became apparent that the WF did not adequately define specific pathologic and clinical entities. The Revised European-American Lymphoma (REAL) classification sys-tem, introduced in 1994, incorporated not only histologic features as described by the WF, but also immunophenotype, cytogenetics, and epidemiologic and etiologic factors. Thus

the REAL classification identified several NHL subtypes that were not easily classified within the WF. These subtypes included the mantle cell lymphomas; the MALT lymphomas and monocytoid B-cell lymphomas, which are both derived from cells in the marginal zone of lymph nodes; and the various T-cell lymphomas, including human T-cell leukemia virus type I (HTLV-I)-associated leukemia and lymphoma, cutaneous T-cell lymphoma (mycosis fungoides or Sézary syndrome), and the biologically aggressive peripheral T-cell lymphomas. The REAL classification was updated in 2001 by the World Health Organization (WHO), and the REAL/WHO classification has replaced all previous classification systems (Table 50–2). The most common NHLs encountered in the United States are the follicular lymphomas, small lym-phocytic lymphoma or leukemia (also known as chronic lymphocytic leukemia [CLL]), mantle cell lymphomas, and diffuse large B-cell lymphomas.

The cause of most NHLs is not known. In the majority of patients with NHL, no apparent genetic predisposition or epidemiologic or environmental factor can be identified. Many of the NHL subtypes carry pathognomonic chromo-somal translocations that often involve an immunoglobulin locus (or *TCR* locus in the case of T cell–derived NHLs) and an oncogene or growth regulatory gene. The cause of these aberrant chromosomal rearrangements is unknown. Patients with congenital immunodeficiency syndromes or auto-immune disorders are at increased risk of developing NHL. Oncogenic human viruses play a causal role in some of the less common NHL variants. Epstein-Barr virus (EBV) is associated with several biologically aggressive NHLs, includ-ing acquired immunodeficiency syndrome (AIDS)-related diffuse aggressive lymphomas, the lymphoproliferative dis-orders that arise in patients who are immunosuppressed after organ transplantation, and the form of Burkitt's lymphoma that is endemic in Africa. HTLV-I is causally linked with an aggressive form of T-cell leukemia or lymphoma that is endemic in areas of Japan and the Caribbean basin. The her-pesvirus of Kaposi's sarcoma has been implicated in a variant of diffuse aggressive NHL that arises in serosal cavities and is encountered almost exclusively in patients infected with HIV. *Helicobacter pylori* infection is causally linked to gastric MALT lymphomas, and eradication of infection with anti-biotics is often associated with regression of the lymphoma.

CLINICAL PRESENTATION, EVALUATION, AND STAGING

As described in the preceding section, the majority of patients with NHL exhibit painless lymphadenopathy involving one or more of the peripheral nodal sites. Addi-tionally, NHL can involve extranodal sites, and thus patients can exhibit a variety of symptoms reflective of the site of involvement. The most common sites of extranodal disease are the gastrointestinal tract, bone marrow, liver, and Waldeyer's ring, although virtually any site potentially can be involved with NHL. In general, the aggressive subtypes of NHL (diffuse large cell, lymphoblastic, and Burkitt's) are more likely than are the indolent lymphomas to involve extranodal sites. Central nervous system involvement, including leptomeningeal spread, rarely occurs in the indolent subtypes but does occur in the aggressive variants. The most aggressive NHLs (Burkitt's and lymphoblastic) have a particular propensity to spread to the leptomeninges.

Table 50–2   REAL/WHO Classification of Lymphoid Neoplasms

B-Cell Neoplasms

Precursor B-cell neoplasm
Precursor B-lymphoblastic leukemia/lymphoma (precursor B-cell acute lymphoblastic leukemia)
Mature (peripheral) B-cell neoplasms
B-cell chronic lymphocytic leukemia/small lymphocytic lymphoma
B-cell prolymphocytic leukemia
Lymphoplasmacytic lymphoma
Splenic marginal zone B-cell lymphoma (± villous lymphocytes)
Hairy cell leukemia
Plasma cell myeloma/plasmacytoma
Extranodal marginal zone B-cell lymphoma of MALT type
Nodal marginal zone B-cell lymphoma of MALT type
Follicular lymphoma
Mantle cell lymphoma
Diffuse large B-cell lymphoma
Mediastinal large B-cell lymphoma
Primary effusion lymphoma
Burkitt's lymphoma/Burkitt cell leukemia

T- and NK-Cell Neoplasms

Precursor T-cell neoplasm
Precursor T-lymphoblastic lymphoma/leukemia (precursor T-cell acute lymphoblastic leukemia)
Mature (peripheral) T-cell neoplasms
T-cell prolymphocytic leukemia
T-cell granular lymphocytic leukemia
Aggressive NK-cell leukemia
Adult T-cell lymphoma/leukemia (HTLV1)
Extranodal NK-/T-cell lymphoma, nasal type
Enteropathy-type T-cell lymphoma
Hepatosplenic gamma-delta T-cell lymphoma
Subcutaneous panniculitis-like T-cell lymphoma
Mycosis fungoides/Sézary syndrome
Anaplastic large cell lymphoma, T/null cell, primary cutaneous type
Peripheral T-cell lymphoma, not otherwise characterized
Angioimmunoblastic T-cell lymphoma
Anaplastic large cell lymphoma, T/null cell, primary systemic type

Note: Only major categories are included. Common entities are shown in **bold type**.
$HTLV1_+$ = human T-cell leukemia virus; MALT = mucosa-associated lymphoid tissue; NK = natural killer.
B- and T-/NK-cell neoplasms are grouped according to major clinical presentations (predominantly disseminated/leukemic, primary extranodal, predominantly nodal).

Table 50–3   Staging Evaluation for Lymphomas

Required Evaluation Procedures

Biopsy of lesion with review by an experienced hematopathologist
History with attention to the presence or absence of *B* symptoms
Physical examination with attention to node-bearing areas (including Waldeyer's ring) and size of liver and spleen
Standard blood work, including:
  Complete blood cell count
  Lactate dehydrogenase and β_2-microglobulin
  Evaluation of renal function
  Liver function tests
  Calcium, uric acid
Radiologic studies, including:
  Chest radiograph (posteroanterior and lateral)
  Chest-abdominal pelvic CT
  Gallium scan (in Hodgkin's and intermediate- and high-grade lymphomas)
  Bilateral bone marrow aspirates and biopsies

Procedures Required under Certain Circumstances

Abdominal ultrasonogram or gastrointestinal contrast studies to supplement CT scans or investigate sites of unexplained symptoms
Bone scan if bone symptoms
Plain bone radiographs of symptomatic or abnormal areas on bone scan
Brain or spinal CT or MRI if neurologic signs and symptoms
Serum and urine protein electrophoresis

CT = computed tomography; MRI = magnetic resonance imaging.

The diagnosis of NHL requires an adequate biopsy of the involved nodal tissue or extranodal site. In patients with bone marrow and peripheral blood involvement, such as small lymphocytic lymphoma or CLL, making the diagnosis from immunophenotyping of peripheral blood lymphocytes by flow cytometry is often possible. Once the diagnosis of a lymphoma has been made, patients should undergo a complete staging evaluation (Table 50–3). Staging determines the extent of involvement, provides prognostic information, and may influence the choice of therapy. The modified Ann Arbor staging classification is used to stage patients with both NHL and Hodgkin's disease (Table 50–4). Standard staging evaluation includes a thorough history to elicit symptoms referable to the lymphoma, including the presence of constitutional symptoms (fevers, night sweats, or weight loss, designated as *B* symptoms); a complete physical examination, with documentation of the size and distribution of enlarged lymph nodes; blood work, including lactate dehydrogenase (LDH) evaluation; computed tomographic (CT) scans of chest, abdomen, and pelvis; and bone marrow aspirate and biopsy. Gallium or positron emission tomo-

Constitutional symptoms such as fevers, weight loss, or night sweats occur in approximately 20% of patients with NHL at the time of onset, and these symptoms are more common in patients with aggressive subtypes of NHL.

Table 50–4	Staging System for Lymphomas

Stage	Description
Stage I	Involvement of a single lymph node region or structure (I) or a single extralymphatic site (IE)
Stage II	Involvement of two or more lymph node regions on the same side of the diaphragm (II) or localized involvement of a contiguous extralymphatic site and lymph node region (IIE)
Stage III	Involvement of lymph node regions on both sides of the diaphragm (III), which may be accompanied by localized involvement of one extralymphatic site (IIIE) or spleen (IIIS) or both (IIISE)
III$_1$	With or without involvement of splenic, hilar, celiac, or portal nodes
III$_2$	With involvement of para-aortic, iliac, and mesenteric nodes
Stage IV	Diffuse or disseminated involvement of one or more extralymphatic organs with or without associated lymph node involvement

Identification of the presence or absence of symptoms should be noted with each stage designation. A = asymptomatic; B = fever, sweats, weight loss >10% of body weight.

graphic (PET) scans can be helpful in assessing response to therapy in lymphomas that are gallium avid or metabolically active (usually the aggressive subtypes such as diffuse large cell lymphoma, lymphoblastic lymphoma, and Burkitt's lymphoma) and is often included in the staging evaluation of the aggressive NHLs. Lumbar puncture for cytologic analysis should be performed only in patients who are at risk for leptomeningeal disease, which includes all patients with Burkitt's and lymphoblastic lymphoma and patients with diffuse large cell lymphoma with involvement of bone marrow, testes, or structures directly abutting the central nervous system (e.g., paranasal sinus, calvarium). A variety of ancillary tests may be performed in specific situations. For example, a test for HTLV-I or HIV should be performed if adult T-cell leukemia or lymphoma or AIDS-related lymphoma is thought to exist, respectively. A gastrointestinal series or endoscopic evaluation may be warranted in all patients with gastrointestinal symptoms or in patients at risk for gastrointestinal tract involvement (lymphomas involving the Waldeyer's ring). Serum protein electrophoresis and determination of β$_2$-microglobulin and quantitative immunoglobulins should be performed in patients who are thought to have plasma cell dyscrasias. A laparotomy for the sole purpose of staging patients with NHL is never performed, because it rarely influences therapeutic decision making.

A variety of prognostic variables have been identified for NHL. In general, the predictors for poor survival in most subtypes of NHL include advanced stage at onset (stage III or IV), involvement of multiple extranodal sites of disease, elevated LDH levels, the presence of B symptoms, and poor performance status.

NATURAL HISTORY, PROGNOSIS, AND TREATMENT

Indolent Non-Hodgkin's Lymphomas

The common low-grade or indolent histologic conditions include the follicular lymphomas (small cleaved cell and mixed cell types) and small lymphocytic lymphoma (the latter is identical to CLL and is discussed later), which account for approximately 30% and 5% of all NHLs, respectively. The low-grade follicular lymphomas are mature clonal B-cell neoplasms with an immunophenotype that is positive for surface immunoglobulin (κ or λ chain restricted) and the mature B-cell markers (CD19, CD20, CD21) and negative for CD5. Follicular lymphomas are characterized cytogenetically by the t(14;18) translocation that juxtaposes the immunoglobulin heavy chain with the antiapoptotic gene *BCL2*; *BCL2* is uniformly expressed in follicular lymphomas. Although the follicular lymphomas are low-grade, indolent neoplasms with a long natural history (median survival approaches 10 years), the majority of patients (80% to 90%) exhibit an advanced stage (stage III or IV), often with bone marrow involvement, and cannot be cured with standard treatment modalities. Factors associated with shortened survival include older age, advanced stage, anemia, multiple lymph node sites (less than four), and elevated LDH. Patients with three or more of these factors have a median survival of 5 years, roughly one half that of patients with zero or one risk factor. Most patients with follicular NHL eventually experience transformation of their disease to a more aggressive lymphoma, characterized pathologically by a diffuse large cell infiltrate and clinically by rapidly expanding nodes or other tumor masses, rising LDH levels, and the onset of disease-related symptoms.

The management of the follicular lymphomas is determined by the stage. For the few patients who are considered to have early-stage (I or nonbulky II) disease after clinical staging, the appropriate treatment is radiation therapy. With the use of subtotal or total lymphoid irradiation, more than one half of patients with early-stage disease will achieve a durable remission and appear to be cured. For patients with advanced-stage disease, the management is more controversial. Although advanced-stage indolent NHL is responsive to a variety of treatment modalities, the incurability and the long natural history has led to the practice of deferring treatment until the patient develops symptoms. This strategy is referred to as the *watch and wait* approach. Indications for treatment include cosmetic or mechanical problems caused by enlarging lymph nodes, constitutional symptoms, and evidence of marrow compromise. The appropriate treatment of advanced-stage disease, when necessary, is systemic chemotherapy. The follicular lymphomas are responsive to a variety of single and multidrug programs. Single alkylating agents (cyclophosphamide or chlorambucil), multidrug regimens containing an alkylating agent (e.g., cyclophosphamide, vincristine, and prednisone [CVP]), or fludarabine-based regimens (i.e., fludarabine and mitoxantrone, fludarabine and cyclophosphamide) are all effective initial regimens for this disease. The addition of the chimeric (mouse-human) anti-CD 20 monoclonal antibody Rituximab to chemotherapy regimens has become commonplace and is associated with improvements in response rate and duration of remission. The majority of patients respond to treatment, and at least one third achieves a clinical complete remission that may last 1 to 3 years. Treatment should be discontinued when the maximum response has been achieved to minimize cumulative toxicity. Once a patient relapses, subsequent remissions may be achieved but are usually less durable compared with the first remission. Therapeutic options for patients who relapse include re-treatment with chemotherapy, often with a different drug or combination than that used initially. Patients in relapse can also be treated with Rituximab as a single agent. Rituximab is a highly effective nontoxic agent for use in patients with relapsed follicular lymphoma, inducing responses that are often durable in over one half of patients. Patients who respond to rituximab are often successfully re-treated with rituximab at subsequent relapse, and, in contrast to the experience with second- or third-line chemotherapy, these patients may experience remissions that actually exceed the duration of their first remission from rituximab. Two radioactively labeled anti-CD20 antibodies, ibritumomab tiuxetan (yttrium-labeled) and 131-iodine tositumomab are now also in use for patients with relapsed or refractory follicular lymphoma and have been associated with a high response rate. For patients who have clinical or pathologic evidence of transformation to a higher grade of lymphoma, treatment that is appropriate for a diffuse aggressive histology should be offered (discussed later). The role of high-dose chemotherapy with autologous or allogeneic stem cell transplant for follicular NHLs remains unclear and should be considered experimental. Long-term follow-up of patients undergoing allogeneic transplantation suggests that some patients are cured with this modality. However, the morbidity associated with allogeneic transplantation has precluded its widespread use for refractory indolent lymphomas.

In addition to the follicular NHLs, the MALT lymphomas and closely related marginal zone lymphomas are also considered low-grade, indolent subtypes. Given the excellent prognosis, localized nature, and long natural history of the MALT lymphomas, they are generally managed conservatively with local treatment modalities (irradiation or surgery) and avoidance of systemic chemotherapy. Importantly, the gastric MALT lymphomas are highly associated with *H. pylori* infection, and remissions can often be achieved with eradication of this infection. Thus antibiotic therapy is the first-line treatment for early gastric MALT lymphoma.

Diffuse Aggressive Non-Hodgkin's Lymphomas

The aggressive NHLs are characterized by effacement of lymph node architecture with a diffuse infiltrate of large lymphocytes and include the diffuse large B-cell lymphoma (accounting for approximately one third of all NHLs), anaplastic large cell lymphoma, and peripheral T-cell lymphoma. The majority of the diffuse aggressive large cell lymphomas are B cell in origin (diffuse large B-cell lymphoma);

the T-cell diffuse aggressive lesions, or peripheral T-cell lymphomas, are managed similarly but have an overall worse prognosis compared with their B-cell counterparts. Burkitt's lymphoma and lymphoblastic lymphoma are among the most aggressive lymphomas and are discussed separately later in this chapter (see High-Grade Non-Hodgkin's Lymphomas).

Diffuse aggressive NHLs exhibit clinically aggressive behavior, and, if left untreated, the median survival is less than 1 to 2 years. Compared with the follicular NHLs, a higher percentage of patients with diffuse aggressive histologies will exhibit early-stage disease (30% to 50%) or with an extranodal site of involvement (50%). The outcome and likelihood of cure of patients with diffuse aggressive histologies is directly related to the total number of adverse prognostic features at onset: age older than 60 years, advanced stage (III or IV), elevated LDH levels, poor performance status, and the presence of two or more extranodal sites of disease. The likelihood of cure and long-term disease-free survival ranges from more than 75% in patients with one or fewer adverse factors to less than 30% in patients with four or more adverse factors.

In contrast to patients with low-grade follicular NHLs, all patients with diffuse aggressive histologies should be offered immediate therapy, because these lymphomas are potentially curable. The standard initial therapy for all patients with diffuse aggressive NHL is a multidrug chemotherapy regimen that includes an anthracycline. The most widely used regimen is a combination of cyclophosphamide, doxorubicin, vincristine, and prednisone (designated as CHOP). This regimen appears to be equivalent to more complex and intensive regimens such as m-BACOD, Pro-MACE, and MACOP-B, and thus CHOP remains the standard. Patients with early-stage disease (I or nonbulky stage II) may be treated with local radiation therapy after a minimum of three cycles of CHOP if exposure to chemotherapy is limited. Patients with advanced-stage disease require six cycles of CHOP; the role of local radiation to sites of bulky disease in the setting of advanced-stage disease is not established. Complete remissions can be achieved with the CHOP or similar regimens, and 30% to 40% of patients are cured. Selected patients with an adverse prognosis may benefit from high-dose chemotherapy and autologous stem cell support in first remission. The addition of rituximab to initial CHOP chemotherapy has been shown to increase the response rate and extend survival in elderly patients with diffuse large B-cell lymphomas compared with CHOP chemotherapy alone. Thus rituximab in combination with CHOP chemotherapy is now used widely as initial therapy for diffuse large B-cell lymphomas. Patients who experience relapse after achieving a remission often can be cured with high-dose chemotherapy with autologous peripheral blood stem cell support, or *transplant*, particularly if their relapsed disease remains responsive to standard doses of chemotherapy. The morbidity and mortality of this procedure have diminished substantially since 1990 with the use of peripheral blood stem cells and colony-stimulating factor support, and it can be safely performed in patients without serious co-morbid conditions. High-dose chemotherapy with autologous stem cell transplant is superior to standard doses of a salvage regimen and is considered standard therapy for patients with relapsed chemosensitive diffuse aggressive NHL.

Mantle Cell Lymphoma

Mantle cell lymphoma has been recognized with increasing frequency since immunophenotyping has become standard practice for classifying NHLs, and it is included in the REAL/WHO classification. Mantle cell NHL was not recognized in the WF and was often designated as a diffuse small cleaved cell or diffuse mixed cell lymphoma in the WF classification. It accounts for 5% to 8% of all NHLs. Mantle cell lymphomas are mature B-cell neoplasms that appear to arise in the mantle zone of the lymphoid follicle and display a highly characteristic immunophenotype. Mantle cells express the CD5 antigen, as well as the mature B-cell markers (CD19, CD20, and CD21), but typically are negative for CD23 expression. Because mantle cell lymphomas can be easily confused pathologically and clinically with CLL, which is the only other B-cell NHL that is CD5$^+$, the absence of CD23 is important for distinguishing mantle cell lymphoma from CLL, which is typically CD23$^+$. Mantle cell lymphomas are also characterized by a pathognomonic t(11;14) chromosomal translocation that juxtaposes the immunoglobulin heavy chain with the *BCL1* or *PRAD1* gene, which encodes the growth-promoting protein cyclin D1. Mantle cell lymphomas are in many ways similar to indolent lymphomas in that patients usually exhibit advanced-stage disease with frequent bone marrow involvement. These lymphomas have a peculiar propensity to involve Waldeyer's ring and the gastrointestinal tract. As with the low-grade follicular lymphomas, mantle cell lymphomas are treatable but not curable. However, in contrast to the indolent lymphomas, these neoplasms are biologically aggressive, with a median survival of only 2 to 3 years. These patients are generally treated with systemic chemotherapy at diagnosis, because of the more aggressive nature of mantle cell lymphomas compared with follicular lymphomas, but durable remissions are difficult to achieve. The optimal therapy for this challenging subtype remains to be established, and these patients should be considered for experimental therapies, including immunotherapy or transplantation.

High-Grade Non-Hodgkin's Lymphoma

The two high-grade subtypes, Burkitt's or small noncleaved cell and lymphoblastic lymphoma, are quite rare in the adult population. Nonetheless, these subtypes are important because they are potentially curable with appropriate therapy and often require urgent, inpatient treatment at the time of diagnosis because of their highly aggressive nature, rapid growth, and tendency to develop tumor lysis on initiation of therapy. Lymphoblastic lymphoma is an aggressive lymphoma that is closely related to T-cell acute lymphocytic leukemia and readily distinguished from most NHLs by its T-cell immunophenotype and the presence of terminal deoxynucleotide transferase. It usually afflicts young adult males and involves the mediastinum and bone marrow, with a propensity to relapse in the leptomeninges. Burkitt's, or small noncleaved cell, lymphoma is a rare B-cell lymphoma in adults that is highly aggressive, with a propensity to involve the bone marrow and central nervous system. Burkitt's lymphoma is characterized cytogenetically by the pathognomonic t(8;14) translocation that juxtaposes the *Ig* locus with the *myc* oncogene. In central Africa, where Burkitt's lymphoma is endemic in children, it is usually

associated with EBV. However, in the United States, it is uncommon for sporadic Burkitt's lymphoma to be EBV positive. Burkitt's lymphoma and lymphoblastic lymphomas both require treatment with intensive multiagent chemotherapy, including intrathecal chemotherapy to prevent leptomeningeal relapse. These lymphomas undergo rapid tumor lysis on initiation of chemotherapy, and all patients must receive prophylaxis against tumor lysis syndrome before and during their first course of chemotherapy. Prophylaxis includes hydration, alkalinization of the urine, and allopurinol.

Hodgkin's Disease

HD is the most common lymphoma in young adults. It has a bimodal age distribution in the United States and industrialized countries, with the larger peak occurring between ages 15 and 35 and a second smaller peak occurring in patients older than 50. The cause of HD remains enigmatic. Although EBV is frequently present in the malignant cell of HD, a direct causal link between EBV and HD has not been established. HD does not appear with increased frequency in patients with congenital immunodeficiency syndromes or in immunosuppressed organ transplant recipients, and the risk of HD does not appear to increase in patients infected with HIV.

The diagnosis of HD is made by identifying the Reed-Sternberg (RS) cell in involved lymphoid tissue. The classic RS cell is large and binucleate, with each nucleus containing a prominent nucleolus, suggesting the appearance of *owl's eyes*. Although the cellular origin of the RS cell was debated for many decades, molecular studies have confirmed that RS cells are B cell in nature with clonal rearrangement of the germline *Ig* locus, despite the absence of cytoplasmic or cell surface immunoglobulin. In contrast to NHL and other malignancies, the bulk of the infiltrate in lymph nodes involved with HD is usually composed of benign reactive inflammatory cells, and often the diagnostic RS cells can be difficult to find. Immunophenotyping of classic RS cells reveals that they are CD30 (Ki-1) and CD15 positive and negative for CD20, CD45, and cytoplasmic or surface immunoglobulin; EBV is identified in the RS cells in approximately one half of patients with HD.

Four pathologic variants of HD have been identified. Nodular sclerosing (NS) is by far the most common (80% of patients with HD) and is characterized by the presence of fibrous bands separating the node into nodules and the *lacunar* type of RS cells. It is the predominant type encountered in adolescents and young adults and typically involves the mediastinum and other supradiaphragmatic nodal sites. In the mixed cellularity (MC) type, which accounts for approximately 15% of patients with HD, band-forming sclerosis is absent, and RS cells are easily identified in a diffuse infiltrate that is more heterogeneous compared with that seen in the NS variant. The MC variant may be encountered in any age group, and advanced-stage disease with subdiaphragmatic involvement is more common with MC-variant HD than it is with NS-variant HD. The lymphocyte-depleted type is rare, accounting for less than 1% of the HD cases, and is characterized by sheets of RS cells with a paucity of inflammatory cells. This variant is most common in older adults, in patients infected with HIV, and in persons in nonindustrialized countries. The lymphocyte-predominant (LP) type has emerged as a distinct entity that may be more closely related to indolent NHL than it is to HD, although it is managed as true HD. The LP type is characterized by a nodular growth pattern with variants of RS cells that have polylobated nuclei and are referred to as *popcorn* cells; classic RS cells are usually absent. The immunophenotype of the atypical cells is distinct from classic RS cells, with expression of B-cell antigens (CD19 and CD20) and CD45 but absence of the classic RS markers CD15 and CD30. The LP type of HD accounts for approximately 5% of cases, has a strong male preponderance, and tends to involve peripheral nodes with sparing of the mediastinum. The prognosis is excellent, although late relapses are more common than they are in the other types of HD.

HD arises in lymph nodes, most commonly in the mediastinum or neck, and spreads to adjacent contiguous or non-contiguous nodal sites, including retroperitoneal nodes and the spleen. As the disease progresses, it spreads hematogenously to involve extranodal sites, including bone marrow, liver, and lung. In contrast to NHL, HD rarely arises in extranodal sites, although HD can involve extranodal sites by contiguous spread from an adjacent lymph node (e.g., involvement of vertebrae from adjacent retroperitoneal lymph nodes, involvement of pulmonary parenchyma from adjacent hilar nodes).

HD usually produces painless enlargement of lymph nodes, most often in the neck. Mediastinal adenopathy may be found incidentally in a patient who is asymptomatic on routine chest radiography. Massive mediastinal or hilar adenopathy, with or without adjacent pulmonary involvement, may cause respiratory symptoms such as cough, shortness of breath, wheezing, or stridor. Approximately one third of patients with HD have constitutional symptoms of fever, night sweats, or weight loss (*B* symptoms), which can be the presenting complaint. In addition to the *B* symptoms, generalized pruritus is also associated with HD and correlates with the NS type. Occasionally, patients give a history of troubling pruritus for months to years before the diagnosis of HD. Although HD is associated with functional T-lymphocyte defects, exhibited as cutaneous anergy to intradermal skin tests, patients rarely have opportunistic infections. If left untreated, the natural history of HD is one of inexorable, albeit often slow, progression to involve multiple nodal sites, followed by hematogenous spread to bone marrow, liver, and other viscera. As the disease advances, patients experience *B* symptoms, malaise, cachexia, and infectious complications, and patients with progressive HD ultimately die of complications of bone marrow failure or infection.

Accurate staging of patients with newly diagnosed HD is important for treatment planning, prognosis, and assessing response to therapy. A modification of the Ann Arbor classification is used (see Table 50–4), and the suffix *A* or *B* is appended to denote the absence or presence, respectively, of fever, night sweats, or weight loss. The staging work-up of a patient with newly diagnosed HD is similar to that for patients with NHL (see Table 50–3). Patients should undergo a thorough history and physical examination; complete blood work, including an erythrocyte sedimentation rate; chest radiography; CT scan of the chest, abdomen, and pelvis; bone marrow aspirate and biopsy; and PET scan or gallium scan. Lymphangiograms have been used historically in assessing subdiaphragmatic adenopathy; however, the expertise to perform and interpret this test is no longer widely available and has been largely replaced by the combination of CT scanning and nuclear imaging techniques. Additional tests, such as bone films, bone scan, and spinal magnetic resonance imaging, should be obtained only if symptoms suggest involvement of these structures. The information derived from this noninvasive work-up defines the clinical stage of a patient with HD. The role of the staging laparotomy to determine involvement below the diaphragm more accurately waned substantially during the 1990s, as therapy for early-stage disease evolved. This procedure entails a laparotomy with splenectomy, liver biopsy, and a sampling of retroperitoneal nodes; the information derived from this procedure defines the pathologic stage of the disease. A staging laparotomy is no longer considered routine, given that treatment has evolved away from the use of primary radiotherapy (discussed later). However, if a patient with clinical stage I or II supradiaphragmatic disease will be treated with radiation therapy as the sole modality, a staging laparotomy is an option to rule out occult involvement of the spleen and retroperitoneal nodes. Occult HD can be found below the diaphragm in as many as 30% of patients with clinical stage I or II disease, mandating treatment with chemotherapy. Patients who do undergo staging laparotomy with splenectomy are at risk for overwhelming bacterial infection with encapsulated organisms and should receive pneumococcal and *Haemophilus influenzae* vaccine before surgery.

A variety of prognostic factors that influence risk of relapse or survival have been identified in HD. The most important adverse prognostic factors are MC or lymphocyte-depleted histologies, male sex, large number of involved nodal sites, advanced stage (age >40), the presence of *B* symptoms, high erythrocyte sedimentation rate, and bulky disease (widening of the mediastinum by more than one third or the presence of a nodal mass measuring more than 10 cm in any dimension). The presence of any of these factors in patients with early-stage disease places them at increased risk of occult abdominal involvement or relapse after primary radiation therapy and thus influences the decision to include chemotherapy in the initial treatment.

The treatment of HD has evolved considerably since 1980. HD is highly curable; the cure rate exceeds 80% with the use of current treatment modalities. Because most patients with HD are young adults and will experience long-term disease-free survival, the emphasis has shifted toward using therapies that minimize treatment-related morbidity and mortality without sacrificing curative potential. Radiation therapy in moderate doses (>35 Gy) to involved sites of disease plus contiguous nodal regions is curative for the majority of patients with low-risk, early-stage disease (nonbulky stages I and IIA without adverse risk factors) and remains a viable treatment option for these patients. However, the long-term follow-up of patients treated with standard doses of radiation therapy has revealed a substantially increased risk of developing a variety of solid tumors within or at the margin of the radiation field more than a decade later. Chest irradiation for HD is associated with a particularly high risk of breast cancer in women and of lung cancer in both men and women. Additional long-term sequelae of standard radiation therapy for HD include thyroid dysfunction (usually hypothyroidism) and accelerated coronary artery disease. Thus enthusiasm for primary radiation therapy in standard doses for low-risk, early-stage Hodgkin's disease is diminishing in patients who will require chest irradiation, which represents the overwhelming majority of patients in the early stage.

In response to the recognition of the long-term carcinogenic effects of standard-dose radiation, the approach to treating patients with low-risk, early-stage HD is evolving. Increasingly, the trend has been to combine chemotherapy (e.g., the doxorubicin [Adriamycin], bleomycin, vinblastine, and dacarbazine, designated as the [ABVD] regimen) with a low dose of radiation therapy (>30 Gy), which has not been associated with an increased risk of secondary solid tumors. The optimal duration of chemotherapy in combination with low-dose irradiation for early-stage HD remains unsettled.

Patients with advanced-stage HD (III or IV) or with early-stage disease with adverse risk factors (e.g., bulky disease, *B* symptoms, MC type) are not candidates for radiation therapy as the sole treatment modality because of the high rate of relapse. These patients should be treated with chemotherapy. The multiagent chemotherapy program nitrogen mustard, vincristine (Oncovin), procarbazine, and prednisone (designated as MOPP) was demonstrated to be highly curative in patients with advanced-stage disease in the 1970s. MOPP remains a highly effective regimen, but it is rarely used in current practice because of the long-term toxic effects associated with MOPP. These effects include sterility in nearly all men and infertility in a significant percentage of women who receive MOPP and a high risk of developing acute myeloid leukemia. The ABVD regimen is now the most widely used program in the United States. ABVD is as effective as is MOPP but does not cause sterility, infertility, or treatment-induced leukemias. ABVD has been associated with pulmonary fibrosis in a small percentage of patients (<5%) because of the inclusion of bleomycin in this regimen; the risk of pulmonary fibrosis is highest in patients who have underlying lung disease or who receive chest irradiation as a part of the treatment program. Patients who have an underlying cardiomyopathy are not candidates for ABVD because of the potential risk of further cardiac injury from doxorubicin, and alternate regimens are required in these patients. Radiation therapy in combination with chemotherapy is not generally used to treat advanced-stage HD. However, in patients with bulky mediastinal disease, consolidative radiation to the mediastinum after completion of chemotherapy has been shown to decrease the rate of relapse. Thus combined modality therapy (chemotherapy plus radiation therapy) is considered standard for patients with bulky mediastinal disease.

Evaluating the patient's response to therapy in HD involves repetition of the staging evaluation (physical examination, CT, gallium or PET scan, and bone marrow biopsy if positive at diagnosis) during and at the completion of treatment. Patients may be cured despite the presence of a residual radiographic abnormality on chest radiography or CT (e.g., enlarged nodes, residual mediastinal mass). Patients with residual radiographic abnormalities after an initial response to therapy should not be subjected to salvage therapy without additional corroborating evidence of

persistent HD, such as biopsy confirmation or radiographic progression over time. A persistently positive gallium or PET scan in patients with residual radiographic abnormalities is associated with a high rate of subsequent relapse, and these patients should be monitored closely or considered for immediate repeat biopsy and/or salvage therapy. The majority of patients destined to relapse will do so within 2 years; relapses after 5 years are exceedingly rare.

Patients who relapse or fail to respond after initial therapy should be offered salvage therapy, given that many of these patients can now be cured if treated appropriately. Approximately 20% of patients with early-stage HD who receive standard-dose radiation therapy (without chemotherapy) will relapse. These patients can be salvaged with standard chemotherapy (e.g., ABVD). Patients who relapse after standard chemotherapy should be treated with high-dose chemotherapy with autologous peripheral stem cell support. More than 50% of patients with recurrent, chemosensitive HD can be cured with this regimen.

Lymphoid Leukemias

ACUTE LYMPHOCYTIC LEUKEMIAS

The acute lymphocytic leukemias that arise from precursor B or T cells are described in detail in Chapter 47.

CHRONIC LYMPHOCYTIC LEUKEMIA

B-cell CLL is a malignant disorder of lymphocytes characterized by expansion and accumulation of small lymphocytes of B-cell origin. CLL is essentially identical to B-cell small lymphocytic lymphoma in the REAL and WF classifications. CLL is the most common form of leukemia in the United States and affects twice as many men as it does women. Although it can occur at any stage of life, the incidence increases with age, and more than 90% of cases are diagnosed in adults older than 50 years of age. The cause of CLL is unknown. No apparent genetic basis for the disease has been found, and environmental factors, such as radiation and exposure to carcinogens, have not been implicated.

The common form of CLL is a clonal proliferation of mature B cells, expressing characteristic mature B-cell markers and low levels of surface immunoglobulin M (IgM) that is light-chain restricted, reflecting the clonal origin of this malignancy. In addition, CLL B cells express the CD5 molecule, which marks a minor subset of normal B cells, and CD23 (the Fc receptor for immunoglobulin E [IgE]). Thus the diagnostic immunophenotype of CLL is that of a mature B-cell population that is clonal (by light-chain restriction or *Ig* gene rearrangement studies) expresses the characteristic mature B-cell markers (CD19, CD20, and CD21) and is positive for both CD5 and CD23. Although a pathognomonic chromosomal abnormality has not been identified in CLL, 30% to 50% of patients have cytogenetic abnormalities. The most frequent abnormalities involve chromosome 12 (often trisomy 12), 13, or 14, and the presence of cytogenetic abnormalities is associated with a poorer prognosis. Smears of the bone marrow or peripheral blood reveal a predominance of small lymphocytes with inconspicuous nucleoli, and involved lymph nodes reveal a diffuse infiltrate of these cells ablating normal architecture.

Table 50–5	**Staging System for Chronic Lymphocytic Leukemia**				
Stage	**Lymphocytosis**	**Lymphadenopathy**	**Hepatomegaly or Splenomegaly**	**Hemoglobin (g/dL)**	**Platelets (×10³/μL)**
RAI System					
0	+	−	−	≥11	≥100
I	+	+	−	≥11	≥100
II	+	±	±	≥11	≥100
III	+	±	±	<11	≥100
IV	+	±	±	Any	<100
BINET System					
A	+	± (<3 lymphatic groups* positive)	±	≥10	≥10
B	+	± (≥3 lymphatic groups* positive)	±	≥10	≥10
C	+	±	±	<10	<10

*Cervical, axillary, inguinal nodes, liver, and spleen are each considered one group whether unilateral or bilateral.

CLL cells accumulate in bone marrow, peripheral blood, lymph nodes, and spleen, resulting in lymphocytosis, decreased bone marrow function, lymphadenopathy, and splenomegaly. CLL is also frequently associated with immune dysregulation, exhibiting as hypogammaglobulinemia with an increased risk of bacterial infections and autoimmune phenomena such as Coombs-positive hemolytic anemia or immune thrombocytopenia. The diagnosis is often made incidentally on a routine blood cell count that shows a leukocytosis with a predominance of small lymphocytes; flow cytometric analysis of peripheral blood or a bone marrow aspirate will reveal the characteristic clonal B-cell population that is CD5 and CD23 positive. Some patients exhibit lymphadenopathy, symptoms related to cytopenias, or, occasionally, recurrent infections. As the disease progresses, patients develop generalized lymphadenopathy, hepatosplenomegaly, and bone marrow failure. Death often results from infectious complications or bone marrow failure in patients who have become refractory to treatment. In approximately 5% of instances, CLL transforms to a highly malignant diffuse large cell lymphoma, which is usually rapidly fatal; this transformation is commonly referred to as Richter's syndrome.

CLL is a low-grade leukemia or lymphoma that is typically characterized by a long natural history with slow progression over years or even decades; the median survival rate is in excess of 6 years. The extent of disease, or stage, at onset is the best predictor of survival. Table 50–5 shows the widely used Rai and Binet staging systems for CLL; the majority of patients exhibit stage 0, I, or II disease. Given that standard therapy is not curative, and because CLL may have a long asymptomatic phase lasting years, specific treatment can be withheld until the patient develops symptoms (e.g., bulky lymphadenopathy, constitutional symptoms such as fevers, cytopenias caused by either bone marrow infiltration or autoimmune phenomenon). When treatment is required, initial therapy is begun either with an alkylating agent such as chlorambucil in combination with prednisone or with the nucleoside-analogue fludarabine. The majority of patients respond to either of these interventions with significant reductions in tumor burden. Fludarabine therapy is associated with a higher rate of complete remissions compared with therapy with chlorambucil and combination regimens (e.g., fludarabine, cyclophosphamide, and rituximab) have shown particularly encouraging results. Patients with recurrent or refractory disease may respond to alemtuzumab, a humanized monoclonal antibody to the CD52 molecule, which is present on most lymphocytes. Rituximab is also an active agent for patients with recurrent CLL. Patients who develop autoimmune phenomena require treatment with corticosteroids, and intravenous gamma globulin may be used to reduce the frequency of infections in patients who have developed hypogammaglobulinemia. The development of a rapidly enlarging mediastinal mass, constitutional symptoms, and high serum LDH suggests transformation of disease to a diffuse large cell lymphoma, which is associated with a poor prognosis.

HAIRY CELL LEUKEMIA

Hairy cell leukemia is a biologically indolent neoplastic lymphoid disorder characterized by an accumulation of neoplastic B cells in the bone marrow, peripheral blood, and spleen that morphologically have a characteristic appearance described as *hairy*. Hairy cells are lymphoid cells with fine cytoplasmic projections that are readily identified by the presence of tartrate-resistant acid phosphatase, B-cell immunophenotype, and rearranged heavy- and light-chain immunoglobulin genes. The diagnosis is made by identifying typical hairy cells in the peripheral blood or on bone marrow biopsy. The bone marrow is often inaspirable because of the extensive reticulin fibrosis typically present.

This disease may resemble CLL superficially, but it has unique clinical features and requires different therapy. Hairy cell leukemia may be diagnosed in a patient who is asymptomatic on routine blood cell count; patients who are symptomatic usually exhibit symptoms referable to splenomegaly, infection caused by impaired host defenses, or associated autoimmune syndromes such as vasculitis or arthritis. Osteolytic bone lesions can occur and may cause pain. *B* symptoms are rare. On examination, splenomegaly is present in more than 80% of patients; hepatomegaly is less common, and lymphadenopathy is distinctly unusual. Pancytopenia is typically present at diagnosis. The course of hairy cell leukemia is generally indolent, with slowly progressive pancytopenia and splenomegaly. However, a considerable variability can be found in severity and rate of disease progression. Before effective therapy, bacterial and fungal infections occurred frequently and were the major cause of death.

Asymptomatic patients without significant cytopenias or other complications of the disease require no immediate therapy and can be monitored closely for progression or infectious complications. Patients who exhibit moderate cytopenias, history of infections, rapidly progressive disease, symptomatic splenomegaly, bone involvement, or autoimmune syndromes should undergo therapy. First-line therapy is the purine nucleoside analogue 2-chlorodeoxyadenosine (2-CDA). In 90% of patients, one course of treatment given as a continuous infusion over 7 days results in a complete response that is usually durable. 2-CDA is considered the treatment of choice and has largely supplanted older therapies such as interferon-α, pentostatin, and splenectomy.

Plasma Cell Disorders

The plasma cell disorders, or *dyscrasias,* comprise a group of B-cell neoplasms that are related to each other by virtue of their production and secretion of monoclonal immunoglobulin (or part of an immunoglobulin molecule), or M protein. The tumor cell of these disorders exhibits features of a differentiated plasma cell that is adapted to synthesize and secrete immunoglobulin at a high rate. The laboratory hallmark of plasma cell dyscrasias is the presence of a homogeneous immunoglobulin molecule (or part of an immunoglobulin molecule) that can be detected in the serum or urine by protein electrophoresis. Clinically, these disorders are often characterized by the systemic effects of the M protein, as well as by the direct effects of bone and bone marrow infiltration. The classification of plasma cell dyscrasias is determined in part by the immunoglobulin class (immunoglobulin G [IgG], immunoglobulin A [IgA], immunoglobulin D, IgE, or IgM) or component of immunoglobulin (heavy chain or light chain) that is produced (Table 50–6). The most common plasma cell neoplasms are multiple myeloma and the closely related plasmacytoma, which is a solitary myeloma of bone and extramedullary soft tissue; other less common plasma cell neoplasms include Waldenström's macroglobulinemia, heavy-chain disease, and primary amyloidosis.

M proteins can be found in benign and malignant conditions other than the plasma cell dyscrasias (see Table 50–6). Approximately 10% of patients with CLL have detectable monoclonal IgG or IgM in their serum. M proteins can be detected in a variety of autoreactive or infectious disorders. In addition, an M protein can be found on serum protein electrophoresis in individuals with no apparent associated disease and in the absence of any other laboratory or clinical evidence of a plasma cell dyscrasia. This finding is designated *monoclonal gammopathy of unknown significance* (MGUS) and is defined by the presence of low levels of serum M protein (<3 g/dL), no urinary Bence Jones protein, less than 10% bone marrow plasma cells, and absence of anemia, hypercalcemia, renal failure, and lytic bone lesions. MGUS is more common than myeloma is and increases in frequency with aging, occurring in 1% to 2% of the population over age 50 years. MGUS is often considered a premalignant condition, and these patients are at increased risk (sevenfold) of developing overt myeloma or related malignant plasma cell neoplasms compared with the general population. Nonetheless, progression of MGUS to a frank plasma cell neoplasm only occurs in approximately 1% of patients per year. Distinguishing patients with stable, nonprogressive MGUS from patients in whom multiple myeloma will eventually develop is difficult. The risk of progression is greater in patients with IgA or IgM M proteins and in patients with initial concentrations of M protein in excess of 1.5 g/dL. Although no definitive evidence has been found that monitoring patients with the diagnosis of MGUS improves survival, patients should undergo annual evaluation, including serum electrophoresis, to detect progression to multiple myeloma before the onset of overt symptoms or complications.

MULTIPLE MYELOMA

Multiple myeloma is a malignant plasma cell disorder characterized by neoplastic infiltration of the bone marrow and bone and the presence of monoclonal immunoglobulin or light chains in the serum or urine. The diagnosis of multiple myeloma is made by identifying an increase in the number of plasma cells in the bone marrow (>30%) and a serum M protein other than IgM exceeding 3 g/dL for IgG or 2 g/dL for IgA or a urine M protein exceeding 1 g/24 hours. Patients with lower levels of M protein or less than 30% bone marrow plasmacytosis may still be diagnosed with myeloma based on the presence of a combination of other features such as hypogammaglobulinemia, lytic bone lesions, or plasmacytoma. For patients lacking these features, the major differential diagnosis is usually between MGUS and myeloma; in some cases, the distinction can only be made by serial follow-up of the patient with evidence of rising M protein levels or the development of associated clinical manifestations of myeloma. Approximately 20% of patients with multiple myeloma do not have detectable serum M protein by standard electrophoresis but have free light chains in the urine (Bence Jones protein) that can be detected in a 24-hour urine collection by urine protein electrophoresis (*light-chain disease*). In rare cases, patients with *nonsecretory* myeloma have neither detectable serum nor urine M protein. However, in these patients, a monoclonal population of plasma cells can be detected by immunohistochemical identification of cytoplasmic light chain–restricted immunoglobulin. Recently, quantitative assays for detection of free light chains in the serum of patients with multiple myeloma have become widely available and may be used to assess disease in a similar fashion to electrophoretic measurements. Free light chains have a relatively short

Table 50–6   Classification of Disorders Associated with Monoclonal Immunoglobulin (M Protein) Secretion

Disorder	M Protein	Antibody Activity of M Protein
Plasma Cell Neoplasms		
Multiple myeloma	IgG > IgA > IgD; ± < free light chain or light chain alone (κ > λ)	
Solitary myeloma of bone	IgG > IgA > IgD; ± free light chain or light chain alone (κ > λ)	
Extramedullary plasmacytoma	IgG > IgA > IgD; ± free light chain or light chain alone (κ > λ)	
Waldenström's macroglobulinemia	IgM ± free light chain (κ > λ)	
Heavy-chain disease	γ, α, or μ heavy chain or fragment	
Primary amyloidosis	Free light chain (λ > κ)	
Monoclonal gammopathy of unknown significance	IgG > IgM > IgA, usually without urinary light chain secretion	
Other B-Cell Neoplasms		
Chronic lymphocytic leukemia	M protein occasionally secreted; IgM > IgG	
B-cell non-Hodgkin's lymphomas; Hodgkin's disease	M protein occasionally secreted; IgM > IgG	
Nonlymphoid Neoplasms		
Chronic myelogenous leukemia	No consistent patterns	
Carcinomas (e.g., colon, breast, prostate)	No consistent patterns	
Autoimmune or Autoreactive Disorders		
Cold agglutinin disease	IgM κ most common	Anti-I antigen
Mixed cryoglobulinemia	IgM or IgA	Anti-IgG
Sjögren's syndrome	IgM	
Miscellaneous Inflammatory, Storage, or Infectious Disorders		
Lichen myxedematosus	IgG λ	
Gaucher's disease	IgG	
Cirrhosis, sarcoid, parasitic diseases, renal acidosis	No consistent pattern	

Modified from Salmon SE: Plasma cell disorders. In Wyngaarden JB, Smith LH Jr (eds): Cecil Textbook of Medicine, 18th ed. Philadelphia, WB Saunders, 1988, p 1026.
IgA = immunoglobulin A; IgD = immunoglobulin D; IgG = immunoglobulin G; IgM = immunoglobulin M.

half-life in the circulation, 2 to 6 hours, in comparison with weeks for intact immunoglobulin molecules and may therefore be used to obtain a more rapid assessment of disease response for patients on therapy.

The clinical manifestations of multiple myeloma relate to the direct effects of bone marrow and bone infiltration by malignant plasma cells, the systemic effects of the M protein, or the effects of the concomitant deficiency in humoral immunity that occurs in this disease. The most common symptom in multiple myeloma is bone pain. Bone radiographs typically show pure osteolytic *punched out* lesions, often in association with generalized osteopenia and pathologic fractures. Bony lesions can show as expansile masses associated with spinal cord compression. Hypercalcemia caused by extensive bony involvement is common in myeloma and may dominate the clinical picture. Anemia

occurs in the majority of patients as a result of marrow infiltration and suppression of hematopoiesis; granulocytopenia and thrombocytopenia are less common. Patients with myeloma are susceptible to bacterial infections because of impaired production and increased catabolism of normal immunoglobulins. Respiratory tract infections from *Streptococcus pneumoniae, Staphylococcus aureus, H. influenzae,* and *Klebsiella pneumoniae* and gram-negative urinary tract infections are common. Renal insufficiency occurs in approximately 25% of patients with myeloma. The cause of renal failure in these patients is often multifactorial; hypercalcemia, hyperuricemia, infection, and amyloid deposition can contribute. However, direct tubular damage from light-chain excretion is invariably present. M proteins can also cause a host of diverse effects because of their physicochemical properties. These effects include cryoglobulinemia,

Table 50–7　Myeloma Staging System

Stage	Criteria
I	All of the following: 1. Hemoglobin >10 g/dL 2. Serum calcium <12 mg/dL 3. Normal bone radiograph or solitary lesion 4. Low M-component production 　a. IgG level <5 g/dL 　b. IgA level <3 g/dL 　c. Urine light chain <4 g/24 hr
II	Fitting neither I nor III
III	One or more of the following: 1. Hemoglobin <8.5 g/dL 2. Serum calcium >12 mg/dL 3. Advanced lytic bone lesions 4. High M-component production 　a. IgG level >7 g/dL 　b. IgA level >5 g/dL 　c. Urine light chains >12 g/24 hr

Subclassification:
A Serum creatinine <2 mg/dL.
B Serum creatinine <2 mg/dL.

hyperviscosity, amyloidosis, and clotting abnormalities resulting from interaction of the M protein with platelets or clotting factors.

The three-tier staging system for myeloma is a functional system that correlates with survival (Table 50–7). In contrast to the anatomic staging systems used for lymphomas and solid tumors, myeloma staging is based on clinical (bone radiographs) and laboratory tests (hemoglobin, serum calcium, serum or urine M protein levels, and serum creatinine) that correlate with tumor burden. Adverse prognostic factors include advanced stage, impaired renal function, elevated LDH levels, abnormal bone marrow cytogenetics, and elevated β_2-microglobulin levels. The last is the single most powerful predictor of survival. Recently, a simplified prognostic scheme, the International Staging System for Myeloma, identified three stages with distinct prognosis based on only two variables, β_2-microglobulin and albumin levels.

The vast majority of patients with myeloma exhibit symptomatic, advanced-stage disease and require therapy. However, approximately 10% of patients have stage I disease and an indolent course. These patients do not require immediate therapy, but they should be monitored for disease progression by serial quantification of the M protein. For patients with solitary bone or extramedullary plasmacytomas, local radiation therapy can induce long-term remissions and is the treatment of choice. Patients with symptomatic, advanced-stage (II or III) myeloma require systemic therapy, as well as meticulous attention to supportive care. Although myeloma is not a curable malignancy,

systemic therapy can prolong survival and dramatically improve quality of life. Standard treatments include chemotherapy regimens, such as the three-drug vincristine, doxorubicin (Adriamycin), and dexamethasone (VAD) regimen, or the nonchemotherapy regimen thalidomide plus dexamethasone. Thalidomide was initially used as a sedative in the United Kingdom in the 1960s but was found to cause birth defects when used to combat nausea during pregnancy. The anti-angiogenic properties of thalidomide subsequently led to its development as an anticancer agent. Although the mechanism of action of thalidomide in myeloma is unclear, one third of patients with recurrent or refractory disease following transplantation responded to thalidomide. In contrast to chemotherapy, thalidomide is infrequently myelosuppressive and has a unique side effect profile, including peripheral neuropathy, constipation, somnolence, and rash. The combination of thalidomide and dexamethasone is highly active as initial therapy in treating myeloma and has the advantage of an all-oral treatment program. A troublesome unique side effect of the combination is the development of deep-vein thrombosis in up to 25% of patients. Alternate initial systemic therapies include dexamethasone as a single agent or alkylator agent–based combination chemotherapy regimens, however, the latter causes stem cell injury and is therefore typically avoided in patients who may be eligible for stem cell transplantation

The majority of patients respond to initial therapy with a reduction in bone pain, hypercalcemia, and anemia in association with a decline in the M protein level. In recent years, the use of high-dose chemotherapy with alkylating agents followed by autologous peripheral stem cell infusion has been shown to improve survival and quality of life compared with standard doses of chemotherapy. Although this approach is not curative, it does represent an important treatment option for some patients and has been shown an association with acceptable toxicity in older patients. Allogenic bone marrow transplantation may represent the only potentially curative treatment for myeloma, but the associated excessive morbidity and mortality in elderly or heavily pretreated patients have limited its use in this disease.

Patients who experience relapse after standard therapy or transplantation may be treated with alternate chemotherapy regimens or with bortezomib, a new novel agent in the class of proteasome inhibitors. Bortezomib was found to induce responses, including some complete responses, in up to a third of heavily treated patients with myeloma. Bortezomib may cause asthenia, thrombocytopenia, or neuropathy. Analogues of thalidomide with higher potency and fewer side effects have also been developed and are under clinical study. High doses of corticosteroids or experimental therapies are also treatment options for patients who have not responded to chemotherapy or transplantation.

Supportive care directed toward anticipated complications of myeloma is an important aspect of the management of this disease. Bone resorption can be reduced with regular injections of the diphosphonates zoledronic acid or pamidronate, reducing pain and pathologic fractures. Bony lesions, particularly those involving weight-bearing bones, may require palliative radiation for controlling pain and preventing pathologic fractures. Vertebral bony lesions may lead to spinal cord compression, with increasing back pain and neurologic symptoms. Any symptoms suggestive of cord compression require prompt evaluation with spinal magnetic resonance imaging and, if necessary, local radiation to involved areas. Avoidance of nephrotoxins, including intravenous dyes, is important to prevent renal failure. Acute renal failure caused by light-chain deposition may improve with plasmapheresis to acutely reduce protein load. All patients should receive pneumococcal and *H. influenzae* vaccine, and intravenous gamma globulin may be useful in preventing recurrent infections in patients with profound hypogammaglobulinemia. Use of erythropoietin may alleviate anemia and decrease the need for blood transfusions.

WALDENSTRÖM'S MACROGLOBULINEMIA

Waldenström's macroglobulinemia is a malignancy of plasmacytoid lymphocytes that secrete large quantities of IgM. It is a chronic disorder affecting elderly patients (median age is 64 years) that shares features of the low-grade lymphomas and myeloma. In contrast to myeloma, Waldenström's macroglobulinemia is associated with lymphadenopathy and hepatosplenomegaly, and, although bone marrow involvement is invariably present, lytic lesions and hypercalcemia are distinctly rare. The major clinical manifestation of Waldenström's macroglobulinemia is usually the hyperviscosity syndrome caused by the physical properties of IgM. In contrast to IgG, IgM remains largely confined to the intravascular space, and, as IgM levels rise, plasma viscosity increases. Epistaxis, retinal hemorrhages, dizziness, confusion, and congestive heart failure are common symptoms of the hyperviscosity syndrome. Approximately 10% of IgM proteins have properties of cryoglobulins, and these patients show symptoms of cryoglobulinemia or cold agglutinin syndrome demonstrated as acrocyanosis, Raynaud's phenomenon and vascular symptoms, or hemolytic anemia precipitated by exposure to cold. Some patients with Waldenström's macroglobulinemia may develop a peripheral neuropathy that may antedate the appearance of the neoplastic process.

The approach to and treatment of Waldenström's macroglobulinemia are similar to that of other low-grade B-cell lymphomas. The use of nucleoside analogues (2-CDA and fludarabine) or an alkylating agent, alone or in combination with prednisone, is effective in decreasing adenopathy and splenomegaly and controlling the M spike but is not curative. Rituximab has also been found to have activity in Waldenström's macroglobulinemia. Plasmapheresis is highly effective in acutely decreasing serum IgM levels and is often needed initially to treat hyperviscosity. Although complete remissions are rare, patients who respond to therapy have median survivals of 4 years, and some patients survive more than a decade.

RARE PLASMA CELL DISORDERS

Heavy-chain disease is a rare lymphoplasmacytoid neoplasm characterized by production of a defective heavy chain of the γ, α, or μ type. The clinical manifestations vary with the type of heavy chain secreted. Gamma heavy-chain disease is associated with lymphadenopathy, Waldeyer's ring involvement with palatal edema, and constitutional symptoms. Alpha heavy-chain disease, also known as Mediterranean lymphoma, is characterized by lymphoid infiltration of the small intestine with associated diarrhea and malabsorption. Mu heavy-chain disease is associated with CLL. Primary amyloidosis is a systemic illness characterized by deposition of immunoglobulin light chain in organs and tissue, resulting in an array of symptoms caused by organ dysfunction. Congestive heart failure, bleeding diathesis, nephrotic syndrome, and peripheral neuropathy are common complications. Patients with primary amyloidosis respond poorly to the treatments used for myeloma. Encouraging results have been reported with high-dose chemotherapy and autologous stem cell support, particularly if patients are treated before the development of significant end-organ dysfunction such as cardiomyopathy.

CONGENITAL AND ACQUIRED DISORDERS OF LYMPHOCYTE FUNCTION

A significant number of congenital disorders affect lymphocyte maturation or function, resulting in immunodeficiency disorders. Acquired disorders of lymphocyte function are far more common compared with congenital disorders. HIV infection is the most important infectious cause of acquired immunodeficiency and is discussed in Chapter 108. Patients with HIV infection are at increased risk of developing NHL. NHLs that occur in the setting of HIV are the diffuse aggressive B-cell histologies, including diffuse large B-cell lymphoma and Burkitt's lymphoma; they are also frequently associated with EBV and are often advanced stage (stage III or IV) at initial diagnosis, with extranodal sites of involvement. Patients with HIV-associated NHL are potentially curable with the multidrug chemotherapy regimens used for treating these NHL subtypes in the general population. In addition, treatment of the underlying HIV infection with highly active antiretroviral therapy has improved the outcome and prognosis of patients with HIV-associated NHL.

Patients who have undergone an allogeneic organ transplant require potent immunosuppressive drugs (e.g., cyclosporine, tacrolimus, azathioprine, corticosteroids, methotrexate) to prevent graft-versus-host disease in the case of bone marrow recipients or allograft rejection in the case of solid organ transplantation. These medications can cause profound defects in T-cell function with an associated acquired immunodeficiency state, and transplant recipients are susceptible to a host of viral and protozoal infections. In addition, patients who receive potent immunosuppressive drugs are at risk for developing a lymphoproliferative disorder (post-transplant lymphoproliferative disorder [PTLD]) that can behave clinically as an aggressive lymphoma. PTLD is an EBV-associated lymphoproliferative disorder characterized by a polymorphous or monomorphous population of B cells that can be monoclonal or polyclonal. Patients who develop PTLD are treated by reducing the doses of immunosuppressive drugs whenever possible; this intervention alone will result in regression of PTLD in approximately one half of the patients, obviating the need for cytotoxic therapy. Patients who are not candidates for withdrawal of immunosuppression because of allograft rejection or who fail to respond to this strategy can be treated with rituximab alone or in combination with chemotherapy.

INFECTIOUS DISORDERS

Lymphocytes play an essential role in the adaptive response to infection. This response can be shown clinically with an increase in lymphocytes in the peripheral blood (reactive lymphocytosis) and lymph node enlargement. Reactive lymphocytosis is always polyclonal, usually predominantly T cell, and is usually easily distinguishable from the common monoclonal B-cell neoplastic processes. Some infections are typically associated with a prominent lymphocytosis (e.g., EBV-associated infectious mononucleosis, cytomegalovirus, toxoplasmosis in immunocompetent hosts, viral hepatitis).

Enlargement of lymph nodes, either local-regional or generalized lymphadenopathy, is a common manifestation of some infections (see Table 50–1). Lymph node enlargement may be striking and associated with tenderness. In most cases, the adenopathy is reactive, and the organism cannot be readily cultured from the node; in other cases (e.g., tuberculosis, fungal disease), culture or appropriate staining in lymph node tissue can identify the organism. Biopsy of the node generally will confirm the non-neoplastic nature of the process, showing a normal architecture and cellular pattern and absence of a monoclonal population of lymphoid cells.

Prospectus for the Future

Further advances in our understanding of lymphoproliferative diseases are likely to come from molecular studies such as DNA microarray analyses used to create profiles of gene expression in malignant cells. Such analyses will aid in further subclassifying lymphoproliferative diseases and will help define prognosis and response to therapy; such data are already available in limited form for diffuse large B-cell lymphoma and CLL. An understanding of gene expression profiles unique to specific disease will also provide additional targets for pharmacologic or immunologically based therapies.

The advent of humanized chimeric monoclonal antibodies targeted to CD20 has changed the therapy of some lymphomas, and antibodies to other cell surface antigens, including radio-labeled antibodies, are in development.

For multiple myeloma, several drugs in development have already shown significant activity in refractory patients, including the thalidomide analogues and the proteasome inhibitor PS-341.

For allogeneic transplantation, reduced-intensity conditioning regimens are improving the therapeutic index of this procedure for curative treatment of multiple myeloma and lymphomas.

References

Armitage JO, Mauch PM, Harris NL, Bierman P: Non-Hodgkin's lymphomas. In DeVita VT Jr, Hellman S, Rosenberg SA (eds): Cancer-Principles and Practice of Oncology. Philadelphia, Lippincott, Williams & Wilkins, 2001, pp 2256–2315.

Canellos GP, Anderson JR, Propert KJ, et al: Chemotherapy of advanced Hodgkin's disease with MOPP, ABVD, or MOPP alternating with ABVD. N Engl J Med 327:1478–1484.

Diehl V, Mauch PM, Harris NL: Hodgkin's disease. In DeVita VT Jr, Hellman S, Rosenberg SA (eds): Cancer-Principles and Practice of Oncology. Philadelphia, Lippincott, Williams & Wilkins, 2001, pp 2339–2388.

Fisher RI, Gaynor ER, Dahlberg S, et al: Comparison of a standard regimen (CHOP) with three intensive chemotherapy regimens for advanced non-Hodgkin's lymphoma. N Engl J Med 328: 1002–1006, 1993.

Gaidano G, Dalla-Favara R: Molecular biology of lymphomas. In DeVita VT Jr, Hellman S, Rosenberg SA (eds): Cancer-Principles and Practice of Oncology. Philadelphia, Lippincott, Williams & Wilkins, 2001, pp 2215–2235.

Harris N, Jaffe E, Diebold J, et al: World Health Organization classification of neoplastic diseases of the hematopoietic and lymphoid tissues: Report of the Clinical Advisory Committee Meeting, Airlie House, Virginia, November 1997. J Clin Oncol 17:3835–3849, 1999.

Kyle RA, Therneau TM, Rajkumar SV, et al: A long-term study of prognosis in monoclonal gammopathy of undetermined significance. N Engl J Med 346:564–569, 2002.

Maloney DG, Grillo-Lopez AJ, White CA, et al: IDEC-C2B8 (rituximab) anti-CD20 monoclonal antibody therapy in patients with relapsed low-grade non-Hodgkin's lymphoma. Blood 90:2188–2195, 1997.

McSweeney PA, Niederwieser D, Shizuru JA, et al: Hematopoietic cell transplantation in older patients with hematologic malignancies: Replacing high-dose cytotoxic therapy with graft-versus-tumor effects. Blood 97:3390–3400, 2001.

Munschi NC, Tricot G, Barlogie B: Plasma cell dyscrasias. In DeVita VT Jr, Hellman S, Rosenberg SA (eds): Cancer-Principles and Practice of Oncology. Philadelphia, Lippincott, Williams & Wilkins, 2001, pp 2465–2498.

Philip T, Guglielmi C, Hagenbeek A, et al: Autologous bone marrow transplantation as compared with salvage chemotherapy in relapses of chemotherapy-sensitive non-Hodgkin's lymphoma. N Engl J Med 33:1540–1545, 1995.

Singhal S, Mehta J, Desikan R, et al: Antitumor activity of thalidomide in refractory multiple myeloma. N Engl J Med 341:1565–1571, 1999.

Normal Hemostasis

Richard Torres

Henry M. Rinder

Normal hemostasis involves the physiologic balance of procoagulant and anticoagulant factors that maintains liquid blood flow and the structural integrity of the vasculature. Vascular damage results in initiation of clotting with the goal of producing a *localized* platelet or fibrin plug to prevent blood loss; this action is followed by processes that lead to clot containment, wound healing, clot dissolution, and tissue regeneration and remodeling. In healthy persons, all of these reactions occur continuously and in a balanced fashion such that bleeding is contained, but blood vessels remain patent and deliver adequate organ blood flow. When one or several of these processes are disrupted because of inherited defects or acquired abnormalities, disordered hemostasis may result in either bleeding or thromboembolic complications.

Blood flow in the arterial and venous systems is disparate and imposes different needs on the coagulation system. In the pressurized arteries, relatively minor vascular damage can rapidly result in massive blood loss; thus the coagulant response in arteries must be capable of arresting bleeding rapidly. Platelets are critical to this response; they initially contain blood loss and then provide an active surface that both localizes and accelerates the fibrin formation that ultimately produces hemostasis. By contrast, in the venous circulation, the lesser flow rates produce slower bleeding, a feature that makes platelets less critical; the pivotal reaction controlling the balance of venous hemostasis is the rate of thrombin generation. These differences are also underscored by the anticoagulant agents used in these settings, that is, antiplatelet agents such as aspirin to prevent coronary artery thrombus and antithrombin-based interventions, such as heparins and warfarin, for prophylaxis against deep-vein thrombosis.

This chapter briefly details the physiologic mechanisms of vascular hemostasis, including the normal balance of procoagulant and anticoagulant functions of the blood vessel wall, platelet physiologic factors and receptor-ligand interactions critical for hemostasis, and the highly complex, interwoven processes that comprise the coagulation cascade.

Vascular Wall Physiology

Vascular endothelial cells (ECs) function as a barrier to contain blood and prevent it from contacting the highly thrombogenic subendothelial contents. In fact, endothelial dysfunction appears to be an important early step in the development of atherosclerotic lesions. Normal intact ECs possess strong anticoagulant functions and secrete prostacyclin, nitric oxide, adenosine diphosphatase (ADPase), and plasminogen activator (Table 51–1). Prostacyclin and nitric oxide have dual mechanisms to prevent thrombosis; both affect smooth muscle cells to induce vasodilation and thereby increase blood flow and minimize platelet contact with the vessel wall. At the same time, prostacyclin and nitric oxide are secreted into the blood stream, where they promote cyclic adenosine monophosphate (cAMP) generation within platelets and thereby inhibit platelet activation and aggregation.

However, when ECs are damaged or activated, the balance of coagulant properties quickly shifts to favor a procoagulant state. This function is mediated both by the ECs themselves and by the subendothelial matrix, which is exposed by vascular injury. Activated ECs express adhesive ligands on their surface, including the selectins (both E selectin and P selectin), β_1 and β_2 integrin, platelet-EC adhesion molecule-1, and von Willebrand factor (vWF) (see Table 51–1). On the EC surface, these proteins localize and promote platelet adhesion and also mediate migration of leukocytes into the tissues. Exposed subendothelial matrix binds vWF (Fig. 51–1) and contains other procoagulant adhesive moieties, including thrombospondin, fibronectin, and collagen. These moieties function both as ligands to capture platelets and as activators of adherent platelets; collagen, in particular, is a strong platelet agonist that causes platelets to undergo dense granule release and to express conformationally active ligands such as glycoprotein IIb/IIIa (GPIIb/IIIa; see later discussion). Another critical procoagulant mediator exposed by EC damage is tissue factor (TF), which is constitutively expressed by subendothelial smooth muscle cells and fibroblasts. As outlined later (see Coagulation Cascade), TF is the

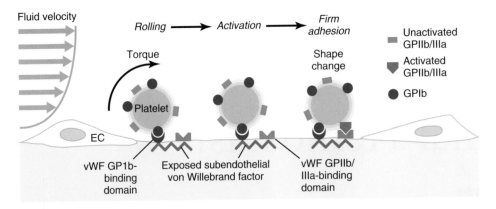

Figure 51–1 The adhesive interactions producing stable platelet attachment to subendothelial von Willebrand factor (vWF). The initial attachment between platelet glycoprotein Ib (GPIb) and its binding domain on vWF is rapid but has a short half-life, and the result is a rolling movement from torque generated by flowing blood. The vWF-GPIb interaction produces transmembrane signaling that activates the platelet to undergo shape change and simultaneously transforms GPIIb/IIIa into an activated conformation capable of binding to a distinct arginine-glycine-aspartate domain on vWF. This secondary adhesion causes the platelet to firmly adhere to the exposed subendothelial vWF. EC = endothelial cell.

Table 51–1	**Endothelial Cell Coagulant Properties**
Procoagulant	**Anticoagulant**
Collagen	Vasodilation
Factor VIII	ADPase
Fibronectin	Heparan sulfates
Integrins	Nitric oxide
Platelet–endothelial cell adhesion molecule-1	Prostacyclin
	Thrombomodulin
Selectins (E and P) von Willebrand factor	Tissue factor pathway inhibitor
	Tissue plasminogen activator
Vasoconstriction	

ADPase = adenosine diphosphatase.

addition, EC constitutive secretion of tissue-type plasminogen activator (t-PA), the primary initiator of fibrinolysis, converts plasminogen to the active enzyme plasmin, which degrades formed fibrin clots. The finding that t-PA must be bound directly to clot to express full activity helps limit the fibrinolytic response to areas of clot formation. ECs also secrete ADPase that degrades platelet-released adenosine diphosphate (ADP) and results in inhibition of additional platelet activation and recruitment, thus limiting clot propagation. Furthermore, ECs release TF pathway inhibitor (TFPI), which is a potent inhibitor of both the TF-VIIa procoagulant complex and the TF-induced Xase complex (see later discussion). By complexing with factor Xa and TF to inhibit their activity, TFPI downregulates thrombin generation. The balance of procoagulant and anticoagulant vascular function localizes and regulates activation of platelets and soluble coagulation factors.

Platelet Physiology

The platelet functions as the cellular-based platform for hemostasis. Platelet membrane receptors mediate primary hemostasis and allow platelets to bind directly to endothelium and subendothelium at sites of damage. Platelet adhesion causes transmembrane signaling through surface receptors to induce platelet activation and to further procoagulant function through translocation of receptors to the membrane surface, receptor conformational change, release of granule contents, and exposure of membrane phospholipid. The procoagulant surface of the platelet then serves as a platform for assembly of the coagulation cascade and formation of thrombin, which (1) feeds back on platelets and the clotting cascade to amplify the procoagulant response and (2) produces fibrin to provide secondary, long-lasting hemostasis. Finally, the platelet assists in clot consolidation and protection from fibrinolysis by contributing factor XIII and platelet factor 4, respectively, to the clot milieu (Table 51–2).

Platelets in the circulation are anucleated cells between 2 and 4 μm in diameter with a volume between 6 and 11 L. Platelets are derived from the megakaryocyte cytoplasm after

major initiator of the soluble coagulation system that results in the formation of a definitive fibrin clot (Fig. 51–2).

These procoagulant properties of the EC and subendothelial matrix ensure plugging of the endothelial injury and cessation of bleeding. At the same time, the normal ECs that surround the site of injury exert anticoagulant properties (see Table 51–1) that prevent propagation of clot beyond the injury, thereby avoiding thrombosis of the entire vessel. These anticoagulant functions may be constitutive, as noted earlier with prostacyclin and nitric oxide, or they may be initiated by vessel damage and the clotting cascade itself. Thrombin generated at the site of endothelial damage or clotting diffuses and binds to normal ECs, where it is bound to surface thrombomodulin. Once bound to thrombomodulin, thrombin acts as an initiator of the natural anticoagulant system, rather than as a primary soluble procoagulant factor. The thrombin-thrombomodulin complex converts protein C to its activated form, APC, which, in conjunction with its coenzyme, protein S, inactivates factors Va and VIIIa to downregulate further thrombin formation (Fig. 51–3). In

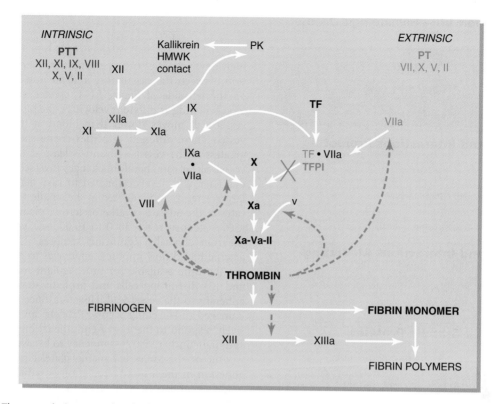

Figure 51–2 The coagulation cascade. The laboratory-defined *extrinsic* and *intrinsic* pathways allow monitoring of anticoagulation by the prothrombin time (PT) and partial thromboplastin time (PTT), respectively. The PT primarily monitors factor VII activity, whereas the PTT is the best measure of the hemophilic factors XI, IX, VIII; both assays will detect deficiency of the common pathway factors (X, V, and II). Initiation of clotting always begins with elaboration of TF, which then combines with small amounts of circulating VIIa to form the extrinsic Xase complex and generate Xa. Xa forms the prothrombinase complex with Va and II, generating small amounts of thrombin, which begin to cleave fibrinogen into weak fibrin monomers. Thrombin's ability to itself activate factors, especially when carried out on the activated platelet surface, is responsible for the amplification of the coagulant response. Thrombin generates XIa, which, in turn, activates IX; the TF-VIIa complex (before its shutdown by TFPI) also generates IXa. Thrombin-activated VIIIa then combines with IXa to from the intrinsic Xase complex, generating large amounts of Xa and prothrombinase complex to further amplify thrombin generation. The large amounts of thrombin now generate enough fibrin monomers to form stable polymers and fibrin clot. HMWK = high–molecular-weight kininogen; PK = prekallikrein; TF = tissue factor; TFPI = tissue factor pathway inhibitor.

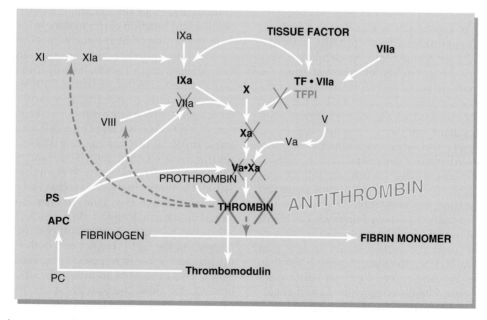

Figure 51–3 Endogenous anticoagulant pathways. In addition to tissue factor pathway inhibitor (TFPI) shutting off tissue factor (TF) stimulation and blocking the TF-VIIa-X complex, the clotting cascade is further downregulated by the natural anticoagulants. This inhibition is partly generated by thrombin itself, which activates thrombomodulin. Circulating antithrombin inhibits thrombin activity and Xa generation of thrombin. The complex of thrombin and thrombomodulin activates protein C (APC), which combines with protein S (PS) to cleave and inactivate VIIIa and Va, further blocking thrombin generation.

Table 51–2   Procoagulant Properties of Platelets

Receptor-Ligand Interactions Promoting Adhesion

GPIb/IX-vWF
GPIIb/IIIa-fibrinogen and GPIIb/IIIa-vWF
GPIa/IIa-collagen
P selectin–P selectin glycoprotein ligand-1

Receptor-Ligand Interactions Mediating Activation

GPV-thrombin
GPVI-collagen

Secreted Alpha-Granule Proteins

Ligands (fibrinogen, fibronectin, thrombospondin, vitronectin, vWF)
Enzymes (α_2-antiplasmin, factors V, VIII, and XI)
Antiheparin (platelet factor 4)

Secreted Dense-Granule Agonists

ADP, serotonin

Secreted Cytosolic Factor XIII—Membrane Components

Thromboxane A_2 formation, phosphatidylserine expression

ADP = adenosine diphosphate; GP = glycoprotein; GPIa/IIa = complex of glycoprotein Ia and CD29; GPIb/IX complex = CD42; GPIIb/IIIa (α_2-β_3) complex = CD41; P selectin = CD62P; P selectin glycoprotein ligand-1 = CD162; vWF = von Willebrand factor.

a maturation time of approximately 4 days, each megakaryocyte contributing approximately 1000 platelets in its lifetime. When platelets are released into the circulation, they survive for 7 to 10 days; platelets are removed from the circulation by a combination of senescence and the normal maintenance of vascular structural integrity. For the latter, approximately 7100 platelets/mcL are required per day when vascular structures have not been breached (as would happen with surgery) and when no additional stressors are causing increased platelet consumption (e.g., sepsis). The normal platelet count range is between 150,000 and 450,000/mcL. With platelet counts in the normal range and normal platelet function, the normal bleeding time, which measures platelet function, is less than 8 minutes. The bleeding time does not usually become prolonged by thrombocytopenia alone until the platelet count is less than 100,000/mcL. However, when the platelet count is less than 100,000/mcL, the bleeding time does not distinguish between bleeding caused by thrombocytopenia and abnormal platelet function or vessel adhesion. The in vitro bleeding time test (Platelet Function Analyzer [PFA]-100) is similarly unable to distinguish between thrombocytopenia and abnormal platelet function when platelet counts are below 100,000/mcL.

Platelet–vessel wall interaction is best illustrated at the high flow velocities of the arterial circulation. The interaction between the vasculature and flowing blood, as shown on the left side of Figure 51–1, creates parallel planes of blood moving at different velocities; the blood closest to the vessel wall moves slower than blood at the center of the vessel. These different velocities create shear stress that is greatest at the vessel wall and is least at the center of the vessel. Shear rate therefore changes inversely with the vessel diameter, with levels estimated to vary between 500/sec in larger arteries and 5000/sec in the smallest arterioles. Shear rates at the surface of atherosclerotic plaques with modest (50%) stenosis reach 3000 to 10,000/sec, with even greater shear in clinically significant stenoses. The high-velocity arterial blood flow opposes tendencies to clot by (1) limiting the time available for procoagulant reactions to occur and (2) disrupting cells and proteins that are not tightly adherent to the vessel wall. However, once the vessel wall is damaged and bleeding occurs, platelets can rapidly and decisively respond to the loss of endothelial integrity while they simultaneously resist the tendency to be swept downstream.

One of the forces enhancing platelet readiness for wall adhesion in the arterial circulation is radial dispersion, the tendency of larger cells (erythrocytes and leukocytes) to stream in the center of the vessel, where shear is lowest; this process effectively pushes the smaller platelets toward the vessel wall and optimally positions them to respond to hemostatic challenges. This size-dependent flow may also explain the seemingly paradoxical ability of red blood cell transfusions to slow or stop bleeding simply by correcting severe anemia, such as noted in patients with severe uremia (see Chapter 52). This effect also underscores the importance of platelets in arterial hemostasis; reductions in platelet number or function may be associated with catastrophic arterial hemorrhage. By contrast, the lesser shear forces experienced in the venous circulation permit more random cell movement and greater time for coagulation reactions to occur and make the minimum requirements for platelet number and function correspondingly less stringent.

In the setting of high-velocity blood flow at an arterial bleeding site, platelets must activate and adhere to the injured vessel nearly instantaneously. Two molecules present in the subendothelium are critical for this process: vWF and collagen. Control of bleeding in vessels under the highest shear stresses absolutely depends on the presence and function of vWF. vWF is a large molecule synthesized as multimeric *strings* in ECs and megakaryocytes, and vWF is both constitutively secreted into blood and stored in Weibel-Palade bodies. The *ultralarge* vWF multimers are the most active at binding platelets and factor VIII, particularly when *unfolded* by either shear stress or after immobilization. The largest multimeric forms of vWF, which are immobilized by adherence to exposed subendothelial collagen, bind to a complex of the GPIb receptor and both GPV and GPIX on the platelet surface in response to high shear stress (see Fig. 51–1). This binding is an extremely rapid but low-affinity binding that slows the platelets at this interface but leaves them only weakly adherent to subendothelial vWF. With platelets no longer streaming by, but instead tumbling over the subendothelium, the high shear stress in tandem with transmembrane signaling produced by the GPIb-V-IX-vWF interaction results in loss of the normal platelet discoid shape (shape change) and conformational change in another platelet receptor, GPIIb/IIIa. The activated GPIIb/IIIa receptor now binds either to fibrinogen or to the larger vWF multimers at a site distinct from the GPIb-binding site. This secondary adhesion is a higher affinity interaction than the GPIb-V-IX-vWF bond and secures the platelet firmly to the subendothelium. An important regulator of this process of platelet binding and activation through vWF is the vWF-cleaving protease: a disintegrin and metalloproteinase with a thrombospondin type 1 motif, member 13 (ADAMTS-13). ADAMTS-13 modulates the activity of vWF by cleaving the ultralarge multimers into smaller fragments that have reduced overall affinity for platelet binding. Loss of the cleaving protease activity results in unchecked platelet binding to ultralarge multimers and microvascular thrombosis (see the discussion of *thrombotic thrombocytopenic purpura* in Chapter 53).

At more moderate shear rates, GPIb-V-IX-vWF adhesion is supplemented by platelet binding to subendothelial collagen, an adhesive moiety that is capable of arresting the platelet by binding to GPIa/IIa (see Table 51–2). Thus subendothelial vWF and collagen act cooperatively to initiate platelet adhesion, with the former predominating at higher shear. Collagen is unique in that it can anchor platelets at one locus by binding to platelet GPIa/IIa and can activate platelets at a second locus by binding to platelet GPVI. The congenital absence of any of the critical platelet adhesion receptors—GPIIb/IIIa, GPIbV/IX, GPVI, or GPIa/IIa—results in a significant hemostatic defect, correctable only by platelet transfusion. Similarly, decreases in vWF, especially the larger multimeric forms, can cause bleeding. Once a layer of platelets is adherent to the site of bleeding, vWF bound to GPIb, V, and IX on the uppermost adherent platelets serves to recruit additional platelets from the flowing blood into the growing platelet plug. The bound platelets then undergo a series of interdependent processes that are collectively referred to as *activation*. Platelet activation has five major effects: (1) local release of ligands essential to stabilizing the platelet-platelet matrix, (2) continued recruitment of additional platelets, (3) vasoconstriction of smaller arteries to slow bleeding, (4) localization and acceleration of platelet-associated fibrin formation, and (5) protection of clot from fibrinolysis.

The basis of the platelet plug is a platelet-ligand-platelet matrix with fibrinogen and vWF serving as bridging ligands (Fig. 51–4). Both fibrinogen and vWF are stored in alpha granules inside the resting platelet and are released with activation, and both can bind to a GPIIb/IIIa receptor on each of two platelets, thereby linking them. As mentioned earlier, platelet GPIIb/IIIa undergoes a calcium-dependent conformational change that allows it to bind to a locus containing the amino acid sequence arginine-glycine-aspartate (RGD) on either fibrinogen or vWF. Each fibrinogen molecule has two RGD sites on its polar ends, and the larger vWF multimers have several RGD sites, all capable of binding to conformationally altered GPIIb/IIIa and creating the platelet-ligand-platelet matrix. GPIIb/IIIa is the most abundant glycoprotein on the platelet surface, with approximately 50,000 copies on the *resting* platelet and additional GPIIb/IIIa receptors within the cytosol that are mobilized to the surface after activation.

Platelets are also recruited and then cemented into the platelet plug by local agonists (collagen, epinephrine, and thrombin) and by platelet release of agonists into the local microenvironment. Both collagen (as noted previously) and thrombin interact with their specific platelet receptors to activate platelets strongly; although epinephrine alone is not a powerful platelet agonist, stimulation of the α-adrenergic receptor on platelets primes them for synergistic activation by even relatively weak agonists such as ADP. Activating compounds released directly from the platelet include thromboxane A_2 (TxA_2), which is formed in the platelet cytosol after cyclooxygenase cleavage of arachidonic acid and then released into the clot milieu. TxA_2 is both a platelet agonist and a vasoconstrictor, and it is rapidly degraded to its inert by-product, thromboxane B_2. Platelet cyclooxygenase-1 (COX-1) activity is *irreversibly* inhibited by aspirin, thereby blocking TxA_2 formation for the lifetime of that platelet. Aspirin irreversibly and covalently binds to a specific serine residue on COX-1 and causes steric hindrance of the active

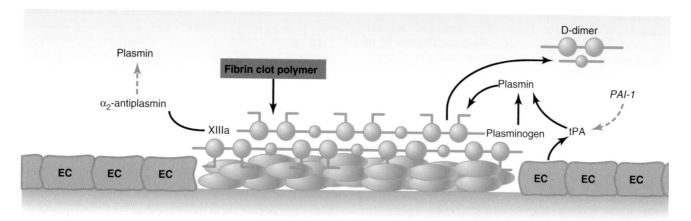

Figure 51–4 Balanced fibrinolysis limiting the platelet-fibrin clot. The platelet plug and fibrin matrices are strengthened by incorporating factor XIIIa into the fibrin clot. Factor XIIIa also binds $α_2$-antiplasmin to the clot to protect it from plasmin-mediated fibrinolysis. At the same time, nearby intact endothelial cells (ECs) secrete tissue-type plasminogen activator (t-PA). t-PA that evades plasminogen activator inhibitor-1 (PAI-1) converts clot-bound plasminogen to plasmin and leads to fibrin clot degradation and release of soluble fibrin peptides and D-dimer. Thus detection of circulating D-dimer indicates active fibrinolysis.

site, a tyrosine molecule across from the serine residue. Nonsteroidal anti-inflammatory drugs (NSAIDs) do not covalently bind through acetylation at serine. Instead, they reversibly and competitively bind at the active, catalytic tyrosine site. Thus NSAID antiplatelet effects are dependent on plasma levels of the drug, unlike aspirin. Mature platelets do not possess COX-2 activity; thus one rationale for development of the highly selective COX-2 inhibitors for inflammatory disease was avoidance of bleeding caused by platelet dysfunction by not affecting platelet COX-1 activity. Unfortunately, clinical trials have now shown that some of the highly selective COX-2 inhibitors increase the likelihood of hypertension and vascular events, including myocardial infarction and stroke, probably through blockade of formation of the antithrombogenic compound, prostacyclin (see Table 51–1 and Chapter 53).

Other platelet agonists are liberated into the extracellular fluid by fusion of the dense and alpha granules with the platelet canalicular membrane, and the result is extrusion of granule contents. The dense granules contain serotonin that, similar to TxA_2, is both a platelet agonist and a vasoconstrictor. Another dense granule constituent, ADP, acts purely as a platelet agonist without vasoactive properties (see Table 51–2). The importance of TxA_2- and serotonin-induced vasoconstriction is not entirely clear. However, vasoconstriction, by decreasing the vessel diameter, may increase shear stress and thereby facilitate recruitment of platelets to the injured site. The importance of dense granule release to the maintenance of hemostasis is underscored by the severe bleeding seen in congenital dense granule deficiencies (e.g., Hermansky-Pudlak syndrome). Platelet activation therefore serves to amplify platelet adhesion and, as detailed later, to optimize the platelet surface for fibrin-generating procoagulant activity by interaction with the coagulation cascade.

Coagulation Cascade

The coagulation cascade is characterized by continuous factor activation and coordinated assembly of enzyme complexes, which are held in check by circulating anticoagulant proteins. These enzyme complexes consist of serine proteases, co-factors, and zymogen substrates assembled on a membrane (phospholipid) surface. Under normal circumstances, formation of these complexes and resultant thrombin generation is relatively slow; inactivation of the complexes by circulating anticoagulants balances their procoagulant activity and prevents clot formation. However, once a procoagulant stimulus occurs that allows a burst of activated factor formation, formation of these enzyme complexes is rapidly amplified and leads to intense thrombin, and subsequent fibrin, formation.

The liver is the major site of synthesis of most of the coagulation factors. In severe liver disease, all coagulation factor levels are diminished except for factor VIII, a finding suggesting that factor VIII is produced not only by the liver, but also by ECs and cells of the reticuloendothelial system. In addition, a subset of factors is vitamin K dependent, that is, prothrombin (factor II) and factors VII, IX, and X. The naturally occurring anticoagulants, proteins C and S, also have vitamin K–dependent synthesis. Post-translational modification (through a vitamin K–dependent carboxylase) of the amino-terminal domain of these proteins adds 10 to 12

γ-carboxyglutamate residues; these residues are critical for calcium binding and for determining the functional three-dimensional structure of the proteins and their proper binding orientation to membrane surfaces. Warfarin blocks liver uptake of vitamin K and inhibits the function of this carboxylase.

From the perspective of laboratory testing, the coagulation cascade is artificially divided into extrinsic (prothrombin time [PT]) and intrinsic (partial thromboplastin time [PTT]) pathways, which converge on a common pathway leading to thrombin and fibrin generation (see Fig. 51–2). However, an important point to understand is that physiologic coagulation is a single pathway of complex factor interactions. The physiologic initiator of coagulation is TF, which is constitutively expressed on subendothelial fibroblasts and smooth muscle cells that are only exposed to blood by EC damage. TF is also expressed on peripheral blood monocytes and vascular ECs after exposure to activating or inflammatory stimuli such as endotoxin. In the laboratory, the *extrinsic* pathway is assessed by measuring the interaction of circulating factor VIIa with exogenously added TF-thromboplastin and is measured as the PT. The PT is highly sensitive to deficiencies of factors VII, V, X, and prothrombin (factor II), and all these deficiencies may be associated with significant bleeding complications. Because factors II, VII, and X are vitamin K-dependent, with factor VII having the shortest half-life, the PT is the most sensitive measurement of the therapeutic efficacy of warfarin (Coumadin). The PT is completely unaffected by deficiencies of factors XII, XI, IX, or VIII. The degree of prolongation of the PT by warfarin partly depends on the strength of the thromboplastin used in the assay, which varies by manufacturer and in its particular activity with each coagulation instrument. Therefore the international normalized ratio (INR) was devised to standardize the variations in the PT induced by warfarin among laboratories so as to allow for global application of anticoagulant recommendations. The INR is based on the international sensitivity index (ISI) of each thromboplastin, standardized to TF, and is calculated for each patient as follows: (patient PT/mean control PT)^{ISI}. Therapeutic INRs with warfarin vary according to the specific disease indication and are covered in Chapter 53. In contrast to warfarin, the PT is relatively insensitive to unfractionated heparin at therapeutic levels.

In vitro contact activation of the coagulation pathway is measured as the PTT in the hematology laboratory; testing is initiated by plasma stimulation with a negatively charged compound such as kaolin. The PTT assay is sensitive to deficiencies of contact factors (prekallikrein [PK], high–molecular-weight kininogen [HMWK], and factor XII), and coagulation factors XI, IX, VIII, V, X, and prothrombin. Deficiencies of PK, HMWK, and factor XII do not result in clinical bleeding, implying that these particular initiators of in vitro coagulation are irrelevant to physiologic hemostasis. By contrast, deficiencies of factor XI, and especially factors IX and VIII, usually cause significant bleeding. The PTT is highly sensitive to unfractionated heparin and is used as a rapid monitoring assay for therapeutic heparin levels. Unlike the INR for warfarin (Coumadin), the range for therapeutic PTT levels with unfractionated heparin is much wider and not as well standardized. Therapeutic unfractionated heparin levels (measured by assays of anti-Xa activity) generally correspond to a PTT of between 1.8 and 2.5 times the patient's initial PTT (before heparin is begun) or times the mean PTT of a control population.

As noted previously, the schema of intrinsic and extrinsic pathways of coagulation reflects a reasonable paradigm only for the purposes of in vitro testing. Physiologic initiation of the clotting cascade is caused by tissue injury and low levels of circulating activated factors, and coagulation events are also bidirectionally linked to inflammation; activated monocytes express functional TF, and factor Xa induces inflammatory responses. The coagulation cascade in vivo is propagated by enzyme complexes that function effectively only on phospholipid membrane surfaces. The appropriate phospholipid surface appears to be predominantly supplied by activated platelets and ECs. Low levels of circulating factor VIIa are generated by thrombin (see Fig. 51–2) and by the factor Xa–phospholipid complex and, to a lesser extent, by factor VIIa–TF itself. TF expressed after EC injury binds to circulating factor VIIa, and the factor VIIa–TF complex subsequently binds to its zymogen substrates, factors IX and X, on the activated platelet membrane to form the TF-dependent tenase complex.

In addition to providing an essential negative phospholipid surface for tenase and the prothrombinase reactions (described later), activated platelets provide specific receptors for factors Xa, IXa, and Va. Factor V is also secreted from the alpha granule of the activated platelet, although evidence indicates that most secreted factor V is derived from the plasma pool. Membrane association of these coagulation factors in their ideal spatial orientation with negatively charged, platelet-expressed phosphatidylserine accelerates procoagulant enzymatic reactions and simultaneously protects the activated factors from circulating inhibitors; this process culminates in accelerated thrombin generation. TF-factor VIIa converts factor X to Xa and factor IX to IXa, both of which are bound to platelet receptors. The platelet factor Xa receptor is closely associated with platelet-bound factor Va; together with free calcium and platelet membrane phosphatidylserine, these factors bind prothrombin (factor II) to form the prothrombinase complex, thereby generating thrombin, albeit in relatively small amounts. This initially formed thrombin may not generate significant fibrin formation but, instead, may activate factor VIII to VIIIa, which binds to membrane-bound factor IXa, factor V to Va, which binds to its platelet receptor, and factor XI to XIa.

Up to this point, the rate of factor Xa and thrombin generation formed is relatively slow. However, once these initial amounts of thrombin generate appreciable quantities of factor XIa and co-factors Va and VIIIa on the platelet surface, activation of factor X through this kinetically favorable pathway becomes dominant, especially after circulating TFPI rapidly blocks TF function. Thrombin feedback activation massively amplifies the clotting cascade, thus increasing the rate of factor Xa and thrombin generation exponentially. This production is mediated initially by the Xase complex formed by TF-induced factors IXa and X, as noted previously, and subsequently by tenase formation via sustained factor XIa–based activation of factor IX. Factor IXa binds to its co-factor, factor VIIIa, and its zymogen substrate, factor X, to further amplify production of factor Xa on the membrane surface (see Fig. 51–2). The burst of factor Xa formation that follows amplifies the formation of the

prothrombinase complex and results in even higher rates of thrombin generation.

With this rapid increase in thrombin generation, fibrinogen is now cleaved to fibrin monomers that rapidly combine to form a fibrin matrix integrated with the platelet plug. Factor XIIIa, a transamidase produced by the action of thrombin on either plasma or platelet-released XIII, converts the soluble fibrin clot into an insoluble fibrin polymer and also binds α_2-antiplasmin to the fibrin to protect the clot from plasmin-mediated dissolution (see Fig. 51–4). Finally, the platelet plug undergoes clot retraction, which protects the platelet-fibrin matrices from lysis by plasmin. These antilytic mechanisms, largely linked to platelet activation, may explain the relative resistance of platelet-rich clots to thrombolysis.

At the same time that tenase and prothrombinase complexes are forming on the platelet and EC membranes, the natural inhibitors of coagulation are activated to downregulate clotting. In the intact circulation and at the perimeter of a newly formed clot, certain endogenous mechanisms, including an intact EC barrier, limit clotting to the area of injury and maintain the surrounding flowing blood in a liquid form. In the arterial circulation, vessel occlusion by the growing clot is counteracted by the high-velocity blood flow that dilutes and disperses coagulation factors. Antiplatelet factors are also part of the anticoagulant activity intrinsic to the healthy EC lining and limit extension of the platelet plug past the area of damage. These factors include the following: (1) net negative surface charge, which repels similarly charged platelets; (2) constitutive release of nitric oxide and prostacyclin, which inhibits platelet aggregation; and (3) constitutive surface expression of an ADPase that inactivates platelet-released ADP and thus limits recruitment of additional platelets (see Table 51–1).

Once the platelet plug and associated fibrin deposition have halted the bleeding and have covered any exposed endothelium, reining in the coagulation cascade becomes critical. Clot limitation occurs by several mechanisms (see Fig. 51–3): (1) tenase and TF–factor VIIa neutralization by TFPI; (2) thrombin and factor IXa, Xa, and XIa neutralization by antithrombin III (ATIII); (3) elimination of thrombin-activated co-factors Va and VIIIa by APC and its co-factor protein S; and (4) dissolution of the formed fibrin clot by t-PA and urokinase (see Fig. 51–4). ATIII and TFPI are circulating, constitutive protease inhibitors. ATIII inhibits the activity of thrombin and factors Xa, IXa, and XIa by complexing with these proteins; both the antithrombin and anti-Xa activity of ATIII are amplified approximately 2000-fold by unfractionated heparin. ECs synthesize an endogenous glycosaminoglycan, heparan sulfate, which associates with the extracellular matrix; heparan sulfate then complexes with blood ATIII to amplify neutralization of locally developed thrombin. Because heparan sulfates are bound to the extracellular matrix associated with neighboring intact endothelium, ATIII-heparan interactions help prevent the clot from extending away from the damaged area. ECs constitutively release TFPI that also inhibits circulating factor Xa activity but mainly acts to downregulate TF-induced tenase function. This task is accomplished through binding of the TFPI–factor Xa complex to the TF–factor VIIa complex and inactivating TF–factor VIIa activity through this quaternary complex formation, thereby shutting down the TF-induced tenase pathway.

Thrombomodulin is another EC surface–associated protein. Thrombin that escapes antithrombin neutralization binds to thrombomodulin on the membranes of nearby intact ECs, and this enzyme complex activates protein C (see Fig. 51–3). APC cleaves non–platelet-associated factors Va and VIIIa and thereby inactivates the respective prothrombinase and tenase complexes and downregulates thrombin formation. The vitamin K–dependent factor, protein S, serves as a co-factor for APC and increases its biologic activity for cleavage of factors Va and VIIIa by 20-fold and 5-fold, respectively. Protein S functions only when it is circulating in the free state and not when it is complexed with the C4b-binding protein; in acute illness, the C4b-binding protein may be increased as an acute-phase reactant. Increased binding of protein S may therefore occur in acute illnesses; this process may decrease free protein S levels and may lead to a relative decrease in natural anticoagulant activity and a procoagulant state.

Endothelial-Associated Fibrinolysis

Intravascular fibrinolytic activity results from a balance between plasminogen activators, such as t-PA and urokinase-type PA (u-PA), and inhibitors, such as plasminogen activator inhibitor-1 (PAI-1) and α_2-antiplasmin (see Fig. 51–4). Regulation of fibrinolysis occurs at the endothelial surface. Vascular ECs synthesize and secrete t-PA and PAI-1. Plasminogen activation to plasmin is boosted by cell surface–associated t-PA, especially in the presence of fibrin clot, and to a lesser extent by the relatively small circulating amounts of u-PA. Plasmin facilitates degradation of fibrin and matrix components in the pericellular environs. PAI-1 is the main blocker of t-PA activity in vivo. It achieves large concentrations relative to t-PA, but significant variability exists in PAI-1 plasma levels in healthy individuals, in part, because of its circadian pattern of secretion. This variability is also associated with polymorphisms of the PAI-1 gene—the 4G promoter region polymorphism is associated with higher PAI-1 levels and perhaps a higher risk of thromboembolism (see Chapter 53). Inhibition of plasmin, a procoagulant effect, is mediated by α_2-antiplasmin and possibly by α_2-macroglobulin. Besides ECs, macrophages are also critical to fibrinolysis. Macrophages degrade fibrin clot through lysosomal proteolysis by a mechanism that does not involve plasmin. The macrophage binds to fibrin(ogen) through its surface integrin receptor, CD11b/CD18; this binding is followed by internalization of the complex into the lysosome, where fibrin(ogen) is degraded.

Tissue repair and regeneration eventually require dissolution of the fibrin-based clot. t-PA and urokinase act on the circulating zymogen plasminogen to generate the active fibrinolytic enzyme plasmin. In addition, the intrinsic pathway activators, kallikrein, XIIa, and XIa, help convert plasminogen to plasmin. Plasminogen binding to cell surface receptors promotes its own activation by placing it in proximity to t-PA and fibrin clot, as well as by protecting plasmin from inactivation by circulating (but not clot-bound) α_2-antiplasmin (see Fig. 51–4). Plasmin dissolves the fibrin matrix and produces soluble fibrin peptides and D-dimer and also activates metalloproteinases that degrade damaged tissue. Fibroblasts and leukocytes migrate into the wound, the latter mediated by E- and P-selectin binding, and these cells act in concert with growth factors secreted by leukocytes and activated platelets (e.g., transforming growth factor-β) to promote vascular repair and tissue regeneration.

Prospectus for the Future

The balance of procoagulant and anticoagulant processes normally achieve hemostasis; in addition, their complex interplay may be regulated by other pathophysiologic conditions. One example is the emerging role of high-density lipoprotein (HDL) in coagulation. Besides removing cholesterol from vascular walls, HDL has some anticoagulant effects mediated through its stimulation of prostacyclin synthesis and inhibition of platelet activating factor production. These observations may explain why low HDL is an independent risk factor for coronary thromboembolism. Whether chronic therapies that improve the HDL-to-cholesterol ratio will affect the risk of arterial vascular events remains to be determined. In a related area, platelets have now been shown to contain high concentrations of vascular endothelial growth factor (VEGF), a critical EC-specific angiogenesis factor. VEGF may also interact with coagulation processes, especially fibrinolysis, through its promotion of urokinase (uPA) production. The role of platelet-derived VEGF is currently being investigated in other processes that involve significant angiogenesis, such as growth and metastasis of carcinomas and postinfarction myocardial remodeling. As we increase our understanding of the molecular processes in hemostasis, we find their assumption of new roles in heretofore unrelated diseases.

References

Antman EM, DeMets D, Loscalzo J: Cyclooxygenase inhibition and cardiovascular risk. Circulation 112:759–770, 2005.

Butenas S, Brummel KE, Branda RF, et al: Mechanism of factor VIIa-dependent coagulation in hemophilia blood. Blood 99:923–930, 2002.

Hoffman M, Monroe DM 3d: A cell-based model of hemostasis. Thromb Haemost 85:958–965, 2001.

Lijnen HR: Pleiotropic functions of plasminogen activator inhibitor-1. J Thromb Haemost 3:35–45, 2005.

Mann K, Kalafatis M: Factor V: A combination of Dr Jekyll and Mr Hyde. Blood 101:20–30, 2003.

Undas A, Brummel K, Musial J, et al: Blood coagulation at the site of microvascular injury: Effects of low-dose aspirin. Blood 98:2423–2431, 2001.

Disorders of Hemostasis: Bleeding

Richard Torres

Henry M. Rinder

Clinical Evaluation of Bleeding

The evaluation of bleeding requires a careful history, physical examination, and laboratory evaluation. The patient's history should include a description of bleeding (e.g., epistaxis, menorrhagia, hematoma formation), the circumstances under which bleeding occurs (e.g., association with trauma, surgery, dental procedures), and whether any blood products (and what kind of products) are required to staunch the bleeding. The clinician should determine whether the temporal addition of medications, such as aspirin, is associated with the bleeding and whether the patient has any concomitant medical illnesses such as infection or liver disease. Finally, determining whether the patient has any family history of bleeding is critical; the physician may need to query several generations and second-degree relations, such as maternal uncles, when hemophilia is suggested in a boy.

The physical examination may yield some clues as to the origin of bleeding and may help distinguish between small-vessel bleeding, such as petechial (pinpoint) hemorrhage, and larger vessel bleeding, which usually produces hematomas and purpura (large bruises). Small-vessel bleeding in the skin, in the mucous membranes, or in the gastrointestinal (GI) tract tends to occur more often in patients with thrombocytopenia, qualitative platelet defects, vascular abnormalities, and von Willebrand disease (vWD). In women, menorrhagia may be the only symptom. Large-vessel bleeding in solid organs, joints, or muscles is more commonly associated with factor deficiencies, such as hemophilia A or B. Screening laboratory assays are often useful in the initial assessment of the patient with bleeding (Table 52–1). Such assays should include the following: (1) *blood cell counts* (especially the platelet count) and examination of the peripheral blood smear; (2) *prothrombin time* (PT), which is highly sensitive to defects in vitamin K–dependent coagulation factors; and (3) *partial thromboplastin time* (PTT), which detects deficiencies in factors VIII, IX, and XI, as well as the contact activators, prekallikrein, high–

molecular-weight kininogen, and factor XII. Abnormalities of factors X, V, and II (prothrombin) result in elevations of both the PT and the PTT. If the PT or the PTT is prolonged, then the patient's plasma should be combined with normal plasma (*mixing study*), and the clotting-time study should be repeated. The mixing study enables one to distinguish between factor deficiency (i.e., the PT or the PTT corrects into the normal range) and a circulating inhibitor (i.e., the clotting time remains prolonged). Another readily available test for the patient with bleeding is the *thrombin time*; this test directly measures the conversion of fibrinogen to fibrin by exogenous thrombin and assays both the fibrinogen level and its functional capability.

Platelet function has been traditionally assessed by the in vivo *bleeding time*, an invasive measure of the time to halt bleeding after an incision is made in the patient's skin. The bleeding time is prolonged by thrombocytopenia (platelet count <100,000/mcL) and by qualitative platelet defects. The technique dependence of the bleeding time test, resulting in low reproducibility, and the difficulty of performing the test in infants and neonates have limited its use. Several commercial instruments are now available for in vitro assessment of platelet function. One such instrument that delivers an *in vitro bleeding time* is the Platelet Function Analyzer-100 (PFA-100); in this instrument, citrate-anticoagulated whole blood is passed through a small orifice in a cartridge impregnated with platelet activators such as collagen, adenosine diphosphate (ADP), and epinephrine. As the platelets activate and adhere, the orifice gradually becomes obstructed, and the time to complete occlusion by the platelet plug is measured as the closure time. The closure time is prolonged by qualitative platelet defects such as aspirin and by decreased platelet adhesive ligands in plasma such as vWD. Although thrombocytopenia affects the closure time similar to the in vivo bleeding time, the in vitro bleeding time tests are gaining favor as a platelet-function screen because they avoid an invasive procedure and lack the variability of manual techniques.

Another laboratory study for evaluation of a prolonged PTT, especially in the inpatient setting, is the PTT plus added

Table 52–1 Screening Hemostasis Assays

Laboratory Test	Aspect of Hemostasis Tested	Causes of Abnormalities
Blood counts and peripheral blood smear	Platelet count and morphologic features	Thrombocytopenia; thrombocytosis; gray platelet and giant-platelet syndromes
Prothrombin time	Factor VII–dependent pathways	Vitamin K deficiency and warfarin; liver disease; DIC; factor deficiency (VII, V, X), factor inhibitor
Partial thromboplastin time	Factor XI–, IX–, and VIII–dependent pathways	Heparin; DIC; lupus anticoagulant*; vWD; factor deficiency (XI, IX, VIII, V, X, XII, HMWK, PK), factor inhibitor
Thrombin time	Fibrinogen	Heparin; DIC; hypofibrinogenemia; dysfibrinogenemia
Bleeding time	Platelet and vascular function	Aspirin; thrombocytopenia; vWD; storage pool disease
Mixing study	Presence of an inhibitor	Abnormal clotting time corrects with a deficiency; does not correct with an inhibitor

*Lupus anticoagulant is not associated with bleeding.
DIC = disseminated intravascular coagulation; HMWK = high–molecular-weight kininogen; PK = prekallikrein; vWD = von Willebrand disease.

polybrene; when concern exists that a sample is contaminated by heparin as a result of drawing it through an indwelling intravenous line, the added polybrene neutralizes the heparin and will correct the prolonged PTT. The polybrene PTT is not useful in patients receiving unfractionated heparin (UFH) therapeutically. A prolonged PTT that does not correct with the mixing study may also be observed in patients with a lupus anticoagulant (often in the context of thrombosis). In this setting, the diagnosis of a lupus anticoagulant can be confirmed by documenting the correction of the PTT with the addition of excess phospholipid to bind antiphospholipid antibodies, as well as other specific tests for lupus anticoagulant (see antiphospholipid syndrome in Chapter 53).

A rapid approach to identifying possible causes of bleeding (Fig. 52–1) should consider the following major disease categories: (1) thrombocytopenia or abnormal platelet function; (2) low levels of multiple coagulation factors resulting from vitamin K deficiency or liver disease; (3) single-factor deficiency, either inherited or acquired; (4) consumptive coagulopathies such as disseminated intravascular coagulation (DIC); and (5) circulating inhibitors to coagulation factors such as antibody to factor VIII. In addition, disorders intrinsic to the blood vessels themselves may cause a bleeding diathesis. The laboratory evaluation is most efficient when performed in the context of these categories.

Vascular Causes of Bleeding

Vascular purpura (bruising) is defined as bleeding caused by intrinsic structural abnormalities of blood vessels or by inflammatory infiltration of blood vessels (*vasculitis*). Although vascular purpura usually causes bleeding in the setting of normal platelet counts and normal coagulation studies, vasculitis and vessel damage may be severe enough to cause secondary consumption of platelets and coagulation factors. Abnormalities of the subcutaneous tissue that overlies blood vessels is often observed in older patients and is termed *senile purpura*; similar skin changes leading to fragile blood vessels are also common effects of steroid therapy. In this setting, collagen breakdown and thinning of subcutaneous tissue lead to bruising as a result of atrophy. Another acquired cause of vascular purpura is scurvy, or vitamin C deficiency. *Scurvy* is characterized by bleeding around individual hair fibers (*perifollicular hemorrhage*) and corkscrew-shaped hairs. Bruising occurs in a classic *saddle* pattern, distributed over the upper thighs. The bleeding gums with scurvy are caused by gingivitis and not by the subcutaneous tissue defect. Thus edentulous patients with scurvy do not have bleeding gums, and scurvy should not be excluded on this basis.

Congenital defects of the vessel wall may cause bruising. These rare syndromes include *pseudoxanthoma elasticum*, a defect of the elastic fibers of the vasculature that is associated with severe GI and genitourinary bleeding, and *Ehlers-Danlos syndrome*, characterized by abnormal collagen molecules in both blood vessels and subcutaneous tissue. Both syndromes exhibit bruising in the skin, but only patients with pseudoxanthoma elasticum develop significant GI bleeding. Another inherited vessel wall defect associated with GI bleeding is *hereditary hemorrhagic telangiectasia (Osler-Weber-Rendu syndrome)*. This disorder is characterized by degeneration of the blood vessel wall that results in angiomatous lesions resembling blood blisters on mucous membranes, including the lips and GI tract. The frequency of bleeding caused by a breakdown of these lesions increases with age, and GI lesions commonly cause significant, chronic bleeding, often resulting in iron deficiency.

The sudden onset of *palpable purpura* (localized, raised hemorrhages in the skin) in association with rash and fever may be caused by vasculitis, either aseptic or septic. *Septic vasculitis* may be caused by meningococcemia and other bacterial infections and is often accompanied by thrombocytopenia and prolongation of clotting times. One cause of aseptic vasculitis in young children and adolescents is *Henoch-Schönlein purpura*, a vasculitis of the skin, GI tract, and kidneys, which is usually accompanied by abdominal pain caused by bleeding into the bowel wall. This syndrome may occur after a viral prodrome and appears to be caused by an immunoglobulin A (IgA) hypersensitivity reaction, as evidenced by serum IgA immune complexes and renal histopathologic features resembling IgA nephropathy. *Drug hypersensitivity,* for example, to allopurinol can exhibit extensive cutaneous purpura as well.

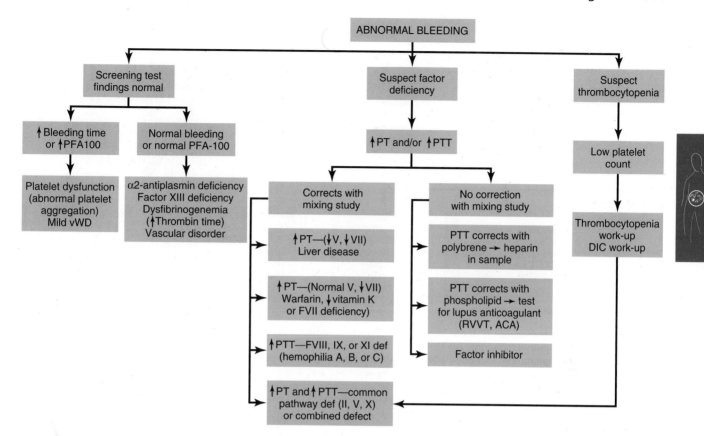

Figure 52–1 Algorithm for the evaluation of bleeding. Screening laboratory tests for platelet and factor deficiencies are used to narrow the work-up for bleeding, followed by specific factor and other coagulation studies (e.g., mixing studies, D-dimer) to confirm the diagnosis. DIC = disseminated intravascular coagulation; FSP = fibrin-split products; PT = prothrombin time; PTT = partial thromboplastin time; Rx = therapy; vWD = von Willebrand disease.

The therapy of bleeding from vascular disorders is straightforward. Senile purpura and steroid-induced purpura do not usually require treatment. Scurvy is corrected by oral ascorbic acid. In the case of congenital disorders, including Ehlers-Danlos syndrome, hereditary hemorrhagic telangiectasia, and pseudoxanthoma elasticum, patients should avoid medications that may aggravate their bleeding tendencies (e.g., aspirin), and they should receive supportive therapy (e.g., iron supplementation). Systemic administration of estrogen in hereditary hemorrhagic telangiectasia may help decrease epistaxis by inducing squamous metaplasia of the nasal mucosa and thereby protecting lesions from trauma. Treatment of septic vasculitis obviously focuses primarily on appropriate antibiotic therapy; in the case of aseptic vasculitis, steroids and/or immunosuppressive agents are most effective. When vasculitis is severe enough to cause consumption of platelets and coagulation factors (see later discussion of DIC), transfusions of platelets, cryoprecipitate, or fresh-frozen plasma may be indicated.

Bleeding Caused by Platelet Disorders: Thrombocytopenia

Thrombocytopenia (platelet count <150,000/mcL) is one of the most common problems in hospitalized patients. The initial diagnostic approach to thrombocytopenia involves classifying whether the low platelet count is caused by (1) decreased platelet production, (2) increased platelet sequestration, or (3) increased peripheral platelet destruction (Fig. 52–2). An evaluation of the number and morphologic features of marrow megakaryocytes has been the traditional diagnostic test for differentiating between decreased platelet production and peripheral sequestration (e.g. splenomegaly) or destruction (e.g., immune thrombocytopenic purpura [ITP]). The reticulated platelet count, similar to the red cell reticulocyte count, is a noninvasive measure of the youngest circulating platelets in the blood (identified via their increased RNA content). Reticulated platelets are being increasingly used as a peripheral blood index of platelet kinetics and can be part of the evaluation of thrombocytopenia.

THROMBOCYTOPENIA CAUSED BY DECREASED MARROW PRODUCTION

Decreased production of platelets in the bone marrow is characterized by decreased or absent megakaryocytes on the bone marrow aspirate and biopsy and a low percentage of reticulated platelets. Suppression of normal megakaryocytopoiesis occurs in the following situations: (1) marrow damage and destruction of stem cells, as exhibited with cytotoxic chemotherapy; (2) destruction of the normal marrow microenvironment and replacement of normal stem cells by

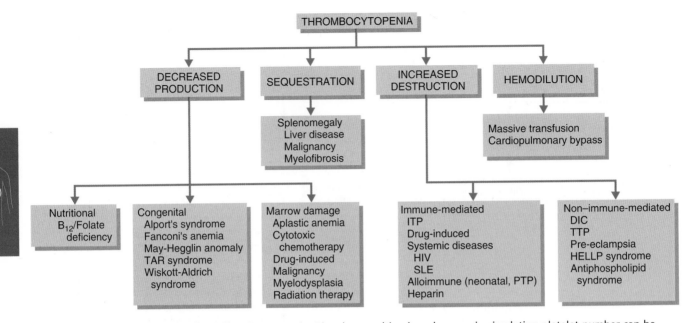

Figure 52–2 Differential diagnosis of thrombocytopenia. Disorders resulting in a decrease in circulating platelet number can be divided into four main pathophysiologic mechanisms: hypoproduction, sequestration, peripheral destruction, and hemodilution. The history, physical examination, and bone marrow evaluation usually narrow the range of possible causes. DIC = disseminated intravascular coagulation; HELLP = hemolysis, elevated liver enzymes, and low-platelet count in association with pre-eclampsia; HIV = human immunodeficiency virus; ITP = immune thrombocytopenic purpura; PTP = post-transfusion purpura; SLE = systemic lupus erythematosus; TAR = thrombocytopenia-absent radius syndrome; TTP = thrombotic thrombocytopenic purpura.

invasive malignant disease, aplasia, infection (e.g., miliary tuberculosis), or myelofibrosis; (3) specific intrinsic defects of the megakaryocytic stem cells; and (4) metabolic abnormalities affecting megakaryocyte maturation.

Thrombocytopenia may result from cytotoxic or immunosuppressive chemotherapy for malignant or auto-immune disease. Thrombocytopenia is usually reversible, and platelet production rebounds as megakaryocytic stem cells recover and regenerate. However, repeated and/or intensive chemotherapy (e.g., stem cell transplantation) may permanently damage the megakaryocytic stem cells and supporting stromal environment and may cause chronic thrombocytopenia. This condition may be accompanied by leukopenia and anemia suggestive of refractory anemia (*myelodysplasia*). Commonly used drugs such as thiazide diuretics, alcohol, and estrogens may also damage bone marrow megakaryocytes. Nutritional disorders, especially alcoholism and abnormal folate or vitamin B_{12} metabolism, are also commonly associated with thrombocytopenia; platelet counts respond to abstinence from alcohol and to appropriate multivitamin replacement therapy.

Platelet production is suppressed by intrinsic malignant diseases of the bone marrow such as leukemia and multiple myeloma and by malignant diseases that secondarily invade the bone marrow (non-Hodgkin's lymphoma, small-cell lung cancer, breast and prostate cancers, and many others). The bone marrow aspirate under these circumstances shows decreased megakaryocytes and, occasionally, malignant cells; bone marrow biopsy has a much higher yield for diagnosing malignant involvement of the marrow. Flow cytometric evaluation for clonal B cells in the marrow aspirate is highly sensitive for detecting lymphoproliferative disease (non-Hodgkin's lymphoma).

Myelofibrosis, an increase in the reticulin fibers (and sometimes collagen) of the marrow, may lead to thrombocytopenia or pancytopenia. Myelofibrosis occurs most commonly in myeloproliferative disorders, in mastocytosis, and in mycobacterial and other infections involving the marrow. It may also occur occasionally in patients with myelodysplasia or acute leukemia, especially megakaryocytic FAB M7 (i.e., the French, American, and British classification scheme for leukemia) and, rarely, on a congenital basis (*osteogenesis imperfecta*). Thrombocytopenia is also observed in patients with severe aplastic anemia, and the bone marrow shows decreased or absent megakaryocytes with other cell lineages similarly affected.

Thrombocytopenia in children can also result from congenital defects of megakaryocyte production as seen with the *thrombocytopenia-absent radii syndrome, congenital amegakaryocytic thrombocytopenia* (secondary to a mutation in the thrombopoietin receptor), and *Fanconi anemia* (congenital aplastic anemia with renal hypoplasia and skin hyperpigmentation). Other disorders that are intrinsic to the bone marrow include the *May-Hegglin anomaly* and related myosin IIa/MYH9 gene diseases, characterized by giant platelets and Döhle's bodies (basophilic inclusions in leukocytes and platelets) on the peripheral blood smear. *Wiskott-Aldrich syndrome* is an X-linked disorder with eczema and immunodeficiency, as well as thrombocytopenia with small platelets that can be diagnosed by the lack of CD43 expression on lymphocytes using flow cytometry. When accompanied by nerve deafness and nephritis, congenital hypoproductive thrombocytopenia is also part of *Alport's syndrome*.

Platelet transfusions are used to support patients with hypoproductive thrombocytopenia of any origin but especially in support of those receiving induction or maintenance chemotherapy for malignant diseases. The *prophylactic* use of platelet transfusions for thrombocytopenia in patients receiving chemotherapy is more common than transfusion for actual bleeding. The platelet count trigger for such prophylactic transfusions is usually set at 10,000/mcL, which is a safe and appropriate threshold in patients with relatively uncomplicated clinical pictures; that is, no fever, sepsis, or GI bleeding. The threshold of 10,000/mcL significantly decreases the frequency of platelet transfusion. If complicating circumstances are present or if patients are about to undergo a procedure, then prophylactic platelet transfusions should be given when counts are lower than 20,000/mcL.

In patients with thrombocytopenia without any cause for increased peripheral platelet destruction, each unit of random donor-platelet concentrate raises the platelet count by about 10,000/mcL. Thus six units of platelets transfused into a patient with a platelet count of 10,000/mcL would be expected to raise the count to nearly 70,000/mcL. However, concomitant fever, sepsis, alloimmunization, use of amphotericin B, graft-versus-host disease, or DIC in patients with thrombocytopenia will increase platelet consumption and blunt the platelet rise. With the exception of alloimmunization, the foregoing conditions generally decrease overall transfused platelet survival but not what is termed *immediate platelet recovery*. Thus the platelet count rises significantly by 1 hour after transfusion and then declines at a steeper rate than in patients with thrombocytopenia but without concomitant complicating factors. In contrast, in an alloimmunized patient, the platelets rise at 1 hour after transfusion may be minimal or absent. Because alloimmunized patients often require donor screening by platelet cross-matching or human leukocyte-antigen matching, obtaining a 1-hour post-transfusion platelet count may be an important test to maximize the response to transfused platelets. In patients with these conditions, efforts should be made to transfuse type-specific platelets, if available, to minimize any clearance caused by ABO determinants carried on the platelet surface. Rh antigens, in contrast, are not present on platelet surfaces; consequently, they play no role in platelet alloimmunization.

THROMBOCYTOPENIA CAUSED BY SEQUESTRATION

Up to 30% of circulating platelets are normally contained within the spleen at any given time. Conditions that lead to splenomegaly cause increased trapping of platelets. This *platelet sequestration* causes thrombocytopenia, often dropping the platelet count into the range of 50,000 to 100,000/mcL but rarely lower. Thrombocytopenia from sequestration is common in advanced liver disease, myeloproliferative disorders accompanied by splenomegaly (e.g., chronic myelogenous leukemia, chronic idiopathic myelofibrosis), and malignant disease involving the spleen. Splenectomy may be indicated in patients with malignant disease. In contrast, splenectomy is rarely used to treat thrombocytopenia resulting from portal hypertension. The decision to perform splenectomy for thrombocytopenia in patients with myeloproliferative syndromes must be individualized and weighed against its complications, both surgical and those related to the specific disease process.

THROMBOCYTOPENIA CAUSED BY PERIPHERAL PLATELET DESTRUCTION

Increased peripheral platelet destruction (caused by immune or nonimmune mechanisms) commonly leads to thrombocytopenia. Autoimmune thrombocytopenia may be a primary immune disorder directed only at platelets or as a secondary complication of another autoimmune disease, such as systemic lupus erythematosus. The pathophysiologic characteristics of immune platelet destruction involve increased levels of polyclonal antiplatelet antibodies in the circulation. These antibodies are usually directed against platelet membrane glycoprotein receptors, most often cryptic neoepitopes of glycoprotein IIb/IIIa (GPIIb/IIIa) and less commonly GPIb. Coating of the platelet with these antibodies leads to opsonization of the platelets by Fc receptors on cells of the reticuloendothelial system (RES). Antibody-coated platelets are cleared by the spleen and, to a lesser extent, by the liver. These disorders generally involve a dramatic increase in marrow platelet production reflected by increased numbers of marrow megakaryocytes. The younger platelets produced have relatively high granule contents, providing increased hemostatic function. Bone marrow examination for the presence of increased or normal megakaryocyte numbers is the traditional means of distinguishing platelet destruction from decreased production. However, as previously mentioned, increased percentages of *reticulated platelets* in the circulation are associated with destructive, especially immune-mediated, thrombocytopenia and may be sufficient for diagnosing platelet destruction. Thrombocytopenia resulting from immune clearance may be severe, and platelet survival is often reduced from the normal 7 to 10 days to less than 1 day. Despite severe thrombocytopenia even in the range of 1000 to 2000/mcL, serious bleeding or hemorrhagic death is rare, partly because the function of young platelets is increased and partly because the number of circulating platelets required to maintain vascular integrity is relatively low, only 7100/mcL per day.

IMMUNE THROMBOCYTOPENIC PURPURA

In children, acute ITP is often preceded by a viral infection, such as varicella. Patients with ITP exhibit petechial hemorrhage, mucosal bleeding, and thrombocytopenia, with counts often lower than 20,000/mcL. The peripheral blood smear shows large platelets and no other abnormal cells such as blasts, which would accompany childhood leukemia. The bone marrow demonstrates increased or occasionally normal numbers of megakaryocytes. The diagnosis of ITP is partly made by exclusion. Fever, organomegaly, pancytopenia, lymphadenopathy, or abnormal peripheral blood cells should prompt an evaluation for malignant disease, such as leukemia, neuroblastoma, or Wilms' tumor, or other bone marrow disorders. Laboratory tests may complement the clinical evaluation, but they are not required to make the diagnosis of ITP. These tests include the demonstration of an increased percentage of reticulated platelets in the peripheral blood or the detection of platelet autoantibodies in serum or on the platelet (*platelet-associated immunoglobulin*). However, assays of platelet-associated antibodies, though sensitive, are not specific for ITP, because immunoglobulins that bind nonspecifically to platelets are often increased in patients with thrombocytopenia secondary to other causes such as liver disease or human immunodeficiency virus (HIV) infection. In contrast, techniques that measure serum antibodies to specific platelet glycoproteins have greater specificity but are relatively insensitive. An increase in mean platelet volume is also a relatively insensitive and nonspecific indicator of destructive thrombocytopenia, in part because of the wide range of normal values. An increase in the reticulated platelet percentage is consistent with increased platelet destruction but cannot distinguish between ITP and other causes of platelet destruction such as heparin-induced thrombocytopenia (HIT) and thrombotic thrombocytopenic purpura (TTP) (both discussed in greater detail in Chapters 52 and 53, respectively). Thus the diagnosis of ITP remains largely clinical.

Acute ITP in children can resolve without therapy, but most clinicians prefer to treat children with steroids or intravenous immunoglobulin (IVIG). IVIG therapy for ITP is thought to work by multiple mechanisms: (1) high immunoglobulin G (IgG) concentrations block Fc receptors on phagocytes of the RES and on cellular effectors of antibody-dependent cytotoxicity; (2) infusion of IgG increases the fractional rate of IgG catabolism and thereby increases the destruction of antiplatelet IgG in direct proportion to its concentration; and (3) clearance of antiplatelet Ig may increase through anti-idiotypic effects (i.e., generating an immunologic response to the ITP antibodies). More than 80% of children with acute ITP have a rapid remission, and ITP does not recur. A subset of 10% to 20% of patients eventually develops recurrent thrombocytopenia (i.e., chronic ITP); however, more than 70% of such children respond completely to splenectomy. For those with chronic courses after splenectomy, episodic IVIG, RhoGAM (see later discussion in this chapter), and, in severe cases, immunosuppressive therapy are used. Hemorrhagic deaths are rare in childhood ITP (<2%), but some mortality (2% to 5%) is associated with chronic, refractory ITP.

As with children, the diagnosis of ITP in adults is made largely by exclusion, but unlike with children, acute ITP in adults rarely remits spontaneously and is more likely to become a chronic disorder, evolving to chronic ITP in more than 50% of patients. Petechial hemorrhage and mucosal bleeding are accompanied by platelet counts commonly lower than 20,000/mcL and often as low as 1000 to 2000/mcL. Hemorrhagic deaths occur in fewer than 10% of adults with ITP. In adults, ITP may be associated with other diseases, such as HIV infection. ITP may be the presenting manifestation of HIV infection, whereas thrombocytopenia in more advanced stages of HIV infection is more often caused by bone marrow failure resulting from megakaryocyte infection with HIV, mycobacterial infection of the bone marrow, and nutritional deficiencies of end-stage HIV disease. ITP also occurs in patients with autoimmune disorders such as systemic lupus erythematosus, inflammatory bowel disease, and hepatitis. As in de novo ITP, increased peripheral platelet destruction, with normal or increased megakaryocytes on bone marrow examination, cause thrombocytopenia in these autoimmune disorders. In some patients, ITP is accompanied by autoimmune hemolytic anemia, otherwise termed *Evans syndrome*. The Coombs' test for erythrocytes is usually positive for a warm-reactive auto-

antibody. Initial treatment may not be significantly different from that for ITP alone, but chronic Evans syndrome is thought to generally respond poorly to splenectomy, unlike ITP alone. In the setting of systemic lupus erythematosus, ITP may be secondary to factors associated with the autoimmune disease itself, including immune-complex deposition on the platelet surface and active vasculitis, both of which may lead to increased platelet clearance and low counts. Therapy of both ITP and the underlying autoimmune disorder is usually complementary. When the lupus anticoagulant or anticardiolipin antibody is present in association with systemic lupus erythematosus and thrombocytopenia, the diagnosis of secondary antiphospholipid antibody syndrome is made; this entity is most commonly associated with thromboembolic complications (see Chapter 53).

Immune-platelet destruction can also be associated with drugs. Quinidine or quinine-based formulations bind to platelets and create a *hapten*, a neoantigen of the platelet and drug together. Antibody is directed against this neoantigen and causes rapid clearance of platelets by the RES. Development of thrombocytopenia is temporally related to exposure to the drug and is usually rapid; discontinuation of the drug causes an equally rapid rise in the platelet count. Other medications that cause ITP include sulfa compounds, gold salts, and psychotropic drugs. Discontinuing medications is always necessary but may need to be accompanied by steroid or IVIG therapy.

The first-line treatment of acute ITP in adults is steroids, usually prednisone, 1 to 2 mg/kg/day. Platelet transfusions are not generally used in ITP because transfused-platelet survival is brief and bleeding complications are uncommon. However, in patients with significant bleeding or requiring surgery, platelet transfusions have been safely used and may transiently increase the platelet count, although usually for less than 24 hours. In patients with acute ITP with severe thrombocytopenia (<5000/mcL) or with life-threatening bleeding, high-dose methylprednisolone (1 g/day for 3 days) may be administered alone or in combination with IVIG (2 g/kg in divided doses over 2 to 5 days). In recurrent ITP, chronic steroid treatment is often necessary but is usually accompanied by significant side effects. Evidence indicates that patients, both children and adults, with chronic ITP who initially respond to IVIG therapy respond well to subsequent splenectomy, whereas those who do not respond to IVIG are less likely to have a disease remission after splenectomy. More than 50% of patients with chronic ITP have some degree of disease remission after splenectomy, although approximately one third of patients who undergo splenectomy will continue to have chronic ITP. If ITP does recur after splenectomy, then the presence of an accessory spleen must be ruled out, usually by liver and spleen scanning, because Howell-Jolly bodies may still be present. Recurrent disease may often be episodic, especially after viral infections, and these patients can be treated with IVIG or RhoGAM in patients who are Rh-positive. *RhoGAM* is antibody to the blood group Rh-D antigen, which induces red cell hemolysis (usually mild), thereby presumably causing Fc receptor blockade of the RES and decreased platelet uptake by the spleen and liver. Some patients with ITP, especially those with HIV infection, have experienced significant hemolysis after RhoGAM, and this therapy should be carefully monitored. RhoGAM is generally ineffective in patients who have undergone splenectomy. In patients who fail to respond to splenectomy, steroid dose may be spared by the addition of danazol, colchicine, or immunosuppressive therapy (e.g., cyclophosphamide). Some patients with chronic ITP have responded to infusions of an anti-CD20 monoclonal antibody. About 5% of adults with ITP die of chronic, refractory disease.

ALLOIMMUNE THROMBOCYTOPENIA

Neonatal alloimmune thrombocytopenia occurs when the mother is homozygous for an uncommon platelet alloantigen, most often Pl(A2) (heparin-associated antibodies [HPA]-1b) on GPIIIa, and the fetus expresses the Pl(A1) (HPA-1a) haplotype inherited from the father. The pathogenesis of alloimmune thrombocytopenia is analogous to the mechanism by which Rh sensitization induces hemolytic disease of the newborn. The mother is exposed to the Pl(A1) antigen during a first pregnancy, and in second and subsequent pregnancies, she produces high-titer IgG antibody against Pl(A1). These antibodies cross the placenta, react with Pl(A1)-positive fetal platelets and cause peripheral-platelet destruction by the RES. Neonatal alloimmune thrombocytopenia may be severe, but this reaction does not necessarily predict whether bleeding will occur in utero, at delivery, or in the first days of life. Maternal platelets (lacking Pl[A1]) and IVIG are used to treat bleeding and to restore platelet count.

Alloimmune thrombocytopenia can also occur in adults after transfusion (*post-transfusion purpura*). As in neonates, this condition is based on exposure to a common platelet alloantigen such as Pl(A1) that is not present on the patient's native platelets. This disorder most commonly occurs after red blood cell or platelet transfusions in a woman who is homozygous for Pl(A2) and who is alloimmunized to Pl(A1) as a result of a previous pregnancy, or, more rarely, in any patient alloimmunized because of prior transfusions. More than 90% of blood donors express Pl(A1), and Pl(A1) is shed by platelets. Consequently, even red blood cell products with little platelet contamination contain Pl(A1). The anamnestic response to the blood product causes destruction of residual donor platelets and, even more interestingly, destruction of native platelets *that do not express the Pl(A1) alloantigen.* The pathophysiologic aspect of post-transfusion purpura

(PTP) is unclear, although evidence suggests that native platelets may be destroyed either nonspecifically by the RES or by adsorption of Pl(A1) onto host platelets. As with neonates, these patients are treated with IVIG, and any further transfusions must be derived from homozygous Pl(A2) donors. Although Pl(A2) is the most common cause of alloimmune thrombocytopenia, other platelet alloantigens have been found to cause this clinical syndrome (Table 52–2).

Thrombocytopenia in neonates can also be caused by maternal ITP. Antiplatelet antibodies are commonly IgG antibodies that may cross the placenta and induce thrombocytopenia in the fetus. However, significant neonatal thrombocytopenia is rare with maternal ITP and occurs in fewer than 10% of those at risk, although some evidence indicates that the incidence of neonatal thrombocytopenia is increased when the mother has ITP and maternal platelet counts lower than 75,000/mcL. Sometimes, the mother needs to be treated for ITP with the goal of decreasing placental transfer of the maternal autoantibody, although in most instances of maternal ITP, fetal thrombocytopenia is uncommon or mild, and safe vaginal delivery may be accomplished.

HEPARIN-INDUCED THROMBOCYTOPENIA

Although also immune in nature, HIT must be distinguished from other drug-induced forms of ITP because of its potentially catastrophic *thrombotic* complications and its unique pathophysiologic features. Nearly 25% of patients who are exposed to UFH will develop antibodies (detected by an enzyme-linked immunosorbent assay [ELISA]) that recognize the complex of heparin and platelet factor 4 (PF4), the latter being released from the alpha granule after platelet activation. When such patients receive heparin again, about 10% to 20% develop HIT, most with platelet counts between 50,000 and 100,000/mcL. Surgery is a specific risk factor for HIT; HIT antibodies occur with high frequency in patients undergoing cardiac surgery with cardiopulmonary bypass and to a lesser extent in patients undergoing hip replacement. In contrast to UFH, the incidence of HIT in patients who have received only low–molecular-weight heparin (LMWH) is far lower—only one fifth to one tenth the rate of patients on UFH. However, the mechanism of thrombocytopenia for

Table 52–2 Molecular Basis for Alloimmune Thrombocytopenia

Glycoprotein	Alleles (Alloantigens)	Phenotype Frequency	Amino Acid and Location
GPIIIa	HPA-1a/1b	0.98/0.25	Leucine/proline; 33
GPIb	HPA-2a/2b	0.99/0.14	Threonine/methionine; 145
GPIIb	HPA-3a/3b	0.91/0.70	Isoleucine/serine; 843
GPIIIa	HPA-4a/4b	0.99/0.01	Arginine/glutamine; 143
GPIa	HPA-5a/5b	0.99/0.21	Glutamic acid/lysine; 505
GPIIIa	HPA-6a/6b	NA	Proline/glutamic acid; 407
GPIIIa	HPA-7a/7b	NA	Proline/glutamic acid; 407
GPIIIa	HPA-8a/8b	NA	Arginine/cystine; 636

GP = glycoprotein; HPA = heparin-associated antibodies; NA = data not available.

both UFH and LMWH appears to be similar: platelet Fc-receptor binding of the heparin-PF4 antibody complex causes signal transduction and induces platelet activation granule release and the enhanced ability for thrombin generation on the platelet surface. Platelet clearance by activation results in thrombocytopenia. The diagnosis is predominantly clinical, but rapid ELISAs will detect heparin-PF4 antibodies. The ELISA's main drawback is that it does not indicate whether the antibody complex is a functional activator of platelets; thus it is sensitive but not specific for HIT. The serotonin release assay is the functional test for HIT, detecting platelet activation after exposure to serum antibody in the presence of heparin. The thrombin-based procoagulant response in HIT clears the platelets and in more than 10% to 20% of patients leads to thrombotic complications which may be severe or life-threatening. Although thrombosis is more frequent in patients with both HIT and concomitant cardiovascular disease and who are receiving full-dose heparin, any heparin dose (even heparin flushes) can result in thrombosis in HIT. Arterial and venous thromboemboli can occur while the patient is receiving heparin and even weeks after heparin has been discontinued, an effect perhaps mediated by the continued circulation of procoagulant platelet microparticles. Discontinuation of heparin, however, is critical; moreover, although the antibody may have been induced by treatment with UFH, more than 80% of these antibodies cross react with LMWHs, and approximately 15% of them react with heparinoid. Thus the preferred therapies for short-term anticoagulation in patients with HIT are the direct thrombin inhibitors, such as lepirudin and argatroban. The heparin-PF4 antibodies do not react with these compounds; warfarin can be added, if needed, for long-term anticoagulation once the platelet count has normalized. Warfarin should not be given on a short-term basis to patients with HIT and especially not without direct thrombin inhibitor coverage. Warfarin alone has resulted in catastrophic limb thrombosis in patients with HIT, probably mediated by acquired protein C deficiency, similar to the warfarin skin necrosis syndrome (see Chapter 53).

DISSEMINATED INTRAVASCULAR COAGULATION

One of the most common and potentially life-threatening causes of nonimmune peripheral platelet destruction is DIC, which is associated with sepsis, malignancy, advanced liver disease, and other disorders that trigger endotoxin release or cause severe tissue damage (Table 52-3). In DIC caused by bacterial sepsis, circulating endotoxin induces expression of tissue factor on circulating monocytes and endothelial cells, a process leading to overwhelming thrombin and fibrin generation. Deposition of fibrin occurs throughout the vasculature, with relatively inadequate concurrent fibrinolysis, and leads to a thrombotic or microangiopathic vasculopathy and subsequent organ damage. Thrombin activation of platelets and circulating factors eventually overwhelms the bone marrow and liver synthetic capability, respectively, and results in thrombocytopenia and prolongation of the PT and PTT. Thus although the primary lesion of DIC is clot generation, the clinical end point is usually *consumptive coagulopathy*. The thrombocytopenia and low factor levels resulting from the consumptive coagulopathy cause mucosal

Table 52-3	**Causes of Disseminated Intravascular Coagulation**
Sepsis or Endotoxin	
Gram-negative bacteremia	
Tissue Damage	
Trauma	
Closed-head injury	
Burns	
Hypoperfusion or hypotension	
Malignant Disease	
Adenocarcinoma	
Acute promyelocytic leukemia	
Primary Vascular Disorders	
Vasculitis	
Giant hemangioma (Kasabach-Merritt syndrome)	
Aortic aneurysm	
Cardiac mural thrombus	
Exogenous Causes	
Snake venom	
Activated-factor infusions (prothrombin-complex concentrate)	

bleeding, especially in the GI tract, and characteristic oozing from intravenous puncture sites.

In the consumptive coagulopathy of DIC, fibrinogen levels are usually low, but they may be normal or slightly high; the acute phase reaction to sepsis or the underlying disorder may actually increase fibrinogen secretion and may lead to normal levels in the midst of DIC. Therefore DIC should not be ruled out because fibrinogen is in the normal range. Fibrinolysis in DIC is triggered by fibrin clot and tissue-type plasminogen activator; laboratory testing usually shows increased levels of fibrin split products to more than 40 mcg/mL (cleavage of fibrin monomers) and D-dimer to more than 0.5 mcg/mL (cleavage of fibrin-fibrin bonds). Although fibrin split products are usually elevated in patients with DIC, this finding is nonspecific; in contrast, an elevated D-dimer is more specific for DIC and is often used to confirm the elevated fibrin split product-screening assay. The peripheral blood smear may also help in the diagnosis of a microangiopathic picture by showing significant numbers of schistocytes; however, this finding is not specific to DIC and is also present in TTP (see the following text).

Chronic DIC may be triggered by consumption of platelets and factors into large clots associated with aneurysms, hemangiomas, and mural thrombi. A unique cause of chronic DIC is malignant disease, often adenocarcinoma or acute promyelocytic leukemia; malignant cells in these disorders secrete substances that either activate factor

X or simulate factor Xa activity. Xa activation leads to the formation of the prothrombinase complex, production of thrombin, and platelet activation and clearance; chronic DIC in this circumstance usually causes enough factor consumption that both the PT and the PTT are slightly prolonged. Clinically, such patients exhibit *migratory thrombophlebitis* (*Trousseau's syndrome*) or *nonbacterial thrombotic (marantic) endocarditis*.

Therapy of DIC should be aimed at the following: (1) treatment of the underlying disorder, such as antibiotics for sepsis or chemotherapy for malignant disease; (2) supportive hemostatic therapy, including platelets, cryoprecipitate (for fibrinogen), and fresh-frozen plasma; and (3) disrupting activation of coagulation factors and platelets. For the last approach, anticoagulation is generally not indicated unless the balance of procoagulant versus anticoagulant activity actively favors clotting, such as arterial thromboemboli with mural thrombus or migratory thrombophlebitis with Trousseau's syndrome. These thrombotic complications of chronic DIC are often resistant to warfarin therapy; resolution of DIC generally requires more intensive anti-Xa therapy (UFH or LMWH), as well as the successful treatment of the underlying malignant disease or consumptive disorder. In addition to anti-Xa agents, new therapies for sepsis and DIC have shown promise; pharmacologic activated protein C has shown to decrease mortality associated with sepsis and/or DIC significantly, and other methods of modulating the coagulation process in DIC are being investigated.

THROMBOTIC THROMBOCYTOPENIC PURPURA

Another nonimmune cause of thrombocytopenia resulting from platelet activation and clearance is TTP. In patients with congenital relapsing TTP, the normal vWF-cleaving protease, known as ADAMTS13, is significantly decreased or absent. Patients with acquired TTP without a family history usually have an antibody, often IgG, that blocks the normal function of this vWF-cleaving protease. Deficient protease function leads to the decreased clearance and higher circulating levels of the larger, high–molecular-weight vWF multimers; these, in turn, cause increased platelet adhesion and clearance *without* activating the coagulation cascade. Therefore both the PT and PTT are normal. TTP after chemotherapy (mitomycin C) and in association with pregnancy or HIV infection seems to have a similar pathogenesis. Thrombocytopenia (often severe) is accompanied by microangiopathy with schistocytes on the peripheral smear and increased serum lactate dehydrogenase. Microvascular occlusions in multiple organs cause many of the symptoms, especially in the kidney and brain. The classic pentad of signs (fever, thrombocytopenia, microangiopathic hemolysis, neurologic symptoms, and renal insufficiency) is present in fewer than 25% of patients with TTP. The diagnosis is generally made on clinical assessment because assays for ADAMTS13 activity and inhibitor are not yet widely available and do not have a rapid turn-around time.

Treatment of TTP is based on the removal of the antibody and replenishment of cleaving protease activity. These goals are generally accomplished by plasma exchange, whereby patient plasma is removed (plasmapheresis) and replaced with fresh-frozen plasma, often "cryo-poor" to reduce vWF

multimer levels in transfused plasma. Steroids and antiplatelet drugs (e.g., aspirin, dipyridamole) are often administered simultaneously, but the relative benefit of both agents remains unclear. Platelet transfusions are relatively contraindicated in TTP but have been used without adverse effects when administered before invasive procedures. Recombinant and/or purified forms of ADAMTS13 hold promise as potential therapeutic agents for the treatment of TTP.

Most authorities consider the *hemolytic uremic syndrome* (HUS) to be part of the TTP spectrum of disease; however, the hemolytic anemia and renal failure of HUS are not usually accompanied by neurologic impairment, and HUS generally does not have the same degree of thrombocytopenia or schistocytosis as TTP. Moreover, HUS is *not* associated with defective vWF-cleaving protease activity. Unlike TTP, HUS is primarily diagnosed in children and less commonly in adults with hemorrhagic colitis caused by Shiga-like, toxin-producing bacteria, especially the *Escherichia coli* 0157.H7 serotype. The similar pathophysiologic features of microvascular platelet thrombi suggests that HUS is part of the TTP continuum, and, indeed, patients with HUS respond to plasmapheresis with plasma exchange, as well as to maintenance dialysis until renal function recovers.

THROMBOCYTOPENIA WITH PREGNANCY-INDUCED HYPERTENSION

Mild thrombocytopenia in pregnant women is most often related to hemodilution and the normal physiologic condition of pregnancy that commonly brings platelet counts into the range of 100,000 to 150,000/mcL; these counts are not associated with maternal or fetal complications. In contrast, autoimmune causes of platelet destruction (as noted earlier) and pregnancy-induced hypertension can result in platelet counts lower than 100,000/mcL with complications. The spectrum of *pregnancy-induced hypertension* includes hypertension progressing to proteinuria and renal dysfunction (*pre-eclampsia*) or to cerebral edema and seizures (*eclampsia*). Thrombocytopenia may appear as a late finding accompanying pregnancy-induced hypertension, most often at the time of delivery or late in the third trimester. The related *HELLP syndrome* in pregnancy is characterized by hemolysis, elevated liver enzymes, and low platelet counts in association with pre-eclampsia. The thrombocytopenia associated with pregnancy-induced hypertension and HELLP is probably caused by abnormal vascular prostaglandin metabolism that leads to platelet consumption, vasculopathy, and microvascular occlusions. These disorders are usually reversed by delivery of the fetus and placenta. Occasionally, IVIG or plasmapheresis has been required to treat the disorder successfully. When thrombocytopenia does not resolve after delivery, other processes, such as TTP, must be considered in the differential diagnosis.

ANTIPHOSPHOLIPID SYNDROME

Distinct from ITP associated with systemic lupus erythematosus, the antiphospholipid syndrome is not associated with bleeding. The antiphospholipid syndrome is characterized by destructive thrombocytopenia, recurrent thrombosis, or fetal loss and is diagnosed by the demonstration of a lupus anticoagulant and/or anticardiolipin antibody. The antiphospholipid syndrome can be a primary disorder without diagnostic criteria for systemic lupus erythematosus, or it can occur secondary to true systemic lupus erythematosus. Thrombocytopenia in the antiphospholipid syndrome is caused by increased peripheral platelet destruction and not as a result of platelet-specific antibodies; rather, vascular angiopathy and increased platelet consumption in the microvasculature are the causes. Long-term, intensive anticoagulation with warfarin or LMWH, sometimes with the addition of aspirin or other antiplatelet drugs, may prevent thrombotic complications and may restore platelet counts to normal (see Chapter 53).

DILUTIONAL THROMBOCYTOPENIA

In addition to sequestration and hypoproductive and destructive causes of thrombocytopenia, thrombocytopenia can also result from *hemodilution*. This circumstance usually follows massive red blood cell and plasma transfusions, especially for trauma or cardiopulmonary bypass, in which significant hemodilution occurs by the addition of the extracorporeal circuit to the normal circulatory system. Moreover, in addition to the hemodilution of bypass, platelets exposed to the cardiopulmonary bypass circuit become temporarily dysfunctional because of activation and loss of membrane receptors; this defect may be mild and transient, but occasionally it is severe and leads to bleeding, especially after long bypass procedures. After the conclusion of bypass or once the acute trauma is resolved, the platelet count rebounds within 48 to 72 hours; however, platelet transfusions may be needed to treat significant bleeding in these patients while the platelet count recovers.

Bleeding Caused by Platelet Disorders: Qualitative Platelet Defects

ASPIRIN AND ACQUIRED CAUSES OF PLATELET DYSFUNCTION

The ability of platelets to adhere to damaged vasculature and to recruit additional platelets into the clot is critical for primary hemostasis, especially when patients are challenged by surgery. One critical question for preoperative screening is whether patients are taking medications that interfere with platelet function, such as aspirin. As noted in Chapter 51, *aspirin* irreversibly blocks normal arachidonic acid metabolism. All exposed platelets are irreversibly affected and do not respond to arachidonic acid even after aspirin is discontinued. The characteristic aspirin-induced platelet aggregation pattern is shown in Table 52–4. In contrast, other *nonsteroidal anti-inflammatory drugs* (NSAIDs) (e.g., indomethacin) *reversibly* inhibit cyclo-oxygenase (COX), and platelet function is restored within 24 to 48 hours after discontinuing the drug. Bleeding associated with aspirin or NSAIDs is usually mild, and aspirin may not need to be discontinued, especially because aspirin-induced platelet dysfunction is desirable in patients at risk of stroke or myocardial infarction. However, when bleeding caused by aspirin requires treatment, infusion of desmopressin acetate (DDAVP) has been shown to be effective at decreasing the bleeding time; occasionally, transfusion of platelets is appropriate. In most cases, a single-platelet transfusion of four to six random donor units contributes enough normal platelets (>10% of total circulating number) to restore primary hemostasis. Similarly, discontinuing the drug and platelet transfusion when needed treats platelet dysfunction and bleeding caused by other drugs (Table 52–5).

Whereas the aspirin effect is nearly restricted to COX-1, the different NSAIDs have variable relative affinity for COX-1 and COX-2. COX-2 is an inducible enzyme synthesized in endothelial cells (but not in platelets) in response to inflammatory cytokines. Suppression of COX-2 results in a reduction of prostaglandin I_2 (prostacyclin, prostacyclin [PGI_2]), a molecule that, among other functions, has antithrombotic effects through inhibition of platelet aggregation. The net effect of NSAIDs on the prothrombotic and/or antithrombotic balance favors bleeding because NSAID-induced COX-1 inhibition means that thromboxane A_2 (TxA_2) production in platelets is blocked. By contrast, the increase in cardiovascular risk seen with the more selective COX-2 inhibitors is attributable to the COX 2–induced lack of endothelial cell PGI_2 production, coupled with intact platelet function (no inhibition of TxA_2 by COX-2 blockade). Recent data also

Table 52–4	**Disorders Causing Abnormal Platelet Aggregation**				
	Response to Agonist				
	Epinephrine	**ADP**	**Collagen**	**Arachidonic acid**	**Ristocetin**
Aspirin and NSAIDs	#	#	NL, ↓*	↓	NL
Glanzmann's disease	Absent	Absent	Absent	Absent	#
Bernard-Soulier syndrome	NL	NL	NL	NL	Absent
Storage pool disease	↓	#	↓	NL, ↓	#
Hermansky-Pudlak syndrome	↓	#	↓	NL	#
Gray platelet syndrome	↓	↓	↓	NL	NL
vWD	NL	NL	NL	NL	↓, NL†

*Aspirin results in decreased aggregation with low-dose collagen, but aggregation is normal with high-dose collagen.
†In vWD type 2B, patients have increased aggregation with low-dose ristocetin, and decreased or normal aggregation with standard doses of ristocetin.
↓ = decreased; # = primary wave aggregation only; ADP = adenosine diphosphate; NL = normal; NSAIDs = nonsteroidal anti-inflammatory drugs; vWD = von Willebrand disease.

Table 52–5 Drugs Affecting Platelet Function

Strong Inhibitors

Abciximab (and other anti-GPIIb/IIIa or anti-RGD compounds)
Aspirin (often contained in over-the-counter medications)
Clopidogrel/ticlopidine (ADP-receptor blockers)
Nonsteroidal anti-inflammatory drugs

Moderate Inhibitors

Antibiotics (penicillins, cephalosporins, nitrofurantoin)
Dextran
Fibrinolytics
Heparin
Hetastarch

Weak Inhibitors

Alcohol
Nitroglycerin
Nitroprusside

ADP = adenosine diphosphate; GP = glycoprotein; RGD = arginine-glycine-aspartate.

show that NSAIDs given before aspirin will compete for COX-1 binding sites and diminish the aspirin's antiplatelet effect, another possible factor in the procoagulant balance of NSAID use.

Uremic platelet dysfunction is caused by proteins that accumulate in renal failure, most importantly guanidinosuccinic acid (GSA), which induces high levels of nitric oxide formation by vascular endothelial cells. Both compounds inhibit platelet function, but data suggest that it is nitric oxide that mediates the inhibitory effect of GSA on platelet function. Control of renal failure with dialysis and maintenance of the hematocrit are usually adequate to preserve platelet function. However, uremic bleeding is a common inpatient problem, especially in the setting of acute renal failure. Short-term treatment of uremic platelet dysfunction includes DDAVP, which has been shown to shorten the bleeding time significantly, and cryoprecipitate. Conjugated estrogens are of some benefit for long-term treatment. Platelet transfusions may be useful in patients with life-threatening bleeding and renal failure, but the effect of this treatment is short-lived because the transfused platelets rapidly acquire the uremic defect.

CONGENITAL PLATELET DYSFUNCTION

Inherited qualitative platelet defects include abnormalities of platelet receptors and granules. Two rare but well-characterized platelet receptor disorders are *Bernard-Soulier syndrome* and *Glanzmann's thrombasthenia*. Bernard-Soulier syndrome is caused by a decreased surface expression of platelet GPIb (the primary vWF receptor) and more rarely by diminished GPIb function. The syndrome is characterized by mild thrombocytopenia, increased bleeding time,

large platelets, and a mild-to-moderate bleeding disorder. The diagnosis is usually made in children, but occasionally the condition may not show symptoms until adulthood. Laboratory testing for Bernard-Soulier syndrome shows an absent platelet aggregation response to ristocetin (see Table 52–4) despite adequate vWF levels and function, such as normal ristocetin co-factor (Rcof) activity. Glanzmann's thrombasthenia is characterized by an increased bleeding time and abnormally low levels of expression of platelet GPIIb/IIIa (the receptor for both vWF and fibrinogen) or, more rarely, normal expression but absent GPIIb/IIIa function. Patients commonly exhibit bleeding in childhood. Platelet aggregation testing in Glanzmann's thrombasthenia shows an absent or a diminished response to all agonists except ristocetin (see Table 52–4). Platelet transfusions correct the bleeding in both Bernard-Soulier syndrome and Glanzmann's thrombasthenia. However, because of the high risk of alloimmunization with frequent platelet transfusions, this therapy should be used sparingly.

Inherited platelet granule disorders are defined by the type of granule that is absent or defective. *Storage pool disease* is characterized by a relative decrease or absence of dense granules and correspondingly moderate-to-severe mucosal bleeding. Because of the defect in dense granules, release of granule constituents that recruit and activate platelets is impaired. Thus storage pool disease is characterized by a diminished or absent secondary wave aggregation in response to most agonists (see Table 52–4). *Hermansky-Pudlak syndrome* is a similar dense granule deficiency associated with oculocutaneous albinism and mild thrombocytopenia. Patients have significant bleeding, which may occur spontaneously but more often in association with surgical procedures. *Chédiak-Higashi* syndrome is a rare general granule disorder characterized by mild bleeding, partial albinism, and recurrent pyogenic infections; large, irregular, gray-blue inclusions are seen in neutrophils and monocytes. Gray platelet syndrome is characterized by colorless or gray platelets that lack normal staining on the peripheral smear; electron microscopy confirms the loss of alpha granules and/or their contents. Patients with gray platelet syndrome have a mild bleeding history, and aggregation testing exhibits diminished responses to epinephrine, ADP, and collagen. All the platelet granule disorders are successfully treated by avoiding aspirin and other antiplatelet drugs, by hormonal control of menses in women, and by platelet transfusions when bleeding occurs.

VON WILLEBRAND DISEASE

Disorders of plasma proteins, which are the functional ligands for platelet adhesion to the vasculature, cause bleeding that clinically resembles the bleeding associated with platelet or vascular disorders (e.g., epistaxis, GI bleeding). vWF is synthesized in endothelial cells and megakaryocytes and functions in plasma to mediate platelet rolling along damaged vessels and subsequent platelet adhesion to the damaged site (see Fig. 51–1). vWF is a large molecule that polymerizes to form multimeric proteins of varying size; the largest multimers contain the greatest number of adhesive sites and thus confer greater hemostatic ability than smaller vWF molecules. In patients with abnormal or low vWF levels, platelet adhesion to damaged vessels is delayed, and

Table 52–6 Classification of von Willebrand's Disease (vWD)

	Type 1	Type 2A	Type 2B	Type 2M	Type 2N	Type 3	Pseudo-vWD	BSS
Inheritance	AD	AD, AR	AD, AR	AD	AR	AR, AD	AD	AR
Platelet count	NL	NL	NL, ↓	NL	NL	NL	↓, NL	↓, NL
Bleeding time	NL, ↑-	↑	↑	↑	NL, ↑	↑↑	↑	↑
PTT	NL, ↑	↑, NL	↑, NL	↑	↑↑	↑↑	↑, NL	NL
VIII	NL, ↓	NL, ↓	↓, NL	NL, ↓	↓↓	↓↓	↓, NL	NL
vWF:Ag	NL, ↓	NL, ↓	↓, NL	NL	NL	Absent	↓, NL	NL
vWF:Rcof	NL, ↓	↓↓	↓, NL	↓↓	NL	Absent	↓, NL	NL
Multimers	NL, ↓	↓ H/I	↓↓ H	NL	NL	Absent	↓↓ H	NL
RIPA	NL, ↓	↓↓	↑*	↓	NL	↓↓	↑*	↓↓

↑ = increased; ↓ = decreased; ↑* = increased agglutination in response to low-dose ristocetin; AD = autosomal dominant; AR = autosomal recessive; BSS = Bernard-Soulier syndrome; H = high–molecular-weight multimers; I = intermediate–molecular-weight multimers; NL = normal; PTT = partial thromboplastin time; RIPA = ristocetin-induced platelet agglutination; vWF:Ag = von Willebrand factor antigen level; vWF:Rcof = von Willebrand factor:ristocetin co-factor activity.

the results are mucosal bleeding and a prolonged bleeding time. vWF also serves as the carrier protein for factor VIII; deficiency of vWF or abnormal vWF-VIII binding leads to rapid clearance of factor VIII, decreased factor VIII levels, and a prolonged PTT. Many mutations in the vWF gene have been described; these have been phenotypically grouped into three major subtypes of vWD (Table 52–6).

Most patients have *type 1 vWD*, a mild-to-moderate *quantitative* decrease in all vWF multimers. This condition is commonly caused by a heterozygous mutation and shows a dominant pattern of inheritance. Type 1 vWD is characterized by equivalent decreases in factor VIII, vWF antigen, and Rcof activity; Rcof measures the ability of patient plasma (which contains vWF) to agglutinate normal platelets in the presence of ristocetin. Patients with type 1 vWD usually have mild-to-moderate bleeding, often only in relation to surgery or dental procedures. Historically, patients with type 1 vWD were treated with cryoprecipitate, which is rich in vWF. However, because cryoprecipitate cannot be virally inactivated, alternatives are now used. DDAVP stimulates endothelial cells to release stored vWF and leads to an increase in plasma vWF antigen, Rcof, and factor VIII levels. DDAVP, at 0.3 mcg/kg given subcutaneously, is commonly used in type 1 vWD with excellent results. However, tachyphylaxis to DDAVP may occur because endothelial cells require time to synthesize new vWF after repeated DDAVP dosing. Thus vWF concentrates must sometimes be used in patients with more severe type 1 vWD or in those who are undergoing a more prolonged hemostatic challenge. Virally-inactivated, *intermediate-purity* factor VIII products (not recombinant or monoclonal antibody purified) contain large amounts of vWF (e.g., Humate-P) and are the preferred therapy after DDAVP. Bleeding in type 1 vWD during pregnancy is exceedingly rare. Because vWF rises significantly in pregnancy, vWF antigen and Rcof levels usually normalize during the second or third trimester and eliminate the bleeding risk for that time. Most pregnant women with type 1 vWD have no bleeding complications with delivery and do not require therapy during pregnancy or in the early postpartum period.

Type 2 vWD is characterized by heterozygous mutations of variable penetrance that produce a *qualitative* defect in the vWF molecule; the most common type 2 disorders are characterized by a relative lack of the larger vWF multimers (see Table 52–6). High– and intermediate–molecular-weight vWF multimers by electrophoresis are absent in *type 2A disease*, and platelet-associated function is moderately decreased; patients with type 2A vWD show disproportionately low Rcof activity compared with those with vWF antigen. Patients with type 2A vWD respond to vWF concentrate and less commonly to DDAVP. The abnormal vWF molecule in *type 2B vWD* has increased affinity for platelets, a situation that causes loss of high–molecular-weight multimers from the circulation and often produces thrombocytopenia. Platelet aggregometry in type 2B vWD (see Table 52–6) shows an abnormal increase in low-dose ristocetin-induced platelet agglutination; in the laboratory the addition of patient vWF to normal platelets similarly increases ristocetin-induced platelet agglutination and confirms the abnormal vWF. DDAVP would induce release of the abnormal vWF in patients with type 2B vWD and therefore is contraindicated in this disorder; vWF concentrate should be used instead.

Type 2M vWD demonstrates decreased platelet-dependent function with laboratory findings similar to those in type 2A, but high–molecular-weight multimers are present through electrophoresis. The defect in this rare type of vWF is most often a mutation in vWF *reducing* binding to its platelet ligand GpIbα. Some patients with type 2M vWD respond to DDAVP, but most require vWF concentrate. In *type 2N vWD*, the abnormal vWF molecule has decreased binding affinity for *factor VIII*, a characteristic that decreases factor VIII survival and produces a phenotype similar to that of hemophilia A. The low factor VIII levels do not respond to high-purity factor VIII infusions, unlike in true hemophilia A, but they improve with vWF concentrate. Rcof and vWF antigen levels are normal in type 2N vWD because the mutation in the factor VIII binding site does not affect vWF function or survival. Phenotypically type 2N can be easily confused for hemophilia A; tests for vWF binding to factor VIII are available in reference laboratories.

The rare patient with *type 3 vWD* has a complete deficiency of vWF, often as a result of the inheritance of two abnormal vWF alleles (compound heterozygote). Patients with type 3 vWD have absent or extremely low levels of both Rcof and vWF antigen and factor VIII levels of 3% to 10% and usually have severe bleeding that may mimic hemophilia. Type 3 vWD does not respond to DDAVP and requires vWF concentrates for bleeding.

vWD can appear as an acquired defect, usually as a severe, type 2A–like defect with absent larger vWF multimers in a patient with no history of bleeding. *Acquired vWD* is caused by abnormal clearance of the larger vWF multimers and is most often associated with monoclonal gammopathies, lymphoproliferative disorders, myeloma, and other malignant and myeloproliferative diseases characterized by thrombocytosis. In these cases, acquired vWD has been successfully treated with IVIG and therapy of the underlying disease. One other cause of abnormal vWF multimer clearance resulting in acquired vWD is critical aortic stenosis, which is corrected with successful surgical repair.

Fibrinogen Disorders

Fibrinogen functions as a bridging ligand for the platelet receptor GPIIb/IIIa in the platelet-platelet matrix at sites of vascular damage. Fibrinogen also functions in the final steps of the coagulation cascade to form fibrin clot. Low fibrinogen levels are most commonly seen with consumptive disorders such as *DIC*, although rare congenital hypofibrinogenemias and afibrinogenemias are recognized. *Dysfibrinogenemia* is defined as an abnormal fibrinogen protein. Patients with dysfibrinogenemia usually bleed because of decreased adhesive function, but some patients have a hypercoagulable state. Dysfibrinogenemia is occasionally inherited, but it is more often acquired with liver disease. Both the PT and the PTT are prolonged by abnormalities of fibrinogen quantity or function (Table 52–7). A prolonged thrombin time is more specific for a low fibrinogen level or abnormal molecule, although inhibitors such as heparin and fibrin split products also prolong the thrombin time. The *reptilase time*, which is insensitive to heparin, can be used to eliminate the possibility of an increased thrombin time resulting from heparin contamination of the sample. Both

hypofibrinogenemia and dysfibrinogenemia are treated with cryoprecipitate, the blood product most enriched for fibrinogen.

Bleeding Caused by Coagulation Factor Disorders

HEMOPHILIA AND OTHER INHERITED FACTOR DEFICIENCIES

With normal platelet function, primary hemostasis initiates plugging of vascular lesions and maintains mucosal integrity. However, if abnormalities of coagulation factors are present, then the initial platelet plug is not solidified by normal secondary hemostasis, and the effects are clot breakdown and bleeding. This bleeding differs from platelet-type bleeding; coagulation deficiencies lead to bleeding in deep tissues and joints, and milder deficiencies may be bleeding in a delayed fashion after surgery. Most patients with significant factor deficiencies exhibit abnormal results of screening laboratory tests (see Table 52–7 and Fig. 52–1), although patients with mild deficiencies can still exhibit bleeding and normal coagulation screens.

The X-linked deficiencies of factor VIII (*hemophilia A*) and factor IX (*hemophilia B*) are the most common factor deficiencies after vWD. Hemophilia A is about six times more frequent than hemophilia B. Approximately 50% or more of patients with severe hemophilia A arise as a result of an inversion of a major portion of the gene that results in complete loss of activity. Other mutations tend to result in milder disease. Most patients with hemophilia B have mutations that result in a functionally abnormal factor IX with absent activity. The combined results of antigenic and functional assays can resolve whether deficiency is due to loss of the protein or loss of its normal function. Both hemophilia A and hemophilia B are categorized by their factor levels: severe deficiency is characterized by absent (<1%) factor VIII

Table 52–7	**Screening Laboratory Results in Coagulation Factor Deficiencies**				
Deficient Factor	**Frequency**	**PT**	**PTT**	**TT**
I (fibrinogen)	Rare	↑	↑	↑
II (prothrombin)	Very rare	↑	↑	↑
V	1:1,000,000	↑	↑	NL
VII	1:500,000	↑	NL	NL
VIII	1: 5,000 (male patient)	NL	↑	NL
IX	1: 30,000 (male patient)	NL	↑	NL
X	1: 500,000	↑	↑	NL
XI	Rare*	NL	↑	NL
XII† or HMWK† or PK†	Rare	NL	↑	NL
XIII	Rare	NL	NL	NL

*Except in those of Ashkenazi Jewish descent (approximately 4% are heterozygous for factor XI deficiency).
†Not associated with clinical bleeding.
↑ = increased over normal range; HMWK = high–molecular-weight kininogen; NL = normal; PK = prekallikrein; PT = prothrombin time; PTT = partial thromboplastin time; TT = thrombin time.

or IX, whereas patients with moderate and mild hemophilia have factor levels of 1% to 5% and more than 5%, respectively. Severe hemophilia A and hemophilia B develop in childhood with bleeding into muscles, joints, and soft tissue. Because they are X-linked disorders, they are observed primarily in male patients; the mother of an affected male patient is a carrier, and 50% of maternal uncles have the disease. About 25% to 30% of cases of hemophilia, however, result from new mutations and hence have no relevant family history. In exceedingly rare instances, a female carrier with extremely skewed X-inactivation may have a mild bleeding disorder with factor levels <30%. Bleeding in severe hemophilia is often spontaneous, as well as common after any type of surgery or even mild trauma.

Bleeding in hemophilia frequently occurs in joints and in the retroperitoneum; hematuria and mucosal and intracranial bleeding also occur. Patients with moderate hemophilia have less spontaneous bleeding, but they are still at significant risk of hemorrhagic complications of surgery or trauma. Patients with mild hemophilia may be undetected into adulthood and may develop only with bleeding after major surgery. The complications of hemophilia stem from chronic bleeding into joints and muscles, which leads to severe deformities, arthritis, muscle atrophy, and contractures; these complications require intensive physical therapy and orthopedic care, often culminating in joint replacement. In addition, patients with hemophilia who received pooled-factor concentrates before the era of viral inactivation have complications related to transfusion-transmitted infections, especially HIV and hepatitis B and C. Current therapy uses factor concentrates that are virally inactivated or recombinant. Rapid factor replacement is the key to effective therapy. Patients with severe hemophilia often infuse themselves with low doses of prophylactic factor on a regular basis (25 to 40 U/kg three times per week) and boost their dose or the frequency of infusion when they sense internal bleeding, sustain trauma, or undergo dental procedures (Table 52–8).

Patients with mild hemophilia A may not need factor infusions for minor surgery; indeed, such patients are often managed with ε-aminocaproic acid, 4 g every 4 to 6 hours, with or without infusions of DDAVP of 0.3 mcg/kg. However, most patients with hemophilia require factor infusions, if not prophylactically, then at times of surgery or trauma. Factor VIII products are infused every 8 to 12 hours, and 1 U/kg of factor VIII concentrate raises plasma factor VIII activity by 2%; thus 50 U/kg of factor VIII theoretically will yield 100% factor VIII activity in a patient with severe hemophilia. Factor IX has a longer half-life and is infused every 18 to 24 hours; factor IX requires 2 U/kg for a 2% increase in factor IX activity (i.e., 100 U/kg for 100% activity). Major surgery in patients with hemophilia requires intensive factor therapy to achieve normal factor levels (>80%) in both the intraoperative period and the early postoperative period to prevent wound hematoma formation. The dosing of factors (see Table 52–8) is adjusted downward from this intensity, depending on the severity of the insult, the patient's response to previous factor infusions, and whether inhibitors to factors have developed.

INHERITED FACTOR DEFICIENCIES OTHER THAN HEMOPHILIA A OR B

Inherited bleeding disorders caused by deficiencies of coagulation factors V, VII, X, and XI (see Table 52–7) are much rarer than hemophilia A and B. Patients with *factor V deficiency* usually lack both plasma factor V and platelet factor V and have joint and muscle bleeding similar to patients with hemophilia. Some patients who are plasma V–deficient are asymptomatic until they are challenged with the stress of surgery or trauma, and these patients are thought to have normal platelet factor V levels. Patients with factor V deficiency can be treated with either fresh-frozen plasma or platelets; platelets are especially useful in patients who have developed inhibitors to factor V after receiving long-term plasma therapy. Rarely, patients inherit factor deficiencies in tandem, such as combined factors V and VIII deficiencies.

Patients with *factor XI deficiency (hemophilia C)* generally have a milder bleeding disorder than do patients with hemophilia A or B (even with factor XI levels <5%), and this patient group is treated with plasma infusions, whereas *factor X deficiency* is usually more severe and is also treated with plasma. *Factor XI deficiency* is an autosomal recessive disorder seen with increased frequency among Ashkenazi Jews; hemophilia C often develops late in adulthood and in clinical settings of increased fibrinolysis such as after prostate surgery. *Acquired factor X deficiency* can occur in association with amyloidosis, a condition in which the abnormal circulating light chains adsorb to and clear factor X and produce low levels and occasional bleeding. The rare *factor VII–deficient patient* with levels of less than 10% can be treated with prothrombin complex concentrate or with recombinant factor VIIa. The development of purified or recombinant factors was important because replacement of factor levels with fresh-frozen plasma is difficult. Factor concentrations in fresh-frozen plasma are variable and, at

Table 52–8	**Factor Replacement Guidelines in Hemophilia A and B**				
	Factor VIII (U/kg)			**Factor IX (U/kg)**	
Injury	**Initial dosing**	**Maintenance**	**Initial dosing**	**Maintenance**
Dental prophylaxis	20	10–20 every 12 hr	10–20	20 every 12 hr
Hemarthrosis	10–20	10–20 every 12 hr	30–60	20 every 24 hr
Muscle hematoma	20–30	20 every 12 hr	30–50	30 every 24 hr
Trauma or surgery	50	20–30 every 8 hr	60–100	40–80

best, similar to in vivo concentrations; thus a patient may require four units or more of fresh-frozen plasma to increase factor levels from 0% to 30%. This high fluid load is problematic in patients with heart disease, liver failure, or renal insufficiency.

ACQUIRED COAGULATION FACTOR DISORDERS

Factor Inhibitors

About 25% of patients with hemophilia A develop autoantibodies to transfused factor VIII. An inhibitor acts functionally in vivo and can be measured in vitro in Bethesda units (BU); 1 BU is designated to be an inhibitor unit that neutralizes 50% of factor activity. High-level inhibitors (>10 BU) neutralize the activity of infused factor concentrates, negating their effectiveness in bleeding episodes. Bleeding therefore requires therapy using different regimens such as factor VIII inhibitor bypass activity (FEIBA) or recombinant factor VIIa. For long-term treatment, suppression of an inhibitor is accomplished by a combination of IVIG, immunosuppressive therapy, plasmapheresis, and induction of immune tolerance using high-dose concentrate infusions. Patients with hemophilia B have a lower incidence of inhibitors (2% to 6%), but otherwise they are treated in a similar fashion with high-dose FEIBA or recombinant VIIa and with similar strategies for long-term suppression of the antibody.

Acquired inhibitors to factor VIII (and more rarely to other coagulation factors) occasionally occur in patients (usually older patients) who do not have a history of bleeding. Acquired factor VIII inhibitor titers in this setting can be extremely high and are commonly associated with malignant diseases, especially lymphoproliferative disorders. Patients with acquired inhibitors to factor VIII are similarly treated with factor VIIa or FEIBA. Intensive immunosuppressive therapy (cyclophosphamide and prednisone) is the mainstay of successful treatment and should be started as soon as possible to eradicate the inhibitor.

Vitamin K Deficiency

Inpatients and outpatients who are severely ill may have bleeding resulting from acquired coagulation factor deficiencies. Foremost among the causes of low factor levels is vitamin K deficiency. Vitamin K deficiency may be caused by any of the following: (1) biliary tract disease interfering with enterohepatic circulation and leading to decreased absorption of vitamin K; (2) drugs, especially antibiotics, that sterilize the gut and reduce bacterial sources of vitamin K or other drugs (cholestyramine) that directly block vitamin K absorption (this category includes cephalosporins, which interfere with intrahepatic metabolism of this fat-soluble vitamin); and (3) poor nutritional status induced by malabsorptive disease (sprue), chronic disease, or poor oral intake in patients who are acutely ill. As noted previously, factors II, VII, IX, and X are vitamin K–dependent procoagulant factors, as are proteins C and S. Warfarin blocks vitamin K–dependent γ-carboxylation of these factors and causes an acute decrease in functional factor VII levels because factor VII has the shortest half-life (6 hours) of all vitamin K–dependent factors *in vivo*. Oral or parenteral replacement

of vitamin K (1 to 10 mg/day for 3 days) restores coagulation factor synthesis in the presence of a normal liver.

Bleeding in Patients with Liver Disease

Patients with mild-to-moderate liver disease have prolongation of the PT and usually normal PTT values. Severe liver disease prolongs both the PT and the PTT. Unlike patients with vitamin K deficiency or those receiving warfarin, patients with liver disease have low levels of nearly all factors, not just the vitamin K–dependent factors; the exception is factor VIII. Although liver transplantation increases factor VIII levels in patients with hemophilia, factor VIII levels usually *rise* with liver disease, a finding corresponding to sources of factor VIII production outside the liver. If factor VIII levels are decreased in patients with liver disease, then consideration should be given as to whether DIC is superimposed. Therefore when a prolonged PT is evaluated for its cause, measurement of factor VII and a nonvitamin K–dependent factor such as factor V is most useful. In vitamin K deficiency, factor VII is low and factor V is normal; in contrast, levels of both factors VII and V should be low in patients with generalized liver disease. The PT is a sensitive measure of liver function and becomes elevated in patients with even mild liver disorders; this elevation precedes a significant decrease in the albumin or prealbumin levels and is usually coincident with transaminase changes. In patients with mild-to-moderate liver disease, the PT is prolonged, but the PTT usually remains within the normal range. When severe liver disease is present, the PT becomes even more prolonged, and the PTT becomes abnormal as well. Causes of bleeding in liver disease other than decreased factor synthesis include (1) decreased clearance of fibrin split products and/or associated DIC, (2) inhibition of platelet function, and (3) increased tissue plasminogen activator levels. Replacement of coagulation factors with fresh-frozen plasma is currently the treatment of choice, but recombinant VIIa shows promise for the treatment or prophylaxis of bleeding in liver disease.

Bleeding in Patients with a Normal Laboratory Screen

Occasionally, patients with bleeding disorders do not exhibit any abnormalities in screening laboratory assays (e.g., PT, PTT, platelet count). As noted previously, these disorders include the vascular purpuras, but other bleeding variants exhibit in this fashion (see Fig. 52–1). Patients with bleeding caused by mild vWD may have a normal PTT, but additional studies usually show mild decreases in factor VIII, vWF antigen, or vWF Rcof; multimeric analysis may also be abnormal in patients with mild type 2A vWD. Similarly, mild factor deficiencies (factor II, V, VII, VIII, IX, or XI) may not prolong the PT or PTT, but specific-factor assays demonstrate levels lower than the normal range. Mild bleeding, often with a delayed onset after surgery or trauma, may occur in patients with clot instability resulting from factor XIII deficiency or dysfibrinogenemia; in neonates, factor

XIII deficiency may develop with late umbilical stump bleeding. Factor XIII deficiency results in increased clot solubility in urea; if the clot dissolves in 8 mol/L urea, then an ELISA for the factor XIII level should be performed. Factor XIII deficiency is treated with fresh-frozen plasma. Low fibrinogen levels or abnormal fibrinogen function will prolong both the thrombin time and the reptilase time. The thrombin time is also prolonged by heparin, but the reptilase time is insensitive to heparin and therefore can enable the presence of contaminating heparin to be ruled out or the testing fibrinogen levels and function to be performed in the presence of heparin. Finally, bleeding in patients with normal platelet counts and clotting times should be evaluated by testing platelet qualitative function; inherited deficiencies of platelet receptors or granules and platelet abnormalities acquired with drugs or uremia can be diagnosed by demonstrating abnormal platelet aggregation or prolonged closure time results.

Prospectus for the Future

Despite advances in the diagnostic modalities available for the identification and classification of vWD, the ability to predict with accuracy the degree of risk for bleeding in specific clinical situations is still limited, particularly with isolated borderline low vWF function. Such assessment becomes even more difficult in the presence of additional risk factors, such as when antiplatelet therapy is instituted. Clinical studies underway may address how to assess de novo bleeding risk, as well as yield insight for such patients. Another area of intense study is the identification of additional settings in which recombinant VIIa may be of clinical use. In addition to its use in congenital hemophilia with an inhibitor and acquired hemophilia, rVIIa is being studied in platelet disorders, in situations requiring rapid reversal of the international normalized ratio (INR), and with unresponsive surgical or traumatic bleeding. Outcomes data, as well as safety and cost-effectiveness studies, will help define the best therapeutic approach in these patients.

References

Bernard GR, Vincent JL, Laterre PF, et al: Efficacy and safety of recombinant human activated protein C for severe sepsis. N Engl J Med 344:699–709, 2001.

Cines DB, Blanchette VS: Immune thrombocytopenic purpura. N Engl J Med 346:995–1008, 2002.

DiNisio M, Middeldorp S, Buller HR: Direct thrombin inhibitors. N Engl J Med 353:1028–1040, 2005.

George JN: How I treat patients with thrombotic thrombocytopenic purpura–hemolytic uremic syndrome. Blood 96:1223–1229, 2000.

Goodnough LT: Utilization of recombinant factor VIIa (rFVIIa) in non-approved settings. ASH Education Program Book, Dec 2004, pp 466–470.

Levesque LE, Brophy JM, Zhang B: The risk for myocardial infarction with cyclooxygenase-2 inhibitors: A population study of elderly adults. Ann Int Med 142:481–489, 2005.

Mannucci PM: How I treat patients with von Willebrand disease. Blood 97:1915–1919, 2001.

Mount JD, Herzog RW, Tillson M, et al: Sustained phenotypic correction of hemophilia B dogs with a factor IX null mutation by liver-directed gene therapy. Blood 99:2670–2676, 2002.

Nick JA et al: Recombinant human activated protein C reduces human endotoxin-induced pulmonary inflammation via inhibition of neutrophil chemotaxis. Blood 104:3878–3885, 2004.

Roberts HR, Monroe DM, White GC: The use of recombinant factor VIIa in the treatment of bleeding disorders. Blood 104:3858–3864, 2004.

Sadler JE: New concepts in von Willebrand Disease. Ann Rev Med 173–191, 2005.

Stasi R, Pagano A, Stipa E, et al: Rituximab chimeric anti-CD20 monoclonal antibody treatment for adults with chronic idiopathic thrombocytopenic purpura. Blood 98:952–957, 2001.

Van't Meer C, Golden NJ, Mann KG: Inhibition of thrombin generation by the zymogen factor VII: Implications for the treatment of hemophilia A by factor VIIa. Blood 95:1330–1335, 2000.

Wang C, Smith BR, Ault KA, et al: Reticulated platelets predict platelet count recovery following chemotherapy. Transfusion 42:368–374; 2002.

Chapter 53

Disorders of Hemostasis: Thrombosis

Richard Torres

Henry M. Rinder

Clinical Evaluation of Thrombosis

The approach to patients with thromboembolism is defined by clinical history, physical findings, and laboratory studies. Events that trigger deep-venous thrombosis (DVT) include immobilization, orthopedic and other surgical procedures, use of oral contraceptives, and pregnancy. Venous thrombosis that is recurrent (thrombophilia), may show at an early age, occurs in unusual sites (e.g., cerebral vessels), or is accompanied by a family history of thromboembolism that may indicate an inherited disorder. In contrast, acquired venous thrombotic risk may be associated with systemic disorders such as hemolysis (paroxysmal nocturnal hemoglobinuria and autoimmune hemolytic anemia), collagen vascular disorders, or various malignant diseases. Arterial thrombotic disease is more commonly superimposed on ruptured atherosclerotic plaque (e.g., coronary artery disease) and atheroembolic disorders (e.g., ischemic stroke). The clinical approach to thrombotic disease is tailored to the location of the disease (arterial vs. venous and the specific vascular bed) and whether abnormalities of the vascular endothelium, platelets, or soluble coagulation factors that predispose the patient to thromboembolism.

Vascular Causes of Thrombosis

Virchow's triad defines the phenotypic mechanisms underlying thrombosis: diminished blood flow, damage to the vascular wall, and an imbalance favoring procoagulant over anticoagulant forces. The first two aspects are clearly localized to specific vascular beds; although the last element of the triad may be systemic, data now show at least partial vascular bed–specific regulation of the hemostatic balance. For example, congenital deficiencies of antithrombin III (ATIII), protein C, or protein S lead to DVT of the lower, but not upper, extremities. In contrast, the inherited hypercoagula-ble disorders associated with factor V Leiden and the prothrombin G20210A mutation produce not only to lower extremity DVT, but also to venous thrombosis of the brain. The interaction of these systemic factors with dynamic signal transduction and the microenvironment of distinct vascular tissues appear to regulate such differences in hypercoagulability. This hemostatic regulation in vascular tissues is mediated by multiple factors that include the following: (1) microenvironmental signals, such as shear stress, that affect endothelial cell (EC) expression of thrombomodulin, tissue factor, and nitric oxide synthase; (2) EC subtype–specific signaling (e.g., shear stress upregulates aortic but not pulmonary artery nitric oxide synthase); and (3) differences in EC transcriptional regulation of proteins such as von Willebrand factor (vWF).

Atherothrombosis

This section briefly discusses factors that lead to thrombosis in the setting of atherosclerotic plaque (atherothrombosis); the pathophysiologic mechanisms of atherogenesis are discussed in Chapter 9. In addition to EC-intrinsic regulation of hemostasis, the interaction of ECs with the fibrinolytic system is important in the development of atherothrombotic disease. Deficiency in EC release of tissue-type plasminogen activator (t-PA) may predispose patients to arterial thrombosis, especially in the coronary arteries. For example, cardiac allografts that were depleted of t-PA had a higher incidence of coronary artery occlusion and lesser graft survival than did allografts with normal t-PA levels. Aprotinin, which decreases blood loss during cardiopulmonary bypass through its antifibrinolytic effects, is associated with increased risk of vein graft occlusion and myocardial infarction after cardiopulmonary bypass. Although cardiovascular risk factors may affect plasminogen activator inhibitor 1 (PAI-1) synthesis, whether increased PAI-1 levels convey an increased risk of atherosclerotic disease or coronary events, with the exception of late restenosis after angioplasty, remains controversial.

HYPERHOMOCYST(E)INEMIA

One disorder linked to atherothrombosis is hyperhomocyst(e)inemia. Investigators recognized early that extremely high plasma homocyst(e)ine (HCY) levels, as are found in rare congenital syndromes characterized by homocystinuria and severe hyperhomocyst(e)inemia syndromes (e.g., cystathionine β-synthase deficiency), are associated with thromboembolism and severe premature atherosclerosis. HCY may damage ECs or may downregulate the normal anticoagulant function of ECs. However, studies support the assertion that even mild elevation in HCY (present in approximately 5% of the general population) leads to increased coronary, peripheral, and cerebral arterial disease. HCY in plasma can be measured after patients have fasted or after they have received a methionine load. Evidence indicates that both measures are important in that they are affected by different abnormalities of HCY metabolism, involving either the remethylation cycle or the trans-sulfuration pathway, respectively. Mildly elevated HCY levels are often associated with a thermolabile form of the N^5, N^{10}-methylene tetrahydrofolate (MTHF) reductase enzyme. This protein results from a point polymorphism (C677T) in the coding region of the MTHF binding site. This mutation occurs in up to 30% to 40% of the general population and is correlated with modest elevations in HCY. Patients who are homozygous for the polymorphism have even higher HCY levels. Furthermore, HCY levels are likely to be elevated when such persons are relatively folate deficient. In fact, deficiency of any of the vitamin co-factors of HCY metabolism (folate, vitamin B_6, and vitamin B_{12}) may lead to mild hyperhomocyst(e)inemia. Reduction in HCY levels by supplementation with vitamin B_6, vitamin B_{12}, and folate is probably the most effective therapy for reducing both the HCY level and the concomitant atherothrombotic risk, regardless of the cause of mild forms of hyperhomocyst(e)inemia. The *MTHFR C677T* mutation and mild hyperhomocyst(e)inemia have not been shown to confer a significantly increased risk for venous thromboembolism (VTE) in North American studies, although international studies show a weak association.

ROLE OF PLATELETS

Although these EC-associated abnormalities clearly influence hemostasis, platelet activation and adhesion are critical to the development of atherothrombosis, especially in patients with myocardial infarction, unstable angina, and ischemic stroke. In addition, both acute and chronic antiplatelet therapies are the primary modalities for maintaining patency after coronary revascularization. Antiplatelet therapy can be targeted against specific platelet functions, including cyclo-oxygenase-mediated thromboxane A_2 formation, interaction of adenosine diphosphate (ADP) with its platelet receptor, and glycoprotein IIb/IIIa (GPIIb/IIIa)-fibrinogen binding for aggregation (Table 53–1). Aspirin has long been a mainstay in treatment of myocardial infarction, angina, and stroke because of its irreversible inhibition of platelet cyclo-oxygenase, a process leading to blockade of thromboxane A_2 release. Aspirin effectively blocks platelet aggregation to weak physiologic agonists (see Table 52–4); however, aspirin is only partially inhibitory to platelet stimulation by thrombin and strong agonists. Thus blockade of

Table 53–1   **Antiplatelet Therapies**
Inhibitors of Cyclo-oxygenase
Aspirin Nonaspirin nonsteroidal anti-inflammatory drugs (not COX-2 selective)
ADP-Receptor Antagonist
Clopidogrel
Phosphodiesterase Inhibitors
Dipyridamole Prostacyclin
GPIIb/IIIa and RGD Blockers
Abciximab Integrilin (or generic Eptifibatide) Lamifiban Tirofiban Xemilofiban

ADP = adenosine diphosphate; COX-2 = cyclo-oxygenase 2; RGD = arginine-glycine-aspartate amino acid sequence.

platelet activation pathways other than through thromboxane A_2 has become an important modality for therapy of patients at risk for arterial thrombosis. Some drugs used to treat stroke and coronary disease specifically block the platelet ADP receptor from interaction with ADP in the clot milieu and thereby blunt platelet recruitment by preventing locally released ADP from activating additional platelets. Two thienopyrimidine derivatives, ticlopidine and clopidogrel, are used to antagonize ADP-induced platelet effects through their metabolites, which block ADP from binding to the platelet ADP receptor. Both drugs are highly inhibitory to platelet function and produce bleeding times that are more prolonged than are those produced with aspirin. Both drugs are effective in combination with aspirin for preventing ischemic stroke and for blocking stent thrombosis after revascularization, although the hematologic side effects of ticlopidine are a concern.

A third avenue for blocking platelet activation has targeted the primary platelet receptor for its binding ligands fibrinogen and vWF, GPIIb/IIIa. One of the first GPIIb/IIIa inhibitors was the modified monoclonal antibody abciximab, which prevents GPIIb/IIIa from binding to fibrinogen and blocks platelet aggregation. Abciximab successfully prevented restenosis after angioplasty, stent placement, or pharmacologic thrombolysis, and it has been used to block infarct extension and to resolve unstable angina. Other GPIIb/IIIa blockers (e.g., eptifibatide [Integrilin] and tirofiban [Aggrastat]) that interfere with the GPIIb/IIIa arginine-glycine-aspartate (RGD) binding sites are also effective in treating acute coronary events. The successful use of such blockers in patients at risk of coronary arterial events further reinforces the importance of platelet receptor–ligand interactions in thrombus formation. Currently, these GPIIb/IIIa inhibitors are indicated for acute intravenous use in patients with unstable angina and myocardial infarction and for maintaining coronary patency after revascularization. Thrombocytopenia is an uncommon (<2%) complication of using all of the GPIIb/IIIa inhibitors, most likely related to exposure of neo-epitopes on the receptor and immune-mediated platelet destruction. Clearance of the drug, with or without platelet transfusion, typically resolves the thrombocytopenia within 1 week. *Oral* anti-GPIIb/IIIa formulations have thus far been unsuccessful in making the leap to large-scale use, in part because of an increased incidence of thrombocytopenia.

Not only is GPIIb/IIIa clearly critical for platelet-dependent atherothrombosis, it also now appears that a specific platelet GPIIb/IIIa allotype, Pl(A2) (see Chapter 52), is an emerging risk factor for coronary thrombosis. Studies have shown that the Pl(A2) allotype of the GPIIIa molecule is associated with an increased incidence of coronary events, both myocardial infarction and unstable angina, as well as with coronary and cerebral injury after cardiac surgery. A large, long-term Danish study has shown that homozygosity for the Pl(A2) allotype confers a three- to fourfold increased risk of myocardial infarction in men. Evidence suggests that Pl(A2) and other platelet receptor allotypes associated with thrombosis may promote increased platelet responsiveness to agonists and shear. (See the "Prospectus for the Future" at the end of this chapter for a discussion of newer strategies for managing coronary thrombosis.)

Inherited Risk Factors for Venous Thrombosis

The balance between thrombin formation and anticoagulant pathways has been extensively studied in patients with inherited deficiencies of naturally occurring anticoagulants (Table 53–2). These patients are predisposed to venous thrombosis and pulmonary embolism (PE).

FACTOR V LEIDEN

The most common inherited disorder leading to DVT is the factor V Leiden mutation. Approximately 5% of the general population is heterozygous for factor V Leiden. The factor V mutation occurs at a site where activated protein C (APC) cleaves and inactivates normal factor Va (Arg506); abolition of this cleavage site results in APC resistance. Failure to inactivate the mutant factor Va allows the prothrombinase complex to be relatively uninhibited and leads to increased thrombin generation and a thrombophilic phenotype. Inheritance of heterozygous factor V Leiden conveys an approximately fivefold increased risk of DVT or PE. Nearly one fourth of patients with an initial occurrence of DVT or PE will have heterozygous factor V Leiden, and this percentage increases to nearly 60% in those with recurrent DVT or a strong family history of DVT. APC resistance can be demonstrated by specialized clotting tests showing that the addition of APC does not adequately prolong the partial thromboplastin time (PTT). Genotyping can then confirm whether the factor V Leiden allele is present and whether it is heterozygous or homozygous.

Factor V Leiden is a weak hypercoagulable risk factor. At 50 years of age, only 25% of persons with heterozygous factor V Leiden have had DVT or PE compared with much higher percentages in persons with other inherited thrombophilias. In addition, DVT or PE in persons with factor V Leiden is typically associated with concomitant *acquired* risk factors such as immobilization, pregnancy, or oral contraceptive use. Occasional reports exist of patients with homozygous factor V Leiden who are asymptomatic into old age, although homozygous factor V Leiden is generally associated with a 90-fold increased risk of DVT compared with persons who have wild-type factor V. In addition, a few patients have demonstrated APC resistance *without* the factor V Leiden mutation. Factor V Cambridge, although much rarer compared with V Leiden, has a similar mutation at an APC cleavage site (Arg306) and is associated with APC resistance and thrombosis. Other factor V defects associated with increased APC resistance and thrombosis have also been described. *Acquired* APC resistance may be caused by the presence of a lupus anticoagulant or cancer and can also be seen in pregnancy, with hormone replacement therapy, and with oral contraceptive use.

PROTHROMBIN G20210A

Another mutation associated with inherited thrombophilia is the prothrombin G20210A mutation, which occurs in the 3′ untranslated region of the prothrombin gene; this mutation leads to higher than normal prothrombin levels and approximately a twofold increased risk of DVT or PE. The heterozygous mutation is present in approximately 3% of European-derived populations. The mutation does not appear to convey any functional difference in the prothrombin molecule, and the elevated prothrombin levels are not sufficiently different from levels in healthy persons to warrant measurement. Thus how this prothrombin mutation exactly affects thrombus development is currently unknown. However, some evidence exists for both an inhibitory action on protein S activity and a decreased fibrinolytic effect through enhanced activation of the thrombin-activatable fibrinolysis inhibitor (TAFI). The diagnosis of the G20210A genotype is made by examining DNA for this specific mutation.

Table 53–2 **Inherited Causes of Thrombophilia**
Activated protein C resistance/factor V Leiden (20–60%)*
Homocyst(e)inemia (10–15%)
Prothrombin 20210A (5–15%)
Antithrombin III deficiency (1–4%)
Protein C deficiency (2–6%)
Protein S deficiency (2–5%)
Tissue plasminogen activator deficiency (rare)
Plasminogen activator inhibitor excess (rare)
Dysfibrinogenemia (rare)
Decreased plasminogen (very rare)

*Prevalence in patients presenting with deep venous thrombosis or pulmonary embolism.

INHERITED DEFICIENCY OF NATURAL ANTICOAGULANT PROTEINS

Deficiencies in the naturally occurring anticoagulants (ATIII, protein C, and protein S) are less common compared with factor V Leiden or prothrombin G20210A, but they are more likely to produce symptomatic venous thrombosis at an earlier age. Only approximately one half the thromboses that occur with these deficiencies are associated with acquired risk factors such as pregnancy, surgery, or immobilization. Deficiencies of ATIII, protein C, or protein S are detected by functional and/or antigenic assays because some mutations cause a quantitative decrease in factors and some produce dysfunctional proteins. Many mutations have been associated with these deficiencies, but none is predominant. Deficiencies of ATIII, protein C, and protein S in the aggregate account for fewer than 5% to 10% of all patients with DVT and/or PE.

ATIII is a naturally occurring anticoagulant that complexes with endogenous heparin sulfates to inhibit both formed thrombin and factor Xa. Heterozygous ATIII deficiency leads to ATIII levels of less than 50% and is associated with thrombosis that occurs exclusively in the venous circulation. However, reports have noted a homozygous mutation in the heparin-binding site of ATIII that results in arterial thrombosis. Thrombosis occurs by the age of 25 years in 50% of patients who are heterozygous. ATIII has a low molecular weight and may be lost through the kidney in the proteinuria of nephrotic syndrome, a process leading to symptomatic acquired ATIII deficiency. Acquired ATIII deficiency (as well as protein C deficiency) may also be associated with severe hepatic veno-occlusive disease after stem cell transplantation; investigators have hypothesized that ATIII and protein C are consumed in the damaged hepatic microvasculature. ATIII replacement with or without heparin appears to be useful in resolving platelet consumption and the fluid disorders of veno-occlusive disease after stem cell transplantation. Successful treatment of symptomatic patients with heterozygous ATIII deficiency has included short-term replacement of ATIII with plasma or concentrate, usually coupled with heparin. Long-term therapy for such patients has consisted primarily of warfarin.

The complex of thrombin and thrombomodulin on the EC surface activates protein C; APC coupled with its cofactor, protein S, cleaves and inactivates factors Va and VIIIa. These actions downregulate the prothrombinase and tenase complexes, respectively, to slow the rate of thrombin generation. Similar to ATIII deficiency, heterozygous protein C and protein S deficiencies are observed with venous, and occasionally arterial, thrombosis at a young age (median occurrence 20 to 40 years). Homozygous protein C deficiency does occur and exhibits in the neonate as *purpura fulminans* with widespread venous thrombosis and skin necrosis. A similar clinical presentation has been reported in adults after instituting warfarin therapy *without* simultaneous heparinization, so-called *warfarin-induced skin necrosis.* Approximately one third of these patients are deficient in protein C on a hereditary basis, whereas the rest of these individuals appear to have an acquired protein C deficiency. Warfarin inhibits production of vitamin K–dependent protein C synthesis, and, because of the factor's short half-life, protein C levels rapidly fall before a decline in the levels of the procoagulant factors II, IX, and X. This imbalance shortly after starting warfarin may favor a procoagulant state and occasionally results in widespread microvascular thrombosis. Although protein C deficiency, either inherited or acquired, is relatively infrequent, most clinicians prefer that a patient with venous thrombosis be fully anticoagulated with heparin (either unfractionated heparin [UFH] or of low–molecular-weight heparin [LMWH]) before concurrent warfarin therapy is begun. Inherited deficiency of protein S has similarly been implicated in warfarin-induced skin necrosis. Protein S deficiency can also be acquired in acute illness. Protein S circulates in a free form and is bound to C4b-binding protein; only free protein S is active as a cofactor for protein C. C4b-binding protein is an acute phase reactant, and increased C4b-binding protein levels with severe illness therefore decrease free protein S levels. A similar effect is seen in normal pregnancy. Short-term therapy for homozygous or doubly heterozygous protein C or S deficiency, especially in the setting of neonatal *purpura fulminans,* has included plasma or protein C concentrate with full-dose heparin anticoagulation. As with ATIII deficiency, long-term treatment with warfarin has been successful in protein C or S deficiency.

A decrease in another natural anticoagulant, tissue factor pathway inhibitor (TFPI), has also been preliminarily associated with an increased risk of DVT. As discussed in Chapter 51, TFPI inhibits the tissue factor-VIIa-tenase complex. Laboratory assays for TFPI activity are not yet widely available.

Acquired Risk Factors for Venous Thrombosis

SURGERY

Many medical and surgical illnesses convey an increased thrombotic risk; these *acquired* risk factors are acknowledged, even though the pathophysiologic features favoring thrombosis are unclear in most instances (Table 53–3). Several of these risk factors, including surgery (especially orthopedic) and trauma, are associated with immobilization with stasis of lower extremity blood flow. When evidence of thrombosis is actively sought, both surgery and trauma can be shown to be associated with extremely high (>50%) incidences of DVT. Besides immobilization, other pathophysiologic factors may contribute to the risk of DVT with surgery and trauma, including fat embolism and tissue damage, the latter especially after closed head injuries that result in massive tissue factor release. In some institutions, prophylactic (and sometimes temporary) inferior vena cava (IVC) filters placed in patients who have undergone trauma have been shown to protect against PE, especially in high-risk patients in whom anticoagulation is contraindicated because of the increased risk of bleeding. Stasis of blood flow in the left atrial appendage with atrial fibrillation is another source of systemic thromboembolism (usually stroke) in untreated patients (see "Prospectus for the Future").

PREGNANCY AND ORAL CONTRACEPTIVE USE

Both pregnancy and oral contraceptive use in general convey an increased risk of DVT and PE. Concomitant

Table 53–3   **Acquired Causes of Thrombosis**

Medical and Surgical Illnesses

Antiphospholipid antibody/lupus anticoagulant
Artificial heart valves
Atrial fibrillation
Hemolytic anemia (sickle cell, thrombotic thrombocytopenic purpura)
Hyperlipidemia
Immobilization
Malignancy
Myeloproliferative disorders/thrombocytosis
Nephrotic syndrome
Orthopedic procedures
Pregnancy
Trauma/fat embolism

Medications

Heparin-induced thrombocytopenia
Oral contraceptives
Prothrombin complex concentrates

heterozygosity for factor V Leiden further increases the risk of DVT and PE in women who take oral contraceptives. Cigarette use in women using oral contraceptives also significantly increases thrombosis risk, and this increase is thought to result from increased platelet reactivity, mediated in part by increased thromboxane synthesis. Epidemiologic evidence clearly points to smoking as the main cardiovascular risk factor but similarly implicates some risk attributable to both the estrogen and progestin components of oral contraceptives; third-generation contraceptives have not erased the thrombosis risk. As stated earlier, acquired protein C resistance can be seen both in pregnancy and with oral contraceptive use, and both free and functional protein S levels decrease throughout pregnancy. Whether additional risk factors for thrombosis, such as hyperhomocyst(e)inemia, have a role in this interplay is unknown.

PROTHROMBOTIC STATES

As noted earlier, thrombosis in nephrotic syndrome appears to be associated with loss of ATIII through the kidneys. Other prothrombotic states appear to be mediated through blood cell destruction, perhaps by increasing exposure to procoagulant membrane phospholipids; these states include artificial heart valves, sickle cell disease, and other hemolytic anemias. Platelet activation and clearance appear to be the primary prothrombotic manifestations of heparin-induced thrombocytopenia and thrombotic thrombocytopenic purpura (see Chapter 52), and abnormal platelet physiologic mechanisms (hyperaggregability) is often present in myeloproliferative disorders associated with thrombosis. Although chronic disseminated intravascular coagulation is present in some malignant diseases (Trousseau's syndrome), malignant diseases in general appear to be associated with an increased risk of DVT and PE that is not related to disseminated intravascular coagulation.

ANTIPHOSPHOLIPID ANTIBODY SYNDROME

Another acquired prothrombotic disorder is antiphospholipid antibody (APA) syndrome. APA syndrome may exhibit as a primary disorder, or it may be secondarily associated with other autoimmune diseases such as systemic lupus erythematosus. All the manifestations of APA syndrome are related to hypercoagulability, including recurrent venous or arterial thrombosis, thrombocytopenia caused by platelet clearance, and recurrent fetal loss resulting from placental vascular insufficiency. The serologic markers of APA syndrome include *anticardiolipin antibodies* and/or the *lupus anticoagulant*. Anticardiolipin antibodies are usually detected by enzyme-linked immunosorbent assay, whereas lupus anticoagulants are defined by prolongation of a phospholipid-dependent clotting test (prothrombin time, PTT, or Russell's viper venom clotting time), which is then corrected by the addition of excess phospholipid. Thus *lupus anticoagulant* is actually a misnomer, because its presence predisposes the patient to clotting rather than to bleeding. Another misleading aspect of this nomenclature is that phospholipid-reactive antibodies are actually directed against phospholipid-binding proteins in plasma, β_2-glycoprotein I (β_2-GPI), and prothrombin. Furthermore, the risk of thrombosis appears to be strongest when antibodies (especially immunoglobulin G but also immunoglobulin M or A) are directed specifically against β_2-GPI and possibly to prothrombin itself.

Hypercoagulability and Platelet Disorders

Essential thrombocythemia, chronic myelogenous leukemia, and polycythemia vera are clonal myeloproliferative disorders that are wholly (essential thrombocythemia) or partially (chronic myelogenous leukemia and polycythemia vera) characterized by an elevated platelet count, so-called *primary thrombocytosis*. Platelet aggregometry in these disorders often shows abnormal responses, especially to weak agonists such as epinephrine and ADP; however, the abnormal aggregation does not correspond well to bleeding risk or thrombosis risk. Patients with myeloproliferative disorders are at increased risk for thrombosis. Patients with polycythemia vera in particular have a high incidence of thrombosis in the mesenteric, portal, and hepatic venous circulation. Thrombotic complications, both arterial and venous, occur in essential thrombocythemia, even in young patients. However, no clear clinical risk factors predict which patients with myeloproliferative disorders will develop thrombosis. High platelet counts, especially more than 1,000,000/µL, are thought to increase the risk of thrombosis, and evidence indicates that increased platelet turnover in thrombocytosis is associated with thromboembolic complications. The latter has been demonstrated by radioactive platelet survival studies and an increase in the percentage of reticulated platelets associated with thrombosis. Antiplatelet agents may cause bleeding in patients with myeloproliferative disorders;

thus aspirin is indicated only in patients with *symptomatic* thrombosis, such as those with erythromelalgia. Successful treatment of symptomatic patients with aspirin increases platelet survival by decreasing platelet clearance. Other therapies to prevent thrombotic complications of thrombocytosis include lowering the platelet count with anagrelide or hydroxyurea. Some evidence suggests that patients with essential thrombocythemia who are at high risk for arterial thrombosis are most effectively treated with the combination of hydroxyurea plus low-dose aspirin. Patients with reactive (secondary) thrombocytosis resulting from iron deficiency anemia, chronic infection, rheumatoid arthritis, or the postsplenectomy state do not generally have significantly increased thrombotic risk.

Laboratory Evaluation of Thrombosis

Recurrent VTE is a strong indication for laboratory testing for causes of thrombophilia, especially in patients younger than 50 years of age, in patients with unexplained DVT, and in those with a family history of venous thrombosis. In these patients, any risk factors that may predispose the individual to recurrence must be defined, as well as any inherited disorders that may necessitate family counseling or avoidance of additional environmental risks. The current assays in the work-up of venous thrombophilia include the following: (1) APC resistance using a dilute factor V method, (2) genotyping for prothrombin G20210A, (3) lupus anticoagulant assay and anticardiolipin antibodies, (4) functional ATIII level, and (5) functional protein C and protein S levels (Table 53–4). Genotyping for the factor V Leiden mutation should be done when APC resistance is present to define whether factor V Leiden is truly present and, if so, to determine whether the patient is heterozygous or homozygous. Testing for antibodies specifically to β_2-GPI can be used to confirm the APA syndrome after positive screening for a lupus anticoagulant or anticardiolipin antibody; anti-β_2-GPI testing is probably not useful when APA screening tests are negative.

The utility of laboratory testing in the setting of atherothrombosis and arterial thromboembolism is unclear. Identification of elevated HCY levels is important because specific therapy (folate, vitamin B_6, and vitamin B_{12} supplementation) is then indicated. Platelet-specific risk factors for both arterial and venous thrombosis have not been defined

adequately for available sophisticated laboratory tests to give meaningful or prognostic data. Therefore platelet aggregation studies and examination of platelet receptor allotypes are not routinely indicated. In the setting of a myeloproliferative disorder, the platelet count and platelet aggregation, as well as platelet closure times, are the only available useful tests. In patients with recurrent thromboses or a strong family history, assays for rarer entities can be justified, including testing for low t-PA levels, high PAI-1 levels, dysfibrinogenemia (prolonged thrombin or reptilase time), and low plasminogen levels, all of which should be done in consultation with specialists in hemostasis.

Therapy for Venous Thromboembolism

Prophylaxis for DVT should be administered in patients undergoing surgical procedures that carry an increased risk of producing venous thrombosis, especially orthopedic procedures or major operations requiring significant postoperative immobilization. Prophylactic therapies include lower extremity intermittent compression and pharmacologic treatment with low doses of UFH or LMWHs. Once thromboembolism is diagnosed, immediate therapy is required. In most patients with venous thrombosis, anticoagulation is accomplished on a short-term basis with heparin compounds and on a long-term basis with warfarin. Thrombolytic therapy is indicated for patients with extensive proximal venous clots or PE. IVC filters are used in patients with contraindications to anticoagulation, complications of anticoagulation (usually active bleeding), or failure of anticoagulation (recurrent PE). IVC filters clearly decrease the incidence of early PE, but their use is also associated with thrombosis at the insertion site and late complications of IVC thrombosis and a 10% to 20% incidence of postphlebitic syndrome; whether simultaneous low-dose anticoagulation will prevent these complications is unknown. Temporary IVC filters are often used in trauma patients and appear to be most efficacious when they are placed for fewer than 7 to 10 days.

UFH is still considered by many experts to be the inpatient therapy of choice for acute anticoagulation because of its low cost, ease of monitoring, and short half-life. Heparin is begun as a bolus intravenous infusion of 80 U/kg, followed by a continuous infusion of 18 U/kg/hr; heparin doses in excess of 30,000 U/day have been shown to be most efficacious at preventing recurrent thrombosis. Heparin is monitored by the PTT. A therapeutic PTT for heparin is between 1.8 and 2.5 times the patient's initial PTT value. This PTT range should correspond to therapeutic anti-Xa levels of 0.4 to 0.7 U/mL. Adjustment of the heparin infusion should be based on the patient's weight and the PTT (Table 53–5); discontinuation of the heparin infusion, even for a brief period, may allow the PTT to normalize because of heparin's short half-life (approximately 4 hours). UFH should be continued for 4 days or more (longer in patients with extensive clots), and UFH can be discontinued when patients are fully anticoagulated with warfarin (international normalized ratio [INR] = 2.0 for 2 consecutive days). Some patients may receive large doses of heparin (usually >40,000 U/day), and yet the PTT does not become therapeutic. This *heparin resis-*

Table 53–4 **Laboratory Evaluation of Venous Thrombosis**
Activated protein C resistance/factor V Leiden
Lupus anticoagulant
Homocyst(e)ine level: fasting or following methionine load
Prothrombin 20210A mutation
Antithrombin III level
Protein C level
Protein S level (total and free)

Table 53–5	Unfractionated Heparin Dose Adjustment Based on Partial Thromboplastin Time (PTT) and Weight*

PTT Value (Times Baseline)	Heparin Adjustment
1.2–1.5	40-U/kg bolus, ↑ infusion by 4 U/kg/hr
>1.5–2.4	No change
>2.4–3.0	↓ infusion by 2 U/kg/hr
>3.0	Hold infusion for 1 hr, ↓ infusion by 3 U/kg/hr

*After initial therapy with 80-U/kg bolus and 18-U/kg/hr infusion.
↑ = increase; ↓ = decrease.

tance is caused by a dissociation of the PTT and the true heparin level (measured as anti-Xa activity); monitoring of anti-Xa levels is generally indicated in heparin resistance. Heparin resistance is only rarely caused by ATIII deficiency; more often, heparin resistance occurs in patients with inflammatory diseases and is caused by increased plasma levels of factor VIII and other heparin-binding proteins.

LMWHs are gradually replacing UFH as the treatment of choice for management of thromboembolism and acute coronary events. The advantages of LMWH over UFH include the following: (1) reduced binding to macrophages and EC, a process that increases the plasma half-life of LMWH; (2) less nonspecific binding to plasma proteins that leads to a more predictable dose response and allows for intermittent fixed dosing; (3) reduced binding to platelets and platelet factor 4, with a resulting lower incidence of heparin-induced thrombocytopenia (10% to 20% of the rate for UFH); and (4) reduced bone loss. Although the incidence of heparin-induced thrombocytopenia is lower with initial use of LMWH when compared with UFH, once heparin-induced thrombocytopenia is established, antibody cross-reactivity with all the LMWH preparations is more than 75% (see Chapter 52). All the LMWH preparations (dalteparin, enoxaparin, nadroparin, and tinzaparin) have been shown to be as safe and effective as UFH is in prophylaxis for DVT, treatment of uncomplicated DVT, and treatment of symptomatic PE when these drugs are given in a subcutaneous, weight-adjusted dose. In particular, outpatient therapy with LMWH for uncomplicated DVT provides a significant cost saving (when compared with hospitalization for intravenous UFH) without compromising patient outcome. Because of its predictable dose-response curve, LMWH therapy in most studies has not required monitoring. LMWH therapy does not prolong the PTT and is monitored, if necessary, by anti-Xa levels. Peak anti-Xa levels generally occur between 3 and 5

hours after subcutaneous LMWH injection and vary according to the dose given. For example, 4000 U of enoxaparin subcutaneously results in a mean peak concentration of 0.4 U/mL of anti-Xa activity 4 hours after injection, and significant anti-Xa activity persists in plasma for 12 hours after subcutaneous injection. As with UFH, switching from LMWH to warfarin for long-term management can be accomplished after therapeutic INR values are present for 2 to 3 days.

Warfarin is still the current treatment of choice for long-term anticoagulation and for preventing early recurrence of thrombus. Warfarin should be begun in the first 24 hours after presentation with VTE and concurrent with heparin treatment. The prothrombin time is prolonged within hours by warfarin because of a rapid decrease in factor VII levels; however, therapeutic warfarin anticoagulation does not occur until other vitamin K–dependent factors (II, IX, and X) also decrease. Therapeutic warfarin anticoagulation usually requires at least 4 to 5 days of adequate warfarin dosing starting at 5 mg daily for 2 to 3 days; UFH or LMWH can be discontinued after at least 4 days of therapy and only when the INR is between 2.0 and 3.0 for at least 2 consecutive days. One long-standing problem with warfarin anticoagulation is the intra-individual drug response such that the same dosing among similar-size individuals may yield widely disparate INR levels. This variation in sensitivity to warfarin may be caused, in part, by genetic differences in the enzymes that metabolize and clear warfarin. Studies are beginning to stratify patients according to enzyme haplotypes, which, in turn, have the potential to predict maintenance dosing ranges for safe warfarin therapy.

The intensity of warfarin dosing, evaluated by the INR, depends on the condition predisposing the patient to thromboembolism. Treatment of uncomplicated DVT in a patient without known risk factors does not require an INR exceeding 3.0; in contrast, prophylaxis for recurrent thrombosis in patients with APA syndrome requires INR values between 3.0 and 4.0 (Table 53–6).

The duration of warfarin treatment also varies depending on the circumstances of the VTE, the estimated clinical risk of bleeding, and the potential for recurrence. In general, the longer the anticoagulation with warfarin is, the less the chance of recurrence will be; short-term warfarin (6 weeks) is not as effective at preventing recurrence compared with longer courses (6 months). Patients with definite, transient risk factors such as orthopedic surgery have low recurrence rates, even with short-term therapy; in contrast, patients with idiopathic thromboembolism have significant recurrence rates, even after 3 to 6 months of warfarin. Evidence indicates that inherited hypercoagulable disorders, such as factor V Leiden, probably confer a lifelong increased risk of DVT or PE. Some studies have shown that the bleeding risks incurred by long-term, but low-intensity, warfarin use are favorably balanced by the decreased incidence of recurrent thrombosis. The presence of inherited thrombophilia, such as factor V Leiden mutation, may warrant continuing warfarin for a longer period, depending on the patient's other medical illnesses and whether certain circumstances may have predisposed the patient to venous thrombosis. Patients who develop recurrent venous thrombosis after discontinuation of warfarin should receive long-term anticoagulation, regardless of whether they have a defined cause of thrombophilia. Table 53–7 suggests guidelines for the duration of

Table 53–6	Therapeutic International Normalized Ratio (INR) Ranges for Warfarin According to Patient Subgroup	

Subgroup	INR Range
Venous Thrombosis	
Treatment	2.0–3.0
Prophylaxis	1.5–2.5
Artificial Heart Valves	
Tissue	2.0–2.5
Mechanical	3.0–4.0
Atrial Fibrillation	
Prophylaxis	1.5–2.5
Lupus Anticoagulant	
Treatment/prophylaxis	3.0–4.0

Table 53–7	Guidelines for Duration of Anticoagulation in Venous Thromboembolism	

Condition	Duration of Therapy
Distal- or superficial-vein thrombus	3 mo
First Proximal DVT/PE	
No risk factors	Long-term*
Correctable risk factor (e.g., surgery, trauma)	3–6 mo
Malignancy	Long-term
Antiphospholipid antibody	Long-term
Inherited risk factor†	6 mo
Recurrent DVT/PE	Lifelong

*Long-term therapy must be adjusted individually according to other diseases, risks of bleeding, presence of transient risk factors, and ease of compliance.
†Inherited risk factors include factor V Leiden; prothrombin 20210A; deficiencies of antithrombin III, protein C, or protein S; and hyperhomocyst(e)inemia.
DVT/PE = deep-venous thrombosis/pulmonary embolism.

Table 53–8	Drugs That Affect Warfarin Levels	

Drugs That Increase Warfarin Levels: Prolonged INR
↓ Warfarin clearance
Disulfiram
Metronidazole
Trimethoprim-sulfamethoxazole
↓ Warfarin-protein binding
Phenylbutazone
↑ Vitamin K turnover
Clofibrate

Drugs That Decrease Warfarin Levels: Subtherapeutic INR
↑ Hepatic metabolism of warfarin
Barbiturates
Rifampin
↓ Warfarin absorption
Cholestyramine

↑ = increased; ↓ = decreased; INR = international normalized ratio.

warfarin therapy in specific patient subgroups. Warfarin is a teratogen; effective contraception should be used concurrently in women of childbearing age.

Supratherapeutic INR levels commonly occur with warfarin therapy, with or without bleeding. In patients with moderately elevated INR values (>5) with little or no bleeding, temporary discontinuation of warfarin and reinstitution of the drug at a lower maintenance dose may be sufficient. Patients with higher INR values (5 to 9) without serious bleeding should have warfarin withheld and should probably receive low doses (1.0 to 2.5 mg/day) of oral vitamin K to reach therapeutic INR levels; parenteral vitamin K can be given if gastrointestinal function is problematic. When serious active bleeding occurs with high INR values, especially if surgery is required to correct the bleeding, a combination of vitamin K and plasma will rapidly correct the INR. The INR can become elevated as a result of concurrent use of drugs that increase free warfarin levels (Table 53–8). Whenever bleeding occurs as a complication of anticoagulation, serious consideration must be given to future bleeding risks and to whether the patient requires IVC filter placement instead of anticoagulation.

Venous Thromboembolism during Pregnancy

The risk of DVT and PE during pregnancy and in the postpartum period is approximately fivefold higher than it is for nonpregnant women. Pregnancy is a hypercoagulable state associated with significant venous stasis, as well as alterations in procoagulant proteins (fibrinogen and vWF). DVT can occur at any time during pregnancy or the puerperium. Heparins, both UFH and LMWH, are the safest therapy for venous thrombosis during pregnancy; neither one crosses the placenta, unlike warfarin, which causes a characteristic fetal embryopathy. Warfarin also causes fetal hemorrhage and placental abruption and should be avoided during pregnancy. DVT or PE during pregnancy should be treated with intravenous UFH for 5 to 10 days, followed by an adjusted-dose regimen of subcutaneous UFH, starting with 20,000 U every 12 hours and adjusted to achieve a PTT higher than 1.5 times baseline at 6 hours after injection. An attractive alternative to UFH during pregnancy is LMWH, which can be given subcutaneously once or twice daily and does not require monitoring. Suprarenal IVC filters have also been used successfully during pregnancy without significant morbidity.

Heparin should be discontinued at the time of labor and delivery, although the risk of hemorrhage is not high during delivery, especially if anti-Xa levels are less than 0.7 U/mL. One concern with residual anticoagulation at delivery is the risk of spinal hematoma with epidural anesthesia; this concern has been reported with both UFH and LMWH. The anti-Xa level that is safe for an epidural procedure is not known. Protamine sulfate can be used to neutralize UFH if the PTT is prolonged during labor and delivery; unfortunately, LMWH is only partially (10%) reversed by protamine.

Anticoagulation during the postpartum period can be carried out with heparin or warfarin; neither drug is contraindicated during breast-feeding. Women who become pregnant and who are at risk of developing a thromboembolism should receive intensive heparin therapy, followed by warfarin in the postpartum period; this category includes women with a history of previous DVT or PE or women with APA syndrome without previous thrombus. Women receiving long-term warfarin therapy (e.g., for valvular heart disease) who wish to become pregnant will need to be switched to a fully anticoagulating dose of UFH or LMWH; warfarin treatment can be restarted postpartum.

Perioperative Anticoagulation

A common clinical problem is the management of anticoagulation in patients who require surgery. The principles of care in this situation reflect the need for adequate hemostasis during and immediately after surgical procedures and the critical importance of restarting anticoagulation as soon as possible postoperatively, especially because surgery itself represents a relative hypercoagulable state. In patients with VTE who are anticoagulated on a short-term basis (<1 month), elective surgical procedures should be postponed; if such patients must undergo surgery, discontinuation of anticoagulation and placement of an IVC filter may be the best option. In most patients receiving long-term anticoagulation for VTE, preoperative heparin is not generally used; warfarin should be discontinued for at least 4 days preoperatively to allow the INR to decrease gradually to less than 1.5, a level that is safe for surgery. Postoperatively, intravenous heparin can be safely used for anticoagulation until therapeutic INR levels are reached after restarting warfarin. These guidelines obviously should be tailored to individual patient care. Patients with arterial thromboembolic disease may need heparin therapy right up until the time of the surgical procedure and shortly thereafter. In contrast, heparin therapy immediately after a major surgical procedure may be contraindicated because of the high risk of hemorrhage; anticoagulation may need to be delayed in this instance for 12 to 24 hours postoperatively.

Prospectus for the Future

The critical roles of platelet adhesion and thrombin generation, especially in arterial thrombogenesis, are providing a rationale for developing antithrombotic strategies:

- Direct thrombin inhibitors (DTIs), unlike heparin, do not require the interaction of antithrombin. DTIs are increasingly finding use in coronary thrombosis and stroke prevention. DTI advantages include: no risk for heparin-induced thrombocytopenia, because they do not interact with platelet factor 4, and reliable pharmacokinetics, because no plasma protein association in vivo has been found. Bivalirudin is one DTI that compares favorably to UFH in patients undergoing angioplasty. Ximelagatran is a long-lived oral DTI with rapid onset of action that may be slightly more effective than is warfarin for stroke prevention in patients with atrial fibrillation, although concerns over liver toxicity have prevented approval in the United States. Cost and lack of established strategies for quick reversal (although rVIIa may be effective) are also limitations of DTIs.
- Another novel class of anticoagulants with potential advantages over current therapy includes the synthetic analogs of the pentasaccharide sequence that mediates the interaction of heparin and LMWH with antithrombin. Fondaparinux and idraparinux are being tested for prevention and therapy of both arterial and venous thrombosis with some promising results. Advantages include no risk for heparin-induced thrombocytopenia (these agents do not bind platelets or platelet factor 4) and predictable pharmacokinetics, which obviates the need for monitoring. These Xa inhibitors also directly inactivate platelet-bound prothrombinase complex, which may further enhance their therapeutic effect. The lack of reversing agents is a consistent drawback, however.
- As we further define the interaction between platelets and coagulation molecules, potential targets for coagulation inhibition appear, including functional platelet receptor allotypes. Drugs to block VII activity are being investigated, including recombinant TFPI and inactivated VIIa (factor VIIai). Synthetic forms of natural anticoagulants such as protein C and thrombomodulin are also in development. Thus tailoring of therapies to individuals at risk of thrombosis may eventually become a reality.

References

Bates SM, Weitz J: New anticoagulants: Beyond heparin, low-molecular-weight heparin, and warfarin. Br J Pharm 144:1017–1028, 2005.

Bauer KA: The thrombophilias: Well-defined risk factors with uncertain therapeutic implications. Ann Intern Med 135:367–373, 2001.

Bojesen SE, Juul K, Schnohr P, et al: Platelet glycoprotein IIb/IIIa PlA2/PlA2 homozygosity associated with risk of ischemic cardiovascular disease and myocardial infarction in young men. J Am Coll Cardiol 42:661–667, 2003.

Butenas S, Cawthern KM, van't Veer C, et al: Antiplatelet agents in tissue factor-induced blood coagulation. Blood 97:2314–2322, 2001.

Dahm A, van Hylckama Vlieg A, Bendz B, et al: Low levels of tissue factor pathway inhibitor (TFPI) increase the risk of venous thrombosis. Blood 101:4387–4392, 2003.

Harrison CN, Campbell PJ, Buck G, et al: Hydroxyurea compared with anagrelide in high-risk essential thrombocythemia. N Engl J Med 353:33–45, 2005.

Hirsh J, Anand SS, Halperin JL, et al: Guide to anticoagulant therapy: A statement for healthcare professionals from the American Heart Association. Circulation 103:2994–3018, 2001.

Levine JS, Branch DW, Rauch J: The antiphospholipid syndrome. N Engl J Med 346:752–763, 2002.

Rieder MJ, Reiner AP, Gage BF, et al: Effect of VKORC1 haplotypes on transcriptional regulation and warfarin dose. N Engl J Med 352:2285–2293, 2005.

Seligsohn U, Lubetsky A: Genetic susceptibility to venous thrombosis. N Engl J Med 344:1222–1231, 2001.

Stam J: Thrombosis of the cerebral veins and sinuses. N Engl J Med 352:1791–1798, 2005.

Streiff MB: Vena caval filters: A comprehensive review. Blood 95:3669–3677, 2000.

Weitz JI: New anticoagulants for treatment of venous thromboembolism. Circulation 110(9 Suppl 1):I19–I26, 2004.

Section IX

Oncologic Disease

Andreoli and Carpenter's
Essentials of Medicine

cecil

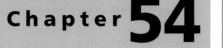

Cancer Biology and Etiologic Factors

Alok A. Khorana

Barbara A. Burtness

Cancer is primarily a genetic disease. For most human cancers, a complex succession of multiple genetic mutations is necessary for a normal cell to transform into a tumor cell. Tremendous strides have been made in understanding the classes of genes responsible for the pathogenesis of cancers, the principles governing aberrant signal transduction in cancer cells, and the hallmarks of the cancer phenotype. In turn, this revolution in the understanding of cancer biology has led to a new wave of research into the design of drugs directed against specific targets and pathways in the cancer cell. This chapter reviews the cancer phenotype and principles of cancer genetics and discusses known etiologic factors that lead to the development of cancer.

Hallmarks of the Cancer Phenotype

Over 100 distinct types and subtypes of human cancer exist, involving nearly every organ and tissue of the body. Pathologically, these cancers may resemble the tissue from which they have arisen; for example, adenocarcinomas of the gastrointestinal tract show glandular formation similar to normal gastrointestinal mucosa. Despite this diversity, most cancers share essential traits that must be acquired for malignant growth. In this sense, tumor cells resemble other tumor cells significantly more than they resemble the normal cells of their tissue of origin. Hanahan and Weinberg have described the six essential acquired capabilities essential for tumor growth (Table 54–1). *Autonomy,* or self-sufficiency in growth signals, is most apparent when cells are grown in culture. Normal cells require the addition of mitogenic growth factors, whereas tumor cells generate many of their own growth signals and proliferate with little dependence on exogenous growth stimulation. In normal tissues, tight control of proliferation is achieved with the use of multiplegrowth inhibitors. Tumor cells, in contrast, display an *insensitivity to antigrowth signals.* In addition, tumor-cell populations maintain continued expansion by reducing the rate of cell attrition, primarily by acquiring *resistance to apoptosis,* or programmed cell death. Normal cells stop growing after a certain number of doublings. Tumor cells, in contrast, are immortalized in culture because of the acquisition of *limitless replicative potential.* The induction of *angiogenesis,* or the establishment of a blood supply, is essential for tumors to grow beyond a size of 1 to 2 mm. Angiogenesis is an increasingly important target for new cancer drugs. Finally, the capacity for *invasion* and *metastasis* allows tumor cells to escape their primary sites and establish colonies at sites where nutrients and space are not limited. Metastatic disease is the cause of death in over 90% of patients with cancer. Separate mutations are not required to acquire each of these characteristics. For example, the loss of the *p53* tumor-suppressor gene can confer both uncontrolled growth and resistance to apoptosis. In the following section, the alterations in genes that are responsible for the acquisition of these common tumor characteristics are discussed.

Cancer Genetics: Pathways to Cancer

The development of most human cancers is a multiple-step process, involving a complex succession of genetic mutations. At each step, the cell undergoing transformation acquires a capability that provides a growth or survival advantage relative to other, normal cells in the population, similar to Darwinian evolution. Most invasive cancers develop only when several genes are mutated; this differentiates cancer from other genetic diseases such as cystic fibrosis in which mutations in one gene alone cause the disease. Studies suggest that four to seven mutational events must occur for progression to the malignant phenotype. Mutations can occur on exposure to environmental carcinogens, in the setting of dysregulated DNA repair, as a consequence of random replication errors, or occasionally in families with hereditary germline mutations in a cancer gene. Broadly, mutations in three classes of genes are responsible for cancer: oncogenes, tumor-suppressor genes, and stability or caretaker genes. Table 54–2 shows the clinical consequences of selected mutations in these classes of genes.

ONCOGENES

Oncogenes are evolutionarily conserved genes that play an important role in normal cellular proliferation. Oncogene activation can result from chromosomal translocations, gene amplifications, or intragenic mutations. Activation of an oncogene leads to an increased amount of the gene product. For example, chronic myelogenous leukemia (CML) occurs when the proto-oncogene, *abl,* from chromosome 9 translocates to the *bcr* gene on chromosome 22. The new protein formed by the union of the *bcr* and *abl* oncogenes, called BCR-ABL, plays a role in coupling cell-surface receptors to the signal transduction pathway with resulting unchecked growth-promoting signals to the nucleus. An activating mutation in one allele of an oncogene is generally sufficient for enhancing tumorigenesis. Oncogene research has led to the use of oncogenes as targets of specifically designed drugs. Oncogenes are also used as biomarkers to predict prognosis and select therapy. The presence of t(8;21) or inv(16)

translocations in patients with acute myeloid leukemia (AML) is usually predictive of a good response to standard antileukemic therapy. In patients with breast cancer, over-amplification of HER-2 is a poor prognostic marker overall, but it is a predictor of response to the anti-HER-2 monoclonal antibody, trastuzumab.

Certain classes of signaling proteins are targeted more frequently by oncogenic mutations. Recent research has focused particularly on *protein tyrosine kinases* (TKs), which are enzymes that catalyze the transfer of phosphate from adenosine triphosphate (ATP) to tyrosine residues in polypeptides. TKs normally regulate important cellular processes including proliferation, survival, differentiation, function, and motility. Mutations in this very small group of genes are responsible for a significant portion of human tumors. TKs can be perturbed in cancer by multiple mechanisms: overexpression of a normal receptor TK or its ligand, constitutive activation of receptor TK (in absence of ligand), or fusion of TK with a partner protein as a consequence of a chromosomal translocation or deletion (common in hematologic malignancies, such as the BCR-ABL translocation in CML as previously discussed). Inhibition of TK activity has emerged as a leading avenue for new cancer drug development. Imatinib, a small molecule directed against the kinase domain of the BCR-ABL oncoprotein, has been remarkably successful in inducing responses in patients with chronic-phase CML (see Chapter 58). Other anti-TK drugs include antibodies against receptor TKs or their ligands to interrupt TK signaling.

TUMOR-SUPPRESSOR GENES

Tumor-suppressor genes are recessive genes that keep cellular growth in check. When tumor-suppressor genes undergo mutation or deletion, the rate of neoplastic transformation is significantly higher. Tumor-suppressor genes are targeted in a different way than oncogenes: mutations in these genes result in a decreased activity of the gene product. One of the best-known tumor-suppressor genes is *p53*. This gene deletion can also be inherited, and progeny have a much higher

Table 54–1	**Hallmarks of the Cancer Phenotype**

Self-sufficiency in growth signals
Insensitivity to antigrowth signals
Evasion of apoptosis
Limitless replicative potential
Induction of angiogenesis
Tissue invasion and metastasis

Table 54–2	**Cancers Associated with Selected Genetic Mutations**	
Gene	**Associated Hereditary Syndrome**	**Major Tumor Types**
Oncogenes		
BCR-ABL translocation	—	Chronic myelogenous leukemia
BCL-2	—	Chronic lymphocytic leukemia
KIT, PDGFRA	Familial gastrointestinal stromal tumors	Gastrointestinal stromal tumors
Tumor-Suppressor Genes		
p53	Li-Fraumeni syndrome	Breast, sarcoma, adrenal, brain, multiple others
APC	Familial adenomatosis polyposis	Colon, stomach, intestine
VHL	Von Hippel-Lindau syndrome	Kidney
Stability Genes		
BRCA1, BRCA2	Hereditary breast cancer	Breast, ovary
MSH2, MLH1	Lynch syndrome	Colon, uterus, stomach

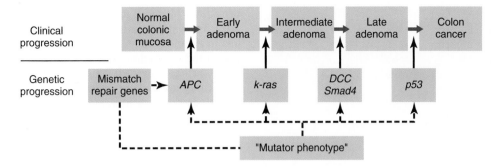

Figure 54–1 Adenoma-to-carcinoma sequence. Development of colon cancer from normal colonic epithelium is an example of multiple-step progression of neoplasia. In a majority of patients, mutation of the tumor-suppressor *APC* gene is the initial step, followed by mutations in *K-ras, DCC,* and *p53* genes. However, defects in DNA mismatch repair genes (hereditary or acquired) *(left)* can create a mutator phenotype that can initiate and possibly accelerate this multiple-step progression.

rate of a variety of cancers, including breast and brain tumors, leukemia, and sarcoma, a pattern termed the *Li-Fraumeni syndrome.* If a loss of function of the remaining normal copy of *p53* occurs through mutation or deletion in a specific organ through an acquired insult, tumors then may occur in that organ, such as in the breast, bladder, and colon. The most commonly mutated gene in sporadic human cancers is *p53.* Suppressor-gene mutations are also the most common cause of hereditary cancer. Unlike oncogene activation, mutations in both alleles of a tumor-suppressor gene are required to induce tumorigenesis. For instance, a germ-line (inherited) mutation in a single retinoblastoma gene (*RB1,* a tumor-suppressor gene) may not by itself cause retinoblastoma in a young child. However, if that child's genome suffers a *second hit* after birth (i.e., an *RB1* somatic mutation), multiple tumors including bilateral retinoblastomas may occur. Single mutations in the *RB1* tumor-suppressor gene may predispose an individual to osteosarcoma, soft tissue sarcoma, melanoma, and brain tumors later in life.

STABILITY GENES

Accumulating evidence suggests that in addition to oncogenes and tumor-suppressor genes, mutations in a third class of genes called *stability* or *caretaker genes* can also promote tumorigenesis. Stability genes are responsible for the repair of errors in normal DNA replication and include mismatch repair genes, base-excision repair genes, and nucleotide-excision repair genes. Mutations in stability genes lead to increased errors in replication. Eventually, mutations in oncogenes and tumor-suppressor genes occur and this drives malignant transformation. The Lynch syndrome, or hereditary nonpolyposis colon cancer, is an example of an inherited syndrome of defects in DNA mismatch repair genes. Colon and endometrial cancers are two of the most commonly observed cancers in families afflicted by the Lynch syndrome. Somatic mutations in these genes are responsible for 10% to 15% of sporadic colon cancers as well. Similar to tumor-suppressor genes, both alleles of stability genes must be inactivated for tumorigenesis to occur.

ADENOMA TO CARCINOMA SEQUENCE

The cascade of genetic events that leads to the transformation of normal colonic mucosa through the development of preneoplastic polyps into colon cancer is the best-studied pathway in human solid tumors and provides an excellent example of tumorigenesis (Fig. 54–1). The earliest change, or *gatekeeper* mutation, associated with adenomatous polyps is in the tumor-suppressor activated protein C (*APC*) gene. K-ras mutations occur relatively early and appear to correlate with early-to-late adenomas. Later in this sequence, *p53* mutations occur and may mark the transition from adenoma to carcinoma. As previously discussed, mutations in DNA mismatch repair genes create a mutator phenotype in which mutations in *APC* can occur, initiating neoplastic transformation and subsequent mutations. The genetic pathway responsible for tumorigenesis has clinical consequences; colon cancers that are initiated by defects in stability genes (the microsatellite instability pathway) are characterized by a better prognosis but possible resistance to adjuvant 5-fluorouracil chemotherapy, in contrast to those primarily initiated by *APC* mutations (the chromosomal instability pathway).

Etiologic Factors

Our understanding of the genetic control of cancer is derived largely from decades of elegant in vitro and preclinical research supplemented by translational studies in human cancers. Our understanding of the causes of human cancers, in contrast, is derived primarily from observations in large-scale epidemiologic studies. The variation between rates of particular sites of cancer between different geographic areas, changes in cancer rates over time, and changes in rates in immigrant families from one location to another and over generations all suggest the importance of *environmental factors* in the development of cancer (Table 54–3). This section outlines known important etiologic factors associated with human cancers.

TOBACCO

Cigarette smoking is the major cause of lung cancer throughout the world. The risk of cancer is 20-fold greater in long-term heavy smokers than it is in nonsmokers. Smoking cessation decreases the risk of cancer to one third the risk observed in continuing smokers after 10 years. Smoking and tobacco chewing are principal causes of head and neck cancers. Tobacco exposure is also a major factor in

Table 54–3	Selected Environmental Factors Associated with Human Cancers
Agent	**Associated Cancer(s)**
Tobacco	Lung, esophagus, head and neck, stomach, pancreas, kidney, bladder and cervix
Asbestos	Mesothelioma, lung
Ionizing radiation	Leukemia, breast, thyroid, lung
Ultraviolet radiation (sun exposure)	Melanoma, squamous and basal cell skin cancers
Human papillomavirus 16 and 18	Uterine cervix
Estrogen	Breast, uterus
Diet	Breast, colon, stomach

the development of cancers of the stomach, pancreas, kidney, bladder, and cervix. Exposure to second-hand smoke is also associated with an increased risk of lung cancer in non-smoking women married to heavy smokers. All told, tobacco is thought to account for nearly one third of all cancers in the United States. Over 1 million deaths occur worldwide every year from tobacco-induced cancers. Polycyclic aromatic hydrocarbons and tobacco-specific nitrosamines are the most potent carcinogens in tobacco smoke. Major public health initiatives have led to declines in smoking prevalence in adult American men from a peak of nearly 60% in the 1950s to approximately 25%. However, producers of tobacco continue to target adolescents and young adults worldwide. Tobacco remains the single largest preventable cause of cancer. Global reductions in the prevalence of tobacco use are possible and imperative for public health.

ALCOHOL

Abuse of alcohol, particularly in conjunction with tobacco, has been implicated in squamous cell cancers of the oral cavity, pharynx, larynx, and esophagus. Alcohol has also been linked to liver, rectal, and breast cancers. Epidemiologic studies suggest that all types of alcoholic beverages are associated with an increased risk of cancer.

OCCUPATIONAL AND ENVIRONMENTAL EXPOSURES

Asbestos exposure, linked with the development of lung cancer and mesothelioma, is the most common cause of occupational cancer. However, rates of asbestos-related cancers are declining with the decrease in workplace-related exposure to asbestos. Miners exposed to radon are at a 20-fold increased risk of lung cancer. Several other chemical compounds have been linked to human cancers including benzene (leukemia),

benzidine (bladder), arsenic, soot and coal tars (lung and skin), and wood dusts (nasal). Carcinogens have been identified in air and water pollution as well. However, quantification of the association of these pollutants with development of cancer has proven difficult. Exposure to ionizing radiation, either accidental or therapeutic, is associated with an increased risk of leukemia, as well as a variety of solid tumors, particularly breast, thyroid, and lung cancers. Exposure to ultraviolet radiation from sun rays is a major cause of basal and squamous cell carcinomas and melanoma.

INFECTIOUS AGENTS

Viral agents are a prominent cause of human cancers. Chronic hepatitis B and C viral infections have been linked with the development of liver cancer. A universal vaccination program directed against hepatitis B has been shown to decrease clearly the incidence of childhood hepatocellular carcinoma in children in Taiwan. Human papilloma viruses 16 and 18 have been linked with cervical and anal cancers, and vaccines against these viruses are in development (see Chapter 55). The immunodeficiency resulting from human immunodeficiency virus (HIV) can lead to Kaposi's sarcoma, certain lymphomas, and anal cancer, but little evidence exists that confirms HIV as directly oncogenic. Other viral agents implicated in cancer include the Epstein-Barr virus (nasopharyngeal cancer and Burkitt's lymphoma) and human T-cell leukemia virus type I (HTLV-1). Chronic infection with the bacterium *Helicobacter pylori* can cause certain gastric lymphomas and gastric adenocarcinoma.

PHARMACOLOGIC AGENTS

Various pharmacologic agents have been associated with an increased risk of specific cancers. Unopposed estrogen given to postmenopausal women increases the risk of endometrial cancer, although rates drop significantly when combined estrogen-progesterone therapy is substituted. Long-term hormonal replacement therapy appears to be associated with an increased risk of breast cancer, but after cessation of hormone replacement therapy, the risk of breast cancer returns to the level of risk in women who had never used replacement therapy. Synthetic estrogens such as diethylstilbestrol, which was given to mothers during pregnancy, may result in the development of vaginal cancer in their offspring. Pharmacologic immunosuppression in organ transplant recipients is associated with a high risk of cervical, lymphoid, and skin cancers. Particularly ironic is the development of *secondary* malignancies 5 to 10 years after the use of chemotherapy or radiation to treat a primary cancer successfully. For instance, long-term survivors of Hodgkin's disease have a 10- to 15-fold increased risk of subsequent leukemia and a 4- to 11-fold increased risk of solid tumors—the unfortunate price of remarkable improvements in outcomes for patients with this disease.

DIETARY FACTORS

Several epidemiologic studies suggest a strong linkage between dietary ingredients or deficiencies and the incidence of certain epithelial cancers. However, the mechanisms underlying this linkage have not been completely elucidated.

Dietary fat in the Western diet has been linked to an increased incidence of breast and colon cancer, but it is unclear whether the component of fat is responsible or whether total caloric intake plays a role. A clear inverse association has been observed between the risk of esophageal and gastric cancers and the intake of fresh fruits and vegetables.

A linkage between dietary fiber and colon cancer has been observed in epidemiologic studies, but dietary fiber intake has not been shown to be of value in reducing the incidence of colonic adenomas in prospective clinical trials. Prospective studies of various micronutrients as cancer preventive agents are ongoing (see Chapter 55).

Prospectus for the Future

The completion of the human genome project and continued advances in technologies for gene discovery will allow further rapid progress in cancer molecular genetics. Transforming these discoveries into meaningful advances in therapies for patients with cancer—the *translational* research—remains, however, an extraordinary challenge for which no clear road map exists. Research endeavors that bridge gaps in knowledge between the bench and bedside will preoccupy oncologists for the next generation. In addition, discoveries in cancer genetics will be used even more effectively to develop sophisticated diagnostic tests, such as fecal DNA analysis, that can lead to discovery of cancers at much earlier, curable stages. In the meantime, cancer-related mortality continues to rise worldwide, and cancer is expected to become the leading cause of death in the United States in the next decade. Despite recent promising successes, we are only at the threshold of understanding and treating the complex and heterogenous group of diseases collectively known as cancer.

References

Bertino JR, Hait W: Principles of Cancer Therapy. In Goldman L, Ausiello D (eds): Cecil Textbook of Medicine. 22nd ed. Philadelphia, WB Saunders, 2004: 1137–1150.

Blot WJ: Epidemiology of Cancer. In Goldman L, Ausiello D (eds): Cecil Textbook of Medicine. 22nd ed. Philadelphia, WB Saunders, 2004: 1116–1120.

Krause SD, van Etten RA: Tyrosine kinases as targets for cancer therapy. N Engl J Med 353(2):172–187, 2005.

Vogelstein B, Kinzler KW: Cancer genes and the pathways they control. Nat Med 10(8):789–799, 2004.

Weinberg RA, Hahn WC: Rules for making human tumor cells. New Engl J Med 347(20):1593–1603, 2002.

IX

Chapter 55

Cancer Epidemiology and Cancer Prevention

Jennifer J. Griggs

Cancer Epidemiology

Cancer incidence rates are expressed as the number of new cases per 100,000 people. Because the incidence of most cancers increases with age, rates are age adjusted to account for the age distribution of the population under study. The risk of developing a particular type of cancer is described as a lifetime risk or as an *age group–specific risk*. For example, the risk of developing breast cancer between the ages of 40 and 59 years is 4%, or 1 in 24, and the lifetime risk is 13%, or 1 in 7 (Table 55–1). *Disease-specific mortality rates* are also expressed as rates per 100,000.

Survival rates are usually expressed as relative survival rates. For example, the survival rate is the percentage of people with the disease who are alive 5 years after the cancer is diagnosed. Survival rates are often broken down by the stage of disease. People who have limited-stage disease (confined to the organ of origin) have higher 5-year survival rates than those with regional disease (involving regional lymph nodes), and people with regional disease have higher survival rates than do people with metastatic disease.

Survival rates for all patients with cancer are consistently poorer among African Americans than among any other ethnic or racial group in the United States. Differences in mortality and survival rates according to the ethnic or racial group are not accounted for by differences in the stage of presentation of the disease; even within the same stage, mortality differences persist. Socioeconomic factors and differences in treatment are probably the greatest determinants of the differences in outcome.

The *prevalence* of a disease is the number of people (e.g., per 100,000) living with the disease. Cancers associated with a longer life expectancy have a higher prevalence than those associated with a shorter life expectancy.

CANCER PREVENTION

The three levels of disease prevention are primary, secondary, and tertiary. *Primary* prevention keeps the disease from occurring by reducing exposure to risk factors. *Sec-ondary* prevention detects the disease before it is symptomatic and when intervention can prevent illness. *Tertiary* prevention reduces the complications of a disease once the disease is clinically evident. Tertiary prevention measures are addressed in Chapters 57 and 58.

Studying the effectiveness of cancer prevention measures requires large numbers of participants in both intervention and control groups, close monitoring for adherence in the intervention group and accurate assessment of screening and lifestyle behaviors in the control group, long-term follow-up, and appropriate ascertainment of disease and disease-free status. Such trials are challenging because of the effort and cost involved in enrollment, retention, and intervention of study participants. Many trials use intermediate endpoints, such as serum markers associated with risk of disease rather than the disease itself. Obviously, such intermediate endpoints do not always translate into reduction in rates of disease.

Primary Prevention

Primary prevention of cancer is achieved either by avoiding a causative agent or by using an agent that prevents the development of the malignant process. Primary prevention includes lifestyle risk reduction measures (e.g., avoidance of tobacco exposure; ingestion of a low-fat, high-fiber diet; use of sunscreen), chemopreventive agents, and, in the case of cervical cancer, cancer vaccination. Chemopreventive agents are drugs or micronutrients (i.e., minerals, vitamins) used to prevent the development of cancer. Many agents are being evaluated through epidemiologic studies and randomized controlled trials for the prevention of breast, ovarian, lung, prostate, and colon cancers (Table 55–2). Chemopreventive agents usually have side effects and associated costs and are generally considered for people at high risk of developing the disease. Cancer vaccines, such as the vaccine directed against the human papilloma virus (HPV), offer the promise of preventing cervical and perhaps other virus-associated cancers.

Table 55–1 Probability of Developing Cancer by Age Group and Sex, 1998–2000

		Lifetime	Ages 40–59 yr	Ages 60–79 yr
All sites	Male	45% (1 in 2)	8% (1 in 12)	35% (1 in 3)
	Female	38% (1 in 3)	9% (1 in 11)	22% (1 in 5)
Lung cancer	Male	8% (1 in 13)	1% (1 in 98)	6% (1 in 17)
	Female	6% (1 in 17)	0.8% (1 in 126)	4% (1 in 25)
Colorectal cancer	Male	6% (1 in 17)	0.8% (1 in 116)	4% (1 in 25)
	Female	6% (1 in 18)	0.7% (1 in 150)	3% (1 in 33)
Breast cancer	Female	13% (1 in 7)	4% (1 in 24)	7.5% (1 in 13)
Prostate cancer	Male	17% (1 in 6)	2% (1 in 44)	14% (1 in 7)

Table 55–2 Cancer Chemopreventive Agents

Malignant Disease	Chemopreventive Agent
Breast cancer	Selective estrogen receptor modulators (e.g., tamoxifen, raloxifene)
	Statin drugs
Ovarian cancer	Oral contraceptives
Colon cancer	Folic acid
	Nonsteroidal anti-inflammatory agents
	Statin drugs
Melanoma	Topical sunscreens
Prostate cancer	Lycopene
	Statin drugs

Table 55–3 Cancer with Demonstrated Benefit Screening Tests

Cancer	Recommendations for People at Average Risk
Breast	Annual mammogram in women ≥50 yr; possible benefit in women ages 40–49 yr
	Annual clinical breast examination
Cervical	Annual Pap test for women within 3 years of beginning sexual intercourse but no later than age 21 years
Colon	Annual fecal occult blood testing (three specimens); flexible sigmoidoscopy and barium enema every 5 yr or colonoscopy every 10 yr

Secondary Prevention

Secondary prevention of cancer is achieved with screening tests to detect disease in asymptomatic patients with early-stage disease. Examples include mammography to detect breast cancer, Papanicolaou (Pap) smears to detect cervical cancer, and sigmoidoscopy to detect colon cancer. Screening tests do not prevent disease and are not diagnostic on their own. Instead, they identify patients who need additional diagnostic tests and may need treatment for the disease. For most types of cancers, no effective screening tests exist. Diseases for which screening tests are available and recommended are listed in Table 55–3.

For screening to be recommended for a disease, these criteria must be met: (1) the disease must be common and severe; (2) the disease must have a long asymptomatic (preclinical) phase, during which time intervention is likely to be beneficial; (3) an effective intervention must be available; (4) early treatment must be more effective than later treatment; and (5) the test should be highly sensitive and specific, inexpensive, and safe.

The *sensitivity* of a screening test is the likelihood of a positive test result in a person with the disease. A 100% sen-sitive test is never negative in a person who has the disease; that is, it has a 0% false-negative rate. The *specificity* of a test is the likelihood of a negative test result in a person who does not have the disease. A 100% specific test is never positive in a person without the disease and has a 0% false-positive rate. The *positive predictive value* (PPV) of a test is the likelihood that a person with a positive test result has the disease, and the *negative predictive value* of a test is the likelihood that a person with a negative test result does not have the disease. Both values depend on the sensitivity and specificity of the test and the prevalence of the disease in the population screened.

Screening tests are used in large numbers of asymptomatic people in whom the prevalence of the disease is usually low. The PPV of screening tests is often low, and many people with abnormal test results but without disease must undergo further testing to determine whether the disease is truly present. The costs and risks of additional testing need to be included in the evaluations of screening tests.

Randomized trials are theoretically the best way to demonstrate the effectiveness of cancer screening, but these trials require large numbers of participants, require years to

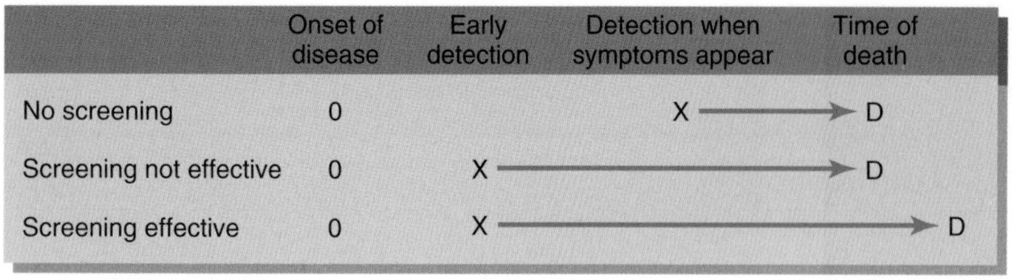

	Onset of disease	Early detection	Detection when symptoms appear	Time of death
No screening	0		X ——————→ D	
Screening not effective	0	X ———————————→ D		
Screening effective	0	X ——————————————→ D		

Figure 55–1 Effect of lead-time bias. Both effective and ineffective screening tests can increase survival time from diagnosis to death without increasing life expectancy. An effective screening test improves life expectancy.

complete, and are vulnerable to errors, such as unplanned screening among participants randomized to the non-screening arm of the study or noncompliance with screening among study participants randomized to the screening arm of the trial. Case-control and cohort studies are alternative study designs, but a suitable control group is essential.

Three types of bias may occur in studies of the effectiveness of screening tests: (1) lead-time bias, (2) length-time bias, and (3) compliance bias. *Lead time* is the time between detection of disease by screening and the actual appearance of symptomatic disease. For rapidly progressive diseases with a short asymptomatic period, such as pancreatic cancer, treatment of disease detected by screening does not alter outcome much more than treatment when symptoms appear. Diagnosing the disease earlier with screening may make it appear that the patient lived longer, but the survival of the patient from the onset of disease is not altered (Fig. 55–1). To avoid lead-time bias, analyses of screening tests must demonstrate improvements in age-specific mortality, rather than improvements in duration of survival after cancer detection among the screened population.

Length-time bias occurs when subsets of the cancer under study have different growth rates. Screening is more likely to detect those cancers that grow more slowly because of the greater prevalence of asymptomatic people with slow-growing tumors than with fast-growing tumors. People with fast-growing tumors receive medical attention before screening can be performed and have shorter life expectancy because of the nature of their tumors. Thus patients with cancer that is detected with screening appear to have longer survival as a result of screening, when in fact the longer course of their disease results from the behavior of the tumor itself (Fig. 55–2). Randomized controlled trials, which will include a mixture of people with slow-growing and fast-growing tumors, will avoid length-time bias.

Selection compliance bias is seen in nonrandomized studies of screening tests in which volunteers are tested. Such studies may suggest that screening tests lead to better health. However, because people who request screening studies tend to be healthier and have longer life expectancy, such a conclusion is flawed. Randomized, controlled studies of screening interventions are needed to circumvent compliance bias.

Screening tests have risks and benefits. False-negative results miss the diagnosis, and the patient does not benefit from having had the screening test. False-positive results are expensive, inconvenient, and may have health risks. False-positive test results can cause the patient to be labeled with a disease that is not truly present. Moreover, true-positive test results for a disease that cannot be treated satisfactorily cause anxiety without health benefit.

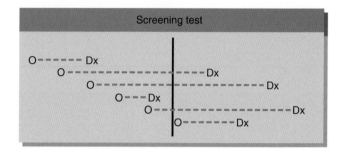

Figure 55–2 Length-time bias. Screening is more likely to detect tumors with longer time from onset of disease (O) to diagnosis (Dx) than it is to detect fast-growing tumors. The conclusion that the screening test has led to an improved survival rate would be erroneous because improved survival is actually the result of the tumor biology.

Table 55–4	**Hereditary Cancer Syndromes for which Genetic Testing Is Available**

Cancer and Involved Gene(s)	Prevention Measures
Breast: *BRCA1, BRCA2*	Prophylactic mastectomy Oophorectomy Tamoxifen Lifestyle measures
Ovarian: *BRCA1, BRCA2*	Prophylactic oophorectomy Oral contraceptives
Colon cancer syndromes Familial adenomatous polyposis coli (APC) Hereditary nonpolyposis colon cancer: *SDH2, MLH1, PMS1, PMS2*	Prophylactic colectomy Nonsteroidal anti-inflammatory drugs Lifestyle risk reduction

Genetic Screening

DNA testing is available for several types of cancer. In general, this testing is reserved for people with a strong family history of the disease (Table 55–4). If a mutation is found in an affected family member, other family members can be tested to assess their risk of developing the disease.

Most genes associated with a predisposition to cancer are large, and mutations can occur anywhere within the gene.

Patients having genetic testing must receive counseling before and after the test to ensure that they know the test limitations, the prevention options available if the test result is positive, and the risks of having a positive test result. Side effects of possible prevention measures, psychosocial issues, and the possibility of discrimination by employers, friends, and family should all be fully discussed with patients before DNA testing. Patients who receive a negative test result must understand that their risk of cancer is not zero but is similar to that of the general population.

Prospectus for the Future

The tools of molecular epidemiology allow for recognition of gene-environmental interactions, thus helping identify markers of disease risk and the steps involved in the development, progression, and response of a disease to treatment. An example of such an application is the recognition of genetic polymorphisms that identify smokers at a particularly high risk of lung cancer. Patients found to be at high risk would then be candidates for screening or chemoprevention-based clinical trials. In addition, genomic medicine allows for the identification of heterogeneity within tumor types. For example, breast cancer, once thought to be one disease, has been shown to have at least four distinct genomic profiles. An understanding of tumor heterogeneity will allow for the identification of distinct risk factors and prevention strategies.

Other advances in cancer prevention include the development of cancer vaccines to prevent cancers associated with the human papilloma virus will be important in decreasing the risk of, for example, cervical cancer.

At the population level, developing cost-effective strategies through which to disseminate behavioral, screening, vaccine, and other chemoprevention measures to those at highest risk are critical in realizing the full potential of such prevention measures.

References

Anthonisen NR, Skeans MA, Wise RA, et al: The effects of a smoking cessation intervention on 14.5-year mortality: A randomized clinical trial. Ann Intern Med 142:233–239, 2005.

Grann VR, Jacobson JS, Troxel AB, et al: Barriers to minority participation in breast cancer prevention trials. Cancer 104:374–379, 2005.

Segnan N, Senore C, Andreoni B, et al: Randomized trial of different screening strategies for colorectal cancer: Patient response and detection rates. J Natl Cancer Inst 97:347–357, 2005.

Villa LL, Costa RL, Petta CA, et al: Prophylactic quadrivalent human papillomavirus (types 6, 11, 16, and 18) L1 virus-like particle vaccine in young women: A randomised double-blind placebo-controlled multicentre phase II efficacy trial. Lancet Oncol 6:271–278, 2005.

Solid Tumors

Jennifer J. Griggs
Christopher E. Desch[†]

Lung Cancer

Lung cancer is a devastating malignant disease. Although the rate of increase of new lung cancers has leveled off more people die of lung cancer than of any other solid tumor.

EPIDEMIOLOGY

Lung cancer is one of the most common malignant diseases in the United States. More than 173,000 new cases of lung cancer are estimated to have occurred in 2005, and more than 163,000 deaths occur each year from lung cancer.

Tobacco smoke accounts for more than 90% of all lung cancers. One metabolite of cigarette smoke, benzopyrene diolepoxide, binds to areas near the *TP53* suppressor gene. This finding provides a link between the genetics of lung cancer and the epidemiologic association between smoking and cancer. Second-hand smoke is also associated with a higher risk of lung cancer than in the general population. A nonsmoking spouse has a relative risk of lung cancer of 1.5 to 2.0 compared with nonexposed control individuals.

In addition to cigarette smoke, household exposure to radon seeping through the ground into enclosed spaces, as well as asbestos exposure, increase cancer risk. Cigarette smoking enhances the risk of cancer from both these toxic exposures.

PATHOLOGY

The two major types of lung cancer are *non–small-cell lung cancer* (NSCLC) and *small-cell lung cancer* (SCLC). NSCLC includes several histologic subtypes, including squamous-cell carcinomas, adenocarcinomas, and large-cell tumors. *Squamous-cell carcinoma* usually exhibits a centrally located endobronchial lesion and is the subtype most commonly associated with paraneoplastic hypercalcemia. *Adenocarcinomas* are the most common lung cancers and are the type most often diagnosed in nonsmokers. Adenocarcinomas often exhibit a peripheral lung nodule. *Bronchioalveolar lung cancer* is a histologic variant of adenocarcinoma, char-

acterized by multiple nodules and interstitial infiltration. Sputum production with this subtype can be prolific. *Large-cell tumors* are the least common; some have histologic features of neuroendocrine tumors. Although differences are noted in the clinical presentation of various subtypes, the natural history and response to treatment are similar.

SCLC is significantly linked to cigarette smoke exposure. The cell of origin is derived from the neuroendocrine family, which probably explains its proclivity to cause paraneoplastic syndromes such as the syndrome of inappropriate antidiuretic hormone production (SIADH) and Cushing's syndrome. SCLC often exhibits a large, central tumor with mediastinal involvement.

GENETICS

Many genetic abnormalities are associated with lung cancer. Mutations in the *ras* gene are common in adenocarcinomas and predict a poorer prognosis. The oncogene *myc* is commonly amplified in SCLC and is also associated with a resistance to therapy. Abnormalities in the tumor suppressor genes on chromosome 3 and *TP53* are both common.

CLINICAL PRESENTATION

Signs and symptoms of all types of lung cancer commonly include cough, hemoptysis, chest pain, radiographic evidence of a mass or pneumonia, and weight loss in the chronic smoker. Approximately 60% of patients with SCLC exhibit metastatic disease. Common metastatic sites include the brain, liver, skeleton, adrenal glands, and bone marrow. SCLC may also cause the superior vena cava syndrome as well as paraneoplastic syndromes. NSCLC exhibits metastatic disease in less than one third of patients, most often in the bone and adrenal glands. NSCLC is associated with paraneoplastic syndromes such as pulmonary hypertrophic osteoarthropathy and hypercalcemia.

STAGING

Table 56–1 describes the tests usually required to thoroughly work-up the patient with lung cancer. Because treatment

[†]deceased

substantially differs between NSCLC and SCLC, the testing strategies are discussed separately.

NSCLC. The goals of staging for NSCLC are to find patients who may be cured by resection. Therefore attention to the mediastinum, a common site of lymph node spread, and a search for metastatic disease are both performed as soon as possible after diagnosis. Testing usually begins with a computed tomographic (CT) scan extending through the liver and adrenal glands, common sites of metastases. Bronchoscopy or fine-needle aspiration is frequently used to make the histologic diagnosis. Patients with NSCLC who have enlarged mediastinal lymph nodes should undergo mediastinoscopy to determine resectability (mediastinal nodes are rarely resectable). If the adrenal gland is enlarged,

then it should be examined by biopsy to determine whether the enlargement is the result of metastases. In patients with resectable disease, surgical treatment may offer a chance for cure. PET is a useful test during the work-up of the patient with NSCLC, but positive findings require pathologic or more precise radiologic corroboration before deciding against lung cancer surgery.

SCLC. Staging for SCLC is slightly different than staging for NSCLC. Because surgical resection is rarely performed, the focus of the staging evaluation is to uncover signs of metastatic disease that would preclude aggressive local therapy to the chest and prophylactic radiation to the brain. Therefore a patient with SCLC should undergo additional tests such as a bone scan and a CT scan or a magnetic resonance image (MRI) of the brain before treatment is initiated.

The staging system for each type of lung cancer is shown in Table 56–2. For the patient with NSCLC, tumor size, proximity to central structures, and location of lymph nodes are the most important features. Because surgery is rarely performed for the patient with SCLC, nodal detail is seldom obtained. The regional extent of the cancer and the ability to encompass the involved areas within a single radiation field determine all treatment planning (Table 56–3).

TREATMENT

Non–Small-Cell Lung Cancer

Because complete removal of the tumor provides the best chance for long-term survival, the focus of the primary treatment for the patient with NSCLC should begin with an assessment of resectability. Resectability depends on the anatomic location of the tumor, as well as the patient's medical condition and pulmonary reserve. In general terms, the risk of pneumonectomy is small if the patient has a forced expiratory volume in 1 second greater than 2 L,

Table 56–1	**Staging Work-up for Lung Cancer**
Tumor	**Staging Tests**
Non–small-cell lung cancer	Computed tomographic scans of chest through adrenal glands
	Bronchoscopy and mediastinoscopy if enlarged lymph nodes
	Positron emission tomography if considering resection
Small-cell lung cancer	Computed tomographic scans of chest, abdomen, and head
	Bone scan
	Positron-emission tomographic scan may also be useful for detecting cancer outside the chest

Table 56–2 Staging System for Lung Cancer

Stage	Criteria
Non–Small-Cell Lung Cancer	
IA	Tumor size is ≤3 cm and located more than 2 cm from the carina. No lymph nodes are involved.
IB	Tumor size is >3 cm or located less than 2 cm from the carina. No lymph nodes are involved.
IIA	Tumor size is ≤3 cm and located more than 2 cm from carina. Peribronchial and/or hilar nodes are involved.
IIB	Tumor size is >3 cm or located less than 2 cm from the carina. Tumor has invaded chest wall or pleura. Peribronchial and/or hilar nodes are involved.
IIIA	Any size tumor is present and may have invaded chest wall but not the heart, great vessels, trachea, and esophagus. Tumor may be close to carina but has not invaded it. Tumor always involves ipsilateral mediastinal nodes and/or subcarinal nodes.
IIIB	Any size tumor is present and may have invaded any structure. Nodal involvement is always present and extends to contralateral mediastinum or supraclavicular or scalene area.
IV	Metastases are present.
Small-Cell Lung Cancer	
Limited	Tumor is confined to one lung. Nodes may involve contralateral lung, but all cancer must be encompassed in one radiation portal.
Extensive	Metastatic disease is present or disease is not limited to one radiation field.

Table 56–3 Treatment and Outcomes for Lung Cancer

Tumor	Standard Treatment by Stage	Outcome
Non–small-cell lung cancer	Early stages: Surgery only (IA); surgery followed by adjuvant chemotherapy (IB, II, IIIA) Later stage (unresectable): Combined chemotherapy and radiation or chemotherapy alone	Early stages: Patients with stage II lung cancer have a 40–50% survival rate with surgery Late stage: Patients with stage IV lung cancer have 1-yr survival rate at near 20% with chemotherapy
Small-cell lung cancer	Limited: Cisplatin-based chemotherapy with concurrent chest radiation Prophylactic cranial radiation is considered Extensive: Chemotherapy palliates symptoms and prolongs survival but is not curative	Limited: 20–30% 5-yr survival rate Extensive: Median survival rate is 10 months with treatment

carbon dioxide diffusing capacity of more than 60%, a maximum voluntary ventilation of more than 50% of predicted values, or the ability to walk up three flights of stairs. Lesser resections (e.g., lobectomy) may require less stringent criteria. Occasionally, patients with severe obstructive disease cannot undergo a curative procedure because they lack pulmonary reserve.

Patients with stage I and II tumors (localized lesions or involvement limited to hilar lymph nodes) should undergo surgical treatment. Peripheral tumors are removed by lobectomy; more central tumors, if resectable, require pneumonectomy. Stage III tumors may be operable in some patients, particularly if they are treated with chemotherapy and radiation therapy (i.e., neoadjuvant therapy) before resection. In patients with significant mediastinal lymph node involvement detected during tumor resection or at the time of mediastinoscopy, the chance of long-term survival is less than 20% even with surgical treatment. Although postoperative radiation therapy is seldom useful, recent reports show a survival benefit when patients with stages IB, II, and IIIA undergo adjuvant chemotherapy. Chemotherapy using a variety of agents combined with cisplatin or carboplatin improves survival after surgery by approximately 5%.

Almost 80% of lung cancers are unresectable. If the tumor cannot be resected and has not spread to distant organs (stages IIIA and IIIB), then chemotherapy is administered concurrently with radiation. This treatment leads to better median survival and 5-year disease-free survival rates than with radiation alone, but combined therapy for unresectable disease should be reserved for patients with good functional status. Aggressive treatment is much less effective in patients who have lost more than 5% of their body weight or who are active less than 50% of the day. The median survival for patients with locally advanced, unresectable lung cancer is approximately 10 months.

Patients with metastatic disease may benefit from chemotherapy. The most active agents are platinum derivatives such as cisplatin and carboplatin, taxanes such as paclitaxel and docetaxel, gemcitabine, vinorelbine, irinotecan, and pemetrexed. Approximately 50% of patients undergo a reduction in their tumor volume after chemotherapy. For patients with advanced-stage lung cancer (stages IIIB and IV), chemotherapy improves survival from an average of 8.5 to 11 months; quality-of-life studies show that chemotherapy delays symptoms and reduces their severity compared

with no treatment. New agents that target neoplastic angiogenesis such as bevacizumab or the epidermal growth factor receptor antagonists such as erlotinib and cetuximab may prove useful in combination with other treatments for these cancers.

Small-Cell Lung Cancer

The cornerstone of treatment of SCLC is combination chemotherapy. Active agents for this cancer include cyclophosphamide, doxorubicin, irinotecan, vincristine, topotecan, cisplatin, and etoposide. Patients with limited-stage SCLC (i.e., limited to the thorax and encompassed in a single radiation-therapy portal) should undergo four to six cycles of chemotherapy as long as they respond to treatment. Approximately 50% of patients have a complete response; another 20% to 30% may have a partial response. Concurrent radiation therapy provides longer survival than either modality alone in patients with limited-stage disease. Because almost 40% of patients with SCLC have brain involvement, prophylactic cranial radiation should be considered for those patients who have a complete response in the lung to primary chemoradiotherapy. Oral etoposide may palliate extremely old or infirm patients with SCLC. Approximately 20% to 30% of patients with SCLC are alive and free of disease 3 years after diagnosis. These patients are, however, still at risk for late relapses and other tobacco-related cancers.

Recurrent Lung Cancer

Both NSCLC and SCLC have high relapse rates. The use of second-line chemotherapy for these patients may palliate symptoms, but its use is not curative. Although these cancers occasionally respond to subsequent agents such as erlotinib, the use of these drugs should be limited to patients with good performance status, preferably on a clinical trial.

Head and Neck Cancers
EPIDEMIOLOGY AND NATURAL HISTORY

The majority of cancers of the head and neck, including cancers of the larynx, oral cavity, oropharynx, and sinuses, are squamous cell carcinomas. Tobacco use, alcohol consumption, and poor oral hygiene have all been linked to the development of cancers of the head and neck. Nasopharyngeal cancers are associated with Epstein-Barr viral infection.

The major determinant of prognosis is the tumor burden, or the thickness of the tumor, and the presence or absence of regional lymph node involvement. The cure rate with small tumors is as high as 75% to 95% with radiation therapy or surgery. Continued use of tobacco after a diagnosis of a head and neck cancer is associated with a poor prognosis. People who have had cancer of the head and neck are at high risk of having a primary lung or esophageal cancer.

SYMPTOMS

Symptoms of cancers of the head and neck are related to the location of the tumor. For example, supraglottic laryngeal cancers cause pain with swallowing and a change in voice quality. Cancers of the oral cavity may exhibit a mass under the tongue or red or white patches in the mouth. Bleeding in the mouth or ill-fitting dentures may also be symptoms of cancer in the oral cavity. Symptoms of cancers of the sinus include sinusitis that does not resolve with appropriate treatment. Ear pain may be present with cancers of the oropharynx or hypopharynx.

DIAGNOSIS

Diagnosis of head and neck cancers require histologic confirmation with biopsy. An MRI or a CT scan of the head and neck are performed to determine a precise estimate of the extent of the tumor. Thorough examination of the entire aerodigestive tract with endoscopy will demonstrate a synchronous second primary tumor, for example, in the esophagus, in up to 15% of patients. Staging of the tumor is based on clinical and radiographic assessment.

TREATMENT

Small tumors that have not spread to regional lymph nodes are treated with radiation or surgery. Primary radiation therapy may allow preservation of organ function of, for example, the larynx, with surgical resection used in the case of recurrence. Locally advanced disease is treated with a combination of surgery, radiation therapy, and cisplatin-containing chemotherapy regimens. Twice-daily (hyperfractionated) radiation therapy in combination with chemotherapy may improve outcomes in patients with locally advanced disease. Most recurrences occur within 2 to 3 years after therapy. Close surveillance is therefore warranted.

Gastrointestinal Cancers

Cancers of the gastrointestinal tract are among the most common tumors. Advances in the treatment of colorectal cancer have improved survival and quality of life for patients with these diseases. Cancers of the esophagus, pancreas, liver, and stomach are less common. Table 56–4 outlines the common signs and symptoms, treatments, and prognosis of gastrointestinal tumors.

ESOPHAGEAL CANCER

Epidemiology and Natural History

The two types of esophageal cancer are squamous cell and adenocarcinoma. *Squamous cell cancers* are most common in the cervical and thoracic esophagus, and *adenocarcinomas* commonly occur in the lower esophagus down to the gastroesophageal junction. Squamous cell cancers are more common in African Americans and are associated with predisposing factors that include smoking, caustic injury, achalasia, and alcohol intake. Squamous cell cancers are associated with other tobacco-related cancers in the upper airways and digestive tract. Adenocarcinomas, conversely, are most common in the lower esophagus. The rate of adenocarcinoma is increasing; this increase is related in part to Barrett's esophagus, an adenomatous metaplasia of the distal esophagus often caused by gastroesophageal reflux disease, but other factors are likely. Almost 25% of patients with severe Barrett's esophagus eventually have esophageal adenocarcinoma. The most useful intervention for patients with Barrett's esophagus is frequent endoscopic screening and biopsy; pharmacologic treatment of acid reflux disease does not prevent neoplastic transformation.

Symptoms

The most common symptom of esophageal cancer is dysphagia. As the lumen of the esophagus narrows, the patient loses normal swallowing capacity and has a sensation that solid food becomes "stuck." Eventually, the patient may be unable to swallow liquids. Patients commonly become afraid to eat because of frequent regurgitation at mealtime, resulting in significant weight loss.

Diagnosis

An upper gastrointestinal radiographic series or endoscopy will demonstrate an esophageal lesion, which should then undergo biopsy. The most effective staging tool is endoscopic ultrasonography, an accurate tool in assessing local depth of penetration and lymph node metastases. CT and positron-emission tomographic (PET) scanning are also required to ensure that the tumor has not already metastasized to the chest or liver, the two most common sites of spread.

Treatment

The most common treatment of esophageal cancer is surgery. Resection of the involved esophagus includes a wide margin on either side. The stomach is then pulled up to join the remainder of the esophagus. Alternatively, part of the intestine may be transposed to the chest to create another digestive pathway. Approximately 10% to 30% of patients with stage II disease who are treated by surgical resection alone are alive and free of cancer at 5 years after diagnosis. If surgical treatment is not possible, then either the cancer is technically unresectable or the patient is medically unfit for surgery; the standard of care for these patients is to provide chemotherapy and radiation. This approach may cure 20% to 30% of patients. Whether the outcomes of combined chemotherapy and radiation are as favorable as surgical resection alone is not clear.

For patients with metastatic esophageal cancer, systemic chemotherapy using platinum-based combination regimens are effective in palliation and extending survival. For patients with severe dysphagia that does not resolve with radiation or surgery, endoscopic placement of a metal or plastic stent may permit adequate nutrition and resumption of a normal lifestyle.

Table 56–4 Gastrointestinal Cancers

Tumor Site	Common Findings	Standard Treatments	Expected Outcome
Esophageal	Dysphagia, chest pain, weight loss	Early stage: Surgery alone Later stages: Combination chemotherapy and radiation therapy and/or surgery	Stage II/III stage: ≈30% 5-yr survival Average survival for metastatic disease is <9 mo
Gastric	Pain, supraclavicular adenopathy, vomiting, melena	Stage I: Surgery alone Stage II and III: Surgery if possible, followed by chemotherapy and/or radiation Metastatic disease: Chemotherapy alone	Early stage: >90% 5-yr survival Positive nodal involvement: 20–75% 5-yr survival for tumors <2 cm
Hepatocellular	Elevated α-fetoprotein; pain or change in liver function test	Resection for early lesions	Always fatal in later stages of disease
Pancreas	Weight loss, boring midline pain through back, jaundice	Early stage: Whipple's procedure and/or radiation therapy Late stage: Chemotherapy with radiation or chemotherapy alone	Resectable: Median survival 10–20 mo Radical surgery: 25% with negative nodal involvement and 10% with positive nodal involvement may be cured by surgery Unresectable: Median survival 4–6 mo
Colon/rectal	Abdominal pain, occult or overt bleeding in stool, change in bowel habits	Early stage: Resection alone If nodal involvement, add chemotherapy Chemotherapy and radiation therapy before and after surgery for patients with rectal cancers	Early stage: >70% at 5 yr Nodal involvement: 50–70% at 5 yr Metastatic: Median 14–24 mo
Anal	Constipation, bleeding, rectal pain and urgency	Early stage: Chemotherapy with radiation therapy Later stage: Abdominoperineal resection	Localized: 70% at 5 yr

GASTRIC CANCER

Epidemiology and Natural History

Gastric cancer rates are highest in poor countries that use smoked meats and meats high in nitrates. Other predisposing conditions include pernicious anemia, achlorhydria, gastric ulcers, and prior gastric surgery. Except for cancers of the gastroesophageal junction, gastric cancer rates have decreased in the United States. A recognized risk factor for gastric cancer is infection with *Helicobacter pylori*. Whether early treatment of *H. pylori* infection changes the rate of cancer in infected populations is not clear.

Diagnosis

Patients with gastric cancer commonly experience abdominal pain, early satiety, anemia, hematemesis, weakness, and weight loss. Frequently, the cancer has already involved local lymph nodes by the time the diagnosis is made. Physical examination may show a gastric mass, an umbilical node (Sister Mary Joseph's node), or a left supraclavicular node (Virchow's node). Pathologic analysis shows an adenocarcinoma that can be localized or spread throughout the gastric lining *(linitis plastica)*. Required staging includes a CT scan to search for obvious nodal or metastatic involvement of the liver, upper gastrointestinal endoscopic examination, and endoscopic ultrasonography to determine depth of invasion and biopsy abnormal lymph nodes.

Treatment

Gastric cancer is most often treated surgically. When the tumor and all relevant lymph nodes have been removed, patients have a 20% to 60% chance of a 5-year survival, depending on the pathologic stage. If gastric cancer recurs, then the most common sites are local extension or hematogenous spread through the portal vein to the liver. Patients undergoing a complete resection for gastric cancer benefit from the addition of 5-fluorouracil (5-FU)/leucovorin chemotherapy and postoperative radiation therapy. This combination improves median survival by about 15 months compared with no adjuvant therapy. Patients with metastatic gastric cancer may elect chemotherapy to palliate symptoms. Chemotherapy provides a 20% to 40% response rate and may extend survival.

COLORECTAL CANCER

Epidemiology and Natural History

Approximately 1 in 20 people in the United States will be diagnosed with colon cancer (lifetime risk is 6%). Known predisposing factors are a history of ulcerative colitis and a strong family history of colon cancer. Several mutations, whether inherited or spontaneous, play a major role in the predisposition to colon cancer (see Chapter 54, Fig. 54–1 and Table 54–2). For example, familial polyposis is transmitted in an autosomal dominant manner. Individuals have mutations in the *APC* gene, which may be associated with peri-ampullary and thyroid cancers or non-neoplastic growth such as osteomas, sebaceous cysts, and gastric polyps. Hereditary nonpolyposis colorectal cancer (HNPCC) is a more common autosomal disorder associated with microsatellite instability and mutations in h*MSH2*, h*MLH1, PMS1, PMS2,* and h*MSH6*. Patients with HNPCC usually have colon or endometrial cancer when under the age of 50 years and have first-degree relatives with colon cancer or other HNPCC-related cancers derived from the stomach, ovary, small bowel, biliary tract, ureter, or renal pelvis.

Whether the predisposing risk for colon cancer is genetically transmitted or sporadically acquired, a clear relationship exists between adenomatous polyps and the later development of colon cancer. Because the removal of polyps is probably the most important way to prevent the development of invasive colon cancer, the most reliable way to reduce colon and rectal cancer mortality is to perform regular screening. Colonoscopy is the most commonly used screening test. Studies using sigmoidoscopy and regular fecal occult blood testing also show reductions in the incidence and mortality of colorectal cancer. For patients with a proven mutation (Gardner's syndrome, HNPCC) or a strong family history (familial adenomatous polyposis) or who acquire other diseases associated with colorectal cancer, such as ulcerative colitis, should begin colonoscopy earlier than suggested for the general population. For patients with familial adenomatous polyposis, screening should start in the teenage years. For patients with HNPCC, screening for colon cancer should start 10 years before the age of diagnosis in the youngest family member with colorectal cancer. Research efforts are underway in the primary prevention of colorectal cancers using interventions such as diet, daily aspirin, cyclo-oxygenase-2 inhibitors, calcium and vitamin D supplementation, and other chemopreventive agents to reduce cancer incidence. Enthusiasm for promoting a high-fiber diet to reduce the risk of colon cancer has waned. Lifestyle changes are still considered important—fresh fruits and vegetables, regular exercise, fewer than two red meat servings per week —based on epidemiologic association.

Symptoms

Rectal bleeding commonly occurs with colon and rectal cancers. Patients with left-sided colon lesions often complain of a change in stool color or caliber or pelvic pain and transient bloating. Right-sided lesions may become friable and may result in occult bleeding. Occasionally, patients with colon and rectal cancers are asymptomatic until the tumor totally obstructs the bowel or perforates the peritoneal cavity. Colon and rectal cancers tend to spread hematogenously to the lungs and liver. Rectal cancer is more likely than colon cancer to recur locally because it is more difficult to get a wide margin of normal tissue and lymph nodes within the tight confines of the pelvis.

Diagnosis

The work-up for colon cancer requires measurement of serum carcinoembryonic antigen; palpation of the liver at operation; or an abdominal CT scan, chest x-ray study, and endoscopic imaging of the colon to ensure that all polyps and cancers are removed near the time of the primary operation. Table 56–5 describes the staging system for colon and rectal cancers.

Treatment

Treatments for colon cancer and rectal cancer differ. Even in patients with metastatic disease, the most appropriate treatment for colon cancer is surgery. Surgical resection treats or prevents obstruction and pain. If cancer has spread to the lymph nodes, then adjuvant chemotherapy reduces the chance of tumor recurrence by approximately 40%. For patients with rectal cancer, any lesion that invades the muscle

---

Table 56–5 **Staging for Colon and Rectal Cancer**

Stage	Tumor Size	Nodal Status	Metastases
0	In situ	No	No
I	Invades mucosa only	No	No
II	May invade muscularis or through serosa	No	No
III	Any size tumor or any level of invasion	Yes	No
IV	Any size or depth	Positive nodal involvement present or absent	Yes

or lymph nodes should be treated with chemotherapy and radiation before or after surgery to reduce the chance of local and distant recurrence of the disease.

Significant advances have been made in the use of chemotherapy for colorectal cancer. Regimens proven successful in prolonging survival for colon cancer include 5-FU with leucovorin or its oral analog, capecitabine, alone. The addition of oxaliplatin to 5-FU–based adjuvant therapy has recently been shown to further improve survival after surgery. In the setting of metastatic cancer, infusions of chemotherapy with FOLFOX (5-FU, leucovorin, oxaliplatin), or FOLFIRI (5-FU, leucovorin, irinotecan) with the addition of the anti-angiogenic antibody bevacizumab prolong median survival beyond 20 months, almost twice the survival expected in the early 1990s. Despite improvements in the mean survival rate, metastatic colon and rectal cancers are incurable unless the metastatic lesions can be surgically resected.

ANAL CARCINOMA

Anal cancers are increasing in frequency. Persons infected with the human papillomavirus (HPV) and human immunodeficiency virus (HIV) are more likely to develop anal cancer. Patients with anal cancer usually experience rectal bleeding or complain of rectal fullness.

Combined chemotherapy with 5-FU and mitomycin and radiation therapy make up the standard approach to a patient with localized anal cancer. Results with combined therapy are superior to those with surgery, with the additional benefit of sparing the anal sphincter. Abdominoperineal resection is reserved for patients who fail chemoradiotherapy.

PANCREATIC CANCER

Epidemiology and Natural History

Pancreatic cancer is strongly associated with cigarette smoking. A small proportion of pancreatic cancers are inherited from mutations in the *p16* and *BRCA2* genes. Epithelial pancreatic cancer is an adenocarcinoma with an extremely high mortality rate because it is usually diagnosed when the tumor is beyond the capability of surgical resection. A less common type of pancreatic cancer, islet cell carcinoma, originates in the endocrine cells. Symptoms related to secretion of peptides such as gastrin, vaso-intestinal polypeptide, and insulin characterize these tumors.

Symptoms

The most common presentation of epithelial pancreatic cancer is abdominal pain accompanied by rapid weight loss. Characteristically, the pain is located in the peri-umbilical region and pierces or stabs through to the back. The pain is often explained by the frequent invasion of the celiac plexus deep in the retroperitoneum. Other symptoms of pancreatic cancer are the recent onset of diabetes, intestinal angina reflecting encasement of the superior mesenteric artery, a palpable gallbladder (Courvoisier's sign), and jaundice from blockage of the distal common bile duct. Migrating thrombophlebitis (Trousseau's sign) is a common paraneoplastic complication of pancreatic adenocarcinoma. The tumor

marker CA-19-9 is elevated in 75% or fewer of all patients with pancreatic cancer.

Treatment

The only curative treatment for pancreatic cancer is pancreaticoduodenectomy (Whipple's procedure), an extensive operation requiring numerous anastomoses and splenectomy that carries a high mortality rate in centers with less experience with the procedure. The 5-year survival for surgically treated patients with localized pancreatic cancer is 25% for node-negative cancer but only 10% when lymph nodes are involved. Patients with unresectable disease may benefit from local radiation therapy with concurrent 5-FU; more than 30% of patients treated with this combination have some improvement in their symptoms. When patients have progressive disease, the use of palliative chemotherapy with weekly gemcitabine has been shown to improve quality of life and survival to a small degree (5.7 months with gemcitabine, 4.4 months without gemcitabine, or 20% 1-year survival versus 5%).

HEPATOCELLULAR CARCINOMA

Although uncommon in the United States, hepatocellular carcinoma (HCC) is one of the most common cancers throughout the world; more than 1 million cases are diagnosed each year. The common causes of HCC are chronic viral hepatitis (both B and C) and cirrhosis related to alcohol use or hemochromatosis. Although this approach is unproved, considerable interest exists in screening patients who are at extremely high risk with serial measurement for α-fetoprotein (AFP) levels. AFP levels are commonly elevated even in early-stage HCC.

Treatment of early-stage HCC is surgery. Cure rates are more than 75% for patients with tumors less than 2 cm. Patients with severe cirrhosis and who have small liver cancers may benefit from liver transplantation. Patients with cancers that are more extensive rarely benefit from chemotherapy or radiation.

Breast Cancer
EPIDEMIOLOGY

Breast cancer is the most common non–skin cancer in women and the second leading cause of cancer death (after lung cancer) among women in the United States. In 2005, an estimated 213,000 women were diagnosed with invasive breast cancer, and over 40,000 died of breast cancer. Breast cancer in men is rare.

Risk factors for breast cancer include older age, family history of breast cancer, early menarche, late menopause, first-term pregnancy after age 25 years, nulliparity, prolonged use of exogenous estrogen, and postmenopausal obesity. Exposure to ionizing radiation, as is used in the treatment of Hodgkin's disease, also increases the risk of breast cancer. Only 5% to 10% of patients with breast cancer are associated with the breast cancer–susceptibility genes, *BRCA1* and *BRCA2*. Patients with multiple affected family members or those with a personal or family history of male breast cancer, bilateral breast cancer, or ovarian cancer should be offered genetic counseling and genetic testing for *BRCA1* and *BRCA2*.

PATHOLOGY

Most breast cancers are infiltrating ductal adenocarcinomas. A smaller proportion of breast cancers are infiltrating lobular adenocarcinomas. Tubular and mucinous carcinomas are associated with a better prognosis. The estrogen- and progesterone-receptor status of the primary tumor should be assessed in all cases of invasive breast cancer. The oncoprotein-oncogene HER-2/neu (*Human Epidermal Growth Factor Receptor*) is important in defining prognosis and treatment. Tumors that are negative for the estrogen and progesterone receptor and for overamplification of the HER-2 oncogene (i.e., the so-called *triple-negative* tumors) are associated with a poorer prognosis. Such tumors are characteristic of those that develop in women who have the *BRCA1* breast cancer–susceptibility gene. Ductal carcinoma in situ (DCIS), or intraductal carcinoma, is increasing in frequency, most likely because of increased mammographic screening.

CLINICAL PRESENTATION

Breast cancer is most often diagnosed through screening mammography or after a patient or her physician notices a palpable mass. Fewer than 10% of women have metastatic disease at diagnosis. Recurrent breast cancer most commonly exhibits metastases in the bone, liver, lung, and central nervous system, but breast cancer can recur in any organ of the body. Women with a history of breast cancer are also at increased risk of breast cancer in the contralateral breast. Inflammatory breast cancer is a clinical diagnosis in a woman with breast induration and erythema, often without a palpable mass. The skin findings are due to tumor emboli in the dermal lymphatics; skin biopsy is negative for cancer in 50% of patients.

STAGING

Breast cancer staging requires removal of the primary tumor and ipsilateral axillary lymph node dissection. Women with tumors more than 5 cm and those with positive axillary lymph node involvement may have additional radiographic tests, including a chest radiograph, bone scan, and CT scan of the abdomen. Patients with smaller tumors and negative lymph node involvement do not need these tests unless they exhibit symptoms (e.g., skeletal pain) suggestive of metastatic involvement.

TREATMENT

For women with small breast tumors, breast-conserving therapy with lumpectomy followed by radiation therapy is standard therapy. Women with large tumors or with two or more tumors in separate quadrants of the breast should undergo mastectomy. Some women also prefer mastectomy, with or without breast reconstruction. Women who have had previous radiation to the breast, either for a previous breast cancer or other malignancies, are generally treated with mastectomy. Chemotherapy administered before surgical treatment (*primary* or *neo-adjuvant chemotherapy*) may

allow breast conservation in women with large tumors who would otherwise not be able to undergo a lumpectomy. Preoperative hormone therapy can be considered in frail patients with hormone receptor–positive tumors, but hormone therapy does not replace surgical treatment for the majority of patients. Adjuvant therapy with chemotherapy and hormonal therapy improves relapse-free and overall survival rates in premenopausal and postmenopausal women who are at high risk of metastatic relapse. The monoclonal antibody trastuzumab, directed at the HER-2 pathway, improves disease-free survival in patients with tumors that have overamplification (or high levels of overexpression) of the HER-2 oncoprotein.

Treatment decisions in women with metastatic disease are based on the hormone-receptor status, sites of disease, presence and severity of symptoms, time since initial diagnosis, and previous treatments. The monoclonal antibody, trastuzumab, may be used in combination with chemotherapy, hormonal therapy, or as a single agent. Life expectancy is longer in women with hormone-responsive disease and with lymph node or bone metastases, rather than liver, lung, or central nervous system metastases. Patients with metastatic breast cancer may live for many years, often responding to hormonal therapy for years before requiring chemotherapy for disease control. Bisphosphonates, such as zoledronate and pamidronate, are given intravenously to decrease the pain associated with bone metastases and the risk of fracture in women with skeletal metastases.

DCIS is treated with either lumpectomy followed by radiation therapy or mastectomy. Women with multifocal or palpable DCIS should have assessment of lymph node status because a small but measurable proportion will have positive lymph node involvement that indicate foci of invasive cancer. In these patients, systemic treatment is identical to that given to women with a clearly invasive breast primary tumor.

Prophylactic bilateral mastectomy is offered to women with the *BRCA1* or *BRCA2* breast cancer–susceptibility genes. An alternative approach is close clinical surveillance, including monthly self-examination, frequent examination by a physician, and regular mammography or MRI. Oophorectomy or anti-estrogen therapy can be used to decrease the risk of breast cancer in these women and in other women at high risk of the disease (see Chapter 55).

Genitourinary Cancers (Table 56–6)

PROSTATE CANCER AND TESTICULAR CANCER

These cancers are addressed in Chapter 71D.

BLADDER CANCER

Epidemiology and Natural History

Approximately 60,000 patients are diagnosed with bladder cancer each year in the United States. The disease is much less common in women than in men. About one fifth of affected patients will die of their disease. The most important risk factor is cigarette smoking, which accounts for at

Table 56–6 **Genitourinary Cancers**

Tumor Site	Common Findings	Standard Treatments	Expected Outcomes
Testicle	Testicular swelling, pain, back pain Cough with metastatic presentation	Inguinal (not scrotal) orchiectomy Node-positive seminoma: Radiation therapy Node-positive NSGCT: RPLND or chemotherapy	Early-stage seminoma: >90% 5-yr survival Stage III NSGCT: ≈75% 5-yr survival Poor risk tumors: <50%
Prostate	Elevated prostate-specific antigen, decreased urinary stream Bone pain with metastatic presentation	Early-stage: Prostatectomy, radiation therapy, or watchful waiting Treatment recommendations depend on age, likelihood of spread and tumor grade Later-stage tumors: Hormone therapy and/or radiation therapy	Early-stage: ≈80–90% 5-yr survival with surgery and radiation Stages C and D2: Worse prognosis, time to relapse is variable
Bladder	Hematuria, cystitis	Superficial cancers: Cystoscopic resection, biopsy, and intravesical chemotherapy Muscle invasion: Radical cystectomy or bladder-sparing chemotherapy and radiation	10–30% of superficial tumors progress to invasive cancer Muscle invasive disease: 20–50% 5-yr survival; <20% of patients with positive nodal involvement live 5 yr
Renal cell	Hematuria, abdominal pain, and flank mass	Early-stage: Radical nephrectomy Advanced or metastatic disease: High IL-2 or low doses of IL-2 plus interferon	Confined to organ: 5-yr survival Metastatic disease: Median survival is 1 yr; 5-yr survival 0–10%

NSGCT = nonseminomatous germ cell tumor; RPLND = retroperitoneal lymph node dissection; IL-2 = interleukin-2.

least two thirds of all cases. Other risk factors include exposure to polycyclic hydrocarbons in the dye, rubber, and paint industries, as well as long-term exposure to cyclophosphamide and phenacetin and chronic infection with *Schistosoma haematobium*.

Transitional cell carcinoma is the most common histologic type of bladder cancer. These tumors can occur anywhere transitional cell urothelial lining exists, from the renal pelvis through the bladder. Squamous cell cancers and adenocarcinomas of the bladder and renal pelvis are less common and account for only 10% of all tumors in this region.

Symptoms

The most common presentation is gross or microscopic hematuria. Approximately 30% of patients with bladder cancers experience symptoms of bladder irritation or spasms. When this cancer extends beyond the confines of the bladder, the symptoms relate to compression of local structures and may include leg swelling, pelvic pain, and compression of the nerves in the pelvic plexus.

Diagnosis

Bladder cancers are divided into superficial, invasive, and metastatic tumors. The evaluation of bladder cancer requires direct imaging and biopsy to determine the level of tumor invasion. Depth of invasion correlates with prognosis and determines the type of treatment required. Therefore cystoscopy is the most important diagnostic tool. In patients at high occupational risk of developing the disease, urine cytologic examination may be helpful in the absence of symptoms that require cystoscopy. Furthermore, an intravenous pyelogram may be needed if cystoscopy does not localize a tumor in the bladder or ureters.

The most important determinant of prognosis and treatment is whether the tumor has invaded the muscular wall of the bladder. Because the relationship between the depth of invasion detected by cystoscopy and that detected by cystectomy is only 50%, other tools such as a CT scan, an MRI, and a bone scan are important to help define the presence of invasion, nodal involvement, or metastasis. Histologic grade is important because low-grade tumors rarely invade muscle, whereas high-grade cancers do so frequently.

Treatment

Superficial tumors are treated by transurethral resection of the bladder (TURB). Cystoscopy is performed every 3 months to assess response and perform resections when required. For frequent relapses or when superficial cancer involves most of the surface of the bladder, intravesical therapy is recommended. For these patients, immunomodulators such as bacille Calmette-Guérin (BCG) vaccine or interferon or chemotherapeutic agents such as thiotepa or mitoxantrone are instilled in the bladder through a Foley catheter, allowed to dwell for a short time, and then voided. This process is repeated every week for 6 weeks and is followed by cystoscopy to assess response.

Tumors that invade the muscle require more aggressive surgical treatment. If the tumor has invaded muscle but is not through the bladder wall, then the standard approach is radical cystectomy. In this procedure the bladder is removed along with the prostate, seminal vesicles, and proximal urethra in men; in women, a hysterectomy is performed along with a bilateral salpingo-oophorectomy and partial removal of the anterior vaginal wall. Because the bladder is removed, a pouch is created from the small bowel, often called an *ileal conduit,* to store and expel urine. Not all patients with tumors that invade the bladder wall require removal of the bladder. Bladder preservation and a combination of TURB followed or preceded by chemotherapy and radiation may be considered for patients with localized tumors away from the trigone or for those who are unable to tolerate aggressive surgery, although the outcomes of this approach may not be equivalent to radical cystectomy. Chemotherapy after surgery is recommended when bladder cancer is found in lymph nodes or when patients have metastatic disease. Patients with metastatic disease frequently respond to combination chemotherapy containing cisplatin or other agents such as gemcitabine and a taxane, but the tumor invariably relapses.

RENAL CELL CARCINOMA

Epidemiology and Natural History

Renal cell carcinoma, one of the least common tumors of the genitourinary system, accounts for about 3% of all cancers. Some relationship exists between kidney cancer and exposure to cadmium, perhaps in cigarette smoke. Renal cell carcinoma occurs commonly in von Hippel-Lindau disease, in which synchronous, bilateral renal carcinomas occasionally occur. Abnormalities of the long arm of chromosome 3 are observed in more than 90% of patients. Most renal cell carcinomas are adenocarcinomas; a subtype called clear-cell carcinoma represents over 75% of all the tumors removed.

The natural history of kidney cancers is erratic. Some tumors progress relentlessly and are refractory to all interventions, whereas some patients can have spontaneous regression of metastases.

Symptoms

The classic presentation, consisting of hematuria, flank pain, and an abdominal mass, is observed in only 10% of patients. More often, hematuria alone or persistent back pain prompts the patient to seek attention. Many renal cell carcinomas are found during a CT scan performed for unrelated reasons. Occasionally, bilateral lower extremity edema occurs when the tumor has completely occluded the inferior vena cava. Renal cell carcinoma is also associated with some unusual paraneoplastic syndromes, including fever, polycythemia from erythropoietin production, and hypercalcemia from ectopic production of parathyroid hormone (PTH).

Diagnosis

The most common tool to diagnose renal cell carcinoma is CT scanning of the abdomen. A large, dense, contrast-enhancing mass occupies a substantial amount of one kidney and is frequently accompanied by nodal or venous involvement. An MRI or direct injection of dye is recommended to assess inferior vena cava involvement. Because renal cell carcinoma commonly spreads to lungs and liver, a CT evaluation of the chest should be included in the staging procedures.

Treatment

Resection is the most common treatment for cancer limited to the kidney. Surgical treatment may be possible even if parts of the renal vein and vena cava are involved.

Renal cell carcinoma is notably resistant to chemotherapy and radiation. However, renal tumors may respond to biologic response modifiers such as IL-2 and interferon-α in approximately 10% to 15% of patients. Occasionally, these agents induce complete responses. Similar dramatic events have spontaneously occurred. Clinical trials have suggested that nonmyeloablative allogeneic bone marrow transplantation may be effective in some patients with renal cell cancer refractory to other conventional immunotherapy, but the usefulness of this approach is limited by its toxicity and by availability of a suitable donor. Other biological agents such as bevacizumab and sorafenib may shrink metastatic lesions, but they are not curative.

OVARIAN CANCER

Epidemiology

Ovarian cancer occurs in 1 in 60 women in the United States. More than 22,000 cases were diagnosed in the United States in 2005, and 16,000 women died of the disease. As with most cancers, the incidence of ovarian cancer increases with age. Other risk factors include nulliparity and a family history of ovarian cancer. Ovarian cancer is more common in women who have one of the breast cancer–susceptibility genes (see Chapter 55). Exposure to talc may increase the risk of ovarian cancer. Use of oral contraceptives decreases the risk of ovarian cancer, as do more than one pregnancy and breast-feeding.

Pathology

Most malignant ovarian tumors arise from celomic epithelium. Tumors can arise in any part of the peritoneal cavity; thus prophylactic oophorectomy reduces but does not eliminate the risk of ovarian cancer. Epithelial ovarian tumors are classified histologically as benign, malignant, or borderline. The most common histologic types of ovarian cancer are serous, mucinous, and endometrioid. Stromal tumors, most often granulosa cell tumors, and germ cell tumors account for fewer than 15% of ovarian tumors. Cancers from other sites such as the breast and gastrointestinal tract can metastasize to the ovaries.

Clinical Presentation

Symptoms of early ovarian cancer include vague pelvic or abdominal pain, early satiety, and indigestion, but the

symptoms are nonspecific; most patients with ovarian cancer are not diagnosed until the disease is advanced. No effective screening tests exist for ovarian cancer, although transvaginal ultrasound may be helpful in women with an affected first-degree relative and in women who carry a breast cancer–susceptibility gene. Advanced ovarian cancer causes abdominal swelling and pain, intestinal obstruction, and vaginal bleeding. Patients with malignant pleural effusions have stage IV disease.

Staging and Treatment

Ovarian cancer is surgically staged with a total abdominal hysterectomy and bilateral salpingo-oophorectomy, omentectomy, lymph node sampling, and peritoneal biopsies. Stage I disease involves only the ovaries; stage II disease involves extension to the uterus or fallopian tubes; and peritoneal or inguinal lymph node involvement is stage III disease. Many patients have clearly visible peritoneal tumor implants; however, in those who do not, representative biopsy specimens from all areas of the peritoneum should be removed for microscopic examination. Disease outside the pelvis, except for implants on the surface of the liver, is stage IV disease.

The mainstay of treatment for ovarian cancer is surgery. Women whose total residual disease after surgery is less than 2 cm in diameter have an improved prognosis as compared with women who have greater amounts of residual disease.

Combination chemotherapy with paclitaxel and carboplatin is administered postoperatively to women with locally advanced but nonmetastatic ovarian cancer. If first-line therapy fails, additional chemotherapy can be given with responses occurring in 60% of women. Women with metastatic disease at presentation should also have *debulking* surgery. Pleural effusions can be palliated with chemotherapy.

ENDOMETRIAL CANCER

Epidemiology

Endometrial cancer is the fourth most common malignant disease among women in the United States; more than 40,000 cases are diagnosed each year. The tumor is usually found with early-stage disease and is usually curable, with 5-year survival rates of more than 80%. Risk factors for endometrial cancer include increasing age, late menopause, nulliparity, obesity, and previous pelvic radiation. Women who are treated with estrogen without concomitant progesterone and those who do not ovulate are also at increased risk of the disease. Most endometrial cancers are adenocarcinomas.

Clinical Presentation

Most women with endometrial carcinoma have abnormal uterine bleeding. Even minimal postmenopausal bleeding should prompt an evaluation for endometrial cancer. Advanced disease can cause urinary symptoms or back or pelvic pain.

Staging and Treatment

Staging is achieved by surgical exploration. Most endometrial cancers are stage I, with invasion into less than half the uterine wall. More advanced tumors involve the cervix, vagina, pelvic or periaortic lymph nodes, bladder, and rectal mucosa. Metastases outside the pelvis (stage IV disease) are unusual.

Treatment of endometrial cancer is with abdominal hysterectomy, bilateral salpingo-oophorectomy, and peritoneal washings for histologic examination. Lymph node sampling is performed in patients with high-grade tumors. Radiation therapy is given to women with histologically high-grade tumors and those with deep myometrial involvement. Women with advanced disease are treated with megestrol acetate and chemotherapy.

CERVICAL CANCER

Because of widespread screening for cervical cancer with the Papanicolaou (Pap) smear, the incidence of invasive cervical cancer and mortality from cervical cancer have continued to decline in the United States. Cervical cancer and its precursor, cervical intraepithelial neoplasia, are more common in women with HIV infection and those infected with HPV subtypes 16, 18, 31, 33, and 35. The cervical cancer vaccine directed against HPV offers promise of preventing cervical cancer worldwide when administered to women before the onset of sexual activity (see Chapter 55). Most women with cervical intraepithelial neoplasia or cervical cancer are asymptomatic and are found to have the disease by Pap smear. Vaginal bleeding, postcoital bleeding, vaginal discharge, and pelvic pain may occur in women with invasive disease. Signs and symptoms of advanced disease are local pelvic involvement, including leg edema, or back and leg pain. Metastatic disease is rare.

Biopsy of the cervix confirms the diagnosis of cervical cancer in a woman with an abnormal Pap smear. Some women may need cone biopsy if the colposcopy-directed biopsy is inconclusive, does not confirm invasive disease, shows cervical dysplasia, or if the sample is inadequate. The use of other staging tests depends on the extent of local involvement, as determined by pelvic and rectal examination.

Treatment of cervical cancer depends on the stage of the disease. Cone biopsy may be sufficient in women with minimal microscopic invasion into the cervix. Women with more advanced disease undergo radical hysterectomy with lymph node dissection. Combination chemotherapy with 5-FU and cisplatin and radiation therapy are recommended for women with locally advanced disease.

Skin Cancer

BASAL CELL AND SQUAMOUS CELL CARCINOMA

Epidemiology and Natural History

Basal cell and squamous cell carcinomas are the most common cancers of the skin. Mortality from these cancers is exceedingly low, however, accounting for less than 0.1% of cancer deaths. Both types of cancer are more common on parts of the body exposed to sun and in people with light complexions. Although the most significant risk factor is exposure to ultraviolet radiation in sunlight, patients with immunosuppressive disorders (e.g., recipients of organ transplantation) or acquired immunodeficiency syndrome (AIDS), as well as those with genetic disorders such as xeroderma pigmentosum, have a rate of skin cancer incidence that is many times higher than the rate of the general population. Unlike basal cell cancers, which rarely metastasize, squamous cell cancers can spread to regional lymph nodes. Thorough examination of regional lymph nodes is therefore necessary in patients with squamous cell cancer, particularly with squamous cell cancers of the lips, ears, and peri-anal and genital regions.

Treatment

Treatment options for basal cell and squamous cell cancers include surgical excision, radiation therapy, and cryosurgery. Topical fluorouracil may be used for treatment of superficial basal cell carcinomas or in situ squamous cell carcinomas. Dermatologists used Mohs' micrographic surgery, which is a technique that examines serial frozen sections to achieve negative margins on each tumor border. This specialized approach offers the highest local control rates and is indicated for tumors with ill-defined borders or for those occurring in areas where maximum preservation of unaffected tissues is desirable, such as the eyes, nose, and genitalia.

MELANOMA

Epidemiology

The incidence of melanoma is increasing at a rate of 4% per year in the United States. Each year, more than 60,000 new cases are diagnosed, and more than 7000 deaths occur. Incidence rates increase with age and are 10-fold higher in white persons than in black individuals. Melanoma risk factors are similar to those of basal cell and squamous cell skin cancers (see previous discussion) but also include a genetic component such as a personal history of dysplastic nevi and a family history of melanoma.

Pathology

Most melanomas are superficial-spreading melanomas. The antigenic markers S-100 and homatropine methylbromide (HMB-45) can be used to confirm the diagnosis of undifferentiated melanomas, although S-100 is nonspecific and HMB-45 is not 100% sensitive. Ulceration indicates a worse prognosis.

Clinical Presentation

Patients with melanoma most often report a change in a pigmented skin lesion on a sun-exposed surface. Characteristic changes include *a*symmetry, *b*order irregularities, *c*olor variation, *d*iameter more than 6 mm, and *e*nlargement (the ABCDE system). Although 90% of melanomas arise in the skin, melanomas can arise from any area where melanocytes reside, including the choroid of the eye. Approximately 5% of melanomas arise from unknown primary sites. Melanoma can exhibit metastatic disease in lymph nodes, lung, bone, liver, and brain.

Staging

Melanoma is staged according to the thickness of the primary tumor, as measured both in millimeters of the tumor and in the depth of invasion into the skin. The tumor thickness is the single most important prognostic factor. Even without nodal involvement, a melanoma over 4 mm thick on the trunk has more than a 50% chance of distant metastasis. Sentinel lymph node analysis is indicated in patients with high-stage melanomas.

Treatment

Surgical excision with wide margins is required for cure of primary cutaneous lesions. The location and thickness of the lesion determine the optimal surgical margin. Locally recurrent lesions are surgically resected if possible; radiation therapy is given if surgical resection is not possible. In patients with regional lymph node involvement, adjuvant immunotherapy with 12 months of interferon-α may improve relapse-free and overall survival rates. Many patients have severe side effects with interferon-α, such as myalgias and fever, and need to discontinue treatment early.

When metastatic melanomas recur, the best treatment is high-dose interleukin-2 (IL-2). Although 5% to 10% of patients receiving this treatment may become long-term survivors, the toxicity of this approach precludes most patients from receiving it. In such patients, lower-dose interleukin treatments, oral temozolomide, intravenous dacarbazine, or multiagent chemotherapy (often administered with biological agents like IL-2 and interferon) may be offered but are not curative. Radiation therapy is used to treat metastases to the brain, spinal cord, and bone, but melanoma is relatively resistant to radiation therapy.

Cancer of Unknown Primary

Approximately 5% of people with cancer have metastatic disease in the absence of an identifiable primary tumor. Cancer of unknown primary most commonly exhibits disease in the bone, liver, lungs, or lymph nodes. Detailed pathologic examination, aided by immunohistochemical stains, electron microscopy, and chromosomal analysis, will usually distinguish between lymphomas and carcinomas. Such a distinction is important to make because lymphomas tend to be more responsive to therapy, and treatment for lymphomas differs from that for carcinomas. In patients with *adenocarcinoma of unknown primary origin*, limited radiographic examination, such as CT scans of the chest and abdomen, may help identify the site of the primary tumor. Other features of the metastatic disease may be revealing as well. For example, bone metastases are common in prostate and breast cancers, axillary lymphadenopathy is commonly seen in a woman with breast cancer, and liver metastases frequently occur in patients with lung, colon, and pancreatic cancers. Most tumor markers are nonspecific; therefore reliance on a tumor marker alone in identifying a primary source of the cancer is not recommended. However, an elevated tumor marker level may provide supporting evidence for a primary cancer if risk factors for the tumor are present and the clinical pattern of spread is consistent.

Treatment of cancer of unknown primary is geared at palliation of symptoms with surgery, radiation therapy, combination chemotherapy with a broad spectrum of activity (active against a variety of cancers), or hormonal therapy (if the tumor is thought to be from an endocrine-responsive primary source such as prostate or breast cancer). Some people with cancer of unknown primary, such as people with only lymph node involvement, may live free of disease for many years and may be considered cured.

Metastases from Solid Tumors

Most patients who die from cancer generally die from metastatic spread of the primary tumor to distant sites. The process of invasion and metastasis requires each of the following steps: (1) development of the tumor's own vascular supply through angiogenesis, (2) tumor cell invasion through the host tissue basement membrane, (3) tumor embolization through either the lymphatic system or the blood stream (hematogenous spread), (4) arrest and invasion into the basement membrane of the distant organ, (5) reestablishment of blood vessels to sustain growth of the metastatic cells, and (6) proliferation within the target organ. The processes of invasion and metastasis are highly selective, with only 0.01% of circulating cells forming a metastatic focus.

Advances in cancer therapeutics, such as the use of antibodies to the angiogenic molecule vascular endothelial growth factor receptor, are targeted at disrupting neovascularization within malignant cells or at interfering with tumor-cell proliferation. The hope is that targeted therapies used alone or with cytotoxic chemotherapy will improve outcome while minimizing the toxicity to normal tissues (see Chapters 54 and 58).

Surgery for metastatic disease is reserved for palliation of symptoms because surgical resection is not curative and is associated with morbidity itself. In selected patients with metastatic colon cancer to the liver or lung, resection of the metastatic disease may offer a chance for cure.

Prospectus for the Future

Advances in our understanding of cancer causation and epidemiology, disease staging, tumor heterogeneity, and tumor and patient factors involved in response to treatment will all increase our ability to prevent and treat cancer. For example, polymorphisms in drug metabolizing enzymes may explain differences in response to chemotherapy and survival among women with breast cancer. Similarly, microarray technology, which allows analysis of hundreds of genes involved in cell proliferation, can elucidate pathways of resistance to treatment and allow for more precise selection of cytotoxic therapy. Advances in imaging techniques may allow for detection of minimal residual disease, identifying patients who are likely to benefit from additional treatment. Finally, the increasing interest in measuring and improving quality of care will expand the reach of cancer therapies, improving cancer-specific outcomes at the population level.

References

Herr HW: Surgical factors in the treatment of superficial and invasive bladder cancer. Urol Clin North Am 32:157–164, 2005.

Jansen EP, Boot H, Verheij M, et al: Optimal locoregional treatment in gastric cancer. J Clin Oncol 23:4509–4517, 2005.

Meyerhardt JA, Mayer RJ: Drug therapy: Systemic therapy for colorectal cancer. NEJM 352:476–487, 2005.

Piccart-Gebhart MJ et al: For the Herceptin Adjuvant (HERA) Trial Study Team. Trastuzumab after adjuvant chemotherapy in HER2-positive breast cancer. NEJM 353:1659–1672, 2005.

Romond EH, Perez EA, Bryant J, et al: Trastuzumab plus adjuvant chemotherapy for operable HER2-positive breast cancer. NEJM 353:1673–1684, 2005.

Spira A, Ettinger DS: Multidisciplinary management of lung cancer. NEJM 350:379–392, 2004.

Winton T, Livingston R, Johnson D, et al. Vinorelbine plus cisplatin vs. observation in resected non-small-cell lung cancer. NEJM 352:2589–2597, 2005.

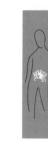

Complications of Cancer and Cancer Treatment

Jennifer J. Griggs

Cancer cells can metastasize to any organ, including the central nervous system. Management of cancer complications requires a multidisciplinary approach. Cancer therapies can also lead to acute and chronic complications.

Venous Thromboembolism

SIGNIFICANCE

Venous thromboembolism (VTE) is one of the most common complications encountered in cancer care. The development of VTE in a patient with cancer is associated with shortened life expectancy. VTE is also the presenting finding in cancer in up to 10% of patients. The hypercoagulable state in patients with cancer is the result of the activation of the coagulation system by neoplastic cells. Cancer chemotherapy further increases the risk of VTE, as does tamoxifen, which is commonly used in the treatment of breast cancer (see Chapter 56). The use of central venous access devices increases the already heightened risk of thrombosis in patients with cancer.

CLINICAL PRESENTATION

The suggestion of VTE should be high in patients with cancer who have dyspnea, cough, wheezing, chest pain, upper abdominal pain, or leg swelling. Even in patients who are ambulatory or on adequate anticoagulation, VTE should remain a consideration. The evaluation of patients with possible VTE is described in Chapter 53.

TREATMENT

In patients with malignant disease, oral anticoagulation is complicated by concurrent and intermittent administration of chemotherapeutic agents, variable nutrition status, and relative resistance to vitamin K antagonists. Low–molecular-weight heparins offer an effective and a safer alternative to oral anticoagulation with warfarin and should be considered

in planning both short- and long-term treatments. Chapter 53 addresses the use of anticoagulation therapy.

Spinal Cord Compression

SIGNIFICANCE

After brain metastases, spinal cord compression is the most common neurologic complication of cancer. Approximately 20,000 patients develop spinal cord compression each year, and most of these patients already have a known diagnosis of a malignant disease. Lung and breast cancers cause approximately 20% of patients to develop spinal cord compression. Lymphoma, sarcoma, multiple myeloma, and prostate and renal cell cancers each account for 6% to 7% of the patients with spinal cord compression. In only 10% of patients is spinal cord compression the first manifestation of cancer. Although the risk of spinal cord compression in a patient with cancer is only 1%, the effects can be devastating. Early recognition of symptoms and intervention usually prevents a complete loss of motor function.

Most compressive tumors occur at the anterior aspect of the spinal cord. Tumor cells disseminate through the blood stream to the bone marrow, where they multiply within the vertebral body and eventually extend posteriorly. Tumors cause necrosis and demyelination of predominantly the lateral and posterior white matter columns. This observation suggests that the obstruction of venous outflow is the cause of the congestion, edema, and hemorrhage within the spinal cord.

CLINICAL PRESENTATION

Approximately 70% of cases of spinal cord compression are thoracic, 20% are lumbosacral, and 10% occur in the cervical region. In 50% of patients, only one vertebral body is involved; in 25% of people, contiguous vertebral bodies are involved. In the remaining patients, multiple noncontiguous vertebral bodies are involved. Most patients complain of back pain that is constant, dull, aching, and progressive. Sneezing, coughing, or neck flexion often exacerbates the pain. In contrast to the pain associated with disc herniation, the pain is usually worse when the patient is in the supine position. Radicular pain may be constant or intermittent and usually localizes to the level of the compression. Bilateral bandlike pain is more common with thoracic disease, whereas unilateral radicular pain is more common with lumbosacral lesions.

Neurologic signs develop insidiously: (1) weakness, particularly exhibiting difficulty with proximal leg function, causes difficulty in climbing stairs, which occurs in about 80% of patients; (2) paresthesias; (3) ataxia, which is the result of proprioceptive impairment; and (4) autonomic dysfunction, including loss of bowel and bladder function. Weakness, sensory loss, ataxia, and autonomic dysfunction can all progress rapidly and may lead to paraplegia if treatment is not rapidly instituted.

DIAGNOSIS

Physical examination can usually suggest the diagnosis and identify the level of spinal cord involvement. Radiologic tests should initially focus on the suspected area of involvement but should also include a thorough evaluation of the entire spine. The rapidity and severity of symptoms and signs determine how quickly diagnostic tests should be performed.

Plain radiographs are abnormal in 70% of patients with spinal cord compression. Among patients with pain, more than 80% will have abnormal radiographs. Typical radiographic findings include destruction of the pedicle and vertebral body collapse. Magnetic resonance imaging and computed tomography (CT) provide more information than do plain radiographs, and CT scans are superior in evaluating vertebral stability and bone destruction in patients undergoing surgical decompression.

TREATMENT

Loss of ambulation or sphincter function before treatment predicts a poor response to treatment. Goals of treatment are to prevent loss of neurologic function, palliate pain, prevent local recurrence, and preserve spinal stability.

Corticosteroids should be administered immediately. An intravenous bolus of dexamethasone, 10 mg, with subsequent doses of 4 to 24 mg every 6 hours, is recommended for most patients. In highly selected patients with a single area of metastatic epidural spinal cord compression, immediate and direct decompressive surgical resection followed by radiation therapy is superior to radiation therapy alone. In patients with multiple sites of spinal cord compression or in those with highly radiosensitive cancers (e.g., lymphoma, multiple myeloma, germ cell tumors), radiation therapy is preferred. Surgical treatment is clearly needed in patients with spinal instability, in those without a histologic diagnosis, and in those who again develop epidural compression after or during radiation therapy.

Superior Vena Cava Syndrome

SIGNIFICANCE

Superior vena cava (SVC) syndrome is the result of obstruction of blood flow caused by compression or invasion of the SVC by tumor thrombi. The SVC is a thin-walled, low-pressure vessel surrounded by rigid structures that make it vulnerable to metastatic disease in adjacent lymph nodes. The SVC collateral vessels, including the azygos vein and the internal mammary, paraspinous, lateral thoracic, and esophageal veins, lessen the obstruction of flow. The azygos vein is the most important of these collateral vessels; SVC obstruction below the level of the azygos vein is not well tolerated.

Cancer is the cause of SVC syndrome in 80% of patients. Lung cancer is responsible for 80% of these cases, and lymphoma, breast cancer, and germ cell tumors account for the majority of the others. Nonmalignant causes include mediastinal fibrosis (e.g., histoplasmosis) and thrombosis of central venous catheters and pacemakers.

CLINICAL FINDINGS

Symptoms begin insidiously and are often worse on bending, stooping, or lying down. Symptoms include dyspnea, occurring in 60% to 70% of patients, and facial fullness, which occurs in 50% of patients. Cough, arm swelling, chest pain, and dysphagia may occur. Physical findings include venous distention of the neck and chest wall (60%), facial edema (50%), plethora and cyanosis (each in 20% of patients), and arm edema (10%).

DIAGNOSIS AND TREATMENT

Chest radiography shows mediastinal widening in two thirds of these patients and a pleural effusion in one fourth. A right hilar mass is observed in up to 15% of patients. CT scans can demonstrate the size, shape, and location of a mass; the extent of obstruction; and options for biopsy. Venography is not routinely obtained, but it may show patency of an SVC initially thought to be completely obstructed.

Treatment of the SVC syndrome requires a histologic diagnosis of the tumor before radiation or chemotherapy. Radiation to an occlusive mass can alter the tumor enough to preclude identification of the tumor type. Biopsy of a palpable supraclavicular or cervical node, thoracentesis, sputum cytologic analysis, mediastinoscopy, thoracoscopy, and percutaneous needle biopsy of the obstructing tumor are options for diagnosis.

The goals of treatment are to alleviate the obstruction and to attempt a cure. SVC occlusion does not change the prognosis of the underlying tumor. Small-cell lung cancer, lymphoma, and germ cell tumors are best treated with chemotherapy alone or chemotherapy combined with radiation therapy. Radiation therapy alone is preferred for tumors of all other histologic types.

Endothelial stents may successfully relieve a venous obstruction, even in patients with SVC thrombus. Corticosteroids may improve symptoms in patients with cancers that respond to the cytolytic effects of steroids, such as breast cancer, lymphoma, and, occasionally, germ cell tumors. Corticosteroids are not effective in relieving symptoms in patients with lung cancer.

Hypercalcemia

SIGNIFICANCE

Hypercalcemia occurs with all types of cancer but most commonly in multiple myeloma and breast cancer. In patients with extensive osteolytic bone disease, the secretion of the parathyroid hormone–related polypeptide by the tumor, along with other cytokines such as transforming growth factor-α, interleukin-6, and tumor necrosis factor, causes hypercalcemia. The possibility of hypercalcemia should be considered in all patients with cancer who exhibit a change in mental status.

CLINICAL FINDINGS

The symptoms of hypercalcemia depend less on the absolute serum calcium level than on the time course over which the hypercalcemia develops. Common symptoms are constipation, polydipsia, polyuria, fatigue, nausea, vomiting, and bradycardia. Most patients with hypercalcemia have volume depletion. Patients are often confused and may be obtunded. Muscle stretch reflexes are often hyperactive.

TREATMENT

Treatment of hypercalcemia uses two strategies: increasing urinary calcium excretion and decreasing bone resorption (Table 57–1). Drugs such as thiazide diuretics, those that decrease renal blood flow (e.g., histamine$_2$-blockers, nonsteroidal anti-inflammatory drugs), calcium-containing drugs, and vitamins A and D should be stopped immediately.

Fluid replacement at a rate of 300 to 400 mL/hr for 3 to 4 hours should be given, with frequent monitoring of electrolytes. Such rapid fluid replacement should be seen as rehydration rather than as primary therapy. Drugs that decrease bone resorption should be administered as soon as the patient is rehydrated. Bisphosphonates are the most commonly used antiresorptive drugs; pamidronate, at a dose of 60 to 90 mg, is administered over 2 to 4 hours. The major side effects of pamidronate are fever and myalgias. Finally, furosemide, which inhibits calcium absorption in the thick ascending loop of Henle, is a useful calciuretic agent.

Gallium nitrate is a more potent inhibitor of bone resorption and induces normocalcemia in 70% to 90% of patients. Calcitonin, at a dose of 6 to 8 U/kg intramuscularly every 6 hours for 48 hours, is a weak hypocalcemic agent but has a rapid onset of action. Calcitonin can be used concurrently with pamidronate and gallium. Corticosteroids can be used to treat hypercalcemia caused by hematologic malignancies; patients with breast cancer occasionally respond to steroids.

Patients can be treated as outpatients if (1) the serum calcium concentration is less than 12 mg/dL, (2) they have no significant nausea and only mild constipation, (3) they are able to take fluids orally, (4) mentation is intact, (5) creatinine levels are normal, (6) they have a stable cardiac rhythm, and (7) a companion is available to observe them. Immediate inpatient management is indicated in all other situations.

Unless the underlying malignant disease is treated, hypercalcemia will persist or recur. Appropriate management of hypercalcemia therefore requires an attempt to control the cancer itself. Hypercalcemia that responds poorly to the previously discussed measures indicates a poor prognosis.

In patients with metastatic breast cancer undergoing effective treatment, hypercalcemia can develop as part of a treatment *flare*. Typically, such a response is characterized by bone pain and hypercalcemia, sometimes severe, occurring within 2 to 6 weeks of starting a new therapy. If symptoms are due to successful treatment, then resolution typically occurs within 12 weeks. Technetium imaging with a bone scan may show greater activity than at baseline and may even demonstrate new bone lesions.

Table 57–1 Management of Hypercalcemia

Outpatient Management of Hypercalcemia

Preferably administer therapy for hypercalcemia with cytotoxic therapy (e.g., chemotherapy, radiation therapy)
Provide clear instructions about oral intake of fluids
Avoid thiazide diuretics; furosemide is acceptable
Administer pamidronate once a week
Administer gallium nitrate subcutaneously daily to minimize rebound hypercalcemia after acute normalization

Inpatient Management of Hypercalcemia

Administer intravenous fluids immediately
Administer antiresorptive therapy once good urine output is established
Administer pamidronate twice every 48–72 hr
Administer gallium nitrate (5-day infusion)
Cross over to another therapy if no response occurs
Administer calcitonin for the comatose patient or for the patient with cardiac irritability
Administer mithramycin for nonresponding patients only
Consider dialysis in patients with renal insufficiency

Paraneoplastic Syndromes

Tumors have disease manifestations through immunologic and metabolic factors that are not the direct result of invasion by neoplastic cells. These *paraneoplastic syndromes* may appear before the diagnosis of cancer is made. Because detection and treatment of the underlying malignant disease may improve the syndrome and occasionally may facilitate cure of the cancer, recognition of paraneoplastic syndromes is important.

Several of the paraneoplastic syndromes are the result of autoantibodies produced in response to the tumor, whereas others are the result of the hormonal production of ectopic peptide by the tumor. Tumor cells may also secrete hormones that are structurally distinct from the normal hormone; some of these are less active biologically than the normal hormone. The most common paraneoplastic syndrome is humoral hypercalcemia of malignancy, a condition usually caused by secretion by the tumor of the parathyroid hormone–related polypeptide. Table 57–2 lists the endocrinologic, neurologic, and hematologic paraneoplastic syndromes. Cutaneous syndromes, such as necrotizing migratory erythema and dermatomyositis, and gastrointestinal syndromes can also occur.

Table 57–2 Paraneoplastic Syndromes

Syndrome	Associated Tumors	Mechanism
Ectopic ACTH production	Small-cell lung cancer, pancreatic cancer, pheochromocytoma	Tumor secretion of ACTH precursor
SIADH	Lung cancer, head and neck tumors, brain tumors	Ectopic production of antidiuretic hormone
Cerebellar degeneration and peripheral neuropathy	Lung, ovarian, breast cancers; lymphoma (especially Hodgkin's disease)	Autoantibodies, including antibodies to Purkinje cells (anti-YO antibodies) and anti-Hu antibodies
Opsoclonus-myoclonus	Lung cancer Neuroblastoma (in children)	No consistent findings; some patients have anti-HU antibodies
Lambert-Eaton myasthenic syndrome	Small-cell lung cancer	Antibody production against calcium channels in presynaptic nerve terminal
Erythrocytosis	Renal cell carcinoma, hepatoma	Tumor production of erythropoietin
Thrombophlebitis	Pancreatic cancer, adenocarcinomas	Uncertain

ACTH = adrenocorticotropic hormone; SIADH = syndrome of inappropriate secretion of antidiuretic hormone; anti-HU = antineuronal.

Table 57–3 Long-Term Complications of Cancer Treatment

Treatment	Examples of Long-Term Complications
Surgery	Loss of vocal function after laryngectomy for laryngeal cancer Malabsorption after bowel resection Erectile dysfunction and incontinence after radical prostatectomy Premature menopause after oophorectomy Postmastectomy pain and upper extremity lymphedema
Radiation therapy	Pulmonary fibrosis after mediastinal or lung radiation Esophageal stricture after esophageal radiation Secondary malignancies (e.g., breast cancer after radiation therapy for Hodgkin's disease) Chronic breast fibrosis after breast radiation Neurocognitive deficits after whole brain radiation Loss of salivary gland function after radiation for cancers of the head and neck Premature atherosclerosis after mediastinal radiation
Chemotherapy	Cardiac dysfunction from prolonged exposure to anthracycline treatments Peripheral neuropathy from taxanes, cisplatin, and vinca alkaloids Pulmonary toxicity from bleomycin Secondary leukemia from cyclophosphamide and etoposide Premature menopause
Hormonal therapy	Endometrial cancer from tamoxifen Thromboembolic events related to tamoxifen Loss of bone mineral density related to aromatase inhibitors and luteinizing hormone–releasing hormone agonists

Long-Term Effects of Cancer and Cancer Treatment

People who have been successfully treated for cancer may experience long-term effects of the cancer and its treatment. Surgery, chemotherapy, radiation therapy, hormonal therapy, and biologic therapies can all have adverse effects that persist long after disease control, remission, or cure is achieved. Such long-term sequelae of cancer treatments are increasingly important as the number of cancer survivors increases and as the indications for chemotherapy and radiation broaden. Table 57–3 lists some of the long-term physical complications of cancer therapies.

In addition to the physical effects of cancer treatments, people who have survived cancer face a number of other issues, such as psychological consequences, sexual dysfunction, and employment and insurance discrimination. Although most people can expect to return to their previous activities, most survivors report being affected in at least one of these areas. The impact of cancer on the family, including parents and siblings, partner, and children, persists long after cancer treatment is complete. Most people who have had cancer indicate that the disease and its treatment are life-changing events.

Prospectus for the Future

Advances in the management of cancer are likely to decrease the risk of catastrophic and permanent complications of cancer treatment. Selection of patients who are likely to reap the survival benefits of treatment will decrease the numbers of patients living with the long-term effects of treatment. Similarly, identifying patients at high risk of complications, such as thromboembolism, will lead to prevention strategies for those most likely to benefit from such strategies.

References

Dropcho EJ: Update on paraneoplastic syndromes. Curr Opin Neurol 18:331–336, 2005.

Hahn SM: Oncologic emergencies. In Bennett JC, Plum F (eds): Cecil Textbook of Medicine, 20th ed. Philadelphia, WB Saunders, 1996, pp 1049–1054.

Lee AY, Levine MN, Baker RI, et al: Low-molecular-weight heparin versus a coumarin for the prevention of recurrent venous thromboembolism in patients with cancer. N Engl J Med 349:146–53, 2003.

Patchell RA, Tibbs PA, Regine WF, et al: Direct decompressive surgical resection in the treatment of spinal cord compression caused by metastatic cancer: A randomized trial. Lancet 366:643–648, 2005.

Chapter 58

Principles of Cancer Therapy

Alok A. Khorana

Barbara A. Burtness

The treatment of cancer is in the midst of a quiet revolution. Chemotherapy continues to be the mainstay of systemic treatment, but the explosion of knowledge regarding cancer biology has allowed research efforts to focus on the development of more specific *targeted* agents. The annual number of new drugs approved for cancer treatment has increased several fold since the 1990s. In addition, nearly 400 anticancer agents are now in clinical trials, more than for any other class of medicine. Surgery and radiation therapy techniques continue to be refined, and these techniques are safe and effective treatments for localized cancers. Despite these advances, cancer is still the second leading cause of death in the United States, and considerable resources are devoted to the palliative care of patients with cancer. The treatment of cancer involves multiple disciplines and requires that surgeons, medical professionals, and radiation oncologists work in an integrated fashion to deliver the best possible care to the patient. This chapter reviews the principles of surgical, radiation, and medical approaches to cancer at various points during its natural history. Prerequisites to starting treatment, such as diagnosis and staging, as well as supportive care interventions that can improve the safety of cancer treatments, are also discussed.

Diagnosis and Staging

Definitive treatment for cancer must not commence without a histologic diagnosis, except under urgent circumstances. This histologic diagnosis generally involves an invasive biopsy that obtains sufficient material to evaluate morphology, invasiveness of the tumor, and expression of various molecular markers using immunohistochemistry. Noninvasive tests, such as radiologic imaging, should not be accepted as substitutes for tissue diagnosis.

Once the diagnosis of cancer has been made, the next step is to determine systematically the extent of tumor spread, a process called *staging*. Tumor staging can be a clinical or pathologic determination. *Clinical staging* involves physical examination and imaging studies, including computed tomographic (CT) scans, whole-body positron-emission tomography (PET) scans, and radionuclide scans. The choice of studies for particular tumors is based on the accepted knowledge of the tumor's propensity to spread to particular organs. *Pathologic staging* is more definitive and follows the tumor-node-metastasis (TNM) method developed by the American Joint Committee on Cancer and the International Union Against Cancer. This system requires a careful evaluation of the primary resection specimen for three measurements: (1) the size and extent of invasion of the primary tumor (the T score), (2) the number and location of histologically involved regional lymph nodes (the N score), and (3) the presence or absence of distant metastases (the M score). The M score is based on information derived from both clinical and pathologic staging. TNM scores are then grouped into categories of stages from I through IV, reflecting an increasing burden of disease. The final TNM stage has both prognostic and therapeutic implications. For instance, a resected colon cancer that invades the muscularis propria involves 2 of the 16 lymph nodes but has no evidence of distant metastases is staged as a T2N1M0 (stage III) colon cancer. The likelihood of tumor recurrence is 40% to 50%, and 6 months of chemotherapy is recommended to the patient after surgery. On the other hand, if no lymph nodes are involved (T2N0M0, stage I), the likelihood of recurrence is less than 10%, and no chemotherapy is recommended.

Biomarkers provide additional prognostic information; as an example, the absence of hormone receptors or expression of HER-2/neu in breast cancer is indicative of a poor prognosis. Such markers can also be predictive; the presence of HER-2/neu predicts for a positive antineoplastic response to trastuzumab and the presence of hormone receptors predicts for a positive antineoplastic response to tamoxifen. Prognostic and predictive biomarkers are available for different cancers, but these are not standardized and most biomarkers have not been integrated into formal staging. Gene expression signatures that provide prognostic information beyond those that are already available from formal staging have been identified for certain cancers. These await clinical standardization as well. For certain tumors, measurement of serum levels of tumor markers (e.g., carcinoembryonic antigen in colon cancer, α-fetoprotein in testicular and liver cancers) can also be of prognostic importance.

An evaluation of the patient's major organ functions and other illnesses must also be conducted before treatment can commence. In addition, when the intent of treatment is palliative and not curative, the patient's functional ability, termed *performance status,* must be assessed. This assessment can be done using various history-based methods, such as the Eastern Cooperative Oncology Group (ECOG) or Karnofsky scales. Patients with poor performance status or significant co-morbid conditions may not derive a benefit from chemotherapy and are at greater risk of significant adverse events.

Principles of Cancer Surgery

The surgeon is involved in the care of the patient with cancer at various times.

- Preventing cancer by removing precancerous lesions or organs at high risk of cancer
- Performing a bilateral mastectomy in the patient with hereditary defects that can lead to breast cancer
- Making the diagnosis of cancer by biopsy
- Providing definitive treatment by removing the primary tumor
- Assisting in staging by sampling lymph nodes
- Reconstructing the sacrificed limb or organ
- Providing palliative treatment of cancer (e.g., intestinal bypass for obstruction, spinal cord decompression, orthopedic procedures to prevent or treat pathologic fractures)

Interventional radiologists rather than surgeons are increasingly performing invasive biopsies and certain minor surgical procedures, such as inserting permanent intravenous access devices or temporary feeding tubes.

When cancer is localized, surgery is the most effective curative treatment available. The intent is to remove the tumor, regional lymph nodes, and adjacent involved tissue completely, with a safe margin of normal tissue. At surgery, the tumor is isolated and almost never opened during the procedure. Refinements in cancer surgery include increased use of laparoscopic procedures in selected patients and the identification of a sentinel lymph node by injecting a dye during surgery and foregoing a full lymph node dissection if the sentinel node is uninvolved by cancer.

Principles of Radiation Therapy

Over one half of all patients with cancer receive radiation therapy at some point during the course of their disease. Radiation therapy can be used as definitive treatment, either alone or in combination with chemotherapy. Unlike surgery, locoregional treatment with radiation can preserve organ structure and function, thereby resulting in enhanced quality of life for patients. For example, the use of radiation with chemotherapy for the treatment of localized laryngeal cancer has similar outcomes compared with surgery, but it allows for the preservation of the larynx. Radiation therapy is also effective in the palliative setting in relieving many symptoms of advanced cancer, particularly pain.

Ionizing radiation damages cellular DNA directly or indirectly through free-radical intermediates. Cells are most susceptible to radiation during the M and G2 phases of the cell cycle. The aim of radiation therapy is to deliver the highest dose possible to the tumor with minimal toxicity to adjacent normal tissues. Dividing the total planned radiation dose into small daily fractions takes advantage of the difference in repair capability between normal and malignant tissues and improves the tolerance of normal tissue. The biologic effects of radiation can be modified by numerous factors, including the amount of oxygen in the irradiated tissue and the use of chemotherapy for sensitizing tissue to radiation.

The goal of treatment planning for radiation therapy is to define precisely the dose and volume irradiated. The dose of radiation is measured in units of absorbed dose; Gray (Gy) has replaced the older unit rad (1 Gy = 100 rads). Conventional radiation treatments deliver 1.8 to 2 Gy per day, 5 days per week for over 5 to 6 weeks. For palliative treatment, higher doses per fraction are used to deliver an effective dose over a shorter period.

Ionizing radiation can be administered as external beam therapy using a linear accelerator to generate electrons or high-energy x-ray beams. Electrons have a limited depth of penetration and are useful for superficial tumors. High-energy x-ray beams deliver the radiation deep into the body, while reducing the dose to the skin as they enter. Brachytherapy uses radioactive sources to deliver ionizing radiation (gamma rays) directly to the tumor. An example of brachytherapy is implantation of iodine-125 seeds into the prostate as definitive therapy for early prostate cancer. Current approaches to improving radiation therapy include the use of advanced software that allows delivery of a higher dose of radiation to specific areas of the tumor while sparing normal tissue (e.g., conformal and intensity-modulated radiation therapy).

Normal tissue response to radiation therapy can be acute or late (Table 58–1). Acute effects occur within days to weeks of irradiation and are observed primarily in rapidly proliferating tissues such as skin and gastrointestinal mucosa. The severity depends on the total dose, but the damage can usually be repaired. Late effects, such as necrosis, fibrosis, or organ failure appear months or years after irradiation and are dependent on fraction size. Another late complication of radiation therapy is the development of secondary malignancies. This development has been documented after radiation for breast cancer and Hodgkin's disease.

Principles of Medical Therapy

The term *chemotherapy* refers to the use of cytotoxic agents, singly or in combination, for the systemic treatment of cancer. Most such agents are general antiproliferative agents that are more effective against rapidly growing tumors and have significant adverse effects on normal tissues that also divide rapidly, such as bone marrow and digestive tract mucosa. Newer agents, including monoclonal antibodies and signal-transduction inhibitors, are directed against targets that are relatively specific to tumor cells and therefore have less toxicity. These drugs are classified separately from chemotherapy as *targeted*-therapeutic agents.

Table 58–1 Acute and Late Effects of Radiation Therapy

Organ	Acute	Late	Dose (Gy) Associated with Adverse Effects
Bone marrow	Aplasia	Leukemia, myelodysplasia	25
Spinal cord	None	Myelopathy	45
Heart	None	Pericarditis, cardiomyopathy, coronary artery disease	45
Rectum	Diarrhea, tenesmus	Stricture, obstruction	60
Eye	Conjunctivitis	Retinopathy	55
Lung	Pneumonitis	Chronic pneumonitis	25

Table 58–2 Commonly Used Chemotherapeutic Agents

Drug	Cancers Treated	Specific Class and Mechanism of Action	Common Side Effects
Cell Cycle–Specific			
5-fluorouracil	Colorectal and other gastrointestinal, head and neck, breast	Antimetabolite, inhibits thymidylate synthase	Myelosuppression, mucositis, diarrhea
Gemcitabine	Pancreas, lung, breast, bladder	Antimetabolite, deoxycytidine analog	Myelosuppression, N/V
Methotrexate	ALL, choriocarcinoma, breast, bladder, head and neck, lymphoma	Antimetabolite, folic acid antagonist	Myelosuppression, mucositis, acute renal failure
Doxorubicin	Breast, lung, NHL	Anthracycline, intercalates into DNA	Myelosuppression, N/V, mucositis, cardiomyopathy
Irinotecan	Colorectal, lung	Camptothecin, topoisomerase I inhibitor	Myelosuppression, diarrhea
Paclitaxel	Breast, lung, Kaposi's sarcoma, ovarian	Plant alkaloid, inhibits microtubule formation	Myelosuppression, hypersensitivity reaction, sensory neuropathy
Vincristine	ALL, lymphomas, myeloma, sarcoma	Plant alkaloid, disrupts microtubule assembly	Peripheral neuropathy, constipation
Cell Cycle–Nonspecific			
Cyclophosphamide	Breast, NHL, CLL, sarcoma	Alkylating agent, cross links DNA	Myelosuppression, hemorrhagic cystitis, N/V, alopecia
Cisplatin	Lung, bladder, ovarian, testicular, cervical, head and neck	Alkylating agent, cross links DNA	Nephrotoxicity, N/V, myelosuppression, sensory neuropathy

ALL = acute lymphoblastic leukemia, N/V = nausea and vomiting, NHL = non-Hodgkin's lymphoma, CLL = chronic lymphocytic leukemia.

MECHANISMS OF CHEMOTHERAPY

Chemotherapeutic agents can be cell cycle–specific or cell cycle–nonspecific. Cell cycle–nonspecific agents have a greater effect on cells traversing the cell cycle, but they also affect noncycling cells, whereas cell cycle–specific agents affect only cycling cells. Chemotherapeutic agents are further classified according to their mechanism of action into alkylating agents, antimetabolites, antitumor antibiotics, and mitotic spindle inhibitors. Commonly used chemotherapeu-

tic agents, their mechanisms of action, major indications, and common side effects are described in Table 58–2. A prominent side effect of most chemotherapeutic agents is bone marrow suppression. This, in turn, can lead to infections from neutropenia and life-threatening bleeding from thrombocytopenia. For most drugs, treatment schedules have been developed during which successive doses are given once every 3 to 4 weeks. This interval between successive doses, called a *cycle* of chemotherapy, allows recovery of blood counts and other side effects before administering the next dose. The concept of *dose intensity* is also important. Cellular killing with chemotherapy follows first-order kinetics; a given dose of drug kills only a fraction of tumor cells. The dose-response curve for chemotherapeutic drugs is steep; that is, the greater the dose administered, the greater the kill. A two-fold increase in dose can lead to a ten-fold increase in tumor cell kill. Unfortunately, this also means that a dose reduction of only 20% may lead to a decrease of up to 50% in the eventual cure rate. Arbitrary reductions in doses of chemotherapy to spare patients anticipated toxicity must therefore be avoided at all costs. Shortening the interval between cycles of chemotherapy to 2 weeks using growth-factor support, termed the *dose-dense* approach, has been shown to improve survival in some patient groups with breast cancer when compared with dosing every 3 weeks.

With rare exceptions, single chemotherapeutic agents cannot cure cancer. Combination chemotherapeutic regimens have therefore been developed for a variety of cancers. Combination therapy provides maximal cell kill, broader coverage of resistant cell lines, and may prevent or slow the development of resistant cells. Drugs used in a combination are chosen on the basis of known efficacy as a single agent but with differing mechanisms of action and nonoverlapping toxicity profiles. These regimens are commonly referred to by acronyms: CHOP (cyclophosphamide, doxorubicin, vincristine and prednisone) for lymphoma and CMF (cyclophosphamide, methotrexate and 5-fluorouracil) for breast cancer.

INDICATIONS FOR CHEMOTHERAPY

Chemotherapy is most often used in the treatment of metastatic disease where surgery or radiation therapy is insufficient in controlling disease. In this setting, chemotherapy can be occasionally curative, such as in certain lymphomas or testicular cancers. Even when it is not curative, however, chemotherapy can often extend survival and improve cancer-related symptoms and the patient's quality of life (Table 58–3). *Adjuvant* chemotherapy refers to its use after the primary tumor has been resected. Chemotherapy is directed against presumed systemic micrometastases in patients believed to be at high risk for recurrence. In the example of stage III colon cancer previously cited, 6 months of adjuvant chemotherapy after colonic resection can reduce the likelihood of recurrent cancer from 50% to 25%. Adjuvant chemotherapy has been shown to increase cure rates in breast and lung cancers as well. *Neoadjuvant* or *primary* chemotherapy refers to the use of chemotherapy before surgery, sometimes in combination with radiation therapy. Neoadjuvant therapy can reduce the size of the tumor and consequently permit less radical surgery if successful (e.g., a lumpectomy instead of a mastectomy in breast cancer, limb-sparing surgery instead of amputation in extremity sarcoma). In certain tumor sites, such as larynx or anal canal, neoadjuvant therapy can be so successful that it can lead to a complete obliteration of the tumor and avoid the need for surgery altogether.

EVALUATION OF RESPONSE

The efficacy of chemotherapy is gauged by various methods and has been granted its own vocabulary. In patients with

Table 58–3	**Efficacy of Medical Therapy in Selected Cancers**

Cure Possible in Advanced Setting

Testicular cancer
Acute leukemias: lymphocytic, promyelocytic, selected myelocytic
Lymphomas: Hodgkin's, selected non-Hodgkin's
Childhood solid tumors: rhabdomyosarcoma, Ewing's sarcoma, Wilms' tumor
Choriocarcinoma
Small-cell lung cancer

Cure Possible in Adjuvant Setting

Breast cancer
Colorectal cancer
Osteosarcoma
Non-small cell lung cancer

Increased Survival and Palliation in Advanced Disease

Colorectal cancer
Breast cancer
Ovarian cancer
Head and neck cancer
Bladder cancer
Small cell lung cancer
Multiple myeloma

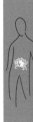

metastatic disease, physical examination and serial radiologic imaging monitor all known sites of disease. Disappearance of all known lesions is called a *complete response,* whereas a 30% or greater reduction in long diameter is called a *partial response.* Appearance of new lesions or an increase in the size of known lesions by 20% is termed *progression* and implies failure of treatment. A cancer that is neither responding nor progressing is termed *stable disease.* The percentage of patients who experience a response is called the *response rate* to the agent or agents being given. New drugs are often evaluated on the basis of response rates. It is important for both patient and physician to realize, however, that response rates do not imply cure. A drug with even a 100% response rate is not curative if all patients relapse within, for example, 6 months. Therefore the gold standard for measuring the efficacy of a drug is considered to be an improvement in *survival* or its surrogate, *disease-free survival*—the time interval when no disease is present. The use of effective second-line therapies may minimize the survival differences between two treatments prescribed as initial therapy; in this context, disease-free survival can serve as an important endpoint in evaluating new regimens. Increasingly, quality of life endpoints, such as the use of pain medications or analysis of patient-filled questionnaires, are being used to assess efficacy of drugs given with palliative intent. In patients receiving adjuvant therapy, response rates cannot be measured because no disease is clinically evident: disease-free and overall survival rates are the only endpoints of efficacy in this setting. Serial measurement of tumor markers can also be useful in identifying recurrence of cancer and monitoring response to therapy.

LIMITATIONS OF CHEMOTHERAPY

Despite the wide use of chemotherapy, it is now understood that chemotherapy can be curative only under certain circumstances. Several reasons exist for the inability of standard doses of chemotherapy to cure cancer. First, tumor-cell kinetics naturally protect against chemotherapy. When chemotherapy was initially developed, it was believed that tumors contained a very high percentage of cells traversing the cell cycle. However, it is now known that most human tumors display Gompertzian growth kinetics (i.e., the rate of tumor-cell doubling *slows* progressively as the tumor size increases). Thus the growth fraction of tumors is greatest when a tumor is clinically undetectable. However, when the patient is symptomatic and has clinically evident disease, the growth fraction of tumors is less than 5%. This partly explains why chemotherapy can be successful in the adjuvant setting (when the burden of disease is minimal) but rarely results in cures in the metastatic setting. Secondly, cancer cells can be resistant to chemotherapy. One of the most important forms of resistance is intrinsic and is mediated by an evolutionarily conserved cell membrane efflux pump called the P-glycoprotein. Resistance can also be acquired after a period of exposure to chemotherapeutic agents by a variety of mechanisms; for example, tumor cells can decrease the uptake of methotrexate by decreasing the expression of the folate transporter or amplifying the expression of the target enzyme thymidylate synthase when treated with 5-fluorouracil. Finally, mutations in the *p53* gene are quite common in various cancers. The *p53* protein causes cell-cycle arrest and mediates apoptosis when DNA damage occurs. In the absence of a functioning *p53*, cancer cells are protected from chemotherapy-induced apoptosis.

STEM CELL TRANSPLANT

One way of overcoming the limitations of chemotherapy is to increase the dose given to patients. A major obstacle to delivering higher doses, however, is the possibility of life-threatening complications that can result from bone marrow suppression. Stem cell transplantation is a procedure whereby patients are given myeloablative doses of chemotherapy (sometimes with radiation therapy), and then "rescued" with infusions of peripheral blood or bone marrow stem cells that reconstitute the ablated bone marrow. The source of stem cells can be the patients themselves (*autologous* transplant) or a human leukocyte antigen-matched related or unrelated donor (*allogeneic* transplant). Stem cell transplant has been shown to improve survival in selected patients with chronic myelogenous leukemia, relapsed Hodgkin's and non-Hodgkin's lymphoma, refractory acute myelogenous leukemia, and multiple myeloma. Allogeneic transplants are more successful in inducing cures than autologous transplants because of the immunologic response mounted by the donor cells, termed *graft-versus-malignancy* effect. Newer approaches to stem cell transplantation take advantage of this phenomenon by using lower, nonmyeloablative doses of chemotherapy and relying on the graft-versus-malignancy effect to achieve tumor remissions. However, allogeneic transplants can only be offered to a minority of patients because of the limited availability of matched donors (particularly in ethnic minorities) and the inability of older patients and those with co-morbid illnesses to tolerate this procedure. To increase the availability of donors, umbilical cord blood is increasingly being studied as a source of stem cells.

The complications of stem cell transplantation are primarily related to the toxicity of chemotherapy and radiation therapy to vital organs, including lungs and liver. Long-term morbidity and mortality in allogeneic transplants can result from *graft-versus-host disease* and from complications of immunosuppressive agents used to treat it.

TARGETED THERAPY

The limitations of chemotherapy, coupled with a greater understanding of cancer cell biology, have led to the development of a new class of drugs that are directed against targets that are relatively specific to cancer cells. These targets include growth factors and signaling molecules that are essential for the proliferation of tumor cells, cell-cycle proteins, regulators of apoptosis, and molecules that promote interactions between the tumor and host tissues, such as angiogenesis. Agents developed against these targets are also quite diverse and include monoclonal antibodies directed against cell-surface antigens or growth factors, specific receptor tyrosine kinase inhibitors, specific pathway signal transduction inhibitors, antisense oligonucleotides, and gene therapies. Many of these agents are still in development. The usual side effects associated with chemotherapy such as myelosuppression, nausea and emesis, and alopecia are not observed with targeted drugs. However, other unique toxicities are seen. Commonly used targeted therapeutic agents, their mechanisms of action, major indications, and common side effects are described in Table 58–4.

The best-known targeted therapeutic agent is imatinib (Gleevec), which inhibits *bcr-abl*, the constitutively active fusion product arising from the Philadelphia chromosome of chronic myelogenous leukemia (CML), and *c-kit* (CD117), which is over-expressed in gastrointestinal stromal tumors (GIST) (Fig. 58–1). The daily oral administration of imatinib results in complete hematologic responses in over 90% of patients with CML and partial responses in over 50% of patients with metastatic GIST. Although a major advance over traditional treatment for these malignancies, imatinib is not considered curative in most patients. Drug resistance to imatinib, in the form of a mutation in the kinase domain of *abl* that leads to poor binding of the drug, has been observed.

The success of imatinib as a single agent is unlikely to be replicated in other malignancies, in which multiple redundant signaling pathways are dysregulated. However, it is increasingly being recognized that targeted therapeutic drugs can increase the efficacy of chemotherapy through various mechanisms. For instance, bevacizumab, an anti-angiogenic agent directed against the pro-angiogenic vascular endothelial growth factor (VEGF), increases both response and survival rates when combined with standard chemotherapy in patients with advanced colon cancer. The availability of these

Table 58–4   Commonly Used Targeted Therapeutic Agents

Drug	Cancers Treated	Mechanism of Action	Common Side Effects
Monoclonal Antibodies			
Rituximab	NHL	Anti-CD-20	Infusional reaction, tumor lysis syndrome, skin reactions
Tositumomab	NHL	Anti-CD-20 radiolabeled with I-131	Infusional reaction, myelosuppression, infections
Bevacizumab	Colorectal, renal, lung, breast	Anti-VEGF	Hypertension, proteinuria, epistaxis, thromboembolism
Cetuximab	Colorectal	Anti-EGFR	Infusional reaction, skin rash
Trastuzumab	Breast	Anti-HER-2/neu	Infusional reaction, congestive heart failure
Signal Transduction Inhibitors (Oral)			
Imatinib	CML, GIST	Inhibits *bcr-abl* and other receptor tyrosine kinases	N/V, diarrhea, fluid retention, myelosuppression
Erlotinib	Lung, pancreas	Anti-EGFR tyrosine kinase	Rash, diarrhea
Gefitinib	Lung	Anti-EGFR tyrosine kinase	Rash, hypertension, mild N/V
Others			
Tretinoin (all-transretinoic-acid)	Acute promyelocytic leukemia	Differentiating agent	Vitamin A toxicity, retinoic acid syndrome, hyperlipidemia

NHL = non-Hodgkin's lymphoma, VEGF = vascular endothelial growth factor, EGFR = epidermal growth factor receptor, CML = chronic myelogenous leukemia, GIST = gastrointestinal stromal tumor, N/V = nausea and vomiting.

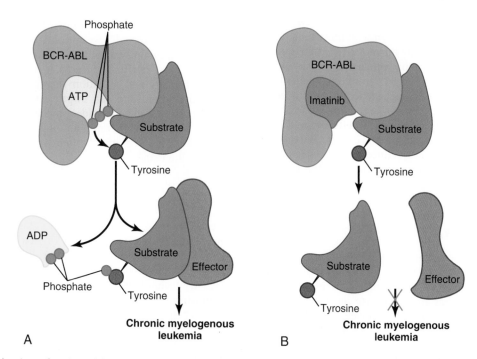

Figure 58–1 Mechanism of action of *bcr-abl* and of its inhibition by imatinib. *A*, The *bcr-abl* oncoprotein is shown with a molecule of adenosine triphosphate (ATP) in the kinase pocket. The substrate is activated by the phosphorylation of one of its tyrosine residues. It can then activate other downstream effector molecules. *B*, When imatinib occupies the kinase pocket, the action of *bcr-abl* is inhibited, preventing phosphorylation of its substrate. ADP denotes adenosine diphosphate. (Reproduced from Savage DG, Antman KH: Imatinib mesylate—A new oral targeted therapy. N Engl J Med 346:683–693, 2002.)

agents has increased the number of drug combinations that can be used to treat particular cancers. Multiple combinations of chemotherapy and targeted therapy are now available for the treatment of advanced colon cancer. Correspondingly, the median survival of patients with advanced colon cancer has doubled. Another heartening aspect of targeted therapeutic agents has been (ironically) their broad applicability, since many cancers use similar processes for growth and metastasis. For instance, bevacizumab may also be effective in renal, lung, and breast cancers.

Despite the excitement surrounding targeted therapy, much work is necessary to understand how and when these agents should be used. An example of how this might be done comes from recent research identifying specific molecular changes in epidermal growth factor receptor (EGFR) mutations, which are present in only 10% of patients with lung cancer. Although gefitinib is ineffective in the large majority of patients with lung cancer, patients with advanced lung cancer with these activating EGFR mutations have an extremely high likelihood of response.

ENDOCRINE THERAPY

Cancers originating from tissues that are regulated by hormones, such as breast and prostate, continue to be susceptible to hormonal control mechanisms even when metastatic. Endocrine therapy includes the use of both hormones and antihormonal agents that work as antagonists or partial agonists. As described in Chapter 56, many patients with metastatic breast cancer express hormone receptors (estrogen or progesterone) in tumor cells. Over 60% of these patients respond either to tamoxifen, an estrogen-receptor modulator, or to aromatase inhibitors (e.g., letrozole, anastrazole, exemestane), which inhibit steroid production within the adrenal glands and adipose tissue. Similar response rates are observed in men with metastatic prostate cancer treated with luteinizing hormone-releasing hormonal agonists leuprolide or goserelin, which decrease testosterone to castrate levels (see Chapter 56). In selected patients with breast and prostate cancers, metastatic disease can be controlled for years with only endocrine therapy. Tamoxifen and the aromatase inhibitors are also highly effective in the adjuvant treatment of resected breast cancer. Furthermore, tamoxifen has been shown to reduce the incidence of breast cancer by 50% in healthy women at high risk for developing breast cancer, making it a highly effective chemopreventive agent (see Chapter 55).

BIOLOGIC THERAPY

A diverse group of cytokines that uses host immunomodulatory effects as their primary mechanism of action is classified as *biologic-response modifiers* or *biologic agents.* Monoclonal antibodies are sometimes classified as biologic agents, although they have been reviewed under targeted therapy in this text. Interferons are used most commonly in patients with chronic myelogenous leukemia, although they are not as successful as imatinib in inducing responses. Interferons are also used for the treatment of hairy-cell leukemia, Kaposi's sarcoma, and selected cases of melanoma and renal cell carcinoma. Interleukin-2 (IL-2) functions as a T-cell growth factor and induces lymphokine-activated and natural killer cell activity. IL-2 can induce responses in 10% to 20% of patients with metastatic melanoma or renal cell carcinoma. In a minority of these patients, responses are complete and last for years. However, IL-2 is associated with considerable toxicity, in particular with a capillary leak syndrome that leads to hypotension, edema, renal insufficiency, and even death.

SUPPORTIVE CARE

Supportive care interventions can improve the safety and tolerability of chemotherapeutic treatments and can reduce the complications of the disease itself. A diverse array of drugs is available for the treatment of chemotherapy-related side effects. Serotonin-receptor antagonists and neurokinin 1–receptor antagonists, in combination with older antiemetic drugs, have made it possible to achieve complete control of chemotherapy-induced nausea and vomiting in nearly all settings. Erythropoietin and darbapoetin stimulate division and differentiation of erythroid precursors and are used for the treatment of cancer- and chemotherapy-induced anemia. Granulocyte-colony stimulating factor (filgrastim) and granulocyte-macrophage stimulating factor (sargramostim) stimulate the proliferation and differentiation of myeloid progenitor cells and are used to shorten the duration of chemotherapy-induced neutropenia. These agents are also used to mobilize and collect stem cells for transplantation. Filgrastim can also be used to shorten the interval between courses of chemotherapy, permitting the *dose-dense* approach in adjuvant treatment of breast cancer previously discussed. Recombinant human keratinocyte growth factor (palifermin) helps protect against chemotherapy and radiation therapy–induced mucositis.

Palliative care is an integral part of the treatment of cancer, particularly in noncurative settings. Palliative aspects of treating cancer address not only the physical symptoms, in particular pain syndromes, but they also address the psychosocial and spiritual concerns. It is important to note that chemotherapy and radiation therapy are often used with palliative intent and can improve the quality of life. The oncologist usually provides palliative care along with active anticancer therapy, although those with expertise in palliative care more often appropriately deal with end-of-life issues.

Drug Development

Currently, it takes $1 billion and 10 years to develop a single new drug. Given the plethora of new agents and limited resources to test them, preclinical validation of drug targets must be improved. The use of ribonucleic acid inference (RNAi) technology, as well as the development of more sophisticated preclinical models, will allow vetting of new agents before they enter clinical trials. A more rational selection of patients based on an understanding of the drug target should also accelerate drug development. Many targeted therapies affect processes important for early tumor development, such as angiogenesis. The paradigm of cancer drug development therefore requires change: instead of first testing drugs in patients with advanced and heavily pretreated disease, clinical trials should focus on testing drugs in patients with early-stage cancers. Finally, optimizing clinical trial endpoints so that the efficacy of the drug can be discovered in real-time using biomarkers or functional imaging techniques (such as PET scans) will hasten the clinical trials process.

Rational Drug Therapy

The selection of agents to treat an individual patient is based primarily on histologic diagnosis and staging. For instance, all patients with stage II breast cancer are treated with adjuvant chemotherapy. Yet, even within a given histologic classification and stage, enormous heterogeneity exists in tumor behavior. Molecular profiling of tumors using newly available genomic and proteomic technology will soon be incorporated into formal staging. This will permit rational, individualized therapy right at the bedside, rather than the "one size fits all" approach currently being used. Patients with stage II breast cancer with gene expression profiles indicative of poor prognosis would continue to be treated aggressively with adjuvant chemotherapy, whereas patients with an excellent prognosis would be spared. Similarly, instead of treating all patients with advanced lung cancer with an EGFR inhibitor, such a methodology would select only patients with activating EGFR mutations.

Quality of Care

Finally, improving the quality of cancer care given to all patients will improve cancer survival at the population level. By delivering appropriate surgical and medical management to all eligible patients, the impact and effectiveness of available treatments can be improved. Well-documented and widespread variations and disparities in the quality of cancer care indicate a tremendous opportunity to improve cancer outcomes with treatment modalities already in common use.

Prospectus for the Future

Advances in cancer biology and the first wave of targeted therapeutic agents are yet to have a significant impact on cancer mortality. Many changes in cancer drug development and use are required if the National Cancer Institute's stated goal, "to eliminate suffering and death due to cancer" by 2015, is to be achieved.

References

Bertino JR, Hait W: Principles of Cancer Therapy. In Goldman L, Ausiello D (eds): Cecil Textbook of Medicine. 22nd ed. Philadelphia, WB Saunders, 2004: 1137–1150.

Chabner BA, Roberts TG, Jr: Chemotherapy and the war on cancer. Nat Rev Cancer 5(1):65–72, 2005.

Lynch TJ et al: Activating mutations in the epidermal growth factor receptor underlying responsiveness of non-small-cell lung cancer to gefitinib. N Engl J Med 350:2129–2139, 2004.

Meyerhardt JA, Mayer RJ: Drug therapy: Systemic therapy for colorectal cancer. N Engl J Med 352:476–487, 2005.

Krause SD, van Etten RA: Tyrosine kinases as targets for cancer therapy. N Engl J Med 353(2):172–187, 2005.

Section X

Metabolic Disease

Cecil

Andreoli and Carpenter's
Essentials of Medicine

Eating Disorders

Reed E. Pyeritz

Introduction

Various abnormalities of body mass, both increased and decreased, are attracting more attention in medicine and general society. Numerous factors affect the body mass over a person's lifetime, and much remains to be learned about the inter-relations of endogenous and exogenous factors. Clinicians most frequently use body weight or, preferably, the body mass index ([BMI]; weight [kg]/(height [m])^2) to judge whether a patient is *overweight* or *underweight*. Studies of twins and other relatives document that the BMI has a strong genetic component across the entire range of body size. Whether a person is classified as *obese* is a subjective assessment, and the use of *standards* based on BMI, promulgated by experts, is the current approach. The criteria in the first column of Table 59–1 are easily remembered; those in the second column represent criteria used in epidemiologic studies. However, the limitations of the standards must be recognized. For example, very muscular persons may be moderately overweight but not obese. Others with small frames and low muscle mass may be obese without fulfilling the criteria for being overweight.

Body fat is stored as triglycerides in adipose tissue, which is distributed under the skin and in the breasts, buttocks, thighs, and abdomen. Adipose tissue accounts for an average of 26% to 42% of the weight of middle-aged American men and women (Table 59–2). The usual tight regulation of the size of the adipose organ indicates that neural or humoral signals from the adipose organ are transmitted to the brain, which in turn regulates food seeking and consumption and energy expenditure (Fig. 59–1).

Obesity

A United States government task force has set a BMI equal to or greater than 27.3 for women and 27.8 for men as defining the term *overweight*. These values correspond to a 20% excess over ideal body weight. Most authorities define *obesity* as a BMI greater than 30 for both sexes. By these criteria, 50 million Americans are overweight and 12 million are severely obese. In the last 30 years of the twentieth century, the fraction of Americans who were overweight increased from 31% to 35%, and the fraction of those who were obese increased from 13% to 26%. Minority populations are disproportionately affected. Almost 50% of African-American women are overweight. The economic costs of obesity are staggering; a recent estimate placed direct annual costs in the United States at $61 billion and indirect costs, such as lost productivity, at $56 billion. Often unrecognized is the added cost of caring for obese patients, especially in hospitals and nursing homes. Individuals can have a mild-to-moderate increase in their BMI, calculated from height and weight alone, that is primarily due to increased muscle mass (i.e., lean body mass). This increase usually occurs in highly trained athletes and can be validated by, for example, densitometry. However, simply being a highly trained athlete is no protection from obesity, as sumo wrestlers and some lineman in American football demonstrate.

Chapter 59

PATHOGENESIS

Obesity is, to a great extent, genetically determined and is strongly influenced by the availability of palatable food and a sedentary lifestyle. A child of two obese parents has about an 80% chance of becoming obese, whereas the risk is only 15% for the offspring of two parents of normal weight. Moreover, a correlation between the BMI of parents and children is found across a broad spectrum of values, which suggests both polygenic inheritance of obesity and several contributing metabolic mechanisms. The precise causative mechanisms remain unknown, but several genetic loci have been mapped. The endocrine system plays a major role in regulating body weight, and the hormone leptin is central through its interaction with both adipose tissue and the hypothalamus.

Table 59–1	**Obesity Classification Based on Body Mass Index**	
Classification	**BMI (kg/m²)**	
Underweight	<20	<18.5
Ideal	20–25	18.5–27.5
Overweight	25–30	27.5–30
Obese	30–40	>30
Severely obese	>40	

BMI = body mass index.

Table 59–2	**Variation of Fat and Lean Body Mass as Percent of Body Weight with Age**			
	Men		**Women**	
Age	**LBM**	**Fat**	**LBM**	**Fat**
25	81	19	68	32
45	74	26	58	42
65	65	35	51	49

LBM = lean body mass.

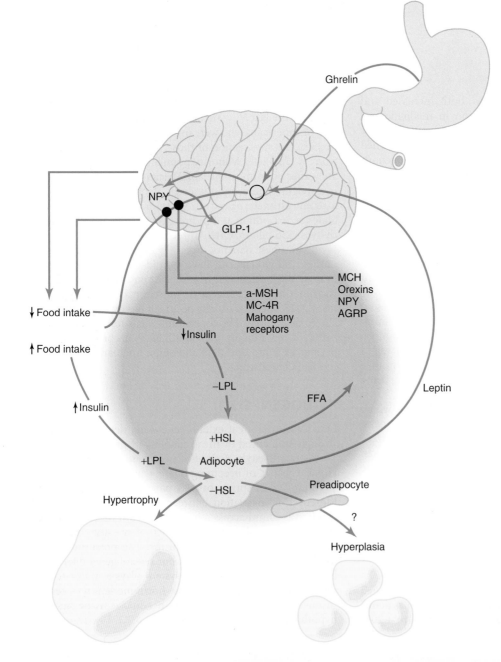

Figure 59–1 Pathogenesis of obesity. Increased food intake stimulates insulin secretion. Insulin, in turn, stimulates lipoprotein lipase (LPL), permitting uptake of circulating triglycerides by the adipocyte, and insulin simultaneously inhibits hormone-sensitive lipase (HSL) and the release of adipocyte free fatty acids (FFA). The overfed adipocyte may hypertrophy, or a stimulus, currently unknown, may trigger differentiation of preadipocytes. The well-fed adipocyte secretes leptin, which circulates and binds to receptors in the hypothalamus, causing glucagon-like peptide-1 (GLP-1) release and inhibiting neuropeptide-Y (NPY), a powerful stimulator of appetite and feeding. Reduced food intake, in contrast, lowers insulin, leading to LPL suppression, activation of HSL, and FFA release. Additionally, fasting stimulates release from the stomach of the peptide hormone, ghrelin. Ghrelin stimulates the release of the growth hormone, but its more important actions are to stimulate food intake, decrease lipid metabolism, and improve carbohydrate use.

Table 59–3 Pathogenetic Factors in Obesity

Neurologic

Reduced sympathetic activity
Increased parasympathetic activity
Leptin-receptor deficiency
Increased neuropeptide Y secretion and neuronal activity
Melanocortin-receptor deficiency
Increased Agouti-related peptide activity
Melanocortin deficiency
Increased activity of melanin-concentrating hormone neurons
Increased activity of orexin neurons
Decreased activity of the *mahogany* receptor

Adipocyte

Increased stimulus and/or response to preadipocyte
  differentiation
Increased lipoprotein lipase activity
Diminished hormone-sensitive lipase
Reduced leptin secretion
β_3-Adrenergic receptor hypofunction

Other

Insulin resistance and/or hyperinsulinemia

At some time in life, the obese individual consumes more calories than he or she expends *and* appetite is not subsequently reduced to compensate for the increase in stored energy. Typically, this pattern begins early in life; large birth weight babies are more likely to be obese as adults, and obesity in childhood is a strong predictor of an elevated BMI later in life. Failure of fat cells to send adequate signals or the failure of the brain to respond to appropriate signals is fundamental to the pathogenesis of obesity (Table 59–3).

Mechanisms controlling fat cell size and numbers are being discovered. Several facts are clear. The enzyme lipoprotein lipase, produced by the adipocyte and residing on its capillary endothelium, permits fat cells to take up fatty acids from circulating chylomicrons (derived from dietary fat) and very low–density lipoproteins (VLDL). Fat cells with enhanced lipoprotein lipase activity may have a competitive advantage in assimilating lipoprotein triglycerides. The enzyme is very active in mesenteric fat and may contribute to abdominal obesity in men and is less active in gluteal fat. Adipocytes can also take up fatty acids bound to albumin.

A second enzyme, hormone-sensitive lipase, which is inhibited by insulin and responds to signals (i.e., circulating or neuronally derived catecholamines, prostaglandins, glucagon, gonadotropins), regulates the breakdown and release of adipocyte triglycerides by increasing intracellular cyclic adenosine monophosphate (cAMP) (see Fig. 59–1). The adipocytes of obese individuals may resist lipolytic stimuli from nerves or circulating catecholamines. Gluteal fat in both men and women, for example, has a lower lipolytic response to β_1-adrenergic stimulation than does abdominal fat. Abdominal fat in men appears to have more α_2-adrenergic receptor function (antilipolytic) than does abdominal fat in women, perhaps accounting for the *beer belly* in men more often than in women.

An adipocyte can engorge to a maximum weight of 1 mcg. Storage of more fat requires an increase in adipocyte number by differentiation of preadipocytes (see Fig. 59–1). The signal for this hyperplasia is unknown and is a critical link if excess caloric consumption can drive an increase in adipocyte number. Some evidence suggests that certain stages of human development are especially susceptible to adipocyte hyperplasia. The converse, that an increased adipocyte number drives increased food intake, is also possible. When fat depot mass results from increased cell numbers, as in gluteal and femoral obesity, fat depots are very resistant to depletion, as evident in the condition called steatopygia and in the so-called cellulite discussed often in periodicals. Fat depots with hyperplastic cells, in contrast, such as those in the abdominal wall and viscera, are much more metabolically active. These are more readily depleted by hypocaloric diets and contribute to the metabolic abnormalities of abdominal obesity. Moderate obesity (BMI < 40) appears more associated with increased fat cell size; severe obesity (BMI > 40) appears associated with a high adipocyte number.

Single-gene effects do not account for most cases of human obesity, but biologically important genes, their products, and their regulators are rapidly being identified. Leptin, a hormone produced primarily by fat cells, circulates to the brain, and inhibits neuropeptide Y and Agouti-related peptide (AGRP), a hormone that binds to central melanocortin receptors. Leptin also stimulates secretion of pro-opiomelanocortin and synthesis of OBR, the leptin receptor. These effects of increased leptin both decrease food intake and increase energy expenditure. Leptin synthesis is induced by hyperglycemia, hyperlipidemia, and a replete fat cell mass, and leptin suppresses insulin production. Mice and humans with congenital leptin deficiency develop hyperphagia and severe obesity. Similarly, mice and humans with homozygous mutations in the leptin receptor gene also develop severe obesity and, in addition, hypogonadotropic hypogonadism. Among most obese individuals, however, leptin levels are high rather than low. Thus common forms of human obesity actually appear to be resistant to leptin. Leptin's primary role in the body economy may be to signal starvation and stimulate feeding when levels are low.

Central mechanisms controlling feeding are localized primarily to the hypothalamus. Output from the ventromedial hypothalamus inhibits feeding, whereas that from the lateral hypothalamus promotes feeding. A number of novel neuropeptides and receptors in the hypothalamus were identified in the 1990s. Activity levels and quantitative interactions among these may eventually explain much of the pathogenesis of obesity. Neuropeptide Y, produced in the arcuate nucleus, is a powerful central nervous system stimulant of appetite. Orexins in the lateral hypothalamus, similar to neuropeptide Y, also increase with starvation and cause hyperphagia and obesity after intracerebroventricular administration. AGRP is highly expressed when leptin levels are low, and it interacts with the melanocortin-4 receptor and antagonizes the effect of α-melanocyte-stimulating hormone; this action, when unopposed, reduces appetite and increases metabolic rate. Finally, melanocortin-concentrating hormone, which does not interact with the melanocortin-4 receptor, is confined to neurons in the lateral hypothalamus, is highly expressed in leptin deficiency and starvation, and may project to higher centers, thereby integrating effects of other neurotransmitters. Many potential targets for pharmacologic control of feeding are now identified, and these should lead to novel drugs for modulating appetite and obesity.

A specific pattern of eating associated with obesity, termed the *night-eating syndrome*, may be more common than generally recognized. Patients have anorexia in the morning and overeating (hyperphagia) in the evening, often making repeated excursions to the kitchen associated with difficulty sleeping. This behavior is associated with a lower-than-normal rise in plasma leptin and melatonin levels at night, although cause and effect are uncertain.

Whatever the cause of a person's obesity, the condition is nearly intractable once it occurs. Increased fat cell size and numbers are maintained, and fat cells, when deprived of calories, seem to communicate their underfed status to the brain, thus stimulating appetite. Moreover, caloric restriction to achieve weight loss is associated with reductions in energy expenditure in the obese to levels far below those in naturally lean individuals.

ANATOMY

Regional depots of body fat, as noted earlier, differ significantly in their metabolic features and in their relation to the adverse health consequences of obesity. The form of obesity that characteristically occurs in men, android or abdominal obesity, is closely associated with metabolic complications such as hypertension, insulin resistance, hyperuricemia, and dyslipoproteinemia (the *metabolic syndrome*, which used to be termed *syndrome X*). Mutation of the ß$_3$-adrenoreceptor gene, which is expressed predominantly in visceral fat depots, has been linked to increased waist-to-hip circumference, glucose intolerance, and high blood pressure. The mechanism involved may be enhanced sensitivity of visceral fat to catecholamine-mediated lipolysis. Increased free-fatty acid release may drive VLDL production by the liver and, by increasing skeletal muscle triglycerides, may promote insulin resistance.

It appears that the typical female or gynecoid obesity with fat deposits in the hips and gluteal and femoral regions has much less metabolic importance. The waist-to-hip circumference ratio has been used to distinguish these forms of obesity. A ratio above 1.0 in men and above 0.6 in women suggests the undesirable android obesity pattern. Thus it is healthier to be shaped like a pear than like an apple.

MEDICAL CONSEQUENCES
Clinically Severe Obesity

Individuals weighing 45 kg (100 lb) or about 60% more than desirable are designated as being severely obese. This corresponds to a weight of 240 lb (109 kg) in a woman 63 inches (157 cm) tall and to a weight of 260 lb (118 kg) in a man 68 inches (173 cm) tall. Cardiorespiratory problems present the greatest risk (Table 59–4). Chronic hypoventilation is common and leads to hypercapnia, pulmonary hypertension, and right ventricular heart failure. Left ventricular dysfunc-

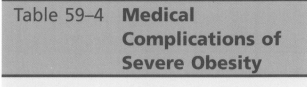

Table 59–4 Medical Complications of Severe Obesity
Sudden death
Obstructive sleep apnea
Pickwickian syndrome: Daytime hypoventilation, somnolence, polycythemia, cor pulmonale
Congestive heart failure
Nephrotic syndrome and/or renal vein thrombosis
Immobility limiting daily activities
Degenerative arthritis

tion also occurs and may be related to both hypertension and hypervolemia. Severe episodic hypoxia can cause arrhythmias, and sudden death is 10 times more common among those who are severely obese as among individuals of normal weight. Most devastating, however, are the psychosocial consequences of the disorder. Self-esteem and body image are impaired, immobility greatly limits work and recreational activities, and humiliation is a daily experience when body size is too large for conventional scales, furniture, vehicles, and clothes.

Moderate Obesity

Body habitus associated with BMIs between 19 and 27 vary widely, and within this broad range little association between BMI and health exists. Adverse health consequences accrue with a BMI of 27. Even a mild overweight level in young individuals is associated with increased total and cardiovascular mortality rates, and the effect is evident at lower BMIs in men than in women (Table 59–5). Risks associated with increased BMI are more pronounced the older the patient. Being moderately overweight in men and women aged 60 years is associated with more than a 20% increase in 12-year mortality, and more than one half of this added mortality is from cardiovascular disease.

Hypertension and diabetes mellitus are clearly related to obesity. Hypertension is more frequent in obese individuals than in those of ideal weight, perhaps because of sympathetic hyperactivity or to hyperinsulinemia, but neither mechanism is clearly established. Type II diabetes mellitus can be unmasked and aggravated by excess weight, and this complication may be the most important medical finding of moderate obesity. The cause appears to be insulin resistance, but many obese individuals never develop hyperglycemia. Obesity is often associated with high triglyceride levels and low levels of high-density lipoproteins, particularly when mild glucose intolerance is also present. Finally, obesity clearly increases the risk of cholelithiasis, endometrial carcinoma, and pseudotumor cerebri.

TREATMENT
Moderate Obesity

Americans spend many billions of dollars annually on weight-loss programs and diet products; and at any time, up to one third of the population is dieting. Low-calorie diets

Table 59–5	Body Mass Index Associated with a 50% Increase in Total and Cardiovascular Mortality Over a 12-Year Period in Men and Women			
	Total Population		**BMI with 50% Increased Mortality**	
Age (yr)	**Absolute Mortality Rate**	**Population Mean BMI**	**Total Mortality**	**CV Mortality**
Men				
30–44	3%	25.6	27.2	26.3
55–64	17%	25.6	29.1	27.5
65–74	40%	25.1	42.1	33.2
Women				
30–44	2%	23.8	32.1	26.5
55–64	10%	25.2	32.0	30.3
65–74	27%	25.0	40.8	38.7

BMI = body mass index (kg/m^2); CV = cardiovascular.
Data for subjects who never smoked; derived from Stevens J, Cai J, Pamuk ER, et al: The effect of age on the association between body-mass index and mortality. N Engl J Med 338:1–7, 1998. A BMI of 21.0 was used as the reference point of comparison.

remain the most widely advocated treatment for obesity. The recommendation to count calories and eat less of everything has intuitive appeal but little success. Behavior modification techniques, focusing on stimulus control, the obese-eating style, group and spouse support, reinforcement procedures, and exercise are probably more effective. These more aggressive programs produce about 6 kg of weight loss over 1 year. Nevertheless, at least 90% of graduates of such plans return to their initial weight within 5 years. More popular but even less successful are innumerable diets based on significant nutritional imbalance (e.g., predominantly rice, grapefruit). These diets are only transiently helpful because a diet very low in either fat or carbohydrate rapidly becomes monotonous and unpalatable. Diets very low in carbohydrates are ketogenic and inhibit appetite. Very low calorie diets that rely on withdrawal of most conventional foods and involve a typically expensive diet supplement may produce dramatic short-term effects but are potentially hazardous. No diet calling for 800 or fewer calories should be undertaken without medical supervision. More than 50 deaths, some from documented ventricular tachycardia and fibrillation, occurred with the early liquid protein, very low calorie diets. No program consisting of caloric restriction alone has been generally successful beyond 12 to 18 months, despite the enormous commercial success of diet books and systems.

Anorectic drugs are potentially addicting, often unsafe, and only marginally effective. The medical profession and the public have been considerably chastened by the recognition that the fenfluramine and phentermine combination marketed in the 1990s caused valvular heart disease. Patients with any history of drug abuse should avoid all amphetamines. Anorectic agents may be useful in the short term when incorporated in a program that includes diet counseling, behavior modification, and close medical supervision.

As the pathophysiologic factors of obesity are better elucidated, more specific and effective measures should emerge.

Clinically Severe Obesity

Severe caloric restriction to 200 to 800 kcal/day, with or without anorectic drugs, should be tried first. A 90% failure rate is the rule. Individuals more than 100 lb (45 kg) overweight in whom medical treatment has failed may be candidates for surgery to reduce stomach size and hence the quantity of food that can be ingested at any one sitting. Vertical-banded gastroplasty consists of constructing a small pouch with restricted outlet, high along the lesser curvature of the stomach. Gastric bypass procedures involve the creation of a similar small pouch but with drainage into a loop of jejunum rather than into the lower stomach. Patients typically lose 40% to 50% of excess weight within 1 year of gastric surgery, but some consume calorie-dense liquids and regain weight. The number of *bariatric* surgeries quadrupled between 1998 and 2002 in the United States. The long-term safety and efficacy of this surgery are not certain. Intestinal bypass surgery for morbid obesity has been abandoned because of unacceptable long-term complications.

Anorexia Nervosa and Bulimia Nervosa

These two psychiatric disorders are characterized by a distorted perception of body image and abnormal eating patterns. Neither has a distinctive pathognomonic feature; the two disorders share some common features, and they may overlap (Table 59–6). Bulimia nervosa is not associated with cachexia, whereas this is the most prominent aspect of anorexia nervosa. The primary treatment of both disorders is psychiatric, although they may exhibit important medical complications.

Table 59–6   Diagnostic Criteria for Anorexia Nervosa and Bulimia Nervosa

Anorexia Nervosa

A. Refusal to maintain body weight at or above a minimally normal weight for age and height (e.g., weight loss leading to maintenance of body weight less than 85% of that expected or failure to make expected weight gain during period of growth, leading to body weight less than 85% of that expected).

B. Intense fear of gaining weight or becoming fat, although underweight.

C. Disturbance in the way in which own body weight or shape is experienced, undue influence of body weight or shape on self-evaluation, or denial of the seriousness of the current low body weight.

D. In postmenarchal women, amenorrhea, (i.e., absence of at least three consecutive menstrual cycles); a woman is considered to have amenorrhea if her periods occur only after hormone administration (e.g., estrogen).

Bulimia Nervosa

A. Recurrent episodes of binge eating; an episode of binge eating is characterized by both of the following:
1. Eating in a discrete period of time (e.g., within any 2-hour period) an amount of food that is definitely greater than most people would eat during a similar period of time and under similar circumstances.
2. A sense of lack of control over eating during the episode (i.e., a feeling that one cannot stop eating or control what or how much one is eating).

B. Recurrent inappropriate compensatory behavior to prevent weight gain, such as self-induced vomiting; misuse of laxatives, diuretics, enemas, or other medications; fasting; or excessive exercise.

C. Binge eating and inappropriate compensatory behaviors both occur, on average, at least twice a week for 3 months.

D. Self-evaluation is unduly influenced by body shape and weight.

E. The disturbance does not occur exclusively during episodes of anorexia nervosa.

From American Psychiatric Association: *Diagnostic and Statistical Manual of Mental Disorders*, 4th ed. Washington, DC: American Psychiatric Association, pp 549–550. Copyright ©1994 by the American Psychiatric Association. Reprinted by permission.

ANOREXIA NERVOSA

Prevalence

The lifetime prevalence of anorexia nervosa in American women is about 0.5%. Among women evaluated for amenorrhea, between 5% and 15% are affected. The disorder affects girls at least 10 times as often as boys. The onset occurs typically during adolescence, but it may occur as late as during menopause. Anorexia nervosa is principally a disorder of societies in which hunger is uncommon but some premium is placed on being thin. Thus individuals who engage seriously in certain activities such as dancing, modeling, and athletics are at increased risk.

Pathogenesis and Clinical Features

In the United States, prepubescent children often voice concern over body image. Some individuals can recall life situations or events that triggered their preoccupation with thinness. The usual pubertal weight increase may be critical in most affected girls. The restriction of food intake is initially voluntary and may not progress to binge eating, self-induced vomiting, abuse of purgatives and diuretics, and exhausting exercise. Patients view their own body dimensions as excessive, but their view of other people is not abnormal. Treated patients with anorexia have high cerebrospinal fluid levels of serotonin, which experimentally reduces feeding, but it is unclear whether this is a cause or an effect of anorexia nervosa.

In typical cases, the diagnosis of anorexia nervosa presents little difficulty. In atypical cases that occur, for example, in men and older women, consideration of malignancy, acquired immunodeficiency syndrome, malabsorption, and hyperthyroidism is warranted. Weight loss in anorexia nervosa usually begins within a few years of menarche, although onset may occur even later than 40 years. Amenorrhea, defined by the absence of three consecutive menstrual cycles, is the rule and is secondary to weight loss and low gonadotropin levels. The latter may in turn be secondary to low leptin levels. Men complain of poor libido and impotence. Stunted growth and pathologic fractures may occur when the disease begins in early adolescence.

Physical examination shows little subcutaneous fat, with gaunt facies, atrophic breasts and buttocks, and extensive growth of fine lanugo-like hair on neck and extremities. The BMI for adult women is less than $18.5\,kg/m^2$. Extremities may be cold, cyanotic, and mildly edematous. Skin is often yellow from hypercarotenemia. Bradycardia and hypothermia may occur, presumably because of low triiodothyronine (T_3) levels. Hypovolemia and mild diabetes insipidus may cause hypotension. The psychologic profile can be key to the correct diagnosis; patients are afraid of gaining weight despite their thinness.

Laboratory findings are not diagnostic but usually include low levels of gonadotropins and gonadal hormones, hypercortisolism, and low T_3 and increased reverse T_3, as in *sick euthyroidism*. Occasionally, pancytopenia occurs but rarely with an increased number of severe infections;

hypoglycemia, occasionally with coma develops; uncommonly, hypoalbuminemia and hypercholesterolemia occur. Hypokalemia is rare in patients who are not purging. Abdominal radiographic studies may show gastric distention and megaduodenum, and echocardiography may show mitral valve motion abnormalities and reduced left ventricular mass.

Treatment and Prognosis

All patients with anorexia nervosa should be evaluated by a psychiatrist or psychologist experienced in those with eating disorders. Patients weighing at least 65% of ideal body weight may be successfully managed as outpatients. Those under 65% of ideal body weight are candidates for inpatient psychiatric and nutritional care. If the patient is unable or unwilling to consume 500 kcal more than needed for daily energy requirements, then peripheral parenteral nutritional supplementation (see Chapter 60) or tube feeding should be considered.

Hypothalamic and endocrine problems generally resolve when 85% of normal body weight is restored. Amenorrhea may persist for several more months, but menses usually return without specific intervention.

The mortality rate among patients with anorexia nervosa is about 6% per decade. At least 50% to 60% regain normal weight and eating habits, and normal menses return. In 20% of patients the condition remains chronic despite therapy. Prognosis is poorer in those with bulimic features or long duration of illness.

BULIMIA NERVOSA

Prevalence

The lifetime prevalence of bulimia in a large Canadian study was 1.1% among women and 0.1% among men. Less comprehensive studies have suggested that up to 20% of college students report bulimic symptoms. Within families of patients with bulimia, serious depression and substance abuse, particularly alcoholism, occur six times more frequently than expected by chance. The increase in weight and adiposity at puberty is probably the stimulus for bulimia,

just as it is for anorexia nervosa. The hallmark of bulimia is repeated binge eating. Binges leave the patient embarrassed, guilty, and focused again on maintaining weight below an arbitrary level. Prolonged fasting, self-induced vomiting, and the use of nonprescription anorectic drugs (e.g., emetics, diuretics, laxatives) achieve this end. In significant contrast to patients with anorexia nervosa, patients with bulimia generally feel out of control and often welcome help.

Patients with bulimia may have normal or even elevated BMI, and physical findings may be subtle or absent. Calluses or scratches on the dorsum of the hand may result from abrasion by teeth during induced gagging. Puffy cheeks from parotid or other salivary gland enlargement are present in up to 50% of patients, and serum salivary amylase levels may be elevated. Erosions occur on the lingual, palatal, and posterior occlusal surfaces of the teeth from acid-induced enamel dissolution and decalcification.

Frequent binge eating and vomiting may cause gastric or esophageal perforation or bleeding, pneumomediastinum, or subcutaneous emphysema. Heavy use of ipecac to induce vomiting may cause myopathic weakness and electrocardiographic abnormalities from emetine toxicity. Loss of gastric fluids can result in metabolic alkalosis with elevated carbon dioxide levels and hypochloremia. Diuretic abuse can produce both hypokalemia and hyponatremia. Menstrual irregularities are common, but amenorrhea is rare.

Treatment and Prognosis

Patients with bulimia, in general, do not need hospitalization for their physical or psychological problems. Psychiatric evaluation and management can be highly effective. Cognitive behavioral therapy, focusing on thought processes and their modification, is probably superior to therapy directed at managing anxiety or to treatment with antidepressant drugs. Prescription of desipramine, followed if necessary by fluoxetine, may be effective. At least one third of patients experience relapse within a 2-year follow-up period, most within the first 6 months, and require additional treatment. Bulimia nervosa is associated with low added mortality, and few patients progress to anorexia nervosa. However, even successfully treated patients with bulimia remain at high risk for alcohol and other drug dependencies.

Prospectus for the Future

- Heightened awareness in the medical and public health communities of the epidemic in overweight and obesity, accompanied by extensive educational campaigns
- Identification of genes that predispose to the common varieties of obesity, anorexia nervosa, and bulimia nervosa
- Initiation of trials to intervene at early stages in individuals identified as having strong predictors of eating disorders later in life
- Development of drugs that act on specific effectors of the physiologic pathways that control fat metabolism, metabolic rate, and appetite

References

Dansinger ML, Gleason JA, Griffith JL: Comparison of the Atkins, Ornish, Weight Watchers, and Zone diets for weight loss and heart disease risk reduction: A randomized trial. JAMA 293:43–53, 2005.

Dietz WH, Robinson TN: Clinical practice. Overweight children and adolescents. N Engl J Med 352:2100–2109, 2005.

Janeckova R: The role of leptin in human physiology and pathophysiology. Physiol Rev 50:443–459, 2001.

Kaplan AS: Psychological treatments for anorexia nervosa: A review of published studies and promising new directions. Can J Psychiatry 47:235–242, 2002.

McTigue KM, Garrett JM, Popkin BM: The development of obesity in young U.S. adults, 1981–1998. Ann Intern Med 136:857–864, 2002.

Nicholls D, Viner R: Eating disorders and weight problems. BMJ 330: 950–953, 2005.

Polivy J, Herman CP: Causes of eating disorders. Ann Rev Psychol 53: 187–213, 2002.

Powers PS, Santana CA: Eating disorders: A guide for the primary care physician. Prim Care 29:81–98, 2002.

Chapter 60

Nutritional Assessment, Malnutrition, and Nutritional Support in Adult Patients

Reed E. Pyeritz

Nutritional Assessment

Every patient deserves objective consideration of nutritional status. The depth of the assessment will vary, considering a host of factors, but the health care team should make a point of including the patient's nutritional status before being forced to by clinical circumstances. Severely malnourished patients have worse outcomes, regardless of the disease entity or reason for hospitalization. Nutritional assessment performed as part of primary care will identify patients who are in need of general or specific nutritional support, and therapy can often be less drastic than might be necessitated by an acute illness or other stress factors. Furthermore, nutritional assessment may uncover disorders (e.g., celiac disease, alcoholism) about which the patient, physician, or both are unaware.

No single measure in isolation is sufficient for defining nutritional adequacy. An adult of 70 kg lean body mass requires stores of fat (~15 kg), protein (~6 kg, in muscle) and glycogen (~0.4 kg) to provide energy when food intake is inadequate to meet immediate metabolic demands. Depletion of these energy stores is one measure of malnourishment and is evidenced by low weight for height, low body mass index (BMI) (weight in kg/[height in m]^2), little subcutaneous adiposity, low muscle mass, and temporal wasting. Depletion of vitamins and minerals, either in general or in specific, can also be suggested by physical findings, the presence of certain diseases, or a dietary history. A number of measurements can be used to assess the adequacy of a person's nutrition (Table 60–1), but the average clinician will have neither the experience nor time to apply quantitative assessments, such as anthropometry, calorimetry, or bioelectric impedance. However, sending a blood specimen to assess the serum albumin level is hardly adequate. A normal level does not exclude serious nutritional deficiencies, and a low level can be the result of a number of reasons short of excess catabolism of protein over its synthesis.

Similarly, lymphopenia has causes other than malnutrition, particularly the adrenocorticotropic hormone (ACTH) and corticosteroid responses to acute stress.

Nutritional Requirements

WATER

Adults require approximately 30 mL of water per kilogram of body weight daily, or approximately 1 mL/kcal of energy. Older patients and other individuals incapable of expressing their thirst require careful attention to their serum osmolality levels. Serum osmolality should be routinely calculated and adjusted, if indicated, by increasing or decreasing total fluid volume (see Chapter 27). Patients with ascites, edema, heart failure, or intrinsic kidney disease may have low urine output and require less water. Those with fistulas, gastrointestinal drainage, or impaired renal water conservation may require large volumes of water and electrolytes.

CALORIES AND PROTEIN

Protein and carbohydrates provide approximately 4 kcal of energy per gram, and fat provides 9 kcal/g. In a typical American diet, about 16% of calories are protein, 37% are fat, and 47% are carbohydrates. A healthy adult requires approximately 30 kcal/kg ideal body weight per day, and protein should constitute at least 15% (1 g/kg/day) of total calories. Stressed patients, such as those with major trauma, burns, inflammatory bowel disease, or infections, require more protein (up to 1.5 g/kg/day) to avoid catabolism of muscle protein. Several amino acids are called *essential* because they are not synthesized and must be consumed or provided in a nutritional supplement. Similarly, two long-chain fatty acids are essential.

Table 60–1	**Elements of the Nutritional Assessment**

History

Decreased oral intake
Alcoholism and other sources of empty calories
Symptoms of gastrointestinal disease
Unintentional loss of 10% or more of body weight
Recent severe illness
Chronic illness, especially malignancy, chronic obstructive pulmonary disease, infection, acquired immunodeficiency syndrome

Physical Examination

Weight < 10% of ideal
Sparse subcutaneous adiposity
Muscle wasting
Dermatitis
Neurologic signs (e.g., Wernicke's encephalopathy, posterior column signs)

Laboratory Findings

Low serum albumin and other serum proteins
Low vitamin and mineral levels
Lymphopenia

Procedures

Creatinine-height index
Calorimetry
Bioelectric impedance
Measurement of nitrogen balance

Table 60–2	**General Causes of Malnutrition**

Decreased oral intake
Anorexia from chronic or acute illness, chemotherapy, depression
Anorexia nervosa, bulimia nervosa
Restrictive diets (personal choice, typically involve specific nutrients)
Socioeconomic deprivation
Abdominal pain induced by eating (abdominal angina)
Decreased absorption
Abnormal gastrointestinal transit
Maldigestion (e.g., pancreatitis, short-gut syndrome)
Malabsorption (e.g., celiac disease, Crohn's disease, cystic fibrosis)
Increased caloric demands
Chronic illness (e.g., malignancy, COPD, AIDS, hyperthyroidism)
Trauma and burns
Acute illness (e.g., infection)
Major surgery
Metabolic aberrations
Acute or chronic liver disease

COPD = chronic obstructive pulmonary disease; AIDS = acquired immunodeficiency syndrome.

VITAMINS AND MINERALS

Metal ions and vitamins are required for most metabolic reactions, often as co-factors for enzymes. Although co-factors are not consumed in reactions, they are lost from the body and must be replaced.

Malnutrition

Based on simple measurements and questions, the physician can develop a high index of suspicion that a patient is malnourished. For example, patients who has lost 10% or more of their usual body weight in recent few months without trying to do so or patients who weigh less than 90% of their ideal weight or who have a BMI less than 18.5 should be carefully evaluated. Any person who weighs less than 85% of ideal should be considered to have malnutrition, even if the weight loss is intentional. Some endurance athletes, with little adiposity and muscle bulk, will qualify using this definition, even though they are otherwise healthy. However, should they suffer trauma or an acute illness, they should be recognized as having little metabolic reserve.

The causes of malnutrition are diverse (Table 60–2), and multiple issues may pertain in any given patient. For example, an older person with heightened energy demands secondary to cancer may have anorexia because of therapy or depression and have an inadequate social support to provide nourishment. Solutions to malnourishment must account for these assorted causes.

Nutritional Support

A number of issues must be addressed when considering the proper application of nutritional support. First, patient selection is important because some patients are more likely to benefit, whereas others might not. Further, nutritional support can be costly and associated with complications, especially when administered parenterally. Second, the timing of support needs attention. Initiating therapy in a malnourished patient in advance of a stress such as major surgery is far better than waiting until the postoperative period. Third, the composition of the support should be individualized, with proper attention given to specific deficiencies that can be identified in a patient. Fourth, the route of administration should be addressed. Finally, the length of therapy should be considered at the outset, even when the actual course depends on numerous factors, including response to support.

Types of patients likely to benefit from nutritional support are listed in Table 60–3. In general, patients who meet the criteria for malnutrition are considered candidates for nutritional support. Patients who will be without

Table 60–3 Indications for Enteral Nutritional Support and Parenteral Nutritional Support in Adults

Strongly Supported by Outcome Studies	Moderately Supported by Research Studies	Recommended by Expert Panels
Acute respiratory failure with mechanical ventilatory support (ENS or PNS)	Acute or chronic alcoholic liver disease (ENS or PNS)	Severely malnourished patients with cancer with time-limited radiation or chemotherapy enteritis (ENS or PNS)
Acute exacerbation of Crohn's disease (ENS)	Acute renal failure (ENS or PNS)	Chronic renal failure (ENS or PNS)
	AIDS (ENS or PNS)	Prolonged (>7 days) acute pancreatitis (ENS)
Short-bowel syndrome (PNS or ENS)	Severe but stable COPD and cystic fibrosis (ENS)	Intensive care or critically ill patients (>7 days) (ENS or PNS)
Patients who are severely malnourished preoperatively (PNS or ENS)	Chronic Crohn's disease (ENS)	Neurologic impairment of oral intake
	Acute ulcerative colitis (ENS or PNS)	Anorexia nervosa with 30% recent weight loss or ≤65% of ideal body weight (ENS or PNS)
	Blunt trauma/head trauma (ENS)	Any patient with predicted severe inadequate nutrition >7 days (ENS or PNS)
	Enterocutaneous fistulas (PNS)	

ENS = enteral nutritional support; PNS = parenteral nutritional support; AIDS acquired immunodeficiency syndrome; COPD = chronic obstructive pulmonary disease.

adequate nutrition for 7 days or longer should be supported from the time of admission. Finally, patients with a variety of specific disease entities have quicker recoveries and shorter hospital stays if nutritional needs are met.

ROUTE OF NUTRITIONAL SUPPORT

The enteral route should be chosen to administer nutritional support unless contraindications (Fig. 60–1) are present. Most critically ill patients tolerate enteral feeding. Using the gut avoids gut starvation, gut atrophy, and undesirable increases in mucosal permeability to bacteria. Absorption through the small intestine presents most nutrients to the enterohepatic circulation, reduces surges of glycemia and lipemia, permits first-pass hepatic extraction of nutrients, and stimulates physiologic endocrine responses to feeding. Conversely, central parenteral nutrition through subclavian or internal jugular veins is plagued by mechanical complications of catheter insertion in 4% to 6% of patients. These complications include pneumothorax and hemothorax, as well as injury to blood vessels, brachial plexus, and thoracic duct. Infectious complications occur in about 5% of patients receiving parenteral nutrition and include tunnel and line sepsis, metastatic abscess, and right-sided endocarditis. Severe hyperglycemia and fluid, acid-base, and electrolyte disturbances, as well as nutritional deficiencies, are more common with parenteral nutrition unless great attention is paid to detail. Many hospitals have a team dedicated to this activity.

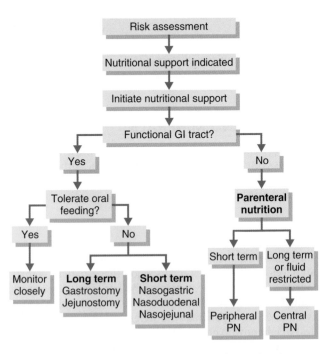

Figure 60–1 Algorithm for selecting type of nutritional support. GI = gastrointestinal; PN = parenteral nutrition.

Table 60–4	**Typical Nutrient Contents of Peripheral Parenteral Nutrition or Central Parenteral Nutrition Solutions**	
Nutrient	**CPN**	**PPN**
Nonprotein calories	1 kcal/mL	0.5 kcal/mL
Dextrose	20% (680 kcal/L)	5.0% (170 kcal/L)
Fat	3% (272 kcal/L)	3.8% (340 kcal/L)
Electrolytes (per liter)		
Cations		
Sodium	45.0 mEq	
Potassium	31.0 mEq	
Calcium	4.5 mEq	
Magnesium	5.0 mEq	
Anions		
Chloride	35.0 mEq	
Phosphate	12.5 mmol	
Acetate	29.5 mEq	
Trace elements (per day)		
Zinc	2.5 mg	
Copper	1.0 mg	
Manganese	0.25 mg	
Chromium	0.01 mg	
Multivitamins (per day) (A, D, E, B$_1$, B$_2$, niacin, B$_6$, C, K, biotin, pantothenic acid)	One vial	

PPN = peripheral parenteral nutrition; CPN = central parenteral nutrition.

Peripheral parenteral nutrition (PPN) through a vein in the arm or hand may be used to provide partial or total nutrition for up to 2 weeks. Thereafter, however, venous access becomes difficult. Solutions for PPN cannot contain more than 10% dextrose, and 5% is typically used (Table 60–4). Solutions of high osmolality cause painful thrombophlebitis. Therefore relatively high volumes of PPN are necessary to deliver a modest number of calories, and patients must be able to tolerate these volumes.

Clinicians frequently have limited options in selecting the route of administration. Nasogastric feeding tubes are never practical for more than 4 to 6 weeks even when small-diameter (6- to 12-French) silicone or polyurethane tubes

are used. Thereafter, insertion of percutaneous endoscopic gastrostomy (PEG) or jejunostomy (PEJ) tubes is necessary. Patients with severe inflammatory bowel disease or those with bowels shortened from superior mesenteric artery infarction or other causes often require parenteral nutrition.

All parenteral nutrition solutions supply amino acids rather than proteins. Two liters of a 5% amino acid solution is equivalent to about 80 g of protein. Disease-specific amino acid mixtures are available, but their superiority over balanced mixtures of essential and nonessential amino acids is uncertain. Preparations for patients with renal disease contain only essential amino acids to limit the nitrogen load, whereas preparations for patients with liver failure, who tend to have low levels of valine, leucine, and isoleucine, are enriched in these branched-chain amino acids.

Most of the calories in parenteral nutrition formulations are derived from dextrose and fat. Dextrose concentrations as high as 25% to 30% can be infused through centrally placed catheters. Lipid emulsions, unless contraindicated by pancreatitis or severe hypertriglyceridemia, can be used to advantage to provide 20% to 40% of total calories. Lipid emulsions are isotonic rather than hypertonic and provide essential fatty acids. In certain patients, lipid emulsions also limit the risk of severe hyperglycemia, hepatic steatosis, and hypercapnia from excessive dextrose administration.

Most commercially available enteral feeding formulas also contain about 1 kcal/mL energy, but products as calorically dense as 1.5 kcal/mL are also available. Calories are generally supplied by soy protein, cornstarch or syrup, and vegetable oil. Because most of their carbohydrates are complex, these formulas have relatively low osmolality (300 to 500 mOsm), and moderate volumes do not cause diarrhea. Most of the formulas are also lactose- and gluten-free and have little residue.

Vitamins and Minerals

Commercial enteral solutions contain sufficient vitamins, electrolytes, and trace minerals to guarantee adequate nutrition when provided in 2- to 3-L volumes each day. The majority contains less than 2 g of sodium and is acceptable when salt intake must be limited.

Parenteral solutions routinely have water-soluble and miscible vitamins, as well as standard additions of trace minerals. Notable exceptions are vitamin B$_{12}$, which should be administered intramuscularly every month during long-term parenteral nutrition, and selenium and molybdenum, which may become deficient after several months. The hospital nutritional support team often recommends a standard electrolyte mix (See Table 60–4), but physicians should monitor these carefully and stipulate different concentrations when indicated. Potassium uptake by cells may be at an abnormally high level during the first 10 days of central parenteral nutrition, thereby necessitating relatively high initial potassium infusion rates during this time.

Home Nutritional Support

More than 300,000 Americans receive home enteral tube feeding (HETF). The major indications cited are malignancy (~40% of patients) and neurologically impaired swallowing (30% of patients). The ease of endoscopic placement of gastrostomy tubes has dramatically increased the demand for HETF.

At least 50,000 Americans receive home parenteral nutrition (HPN); this number exceeds the annual prevalence in the rest of the world. The usual accepted indications are Crohn's disease, ischemic bowel disease, fistulas, and gastrointestinal motility disorders. In the United States, approximately 40% of patients receiving HPN have cancer. The annual cost of HPN is approximately $55,000, whereas the cost for HETF approximates $10,000.

Home nutritional support for those with Crohn's disease has been provided for up to 20 years and generally leads to long-term survival. HETF or HPN is also justified in a few other conditions. The use of home nutritional support to prolong life by weeks or months in the terminally ill patient and in the very old adult, however, is widely debated. Cost aside, physicians must ask whether nutritional support in such patients actually prolongs life or merely prolongs the dying process.

Prospectus for the Future

- Physicians and other health care providers will have gradually improved education about nutrition, disordered nutrition and its implications for health care, and nutritional support at the undergraduate, graduate, and postgraduate levels.
- People with disordered nutrition of specific nutrients or generalized malnutrition will be recognized earlier and considered for therapy.

- Economic analyses will demonstrate that attention to nutritional needs will save health care costs in both the short and long terms.
- The number of patients receiving HETF will grow rapidly in the next few years.

References

Carney DE, Meguid MM: Current concepts in nutritional assessment. Arch Surg 137:42–45, 2002.

Howard L, Malone M: Clinical outcome of geriatric patients in the United States receiving home parenteral and enteral nutrition. Am J Clin Nutr 66:1364–1370, 1997.

Huffman GB: Evaluating and treating unintentional weight loss in the elderly. Am Fam Phys 65:640–650, 2002.

Mechanik JI, Brett EM: Nutrition and the chronically critically ill patient. Curr Opin Clin Nutr Metab Care 8:33–39, 2005.

Nightengale JM: Parenteral nutrition: multidisciplinary management. Hosp Med 66:147–151, 2005.

Simpson F, Doig GS: Parenteral vs. enteral nutrition in the critically ill patient: a meta-analysis of trials using the intention to treat principle. Intensive Care Med 31:12–23, 2005.

Disorders of Lipid Metabolism

Reed E. Pyeritz

Introduction

The term *lipid* refers to substances that can be solubilized by nonpolar solvents. Major classes from human cells include fatty acids, glycolipids, sphingolipids, phospholipids, fat-soluble vitamins (A, D, E and K), and sterols. All lipids with functional roles in the human body, except for some vitamins and long-chain unsaturated fatty acids, can be synthesized endogenously. Important inborn errors of metabolism result from defects in synthesis and, especially, catabolism of these macromolecules. Lipids of various types are ingested; most are broken down to simple moieties that serve as precursors, fuel, or both. The two classes of lipid are discussed in this chapter, triglyceride (TG) and cholesterol. They are both synthesized and ingested and have important clinical relevance primarily because of their role as pathogenetic factors for atherosclerosis.

TGs are composed of three free fatty acid (FFA) chains bound in ester linkage to glycerol. FFAs can also be esterified to cholesterol in high-density lipoprotein (HDL) particles and are essential components of membrane lipids and are oxidized as sources of energy, preferentially in situations of fasting, exercise, or a high-fat diet. Mitochondrial ß-oxidation of FFAs produces acetoacetate, which is preferred by the heart, liver, and kidney to glucose as an energy source. During aerobic exercise, skeletal muscle derives 60% or more of its energy from FFAs. Cholesterol esters and TGs are hydrophobic, are transported in the bloodstream, and are taken up and excreted by cells in combination with phospholipids and apolipoproteins in lipoprotein particles, which are named based on how they separate under density-gradient centrifugation (Table 61–1). More than 20 well-characterized apolipoproteins, unimaginatively named alphabetically and encoded by genes spread across the genome, cluster on the surfaces of various lipoproteins. Apolipoproteins stabilize the lipoprotein micelle, are recognized by cell membrane receptors, and serve as enzyme co-factors.

Most of the clinical interest in the lipoproteins and TGs derives from their epidemiologic association with atherosclerosis. Those whose plasma concentrations are positively associated with the occurrence of atherosclerosis and its complications are TGs, low-density lipoproteins (LDLs), intermediate-density lipoproteins (IDLs), remnant particles, and lipoprotein(a) (Lp[a]); the concentration of HDLs is inversely associated with cardiovascular risk.

Plasma Lipoprotein Physiology

A typical American diet includes 50 to 120 g of fat (mainly TGs) daily; this represents about 40% of caloric intake and is more than necessary or desirable for the vast majority of people. Included in the typical western diet is about 400 to 500 mg/d of cholesterol, which is 50% or so more than ideal.

Dietary TG is hydrolyzed by pancreatic lipase, absorbed by the intestinal mucosal cells, and secreted into the mesenteric lymphatics as chylomicrons (Fig. 61–1). The liver also transforms plasma FFAs, which are unneeded when excess calories are ingested from the diet, into TGs and daily secretes an additional 10 to 30 g of very low–density lipoprotein (VLDL) TGs into the plasma. Both chylomicrons and VLDLs acquire apolipoprotein C-II (apo C-II) from plasma HDLs. Apo C-II is a critical co-factor for lipoprotein lipase, which is located on the capillary endothelium of muscle and adipose tissue. After hydrolysis of chylomicron and VLDL TGs, excess phospholipids, cholesterol, and apoproteins transfer to HDLs and increase HDL mass. The remnants remaining after hydrolysis of chylomicron TGs are cleared very rapidly by the liver and do not normally accumulate in plasma. Apolipoprotein E (apo E) mediates this process on the chylomicron surface, which binds to hepatic heparan sulfate proteoglycans (HSPG) and accounts for the rapid clearance of chylomicron remnants from the bloodstream. Apo E on the chylomicron surface is then specifically

Table 61–1 Properties of Lipoproteins

Lipoprotein Class	Origin	Major Apoproteins	Major Core Lipid
Chylomicrons	Intestine	B-48, C, E	Dietary TG
VLDL	Liver	B-100, C, E	Hepatic TG
IDL	VLDL catabolism	B-100, E	TG, C-esters
LDL	IDL catabolism	B-100	C-esters
Lp(a)	Liver	B-100, (a)	C-esters
HDL	Liver, intestine	A I, A II, E	C-esters

C = cholesterol; HDL = high-density lipoprotein; IDL = intermediate-density lipoprotein; LDL = low-density lipoprotein; Lp(a) = lipoprotein(a); TG = triglyceride; VLDL = very low-density lipoprotein.

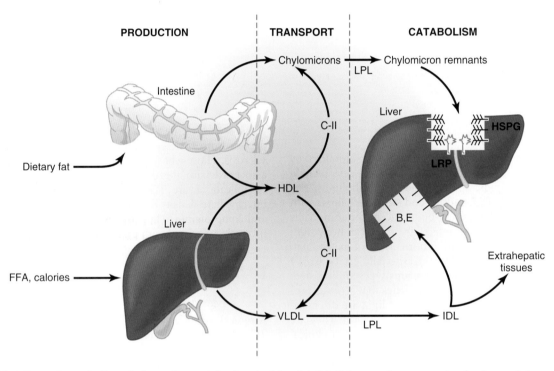

Figure 61–1 Normal metabolism of plasma lipoproteins (see text for details). B,E = membrane receptor for lipoproteins containing apo B and apo E (synonymous with the LDL receptor); apo C-II = apolipoprotein C-II; FFA = free (unesterified) fatty acids; HDL = high-density lipoproteins; HSPG = heparan sulfate proteoglycans; IDL = intermediate-density lipoproteins; LDL = low-density lipoproteins; LPL = lipoprotein lipase; LRP = LDL receptor–related protein; VLDL = very low–density lipoproteins.

bound to both the LDL-receptor and its lipoprotein receptor–related protein (LRP) in the hepatocyte cell membrane and internalized (see Fig. 61–1).

Some VLDL remnants (30% to 50%) are also cleared directly by the liver, and the remainder is converted to IDLs. IDLs are normally short lived and, by the action of lipases, are converted to the final VLDL catabolic product, LDLs (see Fig. 61–1). In contrast to VLDLs, which survives about 20 minutes in plasma, LDL particles circulate for 2 to 4 days depending on the availability of LDL receptors. Although LDLs normally account for 70% of the total plasma cholesterol, the particles are little more than metabolic garbage. Most LDL clearance from plasma takes place when apolipoprotein B (apo B) on the LDL surface binds to the LDL receptor on membranes of many tissues, particularly

the liver. The LDL-receptor pathway clears about 75% of LDLs, and the liver removes approximately two thirds.

Lp(a) lipoproteins are secreted by the liver, constitute 10% or less of the total plasma lipoprotein mass, possess kringle domains homologous to plasminogen, and are associated with a risk of vascular disease. Genetic heterogeneity produces 100-fold concentration differences among individuals, and levels are little affected by diet, habits, and most lipid-lowering drugs.

HDL particles are secreted into plasma by both the intestine and liver. When cholesterol and phospholipid are transported out of cells by an adenosine triphosphate (ATP)–binding cassette (ABC) transporter, HDL particles bind the lipids. Cholesterol is initially absorbed onto the HDL surface, where it is substrate for the plasma enzyme

Table 61–2 Approach to Elevated LDL-Cholesterol Levels in Adults*

Risk Category	LDL-C Goal (mg/dL)	LDL-C to Initiate TLC (mg/dL)	LDL-C Level to Initiate Drug Therapy (mg/dL)
≤1 RF	<160	≥160	≥190
2 + RF, 10-yr risk 0–10%	<130	≥130	≥160
2 + RF, 10-yr risk 10–20%	<130 (optional <100)	≥130	≥130
CAD or CAD-risk equivalent	<100 (optional <70)	≥100	≥130

*Recommendations of the Adult Treatment Panel, National Cholesterol Education Program III, as modified in 2004. CHD risk factors include male patient aged >45 yr, female patient aged >55 yr, or postmenopausal woman without estrogen replacement, family history of CHD before age 55 yr, smoking, hypertension, diabetes mellitus, and HDL-C <35 mg/dL. Subtract a risk factor if HDL-C is >60 mg/dL. 10-year risk of clinical CAD calculated with the Framingham Study equation. CAD-risk equivalents include diabetes mellitus requiring medication.
CAD = coronary artery disease; HDL = high-density lipoprotein; HDL-C = high-density lipoprotein–cholesterol; LDL = log-density lipoprotein; LDL-C = low-density lipoprotein–cholesterol; RF = risk factor; TLC = therapeutic lifestyle changes.

lecithin-cholesterol acyltransferase (LCAT). LCAT transfers a fatty acid from phosphatidyl choline to the 3-hydroxyl group of cholesterol. This produces cholesteryl esters that move from the hydrophilic HDL surface into the hydrophobic HDL core. The HDL surface is then free to accept more cholesterol from cells or other lipoproteins. The cholesteryl esters in the HDL core can be removed and transferred by a plasma protein and are the major source of cholesteryl esters contained in chylomicrons, VLDLs, and LDLs. Cholesterol ester transfer protein (CETP) mediates the transfer of cholesterol from HDLs to VLDLs.

The usefulness of quantifying apolipoproteins as opposed to lipoprotein classes in clinical practice is uncertain. The ratio of apo B to apolipoprotein A1 (apo A1) is a better predictor of cardiovascular risk than the ratio of HDL-cholesterol (HDL-C) to LDL-cholesterol (LDL-C), which has been used for years by physicians and clinical laboratories.

Evaluation of Serum Lipoprotein Concentrations

Elective determinations of plasma lipid concentrations should be made after an overnight fast, preferably of 14 hours. Most clinical laboratories focus on the major classes. Directly measured components include TGs, total LDL-C, and HDL-C. If TG levels are lower than 400 mg/dL, then the VLDL-cholesterol (VLDL-C) can be calculated by dividing the TG concentration by 5.

Primary care physicians repeatedly face the issue of who to screen for abnormalities of lipoproteins and when to initiate assays. Cholesterol levels should be measured in children who have a parent with a lipoprotein abnormality or coronary heart disease (CHD), stroke, or peripheral arterial disease that developed before the age of 55. Routine screening of other children is not recommended. Every adult should have total serum cholesterol and HDL-C levels determined during his or her 20s. A total cholesterol value of less than 200 mg/dL at any time of day does not necessitate retesting for 5 years. A level higher than 200 mg/dL should lead to measurement of total cholesterol, TGs, and HDL-C after a 14-hour fast. Similar testing is indicated in adults who have first-degree relatives with vascular disease or lipid

disorders. HDL-C levels lower than 40 mg/dL in men and women signify increased risk of occlusive arterial disease. If TG levels are over 500 mg/dL, specific treatment of hypertriglyceridemia should be undertaken. The highest levels of total cholesterol commonly encountered (600 to 2000 mg/dL) are usually due to increases in chylomicrons and VLDLs. Elevated cholesterol levels therefore cannot be interpreted without knowledge of TG levels.

A therapeutic strategy based on LDLs is indicated in Table 61–2. Management requires an overall assessment of a patient's risk factors for atherosclerosis (see Chapter 9).

Elevated HDL levels are thought to confer protection against CHD and do not require treatment. A low HDL level is one of the components of the *metabolic syndrome*, which also includes elevated TGs, hypertension, abdominal obesity, hypertension, and glucose intolerance. Growing evidence supports using a low HDL-C to initiate aggressive modification of other factors, including mild LDL elevations (100 to 130 mg/dL).

Lipids and Vascular Disease

Intervention studies in the 1990s showed that cholesterol reduction by means of diet, drugs, or surgery reduces the risk of development or progression of CHD. Subsequent clinical trials using various statin drugs have convincingly shown that, for people at high risk for CHD, the lower the LDL-C, the better the prognosis. Treatment with moderate doses of statins reduces LDL-C levels by an average 30% to 40% beyond that achieved by diet. People with atherosclerosis defined by imaging studies of the vascular wall may show small but definite regressions of atherosclerotic lesions. A wide spectrum of patient populations, including women, patients with diabetes, and older adults, has benefited from statins in primary and secondary heart disease intervention trials (Table 61–3). These impressive results notwithstanding, secondary prevention is far inferior to risk reduction before clinical evidence of occlusive arterial disease emerges.

Considerable debate still exists about the cost effectiveness of screening the general population for lipid disorders and treating individuals without clinical evidence of vascular disease who are found to have cholesterol elevations.

Table 61–3 Populations in Whom Treatment with Statins Has Reduced Coronary Events

Middle-aged men with hypercholesterolemia and without known CHD

Middle-aged men with average cholesterol levels, below-average HDL levels, and no known CHD

Middle-aged men and women with hypercholesterolemic and known CHD

Men and women with diabetes and with CHD

Older men (>60 years) with CHD

Men and women with coronary bypass grafts

CHD = Coronary heart disease.

Table 61–4 Guidelines for Treatment of Hyperlipopro-teinemia

Initiation

Document abnormality twice after a 14-hr fast while on typical American diet. Provisionally classify as cholesterol or TG problem. Test total cholesterol and TG and HDL-C levels.

Evaluate potential for control with diet modification (e.g., fish-vegetarian diet) for 2 wk; retest after 2 wk.

Return to conventional lipid-lowering diet (30% or less fat with equal proportions of polyunsaturated, monounsaturated, and saturated fats) for 4 wk; retest.

If target values are not achieved, add lipid-lowering medicine or food supplements. Retest 4 wk after each change in regimen.

Maintenance

Patient keeps lipid record on flow sheet and has rapid access to test results.

Minimum follow-up test frequency is every 4–6 mo.

HDL-C = High-density lipoprotein–cholesterol; TG = triglyceride.

According to the reference ranges established by the National Cholesterol Education Program (NCEP), about one third of adult Americans would be classified as having *high cholesterol* and another one third as having borderline high values. Indeed, almost one half of all postmenopausal women have total and LDL-C levels over 240 mg/dL and 160 mg/dL, respectively. An estimated 100,000 apparently healthy people must be treated annually to prevent 70 deaths from heart disease.

Nevertheless, full agreement exists that eating less saturated fat and cholesterol and adopting diet and exercise habits to reduce obesity benefits the health of most people. Data indicate a significant fall in American cholesterol levels during the 1990s, and vascular disease rates have been falling since the early 1970s. These and other public health efforts (e.g., smoking cessation, blood pressure awareness) have had a much greater affect than individualized medical interventions. However, a time of diminishing return from population-based efforts has likely been reached. Management of individual patients and their relatives, based on their specific risk factors, including TG, LDL, HDL and Lp(a) levels, will have increasing importance in the current decade.

General Principles of Management of Lipid Disorders

The treatment of the lipid disorders requires a systematic approach (Table 61–4). In general, the abnormality should be documented twice before treatment is undertaken. Approximately one half of affected persons are sensitive to diet, achieving a >10% reduction in TG and/or LDL-C levels. The extent of sensitivity can be defined aggressively (i.e., administering a fish-vegetarian diet for 2 to 3 weeks [Table 61–5]) or gradually (i.e., instituting the NCEP Step 1 diet, evaluating, and if necessary instituting the Step 2 diet). Patients are retested once or preferably twice while on the diet they can tolerate, and the results provide a point of

Table 61–5 Fish-Vegetarian Diet

Permissible Foods and Beverages

Seafood—fish, clams, oysters, lobster, scallops, and shrimp (in moderation)

Bread

Pasta (with vegetable oil, tomato sauce, or clam sauce if desired)

Potato (with margarine)

Rice

Vegetables (all)

Fruits (except avocado) and fruit juices

Vegetable oils

Peanut butter

Nuts (except for coconut and macadamia)

Cereal (except granola-type natural cereals)

Low-fat crackers (matzo, RyKrisp, Stoned Wheat Thins)

Angel food cake (plain)

Skim (not 1%) milk

Coffee, tea, soda

Alcohol

Nondairy creamers (Coffee-Rich, Poly-Rich, Poly-Perx)

Foods to Be Omitted

Meat (including fowl)

Baked goods (including desserts and chips)

Dairy products (including eggs, butter, and cheese)

Fast Food Restaurants

None

Table 61-6 Drugs for Hyperlipoproteinemia

Drug Class	Mechanism	Side Effects
Elevated LDL-C Level		
Resins (cholestyramine, colestipol, colesevelam)	Deplete bile acids, upregulate LDL receptors	Constipation Abdominal discomfort
Fibrates (gemfibrozil, fenofibrate)	Inhibit hepatic VLDL production Increase VLDL metabolism	Gallstones Nausea
Niacin	Unclear; inhibits FFA release from adipocytes Decreased synthesis of VLDLs and LDLs	Flushing and pruritis Elevated LFTs
Statins (atorvastatin, cerivastatin, fluvastatin, pravastatin, simvastatin)	Inhibit cholesterol biosynthesis Upregulate LDL receptors	Elevated LFTs CPK Myalgias Myositis
Ezetimibe	Intestinal cholesterol receptor	Diarrhea Angioedema (rare)
Elevated Triglyceride Level		
Fibrates (clofibrate, gemfibrozil, fenofibrate)	Stimulate lipoprotein lipase activity	Diarrhea, nausea
Niacin	Inhibit FFA release from adipocytes	Skin flushing
Fish oils	Inhibit hepatic VLDL production	Minimal

CPK = creatine phosphokinase; FFA = free fatty acid; LDL = low-density lipoprotein; LDL-C = LDL cholesterol; LFT = liver function test; VLD L = very low-density lipoprotein.

reference for all future diet and drug interventions. If diet reduces cholesterol and LDL levels to target values (see Table 62–2) or TG values to less than 120 mg/dL, then it may be liberalized to give greater menu variety. If target values are not achieved, then drug treatment is considered (Table 61–6). Compliance is best when patients chart their lipid levels, have ready access to test results, and undergo follow-up testing every 3 to 4 months. Assessment of drug effects takes no more than 1 to 2 months, and in general the efficacy of individual agents should be established before combinations are prescribed.

Treatment of Hypertriglyceridemia

DIET

Reduced fat consumption is the only treatment for patients with deficiencies of lipoprotein lipase or apo C-II. The daily fat intake is limited to 25 g by restricting all fat-enriched foods, including those made from vegetable oils. Adults with more common forms of severe hypertriglyceridemia and TG levels over 1000 mg/dL should also follow a low-fat, low-alcohol diet, attain ideal body weight, and exercise regularly to reduce TG levels to less than 500 mg/dL. Patients with milder TG elevations benefit from a diet that is close to a fish-vegetarian diet (see Table 61–5). This very strict diet typically lowers cholesterol levels by 15% to 20% and TG levels by 30% to 40% in patients with hypertriglyceridemia. A second major objective of diet is to reduce body fat content. Most individuals with hypertriglyceridemia show significant improvement while actively losing weight, and a significant proportion, primarily those with insulin resis-

tance, are cured after weight reduction. Finally, alcohol should be restricted to one or two servings a week; on occasion, this restriction alone corrects the problem. If diet, weight loss, and exercise programs do not sustain TG levels of 300 mg/dL or less, then drug therapy is appropriate.

EXERCISE

TG levels are reduced after even a single exercise session, and exercise has been shown to augment lipoprotein lipase activity. The efficacy of regular aerobic exercise in patients with mild-to-moderate hypertriglyceridemia has been repeatedly demonstrated, and exercise has great potential in promoting weight loss. The program goal should be 45 minutes of sub-maximal exercise on 5 days each week. The type of aerobics, duration, and intensity should be explicitly defined by the health professional to promote compliance.

DRUGS

The fibrate class of drugs (see Table 61–6) enhances production of apo A1, enhances lipoprotein lipase activity through peroxisome proliferator activated receptor–alpha (PPAR-a), and stimulates oxidation of FFA in peroxisomes. Drugs such as gemfibrozil and fenofibrate are most effective in patients with dysbetalipoproteinemia and in others with high VLDL levels reflected by high total cholesterol levels (500 to 1000 mg/dL), as well as high TG levels (1000 to 10,000 mg/dL). When hypertriglyceridemia results primarily from chylomicronemia and the cholesterol level is only moderately elevated (250 to 500 mg/dL), the fibrates are less effective than dietary fat restriction. Niacin alone can be effective in patients with moderate hypertriglyceridemia (TG levels, 500 to 1000 mg/dL) and has added beneficial effects on LDL

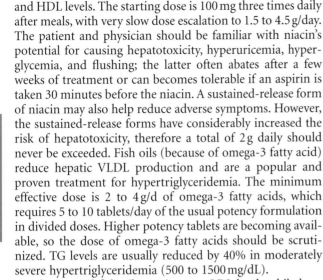

and HDL levels. The starting dose is 100 mg three times daily after meals, with very slow dose escalation to 1.5 to 4.5 g/day. The patient and physician should be familiar with niacin's potential for causing hepatotoxicity, hyperuricemia, hyperglycemia, and flushing; the latter often abates after a few weeks of treatment or can becomes tolerable if an aspirin is taken 30 minutes before the niacin. A sustained-release form of niacin may also help reduce adverse symptoms. However, the sustained-release forms have considerably increased the risk of hepatotoxicity, therefore a total of 2 g daily should never be exceeded. Fish oils (because of omega-3 fatty acid) reduce hepatic VLDL production and are a popular and proven treatment for hypertriglyceridemia. The minimum effective dose is 2 to 4 g/d of omega-3 fatty acids, which requires 5 to 10 tablets/day of the usual potency formulation in divided doses. Higher potency tablets are becoming available, so the dose of omega-3 fatty acids should be scrutinized. TG levels are usually reduced by 40% in moderately severe hypertriglyceridemia (500 to 1500 mg/dL).

Fibrates and fish oils can increase LDL levels while lowering VLDL and chylomicron levels. On occasion, LDL levels are raised above 160 mg/dL (see Table 61–2), and this undesirable effect must be weighed against the potential gain.

Elevated Low-Density Lipoprotein

POLYGENIC HYPERCHOLESTEROLEMIA

Approximately 60% to 70% of a patient's cholesterol or LDL level is genetically determined, with the remaining contribution from age, sex, diet, and other factors. The nature of these genetic effects is incompletely defined. Individuals in the upper range of the normal distribution have an increased risk of CHD, and the upper 50% contribute about 80% of patients with CHD. Modulation of LDL levels is strongly advised for both primary and secondary prevention of vascular disease, and the thresholds for instituting therapy and the goals vary with the risk of clinical events associated with atherosclerosis calculated for the individual patient (see Table 61–2).

FAMILIAL MONOGENIC HYPERCHOLESTEROLEMIA

About 1 in 500 North Americans has a monogenic disorder producing an abnormality of the LDL receptor (see Fig. 61–1). Their cells have approximately one half the normal number of functional receptors, which results in a total cholesterol level around 370 mg/dL and more than twice the average concentration of LDLs. However, relatives with the same mutation in LDL receptor (LDLR) often have widely varying basal LDL levels. An increased LDL level is detectable as early as the first year of life and is associated with corneal arcus, xanthomas of the Achilles tendon and extensor tendons of the hands, and a risk for CHD that is about 25 times that in unaffected relatives. Heterozygous men have a 50% chance of myocardial infarction by 50 years of age, and the comparable risk in women is 10% to 20%. Homozygotes or those heterozygotic individuals with two abnormal alleles (compound heterozygotes) have cholesterol levels of 650 to 1000 mg/dL, severe xanthomatosis, and typically die of cardiovascular disease before age 30.

Treatment of Hypercholesterolemia

DIET

Limitation of dietary saturated fat is central to both cholesterol- and TG-lowering diets. Carbohydrates are often substituted for the saturated fats, but high-carbohydrate diets may increase TGs and reduce HDLs. Polyunsaturated fats are better substitutes for saturated fat. Reduction of dietary cholesterol has a small additional LDL-lowering effect. In practice, the optimal diet approaches the fish-vegetarian diet used to establish diet sensitivity (see Table 61–5). On average, a person with hypercholesterolemia lowers total cholesterol by 12% (range, 0% to 40%) on this diet. When those who initially respond to diet are again found to have hypercholesterolemia, the usual cause is noncompliance, which can be identified by asking patients to complete a 7-day diet diary and reviewing the record with them. Subjects who travel extensively and eat frequently in restaurants have the greatest difficulty with dietary compliance. When large populations have been studied, results with most cholesterol-lowering diets have been disappointing, with mean total cholesterol reductions in the range of 5%. This recognition prompts many clinicians to teach and prescribe dietary management, but not to spend time and effort documenting effectiveness before moving to medications.

EXERCISE

Although trained endurance athletes have LDL levels about 10% lower than those individuals matched for age, diet, and other characteristics, moderate exercise alone is generally not effective in reducing LDL concentrations. However, regular exercise has a beneficial affect on raising HDL-C and lowering TG levels.

DRUGS

For patients who do not achieve goal LDL levels after dietary and exercise modification, several considerations govern the choice of drug therapy. Balancing the potential for adverse effects against the likely benefits takes on added importance because the drugs are usually prescribed for many years, and most are moderately expensive.

Resin agents act by binding bile acids in the gut, thereby increasing fecal excretion, decreasing enterohepatic recycling, and decreasing the pool of cholesterol through increased synthesis of bile acids. The resins (see Table 61–6) are safe and effective and are the only agents extensively evaluated in children. The starting dose is 2 scoops or unit dose packets before supper; this dose is enough in many patients with mild hypercholesterolemia, and more than 6 unit doses a day is rarely worth the cost and inconvenience. A large bowl of wheat or corn bran cereal can prevent constipation during resin use, but some patients still feel bloated. Colesevelam is administered in up to 6 pills daily and has a lower incidence of gastrointestinal side effects. Resins are contraindicated in those with hypertriglyceridemia, and TG levels should be reduced to less than 300 mg/dL before resins are used in patients with mixed or combined hyperlipidemia.

Niacin is useful in patients with LDL elevations, and the same precautions that were noted for niacin use in hypertriglyceridemia apply.

The statins (see Table 61–6) competitively inhibit hydroxymethylglutaryl–coenzyme A (HMG-CoA) reductase, the rate-limiting enzyme in cholesterol biosynthesis. This inhibition induces an increase in hepatic LDL receptors, and LDL levels typically are lowered by 25% to 50%. Statins are now the mainstays of both primary and secondary intervention for atherosclerotic vascular disease (see Table 61–3). They have been shown to both prevent cardiac end points (e.g., myocardial infarction, coronary revascularization) and prolong life in diverse populations. A growing body of evidence suggests that a statin should be started soon after myocardial infarction, regardless of the plasma lipid profile. Statins are appropriate for patients of any age with hypercholesterolemia who have established CHD and for other adults with moderately severe hypercholesterolemia (LDL level, >190 mg/dL). Statins are expensive but well tolerated, and the compliance rate is excellent; generic versions of some of the first statins are entering the market. Statins alone, or especially in combination with niacin, fibrates, or cyclosporine, may cause myositis and even rhabdomyolysis. The risks of elevated hepatic transaminases and muscle creatine phosphokinase (CPK) levels as a result of statins are related to dose, which is cited as an important reason why primary care physicians are reluctant to titrate the dose to 80 mg/day to achieve maximum LDL-lowering results.

Ezetimibe is a drug that blocks intestinal absorption of cholesterol and may be a sufficient treatment of mild LDL elevations that persist after lifestyle adjustments. Ezetimibe can also be combined with a statin to treat two independent aspects of cholesterol metabolism.

The fibrates are not approved for simple hypercholesterolemia. They typically lower LDL levels by only 8% to 10% but may produce dramatic results in some patients.

Many patients, particularly those who have heterozygotic familial hypercholesterolemia, require two or three drugs to achieve adequate control. Resins plus niacin plus a statin or resins plus fibrates have been widely used. A statin plus ezetimibe can be tried. LDL-apheresis also plays a role. Resins or statins plus fish oils are also effective in patients with mixed hyperlipidemia. Homozygotic patients with familial hypercholesterolemia respond inadequately to diet and drugs and may require liver transplantation. Finally, estrogen replacement therapy after the menopause can significantly lower LDL levels while increasing HDLs. However, estrogen alone does not seem to reduce the risk of CAD.

Elevated Chylomicrons, Very Low–Density Lipoprotein, and Intermediate-Density Lipoprotein

DISORDERS IN CHILDHOOD

The occurrence of eruptive xanthomas, lipemia retinalis, hepatosplenomegaly, and abdominal pain in an infant or a small child suggests a primary defect in clearance of chylomicrons and VLDLs. This occurrence may be the result of a deficiency of lipoprotein lipase (assayed in plasma after heparin injection) or of apo C-II, the co-factor for lipoprotein lipase. These abnormalities have a combined prevalence of less than 1 to 2 in 1 million people.

DISORDERS ARISING IN ADULTHOOD

Both chylomicrons and VLDLs are catabolized by lipoprotein lipase, and the enzyme is saturable. The enzyme prefers chylomicrons, so VLDLs usually accumulate first until TG levels exceed 500 mg/dL. At higher levels, both VLDLs and chylomicrons contribute to hypertriglyceridemia. Testing to resolve the independent contribution of these two lipoproteins is rarely indicated, and tests for lipoprotein lipase and apo C-II should be reserved for cases arising in childhood. Most hypertriglyceridemia in adults appears to be associated with insulin resistance or overt diabetes and is due to VLDL overproduction, although defective catabolism is responsible in a subset of patients.

Moderate-to-severe hypertriglyceridemia is relatively common in men and women older than 30 years of age. The disorder is usually genetic and is commonly associated with the *metabolic syndrome* (previously termed *syndrome X*). Recent estimates suggest a prevalence of metabolic syndrome in the United States of 47 million. Obesity, even moderate alcohol consumption, exogenous estrogens, and drugs such as diuretics and β-adrenergic receptor blockers may aggravate hypertriglyceridemia. Common secondary causes of hypertriglyceridemia are renal disease with proteinuria, hyperthyroidism and hypothyroidism, exogenous and endogenous glucocorticoids, and type II diabetes mellitus. A very severe form of hypertriglyceridemia (TG levels 2000 to 6000 mg/dL) can occur in patients with chronic insulin deficiency and very mild acidosis. This abnormality is completely corrected by insulin administration. The hypertriglyceridemia occurring in acute diabetic ketoacidosis is usually milder (TG levels, 250 to 800 mg/dL) and also responds to insulin.

The importance of hypertriglyceridemia in vascular disease risk has been controversial. A National Institutes of Health consensus conference concluded that TG levels less than 250 mg/dL were acceptable, those 250 to 500 mg/dL were borderline elevated, and only higher values were abnormal. Nevertheless, TG levels in the upper normal range (120 to 250 mg/dL) are very prevalent in patient populations with CHD, and within this range the inverse relationship between TG and HDL-C is strongest. The association of hypertriglyceridemia and diabetes mellitus, obesity, and hypertension has long confounded efforts to define its independent role in vascular disease. A recent meta-analysis strongly supports the finding that an elevated TG level independently increases the risk of CAD in both men and women.

DYSBETALIPOPROTEINEMIA

Dysbetalipoproteinemia is characterized by the accumulation of chylomicron remnants and IDLs in plasma. It is caused by homozygosity for a variant of apo E (E$_2$), which binds less avidly to the LDL receptor than do apo E$_3$ and apo E$_4$ (see Fig. 61–1). This accumulation leads to a defective hepatic clearance of chylomicron remnants and an ineffective catabolism of IDLs to LDLs. Less commonly, heterozygosity for a variant apo E results in an autosomal dominant form of dysbetalipoproteinemia.

Apo E_2, which occurs in 12% of Americans, differs from normal apo E_3 and apo E_4 because of a point mutation that causes a single amino acid substitution. Homozygosity for apo E_2 occurs in 1% to 2% of the population, but a minority develops hyperlipidemia solely as a consequence of this polymorphism. Dysbetalipoproteinemia occurs only if the E_2 homozygote also has an additional disorder such as hypothyroidism or familial hypertriglyceridemia, the latter suggested in persons who have both elevated cholesterol and TG levels. Diagnosis requires demonstration of apo E_2 homozygosity or unusual cholesterol enrichment of the VLDL. If the ratio of cholesterol to TG in VLDL, isolated by ultracentrifugation, is higher than 0.40, then dysbetalipoproteinemia is likely to be present. This form of hyperlipoproteinemia causes palmar and tuberoeruptive xanthomas, as well as coronary and peripheral vascular disease. The condition is worth identifying because it is exquisitely sensitive to weight reduction, cholesterol-lowering diets, and drugs such as gemfibrozil, fenofibrate, and HMG-CoA reductase inhibitors (statins).

FAMILIAL COMBINED HYPERLIPOPROTEINEMIA

Familial combined hyperlipoproteinemia describes families with a mixture of lipoprotein abnormalities that appear to segregate as an autosomal dominant trait. Affected members may have high VLDL levels, high LDL levels, or both. The basic abnormality is probably VLDL overproduction. Patients who do not effectively catabolize VLDL exhibit only hypertriglyceridemia. Those who are very efficient in VLDL catabolism exhibit only increased total and LDL-C levels. Others exhibit combined elevations of VLDL TG and LDL-C levels. Family screening is required for a confident diagnosis, but the label is often loosely used to describe the combination of both VLDL and LDL elevations. The abnormality occurs frequently in patients with occlusive vascular disease, and affected patients often require diet and several lipid-lowering drugs to achieve normal lipid concentrations.

Prospectus for the Future

- Heightened emphasis on early treatment of even mildly elevated LDL-C levels with a variety of approaches, especially statins, in primary prevention
- Better understanding of the so-called pleiotropic effects of statins and their putative role in other common disorders of adulthood, such as osteoporosis and dementia
- Development of drugs tailored to increase HDL-C levels
- Improved methods for noninvasively detecting early atherosclerosis, which will create additional indications for aggressive modulation of risk factors, including lipids

References

Grundy SM, Cleeman JI, Merz CN, et al: Implications of recent clinical trials for the National Cholesterol Education Program (NCEP) Adult Treatment Panel III Guidelines. Circulation 110:227–239, 2004.

Lusis AJ et al: Lipoprotein and Lipid Metabolism. In Rimoin DL, Connor JM, Pyeritz RE, Korf BR (eds). Principles and Practice of Medical Genetics, 5th ed, Philadelphia, Churchill-Livingstone, 2007. In press.

Nissen SE et al: Effect of intensive compared with moderate lipid-lowering therapy on progression of coronary atherosclerosis: A randomized controlled trial. JAMA 291:1071–1080, 2004.

Henley E, Chang L, Hollander S: Treatment of hyperlipidemia. J Fam Pract 51:370–376, 2002.

ACKNOWLEDGMENT

I thank Paul D. Thompson, MD, for helpful suggestions.

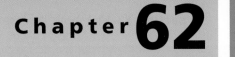

Disorders of Metals and Metalloproteins

David G. Brooks

Wilson's Disease

Wilson's disease, or hepatolenticular degeneration, is the result of the defective excretion of copper. Accumulation of this metal produces damage to multiple organs with the liver and brain being the ones prominently affected. Wilson's disease is an autosomal recessive genetic disorder that affects people worldwide with a frequency approximating 1 in 30,000.

NORMAL COPPER METABOLISM

Copper is an essential dietary trace element. A balance of dietary intake and hepatobiliary excretion meet physiologic requirements. Humans ingest 1 to 5 mg/day, and an adult body contains 100 to 150 mg copper. Copper is absorbed in the proximal small intestine. The liver, which is the main organ for copper homeostasis, rapidly takes up absorbed copper. The liver plays important roles in transport, storage, and excretion of copper. Copper is normally excreted into bile canaliculi in a regulated fashion that is dependent on copper concentration in hepatocytes. Up to 95% of plasma copper is bound to ceruloplasmin, an abundant plasma protein. The putative role of ceruloplasmin as a copper transporter to extrahepatic tissues has been called into question by the absence of copper deficiency in aceruloplasminemia, a genetic disease featuring the absence of apoceruloplasmin. Rather, ceruloplasmin is more likely to play a critical role in recycling iron by oxidation of iron to enable ferric iron to bind to apotransferrin, which is evidenced by the dramatic iron overload in aceruloplasminemia.

PATHOGENESIS

Mutations in patients with Wilson's disease occur in a gene, *ATP7B*, that encodes a copper-transporting adenosine triphosphatase (ATPase). This protein transports copper across cell membranes and is essential for exporting copper from hepatocytes into the bile canaliculi. Wilson's disease protein also transports cytosolic copper into membrane-bound compartments of hepatocytes containing newly synthesized apoceruloplasmin. In the absence of the transporter, copper is not transported and apoceruloplasmin is secreted into the blood where it has a rapid turnover. Thus low plasma ceruloplasmin levels are a helpful diagnostic sign of Wilson's disease (Table 62–1). Copper accumulates slowly in liver (see Table 62–1) and later in other organs. High levels of copper are a risk factor for generating reactive oxygen species, which contribute to end-organ damage. Liver dysfunction, the most common presentation in childhood, usually appears after 6 years of age. Presentations vary from acute hepatitis to chronic, progressive liver failure. Most patients have liver biopsy evidence of some cirrhosis resulting from copper-mediated damage. Neurologic symptoms, in particular as a result of basal ganglia dysfunction, are the initial presentation in up to 60% of patients. Parkinsonian symptoms predominate with dystonia, choreoathetosis, and tremor. A minority of patients experience personality change, depression, or cognitive impairment, all of which indicate that the cerebral cortex is affected by copper deposition. Associated findings include *hemolytic anemia* (negative Coombs test) and kidney damage (*nephrolithiasis* and *Fanconi syndrome* with amino aciduria and glucosuria). Cardiac dysrhythmia, rhabdomyolysis, arthralgia, and endocrine dysfunction have also been reported.

DIAGNOSIS

A combination of laboratory tests strongly supports the diagnosis of Wilson's disease (see Table 62–1). Approximately 95% of patients will have a low ceruloplasmin level with some having normal levels because ceruloplasmin is an acute phase reactant that is high during inflammation. Serum copper is slightly decreased and nonceruloplasmin-bound serum copper is usually elevated. A significant increase in urinary copper excretion (>100 μg/24 hr) is

Table 62–1 Diagnostic Copper Testing in Wilson's Disease

Test	Levels in Healthy Persons	Levels in Wilson's Disease
Liver copper content (µg Cu/g dry weight)	10–50	100–2000
Serum ceruloplasmin (mg/dL)	20–45	0–20
Serum copper (µg/dL)	70–160	25–70
Urinary copper (µg/day)	3–35	100–1000

almost always present, which should increase further with chelator therapy. Liver biopsy often reveals micronodular cirrhosis with nodular regeneration, copper deposition, and elevated copper content. Kayser-Fleischer rings, which are yellow-brown to green deposits at the periphery of the cornea, strongly support the diagnosis. Magnetic resonance imaging (MRI) of basal ganglia may show degeneration or evidence suggestive of copper deposition. Genetic testing is available; however, hundreds of mutations are known, which means that only specialized laboratories offer this service. In defined ethnic groups, identifying genetic mutations that confirm Wilson's disease may be practical and have important genetic counseling implications for family members.

TREATMENT

Wilson's disease is a treatable genetic disorder. Therefore this diagnosis is an important consideration in anyone with unexplained liver, basal ganglia, or psychiatric signs or symptoms. The goal of therapy is to reduce total body copper burden. A diet low in copper is important to limit absorption; however, symptomatic patients require chelation therapy to remove excess copper. Two copper chelators are approved for clinical use: trientine (Syprine) and D-penicillamine (Cuprimine). Historically, penicillamine was the treatment of choice. However, because of frequent treatment-limiting side effects of this therapy, trientine has merit as a first-line therapy. For D-penicillamine, treatment should be initiated with 1 to 3 g/day and is divided into two to four doses. Pyridoxine should be supplemented while taking penicillamine. Urine copper excretion should increase from 1 to 5 mg/day with symptomatic improvement on average after 4 months of therapy. Life-long treatment at reduced doses of penicillamine may be required. Further, under no circumstances should D-penicillamine be abruptly stopped; doing so increases the risk of acute hepatic decompensation. After high-dose chelation therapy has successfully removed the excess copper, a novel dietary strategy may decrease further copper absorption. The diet can be supplemented with zinc acetate or sulfate (150 mg/day) because zinc inhibits net copper absorption by inducing the small intestine to produce the copper-chelating protein, metal-

lothionein. Metallothionein-bound copper is sloughed with small intestinal absorptive cells. Supplementation with the antioxidant vitamin E, taken with meals, may offset some of the organ damage induced by reactive oxygen species. Urinalysis and blood counts should be followed closely during penicillamine therapy. Giving a test dose of penicillamine is important because it triggers hypersensitivity reactions strong enough to prevent up to 10% of patients from taking the medication. Fever, lymphadenopathy, cytopenias, lupus erythematosus–like reactions, and nephrotic syndrome can result. Trientine is an alternative treatment for those with hypersensitivity reactions to penicillamine. An investigational agent, ammonium tetrathiomolybdate, may inhibit copper absorption and chelate-serum copper. Liver transplantation, even from living related donors who carry a single defective gene for Wilson's disease, has been a successful treatment for those with progressive liver failure.

Hemochromatosis

Hemochromatosis is the condition of excessive iron storage causing dysfunction of a characteristic pattern of organs. It may be primary, which mean genetic, or secondary, which may be due, for example, to multiple transfusions. The primary forms, which are known as hereditary hemochromatoses, are the only concerns of this chapter.

NORMAL IRON METABOLISM

The adult male body contains 4 g of iron, over one half of which is in the form of hemoglobin. To meet the daily iron requirement for erythropoiesis, iron is recycled from the reticulo-endothelial system. Iron is absorbed in the duodenum, and the efficiency of absorption is regulated. Thus the duodenum responds to bodily iron requirements and can significantly increase in times of iron deficiency. Iron is not actively excreted. About 1 mg of iron is lost daily through sloughed cells; this amount is increased by menstrual blood loss and pregnancy. These losses are offset by absorption of 1 to 3 mg of iron daily in normal individuals, although this amount is increased in patients with hemochromatosis.

The liver is important for iron storage and transport. Iron is stored in *ferritin* in the liver. Ferritin secretion from the liver is positively correlated with hepatic iron stores. Hepatocytes secrete the iron transport protein transferrin; and transferrin then circulates with approximately 20% to 40% saturation of iron (Table 62–2). Transferrin-bound iron is the major source of iron for extrahepatic tissues that have transferrin receptors. After transferrin receptor–mediated endocytosis, iron may be released in the acidic environment of an intracellular vesicle (endosome) and transferrin is recycled to be released at the cell surface.

PATHOGENESIS OF HEREDITARY HEMOCHROMATOSIS

Four types of hereditary hemochromatosis are known. The genetic bases of these disorders are known in three of the four types, and all defective gene products have a role in cellular iron trafficking. In two of the types, the defective genes encode ferritin or transferrin receptors. In the third type,

Table 62-2	Iron Indices in Healthy Persons and in Patients with Symptomatic Hemochromatosis	
Index	**Levels in Healthy Persons**	**Levels in Hemochromatosis**
Plasma iron (μg/dL)	50–150	180–300
Total iron-binding capacity (μg/dL)	250–375	200–300
Percent transferring saturation	20–40	80–100
Serum ferritin (ng/mL)	10–200	900–6000
Urinary iron after 0.5 g desferrioxamine	0–2	9–23
Liver iron (μg/100 mg dry weight)	30–140	600–1800

which is the common form of hereditary hemochromatosis, discovery of the gene has generated new insight to the basis of iron homeostasis. Only the common form of hereditary hemochromatosis is discussed in this chapter.

The common form of hereditary hemochromatosis is the result of defects in a gene and protein called HFE, hence the name HFE-linked hemochromatosis. This gene is near the major histocompatibility complex (MHC) locus on chromosome 6, in keeping with the long-standing observation that certain MHC isotypes (e.g., human leukocyte–associated antigen [HLA-A3]) are co-inherited with hemochromatosis. The HFE protein is an MHC class I–like molecule that requires association with β_2-microglobulin to function. In the absence of either HFE or β_2-microglobulin, mice develop iron overload, reminiscent of human hemochromatosis. HFE binds tightly to the transferrin receptor and regulates its affinity for transferrin ligand. More than 85% of patients with hemochromatosis of northern European ancestry have two mutations that interfere with HFE function. The most common mutation in patients results in the substitution of tyrosine for the normal cysteine at position 282 (C282Y). This mutation is most concentrated in people of northern European ancestry, a finding that accounts for the Caucasian predilection of hereditary hemochromatosis. The C282Y mutation is found in 1 in 10 Caucasians in the United States. Therefore 1 in 400 Caucasians carries two of these mutations. However, the observed prevalence of hemochromatosis is closer to 1 in 4000. Thus a small minority of individuals with two mutations will develop hemochromatosis, and the positive predictive value of a genetic test is low. This phenomenon, called *reduced penetrance*, explains why genetic testing has limited utility as a screening tool for this disorder. However, testing for C282Y or another common mutant allele, H63D, is useful in patients with iron overload to confirm the diagnosis of hemochromatosis.

The essential defect in hereditary hemochromatosis is increased absorption of dietary iron. A slight increase in the efficiency of iron absorption, coupled with the inability to excrete iron, leads to increasing hepatic iron storage as a function of time. With increasing iron stores, the liver secretes more ferritin and serum transferrin becomes increasingly saturated with iron. Initially, a patient may have general signs such as fatigue. Later, signs of liver disease are apparent. Liver biopsy shows increased iron stores in hepatocytes with sparing of Kupffer cells; a specimen should be analyzed for the amount of iron. High iron stores can lead to a generation of toxic reactive oxygen species, fibrosis, and cirrhosis.

The earliest symptoms of hemochromatosis include fatigue, lethargy, arthralgia, and right upper quadrant discomfort. As the capacity of liver to store iron safely is exceeded, particularly after transferrin saturation reaches 100%, iron is deposited in other tissues. Deposition in the synovium produces iron-induced arthritis. In the pancreatic islets, β cells are damaged, resulting in diabetes as a result of insulin insufficiency. Iron can cause restrictive cardiomyopathy and a predisposition to conduction system abnormalities, resulting in arrhythmias. Hypogonadism, secondary to hypopituitarism, can result in impotence, menstrual irregularities, or premature menopause. Discoloration of the skin, often a grey-brown color and referred to as *bronzing*, is characteristic of late hemochromatosis. The classic triad of *bronze diabetes with liver failure* is a late manifestation that is rarely observed today. Physicians should strive to recognize the early, more general symptoms of fatigue and arthralgia because treatment can prevent permanent organ damage.

DIAGNOSIS

In its earliest stages, hyperferritinemia and transferrin saturation above 50% are the only signs of hemochromatosis (see Table 62-2). Transferrin saturation is calculated as serum iron ÷ total iron-binding capacity (TIBC). Modern laboratory measurements are usually of serum transferrin, and the TIBC is calculated as 1.4 × serum transferrin. If these values are marginally elevated, then a repeat measure on a fasting blood sample is indicated. As the disease progresses, hepatomegaly with elevated serum transaminases may develop. Liver biopsy is the only method to ascertain whether fibrosis is present and to show increased hepatic iron content (see Table 62-2), the gold standard for the diagnosis of hemochromatosis. Genetic testing in an individual with elevated serum iron indices can confirm the diagnosis of hemochromatosis. As previously discussed, genetic testing should not be used to screen patients with unknown liver disease because it has limited positive predictive value. MRI appears useful for detecting hepatic iron overload, and future research will be aimed at making this noninvasive test more quantitative.

TREATMENT

Symptomatic patients without treatment have a 5-year survival of 10%. Early diagnosis is crucial in hemochromatosis because treatment may prevent serious complications such as cirrhosis and hepatocellular carcinoma. Established arthritis, hypogonadism, and liver fibrosis remain resistant to treatment, although proper treatment will slow progression. Therapy consists of phlebotomy to remove iron from the body; this therapy can increase the 10-year survival rate to 75% in patients with cirrhosis. Because the source of excess iron is dietary, removing iron supplements from the diet of a patient with hemochromatosis is imperative. Because vitamin C aids absorption of iron, recommending avoidance of vitamin C supplements is prudent. A unit of blood, containing up to 250 mg of iron, can be removed at more frequent intervals from patients with hemochromatosis than from normal individuals. Patients with severe iron loading can tolerate weekly phlebotomy without anemia for months. Tolerating frequent phlebotomy serves as a confirmation of the diagnosis of hemochromatosis, and a running total of units of blood removed should be maintained. Serum iron indices should be checked periodically during phlebotomy therapy. Goals include maintaining ferritin below 50 ng/mL and transferrin saturation below 30%. After these goals have been reached, maintenance phlebotomy two to five times each year is required to prevent re-accumulation of iron. It is important for patients with evidence of liver disease to avoid other hepatotoxins such as alcohol. Iron-loaded patients are advised to avoid raw seafood and shellfish from warm waters because they are at increased risk for *Vibrio* sepsis. For such pathogens, iron is often a growth-limiting nutrient and therefore iron-loaded patients are at increased risk for severe infection.

Porphyrias

Porphyrias is the name given to a group of genetic or acquired diseases associated with deficient synthesis of heme. Heme is as an essential co-factor for the structure and function of hemoglobin and proteins such as cytochrome P450. Bone marrow produces more than 80% of body heme at a steady state to support erythropoiesis. Liver produces about 15% of total heme, but its synthesis can be increased tenfold. For example, heme synthesis will be induced by ingestion of a drug that relies on a heme-containing enzyme for detoxification. This induction of hepatic heme synthesis underlies the important observation that certain drugs trigger porphyria attacks (Table 62–3).

Porphyrias result from partial deficiency of one of seven enzymes involved in biosynthesis of heme (Figure 62–1). Attacks of porphyria are associated with the accumulation of the biochemical intermediates in the heme synthesis

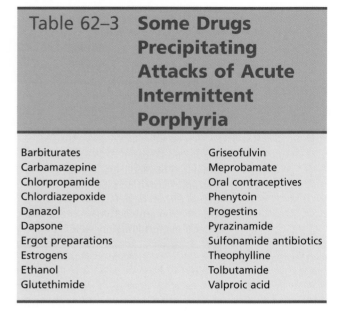

Table 62–3	Some Drugs Precipitating Attacks of Acute Intermittent Porphyria
Barbiturates	Griseofulvin
Carbamazepine	Meprobamate
Chlorpropamide	Oral contraceptives
Chlordiazepoxide	Phenytoin
Danazol	Progestins
Dapsone	Pyrazinamide
Ergot preparations	Sulfonamide antibiotics
Estrogens	Theophylline
Ethanol	Tolbutamide
Glutethimide	Valproic acid

pathway that precede the deficient enzyme (see Figure 62–1). Some of these intermediates are toxic. The two major classes of porphyria are bone marrow and hepatic, depending on the organ accounting for the overproduction of heme synthesis intermediates (Table 62–4). Hepatic porphyrias have acute onset of neurovisceral pain as a result of the accumulation of early intermediates of heme synthesis such as δ-aminolevulinic acid (ALA) (see Figure 62–1). Excess porphyrins, produced in bone marrow porphyrias, deposit in skin and absorb light, which confers photosensitivity and results in cutaneous manifestations such as blistering of sun-exposed skin. This section describes three porphyrias that are the most common and encompass the cardinal biochemical and clinical features of these disorders.

ACUTE INTERMITTENT PORPHYRIA

Acute intermittent porphyria (AIP) is an autosomal dominant disorder due to one half or less normal activity of porphobilinogen (PBG) deaminase. Under most circumstances, half-normal activity of this enzyme is sufficient to prevent porphyria; indeed, up to 90% of people with half-normal enzyme activity never experience attacks. PBG deaminase is the third enzyme in the pathway of heme biosynthesis (see Figure 62–1). When it is limiting, the two intermediates (ALA and PBG) accumulate in the pathway before this enzyme (see Figure 62–1). A high-urinary PBG level during an attack is a critical diagnostic feature. Finding deficient PBG deaminase enzyme activity in red blood cells confirms the diagnosis.

As the names *acute* and *intermittent* imply, acute attacks punctuate prolonged well periods in patients with AIP. The acute presentation of AIP can be dramatic and life threatening. Abdominal pain, largely thought to be the result of neurotoxicity, is present in more than 90% of patients with acute attacks. Abdominal pain may be severe enough to prompt surgical evaluation for an acute abdomen and can be associated with nausea, vomiting, and bowel dysmotility.

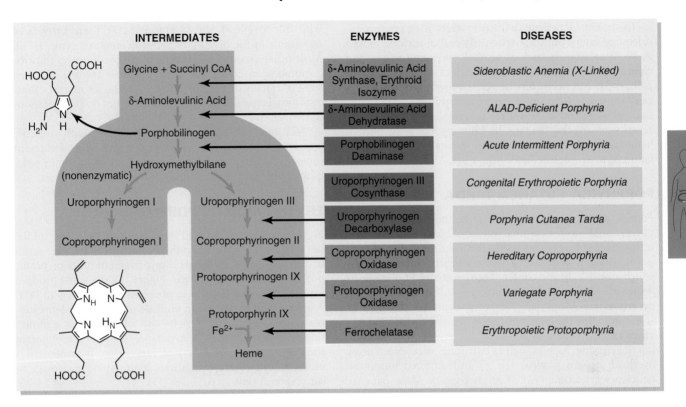

Figure 62–1 The heme biosynthetic pathway and the major diseases of porphyrin metabolism. The initial and last three enzymes *(in red)* are mitochondrial, and the other four *(in blue)* are cytosolic. X-linked sideroblastic anemia is not classically considered a porphyria. (From Anderson KE: The prophyrias. In Goldman L, Bennett JC [eds]: Cecil Textbook of Medicine, 21st ed. Philadelphia, WB Saunders, 2000, p 1124.)

Table 62–4	**Porphyrias Grouped by Organ Source of Excess Heme Precursors**				
Oran Source	**Porphyria**	**Prevalence**	**Neurologic Symptoms**	**Skin Photosensitivity**	**Drug Inducible**
Liver	ALA dehydratase porphyria	Very rare	+	−	+
	Acute intermittent porphyria	5–10/100,000	+	−	+
	Porphyria cutanea tarda	Uncertain, but most common porphyria	+	+	+
	Hereditary coporphyria	Rare	+	+	+
	Variegate porphyria	Not rare	+	+	+
Bone marrow	Congenital erythropoietic porphyria	Rare	−	+	−
	Erythropoietic protoporphyria	Several hundred known worldwide	−	+	−

ALA = δ-aminolevulinic acid.

Neuropathy is evidenced by decreased sensation or muscle weakness that may involve cranial and respiratory nerves. Sympathetic tone is high with hypertension and tachycardia. Central nervous system manifestations include anxiety, paranoia, depression, seizures, and inappropriate secretion of antidiuretic hormone.

Most patients suffer their initial attack after puberty. Triggers of attacks include drugs, particularly those that induce the mitochondrial cytochrome P-450 system such as barbiturates, carbamazepine, and sulfonamides (see Table 62–3). Caloric restriction, fasting, surgery, and infections have precipitated attacks.

Treatment of patients with AIP starts with prevention. Adequate caloric intake, particularly carbohydrates, as well as avoiding triggers such as alcohol, offending drugs, and caloric restriction, is important. Narcotics are safe to control pain, and β-adrenergic blockers can be used to control tachycardia and hypertension. Intravenous formulations of heme, such as hematin, are effective in reducing duration and severity of attacks, perhaps by blunting the induction of heme biosynthesis and thereby abrogating further accumulation of toxic intermediates (e.g., PBG, ALA).

PORPHYRIA CUTANEA TARDA

Porphyria cutanea tarda (PCT) is the most common porphyria and shows the cardinal feature of bullous involvement of sun-exposed skin. This results from accumulation of uroporphyrinogen and related heme-synthetic intermediates, which absorb light and confer photosensitivity. PCT is due to decreased activity of the hepatic enzyme uroporphyrinogen decarboxylase. More than 75% of patients are classified as *sporadic,* in that the family history is negative for affected relatives and there is no mutation in the gene (*UROD*) encoding the enzyme. Factors such as hormones, alcoholism, iron overload, hepatis C virus (HCV) and acquired immunodeficiency syndrome (AIDS) act as triggers. Many patients with iron overload and symptomatic PCT are carriers of mutations in the hereditary hemochromatosis gene (*HFE*). Most other cases of PCT occur in people heterozygous for a mutation in *UROD*. In them, the same triggers as noted for AIP can elicit symptomatic PCT. Rare, severe cases show autosomal recessive inheritance and are not due to mutations in *UROD*.

PCT typically begins in early adulthood with subacute appearance of vesicles, bullae, and fragile skin. Treatment includes avoiding triggers, removing any excess iron by phlebotomy, hematin, and chloroquine for refractory cases.

ERYTHROPOIETIC PORPHYRIA

Erythropoietic porphyria (EPP) results from deficiency of the last enzyme in heme biosynthesis, ferrochelatase. As a result of this late block in the pathway, large amounts of protoporphyrin accumulate (see Figure 62–1) and produce serious cutaneous damage as observed in patients with PCT. A brief exposure to sun can produce redness and edema suggestive of angioedema. Vesicles and bullae are less common than in patients with PCT. Avoidance of sun or use of potent sunscreens are the mainstay of prevention. β-carotene is a useful adjunct therapy that may limit oxidative damage to sun-exposed skin.

Prospectus for the Future

- Identification of factors that will protect a person with a deleterious genotype from developing hemochromatosis, Wilson's disease, or a porphyria. Development of drugs and other therapeutic approaches will be based on this knowledge.

- Effective screening strategies will be expanded, based on biochemical indices for hemochromatosis, with more people entering therapy at earlier stages of the disease.

References

Adams PC: Hemochromatosis. Clin Liver Dis 8:735–753, 2004.

Anderson KE, Bloomer JR, Bonkovsky HL, et al: Recommendations for the diagnosis and treatment of the acute porphyrias. Ann Intern Med 142:439–450, 2005.

Brewer GJ, Askari FK: Wilson's disease: Clinical management and therapy. J Hepatol 42 Suppl(1):S13–S21, 2005.

Beutler E, Felitti VJ, Koziol JA, et al: Penetrance of 845G→A (C282Y) HFE hereditary haemochromatosis mutation in the USA. Lancet. 359:211–218, 2002.

Cizewski Culotta V, Gitlin JD: Disorders of copper transport. In Scriver CR, Beaudet AL, Valle D, et al (eds): The Metabolic and Molecular Basis of Inherited Disease, 8th ed. New York, McGraw-Hill, 2001, pp 3105–3126.

Neimark E, Shilsky ML, Schneider BL: Wilson's disease and hemochromatosis. Adolesc Med Clin 15:175–194, 2004.

Steinberg KK, Cogswell, ME, Chang JC, et al: Prevalence of C282Y and H63D mutations in the hemochromatosis (*HFE*) gene in the United States. JAMA 285:2216–2222, 2001.

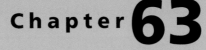

Heritable Disorders of Connective Tissue

Reed E. Pyeritz

The extracellular matrix (ECM), also called connective tissue, provides structural support for all tissues and organs. Additionally, a number of specialized functions, such as migration of cells during embryogenesis, transmission of light through the vitreous, diffusion of oxygen and nutrients through many boundaries, cushioning in the joints and vertebral column, elasticity of ligaments, and force transmission by tendons, require a normal ECM. In the past several years, the importance of the ECM in binding and activating numerous cytokines such as growth factors has been discovered. Thus either congenital or acquired abnormalities of any one of the hundreds of biochemical components of the ECM can have wide-ranging and substantial effects on health. The major components include collagen fibrils, elastic fibers, and amorphous ground substance, each of which varies among tissues and stages of development. The genes that encode the primary structure and post-translational modification of the scores of individual components of the ECM are scattered across the human genome; mutations in these genes account for more than 200 heritable disorders of connective tissue. Discovery of the cause and pathogenesis of these conditions have revealed a great deal about the normal function of the ECM. Many of the conditions are evident in childhood, whereas some are often not diagnosed until adolescence or adulthood.

This chapter reviews four of the most common groups of these disorders that are encountered in adult medicine. Features in multiple organs systems that progress in severity characterize each group.

Osteogensis Imperfecta Syndromes

The various osteogenesis imperfecta (OI) syndromes are mostly the result of mutations in one or the other of two genes that encode the procollagen chains that combine to form the most prevalent protein in the human body, type I collagen. Type I collagen is the archetypal fibrillar molecule, with ends that are globular and a long midsection composed of a triple helix. Two $\alpha_1(I)$ and one $\alpha_2(I)$ procollagen molecules intertwine as they leave the cell and are modified by intrachain bonds, multiple hydroxylations and glycosylations, and cleavage of portions of the N- and C-terminal propeptides. Formation of the collagen triple helix depends on repeating Gly-X-Y triplets in which X and Y are predominantly prolyl and hydroxypropyl residues. The individual triple-helical collagen molecules combine into fibrils that produce the characteristic banded pattern observed on electron microscopy of all fibrous connective tissues. Many of the mutations that cause the most severe collagen disorders, whether of types I, II, or III collagen, result in substitution of Gly, X, or Y with an amino acid that disrupts the triple helix, which in turn prevents formation of normal fibrils.

All forms of OI involve osteopenia that is due to decreased organic matrix of bone, and this in turn leads to the clinical complications of osteoporosis, including fractures. The severity of the various conditions ranges from lethality in the perinatal period to diagnosis in late adulthood. The milder forms are often due to decreased synthesis of one of the $\alpha(I)$ procollagen chains, whereas the more severe forms are due to substitutions of single amino acids that disrupt the triple helix. The former result in a reduced amount of normal type I collagen, whereas the latter causes the production of a preponderance of abnormal collagen fibrils that severely disrupt the ECM of bone and other tissues.

The forms of OI observed in adults potentially involve multiple tissues in addition to the skeleton, including the eye with blue or blue-grey sclerae, hearing loss, and brittle, discolored teeth (dentinogenesis imperfecta) (Table 63–1). The skeletal involvement results in fractures that are especially prominent in childhood, in postmenopausal women, and in individuals of relative short stature, as well as bony deformity in the absence of fractures. Treatment has traditionally

Table 63–1   Some Heritable Disorders of Fibrillar Collagen

Disorder	Inheritance	Basic Defect	Major Clinical Manifestations
Osteogenesis imperfecta			
Type I	AD	Mutations in *COL1A1* & *COL1A2*	Short stature, fractures, boney deformity, blue sclerae, hearing loss, dentinogenesis imperfecta in some families
Type II	Sporadic, due to new mutations	Mutations in *COL1A1*	In utero fractures, neonatal death from respiratory failure
Type III	AD, AR	heterogeneous	Short stature, severe boney deformity
Type IV	AD	Mutations in *COL1A1* & *COL1A2*	Fractures more severe than type I, normal scleral hue
Ehlers-Danlos syndrome			
Classic type	AD	Mutations in *COL5A1*	Hyperextensible, fragile skin with thin and widening scars, joint hypermobility
Vascular type	AD	Mutations in *COL3A1*	Rupture of large arteries, bowel, and uterus; variable thin and fragile skin and easy bruisability; variable joint hypermobility
Hypermobility type	AD	none known	Joint hypermobility; variable but mild skin hyperextensibility; abnormal scarring

AD = autosomal dominant; AR = autosomal recessive.

focused on responding to problems, with orthopedic correction of deformities and intramedullary *rodding* of brittle bones. Agents that inhibit osteoblasts are under study to improve bone density and growth and to prevent complications.

EHLERS-DANLOS SYNDROMES

The variants of Ehlers-Danlos syndrome (EDS; Table 63–1) share abnormalities in the skin and joints. All are caused by abnormalities in either collagen synthesis or the enzymes involved in post-translational processing of collagen. If only the joints are involved, then a diagnosis of familial joint instability or hypermobility syndrome, rather than EDS, should be entertained. The skin of a patient with Ehlers-Danlos syndrome is hyperextensible and can be pulled far away from underlying structures, promptly returning to its original position on release. Minor trauma may cause gaping wounds. Sutures may pull through the edges of a wound. Bruising may occur from unnoticed trauma. Small and large joints are hyperextensible and may be unstable. More serious orthopedic problems include congenital hip dislocation, severe kyphoscoliosis, tendon and muscle rupture, and clubfoot. Some people with EDS are especially prone to hernias.

The most troublesome type of EDS is the vascular form (type IV in the old nomenclature), which is due to a deficiency of type III collagen. Because type III collagen is an important component of the ECM of the walls of the arteries, the uterus, and the intestine, people with vascular EDS are prone to spontaneous rupture of these organs. The average life expectancy is reduced by about one half. Pregnancy is an especially vulnerable time for the woman with vascular EDS.

Therapy of all forms of EDS is largely symptomatic. The rare ocular-scoliotic form may respond to high doses of vitamin C. Patients with the vascular form should avoid strenuous activities and those that risk physical trauma. Genetic counseling should be provided to all patients of childbearing age.

Marfan Syndrome

Marfan syndrome is caused by abnormalities of the ubiquitous extracellular protein fibrillin-1. This cysteine-rich, 350-kd protein forms disulfide-bonded aggregates that are the principal component of the extracellular microfibril. Along with elastin, microfibrils form elastic fibers that give elasticity to vascular walls, tendons, ligaments, and skin. Microfibrils perform other important functions independent of elastin, such as constituting the zonule of the eye, which attaches the lens to the ciliary bodies, providing strength to certain tissues including skin and dura, and serving as a regulator of cytokine expression during development. Fibrillin-1 is encoded by *FBN1*, a larger gene on chromosome 15, in which more than 700 different mutations have been found to cause Marfan syndrome and a number of other related conditions.

Marfan syndrome is inherited in an autosomal dominant pattern, and about 30% of patients have neither parent affected and thus represent new mutations that occurred in either the egg or the sperm. The features affect multiple organs (Table 63–2). Typical patients are disproportionately tall with long arms and legs, have scoliosis and deformity of the anterior chest, are myopic with dislocation of the ocular lens, and have dilation of the aortic root. The latter finding

Table 63–2   Manifestations of Marfan Syndrome and Related Disorders

Disorder	Inheritance	Basic Defect	Major Clinical Manifestations
Marfan syndrome	AD	Mutations in *FBN1*	Dislocated ocular lens, myopia, cataract; aortic root dilation, aortic dissection, mitral valve prolapse; tall disproportionate stature, anterior chest deformity, scoliosis, joint hypermobility, dural ectasia, pneumothorax
Contractural arachnodactyly	AD	Mutations in *FBN2*	Congenital contractures of digits, elbows, and knees; scoliosis; crumpled helix of the ear
Familial aortic aneurysm	AD	Mutations in *FBN1* and *TGFBR2* and at least two other loci	Dilatation of the proximal or abdominal aorta, dissection of proximal or distal thoracic aorta; thoracic cage deformity
MASS phenotype	AD	A few mutations in *FBN1*, unknown how many other loci	Mitral valve prolapse; myopia; tall disproportionate stature, anterior chest deformity, scoliosis, striae atrophicae; aortic root diameter may be upper limits of normal but usually does not progress
Loeys-Dietz syndrome	AD	Mutations in *TGFBR1* and *TGFBR2*	Dissection of the aorta and branch arteries; arterial tortuosity; bifid uvula or cleft palate; hypertelorism

AD = autosomal dominant.

predisposes the patient to aortic dissection, which accounts for much of the precocious mortality. Patients are also prone to spontaneous pneumothorax and enlargement of the neural canal in the lumbosacral region, which can produce radicular pain.

Patients with Marfan syndrome should be followed at least annually with transthoracic echocardiography to monitor the aortic root diameter and valvular function. Aortic regurgitation occurs when the root becomes moderately dilated, and mitral regurgitation can be an important complication of the very common mitral valve prolapse. Patients should be advised to avoid strenuous exertion and contact sports. Chronic treatment with a β-adrenergic blocking drug, such as atenolol, retards the rate of aortic dilation and reduces the risk of dissection. When the root becomes dilated to 50 mm in an adult, consideration should be given to prophylactic root repair, either with a composite graft or with one of the newer approaches that replaces the root while sparing the native valve.

Examination of *FBN1* for mutations has little role in the diagnosis of equivocal cases, because mutations in this gene can also cause some of the conditions often confused with Marfan syndrome, such as MASS phenotype and familial aortic aneurysm. In addition, searching for mutations is expensive and, for unclear reasons, successful in only 90% of people with bona fide Marfan syndrome. Nonetheless, all patients with Marfan syndrome should receive detailed genetic counseling, and some will choose to pursue genetic analysis for the purposes of prenatal diagnosis.

Pseudoxanthoma Elasticum

Pseudoxanthoma elasticum (PXE) is a secondary disorder of the ECM of known cause but unclear pathogenesis. The pathologic hallmark is calcification of elastic fibers. The walls of smaller arteries and arterioles become stiff and thickened. The former leads to difficult hemostasis, especially reflected in gastrointestinal hemorrhage and the latter in ischemic coronary and cerebral vascular disease. Hypertension, perhaps the result of renovascular disease, is common, as is the loss of peripheral pulses often associated with claudication. Breakage of elastic laminae in the skin produces the characteristic "plucked chicken skin" lesions, or pseudoxanthoma, in areas of flexural stress such as the neck, groin, and cubital fossa. Skin changes may occur as early as the in the middle teenage years, and skin may become lax and redundant. Breaks in the elastic Bruch membrane of the retina produce the angioid streak. Progressive loss of vision as a result of microhemorrhages and neovascularization is a major complication. Families that show autosomal recessive inheritance are significantly more common that those who are consistent with autosomal dominance. However, both types are due to mutations in a gene, *ABCC6*, which maps to 16p13.1 and encodes a membrane protein capable of binding adenosine triphosphate (ATP). How mutations in this gene produce the clinical features is unclear. Treatment is focused on traditional approaches to the many organ systems that can be affected.

Prospectus for the Future

- Improved understanding of the biochemical and molecular bases of the heritable disorders of connective tissue and the role of laboratory testing in diagnosis and prognosis
- Clinical trials of agents that treat the cytokine activation that appears to account for many features of Marfan syndrome

- Better understanding of the long-term efficacy of valve-sparing aortic root surgery in patients with Marfan syndrome and other conditions that cause ascending aortic aneurysms
- Better treatments of the metabolic bone disease in osteogenesis imperfecta

References

Beighton P, De Paepe A, Steinmann B, et al: Ehlers-Danlos syndromes: Revised nosology, Villefranche, 1997. Am J Med Genet 77:31–37, 1998.

Pyeritz RE. Marfan syndrome and other disorders of fibrillin. In Rimoin DL, Conner JM, Pyeritz RE, Korf B (eds): Principles and Practice of Medical Genetics, 5th ed. Edinburgh, Churchill Livingstone, 2007. In press.

Royce PM, Steinmann B (eds): Connective tissue and heritable disorders: Molecular, genetic and medical aspects, 2nd ed. New York, Wiley-Liss, 2002.

Section XI

Endocrine Disease

Cecil Andreoli and Carpenter's Essentials of Medicine

Hypothalamic-Pituitary Axis

Vivien S. Herman-Bonert

Anatomy and Physiology

The pituitary gland, weighing 500 to 900 mg, lies at the base of the skull in the sella turcica within the sphenoid bone. The cavernous sinus borders laterally on the pituitary gland. The optic chiasm courses over the superior aspect. Two thirds of the pituitary gland is composed of the anterior lobe and one third is the posterior lobe.

The anterior pituitary gland receives a rich vascular supply, largely from the hypothalamus via a hypothalamic-pituitary portal circulation. Hypothalamic stimulatory and inhibitory hormones are directly transported via the hypothalamic-pituitary portal circulation to specific cells of the anterior pituitary gland, where they regulate synthesis and secretion of pituitary trophic hormones (Fig. 64–1; **Web Fig. 64–1; Web Fig. 64–2**).

A specific pituitary cell type secretes each of the anterior pituitary hormones—adrenocorticotropic hormone (ACTH), growth hormone (GH), prolactin (PRL), and thyroid-stimulating hormone (TSH). In addition, the same cell secretes the gonadotropins luteinizing hormone (LH) and follicle-stimulating hormone (FSH). Arginine vasopressin (AVP), also known as antidiuretic hormone (ADH), is synthesized in the hypothalamus and transported via the pituitary stalk to the posterior lobe of the pituitary gland (Table 64–1), where it is stored and available to be secreted when stimulated. Oxytocin is also stored and secreted by the posterior pituitary lobe.

Pituitary Tumors

Each of the five pituitary cell types, either singly or in combination, can give rise to benign pituitary adenomas, which secrete hormones characteristic of the particular cell type. Prolactinomas are the most common secretory pituitary tumors. Isolated reports of pituitary carcinomas with distant metastases have been described.

The earliest clinical manifestations of pituitary tumors are usually the characteristic signs and symptoms caused by the hormone hypersecretion. Subsequently, if the tumor is large, local manifestations of tumor enlargement may develop. Pressure on surrounding structures can cause signs and symptoms of large pituitary adenomas (secretory or nonsecretory). Headache is a frequent symptom. If the tumor extends into the suprasellar space, then the optic chiasm may be compressed, which classically results in bi-temporal hemianopia. Lateral extension into the cavernous sinus can result in ophthalmoplegia, diplopia, or ptosis as a result of dysfunction of the third, fourth, and sixth cranial nerves. Compression of surrounding normal pituitary tissue by an enlarging tumor mass can cause hyposecretion of one or several pituitary trophic hormones, resulting in signs and symptoms of hypopituitarism. Destructive pituitary lesions result in hormone loss, which follows a particular pattern: initially GH secretion is reduced, followed by LH and FSH, then TSH, and lastly ACTH.

The presence of a pituitary tumor is confirmed by pituitary magnetic resonance imaging (MRI) (**Web Fig. 64–3**). The contrast agent gadolinium is used to help differentiate small pituitary lesions from normal anterior pituitary tissue. Microadenomas are defined as pituitary lesions less than 10 mm in diameter. Macroadenomas are pituitary lesions more than 10 mm in diameter. They may cause significant deviation of the pituitary stalk to the opposite side. Adenomas exceeding 15 mm frequently have suprasellar extension with compression and displacement of the optic chiasm. An MRI may also show lateral extension of large adenomas into the cavernous sinus. A primary congenital defect or herniation of the arachnoid membrane through an incompetent diaphragma sellae, either after pituitary surgery or radiation, can cause empty sella syndrome, the most common cause of an enlarged sella.

Endocrine evaluation should precede imaging studies because about 10% to 20% of the normal population harbors nonfunctional asymptomatic pituitary microadenomas that are incidentally detected by MRI (Table 64–2).

Disorders of Anterior Pituitary Hormones

GROWTH HORMONE

GH is a 191-amino acid peptide with a molecular weight of 22,000 D^a. Secretion is stimulated by the 40-and 44-amino acid hypothalamic growth hormone-releasing hormone (GHRH) and inhibited by the hypothalamic tetradecapeptide somatostatin. These hypothalamic factors bind to pituitary somatotroph cells and regulate GH secretion. GH binds to receptors in the liver and induces secretion of insulin-like growth factor I (IGF-I), which circulates in the blood bound to binding proteins (BPs), the most important of which is IGF-BP3. IGF-I mediates most of the growth-promoting effects of GH. GH also affects carbohydrate metabolism.

Evaluation of Growth Hormone Reserve

Provocative tests that stimulate the somatotroph are necessary to assess GH deficiency because basal GH levels are frequently very low even in normal individuals. Insulin-induced hypoglycemia (insulin tolerance test [ITT]) is the gold standard test for assessing GH reserve. Insulin (0.05 to 0.15 U/kg) is administered intravenously to reduce the patient's blood glucose levels to 50% of initial blood glucose or to 40 mg/dL with serial sampling of serum GH and glucose. Hypoglycemia is a potent stimulus for GH secretion, and a normal response is a peak GH level in excess of

5 ng/mL at 60 minutes. Combined infusion of GHRH and arginine is as sensitive and specific as insulin-induced hypoglycemia in stimulating GH secretion in adulthood. Oral propranolol and L-dopa, a precursor of dopamine and norepinephrine, also stimulate GH secretion from the pituitary somatotroph and are used to evaluate childhood GH deficiency, but they lack sensitivity in adult GH deficiency. Multiple tests are performed to diagnose GH deficiency in a

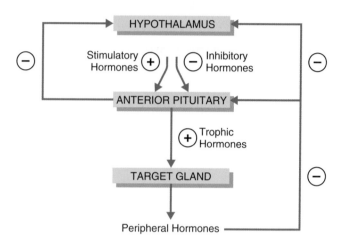

Figure 64–1 Feedback control of the hypothalamic-pituitary target–gland axis.

Table 64–1	**Pituitary-Target Organ Hormone Axis**			
Hypothalamic Hormone	**Pituitary Target Cell**	**Pituitary Hormone Affected**	**Peripheral Target Gland**	**Peripheral Hormone Affected**
Stimulatory				
Anterior Lobe of Pituitary Gland				
Thyrotropin-releasing hormone	Thyrotroph	Thyroid-stimulating hormone	Thyroid gland	Thyroxine (T$_4$) Triiodothyronine (T$_3$)
Growth hormone-releasing hormone (GHRH)	Somatotroph	Growth hormone	Liver	Insulin-like growth factor I (IGF-I)
Gonadotropin-releasing hormone	Gonadotroph	Luteinizing hormone (LH)	Ovary	Progesterone
			Testis	Testosterone
		Follicle-stimulating hormone	Ovary	Estradiol
			Testis	Inhibin
Corticotropin-releasing hormone	Corticotroph	Adrenocorticotrophic hormone	Adrenal gland	Cortisol
Posterior Lobe of Pituitary Gland				
Vasopressin			Kidney	
Oxytocin			Uterus, breast	
Inhibitory				
Somatostatin	Somatotroph	Growth hormone		
	Thyrotroph	Thyroid-stimulating hormone		
Dopamine	Lactotroph	Prolactin	Breast	

Table 64–2 Screening Tests for Pituitary Disorders

Disorder	Tests
Pituitary Tumor	
Acromegaly	IGF-1
	OGTT: Measure BS and GH (0, 60, 120 mins)
Prolactinoma	Basal serum prolactin
ACTH-secreting tumor	24-hr urine-free cortisol and creatinine level
	1 mg overnight dexamethasone suppression test
	2 mg and 8 mg dexamethasone suppression tests
	Serum ACTH
	Dexamethasone-CRH test
	Bilateral inferior petrosal sinus sampling
TSH-secreting tumor	Serum TSH, TFT
Gonadotropin-secreting tumor	FSH, LH alpha subunit
Hypopituitarism	
Growth hormone deficiency	IGF-1
	GH provocative test: ITT Arginine-GHRH
Gonadotropin deficiency	Women: Basal estradiol, LH, FSH
	Men: Testosterone (total; free), LH, FSH
TSH Deficiency	Serum TSH, Free T4,
ACTH Deficiency	ACTH
	Provocative test:
	ITT
	Metyrapone test
	Cortrosyn-stimulation test (1 mcg and 250 mcg)

ACTH = adrenocorticotropic hormone; BS = blood sugar; CRH = corticotropin-releasing hormone; FSH = follicle-stimulating hormone; GH = growth hormone; GHRH = growth hormone-releasing hormone; IGF-1 = insulin-like growth factor I; ITT = insulin tolerance test; LH = luteinizing hormone; OGTT = oral glucose tolerance test; TSH = thyroid-stimulating hormone; TFT = thyroid function test.

single patient because only 90% of normal individuals respond adequately to any single test. IGF-I levels can be used as a screening test for GH deficiency because GH regulates IGF-I levels. GH deficiency is associated with low IGF-I. Low IGF-I levels indicate the need to perform provocative testing of GH secretion.

Evaluation of Growth Hormone Hypersecretion

GH is secreted in a pulsatile manner, and thus dynamic GH testing is more valuable than the measurement of a single random GH level. Moreover, cirrhosis, starvation, anxiety, type 1 diabetes mellitus, and acute illness can be associated with GH hypersecretion. However, measurement of serum IGF-I is a useful indicator of GH hypersecretion because this level does not fluctuate throughout the day. IGF-I levels are elevated in almost all patients with GH hypersecretion. A simple and specific dynamic test for GH hypersecretion is the administration of oral glucose, in which 100 g of glucose administered orally suppresses GH levels to less than 1 ng/mL after 120 minutes in healthy individuals. In patients with acromegaly, GH levels may increase, remain unchanged, or decrease (however, not below 1 ng/mL) after an oral glucose load. If no pituitary mass is detected, then an extrapituitary source of ectopic GH or GHRH should be sought through imaging studies of the chest and abdomen.

Adult Growth Hormone Deficiency

GH deficiency during infancy and childhood is exhibited as growth retardation, short stature, and fasting hypoglycemia. Adult GH deficiency is exhibited as increased abdominal adiposity, reduced muscle strength and exercise capacity, decreased lean body mass and increased fat mass, reduced bone mineral density, glucose intolerance and insulin resistance, abnormal lipid profile, and impaired psychosocial well-being. Adult GH deficiency is frequently accompanied by other symptoms of panhypopituitarism.

Treatment. GH is administered in adulthood as a subcutaneous daily injection (0.1 to 0.3 mg/day). GH replacement therapy in adults decreases fat mass, increases lean body mass and bone mineral density, and is associated with improved cardiovascular risk factors (e.g., lipid profile, waist-hip ratio, central obesity).

Acromegaly and Gigantism

In childhood, GH hypersecretion leads to gigantism; in adults whose long bone epiphyses are fused, GH excess causes acromegaly with local overgrowth of bone in the acral areas. GH hypersecretion is almost always caused by a GH-secreting pituitary adenoma. Approximately 70% of patients with acromegaly have tumors larger than 1 cm. Ectopic GHRH secretion can occur with pancreatic islet cell tumors and bronchial or intestinal carcinoids. Ectopic GH secretion occurs very rarely with pancreas, breast, and lung tumors. Both ectopic GH and GHRH are clinically exhibited with acromegaly but are extremely rare.

Clinical Features. The clinical features of acromegaly are insidious, and it may take several years for the disfiguring features to be diagnosed. Untreated, acromegaly causes increased rates of morbidity and mortality late in the course of the disorder. The most classic clinical feature is acral enlargement, exhibited as a widening of the hands and feet and a coarsening of the facial features—frontal sinuses enlarge, leading to prominent supraorbital ridges, and the mandible grows downward and forward, resulting in prognathism and wide spacing of the teeth. Ring, glove, and shoe sizes increase as a result of soft tissue enlargement of hands and feet (**Web Fig. 64–4**). The bony and soft tissue changes are accompanied by endocrine, metabolic, and systemic manifestations (Table 64–3).

Treatment. Trans-sphenoidal microsurgery is the initial therapy of choice, resulting in rapid reduction of GH levels with a low rate of surgical morbidity. Cure rates are proportional to preoperative tumor size with a 90% success rate for

Table 64–3	Clinical Features of Acromegaly	
Change	**Manifestations**	
Somatic Changes		
Acral changes	Enlarged hands and feet	
Musculoskeletal changes	Arthralgias	
	Prognathism	
	Malocclusion	
	Carpal tunnel syndrome	
	Proximal myopathy	
Skin changes	Sweating	
Colon changes	Polyps	
	Carcinoma	
Cardiovascular symptoms	Cardiomegaly	
	Hypertension	
Visceromegaly	Tongue	
	Thyroid	
	Liver	
Endocrine-Metabolic Changes		
Reproduction	Menstrual abnormalities	
	Galactorrhea	
	Decreased libido	
Carbohydrate metabolism	Impaired glucose tolerance	
	Diabetes mellitus	
Lipids	Hypertriglyceridemia	

patients with microadenomas. Radiotherapy is an effective method of reducing GH hypersecretion; however, it may take as long as 20 years for GH levels to fall after radiotherapy, and the incidence of hypopituitarism is high. Medical management involves the use of drugs that decrease GH secretion from the pituitary tumor (e.g., somatostatin analogs, dopamine agonists) or block the peripheral action of GH at the hepatic receptor (e.g., GH-receptor antagonists). Octreotide acetate, a long-acting somatostatin analog, is effective in reducing GH and IGF-I levels to normal in 40% to 65% of patients and shrinks tumor mass in some cases. A long-acting, slow-releasing depot preparation of octreotide administered once monthly is as effective as short-acting subcutaneous octreotide preparations. Side effects of octreotide include diarrhea, abdominal cramps, flatulence, and gallstone formation. Bromocriptine, a dopamine agonist, is effective in suppressing GH in only a minority of patients with acromegaly. The GH-receptor antagonist, pegvisomant, binds to the GH receptor on the hepatic surface and thus blocks the normal physiologic action of GH. The mechanism of normal GH action at the liver involves binding of the GH to its hepatic receptor, followed by receptor dimerization, which then activates signaling pathways that result in IGF-1 generation. Pegvisomant blocks GH-receptor dimerization and subsequent IGF-1 generation and normalizes IGF-1 levels in 97% of patients with acromegaly. Liver function tests and pituitary adenoma size must be monitored on a long-term basis.

PROLACTIN

PRL, a 198-amino acid, 22,000-D[a] polypeptide, is synthesized and secreted by pituitary lactotrophs. Hypothalamic dopamine provides predominately inhibitory control of PRL secretion, allowing only a low basal rate of secretion. Thyrotropin-releasing hormone (TRH) and vasoactive intestinal polypeptide are putative PRL-releasing factors. PRL secretion is episodic. Estrogens increase basal and stimulated PRL secretion; glucocorticoids and TSH blunt TRH-induced PRL secretion. PRL levels increase during pregnancy. After childbirth, PRL stimulates milk production. However, elevated PRL levels are not needed to maintain lactation, and basal PRL secretion falls as the infant's suckling reflex maintains lactation.

Prolactinomas

Microprolactinomas are more common in women, whereas macroadenomas occur more frequently in men. PRL inhibits pulsatile gonadotropin secretion and suppresses the mid-cycle LH surge with consequent menstrual irregularities. Hyperprolactinemia in women can cause hypogonadotropic hypogonadism, resulting in estrogen deficiency. In men who have hyperprolactinemia, testosterone levels are usually suppressed.

Clinical Features. Prolactinomas are often recognized earlier in women, who have menstrual irregularities and infertility, as opposed to men, who exhibit decreased libido and impotence.

Approximately 90% of women who have hyperprolactinemia have amenorrhea, galactorrhea, or infertility. If the prolactinoma occurs in adolescents before the onset of menarche, then they may have primary amenorrhea. Prolactinomas account for 15% to 20% of secondary amenorrhea. Anovulation is associated with infertility. Galactorrhea may not be clinically obvious and may be discovered only during breast examination.

Estrogen deficiency may cause osteopenia, vaginal dryness, hot flashes, and irritability. PRL stimulates adrenal androgen production, and androgen excess can result in weight gain and hirsutism. Hyperprolactinemia may be associated with anxiety and depression.

Men usually exhibit a loss of libido and impotence as a result of hypogonadism. These symptoms are often attributed to causes other than prolactinoma, which results in frequent delay in diagnosis until visual impairment, headache, and hypopituitarism develop.

Diagnosis. Several physiologic conditions (e.g., pregnancy, stress, nipple stimulation), as well as certain medications (e.g., phenothiazines, methyldopa, cimetidine, metoclopramide) and pathologic states (e.g., hypothyroidism, chronic renal failure, chest wall lesions), increase PRL secretion. These conditions may be associated with mildly elevated PRL levels; however, basal PRL levels in excess of 200 ng/mL usually imply prolactinoma. An MRI should confirm the diagnosis of prolactinoma.

Treatment. Medical management with a dopamine agonist (e.g., bromocriptine, cabergoline) restores gonadal function and fertility in the majority of patients. Dopamine agonists cause tumor shrinkage in a significant number of patients with macroadenomas. Trans-sphenoidal surgery is indicated in patients who are intolerant or resistant to medical treatment.

THYROID-STIMULATING HORMONE

TSH, a 28,000-D[a] glycoprotein hormone, is synthesized and secreted by the pituitary thyrotroph cells. TSH secretion is stimulated by the hypothalamic tripeptide TRH. The inhibitory effect of hypothalamic somatostatin augments the negative feedback inhibition of TSH secretion by peripheral thyroid hormones. TSH attaches to receptors on the thyroid gland and activates adenylyl cyclase, stimulating iodine uptake and the synthesis and release of the thyroid hormones thyroxine (T_4) and triiodothyronine (T_3). T_4 and T_3, in turn, exert negative feedback inhibition on pituitary TSH and hypothalamic TRH secretion.

Evaluation of TSH Secretion

TSH is measured by ultrasensitive assays (immunoradiometric assays), which can accurately distinguish low, normal, and high TSH levels. The ultrasensitive TSH assay has largely replaced the need for any further tests. In a patient with hypothyroidism, a suppressed TSH level indicates central (secondary) hypothyroidism and an elevated level indicates primary hypothyroidism.

TSH Deficiency

TSH deficiency causes thyroid gland involution, hypofunction, and clinical hypothyroidism. Clinical features of hypothyroidism include lethargy, constipation, cold intolerance, bradycardia, weight gain, poor appetite, dry skin, and delayed relaxation time of peripheral reflexes. The presence of low-circulating TSH levels in the presence of low thyroid hormone levels differentiates secondary hypothyroidism as a result of hypothalamic-pituitary dysfunction from primary hypothyroidism.

Treatment. Patients with central hypothyroidism are treated with thyroxine in doses of 75 to 150 mcg/day. Measuring the serum FT4 level, which should be in the mid-to-normal range, assesses the adequacy of thyroid replacement. TSH levels are low-to-normal in central hypopituitarism; thus TSH levels cannot be used to monitor thyroid hormone replacement dosage in secondary hypothyroidism.

Thyrotropin-Secreting Pituitary Tumors

Thyrotropin-secreting pituitary tumors are extremely rare, exhibiting hyperthyroidism, goiter, and inappropriately elevated (or normal) TSH levels in the presence of elevated serum thyroid hormone levels. TSH-secreting tumors are usually plurihormonal, secreting GH, PRL, and the glycoprotein hormone alpha-subunit, as well as TSH. These tumors are often resistant to removal, which necessitates several surgical procedures or radiotherapy. Octreotide acetate, a somatostatin analog, has been found to be useful in decreasing TSH secretion in patients with these tumors and has been shown to shrink the tumor in some cases. Iodine-131 thyroid ablation or thyroid surgery may be needed to control thyrotoxicosis.

ADRENOCORTICOTROPIC HORMONE

ACTH, a 39-amino acid peptide, is synthesized as part of a larger 241-amino acid precursor molecule, pro-opiomelanocortin, which is subsequently cleaved enzymatically into β-lipotropin (β-LPH), ACTH, joining peptide, and an amino-terminal peptide in the anterior lobe of the pituitary gland. ACTH is then cleaved into β-melanocyte–stimulating hormone and corticotropin-like peptide (ACTH [18–39]), whereas β-LPH is split into LPH and β-endorphin.

Hypothalamic corticotropin-releasing hormone (CRH), and to a lesser extent ADH, stimulate ACTH secretion by pituitary corticotroph cells. ACTH stimulates cortisol synthesis and secretion from the adrenal gland. Cortisol exerts a negative feedback on ACTH and CRH secretion. ACTH is secreted in pulses and is under circadian control, reaching maximal levels in the last hours before awakening, followed by a steady decline to a nadir in the evening. Both psychologic and physical stress increases ACTH and cortisol secretion, whereas glucocorticoids inhibit ACTH secretion, as well as CRH and ADH synthesis and release. ACTH also maintains adrenal size by increasing protein synthesis.

Evaluation of ACTH Secretion

Excess ACTH secretion results in hypercortisolemia, which may be caused by an ACTH-secreting pituitary adenoma (Cushing's disease) or by ectopic ACTH secretion. ACTH deficiency results in adrenocortical insufficiency, with decreased secretion of cortisol. Aldosterone secretion is largely regulated by the renin-angiotensin axis; therefore aldosterone secretion remains intact (see Chapter 66).

Basal ACTH Levels. Random basal ACTH measurements are unreliable because of the short plasma half-life and pulsatile secretion of the hormone. Interpretation of plasma ACTH levels requires concomitant assessment of plasma cortisol levels. Because ACTH regulates cortisol secretion, plasma cortisol levels better reflect hypothalamic-pituitary-adrenal function. An 8:00 AM cortisol less than 3 mcg/dL suggests adrenal insufficiency. ACTH levels can be used to differentiate primary from secondary adrenal insufficiency. Plasma ACTH levels are normal to high in adrenal insufficiency because of a primary adrenal disorder and are low to absent in adrenal insufficiency secondary to hypothalamic-pituitary hypofunction (see Chapter 66).

Evaluation of ACTH Reserve. To assess the adequacy of ACTH reserve under conditions of stress, provocative testing is performed. The insulin-induced hypoglycemia test previously described as a stimulus for pituitary GH release also stimulates the hypothalamic-pituitary-adrenal axis. A peak cortisol level of at least 18 mcg/dL confirms normal ACTH reserve. Insulin-induced hypoglycemia is the most reliable test of the ACTH-secretory response to stress. The test is contraindicated in older patients and in patients with cerebrovascular disorders, seizure disorders, or cardiovascular disease. Metyrapone (30 mg/kg orally at midnight) inhibits the 11-beta hydroxylase enzyme in the adrenal gland, which converts 11-deoxycortisol to cortisol. Low cortisol stimulates CRH and ACTH. An 11-deoxycortisol level greater than 7 mg/dL, with a simultaneous serum cortisol less than 5 mcg/dL, the morning after metyrapone administration, indicates an adequate response. If compromised adrenal function is suggested, then the ITT and metyrapone tests are potentially hazardous and a physician should closely monitor patients.

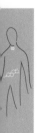

Prolonged ACTH deficiency results in adrenal atrophy, and thus ACTH status can be assessed indirectly by measuring adrenal cortisol reserve. Cortrosyn-stimulation testing correlates well with the ITT. Approximately 250 mcg cosyntropin (Cortrosyn; synthetic ACTH [1–24]) administered intravenously or intramuscularly results in a peak cortisol level of more than 20 mcg/dL within 60 minutes in normal individuals. An inadequate response implies either impaired pituitary ACTH secretion or primary adrenal failure. Numerous recent studies suggest that low-dose (1 mcg) ACTH stimulation provides a more sensitive test than the supraphysiologic 250-mcg dose.

Evaluation of ACTH Hypersecretion. Pituitary corticotroph adenomas in Cushing's disease or ectopic ACTH-secreting tumors result in ACTH hypersecretion and hypercortisolemia.

Initially a diagnosis of hypercortisolemia must first be confirmed by measuring 24-hour urinary-free cortisol levels, midnight plasma cortisol levels, or lack of suppression of an 8:00 AM serum cortisol after 1 mg of dexamethasone administered at 11:00 PM on the evening before (1 mg overnight dexamethasone suppression).

After confirming Cushing's syndrome and hypercortisolemia, plasma ACTH levels are measured to differentiate between ACTH-dependent Cushing's syndrome (pituitary or ectopic ACTH secretion) and ACTH-independent Cushing's syndrome (adrenal adenoma or hyperplasia). This differential diagnosis is discussed in Chapter 66.

ACTH Deficiency

ACTH deficiency results in adrenal failure, causing lethargy, weakness, nausea, vomiting, dehydration, orthostatic hypotension, coma, and, if untreated, death.

Treatment. Patients with adrenal insufficiency should be treated with hydrocortisone, 15 to 25 mg/day in two divided doses or equivalent. Two thirds of the dose is administered in the morning and one third in the late afternoon or evening. The dose should be increased five- to tenfold in times of stress. Stress doses of hydrocortisone should be administered if the patient undergoes surgery with rapid tapering of the dose postoperatively. The dose of hydrocortisone should be doubled when the patient has minor illnesses.

Mineralocorticoid replacement is not required with central adrenal insufficiency because the renin-aldosterone system is intact.

ACTH-Secreting Pituitary Tumors

ACTH-secreting pituitary tumors result in hypercortisolemia associated with obesity, moon facies, cervicodorsal dysplasia, striae, thinning of the skin, hirsutism, hypertension, menstrual irregularities, glucose intolerance, mood changes, proximal myopathy, and osteopenia (Fig. 64–2). The differential diagnosis of hypercortisolemia is discussed in Chapter 66.

Treatment. Treatment modalities used to control ACTH hypersecretion in Cushing's disease include trans-sphenoidal resection, radiation therapy, and medical therapy. Drugs that block steroid synthesis include ketoconazole, metyrapone and aminoglutethimide, RU-486, and trilostane.

Treatment of ectopic ACTH syndrome is designed to remove the ectopic tumor if possible.

GONADOTROPINS (LH AND FSH)

Gonadotroph secretion of LH and FSH is regulated by hypothalamic gonadotropin-releasing hormone (GnRH), a 10-amino acid peptide secreted in a pulsatile manner. Gonadal steroids (estrogen and testosterone) and peptides (inhibin and activin) regulate negative feedback inhibition. Basal LH and FSH are secreted in a pulsatile manner, concordantly with the pulsatile release of GnRH. GnRH release determines the onset of puberty and generates the midcycle gonadotropin surges necessary for ovulation. Gonadal steroids exert both positive and negative feedback effects on gonadotroph secretion. In addition, the gonadal polypeptide inhibin, produced by ovarian granulosa cells and testicular Sertoli cells, negatively inhibits FSH secretion, whereas activins stimulate FSH secretion. LH and FSH bind to receptors in the ovaries and testes and stimulate sex steroid secretion (predominantly LH), as well as gametogenesis (predominantly FSH). LH stimulates gonadal steroid secretion by testicular Leydig cells and by the ovarian follicles. In women, the ovulatory LH surge results in rupture of the follicle and then luteinization. FSH stimulates Sertoli cell spermatogenesis in men and follicular development in women.

Evaluation of Hypothalamic-Pituitary-Gonadal Axis

LH and FSH levels vary with age in patients and with the menstrual cycle in women. Prepubertal gonadotropin levels are low, and postmenopausal women have elevated levels. Male FSH and LH levels are pulsatile but fluctuate less than those in women. During the follicular phase of the menstrual cycle, LH levels rise steadily, with a midcycle spike that stimulates ovulation. FSH rises during the early follicular phase, falls in the late follicular phase, and peaks at midcycle, concurrent with the LH surge. Both LH and FSH levels fall after ovulation. LH and FSH levels in men are measured by three pooled samples drawn 20 minutes apart, which compensates for the normal pulsatile secretion.

Gonadotropin and sex steroid estimation in women are more complex. However, women with regular menstrual cycles and a documented normal luteal-phase serum progesterone concentration are unlikely to have significant gonadotropin dysfunction. In women with amenorrhea, measurement of serum LH, FSH, estradiol, PRL, and human chorionic gonadotropin (hCG) can differentiate among (1) primary ovarian failure, with elevated FSH and LH levels and normal PRL levels; (2) hyperprolactinemia, with elevated PRL and normal-to-low follicular-phase LH, FSH, and estradiol levels; and (3) pregnancy, with a positive hCG, normal-to-high PRL, normal LH, and high estradiol.

Gonadotropin deficiency is best diagnosed by concurrent measurement of serum gonadotropins and gonadal steroid concentrations. Low or normal FSH and LH levels in the presence of a low testosterone level (in men) or a low estradiol level (in women) confirm the diagnosis of gonadotropin deficiency. Low levels of gonadal steroids in the presence of elevated gonadotropin levels suggest primary gonadal failure.

Gonadotropin Deficiency

Central hypogonadism during childhood results in failure to enter normal puberty. Girls have delayed breast develop-

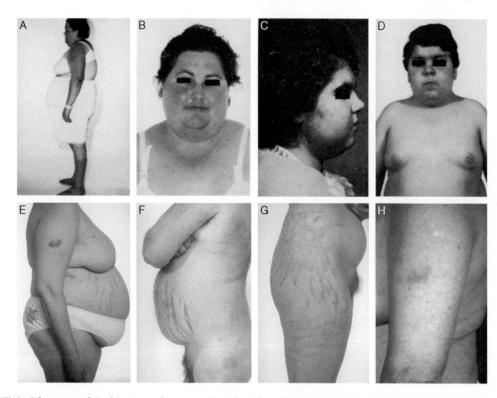

Figure 64–2 Clinical features of Cushing's syndrome. *A,* Centripetal and some generalized obesity and dorsal kyphosis in a 30-year-old woman with Cushing's disease. *B,* Same woman as shown in *A,* depicting moon facies, plethora, hirsutism, and enlarged supraclavicular fat pads. *C,* Facial rounding, hirsutism, and acne in a 14-year-old girl with Cushing's disease. *D,* Central and generalized obesity and moon facies in a 14-year-old boy with Cushing's disease. *E, F,* Typical centripetal obesity with livid abdominal striae observed in a 41-year-old woman *(E)* and a 40-year-old man *(F)* with Cushing's disease. *G,* Striae in a 24-year-old patient with congenital adrenal hyperplasia treated with excessive doses of dexamethasone as replacement therapy. *H,* Typical bruising and thin skin of a patient with Cushing's disease. In this case, the bruising has occurred without obvious injury. (From Larsen PR, Kronenberg H, Melmed S, et al: Williams Textbook of Endocrinology, 10th ed. Philadelphia, WB Saunders, 2003.)

ment, scant pubic and axillary hair, and primary amenorrhea. In boys, the phallus and testes remain small, and body hair is sparse. Sex steroids are required for closure of the epiphyses of the long bones; thus in isolated gonadotropin deficiency, growth continues (as GH is intact) because epiphyseal fusion fails, resulting in tall adolescents with eunuchoid proportions (upper-to-lower segment ratio less than 1:1). In adult women, hypogonadism is exhibited as breast atrophy, loss of pubic and axillary hair, and secondary amenorrhea. Hypogonadal men develop testicular atrophy, decreased libido, impotence, decreased muscle mass and bone-mineral density, loss of body hair, and elevated low-density lipoprotein (LDL) cholesterol levels.

Treatment. Androgen replacement therapy is recommended in men with central hypogonadism. Testosterone can be administered as an intramuscular injection (testosterone enanthanate 200 to 300 mg every 2 or 3 weeks) or as a transdermal patch (2.5 to 5 mg/day) or gel (2.5 to 10.0 mg/day). Adequate replacement results in a midnormal serum testosterone level.

Premenopausal women with central hypogonadism should receive estrogen replacement therapy, and, if they have a uterus, they should receive progesterone either continuously or cyclically to protect the uterine lining. Estrogen-progesterone replacement recommendations for postmenopausal hypopituitary women are the same as for postmenopausal women without hypopituitarism.

Gonadotropin-Secreting Pituitary Tumors

Gonadotropin-secreting pituitary tumors are rare and have been reported mainly in men. The majority of tumors are large at the time of presentation and hypersecrete only FSH. Patients usually have signs and symptoms of local pressure, such as visual impairment. Patients may also exhibit hypogonadism with low or normal testosterone levels or low or normal sperm counts. This results from inhibitory effects of chronically high levels of gonadotropins (LH and FSH) on the testicles. In rare cases, excess LH may stimulate testosterone levels.

Surgical removal of gonadotropin-secreting adenomas is the usual primary treatment; however, patients may require subsequent radiotherapy.

Hypothalamic Dysfunction

In children and young adults, craniopharyngioma is the most frequent cause of hypothalamic dysfunction. Primary central nervous system tumors, pinealomas, and dermoid and epidermoid tumors also cause hypothalamic dysfunction in adulthood. Clinical manifestations of tumors that can cause hypothalamic dysfunction include visual loss, symptoms of raised intracranial pressure (headache and vomiting), hypopituitarism (including growth failure), and diabetes insipidus. Hypothalamic disturbances include disorders of thirst (e.g., polydipsia, polyuria, dehydration), appetite (e.g., hyperphagia, obesity), temperature regulation, and consciousness (e.g., somnolence, emotional lability). Diabetes insipidus is a common manifestation of hypothalamic lesions but rarely occurs with primary pituitary lesions. An MRI can confirm the diagnosis. Because hypopituitarism occurs frequently with hypothalamic lesions, anterior pituitary function should be assessed.

Craniopharyngioma is treated by surgical resection and may require subsequent radiotherapy. Biopsy of other types of hypothalamic tumors is usually required for histologic diagnosis before surgical resection because some, such as dysgerminoma, may be radiosensitive.

Hypopituitarism

Hypopituitarism results from diminished secretion of one or more pituitary hormones. The syndrome results either from anterior pituitary gland destruction or dysfunction secondary to deficient hypothalamic stimulatory-inhibitory factors that normally regulate pituitary function. Congenital or acquired lesions can also cause hypopituitarism (Table 64–4). Pituitary insufficiency is usually a slow, insidious disorder. Pituitary lesions may result in single or multiple hormone losses.

DIAGNOSIS

The diagnosis of pituitary hormone deficiency has been previously discussed in relation to the individual hormones.

TREATMENT

Patients with panhypopituitarism must have adequate replacement of T_4, glucocorticoids, and appropriate sex steroids. Children with short stature resulting from GH deficiency should receive GH replacement therapy. The safety and efficacy of GH replacement therapy for adults who develop GH deficiency is being evaluated. Testosterone therapy in men restores libido and potency, growth of body hair, and muscle strength. Estrogen replacement therapy in women maintains secondary sex characteristics and prevents hot flashes. Human menopausal gonadotropins and hCG given intramuscularly or GnRH administered by infusion pumps may be given to induce ovulation. In patients with combined TSH and ACTH deficiency, glucocorticoids should be replaced before T_4 because T_4 may aggravate adrenal insufficiency and may precipitate acute adrenal failure.

Posterior Pituitary Gland

The posterior pituitary gland secretes ADH and oxytocin. These hormones are synthesized in the hypothalamic nuclei in neuronal cell bodies that extend from the hypothalamus to the posterior pituitary. ADH binds to receptors on the

Table 64–4	Causes of Hypopituitarism
Type of Disorder	**Cause**
Congenital	Septo-optic dysplasia Prader-Willi syndrome Laurence-Moon-Biedl syndrome Isolated anterior pituitary hormone; releasing factor deficiency

Tumors	Pituitary tumors
	  Secretory adenomas
	  Nonsecretory adenomas
	Hypothalamic tumors
	Craniopharyngioma
	Hamartoma
	Pinealoma
	Dermoid
	Epidermoid
	Glioma
	Lymphoma
	Meningioma
	Immunologic cancers

Infiltrative	Hemochromatosis Langerhans cell histiocytosis Sarcoidosis Metastatic carcinoma (breast and bronchus) Amyloidosis
Infectious	Tuberculosis Mycoses Syphilis
Physical trauma	Cranial trauma and hemorrhage Ionizing radiation Stalk section Surgery
Vascular	Postpartum pituitary necrosis (Sheehan's syndrome) Pituitary apoplexy Carotid aneurysm

renal tubule, increasing the water permeability of the luminal membrane of the collecting duct epithelium, thus facilitating reabsorption of water and concentration of the urine. Maximal ADH effect results in a small volume of concentrated urine with a high osmolarity (as high as 1200 mOsm/kg). Deficiency of ADH results in a large volume of very dilute urine (as low as 100 mOsm/kg). In addition to the renal tubular effects, ADH also binds to peripheral arteriolar receptors, causing vasoconstriction and resultant increase in blood pressure. However, a counter effect to the hypertensive effect of ADH is that ADH also causes bradycardia and the inhibition of sympathetic nerve activity.

Deficiency of ADH or insensitivity of the kidneys to ADH results in diabetes insipidus, which is exhibited as polyuria and polydipsia. Inappropriate secretion of ADH in excess amounts results in the syndrome of inappropriate antidiuretic hormone production (SIADH) and causes a hyponatremic state.

Oxytocin causes uterine smooth muscle contraction.

DIABETES INSIPIDUS

Vasopressin deficiency occurs with posterior pituitary dysfunction and leads to diabetes insipidus with polyuria, polydipsia, and nocturia. Diabetes insipidus can be of a central (neurogenic) origin where the posterior lobe of the pituitary fails to secrete adequate amounts of ADH; or it can be of nephrogenic origin, caused by failure of the kidney to respond to adequate amounts of circulating ADH. Regardless of the cause, patients are polyuric, secreting large volumes of dilute urine. This causes cellular and extracellular dehydration, stimulating thirst, which results in polydipsia. The causes of central diabetes insipidus are entirely different from those of nephrogenic diabetes insipidus (Table 64–5).

Table 64–5 Causes of Diabetes Insipidus

Central Diabetes Insipidus

Idiopathic
Familial
Hypophysectomy
Infiltration of hypothalamus and posterior pituitary
Langerhans cell histiocytosis
Granulomas
Infection
Tumors (intrasellar and suprasellar)
Autoimmune

Nephrogenic Diabetes Insipidus

Idiopathic
Familial
V_2 receptor gene mutation
Aquaporin-2 gene mutation
Chronic renal disease (e.g., chronic pyelonephritis, polycystic kidney disease, or medullary cystic disease)
Hypokalemia
Hypercalcemia
Sickle cell anemia
Drugs
Lithium
Fluoride
Demeclocycline
Colchicine

Differential Diagnosis

Diabetes insipidus (central or nephrogenic) must be distinguished from primary polydipsia, a compulsive disorder of thirst in which patients drink in excess of 5 to 10 L of water a day, resulting in decreased ADH secretion and subsequent diuresis. One possible distinguishing clinical feature is that patients with diabetes insipidus prefer cold beverages. Several tests can be performed to confirm the diagnosis of diabetes insipidus and differentiate the syndrome from primary polydipsia. Initially, random simultaneous samples of plasma and urine for evaluation of sodium and osmolarity are obtained. In diabetes insipidus (central or nephrogenic), inappropriate diuresis results in a urine osmolarity that is less than that of plasma osmolarity. Plasma osmolarity may be elevated, depending on the patient's state of hydration. However, in primary polydipsia, both plasma and urine are dilute.

The primary test used to differentiate the causes of polyuria is the water deprivation test (**Web Fig. 64–5**). The patient is denied fluids for 12 to 18 hours, and body weight, blood pressure, urine volume, urine-specific gravity, and plasma and urine osmolarity are measured every 2 hours. Careful supervision is required because patients with diabetes insipidus may become rapidly dehydrated and hypotensive if denied access to water, in which case the test is stopped. A normal response is a decrease in urine output to 0.5 mL/min, as well as an increase in urine concentration to greater than that of plasma. Patients with diabetes insipidus (either central or nephrogenic) maintain a high urine output, which continues to be dilute (specific gravity 1.005) despite water deprivation. In patients with primary polydipsia, urine osmolarity increases to values greater than plasma osmolarity. Water deprivation is continued until the urine osmolarity plateaus (an hourly increase of 30 mOsm/kg for 3 successive hours). At that point, 5 units of aqueous vasopressin are administered subcutaneously, and the urine osmolarity is measured after 1 hour. In patients with complete central diabetes insipidus, urine osmolarity increases above plasma osmolarity, whereas in nephrogenic diabetes insipidus, the urine osmolarity increases less than 50% in response to ADH. Patients with partial central diabetes insipidus also show an increase in urine osmolarity, but it is less than 50%, whereas patients with primary polydipsia have increases of less than 10%. ADH levels should be measured during the water deprivation test. Patients with nephrogenic diabetes insipidus have normal or increased levels of ADH during water deprivation, in contrast to those with complete central diabetes insipidus, who have suppressed levels. Patients with partial central diabetes insipidus show a smaller than normal increase in plasma ADH during water deprivation. Patients should be cautioned not to drink large amounts of fluid until the effects of the aqueous vasopressin have worn off (4 to 8 hours) to avoid symptomatic hyponatremia.

Treatment

Central Diabetes Insipidus. Desmopressin acetate (DDAVP), a synthetic analog of ADH, is usually administered intranasally or orally in the treatment of diabetes insipidus. It has a lower pressor:antidiuretic ratio than does ADH. Frequency of administration is determined by the severity of the disease. Adequacy of replacement is monitored by regular measurement of serum osmolarity and sodium.

Nephrogenic Diabetes Insipidus. As far as possible, the underlying disease process should be reversed. Specific treatment of nephrogenic diabetes insipidus is designed to maintain a state of mild sodium depletion with reduction in the solute load on the kidneys and subsequent increased proximal tubular reabsorption. Diuretics coupled with dietary salt restriction can be used to achieve this goal.

SYNDROME OF INAPPROPRIATE ANTIDIURETIC HORMONE PRODUCTION

See Chapter 27.

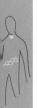

Prospectus for the Future

- U.S. Food and Drug Administration approval and clinical use of several novel therapies for secretory pituitary tumors (e.g., somatostatin receptor subtype and selective analog therapy, universal somatostatin receptor ligand for acromegaly)
- Long-term studies to define indications, safety, and efficacy of GH replacement therapy in adulthood

- Development of novel methods of GH administration including long-acting depot and intranasal preparations
- Clear understanding of the relative roles of surgery, radiation therapy, and novel medical therapies for the treatment of pituitary tumors
- Definition of the role of primary medical therapy in the treatment algorithms for pituitary tumors

References

Arnaldi G, Angeli A, Atkinson AB, et al: Diagnosis and complications of Cushing's syndrome: A consensus statement. J Clin Endocrinol Metab 88(12):5593–602, 2003.

Biller BM, Samuels MH, Zagar A, et al: Sensitivity and specificity of six tests for the diagnosis of adult GH deficiency. J Clin Endocrinol Metab 87(5):2067–2079, 2002.

Boscaro M, Barzon L, Fallo F, Sonino N: Cushing's syndrome. Lancet. 357(9258):783–791, 2001.

Clemmons DR, Chihara K, Freda PU, et al: Optimizing control of acromegaly: integrating a growth hormone receptor antagonist into the treatment algorithm. J Clin Endocrinol Metab 88(10):4759–4767, 2003.

Growth Hormone Research Society: Consensus guidelines for the diagnosis and treatment of adults with GH deficiency. Summary statement of the GH Research Society Workshop on Adult GH Deficiency. J Clin Endocrinol Metab 83:379–381, 1998.

Melmed S, Casanueva FF, Cavagnini F, et al: Acromegaly treatment consensus workshop participants. Guidelines for acromegaly management. J Clin Endocrinol Metab 87(9):4054–4058, 2002.

Schlechte JA: Clinical practice. Prolactinoma. N Engl J Med 349(21): 2035–2041, 2003.

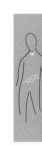

Thyroid Gland

Theodore C. Friedman

Vivien S. Herman-Bonert

The thyroid gland secretes thyroxine (T_4) and triiodo-thyronine (T_3), both of which modulate energy utilization and heat production and facilitate growth. The gland consists of two lateral lobes joined by an isthmus. The weight of the adult gland is 10 to 20 g. Microscopically, the thyroid is composed of several follicles that contain colloid surrounded by a single layer of thyroid epithelium. The follicular cells synthesize thyroglobulin, which is then stored as colloid. Biosynthesis of T_4 and T_3 occurs by iodination of tyrosine molecules in thyroglobulin.

Thyroid Hormone Physiology

THYROID HORMONE SYNTHESIS

Dietary iodine is essential for synthesis of thyroid hormones. Iodine, after conversion to iodide in the stomach, is rapidly absorbed from the gastrointestinal tract and distributed in the extracellular fluids. After active transport from the bloodstream across the follicular cell basement membrane, iodide is enzymatically oxidized by thyroid peroxidase, which also mediates the iodination of the tyrosine residues in thyroglobulin to form monoiodotyrosine and diiodo-tyrosine. The iodotyrosine molecules couple to form T_4 (3,5,3',5-tetraiodothyronine) or T_3 (3,5,3-triiodothyronine). Once iodinated, thyroglobulin containing newly formed T_4 and T_3 is stored in the follicles. Secretion of free T_4 and T_3 into the circulation occurs after proteolytic digestion of thyroglobulin, which is stimulated by thyroid-stimulating hormone (TSH). Deiodination of monoiodotyrosine and diiodotyrosine by iodotyrosine deiodinase releases iodine, which then reenters the thyroid iodine pool (**Web Fig. 65–1**).

THYROID HORMONE TRANSPORT

T_4 and T_3 are tightly bound to serum carrier proteins: thyroxine-binding globulin (TBG), thyroxine-binding pre-albumin, and albumin. The unbound or free fractions are the biologically active fractions and represent only 0.04% of the total T_4 and 0.4% of the total T_3.

PERIPHERAL METABOLISM OF THYROID HORMONES

The normal thyroid gland secretes T_4, T_3, and reverse T_3, a biologically inactive form of T_3. Most of the circulating T_3 is derived from 5'-deiodination of circulating T_4 in the peripheral tissues. Deiodination of T_4 can occur at the outer ring (5'-deiodination), producing T_3 (3,5,3'-triiodothyronine), or at the inner ring, producing reverse T_3 (3,3,5'-triiodothyronine).

CONTROL OF THYROID FUNCTION

Hypothalamic thyrotropin-releasing hormone (TRH) is transported through the hypothalamic-hypophysial portal system to the thyrotrophs of the anterior pituitary gland, stimulating synthesis and release of TSH (Fig. 65–1). TSH, in turn, increases thyroidal iodide uptake and iodination of thyroglobulin, releases T_3 and T_4 from the thyroid gland by increasing hydrolysis of thyroglobulin, and stimulates thyroid cell growth. Hypersecretion of TSH results in thyroid enlargement (goiter). Circulating T_3 exerts negative feedback inhibition of TRH and TSH release.

PHYSIOLOGIC EFFECTS OF THYROID HORMONES

Thyroid hormones increase basal metabolic rate by increasing oxygen consumption and heat production in several body tissues. Thyroid hormones also have specific effects on several organ systems (Table 65–1). These effects are exaggerated in hyperthyroidism and lacking in hypothyroidism, accounting for the well-recognized signs and symptoms of these two disorders.

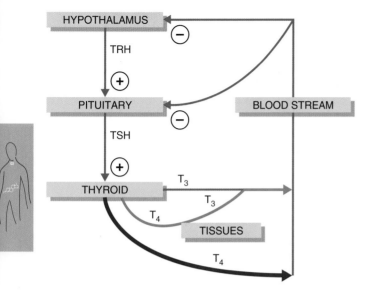

Figure 65–1 Hypothalamic-pituitary-thyroid axis. T_3 = triiodothyronine; T_4 = thyroxine; TRH = thyrotropin-releasing hormone; TSH = thyroid-stimulating hormone.

Thyroid Evaluation

Thyroid gland function and structure can be evaluated by (1) determining serum thyroid hormone levels, (2) imaging thyroid gland size and architecture, (3) measuring thyroid autoantibodies, and (4) performing a thyroid gland biopsy by fine-needle aspiration (FNA).

TESTS OF SERUM THYROID HORMONE LEVELS

Total serum T_4 and T_3 measure the total amount of hormone bound to thyroid-binding proteins by radioimmunoassay. Total T_4 and total T_3 levels are elevated in hyperthyroidism and are low in hypothyroidism. Increase in TBG (as with pregnancy or estrogen therapy) increases the total T_4 and T_3 without actual hyperthyroidism. Similarly, total T_4 and T_3 are low despite euthyroidism in conditions associated with low thyroid-binding proteins (e.g., cirrhosis, nephrotic syndrome). Thus further tests to assess the free hormone level that reflects biologic activity must be performed. Free T_4 level can be estimated by calculating the free T_4 index or can be measured directly by dialysis or ultrafiltration. The free T_4 index is an indirect method of assessing free T_4-derived by multiplying the total T_4 by the T_3 resin uptake, which is inversely proportional to the available T_4 binding sites on TBG. Free T_4 measurement has largely replaced calculation of the free T_4 index.

Serum TSH is measured by a third-generation immunometric assay, which uses at least two different monoclonal antibodies against different regions of the TSH molecule, resulting in accurate discrimination between normal TSH levels and levels below the normal range. Thus the TSH assay can diagnose clinical hyperthyroidism (elevated free T_4 and suppressed TSH) and subclinical hyperthyroidism (normal free T_4 and suppressed TSH). In primary (thyroidal) hypothyroidism, serum TSH is supranormal because of diminished feedback inhibition. The TSH is usually low but may be normal in secondary (pituitary) or tertiary (hypothalamic) hypothyroidism.

Serum thyroglobulin measurements are useful in the follow-up of patients with papillary or follicular carcinoma. After thyroidectomy and iodine-131 (^{131}I) ablation therapy, thyroglobulin levels should be less than 0.5 mcg/L while the patient is on suppressive levothyroxine treatment. Levels in excess of this value indicate the presence of persistent or metastatic disease.

Calcitonin is produced by the C-cells of the thyroid and has a minor role in calcium homeostasis. Calcitonin measurements are invaluable in the diagnosis of medullary carcinoma of the thyroid and for monitoring the effects of therapy for this entity.

Table 65–1	**Physiologic Effects of Thyroid Hormone**

Cardiovascular Effects

Increased heart rate and cardiac output

Gastrointestinal Effects

Increased gut motility

Skeletal Effects

Increased bone turnover and resorption

Pulmonary Effects

Maintenance of normal hypoxic and hypercapnic drive in the respiratory center

Neuromuscular Effects

Increased muscle protein turnover and increased speed of muscle contraction and relaxation

Lipids and Carbohydrate Metabolism Effects

Increased hepatic gluconeogenesis and glycogenolysis, as well as intestinal glucose absorption
Increased cholesterol synthesis and degradation
Increased lipolysis

Sympathetic Nervous System Effects

Increased numbers of β-adrenergic receptors in the heart, skeletal muscle, lymphocytes, and adipose cells
Decreased cardiac α-adrenergic receptors
Increased catecholamine sensitivity

Hematopoietic Effects

Increased red blood cell 2,3-diphosphoglycerate, facilitating oxygen dissociation from hemoglobin with increased oxygen available to tissues

THYROID IMAGING

Technetium-99m (^{99m}Tc) pertechnetate is concentrated in the thyroid gland and can be scanned with a gamma camera, yielding information about the size and shape of the gland and the location of the functional activity in the gland (thyroid scan). The thyroid scan is often performed in conjunction with a quantitative assessment of radioactive iodine uptake by the thyroid with ^{123}I, which quantitates thyroid uptake. Functioning thyroid nodules are called *warm* or *hot* nodules; cold nodules are nonfunctioning. Malignancy is usually associated with a cold nodule; 16% of surgically removed cold nodules are malignant.

Thyroid ultrasound evaluation is useful in the differentiation of solid nodules from cystic nodules. It also may be used to guide the clinician during FNA of a nodule (**see Web Fig. 65–2**).

THYROID ANTIBODIES

Autoantibodies to several different antigenic components in the thyroid gland, including thyroglobulin (TgAb), thyroid peroxidase (TPO Ab, formerly called antimicrosomal antibodies), and the TSH receptor, can be measured in the serum. A strongly positive test for TPO Ab indicates autoimmune thyroid disease. Elevated thyroid receptor-stimulating antibody occurs in Graves' disease (see the discussion under Pathogenesis later in this chapter).

THYROID BIOPSY

FNA of a nodule to obtain thyroid cells for cytologic evaluation is the best way to differentiate benign from malignant disease. FNA requires adequate tissue samples and interpretation by an experienced cytologist.

Hyperthyroidism

Thyrotoxicosis is the clinical syndrome that results from elevated circulating thyroid hormones. Clinical manifestations of thyrotoxicosis are due to the direct physiologic effects of the thyroid hormones, as well as to the increased sensitivity to catecholamines. Tachycardia, tremor, stare, sweating, and lid lag are all due to catecholamine hypersensitivity.

SIGNS AND SYMPTOMS

Table 65–2 lists the signs and symptoms of hyperthyroidism. Thyrotoxic crisis, or *thyroid storm,* is a life-threatening complication of hyperthyroidism that can be precipitated by surgery, radioactive iodine therapy, or severe stress (e.g., uncontrolled diabetes mellitus, myocardial infarction, acute infection). Patients develop fever, flushing, sweating, significant tachycardia, atrial fibrillation, and cardiac failure. Significant agitation, restlessness, delirium, and coma frequently occur. Gastrointestinal manifestations may include nausea, vomiting, and diarrhea. Hyperpyrexia out of proportion to other clinical findings is the hallmark of thyroid storm.

Table 65–2	**Signs and Symptoms of Hyperthyroidism**
Symptoms	
Nervousness	
Heat intolerance	
Fatigue and weakness	
Palpitations	
Increased appetite	
Weight loss	
Oligomenorrhea	
Signs	
Tachycardia	
Atrial fibrillation	
Wide pulse pressure	
Brisk reflexes	
Fine tremor	
Proximal limb-girdle myopathy	
Chemosis	

DIFFERENTIAL DIAGNOSIS

Thyrotoxicosis usually reflects hyperactivity of the thyroid gland resulting from Graves' disease, toxic adenoma, multinodular goiter, or thyroiditis (Table 65–3 and Fig. 65–2). However, it may be the result of excessive ingestion of thyroid hormone or, rarely, thyroid hormone production from an ectopic site as observed in struma ovarii.

GRAVES' DISEASE

Graves' disease, the most common cause of thyrotoxicosis, is an autoimmune disease that is more common in women with a peak age incidence of 20 to 40 years. One or more of the following features are present: (1) goiter; (2) thyrotoxicosis; (3) eye disease ranging from tearing to proptosis, extraocular muscle paralysis, and loss of sight as a result of optic nerve involvement; and (4) thyroid dermopathy, usually observed as significant skin thickening without pitting in a pretibial distribution (pretibial myxedema).

Pathogenesis

Thyrotoxicosis in Graves' disease is due to the overproduction of an antibody that binds to the TSH receptor. These thyroid-stimulating immunoglobulins increase thyroid cell growth and thyroid hormone secretion. Ophthalmopathy is due to inflammatory infiltration of the extraocular eye muscles by lymphocytes, with mucopolysaccharide deposition. The inflammatory reaction that contributes to the eye signs in Graves' disease may be caused by lymphocytes sensitized to antigens common to the orbital muscles and thyroid.

Clinical Features

The common manifestations of thyrotoxicosis (see Table 65–2) are characteristic features of younger patients with

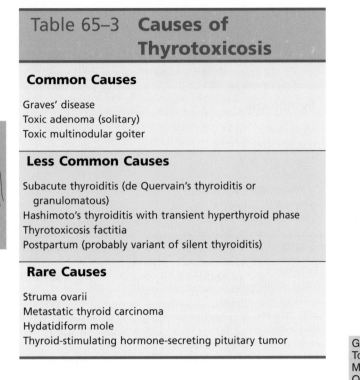

Table 65–3   Causes of Thyrotoxicosis

Common Causes

Graves' disease
Toxic adenoma (solitary)
Toxic multinodular goiter

Less Common Causes

Subacute thyroiditis (de Quervain's thyroiditis or
    granulomatous)
Hashimoto's thyroiditis with transient hyperthyroid phase
Thyrotoxicosis factitia
Postpartum (probably variant of silent thyroiditis)

Rare Causes

Struma ovarii
Metastatic thyroid carcinoma
Hydatidiform mole
Thyroid-stimulating hormone-secreting pituitary tumor

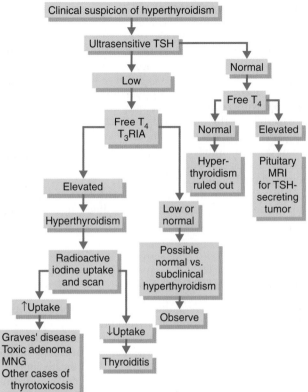

Figure 65–2 Algorithm for differential diagnosis of hyperthyroidism. MNG = multinodular goiter; T_3RIA = triiodothyronine radioimmunoassay; T_4 = thyroxine; TSH = thyroid-stimulating hormone.

Graves' disease. In addition, patients may exhibit a diffuse goiter or the eye signs characteristic of Graves' disease. Older patients often do not have the florid clinical features of thyrotoxicosis, and the condition termed *apathetic hyperthyroidism* is exhibited as flat affect, emotional lability, weight loss, muscle weakness, or congestive heart failure, and atrial fibrillation resistant to standard therapy.

Eye signs of Graves' disease may be either a nonspecific manifestation of hyperthyroidism from any cause (e.g., thyroid stare) or may result from Graves' disease as a result of a specific inflammatory infiltrate of the orbital tissues leading to periorbital edema, conjunctival congestion and swelling, proptosis, extraocular muscle weakness, and/or optic nerve damage with visual impairment (**see Web Fig. 65–3**).

Pretibial myxedema (thyroid dermopathy) occurs in 2% to 3% of patients with Graves' disease and exhibits a thickening of the skin over the lower tibia without pitting. Onycholysis, characterized by separation of the fingernails from their beds, often occurs in the patient with Graves' disease. Thyroid acropachy, or clubbing, may also occur in Graves' disease.

Laboratory Findings

Elevated T_4 and/or T_3 and a suppressed TSH confirm the clinical diagnosis of thyrotoxicosis. Thyroid-stimulating immunoglobulin (TSH-receptor antibody) is usually elevated and may be useful in patients with eye signs who do not have other characteristic clinical features. Increased uptake of ^{123}I differentiates Graves' disease from early subacute or Hashimoto's thyroiditis, in which uptake is low in the presence of hyperthyroidism. Magnetic resonance imaging or ultrasonography of the orbit usually shows orbital muscle enlargement, whether or not clinical signs of ophthalmopathy are observed.

Treatment

Three treatment modalities are used to control the hyperthyroidism of Graves' disease. They are antithyroid drugs, radioactive iodine, and surgery.

Antithyroid Drugs. The thiocarbamide drugs propylthiouracil, methimazole, and carbimazole block thyroid hormone synthesis by inhibiting thyroid peroxidase. Propylthiouracil also partially inhibits peripheral conversion of T_4 to T_3. Medical therapy must be administered for a prolonged period (1 to 2 years) until the disease undergoes spontaneous remission. On cessation of medication, 40% to 50% remain in remission, and the patients who experience relapse must then undergo definitive surgery or radioactive iodine treatment. Side effects of the thiocarbamide regimen include pruritus and rash (in approximately 5% of patients), cholestatic jaundice, acute arthralgias, and, rarely, agranulocytosis (in 0.5% of patients). Patients must be instructed to discontinue the medication and consult a physician if they develop fever or sore throat because these symptoms may indicate agranulocytosis. At the onset of treatment during the acute phase of thyrotoxicosis, β-adrenergic blocking drugs help alleviate tachycardia, hypertension, and atrial fibrillation. As the thyroid hormone levels return to normal, treatment with β-blockers is tapered.

Radioactive Iodine. In terms of cost, efficacy, ease, and short-term side effects, radioactive iodine has benefits that exceed both surgery and antithyroid drugs. ^{131}I is the treatment of choice in most adults with Graves' disease. It is contraindicated in women who are pregnant, but it does not increase the risk of birth defects in offspring conceived after ^{131}I therapy. Patients with severe thyrotoxicosis, very large glands, or underlying heart disease should be rendered euthyroid with antithyroid medication before receiving radioactive iodine because ^{131}I treatment can cause a release of preformed thyroid hormone from the thyroid gland into the circulation; this release can precipitate cardiac arrhythmias and exacerbate symptoms of thyrotoxicosis. After administering radioactive iodine, the thyroid gland shrinks and patients become euthyroid over a period of 6 weeks to 3 months. Between 10% and 20% of patients become hypothyroid within the first year of treatment, and thereafter hypothyroidism occurs at a rate of 3% to 5% per year. Ultimately, 50% to 80% of patients become hypothyroid after radioactive iodine treatment. Serum-free T_4 and TSH levels should be monitored and replacement with levothyroxine instituted if hypothyroidism occurs. Hypothyroidism may also develop after surgery or antithyroid medication, mandating lifelong monitoring of all patients with Graves' disease.

Surgery. Either subtotal or total thyroidectomy is the treatment of choice for patients with very large glands and obstructive symptoms or multinodular glands, or for patients desiring pregnancy within the next year. It is essential that the surgeon be experienced in thyroid surgery. Preoperatively, patients receive 6 weeks of treatment with antithyroid drugs to ensure that they are euthyroid at the time of surgery. Two weeks before surgery, oral-saturated solution of potassium iodide is administered daily to decrease the vascularity of the gland. Permanent hypoparathyroidism and recurrent laryngeal nerve palsy occur postoperatively in less than 2% of patients.

TOXIC ADENOMA

Solitary toxic nodules, which are usually benign, occur more frequently in older patients. Clinical manifestations are those of thyrotoxicosis. Physical examination shows a distinct solitary nodule. Laboratory investigation shows suppressed TSH and significantly elevated T_3 levels, often with only moderately elevated T_4. Thyroid scan shows a *hot* nodule of the affected lobe with complete suppression of the unaffected lobe. Solitary toxic nodules are treated with radioactive iodine. However, unilateral lobectomy after the administration of antithyroid drugs to render the patient euthyroid may be required for large nodules.

TOXIC MULTINODULAR GOITER

Toxic multinodular goiter occurs in older patients with long-standing multinodular goiter, especially in patients from iodine-deficient regions. The presenting clinical features are frequently tachycardia, heart failure, and arrhythmias.

Physical examination shows a multinodular goiter. The diagnosis is confirmed by laboratory features of suppressed TSH, elevated T_3 and T_4, and a thyroid scan with multiple functioning nodules. The treatment of choice is often ^{131}I ablation. It is especially effective in patients with small glands and a high radioactive uptake.

SUBCLINICAL HYPERTHYROIDISM

In subclinical hyperthyroidism, T_4 and T_3 levels are normal with a suppressed TSH. The causes of this condition include early presentation of all forms of hyperthyroidism, including Graves' disease, toxic adenoma, and toxic multinodular goiter. Because these patients, especially those who are older, are at an increased risk for developing cardiac dysrhythmias, many patients with a persistently suppressed TSH should be treated with thiocarbamide drugs or radioactive iodine.

Thyroiditis

Thyroiditis may be classified as acute, subacute, or chronic. Although thyroiditis may eventually result in clinical hypothyroidism, the initial presentation is often that of hyperthyroidism as a result of acute release of T_4 and T_3. Hyperthyroidism caused by thyroiditis can be readily differentiated from other causes of hyperthyroidism by suppressed uptake of radioactive iodine, reflecting decreased hormone production by damaged cells.

A rare disorder, acute suppurative thyroiditis, exhibits high fever, a redness of the overlying skin, and thyroid gland tenderness; it may be confused with subacute thyroiditis. If blood cultures are negative, then needle aspiration should identify the organism. Intensive antibiotic treatment and, occasionally, incision and drainage are required.

SUBACUTE THYROIDITIS

Subacute thyroiditis (de Quervain's thyroiditis or granulomatous thyroiditis) is an acute inflammatory disorder of the thyroid gland, probably secondary to viral infection, which resolves completely in 90% of cases. Patients with subacute thyroiditis complain of fever and anterior neck pain. The patient may have symptoms and signs of hyperthyroidism. The classic feature on physical examination is an exquisitely tender thyroid gland. Laboratory findings vary with the course of the disease. Initially, the patient may be symptomatically thyrotoxic with elevated serum T_4, depressed serum TSH, and very low radioactive iodine uptake on scan. Subsequently, the thyroid status will fluctuate through euthyroid and hypothyroid phases and may return to euthyroidism. An increase in radioactive iodine uptake on the scan reflects recovery of the gland. Treatment usually includes nonsteroidal anti-inflammatory drugs, but a short course of prednisone may be required if pain and fever are severe. During the hypothyroid phase, replacement therapy with levothyroxine may be indicated.

Postpartum thyroiditis resembles subacute thyroiditis in its clinical course. It usually occurs within the first 6 months after delivery and goes through the triphasic course of hyperthyroidism, hypothyroidism, and then euthyroidism, or it may develop with only hypothyroidism. Some patients have an underlying chronic thyroiditis.

CHRONIC THYROIDITIS

Chronic thyroiditis (Hashimoto's thyroiditis or lymphocytic thyroiditis) from destruction of normal thyroidal architecture by lymphocytic infiltration results in hypothyroidism and goiter. Riedel's struma is probably a variant of Hashimoto's thyroiditis, characterized by extensive thyroid

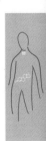

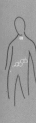

fibrosis resulting in a rock-hard thyroid mass. Hashimoto's thyroiditis is more common in women and is the most common cause of goiter and hypothyroidism in the United States. Occasionally, patients with Hashimoto's thyroiditis may have transient hyperthyroidism with low radioactive iodine uptake, owing to the release of T_4 and T_3 into the circulation. Chronic thyroiditis can be differentiated from subacute thyroiditis in that the gland is nontender to palpation and antithyroid antibodies are present in high titer. Early in the disease, TgAb is significantly elevated, but it may disappear later. TPO Ab also is present early and generally remains present for years. Radioactive iodine uptake may be high, normal, or low. Serum T_3 and T_4 levels are either normal or low; when low, the TSH is elevated. FNA of the thyroid shows lymphocytes and Hürthle cells (enlarged basophilic follicular cells). Hypothyroidism and significant glandular enlargement (goiter) are indications for levothyroxine therapy. Adequate doses of levothyroxine are administered to normalize TSH levels and shrink the goiter.

Thyrotoxicosis Factitia

Thyrotoxicosis factitia exhibits typical features of thyrotoxicosis from ingestion of excessive amounts of thyroxine, often in an attempt to lose weight. Serum T_3 and T_4 levels are elevated and TSH is suppressed, as is the serum thyroglobulin concentration. Radioactive iodine uptake is absent. Patients may require psychotherapy.

Rare Causes of Thyrotoxicosis

Struma ovarii occurs when an ovarian teratoma contains thyroid tissue, which secretes thyroid hormone. A body scan confirms the diagnosis by demonstrating uptake of radioactive iodine in the pelvis.

Hydatidiform mole is due to proliferation and swelling of the trophoblast during pregnancy, with excess production of chorionic gonadotropin, which has intrinsic TSH-like activity. The hyperthyroidism remits with surgical and medical treatment of the molar pregnancy.

Hypothyroidism

Hypothyroidism is a clinical syndrome caused by deficiency of thyroid hormones. In infants and children, hypothyroidism causes retardation of growth and development and may result in permanent motor and mental retardation. Congenital causes of hypothyroidism include agenesis (complete absence of thyroid tissue), dysgenesis (ectopic or lingual thyroid gland), hypoplastic thyroid, thyroid dyshormogenesis, and congenital pituitary diseases. Adult-onset hypothyroidism results in a slowing of metabolic processes and is reversible with treatment. Hypothyroidism is usually primary (thyroid failure), but it may be secondary (hypothalamic or pituitary deficiency) or the result of resistance at the thyroid hormone receptor (Table 65–4). In adults, autoimmune thyroiditis (Hashimoto's thyroiditis) is the most common cause of hypothyroidism. This condition may be isolated or part of the polyglandular failure

Table 65–4 Causes of Hypothyroidism
Primary Hypothyroidism
Autoimmune
Hashimoto's thyroiditis
Part of polyglandular failure syndrome, type II
Iatrogenic
^{131}I therapy
Thyroidectomy
Drug-induced
Iodine deficiency
Iodine excess
Lithium
Amiodarone
Antithyroid drugs
Congenital
Thyroid agenesis
Thyroid dysgenesis
Hypoplastic thyroid
Biosynthetic defect
Secondary Hypothyroidism
Hypothalamic dysfunction
Neoplasms
Tuberculosis
Sarcoidosis
Langerhans cell histiocytosis
Hemochromatosis
Radiation treatment
Pituitary dysfunction
Neoplasms
Pituitary surgery
Postpartum pituitary necrosis
Idiopathic hypopituitarism
Glucocorticoid excess (Cushing's syndrome)
Radiation treatment

syndrome type II (Schmidt's syndrome), which also includes insulin-dependent diabetes mellitus, pernicious anemia, vitiligo, gonadal failure, hypophysitis, celiac disease, myasthenia gravis, and primary biliary cirrhosis. Iatrogenic causes of hypothyroidism include ^{131}I therapy, thyroidectomy, and treatment with lithium or amiodarone. Iodine deficiency or excess can also cause hypothyroidism.

CLINICAL MANIFESTATIONS

The clinical presentation of hypothyroidism (Table 65–5) depends on the age of onset and severity of thyroid deficiency. Infants with congenital hypothyroidism (also called

Table 65–5 Clinical Features of Hypothyroidism

Children

Learning disabilities
Mental retardation
Short stature
Delayed bone age
Delayed puberty

Adults

Fatigue
Cold intolerance
Weight gain
Constipation
Menstrual irregularities
Dry, coarse, cold skin
Periorbital, peripheral edema
Delayed reflexes
Bradycardia

cretinism) may exhibit feeding problems, hypotonia, inactivity, an open posterior fontanelle, and/or edematous face and hands. Mental retardation, short stature, and delayed puberty occur if treatment is delayed.

Hypothyroidism in adults usually develops insidiously. Patients often complain of fatigue, lethargy, and gradual weight gain for years before the diagnosis is established. A delayed relaxation phase of deep tendon reflexes (*hung-up* reflexes) is a valuable clinical sign characteristic of severe hypothyroidism. Subcutaneous infiltration by mucopolysaccharides, which bind water, causes the edema (termed *myxedema*) and is responsible for the thickened features and puffy appearance of patients with severe hypothyroidism (**see Web Fig. 65–4**).

Severe untreated hypothyroidism can result in myxedema coma, characterized by hypothermia, extreme weakness, stupor, hypoventilation, hypoglycemia, and hyponatremia and is often precipitated by cold exposure, infection, or psychoactive drugs.

LABORATORY TESTS

Laboratory abnormalities in patients with primary hypothyroidism include elevated serum TSH and low total and free T_4. A low or low-normal morning serum TSH in the setting of hypothalamic or pituitary dysfunction characterizes secondary hypothyroidism. Often, the serum total and free T_4 levels are at the lower limits of normal.

Hypothyroidism is often associated with hypercholesterolemia and elevated creatine phosphokinase skeletal muscle (MM) fraction (the fraction representative of skeletal muscle). Anemia is usually normocytic, normochromic but may be macrocytic (vitamin B_{12} deficiency resulting from associated pernicious anemia) or microcytic (caused by nutritional deficiencies or menstrual blood loss in women).

DIFFERENTIAL DIAGNOSIS

Because the initial manifestations of hypothyroidism are subtle, the early diagnosis of hypothyroidism demands a high index of suggestion in patients with one or more of the signs or symptoms (Table 65–5). Early symptoms that are often overlooked include menstrual irregularities (usually menorrhagia), arthralgias, and myalgias.

Laboratory diagnosis may be complicated by the finding of a low total T_4 in euthyroid states associated with low TBG, such as nephrotic syndrome, cirrhosis, or TBG deficiency. TSH and free T_4 levels are normal in these instances. A low total T_4 may also be found in the *euthyroid sick syndrome,* a condition occurring in acutely ill patients. In such patients, total and occasionally free T_4 levels are low and the serum TSH level is usually normal but may be mildly elevated. This condition may be differentiated from primary hypothyroidism by absence of a goiter, negative antithyroid antibodies, and elevated serum reverse T_3 levels, as well as by clinical presentation. The thyroid hormone levels return to normal with resolution of the acute illness, and the patients do not require levothyroxine therapy.

TREATMENT

Patients with hypothyroidism should be initially treated with synthetic levothyroxine. Although T_3 is the more bioactive thyroid hormone, peripheral tissues convert T_4 to T_3 to maintain physiologic levels of the latter. Thus administration of levothyroxine results in bioavailable T_3 and T_4. Levothyroxine has a half-life of 8 days; consequently, it needs to be given only once a day. The average replacement dose of levothyroxine for adults is 75 to 150 mcg/day. In healthy adults, 1.6 mcg/kg/day is an appropriate starting dose. In some older patients or patients with cardiac disease, levothyroxine should be increased gradually, starting at 25 mcg daily and increasing this dose by 25 mcg every 2 weeks, although most patients can safely be started on a full replacement dose. The therapeutic response to levothyroxine therapy should be monitored clinically and with serum TSH levels, which should be measured 6 weeks after a dose adjustment. TSH levels between 0.5 and 2.0 mU/L are optimal. Patients with secondary hypothyroidism (pituitary or hypothalamic dysfunction) should be treated with levothyroxine until their free T_4 is in the midnormal range because TSH measurements are not useful to guide therapy in this condition.

In patients with myxedema coma, 300 to 400 mg of levothyroxine is administered intravenously as a loading dose, followed by 50 mg daily and hydrocortisone (100 mg intravenously three times a day) and intravenous fluids. The underlying precipitating event should be corrected. Respiratory assistance and treatment of hypothermia with warming blankets may be required. Although myxedema coma carries a high mortality rate despite appropriate treatment, many patients improve in 1 to 3 days.

Subclinical Hypothyroidism

In subclinical hypothyroidism, T_4 and/or T_3 levels are normal or low normal, with a mildly elevated TSH. Some but not all of these patients will develop overt hypothyroidism. The decision about when to treat patients with a mildly elevated TSH is controversial; it is frequently recommended that patients should be treated with levothyroxine if they have a TSH greater than 5 mU/L on two occasions and either positive anti-TPO Ab test results or a goiter. If the patient does not have an appreciable goiter and has negative anti-TPO Ab results, then the patient should be treated with levothyroxine only if he or she has a TSH greater than 10 mU/L on two occasions.

Goiter

Enlargement of the thyroid gland is called goiter. Patients with goiter may be euthyroid (simple goiter), hyperthyroid (toxic nodular goiter or Graves' disease), or hypothyroid (nontoxic goiter or Hashimoto's thyroiditis). Thyroid enlargement (often focal) may also be the result of a thyroid adenoma or carcinoma. In nontoxic goiter, inadequate thyroid hormone synthesis leads to TSH stimulation with resultant enlargement of the thyroid gland. Iodine deficiency (endemic goiter) was once the most common cause of nontoxic goiter. With the use of iodized salt, it is now almost nonexistent in North America.

Dietary goitrogens can cause goiter, and iodine is the most common goitrogen. Other goitrogens include lithium and vegetable products such as thioglucosides found in cabbage. Thyroid hormone biosynthetic defects can cause goiter associated with hypothyroidism or, with adequate compensation, euthyroidism.

A careful thyroid examination coupled with thyroid hormone tests can delineate the cause of the goiter. A smooth, symmetrical gland, often with a bruit, and hyperthyroidism are suggestive of Graves' disease. A nodular thyroid gland with hypothyroidism and positive antithyroid antibodies is consistent with Hashimoto's thyroiditis. A diffuse, smooth goiter with hypothyroidism and negative antithyroid antibodies may be indicative of iodine deficiency or a biosynthetic defect. Goiters may become very large, extend substernally, and cause dysphagia, respiratory distress, or hoarseness. An ultrasound evaluation or radioactive iodine scan delineates the thyroid gland, and a thyroid uptake scan can determine the functional activity of the goiter.

Hypothyroid goiters are treated with thyroid hormone at a dose that normalizes TSH. Euthyroid goiters may be treated with levothyroxine therapy; however, in most cases, especially with longstanding goiters, regression is unlikely. Surgery is indicated for nontoxic goiter only if obstructive symptoms develop or substantial substernal extension is present.

Solitary Thyroid Nodules

Thyroid nodules are common. They can be detected clinically in about 4% of the population and are found in about 50% of the population at autopsy. Benign thyroid nodules are usually follicular adenomas, colloid nodules, benign cysts, or nodular thyroiditis. Patients with Hashimoto's thyroiditis may have one prominent nodule on clinical examination, but thyroid ultrasound evaluation may reveal multiple nodules. Although the majority of nodules are benign, a small percentage is malignant. In addition, most thyroid cancers are low-grade malignancies. History, physical examination, and laboratory tests can be helpful in differentiating benign from malignant lesions (Table 65–6). For example, lymph node involvement or hoarseness is strongly suggestive of a malignant tumor.

The major etiologic factor for thyroid cancer is childhood or adolescent exposure to head and neck radiation. Previously, radiation was used to treat an enlarged thymus, tonsillar disease, hemangioma, or acne. Recently, exposure to radiation from nuclear plants (e.g., Chernobyl, Ukraine) has contributed to an increased incidence of thyroid cancer. Patients with a history of irradiation should have a baseline thyroid ultrasound and their thyroid carefully palpated every 1 to 2 years.

A dominant nodule or nodules with ultrasound features compatible with neoplasia should undergo an FNA, which is a safe procedure that has reduced the need for surgical excision. An expert cytologist can identify most benign lesions (75% of all biopsies). In addition, malignant lesions (5% of biopsies), such as papillary, anaplastic, and medullary carcinoma, can be specifically identified. Follicular neoplasms, however, cannot be diagnosed as benign or malignant by FNA; a cytology report of follicular neoplasia, along with "suspicious" cytology, requires surgical excision. However, if the patient has a follicular lesion and a suppressed TSH, a thyroid scan should be performed because *hot* nodules are rarely malignant.

Although previously benign thyroid nodules were treated with levothyroxine suppression, this is no longer recommended because it is uncommon for thyroid nodules to shrink substantially with levothyroxine.

Table 65–6 **High-Risk Factors for Malignancy in a Thyroid Nodule**

History

Head and neck irradiation
Exposure to nuclear radiation
Rapid growth
Recent onset
Young age
Male sex
Familial incidence (medullary and ~5% of papillary)

Physical Examination

Hard consistency of nodule
Fixation of nodule
Lymphadenopathy
Vocal cord paralysis
Distant metastasis

Laboratory and Imaging

Elevated serum calcitonin
Cold nodule on technetium scan
Solid lesion on ultrasonography

Table 65–7 Characteristics of Thyroid Cancers

Type of Cancer	Percentage of Thyroid Cancers	Age of Onset	Treatment	Prognosis
Papillary	80	40–80	Thyroidectomy, followed by radioactive iodine ablation	Good
Follicular	15	45–80	Thyroidectomy, followed by radioactive iodine ablation	Fair to good
Medullary	3	20–50	Thyroidectomy and central compartment lymph node dissection	Fair
Anaplastic	1	50–80	Isthmusectomy followed by palliative x-ray treatment	Poor
Lymphoma	1	25–70	X-ray therapy and/or chemotherapy	Fair

Thyroid Carcinoma

The types and characteristics of thyroid carcinomas are presented in Table 65–7. Papillary carcinoma is associated with local invasion and lymph node spread. Poor prognosis is associated with thyroid capsule invasion, size greater than 2.5 cm, age at onset older than 45 years, tall-cell variant, and lymph node involvement. Follicular carcinoma is slightly more aggressive than papillary carcinoma and can spread by local invasion of lymph nodes or hematogenously to bone, brain, or lung. Patients may exhibit metastases before diagnosis of the primary thyroid lesion. Anaplastic carcinoma tends to occur in older individuals, is very aggressive, and rapidly causes pain, dysphagia, and hoarseness.

Medullary thyroid carcinoma is derived from calcitonin-producing parafollicular cells and is more malignant than papillary or follicular carcinoma. It is multifocal and spreads both locally and distally. It may be either sporadic or familial. When familial, it is inherited in an autosomal dominant pattern and is part of multiple endocrine neoplasia type IIA (medullary carcinoma of the thyroid, pheochromocytoma, and hyperparathyroidism) or multiple endocrine neoplasia type IIB (medullary carcinoma of the thyroid, mucosal neuromas, intestinal ganglioneuromas, marfanoid habitus, and pheochromocytoma). Elevated basal serum calcitonin levels confirm the diagnosis. Evaluation for *RET* proto-oncogene mutations should be performed in patients with medullary carcinoma, and, if present, all first-degree relatives of the patients should be examined.

TREATMENT

Lobectomy may be performed for isolated papillary microcarcinoma. However, most papillary or follicular tumors require thyroidectomy with a central compartment lymph node dissection, as well as a modified neck dissection if evidence of lateral lymph node metastases is found. After surgery, patients with low risk, small carcinomas may be placed on doses of levothyroxine sufficient to suppress the TSH level and monitored with serum thyroglobulin determinations and neck ultrasound examinations. Patients with large lesions or who are at high risk of persistence or metastatic disease should be treated with radioactive iodine. Sufficient levothyroxine is then administered to suppress serum TSH to subnormal levels. Frequent neck examinations for masses should be accompanied by measurement of serum thyroglobulin levels. Recurrence and metastases are also evaluated by ^{131}I total-body scans carried out under conditions of TSH stimulation, which increase ^{131}I uptake by the thyroid tissue. Elevated TSH levels can be achieved by withdrawal of thyroxine supplementation for 6 weeks. As an alternative, to avoid the resultant symptomatic hypothyroidism, recombinant human TSH can be administered while the patient remains on thyroid hormone replacement. A rise in serum thyroglobulin levels suggests recurrence of thyroid cancer. Local or metastatic lesions that take up [131]I (whole-body scan) can be treated with radioactive iodine after the patient has stopped thyroid hormone replacement, whereas those that do not take up ^{131}I can be treated with surgical excision or local x-ray therapy. Medullary carcinoma of the thyroid requires total thyroidectomy with removal of the central lymph nodes in the neck. Completeness of the procedure is determined by measurement of serum calcitonin, which is also used in monitoring for recurrence.

Anaplastic carcinoma is treated with isthmusectomy to confirm the diagnosis and to prevent tracheal compression, followed by palliative x-ray treatment. Thyroid lymphomas are also treated with x-ray therapy and/or chemotherapy.

The prognosis for well-differentiated thyroid carcinomas is good. The patient's age at the time of diagnosis and sex are the most important prognostic factors. Men older than 40 years of age and women older than 50 years of age have a higher recurrence and death rates than do younger patients. The 5-year survival rate for invasive medullary carcinoma is 50%, whereas the mean survival for anaplastic carcinoma is 6 months.

Prospectus for the Future

- Use of recombinant TSH in combination with radioactive iodine to treat euthyroid goiters and recurrences and metastases of thyroid cancers

- Genetic identification of patients at risk for autoimmune thyroid disease
- Differentiation of benign from malignant follicular neoplasms on FNA tissue by immunogenetic methodology

References

Cooper DS: Hyperthyroidism. Lancet 362:459–468, 2003.

Hegedus L: Clinical practice. The thyroid nodule. N Engl J Med 351: 1764–1771, 2004.

Roberts CGP, Ladenson PW: Hypothyroidism. Lancet 363:793–803, 2004.

Sherman SI: Thyroid carcinoma. Lancet 361:501–511, 2003.

Surks MI, Ortiz E, Daniels GH, et al: Subclinical thyroid disease. Scientific review and guidelines for diagnosis and management. JAMA 291: 228–238, 2004.

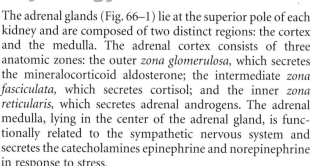

Adrenal Gland

Theodore C. Friedman

Physiology

The adrenal glands (Fig. 66–1) lie at the superior pole of each kidney and are composed of two distinct regions: the cortex and the medulla. The adrenal cortex consists of three anatomic zones: the outer *zona glomerulosa,* which secretes the mineralocorticoid aldosterone; the intermediate *zona fasciculata,* which secretes cortisol; and the inner *zona reticularis,* which secretes adrenal androgens. The adrenal medulla, lying in the center of the adrenal gland, is functionally related to the sympathetic nervous system and secretes the catecholamines epinephrine and norepinephrine in response to stress.

The synthesis of all steroid hormones begins with cholesterol and is catalyzed by a series of regulated, enzyme-mediated reactions (Fig. 66–2). Glucocorticoids affect the metabolism, cardiovascular function, behavior, and inflammatory and immune response (Table 66–1). Cortisol, the natural human glucocorticoid, is secreted by the adrenal glands in response to ultradian, circadian, and stress-induced hormonal stimulation by adrenocorticotropic hormone (ACTH). Plasma cortisol has significant circadian rhythm; levels are highest in the morning. ACTH, a 39-amino acid neuropeptide, is part of the pro-opiomelanocortin (POMC)–precursor molecule, which also contains β-endorphin, β-lipotropin, corticotropin-like intermediate-lobe peptide (CLIP), and various melanocyte-stimulating hormones (MSH). The secretion of ACTH by the pituitary gland is regulated primarily by two hypothalamic polypeptides: the 41-amino acid corticotropin-releasing hormone (CRH) and the decapeptide vasopressin. Glucocorticoids exert negative feedback on CRH and ACTH secretion. The brain hypothalamic-pituitary-adrenal (HPA) axis (Fig. 66–3) interacts with and influences the function of the reproductive, growth, and thyroid axes at multiple levels, with major participation of glucocorticoids at all levels.

The renin-angiotensin-aldosterone system (Fig. 66–4) is the major regulator of aldosterone secretion. Renal juxta-glomerular cells secrete renin in response to a decrease in circulating volume and/or a reduction in renal perfusion pressure. Renin is the rate-limiting enzyme that cleaves the 60-kD angiotensinogen, synthesized by the liver, to the bio-inactive decapeptide angiotensin I. Angiotensin I is rapidly converted to the octapeptide angiotensin II by angiotensin-converting enzyme in the lungs and other tissues. Angiotensin II is a potent vasopressor and stimulates aldosterone production but does not stimulate cortisol production. Angiotensin II is the predominant regulator of aldosterone secretion, but plasma potassium concentration, plasma volume, and ACTH levels also influence aldosterone secretion. ACTH also mediates the circadian rhythm of aldosterone; as a result, the plasma concentration of aldosterone is highest in the morning. Aldosterone binds to the type I mineralocorticoid receptor. In contrast, cortisol binds to both the type I mineralocorticoid and type II glucocorticoid receptors, although the intracellular enzyme 11β-hydroxysteroid dehydrogenase (11β-HSD) type II, which catabolizes cortisol to inactive cortisone, limits the functional binding to the former receptor. The availability of cortisol to bind to the glucocorticoid receptor is modulated by 11β-HSD type I, which interconverts cortisol and cortisone. Binding of aldosterone to the cytosol mineralocorticoid receptor leads to sodium (Na^+) absorption and potassium (K^+) and hydrogen (H^+) secretion by the renal tubules. The resultant increase in plasma Na^+ and decrease in plasma K^+ provide a feedback mechanism for suppressing renin and, subsequently, aldosterone secretion.

Approximately 5% of cortisol and 40% of aldosterone circulate in the free form; the remainder is bound to corticosteroid-binding globulin and albumin.

Adrenal androgen precursors include dehydroepiandrosterone (DHEA) and its sulfate and androstenedione. These are synthesized in the zona reticularis under the influence of ACTH and other adrenal androgen-stimulating factors. Although they have minimal intrinsic androgenic activity, they contribute to androgenicity by their peripheral conversion to testosterone and dihydrotestosterone. In men, excessive adrenal androgens have no clinical consequences;

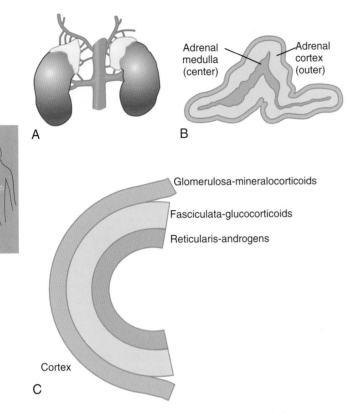

A

B   Adrenal medulla (center)   Adrenal cortex (outer)

Glomerulosa-mineralocorticoids

Fasciculata-glucocorticoids

Reticularis-androgens

Cortex

C

Figure 66–1 *A,* Anatomic location of the adrenal glands. *B,* Distribution of adrenal cortex and medulla. *C,* Zones of the adrenal cortex.

Table 66–1 Actions of Glucocorticoids

Metabolic Homeostasis

Regulate blood glucose level (permissive effects on gluconeogenesis)
Increase glycogen synthesis
Raise insulin levels (permissive effects on lipolytic hormones)
Increase catabolism, decrease anabolism (except fat), inhibit growth hormone axis
Inhibit reproductive axis
Stimulate mineralocorticoid receptor by cortisol

Connective Tissues

Cause loss of collagen and connective tissue

Calcium Homeostasis

Stimulate osteoclasts, inhibit osteoblasts
Reduce intestinal calcium absorption, stimulate parathyroid hormone release, increase urinary calcium excretion, decrease reabsorption of phosphate

Cardiovascular Function

Increase cardiac output
Increase vascular tone (permissive effects on pressor hormones)
Increase sodium retention

Behavior and Cognitive Function

Immune System

Increase intravascular leukocyte concentration
Decrease migration of inflammatory cells to sites of injury
Suppress immune system (thymolysis; suppression of cytokines, prostanoids, kinins, serotonin, histamine, collagenase, and plasminogen activator)

however, peripheral conversion of excess adrenal androgen precursor secretion in women results in acne, hirsutism, and virilization. Because of gonadal production of androgens and estrogens and the secretion of norepinephrine by sympathetic ganglia, deficiencies of adrenal androgens and catecholamines are not clinically recognized.

Adrenal Insufficiency

Glucocorticoid insufficiency can be primary, resulting from the destruction or dysfunction of the adrenal cortex, or secondary, resulting from ACTH hyposecretion (Table 66–2). Autoimmune destruction of the adrenal glands (Addison's disease) is the most common cause of primary adrenal insufficiency in the industrialized world, accounting for approximately 65% of cases. Usually both glucocorticoid and mineralocorticoid secretions are diminished in this condition and, if untreated, may be fatal. Isolated glucocorticoid or mineralocorticoid deficiency may also occur, and it is becoming apparent that mild adrenal insufficiency (similar to subclinical hypothyroidism, discussed in Chapter 65) should also be diagnosed and treated. Adrenal medulla function is usually spared. Approximately 70% of the patients with Addison's disease have anti-adrenal antibodies.

Tuberculosis used to be the most common cause of adrenal insufficiency. However, its incidence in the industrialized world has decreased since the 1960s, and it now accounts for only 15% to 20% of patients of adrenal insufficiency; calcified adrenal glands can be observed in 50% of

these patients. Rare causes of adrenal insufficiency are provided in Table 66–2. Many patients with human immunodeficiency virus infection have decreased adrenal reserve without overt adrenal insufficiency.

Addison's disease may be part of two distinct autoimmune polyglandular syndromes. The triad of hypoparathyroidism, adrenal insufficiency, and mucocutaneous candidiasis characterize type I polyglandular autoimmune syndrome, also termed *autoimmune polyendocrine-candidiasis-ectodermal dystrophy* or *autoimmune polyglandular failure syndrome.* Other, less common manifestations include hypothyroidism, gonadal failure, gastrointestinal malabsorption, insulin-dependent diabetes mellitus, alopecia areata and totalis, pernicious anemia, vitiligo, chronic active hepatitis, keratopathy, hypoplasia of dental enamel and nails, hypophysitis, asplenism, and cholelithiasis. This syndrome develops in childhood. Type II polyglandular autoimmune syndrome, also called Schmidt's syndrome, is characterized by Addison's disease, autoimmune thyroid

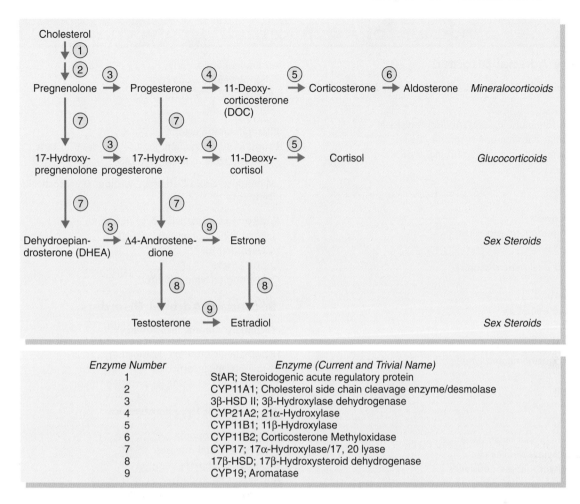

Enzyme Number	Enzyme (Current and Trivial Name)
1	StAR; Steroidogenic acute regulatory protein
2	CYP11A1; Cholesterol side chain cleavage enzyme/desmolase
3	3β-HSD II; 3β-Hydroxylase dehydrogenase
4	CYP21A2; 21α-Hydroxylase
5	CYP11B1; 11β-Hydroxylase
6	CYP11B2; Corticosterone Methyloxidase
7	CYP17; 17α-Hydroxylase/17, 20 lyase
8	17β-HSD; 17β-Hydroxysteroid dehydrogenase
9	CYP19; Aromatase

Figure 66–2 Pathways of steroid biosynthesis.

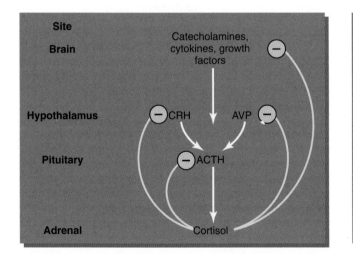

Figure 66–3 Brain hypothalamic-pituitary-adrenal axis. ACTH = adrenocorticotropic hormone; AVP = arginine vasopressin; CRH = corticotropin-releasing hormone.

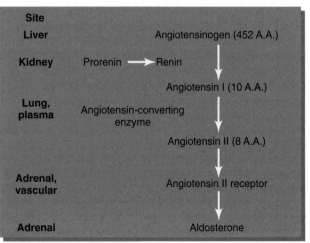

Figure 66–4 Renin-angiotensin-aldosterone axis. AA = amino acids.

Table 66–2 Syndromes of Adrenocortical Hypofunction

Primary Adrenal Disorders

Combined Glucocorticoid and Mineralocorticoid Deficiency

Autoimmune
Isolated autoimmune disease (Addison's disease)
Polyglandular autoimmune syndrome, type I
Polyglandular autoimmune syndrome, type II

Infectious
Tuberculosis
Fungal
Cytomegalovirus
Human immunodeficiency virus

Vascular
Bilateral adrenal hemorrhage
Sepsis
Coagulopathy
Thrombosis; embolism
Adrenal infarction

Infiltration
Metastatic carcinoma and lymphoma
Sarcoidosis
Amyloidosis
Hemochromatosis

Congenital
Congenital adrenal hyperplasia
  21-hydroxylase deficiency
  3β-ol dehydrogenase deficiency
  20,22-desmolase deficiency
Adrenal unresponsiveness to ACTH
Congenital adrenal hypoplasia

Adrenoleukodystrophy
Adrenomyeloneuropathy

Iatrogenic

Bilateral adrenalectomy
Drugs: Metyrapone, aminoglutethimide, trilostane,
  ketoconazole, o,p'-DDD, RU-486

Mineralocorticoid Deficiency without Glucocorticoid Deficiency

Corticosterone methyloxidase deficiency
Isolated zona glomerulosa defect
Heparin therapy
Critical illness
Converting-enzyme inhibitors

Secondary Adrenal Disorders

Secondary Adrenal Insufficiency

Hypothalamic-pituitary dysfunction
Exogenous glucocorticoids
After removal of an ACTH-secreting tumor

Hyporeninemic Hypoaldosteronism

Diabetic nephropathy
Tubulointerstitial diseases
Obstructive uropathy
Autonomic neuropathy
Nonsteroidal anti-inflammatory drugs
β-Adrenergic drugs

ACTH = adrenocorticotropic hormone.

disease (Graves' disease or Hashimoto's thyroiditis), and insulin-dependent diabetes mellitus. Other associated diseases include pernicious anemia, vitiligo, gonadal failure, hypophysitis, celiac disease, myasthenia gravis, primary biliary cirrhosis, Sjögren's syndrome, lupus erythematosus, and Parkinson's disease. This syndrome usually develops in adults.

Common manifestations of adrenal insufficiency are anorexia, weight loss, increasing fatigue, occasional vomiting, diarrhea, and salt craving. Muscle and joint pain, abdominal pain, and postural dizziness may also occur. Signs of increased pigmentation (initially most significantly on the extensor surfaces, palmar creases, and buccal mucosa) often occur secondarily to the increased production of ACTH and other POMC-related peptides by the pituitary gland (**Web Fig. 66–1**). Laboratory abnormalities may include hyponatremia, hyperkalemia, mild metabolic acidosis, azotemia, hypercalcemia, anemia, lymphocytosis, and eosinophilia. Hypoglycemia may also occur, especially in children.

Acute adrenal insufficiency is a medical emergency, and treatment should not be delayed pending laboratory results. In a critically ill patient with hypovolemia, a plasma sample for cortisol, ACTH, aldosterone, and renin should be obtained, and then treatment with an intravenous bolus of 100 mg of hydrocortisone and parenteral saline administration should be initiated. A plasma cortisol concentration of more than 34 mcg/dL rules out the diagnosis of adrenal crisis, whereas a value of less than 20 mcg/dL in the setting of shock is consistent with adrenal insufficiency. A plasma cortisol value between 20 mcg/dL and 34 mcg/dL in the setting of a severely ill patient may indicate partial adrenal insufficiency. In severe illness, albumin and cortisol-binding globulin (CBG) are low, resulting in a low total but not free cortisol level; thus a low total cortisol level may not be diagnostic of adrenal insufficiency in this setting.

In a patient with chronic symptoms suggestive of adrenal insufficiency, a 1-hour cosyntropin test should be performed. In this test, 0.25 mg ACTH (1–24) (cosyntropin) is given intravenously, and plasma cortisol is measured 0, 30, and 60 minutes later. A normal response is a plasma cortisol concentration higher than 20 mcg/dL at any time during the test. A patient with a basal morning plasma cortisol concentration of less than 5 mcg/dL and a stimulated cortisol concentration below 18 mcg/dL probably has evident adrenal insufficiency and should receive treatment. A basal morning plasma cortisol concentration between 10 and 18 mcg/dL in association with a stimulated cortisol concentration lower than 18 mcg/dL probably indicates impaired adrenal reserve and a requirement for receiving cortisol replacement under stress conditions (as described in a later discussion under Treatment in this chapter). Recently, a 1-mcg cosyntropin test to assess partial adrenal insufficiency has been described. This test may identify more patients who need cortisol replacement under stress conditions but should not be used to determine which patients need daily cortisol replacement.

Once the diagnosis of adrenal insufficiency is made, the distinction between primary and secondary adrenal insufficiency needs to be made. Secondary adrenal insufficiency results from inadequate stimulation of the adrenal cortex by ACTH. This can result from lesions anywhere along the hypothalamic-pituitary axis or as a sequela of prolonged suppression of the HPA axis by exogenous glucocorticoids. The presentation of secondary adrenal insufficiency is similar to that of primary adrenal insufficiency with a few important differences. Because ACTH and other POMC-related peptides are reduced in secondary adrenal insufficiency, hyperpigmentation does not occur. In addition, because mineralocorticoid levels are normal in secondary adrenal insufficiency, symptoms of salt craving, as well as the laboratory abnormalities of hyperkalemia and metabolic acidosis, are not present. However, hyponatremia is often observed as a result of increased secretion of the antidiuretic hormone (ADH) (resulting from volume depletion and ADH cosecretion with CRH), which accompanies glucocorticoid insufficiency, resulting in impaired water excretion. Because corticotropin is the most preserved of the pituitary hormones, a patient with secondary adrenal insufficiency caused by a pituitary lesion usually has symptoms and/or laboratory abnormalities consistent with hypothyroidism, hypogonadism, or growth hormone deficiency. To distinguish primary from secondary adrenal insufficiency, a basal morning plasma ACTH value and a standing (upright for at least 2 hours) serum aldosterone level and plasma renin activity should be measured. A plasma ACTH value of more than 20 pg/mL (normal value is 5 to 30 pg/mL) is consistent with primary adrenal insufficiency, whereas a value less than 20 pg/mL probably represents secondary adrenal insufficiency. An upright plasma renin activity of more than 3 ng/mL/hr in the setting of a suppressed aldosterone level is consistent with primary adrenal insufficiency, whereas a value less than 3 ng/mL/hr probably represents secondary adrenal insufficiency. The 1-hour cosyntropin test is suppressed in both secondary and primary adrenal insufficiency.

Secondary adrenal insufficiency occurs commonly after the discontinuation of glucocorticoids. Alternate-day glucocorticoid treatment, if feasible, results in less suppression of the HPA axis than does daily glucocorticoid therapy. The natural history of recovery from adrenal suppression is first a gradual increase in ACTH levels, followed by the normalization of plasma cortisol levels and then normalization of the cortisol response to ACTH. Complete recovery of the HPA axis can take up to 1 year, and the rate-limiting step appears to be recovery of the CRH neurons.

TREATMENT

After stabilization of acute adrenal insufficiency, patients with Addison's disease require lifelong replacement therapy with both glucocorticoids and mineralocorticoids. Unfortunately, most patients are overtreated with glucocorticoids and undertreated with mineralocorticoids. Because overtreatment with glucocorticoids results in insidious weight gain and osteoporosis, the minimal cortisol dose tolerated without symptoms of glucocorticoid insufficiency (usually joint pain) is recommended. An initial regimen of 15 to 20 mg hydrocortisone first thing in the morning and 5 mg hydrocortisone at around 4:00 PM mimics the physiologic dose and is recommended. Whereas glucocorticoid replacement is fairly uniform in most patients, mineralocorticoid replacement varies greatly. The initial dose of the synthetic mineralocorticoid fludrocortisone should be 100 mcg/day, and dosage should be adjusted to keep the standing plasma renin activity between 1 and 3 ng/mL/hr. A standing plasma renin activity higher than 3 ng/mL/hr, while the patient is taking the correct glucocorticoid dosage, is suggestive of undertreatment with fludrocortisone.

Under the stress of a minor illness (e.g., nausea, vomiting, fever higher than 100.5° F), the hydrocortisone dose should be doubled for as short a period as possible. The inability to ingest hydrocortisone pills may necessitate parenteral hydrocortisone administration. Patients undergoing a major stressful event (i.e., surgery necessitating general anesthesia, major trauma) should receive 150 to 300 mg parenteral hydrocortisone daily (in three divided doses) with a rapid taper to normal replacement during recovery. All patients should wear a medical information bracelet and should be instructed in the use of intramuscular emergency hydrocortisone injections.

Hyporeninemic Hypoaldosteronism

Mineralocorticoid deficiency can result from decreased renin secretion by the kidneys. Resultant hypoangiotensinemia leads to hypoaldosteronism with hyperkalemia and hyperchloremic metabolic acidosis. Plasma sodium concentration is usually normal, but total plasma volume is often deficient. Plasma renin and aldosterone levels are low and unresponsive to stimuli, including hypokalemia. Diabetes mellitus and chronic tubulointerstitial diseases of the kidney are the most common underlying conditions leading to the impairment of the juxtaglomerular apparatus. A subset of hyporeninemic hypoaldosteronism is caused by autonomic insufficiency and is a frequent cause of orthostatic hypotension. Stimuli such as upright posture or volume depletion, mediated by baroreceptors, do not cause a normal renin response. Administration of pharmacologic agents such as nonsteroidal anti-inflammatory agents, angiotensin-converting enzyme inhibitors, and β-adrenergic antagonists can also produce conditions of hypoaldosteronism. Fludro-

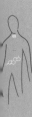

cortisone and/or the α_1-agonist midodrine are effective in correcting the orthostatic hypotension and electrolyte abnormalities caused by hypoaldosteronism.

Congenital Adrenal Hyperplasia

Congenital adrenal hyperplasia (CAH) refers to disorders of adrenal steroid biosynthesis that result in glucocorticoid and mineralocorticoid deficiencies. Because of deficient cortisol biosynthesis, a compensatory increase in ACTH occurs, inducing adrenal hyperplasia and overproduction of the steroids that precede blockage of enzyme production (see Fig. 66–2). Five major types of CAH exist, and the clinical manifestations of each type depend on which steroids are in excess and which are deficient. All these syndromes are transmitted in an autosomal recessive pattern. 21-Hydroxylase (CYP21) deficiency is the most common of these disorders and accounts for approximately 95% of patients of CAH. In this condition, there is a failure of 21-hydroxylation of 17-hydroxyprogesterone and progesterone to 11-deoxycortisol and 11-deoxycorticosterone, respectively, with deficient cortisol and aldosterone production. Cortisol deficiency leads to increased ACTH release, causing overproduction of 17-hydroxyprogesterone and progesterone. Increased ACTH production also leads to increased biosynthesis of androstenedione and DHEA, which can be converted to testosterone. Patients with 21-hydroxylase deficiencies can be divided into two clinical phenotypes: classic 21-hydroxylase deficiency, usually diagnosed at birth or during childhood, and late-onset 21-hydroxylase deficiency, which develops during or after puberty. Two thirds of the patients with classic 21-hydroxylase deficiency have various degrees of mineralocorticoid deficiency (salt-losing form); the remaining one third is not the salt-losing form (simple virilizing form). Both decreased aldosterone production and increased concentrations of precursors that are mineralocorticoid antagonists (progesterone and 17-hydroxyprogesterone) contribute to salt loss in the salt-losing form, in which the enzymatic block is more severe.

The most useful measurement for the diagnosis of classic 21-hydroxylase deficiency is that of plasma 17-hydroxyprogesterone. A value greater than 200 ng/dL is consistent with the diagnosis. Late-onset 21-hydroxylase deficiency represents an allelic variant of classic 21-hydroxylase deficiency and is characterized by a mild enzymatic defect. This deficiency is the most frequent autosomal recessive disorder in humans and is present especially in Ashkenazi Jews. The syndrome usually develops around the time of puberty with signs of virilization (hirsutism and acne) and amenorrhea or oligomenorrhea. This diagnosis should be considered in women with unexplained hirsutism and menstrual abnormalities or infertility. The diagnosis is made from the finding of an elevated level of plasma 17-hydroxyprogesterone (>1500 ng/dL) 30 minutes after administration of 0.25 mg of synthetic ACTH (1-24).

The aim of treatment for classic 21-hydroxylase deficiency is to replace glucocorticoids and mineralocorticoids, suppress ACTH and androgen overproduction, and allow for normal growth and sexual maturation in children. A proposed approach to treating classic 21-hydroxylase deficiency

recommends physiologic replacement with hydrocortisone and fludrocortisone in all affected patients, including those with the simple virilizing form. The deleterious effects of excess androgens can then be prevented by the use of an antiandrogen agent (flutamide) and an aromatase inhibitor (testolactone) that blocks the conversion of testosterone to estrogen.

Although the traditional treatment for late-onset 21-hydroxylase deficiency is dexamethasone (0.5 mg/day), the use of an anti-androgen such as spironolactone (100 to 200 mg/day) is probably more effective and has fewer side effects. Mineralocorticoid replacement is not needed in late-onset 21-hydroxylase deficiency.

11β-Hydroxylase (CYP11B1) deficiency accounts for approximately 5% of the patients with CAH. In this syndrome, the conversions of 11-deoxycortisol to cortisol and 11-deoxycorticosterone to corticosterone (the precursor to aldosterone) are blocked. Affected patients usually have hypertension and hypokalemia because of increased amounts of precursors with mineralocorticoid activity. Virilization occurs, as with 21-hydroxylase deficiency, and a late-onset form exhibiting as androgen excess also occurs. The diagnosis is made from the finding of elevated plasma 11-deoxycortisol levels, either basally or after ACTH stimulation.

Rare forms of CAH are 3β-HSD type II, 17α-hydroxylase (CYP17), and steroidogenic acute regulatory protein deficiencies.

Syndromes of Adrenocorticoid Hyperfunction

Hypersecretion of the glucocorticoid hormone cortisol results in Cushing's syndrome, a metabolic disorder affecting carbohydrate, protein, and lipid metabolism. Hypersecretion of mineralocorticoids such as aldosterone results in a syndrome of hypertension and electrolyte disturbances.

CUSHING'S SYNDROME

Pathophysiology

Increased production of cortisol is seen in both physiologic and pathologic states (Table 66–3). Physiologic hypercortisolism occurs in stress, during the last trimester of pregnancy, and in persons who regularly perform strenuous exercise. Pathologic conditions of elevated cortisol levels include exogenous or endogenous Cushing's syndrome and several psychiatric states, including depression, alcoholism, anorexia nervosa, panic disorder, and alcohol or narcotic withdrawal.

Cushing's syndrome may be caused by exogenous ACTH or glucocorticoid administration or by endogenous overproduction of these hormones. Endogenous Cushing's syndrome is either ACTH dependent or ACTH independent. ACTH dependency accounts for 85% of patients and includes pituitary sources of ACTH (Cushing's disease), ectopic sources of ACTH, and, in rare instances, ectopic sources of CRH. Pituitary Cushing's disease accounts for

Table 66–3 Syndromes of Adrenocortical Hyperfunction

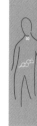

States of Glucocorticoid Excess

Physiologic States

Stress
Strenuous exercise
Last trimester of pregnancy

Pathologic States

Psychiatric conditions (pseudo-Cushing's disorders)
  Depression
  Alcoholism
  Anorexia nervosa
  Panic disorders
  Alcohol and drug withdrawal
ACTH-dependent states
  Pituitary adenoma (Cushing's disease)
  Ectopic ACTH syndrome
    Bronchial carcinoid
    Thymic carcinoid
    Islet-cell tumor
    Small-cell lung carcinoma
  Ectopic CRH secretion
ACTH-independent states
  Adrenal adenoma
  Adrenal carcinoma
  Micronodular adrenal disease

Exogenous Sources

Glucocorticoid intake
ACTH intake

States of Mineralocorticoid Excess

Primary Aldosteronism

Aldosterone-secreting adenoma
Bilateral adrenal hyperplasia
Aldosterone-secreting carcinoma
Glucocorticoid-suppressible hyperaldosteronism

Adrenal Enzyme Deficiencies

11β-hydroxylase deficiency
17α-hydroxylase deficiency
11β-hydroxysteroid dehydrogenase, type II

Exogenous Mineralocorticoids

Licorice
Carbenoxolone
Fludrocortisone

Secondary Hyperaldosteronism

Associated with hypertension
  Accelerated hypertension
  Renovascular hypertension
  Estrogen administration
  Renin-secreting tumors
Without hypertension
  Bartter's syndrome
  Sodium-wasting nephropathy
  Renal tubular acidosis
  Diuretic and laxative abuse
  Edematous states (cirrhosis, nephrosis, congestive heart
    failure)

ACTH = adrenocorticotropin hormone; CRH = corticotropin-releasing hormone.

80% of patients with ACTH-dependent Cushing's syndrome. Ectopic secretion of ACTH occurs most commonly in patients with small-cell lung carcinoma. These patients are older, usually have a history of smoking, and primarily exhibit signs and symptoms of lung cancer rather than those of Cushing's syndrome. Patients with the clinically apparent ectopic ACTH syndrome, in contrast, have mostly intrathoracic (lung and thymic) carcinoids. The remaining patients have pancreatic, adrenal, or thyroid tumors that secrete ACTH. ACTH-independent causes account for 15% of patients with Cushing's syndrome and include adrenal adenomas, adrenal carcinomas, micronodular adrenal disease, and autonomous macronodular adrenal disease. The female-to-male ratio for noncancerous forms of Cushing's syndrome is 4 to 1.

Clinical Manifestations

The clinical signs, symptoms, and common laboratory findings of hypercortisolism observed in patients with Cushing's syndrome are listed in Table 66–4 (see also Fig. 64–2). Typically, the obesity is centripetal, with a wasting of the arms and legs, which is distinct from the generalized weight gain observed in idiopathic obesity. Rounding of the face (called *moon facies*) and a dorsocervical fat pad *(buffalo hump)* may occur in obesity that is not related to Cushing's syndrome, whereas facial plethora and supraclavicular filling are more specific for Cushing's syndrome. Patients with Cushing's syndrome may have proximal muscle weakness; consequently, the physical finding of the inability to stand up from a squat or out of a car seat can be quite revealing. Sleep disturbances, mood swings, and other psychological abnormalities are frequently seen. Cognitive dysfunction and severe fatigue are often found. Menstrual irregularities often precede other cushingoid symptoms in affected women. Patients of both sexes complain of a loss of libido, whereas affected men frequently complain of erectile dysfunction. Adult-onset acne or hirsutism in women should also suggest Cushing's syndrome. The skin striae observed in patients with Cushing's syndrome are violaceous (i.e., purple, dark red) with a width of at least 1 cm. Thinning of the skin on the top of the hands is a very specific sign in younger adults with Cushing's syndrome. Old pictures of patients are extremely helpful for evaluating the progression of the physical stigmata of Cushing's syndrome.

Table 66–4 Signs, Symptoms, and Laboratory Abnormalities of Hypercortisolism

Fat redistribution (dorsocervical and supraclavicular fat pads, temporal wasting, centripetal obesity, weight gain) (95%)
Menstrual irregularities (80% of affected women)
Thin skin and plethora (80%)
Moon facies (75%)
Increased appetite (75%)
Sleep disturbances (75%)
Hypertension (75%)
Hypercholesterolemia and hypertriglyceridemia (70%)
Altered mentation (poor concentration, decreased memory, euphoria) (70%)
Diabetes mellitus and glucose intolerance (65%)
Striae (65%)
Hirsutism (65%)
Proximal muscle weakness (60%)
Psychologic disturbances (emotional lability, depression, mania, psychosis) (50%)
Decreased libido and impotence (50%)
Acne (45%)
Osteoporosis and pathologic fractures (40%)
Virilization (in women) (40%)
Easy bruisability (40%)
Poor wound healing (40%)
Edema (20%)
Increased infections (10%)
Cataracts (5%)

Associated laboratory findings in Cushing's syndrome include elevated plasma alkaline phosphatase levels, granulocytosis, thrombocytosis, hypercholesterolemia, hypertriglyceridemia, and glucose intolerance and/or diabetes mellitus. Hypokalemia or alkalosis usually occurs in patients with severe hypercortisolism as a result of the ectopic ACTH syndrome.

Diagnosis

If the history and physical examination findings are suggestive of hypercortisolism, then the diagnosis of Cushing's syndrome can usually be established by collecting urine for 24 hours and measuring urinary-free cortisol (UFC). UFC excretion reflects plasma-unbound cortisol that is filtered and excreted by the kidney. This test is extremely sensitive for the diagnosis of Cushing's syndrome because in 90% of affected patients, the initial UFC level is greater than 50 mcg/24 hours when measured by high-pressure liquid chromatography (HPLC) or mass spectroscopy cortisol assays. Patients with Cushing's disease usually have UFC levels between 50 and 200 mcg/24 hours, whereas patients with the ectopic ACTH syndrome and cortisol-secreting adrenal adenomas or carcinomas frequently have UFC levels greater than 200 mcg/24 hours (Fig. 66–5).

Cortisol is normally secreted in a diurnal manner; the plasma concentration is highest in the early morning (between 6:00 and 8:00 AM) and lowest around midnight. The normal 8:00 AM plasma cortisol level ranges between 8 and 25 mcg/dL and declines throughout the day. By 11:00 PM, the values are usually less than 5 mcg/dL. Most patients with Cushing's syndrome lack this diurnal variation. Thus although their morning cortisol levels may be normal, their evening concentrations are significantly higher. Evening or night values greater than 50% of the morning values are consistent with Cushing's syndrome. Measurement of random morning cortisol levels is not particularly helpful.

The overnight dexamethasone suppression test has been widely used as a screening test to evaluate patients who may have hypercortisolism. Dexamethasone 1 mg is given orally at 11:00 PM, and plasma cortisol is measured the following morning at 8:00 AM. A morning plasma cortisol level greater than 3 mcg/dL suggests hypercortisolism. This test produces a significant number of both false-positive and false-negative results.

Because of the difficulty of obtaining night-time plasma cortisol levels, measurement of late-night salivary cortisol has been developed to assess hypercortisolism. Late-night salivary cortisol reflects circulating free cortisol and can be obtained by the patient on one or more occasions and mailed to a reference laboratory. This test appears to have a high degree of sensitivity and specificity for the diagnosis of Cushing's syndrome. Growing evidence suggests that a large number of patients found to have Cushing's syndrome have cortisol levels that are elevated on some occasions but not on all occasions. For this reason, multiple measurements of UFC or salivary cortisol may be needed to both diagnose and exclude Cushing's syndrome.

Differential Diagnosis

Once the diagnosis of Cushing's syndrome is established, the cause of the hypercortisolism needs to be ascertained, which is accomplished by biochemical studies that evaluate the feedback regulation of the HPA axis, by venous sampling techniques, and by imaging procedures. The initial approach is to measure basal ACTH levels that are normal or elevated in Cushing's disease and the ectopic ACTH syndrome, but are suppressed in primary adrenal Cushing's syndrome. Patients with a suppressed ACTH level can proceed to adrenal imaging studies. To distinguish between Cushing's disease and the ectopic ACTH syndrome, the high dose or 8 mg overnight dexamethasone suppression test, ovine CRH (oCRH) test, and/or bilateral simultaneous inferior petrosal sinus sampling are used.

In the dexamethasone suppression test (Liddle test), 0.5 mg of dexamethasone is given orally every 6 hours for 2 days, followed by 2 mg of dexamethasone every 6 hours for another 2 days. On the second day of the high dose of dexamethasone, UFC is suppressed to less than 10% of that of the baseline collection in patients with pituitary adenomas but not in patients with the ectopic ACTH syndrome or adrenal cortisol-secreted tumors. Although the Liddle test is often helpful in establishing the cause of Cushing's syndrome, it has some disadvantages. The test requires accurate measurement of urine collections, often necessitating inpatient hospitalization. In approximately 50% of patients with bronchial carcinoids causing ectopic ACTH production, cor-

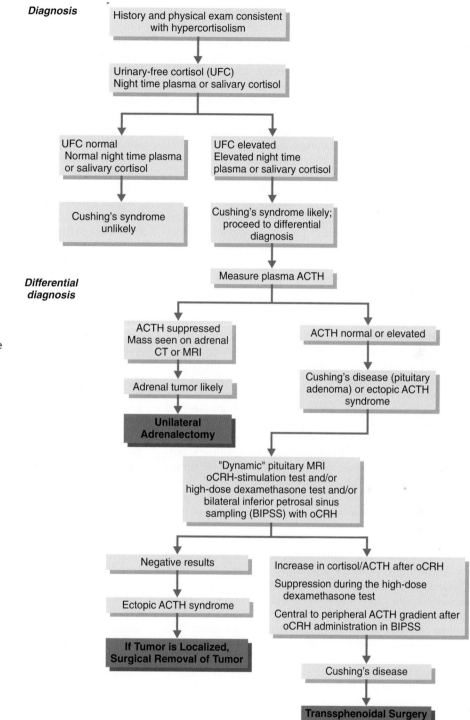

Diagnosis

History and physical exam consistent
with hypercortisolism

↓

Urinary-free cortisol (UFC)
Night time plasma or salivary cortisol

UFC normal
Normal night time plasma
or salivary cortisol

↓

Cushing's syndrome
unlikely

UFC elevated
Elevated night time
plasma or salivary cortisol

↓

Cushing's syndrome likely;
proceed to differential
diagnosis

*Differential
diagnosis*

Measure plasma ACTH

ACTH suppressed
Mass seen on adrenal
CT or MRI

↓

Adrenal tumor likely

↓

**Unilateral
Adrenalectomy**

ACTH normal or elevated

↓

Cushing's disease (pituitary
adenoma) or ectopic ACTH
syndrome

"Dynamic" pituitary MRI
oCRH-stimulation test and/or
high-dose dexamethasone test and/or
bilateral inferior petrosal sinus
sampling (BIPSS) with oCRH

Negative results

↓

Ectopic ACTH syndrome

↓

**If Tumor is Localized,
Surgical Removal of Tumor**

Increase in cortisol/ACTH after oCRH

Suppression during the high-dose
dexamethasone test

Central to peripheral ACTH gradient after
oCRH administration in BIPSS

↓

Cushing's disease

↓

Transsphenoidal Surgery

Figure 66–5 Flowchart for evaluating a patient with probable Cushing's syndrome. *ACTH* = adrenocorticotropic hormone; *oCRH* = ovine corticotropin-releasing hormone.

tisol secretion is suppressible by high-dose dexamethasone, which yields a false-positive result. In addition, because patients with Cushing's syndrome are often episodic secretors of corticosteroids, considerable variation in daily UFC excretion can occur and false results can be obtained. Therefore the Liddle test should be interpreted cautiously and other confirmatory tests should be performed before surgery is recommended.

An overnight high-dose dexamethasone suppression test is helpful in establishing the cause of Cushing's syndrome. In this test a baseline 8:00 AM cortisol level is measured, and

then 8 mg of dexamethasone is given orally at 11:00 PM. At 8:00 AM the following morning a plasma cortisol measurement is obtained. Suppression, which would occur in patients with pituitary Cushing's disease, is defined as a decrease in plasma cortisol to less than 50% of the baseline level. Few patients with bronchial carcinoid have been examined; as a result, the suppressibility of these tumors by high-dose overnight dexamethasone is not well established.

The oCRH test can also be used to establish the cause of Cushing's syndrome. Pituitary corticotrophs of normal individuals and of patients with pituitary Cushing's disease

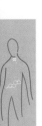

respond to oCRH by increasing the secretion of ACTH and therefore cortisol. Thus the oCRH test cannot be used to distinguish normal persons from patients with pituitary Cushing's disease. Patients with cortisol-secreting adrenal tumors have low or undetectable concentrations of ACTH that do not respond to the oCRH test. Patients with ectopic ACTH secretion have high basal ACTH levels that do not increase with the oCRH test. In patients with both the ectopic ACTH syndrome and primary adrenal hypercortisolism, cortisol levels do not change in response to the oCRH test. Discrepancies between the oCRH and dexamethasone tests necessitate further work-up to ascertain the diagnosis.

Bilateral inferior petrosal sinus sampling (BIPSS) is an accurate and safe procedure for distinguishing pituitary Cushing's disease from the ectopic ACTH syndrome. Venous blood from the anterior lobe of the pituitary gland empties into the cavernous sinuses and then into the superior and inferior petrosal sinuses. Venous plasma samples for ACTH determination are obtained from both inferior petrosal sinuses, along with a simultaneous peripheral sample, both before and after intravenous bolus administration of CRH. In baseline measurements an ACTH concentration gradient of 1.6 or more between a sample from either of the petrosal sinuses and the peripheral sample is strongly suggestive of pituitary Cushing's disease, whereas patients with the ectopic ACTH syndrome or adrenal adenomas have no ACTH gradient between their petrosal and peripheral samples. After CRH administration, a central-to-peripheral gradient of more than 3.2 is consistent with pituitary Cushing's disease. The use of CRH has enabled complete distinction of pituitary Cushing's disease from nonpituitary Cushing's syndrome. An ACTH gradient ipsilateral to the side of the tumor is found in 70% to 80% of patients sampled. Although BIPSS requires an experienced radiologist in petrosal sinus sampling, this procedure is currently available at many tertiary care facilities.

Imaging of the pituitary gland by magnetic resonance imaging (MRI) with gadolinium is the preferred procedure for localizing a pituitary adenoma. In many centers, a *dynamic* MRI is performed, which visualizes the pituitary as the gadolinium enters and leaves the gland. This test detects approximately 60% to 90% of pituitary ACTH-secreting tumors and can detect many pituitary tumors as small as 2 mm in diameter. Approximately 10% of normal individuals may have a nonfunctioning pituitary adenoma found on a pituitary MRI. It is therefore recommended that pituitary imaging not be the sole criterion for the diagnosis of pituitary Cushing's disease.

Treatment

The preferred treatment for all forms of Cushing's syndrome is appropriate surgery. Pituitary Cushing's disease is best treated by trans-sphenoidal surgery. When the operation is performed by an experienced neurosurgeon, the cure rate is higher than 80%. Trans-sphenoidal surgery carries very low rates of morbidity and mortality. Growth hormone and/or androgen deficiency in both sexes are the most common complications of surgery. Other complications (e.g., meningitis, cerebrospinal fluid leakage, optic nerve damage, isolated thyrotropin deficiency) are uncommon. Patients who have failed initial pituitary surgery or have recurrent Cushing's disease may be treated with either pituitary irra-

diation or bilateral adrenalectomy. Irradiation has more long-term complications than does trans-sphenoidal surgery and results in curing approximately 60% of patients, but it may take up to 5 years to render a person eucortisolemic. Panhypopituitarism eventually develops in almost all these patients; consequently, growth hormone, thyroid, gonadal, and even steroid replacement may be needed. A more appealing option for patients with Cushing's disease who remain hypercortisolemic after pituitary surgery is bilateral adrenalectomy, followed by lifelong glucocorticoid and mineralocorticoid replacement therapy. About 10% of patients with Cushing's disease who undergo bilateral adrenalectomy develop Nelson's syndrome, which is an ACTH-secreting macroadenoma that often causes visual field deficits and hyperpigmentation. The incidence of Nelson's syndrome is reduced if patients undergo pituitary irradiation.

In patients with the ectopic ACTH syndrome, it is hoped that the tumor is localized by appropriate scans and can be removed surgically. A unilateral adrenalectomy is the treatment of choice in patients with a cortisol-secreting adrenal adenoma. Patients with cortisol-secreting adrenal carcinomas initially should also be managed surgically; however, they have a poor prognosis with only 20% surviving more than 1 year after diagnosis.

Medical treatment for hypercortisolism may be needed to prepare patients for surgery, in patients who are undergoing or have undergone pituitary irradiation and are awaiting its effects, or in patients who are not surgical candidates or who elect not to have surgery. Ketoconazole, o,p'-DDD, metyrapone, aminoglutethimide, RU-486, and trilostane are the most commonly used agents for adrenal blockade and can be used alone or in combination.

PRIMARY MINERALOCORTICOID EXCESS

Pathophysiology

Increased mineralocorticoid activity is exhibited by salt retention, hypertension, hypokalemia, and metabolic alkalosis. The causes of primary aldosteronism (see Table 66–3) are aldosterone-producing adenoma (75%), bilateral adrenal hyperplasia (25%), adrenal carcinoma (1%), and glucocorticoid-remediable hyperaldosteronism (<1%). The adrenal enzyme defects-11β-HSD type II, 11β-hydroxylase, and 17α-hydroxylase deficiencies and apparent mineralocorticoid excess (from licorice or carbenoxolone ingestion, which inhibits 11β-HSD type II, or from a congenital defect in this enzyme) are also states of functional mineralocorticoid overactivity. Secondary aldosteronism (see Table 66–3) results from an overactive renin-angiotensin system.

Primary aldosteronism is usually recognized during evaluation of hypertension or hypokalemia and represents a potentially curable form of hypertension. Up to 5% of patients with hypertension have primary aldosteronism. These patients are usually between the ages of 30 and 50 years, and the female-to-male ratio is 2:1.

Clinical Manifestations

Hypertension, hypokalemia, and metabolic alkalosis are the main clinical manifestations of hyperaldosteronism; most of the presenting symptoms are related to hypokalemia. Symptoms in patients with mild hypokalemia are fatigue, muscle weakness, nocturia, lassitude, and headaches. If more severe hypokalemia exists, then polydipsia, polyuria, paresthesias, and even intermittent paralysis and tetany can occur. Blood pressure can range from being minimally elevated to very high. A positive Trousseau's or Chvostek's sign may occur as a result of metabolic alkalosis.

Diagnosis and Treatment

Initially, hypokalemia in the presence of hypertension must be documented (Fig. 66–6). The patient must have adequate salt intake and discontinue diuretics before potassium measurement. If hypokalemia is found under these conditions and the patient is taking spironolactone, then it should be stopped and a morning plasma aldosterone level and a plasma renin activity (PRA) should be measured. A serum aldosterone/PRA ratio greater than 20 ng/dL per ng/mL/hour and a serum aldosterone level greater than 15 ng/dL suggest the diagnosis of hyperaldosteronism.

Once the diagnosis of primary aldosteronism has been demonstrated, distinguishing between an aldosterone-producing adenoma and a bilateral hyperplasia is important because the former is treated with surgery and the latter is treated medically. In the initial test (a postural challenge), an 8:00 AM supine blood sample is drawn for plasma aldosterone, 18-hydrocorticosterone, renin, and cortisol measurement. The patient then stands for 2 hours, and an upright sample is drawn for measurement of the same hormones. A basal plasma aldosterone level of less than 20 ng/dL is usually found in patients with bilateral hyperplasia, and a value greater than 20 ng/dL suggests the diagnosis of adrenal adenoma. In bilateral hyperplasia, plasma aldosterone often increases as a result of the increase in renin in response to the upright position, whereas in adenoma, plasma aldosterone levels usually fall as a result of decreased stimulation by ACTH at 10:00 AM in comparison with ACTH stimulation at 8:00 AM. At 8:00 AM a plasma 18-hydroxycorticosterone level of greater than 50 ng/dL that falls with upright posture occurs in most patients with an adenoma, whereas an 8:00 am level less than 50 ng/dL that rises with upright posture occurs in most patients with bilateral hyperplasia.

A computed tomographic (CT) scan of the adrenal glands should be performed to localize the tumor. The patient should undergo unilateral adrenalectomy if a discrete adenoma is observed in one adrenal gland, if the contralateral gland is normal, and if biochemical test results are consistent with an adenoma. Patients in whom biochemical study findings are consistent with an adenoma but CT results are consistent with bilateral disease should undergo adrenal venous sampling for aldosterone and cortisol measurement. Patients in whom biochemical and localization study findings are consistent with bilateral hyperplasia should be treated medically, usually with epleronone or spironolactone. Those in whom biochemical study results are consistent with bilateral hyperplasia should also be evaluated for dexamethasone-suppressible hyperaldosteronism by receiving a trial of dexamethasone, which reverses the hyperaldosteronism in this rare autosomal dominant disorder.

Hyperaldosteronism and hypertension secondary to activation of the renin-angiotensin system can occur in patients with accelerated hypertension, in those with renovascular hypertension, in those receiving estrogen therapy, and rarely in patients with renin-secreting tumors. Hyperaldosteronism without hypertension occurs in patients with Bartter's syndrome, sodium-wasting nephropathy, and renal tubular acidosis, as well as those who abuse diuretics or laxatives.

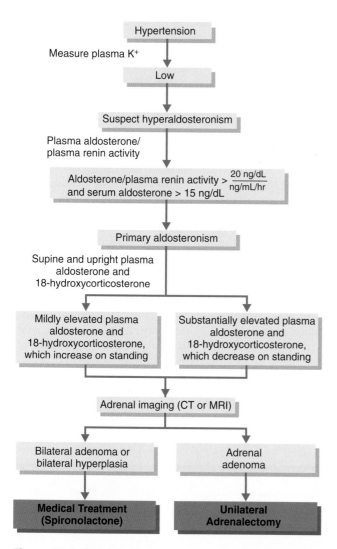

Figure 66–6 Flowchart for evaluating a patient with probable primary hyperaldosteronism.

Adrenal Medullary Hyperfunction

The adrenal medulla synthesizes the catecholamines norepinephrine, epinephrine, and dopamine from the amino acid tyrosine. Norepinephrine, the major catecholamine produced by the adrenal medulla, has predominantly α-agonist actions, causing vasoconstriction. Epinephrine acts primarily on the β-receptors, having positive inotropic and chronotropic effects on the heart, causing peripheral vasodilation and increasing plasma glucose concentrations in response to hypoglycemia. The action of circulating dopamine is unclear. Whereas norepinephrine is synthesized in the central nervous system and sympathetic postganglionic neurons, epinephrine is synthesized almost entirely in the adrenal medulla. The adrenal medullary contribution to norepinephrine secretion is relatively small. Bilateral adrenalectomy results in only minimal changes in circulating norepinephrine levels, although epinephrine levels are dramatically reduced. Thus hypofunction of the adrenal medulla has little physiologic affect, whereas hypersecretion of catecholamines produces the clinical syndrome of pheochromocytoma.

PHEOCHROMOCYTOMA

Pathophysiology

Although pheochromocytomas can occur in any sympathetic ganglion in the body, more than 90% of pheochromocytomas arise from the adrenal medulla. The majority of extra-adrenal tumors occur in the mediastinum or abdomen. Bilateral adrenal pheochromocytomas occur in approximately 5% of the cases and may occur as part of familial syndromes. Pheochromocytoma occurs as part of multiple endocrine neoplasia type IIA or IIB. The former (Sipple's syndrome) is marked by medullary carcinoma of the thyroid, hyperparathyroidism, and pheochromocytoma; the latter is characterized by medullary carcinoma of the thyroid, mucosal neuromas, intestinal ganglioneuromas, marfanoid habitus, and pheochromocytoma. Pheochromocytomas are also associated with neurofibromatosis, cerebelloretinal hemangioblastosis (von Hippel-Lindau disease), and tuberous sclerosis.

Clinical Manifestations

Because a majority of pheochromocytomas secrete norepinephrine as the principal catecholamine, hypertension (often paroxysmal) is the most common finding. Other symptoms include the triad of headache, palpitations, and sweating, as well as skin blanching, anxiety, nausea, fatigue, weight loss, and abdominal and chest pain. Emotional stress, exercise, anesthesia, abdominal pressure, or intake of tyramine-containing foods may precipitate these symptoms. Orthostatic hypotension can also occur. Wide fluctuations in blood pressure are characteristic, and the hypertension associated with pheochromocytoma usually does not respond to standard antihypertensive medicines. Cardiac abnormalities, as well as idiosyncratic reactions to medications, may also occur.

Diagnosis and Treatment

Although measurement of fractionated catecholamine and metanephrine levels in the urine are the most used screening tests, plasma-free metanephrine and normetanephrine levels are the best test for confirming or excluding pheochromocytoma because the metabolism of catecholamines to free metanephrines is independent of catecholamine release and can be performed in the absence of hypertension and other symptoms. A plasma-free metanephrine level greater than 0.61 nmol/L and a plasma-free normetanephrine level greater than 0.31 nmol/L are consistent with the diagnosis of a pheochromocytoma. If the values are only mildly elevated, then a clonidine suppression test could be performed. In this test, clonidine (0.3 mg) is given orally and plasma catecholamines (including free metanephrine and normetanephrine) are measured before and 3 hours after administration. In normal persons, catecholamine levels decrease into the normal range, whereas in patients with a pheochromocytoma, levels are unchanged or increase. Once the diagnosis of pheochromocytoma is made, a CT scan of the adrenal glands should be performed. Most intra-adrenal pheochromocytomas are readily visible on this scan. If the CT scan is negative, then extra-adrenal pheochromocytomas can often be localized by iodine 131–labeled metaiodobenzylguanidine (^{131}I-MIBG), positron emission tomography, octreotide scan, or abdominal MRI.

The treatment of pheochromocytoma is surgical if the lesion can be localized. Patients should undergo preoperative α-blockade with phenoxybenzamine 1 to 2 weeks before surgery. β-Adrenergic antagonists should be used before or during surgery. Approximately 5% to 10% of pheochromocytomas are malignant. ^{131}I-MIBG or chemotherapy may be useful, but the prognosis is poor. α-Methyl-p-tyrosine, an inhibitor of tyrosine hydroxylase, the rate-limiting enzyme in catecholamine biosynthesis, may be used to decrease catecholamine secretion from the tumor.

INCIDENTAL ADRENAL MASS

Clinically inapparent adrenal masses are discovered inadvertently in the course of diagnostic testing or treatment for other clinical conditions that are not related to the suggestion of adrenal disease and thus are commonly known as *incidentalomas* (**Web Fig. 66–2**). Some of these tumors secrete a small amount of excess cortisol, leading to a condition called *subclinical Cushing's syndrome.* A morning ACTH level and an overnight 1 mg-dexamethasone test are recommended for patients with an adrenal incidentaloma. Patients with hypertension should also undergo measurement of serum potassium level, plasma aldosterone concentration and/or plasma renin activity ratio, and measurement of urine or plasma-free metanephrines. Surgery should be considered in all patients with functional adrenal cortical tumors that are hormonally active or greater than 5 cm. Tumors not associated with hormonal secretion of less than 5 cm can be monitored with repeat imaging and hormonal assessment.

Prospectus for the Future

- Appreciation of the role tissue-specific, intracellular glucocorticoid excess plays in common diseases such as osteoporosis, depression, cardiovascular disease, diabetes, and hypertension

- Selective adrenal adenomectomy, sparing normal adrenal tissue
- Appreciation of the importance of mild (subclinical) adrenal insufficiency and excess

References

Arnaldi G, Angeli A, Atkinson AB, et al: Diagnosis and complications of Cushing's syndrome: A consensus statement. J Clin Endocrinol Metab 88:5593–5602, 2003.

Falorni A, Laureti S, DeBellis A, et al: Italian Addison network study: Update of diagnostic criteria for the etiological classification of primary adrenal insufficiency. J Clin Endocrinol Metab 89:1598–1604, 2004.

Grumbach MM, Biller BM, Braunstein GD, et al: Management of the clinically inapparent adrenal mass ("incidentaloma"). Ann Intern Med 138:424–429, 2003.

Pacak K, Ilias I, Adams KT, Eisenhofer G: Biochemical diagnosis, localization and management of pheochromocytoma: Focus on multiple endocrine neoplasia type 2 in relation to other hereditary syndromes and sporadic forms of the tumour. J Intern Med 257:60–68, 2005.

Vaughan ED Jr: Diseases of the adrenal gland. Med Clin N Am 88:443–466, 2004.

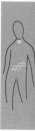

Male Reproductive Endocrinology

Glenn D. Braunstein

The testes are composed of Leydig (interstitial) cells that secrete testosterone and estradiol and the sperm-producing seminiferous tubules. They are regulated by the gonadotropins luteinizing hormone (LH) and follicle-stimulating hormone (FSH), which are secreted by the anterior pituitary under the influence of the hypothalamic decapeptide gonadotropin-releasing hormone (GnRH) (Fig. 67–1). LH stimulates the Leydig cells to secrete testosterone, which feeds back in a negative fashion at the level of the pituitary and hypothalamus to inhibit further LH production. FSH stimulates sperm production through interaction with the Sertoli cells in the seminiferous tubules. Feedback inhibition of FSH is through gonadal steroids, as well as through inhibin, a glycoprotein produced by Sertoli cells.

Biochemical evaluation of the hypothalamic-pituitary-Leydig axis is carried out by the measurement of serum LH and testosterone concentrations, whereas a semen analysis and a serum FSH determination provide an assessment of the hypothalamic-pituitary-seminiferous tubular axis. The ability of the pituitary to release gonadotropins can be tested dynamically through GnRH stimulation, and the ability of the testes to secrete testosterone can be evaluated through injections of human chorionic gonadotropin (hCG), a glycoprotein hormone that has biologic activity similar to that of LH.

Hypogonadism

Either testosterone deficiency or defective spermatogenesis constitutes *hypogonadism*. Often both disorders co-exist. The clinical manifestations of androgen deficiency depend on the time of onset and the degree of deficiency. Because testosterone is required for wolffian duct development into the epididymis, vas deferens, seminal vesicles, and ejaculatory ducts, as well as for virilization of the external genitalia through the major intracellular testosterone metabolite,

dihydrotestosterone, early prenatal androgen deficiency leads to the formation of ambiguous genitalia and to male pseudohermaphroditism. Androgen deficiency occurring later during gestation may result in micropenis or *cryptorchidism*, the unilateral or bilateral absence of testes in the scrotum resulting from the failure of normal testicular descent. During puberty, androgens are responsible for male sexual differentiation, which includes growth of the scrotum, epididymis, vas deferens, seminal vesicles, prostate, penis, skeletal muscle, and larynx. Additionally, androgens stimulate the growth of axillary, pubic, facial, and body hair, as well as increased sebaceous gland activity, and they are responsible through conversion to estrogens for the growth and fusion of the epiphyseal cartilaginous plates clinically seen as the *pubertal growth spurt*. Thus prepubertal androgen deficiency leads to poor muscle development, decreased strength and endurance, a high-pitched voice, sparse axillary and pubic hair, and the absence of facial and body hair. The long bones of the lower extremities and arms may continue to grow under the influence of growth hormone, a condition leading to eunuchoidal proportions in which the arm span exceeds the total height by 5 cm or more, and growth of the lower extremities is greater relative to total height. Postpubertal androgen deficiency may result in a decrease in libido, impotence, low energy, fine wrinkling around the corners of the eyes and mouth, and diminished facial and body hair.

Male hypogonadism may be classified into three categories according to the level of the defect (Table 67–1). Diseases directly affecting the testes result in *primary* or *hypergonadotropic hypogonadism,* characterized by oligospermia or azoospermia and low testosterone levels but with elevations of LH and FSH because of a decrease of the negative feedback regulation on the pituitary and hypothalamus by androgens and inhibin. In contrast, hypogonadism from lesions in the hypothalamus or pituitary gives rise to *secondary* or *hypogonadotropic hypogonadism* because the low testosterone level or ineffective spermatogenesis is a result of inadequate stimulation of the testes by insufficient

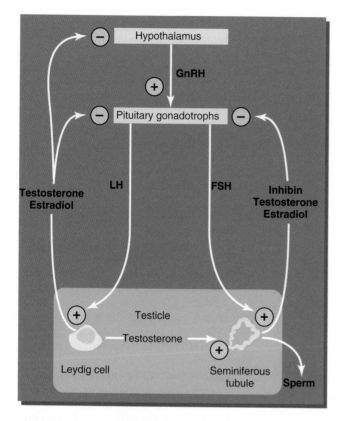

Figure 67–1 Regulation of the hypothalamic-pituitary-testicular axis. + = positive feedback; – = negative feedback; FSH = follicle-stimulating hormone; GnRH = gonadotropin-releasing hormone; LH = luteinizing hormone.

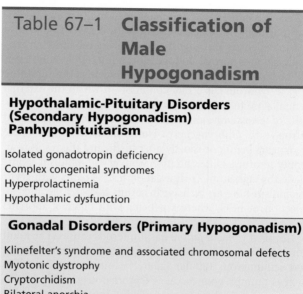

Table 67–1	**Classification of Male Hypogonadism**

Hypothalamic-Pituitary Disorders (Secondary Hypogonadism) Panhypopituitarism

Isolated gonadotropin deficiency
Complex congenital syndromes
Hyperprolactinemia
Hypothalamic dysfunction

Gonadal Disorders (Primary Hypogonadism)

Klinefelter's syndrome and associated chromosomal defects
Myotonic dystrophy
Cryptorchidism
Bilateral anorchia
Seminiferous tubular failure
Adult Leydig cell failure
Androgen biosynthesis enzyme deficiency

Defects in Androgen Action

Testicular feminization (complete androgen insensitivity)
Incomplete androgen insensitivity
5α-Reductase deficiency

or inadequate concentrations of the gonadotropins. The third category of hypogonadism is the result of defects in androgen action.

HYPOTHALAMIC-PITUITARY DISORDERS

Panhypopituitarism occurs congenitally from structural defects or from inadequate production or the release of the hypothalamic-releasing factors. The condition may also be acquired through replacement by tumors, infarction from vascular insufficiency, infiltrative disorders, autoimmune diseases, trauma, and infections.

Kallmann's syndrome is a form of hypogonadotropic hypogonadism associated with problems in the ability to discriminate odors, either incompletely (*hyposmia*) or completely (*anosmia*). This syndrome results from a defect in the migration of the GnRH neurons from the olfactory placode into the hypothalamus. Thus it represents a GnRH deficiency. Patients remain prepubertal, with small, rubbery testes, and they develop eunuchoidism (**Web Fig. 67–1**).

Hyperprolactinemia may result in hypogonadotropic hypogonadism because prolactin elevation inhibits normal GnRH release, decreases the effectiveness of LH at the Leydig cell level, and also inhibits some of the action of testosterone at the target organ level. Normalization of prolactin levels through withdrawal of an offending drug, by surgical

removal of the pituitary adenoma, or with the use of dopamine agonists reverses this form of hypogonadism.

Weight loss or systemic illness in male patients can cause another form of secondary hypogonadism, *hypothalamic dysfunction*. This weight loss or illness induces a defect in the hypothalamic release of GnRH and results in low gonadotropin and testosterone levels. This condition is commonly observed in patients with cancer, acquired immunodeficiency syndrome, and chronic inflammatory processes.

PRIMARY GONADAL ABNORMALITIES

The most common congenital cause of primary testicular failure is *Klinefelter's syndrome,* which occurs in approximately 1 of every 600 live male births and is usually caused by a maternal meiotic chromosomal nondisjunction that results in an XXY genotype. At puberty, clinical findings include the following: varying degrees of hypogonadism; gynecomastia; small, firm testes measuring less than 2 cm in the longest axis (normal testes measure 3.5 cm or greater); azoospermia; eunuchoidal skeletal proportions; and elevations of FSH and LH (**Web Fig. 67–2**). Primary gonadal failure is also found in patients with another congenital condition, *myotonic dystrophy,* which is characterized by progressive weakness; atrophy of the facial, neck, hand, and lower extremity muscles; frontal baldness; and myotonia.

Approximately 3% of full-term male infants have *cryptorchidism,* which spontaneously corrects during the first year of life in most of these children; consequently, by 1 year of age, the incidence of this condition is approximately

0.75%. When the testes are maintained in the intra-abdominal position, the increased temperature leads to defective spermatogenesis and oligospermia. Leydig cell function generally remains normal, and therefore adult testosterone levels are normal. *Bilateral anorchia*, also known as the vanishing testicle syndrome, is a rare condition in which the external genitalia are fully formed, thus indicating that ample quantities of testosterone and dihydrotestosterone were produced during early embryogenesis. However, the testicular tissue disappears before or shortly after birth, and the result is an empty scrotum. Differentiation from cryptorchidism can be made through an hCG stimulation test. Patients with cryptorchidism have an increase in serum testosterone after an injection of hCG, whereas patients with bilateral anorchia do not.

Acquired gonadal failure has numerous causes. The adult seminiferous tubules are susceptible to a variety of injuries, and seminiferous tubular failure is found after infections such as mumps, gonococcal or lepromatous orchitis, irradiation, vascular injury, trauma, alcohol ingestion, and use of chemotherapeutic drugs, especially alkylating agents. The serum FSH concentrations may be normal or elevated, depending on the degree of damage to the seminiferous tubules. The Leydig cell compartment may also be damaged by these same conditions. In addition, some men experience a gradual decline in testicular function as they age, possibly because of microvascular insufficiency. The decreased testosterone production may clinically exhibit lowered libido and potency, emotional lability, fatigue, and vasomotor symptoms such as hot flushes. The serum LH concentration is usually elevated in this situation.

DEFECTS IN ANDROGEN ACTION

When either testosterone or its metabolite, dihydrotestosterone, binds to the androgen receptor in target cells, the receptor is activated and binds DNA with resulting stimulation of transcription, protein synthesis, and cell growth, which collectively constitutes androgen action. An absence of androgen receptors causes the syndrome of *testicular feminization*, a form of male pseudohermaphroditism. These genetic males have cryptorchid testes but appear to be phenotypic females. Because androgens are inactive during embryogenesis, the labial-scrotal folds fail to fuse, and a short vagina results. The fallopian tubes, uterus, and upper portion of the vagina are absent because the testes secrete müllerian duct inhibitory factor during early fetal development. At puberty, these patients have breast enlargement because the testes secrete a small amount of estradiol, and the peripheral tissues convert testosterone and adrenal androgens to estrogens. Axillary and pubic hair does not grow because androgen action is required for development. The serum testosterone concentrations are elevated as a result of continuous stimulation by LH, the concentrations of which are raised because of the inability of the testosterone to act in a negative feedback fashion at the hypothalamic level. Patients may have incomplete forms of androgen insensitivity caused by point mutations affecting the androgen receptor gene, and clinically these patients show varying degrees of male pseudohermaphroditism.

Patients who lack the 5α-reductase enzyme required to convert testosterone to dihydrotestosterone are born with a *bifid scrotum,* which reflects abnormal fusion of the labial-scrotal folds, and *hypospadias,* in which the urethral opening is in the perineal area or in the shaft of the penis. At puberty, androgen production is sufficient to partially overcome the defect; the scrotum, phallus, and muscle mass enlarge, and these patients appear to develop into physiologically normal men.

DIAGNOSIS

Figure 67–2 illustrates an algorithm for the laboratory evaluation of hypogonadism in a phenotypic man. Serum concentrations of LH, FSH, and testosterone should be obtained, and a semen analysis should be performed. A low testosterone level with low concentrations of gonadotropins indicates a hypothalamic-pituitary abnormality, which needs to be evaluated with serum prolactin determination and radiographic examination. Elevated concentrations of gonadotropins with a normal or low testosterone level reflect a primary testicular abnormality. If no testes are palpable in the scrotum and careful *milking* of the patient's lower abdomen does not bring retractile testes into the scrotum, then an hCG stimulation test should be performed. A rise in serum testosterone concentrations indicates the presence of functional testicular tissue, and a diagnosis of cryptorchidism can be made. An absence of a rise in testosterone levels suggests bilateral anorchia. Small, firm testes in the scrotum are highly suggestive of Klinefelter's syndrome; this diagnosis needs to be confirmed with a chromosomal karyotype. Testes more than 3.5 cm in the longest diameter that are of normal consistency or are soft indicate postpubertal acquired primary hypogonadism. If the major abnormality is a deficient sperm count with or without an elevation of FSH, then differentiation between a ductal problem and acquired primary hypogonadism must be made. When spermatozoa are present, then at least the ducts emanating from one testicle are patent; this condition indicates an acquired testicular defect. If the patient has no sperm in the ejaculate, then a primary testicular or ductal problem may cause this condition. The seminal vesicles secrete fructose into the seminal fluid. Therefore the presence of fructose in the ejaculate should be followed by a testicular biopsy to determine whether the defect results from spermatogenic failure or from an obstruction of the ducts leading from the testes to the seminal vesicles. Absence of seminal fluid fructose indicates a congenital absence of the seminal vesicles and vas deferens.

MALE INFERTILITY

Infertility affects approximately 15% of couples, and male factors appear to be responsible in approximately 40% of cases. Female factors account for another 40%, whereas a couple factor is present in approximately 20% of cases. In addition to the defects in spermatogenesis that occur in patients with hypothalamic, pituitary, testicular, or androgen action disorders, hyperthyroidism, hypothyroidism, adrenal abnormalities, and systemic illnesses may also result in defective spermatogenesis, as can microdeletions of genetic material on the Y chromosome. Disorders of the vas deferens, seminal vesicles, and prostate may also lead to infertility, as can diseases affecting the bladder sphincter that may

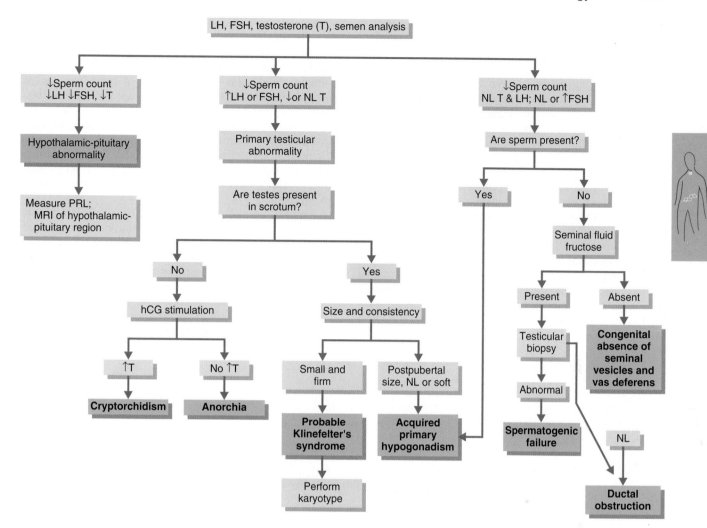

Figure 67–2 Laboratory evaluation of hypogonadism. − = elevated; ↓ = decreased or low; FSH = follicle-stimulating hormone; hCG = human chorionic gonadotropin; LH = luteinizing hormone; MRI = magnetic resonance imaging; NL = normal; PRL = prolactin.

result in *retrograde ejaculation*, in which the sperm passes into the bladder rather than through the penis. Anatomic defects of the penis as observed in patients with hypospadias, poor coital technique, and the presence of antisperm antibodies in the male or female genital tract also are associated with infertility.

THERAPY FOR HYPOGONADISM AND INFERTILITY

Treatment of androgen deficiency in patients who have hypothalamic-pituitary or primary testicular abnormalities is best accomplished with exogenous testosterone administration, either through intramuscular injection of intermediate-acting testosterone esters or with transdermal testosterone patches or gel. Testosterone therapy increases libido, potency, muscle mass, strength, athletic endurance, and hair growth on the face and body. Side effects include acne, fluid retention, erythrocytosis, and, rarely, sleep apnea. This therapy is contraindicated in patients with cancer of the prostate.

If fertility is desired, then patients with hypothalamic abnormalities may develop virilization and spermatogenesis with the use of GnRH given in a pulsatile fashion subcutaneously with an external pump. Direct stimulation of the testes in patients with hypothalamic or pituitary abnormalities may be accomplished with the use of exogenous gonadotropins, which increase testosterone and sperm production. If primary testicular failure is present and the patient has oligospermia, then an attempt can be made to concentrate the sperm for intrauterine insemination or in vitro fertilization. If the azoospermia is due to ductal obstruction, then repair of the obstruction may be undertaken, or aspiration of sperm from the epididymis may be accomplished for in vitro fertilization.

Gynecomastia

Gynecomastia refers to a benign enlargement of the male breast resulting from proliferation of the glandular component. This common condition is found in as many as 70% of pubertal boys and in approximately one third of adults 50 to 80 years old. Estrogens stimulate and androgens inhibit breast glandular development. Thus gynecomastia is the result of an imbalance between estrogen and androgen action at the breast tissue level. This condition may result from an absolute increase in free estrogens, a decrease in endogenous free androgens, androgen insensitivity of the tissues, or enhanced sensitivity of the breast tissue to estrogens. Table 67–2 lists the common conditions associated with gynecomastia.

Gynecomastia must be differentiated from fatty enlargement of the breasts without glandular proliferation and other disorders of the breasts, especially breast carcinoma. *Male breast cancer* is usually seen as a unilateral, eccentric, hard or firm mass that is fixed to the underlying tissues. It may be associated with skin dimpling or retraction, as well as crusting of the nipple or nipple discharge. In contrast, gynecomastia occurs concentrically around the nipple and is not fixed to the underlying structures.

Painful and tender gynecomastia in a pubertal adolescent should be monitored with periodic examinations because, in most patients, pubertal gynecomastia disappears within 1 year. Incidentally discovered, asymptomatic gynecomastia in an adult requires a careful assessment for the following: alcohol, drug, or medication use; liver, lung, or kidney dysfunction; and signs and symptoms of hypogonadism or hyperthyroidism. If these conditions are not present, then only follow-up is required. In contrast, in an adult with recent onset of progressive painful gynecomastia, thyroid, liver, and renal function should be determined. If test results are normal, then serum concentrations of hCG, LH, testosterone, and estradiol should be measured. Further evaluation should be carried out according to the scheme outlined in Figure 67–3.

Removal of the offending drug or correction of the underlying condition causing the gynecomastia may result in regression of the breast glandular tissue. If the gynecomastia persists, then a trial of antiestrogens such as tamoxifen may be given for 3 months to see whether regression occurs. Gynecomastia that has been present for more than 1 year usually contains a fibrotic component that does not respond to medications. Therefore correction usually requires surgical removal of the tissue.

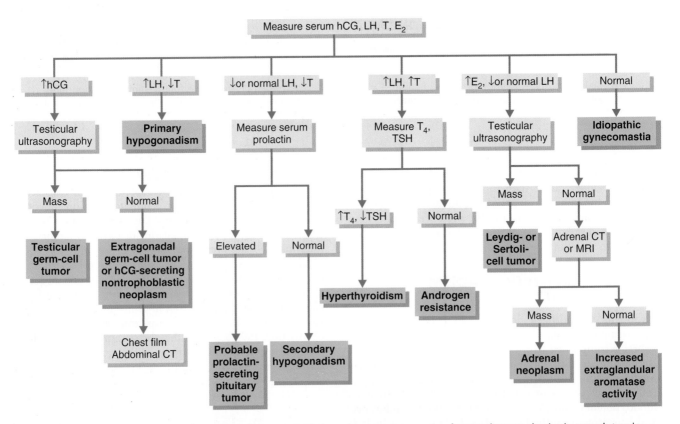

Figure 67–3 Diagnostic evaluation for causes of gynecomastia based on measurements of serum human chorionic gonadotropin (hCG), luteinizing hormone (LH), testosterone (T), and estradiol (E_2). ↑ = increased; ↓ = decreased; CT = computed tomography; MRI = magnetic resonance imaging; T_4 = thyroxine; TSH = thyroid-stimulating hormone. (From Braunstein GD: Gynecomastia. N Engl J Med 328:490–495, 1993. Copyright © 1993, Massachusetts Medical Society.)

Table 67–2 Conditions Associated with Gynecomastia

Physiologic Conditions

Neonatal
Pubertal
Involutional

Pathologic Conditions

Neoplasms
Testicular
Adrenal
Ectopic production of human chorionic gonadotropin
Primary gonadal failure
Secondary hypogonadism
Enzyme defects in testosterone production
Androgen insensitivity syndromes
Liver disease
Malnutrition with refeeding

Dialysis
Hyperthyroidism
Excessive extraglandular aromatase activity
Drugs
  Estrogens and estrogen agonists
  Gonadotropins
  Antiandrogens or inhibitors of androgen synthesis
  Cytotoxic agents
  Alcohol
  Idiopathic

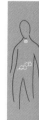

Prospectus for the Future

- Prospective, randomized, double-blind studies that examine the risks and benefits of testosterone replacement in aging men with a low level of testosterone
- Improved definition of the molecular basis for unexplained infertility
- New genetic tools for evaluating the androgen receptor

- Improved gonadotropin assays to differentiate hypogonadotropic hypogonadism from the low serum gonadotropin concentrations found at times in normal men
- Elucidation of the roles of inhibin and leptin in gonadal function and fertility
- Improved definition of environmental toxins that affect testicular function

References

Allan CA, McLachlan RI: Age-related changes in testosterone and the role of replacement therapy in older men. Clin Endocrinol 60:653–670, 2004.

Barthold JS, Gonzalez R: The epidemiology of congenital cryptorchidism, testicular ascent and orchiopexy. J Urol 170:2396–2401, 2003.

Braunstein GD: Aromatase and gynecomastia. Endocr Relat Cancer 6:315–324, 1999.

Khorram O, Patrizio P, Wang C, Swerdloff R: Reproductive technologies for male infertility. J Clin Endocrinol Metab 86:2373–2379, 2001.

Lanfranco F, Kamischke A, Zitzmann M, Nieschlag E: Klinefelter's syndrome. Lancet 364:273–283, 2004.

Rhoden EL, Mortgentaler A: Risks of testosterone-replacement therapy and recommendations for monitoring. N Engl J Med 350:482–492, 2004.

Chapter 68

Diabetes Mellitus

Philip S. Barnett

Glenn D. Braunstein

Abbreviations

ACEI	angiotensin II-converting enzyme inhibitor
ARB	angiotensin II-receptor blocker
BMI	body mass index
Cr	creatinine (serum)
CSII	continuous subcutaneous insulin infusion
DKA	diabetic ketoacidosis
DPP-4	dipeptidyl peptidase-4
ESRD	end-stage renal disease
FFA	free fatty acid
FPG	fasting plasma glucose
GDM	gestational diabetes mellitus
GFR	glomerular filtration rate
GIP	glucose-dependent insulinotropic polypeptide
GLP-1	glucagon-like peptide-1
HbA$_{1c}$	glycosylated hemoglobin
HDL	high-density lipoprotein
HGP	hepatic glucose production
HLA	human leukocyte antigen
HNKS	hyperosmolar nonketotic syndrome
hs-CRP	highly selective creatine phosphokinase
IFG	impaired fasting glucose
IGT	impaired glucose tolerance
IMT	intima medial thickness
IR	insulin resistance
LDL	low-density lipoprotein
MI	myocardial infarction
NYHA	New York Heart Association
OGTT	oral glucose tolerance test
PAI-1	plasminogen activator inhibitor-1
PCG	postchallenge glucose
PCOS	polycystic ovarian syndrome
PPAR	peroxisome proliferator activated receptor
PPG	postprandial glucose
SMBG	self-monitoring of blood glucose
T1DM	type 1 diabetes mellitus
TZD	thiazolidinedione
T2DM	type 2 diabetes mellitus
TG	triglyceride
VLDL	very low-density lipoprotein
USDA	U.S. Department of Agriculture

Definition

Diabetes mellitus comprises a heterogeneous group of metabolic diseases that are characterized by chronic hyperglycemia and disturbances in carbohydrate, lipid, and protein metabolism resulting from defects in insulin secretion and/or insulin action. Fasting (chronic) and postprandial hyperglycemia are mainly responsible for the acute, short-term, and late complications, which affect all body organs and systems.

United States population statistics for 2005 show that the total prevalence of diabetes in all ages was an estimated 20.8 million people (7% of the population); 14.6 million diagnosed, 6.2 million undiagnosed, and 41 million between the ages of 40 and 74 years with prediabetes. In people 20 years or older, the prevalence was 20.6 million (9.6%), and in those 60 years or older, the prevalence rose to 10.3 million (20.9% of all people in this age group). The incidence of diabetes in people 20 years or older in 2005 was 1.5 million. The total cost of diabetes in the United States in 2002 was estimated to be $132 billion (direct medical costs $92 billion, and indirect costs $40 billion), with a per capita annual health care cost of $13,243, compared with $2,560 in people without diabetes. Diabetes, the sixth leading cause of death by disease in the United States, accounts for almost 18% of all deaths in people over 25 years of age, and it is the leading cause of end-stage renal disease (ESRD), new cases of blindness, and nontraumatic lower limb amputations. Cardiovascular disease is the major cause of diabetes-related death and is two to five times more common in patients with diabetes than in the general population. Life expectancy in middle-aged patients is reduced by 5 to 10 years. The prevalence of diabetes worldwide is reaching pandemic proportions, currently more than 150 million (300 million people by 2025), in large part because of increased obesity (65% of U.S. adults are overweight or obese) and sedentary lifestyles in both adults and children.

Diagnosis

Presentation of patients with diabetes depends on the type of diabetes and the stage of the pathologic process. Patients with *type 1 diabetes mellitus* (T1DM) commonly present with classic acute symptoms of hyperglycemia: polydipsia, polyuria, weight loss, and, less frequently, polyphagia, blurred vision, and pruritus, 25% for the first time in diabetic ketoacidosis (DKA). In patients with *type 2 diabetes mellitus* (T2DM), the disease is often present for many years (average 4 to 7 years) before diagnosis, and as many as 50% have an established cardiovascular complication at the time of diagnosis. The symptoms are usually less acute than those in T1DM, and they may be accompanied by lethargy and fatigue in what was, until recently, a generally older population. With the current epidemic of obesity, a significant increase occurs in the incidence and prevalence of T2DM in childhood and adolescence. Chronic hyperglycemia may be associated with impairment of growth, susceptibility to infections (e.g., balanitis, vaginitis), and slow wound healing. Risk factors for T2DM are listed in Table 68–1 and include sedentary lifestyle, poor nutrition, and overweight and obesity.

Diagnostic criteria for diabetes are listed in Table 68–2. Any of the three serum glucose measurements may be used for diagnosis, and must be confirmed, on a subsequent day, by any one of the three. The diagnostic *fasting plasma glucose* (FPG) correlates with the 2-hour postchallenge glucose (PCG) cut-point, resulting in fewer people with undiagnosed and misdiagnosed diabetes. These low cut-off diagnostic values identify critical levels at which the prevalence of microvascular complications increases dramatically, and set new levels for earlier and aggressive diabetes therapy, in an attempt to prevent these complications.

Although the *oral glucose tolerance test* (OGTT) remains the standard for diagnostic purposes, measurement of FPG by comparison, which is simpler, cheaper, equally accurate, faster to perform, more reproducible, and convenient, is used for routine diagnosis. Measurement of *glycosylated hemoglobin* (HbA$_{1c}$) is a useful tool for monitoring glycemic control and for making therapeutic decisions but is not recommended for diagnostic purposes. The OGTT is still used for diagnosing gestational diabetes (Table 68–3).

In the United States, estimates indicate that at least 41 million people have blood glucose levels greater than normal

---

Table 68–1   Screening Criteria for Diabetes in Asymptomatic, High-Risk Adults

1. Testing for diabetes should be considered in all persons ≥45 years and, if normal, should be repeated at 3-year intervals.
2. Testing should be considered at a younger age (≥30 years) or performed more frequently in individuals who:
   a. Are overweight (BMI >25) or who have central obesity with normal BMI (18.5–24.9)
   b. Have a habitually sedentary lifestyle
   c. Have a first-degree relative with diabetes (i.e., parent or sibling, 45–80% in T2DM, 5% in T1DM; equates to a 40% risk)
   d. Are members of a high-risk ethnic population (e.g., African American, Latino, Hispanic American, Native American, Asian American, Pacific Islander)
   e. Have delivered a baby weighing >9 lb (4 kg), have experienced unexplained perinatal death, or who have been diagnosed with gestational diabetes
   f. Are hypertensive (≥140/90 mm Hg)
   g. Have an HDL cholesterol level ≤35 mg/dL (0.9 mmol/L) and/or a triglyceride level ≥250 mg/dL (2.82 mmol/L)
   h. Had, on previous testing, impaired glucose tolerance (plasma glucose ≥140 mg/dL [7.8 mmol/L] but <200 mg/dL [11.1 mmol/L] during 2 hr after 75-g oral glucose tolerance test) or impaired fasting glucose (plasma glucose 100–125 mg/dL [5.6–6.9 mmol/L])
   i. Have other clinical conditions associated with insulin resistance (e.g., PCOS, acanthosis nigricans [60–90% in T2DM])
   j. Have a history of vascular disease, particularly cardio- and cerebrovascular

Adapted from the American Diabetes Association: Clinical Practice Guidelines 2006. Diabetes Care 29(Suppl. 1):S6, 2006.
BMI = body mass index (weight [kg]/height [m²]); HDL = high-density lipoprotein; PCOS = polycystic ovary syndrome; T1DM = type 1 diabetes mellitus; T2DM = type 2 diabetes mellitus.

Table 68–2   Criteria for the Diagnosis of Diabetes Mellitus

Plasma Glucose	Normal	Impaired Fasting Glucose§	Impaired Glucose Tolerance§	Diabetes Mellitus
Fasting*	>100 (5.6)	≥100 and <126	—	≥126 (7.0)
2-hour postload	>140 (7.8)	—	≥140 and <200	≥200 (11.1)
Random†	—	—	—	≥200 with symptoms

Data from the American Diabetes Association: Clinical Practice Guidelines 2006. Diabetes Care 28(Suppl. 1):S5, 2005.
*Fasting; no solid or liquid food, except water, for at least 8 hours.
†Random; refers to any time of day, unrelated to meals.
§Prediabetes refers to impaired fasting glucose and/or impaired glucose tolerance.
The standard oral glucose tolerance test, defined by the World Health Organization, requires a 75-g anhydrous glucose load.
Numbers represent venous plasma glucose values in mg/dL. Numbers in parentheses represent venous plasma glucose values in mmol/L.

Table 68–3 **Screening and Diagnostic Criteria for Gestational Diabetes Mellitus**

Plasma Glucose	50-g Screening Test	75-g Diagnostic Test	100-g Diagnostic Test
Fasting	—	≥95	≥95 (5.3)
1 hr	≥140	≥180	≥180 (10.0)
2 hr	—	≥155	≥155 (8.6)
3 hr	—	—	≥140 (7.8)

Data from the American Diabetes Association: Clinical Practice Guidelines 2006. Diabetes Care 29(Suppl. 1):S48, 2006.
50-g, 75-g, and 100-g refer to oral glucose loads.
Numbers represent venous plasma glucose values in mg/dL. Numbers in parentheses represent venous plasma glucose values in mmol/L.

but less than those diagnostic for diabetes, a state referred to as *prediabetes*. These people are generally euglycemic and have abnormal glucose responses only when challenged with an OGTT. Depending on the diagnostic test, this group or metabolic stage is referred to as having either *impaired fasting glucose* (IFG) or *impaired glucose tolerance* (IGT) (see Table 68–2). These people are at increased risk of developing T2DM (7% per year) and its complications, particularly cardiovascular (50% increased risk), and need to be identified for early counseling and treatment.

Screening for Diabetes

Screening for T1DM involves the measurement of autoantibody markers (antibodies to islet cells, insulin, glutamic acid decarboxylase, and tyrosine phosphatase). Several reasons mitigate against the routine screening of both healthy children in the general population, and those at high risk of developing T1DM (siblings of patients with T1DM); these include lack of established cut-off values for immune markers, lack of consensus regarding effective therapy for patients with positive test results, and lack of cost effectiveness.

Screening of certain high-risk populations for T2DM (see Table 68–1) is considered cost effective. More than one third of people with T2DM are undiagnosed. Twenty-five to 33% of patients with T2DM have family members with diabetes. Because of the insidious nature of T2DM, patients have a high risk of developing complications by the time of clinical diagnosis (see Complications, later in this chapter). Early diagnosis and treatment may reduce the burden of this disease, its complications (particularly micro- and macrovascular disease), and associated co-morbidities, such as dyslipidemia, hypertension, and obesity.

Gestational diabetes mellitus (GDM) refers to the presence of glucose intolerance that develops during pregnancy and usually returns to normal after delivery. GDM occurs in 2% to 5% of all pregnancies, but it may complicate as many as 14% in certain populations (see Table 68–1, criterion 2c), and accounts for approximately 90% of diabetes during pregnancy. If this condition is not diagnosed, or left untreated, the consequences for both mother and fetus may be severe. Screening for GDM is routinely performed between 24 and 28 weeks gestation in women older than 25 years, and younger women who fulfill one or more of the criteria in Table 68–1 (2a through 2d and 2g). Women at high risk (obese, personal history of GDM, glycosuria, first-degree relative with diabetes) should be screened at their initial obstetric or prenatal visit. A positive screening test (plasma glucose ≥140 mg/dL [7.8 mmol/L] 1 hour after a 50-g glucose challenge administered to a nonfasting patient) dictates the need for diagnostic testing with a 3-hour, 100-g OGTT performed in the fasting state (≥8 hrs). Meeting or exceeding any two or more of the plasma glucose values listed in Table 68–3 is diagnostic of GDM. Women with GDM should be reclassified 6 or more weeks postpartum (see Table 68–2). Approximately 25% of lean women and up to 50% of obese women will go on to develop overt diabetes (types 1 or 2), IFG, or IGT over a 20-year period. Pregnancy serves as a provocative test and not as a risk factor for the future development of diabetes.

Classification

Improved understanding of the origins and pathogenesis of diabetes facilitated revision of the classification of diabetes mellitus (Table 68–4) from one based mainly on therapeutic considerations, such as insulin dependence or insulin independence, to one based on the etiology. Any patient with diabetes may require insulin therapy at some stage of the disease, irrespective of the classification.

TYPES 1 AND 2 DIABETES

The underlying pathologic process in most patients with T1DM (5% to 10% of people with diabetes) is autoimmune destruction of the pancreatic islet β cells with absolute loss of insulin secretion. The disease has strong human leukocyte antigen (HLA) associations and numerous antibody markers of immune destruction (Table 68–5). In a few patients with T1DM, the pathogenesis remains idiopathic. Patients with β-cell destruction or failure resulting from identifiable non-autoimmune causes are not included in this class. T2DM (90% to 95% of people with diabetes) results from variable combinations of insulin resistance and insulin secretory defects (β-cell dysfunction), with one or the other abnormality predominating in a given patient.

Distinguishing between T1DM and T2DM is not always a simple process. T2DM is diagnosed in children as young as 6 years and may account for as many as 25% to 33% of

Table 68–4	**Etiologic Classification of Diabetes Mellitus**

Type 1 Diabetes Mellitus

Immune mediated
Idiopathic
LADA

Type 2 Diabetes Mellitus

Other specific types
    Genetic defects of β-cell function
    Genetic defects in insulin action
    Diseases of the exocrine pancreas
    Endocrinopathies
    Drug- or chemical-induced
    Infections
    Uncommon forms of immune-mediated diabetes
    Other genetic syndromes sometimes associated with
        diabetes
Gestational diabetes mellitus

Data from the American Diabetes Association: Clinical Practice Guidelines 2006. Diabetes Care 29(Suppl. 1):S46, 2006.
LADA = latent autoimmune diabetes of adults.

all new cases of diabetes diagnosed in adolescents 9 to 19 years of age, often associated with an increase in weight and parallel decrease in physical activity. These adolescents may even present in DKA before they ultimately achieve control of their disease with diet and oral antihyperglycemic agents. T1DM can also occur in elderly patients. This condition has been described as *latent autoimmune diabetes of adulthood* (also known as late-onset autoimmune diabetes, or *type 1¹/₂*) and may account for many insulin-requiring patients previously misclassified as T2DM. Patients with T1DM who later develop obesity, insulin resistance, and possibly metabolic syndrome and T2DM are said to have *double double, hybrid,* or *type 3* diabetes.

Hyperglycemia, the hallmark of diabetes, changes in degree over time, which reflects the severity and stage of the underlying pathologic process, which may progress, regress, or remain static, and the effectiveness of its treatment, but does not signal an alteration in the *nature* of the process.

OTHER SPECIFIC TYPES OF DIABETES

These groups together account for 1% to 2% of patients with diabetes. Inheritance of *maturity-onset diabetes of the young* (MODY types 1 to 5) is autosomal dominant, and hyperglycemia appears before the age of 25 years.

Within the small group of *genetic insulin-resistance states,* impaired insulin action is the result of either a defective insulin receptor molecule (type A insulin resistance, leprechaunism, or Rabson-Mendenhall syndrome) or abnormalities in postreceptor signal transduction pathways (lipoatrophic diabetes).

Destruction of the pancreas results in reduced insulin secretion, with subsequent development of diabetes.

Several *insulin counter-regulatory hormones* (glucagon, catecholamines, cortisol, and growth hormone) that antagonize insulin action and increase insulin resistance precipitate diabetes when they are produced in excess. Excess *aldosterone* production by a tumor, through induction of hypokalemia and increased production of *somatostatin,* may impair insulin secretion and cause diabetes. The hyperglycemia in these cases resolves following successful removal of the responsible tumor.

The mechanism of *drug-* or *chemical-induced diabetes* depends on the offending agent: β-cell destruction (by the rodenticide vacor, intravenous pentamidine, or α-interferon with autoantibodies), impaired insulin action (nicotinic acid and glucocorticoids), or peripheral insulin resistance and impaired conversion of proinsulin to insulin (protease inhibitors). In some forms of immune-mediated diabetes, anti-insulin receptor antibodies may cause insulin resistance.

METABOLIC SYNDROME

Also known as the *insulin resistance syndrome, Reaven's syndrome, dysmetabolic syndrome,* and *syndrome X,* metabolic syndrome is not a subclass of diabetes mellitus, although it is extremely common in patients with diabetes and affects at least 50 million people in the United States (one in three to four adults). It consists of a cluster of clinical findings and laboratory abnormalities that include obesity (central, abdominal, or visceral), increased sympathetic nervous system activity, hypertension, glucose intolerance, insulin resistance (the common etiologic factor), hyperinsulinemia (compensatory), T2DM, dyslipidemia (hypertriglyceridemia, increased small dense low-density lipoprotein [LDL₃], and/or decreased high-density lipoprotein [HDL]), fatty liver, enhanced postprandial lipemia, disordered fibrinolysis (elevated plasminogen activator inhibitor-1 [PAI-1], tissue-type plasminogen activator, clotting factors VII and XII, and fibrinogen, with decreased levels of antithrombotic factors C and S and antithrombin III), hyperuricemia, systemic inflammation (especially vascular), and endothelial dysfunction (**Web Table 68–1**). To date, no national or international agreement exists on the cut points for these various components, nor a consensus regarding the definition or actual existence of a *syndrome.* Abdominal adiposity, regarded by most authorities as a prerequisite for the diagnosis, is associated with increased lipolysis, increased free fatty acids (FFAs), and tumor-necrosis factor alpha (TNF-α), with decreased adiponectin. This syndrome is associated with a greatly increased risk of atherosclerotic vascular disease, specifically coronary artery disease, diabetes, and polycystic ovarian syndrome (PCOS).

Pathogenesis

TYPE 1 DIABETES

Generally, T1DM is an autoimmune disease in which some environmental insult (microbial, chemical, or dietary) triggers an autoimmune reaction in a genetically susceptible individual. HLA-DR3 and/or HLA-DR4 is present in 90% to

Table 68–5 General Comparison of the Two Most Common Types of Diabetes Mellitus

	Type 1	Type 2
Previous terminology	Insulin-dependent diabetes mellitus, type I, juvenile-onset diabetes	Non–insulin-dependent diabetes mellitus, type II, adult-onset diabetes
Age of onset	Usually <30 yr, particularly childhood and adolescence, but any age	Usually >40 yr, but increasingly at younger ages
Genetic predisposition	Moderate; environmental factors required for expression; 35–50% concordance in monozygotic twins; several candidate genes proposed	Strong; 60–90% concordance in monozygotic twins; many candidate genes proposed; some genes identified in maturity-onset diabetes of the young
Human leukocyte antigen associations	Linkage to DQA and DQB, influenced by DRB3 and DRB4 (DR2 protective)	None known
Other associations	Autoimmune; Graves' disease, Hashimoto's thyroiditis, vitiligo, Addison's disease, pernicious anemia	Heterogenous group, ongoing subclassification based on identification of specific pathogenic processes and genetic defects
Precipitating and risk factors	Largely unknown; microbial, chemical, dietary, other	Age, obesity (central), sedentary lifestyle, previous gestational diabetes (see Table 68–1)
Findings at diagnosis	85–90% of patients have one and usually more autoantibodies to ICA512, IA-2, IA-2β, GAD$_{65}$, IAA	Possibly complications (microvascular and macrovascular) caused by significant hyperglycemia in the preceding asymptomatic period
Endogenous insulin levels	Low or absent	Usually present (relative deficiency), early hyperinsulinemia
Insulin resistance	Only with hyperglycemia	Mostly present
Prolonged fast	Hyperglycemia, ketoacidosis	Euglycemia
Stress, withdrawal of insulin	Ketoacidosis	Nonketotic hyperglycemia, occasionally ketoacidosis

GAD = glutamic acid decarboxylase; IA-2, IA-2β = insuloma-associated protein 2 and 2β (tyrosine phosphatases); IAA = insulin autoantibodies; ICA = islet cell antibody; ICA512 = islet cell autoantigen 512 (fragment of IA-2).

95% of patients with T1DM compared with 45% to 50% in the general population. Predominantly cell-mediated (mononuclear cells; mainly macrophages and CD8+ T lymphocytes) destruction of the β cells of the islets of Langerhans is associated with several autoantibodies to islet cell constituents (see Table 68–5). These antibodies, some of which may occur secondary to release of antigens following β-cell death, serve as markers of the immune destruction. Figure 68–1 illustrates how the autoimmune process may be present for several years, with competing destruction and regeneration of β cells, before the disease becomes clinically apparent. At this time, the critical mass of remaining β cells (10% to 20%) is unable to sustain compensatory insulin secretion at a level sufficient to maintain normal blood glucose values. After diagnosis and institution of insulin therapy, patients usually have some degree of recovery of β-cell function to the extent that exogenous insulin requirements drop to extremely low levels (*honeymoon* period). This period usually lasts for a couple of months but may be as long as a year. Patients should continue insulin administration throughout this time, even at these low doses. β-cell insulin secretion eventually fails completely, and, at this point, patients become insulin dependent, with DKA developing in the absence of insulin replacement.

TYPE 2 DIABETES

A significant but poorly defined genetic predisposition exists to the development of T2DM, complicated by the heterogeneous nature of the disease and the influence of acquired factors. Five main elements characterize the pathophysiology: (1) insulin resistance, (2) β-cell dysfunction, (3)

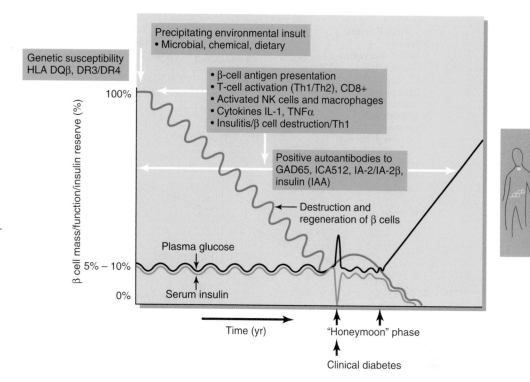

Figure 68–1 Natural history of type 1 diabetes mellitus. The *honeymoon* period with temporary improvement in β-cell function occurs with the initiation of insulin therapy at the time of clinical diagnosis. ICA512 = islet cell autoantigen 512 (fragment of IA-2); IA-2, IA-2β = tyrosine phosphatases; GAD = glutamic acid decarboxylase; HLA = human leukocyte antigen; ICA = islet cell antibody; IL-1 = interleukin-1; NK = natural killer; Th1 = subset of CD4+ T-helper cells responsible for cell-mediated immunity; Th2 = subset of CD4+ T-helper cells responsible for humoral immunity; TNF-α = tumor-necrosis factor alpha.

dysregulated hepatic glucose production (HGP), (4) abnormal intestinal glucose absorption, and (5) obesity. Insulin resistance results from defective intracellular signaling following binding of insulin to its receptor. This defect results in decreased intracellular glucose transporter activity. In the preclinical phase, the pancreatic β cells compensate for a genetically predetermined peripheral (skeletal muscle, adipose tissue, and liver) *insulin resistance* by producing more insulin (hyperinsulinemia) to maintain euglycemia. Some patients are identified at this stage while they are clinically asymptomatic.

With time, the β cells gradually fail to compensate for the progressive increase in insulin resistance (stage of IGT or IFG; 40% reduction of β-cell mass), and eventually hyperglycemia becomes clinically manifest as diabetes mellitus (80–90% reduction of β-cell mass) (Fig. 68–2). Insulin secretion continues, albeit not in the hyperinsulinemic range, with resultant relative insulin deficiency. Classically, early loss of the first phase of glucose-stimulated insulin secretion occurs (peaking at 10 minutes), with subsequent gradual loss of the second phase (starting 30 minutes after glucose stimulus and peaking at 60 minutes). Other features of β-*cell dysfunction* include dysrhythmic pulsatile insulin secretion, defective glucose potentiation of nonglucose insulin secretagogues (the incretins: glucose-dependent insulinotropic polypeptide [GIP] and glucagon-like peptide-1 [GLP-1]), increased proinsulin-to-insulin ratio (from defective protease activity), accumulation of islet amyloid polypeptide, increased glucagon secretion from islet α cells, and *glucotoxicity*. Glucotoxicity refers to the effect of chronic hyperglycemia in decreasing insulin secretion (through impaired β-cell sensitivity) and insulin activity (by increasing insulin resistance and insulin receptor tyrosine kinase activity). Glucotoxicity is a function of the duration and magnitude of the hyperglycemia and contributes to the progressive worsening of hyperglycemia. Elevated FFA levels, the result of unre-

strained adipose tissue lipolysis in the relative absence of insulin, also have a toxic effect on β-cells *(lipotoxicity)* and, together with intracellular protein glycation, contribute further to the failure of these cells. FFAs exacerbate hyperglycemia through increased oxidation in skeletal muscle and liver, where they decrease glucose utilization and increase gluconeogenesis, respectively. In obesity, the increased FFAs released from visceral fat stimulate increased hepatic synthesis of triglycerides and may impair first-pass hepatic metabolism of insulin, contributing to hyperinsulinemia.

Before the appearance of fasting hyperglycemia (elevated FPG), in the latter stages of compensatory hyperinsulinemia, it is possible to demonstrate *abnormal postprandial glucose (PPG) metabolism,* IGT, that is not evident clinically. Therapeutic intervention at this point may prevent or delay the onset of T2DM. The relative contributions of insulin resistance and insulin secretory defect to the pathogenesis in individual patients vary, with insulin resistance playing a dominant role in most patients who are obese (~80% to 90% of patients in the United States) and failure of insulin secretion being more important in patients of normal weight.

Excessive HGP (25% to 50% higher than normal) results from inadequate suppression of hepatic gluconeogenesis, the result of hepatic insulin resistance, exacerbated by waning insulin secretion from failing β cells. Postprandial HGP is markedly increased, with a variable increase in the basal rate. Within the diabetic liver, decreased glycogen synthesis and increased fat synthesis also occur.

Hyperglycemia, with or without autonomic nerve involvement, may contribute to *gastric dysmotility* (symptomatic or not) and alterations in the rate and timing of glucose absorption (usually increased), with consequent exacerbation of hyperglycemia, resulting in a vicious cycle.

Endothelial dysfunction is the precursor of the extensive vasculopathy seen in patients with diabetes. FFAs that are

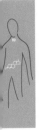

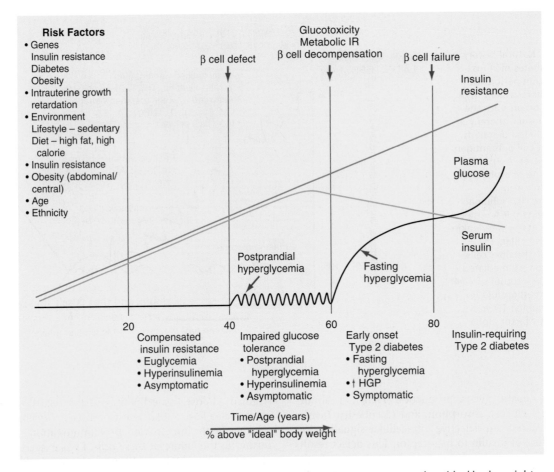

Figure 68–2 Natural history of type 2 diabetes mellitus. The numbers for percentage greater than *ideal* body weight are only approximate. Similarly, the age markers for the different phases of β-cell decompensation toward overt diabetes and an insulin-requiring state are approximate guides. Certain groups are more insulin sensitive and require a greater loss of β-cell function to precipitate diabetes than do obese insulin-resistant people, who develop diabetes after small declines in β-cell function. Use of insulin in patients with type 2 diabetes varies considerably and is not age dependent. Insulin resistance increases proportionately to adiposity, represented here by weight. HGP = hepatic glucose production; IR = insulin resistance.

increased in T2DM acutely impair endothelial function, as well as raise blood pressure. Insulin improves endothelium-dependent vasodilation, but with insulin resistance and hyperinsulinemia, impairment of vascular nitric oxide production and insulin-induced vasodilation occur, with proliferation of vascular smooth muscle cells. Several markers of acute *inflammation* (including interleukin [IL]-6, C-reactive protein, and TNF-α) have been demonstrated in people with IGT, newly diagnosed diabetes, and atherosclerosis. Low-grade chronic inflammation, in this group of patients, is associated with insulin resistance through interference with insulin signal transduction.

Other endocrine associations in people with T2DM are subclinical hypercortisolism (7%), mainly adrenal in origin, and lowered levels of testosterone in males.

Management

GOALS

The goals of management can be divided into three stages: (1) short-term, involving immediate treatment to relieve symptoms such as polydipsia, polyuria, or acute infections;

(2) intermediate-term, to return the patient to a physiologic state and social life that are as normal as possible; and (3) long-term, to prevent the development, or delay the progression, of the complications of diabetes. People diagnosed with this chronic disease experience a range of emotions, including denial, anger, guilt, and depression, and most require some form of psychological support.

The cornerstones of a comprehensive diabetes management plan include patient education, healthy nutrition, weight control, physical activity, self-monitoring of blood glucose (SMBG), and antihyperglycemic agents when necessary. Patient education aims to *empower patients* by equipping them with the necessary knowledge about diabetes and self-management skills with which to make meaningful decisions about their health on a daily basis. Treatments need to be individualized, addressing medical, psychosocial, and lifestyle issues.

BLOOD GLUCOSE MONITORING

Control of blood glucose levels is a crucial component of the diabetes management plan because hypo- and hyperglycemia are major contributors to the complications of

Table 68–6 Blood Glucose Goals for Glycemic Control in Patients with Diabetes*

Biochemical Index	Normal	Goal	Action Suggested
Preprandial fasting glucose (mg/dL)[†]	60–100 (3.3–5.6)	<100 (6.1)	<80 or >140 (<4.4 or >7.8)
Postprandial glucose (mg/dL)[†]	<140	<140	>180 (10.0)
Bedtime glucose (mg/dL)[†]	<110	100–140	<100 or >160 (<5.6 or >8.9)
HbA$_{1c}$ (%)	<6	<6.5	>8

Data from American Diabetes Association: Clinical practice recommendations 2006. Diabetes Care 29(Suppl. 1):S10, 2006, and Endocrine Practice 8(Suppl. 1):5–11, 2002.
*These values are generalized to the entire population of nonpregnant adults with diabetes. Glycosylated hemoglobin (HbA$_{1c}$) is referenced to a nondiabetic range of 4.0 to 6.0% (mean, 5.0%; standard deviation, 0.5%).
[†]Measurement of capillary blood glucose. Postprandial blood glucose refers to the level 2 hours after the beginning of a meal.
Numbers represent venous plasma glucose values in mg/dL. Numbers in parentheses represent venous plasma glucose values in mmol/L.

diabetes. *SMBG* with blood glucose meters, by all patients, facilitates adjustments in treatment and also acts as an educational tool for the patient. Ideally, SMBG should be performed as frequently as practicable—fasting, preprandial, 2 hours postprandial (especially in GDM; measure at 1 hour postprandial), at bedtime, and occasionally at 2:00 AM to 3:00 AM—and values should be recorded. Continuous glucose monitoring systems (measurement of interstitial fluid, or intravenous, glucose levels at 5-minute intervals for 72 hours) detect trends in glucose levels not possible with regular SMBG. This approach facilitates fine-tuning of diabetes treatments.

The *HbA$_{1c}$* value,[‡] by providing a measure of the average blood glucose level (**Web Table 68–2, Web Fig. 68–1**) over the preceding 2 to 3 months, serves as an indicator of diabetes control (Table 68–6). Testing frequency is two or more times per year in patients with T2DM with stable glycemic control and meeting treatment goals, and four or more times per year for patients with T1DM, those with poor glycemic control, or in those after therapy change. Caution must be exercised in using HbA$_{1c}$ as the only gauge of diabetes control. Patients with wide fluctuations in blood glucose levels may sometimes have normal, average blood glucose levels and HbA$_{1c}$. Elevated HbA$_{1c}$ despite normal FPG (*good control*) is frequently the result of elevated PPG (>200 mg/dL in 75% of patients with T2DM with HbA$_{1c}$ values ≥7%; HbA$_{1c}$ = FPG + PPG) (see Tight Control, later in this chapter). Records of SMBG are often more informative and useful for making therapeutic decisions. The importance of PPG cannot be overestimated. Elevated PPG, not FPG, is an independent risk factor for cardiovascular disease and all-cause mortality.

Spuriously low levels of HbA$_{1c}$ may be seen in patients with hemoglobinopathies such as homozygous or heterozygous HbS, C, G, or H. Variable levels of HbA$_{1c}$ may be noted with HbE or persistent HbF. β-Thalassemia and sickle cell trait, with increased frequency of hemolysis, result in short-

ened red blood cell life span, reduced time available for glycosylation of hemoglobin, and thus falsely low HbA$_{1c}$ levels.

Measurement of serum *fructosamine* may be a useful marker for shorter-term assessment of integrated glucose concentrations (2 to 4 weeks), for example, during pregnancy.

STANDARDS OF CARE AND SPECIFIC TREATMENT GOALS

Regular patient assessment includes weight, blood pressure, pulse, SMBG records, foot examination, and discussion about smoking cessation at every office visit, with quarterly assessment of HbA$_{1c}$. Determination of micro-albuminuria, serum creatinine levels, dilated retinal examination, general physical, neurologic (with autonomic testing), cardiac, nephrology, and dental examinations, with comprehensive foot evaluation, should be performed yearly, provided all are normal. Influenza vaccine should be administered yearly and Pneumovax every 5 years. Following the initial measurement of serum lipids, the frequency of reevaluation is dictated by results and treatment and should be done at least yearly. **Web Table 68–3** lists the optimal evaluation frequencies in people with diabetes. Regular diabetes education should be an integral part of every patient's management plan. Patients should be advised to carry some documentation regarding their diabetes status (e.g., Medic Alert bracelet).

Blood glucose goals for glycemic control are listed in Table 68–6.

Aspirin therapy should be considered in every patient with diabetes, provided that no contraindications exist.

Goals for lipid levels are influenced by cardiovascular risk factors (see Chapter 9). Optimal values are LDL cholesterol under 100 mg/dL (2.6 mmol/L) (<70 mg/dL in patients with established cardiovascular disease), HDL cholesterol over 45 mg/dL (1.15 mmol/L) for men and over 55 mg/dL (1.4 mmol/L) for women, and triglycerides under 150 mg/dL (1.7 mmol/L). Hydroxymethylglutaryl coenzyme-A reductase inhibitors, *statins*, are highly effective in the management of diabetic dyslipidemia and, together with their anti-inflammatory actions and improvement in endothelial function, may reduce the risk of cardiovascular events by approximately 30%. Fibrates or niacin (used with caution in patients with T2DM) may be required for lowering triglyc-

---

[‡]Nonenzymatic irreversible glycosylation of the hemoglobin molecule, HbA$_{1c}$, depends on ambient plasma glucose levels. The average lifespan of a red blood cell, and hence its HbA$_{1c}$, is 120 days.

erides or elevating HDL, respectively (see Chapter 61). Combined use of several classes of agents may be necessary for lipid control. Combination tablets of ezetimibe and simvastatin, fibrates with statins and niacin with statins are the way forward.

Normal urinary albumin/creatinine ratio is under 30 mcg/mg. Micro-albuminuria refers to an albumin-creatinine ratio of 30 to 299 mcg/mg and macro-albuminuria greater than 300 mcg/mg.

Blood pressure management is discussed under Macrovascular Complications.

The previous paragraphs address the problems of β-cell failure, insulin resistance, and co-morbidities. The other major contributors to the modern epidemic of diabetes are excess weight, obesity, and a sedentary lifestyle. These conditions are managed through lifestyle changes including weight loss, healthy nutrition, and exercise (see later discussion).

MEDICAL NUTRITION THERAPY

Medical nutrition therapy should be individualized to the patient's lifestyle, exercise regimen, eating habits, culture, and financial resources. A prescription for a *diabetic diet* no longer exists, nor is there a need to purchase *diabetic foods*. Dietary recommendations are generally in line with those for the general population: increased intake of fruit and vegetables, whole grains and fish, and maintaining moderate calorie restriction. Daily energy requirements include consumption of a balanced, healthy diet composed of 10% to 20% protein (1 g/kg body weight, provided no nephropathy exists) less than 35% total fat (>10% saturated, ≤10% polyunsaturated, 10% to 20% monounsaturated and transunsaturated, and <200 to 300 mg cholesterol), and 45% to 60% carbohydrate (see Chapter 60).

Soluble fiber (>15 g/1000 kcal) in the diet delays carbohydrate absorption (dampening the PPG peak) and improves serum lipid profiles. Insoluble fiber contributes to satiety (especially important if overweight) and *gastrointestinal homeostasis.*

Salt (NaCl) intake should be restricted to less than 6 g/day. Partial substitution of potassium chloride or magnesium chloride may be beneficial.

In addition to dietary counseling, reference to the food pyramid, generated by the U.S. Department of Agriculture (USDA), will provide general guidance for all individuals to daily nutritional requirements and the foods that provide these requirements.

Dietary adjustments are based on nutritional assessment, blood pressure, renal function, and HbA_{1c}, as well as on diabetic treatment goals. The *glycemic index* refers to the increase in blood glucose after ingestion of a particular food, expressed as a percentage of the increase in blood glucose following ingestion of the equivalent amount of glucose. For a given food, the glycemic index will vary according to the method of preparation and the concurrently ingested foods. Current recommendations encourage consumption of foods with a low glycemic index. *Carbohydrate counting* involves using either a simple system of exchanges, or *carbs* (15-g carbohydrate portions) or the more precise carbohydrate gram counting. This method allows for fine-tuning of insulin dosing during mealtimes. Training in nutrition self-management empowers patients to make correct food choices, plan meals, exercise, and calculate bolus doses of insulin.

Alcohol is allowed in moderation (≤2 drinks for men and ≤1 drink for women per day [21 units/week for men, 14 units/week for women]; one alcoholic beverage is equivalent to 12 oz beer, 5 oz wine, or 1.5 oz spirits) and should always be taken with food. Alcohol is not metabolized to glucose and inhibits gluconeogenesis, an effect that may result in hypoglycemia as late as 8 to 16 hours following consumption. Alcohol should not be substituted for food, but, when alcohol calorie content needs to be calculated as part of a meal plan, it should be counted as fat calories (one alcoholic beverage = two fat exchanges).

WEIGHT-MANAGEMENT THERAPY

Overweight (body mass index [BMI]* of 25.0 to 29.9) and obesity (BMI >30) are major risk factors for T2DM and cardiovascular disease. *Healthy, reasonable, achievable,* and *sustainable* body weights are more realistic terms than *desirable* or *ideal* body weight. A strong correlation exists between increasing BMI and the risk of T2DM. As little as 5% to 10% weight loss in overweight and obese patients reduces the risk of diabetes and leads to increased insulin sensitivity, with improvement in glycemic control, and the possibility of a reduction or cessation of antihyperglycemic therapy. This degree of weight loss also leads to significant improvements in dyslipidemia and blood pressure, as well as an increase in longevity. Behavioral modification and meal replacements, including low- or very low–calorie diets, in a structured weight-reduction or maintenance program, are of proven efficacy in patients who are unable to lose weight on their own or with the support of a qualified nutritionist. Portion control and self-monitoring are necessary behavioral adjuncts.

The pharmaceutical agents approved by the U.S. Food and Drug Administration (FDA) for adjuvant use in weight reduction, with close medical supervision, are sibutramine (1 year; longer at physician discretion), orlistat (unrestricted long term), phentermine (limited to 3 months), and diethylpropion, benzphetamine, and phendimetrazine (short term).

BARIATRIC SURGERY

Several highly successful gastrointestinal surgical procedures exist for the management of obese patients with a BMI above 35. These procedures are either *restrictive,* reducing bowel lumen circumference (e.g., lap-band procedure), or *bypass,* usually circumventing stomach and upper small bowel (e.g., Roux-en-Y gastric bypass). Results in patients with T2DM with BMI above 35 undergoing bariatric surgery are extremely promising. Eighty-three percent of patients undergoing gastric bypass surgery exhibit resolution of their diabetes, and 86% show resolution at 5 years. Patients having the gastric banding procedure have 64% resolution at 1 year. Resolution involves up to a threefold reduction in mortality, reduced HbA_{1c}, normal FPG, improvement in insulin sensitivity and action, improvement in glucose tolerance, and cessation of antihyperglycemic agents. Obviously, significant

---

*Body mass index (BMI) = weight (kg)/height (m²)

risks exist with these surgical procedures, but in well-selected patients, this approach to treating *diabesity* is gaining momentum.

EXERCISE THERAPY

As with nutrition and weight management, physical activity is recognized as a specific therapy for patients with diabetes and is an independent risk factor for death. Benefits, many independent of associated weight loss, include improvements in the sense of well being, blood pressure, endothelial function, insulin sensitivity, lipid profile (consistent reduction in VLDL), cardiorespiratory fitness, and glycemic control, with reduction in HbA$_{1c}$.

Notably, exercise itself, unless extreme, will not contribute to significant weight loss, but will, however, help in weight maintenance and prevention of weight gain. Ideally, this regimen involves moderate aerobic exercise (e.g., walking) for 60 to 90 min/day or vigorous exercise for 35 min/day. (Specifically, the USDA advocates that everyone should be physically active for at least 30 minutes most days of the week; 60 min/day of physical activity to prevent weight gain; 60 to 90 min/day of physical activity to sustain weight loss.) Resistance exercises do not burn as many calories as an equivalent time of aerobic exercise, and how effective this form of exercise is compared with aerobic exercise is unknown at present. Physical activity can be measured by duration, distance, and intensity. Using a pedometer, recommendations are that 8,000 to 10,000 steps/day are necessary for weight maintenance. Medical evaluation is advised to determine the target level of fitness and appropriate exercise based on the presence and degree of microvascular and/or cardiovascular complications. Blood glucose levels should be measured before any exercise activity is initiated. Exercise should not be undertaken in patients with FPG greater than 250 mg/dL (13.8 mmol/L) with ketones or greater than 300 mg/dL (16.6 mmol/L) without ketones, because this may paradoxically precipitate DKA. If FPG is less than 100 mg/dL (5.5 mmol/L), exercise may result in hypoglycemia, and carbohydrate should be consumed in advance. With the initiation of an exercise program, SMBG should be performed every 30 minutes during exercise lasting longer than 30 to 45 minutes; glucose or carbohydrate may need to be consumed, depending on glucose levels.

TIGHT CONTROL

With few exceptions, the aim of achieving euglycemia, or *tight control* (see Table 68–6, "Goal" column) in all patients with diabetes is now supported by several large studies. In patients with T1DM, when compared with patients receiving standard care, intensive treatment prevented or slowed the onset and/or progression of the microvascular complications of diabetes: retinopathy by 76%, neuropathy by 60%, and proteinuria by 54%. The threefold increase in the incidence of significant hypoglycemia should not deter attempts to achieve euglycemia. In patients with T2DM, an overall reduction in microvascular complications of 25% occurs with tight control. Tight glycemic control in several other studies has been associated with statistically significant reductions in cardiovascular morbidity and mortality.

A continuum of risk of complications and the level of glycemia exists, with no glycemic threshold for complications within or above the normal glucose range. Every percentage point reduction in HbA$_{1c}$ is associated with a 40% reduction in the risk of complications in patients with T1DM and a 35% reduction in patients with T2DM. A target HbA$_{1c}$ value of less than 6.5% is recommended. Pregnant women with diabetes should aim for an HbA$_{1c}$ value of 6%. Tight control of blood pressure significantly reduces the incidence of stroke, heart failure, microvascular complications, loss of vision, and diabetes-related deaths, supporting the aggressive treatment of even mild to moderate hypertension in patients with diabetes in an attempt to reduce blood pressure to less than 130/80 mmHg (or 125/75 mmHg in patients with renal insufficiency and proteinuria >1 g/24-hr period). The reduction in microvascular complications with improved blood pressure control is independent of glycemic control.

Achieving tight control through intensive therapy of all metabolic derangements, and co-morbidities, including blood pressure and serum lipids, requires regular, close follow-up with a comprehensive diabetes health care team. In patients with T1DM, the use of multiple daily insulin injections or the use of a programmable insulin infusion pump (continuous subcutaneous insulin infusion [CSII]) is necessary to achieve glycemic control. In patients with T2DM, exercise, medical nutrition therapy, weight reduction, and combination oral antihyperglycemic agents may suffice, although failure to achieve glucose targets necessitates the use of insulin in combination with oral agents or alone (~58% of patients). This regimen should be started sooner rather than later. Seventy-six percent of all patients taking insulin have T2DM. In women with gestational diabetes, when proper diet and exercise fail to achieve acceptable blood glucose control, insulin is required. Until recently, oral antihyperglycemic agents have been contraindicated in pregnancy. New data suggest that use of metformin in women with gestational diabetes is safe and effective. Insulin may be required temporarily in some patients during serious infections or surgery. CSII reduces the frequency and severity of hypoglycemia, especially nocturnal, and allows greater freedom of lifestyle (with exclusion of fixed mealtimes), and its use is equally applicable in patients with T2DM.

Normalization of FPG has been the focus of tight control. Studies now confirm that elevated PCG levels are associated with increased cardiovascular morbidity and mortality, and all-cause mortality in patients with T2DM, and may have greater predictive power than FPG levels. Correction of PCG values may reduce cardiovascular disease and mortality in these patients. Several therapies specifically target PPG and include the rapid-acting insulin analogues (lispro, aspart, glulisine), meglitinides, D-phenylalanine derivatives, α-glucosidase inhibitors, and dietary fiber. The availability of continuous glucose monitoring facilitates continuous correction of blood glucose levels through a *closed-loop glucose sensing and insulin infusion system*.

Tight control may be inappropriate in infants and children under 13 years of age (no long-term studies have been conducted), in patients with a shortened life expectancy, severe cardiovascular disease (in whom hypoglycemia may be deleterious), end-stage microvascular disease, or minimal complications of diabetes after 20 to 25 years, and

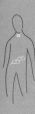

in those with recurrent hypoglycemia and/or hypoglycemia unawareness.

It is now well-established that tight control of blood glucose, by means of intensive insulin infusion therapy, in patients with hyperglycemia undergoing surgery, or in intensive care units, significantly reduces morbidity (e.g., wound infections, time on ventilator) and mortality by 30% to 50%, as well as reducing length of hospital stay. This benefit of blood glucose control in acute situations is not limited to people with diabetes; it has also been documented in all patients with stress-induced hyperglycemia who do not have diabetes or in people not previously known to have diabetes (newly discovered diabetes).

TYPE 1 DIABETES

Prevention of T1DM, using immune modulation, in people at high risk or in newly diagnosed patients is not yet possible.

Patients with T1DM have an absolute requirement of *insulin* for survival. This requirement also applies to patients with diabetes resulting from total or near-total β-cell depletion, as in chronic pancreatitis. Most insulin preparations are manufactured enzymatically or by recombinant DNA technology (including insulin analogues), and most are available at a concentration of 100 U/mL (U-100). Based on pharmacodynamic properties, the types of insulins currently available are rapid-acting (ultrashort), short-acting (regular), intermediate-acting, and long-acting preparations (Table 68–7). Insulin therapy is usually started in the outpatient setting unless DKA is the initial presentation. Multiple different insulin regimens exist.

Standard insulin therapy consists of one to two injections per day using intermediate- or long-acting insulin with or without short- or rapid-acting insulin. This approach provides simplicity, relative safety, and ease of compliance. Premixed insulins such as 70/30 (70% neutral protamine Hagedorn [NPH]/30% regular), 75/25 (75% neutral protamine lispro [NPL]/25% lispro or aspart or glulisine), or 50/50 (50% NPH/50% regular), usually administered twice daily, provide ease of use but are less likely to achieve good glycemic control. A split or mixed regimen of NPH/regular or NPL/lispro (or aspart or glulisine) twice daily (two thirds of the calculated total daily dose before breakfast and one third before dinner; at each time two-thirds NPH or NPL and one-third regular or lispro or aspart or glulisine) dictates regular mealtimes and insulin injections.

Intensive insulin therapy refers to multiple (three or more) daily injections or CSII. Multiple-injection regimens include use of regular or rapid-acting insulins three times daily (adjusted before meals) in combination with NPH twice daily or at bedtime or glargine insulin once daily at bedtime. By approximating normal physiologic timing of insulin delivery, patients are able to achieve better glycemic control and improve lifestyle flexibility. NPH should be given at least 30 minutes before a meal and can be mixed with regular insulin in the same syringe. Relatively *peakless,* long-acting, once-daily glargine should be administered at the same time each day and should not be mixed with other insulins.

Three new insulin formulations have been developed for patients with types 1 and 2 diabetes.

Glulisine

Glulisine is s rapid-acting, recombinant DNA–derived human insulin with a similar pharmacodynamic profile to insulin lispro. It should be injected no longer than 15 minutes before a meal or within 20 minutes of starting a meal.

Detemir

The recombinant DNA insulin analogue, detemir, is another very–long-acting insulin preparation that can be subcutaneously injected once (with evening meal or at bedtime) or twice daily (12 hours after the morning dose), providing a *peakless* basal insulin. This level is achieved through albumin binding subcutaneously and in the circulation. Detemir may be used alone, with oral antihyperglycemic agents, or in combination with mealtime insulins, and is associated with little weight gain.

Exubera

Exubera is a recombinant human inhaled insulin powder. It is taken before meals and appears to achieve blood glucose levels comparable to levels achieved with injected insulins. The bioavailability is only approximately 10% of subcutaneus administered insulin, with losses of insulin caused by deposition in the administration device, mouth, and throat, with 30% to 50% of the insulin deposited in the lungs being absorbed. This inhaled insulin is better than regular insulin in reducing postprandial glucose values and causes less weight gain. Inhaled insulin has been demonstrated to produce a decline in lung function in some patients that may be reversible. The limitations that certain lung pathologies will place on the effective use of inhaled insulin remains to be determined. The efficacy of inhaled insulin in people with chronic lung disease or those exposed to second-hand smoke is not fully appreciated. Studies indicate that chronic smokers absorb more of this insulin than nonsmokers. This may increase the risk of hypoglycemia. Inhaled insulin use may cause or exacerbate asthma and is contraindicated in people with chronic obstructive pulmonary disease, emphysema, and most respiratory disorders. Use of Exubera is contraindicated in smokers and patients who have stopped smoking for less than 6 months. Use in patients under the age of 18 years is also contraindicated because no clinical trials examining its use have been conducted in this patient population. Lung function testing is advocated in all patients before use of Exubera. Side effects include allergic reactions, cough, dry mouth, and chest discomfort. Exubera is approved for use in types 1 and 2 diabetes and is supplied as 1-mg and 3-mg dose *blisters.* It should be administered 10 minutes before a meal.

Calculating insulin doses is still somewhat empirical but may be improved through carbohydrate counting and calculation of insulin-to-carbohydrate ratios and insulin sensitivity. Starting doses of insulin vary from 0.15 to 0.5 U/kg/day, depending on patient size and degree of glycemia, and may be as high as 1.5 U/kg in patients with severe insulin resistance (commonly patients with T2DM). The calculated total daily insulin requirement is then divided according to the administration regimen chosen. In general, 40% to 50% of the total daily dose provides basal requirements, and the remainder is divided between meals in a

Table 68–7 Types of Insulin

Insulin Type	Generic Name	Preprandial Injection Timing* (hr)	Onset* (hr)	Peak* (hr)	Duration* (hr)	Blood Glucose (BG) Nadir* (hr)
Rapid-acting	Lispro†	0–0.2	0.1–0.5	0.5–2	<5	2–4
	Aspart‡	0–0.2	0.1–0.3	0.6–3	3–5	1–3
	Glulisine*	0–0.25 (15 min before a meal or within 20 min of starting a meal)	0.15–0.3	0.5–1.5	1–5.3	2–4
Short-acting	Regular	0.5–(1)	0.3–1	2–6	4–8	3–7
Intermediate-acting	Lente	0.5–(1)	1–2	4–12	(≤16)	Before next meal
	NPH	0.5–(1)	1–3	6–15	16–26	6–13
Long-acting	Ultralente	0.5–(1)	4–6	8–30	24–36	10–28
	Glargine§	‖Once daily; evening meal or bedtime: twice daily; 12 hourly	1.1–4	No peak	10.8–>24	Before next dose
	Detemir	‖Once daily; evening meal or bedtime: twice daily; 12 hourly	1.1–4	No peak	12–24	Before next dose
Human Premixed						
NPH/regular	70/30	0.5–(1)	0.5–1	2–12	14–24	3–12
NPH/regular	50/50	0.5–(1)	0.5–1	2–5	14–24	3–12
Insulin Analog Premixed						
Lispro protamine/ lispro	75/25	0.25	0.15–0.25	1	14–24	—
Aspart protamine/ aspart	70/30	0.25	0.15–0.3	2–4	24	—
Inhaled insulin	Exubera	0–0.2	~0.1–0.5	~0.5–2	~3–5	—

*Time profiles depend on several factors, including dose, anatomic site of injection, method (subcutaneous, intramuscular, or intravenous; above profiles are for subcutaneous injections), duration of diabetes, type of diabetes, degree of insulin resistance, level of physical activity, presence of obesity, and body temperature. Some time ranges are wide to include data from several separate studies. Preprandial injection timing depends on premeal BG values and insulin type. If BG is low, it may be necessary to inject insulin and eat immediately (carbohydrate portion of meal first). If BG is high, it may be necessary to delay meal after insulin injection and eat carbohydrate portion last.
†Insulin analogue with reversal of lysine and proline at positions 28 and 29 on the B chain of the insulin molecule.
‡Insulin analogue with substitution of aspartic acid for proline at position 28 on the B chain of the insulin molecule.
§Insulin analogue with substitution of glycine for asparagine at position 21 on the A chain and addition of two arginines to the carboxyl terminus of the B chain of the insulin molecule.
*Insulin analogue with substitution of lysine for asparagine at position 3 on the B chain and glutamic acid for lysine at position 29 on the B chain of the insulin molecule.
‖Administer at same time each day, unrelated to meals. Morning administration may result in greater glucose lowering and less nocturnal hypoglycemia. Do not mix glargine, detemir, or ultralente insulins with other insulins.
70/30 = 70% NPH, 30% regular or 70% NPL/30% aspart; 50/50 = 50% NPH, 50% regular; 75/25 = 75% NPL, 25% lispro; 70/30 = 70% NPA, 30% aspart; NPH = neutral protamine Hagedorn; NPL = neutral protamine lispro; NPA = neutral protamine aspart.

manner proportionate to the relative carbohydrate and lipid contents of the meal or using the approximate ratio of 0.8 to 1.2 U (insulin) to 10 g carbohydrate (slightly more at breakfast): for example, prebreakfast (rapid or regular insulin), 15% to 25%; prelunch (rapid-acting or regular insulin), 15%; and predinner (rapid-acting or regular insulin), 15% to 20%. Requirements are increased during intercurrent illness, pregnancy, and the adolescent growth spurt. On average, insulin dose adjustments are made every 2 to 3 days,

and increments can be by as much as 10% to 20% of the total daily dose. When blood glucose values rise to greater than 250 mg/dL, patients should check for ketones, which are readily detected in the urine.

Several factors may cause elevations of FPG. The *Somogyi effect* refers to rebound hyperglycemia that follows undetected hypoglycemia, commonly nocturnal, in the early hours of the morning. The elevated FPG in this situation is treated by decreasing the preceding evening dose of insulin

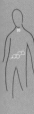

and/or by altering the timing of administration (from predinner to bedtime) and/or altering the type of insulin used, based on the expected time to maximal effect of the insulin. This approach reduces hypoglycemia and prevents the rebound. In the *dawn phenomenon,* the nocturnal secretion of growth hormone is responsible for a nighttime-to-morning rise in blood glucose. This condition is treated by increasing the evening dose of insulin and/or by altering the timing of administration and/or the type of insulin used. In both of these situations, meal composition and quantity should also be evaluated. Poor insulin injection technique is an extremely common reason for increasing insulin requirements or unexplained fluctuations in blood glucose values, despite adherence to a strict exercise and nutrition program. Rotating use of different anatomic sites for injection may be responsible for variable and erratic insulin absorption, and repeated injection into a single site leads to local *resistance* through lipohypertrophy and tissue fibrosis. Rotation of injection sites exclusively into the abdominal subcutaneous tissue is optimal.

TYPE 2 DIABETES

Prevention of T2DM has been achieved through *lifestyle changes* (healthy diet, weight reduction, and regular exercise) in people at high risk (e.g., IGT), with the incidence of T2DM reduced by as much as 58%, whereas the use of *metformin* reduced the incidence by only 31%.

The aim of treatment in T2DM is to reverse insulin resistance, control intestinal glucose absorption, normalize HGP, improve β-cell glucose sensing and insulin secretion, and ultimately prevent the occurrence of long-term complications. Provided that pharmacologic therapy is not required immediately (FPG >250 mg/dL), all newly diagnosed patients should be given at least a 1-month trial of diet, exercise, and weight management. If this regimen does not lead to adequate blood glucose control, the physician will need to prescribe oral or subcutaneous antihyperglycemic agents and/or insulin. After FPG is controlled, substituting a non-insulin agent in patients who were initiated on insulin may be possible. Maximal-dose sulfonylurea therapy has been used effectively as initial treatment in patients with marked hyperglycemia, with doses decreasing as control improves. The regimen of bedtime insulin, NPH, and daytime sulfonylurea therapy (bedtime insulin and daytime sulfonylurea [BIDS]) has been successful in patients with T2DM as regular therapy or as a transition stage from noninsulin antihyperglycemic therapy to total insulin therapy. Metformin could be substituted for the sulfonylurea in BIDS.

The eight classes of *noninsulin antidiabetic agents* currently available are listed in Table 68–8. The insulin secretagogues (sulfonylureas, meglitinides, and D-phenylalanine derivatives) have similar mechanisms of action and may cause hypoglycemia, hence the term *oral hypoglycemic agents.* The other classes of noninsulin agents each target a different pathologic process and are referred to as *antihyperglycemic agents.* T2DM is a progressive disease, and monotherapy is seldom permanently successful.

Combination drug therapy using submaximal doses of two or more agents, including insulin, each targeting a different metabolic abnormality, has synergistic effects that may be far greater than the effects of any agent used alone at maximal dose. The incidence and severity of adverse events are also reduced with combination therapy, and, in addition, improved compliance and, in many instances, a cost savings takes place. Although some physicians still use a stepped-care approach, many now initiate therapy with drugs from more than one class of antihyperglycemic agents, depending on the patient's profile and the predominant pathologic defects (see Table 68–8). Additional agents are added (not substituted) if adequate glycemic control is not achieved at 25% to 75% of the maximal dose. Only one agent from each class should be used in an individual patient at any one time. Regular blood glucose estimations allow timely increases in drug doses and the addition of other agents as necessary. Comprehensive combination therapy requires a multipronged approach to the treatment of hyperglycemia, dyslipidemia, obesity, hypertension, and the associated co-morbidities, with proactive preventive measures when appropriate.

Sulfonylureas

For many years, the only class of oral hypoglycemic (antihyperglycemic) agents available has as its principal action the stimulation of endogenous insulin secretion from the pancreatic β cells. The drugs in this class also increase β-cell sensitivity to glucose and exert some influence in diminishing insulin resistance. These agents have vasoconstrictive properties, raise blood pressure (chlorpropamide), prevent ischemic preconditioning in the heart, and increase plasma levels of PAI-1. The drugs differ in potency, time of onset, duration of action, plasma protein binding, absorption characteristics, and route of metabolism and excretion, and some involve novel delivery systems. At maximal dose, these drugs are all equally effective (except tolbutamide) in lowering blood glucose levels. Primary failure to respond to sulfonylureas occurs in 20% to 25% of patients. Secondary failure occurs at the rate of 10% to 15% per year, in part because of progressive β-cell failure and insulin resistance and in part because of poor patient compliance. Replacing one agent with another in this class is unlikely to produce a substantially different effect and is not recommended unless for reasons of patient compliance. The risk of hypoglycemia, the major adverse effect, increases with increasing patient age, use of a preparation with a long half-life (e.g., chlorpropamide), and renal dysfunction. Weight gain is also a recognized side effect. Characteristics of patients best suited for sulfonylurea therapy include diagnosis at greater than 30 years of age, disease presence for less than 5 years, residual β-cell function, relative lack of obesity, and FPG less than 300 mg/dL (see Table 68–8).

Biguanides (Metformin)

The major mechanism of action of this insulin sensitizer is in reducing HGP by inhibiting gluconeogenesis. This drug also increases anaerobic glycolysis with resultant increased lactate production, enhances glucose uptake and utilization by muscle, and decreases intestinal glucose absorption. In addition to its glucose-lowering effect, this drug is associated with weight loss (5 to 10 lb), possibly related to mild nausea and anorexia, a decrease in plasma insulin levels, and significant lipid-lowering effects (decreasing total cholesterol, LDL, and triglyceride by 10% to 20% and increasing HDL). Metformin improves endothelial function, lowers PAI-1 levels, and reduces cardiovascular events. It is well suited for use in obese, hyperlipidemic patients with T2DM.

Metformin's use in patients with IGT and the metabolic syndrome, as prophylaxis against development of diabetes, has proved successful. Primary failure rates are approximately 12%, and secondary failure rates are between 5% and 10%. Strong evidence-based support can be found for using metformin as initial therapy, especially in overweight or obese individuals, and often in combination with an agent or agents from another class.

Major adverse effects are gastrointestinal and metabolic. Gastrointestinal side effects include metallic taste, anorexia, nausea, abdominal discomfort, and diarrhea; these are usually mild and transient and improve with temporary reduction in dose and administration with meals. The major metabolic side effect is lactic acidosis, which occurs most often in patients with renal disease (creatinine ≥1.5 mg/dL in men and ≥1.4 mg/dL in women), low cardiac output, impaired hepatic function, excessive alcohol intake, or concomitant use of radiographic contrast.

α-Glucosidase Inhibitors (Acarbose and Miglitol)

Within the small bowel lumen, α-glucosidase inhibitors competitively inhibit the breakdown of complex carbohydrates by antagonizing pancreatic α-amylase and the microvillar brush border α-glucosidase enzymes, thereby delaying glucose absorption and dampening the PPG (and insulin) peaks, with modest effect on FPG levels. When acarbose is taken with the first bite of a carbohydrate-containing meal, only 1% to 2% of the drug is absorbed. Major common side effects are gastrointestinal, including bloating, abdominal discomfort, diarrhea, and flatulence. These effects occur at the initiation of therapy and/or with dose increases, but they commonly disappear with continued use. The side effects can be minimized by starting with a low dose (12.5 to 25.0 mg once daily) and increasing it gradually over several weeks to a maintenance dose of 50 to 100 mg three times daily, depending on the patient's body weight (see Table 68–8). These agents do not cause hypoglycemia when used alone, but hypoglycemia may occur when they are used in combination with insulin, a sulfonylurea, a meglitinide, or a D-phenylalanine derivative. Oral treatment of hypoglycemia during therapy with these agents requires administration of pure glucose, fructose, or lactose (not sucrose, maltose, or starch).

Thiazolidinediones (Rosiglitazone and Pioglitazone)

Thiazolidinediones, which are peroxisome proliferator activated receptor-γ (PPAR-γ) agonists, reduce insulin resistance, improve the peripheral action of insulin (insulin sensitizers), and reduce hyperglycemia by increasing glucose uptake and utilization in peripheral tissues and reducing HGP. These agents increase the differentiation of preadipocytes to adipocytes and may cause an increase in total body fat mass, with remodeling (increased number of small, insulin-sensitive adipocytes) and redistribution (visceral to subcutaneous) of body fat. Improvements in serum lipids (decrease in TGs and FFAs, increase in HDL, and increase in large buoyant LDL [LDL$_1$]) depend on each particular agent and may occur via nuclear-PPAR-γ activation. Thiazolidinediones have little effect in the presence of euglycemia and thus tend not to produce hypoglycemia when used as monotherapy. They bind to PPAR-γ to induce transcription of several genes involved in glucose and lipid metabolism. Because of their mechanism of action on receptors in the cell nucleus, 3 to 4 weeks may be required to produce a clinical effect and 10 to 12 weeks for a full effect. Dosage adjustments should therefore only be made every 3 months.

Activation of PPAR-γ, found predominantly in fat, results in a decrease in FFAs and an increase in insulin sensitivity and glucose uptake, resulting in lowering of plasma glucose levels. Activation of PPAR-α, in liver and muscle, lowers plasma TG levels and raises HDL levels by stimulating fatty acid oxidation and lowering apolipoprotein (apo) CIII and apo AI. In addition to their glucose-lowering properties, their actions include anti-inflammatory effects (especially on the vasculature, with reduction in macrophage migration, macrophage foam cell formation, IL-6, highly sensitive C-reactive protein [hs-CRP], monocyte chemotactic protein-1, and white blood cell count), mild blood pressure reduction, increased thrombolysis (reduction in PAI-1 activity, as well as antigen levels), reduced vascular smooth muscle proliferation (improvement in carotid intima medial wall thickness [IMT], a useful index for monitoring atherosclerosis progress), improved endothelial function and vascular activity, reduced urinary albumin excretion, and preservation of β-cell function (partly through a reduction in the rate of β-cell apoptosis). These agents increase adipose-derived adiponectin levels, thereby enhancing liver and muscle insulin sensitivity and fat oxidation and inhibiting endothelial inflammation. The anti-inflammatory action helps restore insulin sensitivity and reverse the atherosclerotic process. Restoration of endothelial integrity is demonstrated by improvement in endothelium mediated brachial vasodilation.

Severity of cardiovascular disease is often assessed by determination of IMT, as already mentioned. Some of the therapies used in the management of diabetes are responsible for a reduction in IMT and may in fact act synergistically, namely exercise, thiazolidinediones, and hydroxymethylglutaryl–coenzyme A (HMG-CoA) reductase inhibitors. These agents may also improve cardiovascular risk markers.

Pioglitazone, when part of standard therapy, has been shown to reduce the combined risk of heart attacks, strokes, and death by 16% in high-risk patients with T2DM.

Thiazolidinediones (TZD) do not have to be taken with food. Combination with insulin therapy may facilitate a reduction in insulin dose or even its discontinuation. A 25% primary failure rate is probably caused by inappropriate use in patients with minimal endogenous insulin secretion. Rosiglitazone may be given as monotherapy or in combination with metformin or a sulfonylurea. Pioglitazone may be used as monotherapy or with insulin, sulfonylureas, or metformin. Side effects include dilutional anemia, edema, and mild weight gain. These drugs should be used with caution in patients at risk for heart failure. Hypoglycemia is a risk when these drugs are used in combination with oral hypoglycemia agents, amylin, or incretin mimetics. Therapy with this class of drugs should be initiated early while reasonable β-cell function still exists.

Although pioglitazone and rosiglitazone do not appear to cause liver dysfunction, as did their predecessor troglitazone, the FDA recommends that therapy with TZDs should not be initiated if the alanine aminotransferase level is greater than

Table 68–8 Noninsulin Antidiabetic Agents

	Sulfonylureas	Biguanides	α-Glucosidase Inhibitors	Thiazolidinediones	Meglitinides	D-Phenyl Alanine Derivatives
Generic name	Glimepiride	Metformin	Acarbose	Rosiglitazone	Repaglinide	Nateglinide
	Glyburide: micronised, nonmicronised. Glipizide, glipizide XL Chlorpropamide Tolbutamide	Metformin XR	Miglitol	Pioglitazone		
Mode of action	↑↑ Pancreatic insulin secretion chronically ↑ Tissue insulin sensitivity	↓↓ HGP ↓ peripheral IR ↓ intestinal glucose absorption	Delays PP digestion of carbohydrates and absorption of glucose leading to ↓↓ PP hyperglycemia	↓↓ Peripheral IR ↑↑ Glucose disposal ↓ HGP	↑↑ Pancreatic insulin secretion acutely	↑↑ Pancreatic insulin secretion acutely
Preferred patient type	Diagnosis age >30 yr, lean, diabetes >5 yr, insulinopenic	Overweight, IR, fasting hyperglycemia, dyslipidemia	PP hyperglycemia	Overweight, IR, dyslipidemia, renal dysfunction	PP hyperglycemia, insulinopenic	PP hyperglycemia insulinopenic

Therapeutic Effects

	Sulfonylureas	Biguanides	α-Glucosidase Inhibitors	Thiazolidinediones	Meglitinides	D-Phenyl Alanine Derivatives
↓ HbA$_{1c}$[†] (%)	1–2	1–2	0.5–1	0.8–1.6 (2.6 with 45 mg pioglitazone monotherapy, in newly diagnosed)	1–2	1–2
↓ FPG* (mg/dL)	50–70	50–80	15–30	25–50	40–80	40–80
↓ PPG* (mg/dL)	~90	80	40–50	—	30	30
Insulin levels	↑	—	—	—	↑	↑
Weight	↑	↓	—	↑	↑	↑
Lipids		↓ LDL ↓↓ TG	↓ TG	LDL$_3$, TC (rosi) ↓↓ TG (pio) ↑ HDL (both)		

DPP-4 Inhibitors	Amylin Mimetics	Incretin Mimetics	Combination Preparations			
Sitagliptin phosphate	Pramlintide	Exenatide (GLP-1 agonist)	Glyburide/ metformin	Glipizide/ metformin	Rosiglitazone/ metformin	Rosiglitazone/ glimepiride
Inhibits DPP-4 resulting in ↑ levels of incretins (GLP-1, GIP)	↓ Glycemic surges ↓ PP glucagon secretion ↓ TG fluxes Delays gastric emptying Inhibits ghrelin	↑ Glucose dependent pancreatic β-cell insulin synthesis and secretion ↓ Glucagon secretion Restores first phase insulin release ↓ FPG ↓ Gastric emptying ↓ PPG β-cell preservation (induction of β-cell neogenesis → Anti-apoptosis →↑ β-cell mass)	As for individual agents	As for individual agents	As for individual agents	As for individual agents
In combination with diet and exercise, metformin or TZD	Insulin-treated DM (as adjunctive therapy) wide glycemic fluctuations, insulin resistant, predominant PPG, obese	Advanced T2DM Obese Inadequate response to metformin and/or sulfonylurea Adjunct to oral medications				
0.6–1.4	0.6–0.9	0.8–1.3				
25	–	14–25 (at 1 year)	1.5	2.1	1.2	1.6
51	↓	63–71				
↑	↓	↓				
	↓	↓				
	↓ TG					

Table 68–8   **Noninsulin Antidiabetic Agents—Cont'd**

	Sulfonylureas	**Biguanides**	**α-Glucosidase Inhibitors**	**Thiazolidinediones**	**Meglitinides**	**D-Phenyl Alanine Derivatives**
Side effects	Hypoglycemia, weight gain, GI side effects	Diarrhea, abdominal discomfort, lactic acidosis Contraindicated: Cr >1.5 mg/dL (men), >1.4 mg/dL (women), hepatic disease, CHF, alcoholism	Abdominal pain, bloating, flatulence, diarrhea. Contraindicated: inflammatory bowel disease, bowel obstruction, cirrhosis Cr >2.0 mg/dL	Edema, anemia, weight gain. Contraindicated: ALT > 2.5 upper limit of normal, NYHA class 3 or 4, hepatic disease, alcoholism	Hypoglycemia (low risk), caution if moderate /severe liver disease, slight weight gain	Hypoglycemia (low risk), caution if moderate/ severe liver disease
Route of administration	Oral	Oral	Oral	Oral	Oral	Oral
Dose(s)/day	1–3	2–3	1–3	1–2	1–4+	1–4+
Maximum daily Dose (mg)	Depends on agent	2550	150 (>60 kg BW) 300 (>60 kg BW)	45 (pioglitazone) 8 (rosiglitazone)	16	360
Range/dose (mg)	Depends on agent	500–1000	25–50 (>60 kg BW) 25–100 (>60 kg BW), slow titration of dose	15–45 (pioglitazone) 4–8 (rosiglitazone)	0.5–4	60–120
Optimal administration time	~30 min premeal (some with food, others on empty stomach)	With meal	With first bite of meal	With/without meal (breakfast)	Preferably <15 min premeal; (omit if no meal)	Preferably <15 min premeal (omit if no meal)
Main site of metabolism/ excretion	Hepatic/renal, fecal	Not metabolized/ renal excretion	2% of acarbose absorbed/fecal, 50–100% of migitol absorbed/not metabolized/ renal	Hepatic/fecal	Hepatic/fecal, renal	Renal 80%, hepatic/fecal 10%

*Not yet FDA approved
†Values combined from numerous studies; values are also dose dependent.
↑ = increased; ↓ = decreased; — = unchanged; ALT = alanine aminotransferase; BW = body weight; CHF = congestive heart failure; CHO = carbohydrate; Cr = creatinine; DKA = diabetic ketoacidosis; FPG = fasting plasma glucose; GLP-1 = glucagon-like peptide-1; HbA$_{1c}$ = glycosylated hemoglobin; HDL = high-density lipoprotein; HGP = hepatic glucose production; IR = insulin resistance; LDL = low-density lipoprotein; LDL$_3$ = large buoyant LDL; NYHA = New York Heart Association; PP = postprandial; PPAR = peroxisome proliferator activated receptor; PPG = postprandial plasma glucose; T1DM = type 1 diabetes mellitus; T2DM = type 1 diabetes mellitus; TG = triglyceride.
XR,XL = extended release.

DPP-4 Inhibitors	Amylin Mimetics	Incretin Mimetics	Combination Preparations			
Nasopharyngitis Upper respiratory tract infections Headache	Nausea, headache, anorexia, early satiety, weight loss (↓ calorie intake; ↓ fat, protein, CHO), vomiting, indigestion, abdominal pain, tiredness, dizziness, hypoglycemia (in combination with insulin and/or sulfonylurea) More common in T1DM	Nausea, vomiting, diarrhea, headache, dose dependent anorexia, ↓ food intake, weight loss Hypoglycemia when in combination with sulfonylurea (dose dependent) DO NOT use in T1DM or DKA	As for individual agents (may be reduced because of lower individual component doses)	As for individual agents (may be reduced because of lower individual component doses)	As for individual agents (may be reduced because of lower individual component doses)	As for individual agents (may be reduced because of lower individual component doses)
Oral	Subcutaneous injection (abdomen, thigh)	Subcutaneous injection (abdomen, thigh, arm)				
1	1–3	1–2	1–2	2	2	1
100	Type 1 (180 mcg) Type 2 (360 mcg)	10 mcg	20/2000	20/2000	8/2000	8/8
25–100 dependent on renal function	Type 1 (15–60 mcg) Type 2 (60–120 mcg)	5–10 mcg (start with 5 mcg; ↑ to 10 mcg after 1 month if necessary)	1.25/250–20/2000	2.5/250–20/2000	1/500–8/2000	4/1–8/8
Daily with or without food	Immediately prior to major meals (≥ 250 cal or ≥30 g CHO) Do not mix with insulin Halve dose of rapid/short-acting or fixed-mixed insulin	Within 60 min of breakfast and dinner	With meals	With meals	With meals	With first meal of the day
	Renal	Renal excretion (proteolytic degradation)	As for individual agents	As for individual agents	As for individual agents	As for individual agents

2.5 times the upper limit of normal. Patients should have liver function tests performed every 2 months for the first year and periodically thereafter. No restrictions in renal insufficiency are recommended.

DIPEPTIDYL PEPTIDASE-4 (DPP-4) INHIBITORS

DPP-4 inhibitors selectively (no effect on DPP-8 or DPP-9) and reversibly block GLP-1 and other incretin degradation, thereby prolonging the activity of natural incretins. They increase insulin synthesis and release, while suppressing the release of glucagon in a glucose dependent manner, lowering the potential for hypoglycemia. In patients with T2DM there is an improvement in β-cell function and insulin sensitivity.

Meglitinides (Repaglinide) and D-phenylalanine Derivatives (Nateglinide)

The mechanism of action of meglitinides and D-phenylalanine derivatives is similar to that of the sulfonylureas in stimulating insulin secretion from the pancreas. The advantages of these classes over the sulfonylureas are the rapid onset and short duration of action, which suppress postprandial hyperglycemia. They should be taken with meals and omitted in the absence of a meal, a feature that permits flexibility of lifestyle. The stimulation of prandial insulin secretion avoids chronic stimulation of β cells and results in reduced between-meal and nocturnal hyperinsulinemia, a feature of sulfonylurea therapy. The insulin secretagogue action is glucose dependent, sensitizing β cells to secrete more insulin in response to elevated glucose levels. For this reason, hypoglycemia is seen less often than with sulfonylureas. Clinical response to these agents is seen within approximately 1 week. These drugs may be prescribed in the presence of renal dysfunction. Combination therapy of a sulfonylurea with either of these agents is not FDA approved.

Combination Preparations of Antihyperglycemic Agents

Increasingly, pharmaceutical companies are manufacturing combinations of oral agents (e.g., glyburide and metformin, glipizide and metformin, rosiglitazone and metformin, rosiglitazone and glimepiride), which, although in fixed doses, may help improve patient compliance when faced with increasing numbers of drugs to swallow each day (see Table 68–8). Combination therapy, while promoting synergistic effects, also allows for lower doses of each agent with a reduced risk of side effects.

To enhance patient compliance, certain oral agents are formulated as long-acting or slow, or extended-release preparations (e.g., glipizide XL, metformin XR) and in solution (e.g., metformin) for children.

Currently available antihyperglycemic therapeutic agents, other than insulin, each treat separate metabolic problems in patients with diabetes. Combinations of these drugs target some of the functions in the spectrum performed by insulin. Current research is directed at manipulating endogenous compounds to produce agents able to approximate normal physiologic homeostatic control of hyperglycemia as closely as possible.

Incretin Mimetics

Incretin mimetics constitute a novel class of antidiabetic agents that mimic the actions of naturally occurring incretins (gut hormones) involved in the enteroinsular axis. The importance of this class of hormones with respect to plasma glucose levels following food ingestion is noted in the *incretin effect:* a greater insulin secretory response after similar increases in plasma glucose concentrations following oral, compared with intravenous, routes of glucose administration. The hormones GLP-1 (accounting for 70% to 80% of the insulin effect), GLP-2, and the gastric inhibitory peptide GIP are secreted from the small intestine (GLP-1 from enteroendocrine L cells of the distal ileum, GIP from enteroendocrine K cells of the proximal jejunum) following nutrient ingestion. Serum GLP-1 levels are generally lower in people with diabetes compared with those without. GLP-1 regulates blood glucose through several mechanisms: enhancing glucose dependent pancreatic β-cell insulin secretion with subsequent promotion of insulin-mediated tissue glucose uptake, inhibition of glucagon secretion from pancreatic α cells, during hyperglycemia or the fed state (leading to reduced HGP, insulin requirements, and PPG excursions), restoration of first-phase insulin release (lost early in T2DM), increased second-phase insulin secretion, insulin-sensitizing effect, and delayed gastric emptying (limiting PPG excursions). GLP-1 also protects and preserves β cells from damage by FFAs and cytokines. It does not impair the glucagon response to hypoglycemia. Other effects include depressed appetite and increased satiety, resulting in reduced food intake with subsequent weight loss. Prevention of pancreatic β-cell deterioration (a central feature of T2DM) and expansion of β cells (increasing β-cell mass) involves regeneration through proliferation and differentiation, neogenesis, and anti-apoptosis of β cells by GLP-1.

The incretin mimetic available at present is exenatide (structurally identical to exendin-4, derived from the saliva of the Gila monster lizard), the naturally occurring GLP-1 analog. This preparation is resistant to inactivation. Used as an adjunct in T2DM when sulfonylureas and/or metformin do not adequately control blood glucose, exenatide is administered subcutaneously before breakfast and dinner (see Table 68–8). A long-acting GLP-1 analog, liraglutide, is currently in clinical trials. Compared with a sulfonylurea, this agent, given subcutaneously once daily, produced less hypoglycemia.

Amylin Mimetics

Amylin, a peptide hormone, is synthesized in pancreatic β cells and stored with insulin within secretory granules. It is cosecreted with insulin, in equimolar amounts, in response to nutrient stimuli. Biochemical characteristics are similar to insulin except that it is metabolized and excreted mainly by the kidneys. The main function of amylin is to control postprandial glucose levels through inhibition of postprandial glucagon secretion, with subsequent decreased HGP, delayed gastric emptying and thus carbohydrate absorption, and reduced food intake through centrally mediated early satiety.

Amylin also acts in an autocrine fashion to inhibit pancreatic β-cell insulin secretion.

With β-cell destruction (T1DM), or atrophy and *exhaustion* (T2DM), the secretion of insulin and amylin is absent and reduced, respectively.

Pramlintide, a stable analog of amylin, is approved for use in both T1DM and T2DM as adjunctive therapy. Concurrent insulin doses should be halved at the initiation of pramlintide therapy. In addition to dampening PPG peaks, pramlintide is also effective in reducing glucose fluctuations throughout the day. It is given subcutaneously and at lower doses in patients with T1DM than those with T2DM (see Table 68–8). Side effects include nausea, vomiting, and transient headaches. Hypoglycemia may result when used in combination with sulfonylureas.

TREATMENT OF THE METABOLIC SYNDROME

Lifestyle modification, including weight reduction and enhanced physical activity, are the most important aspects of treatment in this group of patients. Obviously, each of the dysmetabolic factors present needs to be managed in its own right. All treatments are greatly facilitated by weight reduction, a 10% weight loss being associated with major metabolic improvements. Useful adjunctive pharmacotherapy includes the insulin sensitizers, metformin, and TZDs, with beneficial elevation of adipose tissue–specific adiponectin.

Complications

ACUTE COMPLICATIONS

Hypoglycemia

Hypoglycemia is discussed in Chapter 69.

Lactic Acidosis

A rare event, lactic acidosis is discussed in Chapter 27.

Diabetic Ketoacidosis

Although DKA develops most commonly in patients with T1DM, it can be seen in patients with T2DM, especially during acute illness. DKA is defined as being present in patients with absolute or relative insulin deficiency when the following criteria are met:

1. *Hyperglycemia:* plasma glucose levels greater than 250 mg/dL
2. *Ketosis:* moderate to severe ketonemia (ketone levels positive at a serum dilution of ≥1:2, or serum β-hydroxybutyrate concentration >0.5 mmol/L) and moderate ketonuria (2+ to 3+ by the nitroprusside method). The nitroprusside reagent reacts primarily to acetoacetate and, to a lesser extent, acetone, but does not detect β-hydroxybutyrate. When lactic acidosis co-exists with DKA, there is a shift towards more β-hydroxybutyrate production, which decreases the reactivity with the nitroprusside reagent.

3. *Acidosis:* pH less than or equal to 7.3 and/or bicarbonate less than or equal to 15 mEq/L
Associated metabolic and plasma abnormalities include dehydration, increased osmolality (usually >320 mOsm/kg), increased anion gap (>12 mEq/L), increased serum amylase, elevated white blood cell count, and hypertriglyceridemia.

Precipitating factors for DKA are infection (30%), often minor (respiratory or urinary tract) new-onset diabetes (25%), problems with insulin administration (20%), *stress,* and many less frequent causes. Insulin deficiency and raised insulin counter-regulatory hormones result in increased HGP and decreased peripheral glucose utilization, leading to hyperglycemia and hyperosmolality with consequent osmotic diuresis, electrolyte loss (sodium, potassium, phosphate, magnesium, calcium, and chloride), and dehydration. Activation of insulin-sensitive lipase stimulates release of FFAs from adipose tissues, which are oxidized in the liver to produce ketone bodies. Diminished peripheral utilization of ketones during insulin deficiency results in ketosis and metabolic acidosis.

DKA develops within hours to days. The ill feeling associated with the metabolic acidosis leads patients to seek early medical attention, a feature that accounts for the lower levels of glucose and osmolality compared with those in hyperosmolar nonketotic syndrome (HNKS) (Table 68–9). DKA may not always be obvious at the time of presentation because early signs and symptoms are subtle. Symptoms include nausea, vomiting, thirst, polydipsia, polyuria, abdominal pain, weakness, fatigue, and anorexia. Signs include tachycardia, orthostatic hypotension, poor skin turgor, warm or dry skin and mucous membranes, hyperventilation or Kussmaul's respiration, hypothermia or normothermia, ketones on the breath, weight loss, and altered mental status or coma.

Initial assessment includes mental status, presence of gag or cough reflex, abdominal succussion splash (requiring a nasogastric tube), and urinary output. The search for a precipitating cause (e.g., infection or sepsis, myocardial infarction, pregnancy, cerebrovascular accident, trauma, psychosocial factor) is crucial, both to treating the underlying disorders and to facilitating resolution of the DKA. Baseline investigations should include plasma glucose, plasma acetone, serum electrolytes, serum lipid profile, serum amylase and lipase, full blood count with differential, arterial blood gas determination, blood cultures, culture of abscess or infected site, urine glucose and ketones, urine microscopy and culture, chest radiograph, abdominal radiograph (with abdominal pain), electrocardiogram, cardiac enzymes (if appropriate), lumbar puncture (if appropriate), serum osmolality, and anion gap.*

Most important in the therapy of DKA is the restoration of circulating plasma volume, with maintenance of cardiac output and renal function (**Web Table 68–4**). Intravenous fluid lowers blood glucose through serum dilution and

---

*Calculation of serum osmolality: $2[Na^+ \ (mEq/L)] + 2[K^+ \ (mEq/L)] + glucose \ (mg/dL)/18 + BUN \ (mg/dL)/2.8$; calculation of anion gap: $Na^+ - (Cl^- + HCO_3^-)$.

Table 68–9	The Hyperglycemic Crises: A Comparison of Diabetic Ketoacidosis and Hyperosmolar Nonketotic Syndrome	

Feature	Diabetic Ketoacidosis	Hyperosmolar Nonketotic Syndrome
Age of patient	Usually <40 yr	Usually >60 yr
Duration of symptoms	Usually <2 days	Usually >5 days
Plasma glucose	Usually <600 mg/dL	Usually >600 mg/dL
Serum sodium	Normal or low (130–140 mEq/L)	Normal or high (145–155 mEq/L)
Serum potassium	Normal or high (5–6 mEq/L)	Normal (4–5 mEq/L)
Serum bicarbonate	<15 mEq/L	>15 mEq/L
Ketone bodies	Positive at ≥1:2 dilution	Negative at 1:2 dilution
Ph	<7.35	>7.3
Serum osmolality	Usually <320 mOsm/kg	Usually >320 mOsm/kg
Fluid deficit	≤10% body weight	≤15% body weight
Cerebral edema	Subclinical asymptomatic, rare clinically	Very rare
Prognosis	3–10% mortality (>20% for people >65 yr)	10–20% mortality
Subsequent course	Insulin therapy required in most cases	Insulin therapy not usually required

enhanced urinary glucose loss, lowers osmolality and ketones, and improves the peripheral utilization of ketones and glucose. Insulin administration facilitates the peripheral uptake of ketones and glucose, thereby decreasing urinary glucose loss, and, significantly, inhibits hepatic glucose production. Electrolyte imbalances should be corrected concurrently with fluid and insulin replacement and treatment of the precipitating cause. To track the course of treatment, several parameters require regular monitoring:

1. Hourly: Vital signs (temperature, pulse rate, respiratory rate, blood pressure), mental status, fluid intake and output, plasma glucose, insulin infusion rate, arterial blood gases, electrocardiogram (initially, and if in the intensive care unit, preferably continuous monitoring)
2. Every 1 to 2 hours: Serum electrolytes (sodium, potassium, chloride, and bicarbonate), electrocardiogram until stable
3. Every 6 hours: Serum phosphate, magnesium, calcium, blood urea nitrogen, and creatinine

With correction of the metabolic abnormalities, the frequency of their measurements should be reduced appropriately. Weight should be measured initially and then daily. Note that ketones are only measured to help confirm the diagnosis of DKA and subsequently to establish its resolution. With changes in the ratios of the different serum ketones, the routine methods used to measure these may falsely suggest transient elevation in ketones. Tracking the decrease in the anion gap will provide information regarding control of DKA.

Hyperosmolar Nonketotic Syndrome (Hyperglycemic Hyperosmolar State)

HNKS occurs almost exclusively in patients with T2DM, who are usually elderly and physically impaired, with limited access to free water. The pathogenesis of HNKS is similar to that of DKA but may be distinguished from it by the more marked hyperglycemia, the relative absence of acidosis and ketonemia, and the greater degree of dehydration (see Table 68–9). Low FFA levels result in the absence of ketone bodies, with reduced nausea and vomiting. Increased lactic acid levels result from poor tissue perfusion and are more marked than in DKA. Insulin resistance is usually present, with normal or elevated levels of serum insulin. As many as 30% to 40% of patients over 65 years of age with HNKS may have previously undiagnosed diabetes. HNKS usually develops insidiously over days to weeks. Precipitating and/or complicating factors may include infection, intestinal obstruction, mesenteric thrombosis, pulmonary embolism, peritoneal dialysis, heat stroke, hypothermia, subdural hematoma, severe burns, and an extensive list of drugs. Some of these conditions may themselves result from the severe dehydration and poor tissue perfusion of HNKS.

Therapy of HNKS follows the same general principles as that of DKA, with particular emphasis on intravenous fluid therapy and potassium replacement. Fluid replacement should follow the same pattern as in DKA, but a greater total volume is usually required. Careful monitoring is necessary because patients often have cardiac and other co-morbid conditions. Restoration of the fluid deficit should proceed more slowly than in DKA, ideally over 36 to 72 hours. Insulin therapy should only be started after rehydration is in progress. These patients may be sensitive to insulin and may require reduced doses. In view of the severe dehydration and predisposition to vascular thrombosis, these patients should receive heparin (unfractionated or low molecular weight) prophylaxis (5000 U heparin subcutaneously, usually twice daily).

CHRONIC COMPLICATIONS

Chronic complications include microvascular complications (nephropathy, retinopathy, and neuropathy) and macrovascular or cardiovascular complications (hypertension, coronary artery disease, peripheral vascular disease, and cerebrovascular disease). Several different mechanisms are responsible for the development of chronic complications and include activation of the polyol pathway (with accumulation of sorbitol), formation of glycated proteins and advanced glycation end products (cross-linked glycated proteins), abnormalities in lipid metabolism, increased oxidative damage, hyperinsulinemia, hyperperfusion of certain tissues, hyperviscosity, platelet dysfunction (increased aggregation), endothelial dysfunction, and activation of various growth factors.

MICROVASCULAR COMPLICATIONS

The incidence of microvascular complications is significantly higher in patients with T1DM than in those with T2DM.

Nephropathy

Diabetic nephropathy is the most common cause of ESRD in developed countries (~30% of cases). Approximately 20% to 30% of people with T1DM and T2DM develop nephropathy, and the incidence increases with duration of diabetes. Fewer people with T2DM than with T1DM progress to ESRD (20% vs. 75%, respectively, after 20 years). Certain ethnic and racial groups have high prevalence rates of severe nephropathy (Native Americans, Mexican Americans, and African Americans).

Initially, increased glomerular filtration rate (GFR) and renal blood flow occur in all patients and are not associated with any histologic changes. This condition progresses to glomerular hypertrophy, renal enlargement, expansion of the mesangial matrix, and thickening of the glomerular basement membrane, resulting in glomerulosclerosis (**Web Figs. 68–2, 68–3, 68–4**). Subsequently, the GFR returns to normal, with an associated increase in intraglomerular pressure and the appearance of micro-albuminuria (20 to 200 mcg/min, 30 to 300 mg/24 hours) 10 to 15 years after the diagnosis of diabetes (present in 30% of middle-age patients with T1DM or T2DM). This *incipient* or *preclinical diabetic nephropathy* is followed by a decline in GFR as the albumin excretion rate increases.

Micro-albuminuria is a risk factor for cardiovascular events and is associated with a 10- to 20-fold increased risk of progression to diabetic nephropathy. Rigorous control of blood glucose and blood pressure (using angiotensin II-converting enzyme [ACE] inhibitors and/or angiotensin II-receptor blockers [ARBs]) or use of ACE inhibitors and/or ARBs in nonhypertensive patients with micro-albuminuria can prevent or even reverse the progression toward renal failure. β-Blockers and nondihydropyridine calcium-channel antagonists, effective in reducing cardiovascular events, may also be considered, as may thiazide diuretics.

By approximately 15 years after the onset of diabetes, macro-albuminuria (>200 mcg/min, >300 mg/24 hours; dipstick positive) is generally present. Continued blood pressure control is essential, and some dietary protein restriction (0.6 to 0.8 g/kg/day) is probably helpful, but meticulous blood glucose control is unlikely to prevent the inexorable progression of overt diabetic nephropathy to ESRD. The rate of decline in GFR, however, may be slowed, but not halted, by blood pressure and glucose control with protein restriction. Measurement of serum creatinine is an inaccurate guide to the degree of GFR impairment. Within 5 years of the appearance of macro-albuminuria, GFR will have declined by 50% in approximately 50% of patients; within a further 3 to 4 years, one half of these patients will have ESRD. Dialysis (hemo- or peritoneal) or renal transplantation is initiated when the GFR is less than 15 mL/min (serum creatinine ≥10 mg/dL) (see Chapter 27).

Screening for proteinuria should be performed annually in all patients, starting at the time of diagnosis in patients with T2DM and 5 years after the diagnosis in patients with T1DM. The simplest method of screening for micro-albuminuria is measurement of the ratio of protein (albumin) to creatinine in a random spot urine specimen. This measurement correlates closely with 24-hour urinary protein estimations.

Retinopathy

The presence and severity of diabetic retinopathy are related to age at diagnosis and the duration of diabetes; 100% of patients with T1DM and 60% to 80% of those with T2DM are affected by 20 years. Retinopathy is the most common cause of blindness in persons between the ages of 20 and 74 years in the developed world. Approximately 25% of patients with T2DM may already have evidence of retinopathy at the time of diagnosis. The incidence of this complication is increased in Mexican Americans and African Americans.

Diabetic retinopathy is a progressive condition of increasing severity, accelerated by poor glycemic control (**Web Fig. 68–5**). *Background,* or *nonproliferative, retinopathy* consists of increased capillary permeability, dilation of venules, and the presence of micro-aneurysms (focal, saccular, and fusiform dilations of capillary walls as sequelae of loss of supporting pericytes and ischemic occlusion of retinal capillaries). At this stage, hemorrhages deep in the retina appear as dots, whereas more superficial nerve fiber layer hemorrhages are linear or resemble flames or *blots.* Leakage of plasma through permeable and ischemic capillary walls leads to the formation of hard exudates as the water is reabsorbed, leaving behind deep, intraretinal yellow deposits of proteins and lipids. These deposits may be present at any stage of diabetic retinopathy. Collections of hard exudates in a circular pattern (*circinates*) reflect the presence of retinal edema that pushes these exudates peripherally. When these exudates surround the macula, they highlight macular edema (*maculopathy*), a sight-threatening condition requiring urgent attention.

Retinal venous occlusion results in beading, reduplication, and venous loops. *Intraretinal microvascular abnormalities,* which are abnormal dilated capillaries within the retina, result from widespread capillary occlusion. Superficial retinal microinfarcts result in hypoxic necrosis of retinal nerve fibers and appear as white, *cotton-wool spots* with irregular margins. These changes signify a worsening of the retinopathy into the *preproliferative stage.* The widespread retinal ischemia and hypoxia represented by these changes result in the release of several angiogenic growth factors, which lead to the development of new vessels (*neovascularization*) on the retina, optic disc, or iris (*rubeosis iridis*). Inhibitors of protein kinase C, which block the production of vascular endothelial growth factor, are potentially beneficial. This stage is referred to as *proliferative retinopathy* and is also characterized by scarring. The new vessels are extremely fragile, extending through the internal limiting membrane, where they lie between the retina and vitreous, or attaching to the vitreous and extending into it. Bleeding into the preretinal (subhyaloid) space results in a boat-shaped hemorrhage. Hemorrhage from new vessels in the vitreous may cause sudden loss of vision. Neovascularization and fibrosis at the angle of the anterior chamber prevent normal drainage of aqueous and lead to *neovascular glaucoma* and a blind, painful eye. Shrinkage and retraction of the vitreous from the retina, which occurs with age, may result in hemorrhage from neovascularization, and traction on the retina from associated fibrous tissue. Further proliferation of fibrous tissue may lead to a traction retinal detachment with visual loss, most marked with macular involvement.

Premature development of *senile cataracts* occurs in patients with diabetes. *Snowflake lens opacities* develop in younger patients, particularly during periods of poor glycemic control. Referral to an ophthalmologist for urgent argon laser therapy is mandatory in patients with proliferative retinopathy, diabetic maculopathy, and possibly pre-proliferative retinopathy. This therapy can be sight-saving. *Vitrectomy* may be performed in patients with extensive, long-standing, unresolving vitreal hemorrhage or when new traction retinal detachment affects the macula or is associated with a retinal tear.

Annual dilated funduscopic examination by an ophthalmologist should be performed in all patients with diabetes, starting 5 years after diagnosis in patients with T1DM. Improvement of glycemic control may transiently worsen retinopathy, before ultimately improving it over a longer period.

Neuropathy

The likelihood of involvement of the nervous system by diabetes increases with duration of disease and is influenced by the degree of glycemic control (occurring in up to 70% of people with diabetes). Any part of the peripheral or autonomic nervous system may be affected. *Peripheral polyneuropathy* occurs most commonly, which usually presents as a bilaterally symmetrical, distal, primarily sensory (with or without motor) polyneuropathy, with a *glove and stocking* distribution. Pain, numbness, hyperesthesias, and paresthesias progress to sensory loss. This condition, together with loss of proprioception, leads to an abnormal gait, with repeated trauma and fractures of the tarsal bones, sometimes resulting in the development of Charcot's joints. These changes lead to abnormal pressures in the feet that, together with the soft tissue atrophy related to peripheral arterial insufficiency, result in foot ulcers that may progress to osteomyelitis and gangrene. Detailed, regular neurologic examination of all patients is essential, to elicit the early loss of light touch (using a 5.07/10 gram monofilament), reflexes, and vibratory sensation. Painful neuropathies are difficult to treat, and, although they are self-limiting, they may persist for years. Improvement in glycemic control should be the primary therapeutic goal. Analgesia should start with aspirin, acetaminophen, and nonsteroidal anti-inflammatory agents before codeine and addictive drugs such as pentazocine or narcotics are prescribed. Anticonvulsants, including phenytoin, carbamazepine, gabapentin, and pregabalin, as well as the antidepressant amitriptyline, may provide moderate relief. Burning pain may respond to the topical application of capsaicin cream. Use of plastic skin (e.g., OpSite film), transcutaneous nerve stimulation, and nerve block are sometimes effective for chronic pain.

Mononeuropathies usually present acutely, may involve any nerve in the body, and are generally self-limiting. The cranial nerves most commonly involved are the third, sixth, and fourth, in that order. *Radiculopathies* are self-limiting painful sensory syndromes of one or more spinal nerves, usually of the chest or abdomen. *Diabetic amyotrophy* causing muscle atrophy and weakness commonly involves the anterior thigh muscles and pelvic girdle and may also be self-limiting, resolving after several months.

Potential new therapies for diabetic peripheral neuropathy include aldose reductase inhibitors (inhibit excessive activity of the polyol pathway), aminoguanidine (inhibit formation of AGES), γ-linoleic acid (replacement is needed because of impaired production), antioxidants (e.g., α-lipoic acid), vasodilators, and recombinant human nerve growth factor.

Autonomic neuropathy of the sympathetic and/or parasympathetic systems has numerous presentations. Most commonly involved is the gastrointestinal tract, with gastric dysmotility (30% to 50%), gastroparesis and small bowel bacterial overgrowth, responsible for delayed gastric emptying, early satiety, postprandial nausea, abdominal fullness, bloating and discomfort, constipation, and diarrhea (usually nocturnal). Gastropathy is frequently responsible for erratic and unpredictable blood glucose levels, with hyperglycemia itself exacerbating the dysmotility, even in people without diabetes. *Gastroparesis* may respond to treatment with metoclopramide or domperidone (dopamine D2 antagonists), erythromycin (motilin agonist) for bacterial overgrowth, cisapride (cholinergic agonist), or mosapride (selective serotonin 5-HT4 receptor agonist). *Diarrhea* may respond to loperamide or diphenoxylate and atropine. *Orthostatic hypotension* can be treated by attention to mechanical factors such as elevation of the head of the bed, gradual rising from a lying to standing position, use of support stockings, and sometimes use of fludrocortisone. *Cardiac rhythm disturbances* can result in syncope and cardiorespiratory arrest. *Bladder involvement* may result in urinary retention or incontinence. In men, *erectile dysfunction* is multifactorial and may also be related to vascular insufficiency or venous leaks. Arousal is the main problem in the sexual dysfunction of women with diabetes.

DIABETIC FOOT

Care of the feet of patients with diabetes is extremely important to prevent foot ulcers and amputations. Risk factors include distal symmetrical polyneuropathy, peripheral arterial insufficiency, areas of increased pressure, limited joint mobility and bony deformities, obesity, and chronic hyperglycemia. Patient education about foot care includes advice on daily foot inspection, appropriate footwear, drying and nail cutting, and referral to a podiatrist when necessary. Early detection and treatment of blisters, ulcers, trauma, and cellulitis may prevent progression to osteomyelitis and amputation. Treatment of ulcers may include débridement, antibiotics, growth-stimulating factors, reduction of weight bearing (elevation, casting), and improvement in arterial supply (surgical and/or medical).

MACROVASCULAR COMPLICATIONS

Cardiovascular and cerebrovascular diseases include hypertension, myocardial ischemia and infarction, transient ischemic attacks and strokes, and peripheral vascular disease. Seventy to 80% of people with diabetes die from a macrovascular event. The risk of such an event (two to four times increased in patients with T2DM or >20% over 7 years) in people with diabetes is equivalent to that of nondiabetic patients with established cardiovascular disease (i.e., those who have already had a macrovascular event, for example, postmyocardial infarction). Thus all patients with diabetes and no prior cardiovascular event are considered *coronary heart disease, or cardiovascular disease, risk equivalents.* Following a first cardiac event in people with diabetes, the chance of a second event increases dramatically to 45%. The pathogenesis of *atherosclerosis* (increasingly recognized as an inflammatory disease) and *vascular thrombosis* in people with diabetes is similar to that in people without diabetes, albeit markedly accelerated in the former. Tight glucose control, including acutely postmyocardial infarction, results in improvement in cardiovascular disease. Women with diabetes have the same risk profile as men at all ages. *Hypertension* (50% of patients with T2DM), dyslipidemia (40% of patients with T2DM at diagnosis), obesity, hyperglycemia, and smoking are major risk factors.

In people with diabetes, the risk of death from hypertension is greater than from hyperglycemia. Aggressive treatment of hypertension, to less than 130/80 mm Hg, reduces both macro- and microvascular complications and should preferably start with an ACE inhibitor or ARB, for added renal protection. All other classes of antihypertensive agents may be used, including selective β_1-blocking drugs, which are also used in the secondary prevention of myocardial infarction. β-Blockers may increase the severity of hypoglycemia by inhibiting glycogenolysis and gluconeogenesis and may mask the warning symptoms and signs of hypoglycemia by blunting the adrenergic response to hypoglycemia. However, the potential adverse effects of β-blockers in patients with diabetes have not been consistently observed in the clinical setting. Most hypertensive patients require combination antihypertensive therapy, using, on average, three different classes of agents, including diuretics. In hypertensive patients with micro- or macroalbuminuria, nondihydropyridine calcium-channel blockers may be added to the list of other drugs.

The procoagulant state of the blood in patients with diabetes is caused by *platelet hypersensitivity* to the aggregating properties of thromboxane (synthesized in excess), as well as disordered fibrinolysis and increased levels of the prothrombotic mediator, PAI-1 (see The Metabolic Syndrome, earlier in this chapter). Low-dose aspirin (81 to 162 mg/day) is recommended as primary prevention in patients with diabetes who are at high risk of cardiovascular disease, as well as secondary prevention in those with evidence of large vessel disease. Additionally, smoking cessation and management of obesity, dyslipidemia, hypertension, and hyperglycemia, together with initiation of safe exercise, all decrease the risk and severity of macrovascular disease. Lifestyle modification is the single most important therapeutic intervention in addressing insulin resistance, glucose control, and overall cardiovascular risk. Glycemic control is a stronger risk factor for microvascular disease than for macrovascular.

CURE AND PREVENTION OF DIABETES

The concepts of prevention, cure, and treatment of diabetes are all part of a continuum without absolute borders. The influence of any intervention will depend on what point in time action is taken.

Cure of diabetes is possible in certain situations through replacement of insulin, especially in T1DM. In T2DM, the multifactorial pathogenesis prevents a simple cure through insulin replacement. Insulin replacement may be in the form of exogenous insulin (injections, insulin pump; open or closed [artificial pancreas] loop), endogenous insulin (transplantation of pancreas, islets of Langerhans, or β cells), or insulin gene therapy.

Primary prevention of diabetes is the holy grail of diabetes research. Although still limited, the improved ability to predict the development of types 1 and 2 diabetes in certain select high-risk groups has resulted in several separate national and international clinical trials to study whether certain therapies administered to asymptomatic high-risk individuals may prevent the appearance of either type of diabetes. In people at high risk for developing T1DM, preventing or altering the autoimmune process has included avoidance of intact dairy proteins, use of nicotinamide, immune modulators, and administration of intravenous and oral insulins. To date, none of these approaches has proved successful. Several clinical trials are still ongoing. Prevention of T2DM in high-risk individuals (e.g., prediabetes, prior GDM, PCOS [see Table 68–1]) has focused on lifestyle modifications to increase exercise, improve healthy nutrition, and control weight. This approach has proved highly successful in reducing the incidence of T2DM by as much as 58% compared with a 31% reduction in incidence using pharmacotherapy (specifically metformin). Pharmacotherapy to reduce insulin resistance and improve β-cell function, including use of currently available oral antidiabetic agents, is also being investigated.

Secondary prevention of the development of complications of diabetes and tertiary prevention of progression of established complications to end-stage disease is discussed previously.

Prospectus for the Future

The pathogeneses of diabetes and its complications continue to be elucidated, opening original avenues for targeted therapy. New approaches to controlling and modifying this disease, using endogenous physiologic pathways, include use of amylin and incretin mimetics. The glitazars constitute a group of combination preparations of PPAR agonists: α (target of T2Ds) with γ (target of fibrates), and α with γ and δ. The combination of PPAR-α and -γ in a single compound delivers dual management of hyperlipidemia (dose-dependent decrease in TG, increase in HDL, and decrease in apo B) and improved tissue insulin sensitivity, with additional benefits in the metabolic syndrome. They are also responsible for reductions in albumincreatinine ratio, hs-CRP, PAI-1, and fibrinogen. The improvements in plasma lipid and glucose levels, particularly in the postprandial state, hold promise for cardiovascular risk reduction. The list of additional benefits proposed for these combination agents includes an *antiproliferative* role, angiotensin II antagonism, antioxidant, antihypertensive, correction of endothelial dysfunction, reduction in hypertensive and postmyocardial infarction cardiac fibrosis, reduction in visceral, hepatic, and myocellular adipose accumulation, and upregulation of macrophage lipoprotein lipase. These agents may be responsible for weight gain or dyspnea, and should not be used in patients with NYHA classes III/IV heart failure, and those already taking TZDs and fibrates. At this time, no member of this class has received FDA approval.

In the evolving pharmacotherapeutic approaches to treating disease, diabetes, hyperlipidemia, and cardiovascular diseases in particular, the concept of *polypills* to manage several separate but connected metabolic problems is taking hold (e.g., a combination of antihypertensive, antilipid, anti-oxidant, antihyperglycemic, antiplatelet, and possibly anti-inflammatory agents).

Adipose cell–derived adiponectin and adipokines will play increasingly important roles in the management of T2DM. The order of prescribing oral agents for blood glucose control is changing in the light of new therapies such that drugs responsible for β-cell preservation and regeneration will be advocated as first line treatments prior to β-cell stimulators and the other currently available antihyperglycemic agents.

Evaluation of alternate insulin formulations and analogues, delivery routes, and devices, includes oral, buccal, nasal, pulmonary, dermal, rectal, and conjunctival. A long-acting polyethyleneglycol (PEGylated) inhaled insulin is currently under development.

Research proceeds on mechanical devices such as an implantable artificial pancreas, continuous glucose monitoring, and noninvasive glucose sensors.

Inflammatory markers in diabetes are now well established. The role of anti-inflammatory therapy is still a matter for discussion and clinical trial evaluation.

Cure of this multifaceted chronic disease grows closer. Improvements in islet cell transplantation technology and anti-rejection protocols are improving prognosis in these patients. β-cell preservation, regeneration, and proliferation, as well as pancreatic ductal cell differentiation to restore pancreatic β-cell mass with the aid of incretins and islet neogenesis gene-associated protein, are promising lines of investigation. Stem cell and gene therapy, too, hold the potential prospects of cure.

The status of bariatric surgery in the management algorithm of diabetes is currently under review.

Prediction and ultimately prevention still depend on elucidation of the exact genetic, constitutional, and environmental factors responsible for the group of diseases called diabetes mellitus.

References

American Diabetes Association: Clinical practice recommendations 2006. Diabetes Care 29(Suppl. 1):S1–S85, 2006.

Diabetes Control and Complications Trial Research Group: The effect of intensive treatment of diabetes on the development and progression of long-term complications in insulin-dependent diabetes mellitus. N Engl J Med 329:977–986, 1993.

Diabetes Prevention Research Group: Reduction in the evidence of type 2 diabetes with life-style intervention or metformin. N Engl J Med 346:393–403, 2002.

Einhorn D, Rosenstock J (eds): Type 2 diabetes and cardiovascular disease. Endocrinol Metab Clin North Am 34(1):1–235, 2005.

UK Prospective Diabetes Study (UKPDS) Group: Intensive blood-glucose control with sulphonylureas or insulin compared with conventional treatment and risk of complications in patients with type 2 diabetes (UKPDS 33). Lancet 352:854–865, 1998.

UK Prospective Diabetes Study (UKPDS) Group: Effect of intensive blood-glucose control with metformin on complications in overweight patients with type 2 diabetes (UKPDS 34). Lancet 352:837–853, 1998.

http://www.diabetes.org

http://www.mypyramid.gov

Hypoglycemia

Philip S. Barnett

Definition

Hypoglycemia is defined as a recorded blood glucose concentration lower than normal. Plasma glucose is maintained on a day-to-day basis within a narrow range of 72 to 144 mg/dL (4.0 to 8.0 mmol/L) by several hormonal and neural factors. Failure of any of these glucoregulatory mechanisms may result in hypoglycemia. Clinically significant hypoglycemia is rare and is based on the demonstration of Whipple's triad: signs and symptoms of hypoglycemia, in the presence of a low plasma glucose concentration (<45 mg/dL), that are relieved by restoration of plasma glucose to normal concentrations. Low plasma glucose values without signs and symptoms, or vice versa, do not constitute clinical hypoglycemia.

Physiology Of Glucose Homeostasis

Normal fasting and preprandial plasma glucose values are less than 110 mg/dL (6.1 mmol/L). Postprandially, increases in blood glucose and insulin concentrations, influenced by meal composition, size, and time of day, peak at 1 hour and return to normal after 3 to 4 hours. Two-hour postprandial glucose values do not exceed 140 mg/dL (7.8 mmol/L). The postprandial state comprises the first 4 to 5 hours after a meal. Insulin is the predominant hormone, suppressing hepatic glucose production, promoting glycogen storage, and stimulating extrahepatic glucose utilization. The postabsorptive state begins 4 to 5 hours after a meal.

The response to low plasma glucose levels, *glucose counter-regulation,* occurs on several levels. Central nervous system detection of low glucose levels stimulates the hypothalamus and pituitary to release growth hormone and adrenocorticotropin. Catecholamines, particularly epinephrine, are released from the adrenal medulla, and cortisol is released from the adrenal cortex. Insulin secretion is reduced and glucagon secretion is augmented as a direct effect of low blood glucose concentration on pancreatic islets and in response to central neurogenic stimulation. Of the four counter-regulatory hormones (glucagon, epinephrine, growth hormone, and cortisol), glucagon is the most important in the acute response to hypoglycemia. It acts rapidly to increase hepatic glucose production through *glycogenolysis,* the major source of fasting glucose, and *gluconeogenesis,* which becomes increasingly important as glycogen stores are depleted. In patients with type 1 diabetes mellitus (T1DM) of more than 3 to 5 years duration, the glucagon response is lost. Epinephrine is also part of the rapid counter-regulatory hormone response to hypoglycemia and plays a major role when it replaces the lost glucagon response in patients with T1DM. Epinephrine is also subsequently lost as a response to hypoglycemia 10 to 15 years after diagnosis in approximately 25% of patients with diabetes. Epinephrine inhibits insulin secretion and thereby inhibits glucose uptake by muscle. It stimulates glycogenolysis and lipolysis, and the resultant increase in free fatty acids (FFAs) acts as a stimulus for hepatic gluconeogenesis. Growth hormone and cortisol characterize the delayed response to hypoglycemia (2 to 3 hours), enhancing glucagon's effect and antagonizing the action of insulin by accelerating hepatic gluconeogenesis, suppressing muscle glucose utilization, and stimulating lipolysis, ketogenesis, and proteolysis. With prolonged hypoglycemia, the liver itself responds through autoregulation with an increase in glucose production.

SIGNS AND SYMPTOMS OF HYPOGLYCEMIA

The various signs and symptoms of hypoglycemia appear at different glycemic thresholds and in response to different mechanisms. They can be divided into *neurogenic* (increased autonomic nervous system activity) and *neuroglycopenic* (depressed activity of the central nervous system) (Table 69–1). Signs and symptoms may vary among patients but are fairly constant for a given person. Accommodation to hypoglycemia results from a resetting of glycemic thresholds. As many as 25% of patients with diabetes, mainly type 1, may suffer from *hypoglycemic unawareness,* with serious

Table 69–1	**Signs and Symptoms of Hypoglycemia**

Neuroglycopenic

Warmth, weakness
Headache
Tiredness, drowsiness
Fainting, dizziness
Blurred vision
Mental dullness, confusion
Abnormal behavior
Amnesia
Seizures

Neurogenic

Sweating
Pallor
Tachycardia or hypertension
Palpitations
Tremor, shaking
Nervousness, anxiety
Irritability
Tingling, paresthesias (mouth and fingers)
Hunger
Nausea, vomiting

consequences. Loss of warning symptoms and signs results from progressive loss of glucagon and epinephrine responses over time, lowering of the glycemic threshold by intensive therapy and/or repeated hypoglycemic episodes, and autonomic dysfunction resulting from the diabetic process. The delayed counter-regulatory responses of growth hormone and cortisol are usually too late to prevent neuroglycopenia. A prior episode of hypoglycemia often impairs detection of a subsequent one, especially if it occurs soon after the first. In some patients, hypoglycemia awareness may be restored if hypoglycemia is rigorously prevented.

The definition of a normal blood glucose level depends on the circumstances, the sex of the patient, and the sample tested: arterial, venous, or capillary blood, and whole blood versus plasma or serum. Venous plasma is the usual sample measured, and its glucose concentration is approximately 15% higher than that of whole blood. Patients with diabetes use capillary whole blood for daily self-monitoring purposes. Some newer glucose-sensing devices sample interstitial fluid. Normal plasma glucose values during a fast are different in men and women; in men, the fasting plasma glucose concentration is 55 mg/dL (3.1 mmol/L) at 24 hours and 50 mg/dL (2.8 mmol/L) at 48 and 72 hours, whereas, in premenopausal women, it may be as low as 35 mg/dL (1.9 mmol/L) at 24 hours without symptoms of hypoglycemia. Exercise in healthy persons generally does not lead to a fall in glucose levels.

Concern about hypoglycemia stems from its possible devastating effects on the brain. The central nervous system cannot synthesize glucose or store enough glycogen for more than a few minutes' glucose supply. The brain cannot use FFAs as an energy source, and ketone bodies, which are generated late, are not useful in acute hypoglycemia. Because glucose is the predominant metabolic fuel for the central nervous system, significant hypoglycemia can cause acute and/or permanent brain dysfunction, and, if prolonged, it may result in brain death.

GLYCEMIC THRESHOLDS

Despite the ranges of normality discussed previously, the glycemic thresholds discussed in this paragraph apply to the general population. Falling plasma glucose concentrations trigger a set sequence of events. Within the physiologic plasma glucose range, a drop in glucose to less than 81 to 83 mg/dL (4.5 to 4.6 mmol/L) results in decreased insulin secretion. At levels slightly lower than the normal range, 65 to 68 mg/dL (3.6 to 3.8 mmol/L), secretion of the insulin counter-regulatory hormones occurs: glucagon and epinephrine at 68 mg/dL, growth hormone at 67 mg/dL, and cortisol at 58 mg/dL (3.2 mmol/L). The glycemic threshold for symptoms of hypoglycemia is approximately 54 mg/dL (3.0 mmol/L), and for cognitive dysfunction, approximately 47 mg/dL (2.6 mmol/L). These glycemic thresholds vary in response to the level of glucose control, particularly in patients with diabetes; poorly controlled diabetes with persistent hyperglycemia results in higher glucose thresholds, whereas lower glucose thresholds are reset after single or repeated hypoglycemic episodes. In some people, major symptoms of central nervous system dysfunction may not occur until the plasma glucose concentration reaches 20 mg/dL, because these people have a compensatory increase in cerebral blood flow.

Clinical Classification Of Hypoglycemia

Hypoglycemia occurs most commonly as a side effect of the treatment of diabetes mellitus, usually associated with impairment of insulin counter-regulatory responses. Severe hypoglycemia occurs in as many as 25% of patients with diabetes. It is more frequently associated with young patients and older adults, especially if the patient is fasting, has erratic meal times, has alcohol on an empty stomach, following strenuous exercise (up to 12 hours), has renal impairment (reducing insulin excretion), low glycosylated hemoglobin (HbA$_{1c}$), short duration of diabetes, or prior severe hypoglycemic episode, and is more common during sleep. The incidence increases with attempts to achieve euglycemia through tight control of glucose concentrations; 65% of patients with T1DM in the Diabetes Control and Complications Trial, and 11% of patients with type 2 diabetes mellitus (T2DM) in the United Kingdom Prospective Diabetes Study, had episodes of hypoglycemia that required assistance of a second party to administer therapy with either intramuscular or subcutaneous glucagon or intravenous glucose. Men tend to suffer from hypoglycemia more commonly than women. Patients with T1DM have longer hypoglycemic episodes and greater frequency than patients with T2DM treated with insulin or oral hypoglycemic agents. In patients with T2DM, duration of hypoglycemia is greater at night, especially after midnight, than during the day.

Other causes of hypoglycemia in patients with diabetes include overdose of insulin or oral insulin secretagogues, missed or delayed meals, and uncompensated (without supplemental calories or a decrease in insulin dose) exercise (immediate and/or delayed, up to 24 hours). *Nocturnal hypoglycemia,* exhibited by night sweats, snoring, vivid dreams, and deep sleep, occurs in as many as 50% of patients receiving insulin. Maximal insulin sensitivity at 2 or 3 AM may coincide with peak exogenous insulin action. Treatment usually includes changing one or more of the following: timing of intermediate-acting insulin from dinner to bedtime, insulin dose, type of insulin (e.g., glargine), type of insulin delivery (e.g., insulin pump), time of meal, and meal composition. In addition, adding a snack and using uncooked cornstarch can be considered.

The following discussion addresses the separate causes of hypoglycemia listed in Table 69–2.

FASTING (POSTABSORPTIVE) HYPOGLYCEMIA

Fasting (postabsorptive) hypoglycemia results from an imbalance between hepatic glucose production (decreased) and peripheral glucose utilization (increased).

Drugs

Insulin, sulfonylureas, meglitinides, and alcohol are the most common causes of fasting hypoglycemia. Insulin is a well-recognized cause of hypoglycemia in the treatment of diabetes. Elevated serum insulin levels in the absence of elevated C-peptide levels can detect *factitious hypoglycemia* resulting from the covert use of insulin by persons with and without diabetes.

Overdose with sulfonylureas occurs commonly in elderly patients taking long-acting and highly potent agents such as chlorpropamide or glyburide. This overdose is usually inadvertent but occasionally intentional (factitious), and it may be determined by measuring serum or urine sulfonylurea levels. Because of the mechanism of sulfonylurea action (insulin secretagogue), insulin and C-peptide levels are elevated. Patients with sulfonylurea-induced hypoglycemia should not be discharged from the emergency room after initial normalization of plasma glucose concentrations because hypoglycemia recurs soon afterward as a result of the long half-life of many of these agents, which may be even longer in patients with co-morbid conditions such as renal dysfunction. Several days of continuous glucose treatment may be required before the hypoglycemia resolves. Hypoglycemia related to meglitinide therapy or overdose would not be expected to be as severe as that caused by sulfonylureas because of its short duration of action.

Excessive alcohol consumption is a common cause of hypoglycemia. In patients with diabetes treated with oral agents and/or insulin, the combination with alcohol can be dangerous. Hypoglycemia may occur many hours after ingestion of alcohol (*morning after the night before*). Alcohol suppresses hepatic gluconeogenesis, and hypoglycemia occurs in malnourished patients with chronic alcoholism or following a several-day binge of alcohol consumption with minimal food intake (depleted hepatic glycogen reserves).

Table 69–2 **Clinical Classification of Hypoglycemia**
Fasting (Postabsorptive) Hypoglycemia
Drugs
Insulin, sulfonylureas,* meglitinides,* alcohol
β-Adrenergic antagonists (nonselective)
Quinine, pentamidine*
Salicylates, sulfonamides, phenylbutazone, bishydroxycoumarin, ranitidine, doxepin, imipramine, cimetidine
Others
Critical illness
Hepatic, renal, and cardiac dysfunction
Adrenal insufficiency†
Sepsis or shock
Malnutrition or anorexia nervosa
Hormone deficiencies
Hypopituitarism (growth hormone)
Adrenal insufficiency (cortisol)†
Catecholamine deficiency (epinephrine)
Glucagon deficiency
Endogenous hyperinsulinemia
Pancreatic β-cell disorders
Tumor (insulinoma)
Nontumor
β-Cell secretagogue (e.g., sulfonylurea, meglitinide)
Autoimmune hypoglycemia
Insulin autoantibodies
Insulin receptor autoantibodies
Islet β-cell antibodies
Addison's disease†
Ectopic insulin secretion (rare)
Exogenous hyperinsulinemia
Hypoglycemia of infancy and childhood
Non–β-cell tumors
Reactive (Postprandial) Hypoglycemia
Alimentary hypoglycemia
Idiopathic (functional) hypoglycemia
Congenital enzyme deficiencies in adults
Hereditary fructose intolerance
Galactosemia

Adapted from Cryer PE: Hypoglycemia: Pathophysiology, Diagnosis and Management. New York, Oxford University Press, 1997.
*Responsible for endogenous hyperinsulinemia.
†Cortisol deficiency may result from adrenal insufficiency from numerous causes, including infection, hemorrhagic destruction, and autoimmune disease.

Nonselective β$_2$-adrenergic antagonists may cause hypoglycemia in patients with diabetes (especially type 1) who do not have a normal glucagon counter-regulatory response and depend on the adrenergic response to hypoglycemia. β$_2$-Adrenergic antagonists mask the adrenergic symptoms and impair recovery from hypoglycemia. These agents also reduce the glycogenolytic response to epinephrine in muscle. Low doses of β_1-selective adrenergic antagonists do not produce these effects, although their selectivity is incomplete in high doses.

Pentamidine (particularly parenteral), through β-cell destruction, causes acute insulin release with hypoglycemia. Following this acute phase, the destroyed β cells fail to produce insulin, and hyperglycemia ensues. In children, salicylates may lead to increased insulin secretion through prostaglandin inhibition. Quinine can cause excessive pancreatic insulin release.

Critical Illness

In hospitalized patients, the most common cause of hypoglycemia is use of drugs, especially insulin. Single or multiple organ system failures (particularly hepatic, renal, cardiac, and adrenal), malnutrition, sepsis, and shock are next. The mechanism of hypoglycemia in each setting is multifactorial and not always entirely clear. Disease or failure of one organ system may affect another system, resulting in hypoglycemia, such as that seen in right ventricular cardiac failure causing hepatic congestion. Hepatic failure results in impaired gluconeogenesis, as well as an inability to store and release glycogen. Renal failure may lead to prolongation of the half-life of hypoglycemia-inducing agents (sulfonylureas, meglitinides, and insulin). Malnutrition also plays a major role in renal failure as a cause of hypoglycemia. Insulin antibodies and hypothyroidism may delay insulin clearance and increase the risk of hypoglycemia. In adrenal insufficiency, lack of cortisol, which normally supports gluconeogenesis, may result in hypoglycemia. Sepsis is associated with increased glucose utilization in excess of glucose production. Severe malaria may be associated with hypoglycemia resulting from increased glucose utilization by parasitized red blood cells.

Insulinoma

Insulinoma is a rare pancreatic β-cell tumor that has an incidence of 1 in 250,000 patient-years and is more common in women (60%) than in men. It occurs at all ages; the median age at diagnosis is 50 years in sporadic instances and 23 years in patients with multiple endocrine neoplasia type I syndrome (8% to 10% of patients). Most of these tumors are benign (90% to 95%), solitary (93%), confined to the pancreas (99%), and small (average 1 to 2 cm). Characteristically, insulinomas remain undiagnosed or misdiagnosed (20%) as psychiatric or neurologic disorders for several years. Long-term excessive insulin secretion, or *hyperinsulinemia*, which is not responsive to falling glucose concentrations in the fasting state, results in persistent hypoglycemia. Patients eat frequently to stave off the hypoglycemia and may gain weight (20%). Adaptation to the hypoglycemia over time results in manifestation of neuroglycopenic symptoms far more commonly than neurogenic symptoms. Most patients have fasting hypoglycemia (plasma glucose less than 45 mg/dL), demonstrated by a 72-hour fast (Table 69–3), and inappropriately elevated serum insulin, C-peptide, and proinsulin levels (<20% of total insulin). Some patients have reactive hypoglycemia as well. A C-peptide suppression test, in which endogenous insulin and C-peptide are normally suppressed during an insulin infusion, is impaired in the presence of an insulinoma. This test is not routinely performed.

Table 69–3	**Protocol for Performing a 72-Hour Fast**

1. Patient admitted to hospital. Start fast after evening meal at 1800 hr.
2. Blood glucose level monitored by bedside reflectance glucose meter q4h and when symptoms of hypoglycemia develop. The presence of urinary ketones confirms that the patient is fasting.
3. When symptoms of hypoglycemia develop accompanied by a blood glucose level of ≤50 mg/dL (plasma glucose of ≤45 mg/dL), draw *diagnostic labs*, consisting of a fasting plasma glucose concentration; serum insulin, C-peptide, and proinsulin levels; and a serum sample for sulfonylurea agents and insulin-like growth factor I (IGF-I) and IGF-II levels (the latter three to be sent only once per fast). The fast is terminated at this time.
4. In the absence of documented hypoglycemia at the end of 72 hr, the fast is terminated. Vigorous exercise for 2 hr may result in a fall in blood glucose.
5. The patient is fed a meal and is discharged from the hospital.
6. If severe, persistent hypoglycemia is documented, the patient may need to be started on medication, such as diazoxide, to prevent further episodes of hypoglycemia while the work-up is proceeding.

q4h = every 4 hours.

After the biochemical diagnosis of an insulinoma, surgical resection by an experienced surgeon is generally recommended, irrespective of negative tumor localization studies. Localization of insulinomas using computed tomography, ultrasound (including endoscopic), magnetic resonance imaging, celiac axis angiography, aortography, or transhepatic portal venous sampling may be unsuccessful because of the generally small size of these tumors. An octreotide scan may prove useful. At operation, tumors are often found by intraoperative ultrasound or palpation of the pancreas. Distal pancreatectomy is sometimes performed if no tumor is found during the surgical procedure.

In patients who are unwilling to undergo surgical treatment, in patients awaiting surgery, or in those in whom surgical treatment has failed, medical therapy using diazoxide, which inhibits insulin secretion, or octreotide is indicated. Continuous subcutaneous infusion of glucagon prevents hypoglycemia. In patients with malignant insulinoma, streptozotocin, with or without doxorubicin or fluorouracil, has been used.

Non–β-Cell Tumors

Fasting hypoglycemia may be caused by a wide variety of rare, non–β-cell tumors. Many (~50%) are large, slow-growing mesenchymal tumors, which are often malignant. More than one third of these tumors are retroperitoneal, one third intra-abdominal, and the rest intrathoracic. Epithelial tumors include hepatocellular carcinomas (~25%), adrenocortical carcinomas (5% to 10%), and gastrointestinal (carcinoid) tumors (5% to 10%). Lymphomas account for 5% to 10%. In most patients, overproduction of insulin-like growth factor II (IGF-II) and, more particularly, the incompletely processed form, *big* IGF-II, is responsible for hypoglycemia as a result of their direct insulin-like actions, as well as their suppression of glucagon and growth hormone and hence IGF-I levels.

Diagnosis is made based on hypoglycemia in a patient with a known tumor or elevated IGF-II levels. A 72-hour fast reveals hypoglycemia with appropriately suppressed serum insulin, C-peptide, and proinsulin levels. Treatment involves tumor resection. If surgical treatment is not completely successful, glucocorticoids may be beneficial.

Insulin and Insulin-Receptor Autoantibodies

Hypoglycemia may result from production of insulin autoantibodies and insulin-receptor autoantibodies, which are extremely rare situations that may be associated with other autoimmune disorders. Antibody binding to insulin may result in hypoglycemia by releasing insulin at an inappropriate time or by preventing its degradation. Insulin-receptor antibodies may be *blocking,* causing insulin resistance. Alternatively, antibodies with receptor-agonist activity may produce hypoglycemia with elevated C-peptide levels.

REACTIVE (POSTPRANDIAL) HYPOGLYCEMIA

Reactive (postprandial) hypoglycemia typically occurs within 4 hours of food consumption; glucose levels fall more rapidly than insulin levels. Some people with impaired glucose tolerance initially have a delayed excessive insulin response to a meal that results in reactive hypoglycemia. In all forms of fasting hypoglycemia, patients may also demonstrate reactive hypoglycemia.

Alimentary Hypoglycemia

Alimentary hypoglycemia occurs in people who have undergone gastric surgery (gastrectomy, gastrojejunostomy, pyloroplasty, gastric bypass, or vagotomy) and consists of postprandial vasomotor symptoms: palpitations, tachycardia, lightheadedness, sweating, postural hypotension, and sometimes abdominal discomfort and vomiting. This *early dumping syndrome* occurs within 30 minutes of eating and is caused by rapid emptying of food from the stomach into the duodenum, associated with a large fluid shift into the gut lumen. The *late dumping syndrome* occurs between 90 and 180 minutes after eating, resulting in dizziness, lightheadedness, palpitations, sweating, confusion, and rarely syncope. Rapid emptying into the upper small bowel of a meal rich in simple carbohydrates results in abrupt hyperglycemia, enhanced secretion of insulinotropic incretins, early marked hyperinsulinemia, and subsequent hypoglycemia. Treatment of both syndromes includes frequent small meals and elimination of simple sugars and liquids at mealtime.

Idiopathic Hypoglycemia

The existence of idiopathic hypoglycemia, an overdiagnosed condition, is still in dispute. In most patients, adrenergic symptoms, which are usually vague, do not occur simultaneously with biochemical hypoglycemia and are not relieved by consuming food. Occasionally, artificial testing situations (5-hour oral glucose tolerance test [OGTT]; 72-hour fast) may suggest the diagnosis, but these findings are not borne out following consumption of a mixed meal.

Diagnostic Work-up of Hypoglycemia

A thorough history and physical examination are crucial. Hypoglycemia occurs most commonly in patients with drug-treated diabetes mellitus. Confirmation of hypoglycemia is essential before any work-up. Ambulatory patients can be trained in self-monitoring of blood glucose (SMBG), particularly during symptomatic episodes. However, frequent SMBG may miss as many as 50% of hypoglycemic episodes. Use of a continuous glucose monitoring system (CGMS) may be helpful in this setting, with the patient recording symptoms. If blood glucose levels are low (50 mg/dL) and the symptoms resolve after carbohydrate ingestion, the patient probably has true hypoglycemia. If symptoms are present without documentation of hypoglycemia, an alternate explanation must be sought. If hypoglycemia occurs in the fed state, after excluding a history of gastric surgery, the likely cause is impaired glucose tolerance (confirmed by OGTT) or, in rare cases, idiopathic reactive hypoglycemia (diagnosis by exclusion). If reactive hypoglycemia is diagnosed, the patient should consult a dietitian for a diet plan designed to ameliorate these episodes (e.g., frequent low-carbohydrate meals).

Fasting hypoglycemia is more likely to be caused by an organic medical problem, although some of the underlying disorders (such as insulinoma and adrenal insufficiency) can produce both fasting and reactive hypoglycemia (see Table 69–2). When patients are hospitalized and are acutely ill, the distinction between fasting and reactive hypoglycemia is less clear; the work-up is then based on an understanding of the patient's underlying medical problems and therapies and the influence of these factors on blood glucose homeostasis.

The standard evaluation of hypoglycemia attributable to any other underlying cause includes hospital admission for a supervised 72-hour fast (see Table 69–3). During the fast, patients are only allowed noncaloric, noncaffeinated beverages and essential medications. These patients should be active during the day. Approximately 75% of patients with an insulinoma develop symptomatic hypoglycemia within the first 24 hours, 10% in the next 24 hours, and only 5% in the final 24 hours. Difficulties in performing the fast arise when blood glucose levels fall to less than 50 mg/dL and the patient has no symptoms of hypoglycemia or when the patient develops symptoms with normal blood glucose levels. In the former situation, continued measuring blood glucose levels should be performed, with the patient under close medical observation, until the concentration falls to less than 50 mg/dL. In the latter instance, the fast can be continued as long as is clinically warranted to convince both patient and physician that the symptoms are not associated with hypoglycemia. Table 69–4 summarizes the expected findings in various conditions at the completion of the fast.

Table 69–4   Interpretation of Results from a 72-Hour Fast

Condition	Plasma Glucose (mg/dL)	Insulin (μU/mL)	C-Peptide (nmol/L)	Proinsulin (pmol/L)	Plasma Sulfonylurea Level (nmol/L)	Insulin-like Growth Factor II
Normal*	≥45 in men, <36 in women	<6	<0.2	<5	—	—
Insulinoma	≤45	<6	<0.2	<5	—	—
Exogenous insulin	≤45	6[†]	<0.2	<5	—	—
Sulfonylurea agents	≤45	≥6	≥0.2	≥5	>0.2	—
Tumor secreting	≤45	≤6	≥0.2	<5	—	+(↓ IGF-I)

Adapted from Service FJ: Hypoglycemic disorders. N Engl J Med 332:1144–1152, 1995.
*Normal insulin, C-peptide, and proinsulin levels may be higher if blood glucose levels are not less than 60 mg/dL.
[†]Insulin levels may be very high (100 mcU/mL) in these patients.
IGF = insulin-like growth factor; – = present; + = elevated.

Artifactual or pseudohypoglycemia is a test-tube phenomenon caused by excessive glucose utilization by elevated leukocytes in certain chronic leukemias, hemolytic anemia, and polycythemia. Concern about technical problems with sample collection, storage, and analysis warrants repeat testing.

Treatment

The diagnosis of hypoglycemia should be considered in every unconscious patient. The initial treatment of a confused or comatose patient is to infuse a 50-mL intravenous bolus of 50% glucose, preferably after obtaining a blood sample for laboratory analysis. If hypoglycemia is documented, blood should then be tested for electrolytes, blood urea nitrogen and creatinine, ketones (urine and plasma), insulin (<6 mU/mL), C-peptide, cortisol, drugs, toxins, hypoglycemic agents (e.g., sulfonylurea [<0.2 nmol/L] or meglitinide), and alcohol. A plasma insulin:glucose ratio greater than 0.4 is significant. A portion of the sample should be kept for later analysis of proinsulin, carnitine, insulin antibodies, and lactate, when necessary.

Intravenous, intramuscular, or subcutaneous glucagon (1 mg) can be used in the absence of an intravenous glucose preparation. The bolus of glucose should be followed by the continuous infusion of 5% to 10% glucose (rarely 20% to 30%) at a rate sufficient to keep the plasma glucose level greater than 100 mg/dL (starting at 100 mL/hr). The requirement of 8 to 10 g of glucose per hour to prevent recurrent hypoglycemia suggests diminished glucose production as a cause of the hypoglycemia, with higher requirements reflecting increased peripheral glucose utilization. When the patient is capable of eating, a diet with a minimum of 300 g of carbohydrate per day should be supplied. In many situations, especially after administration of long-acting insulin or oral hypoglycemic agents, hypoglycemia persists for an extended time. Treatment and close observation should continue during this time to prevent a relapse. Mild hypoglycemia can be managed with oral glucose tablets (4 or 5 g), fruit juice, or the equivalent, followed by a snack containing carbohydrate and protein, if the patient has to wait more than 30 minutes for the next meal. Thiamine should be administered when alcohol consumption is suggested.

Long-term therapy depends on the cause of the hypoglycemia. If the hypoglycemia is a secondary process, such as from hepatic or renal failure, or sepsis, then treatment of the underlying disorder will resolve the hypoglycemia. If the hypoglycemia results from an insulinoma, then surgical removal of the tumor is the treatment of choice.

Recurrent hypoglycemia in patients with diabetes requires a multidisciplinary intervention with attention to detail at every level of management, including education, nutritional advice, frequent glucose monitoring (including CGMS), and physiologic insulin and oral agent therapy (including administration technique).

Dietary therapy is the cornerstone of the management of all types of reactive hypoglycemia. Patients should avoid simple or refined carbohydrates. Some patients also benefit from frequent, small meals or snacks that contain a mixture of carbohydrate, fat, and protein. If a regimen of avoidance of simple carbohydrates and eating more frequently is ineffective, restricting the daily carbohydrate intake to 35% to 40% of total calories and increasing protein intake can be helpful. Drug therapy with propantheline bromide or phenytoin may sometimes be helpful, but it should be reserved for severe cases. If the disorder results from alimentary hypoglycemia, dietary therapy is usually helpful; in refractory instances (rare), surgical treatment to slow gastric transit time may be successful.

Prospectus for the Future

Successful islet transplantation, β-cell regeneration, or implantable artificial pancreas will result in *physiologic* insulin levels and eliminate the curse of hypoglycemia related to mismatches between insulin and serum glucose levels in patients with diabetes mellitus.

New therapeutic approaches in the management of diabetes should reduce the frequency and severity of hypoglycemic episodes (previous chapter), especially as we aim for tight glycemic control.

Heightened awareness of the causes, sequelae, and treatment of hypoglycemia will hopefully reduce its frequency and severity.

References

American Diabetes Association Workgroup on Hypoglycemia: Defining and reporting hypoglycemia in diabetes: A report from the American Diabetes Workgroup on Hypoglycemia. Diabetes Care 28:1245–1249, 2005.

Banarer S, Cryer PE: Hypoglycemia in type 2 diabetes. Med Clin North Am 88:1107–1116, 2004.

Cryer PE, Davis SN, Shamoon H: Hypoglycemia in diabetes. Diabetes Care 26:1902–1912, 2003.

Marks V, Teale JD: Investigation of hypoglycemia. Clin Endocrinol 44:133–136, 1996.

Saleh M, Grunberger G: Hypoglycemia: An excuse for poor glycemic control? Clin Diabetes 19:161–167, 2001.

Service FJ: Hypoglycemic disorders. N Engl J Med 332: 1144–1152, 1995.

Section XII

Women's Health

cecil Andreoli and Carpenter's Essentials of Medicine

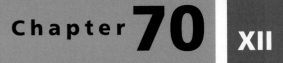
Women's Health Topics

Anne L. Taylor

Sharon S. Allen

Nancy L. Raymond

Sally L. Hodder

Karyn D. Baum

A. General Concepts and Health Maintenance Guidelines

In the past, women's health had traditionally been understood to mean reproductive and gynecologic health, areas in which women's health needs are easily perceived to be distinct. Examination of causes of mortality in women, however, emphasizes the problem of equating only reproductive or gynecologic health with women's overall health. Cardiovascular disease, cancer (cancer of the lung causes more deaths in women than breast cancer), cerebrovascular diseases, pneumonia, chronic lung disease, and accidental deaths are the major causes of mortality in women. Disability in women is far more likely to be caused by nongynecologic diseases such as osteoporosis and stroke than by gynecologic diseases. Sex and gender are significant modulating factors for diseases of nonreproductive organs, including the heart, bone, and brain. Consideration of the role that sex differences play in both disease and treatment processes is critical to an understanding of health and disease. An excellent and more inclusive description of the necessary components of women's health (Table 70–1) has been proposed by the National Academy on Women's Health Medical Education and is useful in examining the broad spectrum of women's health.

Studies of the natural history of diseases prevalent in both men and women, as well as clinical trials of therapeutic agents, have been performed mainly in men. Such studies may not therefore reflect the full expression of diseases, nor do they provide treatment decisions that may always be extrapolated to women. Indeed, after the thalidomide and diethylstilbestrol (DES) results came to light, the U.S. Food and Drug Administration (FDA) excluded pregnant and potentially pregnant women from drug trials. For example, cardiovascular disease is the number one cause of mortality in both men and women, but the impact of risk factors, treatment, and outcomes differ in men and women. Although investigational efforts designed to define the effects of sex and gender on health and disease are critical for the optimal medical care of both men and women, women have historically been poorly represented in clinical trials because of (1) fears of harming pregnant women and fetuses, (2) potential variables introduced by hormone cycles, and (3) increased cost resulting from subgroup analysis. Therefore data guiding optimal evidence-based medical care for many illnesses are less complete for women than for men.

Public outcry, advocacy, and congressional mobilization have since led to a shift in policy regarding the inclusion of women in clinical trials. The National Institutes of Health (NIH), through the NIH Revitalization Act of 1993, now specifies that women, as well as underrepresented minorities, be included in study populations, unless a *compelling* reason for their exclusion exists.

Table 70–1	**Women's Health Knowledge Base**

Knowledge of conditions unique to women (i.e., gynecologic and obstetric conditions)

Knowledge of conditions more common in women (i.e., autoimmune diseases, depression, breast cancer)

Knowledge of conditions with serious impact for women (e.g., osteoporosis)

Knowledge of conditions with manifestations, risk factors, interventions, or outcomes different in women (e.g., coronary heart disease)

Knowledge of changes in women's health and wellness needs over women's life spans (i.e., nutritional requirements, hormonal changes)

Adapted from Donoghue GD (ed): Women's Health in the Curriculum: A Resource Guide for Faculty. Philadelphia, National Academy on Women's Health Medical Education (NAWHME), 1996.

Sex Differences in the Causes of Disease by Age Group

Although women have longer life spans than men, they have higher rates of disability. Overall, considering all races and ages, the major causes of mortality for men and women are identical: heart disease, malignant neoplasms, and cerebral vascular disease. At the extremes of age, few sex differences in causes of morbidity and mortality exist. After adolescence, significant sex differences in morbidity and mortality begin to emerge.

For both women and men age 20 to 34 years, accidents are the leading cause of death. Second and third most frequent causes of death in this age group differ for the two sexes, with assault and suicide most frequent in men, whereas malignancies and heart diseases are most frequent in women. Of interest, human immunodeficiency virus infection in both sexes of this age group has declined over the last decade to the sixth or seventh cause of death (see Chapter 107). From age 35 to 54 years, accidents and heart disease are leading causes of mortality in men, and malignancies lead in women. Beyond age 55 years, causes of mortality for the two sexes are identical: cancer and heart disease from age 55 to 64 years and heart disease, malignancies, and cerebral vascular disease beyond age 65 years.

Preventive Care for Women

Health screening and aggressive preventative health interventions would significantly reduce the chronic illness and debilitation suffered by many women. Although screening and prevention guidelines vary both by age and by risk stratifications, health care professionals should identify ways to consistently track these parameters and to intervene and educate patients in ways likely to result in more positive health outcomes. As new and better clinical trial and epidemiologic evidence emerges, preventative health guidelines will continually evolve. The current recommendations, largely adapted from the U.S. Preventative Services Task Force's 2005 Guide to Clinical Preventive Services, are summarized in **Web Table 70–1**.

Exercise Through the Life Cycle

Regular exercise (both aerobic and resistive) has salutary effects on cardiovascular health, lipid profiles, blood pressure control, maintenance of bone density, insulin and glucose metabolism, breast cancer incidence, and maintenance of normal body mass index. Although the health benefits are substantial, fewer than 10% of women 18 to 65 years of age exercise regularly and appropriately. During adolescence, less than one third of girls are involved in organized athletics. The number of women involved in regular exercise activities decline further with advancing age, whereas the health benefits of exercise increase with age.

Aerobic exercise capacity is measured by maximal oxygen uptake. *Resistive exercise capacity* is measured by the amount of weight that can be lifted under standardized conditions. Both aerobic exercise and resistive exercise are necessary for optimal health benefits. Maximal oxygen uptake is greater in men than in women, a difference attributable to higher body fat content, lower muscle mass, lower hemoglobin concentrations, smaller lung capacities, and cardiac stroke volumes in women. Gender differences in maximal oxygen uptake decrease when comparing male and female endurance athletics as the result of changes in muscle and body fat composition of elite female athletes.

For maximal benefit, aerobic exercise should include 30 to 40 minutes of an aerobic activity at least three times weekly at 60% to 90% of the age-predicted maximal heart rate. Running, stair climbing, using cross-country ski machines, cycling, or swimming can accomplish this goal. Although swimming is suitable for older women with musculoskeletal problems, it lacks the positive effect of weight-bearing exercise on bone density. Intense aerobic exercise in young women may be associated with small size and delayed menarche. This effect has been observed largely in gymnasts and ballerinas, and it has not been consistently noted in other competitive female athletes such as swimmers, basketball players, and volleyball players; this finding suggests that the observed abnormalities may reflect the other behaviors (i.e., eating habits, smoking) of young women who select certain sports, rather than a general training effect.

Strength training (resistive exercise) results in increased muscle mass, increased bone density, and improved functional capacity. Measurement of strength training includes the amount of resistance and the frequency of repetitions of each muscle motion against the resistance. Skeletal muscle enlargement resulting from resistive exercise is considerably less in women than in men.

Exercise during pregnancy contributes to the maintenance of normal blood pressure, glucose tolerance, and weight gain. However, special considerations exist. Intense exercise should be avoided because imbalances in the distribution of blood flow to the placenta may occur. Exercise in the supine position is also to be avoided because pressure by the gravid uterus on the vena cava and aorta may cause circulatory impairment. Women who exercise regularly before pregnancy should continue to exercise during pregnancy, but they should avoid extremes of temperature and of exercise levels. Pregnant women who have not exercised before pregnancy should initiate only a low-intensity exercise regimen.

Sex and The Patient–Physician Interaction

In addition to physiologic variables, the interaction between patient and physician influences health status. Improved communication between physician and patient results in improved patient adherence to treatment plans and in better outcomes. Women tend to ask more questions of and provide more information to their health care providers and exhibit more emotion than men. Women are more commonly perceived by physicians to make excessive demands on a physician's time and to lack understanding of medical terminology. Men are more likely than women to receive technically detailed information from physicians. Some physicians are more likely to ascribe a psychosomatic origin to women's complaints. Women seek more information, communication, and partnership building from their health care providers than men, actions that may be interpreted by health care providers as making excessive time demands. Concentration by the physician on efficiency may compromise a woman's ability to ask questions and to receive information, which often has a negative impact on her satisfaction with her health care.

Effective medical history taking must consider sex differences in communication style. Questions should be actively solicited from women. If the physician is unable to spend the necessary time with a patient during a busy office session, then the patient may be asked to return for an additional appointment to supply additional technical information while more fully addressing the patient's concerns and questions. Ancillary personnel may provide the necessary technical information that women seek. The time taken to understand a patient's concerns and expectations greatly enhances patient adherence to treatment and follow-up.

B. Hormonal Influences on Women's Health and the Major Outcomes of the Women's Health Initiative

Normal Physiology

Three distinct hormonal phases occur during a woman's life. In *childhood,* estradiol levels are low, and both the hypothalamus and the pituitary are exquisitely sensitive to the inhibitory effects of circulating hormone. At *puberty,* as the hypothalamus becomes less sensitive and pulsatile, gonadotropin-releasing hormone levels initiate puberty, with increased gonadotropin secretion enhancing ovarian production of estrogen. Prolactin levels rise during puberty, and the pituitary episodically releases growth hormone. With establishment of regular ovulation, women experience monthly cycles of estrogen and progesterone secretion from the ovary. Estrogen and progesterone act by binding to specific receptor proteins that subsequently bind to DNA to regulate transcription. Target tissues of steroid hormones produce a measurable response when hormone exposure occurs. In adults, both reproductive and nonreproductive tissues contain measurable levels of estrogen receptors. Non-reproductive tissue that binds with detectable, active estrogen receptors includes bone, arterial endothelium and smooth muscle, brain, and urethral mucosa. Estrogen plays an important role in the healthy maintenance of these and other tissues.

In the *perimenopausal period,* ovarian responsiveness to gonadotropins decreases, and levels of estrogen and progesterone fall over time, whereas levels of luteinizing hormone and levels of follicle-stimulating hormone increase. Various symptoms such as hot flashes, insomnia, weight gain, and anxiety may occur at this time. Ovaries in postmenopausal women continue to secrete testosterone and androstenedione. Peripheral conversion of androgens result in the low circulating levels of estrogen observed in postmenopausal women. Higher estrogen levels are observed in obese women because of the increased androgen conversion in adipose tissue; this phenomenon places obese women at increased risk for endometrial hyperplasia and carcinoma. Because women currently live approximately one third of their lives

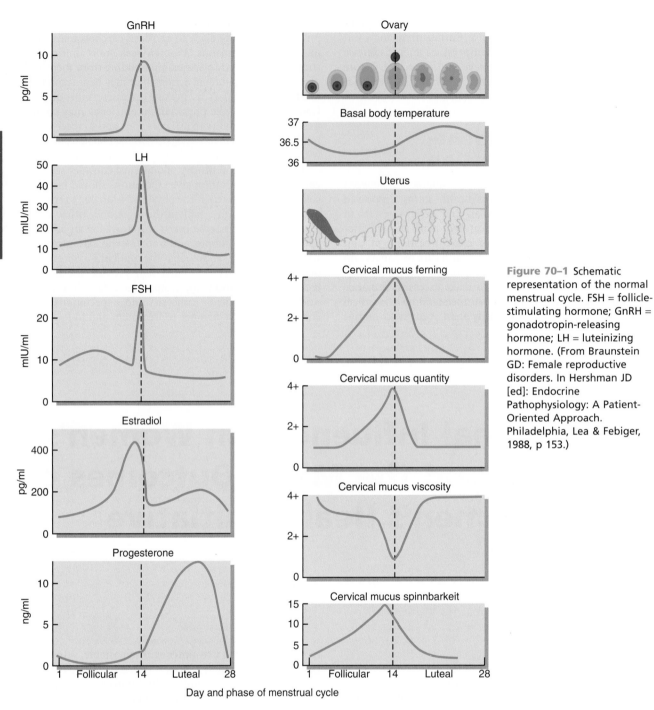

Figure 70–1 Schematic representation of the normal menstrual cycle. FSH = follicle-stimulating hormone; GnRH = gonadotropin-releasing hormone; LH = luteinizing hormone. (From Braunstein GD: Female reproductive disorders. In Hershman JD [ed]: Endocrine Pathophysiology: A Patient-Oriented Approach. Philadelphia, Lea & Febiger, 1988, p 153.)

after menopause, the health consequences of endogenous estrogen loss and the potential risks and benefits of long-term hormone replacement have been critical issues in clinical medicine. Publication of the results of the NIH-sponsored Women's Health Initiative have provided much-needed information on the effects of postmenopausal hormone replacement therapy (HRT).

The normal menstrual cycle is a series of hormonal events that result in changes in the endometrium. The normal cycle is usually 21 to 35 days in duration and consists of three phases: (1) the *follicular or proliferative phase,* (2) the *ovulatory phase,* and (3) the *luteal or secretory phase* (Fig. 70–1). During the first half of the cycle, gonadotropin-releasing

hormone secreted by the hypothalamus stimulates pituitary secretion of follicle-stimulating hormone and luteinizing hormone. Circulating follicle-stimulating hormone stimulates estrogen secretion by ovarian follicles that, in turn, prompts endometrial proliferation. During the follicular phase, one ovarian follicle becomes dominant. At midcycle, ovulation occurs when a surge in luteinizing hormone results in release of the oocyte from the dominant follicle. Remaining follicular cells form the progesterone-producing corpus luteum. If fertilization does not occur, then the corpus luteum secretes progesterone only for approximately 14 days and subsequently involutes. Both estrogen and progesterone levels decrease as the corpus luteum is progressively broken down. Falling progesterone levels result in shedding of the endometrium and the onset of menstruation. A normal menstrual period lasts 7 days or less. In the perimenopausal period, cycle length may decrease because of a shortened follicular phase and decreased progesterone secretion. Cycles lasting less than 21 days are considered abnormal.

Dysmenorrhea and Premenstrual Syndrome

Dysmenorrhea is a group of symptoms most prominently manifested by pelvic pain that occur just before and during menstruation. Dysmenorrhea occurring without the presence of disease is known as *primary dysmenorrhea*. The pelvic pain results from uterine contractions mediated by prostaglandins. Nonsteroidal anti-inflammatory agents that inhibit prostaglandin synthesis effectively control pelvic pain in most women. *Secondary dysmenorrhea* occurs when pelvic disorders such as *endometriosis* (the presence of endometrial tissue outside the uterus), *adenomyosis* (endometrial tissue within the uterine wall), or *fibroids* are present.

Premenstrual syndrome (PMS) is a collection of symptoms that are typically present in the 1 to 2 weeks preceding the onset of menstruation and resolve in the first 1 to 2 days of menstruation. Although most women have mild symptoms, approximately 5% to 10% have significant symptoms that interfere with daily functioning. Symptoms are diverse and may include irritability, low self-esteem, insomnia, fatigue, lightheadedness, food cravings, thirst, breast tenderness, edema, and weight gain. Some women even report changes in cognitive function, with difficulty in concentrating and short-term memory problems. The precise cause of PMS remains unknown; however, ovulation is a prerequisite for its occurrence.

The challenge for physicians is to identify PMS and to distinguish it from noncyclic disorders or from perimenstrual intensification of symptoms of other disorders. Evaluation must include a thorough history of symptoms with establishment of their timing. Daily symptom charts, completed over two menstrual cycles, may be helpful to analyze different symptom patterns. As Figure 70–2 illustrates, symptoms of PMS resolve completely during menstruation. Figure 70–2 also illustrates that diagnosis may be difficult when premenstrual intensification of symptoms of an underlying disorder occurs or when PMS is superimposed on another ailment. Unless the patient's history clearly suggests PMS, the clinician must first diagnose and treat any suggested underlying disorders.

Many treatment options are available for patients with PMS. Regular exercise and dietary alterations, including decreased caffeine intake and increased complex carbohydrate intake, may alleviate PMS symptoms. Daily supplementation with 1000 mg of calcium carbonate, available without prescription, has been effective in decreasing a variety of premenstrual symptoms, including dysphoria, fatigue, and back pain. Relaxation and cognitive psychotherapy may help women cope better with cyclic symptoms. Patient selection for PMS treatment should be undertaken when symptoms are severe enough to affect a woman's lifestyle and well being. Therapy should be targeted

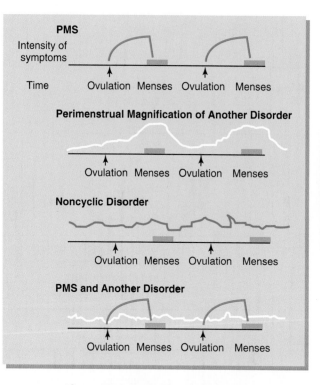

Figure 70–2 Premenstrual syndrome.

to relief of specific symptoms. For example, selective serotonin reuptake inhibitors should be prescribed for patients in whom premenstrual dysphoria is paramount, whereas spironolactone may be useful for fluid retention and bromocriptine for breast pain.

Amenorrhea

Amenorrhea is the absence of menstrual bleeding. *Primary amenorrhea* is the failure of menstruation to occur in an adolescent by age 16 years, regardless of whether secondary sexual characteristics are present. *Secondary amenorrhea* is the cessation of menses for at least 3 months. *Physiologic causes* of amenorrhea include pregnancy, the most common cause of secondary amenorrhea. Amenorrhea also occurs during lactation and, of course, after menopause. Amenorrhea occurring at other times is pathologic and requires evaluation.

Broadly, amenorrhea may be classified into seven areas as outlined in Table 70–2. Genetic abnormalities include *Turner's syndrome* (45, X gonadal dysgenesis), a disorder in which the ovary is replaced by a fibrous streak without germ cells. Occurring in 1 in 3000 to 5000 female infants, Turner's syndrome is the most common genetic disorder resulting in primary amenorrhea. Persons with this disorder are characteristically short and may have associated somatic anomalies such as webbed neck. Gonadal dysgenesis marked by presence of fibrous streak gonads may also occur in persons with chromosomal mosaicism or in individuals having either a normal 46, XY or 46, XX karyotype. A minority of individuals with 46, XY exhibit signs of virilization. The incidence of gonadal streak tumors is increased in persons possessing a Y chromosome, prompting the recommendation for

Table 70–2	Causes of Amenorrhea	
Physiologic	Pregnancy	
	Lactation	
	Menopause	
Genetic	Turners syndrome, (45, X)	
	46, XY	
	Trisomy (46, XXX)	
	Mosaics	
	17-Hydroxylase deficiency	
	Galactosemia	
Structural	Congenital vaginal defects	
	Müllerian agenesis	
	Imperforate hymen	
	Endometrial destruction	
Hypothalamic	Anorexia nervosa	
	Excessive exercise	
	Inactive gonadotropin secretion	
	Emotional stress	
	Chronic disease	
Ovarian	Chronic anovulation	
	Neoplasms (e.g., androgen producing tumors)	
Other endocrinologic	Hypopituitarism	
	Pituitary adenoma	
	Hyperthyroidism	
	Hypothyroidism	
	Cushing's syndrome	
	Adrenal hyperplasia	
External	Chemotherapy	
	Drugs (e.g., phenothiazines)	
	Pelvic irradiation	

abnormality is corrected. Adolescent girls with minimal body fat who exercise and diet excessively, such as gymnasts and ballerinas, may also have primary amenorrhea caused by hypothalamic perturbations. Normal menarche follows when exercise is decreased and body fat is increased. *Constitutional delay* in the onset of menses occurs in girls with family histories of late menarche. Although some secondary sexual characteristics may be present in these girls, menses may not begin until they are older than 16 years of age. Finally, amenorrhea caused by abnormal *hypothalamic dysfunction* may result from emotional stress or systemic illness.

The most common cause of ovarian-mediated secondary amenorrhea is *chronic anovulation,* formerly known as *polycystic ovary syndrome. Chronic anovulation* may also be a cause of oligomenorrhea (menses at intervals of more than 40 days); although this condition is classically associated with obesity, hirsutism, and infertility, many women with *chronic anovulation* are of normal body weight. Recent data suggest an association of insulin resistance and increased atherosclerosis risk with this disorder. *Ovarian tumors* are rarely associated with amenorrhea, but amenorrhea may occur when androgen-secreting tumors are present.

Miscellaneous endocrinologic causes of amenorrhea include *hyperthyroidism* and *hypopituitarism,* both of which may result in sexual infantilism and primary amenorrhea if present in adolescence. *Hyperthyroidism* is a major cause of secondary amenorrhea, whereas polymenorrhea, in which cycles last fewer than 21 days, is more often associated with hypothyroidism. Pituitary destruction resulting in secondary amenorrhea may occur from certain disorders, including tumors, infections, infiltrative disorders (e.g., sarcoidosis), and vascular or immunologically mediated destruction. Prolactin-producing pituitary tumors resulting in *hyperprolactinemia* interfere with normal cyclic gonadotropin release and ultimately lead to amenorrhea. Additionally, amenorrhea may occur with *Cushing's syndrome* and *congenital adrenal hyperplasia.*

Administration of pharmacologic agents may result in amenorrhea by a variety of mechanisms. Phenothiazines, narcotics, and monoamine oxidase inhibitors may cause *hyperprolactinemia* with resultant amenorrhea. *Ovarian follicle destruction* may result from chemotherapeutic agents, particularly alkylating agents, and pelvic irradiation.

A history and physical examination should be performed in all patients with primary amenorrhea assessing for physical evidence of a possible genetic disorder. Presence of weight loss from excessive exercise, eating disorder, or systemic illness should be sought and treated if present. Laboratory studies including follicle-stimulating hormone (FSH), thyroid-stimulating hormone (TSH), and prolactin levels should be assessed. Estrogen replacement therapy should be initiated in patients with hypogonadism or untreatable hypothalamic-pituitary disorders to prevent the development of osteopenia that occurs in women with long-standing estrogen deficiency.

Pregnancy must first be ruled out in patients with secondary amenorrhea. Levels of luteinizing hormone (LH) and FSH are useful to separate hypothalamic and pituitary causes from ovarian failure. Progesterone may be administered in an effort to determine whether appropriate estrogen priming of the endometrium is present; failure of menstrual bleeding to occur within several days of progesterone

gonadal streak removal in these individuals. A deficiency of 17-hydroxylase results in primary amenorrhea and sexual infantilism in those surviving to the second decade.

Structural abnormalities of the lower female genital tract, including congenital vaginal defects or an imperforate hymen, are observed in primary amenorrhea patients with normal secondary sexual development and are often associated with cyclic symptoms such as pelvic pain and PMS. Müllerian agenesis may occur with vaginal absence and a rudimentary uterus but with normal cyclic ovarian function. Uterine infection or surgical manipulation may result in endometrial destruction and subsequent hormonal unresponsiveness.

Endocrinologic causes of amenorrhea may be divided into *hypothalamic causes, ovarian causes,* and *other causes. Anorexia nervosa, bulimia,* and *excessive dieting* may result in primary amenorrhea as a result of hypothalamic dysfunction, however, normal menarche occurs when the nutritional administration indicates estrogen deficiency or abnormal endometrium. However, this test is not completely reliable because some women with premature ovarian failure may exhibit progestin withdrawal bleeding. Estrogen administration for 1 to 2 months is followed by menstrual bleeding in persons with estrogen deficiency but not in women with an endometrial abnormality. Treatment of secondary amenorrhea depends on the cause. Women with a suggested endometrial abnormality should be referred to a gynecologist for further work-up. Patients with ovarian failure resulting from underlying pituitary or hypothalamic dysfunction should be evaluated for estrogen replacement therapy. Ovarian and adrenal neoplasms should be surgically removed. Patients with chronic anovulation may be treated with progesterone every 1 to 3 months to ensure adequate shedding of the endometrium. Oral contraceptives may be used to treat hirsutism and virilization. Additionally, women with chronic anovulation may benefit from diet and exercise therapies to improve insulin sensitivity. Some authorities also recommend the use of an insulin-sensitizing agent, metformin, for some patients.

Abnormal Uterine Bleeding

Abnormal uterine bleeding includes oligomenorrhea, characterized by menses at intervals of more than 40 days, and polymenorrhea, characterized by menses at intervals of less than 21 days. *Menorrhagia* refers to excessive bleeding (either in amount or in duration), and *metrorrhagia* indicates irregular intervals between menses. Table 70–3 categorizes some of the causes of abnormal uterine bleeding. *Anovulation* is a common cause of abnormal uterine bleeding in both adolescents and perimenopausal women. In perimenopausal women, declining ovarian function may result in abnormal bleeding, and careful evaluation is essential to rule out neoplasia. In addition, pregnancy must be excluded.

Anovulatory or *oligovulatory bleeding* may occur as the result of hypothalamic, pituitary, ovarian, adrenal, or thyroid dysfunction. In *chronic anovulation,* the ovary secretes estrogen, but ovulation does not occur, and thus progesterone is not secreted. High tonic estrogen levels are also present in the setting of estrogen-secreting ovarian tumors. Long-term endometrial exposure to estrogen without opposing progesterone may result in endometrial hyperplasia or carcinoma. Therefore prompt and accurate diagnosis of anovulatory bleeding and appropriate treatment are crucial.

Evaluation requires a thorough history in an attempt to identify whether ovulation is occurring. Menses at regular intervals, preceded by breast tenderness or other premenstrual symptoms, usually indicate the presence of ovulation. Examination should include careful inspection for signs of androgen excess and of potentially associated disorders (see Table 70–3). Pregnancy must always be excluded. Further evaluation is largely determined by the patient's age and by whether the patient's history indicates the presence or absence of ovulation. Adolescents in whom pregnancy and infection have been excluded and in whom the history suggests anovulatory bleeding may not require further invasive testing. On the other hand, perimenopausal women who often have bleeding related to declining ovarian function require further evaluation, including ultrasonography and/or endometrial biopsy to exclude uterine disease.

Table 70–3	Abnormal Uterine Bleeding	
Cause	**Clinical Findings**
Hormonal abnormalities	Failure to release gonadotropin-releasing hormone Hyperprolactinemia Hypothyroidism Waning ovarian function Estrogen-secreting ovarian tumors Chronic anovulation
Structural abnormalities	Leiomyoma Polyps Adenomeiosis Uterine cancer Cervical cancer Endometritis
Bleeding diatheses	Thrombocytopenia Platelet dysfunction
Miscellaneous	Pregnancy

Treatment depends on accurate diagnosis. Adolescents may benefit from estrogen therapy to ensure adequate endometrial proliferation. Perimenopausal women with abnormal uterine bleeding not associated with neoplasia may benefit from cyclic estrogen and progesterone therapy. Removal of uterine polyps or leiomyomas, if present, may also be curative. Complete evaluation may not reveal a cause of the abnormal bleeding. In severe, refractory cases, hysterectomy or endometrial ablation may be considered.

Hormone Therapy

Premenopausal hormone therapy is often used for control of conception. Hormonal contraceptives can be administered as oral medications or as injectable or implantable preparations. *Oral contraceptive agents* are the most widely used form of contraception in the industrialized world. Table 70–4 describes the potential benefits of oral contraceptives, and Table 70–5 describes contraindications to their use.

Current oral contraceptive formulations contain combinations of estrogen in doses ranging from 20 to 50 mcg and progestin in varying types and dose strengths. Additionally, some oral contraceptives contain only progestin. When oral contraceptives are used properly, the failure rate for combination pills is 1% to 2%, and that for progestin-only pills is 4% to 9%. Injectable or implantable contraceptives such as medroxyprogesterone and levonorgestrel have a contraceptive effect that lasts for months. Newer delivery systems for combination (estrogen and progestin) hormonal contraception include a patch, vaginal ring, and monthly injection. Emergency (postcoital) contraception is effective within 72 hours of coitus; effective medications include high-dose

Table 70–4 Benefits Associated with Oral Contraceptives

Reduced Pregnancy Risk

Morbidity and mortality
Ectopic pregnancy
Anemia
Spontaneous and induced abortions

Reduced Risk of Hospitalizations and Gynecologic Surgery

Pelvic inflammatory disease, salpingitis, infertility
Ovarian cancer
Functional ovarian cysts
Uterine fibroids
Endometrial cancer
Abnormal bleeding

Other Benefits

Reduced dysmenorrhea
Fewer mood swings and less premenstrual syndrome
Increased bone mass
Decreased benign breast disease

Data from Shoupe D: Contraception-conception control. In Wallis LA (ed): Textbook of Women's Health. Philadelphia, Lippincott-Raven, 1998, p 632.

Table 70–5 Contraindications to Oral Contraceptive Use

Age >35 yr and smoker or hypertensive
Current or past history of cerebral vascular or cardiovascular disease
Significant impairment of liver function
Present or history of thromboembolic disorders of coagulopathies
Known or suggested carcinoma of the breast
Known or suggested estrogen-dependent neoplasia
Undiagnosed abnormal genital bleeding
Pregnancy
Severe hyperlipidemia
Severe migraine headaches with localizing signs
Uncontrolled hypertension
Symptomatic gallbladder disease
Uncontrolled diabetes mellitus
Sickle cell disease

Data from Carlson KJ, Osathanondh R, Stelluto MR: Contraception. In Carlson KJ, Eisenstat SA (ed): Primary Care of Women, 2nd ed. St. Louis, Mosby, 2002, pp 421–427.

Table 70–6 Indications for Hormone Replacement Therapy

Premature menopause
Spontaneous or induced menopausal symptom relief
Genitourinary atrophy
Prevention of osteoporosis (consider other treatment choices)
Urogenital atrophy
Dryness
Dyspareunia
Dysuria and frequency
Urge incontinence
Stress incontinence
Bleeding

Data from Martin KA. Menopause. In Carlson KJ, Eisenstat SA (ed): Primary Care of Women, 2nd ed. St. Louis, Mosby, 2002, pp 358–365.

estrogen to block implantation, progestins alone, danazol, and mifepristone (RU 486).

Before prescribing contraceptive hormone therapy, the physician should obtain a detailed medical history, particularly with respect to past or current malignant diseases, liver disease, thrombophlebitis, coagulopathies, hypertension, migraine headache, stroke, diabetes, and smoking. A menstrual history should also be taken, and the presence of abnormal uterine bleeding should prompt appropriate investigation before initiating hormonal contraceptive therapy. Thorough thyroid, breast, pelvic, and abdominal examinations should be performed.

When considering prescriptions of oral contraceptive agents in women older than age 35 years, the physician must review several issues. The combination of oral contraceptives and smoking significantly increases the risk of myocardial infarction and ischemic stroke because of the interaction of the procoagulant effects of oral contraceptives and abnormal endothelial function induced by cigarette smoking. Oral contraceptives have not been associated with increases in the incidence of breast cancer. Decreases in malignant tumors of the ovary and endometrium are seen in oral contraceptive users. Perimenopausal women taking oral contraceptives have less bone loss than women receiving replacement estrogen therapy.

Postmenopausal Hormone Replacement Therapy (*HRT*) has been given for many reasons (Table 70–6). HRT may consist of estrogen alone in women without a uterus or combination of estrogen and progesterone in women with an intact uterus. At the time of natural menopause, current guidelines based on the outcomes of the Women's Health Initiative recommend that HRT may be administered for short-term amelioration of menopausal symptoms at the lowest dose and briefest duration.

Although estrogen therapy has many beneficial effects in women with estrogen-deficient states, unopposed estrogen use stimulates the endometrium and may result in uterine hyperplasia or, rarely, carcinoma. Therefore postmenopausal women with intact uteri who receive HRT require progestins in either a cycled fashion or as a small daily dose. Progestins

Table 70–7 Contraindications to Hormone Replacement Therapy

Absolute Contraindications	Relative Contraindications
Presence or history of breast cancer	Family history of breast cancer
Breast mass, unevaluated	History of thromboembolism
Presence of noneradicated endometrial cancer	Enlarging or excessively bleeding fibroids
Active thromboembolic disease	Severe endometriosis, untreated
Acute and chronic liver disease	
Unexplained vaginal bleeding	
Pregnancy	

Data from Wallis, LA Barbo DM: Hormone replacement therapy (HRT). In Wallis LA (ed): Textbook of Women's Health. Philadelphia, Lippincott-Raven, 1998, p 732.

have opposing effects to estrogen on high-density lipoprotein cholesterol and have vasoconstrictor effects on vascular smooth muscle. Progestins are not indicated in women who have had hysterectomies. Contraindications to HRT are shown in Table 70–7.

Outcomes of the Women's Health Initiative Trial

Although HRT has been widely prescribed since the 1960s, sound clinical trial data examining benefits and risks emerged only recently. The Women's Health Initiative (WHI) trial is the largest randomized, double-blind, placebo-controlled, long-term trial designed to evaluate major health benefits and risks of HRT (estrogen plus progestin). The WHI enrolled 16,608 postmenopausal women in the age range of 50 to 79 years with an intact uterus. Forty U.S. clinical centers were involved. The study regimen used combined estrogen and progestin in one daily tablet containing 0.625 mg of oral conjugated equine estrogen and 2.5 mg of medroxyprogesterone acetate. The primary outcome was evaluation of primary prevention of coronary heart disease by HRT, with invasive breast cancer as the primary adverse outcome. Potential cardioprotection was based on supportive data from studies using lipid levels as cardiovascular disease surrogates and a large body of observational data suggesting a 40% to 50% reduction in risk in users of postmenopausal hormone replacement. The trial was stopped early at 5.2 years because the health risks significantly outweighed the benefits. A parallel trial of estrogen alone in women with a hysterectomy was continued through February 2004. In the estrogen-only arm, the WHI enrolled 10,739 postmenopausal women age 50 to 79 with prior hysterectomy. The major findings of this landmark trial are summarized here.

ESTROGEN PLUS PROGESTIN AND RISK OF CORONARY DISEASE

Although previous observational studies had suggested that HRT was associated with a 40% to 50% reduction of risk in coronary heart disease (CHD), baseline risk factors for CHD were significantly lower in HRT users versus nonusers. The primary findings of the WHI trial demonstrated a significantly increased hazard ratio for subsequent CHD for estrogen plus progestin relative to placebo. The increased risk occurred predominantly for myocardial infarction, with no increase in the risk of angina or congestive heart failure.

ESTROGEN PLUS PROGESTIN AND RISK OF BREAST CANCER

Earlier observational studies had suggested an increase in breast cancer risk with long-term HRT use, but the magnitude has been controversial. The WHI trial demonstrated that combined estrogen plus progestin use significantly increased the risk of invasive breast cancer (hazard ratio [HR] = 1.26). The invasive breast cancers in estrogen-progestin users compared with woman taking placebo were larger and at a more advanced stage (regional and metastatic 25% vs. 16%). Furthermore, after 1 year, the estrogen-progestin group had a significantly higher percentage of abnormal mammograms compared with the placebo group. The WHI trial thus supported the observational findings that relatively short-term use of estrogen plus progestin increases the incidence of breast cancers.

ESTROGEN PLUS PROGESTIN AND RISK OF STROKE

Stroke is the third leading cause of death and the leading cause of disability in women. The World Health Organization demonstrated an increased overall risk of stroke (fatal and nonfatal) in the estrogen plus progestin group (HR = 1.41). All age groups experienced increased risk for stroke, as well as those in all categories of baseline stroke risk, that is, in women with or without hypertension, history of cardiovascular disease, and use of hormones, statins, or aspirin. Other stroke risk factors (i.e., smoking, blood pressure, diabetes, lower use of vitamin C supplement, blood based biomarkers of inflammation) did not modify effect of estrogen plus progestin on stroke.

ESTROGEN PLUS PROGESTIN AND RISK OF VENOUS THROMBOEMBOLIC DISEASE

Venous thrombosis in the form of deep-vein thrombosis and pulmonary embolism has an incidence of 1 to 2 in every 1000 person-years in adults. Venous thrombosis is increased in men, people of older age, African Americans, and in obese persons but not generally associated with atherogenic risk factors. The overall HRs for venous thromboembolic disease associated with HRT events was 2.11. The risk associated with HRT was higher both with weight, age, and with increasing body weight. Factor V Leiden further enhanced the HRT risk with a 6.69-fold increased risk.

ESTROGEN PLUS PROGESTIN AND RISK OF GYNECOLOGIC CANCERS

The link between unopposed estrogen and endometrial hyperplasia and endometrial cancer is well recognized. To reduce the risk, progestin was added, but randomized trials to confirm the benefit of progestin have been limited. The WHI found in 5.6 years of follow-up 32 cases of ovarian cancer, 58 cases of endometrial cancer, 1 case of nonendometrial uterine cancer, 13 cases of cervical cancer, and 7 cases of other gynecologic cancers. The HR for ovarian cancer was 1.58, and the HR for endometrial cancer was 0.81. No appreciable difference was found in tumor histology, stage, or grade for any of the cancer types. This data suggest that HRT may increase the risk of ovarian cancer but does not increase risk for uterine cancer.

ESTROGEN PLUS PROGESTIN AND RISK FOR GLOBAL COGNITIVE EFFECT

A growing public health concern is the well-documented age-associated patterns of decline in cognitive function. With the studies showing modulating effects of estrogen and progestin on neurotransmitters and neuroconnectivity and the wide distribution of estrogen receptors within the brain, a role of estrogen in memory function had been suggested. The Women's Health Initiative Memory Study (WHIMS), an ancillary study of the WHI trial, enrolled 4532 geographically diverse, community-dwelling women age 65 years and older. Cognitive function score was measured annually with a *modified mini-mental status* examination. No overall significant difference was found in cognitive function between the HRT and placebo groups.

ESTROGEN PLUS PROGESTIN AND RISK FOR FRACTURE

Lifetime risk of fracture at common sites (hip, wrist, and vertebral) for white women is 40%, approximately the same risk as for breast, ovarian, and colon cancer combined. The WHI trial demonstrated that HRT significantly increases bone mineral density and reduces risk of fracture in healthy postmenopausal women in all subgroups examined. The HR for hip fracture and for vertebral fracture was 0.66.

ESTROGEN PLUS PROGESTIN RISK FOR COLORECTAL CANCER

The WHI data demonstrated that HRT was associated with a significant decrease in the incidence of colorectal cancer (0.63). However, the HRT group had more advanced (original and metastatic) disease at the time of diagnosis.

ESTROGEN-ONLY ARM OF THE WOMEN'S HEALTH INITIATIVE

The ancillary parallel randomized, double-blind, placebo-controlled clinical trial on postmenopausal women who had a hysterectomy and were placed on estrogen alone enrolled 10,739 women between the ages of 50 and 79 years with prior hysterectomy. Women received 0.625 mg of conjugated equine estrogen. The estrogen-only arm of the WHI demonstrated decreased risk of hip fracture (0.61) and no effect on the incidence of CHD in postmenopausal women with a hysterectomy over an average of 6.8 years. Given the same burden of incident disease events in the estrogen-only arm and the placebo group, no indicated benefit was found, and estrogen therapy alone should not be recommended for chronic disease prevention.

SUMMARY

The benefits of HRT from the combined group include prevention of osteoporotic fractures and colorectal cancer. No improvement was found in cognitive function compared with placebo. Adverse consequences included CHD, stroke, thromboembolic events, and breast cancer with 5 or more years of use. In the estrogen-only group, the only benefit was decreased risk of hip fracture. Although most women did not experience clinically relevant adverse effects on cognition, a small increased risk of clinically meaningful cognitive decline occurred in the combined group.

New evidence-based practice standards are emerging that clearly limit the role of estrogen use. The U.S. Preventive Services Task Force and the FDA have issued new recommendations against the use of estrogen and progestin for preventing chronic disease. However, treatment of menopausal symptoms does remain an indication for HRT. The FDA advises physicians to use the smallest effective dose for the shortest duration possible. Most menopausal women experience symptoms at menopause such as hot flashes, sleep disturbances, mood changes, urogenital atrophy, and other adverse events that diminish life quality. Most of the time, these symptoms are mild and transient, but for some women, these symptoms are disruptive. Short-term use of hormone therapy can be beneficial.

Although estrogen and progesterone should not generally be used for preventing chronic disease, overall, women deserve an individualized risk assessment for hormone therapy, keeping in mind the known risks and benefits.

C. Special Women's Health Considerations

Cardiovascular Diseases

Cardiovascular diseases kill more women annually than all forms of cancer, chronic lung disease, pneumonia, and diabetes, but the prevalence and consequences of heart disease in women are often underestimated. The widely held belief is that male gender is associated with susceptibility to cardiovascular morbidity and mortality and that female gender is associated with protection from cardiovascular disease. These generalizations are true for men and women in early adulthood but become progressively less relevant with each decade of life. By the seventh and eighth decades, heart disease is almost equally prevalent in men and women, and the absolute number of women dying from heart disease and stroke is greater than the number of men. Significant differences exist between men and women with respect to the impact of risk factors in the development of coronary atherosclerosis, the presentation and clinical features of CHD, and the morbidity and mortality of coronary events. Women develop the disease approximately 10 years later than men; however, when women have a myocardial infarction, their outcome is substantially poorer than that of their male counterparts. Women with myocardial infarction are less likely to be managed aggressively by their physicians. Comparison of women by ethnicity shows that cardiovascular mortality in African-American women is 34% higher than in white women.

Risk factors for CHD in women are generally the same as those in men (see Chapter 9). However, the *impact* of many risk factors differs between men and women. For example, diabetes mellitus increases the risk of developing CHD by threefold to sevenfold in women compared with twofold to threefold in men. A low high-density lipoprotein cholesterol level is a stronger predictor of CHD in women than in men, and an elevated triglyceride level in the presence of low high-density lipoprotein cholesterol may also be a more important risk factor in women. Hypertension has an equal effect on coronary disease risk in men and women, and control of hypertension results in equivalent reductions in CHD risk in men and women. Reduction of cholesterol in women with established CHD has substantial secondary preventive effects; however, women tend to be less often treated than men for hyperlipidemias. Cigarette smoking, an especially important risk factor for women taking oral contraceptives, has been increasing at higher rates among young women than among young men. The effects of psychosocial factors such as depression (five times more common in women than in men), social and economic support (diminished in older women), and sex–specific responses to stress all require further study.

Because of the underutilization of cardiovascular preventive strategies in women, the American Heart Association and American College of Cardiology published evidence-based guidelines for preventing cardiovascular disease in women in 2004. New conceptual foundations for these guidelines include the following: (1) Cardiovascular risk is addressed as a continuum, an important approach given that atherosclerosis develops from childhood onward and is expressed in maturity, and (2) the intensity of risk intervention is determined by the baseline level of cardiovascular disease risk. The guidelines assign level of risk based on the Framingham global risk assessment (high [>20%] 10-year risk, intermediate [10% to 20%] 10-year risk, and low/optimal [<10%] 10-year risk). Evidence for the recommendations was weighted based on the strength of evidence found on review of clinical trials. The limitations of this approach include poor representation of women and ethnic minorities in many important clinical trials, the fact that clinical trial populations do not precisely match treatment populations, and the omission of such endpoints as quality of life, functional status, hospitalizations, and health care resource utilization.

The guidelines addressed five major areas: (1) lifestyle interventions (exercise, diet, tobacco avoidance, weight management, and psychosocial factors), (2) major risk-factor intervention (lipids, blood pressure, diabetes mellitus), (3) preventative drug interventions (aspirin, β-blockers, blockade of angiotensin system), (4) atrial fibrillation and stroke prevention, of particular importance because mortality and morbidity associated with atrial fibrillation is increased in women, and (5) interventions with no benefit or potential harm (HRT and antioxidant supplements).

The recommended cardiovascular risk strategy would include assessment of risk factors and stratification into high, intermediate, or low risk. Lifestyle interventions are recommended for all women, whereas other risk reduction interventions are based on level of risk and the level of evidence of efficacy of the risk reduction strategy.

Significant differences exist between men and women in the clinical presentation of coronary artery disease. Myocardial infarction is more often the initial presentation in men, whereas angina is more frequently the initial presentation in women. Of particular interest are the results of a study of 515 women with an acute myocardial infarction. Symptoms reported by these women in the month before their infarct included unusual fatigue (70%), sleep disturbance (48%), dyspnea (42%) and chest pain (30%). Acute symptoms at the time of the infarct included dyspnea (58%), chest pain (57%) but often in atypical locations, weakness (55%), unusual fatigue (55%), cold sweats (39%), and dizziness (39%). This study established the importance of recognition that women with coronary syndromes often exhibit subtle, *atypical* pain symptoms. Women with established CHD have significantly increased short- and long-term mortality rates after myocardial infarction. After myocardial infarction, women are twice as likely as men to have congestive heart failure, recurrent angina, and recurrent infarction. Factors possibly related to the poorer outcome of women include older age at diagnosis and higher prevalence rates of diabetes and hypertension. Treatment patterns for men and women also differ, with women significantly less likely to receive aggressive management that includes cardiac catheterization and revascularization procedures. Significant differences in physician interpretation of a patient's symptoms and the patient's assessment of risk of symptoms may also contribute to sex differences in outcomes.

Congestive heart failure, the most common cause of hospitalization in older adults, has gender differences in the pattern of outcomes. When the cause of heart failure is ischemic, men and women fare equally poorly. When men and women with nonischemic cardiomyopathies are compared, women have a significantly better outcome. Approximately 40% of those with congestive heart failure symptoms have preserved left ventricular function, frequently associated with hypertension.

Stroke is the third leading cause of death and the most important cause of severe disability in the United States. Although men have a higher prevalence and a higher case fatality rate from stroke, more women die from stroke because of the overrepresentation of women in elderly age groups. African-American women have an increased prevalence of stroke when compared with white women. Of the recognized risk factors for stroke in both men and women, the most important factors, hypertension and diabetes mellitus, are more prevalent in women.

Benign Breast Disease

Evaluating breast complaints aggressively in women is important to avoid delays in the diagnosis of breast cancer. The incidence of breast cancer (see Chapter 56) as the underlying cause of a breast mass increases with increasing age. Breast masses in adolescents are commonly caused by fibroadenomas. Ten percent of breast masses are malignant in women age 25 to 40 years, whereas 35% are malignant in the 35- to 55-year age group, and 85% of breast masses in women older than the age of 55 are caused by carcinoma. Fibroadenomas constitute 25% of breast masses in women age 25 to 40 years and 10% in women age 35 to 55 years. Fibrocystic breast disease accounts for 55% of breast masses in the 25- to 40-year age group and 30% in the 35- to 55-year age group. Cystic masses are easily distinguished from solid masses with fine-needle aspiration. Cysts that yield bloody fluid or fail to resolve completely with aspiration should be further evaluated with biopsy. Presence of breast erythema or skin dimpling requires biopsy to rule out carcinoma even if breast examination and mammogram fail to show a defined mass. Paget's carcinoma should be considered in cases of nipple scaling and ruled out by punch biopsy. Staging and treatment strategies are discussed in Chapter 56.

Breast pain is a common complaint. An associated breast mass must be thoroughly evaluated to exclude the presence of breast cancer. Dietary modulation to decrease caffeine ingestion may be beneficial in some patients with breast pain. Although oral contraceptive agents do not appear to cause breast pain, HRT may do so; in such cases, estrogen dose alteration may be helpful.

Pelvic Inflammatory Disease

Pelvic inflammatory disease (PID) is a spectrum of upper genital tract inflammatory disorders that can include any combination of endometritis, salpingitis, tubo-ovarian abscess, and pelvic peritonitis (see Chapter 106). Sexually transmitted infectious organisms are implicated in most cases. Adolescents are at greater risk than women of other ages. Other recognized risk factors include multiple sexual partners and new sexual partners within the previous 30 days. PID is the leading cause of preventable infertility. A single episode of PID results in infertility in 13% of affected women. Infertility rates increase rapidly with subsequent PID episodes, with approximately 30% of women becoming infertile after two PID episodes and 50% to 75% becoming infertile after three or more episodes. Subsequent ectopic pregnancy, the leading cause of pregnancy-related deaths in African-American women, is a major complication.

Diagnosis of PID is made difficult by the diversity of signs and symptoms that may be present. Many patients may be asymptomatic; two thirds of patients with laparoscopic evidence of old PID cannot recall a history of the disease. Moreover, some women may have mild symptoms, such as a vaginal discharge and dyspareunia. Although laparoscopy may be used to diagnose salpingitis, it is not readily available for use in many acute cases. The diagnosis of PID is therefore based on clinical findings, but no single historical, physical, or laboratory finding is both sensitive and specific for the diagnosis of PID. Empirical treatment for PID should be initiated in any patient at risk for PID in whom all of the following criteria are present and for which no other diagnosis is identified: (1) lower abdominal tenderness, (2) adnexal tenderness, and (3) cervical motion tenderness. Further confirmatory support for the clinical diagnosis is provided by abnormal cervical discharge and documentation of infection with *Neisseria gonorrhoeae* or *Chlamydia trachomatis*. Definitive criteria for diagnosing PID include (1) histopathologic evidence of endometritis on endometrial biopsy, (2) thickened fluid-filled fallopian tubes with or without free pelvic fluid or tubo-ovarian abscess demonstrated by abdominal imaging, and (3) laparoscopic abnormalities consistent with PID. A low threshold for considering this diagnosis and for initiating empirical treatment in women with atypical symptoms is essential.

Table 70–8 presents treatment regimens recommended by the Centers for Disease Control and Prevention. No definitive data comparing the efficacy either of parenteral with oral treatment regimens or inpatient and ambulatory treatment settings have been found. Table 70–9 contains currently recommended criteria for hospitalization of patients with PID. Patients should show marked clinical improvement within 3 days after treatment is initiated. Patients who remain febrile or fail to show diminished abdominal, adnexal, and cervical motion tenderness usually require additional diagnostic studies or surgical intervention. Sexual partners of PID patients should be evaluated for sexually transmitted diseases and treated for *C. trachomatis* and *N. gonorrhoeae* infection even if evidence is not found by diagnostic studies.

Table 70–8 Treatment Regimens for Pelvic Inflammatory Disease

Intravenous Regimens

Cefotetan 2 g q12h or cefoxitin; 2 g q6h plus doxycycline; 100 mg q12h

Clindamycin, 900 mg q8h plus gentamicin; 2 mg/kg loading dose followed by 1.5 mg/kg q8h*

Other Regimens

Ofloxacin 400 mg IV q12hr or levofloxacin 500 mg IV qd with or without metronidazole 500 mg IV q8h

Ampicillin/sulbactam 3 g IV q6h plus doxycycline 100 mg PO or IV q12h

*Although single-daily-dose gentamicin has not been evaluated for the treatment of pelvic inflammatory disease, it is efficacious in other analagous situations.
From Centers for Disease Control and Prevention: 2006 Guidelines for treatment of sexually transmitted diseases. MMWR Morbid Mortal Wkly Rep 55(RR-11), 58–59, 2006.
IV = intravenous; PO = by mouth; q12h = every 12 hours; q6h = every 6 hours; q8h = every 8 hours; qd = every day.

Table 70–9 Criteria for Hospitalization of Persons with PID

Surgical emergencies such as appendicitis cannot be excluded.

Patient is pregnant.

Patient does not respond clinically to oral antimicrobial therapy.

Patient is unable to follow or tolerate an outpatient oral regimen.

Patient has severe illness, nausea and vomiting, or high fever.

Patient has a tubo-ovarian abscess.

Patient is immunodeficient (i.e., has human immunodeficiency virus infection with low CD4 counts, is taking immunosuppressive therapy, or has another disease).

From Centers for Disease Control and Prevention: 2006 Guidelines for treatment of sexually transmitted diseases. MMWR Morbid Mortal Wkly Rep 55(RR-11), 58, 2006.

Urinary Incontinence

Incontinence, an involuntary loss of urine, occurs when bladder pressure exceeds urethral pressure. It may be further categorized as stress incontinence (related to position changes or Valsalva's maneuver when coughing or sneezing), urge incontinence (loss of urine with urgency to urinate), overflow incontinence (pressure in maximally distended bladder is relieved by flow of urine out of bladder), and functional incontinence (loss of urine caused by extrinsic factors such as stroke or immobility). Incontinence is common in women; in fact, the incidence may approach 25% in postmenopausal women. This incidence contrasts to its uncommon occurrence in men. The normal female urethra has many folds that result in a mucosal seal. Urethral mucosa cells possess estrogen receptors, and estrogen is necessary for maintaining a highly functional urethral mucosa. In the perimenopausal period, stress incontinence may occur because of a loss of the elasticity and tone of the urethral epithelium. In addition to mucosal abnormalities caused by hypoestrogen states, bladder outlet dysfunction may also result from presence of cystourethrocele (relaxation of the bladder and urethra into the vagina), weakness of the external sphincteric mechanism (e.g., pudendal nerve damage), and bladder neck incompetence (usually caused by a previous invasive procedure such as urethropexy).

Evaluation of women with incontinence should include a history that clearly characterizes the type of incontinence, as well as its frequency. Current medications, coexistent medical problems (e.g., diabetes mellitus, primary neurologic disease), and current hormonal status are also important components of the history. Physical examination should include a complete pelvic examination with careful observation of vaginal and urethral mucosa. In addition, a complete neurologic examination should be performed. Rectal examination that specifically assesses resting anal sphincter tone, presence or absence of rectocele, presence of an anal wink, and ability to voluntarily contract sphincters is also required. Further evaluation should include urinalysis and cultures to rule out urinary tract infection and to determine postvoid residual urine volume. Referral to a urologist or urogynecologist for performance of urodynamics is indicated in patients with previous pelvic surgery, nocturnal enuresis, continuous incontinence, increased postvoid residuals, or history or signs of neurologic disease. Experts disagree on whether urodynamic evaluation is required before surgery for all women with stress incontinence without other symptoms or signs.

Treatment depends on the cause of the incontinence. Anticholinergic medications are effective for urge incontinence. Topical estrogen therapy is often helpful in postmenopausal women with incontinence. Other medical therapies are listed in Table 70–10. In addition to pharmacologic therapy, pelvic muscle exercises may improve pelvic floor muscle strength. Regular voiding without waiting for the urinary urge may also be helpful. Surgery may be indicated when conservative therapies fail.

Domestic Violence

Violence against women is a major health care issue. In the United States, domestic violence is the leading cause of injury to women age 15 to 44 years. Estimates suggest that 2 to 4 million women in the United States are physically abused every year and that violence may occur in up to one of every four families. Domestic violence occurs across all cultural, ethnic, and socioeconomic boundaries. Frequent physician visits for multiple physical complaints may be an indication that a woman is a victim of violence, inasmuch as

Table 70–10	**Treatment for Urinary Incontinence**	
Medication	**Indication**	**Starting Dosage**
Oxybutynin chloride	Urgency incontinence Frequency/urgency	2.5 mg one to three times daily
Hyoscyamine sulfate	Urgency incontinence Frequency/urgency	$^1/_2$ of a 0.375 mg pill one to two times daily
Propantheline bromide	Urgency incontinence Frequency/urgency	15 mg one to three times daily
Imipramine hydrochloride	Urgency incontinence Mixed incontinence	10 mg one to three times daily
Pseudoephedrine*	Stress incontinence	30 mg one to three times daily
Phenylpropanolamine*	Stress incontinence	50 mg one to three times daily

*These medications are administered in sustained-release formulas, such as Rondec TR, Entex LA, or Ornade.
Data from Bavendan TG: Urinary tract health and disorders of women. In Wallis LA (ed): Textbook of Women's Health. Philadelphia, Lippincott-Raven, 1998, p 431.

women often complain of multiple somatic illnesses rather than the abuse. In families in which women are victims of violence, children are also frequently assaulted. Thus physicians must identify all patients who are victims of domestic violence.

Domestic violence encompasses violence not only in marital relationships, but also in other significant relationships such as dating and cohabitation. Although all female patients should be asked about the possibility of physical, sexual, and emotional abuse, few primary care physicians consistently attempt to elicit such information. Sensitive screening of women for a history of family violence is essential. Although revealing information about her history or current situation of abuse is often emotionally difficult for an abused woman, they may respond honestly to personal history questions when alone with their physicians. If she does not respond the first time out of fear or embarrassment, then she may be able to do so on a subsequent visit, or she may be able to bring up the subject later on her own later.

Although no singular symptom has been found that indicates domestic violence, red flags and signs of abuse do exist, including multiple fractures, multiple bruises in varying stages of healing, fractured mandible or nasal bones, perforated tympanic membrane, vulvar and rectal scarring, and suicidal ideation. More subtle signs of abuse may include delay between injury and treatment, discrepancy between the patient's statements and appearance of injury. In many instances, abusers do not want women to be alone with health care providers and will accompany women to their appointments to prevent them from discussing the abuse. Providers must insist that women be seen alone for some part of the visit. If necessary, an excuse can be used such as the woman needs to have some test done that requires that she go alone with the nurse or physician. When asking about domestic violence, ensure concern for the patients' health

and safety, and remind them that the office visit is confidential. Screening questions may include asking if the patient is or has been in a relationship in which she has been abused or if she ever feels afraid of a current partner.

Despite risk of serious injury or death, women with a history of domestic violence often visit primary care physicians with other somatic complaints. Illness associated with domestic violence may exhibit in a variety of health care settings and in numerous physical and psychological ways. Women who are victims of domestic abuse often use the emergency department. Treatment of domestic violence includes immediate assessment and management of injuries. Provision for emotional and psychological support, as well as counseling regarding safe havens for the patient and her children, are essential elements in managing victims of domestic violence. Physicians must have available shelter and telephone numbers of support services for prompt referrals.

Eating Disorders (See also Chapter 59)

The eating disorders anorexia nervosa and bulimia nervosa affect primarily young women, occurring ten times more often in women compared to men. Approximately 0.5% of women are affected by anorexia nervosa and 1 to 3% are affected by bulimia nervosa. Probably twice as many women have serious disturbances of eating patterns, body image and weight that lead to negative physical and psychosocial consequences but do not quite meet criteria for one of the eating disorders. These women would be diagnosed with an eating disorder, not otherwise specified. There is significant medical and psychiatric morbidity and mortality associated with both of these disorders. Thirty to 50% of women with eating disorders suffer from another psychiatric disorder such as depression, obsessive compulsive disorder or a substance use disorder. Multiple factors have been implicated in the etiology of eating disorders. Early theories stressed the sociocultural pressures to achieve thinness in order to be beautiful, dysfunctional families and premorbid personality problems suffered by the individual who developed the disorder. Family, twin, adoption, and genetic linkage studies have provided evidence for genetic bases for these disorders. As with many medical disorders, the etiology of eating disorders is based on complex interactions of genetic and biological factors interacting with environmental/sociocultural factors (See Chapter 59).

Anorexia nervosa is characterized by an inability to maintain body weight at or above a minimally normal weight for age and height. Young women fear weight gain and think they are fat, or that certain parts of their body are fat, even when they are emaciated. Patients also become amenorrheaic, although onset of the disorder is becoming frighteningly more common in prepubescent girls. Low weight is achieved and maintained most often by caloric restriction and excessive exercise, although some women have a variant of anorexia nervosa where they also exhibit the binge eating and purging behavior that is common in bulimia nervosa. Presence of these bulimic symptoms is predictive of poorer response to treatment (See Table 59-6).

Women with bulimia nervosa are usually normal weight. Their disorder is characterized by repeated episodes of binge eating (eating large amounts of foods with a sense that one cannot control what or how much one is eating). These episodes are followed by purging, either by self-induced vomiting, excessive exercise, overuse of laxatives or diuretics, or some combination of the above. Unlike anorexia nervosa, women can suffer from bulimia nervosa for years without anyone knowing they are ill. Despite increased public awareness of the syndrome and the dangers of the behavior, women are usually ill for many years before they seek treatment.

Patients do not often present complaining of an eating disorder. In fact, denial of the significance of the behaviors and the illness are cardinal symptoms of the disorders. Common presenting complaints and symptoms include: anxiety, depression, fatigue, irritability, withdrawal, constipation (usually in the absence of any objective findings), abdominal bloating/discomfort, irregular menses or amenorrhea, and headaches. Common findings of anorexia nervosa include: low weight, bradycardia, hypotension with or without orthostasis, hair loss, formation of lanugo, low body temperature, dry skin and hair, and peripheral edema in severe cases. In contrast, women with bulimia nervosa usually appear healthy. A dentist may notice erosion of the dental enamel on the inner surface of the teeth caused by repeated vomiting. Parotid or salivary glands may be enlarged. A callous may be found on the index finger of the dominate hand, again caused by the effect of vomitus on the skin from repeated use of the finger to induce vomiting (Russell's sign). However, many patients learn over time to induce vomiting without physically stimulating their gag reflex.

The medical complications of these disorders are enormous, making these among the most difficult psychiatric patients to manage from a medical perspective. Nearly every body system is affected. Some of the most dangerous complications are the cardiac arrhythmias (both ventricular and sinus) and QT prolongation that can lead to sudden cardiac death. Ipecac myocarditis can also lead to death in patients who use ipecac to induce vomiting. Both eating disorders can lead to delayed gastric emptying. Women with anorexia can suffer from superior mesenteric artery syndrome and can develop pancreatitis during refeeding. Repeated vomiting can lead to esophagitis in women with bulimia nervosa. This can progress to esophageal perforation or Mallory-Weiss tears. In rare cases, gastric rupture has occured. Both disorders can result in disturbances of the hypothalamic adrenal, gonadotropin and thyroid axes. The resulting hormonal abnormalities can result in hypothyroidism or euthyroid sick syndrome, infertility, osteopenia and particularly, in anorexia nervosa, growth retardation. Volume depletion must be corrected, but administering fluid to a compromised patient must be carefully managed. Hypokalemia, refeeding hypophosphatemia and hypokalemic "contraction" alkalosis must all be treated appropriately. During the refeeding process, excess fluid retention leading to low sodium levels is common. Replacement of potassium, calcium, phosphorus, magnesium, and zinc during refeeding is often required. Some severely ill patients need to be stabilized on a medical unit or in an intensive care unit. However, the surreptitious attempts to sabotage efforts to re-feed and rehydrate them can make these patients very difficult to manage on a medical unit.

Once the patient is medically stable, treatment consists of adequate nutrition, psychotherapy, and sometimes medications to treat co-morbid depression and anxiety. Psychotherapy is an essential component to treatment. Family therapy is a useful and possibly essential adjunct when one is treating a prepubertal or adolescent patient who is still living at home.

Disorders of Affect, Cognition, and Perception

The incidence, patterns of onset, and symptoms of disorders of cognition and affect are different in men and women. Mood disorders such as depression and seasonal affective disorders are two to three times more common in women than men. Variations in levels of hormones such as estrogen and progesterone over a woman's life cycle also lead to increased risk of depression during menarche, the postpartum period, and menopause. Bipolar disorder is equally prevalent in men and women, but women have more depressive episodes and more rapid cycling of moods. In addition, drug-induced and hyperthyroid-induced rapid cycling is extremely common in women. Although the incidence of schizophrenia is equal in men and women, the onset is approximately 5 years later in women. Estrogen may be a protective factor with regard to the development of schizophrenias, and low estrogen states may lead to exacerbations of psychotic illnesses. Hormonal effects on neurotransmitter activity may, in part, mediate the greater prevalence of depression and anxiety. Estrogen produces serotonergic, dopaminergic, and noradrenergic-enhancing effects, in part, because it inhibits monoamine oxidase activity, the primary enzyme that metabolizes these neurotransmitters. Studies in animals have also shown that estrogen increases the serotonin-receptor density in the brain. Low serotonin levels and low noradrenaline levels are thought to be associated with depression. In contrast, progesterone metabolites affect γ-aminobutyric acid (GABA) receptors. Medications that mimic GABA reduce anxiety.

Mood and psychological state change with hormonal fluctuations of the reproductive cycle. Premenstrual dysphoric disorder (PMDD) occurs during the luteal phase of the menstrual cycle and abates within a few menstruation cycles. A few studies show that contraceptives may help reduce some symptoms of PMDD. However, oral contraceptives may also precipitate recurrences of depression in women with a history of depression. If a woman has a history of depression or develops depression while taking oral contraceptives, then a specialist who is experienced with prescribing different preparations of oral contraceptives should make recommendation to the patient.

The risk of depression or other major psychiatric illness is low during pregnancy but high in the postpartum period. Approximately 10% of women develop significant postpartum depression, with a peak incidence 4 to 5 months after delivery. Postpartum depression has been associated with emotional and intellectual deficits in children; thus recognition and appropriate treatment may benefit both mothers and children. Estrogen treatment has been associated with relief of postpartum depression, but it may induce rapid cycling in patients with a history of bipolar disorder.

During menopause, a variety of neurophysiologic and cognitive changes occur. Women with a history of reproductive cycle–related mood disorders appear to have an increased risk for perimenopausal depression. In elderly populations, the incidence of Alzheimer's dementia is 2.7-fold higher in women than in men, whereas the incidence of multi-infarct dementia is the same in the two sexes.

Other major disease entities that occur exclusively or with relatively high frequency in women are discussed in the relevant system-oriented section of the text. These conditions include cancer of the breast, uterus, and ovary (Chapter 56), eating disorders (Chapter 59), osteoporosis (Chapter 75), and sexually transmitted diseases (Chapter 106).

Prospectus for the Future

- Understanding how the sex hormones modulate the health and disease of other organ systems, including the cardiovascular, immune, neuropsychiatric, musculoskeletal, and gastrointestinal systems

- Continuing decrease in incidence of cervical cancer, as increasing number of women receive the human papillomavirus vaccine as adolescents or young adults

References

Agency for Healthcare Research and Quality: Guide to clinical preventive services, 2005, Rockville, Md. http://www.ahrq.gov/clinic/pocketgd.htm

Bavendam TG: Urinary tract health and disorders of women. In Wallis LA (ed): Textbook of Women's Health. Philadelphia, Lippincott-Raven, 1998, pp 421–432.

Centers for Disease Control and Prevention: 2006 guidelines for treatment of sexually transmitted diseases. MMWR Morbid Mortal Wkly Rep 55:RR-11, 56–61, 2006.

Donoghue GD (ed): Women's Health in the Curriculum: A Resource Guide for Faculty. Philadelphia, National Academy on Women's Health Medical Education (NAWHME), 1996.

Heer T, Schiele R, Schneider S, et al: Gender differences in acute myocardial infarction in the era of reperfusion (the MITRA registry). Am J Cardiol 89:511–517, 2002.

McSweeney JC, Cody M, O'Sullivan P, et al: Women's early warning symptoms of acute myocardial infarction. Circulation 108:2619–2623, August 2003.

Mosca L, Appel LJ, Benjamin EJ, et al: Evidence-based guidelines for cardiovascular disease prevention in women. Circulation 109:672–693, February 2004.

National Vital Statistics Report, Vol. 49, No. 11, October 2001.

Stefanick M, Manson J, Greenland P, et al: Walking compared with vigorous exercise for the prevention of cardiovascular events in women. N Eng J Med 347:1545, 2002.

Ulman KH, Carlson KJ: Premenstrual syndrome. In Carlson KJ, Eisenstat SA (eds): Primary Care of Women, 2nd ed. St. Louis, Mosby, 2002, pp 410–414.

Wyshak, G: Violence, mental health, substance abuse—problems for women worldwide. Health Care Women Int 21:631–639, 2000.

Section XIII

Men's Health

Andreoli and Carpenter's

Essentials of Medicine

Cecil

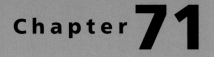

Men's Health Topics

Johnathan S. Starkman

Douglas F. Milam

Joseph A. Smith, Jr.

This chapter addresses disorders unique to men because of involvement of the male genitalia and reproductive system. It incorporates aspects of voiding, oncology, reproductive function, and infection.

A. Benign Prostatic Hyperplasia

Benign prostatic hyperplasia (BPH), a nonmalignant enlargement of the prostate gland, is a common condition in the aging male patient. Estimates are that over 90% of all men will develop histologic evidence of BPH during the course of their lifetime; of those, at least 50% will develop lower urinary tract symptoms (LUTS) that prompt them to seek medical care. Broadly speaking, LUTS can be divided into two groups: (1) obstructive voiding symptoms and (2) irritative voiding symptoms (Table 71–1).

Although the majority of patients who seek medical care for BPH do so because of the associated LUTS, these same symptoms can be the result of several different factors, including systemic illnesses such as diabetes mellitus, as well as neurologic conditions, including spine disease, Parkinsonism, multiple sclerosis, and cerebrovascular disease (Fig. 71–1). Evaluating the patient for these non–BPH-related conditions is important to ensure optimal management. Also important is to pay close attention to medication usage because a large number of medications used in the elderly population can result in various urologic symptoms, including both obstructive and irritative voiding symptoms.

Pathophysiology

Prostate growth and the subsequent development of BPH occur under the influence of testosterone and the more metabolically active dihydrotestosterone. Testosterone, which is produced by the testes and controlled via the hypothalamic-pituitary gonadal axis, is converted to dihydrotestosterone by the action of the enzyme 5a-reductase. Dihydrotestosterone is the major intracellular androgen and is believed to be responsible for the development and maintenance of the hyperplastic cell growth characteristic of BPH.

The development of BPH occurs predominantly in the periurethral prostatic tissue referred to as the *transition zone* (Fig. 71–2). Tissue growth in this area leads to the phenomenon of bladder outlet obstruction (BOO), which leads to LUTS. BOO occurs as a result of two mechanisms: (1) mechanical obstruction, resulting from an increased tissue volume in the periurethral zone of the prostate, and (2)

Table 71–1	**Lower Urinary Tract Symptoms**
Irritative	**Obstructive**
Frequency	Hesitancy
Nocturia	Slow stream
Urgency	Stop-and-start voiding
Urge incontinence	Sensation of incomplete emptying

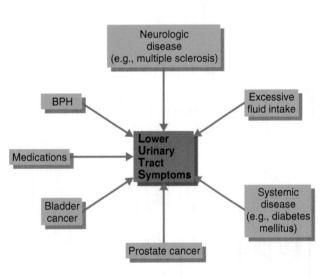

Figure 71–1 Causes of lower urinary tract symptoms (LUTS).

dynamic obstruction, which is the result of increased smooth muscle tone in the bladder neck and prostate gland. Also important but less well characterized is the response of the bladder muscle to the increase in outlet resistance provided by the combination of mechanical obstruction and increased prostatic and bladder-neck–smooth-muscle tone. As bladder outlet resistance increases, the bladder responds by increasing the force of contraction. This added work results in physical and mechanical changes in bladder function.

Early in the course of the development of BOO, the bladder is able to compensate; however, with persistent obstruction, the patient will typically develop LUTS, particularly irritative voiding symptoms such as nocturia, frequency, and urgency. These symptoms frequently drive patients to seek medical care. Later during the course of the obstructive process, the bladder wall becomes thickened and loses compliance. The subsequent loss of compliance results in a decrease in the functional capacity of the bladder, which exacerbates the patient's irritative voiding symptoms.

Diagnosis

The initial evaluation of a patient with LUTS suggestive of BPH should include a detailed medical history, focusing on the patient's urinary symptoms, as well as the patient's medical history that includes co-morbid conditions and any previous surgical procedures, general health conditions, and alcohol and/or tobacco use. The assessment of a patient's symptoms can be facilitated with the use of the American Urological Association (AUA) symptom index. This index is a self-administered, validated questionnaire consisting of seven questions related to the symptoms of BPH and BOO. Using the AUA symptom index, symptoms can be classified as mild (0 to 7), moderate (8 to 19), or severe (20 to 35). Validated instruments such as the AUA symptom index are useful during the initial evaluation as an overall assessment of symptom severity and during follow-up visits to assess the effectiveness of any interventions, medical or surgical.

A general physical examination should also be performed that includes a digital rectal examination (DRE), as well as a focused neurologic examination. Urinalysis, either by dipstick or microscopic examination of urine sediment, is also

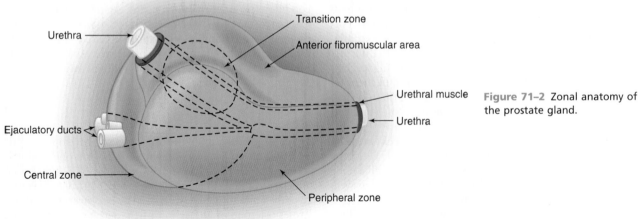

Figure 71–2 Zonal anatomy of the prostate gland.

Zonal anatomy of the prostate gland

mandatory to rule out hematuria or evidence of urinary tract infection. Glycosuria can also be a significant finding, particularly if not previously identified. The initial clinical practice guidelines for the diagnosis of BPH recommended a serum creatinine to assess renal function in all patients with signs or symptoms suggestive of BPH. However, this recommendation has come under some scrutiny as a result of its low yield for detecting renal insufficiency secondary to obstructive uropathy. Serum creatinine is no longer a routine part of the BPH work-up. According to the same clinical practice guidelines, measurement of prostate-specific antigen (PSA) is optional during the initial evaluation. PSA can function as a surrogate for prostate volume measurement in addition to being a screening test for prostate cancer. A recent National Institutes of Health (NIH)-sponsored study, Medical Therapy of Prostatic Symptoms (MTOPS), demonstrated that PSA increases linearly with prostate volume and that PSA greater than 4.0 ng/ml conveyed a 9% risk of requiring surgical therapy over a 4.5-year period.

The following additional diagnostic tests are also considered to be optional; however, they may be useful, particularly in patients with moderate to severe AUA symptom scores, in determining whether the patient's symptoms are compatible with obstruction from BPH. Uroflowmetry is a noninvasive method of measuring urinary flow rate. It is generally considered the most useful method of identifying patients with BOO. However, patients with diminished flow rates may also have impaired bladder contraction. Measurement of postvoid residual urine may be accomplished via urethral catheterization or, preferably, by ultrasonography. Elevated postvoid residual urine volumes indicate an increased risk of acute urinary retention and eventual need for surgical intervention. The NIH-sponsored MTOPS study demonstrated that 7% of men with postvoid residual urine volume greater than 39 mL required surgical intervention over a 4.5-year period.

Urodynamic evaluation involves the introduction of pressure monitoring transducers into the bladder and rectum and the subsequent measurement of intravesical and intra-abdominal pressures. These relationships, particularly those relating to intravesical pressure and flow rate while voiding (pressure-flow studies), can provide significant information about the nature of the patient's symptoms and the presence or absence of BOO. Pressure-flow studies are most useful in distinguishing BOO caused by BPH from impaired bladder contraction (hyper or hypo). However, urodynamic evaluation is an invasive modality that requires specific urologic expertise for its optimal utilization. Routine cystoscopic examination is optional in the evaluation of the patient with BPH. It is most frequently performed either in the course of evaluating the patient for a potentially invasive therapy, such as surgical resection, or for evaluating a co-existing condition, such as hematuria.

Routine evaluation of the upper tracts (kidneys and ureters) with excretory urography or ultrasonography is not recommended for the average patient with BPH unless a concomitant urinary pathologic abnormality (i.e., hematuria, urinary tract infection, renal insufficiency, a history of prior urologic surgery, a history of nephrolithiasis) exists. Similarly, transrectal ultrasonography (TRUS) is not routinely recommended unless it is used for preoperative assessment of prostate gland size while planning surgical intervention.

Differential Diagnosis

Many conditions can cause LUTS in the aging male. DRE and PSA testing are helpful in distinguishing between BPH and prostate cancer. Typically, early-stage prostate cancer is asymptomatic. Therefore patients may have both conditions concurrently. Although PSA testing is not sufficiently sensitive or specific enough to differentiate BPH from prostate cancer reliably, it is a useful tool to stratify a patient's risk for the presence of prostate cancer. Prostatitis is another condition that can cause LUTS. It may result from bacterial infection or from an inflammatory process, and the symptoms may substantially overlap those of BPH, particularly in the older man. Diabetes mellitus, neurologic diseases such as Parkinson's disease or cerebrovascular disease or other conditions of the urinary tract such as urethral strictures may result in LUTS seen in patients with BPH. Finally, many medications, particularly those with significant anticholinergic side effects, may mimic the symptoms associated with BPH.

Management

MEDICAL THERAPY

Medical management is the preferred first-line treatment option for patients diagnosed with LUTS from BPH. Most patients can be managed effectively with a minimum of side effects using the medications discussed later in this chapter. The NIH MTOPS study conclusively demonstrated that combination therapy with both a long-acting α-blocker and a 5a-reductase inhibitor was more effective than single-agent therapy alone. In general, medical management is initiated for patients with moderate to severe AUA symptom scores. However, notably, in the absence of indications for surgery (refractory urinary retention, hydronephrosis with or without renal impairment, recurrent urinary tract infections, recurrent gross hematuria, or bladder calculi), the decision to embark on any course of therapy, medical or otherwise, is principally driven by the degree of bother of the patient's symptoms. Every patient has a different perception of his symptoms; therefore nocturia twice nightly, though a minor nuisance to some people, may represent a significant problem for others. No absolute AUA symptom score or other objective measure exists that dictates the need for initiation of therapy for symptomatic BPH. Each patient must be evaluated individually, and his treatment course must be tailored to his individual situation.

α-Adrenergic Antagonists

α-Adrenergic antagonists, or α-blockers, are the most commonly prescribed medications for the treatment of LUTS associated with BPH. The bladder neck and prostate are richly innervated with α-adrenergic receptors, specifically α_{1a}-receptors, which constitute approximately 70% to 80% of the total number of α-receptors in these areas. α_{1b}-Receptors modulate vascular smooth muscle contraction and are located in the bladder neck and prostate to a lesser degree.

Doxazosin, terazosin, tamsulosin, and extended-release alfuzosin are long-acting α-receptor antagonists. They are generally administered once daily, usually at bedtime, to minimize the potential for orthostatic hypotension. These medications act via α_1-receptors and can cause vasodilation resulting in transient hypotension and light-headedness. Blood pressure reduction is greater in patients with hypertension (average reduction of 10 to 15 mm Hg) relative to normotensive patients (average reduction 1 to 4 mm Hg). Overall, 10% to 20% of patients experience some often-transient side effects from these medications, including dizziness, asthenia, headaches, peripheral edema, and nasal congestion. Dose titration is recommended for doxazosin and terazosin to minimize occurrence of these adverse effects and optimize therapeutic response. Doxazosin and terazosin require at least 4 or 5 mg, respectively, to achieve a therapeutic effect. Maximal response is usually seen within 1 to 2 weeks with doxazosin and 3 to 6 weeks with terazosin. Overall, these drugs reduce symptom scores by 40% to 50% and improve urinary flow rates by 40% to 50% in approximately 60% to 65% of patients treated.

Tamsulosin is a selective α_{1a}-receptor antagonist with a long half-life. It has a significantly lower degree of nonspecific α-receptor binding compared with other α-receptor antagonists. Therefore side effects such as postural hypotension and dizziness are less common. Tamsulosin does not appreciably affect blood pressure in hypertensive or normotensive patients. Maximal response is usually seen within 1 to 2 weeks of initiating therapy.

5a-Reductase Inhibition (Finasteride and Dutasteride)

Finasteride and dutasteride block the intracellular conversion of testosterone to 5-dihydrotestosterone by inhibiting the action of the enzyme 5a-reductase. This action results in an approximate 18% reduction in prostate gland size and improvement in LUTS. This regimen is most effective in reducing symptoms and preventing disease progression in patients with large prostate glands (>40 g). 5a-Reductase inhibition has also been shown to decrease the risk of urinary retention and the risk of subsequent surgical intervention, again, predominantly in patients with larger glands. Maximal response is seen in 6 to 12 months following the initiation of therapy.

Finasteride and dutasteride reduce serum PSA by approximately 50%. This reduction must be taken into consideration when interpreting PSA values in men taking these agents. After 6 months of therapy, the effective PSA level in a patient taking finasteride or dutasteride may be calculated by multiplying the measured PSA times 2. Free PSA (the percentage of non–protein-bound PSA) is also reduced by approximately 50%. Use of finasteride or dutasteride may result in sexual dysfunction, including decreased erectile rigidity, decreased libido, and ejaculatory dysfunction.

Phytotherapy

A growing body of evidence suggests that various plant extracts may have a therapeutic effect in the treatment of LUTS associated with BPH. Saw palmetto berry (*Serenoa repens*) extracts are the most widely used and studied. Use of saw palmetto has been shown to improve symptom scores in randomized trials in Europe. The therapeutic action of saw palmetto is believed to be derived from the action of lipid-soluble phytosterols, β-sitosterol being the most significant. African plum (*Pygeum africanum*) extract has also been used to treat symptoms associated with BPH. However, less is known about its overall efficacy and mechanism of action.

Use of herbal or plant extracts for the therapeutic management of symptomatic BPH remains somewhat controversial in the United States, despite their widespread use in Europe, particularly Germany. However, interest in evaluating these compounds is growing in the United States. Clinical trials are currently ongoing; however, results will not be available for several years.

SURGICAL MANAGEMENT

Minimally Invasive Therapy

Although transurethral resection of the prostate (TURP) remains the *gold standard* for the surgical treatment of BPH, substantial effort has been devoted to the development of less invasive and less morbid methods of treating patients with symptomatic BPH. This effort has led to a proliferation of minimally invasive therapies, primarily using different methods of generating heat within the prostate gland that results in tissue destruction.

Transurethral microwave thermotherapy (TUMT) is one of the most widely studied minimally invasive methods of treating patients with symptomatic BPH. Catheter-mounted transducers use microwave energy (30 to 300 Hz) to heat prostatic tissue, resulting in coagulative necrosis and shrinkage of the prostate gland. The subsequent reduction in prostate transition zone volume results in an improvement in flow rates and symptom scores. Transurethral needle ablation (TUNA) uses low-level radio-frequency energy to effect similar changes within the prostate gland. Other therapies currently available or in development include interstitial lasers and high-intensity focused ultrasound. All of these therapies are designed to deliver sufficient energy to the prostate to cause tissue destruction, resulting in smaller prostate glands and an attendant reduction in patient symptoms.

The most common side effects of these treatments are temporary increases in irritative voiding symptoms, transient urinary retention, hematuria, and ejaculatory dysfunction (primarily retrograde ejaculation). Late complications, such as urethral strictures and erectile dysfunction, have been reported but are significantly less common than those with traditional surgical approaches. The major benefits of these less invasive therapies are the reduction in traditional surgical morbidities such as bleeding, fluid absorption (TUR syndrome), and the risks associated with general or spinal anesthesia, as well as decreased rates of long-term complications such as incontinence, erectile dysfunction, bladder neck contractures, and urethral strictures. Additional advantages include decreased anesthetic requirements and decreased hospital stays resulting from the fact that the majority of these procedures can be accomplished safely on an outpatient basis, either in the office or in an ambulatory surgical setting.

Success rates for the heat-based minimally invasive therapies are intermediate between those achieved with medical management and those achieved with traditional surgical

Table 71–2	**Success in Medical Versus Surgical Management of Benign Prostatic Hyperplasia**				
	α₁-Blockers	**Finasteride**	**TURP**	**TUIP**	**Open Surgery**
Symptom improvement (%)	48	31	82	73	79
Flow rate improvement (%)	40–50	17	120	100	185
Mean probability of achieving the above improvement (%)	74	67	88	80	98

TUIP = transurethral incision of the prostate; TURP = transurethral resection of the prostate.

therapy, with 65% to 75% of patients experiencing symptomatic reduction and flow rate improvement. The long-term durability of these therapies is presently being evaluated.

Traditional Surgical Management

TURP remains the gold standard for the surgical management of symptomatic BPH. This procedure produces the greatest improvement in both urinary flow rates and symptom score. It is the preferred method of surgical management for all but the largest prostate glands (>100 g), which are best managed with open surgical enucleation. However, complications following TURP are higher than those following the minimally invasive approaches. Urinary incontinence, retrograde ejaculation, and urethral stricture rates are all higher following TURP than they are with office-based therapies. Peri-operative morbidity, including the need for blood transfusion, though substantially decreased by technical improvements, is similarly increased after TURP.

These complication rates have been reduced with modifications of the procedure, including the use of lasers as an energy source (reducing blood loss and fluid absorption) and the use of specially designed electrodes that can function in an isotonic saline environment (eliminating the risk of dilutional hyponatremia). However, standard electrosurgical resection of the prostate, TURP, is the most effective surgical treatment for symptomatic BPH, short of open surgical enucleation. Success rates, as measured by improvements in symptom score and increases in urinary flow rates, are 80% to 90% following TURP.

Transurethral incision of the prostate (TUIP) is another more limited surgical procedure consisting of incision of the bladder neck and proximal prostatic urethra. Although more invasive than the heat-based therapies, in properly selected patients (i.e., those with prostate glands less than 30 g in size), success rates approach those seen following TURP. Morbidity following TUIP is significantly less than that following TURP, but long-term durability of symptom relief is less than that seen with TURP.

Open surgical enucleation, or simple prostatectomy, is reserved for patients with severely large glands. Success rates are high following this approach; however, the rate of complications following open surgical resection is highest of all the traditional surgical approaches (Table 71–2).

The management of LUTS resulting from BPH has undergone a dramatic shift from principally a surgical approach to a medical approach. The vast majority of patients with LUTS believed to be secondary to BPH are initially managed medically as discussed previously. This trend, coupled with the aging of the U.S. population, has resulted in a shift of the care of these patients from the urologist to the primary care physician. In the absence of severe LUTS or indications for early surgical intervention, the primary care physician can now successfully manage the majority of patients with mild to moderate BPH.

B. Prostatitis

Prostatitis is an extremely common clinical condition, estimated to account for one in four office visits to urologists. It is the most common urologic diagnosis in men younger than 50 years of age and is the third most common diagnosis in men older than 50 years of age. Prostatitis is associated with a multitude of symptoms ranging from pelvic pain to voiding dysfunction. Until recently, the diagnosis of prostatitis was poorly defined and based primarily on clinical history. Treatment of the prostatitis syndromes remains equally problematic, with the efficacy of the most common therapies lacking evidence-based guidelines. Recently, the NIH has developed a standardized classification of prostatitis syndromes:

NIH category I: Acute bacterial prostatitis (ABP)
NIH category II: Chronic bacterial prostatitis (CBP)
NIH category III: Chronic pelvic pain syndrome (CPPS)

NIH category IIIa: Inflammatory CPPS
NIH category IIIb: Noninflammatory CPPS
NIH category IV: Asymptomatic prostatitis

Chronic nonbacterial prostatitis–CPPS (category IIIa and IIIb) is the most common symptomatic type of prostatitis and may be the most prevalent of all prostate disorders, including BPH. Despite this fact, chronic nonbacterial prostatitis–CPPS remains enigmatic and has not been conclusively demonstrated to be primarily a disease of the prostate or the result of a defined inflammatory process.

Acute Bacterial Prostatitis

ABP is a relatively rare serious systemic illness requiring aggressive treatment with intravenous antibiotics. Patients typically exhibit fever, chills, dysuria, and perineal and low back pain. Advanced cases may produce signs of sepsis. Physical examination may reveal a distended bladder, and DRE usually reveals a warm, boggy, and tender prostate. Rectal examination should be performed with caution to minimize the risk of inducing bacteremia as a result of overaggressive manipulation of the gland. Some urologists recommend deferring a rectal examination if the clinical presentation is highly suggestive of acute prostatitis.

Laboratory analysis typically reveals an elevated white blood cell (WBC) count and a positive urine culture. Localization examination is not useful because the pathogen is identified in the midstream urine. If the patient has evidence of urinary retention, a suprapubic cystostomy tube is recommended for bladder drainage to minimize transurethral instrumentation. Acutely ill patients are typically hospitalized for treatment with parenteral antibiotics and supportive care. Patients should be treated for a total of 30 days with combined parenteral and oral antibiotics to reduce the risk of development of chronic prostatitis. Fluoroquinolones are recommended because they achieve excellent tissue levels within prostate tissue. Although bacterial persistence or conversion to CBP is low, follow-up urine cultures should be obtained to document clearance of the infection. In rare instances, a prostatic abscess may form, especially in immunocompromised patients (i.e., those with diabetes and human immunodeficiency virus infection). The presence of a prostatic abscess can be evaluated with TRUS or contrast-enhanced pelvic computed tomographic (CT) scan and is treated with surgical transurethral unroofing of the abscess cavity and supplementary antibiotics.

Chronic Bacterial Prostatitis

CBP is associated with inflammation of the prostate gland and recurrent urinary tract infections with bacteria localized to the prostate via standardized localization testing. Etiologic agents range from common uropathogens to cryptic organisms that are difficult to culture. The differential diagnosis includes cystitis, urethritis, and the CPPSs IIIa and IIIb. Symptoms are nonspecific and include LUTS, pelvic pain, and sexual dysfunction, either alone or in combination. Physical examination may reveal abdominal tenderness, testicular or epididymal tenderness, prostate tenderness, or tenderness associated with DRE. The prostate is often normal to palpation, although it may be enlarged secondary to concomitant BPH.

Traditional testing of the urine in this patient population is accomplished by evaluation of urine in the following manner. The first voided urine (VB-1) is collected, followed by collection of midstream urine (VB-2). Following this procedure, a DRE is performed, and the prostate is massaged. Expressed prostatic secretions (EPS) are then collected. The patient is then asked to void again, and the postmassage urine (VB-3) is collected. Evaluation of each of these fractions can provide evidence of the source of any infection. CBP is diagnosed when 10 times the number of WBCs are present in the EPS or VB-3 relative to the VB-1 or VB-2. Alternatively, culture of the EPS or VB-3 must grow 10-fold more organisms than the VB-1 or VB-2. Pre- and postprostatic massage urine can also be compared for the presence of WBCs and/or uropathogenic organisms. Although these measures are commonly described for the accurate diagnosis of prostatitis, a presumptive diagnosis is often made based on clinical symptoms, EPS, and urinalysis findings.

Treatment involves a 4- to 8-week course of antimicrobial therapy. This period can be extended to 12 weeks in persons who respond initially but fail to eradicate the organism from the gastrourinary tract. Broad-spectrum antibiotics such as trimethoprim-sulfamethoxazole (TMP-SMX) or a fluoroquinolone are indicated for the treatment of CBP and must be tailored to the suspected pathogen. Studies have shown excellent tissue levels of these drugs within the prostate. Typically, between 60% and 80% of patients are cured with 1- to 3-month treatment courses. One third of patients will relapse with recurrent symptoms and bacteriuria. For patients who have relapsing infections, long-term suppressive therapy may be indicated, whereas patients who have recurrent infections with different organisms are best treated with low-dose prophylactic antibiotics. Surgery is rarely indicated in patients with CBP because cure rates of only 33% are achieved with aggressive transurethral prostatectomy (e.g., TURP). This low rate of cure is thought to be caused by the fact that most of the infected tissue lies in the peripheral zone of the prostate, as opposed to the transition zone. Treatment end points are the clearance of appropriate cultures and the resolution of the patient's symptoms.

Chronic Nonbacterial Prostatitis–Chronic Pelvic Pain Syndrome

The NIH category III chronic nonbacterial prostatitis–CPPS makes up the largest percentage of patients with clinical prostatitis. These syndromes are the most difficult to diagnose, treat, and are the most poorly understood pathophysiologically. In addition, a substantial economic impact is associated with CPPS, which warrants further research to determine more effective treatment strategies. Patients with CPPS typically exhibit a combination of pain (perineal, low back, suprapubic, groin, or scrotal), voiding dysfunction (dysuria, weak stream, frequency, urgency, or nocturia), and/or sexual dysfunction (painful ejaculation or low libido). The presence of pelvic pain, regardless of the degree of associated symptoms, is mandatory for the diagnosis of category III prostatitis. Because of varied symptoms and interpatient variability, the NIH created a validated chronic prostatitis symptom index (NIH-CPSI) that is now available for the initial assessment and subsequent follow-up of patients with chronic prostatitis. The index is a 13-item questionnaire with three domain scores: (1) pain, (2) urinary symptoms, and (3) quality of life. The clinical evaluation of patients with chronic prostatitis–CPPS (CP-CPPS) often includes clinical history and examination, administration of the NIH-CPSI, urinary tract localization studies, and urinary flow rate with postvoid residual.

Inflammatory CPPS (NIH category IIIa) is associated with the same symptoms seen in CBP; however, no causative organism is typically identified. Pelvic pain is a frequent symptom that may be exacerbated by stress, certain dietary factors, or vigorous physical exercise. The cause of the symptoms is unclear; however, clearly, patients' quality of life is significantly affected by the presence of this disorder. On physical examination, rectal examination typically reveals nonspecific findings, and the prostate may be tender or indurated, although, more frequently, the examination findings are within normal limits. Urinalysis should be normal, and urine cultures should be sterile. The EPS often reveal significant numbers of WBCs, but, again, the EPS should be sterile. Treatment can be frustrating for both patients and providers and includes measures such as warm baths and nonsteroidal anti-inflammatory drugs (NSAIDs), with some urologists recommending prostatic massage for patients who ejaculate infrequently. The routine use of antibiotics is common but controversial. Generally, antibiotic therapy should be limited to an empirical 2-week course of an appropriate antibiotic and terminated if no clinical response to treatment occurs. If the patient responds, extension to a full 6-week course may be indicated.

Noninflammatory Chronic Pelvic Pain Syndrome

Noninflammatory CPPS, also known as prostatodynia, is typically seen in younger male patients age 20 to 50 years.

These patients typically show symptoms suggestive of prostatitis, including pelvic pain and voiding symptoms, but have negative urine cultures, normal EPS, and a normal prostate on DRE. Stress is a frequent component of the symptom complex.

Treatment in this population again includes the same supportive measures mentioned previously. α-Adrenergic antagonists are the primary pharmacologic agent used to treat this condition, though efficacy data is scant. NSAIDs are also useful and may be used in conjunction with tricyclic antidepressants for the management of chronic pain. The anticholinergic side effects of the tricyclics can also help with the associated frequency and urgency often experienced by these patients. Biofeedback and other stress-management techniques have been used with limited success.

Recently, small studies have suggested that the heat-based, minimally invasive methods used to treat BPH may have some role in treating noninflammatory CPPS. TUMT has been shown to decrease pain and voiding symptoms in small series of patients. Larger studies are needed to confirm the utility and safety of this approach.

Noninflammatory CPPS is a difficult and demanding problem for both patients and physicians. Patients have frequently seen multiple physicians, and some have chronic pain and other psychiatric problems, such as depression or anxiety disorders. An important point to remember, however, is that, despite our poor understanding of the pathophysiology of this condition, noninflammatory CPPS is common and has a major impact on quality of life. Appropriate clinical concern coupled with good patient communication and rational treatment strategies are the foundation for the successful management of this challenging group of patients.

C. Erectile Dysfunction

Impotence is a condition defined by the inability to attain and or maintain adequate penile rigidity sufficient for intercourse. Impotence is the most common cause of erectile dysfunction (ED) in the United States. Other important, though less common, causes of ED include Peyronie's disease, trauma, and rapid ejaculation. Approximately 10 million Americans are affected by ED. Table 71–3 illustrates the prevalence of ED measured in the Massachusetts Male Aging Study. As this study shows, at age 40, approximately 5% of men never have penile rigidity sufficient for vaginal penetration. By age 70, at least 15% of men experience complete ED, whereas approximately 50% have varying degrees of ED. Age and physical health are the most important predictors of the onset of ED. The study showed that smoking was the most important lifestyle variable, and ED did not correlate with male hormone levels.

Mechanism of Erection

Psychogenic or tactile sexual stimulation, or both, is the initial point in the pathway leading to penile erection. Nerve

Table 71–3	**Relationship of Risk Factors to Erectile Dysfunction: Prevalence (%) of Complete Erectile Dysfunction**			
		Risk Factor Plus Smoking Status		
Risk Factor	**Prevalence**	**Smoker**	**Former Smoker**	**Nonsmoker**
Age 40	5.1			
Age 70	15			
Diabetes*	28			
Heart Disease*	39	56	21	8.5
Hypertension*	15	20		
All patients	9.6			

Data from Feldman HA, Goldstein I, Hatzichristou DG, et al: Impotence and its medical and psychosocial correlates: Results of the Massachusetts Male Aging Study. J Urol 151:54–61, 1994.
*Patients diagnosed with and undergoing treatment for these conditions.

signals are carried through the pelvic plexus, a portion of which condenses into the cavernous nerves of the penile corpora cavernosa. The pelvic plexus receives input from both the sympathetic and parasympathetic nervous system. Sympathetic fibers originate in the thoracolumbar spinal cord, condense into the hypogastric plexus located immediately below the aortic bifurcation, and course into the pelvic plexus. Parasympathetic fibers originate in sacral spinal cord segments 2 through 4 and join the pelvic plexus. Discrete nerves carrying both sympathetic and parasympathetic fibers innervate the organs of the pelvis. In 1982, Walsh and Donker demonstrated that nerves coursing immediately lateral to the urethra continue on to innervate the corpora cavernosa. The fact is now known that branches of these nerves are the principle innervation of the neuromuscular junction where arterial smooth muscle controls penile blood flow.

Sexual stimulation causes the release of nitric oxide (NO) by the cavernous nerves into the neuromuscular junction (Fig. 71–3). NO activates guanylyl cyclase, which converts guanosine 5′-triphosphate (GTP) into cyclic guanosine monophosphate (cGMP). Protein kinase G is activated by cGMP and, in turn, activates several proteins that decrease intracellular calcium (Ca_2^+) concentration. Decreased smooth-muscle Ca_2^+ concentration causes muscular relaxation, cavernosal artery dilation, increased blood flow, and subsequent penile erection. The control of blood flow on the venous outflow side is less well understood.

Causes of Erectile Dysfunction

Psychogenic ED was formerly thought to be the most common cause of ED. Progressive advances in understanding of the mechanics and neurophysiologic factors of erectile function have identified other more common causes of ED. Psychogenic ED is now thought to represent less than 15% of patients seen by ED specialists. The anatomic site now believed to be the most common cause of ED is the neuromuscular junction where the cavernosal nerves meet

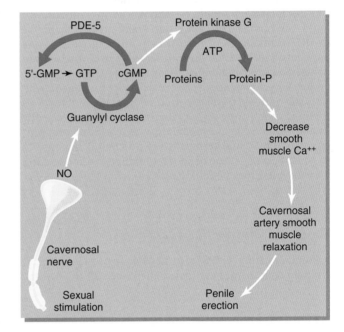

Figure 71–3 Sexual stimulation causes the release of nitric oxide (NO) by the cavernous nerve into the neuromuscular junction.

the smooth muscle and endothelium of the deep cavernous penile arteries. This site is where NO and cGMP play a critical role in regulating penile blood flow. This so-called endothelial dysfunction may be an early tip-off of evolving systemic arterial disease. Other less-common causes of decreased erectile rigidity include endocrine disorders, vascular disease, central and peripheral nerve disorders, drug-induced ED, and venogenic ED.

NEUROMUSCULAR JUNCTION DISORDERS

NO is released from cavernosal nerves, causing activation of guanylyl cyclase within the corpus cavernosum. Figure 71–3 illustrates several steps that, if not functioning properly, can impede erectile function. Most research at this time is focused on generation of NO by the cavernous nerves. Further understanding of all the steps in the erectile pathway will likely implicate other biochemical reactions as causing ED. The fact that at least 60% of patients with ED from all causes other than trauma or medical treatment respond to phosphodiesterase type 5 (PDE-5) inhibition is strong evidence supporting the inference that biochemical dysfunction at the neuromuscular junction is by far the most common cause of ED.

ENDOCRINE DISORDERS

Testosterone plays a permissive role in erectile function. Endocrine disorders may directly or indirectly decrease plasma-free or bound testosterone. The most obvious, but one of the least prevalent, causes of ED is hypogonadism. Erectile ability is partially androgen-dependent. These patients exhibit decreased or absent libido in addition to loss of erectile rigidity. Physical examination of the testes in patients afflicted with primary or secondary hypogonadism often reveals soft, atrophic gonads. Androgen replacement (testosterone cypionate, 200 mg every 2 to 3 weeks, or daily topical testosterone gel or patch preparations) is expected to induce return of erectile function in patients with very low or undetectable serum testosterone concentrations resulting from hypogonadism. These instances are relatively uncommon, however. More commonly, the impotent patient will have normal or mildly decreased levels of circulating androgens. Testosterone replacement rarely restores erectile function in patients with mildly decreased serum testosterone levels and should not be routinely given for this indication. Testosterone supplementation is never indicated for patients with normal circulating androgen levels.

The most common endocrine disorder affecting erectile ability is diabetes mellitus. Diabetes affects both the autonomic and somatic nervous system in addition to causing atherosclerotic vascular disease. The most important effect diabetes has on erectile ability appears to relate to loss of function of long autonomic nerves. Erection is partially mediated by efferent parasympathetic cholinergic neural stimuli. Loss of long cholinergic neurons results in interruption of the efferent side of the erectile reflex arc. Diabetes also appears to produce dysfunction of the neuromuscular junction at the level of arterial smooth muscle in the penile corpora cavernosa. Studies have indicated markedly decreased acetylcholine and NO concentrations in the trabeculae of the corpora cavernosa in diabetics. These findings probably represent a combination of neural loss and neuromuscular junction dysfunction.

Other endocrine disorders, including hypothyroidism, hyperthyroidism, and adrenal dysfunction, may uncommonly cause ED. Because of the uncommon occurrence of thyroid and adrenal conditions in persons seeking treatment of ED, testing of these axes is not a part of the routine work-up of ED.

VASCULAR DISEASE

Vascular disease is a frequent cause of ED in the United States, primarily because of the high prevalence and often severe nature of peripheral vascular disease. Penile erection is obtained by a combination of relaxation of arteriolar smooth muscle and increasing venous resistance of channels penetrating the wall of the corpora cavernosa. Arterial disease may interfere with or decrease erectile ability either by mechanical obstruction of the vascular lumen or more commonly by endothelial dysfunction, which, as discussed previously, interrupts the neural control mechanism of vascular smooth-muscle function. This process leads to complete filling of the corpora cavernosa with blood at systemic blood pressure. The principle blood vessels supplying the corpora cavernosa are the cavernosal arteries. These vessels are terminal branches of the pudendal artery, which itself is the terminal branch of the internal iliac artery. Either large or small vessel arterial disease may decrease corporal blood pressure, leading to failure to achieve penile lengthening and rigidity.

Normal penile erection requires a functioning vascular tree upstream from the cavernosal arteries. Many cases of ED were formerly attributed to anatomic vascular disease when the problem actually was with control of cavernosal artery smooth muscle. Pharmacologic injection therapy involves injecting vasodilator agents (prostaglandin-E_1 [PGE_1], papaverine, phentolamine, or combinations of these agents) into the corpora cavernosa to produce erection by dilating the corporal artery smooth muscle. Over 90% of patients with ED respond to this type of therapy, indicating that atherosclerotic arterial narrowing is not the cause of most cases of ED.

Veno-occlusive disease in the penis is also a significant cause of ED. These patients often experience normal initial rigidity but quickly, and before ejaculation, lose their erection.

NEUROGENIC ERECTILE DYSFUNCTION

Pure neurogenic ED is a frequent cause of erectile failure. Interruption of either somatic or autonomic nerves or their end units may cause ED. These nerves control the flow of blood into and likely out of the corpora cavernosa. Afferent somatic sensory signals are carried from the penis via the pudendal nerve to S2 through S4. This information is routed both to the brain and to spinal cord autonomic centers. Parasympathetic autonomic nerves originate in the intermediolateral gray matter of S2 through S4. These preganglionic fibers exit the anterior nerve roots to join with the sympathetic fibers of the hypogastric nerve to form the pelvic plexus and cavernosal nerves. The paired cavernosal nerves penetrate the corpora cavernosa and innervate the cavernous artery and veins. Parasympathetic ganglia are located distally near the end organ.

Sympathetic innervation also originates in the intermediolateral gray matter but at thoracolumbar levels T10 through L2. Sympathetic efferents course through the retroperitoneum and condense into the hypogastric plexus located anterior and slightly caudal to the aortic bifurcation. A concentration of postganglionic sympathetic fibers forms the hypogastric nerve, which is joined by parasympathetic efferents. Adrenergic innervation appears to play a role in the process of detumescence. High concentrations of norepinephrine have been demonstrated in the tissue of the corpora cavernosa and tributary arterioles. Additionally, the α-adrenergic antagonist phentolamine is routinely used for intracorporal injection therapy to produce erection.

Table 71–4	Frequency of Decreased Erectile Rigidity and Ejaculatory Dysfunction by Medication Class	
Medication Class	**Decreased Erectile Rigidity**	**Ejaculatory Dysfunction**
β-Adrenergic antagonists	Common	Less common
Sympatholytics	Expected	Common
α_1-Agonists	Uncommon	Uncommon
α_2-Agonists	Common	Less common
α_1-Antagonists	Uncommon	Less common*
Angiotensin-converting enzyme inhibitors	Uncommon	Uncommon
Diuretics	Less common	Uncommon
Antidepressants	Common†	Uncommon‡
Antipsychotics	Common	Common
Anticholinergics	Less common	Uncommon

*Patients able to ejaculate but retrograde ejaculation seen in 5% to 30%.
†Uncommon with serotonin reuptake inhibitors.
‡Delayed or inhibited ejaculation with serotonin reuptake inhibitors.

Afferent signals capable of initiating erection can either originate within the brain, as is the case with psychogenic erections, or result from tactile stimulation. Patients with spinal cord injury often respond to tactile sensation but usually require medical therapy to maintain the erection through intercourse. No discreet center exists for psychogenic erections. The temporal lobe appears to be important; however, other locations such as the gyrus rectus, the cingulate gyrus, the hypothalamus, and the mammillary bodies also appear to be important.

MEDICATION-INDUCED ERECTILE DYSFUNCTION

Commonly prescribed medications often cause or contribute to decreased erectile function. A complete list of these agents and their mechanisms of action is beyond the purview of this text. Table 71–4 lists the major classes of medications implicated in ED and suggests how commonly these medications interfere with erectile function. In clinical practice, patients are frequently on specific classes of medications for important purposes. For this reason, substituting a different medication is usually unsuccessful in restoring erectile function in patients who often have several risk factors for ED. Proceeding directly to treatment of ED is usually the preferred option in all but the most straightforward cases.

Medical and Surgical Treatment

Since the introduction of sildenafil in 1998, the Process of Care Model for the Evaluation and Treatment of ED has been adopted and targets the primary care provider as the initial source of care for patients with ED (Fig. 71–4). Currently available therapies for ED include oral PDE-5 inhibitors, intra-urethral alprostadil, intracavernous vasoactive injection therapy, vacuum constriction devices, and penile pros-

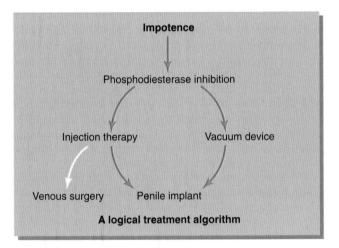

Figure 71–4   A logical treatment algorithm for impotence.

thesis implantation. A stepwise treatment approach is adopted, starting with oral agents and progressing to more invasive therapeutic interventions as indicated. Informed patient decision making is critical toward successful progression along the plan of care pathway. Patient referral is primarily based on failure of specific medical therapy, as well as the need or desire for specialized diagnostic testing and management. As a result, the majority of prescriptions for oral PDE-5 inhibitors are written by primary care providers, and specialized diagnostics such as Doppler ultrasound of the penile arteries and nocturnal penile tumescence (NPT) testing are used by urologists to work-up select cases.

Oral Phosphodiesterase Type 5 Inhibitors

Current medical therapy is based on inhibition of PDE-5. Figure 71–3 illustrates that cGMP is broken down to inactive

5′-GMP by PDE-5. Sildenafil, vardenafil, and tadalafil competitively inhibit PDE-5 breakdown of cGMP by binding to the catalytic domain of PDE-5. Use of a PDE-5 inhibitor results in improved erectile rigidity even in patients with decreased NO or cGMP synthesis. Not all patients respond to PDE-5 inhibition, however. Adequate sexual stimulation and intact neural and vascular pathways are necessary to produce an adequate amount of NO and cGMP to increase deep penile artery blood flow. PDE-5 inhibitors are effective in men with organic, psychogenic, neurogenic, and mixed cases of ED. The overall response rate is 70%, with placebo response rates of 20% to 30%. In terms of disease-specific response to oral agents, improved erections were observed in 70% of patients with hypertension, 80% of patients with spinal cord injury, 56% of patients with diabetes, and 42% of patients who have had radical prostatectomy.

PDE-5 inhibition should be considered first-line therapy, unless contraindicated. At the present time, no evidence-based data exist or randomized trials have been conducted supporting superior efficacy of one drug over another. All of the agents are hepatically metabolized. Initial concerns about concomitant use of PDE-5 inhibitors and α-blockers have been resolved. PDE-5 inhibitors should not be used concurrently with nitrate medications because a large (≥ 25 mm Hg) synergistic drop in blood pressure is observed in many patients. Periodic follow-up is necessary to determine therapeutic efficacy, side effects related to PDE-5 inhibition, and a change in health status, including medications.

PHARMACOLOGIC INJECTION THERAPY

Several vasoactive agents can be safely injected directly into the corpora cavernosa to produce penile erection. Commonly used agents include PGE$_1$, papaverine, and phentolamine. These agents can be used either alone or in combination. As monotherapy, PGE$_1$ is most commonly used, and of the three, only PGE$_1$ has been evaluated in rigorous clinical trials and has specific marketing approval from the U.S. Food and Drug Administration for the treatment of ED. PGE$_1$ and papaverine are often used alone. Phentolamine, in contrast, is used to potentiate the action of papaverine or is used in combination with both PGE$_1$ and papaverine. These vasoactive drugs are frequently combined (bimix and trimix) to achieve increased efficacy and decreased side effects.

Injection therapy has two principal risks, (1) priapism and (2) corporal scarring, causing penile curvature. Priapism has been reported to occur in 1% to 4% of patients. Prolonged erections occur more commonly in patients with neurogenic ED, especially young men with spinal cord injury. Significant acquired penile curvature is seen uncommonly and usually follows several years of injection therapy. Penile curvature appears to be less common with use of PGE$_1$ than papaverine. The most common problem with pharmacologic injection therapy is not complications from therapy, but rather that 50% to 60% of patients stop using the technique by 1 year.

INTRAURETHRAL DRUG THERAPY

PGE$_1$ can be inserted into the urethra using a pellet applicator. This method of delivery assumes substantial venous communications between the corpus spongiosum surrounding the urethra and the corpus cavernosum. As a consequence, the technique is considerably less effective than intracavernous injection.

VACUUM CONSTRICTION DEVICES

These devices enclose the penis in a plastic tube with an air-tight seal at the penile base. Air is pumped out of the cylinder, creating a vacuum. Blood flows into the corporal bodies, leading to penile erection. A constriction band remains on the base of the penis to maintain erection. Simultaneous use of a vacuum device and a PDE-5 inhibitor is safe. Many patients couple the two techniques to achieve satisfactory results.

PENILE PROSTHESIS

A penile prosthesis is implanted in the operating room. Two general types of devices can be implanted: semirigid and inflatable. Most patients prefer the inflatable devices because they provide a more natural erection when inflated and a flaccid penis when deflated. Though more invasive than the other techniques, a penile prosthesis is the most effective long-term option for impotence treatment. Ninety percent of patients and partners are satisfied with the result.

Future Treatments

A period of rapid expansion in the understanding and treatment of ED has just been completed. Much of the biochemical pathway leading to erection has been elucidated, and several effective oral medications have been introduced. Future medical treatments will depend on identification of specific biochemical events in the erection pathway that are unique to penile function. PDE-5 is a good example of this identification. To this point, other biochemical events such as production of cGMP are ubiquitous in other important systems of the body and do not make good targets for drugs designed to enhance erectile function. That other classes of oral medications will have to await further advances in the basic understanding of erectile function is anticipated.

Important interval improvements have been made in the design of implantable penile prostheses that make the devices more durable and resistant to infection. Improvements in the connection between tubing and corporal cylinders have cut the mechanical failure rate to less than 5% in 5 years. Components also have special coatings that either contain antibiotics or absorb antibiotics applied topically at the time of implantation. These improvements have cut the rate of postoperative infection by one half.

D. Carcinomas of Men

Prostate Cancer

Carcinoma of the prostate is the most common cancer that occurs in men and the second leading cause of cancer death. Prostate cancer incidence increases with advancing age. Clinical diagnosis of prostate cancer is unusual made before the latter half of the fifth decade of life but increases progressively thereafter.

Risk factors for prostate cancer are poorly understood (Table 71–5). Some racial correlation exists because prostate cancer is more common in African-American men than in whites. A high-fat diet has been implicated in some studies. The role of lycopenes and selenium is under investigation. No association has been demonstrated between prostate cancer and cigarette smoking, sexual activity, or a prior history of prostatitis or BPH.

Considerable disparity can be found between the autopsy incidence of prostate cancer and clinical detection of the disease. Pathologic examination of step-sectioned prostate specimens shows histologic evidence of prostate cancer in more than 50% of men over the age of 60 years. The overwhelming majority of these *autopsy* or *latent* cancers are less than 0.2 mL in volume and of a low pathologic grade. These tumors are distinctly different from their clinically diagnosed counterparts. The reasons for this disparity or the factors that may trigger development of clinically aggressive disease are unknown.

DETECTION AND DIAGNOSIS

Controversy about the value of prostate cancer screening is ongoing. Much of this debate is fueled by the failure to take into account age and co-morbidity. Whereas men with a less than 10-year life expectancy may not benefit from prostate cancer screening, those younger than 70 to 75 years of age who are otherwise in good health have a substantial risk of morbidity or mortality from untreated prostate cancer. Most experts recommend routine screening in this group.

Both the DRE and serum PSA determination have a role in the early diagnosis of prostate cancer. Prostate cancer typically arises from the peripheral portion of the prostate, which can be palpated on DRE. Induration or nodularity of the prostate on DRE should be considered suggestive of prostate cancer.

PSA is a protein produced by both benign and malignant prostate cells. Serum PSA may be elevated in the presence of prostate enlargement, inflammation, or cancer (Table 71–6). Although an elevated PSA is not diagnostic of prostate cancer, it may lead to a prostate biopsy to exclude cancer. Probably because of progressive enlargement in prostate size, serum PSA values increase as men age. A value of 4.0 ng/mL historically has been considered a *normal* cut-off for PSA. However, values as low as 2.5 or 3.0 ng/mL may prompt biopsy in men younger than 60 years of age. The rate of increase in PSA over time is probably the most important piece of diagnostic information. Specifically, a rise in PSA of greater than 0.75 ng/mL per year may be cause for concern.

Whenever prostate cancer is suggested, either because of an abnormality in DRE or PSA rise, prostate biopsy is performed. TRUS imaging of the prostate is used to guide prostate biopsy. Prostate cancers typically have a hypoechoic appearance. However, TRUS is of limited value for diagnosis and is used primarily to direct biopsies. Transrectal cores of prostate tissue are obtained. This procedure is an office-based procedure, and local infiltration of lidocaine (Xylocaine) around the prostate minimizes discomfort. In most instances, 8 to 12 tissue cores are taken systematically from the entire prostate.

Prostate cancer is most often graded according to the Gleason system. This scoring system uses two numbers based on the primary and secondary histologic pattern. Gleason sums of 2, 3, or 4 are uncommon with clinically detected cancers. Gleason 5 or 6 tumors are most common, whereas sums of 8, 9, and 10 imply an aggressive tumor behavior.

DRE is the most useful test for determining local tumor extent. CT scanning is of limited value and usually not indicated clinically for determining either local extent or nodal metastasis. In patients with high-grade tumors or a substantially elevated PSA, a bone scan is indicated because bone is the most common site of distant spread. Soft tissue metastasis is unusual with a normal bone scan.

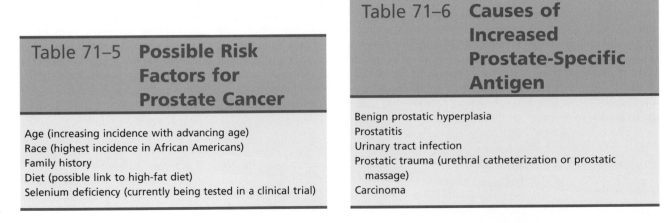

Table 71–5	**Possible Risk Factors for Prostate Cancer**
Age (increasing incidence with advancing age)	
Race (highest incidence in African Americans)	
Family history	
Diet (possible link to high-fat diet)	
Selenium deficiency (currently being tested in a clinical trial)	

Table 71–6	**Causes of Increased Prostate-Specific Antigen**
Benign prostatic hyperplasia	
Prostatitis	
Urinary tract infection	
Prostatic trauma (urethral catheterization or prostatic massage)	
Carcinoma	

Table 71–7	**Treatment Options for Localized Prostate Cancer**

Radical prostatectomy
Brachytherapy (I$_{125}$, etc., seeds)
External beam irradiation
Cryotherapy
Hormonal therapy
Watchful waiting

TREATMENT OF LOCALIZED DISEASE

Considerable controversy exists about the best treatment for clinically localized prostate cancer, and patients should enter into an informed decision-making process (Table 71–7). For people with a less than 10-year life expectancy otherwise, a policy of no initial treatment, often termed *watchful waiting*, is appropriate. Most older men or those with significant co-morbidity die from causes other than prostate cancer even without curative therapy when the tumor is detected at a clinically localized stage.

For men with a greater than 10-year life expectancy otherwise, curative therapy is usually indicated. Surgical removal of the prostate (radical prostatectomy) is the treatment with the most proven ability for long-term cure of prostate cancer. Contemporary radical prostatectomy is an operation with limited peri-operative morbidity. The greatest drawbacks to the procedure are the risks of long-term consequences. Significant incontinence occurs in only approximately 2% of men, but up to 10% may have at least some degree of mild stress incontinence. The cavernosal nerves, which are responsible for dilation of the blood vessels that lead to penile tumescence, lie immediately adjacent to the prostate. Dissection of these nerves from the prostate (nerve-sparing radical prostatectomy) is appropriate in patients with tumors localized to the prostate. The success of nerve-sparing prostatectomy is related to patient age and preoperative erectile function. Preservation of potency can be achieved in up to 60% to 80% of patients.

After radical prostatectomy, serum PSA should decline to an undetectable range. No measurable PSA is produced from any source other than prostate cells. Metastatic foci of cancer continue to produce PSA, therefore an undetectable value is an excellent prognostic sign. Furthermore, an increase in PSA to a detectable range precedes other signs or symptoms of prostate cancer recurrence after radical prostatectomy almost 99% of the time. Thus PSA is an extremely sensitive and specific marker for monitoring men after radical prostatectomy.

Radiation therapy, delivered either by external beam therapy or by interstitial brachytherapy, is the primary alternative to surgery for localized prostate cancer. External beam therapy is delivered over 7 to 8 weeks and is associated with a risk of radiation cystitis or proctitis. Impotence is progressive and by 2 years after radiation therapy occurs in one half of patients, depending on age.

Brachytherapy is performed by interstitial implantation of radioactive isotopes. Iodine-125 is used most commonly

Table 71–8	**Long-Term Side Effects of Androgen Deprivation Therapy**

Hot flashes
Loss of libido
Impotence
Osteoporosis
Decreased facial hair
Loss of muscle mass
Weight gain

and is often supplemented with external beam radiation known as a boost. Brachytherapy requires administration of an anesthetic but has minimal short-term morbidity, and patients return rapidly to preoperative activities. However, questions remain about the long-term durability of this treatment in curing prostate cancer. Difficulty voiding and impotence are risks of brachytherapy, whereas radiation proctitis is relatively unusual.

TREATMENT OF ADVANCED DISEASE

Endocrine manipulation remains the primary form of treatment for patients with advanced or metastatic carcinoma of the prostate. The goal of therapy is to deprive the prostate cancer cells of serum androgens. This goal can be accomplished by either surgical or medical castration. Surgical orchiectomy removes both testes, the source of testosterone production. Luteinizing hormone–releasing hormone (LHRH) analogues are administered by a slow-release depot injection every 3 to 4 months. These drugs have the paradoxical effect of decreasing serum LH release from the pituitary gland and, consequently, diminishing testosterone production from the testis. Testosterone declines to castrate values within a few days after surgical orchiectomy and a few weeks after administering an LHRH analogue.

In response to androgen deprivation, prostate cancer typically undergoes rapid regression. This regression is demonstrated by a decrease in prostate size, improvement in any disease symptoms such as bone pain, and a rapid decline in serum PSA. The duration of response varies but is usually on the order of a couple of years for patients who have metastatic disease. Hormonal therapy generally is well tolerated but frequently causes hot flushes and is associated with some degree of osteoporosis, weight gain, and loss of muscle mass with long-term use (Table 71–8).

Antiandrogens may also be used in hormonal therapy of patients with prostate cancer. These oral medications exert their effect by blocking the metabolism of androgens at the cellular level rather than by decreasing serum values. Antiandrogens may be used in combination with LHRH analogues to block the effect of adrenal androgens in addition to testosterone. Despite multiple randomized studies, the value of combination treatment compared with LHRH analogues alone is still a matter of debate.

Once prostate cancer shows evidence of progression despite hormonal therapy, the prognosis for patients is poor. Bone pain is managed with appropriate analgesics and irradiation. Chemotherapy can sometimes provide palliation but has not been shown to extend survival.

Penile Carcinoma

Squamous cell carcinoma of the penis is an uncommon tumor in the United States and the rest of the developed world, with a rate of less than one case per 100,000 men and an estimated 1470 cases in the United States for 2005. Penile carcinoma is diagnosed almost exclusively in uncircumcised men. Neonatal circumcision seems to have a protective effect. Circumcision in adulthood or late childhood does not appear to confer the same level of protection. Chronic irritation and inflammation are key etiologic factors, given that most men have poor hygiene, leading to phimosis of the foreskin. Further evidence links the development of penile cancer with some serotypes of the human papillomavirus (HPV types 16 and 18). Smoking and other forms of tobacco use have also been a consistent finding in several epidemiologic studies of penile cancer risk factors.

Squamous cell carcinoma typically produces a painless, nonindurated, ulcerated mass involving the glans penis and coronal sulcus. Infection of the primary lesion is common and may produce foul-smelling, purulent discharge and reactive inguinal lymphadenopathy. Delay in diagnosis is common because patients often do not seek immediate treatment secondary to fear and embarrassment, whereas prolonged treatment with antibiotics may delay confirmatory biopsy of the lesion.

Diagnosis and Treatment

Evaluation of suspicious lesions begins with clinical assessment of both the tumor and the inguinal lymph nodes. Imaging studies are not routinely recommended because physical examination has proven to be the most accurate predictor of tumor stage. A diagnosis of carcinoma of the penis is confirmed by histologic evaluation of an excisional biopsy. Prognosis is directly correlated with grade of the tumor and the extent of invasion. Adverse prognostic factors include high histopathologic grade, vascular invasion, and advanced pathologic stage ($\geq$T2).

The classic operation for squamous cell carcinoma of the penis is partial penectomy with a 2-cm negative margin. If the tumor is confined to the distal penis, a sufficient length of proximal penile shaft can be preserved so that the patient can still void in a standing position.

Larger tumors that invade the more proximal penile shaft require total penectomy. The entire corpora cavernosa are excised back to the ischial tuberosity. A perineal urethrostomy is created that allows voiding in a sitting position.

Contemporary studies are now attempting to stratify patients who would benefit from organ-preserving therapies, with improved functional and cosmetic results. These treatment approaches include topical treatments (5-fluorouracil), external beam radiation therapy, Moh's microsurgery, laser ablation (carbon dioxide and neodymium: yttrium-aluminum-garnet [Nd: YAG]), and complete tumor excision with phallic reconstruction. Patients with Tis, Ta, and T1 (grade 1 and 2) tumors who are at low risk for metastasis seem to be ideal candidates for this approach. The main drawback is the increased risk of local tumor recurrence.

Inguinal lymph node dissection is indicated in patients with palpable inguinal nodes that persist after antibiotic therapy or in those with nonpalpable nodes with risk factors for regional metastasis (histopathologic grade 3, vascular invasion, and T stage $\geq$2). Traditionally, significant morbidity has been associated with inguinal lymph node dissection (lymphedema, skin necrosis, deep-vein thrombosis). However, several contemporary studies have shown a decreased incidence and severity of complications. Modified lymphadenectomy and sentinel node biopsy aim at detecting occult metastases while minimizing patient morbidity.

The prognosis for patients with distant metastatic disease or nodal metastasis above the inguinal ligament is poor. Squamous cell carcinoma of the penis is moderately chemotherapy sensitive, and numerous regimens have been studied, reflecting the lack of superior efficacy of one combination over another. A durable response to chemotherapy is unusual, and further studies with novel agents and multimodal therapy are currently being investigated.

Testis Cancer

The management of patients with testicular carcinoma has become a model for the multidisciplinary approach to solid tumors. As a result of effective surgery, radiation therapy, and combination chemotherapy, survival approaches 99% for low-risk disease and 80% for high-risk disease. Testicular tumors are the most common solid malignancy in men age 15 to 34 years. In 2003, 7500 new cases of testicular cancer and 350 deaths were reported, and data from the Surveillance, Epidemiology, and End Results (SEER) database have shown that the incidence of testicular germ cell tumors (TGCT) has increased over the last 25 years.

Cryptorchidism (undescended testicle) is a well-accepted risk factor for subsequent development of carcinoma. Abnormalities in spermatogenesis are well documented (thought to be the primary effect of the tumor), and up to 15% of patients are diagnosed with testicular cancer during a work-up for male-factor infertility. Two to 3% of patients exhibit bilateral tumors, and 5% to 10% of patients develop cancer in the normal contralateral testicle. Despite impairments in spermatogenesis, most men with testicular cancer are capable of fathering children, and a discussion of fertility issues is extremely important, especially in patients who may require adjuvant therapies such as external beam radiation and systemic chemotherapy.

The most common presenting sign or symptom of testis cancer is a firm, painless mass arising from the testis. Patients may exhibit an acute scrotum as a result of tumor hemorrhage, and up to 33% of patients are treated for presumed epididymitis. Scrotal ultrasonography is diagnostic because testis cancer is usually distinguishable from benign scrotal disease owing to the clear involvement of the testicular parenchyma rather than the paratesticular tissues. Signs and symptoms of advanced disease include cough, gastrointestinal symptoms (mass), back pain (retroperitoneal metastasis), neurologic symptoms (brain metastasis), lower

Table 71–9 Testis Cancer Staging Studies

Tumor markers

AFP—elevated only with nonseminomatous tumors

β-hCG—may be increased with either seminoma or nonseminomatous tumor

Abdominal CT scan—retroperitoneal nodes most common site of regional nodal metastasis

Chest radiograph or CT scan—lung most frequent site of distant metastasis

AFP = α-fetoprotein; β-hCG = β-human chorionic gonadotropin; CT = computed tomography.

extremity swelling (iliac and inferior vena cava thrombus), and supraclavicular lymphadenopathy.

DIAGNOSIS AND STAGING

Initial management of the primary tumor is inguinal orchiectomy with high ligation of the spermatic cord. Histopathologic assessment distinguishes germ cell tumors (GCT) from stromal tumors. Seminoma is the most common GCT occurring in pure form. Teratoma, yolk sac tumors, embryonal carcinoma, and choriocarcinoma are classified as nonseminomatous GCT and frequently occur as mixed GCT (more than one histologic pattern within the primary tumor).

Testicular cancer is unique in that serum tumor markers (STM) play an important role in tumor staging. STM include β-human chorionic gonadotropin (β-hCG), α-fetoprotein (AFP), and serum lactate dehydrogenase (LDH). Elevations of the serum hCG may be seen in choriocarcinoma, embryonal carcinoma, and in 15% of seminomas. Elevated AFP can be seen in yolk sac tumors and embryonal carcinoma and excludes a diagnosis of seminoma. These markers may be secreted either by the primary tumor or by metastatic foci (Table 71–9).

The retroperitoneal lymph nodes are the most common initial site of metastasis. Therefore staging of the retroperitoneum with an abdominal CT scan is important in evaluating the extent of disease. However, accurate staging of the retroperitoneum remains problematic with the literature quoting a 20% to 30% false-negative and false-positive rate with CT scanning. Common landing zones for lymph node metastasis include the precaval, interaortocaval, and pre-aortic lymph nodes below the renal hilum and above the aortic bifurcation. Chest x-ray or thoracic CT scanning completes the clinical staging because the lungs and posterior mediastinum are the most common sites of distant metastatic disease.

TREATMENT

Histopathology, pathologic stage, and STM status are used to determine subsequent treatment following inguinal orchiectomy. All patients with elevated STM postorchiectomy receive cisplatin-based chemotherapy, regardless of histologic findings. Radiation therapy and retroperitoneal lymph node dissection (RPLND) have a high likelihood of failure in the presence of elevated serum markers.

Seminoma exhibits as clinical stage I in 70%, stage II in 20%, and stage III in 10% of patients. Although surveillance and single-agent carboplatin are options in patients with stage I seminoma, most experts recommend radiation therapy to the retroperitoneum in patients with stage I and II disease because of the radiosensitivity of seminomas. Patients with bulky stage II (lymph nodes >5 cm) and stage III disease receive combination chemotherapy.

Nonseminomatous GCT exhibit more frequently with advanced stage (stage I 30%, stage II 40%, and stage III 30%). RPLND is frequently recommended in patients with clinical stage I or low-volume stage II disease. Reasons for recommending RPLND include accurate pathologic staging of the retroperitoneum, low relapse rate (<2%) following properly performed RPLND, curative potential in the face of viable GCT, and the potential for retroperitoneal teratoma that is resistant to chemotherapy. Side effects associated with RPLND include lymphocele, chylous ascites (0.4%), and small bowel obstruction (<1%). Nerve-sparing RPLND is able to preserve antegrade ejaculation in greater than 80% of patients. Patients with stage I disease and who are highly motivated and compliant may be candidates for surveillance protocols. Recurrence following surveillance usually occurs within 2 years, and the majority of patients are salvaged with chemotherapy.

Platinum-based chemotherapy is the standard for patients with advanced disease. Cure rates of 70% to 80% are achieved even in patients who have relatively bulky metastatic disease. Side effects of chemotherapy include renal dysfunction, neuropathy, Raynaud's phenomenon, hematologic toxicity, cardiovascular toxicity, and 0.5% risk of secondary leukemias.

Benign Scrotal Diseases

VARICOCELE

Varicoceles are classically described as abnormal dilation of the veins of the pampiniform plexus. Subclinical varicocele can be present in up to 15% of the male population, whereas the prevalence increases to 30% to 50% of men with primary infertility and as high as 70% to 80% of patients with secondary infertility. Varicoceles are diagnosed during workup for male-factor infertility, scrotal pain syndromes, and asymptomatic testicular atrophy. Physical examination can reveal the classic *bag of worms,* testicular atrophy, and tender scrotal contents. Semen analysis reveals multiple abnormalities, reflecting a characteristic *stress pattern,* although this state is not pathognomonic. The diagnosis of varicocele remains a clinical one, although scrotal ultrasound with Doppler is helpful in certain situations. The presence of two to three veins with diameter larger than 3 mm and retrograde flow with Valsalva's maneuver is consistent with clinical varicocele. Surgical intervention for subclinical varicoceles is not indicated. The pathophysiologic mechanism of varicocele has historically been poorly understood. Regardless, dilation of the internal spermatic vein and transmission of increased hydrostatic pressure across dysfunctional venous valves occur. Stasis of blood in the venous system disturbs countercurrent heat exchange responsible for maintaining testicular temperature and results in testicular parenchymal damage and impaired spermatogenesis. Because of anatomic considerations, varicoceles are commonly left-sided. However, unilateral varicoceles have a bilateral effect on spermatogenesis and local testicular steroidogenesis. Indications for surgical correction of a clinical varicocele include male-factor infertility, testicular atrophy in adolescents with ipsilateral varicocele, and intractable pain attributed to the varicocele. Notably, pain is rarely caused by clinical varicoceles, and surgical varicocelectomy often does not produce symptomatic relief for the patient. Common surgical techniques include high retroperitoneal ligation of the internal spermatic vein, microsurgical inguinal and subinguinal varicocelectomy, and laparoscopic varicocelectomy. The inguinal approach using surgical magnification has the highest success and lowest complication and recurrence rates. Semen parameters improve in 60% to 80% of men, with pregnancy rates of 20% to 60%. The most common complication is hydrocele formation. Inadvertent ligation of the testicular artery is a rare complication but may result in testicular atrophy and loss.

EPIDIDYMITIS

Acute epididymitis is a clinical syndrome that produces fever, acute scrotal pain, and swelling as a result of inflammation and infection of the epididymis. Pathophysiologically, epididymitis is caused by retrograde bacterial spread from the bladder or urethra. In men younger than 35 years of age, the most common cause involves organisms associated with urethritis, namely *Gonococcus* and *Chlamydia trachomatis*. In older men, *Escherichia coli* and other coliform bacteria are the causative organisms, usually in association with lower urinary tract infection associated with symptoms of BOO. Patients with acute epididymitis have significant inflammation, and the causative organism can be determined by a Gram stain and culture of a urethral swab or midstream urine specimen. Interestingly, the anti-arrhythmic amiodarone is associated with a noninfectious cause of epididymitis secondary to concentration of the drug in the epididymis. The most important consideration in diagnosing acute epididymitis is differentiating this disease from acute testicular torsion. Physical examination can be nonspecific, although focal epididymal swelling and tenderness is suggestive, and the presence of WBCs in the urine or urethral swab is indicative of an infectious origin. Scrotal ultrasound with Doppler flow can be extremely helpful in differentiating acute epididymitis from torsion in difficult cases. Treatment is generally supportive, including narcotic analgesics, NSAIDs, scrotal support with an athletic supporter, cold ice packs, and targeted antimicrobial therapy. In general, patients younger than age 35 years should be treated with Rocephin and doxycycline or a single dose of Zithromax. Older patients are empirically treated with a fluoroquinolone or TMP-SMX for 2 to 4 weeks. Complications associated with acute epididymitis include abscess formation, testicular infarction, infertility, and chronic epididymitis or orchialgia. Surgical intervention is rarely necessary, although in select cases, orchiectomy and epididymectomy can be therapeutic when solid indications are present.

HYDROCELE

A hydrocele is a serous fluid collection within the parietal and visceral layers of the tunica vaginalis of the scrotum. Hydroceles may surround the testicle and spermatic cord, or communicate with the peritoneal cavity via a patent processus vaginalis. These communicating hydroceles are uncommon in the adult population and are more commonly identified in the pediatric age group in association with an indirect hernia. Patients usually come to the physician with complaints of heaviness in the scrotum, scrotal pain, and an enlarging scrotal mass. Diagnosis is easily made with physical examination and transillumination of the hydrocele. If the testis is not easily palpable in a young patient, ultrasound can rule out an occult testicular tumor with secondary or reactive hydrocele. Hydroceles are caused by increased secretion and/or decreased reabsorption of serous fluid by the tunica vaginalis. Infection, trauma, neoplastic disease, and lymphatic disease are causative in most adults, whereas the remainder of cases are idiopathic. Treatment of symptomatic hydroceles is surgical. Although the recurrence rate is significantly increased with aspiration and sclerotherapy, this can be a good option in patients who are considered poor surgical candidates. Hydrocelectomy procedures involve either some form of excision of the redundant tunica vaginalis versus a plication of the sac without excision. Overall complications occur in up to 20% of patients, with hematoma seen in 15%, infection or abscess and hydrocele recurrence in 9%, and chronic pain in 1%.

TESTICULAR TORSION

Testicular torsion is considered a true urologic emergency. The testicular blood supply is via the testicular artery (aorta), the vasal artery (inferior vesicle artery), and the cremasteric artery (inferior epigastric artery). All three vessels are transmitted to the testicle via the spermatic cord. Torsion of the spermatic cord impairs arterial inflow, as well as venous outflow, producing the characteristic symptoms of acute scrotal pain, swelling, and nausea and vomiting. If detorsion is not performed within 6 to 8 hours, testicular infarction and hemorrhagic necrosis are likely to occur. Typically, patients are younger than 21 years of age, although testicular torsion can occur into early adulthood. Symptoms usually include the acute onset of testicular and scrotal pain, scrotal swelling, and nausea and vomiting. Ecchymosis and involvement of the scrotal skin occur in more advanced cases, but the testis has infarcted by this point. Delay in presentation and delayed diagnosis are more common in the adult patient population and is related to patient and physician factors. An antecedent history of trauma or physical activity is often present. The diagnosis of testicular torsion remains a clinical one, and surgical exploration is undertaken when the index of its presence is high. Doppler ultrasonography is extremely useful in differentiating testicular torsion from other causes of the acute scrotum, such as acute epididymitis, torsion of the appendix testis, and trauma. Important surgical principles include surgical detorsion and assessment of testicular viability in the operating room. If the testis is determined to be viable, bilateral orchiopexy is performed using the technique of three-point fixation (sutures placed medially, laterally, and inferiorly). Otherwise, in the presence of infarction, orchiectomy is recommended. Orchiopexy of the contralateral testicle is always performed simultaneously. When diagnosis and surgery occur in a timely fashion, testicular salvage rates approach 70%. Delayed surgical therapy, for whatever reason, results in the salvage rate dropping off to 40%.

Prospectus for the Future

- Improved basic science understanding of the molecular biology of benign prostate growth
- Improved understanding of the neurophysiologic factors of detrusor function associated with BOO
- Refined methods for the minimally invasive management of symptomatic BPH
- Improved outcomes research regarding long-term benefits of less invasive therapy for BPH, both medical and surgical
- Improved understanding of the immunourologic characteristics and mechanisms of the prostate and urethra

- Enhanced understanding of the neuroanatomic and neurophysiologic aspects of the prostate and bladder, with an emphasis on pain and sensory mechanisms in the prostate, bladder, and surrounding tissues
- Better standardized protocols for therapeutic intervention trials for the treatment of noninflammatory CPPS
- Novel therapies for noninflammatory CPPS (e.g., thermotherapy, phytotherapy)

References

Benign Prostatic Hyperplasia

Blute ML, Larson T: Minimally invasive therapies for benign prostatic hyperplasia. Urology 58(6 Suppl. 1):33–40; discussion 40–41, 2001.

Fagelman E, Lowe FC: Herbal medications in the treatment of benign prostatic hyperplasia (BPH). Urol Clin North Am 29(1):23–9, vii, 2002.

Lepor H, Lowe FC: Evaluation and nonsurgical management of benign prostatic hyperplasia. In Walsh PC, Retik AB, et al (eds): Campbell's Urology, 8th ed. Philadelphia, WB Saunders, 2002, pp 1337–1378.

Lowe FC, McConnell JD, Hudson PB, et al: Finasteride Study Group. Long-term 6-year experience with finasteride in patients with benign prostatic hyperplasia. Urology 61(4):791–796, 2003.

Lummus WE, Thompson I: Prostatitis. Emerg Med Clin North Am 19:691–707, 2001.

McConnell JD, Roehrborn CG, Bautista OM, et al: Medical Therapy of Prostatic Symptoms (MTOPS) Research Group. The long-term effect of doxazosin, finasteride, and combination therapy on the clinical progression of benign prostatic hyperplasia. N Eng J Med 349(25):2387–2398, 2003.

Roehrborn CG, Bartsch G, Kirby R, et al: Guidelines for the diagnosis and treatment of benign prostatic hyperplasia: A comparative, international overview. Urology 58:642–650, 2001.

Roehrborn CG, Bruskewitz R, Nickel JC, et al: Proscar Long-Term Efficacy and Safety Study Group. Sustained decrease in incidence of acute urinary retention and surgery with finasteride for 6 years in men with benign prostatic hyperplasia. J Urol 171(3):1194–1198, 2004.

Sarma AV, Jacobson DJ, McGree ME, et al: A population-based study of incidence and treatment of benign prostatic hyperplasia among residents of Olmsted County, Minnesota: 1987 to 1997. [See comment.] J Urol 173(6):2048–2053, 2005.

Trock BJ, Brotzman M, Utz WJ, et al: Long-term pooled analysis of multicenter studies of cooled thermotherapy for benign prostatic hyperplasia results at three months through four years. Urology 63(4):716–721, 2004.

Prostatitis

Calhoun EA, Collins MM, Pontari MA, et al: The economic impact of chronic prostatitis. Arch Intern Med 164: 1231–1236, 2004.

Carver BS, Bozeman CB, Williams BJ, et al: The prevalence of men with National Institutes of Health category IV prostatitis and association with serum prostate specific antigen. J Urol 169: 589–591, 2003.

Cheah PY, Liong ML, Yuen KH, et al: Terazosin therapy for chronic prostatitis/chronic pelvic pain syndrome: A randomized, placebo controlled trial. J Urol 169:592–596, 2003.

Hau VN, Schaeffer AJ: Acute and chronic prostatitis. Med Clin N Am 88:483–494, 2004.

Lummus WE, Thompson I: Prostatitis. Emerg Med Clin North Am 19:691–707, 2001.

Nickel JC, Downey J, Ardern D, et al: Failure of monotherapy strategy for the treatment of difficult chronic prostatitis/chronic pelvic pain syndrome patients. J Urol 172:551–554, 2004.

Nickel JC, Pontari M, Moon T, et al: A randomized, placebo controlled, multicenter study to evaluate the safety and efficacy of rofecoxib in the treatment of chronic nonbacterial prostatitis. J Urol 169:1401–1405, 2003.

Nickel JC: The three A's of chronic prostatitis therapy: Antibiotics, alpha-blockers, and anti-inflammatories. What is the evidence? BJU Int 94:1230–1233, 2004.

Nickel JC: Prostatitis syndromes: An update for urologic practice. Can J Urol 7:1091–1098, 2004.

Schaeffer AJ: Etiology and management of chronic pelvic pain syndrome in men. Urology 63:75–84, 2004.

Schaeffer AJ: NIDDK-sponsored chronic prostatitis collaborative research network (CPCRN) 5-year data and treatment guidelines for bacterial prostatitis. Int J Antimicrob Agents 24: S49–S52, 2004.

Shoskes DA, Hakim L, Ghoniem G, et al: Long-term results of multimodal therapy for chronic prostatitis/chronic pelvic pain syndrome. J Urol 169:1406–1410, 2003.

Turner JA, Ciol MA, Von Korff M, et al: Validity and responsiveness of the National Institutes of Health chronic prostatitis symptom index. J Urol 169:580–583, 2003.

Erectile Dysfunction

Cappelleri JC, Rosen RC: The Sexual Health Inventory for Men (SHIM): A 5-year review of research and clinical experience. Int J Impotence Res 17(4):307–319, 2005.

Carson CC, Lue TF: Phosphodiesterase type 5 inhibitors for erectile dysfunction. BJU Int 96(3):257–280, 2005.

Feldman HA, Goldstein I, Hatzichristou DG, et al: Impotence and its medical and psychosocial correlates: Results of the Massachusetts Male Aging Study. J Urol 151:54–61, 1994.

Kostis JB, Jackson G, Rosen R, et al: Sexual dysfunction and cardiac risk (the Second Princeton Consensus Conference). Am J Cardiol 96(2):313–321, 2005.

Milbank AJ, Montague DK: Surgical management of erectile dysfunction. Endocrine 23(2–3):161–165, 2004.

Montague DK, Jarow JP, Broderick GA, et al: Erectile Dysfunction Guideline Update Panel. Chapter 1: The management of erectile dysfunction: An AUA update. J Urol 174(1):230–239, 2005.

Prostate Cancer

Bostwick DG, Qian J, Civantos F, et al: Does finasteride alter the pathology of the prostate and cancer grading? Clin Prostate Cancer 2(4):228–235, 2004.

D'Amico AV, Chen MH, Roehl KA, et al: Preoperative PSA velocity and the risk of death from prostate cancer after radical prostatectomy. N Eng J Med 351(2):125–135, 2004.

Eggener SE, Roehl KA, Catalona WJ: Predictors of subsequent prostate cancer in men with a prostate specific antigen of 2.6 to 4.0 ng/ml and an initially negative biopsy. J Urol 174(2):500–504, 2005.

Roehl KA, Han M, Ramos CG, et al: Cancer progression and survival rates following anatomical radical retropubic prostatectomy in 3,478 consecutive patients: Long-term results. J Urol 172(3):910–914, 2004.

Stephenson AJ, Scardino PT, Eastham JA, et al: Postoperative nomogram predicting the 10-year probability of prostate cancer recurrence after radical prostatectomy. J Clin Oncol 23(28):7005–7012, 2005.

Zhou P, Chen MH, McLeod D, et al: Predictors of prostate cancer-specific mortality after radical prostatectomy or radiation therapy. J Clin Oncol 23(28):6992–6998, 2005.

Penile Cancer

Busby JE, Pettaway CA: What's new in the management of penile cancer? Curr Opin Urol 15:350–357, 2005.

d'Ancona CA, de Lucena RG, Querne FA, et al: Long-term followup of penile carcinoma treated with penectomy and bilateral modified inguinal lymphadenectomy. J Urol 172:498–501, 2004.

Joerger M, Warzinek T, Klaeser B, et al: Major tumor regression after paclitaxel and carboplatin polychemotherapy in a patient with advanced penile cancer. Urology 63:778–780, 2004.

Kroon BK, Horenblas S, Lont AP, et al: Patients with penile carcinoma benefit from immediate resection of clinically occult lymph node metastases. J Urol 173:816–819, 2005.

Nelson BA, Cookson MS, Smith JA Jr, et al: Complications of inguinal and pelvic lymphadenectomy for squamous cell carcinoma of the penis: A contemporary series. J Urol 172:494–497, 2004.

Rippentrop JM, Joslyn SA, Konety BR: Squamous cell carcinoma of the penis: Evaluation of data from the Surveillance, Epidemiology, and End Results Program. Cancer 101:1357–1363, 2004.

Sanchez-Ortiz RF, Pettaway CA: The role of lymphadenectomy in penile cancer. Urol Oncol 22:236–244, 2004.

Testicular Cancer

Amato RJ, Ro JY, Ayala AG, et al: Risk-adapted treatment for patients with clinical stage I nonseminomatous germ cell tumors of the testis. Urology 63:144, 2004.

Atsu N, Eskicorapci S, Uner A, et al: A novel surveillance protocol for stage I nonseminomatous germ cell testicular tumors. BJU Int 92:32–35, 2003.

Classen J, Schmidberger H, Meisner C, et al: Radiotherapy for stages IIA/B testicular seminoma: Final report of a prospective multicenter clinical trial. J Clin Oncol 21:1101–1106, 2003.

MacVicar GR, Pienta KJ: Testicular cancer. Curr Opin Oncol 16:253–256, 2004.

Oldenburg J, Alfsen GC, Lien HH, et al: Postchemotherapy retroperitoneal surgery remains necessary in patients with nonseminomatous testicular cancer and minimal residual tumor masses. J Clin Oncol 17:3310–3317, 2003.

Schmoll HJ, Kollmannsberger C, Metzner B, et al: Long-term results of first line sequential high dose etoposide, ifosfamide, and cisplatin chemotherapy plus autologous stem cell support for patients with advanced metastatic germ cell cancer: An extended phase I/II study of the German Testicular Cancer Study Group. J Clin Oncol 15:4083–4091, 2003.

Stephenson AJ, Sheinfeld J: The role of retroperitoneal lymph node dissection in the management of testicular cancer. Urol Oncol 22:225–235, 2004.

Benign Scrotal Disorders

Hopps CV, Goldstein M: Varicocele: Unified theory of pathophysiology and treatment. AUA Update 23(12):90–95, 2004.

Karmazyn B, Steinberg R, Kurareid L, et al: Clinical and radiographic criteria of the acute scrotum in children: A retrospective study in 172 boys. Pediatr Radiol 35(3):302–310, 2005.

Kiddoo DA, Wollin TA, Mador DR: A population-based assessment of complications following outpatient hydrocelectomy and spermatocelectomy. J Urol 171:746–748, 2004.

Kruska JD, Culkin DJ: Outpatient scrotal surgery: Management of benign scrotal diseases. AUA Update 24(11):88–97, 2005.

Lavallee ME, Cash J: Testicular torsion: Evaluation and management. Curr Sports Med Rep 4(2):102–104, 2005.

Neiderberger C: Microsurgical treatment of persistent or recurrent varicocele. J Urol 173(6):2079–2080, 2005.

Raman JD, Walmsley K, Goldstein M: Inheritance of varicoceles. Urology 65(6):1186–1189, 2005.

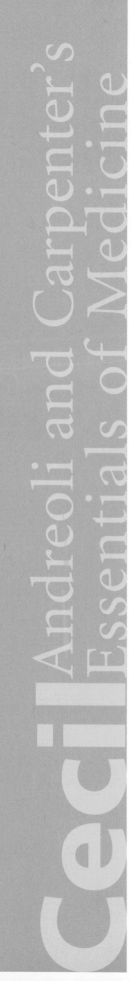

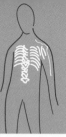

Section XIV

Diseases of Bone and Bone Mineral Metabolism

Normal Physiology of Bone and Mineral Homeostasis

Andrew F. Stewart

Calcium Homeostasis

The maintenance of normal calcium homeostasis is critical to survival for at least three reasons. First, serum calcium concentrations regulate the degree of membrane excitability in muscle and nervous tissue. Increases in serum calcium lead to refractoriness to stimulation of neurons and muscle cells, which translates clinically into coma and muscular weakness. Conversely, reductions in serum calcium lead to increases in neuromuscular excitability that translate clinically into convulsions and spontaneous muscle cramps and contractions referred to as *carpopedal spasm* or *tetany*. Second, terrestrial life requires the existence of a skeleton, and calcium is the major structural cation in the skeleton. Specifically, the mineral phase of the skeleton is composed of a calcium salt called *hydroxyapatite,* and reductions in bone mineral content lead to spontaneous fractures. Third, intracellular calcium has a major intracellular signaling role, and control of intracellular calcium is essential to the survival of all cells. This mechanism is used to advantage pharmacologically through the widespread clinical use of drugs that regulate intracellular calcium concentrations and calcium-channel activity for the treatment of a wide variety of human diseases. Thus physicians, regardless of their specialty, will encounter disorders of calcium homeostasis on a regular basis.

The serum total calcium concentration is normally maintained at approximately 9.5 mg/dL. Of this amount, approximately 4.5 mg/dL is bound to serum proteins, principally albumin, and approximately 0.5 mg/dL circulates as insoluble complexes such as calcium sulfate, phosphate, and citrate. The remaining approximately 4.5 mg/dL circulates as free or unbound or ionized calcium. This free, ionized serum calcium is important clinically and physiologically. This

calcium is available to be filtered at the glomerulus to interact with cell membranes to regulate their electrical potential or excitability and to enter and exit the skeletal hydroxyapatite crystal lattice. Thus the *name of the game* is to maintain a normal ionized serum calcium, although total serum calcium is customarily measured in most clinical laboratories. From a clinical standpoint, recognizing that, in some instances, total serum calcium can change without a change in the ionized calcium is also important. For example, if a decline in serum albumin occurs as a result of hepatic cirrhosis or the nephrotic syndrome, then a corresponding decline in the total serum calcium will ensue, but the ionized serum calcium concentration will remain normal. Thus at times, measuring the ionized serum calcium directly is important.

Given the central importance of calcium homeostasis to terrestrial life, the fact that a complex group of regulatory processes have evolved to protect the integrity of this system is not surprising. A corollary of this concept is that, when a physician encounters patients in whom hypercalcemia, hypocalcemia, or disorders of skeletal mineralization have occurred, multiple safety control points have been breached. These control points are discussed here.

From a homeostatic control point of view, the calcium ion interfaces with three important compartments, as shown in the calcium *physiologic black box* in Figure 72–1. An important point to recall is that, although intracellular calcium is important in intracellular signaling, it is quantitatively unimportant in overall systemic calcium homeostasis, largely because intracellular calcium concentrations are tiny (nanomolar) as compared with extracellular calcium concentrations (millimolar). Thus the three critical regulatory fluxes that maintain normal serum calcium concentration are with the intestine, the kidney, and the skeleton.

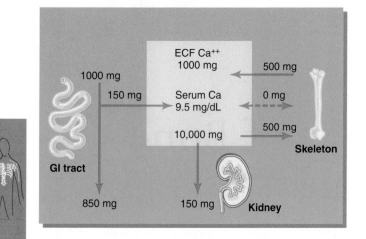

Figure 72–1 The calcium *physiologic black box*. The central box represents extracellular fluid (ECF), which contains a total of approximately 1000 mg of calcium. This black box has three interfaces with the GI tract, the skeleton, and the kidney, as discussed in detail in the text. The fluxes into and out of the ECF are measured in milligrams per day.

CALCIUM FLUXES INTO AND OUT OF EXTRACELLULAR FLUID

Intestinal Calcium Absorption

The normal dietary calcium intake for an adult human is approximately 1000 mg/day. Of this amount, approximately 300 mg is absorbed (i.e., unidirectional absorption is approximately 30%), and this absorption occurs in the duodenum and proximal jejunum. Interestingly, approximately 150 mg/day of calcium is secreted by the liver (in bile), the pancreas (in pancreatic secretions), and the intestinal glands such that net absorption (so-called *fractional absorption*) of calcium is approximately 15% of intake. The mechanisms that regulate the 150 mg/day of calcium secreted by the gastrointestinal (GI) tract have not been well studied, despite their obvious quantitative importance. The efficiency of calcium absorption is regulated at the level of the small intestinal epithelial cell, the enterocyte, by the active form of vitamin D, 1,25-dihydroxyvitamin D (1,25[OH]$_2$D), with increases in 1,25(OH)$_2$D leading to enhanced calcium absorption and decreases in 1,25(OH)$_2$D causing reduced absorption of dietary calcium. Thus dietary calcium absorption can be increased, at least over the short term, by increasing calcium intake, by increasing plasma 1,25(OH)$_2$D concentrations, or by both measures. Pathologic increases in serum calcium (hypercalcemia) can be caused by increases in circulating 1,25(OH)$_2$D (as in sarcoidosis) or by excessive calcium intake (the milk-alkali syndrome). Conversely, hypocalcemia can occur as a result of a decline in 1,25(OH)$_2$D (chronic renal failure and hypoparathyroidism are examples). Thus an overall view of the impact of the GI tract can be summarized as follows: If an individual consumes 1000 mg of calcium per day, and if net absorption is 150 mg/day, then he or she will excrete 850 mg of calcium in feces per day.

Renal Calcium Handling

The normal ionized serum calcium concentration, as noted previously, is approximately 4.5 mg/dL. The normal

glomerular filtration rate is 120 mL/min. Multiplying these two numbers produces the filtered load of calcium, which proves to be approximately 10,000 mg/day. In terms of overall regulation of calcium homeostasis, this number is a very large, making the point that the kidney is the most important moment-to-moment regulator of the serum calcium concentration. The amount also emphasizes that disorders of renal calcium handling (e.g., thiazide diuretic use, hypoparathyroidism) can be expected to lead to significant abnormalities in serum calcium homeostasis.

Of the 10,000 mg filtered at the glomerulus each day, approximately 9000 mg (90%) is reabsorbed *proximally*, meaning in the proximal convoluted tubule, the pars recta, and the thick ascending limb of Henle's loop. This 90% is absorbed in conjunction with sodium and chloride reabsorption and is not subject to regulation by parathyroid hormone (PTH). In contrast, the remaining 10%, or 1000 mg, that arrives at the distal tubule on a daily basis is subject to regulation, with PTH stimulating renal calcium reabsorption. This anticalciuric effect of PTH can be extremely efficient, and elevated PTH concentrations can essentially eliminate calcium excretion into the urine. This action is a potent mechanism for retaining calcium under conditions of calcium deprivation (e.g., a low-calcium diet, vitamin D deficiency, intestinal malabsorption) and can contribute to hypercalcemia under pathologic conditions, as in primary hyperparathyroidism.

Approximately 150 mg of calcium is excreted by the kidney in the final urine on a daily basis in a healthy individual. If the kidney filters 10,000 mg of calcium each day, and if 150 mg is excreted in the final urine, then 9850 mg is reabsorbed at proximal and distal sites. Thus 98.5% of filtered calcium is reabsorbed by the nephron. Conversely, the normal fractional excretion of calcium is approximately 1.5%.

Viewed from a whole-organism standpoint, a healthy person is in zero calcium balance with respect to the outside world: intake (1000 mg/day) − output [(850 mg in feces per day) + (150 mg in urine per day)] = 0.

Skeletal Biology and Calcium Homeostasis

The skeletal compartment contains approximately 1.2 kg of calcium in a male adult and 1.0 kg in a female adult. As noted earlier, the majority of this calcium is in the crystal hydroxyapatite, a calcium phosphate salt. Although calcium contributes in an important way to the structural integrity of the skeleton, as noted previously, the skeleton also serves as a quantitatively large reservoir, as well as a sink, for adding and removing calcium to the extracellular fluid (ECF) compartment at appropriate times.

The adult skeleton is composed of two fundamental types of bone, (1) cortical (or lamellar) bone and (2) trabecular (or cancellous) bone (Fig. 72–2). Cortical bone predominates in the skull and the shafts of long bones, and trabecular bone predominates at other sites, such as the distal radius, the vertebral bodies, and the trochanters of the hip. Bone is not an inert tissue, as might be imagined from visiting the dinosaur room at a natural history museum; instead, bone is a vital tissue that is continually turning over. The adult skeleton is completely remodeled every 3 to 10 years. This remodeling is perhaps best appreciated by recalling that

Figure 72–2 The structure of human bone. This figure depicts a human proximal femur examined using a gross pathologic specimen *(left panel)* and a radiograph of the same section *(right panel)*. Note that two different types of bone are represented. One type is called cortical bone (also called lamellar bone) and the other cancellous bone (also called trabecular bone). Note that the proportion of trabecular and cortical bone differs by location. For example, the shaft of the femur contains mostly cortical bone, whereas the proximal end of the femoral neck and the greater trochanter contain little cortical bone and almost exclusively trabecular bone. This distinction is important because most osteoporotic fractures occur at sites in which trabecular bone predominates, including the greater trochanter, the femoral neck, the vertebrae, and the distal radius. (Courtesy of Webster S. S. Jee, MD, University of Utah.)

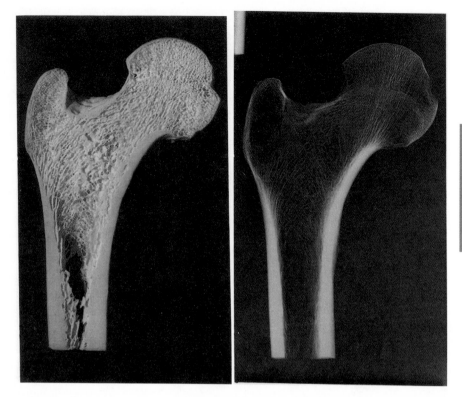

orthopedic surgeons routinely and intentionally set fractures imperfectly, knowing that the normal processes of bone remodeling will lead to restoration of the original shape of a given bone with the passage of time.

The cells that regulate bone turnover can be divided into those that remove old bone and those that provide new bone (Fig. 72–3; see also Chapter 74). Cells that remove (or *resorb*) old bone are osteoclasts. These cells are large, metabolically active, multinucleated cells derived from the fusion of circulating macrophages. They deposit themselves on the surface of bone and form a *sealing zone* over the bone surface into which they secrete protons (acid), proteases (such as collagenase), and proteoglycan-digesting enzymes (such as hyaluronidase). The acid solubilizes hydroxyapatite crystals, releasing calcium, and the enzymes digest bone proteins and proteoglycans (e.g., collagen, osteocalcin, osteopontin), which comprise the nonmineral or *osteoid* component of bone. Osteoclasts literally move along the surface of trabecular bone plates and drill tunnels in cortical bone, periodically releasing the digested contents within their sealed zones into the bone marrow space and thereby creating resorption lacunae, so-called Howship's lacunae, on the trabecular bone surface. The released calcium contributes to the ECF calcium pool, and the released proteolytic products, such as deoxypyridinoline cross-links—collagen fragments and hydroxyproline—can be used clinically as indices of bone resorption.

On the other side of the bone turnover equation is new bone formation. This task is accomplished by osteoblasts, which, in turn, are derived from marrow stromal cells or bone surface lining cells. Osteoblasts synthesize and secrete the components of the nonmineral phase of bone, so-called osteoid. These components are mostly proteins and include

collagen, osteopontin, osteonectin, osteocalcin, and a plethora of growth factors, including transforming growth factor-β and insulin-like growth factor-1, as well as proteoglycans. This complex serves as the scaffolding into which the mineral crystal hydroxyapatite forms its lattices.

Through this process of bone turnover, or bone remodeling, osteoclasts continually remove old bone, and osteoblasts continually produce new osteoid that mineralizes, in the end, replacing the old bone removed by osteoclasts with new bone. Teleologically, this process is viewed as serving to replace old bone (and by implication defective or damaged bone with microfractures and reduced mechanical strength) with new, mechanically strong bone, although the evidence for this action is limited. Indeed, the principal therapy for osteoporosis at present is with so-called antiresorptives such as estrogens, estrogen-like drugs, and bisphosphonates, which dramatically reduce bone turnover and yet appear to improve not only bone mass, but also bone mechanical properties.

From a systemic calcium homeostatic standpoint, however, this process is important. Osteoclasts can be used to access calcium from the skeleton in times of need to maintain a normal serum calcium concentration. Conversely, unmineralized osteoid produced by osteoblasts can be used at appropriate times as a sink into which excess serum calcium can be deposited. Under normal circumstances, estimates are that osteoclasts resorb bone at a rate such that approximately 500 mg of calcium is removed per day from the skeleton and delivered into the ECF compartment. At the same time, osteoblasts produce osteoid that mineralizes at a rate such that approximately 500 mg of calcium leaves the ECF and enters the skeleton at new sites. Seen from the perspective of the *black box* in Figure 72–1, the skeleton is in

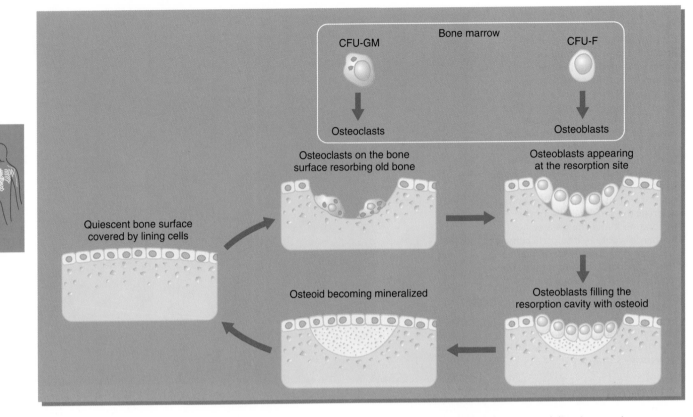

Figure 72–3 The cellular components of bone remodeling. As described in the text in detail, bone remodeling is a continuous process that involves the activation of osteoclast precursors in the macrophage lineage (abbreviated here as CFU-GM) to become actively resorbing osteoclasts, which literally tunnel into the bone surface to dig *resorption lacunae*. Osteoblast precursors in the fibroblast-bone marrow stromal cell lineage (abbreviated here as CFU-F) then appear and become active at the sites of prior resorption, and secrete new osteoid, which later mineralizes to *fill* the lacunae created by osteoclastic bone resorption. (From Manolagas SC, Jilka RL: Bone marrow, cytokines, and bone remodeling: Emerging insights into the pathophysiology of osteoporosis. N Engl J Med 332:305–311, 1995.)

zero calcium balance with the ECF, and the whole organism is in zero calcium balance with the external world, as described previously.

Considering the complexity of this calcium homeostatic system and the importance of maintaining tight control over serum calcium, an obvious need exists for systemic regulation and integration of the fluxes across the GI tract, the skeletal compartment, and the kidney. The two key metabolic regulatory hormones that coordinate these activities are PTH and the active form of vitamin D, $1,25(OH)_2D$.

REGULATORY HORMONES

Parathyroid Hormone

PTH is a peptide hormone produced by the four parathyroid glands (Fig. 72–4). These glands are located behind the normal thyroid lobes, two on the right, and two on the left. Through the calcium sensor—a G protein–coupled receptor for calcium that is located on the surface of the parathyroid cell—the serum ionized calcium concentration is continuously monitored. This exquisitely sensitive system functions such that minor (e.g., 0.1 mg/dL) reductions in serum ionized calcium lead to PTH secretion, and, similarly, minor

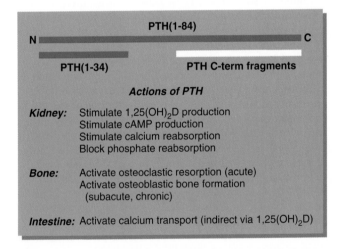

Figure 72–4 The structure and actions of parathyroid hormone. PTH is secreted as an 84-amino-acid protein, which is cleaved in the liver to derivative amino- and carboxy-terminal forms. The actions of the amino-terminally intact forms of PTH are listed here and discussed in detail in the text.

increments in serum calcium lead to suppression of PTH secretion.

PTH is secreted as an 84-amino-acid peptide hormone and is rapidly (half-life of approximately 3 to 5 minutes) cleaved by the Kupffer cells in the liver into amino-terminal and carboxy-terminal species. Of these forms, the intact 84-amino-acid peptide and the amino-terminal species are biologically active. The amino terminal form of PTH is also cleared rapidly (half-life of approximately 5 minutes) in this case in the kidney through glomerular filtration and proteolytic destruction by apical proteases. The continuous monitoring of the serum calcium concentration by the parathyroid glands, the immediate secretion of PTH in response to hypocalcemia, and the rapid clearance of PTH after secretion allow the parathyroid gland and PTH to act as critical, moment-to-moment regulators of the serum calcium. This tight regulatory control maintains the serum calcium at a normal level with rather remarkable precision.

PTH has three target organs, two direct and one indirect. The first direct target organ is the kidney, where renal calcium excretion is inhibited. Additional renal effects of PTH are to inhibit phosphate and bicarbonate reabsorption, which produces phosphaturia and hypophosphatemia and as a proximal renal tubular acidosis, respectively. These renal actions of PTH are essentially immediate. PTH has an additional direct effect on the proximal tubule to stimulate the production of the active form of vitamin D, $1,25(OH)_2D$, as described later. The second direct target organ of PTH is the skeleton. Here, PTH has the ability to mobilize calcium immediately from the skeleton via activation of osteoclastic bone resorption and perhaps via osteocytic release of calcium into the circulation. Over the longer term (days to weeks), PTH also stimulates the activity of osteoblasts to produce new bone and thereby removes calcium from the circulation. The skeletal effects of PTH are discussed in more detail later. The ability to stimulate osteoclasts acutely without activating bone formation is important for the rapid delivery of calcium to the ECF. Finally, PTH has the indirect effect of increasing intestinal calcium absorption through its ability to increase renal synthesis of $1,25(OH)_2D$. This action, too, is described in more detail in the following section on vitamin D absorption. Seen in concert, PTH is secreted in response to hypocalcemia, and the actions of PTH combine to restore a low serum calcium to normal by preventing renal calcium losses, by adding calcium to the ECF from the skeleton, and by stimulating, indirectly via $1,25(OH)_2D$, increases in intestinal calcium absorption.

Vitamin D Metabolism

Vitamin D is really two different compounds, ergocalciferol (vitamin D_2) and cholecalciferol (vitamin D_3) (Fig. 72–5). These compounds were identified through their ability to prevent rickets in humans and laboratory animals. In fact, both substances are actually inactive precursors, one (D_3) derived principally from skin exposed to sunlight, and the other (D_2) derived from plant sterols. Both D_2 and D_3 are present in multivitamins and commercial dietary supplements. These two precursors are converted passively by the enzyme vitamin D-25-hydroxylase in the liver to the respective 25-hydroxyvitamin D (25-OH D) derivatives. These derivatives, too, are inactive precursors, but they have clinical significance of two types. First, severe liver disease such

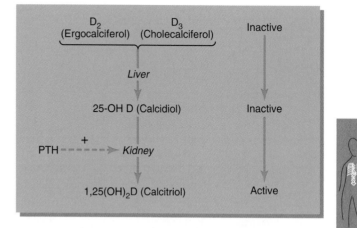

Figure 72–5 The vitamin D metabolic pathway. Vitamin D exists in two forms, D_2 and D_3, that pass through two steps in the liver and kidney to yield the biologically active form of vitamin D, $1,25(OH)_2D$. See text for details.

as cirrhosis prevents this essential step and leads to vitamin D–deficient syndromes collectively called *hepatic osteodystrophy*. Second, 25-OH D is the standard measure of the vitamin D status (repletion vs. deficiency) in a patient with hypocalcemia, osteomalacia or rickets, osteoporosis or intestinal malabsorption, and other similar conditions.

25-OH D is next converted, or activated, in the renal proximal tubule by the enzyme 25-hydroxyvitamin D 1-α-hydroxylase to the active form of the vitamin, $1,25(OH)_2D$. This substance is also called calcitriol, in contrast to 25-OH D, which some call calcidiol. Because $1,25(OH)_2D$ is the active form of vitamin D, its production is necessarily regulated, and this is accomplished primarily by PTH, with increases in PTH-stimulating $1,25(OH)_2D$ production and decreases in PTH-diminishing $1,25(OH)_2D$ synthesis. As noted previously, the primary action of $1,25(OH)_2D$ is to regulate intestinal calcium absorption. Thus PTH, via $1,25(OH)_2D$, indirectly regulates calcium absorption from the diet by the intestine. This action has importance clinically, because the hypocalcemia of hypoparathyroidism is, in an important way, a result of inadequate intestinal calcium absorption. Conversely, hyperparathyroidism is associated with hypercalciuria and nephrolithiasis, both of which are direct results of increases in circulating $1,25(OH)_2D$. Finally, as should be clear from the previous discussion, measurement of $1,25(OH)_2D$ can be used as an index of both parathyroid function and of intestinal calcium absorption.

Calcitonin

Calcitonin is produced by the parafollicular or C cells of the thyroid gland in response to hypercalcemia. It was once viewed as an essential calcium-regulating hormone. Clearly, pharmacologic doses of calcitonin may reduce the serum calcium, and although everyone agrees that it is secreted in response to hypercalcemia, little evidence exists that calcitonin has homeostatic relevance in humans. Indeed, compelling evidence suggests that calcitonin is unimportant in human physiology. First, malignant tumors of the parafollicular cell (medullary carcinomas of the thyroid) routinely overproduce calcitonin and lead to enormous, long-term (years or decades) elevations in circulating calcitonin

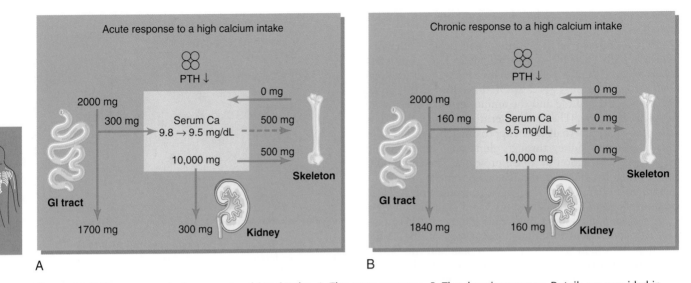

Figure 72–6 The response to increases in calcium intake. *A,* The acute response. *B,* The chronic response. Details are provided in the text.

concentrations. This has no effect on serum calcium or any apparent skeletal effect. Conversely, thyroidectomy, whether achieved surgically or medically using radioiodine ablation, removes calcitonin, but this, too, has no apparent adverse effect on serum calcium or skeletal homeostasis. Thus calcitonin is a hormone in search of a function, at least in humans.

INTEGRATION OF CALCIUM HOMEOSTASIS

The forgoing regulatory system would be all that is needed to control calcium homeostasis if humans received continuous GI infusions of calcium. Of course, all normal people experience periods of high calcium intake (e.g., diets including cheese, milk, ice cream, yogurt), as well as periods of low calcium intake (diets without these dairy products). Even on a daily basis, normal people eat at times and fast at other times between meals. Given the importance of maintaining the serum calcium concentration in a very narrow range, all of these regulatory processes must be, and are, coordinated during periods of high calcium intake and of low calcium intake.

Ingestion of a greater than normal dietary calcium load (Fig. 72–6A) leads to a mild rise in serum calcium followed by immediate suppression of PTH. This action leads to an immediate *opening* of the renal distal tubular calcium *floodgates.* It also leads to an immediate reduction in osteoclastic activity. This latter effect not only prevents continued bone resorption, but also allows continuation of calcium entry from ECF to an unmineralized osteoid *sink.* These two effects lead to a rapid and short-term reduction in serum calcium to normal. However, if the high-calcium diet is maintained over the long term, then these adaptations are insufficient; continued renal calcium wasting would lead to hypercalciuria (with nephrolithiasis and nephrocalcinosis) and to excessive skeletal mineralization (osteopetrosis). Hence two additional responses (see Fig. 72–6B) are required to prevent these potential long-term adverse effects of a high-calcium diet. First, subacute or chronic suppression of PTH results in a reduction in circulating $1,25(OH)_2D$. This

action, in turn, leads to a reduction in the efficiency of calcium absorption from the intestine and a reduction of calcium entry into the ECF and hence a reduction of urinary calcium excretion. Second, a chronic decrement in PTH leads to a chronic decline in osteoblastic activity such that no osteoid is formed, and the ability to deposit calcium into the skeletal sink is lost.

Conversely, during brief periods of dietary calcium deficiency (Fig. 72–7A), as occurs between meals, for example, the serum calcium declines almost imperceptibly, the PTH rises, and this increase immediately prevents renal calcium losses from continuing. At the same time, an acute activation of osteoclasts occurs, and this action delivers calcium into the ECF. Thus the acute response to low calcium intake is the appropriate elimination of renal calcium losses and the development of a new source of calcium entry into the ECF. Over the longer term, however, this response is inadequate and would lead to skeletal demineralization. Hence a longer-term solution is required. This adaptation is again twofold (see Fig. 72–7B). First, a chronic low calcium intake, as would occur in a person with lactose intolerance, for example, leads to a chronic elevation in PTH, and this, over a matter of days to weeks, leads to an increase in $1,25(OH)_2D$. This increase, in turn, leads to an increase in the efficiency of calcium absorption from the intestine (an increase in the fractional absorption of calcium) to compensate for the reduction in dietary intake. Second, a chronic elevation in PTH will lead to an increase in osteoblast activity and osteoid synthesis, with resultant increases in skeletal calcium deposition. In this new steady-state adaptation to a low-calcium diet, PTH will be elevated, and coupled increases in both osteoclastic and osteoblastic activities will take place (i.e., an increase in bone turnover), but net skeletal calcium losses will be negligible or normal.

In summary, from an evolutionary standpoint, as life moved from a calcium-rich marine environment to terrestrial life, in which calcium availability is variable and unpredictable, a complex, but rather beautiful, regulatory mechanism has evolved that permits survival without requiring intentional behavioral adaptations for the vagaries

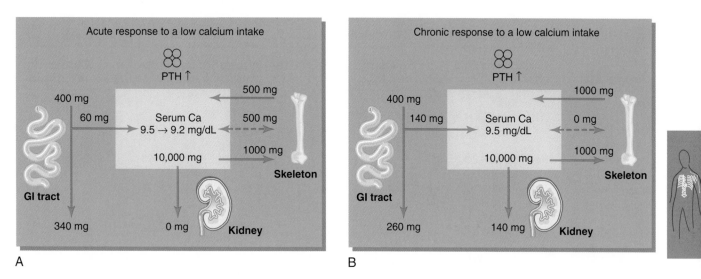

Figure 72–7 The response to decreases in calcium intake. *A*, The acute response. *B*, The chronic response. Details are provided in the text.

of calcium availability. This evolution was essential in evolutionary terms because calcium is so essential for all aspects of mammalian, indeed all eukaryotic, life. As discussed in Chapter 73, disorders that cause hypercalcemia or hypocalcemia are always caused by abnormalities at the interface of the ECF with the intestine, the kidney, or the skeleton, and in several of these interfaces. Moreover, given the robustness of these homeostatic adaptive processes, disorders that cause hypo- or hypercalcemia are rarely subtle: The physician need only recall these homeostatic premises to dissect the pathophysiologic process with precision and accuracy and treat the underlying disorder effectively.

Phosphate Homeostasis

The terms *phosphorus* and *phosphate* are often used interchangeably. To be parochial, phosphorus is an inorganic element, abbreviated as *P* in physical chemistry literature and as *Pi* in physiologic usage. Of course, the biologically relevant molecule is the negatively charged, trivalent phosphate ion PO_4. Phosphorus is the form that most clinical laboratories measure rather than the more biologically relevant phosphate ion. To make matters more complex, phosphate is an important physiologic buffer, and, at neutral pH in blood, phosphate is apportioned between HPO_4 (divalent) and H_2PO_4 (monovalent). The practical effect of this dichotomy is that, whereas physicians receive phosphorus measurements in milligram per deciliter (mg/dL) units, pharmaceutical preparations contain phosphorus in millimoles (mmol). Many physicians are unable to convert milligrams to millimoles, and dosing errors are common. An example is the replacement of potassium-using K-Phos, in which relatively standard amounts of potassium ion (e.g., 40 mEq) given intravenously are coupled with potentially life-threatening amounts of phosphate (30 mmol, or 900 mg). A chart converting milligrams to millimoles in common phosphate-containing preparations is provided in Table 72–1.

Phosphate regulates or participates in the regulation of an enormous number of biologic processes. These actions of

phosphate are fundamental to life itself and range from (1) being an integral component of the DNA double helix, to (2) shuttling oxygen from hemoglobin to cells and vice versa using 2,3-diphosphoglycerate (2,3-DPG), to (3) intracellular signaling via kinases that attach phosphate groups to other molecules, to (4) facilitating critical intracellular messenger systems such as cyclic monophosphate (cAMP) and inositol phosphates, to (5) maintaining basic intracellular redox status via the nicotinamide adenine dinucleotide phosphate (NADP-NADPH) system, to (6) serving as the gateway to the glucose metabolic pathway through glucose 6-phosphate. These actions are but a handful of examples, and, although they illustrate the central importance of adequate phosphorus supplies for life, they also underscore the point that phosphorus is primarily an intracellular ion. Extracellular concentrations are less important because the ECF functions mainly as a transport conduit through which phosphorus must travel from the skeleton or intestine to reach the cell interior. In addition to these critical intracellular roles, phosphate does have a key extracellular role as well: The anion pairs with calcium in the hydroxyapatite crystal lattice that provides structural integrity to the skeleton (see previous discussion). Thus as with calcium, phosphate is critical to skeletal strength, and disorders of phosphorus homeostasis, such as hypophosphatemic rickets, lead to pathologic skeletal fractures. Also in parallel with calcium, the skeleton serves as a major storage site for phosphate that can be, and is, accessed in times of severe phosphate deficiency.

Two corollaries of these broad and critical intracellular roles for phosphate are that: (1) Clinically significant intracellular phosphate deficiency may exist without marked hypophosphatemia (ideally, assessing intracellular phosphorus concentrations would be preferred, but this is not clinically possible); and (2) Importantly, severe, life-threatening phosphate deficiency is often unrecognized because its manifestations are so completely nonspecific yet common in intensive care unit settings (reduced levels of consciousness, hypotension, respirator dependence, and weakness). Astute clinicians learn to recognize general debility as a potential

Table 72–1 Examples of Therapeutic Phosphorus Preparations

Preparations	Composition* (per mL)	pH	mOsm/ kg H_2O	Phosphate (mmol/mL)	Phosphorus (mg/mL)	Sodium (mEq/mL)	Potassium (mEq/mL)
Oral							
Cow's milk (whole)	—	—	288	0.029	0.9	0.025	0.035
Neutra-Phos[†]	Na_2HPO_4, NaH_2PO_4, K_2HPO_4, KH_2PO_4	7.3	—	0.107	3.33	0.095	0.095
Phospho-Soda[†]	180 mg $Na_2HPO_4 \cdot 7H_2O$ + 480 mg $NaH_2PO_4 \cdot H_2O$	4.8	8240	4.150	128.65	4.822	0
Acid sodium phosphate	136 mg $Na_2HPO_4 \cdot 7H_2O$ + 58.8 mg H_3PO_4 (NF 85%)	4.9	1740	1.018	35.54	1.015	0
Neutral sodium phosphate	145 mg $Na_2HPO_4 \cdot 7H_2O$ + 18.2 mg $NaH_2PO_4 \cdot H_2O$	7.0	1390	0.673	20.86	1.214	0
Parenteral							
Neutral sodium phosphate	10.07 mg Na_2HPO_4 + 2.66 mg $NaH_2PO_4 \cdot H_2O$	7.35	202	0.090	2.80	0.161	0
Neutral sodium, potassium phosphate	11.5 mg Na_2HPO_4 + 2.58 mg KH_2PO_4	7.4	223	0.100	3.10	0.162	0.019
Na phosphate[†]	142 mg Na_2HPO_4 + 276 mg $NaH_2PO_4 \cdot H_2O$	5.7	5580	3.000	93.00	4.000	0
K phosphate[†]	236 mg K_2HPO_4 + 224 mg KH_2PO_4	6.6	5840	3.003	93.11	0	4.360

*Hydration states are important. For example, 268 mg $Na_2HPO_4 \cdot 7H_2O$ (molecular weight 268) equals 1.00 mmol, whereas 268 mg Na_2HPO_4 (molecular weight 142) equals 1.89 mmol.
[†]Commercial preparations: Neutra-Phos, Willen Drug Company, Baltimore (Neutra-phos K has twice as much potassium and no sodium); Phospho-Soda, C.B. Fleet Company, Lynchburg, Virginia (enema is one third the strength of Phospho-soda and can be used orally); Na phosphate, Abbott Laboratories, North Chicago, Illinois; K phosphate, Invenex Pharmaceuticals, Grand Island, New York, or Abbott Laboratories. Because Neutra-Phos was not readily dissolved and its specific composition is unknown, data shown are those provided by the manufacturer.
From Lentz RD, Brown DM, Kjellstrand CM: Treatment of severe hypophosphatemia. Ann Intern Med 89:941–944, 1978.
H_2O = water; K_2HPO_4 = dipotassium hydrogen phosphate; KH_2PO_4 = potassium dihydrogen phosphate; Na_2HPO_4 = disodium hydrogen phosphate; NaH_2PO_4 = sodium dihydrogen phosphate.

sign of phosphorus deficiency. Phosphate repletion in this setting may produce dramatic results.

In contrast to the regulation of serum calcium concentration, which is very tight, the regulation of serum phosphate concentrations is relatively lax. The serum phosphorus is maintained in a broad range between approximately 3.0 and 4.5 mg/dL. At least two reasons for this lax maintenance exist. First, as noted previously, in contrast to extracellular calcium concentrations, the precise maintenance of which are critically important to survival, extracellular phosphate concentrations are not critically important. Thus room can be found for laxity in the system. Second, because phosphate is so abundant inside plant and animal cells, phosphate is abundant in almost any diet such that evolutionary pressure has not been intense to develop a systemic regulatory mechanism for phosphate.

As with calcium, a *black box* can be developed for phosphate metabolism as well (Fig. 72–8). This black box represents ECF and, as with calcium, has interfaces with the GI tract, the kidney, and the skeleton. In addition, because the majority of phosphate is contained within cells, the phosphate black box has a quantitatively significant interface with the intracellular compartment.

INTESTINAL PHOSPHATE ABSORPTION

A normal diet contains approximately 1200 to 1600 mg of phosphorus, and approximately two thirds of this amount, or 800 to 1200 mg, is absorbed each day. Absorption occurs in the duodenum and jejunum. Although vitamin D compounds can increase the intestinal absorption of phosphorus, this effect is modest, and phosphate absorption in the

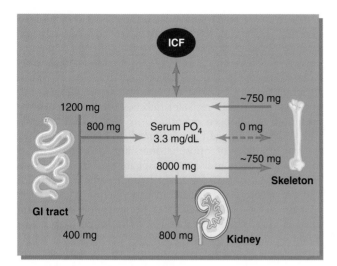

Figure 72–8 The phosphate *physiologic black box*. See Figure 72–1 for nomenclature and the text for details.

intestine can be considered as occurring with a fixed fractional absorption of approximately 67%. In the normal world of phosphate abundance, this amount is more than ample. Conversely, under conditions of dietary phosphorus deficiency, as occurs in chronic alcoholism (alcoholic beverages generally do not contain phosphorus), intensive care units (without adequate oral or parenteral alimentation), intestinal malabsorption, or phosphate-binding antacid use, this amount presents a significant physiologic challenge for which no physiologic remedy exists.

SKELETAL PHOSPHATE FLUXES

As with calcium, osteoclastic bone resorption and osteoblastic new bone formation (see Figs. 72–1 and 72–3) lead to phosphate exit and entry, respectively, from the skeleton. Although the skeleton can thus be used as a source of phosphorus, in general, phosphorus can be viewed as a passive passenger with calcium in the calcium regulatory process described previously in the section on calcium. Again, however, under pathophysiologic conditions, skeletal calcium fluxes may become important. Skeletal destruction in multiple myeloma or severe immobilization syndromes leads not only to hypercalcemia, but also to hyperphosphatemia, which, with the concomitant hypercalcemia, leads to nephrocalcinosis and renal failure. Conversely, osteoblastic metastases in prostate cancer and breast cancer and the hungry bone syndrome following parathyroidectomy all lead to clinically significant hypophosphatemia.

INTRACELLULAR-EXTRACELLULAR PHOSPHATE FLUXES

As noted previously, phosphate shuttles from extracellular to intracellular compartments. In general, the control of these fluxes can best be envisioned as being performed at the cellular level by as yet incompletely understood cellular mechanisms. From a clinical standpoint, these issues become important under certain settings. For example, in the setting

of metabolic acidosis, phosphate leaves the intracellular compartment and may lead to hyperphosphatemia, whereas, under conditions of alkalosis, serum phosphate concentrations decline, and hypophosphatemia develops as phosphate enters the intracellular compartment. Other clinical situations in which intracellular phosphate has important clinical implications are in the settings of crush injury (rhabdomyolysis) and the tumor lysis syndrome, in both of which large intracellular loads of phosphate are delivered into the ECF and result in hypocalcemia, seizures, nephrocalcinosis, and renal failure. Finally, glucose shifts phosphate into cells as glucose-6-phosphate, and overzealous intravenous or oral caloric restitution in the undernourished patient can result in severe hypophosphatemia and sudden death.

RENAL PHOSPHATE HANDLING

By far the most important mechanism for maintaining a normal serum phosphorus concentration is renal phosphorus handling. As with calcium, phosphate is filtered by the glomerulus. Tubular reabsorption of filtered phosphate (TRP) occurs at a rate such that approximately 90% of phosphate is reabsorbed (i.e., the TRP is normally approximately 90%), and the remaining 10% is excreted. This 10% represents the fractional excretion of phosphorus (Fe_{Pi}). The Fe_{Pi} can be calculated in a spot urine sample as follows:

$$Fe_{Pi} = \text{(urine Pi [in mg/dL]/urine creatinine [in mg/dL])} \times \text{(serum creatinine [in mg/dL]/serum phosphorus [in mg/dL])}$$

The TRP is simple to calculate:

$$TRP = 1 - Fe_{Pi}$$

The renal handling of phosphorus is best considered as a tubular maximum (Tm)-regulated process. For example, a renal Tm for glucose exists and is set at approximately 180 mg/dL. When the serum glucose rises above 180 mg/dL, glycosuria occurs. Of course, the serum glucose normally does not rise above 180 mg/dL, therefore glucose does not normally appear in the urine. A similar process occurs with the Tm for phosphorus (TmP), with one exception. The TmP is normally identical to a normal serum phosphorus concentration in blood, approximately 3.3 mg/dL. If the serum phosphate concentration rises above this level, then phosphaturia occurs, and the serum phosphorus declines to 3.3 mg/dL. If the serum phosphate concentration declines below 3.3 mg/dL, then filtered phosphate is entirely reabsorbed, and urinary phosphate excretion declines to zero. Thus the TmP can be considered as a *dam* in the *phosphate reservoir,* over which excess phosphate *spills,* and whose level controls the *level* or concentration of serum phosphorus.

The one exception to this concept is that, unlike the glucose Tm, which is fixed at 180 mg/dL, the TmP is not fixed but can be moved upward or downward, depending on metabolic needs and prevailing metabolic conditions, as described in the following section.

The TRP or Fe_{Pi}, as described previously, can be readily calculated, and then the TmP can be derived from the nomo-

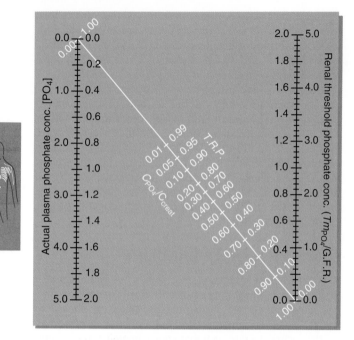

Figure 72–9 The tubular maximum for phosphorus–glomerular filtration rate (TmP-GFR) nomogram. This nomogram allows the conversion of the fractional excretion of phosphorus (or its inverse, the tubular reabsorption of filtered phosphate [TRP]) into the TmP-GFR. The TRP is calculated, as described in the text, and a line is drawn extending from the serum phosphorus *(leftmost line),* through the TRP *(middle, diagonal line),* to the left line, which represents the TmP/GFR. TmP values are provided in both millimolar (mmol) and milligram per deciliter (mg/dL) units. TmP values below 1.0 mmol or 2.5 mg/dL are abnormal and indicate phosphaturia. (From Walton RJ, Bijvoet OLM: Nomogram for derivation of renal threshold phosphate concentration. Lancet 2:309–310, 1975.)

gram of Bijvoet, shown in Figure 72–9. This process proves enormously useful in clinical practice because it is the central starting point for determining whether hypophosphatemia is principally renal or nonrenal in origin.

PARATHYROID HORMONE AND *PHOSPHATONIN*

PTH has long been appreciated to be phosphaturic, that is, to lower the TmP or, more accurately, to inhibit proximal renal tubular phosphate reabsorption. Indeed, the initial bioassay for PTH action in humans, the Ellsworth-Howard test, assessed the responsiveness of the TRP to infusion of bovine parathyroid gland extract. This characteristic also explains the hypophosphatemia associated with primary and secondary hyperparathyroidism and, conversely, the hyperphosphatemia associated with hypoparathyroid states. Thus in TmP terms, excessive PTH lowers the TmP, whereas low PTH values allow the TmP to rise to supranormal levels.

It has been clear for many years, however, that other factors regulated the level of the TmP. For example, experimental dietary phosphorus deprivation in laboratory animals and humans leads to a PTH-independent increase in the TmP, and high-phosphate feeding results in a PTH-independent decline in the TmP. Thus for decades, investi-

gators in this area have postulated the existence of a phosphaturic hormone that has been called *phosphatonin.* Despite decades of research, phosphatonin has remained elusive. This area has become one of intense focus recently with the discovery of the cause of three disorders. In one of these disorders, X-linked hypophosphatemic rickets, also known as vitamin D–resistant rickets, causative inactivating mutations have been identified in the *PHEX* enzyme. Current models suggest that mutant *PHEX* fails to inactivate normal amounts of phosphatonin, and this failure leads to phosphaturia and hypophosphatemia. In two other disorders, autosomal-dominant hypophosphatemic rickets and oncogenic osteomalacia, overproduction of fibroblast growth factor-23 (FGF-23) has been demonstrated, and many clinicians believe that FGF-23 is the long-sought phosphatonin. Other investigators have suggested that matrix extracellular phosphoglycoprotein *(MEPE)* or secreted frizzled-related protein 4 *(sFRP4)* may serve as phosphatonins as well. Much remains to be worked out in this arena, but clearly, a hormonal system that regulates renal phosphorus handling exists, and the kidney is the prime regulatory organ for phosphate homeostasis.

Regulation of Serum Magnesium

Magnesium is a divalent cation, as is calcium, with this exception—magnesium homeostasis has closer parallels with phosphorus homeostasis. Both magnesium and phosphate are principally intracellular, with concentrations inside the cell that far exceed those outside the cell. Both substances govern key intracellular regulatory processes. In the case of magnesium, these processes include such fundamental events as DNA replication and transcription, translation of RNA, the use of adenosine triphosphate as an energy source, and regulated peptide hormone secretion. Both magnesium and phosphate are abundant in the marine environment and therefore became incorporated into basic life processes early in the evolution of single-celled organisms. Both substances are abundant in terrestrial diets, whether vegetarian or carnivorous, given their abundance inside all kinds of cells. Given this abundance, little evolutionary pressure to develop a complex regulatory network exists. As with phosphate, because the important site of magnesium availability is within the cell, ECF serves only as a conduit for magnesium, and serum magnesium concentrations are not tightly regulated. As with phosphate, because magnesium is principally intracellular, measurement of serum magnesium may provide false estimates of actual total body and intracellular magnesium status. Finally, as with phosphate, because magnesium is so essential for fundamental processes such as gene transcription and cellular energy usage, life-threatening magnesium deficiency is often unrecognized because its symptoms are frustratingly nonspecific: weakness, respirator dependence, diffuse neurologic syndromes including seizures, and cardiovascular collapse.

Magnesium, as noted previously, is a divalent cation. Its molecular weight is 24, which is to say that 1 mole is 24 g, and, because it is divalent, one equivalent is 12 g. These considerations are significant clinically because magnesium measurements in blood are often provided in mg/dL or

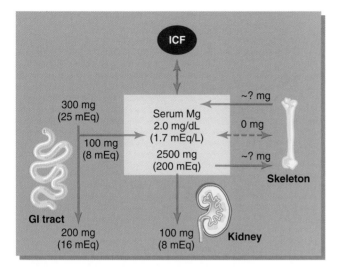

Figure 72–10 The magnesium *physiologic black box*. See Figure 72–1 for nomenclature and the text for details. Magnesium values are provided in both milligram (mg) and milliequivalent (mEq) units.

milliequivalents per liter (mEq/L), oral magnesium supplements in milligrams per tablet or milliequivalents per vial, and urinary magnesium excretion in milliequivalents or milligrams per 24 hours. Quantitative perspective in this clinical world of variable units can easily be lost. Constructing a *black box* for magnesium is helpful, as shown in Figure 72–10, in which magnesium is provided in both milligram and milliequivalent units.

As with phosphorus, magnesium has quantitatively important interfaces with the intestine, the skeleton, intracellular supplies, and the kidney. At the level of the intestine, as noted previously, magnesium is widely available in normal diets, and regulation here is limited: the body absorbs approximately one third of what is ingested. Under normal circumstances, dietary magnesium is abundant, absorption

is ample, and magnesium deficiency does not occur. However, with alcoholism (a pure alcohol diet contains no magnesium), in intensive care unit settings in which adequate nutrition often is not provided, and/or with intestinal malabsorption, magnesium deficiency may occur.

At the level of the skeleton, magnesium is incorporated into the hydroxyapatite crystal as mineralization of osteoid occurs, and it is released by osteoclastic bone resorption (see Figs. 72–1 and 72–3). In quantitative terms, these fluxes are small.

Many instances of magnesium deficiency are caused by excessive renal losses. Examples include the magnesuria that accompanies saline infusions, diuretic use, alcohol use, and secondary hyperaldosteronism states such as cirrhosis and ascites. As with calcium and phosphorus, the fractional excretion of magnesium (FeMg) can be calculated, and this should be used as an index as to whether the kidney is appropriately conserving magnesium in states of hypomagnesemia or whether renal magnesium wasting is the cause of the hypomagnesemia. The normal FeMg is 2% to 4%. Hypomagnesemic individuals should display FeMg values below 1% to 2%.

With regard to homeostatic regulation, magnesium homeostasis can best be viewed as a renal Tm-regulated process (see the general principles described previously for the TmP in the Renal Phosphate Handling section), with the renal Tm for magnesium set at a fixed level of approximately 2.2 mg/dL. In this scenario, abundant dietary magnesium exists, and excessive magnesium intake is managed by spillage of excess magnesium, over the Tm set at 2.2 mg/dL, into the urine. Conversely, in settings of dietary magnesium deficiency, which equate evolutionarily with caloric deficiency, short-term magnesium deficiency is prevented when serum levels fall below the renal Tm of 2.0 mg/dL, and long-term deficiency is associated with, and becomes of lesser importance than, death via starvation. With regard to hormonal regulation, no known independent regulatory system for magnesium exists.

Prospectus for the Future

Although it may seem from this chapter that calcium, PTH, vitamin D, magnesium and phosphorus homeostasis, and skeletal biology are well understood, it should be clear that many of the details of the physiology as described in this chapter have been elucidated over the last 10 to 15 years, and indeed, new hormones (e.g., FGF-23) and diseases continue to accumulate at a rapid rate. The truth is that this area of research is dynamic, with many central unanswered questions. For example, although we know that the GI tract (pancreas, biliary system, and intestinal glands) secretes calcium and that this action is important quantitatively (150 mg/day), we know nothing about how this process is regulated or whether daily losses can be prevented. Similarly, although we now appreciate that phosphate has direct effects on the parathyroid gland and that these effects may be important in chronic renal failure, we do not know precisely what constitutes the parathyroid phosphorus sensor. Moreover, we know that hypomagnesemia and hypophosphatemia result in substantial intensive care unit morbidity and mortality, yet we remain inadequate at recognizing the nonspecific signs and symptoms of these diseases. We know

that bone density is a critical determinant of osteoporotic fracture, but we also know that *bone mass* accounts for only approximately 50% of fracture risk, with the other 50% representing issues of *bone quality*. Yet we have little understanding of what, at a molecular or structural level, determines or defines *bone quality*. In osteoporosis, most of the currently available pharmacologic agents inhibit osteoclast activity and are therefore *antiresorptives* or *anticatabolic agents*. What we really need for osteoporosis are agents that can potently stimulate osteoblasts to synthesize new bone, so-called *skeletal anabolic agents*. One agent, recombinant PTH, has recently been approved, and others are in the pharmaceutical pipeline. Another example of the limitations of our current understanding is a debate over the pulsatile secretion of PTH. Is the secretion pulsatile, and if so, how frequent are the pulses? Is pulsatile secretion important for PTH physiology as it obviously is for gonadotropin-releasing hormone biology, and is it important in pathophysiology? Whereas to the new initiate in mineral and bone physiology, everything has seemingly been discovered already, this assumption is far from the truth!

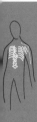

References

DeGroot L, Jameson LJ (eds.): Endocrinology, 5th ed. Philadelphia, W.B. Saunders, 2006.

Favus MF (Ed): The American Society for Bone and Mineral Research Primer on Metabolic Bone Diseases and Disorders of Mineral Metabolism, 5th ed. Washington DC, American Society for Bone and Mineral Research, 2004.

Lentz RD, Brown DM, Kjellstrand CM: Treatment of severe hypophosphatemia. Ann Int Med 89:941–944, 1978.

Marx SJ: Mineral and bone homeostasis. In Goldman L, Bennett JC: Cecil Textbook of Medicine, 21st ed. Philadelphia, WB Saunders, 2000, pp. 1383–1389.

Schiavi SC, Kumar R: The phosphatonin pathway: New insights in phosphate homeostasis. Kidney Int 65:1–14, 2004.

Disorders of Serum Minerals

Andrew F. Stewart

In this chapter, disorders that lead to increases or decreases in the circulating concentrations of calcium, phosphorus, and magnesium are considered. The reader is urged, in considering these disorders, to review the appropriate section in the Chapter 72 describing the normal physiology of calcium, phosphorus, and magnesium metabolism. The optimal approach to diagnosing and treating these disorders is to understand their underlying physiology and pathophysiology. Beginning here, coherent diagnostic and successful therapeutic plans can best be developed. Although obvious at one level, years of experience suggests a common and persistent propensity to jump to the common items on the differential diagnosis list without fully considering the other options, and, in so doing, overlooking the correct, and often easily treatable, diagnosis. For example, hypercalcemia in the setting of a pulmonary nodule may indicate the presence of humoral hypercalcemia of malignancy, and many physicians will jump to this diagnosis with its grim prognosis. However, this complex might also represent hypercalcemia in a patient with treatable tuberculosis (TB) or primary hyperparathyroidism (HPT) in a person with a long-standing and inactive pulmonary scar.

Complete differential diagnoses are provided in the tables that follow. The author's practice is to consider every diagnosis in the appropriate table in every patient with a disorder of mineral metabolism. Hypercalcemia attributed by some physicians to *cancer* has proven in many instances to be due to sarcoid, HPT, hyperthyroidism, milk-alkali syndrome, and a host of other conditions, and hypocalcemia attributed by some physicians to *hypoparathyroidism* has proven to be due to easily treatable causes such as hypomagnesemia resulting from sprue or chemotherapy with cisplatin in some cases and in others to reductions in albumin in patients with the nephrotic syndrome. Each of these examples was incorrectly diagnosed initially but became obvious with appropriate consideration and testing.

Hypercalcemia

SYMPTOMS AND SIGNS

Hypercalcemia causes hyperpolarization of neuromuscular cell membranes and therefore refractoriness to stimulation (see Chapter 72). This condition presents clinically as skeletal muscular weakness, smooth-muscle hypoactivity with constipation and ileus, and the full spectrum of mental dysfunction, progressing from lassitude to mild confusion to deep coma. Hypercalcemia also leads to renal failure. It causes a reduction in the glomerular filtration rate (GFR) via afferent arteriolar vasoconstriction and, via activation of the calcium receptor in the distal nephron, causes a form of nephrogenic diabetes insipidus, associated with polydipsia and polyuria. These events lower the extracellular fluid (ECF) volume and lower the GFR as well. Hypercalcemia may lead to interstitial calcium phosphate crystal deposition in the kidney (nephrocalcinosis or interstitial nephritis) and nephrolithiasis with obstructive uropathy. Hypercalcemia may also lead to shortening of the QTc interval on the electrocardiogram. Frequently, however, hypercalcemia is discovered on routine laboratory testing.

Whether a person develops symptoms depends on several factors. One of these factors is the degree of hypercalcemia. People with serum calcium values above 13 mg/dL are generally symptomatic. Also important is the duration of hypercalcemia. A gradual increase in serum calcium, even into the severe 15- to 17-mg/dL range, may cause little in the way of symptoms if it occurs slowly enough. Finally, the overall health, age, and general status of the person in whom hypercalcemia occurs will influence the severity of symptoms. For example, a child with severe immobilization-induced hypercalcemia in the 15-mg/dL range may be completely alert, whereas an elderly person with underlying Alzheimer's disease and narcotic use may become comatose with a serum calcium of 11.5 mg/dL.

PATHOPHYSIOLOGY

The physiologic *black box* described in Chapter 72 can and should be considered when attempting to diagnose or treat hypercalcemia. These disorders can be grouped into factitious disorders (e.g., caused by abnormalities in serum proteins), renal disorders (e.g., thiazide diuretic or lithium use), gastrointestinal disorders (e.g., sarcoid or the milk-alkali syndrome), skeletal disorders (e.g., hypercalcemia of malignancy, immobilization hypercalcemia), and combined disorders (primary HPT is a good example, with important gastrointestinal [GI] and renal components). Considering each diagnosis in Table 73–1 in the context of the mechanism that might be operative in a given patient brings clarity of diagnosis and corresponding appropriateness to therapy.

DIFFERENTIAL DIAGNOSIS

Malignancy-Associated Hypercalcemia

The most common cause of hypercalcemia among hospitalized patients is cancer. Hypercalcemia occurs late in the course of cancer, and rapid progression to more severe hypercalcemia and rapid death is the rule. The 50% survival rate among patients with cancer following the development of hypercalcemia is approximately 30 days. In general, hypercalcemia is only encountered in patients with large tumor burdens. Conversely, small, occult cancers rarely cause hypercalcemia. The exceptions to this rule are small tumors of the neuroendocrine variety, such as islet cell tumors and bronchial carcinoids. Certain tumors are common causes of hypercalcemia, including breast, renal, squamous, and ovarian carcinomas, as well as multiple myeloma and lymphoma. Conversely, certain other common cancers are not commonly associated with hypercalcemia, exemplified by colon, prostate, and gastric carcinoma. The occurrence of hypercalcemia should always provoke a complete search for the entities described in Table 73–1, particularly in patients with these latter types of cancer, given the likelihood that a vigorous search will reveal a second, more treatable form of hypercalcemia.

Cancer may lead to hypercalcemia through several mechanisms, the most common of which is *humoral hypercalcemia of malignancy* (HHM). HHM accounts for approximately 80% of patients with malignancy-associated hypercalcemia (MAHC) and is the result of secretion by tumors of parathyroid hormone–related protein (PTHrP). PTHrP mimics the actions of parathyroid hormone (PTH) on the kidney to prevent calcium excretion and on the skeleton to activate osteoclasts and induce bone resorption. PTHrP is the product of many normal cell types and is normally produced at low levels. The cause of the increase in PTHrP synthesis in cancer is most often not known but has been demonstrated to be due to PTHrP gene duplication or transcriptional upregulation of the PTHrP gene in some patients. Tumors classically associated with the HHM mechanism are squamous carcinomas of any site (including larynx, lung, cervix, and esophagus), renal carcinomas, ovarian carcinomas, and lymphomas associated with human T-cell lymphotropic virus type I (HTLV-I). More recently, the fact that breast cancer commonly produces hypercal-

---

Table 73–1 Disorders Associated with Hypercalcemia

Malignancy-associated hypercalcemia
  Humoral hypercalcemia of malignancy
  Hypercalcemia caused by 1,25(OH)$_2$D-secreting lymphomas
  Hypercalcemia caused by direct skeletal invasion
  True ectopic hyperparathyroidism
Primary and tertiary hyperparathyroidism
Familial hypocalciuric hypercalcemia or familial benign hypercalcemia
Granulomatous disorders
  Sarcoid
  Berylliosis
  Foreign body
  Tuberculosis
  Coccidioidomycosis
  Blastomycosis
  Histoplasmosis
  Granulomatous leprosy
  Eosinophilic granuloma
  Histiocytosis
  Inflammatory bowel disease
Endocrine disorders other than hyperparathyroidism
  Hyperthyroidism
  Pheochromocytoma
  Addisonian crisis
  VIPoma (WDHA syndrome)
Medications
  Thiazides
  Aminophylline
  Lithium
  Estrogen/antiestrogen in breast cancer with bone
    metastases (*estrogen flare*)
  Vitamin D and derivatives (calcitriol, dihydrotachysterol)
  Vitamin A (including retinoic acid derivatives)
  Foscarnet
Milk-alkali syndrome
Immobilization plus high bone turnover
  Juvenile skeleton
  Paget's disease
  Myeloma and breast cancer with bone metastases
  Prehumoral hypercalcemia of malignancy
  Mild primary hyperparathyroidism
  Secondary hyperparathyroidism (e.g., from continuous
    ambulatory peritoneal dialysis)
Chronic and acute renal failure
  Recovery phase of rhabdomyolysis-induced acute renal
    failure
  Chronic hemodialysis
  Calcitriol
  Immobilization
  Decreased calcium clearance
  Calcium carbonate
Total parenteral nutrition (TPN)
  Calcium-containing TPN in patients with decreased
    glomerular filtration rate
  Chronic TPN in patients with short bowel syndrome
Hyperproteinemia
  Volume contraction with hyperalbuminemia
  Myeloma with calcium-binding immunoglobulin
End-stage liver disease
Manganese intoxication

1,25(OH)$_2$D = 1,25-dihydroxyvitamin D; VIPoma = vasoactive intestinal peptide–producing tumor; WDHA = watery diarrhea, hypokalemia, and achlorhydria.

cemia via this mechanism, as well, has become known. In general, hypercalcemia in HHM occurs in the absence of skeletal metastases or in the presence of a limited number of skeletal metastases, and, if tumor resection or ablation is possible, hypercalcemia reverses. These observations, together with histologic evidence for aggressive bone resorption at sites within the skeleton not involved by tumor, make clear that HHM is indeed the result of a tumor-derived *humor* or hormone. This example is perhaps the only one in which PTHrP acts in an *endocrine* fashion, more typically behaving as a paracrine, autocrine, or intracrine growth and developmental factor. In addition to hypercalcemia, these patients display reductions in PTH, reductions in 1,25-dihydroxyvitamin D (1,25(OH)$_2$D), elevations in PTHrP, and reductions in serum phosphorus and the tubular maximum for phosphorus (TmP) (see Chapter 72).

A second form of MAHC is that caused by local tumor invasion of the skeleton, a process referred to as *local osteolytic hypercalcemia* (LOH). LOH accounts for approximately 20% of patients with MAHC. In these patients, in contrast to those with HHM, the skeletal metastatic or primary tumor burden is large, and the offending tumor is most often a breast cancer or a hematologic neoplasm such as multiple myeloma, leukemia, or lymphoma. The local factors within the skeleton that are secreted by tumors to induce osteoclastic bone resorption include PTHrP, macrophage inflammatory protein-1-α (MIP1α), receptor-activating nuclear factor kappa B ligand (RANKL), interleukin-6, interleukin-1, and likely others as well. These patients display reductions in both PTH and PTHrP, as well as 1,25(OH)$_2$D, and generally have normal to elevated serum phosphorus values.

A third form of MAHC is due to *secretion of 1,25(OH)$_2$D by lymphomas and dysgerminomas*. These instances are unusual and are interesting from a mechanistic standpoint. Although direct bone involvement may occur and may contribute to hypercalcemia, the increase in 1,25(OH)$_2$D leads to intestinal calcium hyperabsorption, as well as to systemically driven bone resorption. Thus this condition is in essence a malignant version of the hypercalcemia that occurs in sarcoidosis (see "Granulomatous Disorders" later). The fact that macrophages produce 1,25(OH)$_2$D and that overproduction of 1,25(OH)$_2$D occurs in some lymphomas is now well documented. Under normal circumstances, 1,25(OH)$_2$D behaves as an immunomodulatory cytokine, produced locally in small amounts by lymphoreticular cells but not contributing significantly to systemic concentrations of 1,25(OH)$_2$D. However, under certain conditions, large amounts of 1,25(OH)$_2$D are produced by a given lymphoma, and hypercalcemia ensues. Thus lymphomas are particularly interesting in that they may cause hypercalcemia through an HHM mechanism with systemic PTHrP secretion through a local skeletal invasion mechanism and through systemic production of 1,25(OH)$_2$D. Recently, the syndrome has been observed in association with ovarian dysgerminomas.

Finally, although the vast majority of instances of HHM are due to PTHrP, several well-documented case reports of *ectopic secretion of authentic PTH* have come to light. These case reports have included a colon carcinoma, a squamous carcinoma of the lung, a small-cell carcinoma of the ovary, and a neuroendocrine tumor.

Primary and Tertiary Hyperparathyroidism

Although MAHC is the most common cause of hypercalcemia among inpatients, primary HPT is by far the most common cause among healthy outpatients. Together, MAHC and HPT account for approximately 90% of cases of hypercalcemia. Most often, the hypercalcemia is mild, with serum calcium values in the 10.6- to 11.5-mg/dL range. However, HPT can occasionally produce spectacular hypercalcemia in the 20-mg/dL range. Approximately 85% of the time, hypercalcemia results from a single parathyroid adenoma that overproduces PTH, and in approximately 15% of patients, it is due to multiple-gland hyperplasia. In less than 1% of patients, HPT may result from parathyroid carcinoma. The diagnosis is made by the discovery of an elevated serum PTH in a patient with hypercalcemia. Hypophosphatemia, a reduction in the TmP, increased plasma 1,25(OH)$_2$D, an increase in serum chloride, and a reduction in serum bicarbonate are also typical features.

Most often, primary HPT is asymptomatic. However, some patients develop hypercalciuria and calcium nephrolithiasis, most often as a result of calcium oxalate and, less commonly, calcium phosphate stones. In addition, some patients with HPT, especially those with more severe HPT, experience a reduction in bone mineral density characterized histologically as hyperparathyroid bone disease or *osteitis fibrosa cystica* (see Chapter 74). Other patients may develop mild to severe renal failure as a result of the considerations described under Symptoms and Signs of hypercalcemia earlier. Each of the previously mentioned conditions—significant osteopenia, hypercalciuria, kidney stones, reduced renal function, and/or a serum calcium greater than 1.0 mg/dL above normal—is considered to be an indication for parathyroidectomy. Other patients may be monitored conservatively. Some authors believe that cognitive dysfunction, peptic ulcers, and hypertension may result from HPT, but many disagree. Most people would regard these indications as *soft* indications for surgery at best.

The cause of parathyroid adenomas is most often not known, but mutations of the cyclin D1 and parafibromin genes have been described in some patients, and mutations in other genes have been identified in the adenomas of others. Mutations in *pRb*, the retinoblastoma gene, and in the parafibromin gene, have been identified in some parathyroid carcinomas.

HPT can occur as part of one of the multiple endocrine neoplasia (MEN) syndromes, in association with pituitary and/or islet tumors (MEN-I) or with pheochromocytomas and medullary carcinoma of the thyroid (MEN-II).

Secondary HPT, by definition, is an appropriate increase in circulating PTH associated with eucalcemia or hypocalcemia, occurring in an attempt to correct hypocalcemia resulting for example from vitamin D deficiency or chronic renal failure. *Tertiary* HPT refers to HPT associated with hypercalcemia that appears in the setting of prolonged stimulation of the parathyroid glands, such as chronic renal failure with hypocalcemia or chronic vitamin D deficiency resulting from malabsorption. Chronic parathyroid stimulation leads to parathyroid hyperplasia and at times adenomas, and these may, if they fail to suppress with the development of hypercalcemia, cause hypercalcemia. The classic example is the development of PTH-dependent hypercalcemia following successful renal transplantation.

Familial Hypocalciuric Hypercalcemia

Familial hypocalciuric hypercalcemia (also known as benign hypercalcemia) is an autosomal-dominant, inherited disorder that is due to heterozygous inactivating mutations in the calcium receptor. Thus parathyroid glands that bear this receptor on their surface (see Chapter 72) inappropriately perceive circulating calcium concentrations to be low, therefore behaving as though the patient is hypocalcemic, and appropriately secrete additional PTH. This action causes the serum calcium to rise, and, with an elevated calcium, the PTH returns to a high-normal level. The hypercalcemia is usually mild, in the 11- to 12-mg/dL range, but may be higher. Importantly, because the calcium receptor is also expressed in the kidney, the kidney inappropriately conserves calcium, leading to hypocalciuria and contributing to hypercalcemia. Urine calcium excretion is in the 20- to 100-mg/day range. Finally, because the defective calcium receptor is also expressed in the central nervous system (CNS), the hypercalcemia goes unperceived by the CNS, and affected individuals are therefore asymptomatic. Thus the two names of this syndrome describe it accurately.

With the exception of the hypocalciuria and the autosomal-dominant pattern of inheritance, these individuals are similar to patients with primary HPT; they have mildly elevated calcium concentrations in the setting of a high-normal to mildly elevated PTH. Because affected individuals are asymptomatic and do not develop adverse sequelae from the syndrome, its primary importance is that affected individuals be properly identified and protected from unnecessary parathyroidectomy. Partial or subtotal parathyroidectomy has no effect on these individuals, and total parathyroidectomy causes hypoparathyroidism.

In some patients, two defective alleles of the calcium sensor are inherited. These individuals may have complete inability to sense calcium and therefore develop severe and symptomatic hypercalcemia, with serum calcium values in the 15- to 20-mg/dL range. Because of the severity of this disorder, homozygous individuals usually present in infancy with so-called neonatal severe hyperparathyroidism. In contrast to the mild heterozygous condition described previously, homozygous individuals require urgent total parathyroidectomy in infancy.

Granulomatous Disorders

Almost all granulomatous disorders can lead to hypercalcemia, as noted in Table 73–1. The prototypes are sarcoidosis, TB, and the fungal diseases listed. Briefly, as previously described for lymphomas, granulomas, as with the kidney, have the ability to convert inactive 25-hydroxyvitamin D to the active metabolite, 1,25(OH)$_2$D. Thus individuals with these disorders, when exposed to sunlight, ultraviolet radiation, or relatively trivial quantities of dietary vitamin D, may develop mild to severe hypercalcemia. Examples include sunlight-induced (i.e., summertime) hypercalcemia in patients with sarcoidosis and hypercalcemic flares in patients with TB given dietary supplements with multivitamins after hospitalization. Hypercalcemia results from components of both intestinal calcium hyperabsorption and 1,25(OH)$_2$D-induced bone resorption, with the former being

the most important in most cases. Because of the hypercalcemia, PTH is suppressed, and serum phosphorus is elevated. The combination of hypercalcemia and hyperphosphatemia leads to nephrocalcinosis and renal failure. The treatment is a low dietary calcium intake, a low vitamin D intake, limiting sun exposure, hydration and loop diuretics to accelerate calcium clearance, and, if the hypercalcemia is severe, glucocorticoids. Of course, treatment of the underlying granulomatous disorder is the most effective and prudent long-term therapy.

Endocrine Disorders Other Than Hyperparathyroidism

In addition to HPT, four other endocrine disorders have been associated with the development of hypercalcemia. One of these disorders is hyperthyroidism. As many as 50% of people with hyperthyroidism have been described as having at least mild hypercalcemia. The hypercalcemia is only rarely greater than 11.0 mg/dL but may be as high as 13.0 mg/dL. The mechanism is believed to be an increase in osteoclast activation by thyroid hormone. A second disorder is pheochromocytoma. Some of these individuals are hypercalcemic as a result of primary HPT occurring as part of the MEN-II syndrome (discussed previously under "Hyperparathyroidism"), but others have been reported to become hypercalcemic as a result of PTHrP secretion by their pheochromocytoma. Severe hypoadrenalism with hypotension, so-called Addisonian crisis, has been reported to lead to hypercalcemia that responds to volume replacement and glucocorticoids. The mechanism is not known. Finally, islet cell tumors that produce vasoactive intestinal polypeptide (VIP), so-called VIPomas, although rare, are regularly associated with hypercalcemia. VIPomas lead to the watery diarrhea, hypokalemia, achlorhydria (WDHA) syndrome, also referred to as pancreatic cholera.

Medications

Certain medications may cause hypercalcemia. These drugs include thiazide diuretics and lithium, which appear to increase renal tubular calcium reabsorption, and the phosphodiesterase inhibitors aminophylline and theophylline, for which the hypercalcemic mechanism is unknown. Both vitamins D and A and their more active congeners, such as 1,25(OH)$_2$D and *cis*-retinoic acid, respectively, may also cause hypercalcemia. Vitamin D causes hypercalcemia primarily by stimulating intestinal calcium absorption but can also stimulate osteoclastic bone resorption. Vitamin A stimulates bone resorption. The antiviral agent, foscarnet, has been reported to cause hypercalcemia via unknown mechanisms. Finally, estrogens and tamoxifen have been described to cause hypercalcemia in the setting of breast cancer with extensive skeletal metastases, the so-called estrogen flare.

Milk-Alkali Syndrome

The normal intake of calcium is in the range of 600 to 1200 mg/day for most people, and, as reviewed in Chapter 72, absorption of calcium from the diet is tightly controlled. However, ingestion of very large quantities of calcium may overwhelm this system and lead to hypercalcemia. This condition was originally described in the 1940s in patients ingesting enormous quantities of milk, cream, and antacids but is still encountered today with some regularity in patients ingesting large quantities of calcium carbonate or other calcium-containing antacids for peptic disease. In general, for hypercalcemia to occur, calcium intake must exceed 4 g/day and is often in the 10- to 20-g/day range. Severe hypercalcemia is common and may lead to renal failure.

Immobilization

Beginning with the polio epidemic in the 1950s, continuing with space missions in the 1970s, and now most commonly observed in the setting of quadriplegia in young adults or children, immobilization hypercalcemia is common and often severe. Development of the syndrome requires two conditions: essentially *complete immobilization* or weightlessness for a period of at least weeks and occurring on a *background of high bone turnover,* as occurs in young adults or children, mild primary or secondary HPT, Paget's disease, and malignant skeletal disease such as breast cancer with bone metastases or multiple myeloma. The basis for the syndrome is that immobilization or weightlessness activates osteoclastic bone resorption and at the same time inhibits osteoblastic activity, producing a severe uncoupling of bone resorption from formation, with rapid and enormous net losses of calcium from the skeleton into the ECF. Left untreated, the condition results in severe demineralization. The syndrome is associated with hypercalciuria as well, and this, together with chronic urinary catheterization, leads to urinary tract infection and severe calcium nephrolithiasis. The most effective treatment for the hypercalcemia is active weight bearing. Hydration and antiresorptive drugs such as the bisphosphonates may be used.

Chronic and Acute Renal Failure

Chronic and acute renal failure have been associated with hypercalcemia. Of course, the more common initial abnormality is hypocalcemia induced by a reduction in kidney-derived $1,25(OH)_2D$ and an increase in serum phosphate as a result of diminished glomerular filtration. However, hypercalcemia may occur in patients with chronic renal failure as a result of calcium antacid use or as a result of $1,25(OH)_2D$ or paracalcitol treatment to prevent renal osteodystrophy. Moreover, immobilization in the setting of chronic renal failure—for example, for peritonitis in the setting of peritoneal dialysis—may also lead to hypercalcemia. In the setting of acute renal failure resulting from rhabdomyolysis (crush injury), transient rebound hypercalcemia has been described as renal failure resolves and serum phosphate concentrations decline.

Parenteral Nutrition

Enteric and parenteral nutrition have both been associated with hypercalcemia. Large doses of oral calcium provided in hypercaloric enteric feeding regimens, particularly in the setting of reduced renal function, may lead to what is in essence a form of the milk-alkali syndrome. More mysterious is the well-described hypercalcemic syndrome occurring in patients treated with total parenteral nutrition (TPN). These patients typically have short bowel syndrome and are on long-term TPN. In some patients, the hypercalcemia can be traced to large amounts of calcium, vitamin D, or aluminum in the TPN solution. In other patients, however, these factors do not appear to be operative, and the pathophysiologic mechanisms remain unexplained.

Hyperproteinemia

Approximately 50% of circulating calcium is bound to serum albumin and other proteins. Thus increases in serum proteins will naturally lead to an increase in total, but not ionized, serum calcium concentrations. This increase is commonly observed in settings of volume depletion and dehydration and may account for the hypercalcemia observed in patients with Addisonian crisis described previously under "Hypercalcemia." A more unusual form of this syndrome occurs in patients with myeloma or Waldenström's macroglobulinemia, whose abnormal immunoglobulin specifically binds calcium and leads to an increase in total, but not ionized, serum calcium. This action, of course, is not the norm in patients with myeloma and hypercalcemia, who have increases in the ionized component of serum calcium. Patients with this syndrome do not display features typical of authentic hypercalcemia: reduced mental status, prolonged QTc interval on electrocardiogram, and hypercalciuria.

End-Stage Liver Disease

Patients with end-stage liver disease awaiting transplant have been described as being hypercalcemic. The pathophysiologic mechanism underlying this syndrome is not known.

Manganese Intoxication

Manganese intoxication in individuals who drink water from contaminated wells has been described. Again, the pathophysiologic mechanism is not understood.

TREATMENT OF HYPERCALCEMIA

Therapy for hypercalcemia is optimally directed at reversing the underlying pathophysiologic abnormality. Although this principle may seem obvious, it is often overlooked in practice. Thus reversal of hypercalcemia associated with cancer is most effectively treated over the long term by effective antineoplastic therapy; correction of hypercalcemia in sarcoidosis is best treated using affective antisarcoid therapy. Seen from this perspective, all other therapies are temporizing, intended to lower calcium while waiting for a response to more definitive therapy. In general, disorders associated with increased intestinal calcium absorption (e.g., sarcoid, milk-alkali syndrome, $1,25(OH)_2D$-secreting lymphomas) are best treated by consuming a low-calcium diet and avoiding vitamin D. Hypercalcemia in the setting of volume depletion and diminished renal function is best treated by expanding the ECF volume and GFR with saline and encouraging diuresis with loop diuretics. Medication-induced hypercalcemia, such as thiazide-induced hypercalcemia, is best treated by discontinuation of the offending medication. Disorders associated with increased osteoclastic bone resorption, such as MAHC and immobilization hypercalcemia, are best treated using inhibitors of bone resorption such as the bisphosphonates, pamidronate, or zoledronate. Of course, disorders with multiple abnormalities will require combinations of these measures. Resection of parathyroid tissue in patients with parathyroid disease is effective. A point worth emphasizing is that not everyone requires treatment for hypercalcemia: Patients with mild HPT with borderline serum calcium values and without other complications may be observed. Patents with end-stage refractory cancer with severe hypercalcemia may arguably be best served by withholding therapy. Familial hypocalciuric hypercalcemia is best left untreated.

Hypocalcemia

SYMPTOMS AND SIGNS

As described in Chapter 72, hypocalcemia leads to a reduction in the potential difference across cell membranes, which leads to hyperexcitability, particularly of cells of the neuromuscular class. Hence neuromuscular cells spontaneously fire and produce spontaneous seizures, paresthesias, and skeletal muscle contractions (referred to as carpal spasm, pedal spasm, or tetany). Two physical signs are observed on examination: Trousseau's sign, which is spontaneous contraction of the forearm muscles in response to application of a blood pressure cuff around the upper arm and inflation to above systolic pressure, and Chvostek's sign, which is twitching of the facial muscles with gentle tapping of the facial nerve as it exits the parotid gland. An electrocardiographic sign is a prolonged QTc interval. Rarely, severe hypocalcemia has been reported to cause hypocontractility of the myocardium and congestive heart failure because calcium is required for muscle contraction. Finally, prolonged hypoparathyroidism may be associated with basal ganglia calcification, which is asymptomatic but impressive on computed tomography scans and plain x-ray films of the skull.

PATHOPHYSIOLOGY

Hypocalcemia may result from five general mechanisms: (1) a reduction in serum binding proteins (albumin), (2) an increase in serum phosphate with a resultant increase in the calcium-phosphate solubility product, (3) an increase in renal calcium excretion, (4) a reduction in intestinal calcium absorption, or (5) a loss of calcium into the skeleton. The reader is referred to Chapter 72 for more details regarding normal calcium homeostasis. In practice, several of these factors are operative in several disorders. For example, in hypoparathyroidism, a reduction in intestinal calcium absorption combines with an inability to reabsorb calcium from the distal tubule to cause hypocalcemia; or, in breast cancer with extensive osteoblastic metastases, increases in osteoblast activity remove calcium from the ECF, and anorexia leads to a reduction in intestinal calcium intake. From a diagnostic perspective, understanding pathophysiologic mechanisms is important because the clinical setting and routine biochemistry analyses will help include or exclude certain diagnoses. From a therapeutic standpoint, this knowledge is important as well because effective therapy requires that the underlying disorder be appropriately managed. Thus giving oral vitamin D supplements to a patient with sprue may not be effective unless the underlying malabsorption is treated; parenteral vitamin D may be more effective.

DIFFERENTIAL DIAGNOSIS

The disorders that may lead to hypocalcemia are summarized here and in Table 73–2.

Table 73–2 Differential Diagnosis of Hypocalcemia

Hypoparathyroidism
  Surgical
  Idiopathic and autoimmune
  Infiltrative diseases
  Wilson's disease (copper)
  Hemochromatosis
  Sarcoidosis
  Metastatic (breast) cancer
  Congenital
  Isolated/sporadic
  DiGeorge syndrome
  Infant of mother with hyperparathyroidism
  Hereditary
  X-linked
  Parathyroid gland calcium receptor-activating mutations
  PTH signal peptide mutation
  GCMB mutation
Pseudohypoparathyroidism
  Type Ia—multiple hormone resistance, Albright's hereditary
    osteodystrophy
  Type Ib—PTH resistance without other abnormalities
  Type Ic—specific PTH resistance, resulting from defect in
    catalytic subunit of PTH-receptor complex
  Type II—specific PTH resistance, postreceptor/adenylyl
    cyclase defect, undefined
Vitamin D disorders
  Absent ultraviolet exposure
  Vitamin D deficiency
  Fat malabsorption
  Vitamin D–dependent rickets, renal 1-α-hydroxylase
    deficiency, 1,25-dihydroxyvitamin D–receptor defects
  Chronic renal failure
  Hepatic failure
Hypoalbuminemia
Sepsis
Hypermagnesemia and hypomagnesemia
Rapid bone formation
  Hungry bone syndrome after parathyroidectomy or
    thyroidectomy
  Osteoblastic metastases
  Vitamin D therapy of osteomalacia/rickets
Hyperphosphatemia
  Crush injury/rhabdomyolysis
  Renal failure
  Tumor lysis
  Excessive PO_4 administration (PO, IV, PR)
Medications
  Mithramycin/plicamycin
  Bisphosphonates
  Calcitonin
  Fluoride
  EDTA
  Citrate
  Intravenous contrast
  Foscarnet
Pancreatitis
  Hypoalbuminemia
  Hypomagnesemia
  Calcium soap formation

EDTA = ethylenediaminetetraacetic acid; IV = intravenous; PO = by mouth; PO_4 = phosphate; PR = per rectum; PTH = parathyroid hormone.

Hypoparathyroidism

Hypoparathyroidism causes hypocalcemia as a result of a decrease in intestinal calcium absorption (a result of low circulating $1,25[OH]_2D$ concentrations, which are a result of low circulating PTH), combined with reduced renal calcium reabsorption in the distal tubule (as a result of decreased circulating PTH). Hypoparathyroidism may be idiopathic or autoimmune, occurring either in isolation or as part of the polyglandular failure syndrome in association with Graves' hyperthyroidism, Hashimoto's thyroiditis, Addison's disease, Type 1 diabetes, vitiligo, mucocutaneous candidiasis, and other autoimmune disorders. Hypoparathyroidism may also be commonly encountered as surgical hypoparathyroidism in patients who have undergone thyroid, parathyroid, or laryngeal surgery for multinodular goiter or Graves' disease, for parathyroid hyperplasia, or for carcinoma of the larynx or esophagus. Surgical and autoimmune hypoparathyroidism together account for the vast majority of patients with hypoparathyroidism. Less common causes include congenital hypoparathyroidism caused by DiGeorge syndrome, isolated parathyroid failure, or mutations in the calcium-receptor gene, the PTH gene, or the glial cell missing-B *(GCMB)* gene. Finally, rarely, tissue infiltrative diseases such as breast cancer, Wilson's disease (copper deposition), hemochromatosis (iron deposition), or sarcoidosis may destroy or replace normal parathyroid tissue.

The diagnosis is made by finding a low serum ionized calcium level in a patient with an inappropriately reduced serum PTH concentration. In general, the phosphorus concentration is high normal or frankly elevated, and plasma $1,25(OH)_2D$ concentrations are reduced (see Chapter 72 for the underlying physiologic factors).

One potential treatment for hypoparathyroidism is subcutaneous injection of PTH. Although this treatment has been accomplished successfully in clinical trials, PTH is not approved for this indication. Thus treatment is normally directed at increasing intestinal calcium absorption through the use of large doses of calcium (~2000 mg/day) in conjunction with vitamin D (typically, large doses of vitamin D_2 in the range of 50,000 to 200,000 IU/day) or the active form of vitamin D, $1,25(OH)_2D$, in normal replacement amounts (0.25 to 1.0 mcg/day). The goal is to induce sufficient intestinal calcium hyperabsorption to overwhelm the ability of the kidney to excrete it. Although this method is the only tenable therapy, it carries the risk of inducing significant hypercalciuria and therefore nephrocalcinosis and nephrolithiasis. Accordingly, 24-hour urinary calcium must be measured regularly, and hypercalciuria minimized, which generally means maintaining the serum calcium in the low-normal range, approximately 8.5 to 9.0 mg/dL. In some instances, calcium and vitamin D alone may be ineffective or may induce severe hypercalciuria. In such cases, addition of a thiazide diuretic such as hydrochlorothiazide, which stimulates renal calcium reabsorption, may be effective in preventing hypercalciuria and at the same time raising the serum calcium.

Pseudohypoparathyroidism

Pseudohypoparathyroidism refers to a group of disorders that have in common resistance to the actions of PTH. In most cases, the resistance is due to different types of inactivating mutations in the signal-transducing protein Gs-α. Patients may be resistant only to PTH, or they may be resistant to multiple peptide hormones, including thyroid-stimulating hormone (with hypothyroidism) and follicle-stimulating hormone and luteinizing hormone (with hypogonadism). The most common form of the syndrome, type Ia, is associated with multiple hormone resistance and a phenotype referred to as Albright's hereditary osteodystrophy, which includes short stature, shortened fourth and fifth metacarpals and metatarsals, obesity, mental retardation, subcutaneous calcifications, and café-au-lait spots. Because the disorder is hereditary, a clear family history of this phenotype is often present, as well as a family history of hypocalcemia and/or seizures.

Biochemically, these patients resemble those with hypoparathyroidism; they are hypocalcemic and have hyperphosphatemia. The diagnosis is made by the finding of an elevated circulating PTH in a patient with hypocalcemia and hyperphosphatemia in whom other causes of hypocalcemia and secondary hypoparathyroidism have been excluded. The diagnosis can be confirmed by infusing PTH and failing to observe the normal phosphaturic, cyclic monophosphate, and calcemic responses.

The treatment is similar to that of hypoparathyroidism.

Vitamin D Disorders

Active vitamin D, $1,25(OH)_2D$, is required to absorb calcium from the intestine. Activation of vitamin D requires adequate exposure to vitamin D from diet or by sunlight exposure, an intact intestine through which to absorb calcium and vitamin D, an intact liver with which to convert vitamin D to 25-hydroxyvitamin D, and an intact kidney to convert 25-hydroxyvitamin D to $1,25(OH)_2D$ (see Chapter 72). Therefore developing hypocalcemia and osteomalacia or rickets (see Chapter 74) in settings in which one or more of these steps is disrupted is common. Specifically, malabsorption syndromes, such as short bowel syndrome and celiac sprue, lead to hypocalcemia as a result of calcium and vitamin D malabsorption. Chronic liver diseases, particularly primary biliary cirrhosis, lead to hypocalcemia and osteomalacia. Chronic renal insufficiency leads to failure to produce $1,25(OH)_2D$, with reductions in serum calcium and inefficient absorption of intestinal calcium. Normal diets contain little in the way of vitamin D. Although Western diets are supplemented with vitamin D in milk and multivitamins, diets composed of no milk, human milk, or unsupplemented bovine milk are vitamin D deficient. Relatively trivial exposure to sunlight can provide ample vitamin D and replace dietary needs for vitamin D. However, in settings in which both sun exposure and dietary intake of vitamin D are poor (cloudy climates, excessive clothing or body covering, prolonged nursing in infants, and the standard *tea and toast* diet of older adults), vitamin D deficiency is the rule rather than the exception.

Certain genetic syndromes occur in which the enzyme vitamin D-1-α hydroxylase is mutated (vitamin D–dependent rickets type I) or in which the vitamin D receptor is mutated (vitamin D–dependent rickets type II). Affected individuals have severe hypocalcemia, alopecia, severe rickets and dental abnormalities, and are easy to recognize and confirm if the diagnosis is considered.

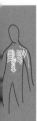

Finally, long-term, high-dose treatment with anticonvulsants such as phenytoin or phenobarbital or their derivatives may lead to hypocalcemia and osteomalacia.

Hypoalbuminemia

Reductions in serum albumin, as occur in burn patients, the nephrotic syndrome, malnutrition, and cirrhosis, lead to reductions in serum total calcium without a reduction in the ionized serum calcium. Of course, these disorders may also be associated with other conditions that lead to bona fide reductions in the ionized serum calcium as well. Several formulas exist for correcting total calcium for albumin, but none is entirely accurate. Therefore measuring ionized calcium directly is important if the authentic ionized serum calcium concentration level is needed.

Sepsis

Gram-positive and gram-negative sepsis have been associated with hypocalcemia that is generally mild. The mechanisms are poorly understood. Hypocalcemia occurring in the setting of sepsis appears to confer a particularly adverse prognosis.

Hypermagnesemia

Magnesium is a divalent cation, as is calcium, and in very high concentrations may therefore mimic the actions of calcium to suppress PTH and, in so doing, lead to a functional type of hypoparathyroidism and hypocalcemia. In practice, this condition is uncommon and is seen typically in patents with severe hypermagnesemia (serum magnesium concentrations in the 10-mg/dL range) caused by renal failure accompanied by magnesium antacid ingestion or following the treatment of eclampsia with large doses of intravenous magnesium.

Hypomagnesemia

Hypomagnesemia is one of the most common causes of hypocalcemia. It is encountered often in patients with alcoholism, malnutrition, cisplatin therapy for cancer, and intestinal malabsorption syndromes. Hypomagnesemia both inhibits PTH secretion (a magnesium adenosine triphosphatase is required for PTH secretion) and prevents the calcemic actions of PTH on the kidney and skeleton. Thus magnesium deficiency causes a functional form of hypoparathyroidism, as well as resistance to PTH. The treatment is straightforward: magnesium replacement (see "Hypomagnesemia"). This treatment corrects the syndrome in minutes to hours. The clinical reality, however, is that this common syndrome is often overlooked and mistreated with intravenous calcium or vitamin D, which are unnecessary and, unless the hypomagnesemia is corrected, ineffective.

Rapid Bone Formation

Increased rates of bone mineralization, out of proportion to the rate of bone resorption, will lead to net calcium entry into the skeleton and, if these rates are large, hypocalcemia. This state occurs in several clinical settings. One condition is the *hungry bones* syndrome that may follow parathyroidectomy. In this syndrome, a patient, usually with severe primary or secondary HPT, undergoes parathyroidectomy. Preoperatively, the rates of bone turnover, both resorption and formation, are very high but are approximately coupled.

Postoperatively, the rate of osteoclastic bone resorption abruptly declines with the decline in PTH, but the rate of bone formation and mineralization remains the same as it was preoperatively for days to a week or more (see Chapter 72 for mechanisms). Because of this acute postoperative imbalance, the skeleton becomes a *sink* for calcium, and hypocalcemia ensues. Another example of this phenomenon may occur in patients with vitamin D deficiency who have severe osteomalacia or rickets and large amounts of unmineralized osteoid. When these patients are treated with vitamin D, rapid mineralization of unmineralized osteoid occurs, and, again, the skeleton becomes a *sink* for calcium, and hypocalcemia ensues. A final example of rapid bone formation leading to hypocalcemia occurs in the setting of extensive osteoblastic bone metastases, as may occur in prostate cancer or breast cancer and occasionally other types of malignancy.

Hyperphosphatemia

Disorders that lead to hyperphosphatemia (see the later section on Hyperphosphatemia) may cause hypocalcemia as a result of exceeding the calcium-phosphate solubility product in serum. Examples of disorders that may cause the kind of severe hyperphosphatemia required include rhabdomyolysis (from crush injuries), renal failure, and the tumor lysis syndrome. Severe hyperphosphatemia may also be seen following the ingestion of large amounts of phosphate-containing purgatives in preparation for colonoscopy, by the inadvertent perforation of the rectum during the administration of phosphate enemas, and with overzealous administration of intravenous phosphate. In all of these examples, the onset of hyperphosphatemia is relatively abrupt, and the hypocalcemia is immediate and severe. Commonly, the first sign of this sequence of events is a seizure. The treatment involves reducing the serum phosphorus by whatever means necessary. Giving intravenous calcium should be avoided because it will simply be precipitated into soft tissues.

Medications

Certain medications may cause hypocalcemia, including those used to treat hypercalcemia, such as mithramycin (plicamycin), the bisphosphonates (e.g., pamidronate, zoledronate), and calcitonin. Hypocalcemia induced by these agents is rare but has been reported. Fluoride intoxication from ingestion of sodium fluoride, inhalation of fluoride-containing anesthetic gases, or drinking of fluoride-contaminated water may cause hypocalcemia. Ethylenediaminetetraacetic acid is a calcium chelator that causes hypocalcemia if infused intravenously. Citrate, as is used in citrated blood for transfusion, is also a calcium chelator and may cause hypocalcemia in the setting of large-volume transfusions. Radiographic intravenous contrast agents may also cause hypocalcemia, as may the antiviral drug foscarnet.

Pancreatitis

Pancreatitis commonly causes hypocalcemia. The classic mechanism is the formation of calcium-free fatty acid soaps, according to the following scenario. Pancreatitis occurs and releases lipase into the retroperitoneum and peritoneum, which leads to the autodigestion of retroperitoneal and omental fat. This action releases free fatty acids such as palmitate, linoleate, and stearate from triglyceride fat stores, and these negatively charged ions tightly bind (chelate) calcium in ECF. This binding leads to the formation of insoluble calcium-free fatty acid salts in the retroperitoneum and rapidly depletes the extracellular calcium, causing hypocalcemia. The hypocalcemia is reversible by calcium infusion and will self-terminate when the pancreatitis improves. Hypocalcemia is a poor prognostic sign among patients with pancreatitis. An important point to remember is that other causes of hypocalcemia occur in patients with pancreatitis, including hypoalbuminemia, hypomagnesemia, and vitamin D deficiency, and these causes should be specifically excluded.

Hyperphosphatemia

SYMPTOMS AND SIGNS

Hyperphosphatemia produces no specific signs per se. It is usually identified incidentally on routine chemical screens or as a result of the induction of hypocalcemia, as described in the preceding section.

PATHOPHYSIOLOGY

Hyperphosphatemia develops as a result of two general mechanisms. One mechanism is a large load of phosphate into the ECF, delivered via the GI tract, via intravenous medications, or via endogenous sources such as muscle or tumor. The second mechanism is the inability to excrete phosphate, as occurs in renal failure (acute or chronic). As noted in Chapter 72, essentially all natural foods contain phosphate, and therefore almost any diet will contain substantial quantities of phosphate. Normally, this phosphate is easily cleared by the healthy kidney, but this ability is lost as the GFR declines below approximately 20 to 30 mg/dL.

DIFFERENTIAL DIAGNOSIS

Differential diagnosis of hyperphosphatemia is listed here and in Table 73–3.

Artifactual

Hyperphosphatemia may occur artifactually as a result of hemolysis in blood collection tubes. Red cells, as with all cells, are rich in phosphate, and, if they are allowed to remain for prolonged periods at room temperature or if blood is obtained too rapidly or through too narrow a needle, they will lyse and release their contents into serum, which will then be reported as being hyperphosphatemic. One clue is that the same phenomenon occurs with potassium. Thus the occurrence of unexplained hyperkalemia and hyperphosphatemia should trigger the collection of a fresh sample and immediate repeat determination of serum phosphate.

Increased Gastrointestinal Intake

Hyperphosphatemia may occur in patients receiving large oral phosphate loads. In a recent literature review, most cases of phosphate-induced hypocalcemia were caused by the administration of phosphate-containing purgatives as

Table 73–3	**Causes of Hyper-phosphatemia**
Artefactual
Hemolysis
Increased Gastrointestinal (GI) Intake
Rectal enemas
Oral Phospho-Soda purgatives
GI bleeding
Intravenous Phosphate Loads
K-Phos
Blood transfusions
Endogenous Phosphate Loads
Tumor lysis syndrome
Rhabdomyolysis (crush injury)
Hemolysis
Reduced Renal Clearance
Chronic or acute renal failure
Hypoparathyroidism
Acromegaly
Tumoral calcinosis

preparation for colonoscopy. Another underappreciated cause of this phenomenon is the inadvertent perforation of the rectum during the administration of a rectal Phospho-Soda enema, with delivery of large amounts of phosphate directly into the peritoneal cavity, from which it is rapidly absorbed. Finally, upper GI tract bleeding from ulcers of gastritis provides a large GI phosphate load and may be associated with hyperphosphatemia.

Intravenous Phosphate Loads

Large amounts of phosphate may be administered as part of a means to replete potassium using potassium phosphate preparations. What appear to be trivial quantities of potassium preparation (e.g., 20 to 40 mEq of K-Phos) actually contain large amounts of phosphate and may lead to severe hyperphosphatemia and hypocalcemia (see Chapter 72). A second vehicle for delivering phosphate intravenously is transfusions of red blood cells, which ultimately hemolyze and release their copious phosphate stores.

Endogenous Phosphate Loads

Hyperphosphatemia may result from the destruction of large amounts of tissue. This destruction is encountered in three situations. Tumor lysis syndrome is one such situation, typified by a large Burkitt's lymphoma responding promptly to chemotherapy with massive cell death. A second phenomenon is acute rhabdomyolysis resulting from a crush injury or drug overdose, which leads to massive release of phosphate from within skeletal muscle cells. A third example is severe hemolysis resulting from autoimmune causes or blood group mismatch. In each of these cases, a large phosphate load is delivered into the ECF, and, in addition, other nephrotoxic molecules such as hemoglobin, myoglobin, and uric acid are released, which reduces the ability of the kidney to clear the large phosphate load. This combination is potentially lethal, resulting in renal failure, severe hypocalcemia, seizures, and sometimes death.

Reduced Renal Clearance

As noted in Chapter 72, renal clearance of phosphate is the main mechanism for maintaining phosphate homeostasis. Thus the fact that disorders of the kidney lead to hyperphosphatemia is not surprising. These disorders include both acute and chronic forms of renal failure. In addition, functional renal abnormalities occur that may lead to hyperphosphatemia. First, because PTH prevents phosphate reabsorption in the proximal nephron, hypoparathyroidism is typically associated with high-normal to frankly elevated serum phosphorus values. Second, acromegaly is associated with hyperphosphatemia. The mechanisms for this association are not well understood, but it appears to be renal in origin. A condition called tumoral calcinosis, in which the ability of the kidney to clear phosphate is specifically defective, leads to chronic hyperphosphatemia and accumulation of calcium-phosphate salts around large joints of the appendicular skeleton. Recently, this syndrome has been shown to be due to inactivating mutations in the *FGF-23* or *GALNT3* genes. Finally, children, particularly adolescents, have higher serum phosphate concentrations than adults.

Hypophosphatemia

SYMPTOMS AND SIGNS

As noted in Chapter 72, phosphate participates in a vast array of key cellular processes, from DNA synthesis and replication, to energy generation and use, to oxygen uptake and delivery by erythrocytes, to maintaining the redox state of every cell in the body. The signs of phosphate depletion are therefore nonspecific, diffuse, and often life threatening. These signs may include respirator dependence, congestive heart failure, coma, hypotension, and generalized weakness and malaise. Because the signs and symptoms are so nonspecific, they are frequently attributed to other causes and are left untreated. They typically occur in intensive care unit (ICU) settings, in which oral nutrition is nonexistent and intravenous phosphate repletion inadequate and in which diuretics and saline infusion accelerate renal phosphate losses. Appropriate therapy can produce startling results, with patients suddenly returning from being moribund to being ambulatory, extubated, and conversant.

Chronic hypophosphatemia leads to defects in skeletal mineralization, a phenomenon called rickets in children or osteomalacia in adults. These syndromes produce weakness, bone pain, bowing of the long bones, and fractures or pseudofractures (see Chapter 74).

DIFFERENTIAL DIAGNOSIS

Disorders can be divided into hypophosphatemia resulting from inadequate intake, from excessive renal losses, from

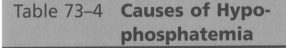

Table 73–4	Causes of Hypophosphatemia

Inadequate PO$_4$ Intake

Starvation
Malabsorption
PO$_4$-binding antacid use
Alcoholism

Renal PO$_4$ Losses

Primary, secondary, or tertiary hyperparathyroidism
Humoral hypercalcemia of malignancy (parathyroid hormone-related protein)
Diuretics, calcitonin
X-linked hypophosphatemic rickets
Autosomal dominant hypophosphatemic rickets
Oncogenic osteomalacia
Fanconi syndrome
Alcoholism

Excessive Skeletal Mineralization

Hungry bone syndrome after parathyroidectomy
Osteoblastic metastases
Healing osteomalacia/rickets

PO$_4$ Shifts into Extracellular Fluid

Recovery from metabolic acidosis
Respiratory alkalosis
Starvation refeeding, intravenous glucose

PO$_4$ = phosphate.

excessive skeletal uptake, or from shifts of phosphate from the ECF into cells (Table 73–4). These abnormalities are discussed individually later. From a diagnostic standpoint, measuring the TmP, as described in Chapter 72, is important because it provides rapid determination of which class of hypophosphatemia the patient is confronting.

Inadequate Phosphate Intake

Disorders that involve inadequate phosphate intake are associated with a high TmP. Because essentially all foods are rich in phosphate, becoming phosphate depleted based on inadequate dietary intake is difficult. However, in settings of severe caloric deprivation, inadequacies can occur. Examples include anorexia nervosa, prisoner-of-war camps, prolonged ICU care, malabsorption syndromes, and chronic alcoholism. In the first three disorders, caloric intake is scant, and therefore little phosphate is consumed. In alcoholism, caloric intake may be high, but alcohol is devoid of phosphate. Finally, the use of phosphate-binding antacids such as aluminum hydroxide gels may lead to severe phosphate deficiency, hypophosphatemia, and osteomalacia.

Excessive Renal Phosphate Losses

Disorders involving excessive losses are associated with a low TmP. PTH is phosphaturic, and therefore all types of HPT are associated with hypophosphatemia, as long as renal function is normal. This state is widely appreciated for primary HPT but is less well appreciated for secondary HPT, particularly occurring in the setting of vitamin D and calcium malabsorption. Indeed, a low serum phosphate may be the first and only noticeable clue to severe vitamin D deficiency. In the author's experience, this fact has led to the diagnosis of celiac sprue in unsuspected cases on many occasions.

PTH-related protein (PTHrP, see earlier section on "Malignancy-Associated Hypercalcemia") is also phosphaturic, as is PTH, and patients with humoral hypercalcemia of malignancy are commonly hypophosphatemic for this reason, as long as their renal function is intact. They frequently become more hypophosphatemic during hospitalization as a result of saline infusion, diuretics, and inadequate oral or intravenous phosphate nutrition.

Medications such as calcitonin, as well as thiazide and loop diuretics, are potent phosphaturic agents, and their use without phosphate replacement therapy will lead to hypophosphatemia. Ethanol is also in this category.

Certain genetic disorders may lead to severe renal phosphate wasting (see Chapter 74). These disorders include X-linked hypophosphatemia (XLH), also referred to as vitamin D–resistant rickets, and autosomal-dominant hypophosphatemic rickets (ADHR). In ADHR, the disorder appears to be due to the overproduction of fibroblast growth factor-23 (FGF-23), the long-sought *phosphatonin* (see Chapter 72), and, in XLH, the cause is an inactivating mutation in the *PHEX* gene, which encodes an extracellular protease. Another renal phosphate–wasting syndrome is oncogenic osteomalacia, also referred to as tumor-induced osteomalacia. Now appreciated is that this disorder, as in ADHR, is due to overproduction of FGF-23, secreted frizzled-related protein 4 (sFRP4), and/or matrix extracellular phosphoglycoprotein (MEPE) (see Chapter 72), by small, often occult, mesenchymal tumors such as hemangiopericytomas.

Acquired or inherited diffuse renal proximal tubular disorders, such as Fanconi's syndrome, may lead to hypophosphatemia as a result of renal phosphate wasting.

Excessive Skeletal Mineralization

In metabolic situations under which the rate of bone formation, or more specifically bone mineralization, is increased with respect to the rate of bone resorption by osteoclasts, large amounts of phosphate may enter the skeleton, leading to hypophosphatemia. One example is the hungry bone syndrome that occurs following parathyroidectomy, as described in the previous section on Hypocalcemia. Other examples are osteoblastic metastases and the treatment of vitamin D–deficient rickets of osteomalacia with vitamin D (see the previous section on Hypocalcemia for additional details). In each of these settings, phosphate enters the mineralizing phase of osteoid as calcium phosphate (hydroxyapatite) and does so at rates such that hypophosphatemia ensues.

Phosphate Shifts into Extracellular Fluid

Phosphate can be shifted from serum into the intracellular compartment by a rise in ECF pH from low to normal or from normal to high. Thus recovery from a metabolic acidosis, such as diabetic ketoacidosis, and the development of a respiratory alkalosis both lead to hypophosphatemia. One of the most stunning examples of this phenomenon is the shift of phosphate into cells following the administration of oral carbohydrate or parenteral glucose to victims of starvation or anorexia nervosa. Insulin increases the rate of glucose uptake into cells and its subsequent phosphorylation to glucose-6-phosphate. A person with no phosphate reserves so treated will abruptly become more severely hypophosphatemic and may die suddenly of respiratory or circulatory failure. Hence refeeding of starvation victims should be accomplished slowly and with attention to phosphate repletion.

TREATMENT

Phosphorus replacement is best accomplished through the oral route and is generally given in divided doses two to four times per day in the range of 2000 to 4000 g/day. Doses above 1000 to 2000 mg/day will often cause diarrhea initially (phosphate is used as a purgative), but, with gradual increments, larger doses may be well tolerated. Intravenous phosphate should only be given with a clear understanding of the quantities involved (see Chapter 72) and in patients in whom oral administration is not an option. Frequent monitoring of serum phosphorus, calcium, and creatinine are required. Doses up to 500 to 800 mg/day intravenously may be required.

Hypermagnesemia

SYMPTOMS AND SIGNS

Clinically significant hypermagnesemia is uncommon. The symptoms are drowsiness, and the signs are hyporeflexia and eventually neuromuscular, respiratory, and cardiovascular collapse. It may also lead to hypocalcemia (see the previous section on Hypocalcemia). Hypermagnesemia is seen in essentially two settings: (1) severe renal failure accompanied by the administration of magnesium-containing antacids and (2) following the intravenous administration of large doses of magnesium sulfate for eclampsia or preeclampsia.

DIFFERENTIAL DIAGNOSIS

The differential diagnosis of hypermagnesemia is brief and is limited to the two disorders noted previously (Table 73–5). Mild hypermagnesemia is common in patients on dialysis, but severe hypermagnesemia is less common in renal failure and occurs in the settings of renal failure accompanied by parenteral or oral magnesium salt administration, such as the use of magnesium-containing antacids or phosphate binders. Hypermagnesemia still occurs commonly, but in a controlled fashion, in the treatment of eclampsia, wherein obstetricians administer large doses of intravenous magnesium sulfate, while observing the blood pressure and reflexes,

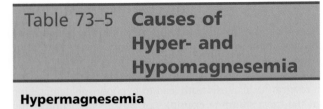

Table 73–5	Causes of Hyper- and Hypomagnesemia

Hypermagnesemia

Renal failure accompanied by magnesium antacid use
Parenteral magnesium sulfate administration for eclampsia

Hypomagnesemia

Inadequate intake
Starvation
Malabsorption
Alcoholism
Vomiting, nasogastric suction
Excessive renal losses
Diuretics
Saline infusion
Secondary aldosteronism
Cirrhosis
Congestive heart failure
Osmotic diuresis, hyperglycemia
Cisplatin, aminoglycoside antibiotics, amphotericin
Hypokalemia
Hypercalcemia, hypercalciuria
Proximal tubular diseases
Genetic defects

to pregnant women with eclampsia. Indeed, a therapeutic end point is when the reflexes diminish or disappear.

Hypomagnesemia

SYMPTOMS AND SIGNS

Hypomagnesemia is common but, as with hypophosphatemia, is often overlooked or ignored. Magnesium is essential for a broad range of biologic processes, and thus hypomagnesemia may cause a broad array of systemic abnormalities (see Chapter 72 for details). Hypomagnesemia may cause hypocalcemia, seizures, and paresthesias independent of hypocalcemia and may cause a broad array of neuromuscular, cardiovascular, or respiratory symptoms. Commonly, hypomagnesemia occurs in an ICU setting in which magnesium administration and diet are inadequate, magnesuric intravenous saline is administered along with diuretics, and serum magnesium is never measured. It responds rapidly and dramatically to parenteral magnesium replacement.

DIFFERENTIAL DIAGNOSIS

Differential diagnoses are listed here and in Table 73–5.

Inadequate Intake

Inadequate intake of magnesium is common among alcoholics and the generally undernourished. It may occur as part of an intestinal malabsorption syndrome and may result from continuous vomiting or nasogastric suctioning. Again, these situations are all common in ICU settings and are often overlooked.

Excessive Renal Losses

Excessive renal losses of magnesium are also common in clinical practice; thiazide and loop diuretics both cause renal magnesium losses, and saline infusion has a similar effect. Magnesium is also lost by the kidney in response to aldosterone in primary hyperaldosteronism but more commonly in the secondary hyperaldosteronism associated with cirrhosis, volume depletion, congestive heart failure, and other common disorders. Osmotic diuresis, as occurs, for example, with poorly controlled diabetes mellitus, causes renal magnesium loss. Certain nephrotoxic drugs such as cisplatin, aminoglycoside antibiotics, and amphotericin induce proximal tubular injury and a severe form of renal magnesium wasting. Hypokalemia may lead to magnesium wasting by the kidney, and the reverse is true as well. Hypercalcemia and hypercalciuria lead to renal magnesium excretion as well, although the cellular basis for this excretion is not fully understood. Genetic or inherited causes of renal magnesium wasting such as mutations in the paracellin-1 gene also occur but are rare. Finally, many diseases that lead to proximal tubular injury, such as Fanconi's syndrome and interstitial nephritis, may lead to magnesium wasting.

TREATMENT

Magnesium can be replaced intramuscularly or intravenously. In general, 24 to 48 mEq/24 hours as magnesium sulfate is provided (see Chapter 72 for unit conversion). Oral magnesium salts such as magnesium oxide are also available, but administering large doses of magnesium orally is difficult because of the cathartic effects of magnesium.

Prospectus for the Future

As is the case with normal mineral and bone physiology, much remains to be learned regarding disorders of serum minerals. What are the genetic defects that underlie the majority of parathyroid adenomas? What additional disease of the calcium-sensing receptor remains to be defined? Will novel calcium receptor agonists and antagonists be useful to better repress or stimulate PTH secretion on primary and secondary hyperparathyroidism and hypoparathyroidism? Can we develop a long-term regimen for treating hypoparathyroidism that does not result in hypercalciuria, kidney stones, nephrocalcinosis, and renal failure over time? What will prove to be the most clinically and cost-effective agents in treating hypercalcemia of malignancy: the current round of intravenous bisphosphonates or monoclonal antibodies being developed against osteoclasts or their developmental pathways? Finally, what is the real *phosphatonin* or *phosphatonins*, how do they work, and how can we best diagnose and treat rickets and osteomalacia resulting from renal phosphorus losses in disorders such as XLH? These questions and many more will occupy researchers in this area for decades to come.

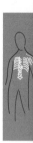

References

DeGroot L, Jameson LJ (eds): Endocrinology, 5th ed. Philadelphia, WB Saunders, 2006.

Favus MF (ed): The American Society for Bone and Mineral Research Primer on Metabolic Bone Diseases and Disorders of Mineral Metabolism, 5th ed. Washington DC, American Society for Bone and Mineral Research, 2004.

Ichikawa S, Lyles KW, Econs MJ: A novel GALNT3 mutation in a pseudoautosomal dominant form of tumoral calcinosis: Evidence that the disorder is autosomal recessive. J Clin Endocrinol Metab 90:2469–2471, 2005.

Konrad M, Schlingmann KP, Gudermann T: Insights into the molecular mechanisms of magnesium homeostasis. Am J Physiol Renal Physiol 286:F599–605, 2004.

Speigel AM: The parathyroid glands, hypercalcemia and hypocalcemia. In Goldman L, Bennett JC: Cecil Textbook of Medicine, 21st ed. Philadelphia, WB Saunders, 2000, pp. 1391–1420.

Stewart AF: Hypercalcemia associated with cancer. N Engl J Med 352:373–279, 2005.

Stewart AF: Translational Implications of the parathyroid calcium receptor. N Engl J. Med 351:324–326, 2004.

Chapter 74

Metabolic Bone Diseases

Andrew F. Stewart

Metabolic bone disease is a term used to describe a host of skeletal diseases (Table 74–1). Most of these disorders are those associated with low bone mass, but some are not. In a sense, the term is misleading because many of these disorders are not *metabolic* at all; rather, they have genetic, viral, or other causes. Still, *metabolic bone disease* is useful as an umbrella term for all diffuse skeletal disorders. The term in its broadest sense includes osteoporosis and Paget's disease of bone, which are discussed in Chapters 75 and 76, respectively. In this chapter, the focus is on the other common members of this family, as listed in Table 74–1. Perhaps the most important message to be gleaned from this chapter, in this era of widespread access to bone density measurements using dual-energy x-ray absorptiometry (DXA), is the concept that low bone mass identified by DXA is not equivalent to a diagnosis of osteoporosis (see Chapter 75). This concept is not broadly appreciated among internists or even among radiologists who may perform DXA measurements. For example, DXA cannot determine whether a patient has low bone mass as a result of osteoporosis, versus osteomalacia or multiple myeloma, yet commonly, DXA reports refer to *osteoporosis*. Every patient assigned a diagnosis of osteoporosis by DXA warrants full consideration for one of the other diagnoses in Table 74–1. Thus the primary physician must determine whether a patient with a low bone mass revealed by DXA actually has *osteoporosis* or whether he or she might actually have a distinct metabolic bone disease.

Differential Diagnosis

HYPERPARATHYROID BONE DISEASE (OSTEITIS FIBROSA CYSTICA)

Hyperparathyroid bone disease, or osteitis fibrosa cystica (OFC), results from chronically elevated parathyroid hormone (PTH) concentrations. Elevated PTH concentrations, in turn, may result from primary hyperparathyroidism that is due, for example, to a parathyroid adenoma, carcinoma, or hyperplasia; to secondary hyperparathyroidism caused by malabsorption, vitamin D deficiency, or chronic renal failure; or to tertiary hyperparathyroidism in the setting of renal failure (see Chapter 73 for details). Patients with primary and tertiary hyperparathyroidism are characterized by hypercalcemia, whereas those with secondary hyperparathyroidism by definition are eucalcemic or hypocalcemic. PTH elevations are commonly severe.

Patients may complain of bone pain or diffuse aches and pains. The skeletal disease is characterized by *high turnover,* meaning coupled increases in both osteoclastic bone resorption and osteoblastic synthesis of osteoid and accelerated rates of bone mineralization (Fig. 74–1). Markers of bone formation, such as alkaline phosphatase and osteocalcin, are increased, as are markers of bone resorption, such as N-telopeptide, hydroxyproline, and deoxypyridinolines. These changes are reflected on undecalcified bone biopsy, which reveals increases in the number and activity of osteoclasts and osteoblasts, increased quantities of unmineralized osteoid, accelerated rates of osteoid mineralization (determined using tetracycline labeling), microcysts in cortex and trabeculae (the *cystica* of OFC), and increased numbers of fibroblasts and marrow stroma (the *fibrosa* of OFC).

Bone density may be normal, as assessed using DXA, or it may be low. The pathognomonic radiologic signs of severe hyperparathyroid bone disease are a *salt-and-pepper* appearance of the calvarium, resorption of the tufts of the terminal phalanges and distal clavicles, subperiosteal resorption of the radial aspect of the cortex of the second phalanges, and *Brown's tumors* (actually collections of osteoclasts that produce gross lytic lesions) of the pelvis and long bones (Fig. 74–2). All of these radiologic signs disappear with parathyroidectomy, and bone mass, assessed by DXA, typically increases rapidly and markedly following parathyroidectomy.

Table 74–1 Metabolic Bone Disease

Osteoporosis (Chapter 75)
Paget's disease of bone (Chapter 76)
Hyperparathyroid bone disease (osteitis fibrosa cystica)
Osteomalacia and rickets
  Hypophosphatemic syndromes
  Vitamin D syndromes
  Anticonvulsants
  Aluminum
  Metabolic acidosis
Renal osteodystrophy
Genetic diseases
  Osteogenesis imperfecta
  Hypophosphatasia
  Osteoporosis-pseudoglioma syndrome
  Miscellaneous
Infiltrative diseases
  Multiple myeloma
  Lymphoma/leukemia
  Sarcoid
  Malignant histiocytosis
  Mastocytosis
  Gaucher's disease
  Hemolytic diseases (thalassemia, sickle cell)
Transplant osteodystrophy

The treatment of hyperparathyroid bone disease involves remediation of the chronically elevated PTH concentrations, either through parathyroidectomy in primary or tertiary hyperparathyroidism or through correction of the underlying cause of secondary hyperparathyroidism. More recently, suppression of PTH using the parathyroid calcium–receptor mimetic drug cinacalcet has been added to this armamentarium. If mild and if bone mass is normal, then no treatment may be required.

Moderate-to-severe hypocalcemia may postoperatively accompany parathyroidectomy. This condition is referred to as the *hungry bones* syndrome and results from the sudden removal of the drive to osteoclastic activity by removing excess PTH in the setting of increased osteoblastic activity with unmineralized, but continuously mineralizing, osteoid. The syndrome abates when the osteoid mineralizes. Of course, postoperative hypocalcemia may also be due to intentional or inadvertent surgical hypoparathyroidism.

Finally, hyperparathyroid bone disease may be *pure*, as in a patient with severe primary hyperparathyroidism caused by a parathyroid adenoma, or it may be mixed, occurring as a component of the bone disease in vitamin D–deficient osteomalacia, in glucocorticoid-induced osteoporosis, in immunosuppressant-induced transplant bone disease, or in renal osteodystrophy (see later discussion).

OSTEOMALACIA AND RICKETS

Osteomalacia and rickets are common both in the United States and in the rest of the world and are commonly over-looked. Two definitions are important. First, osteomalacia and rickets are essentially the same disorders, with the difference being semantic; by definition, rickets occurs in children with open growth plates (epiphyses), whereas osteomalacia occurs in adults with closed epiphyses. Second, the fundamental abnormality in these disorders is an inability to mineralize (i.e., form hydroxylapatite crystals within) *osteoid seams* (see Chapter 72); these patients have osteoblasts and can synthesize osteoid, but they mineralize it inefficiently or not at all. This fundamental inability to mineralize osteoid results in the accumulation of the characteristic thick osteoid seams seen on bone biopsy (Fig. 74–3) and a reduction in the mineral component of bone so that it is deficient mechanically, which leads to bone pain, pseudofractures, fractures, bowing of the long bones, and other skeletal deformities (Fig. 74–4). In children (i.e., in rickets), the inability to mineralize the growth plate leads, in addition, to bulbous knobby deformities of the knees, ankles, and costochondral junctions (the *rachitic rosary*) and dental abnormalities. The characteristic radiologic signs of osteomalacia are Looser's zones or Milkman's pseudofractures. Rickets also shows gross defects in epiphyseal mineralization and compensatory increases in size of the joints and periarticular bone.

Understanding that the disorder is caused by a failure of mineralization, the underlying pathophysiologic mechanism can clearly be understood. These disorders result from an inability to form hydroxyapatite (calcium phosphate) crystals in osteoid, the nonmineralized phase of bone (see Chapter 72). This inability may result from hypophosphatemia (a common cause), a deficiency of calcium (an extremely rare cause), a deficiency of vitamin D (a common cause), or the presence of toxins that interfere with mineralization, such as aluminum, incompletely defined inhibitors of mineralization in uremic plasma, and long-term high-dose anticonvulsant use. Finally, because calcium salts are acid soluble, chronic metabolic acidoses (e.g., as occurs with the chronic bicarbonate wasting seen in patients with ureteral implants into ileal conduits) can result in osteomalacia or rickets. Thus the causes of these mineralization disorders are, in essence, vitamin D disorders (malabsorption, liver disease, genetic disorders; see Chapter 73), hypophosphatemic disorders (X-linked hypophosphatemic rickets, autosomal-dominant hypophosphatemia, and oncogenic osteomalacia; see Chapter 73), metabolic acidoses, and drug-related and genetic (vitamin D–dependent rickets types I and II, and hypophosphatasia; see Chapter 73) conditions.

The diagnosis is suggested in the setting of low bone mass, the characteristic radiologic signs noted previously, and/or unexplained bone pain or weakness. Of course, all of these signs are late signs, and the disorder is optimally considered early in the course of the diseases described previously. The diagnosis is supported by demonstrating reductions of plasma 25-hydroxyvitamin D or its active form, 1,25-dihydroxyvitamin D ($1,25(OH)_2D$), hypophosphatemia, and/or increases in alkaline phosphatase, occurring in an appropriate clinical setting. The diagnosis can often be made clinically but can also be confirmed using undecalcified bone biopsy following oral double tetracycline labeling techniques, which are used to quantitate the degree of failure of mineralization.

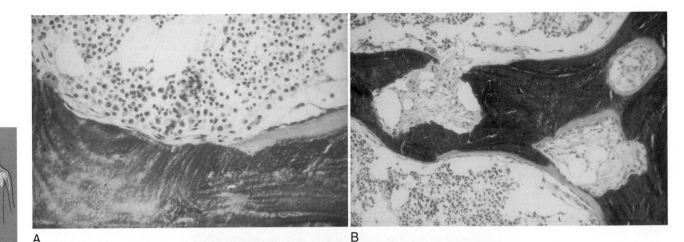

Figure 74–1 *A,* A normal bone-remodeling unit (see Chapter 72) provides an example of normal bone histologic mechanisms. At the bottom half of the figure is a normal mineralized trabecular bone surface *(dark blue).* The top half of the slide shows normal bone marrow. In between is the trabecular bone surface. On the bone surface on the extreme left is a binucleated osteoclast that has moved across the bone surface over the previous week or two, resorbing (removing) old bone. On the extreme right surface, the bone surface is covered by osteoid *(light blue)* secreted by the overlying osteoblasts. In between the osteoclast- and osteoblast-covered surfaces of the trabecular bone are a large number of flat, fibroblastoid cells referred to as *lining cells* or *marrow stromal cells.* These cells are inactive precursors of osteoblasts. *B,* Bone histologic display in a patient with primary hyperparathyroidism showing the classic features of *osteitis fibrosa cystica.* Note that far more osteoid and far more osteoblasts and osteoclasts exist than in the normal example *(A).* Note also that three large microcysts are present that have been created by aggressive osteoclastic bone resorption. These microcysts account for the *cystica* component of osteitis fibrosa cystica. Finally, note that the marrow space, particularly within the microcysts, is filled with fibroblasts. These fibroblasts comprise the *fibrosa* component of osteitis fibrosa cystica. *C,* Tetracycline labeling of a bone biopsy from a patient with hyperparathyroid bone disease. Note the bright yellow parallel lines on the trabecular bone surface. These lines represent the two sets of tetracycline labeling, which occurred 14 days apart. From these sets, the mineralization rate can actually be described in microns per day, the so-called *mineral apposition rate,* and is increased dramatically in this example, as is typical of hyperparathyroid bone disease. Contrast with Figure 74–3B, in which no tetracycline labeling is present.

Treatment depends on the underlying cause and includes an appropriate vitamin D compound, calcium, and/or phosphate, as appropriate, and removal of the inhibitor of mineralization, when appropriate and possible. These diseases are gratifying to treat because the responses are often dramatic, and patients change rapidly from being chronically ill to feeling robust and healthy.

RENAL OSTEODYSTROPHY

Renal osteodystrophy is actually a collection of disorders that in moderate to severe forms lead to bone pain, pathologic fractures, and demineralization, all occurring in the setting of end-stage renal disease or dialysis. Subclinical renal osteodystrophy is common. The syndrome includes pure secondary hyperparathyroidism (see Fig. 74–1B), occurring as a result of defective renal production of $1,25(OH)_2D$ combined with an increase in serum phosphate, which lead to hypocalcemia as a result of reduced intestinal calcium absorption and calcium phosphate precipitation into soft tissues, respectively (see Chapter 72). This circumstance, in turn, evokes a severe increase in PTH secretion that then causes dramatic increases in bone turnover, demineralization, and fracture. These patients may respond dramatically

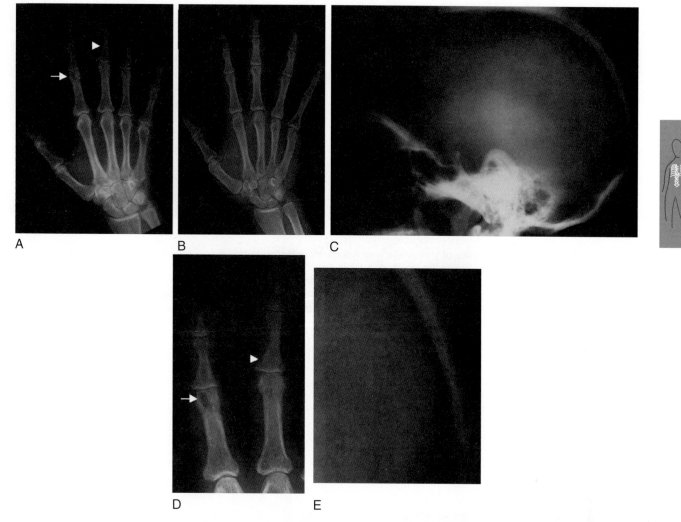

Figure 74–2 Skeletal radiographic changes of hyperparathyroidism. *A,* A hand film from a patient with primary hyperparathyroidism. The arrow indicates a typical Brown's tumor, or giant cell tumor, which is a collection of osteoclasts that lead to macrocystic changes in bone. The arrowhead indicates the irregular radial surface of a phalanx resulting from subperiosteal bone resorption, also typical of hyperparathyroidism. Both the Brown's tumor and the subperiosteal resorption refill and disappear when the offending parathyroid tumor or hyperplasia is resected. *B,* A normal hand film for comparison. No Brown's tumors are present, and the phalangeal periosteal surfaces are smooth. *C,* The classic *salt-and-pepper* appearance of the skull observed in hyperparathyroidism. The periosteal surfaces of the inner and outer cortices or tables of the calvarium are indistinct as a result of subperiosteal bone resorption. In addition, the lateral view of the calvarium is hazy and indistinct, with micropunctations. *D* and *E,* Expanded views of *A* and *C* for greater detail. (Courtesy of Drs. J. Towers and D. Armfield, University of Pittsburgh.)

to oral or parenteral replacement of $1,25(OH)_2D$ and the calcium receptor agonist cinacalcet. Other patients with *renal osteodystrophy* have adequately controlled serum calcium and phosphate, and therefore PTH, as a result of adequate oral calcium supplementation and phosphate binders, but they display severe osteomalacia (bone pain, reduced bone mineral density by DXA and/or bone biopsy, and thickened osteoid seams on bone biopsy with a mineralization defect apparent from tetracycline labeling [see Fig. 74–3]). The precise cause of the mineralization defect is uncertain. These patients, too, may respond dramatically to vitamin D replacement. Still other patients with *renal osteodystrophy* have combinations of secondary hyperparathyroidism and osteomalacia (Fig. 74–5); still others have *low turnover* or *aplastic bone disease.* These terms are intended to describe patients on dialysis who have the oppo-

site of secondary hyperparathyroidism and osteomalacia: little or no osteoblastic activity, osteoid, or osteoclastic activity. The condition may result from inhibitors of bone turnover, such as aluminum intoxication in the past, or from excessive treatment with $1,25(OH)_2D$, with suppression of PTH, causing low bone turnover, or from as yet unidentified causes. As with other bone diseases, understanding the cause is critical for effective treatment. Being aware of the syndrome so that it is recognized early and treated before bone pain and fractures occur is optimal.

GENETIC DISEASES

Genetic diseases that lead to reductions in bone mass are not common but are seen with some frequency in practices devoted to skeletal disease. Perhaps the most common

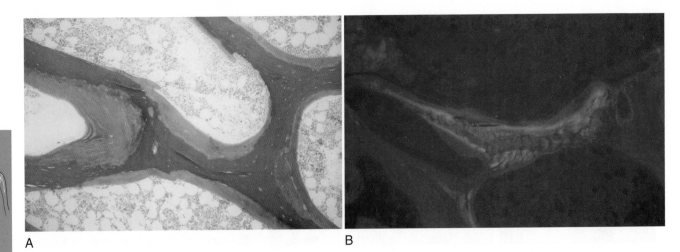

Figure 74–3 *A,* Bone histologic display of osteomalacia or rickets. Note the abundant quantities of partially and chaotically mineralized osteoid *(orange)*. These seams are the thick *osteoid seams* and represent osteoid that has been produced by osteoblasts but that cannot mineralize—the signature defect in osteomalacia and rickets. *B,* To confirm that the increase in osteoid seen in *A* is due to a defect in mineralization, tetracycline labeling can be performed. In this example, no tetracycline labeling exists whatsoever. This example unequivocally confirms the presence of a mineralization defect. Compare with the rapid and aggressive mineralization observed in Figure 74–1C.

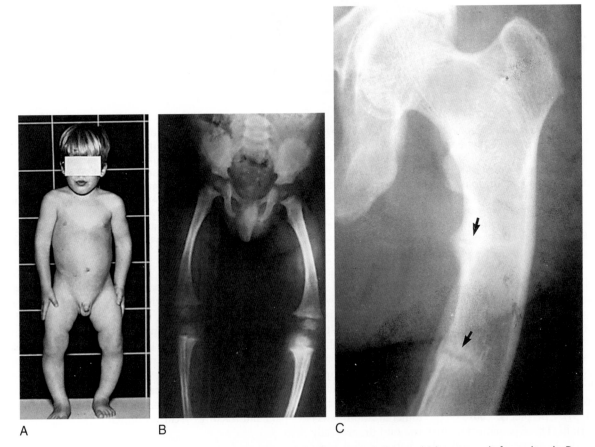

Figure 74–4 *A,* A typical example of rickets. Note the bowing of the femurs and tibiae, which may result from vitamin D deficiency, phosphate deficiency, or other causes. *B,* A skeletal radiograph of a child with rickets. Note that the weight-bearing bones of the lower extremities are bowed and that the epiphyses are open, mottled, and overgrown. *C,* Looser's zones or pseudofractures characteristic of osteomalacia or rickets. Because the epiphyses are closed, the patient is an adult. This radiograph is diagnostic of osteomalacia.

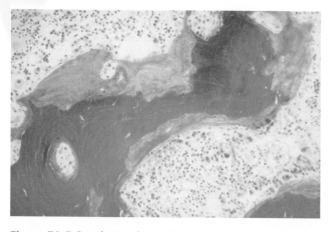

Figure 74–5 Renal osteodystrophy. This photomicrograph of a biopsy from a patient on dialysis demonstrates many of the classic features of renal osteodystrophy. These features include evidence of aggressive osteoclastic bone resorption (see numerous osteoclastic lacunae on the bone surface, as compared with the smooth surfaces in Figure 74–1A) and abundant partially and chaotically mineralized areas of osteoid (orange).

among these uncommon disorders is osteogenesis imperfecta, which may be mild or severe and may be present in neonates or older people, depending on the severity and the mutation involved. Mutations in the collagen I gene most often cause these disorders. Hypophosphatasia is due to a mutation in the tissue-nonspecific alkaline phosphatase gene. These patients also display demineralization, fracture, and bone pain and have little or no measurable alkaline phosphatase. In the last several years, a new genetic disorder has been defined, called the *osteoporosis-pseudoglioma syndrome* (severe autosomal-dominant osteoporosis with blindness). This disorder is due to inactivating mutations in the low-density lipoprotein-related protein-5 *(LRP5)* gene and, although very rare, is particularly interesting because activating mutations in the same gene have been shown in the last year to lead to an autosomal-dominant form of very high bone mass. A myriad of other genetic disorders exists that lead to low bone mass; some are treatable, others less so.

INFILTRATIVE DISEASES

Patients with multiple myeloma or Waldenström's macroglobulinemia classically develop skeletal demineralization, and this is true as well for some patients with leukemia and marrow lymphomas. Other disorders associated with diffuse marrow infiltration by benign, or at least less malignant, processes can also lead to diffuse osteopenia, bone pain, and fracture, and all of these disorders should be considered in the setting of unexplained *osteoporosis*. Examples include

hemolytic anemias such as thalassemia or sickle cell disease, sarcoidosis with diffuse marrow involvement, Gaucher's disease with lipid-laden marrow giant cells, malignant mastocytosis, and diffuse histiocytosis.

TRANSPLANT OSTEODYSTROPHY

Patients who have undergone or are undergoing organ transplantation commonly have severe *osteoporosis*. In some patients, this condition is due to treatment with immunosuppressive drugs such as glucocorticoids, tacrolimus, or cyclosporine, all of which are potent inhibitors of bone formation and regularly lead to reductions in bone mass. In other patients—for example, those with primary biliary cirrhosis—a component of calcium or vitamin D deficiency may exist as well. In patients, such as those with end-stage lung or cardiac disease, contributing components of physical inactivity and generalized malnutrition may be present as well. In yet other patients with end-stage renal disease, all of the components of renal osteodystrophy, as discussed previously, may be operative. This group of patients is particularly vexing because they often have severe, but retrospectively preventable, disease by the time they see an expert in metabolic bone disease, and therapy in late stages is incompletely effective. In addition, these patients may be in the catch-22 situation of being denied organ transplantation because of *severe osteoporosis* that, in retrospect, was preventable. This disorder can be expected to become increasingly common as organ transplantation becomes more common.

Treatment

Treatment of all of these conditions depends on the underlying disorder. Vitamin D deficiency can be treated with the active form of vitamin D, $1,25(OH)_2D$ (calcitriol), or by oral or intramuscular injections of the much less expensive parent compound, vitamin D. Secondary hyperparathyroidism in patients on dialysis can be treated with cinacalcet. Phosphate is best replaced using oral phosphate salts such as Neutra-Phos (see Chapter 72). Other items in Table 74–1 require attention to the underlying disorder.

The most important therapeutic point is that these disorders are commonly amenable to treatment and can have dramatic and satisfying responses to therapy, both for the physician and for the patient. The main stumbling block is that these diagnoses are commonly never considered, and the DXA report of *osteoporosis* is passively accepted and never investigated. The key clinical message, then, is that, whenever a patient is designated as having *osteoporosis*, the physician should mentally run through the checklist in Table 74–1 and eliminate, or investigate, these disorders as appropriate.

Prospectus for the Future

Better understanding of metabolic bone diseases, including but not limited to, osteoporosis, represents one of the largest challenges facing researchers as the population ages. We know so little about how bone is made (we do not even know how it mineralizes) or why some people develop osteoporosis while others with identical risk factors do not. We recognize that postmenopausal women with osteoporotic fracture have bone densities some 50% of normal, yet the current generation of osteoporosis drugs increases bone density by only 2% to 9%. Clearly, we have a long way to go in this arena. Moreover, what is the cause of *low turnover renal osteodystrophy* or *adynamic bone disease* in patients on dialysis? Why do some of these patients get this disorder while others do not, and what are the additional cytokines that cause bone resorption in breast cancer and myeloma, and what drugs can be developed to block these events? Why is rickets still so prevalent in the third world and in U.S. cities as well, and what can we do at a public health level to prevent this unnecessary disease? How can we teach physicians that, just because low bone density found in a bone density study is interpreted to mean *osteoporosis,* that it might equally well represent multiple myeloma, osteitis fibrosa cystica, or osteomalacia? Thus basic, clinical, and public health issues abound in this area, and the coming decade will see answers to at least some of these questions.

References

DeGroot L, Jameson LJ (eds): Endocrinology, 5th ed. Philadelphia, WB Saunders, 2006.

Favus MF (ed): The American Society for Bone and Mineral Research Primer on Metabolic Bone Diseases and Disorders of Mineral Metabolism, 5th ed. Washington DC, American Society for Bone and Mineral Research, 2004.

Goldman L, Bennett JC: Cecil Textbook of Medicine, 21st ed. Philadelphia, WB Saunders, 2000, pp. 1391–1420.

Maalouf NM, Shane E: Osteoporosis after solid organ transplantation. J Clin Endocrinol Metab 90:2456–2465, 2005.

Stewart AF: Translational Implications of the parathyroid calcium receptor. N Engl J. Med 351:324–326, 2004.

Osteoporosis

Susan L. Greenspan

Osteoporosis, the most common disorder of bone and mineral metabolism, affects approximately 40% of women over the age of 50 years. The National Institutes of Health Consensus Development Panel on Osteoporosis Prevention defines osteoporosis as a skeletal disorder characterized by compromised bone strength, predisposing a person to an increased risk of fracture. Bone strength reflects primarily the integration of two main features: (1) bone density and (2) bone quality. Bone density reflects the peak adult bone mass and the amount of bone lost in adulthood. Bone quality is determined by bone architecture, bone geometry, bone turnover, mineralization, and damage accumulation (i.e., microfractures) (Fig. 75–1).

Epidemiologic Factors

In the United States, 1.5 million osteoporotic fractures occur each year, comprising 700,000 vertebral fractures, 250,000 radial fractures, 250,000 hip fractures, and 300,000 other fractures. Hip fractures have the most serious consequences by far, with a mortality rate of more than 20% within the first year. Over 50% of patients with hip fracture will be unable to return to their previous ambulatory state, and approximately 10% of them will be placed in long-term care facilities. Three quarters of all hip fractures occur in women. After the age of 50 years, the lifetime risk of hip fracture is 17% for white women versus 6% for white men. When defined by bone mineral densitometry, 13 to 17 million women have *low bone mass* at the hip, and 4 to 6 million postmenopausal white women have osteoporosis. Although morbidity is decreased with vertebral fractures, mortality is increased as a result of the risk of cardiovascular and pulmonary disease that is associated with an escalating number of vertebral fractures. Only one third of radiologically diagnosed vertebral fractures receive medical attention.

Risk Factors

The major risk factors for osteoporosis have been previously outlined by the National Osteoporosis Foundation (NOF) and include personal history of fracture in adulthood, fracture history in a first-degree relative, low body weight (<127 lb), current smoking, and use of oral corticosteroid therapy for longer than 3 months. Additional risk factors include impaired vision, early estrogen deficiency (younger than 45 years of age), dementia, poor health and/or frailty, recent falls, low calcium intake (lifelong), low physical activity, and alcohol consumption (>2 drinks per day). Risk factors specific to hip fracture were identified by the Study of Osteoporotic Fractures, an epidemiologic trial that prospectively monitored 9704 postmenopausal women over the age of 65. Risk factors for hip fracture included age, history of maternal hip fracture, weight, height, poor health, previous hyperthyroidism, current use of long-acting benzodiazepines, poor depth perception, tachycardia, previous fracture, and low bone mineral density. Investigators found that the more risk factors a woman had, the greater was her risk of fracture.

Peak Bone Mass and Bone Loss

Peak bone mass is determined primarily by genetic factors. Men have a higher bone mass than women, and African Americans and Hispanics have a higher bone mass than whites (Fig. 75–2). Multiple genes, including vitamin D–receptor alleles, estrogen receptor genes, and the *high bone mass* gene, are thought to be associated with bone mass, but studies are ongoing. Other factors that contribute to the development of peak bone mass are the use of gonadal steroids, timing of puberty, calcium intake, exercise, and growth hormone.

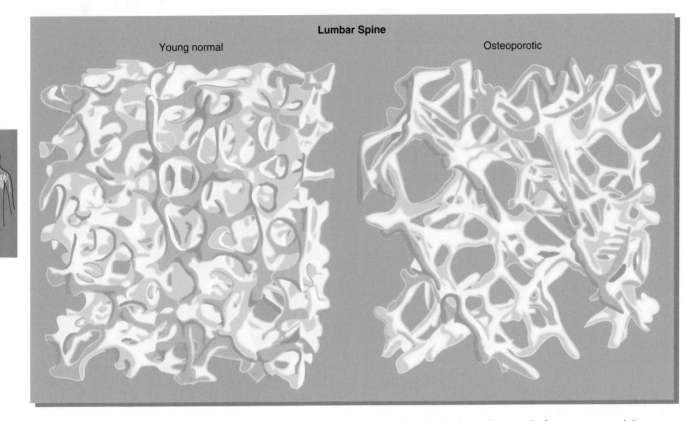

Figure 75–1 Three-dimensional reconstruction by microcomputed tomography of a lumbar spine sample from a young adult normal woman and from a woman with postmenopausal osteoporosis. In the osteoporotic woman, not only is bone mass reduced, but also microarchitectural deterioration of bone structure occurs. Whereas the rodlike structure in the normal case is very isotropic, the structure in the osteoporotic case shows preferential loss of horizontal struts and a concomitant loss of trabecular connectivity. These changes lead to a reduction in bone strength that is more than would be predicted by the decrease in bone mineral density. (From Riggs BL, Khosla S, Melton LJ 3rd: Sex steroids and the construction and conservation of the adult skeleton. Endocr Rev 23:279–302, 2002. Images courtesy of Ralph Mueller, PhD, Swiss Federal Institute of Technology [ETH] and University of Zurich, Zurich, Switzerland.)

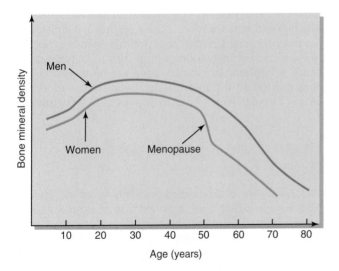

Figure 75–2 Cortical bone mineral density versus age in men and women. Women have lower peak cortical bone density than men and experience a period of rapid bone loss during menopause.

The causes of bone loss in adults are multifactorial. Estrogen deficiency during menopause contributes significantly to bone loss in women because they may lose 1% to 5% of bone mass per year in the first few years after menopause. Women continue to lose bone mass throughout the remainder of their lives, with another acceleration of bone loss occurring after age 75 years. The mechanism of this accelerated loss in old age is not clear. Estrogen deficiency influences a host of local cytokines, which affect osteoblastic and osteoclastic activity, as well as bone turnover. In an adult, skeletal integrity is further influenced by calcium intake, vitamin D, physical activity, and body weight. Finally, multiple causes of secondary bone loss have been found. Medications that commonly cause bone loss include excess thyroid hormone, glucocorticoids, anticonvulsants, heparin, and gonadotropin-releasing hormone agonists. Endocrine diseases resulting in female or male hypogonadism also lead to bone loss. Hyperparathyroidism, hyperthyroidism, and hypercortisolism also commonly cause bone loss, as well as vitamin D deficiency. Gastrointestinal problems can contribute to decreased absorption of calcium and vitamin D (Table 75–1).

Table 75–1	**Secondary Causes of Low Bone Mass**

Endocrine Diseases

Female hypogonadism
Hyperprolacinemia
Hypothalamic amenorrhea
Anorexia nervosa
Premature and primary ovarian failure
Female athlete triad
Male hypogonadism
Primary gonadal failure (e.g., Klinefelter's syndrome)
Secondary gonadal failure (e.g., idiopathic
　hypogonadotropic hypogonadism, androgen deprivation
　therapy for prostate cancer)
Hyperthyroidism
Hyperparathyroidism
Hypercortisolism
Vitamin D insufficiency or deficiency

Gastrointestinal Diseases

Subtotal gastrectomy
Gastric bypass surgery
Malabsorption syndromes
Chronic obstructive jaundice
Primary biliary cirrhosis and other cirrhoses

Bone Marrow Disorders

Multiple myeloma
Monoclonal gammopathy of unknown significance (MGUS)
Lymphoma
Leukemia
Hemolytic anemias
Systemic mastocytosis
Disseminated carcinoma

Connective Tissue Diseases

Osteogenesis imperfecta
Ehlers-Danlos syndrome
Marfan syndrome
Homocystinuria

Drugs

Alcohol
Heparin
Glucocorticoids
Excess thyroid hormone
Anticonvulsants
Gonadotropin-releasing hormone agonists
Cyclosporine
Chemotherapy

Miscellaneous Causes

Immobilization
Rheumatoid arthritis
Chronic obstructive pulmonary disease
Weight loss

Clinical Manifestation

Unlike many other chronic diseases with multiple signs and symptoms, osteoporosis is considered a *silent* disease until fractures occur. Whereas 90% of hip fractures occur following a fall, two thirds of vertebral fractures are silent and occur with minimal stress such as lifting, sneezing, and bending. An acute vertebral fracture may result in significant back pain, which decreases gradually over several weeks with analgesics and physical therapy. Patients with significant vertebral osteoporosis may have height loss, kyphosis, and severe cervical lordosis (known as a dowager's hump).

Diagnosis

The diagnosis of osteoporosis is made following an acute clinical fracture or with bone mineral densitometry assessment. Radiographs can reveal a vertebral compression fracture (Fig 75–3), however, radiologic evidence of low bone mass may not be present until 30% of bone mass has been lost. In addition, when assessing bone mass, radiographs are often read inappropriately as a result of over- or underpenetration of the film. Therefore radiographs are a poor indicator of osteoporosis, and the diagnosis is often made based on bone mineral densitometry.

Bone Mineral Density

Bone mineral density can be assessed through a variety of techniques. In 1994 the World Health Organization developed a classification system for osteoporosis and osteopenia (low bone mass) based on data from white postmenopausal

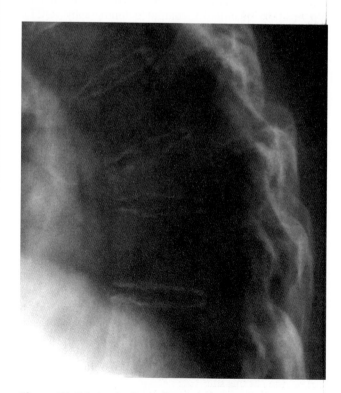

Figure 75–3 Lateral spine radiograph demonstrating a thoracic anterior wedge compression fracture.

Table 75–2	World Health Organization Classifications for Osteoporosis
Classification	**Criteria for Bone Mineral Density**
Normal	Above –1.0 SD of young adult peak mean value
Osteopenia (low bone mass)	Between –1.0 and –2.5 SD of young adult peak mean value
Osteoporosis	Below –2.5 SD of young adult peak mean value

SD = standard deviation.

women (Table 75–2). Osteoporosis was defined as a bone mineral density less than or equal to 2.5 standard deviations below young adult peak bone mass. Osteopenia is defined as a bone mass measurement between 1.0 and 2.5 standard deviations below adult peak bone mass. Normal bone mineral density is defined as assessments above 1.0 standard deviation below adult peak bone mass. The *gold standard* for assessing bone mineral density is dual-energy x-ray absorptiometry (DXA), which has excellent precision and accuracy. Measurements are made of the hip and spine, and approximately 30% of the time, discordance is found between these measurements (Fig. 75–4). Therefore classification is based on the lowest value (total spine, total hip, femoral neck, or trochanter). Bone mineral density can also be measured by hip or spine quantitative computed tomography (QCT). However, few normative data have been found for hip QCT, vertebral precision is inferior to that of DXA, and radiation doses are significantly higher than those of DXA. Finally, single-photon absorptiometry of the forearm and peripheral measures, such as finger DXA and heel ultrasound, have also been used to assess bone mass (Table 75–3).

Classification can vary significantly by the skeletal site and the device used for assessment. For example, the average woman would be diagnosed with osteoporosis at age 60 years when assessing the lateral spine but not until she is over 100 years of age if heel ultrasound is used. Although all of these measurements have an accuracy of 1% to 3%, precision is best with forearm or spine DXA (approximately 1%).

Experts recommend that bone mineral density be monitored approximately every 2 years, depending on the site to be assessed and the type of therapy prescribed. For example, trabecular bone, which is more metabolically active than cortical bone, is more likely to show improvements with stronger-acting antiresorptive agents. Changes in bone mass with potent antiresorptive therapy are more prominent in the spine compared with other areas. Seeing no changes in forearm bone mineral density over time is common, despite good precision. Although the heel has a high percentage of trabecular bone, precision is poor, and monitoring should not be done at this site.

The NOF recommends obtaining a bone mineral density assessment in all women over 65 years of age, postmenopausal women younger than age 65 years with one risk factor, and women who have had a fracture (Table 75–4). The United States Preventive Services Task Force recommends bone density tests in all women over age 65 and women between 60 and 64 years of age with a risk factor. Recommendations for bone mass measurements in men are currently unavailable, but ongoing studies examining risk factors should assist with future recommendations. Currently, databases are available for white, African-American, and Hispanic men and women. Similar T-score assessments for osteopenia and osteoporosis are used for men and women of other races. However, data are lacking to support T-score cut-offs that are similar to those of white postmenopausal women.

In general, bone mass measurements by DXA examine the spine and hip. However, in patients with hyperparathyroidism, in which cortical bone loss is often seen, forearm DXA should also be assessed. Older patients with osteoporosis often to have falsely elevated bone mineral density measurements at the spine as a result of atypical calcifications from degenerative joint disease, sclerosis, or aortic calcifications. Although lateral bone mineral density measurements eliminate these artifacts, they are often difficult to perform because of overlap of the ribs on L2 and overlap of the pelvic brim on L4. Classification should only be made if two or more vertebrae are available for analysis because of the high error rate when only one vertebra is assessed. QCT is recommended less often than DXA because of the former's high radiation exposure and cost.

Treatment is recommended for all patients with a bone mineral density T-score at least 2.5 standard deviations below peak bone mass. Only preventive measures are recommended for patients with T-scores at –1.5 or above. For patients with T-scores between –1.5 and –2.5, treatment depends on the number and severity of risk factors.

Prevention

General preventive measures for all patients include calcium and vitamin D supplementation, exercise, and fall prevention techniques. The recommended daily allowance of calcium was recently reviewed by the National Academy of Science and increased to 1200 mg daily for postmenopausal women. Calcium increases can be accomplished by dietary intake or supplementation. The supplements should generally be pure calcium carbonate or pure calcium citrate, taken in divided doses of approximately 500 to 600 mg twice daily. Calcium carbonate must be taken with meals for best absorption, whereas calcium citrate may be taken with or without food. Calcium supplements are currently available as tablets and in chewable and liquid forms. Many foods, such as orange juice and some cereals, are now calcium fortified.

Vitamin D is important for calcium absorption and bone mineralization. Vitamin D comes from two sources: diet and photosynthesis. Because dietary sources of vitamin D are limited (e.g., fortified milk) and patients are often advised to avoid sun exposure for prevention of skin cancer and wrinkles, many studies have now documented vitamin D deficiency and insufficiency in older adults. In addition, older patients have reduced ability to synthesize vitamin D in the skin. Low vitamin D levels can lead to secondary hyperparathyroidism.

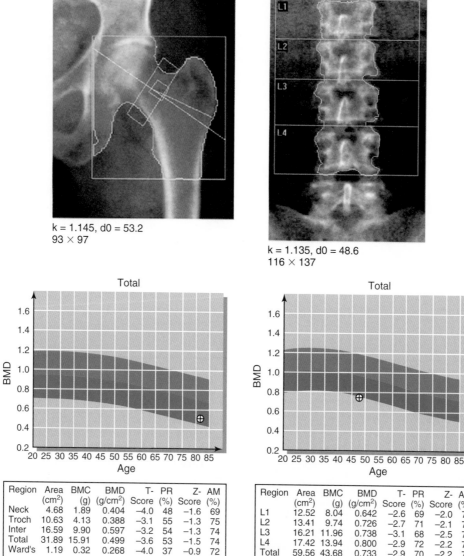

k = 1.145, d0 = 53.2
93 × 97

k = 1.135, d0 = 48.6
116 × 137

Region	Area (cm²)	BMC (g)	BMD (g/cm²)	T-Score	PR (%)	Z-Score	AM (%)
Neck	4.68	1.89	0.404	−4.0	48	−1.6	69
Troch	10.63	4.13	0.388	−3.1	55	−1.3	75
Inter	16.59	9.90	0.597	−3.2	54	−1.3	74
Total	31.89	15.91	0.499	−3.6	53	−1.5	74
Ward's	1.19	0.32	0.268	−4.0	37	−0.9	72

Total BMD CV 1.0%, ACF = 1.028, BCF = 1.006, TH = 5.163
WHO Classification: Osteoporosis
Fracture Risk: High

Region	Area (cm²)	BMC (g)	BMD (g/cm²)	T-Score	PR (%)	Z-Score	AM (%)
L1	12.52	8.04	0.642	−2.6	69	−2.0	74
L2	13.41	9.74	0.726	−2.7	71	−2.1	76
L3	16.21	11.96	0.738	−3.1	68	−2.5	73
L4	17.42	13.94	0.800	−2.9	72	−2.2	77
Total	59.56	43.68	0.733	−2.9	70	−2.2	75

Total BMD CV 1.0%, ACF = 1.028, BCF = 1.006, TH = 5.848
WHO Classification: Osteoporosis
Fracture Risk: High

Figure 75–4 *Right,* This patient has a lumbar spine (L1 through L4) bone mineral density (BMD) of 0.733 g/cm² *(white circle with cross)* as measured by DXA and a T-score of −2.9. The reference database graph displays age- and sex-matched mean BMD levels ±2 standard deviations (SDs) *(shaded areas)* derived from a normative database from the manufacturer (Hologic, Inc., Bedford, Mass). The T-score indicates the difference in SD between the patient's BMD and the predicted sex-matched mean peak young adult BMD; z-value, the difference in SD between the patient's BMD and the sex- and age-matched mean BMD; and percentage of mean, the patient's BMD as a percentage of the mean peak young adult BMD or age-matched BMD level. *Left,* This patient has a total hip BMD of 0.499 g/cm² *(white circle with cross)* as measured by DXA, a femoral neck T-score of −4.0, and a total hip T-score of −3.6. The reference database graph displays age- and sex-matched mean BMD levels ±2 SDs *(shaded areas)* derived from the third National Health and Nutrition Examination Survey. The T-score indicates the difference in SD between the patient's BMD and the predicted sex-matched mean peak young adult BMD; z-score, the difference in SD between the patient's BMD and the sex- and age-matched mean BMD; and percentage of mean, the patient's BMD as a percentage of the mean peak young adult BMD or age-matched BMD level. (Adapted from bone densitometry report, QDR-4500A bone densitometer, Hologic, Inc., Bedford, Mass.)

Studies have shown that vitamin D in doses of 400 to 800 IU/day can normalize serum vitamin D. Vitamin D can be taken in a multivitamin, in a calcium supplement, or in pure form. In pure form, cholecalciferol (D3) is preferable to ergocalciferol (D2). Most multivitamins often contain 400 IU of vitamin D. The current recommended dose is 400 IU/day for most adults and 600 and 800 IU/day for older adults. Older patients with severe vitamin D deficiency may be given 50,000 IU of vitamin D once per week for 3 months to bring serum vitamin D into the normal range. Activated vitamin D is rarely needed and should not be given on a regular basis for postmenopausal osteoporosis.

Weight-bearing exercise is important for maintaining skeletal integrity. Results are controversial concerning

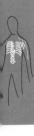

Table 75–3	Techniques for Measuring Bone Mass			
Sites Measured	Precision (%)	Accuracy (%)	Scan Time	Radiation Dose Entrance Exposure (mrem)
Quantitative computed tomography	2–10	5–20	10–15 min	100–2000
Lumbar spine				
Total hip				
Total radius				
Single photon absorptiometry	1–3	4–6	3–5 min	10–20
Proximal radius				
Distal radius				
Calcaneus				
Dual photon absorptiometry	2–6	4–10	20–40 min	10–15
Posteroanterior lumbar spine				
Lateral lumbar spine				
Proximal femur				
Total body				
Dual-energy x-ray absorptiometry	1–3	3–15	2–5 min	1–35
Posteroanterior lumbar spine				
Lateral lumbar spine				
Proximal femur				
Total body				
Calcaneal ultrasound	1.4	3	10 sec	N/A

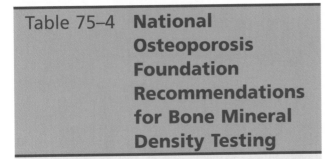

Table 75–4	National Osteoporosis Foundation Recommendations for Bone Mineral Density Testing

1. All postmenopausal women under age 65 who have one or more additional risk factors for osteoporosis (besides menopause)
2. All women ages 65 and older regardless of additional risk factors
3. Postmenopausal women who present with fractures (to confirm diagnosis and determine disease severity)

studies on different types and duration of exercise in postmenopausal women and men. In general, however, weight-bearing or resistance training exercises are suggested and have been shown to improve bone mass or maintain skeletal integrity. In patients with new vertebral fractures, physical therapy is important for improving posture and increasing strength in back muscles.

Because 90% of hip fractures and a significant number of vertebral fractures occur during a fall, fall prevention modalities are suggested for frail older patients. Fall-proofing the household includes installing grab bars in the bathroom and hand rails on stairways, avoiding loose throw rugs and cords, ensuring good lighting by the bedside, and moving objects within easy reach in the kitchen. Other fall prevention modalities include eliminating medications that cause dizziness or postural hypotension (if possible), assessing the need for assistive devices (e.g., canes, walkers), and ensuring appropriate footwear and good vision. In addition, several studies have now demonstrated that hip protectors significantly reduce hip fractures in residents in nursing homes. However, compliance is often poor with these products.

Treatment

BISPHOSPHONATES

Bisphosphonates are the mainstay of osteoporosis prevention and treatment. They inhibit the cholesterol synthesis pathway in the osteoclasts, thereby causing early apoptosis and inhibiting osteoclast migration and attachment. In the United States, the bisphosphonates alendronate, risedronate, and ibandronate have been approved for the prevention and treatment of osteoporosis. Alendronate has been shown to increase bone mass by approximately 8% at the spine and 4% at the hip over 3 years. This increase has been associated with an approximately 50% reduction in spine, hip, and forearm fractures (Table 75–5). Alendronate is prescribed at 5 mg daily or 35 mg once weekly for osteoporosis prevention and 10 mg daily or 70 mg once weekly for the treatment of osteoporosis. Alendronate has been approved for use in men and patients with glucocorticoid-induced osteoporosis.

Risedronate is approved for the prevention and treatment of osteoporosis at a dose of 5 mg/day or 35 mg/week. Large-scale, multicenter studies have shown improvements in bone

Table 75–5	**FDA Approved Therapies for Prevention and Treatment of Osteoporosis**

Agent	Prevention	Treatment	Dose	Vertebral Fracture Reduction	Hip Fracture Reduction
Alendronate	Yes	Yes	Prevention: 5 mg daily, 35 mg weekly Treatment: 10 mg daily, 70 mg weekly	Yes	Yes
Risedronate	Yes	Yes	Prevention and treatment: 5 mg daily, 35 mg weekly	Yes	Yes
Ibandronate	Yes	Yes	2.5 mg daily, 150 mg monthly	Yes	No
Raloxifene	Yes	Yes	60 mg PO daily	Yes	No
HRT	Yes	*Management*	0.625 mg PO daily conjugated estrogen or equivalent (0.45, 0.3 mg also available)	Yes	Yes
Calcitonin	No	Yes	200 IU daily intranasal	Yes	No
Teriparatide (PTH [1–34])	No	Yes	20 mcg SC daily	Yes	No

FDA = Food and Drug Administration; HRT = hormone replacement therapy; PO = orally; SC = subcutaneously.

mass of approximately 6% to 7% at the spine and 3% at the hip over 3 years. In addition, these studies revealed an approximately 50% reduction in vertebral fractures and 40% reduction in femoral fractures (see Table 75–5). Risedronate is also approved for patients with glucocorticoid-induced osteoporosis.

Ibandronate is approved for the prevention and treatment of postmenopausal osteoporosis. After 3 years of treatment, ibandronate increased bone density by 6.5 % at the spine, 3.4% at the hip, and reduced new vertebral fractures by 62%. No reductions in nonvertebral or hip fractures were noted. Ibandronate is approved at an oral dose of 2.5 mg daily or 150 mg monthly. Ibandronate is approved for treatment at an intravenous dose of 3 mg every 3 months.

Because bisphosphonates are poorly absorbed, they must be taken first thing in the morning on an empty stomach with a full glass of water. Patients must wait 30 minutes (when taking alendronate and risedronate) to 60 minutes (when taking ibandronate) before eating and must not lie down. Potential side effects of bisphosphonates include epigastric distress, heartburn, and esophagitis.

SELECTIVE ESTROGEN-RECEPTOR MODULATORS

Selective estrogen-receptor modulators (SERMs) have some estrogen-like and antiestrogen-like benefits. Raloxifene, a SERM, is currently approved for the prevention and treatment of osteoporosis. The Multiple Outcomes of Raloxifene Evaluation (MORE) trial found that bone

mass was increased by 4% at the spine and 2.5% at the femoral neck over 3 years. This increase was associated with an approximately 50% reduction in vertebral fractures. Again, no change in nonvertebral or hip fractures was seen (see Table 75–5). Treatment was also associated with improved lipid status, as shown by decreased total and low-density lipoprotein cholesterol. No change in triglycerides was noted. In addition, early reports suggest a 30% reduction in breast cancer. Raloxifene is not associated with endometrial hyperplasia, thus patients do not have bleeding or spotting, nor do they have breast tenderness or swelling. Patients do have the same small risk of deep-venous thrombosis or pulmonary embolus that is found with hormone replacement therapy (HRT). Raloxifene will not relieve postmenopausal symptoms, such as hot flushes. Raloxifene can be given with or without food in a daily oral form at 60 mg/day. Ongoing studies are examining raloxifene with respect to outcomes on cardiovascular disease and prevention of breast cancer in high-risk patients.

Tamoxifen is a SERM that is used to treat breast cancer. Some epidemiologic studies have suggested decreased fracture risk in these patients, but tamoxifen is not approved for the prevention or treatment of osteoporosis.

HORMONE REPLACEMENT THERAPY

Investigators of the Women's Health Initiative, a large, randomized, placebo-controlled, multicenter trial evaluating HRT, reported a 36% reduction in hip and vertebral fractures after 5.2 years. In addition to improvements in bone mass, other benefits include improved lipid profile, decreased colon cancer, and decreased menopausal symptoms. However, because of the potential risks of HRT, (cardiovascular events, breast cancer, deep-venous thrombosis, pulmonary embolus, and gallbladder problems) HRT should only be used for relief of menopausal symptoms, and other agents should be used for the prevention or treatment of osteoporosis.

CALCITONIN

Calcitonin is a 32-amino-acid peptide produced by the parafollicular cells of the thyroid gland. It is currently approved in a subcutaneous dose but is rarely used because of its expense and potential side effects. The U.S. Food and Drug Administration (FDA) approved the use of calcitonin for the treatment of postmenopausal osteoporosis in a nasal form at a dose of 200 IU/day, taken in alternating nostrils. The Prevent Recurrence of Osteoporotic Fractures (PROOF) study, a large, multicenter trial, did not show any significant changes in bone mineral density following 3 years of treatment. However, the 200-IU dose was associated with an approximately 50% reduction in vertebral fractures (see Table 75–5). No effect on nonvertebral or hip fractures was noted.

PARATHYROID HORMONE

Parathyroid hormone (PTH), an anabolic agent, has been shown to significantly increase bone mineral density and reduce both vertebral and nonvertebral fractures over 18 months. In a large study of postmenopausal women, teriparatide (PTH amino acid sequence 1 through 34), 20 mcg, increased spinal bone mineral density by 9.7%, hip bone mineral density by 2.6%, and was associated with a 65% reduction in vertebral fractures and a 53% reduction in nonvertebral fractures. Teriparatide is taken as a subcutaneous, daily dose and is approved by the FDA. Other forms of PTH (e.g., PTH amino acid sequence 1 through 84) and other anabolic agents (e.g., parathyroid hormone–related protein [PTHrP]) are also under investigation.

FUTURE THERAPIES

Studies with new antiresorptive agents are currently ongoing, including longer-acting and intravenous bisphosphonates and new SERMs. The receptor activator of nuclear factor kappa B (RANK) and its ligand (RANKL) are mediators of osteoclast activity. An antibody to RANKL has been shown to reduce osteoclast activity, decrease bone resorption, and improve bone mass. Strontium has recently been shown to be a potential agent for the treatment of osteoporosis. The exact mechanism of action is not fully understood, but strontium is thought to stimulate osteoblast proliferation and inhibit osteoclast formation. Early studies in postmenopausal women have demonstrated an increase in bone mass and a decrease in new vertebral fractures.

Combination therapy has been examined with two antiresorptive agents or antiresorptive and anabolic agents together. Studies examining two antiresorptive agents have included HRT plus alendronate, HRT plus risedronate, and alendronate plus raloxifene. Overall, studies with combination therapy have suggested greater improvements in bone mass over therapy with single agents. Although dual treatment with antiresorptive agents appears to be safe and well tolerated, studies have not shown greater fracture reduction. Studies have suggested greater improvements in bone mineral density with PTH plus HRT than with HRT alone. The combination of PTH plus alendronate provides no greater benefit than monotherapy with PTH. However, following PTH therapy, patients will benefit from antiresorptive therapy with alendronate rather than calcium supplementation alone.

VERTEBROPLASTY AND KYPHOPLASTY

Vertebroplasty involves injection of cement (polymethylmethacrylate) into a compressed vertebra to prevent the vertebral body from further collapse. Alternatively, kyphoplasty introduces a balloon into the vertebral body to expand it, followed by cement placement inside the balloon. This approach not only expands the vertebral body, but also increases some of the height. Although no controlled trials of these procedures have been conducted, studies suggest that they result in significant reductions in pain. Ongoing studies are needed to determine whether differences in outcomes can be found between vertebroplasty and kyphoplasty or whether potential risks exist to adjacent vertebrae after the procedure. Currently, these procedures are only recommended for patients with significant pain from vertebral fractures and are not routinely performed in asymptomatic patients with vertebral osteoporosis.

Prospectus for the Future

Osteoporosis affects approximately 40% of women over 50 years of age. Although many risk factors exist for low bone mass, the major risk factors for osteoporosis include a personal history of fracture in adulthood, fracture history in a first degree relative, low body weight, current smoking, and use of oral corticosteroid therapy. Because osteoporosis is largely a silent disease until manifestation of fracture, bone mineral density can be used to assess bone mass before a clinical fracture and is also used to monitor the disease. Osteoporosis is classified as a bone mineral density measurement of the hip or spine of equal to or less than –2.5 standard deviations below young adult peak bone mass. National guidelines suggest that all women over the age of 65 years have a bone mass measurement, and those younger than 65 years of age have a bone mass measurement if they have additional risk factors. General preventive measures for all patients include calcium of approximately 1200 mg daily in divided doses, vitamin D supplementation of 400 to 800 IU/day, weight-bearing exercise, and fall prevention for older adults. The mainstays of prevention and treatment include daily, once-weekly, or once-monthly bisphosphonates. A SERM and calcitonin have also been approved as therapy for osteoporosis. PTH, an anabolic agent, is approved for treatment of patients at high risk for osteoporosis. Future therapies include intravenous bisphosphonates, new SERMS, other forms of PTH, other anabolic agents, and antibodies to RANKL (a mediator of osteoclast activity). Monotherapy with PTH appears to be of greater benefit than combination therapy with an antiresorptive.

References

Delmas PD: Treatment of postmenopausal osteoporosis. Lancet 359: 2018–2026, 2002.

Kanis JA: Diagnosis of osteoporosis and assessment of fracture risk. Lancet 359:1929–1936, 2002.

National Osteoporosis Foundation: Physician's Guide to Prevention and Treatment of Osteoporosis. Washington DC, The Foundation, 2003.

U.S. Department of Health and Human Services: Bone Health and Osteoporosis (USHHS): A Report of the Surgeon General. Rockville, Md, USHHS, Office of the Surgeon General, 2004.

U.S. Preventive Services Task Force: Screening for osteoporosis in postmenopausal women: Recommendations and rationale. Ann Intern Med 137:526–528, 2002.

Chapter 76

Paget's Disease of Bone

Mara J. Horwitz

G. David Roodman

Paget's disease is the second most common bone disease after osteoporosis. In contrast to most other metabolic bone diseases (discussed in previous chapters), which are diffuse and involve the entire skeleton, Paget's disease is a focal bone disorder. It can be monostotic (involving a single bone) or polyostotic (involving multiple bones). Although Paget's disease is a chronic condition, over the long course of the disease, new lesions rarely develop. The clinical description of Paget's disease by Sir James Paget over 100 years ago is still accurate today. The primary cellular abnormality of Paget's disease is increased osteoclastic bone resorption. This intense bone resorption is followed by exuberant formation of new bone that is of poor quality. The majority of patients with Paget's disease are asymptomatic, and the disorder is detected by an increased serum alkaline phosphatase level or unexpectedly on a routine radiograph. However, a significant proportion of patients can have bone pain, skeletal deformity, fractures, high-output cardiac failure, or nerve compression syndromes. The most dreaded complication of Paget's disease is development of osteosarcoma in the pagetic lesion. Although this development is extremely rare (<1%), the incidence of osteosarcoma in patients with Paget's disease is approximately 1000-fold greater than in age-matched normal controls.

Incidence and Prevalence

Paget's disease affects approximately 2% of the population over the age of 45 years in the United States. It is common in Great Britain, Germany, France, Australia, and New Zealand but is extremely rare in Scandinavia, Asia, sub-Saharan Africa, and the Arab Middle East. In some areas of Great Britain, the incidence of Paget's disease may reach 5% to 6%. However, the incidence of Paget's disease appears to be decreasing over the last 20 years for unknown reasons. Paget's disease is most commonly diagnosed in patients over the age of 50 and has only rarely been reported under the age of 40 years. Estimates are that the incidence nearly doubles with every decade past the age of 50 years. Both men and women are affected, but it has a slight male predominance.

Etiologic Factors

The cause of Paget's disease is unknown. Studies over the last 30 years, including immunohistochemical, ultrastructural, and in situ hybridization studies, have suggested a possible viral origin for Paget's disease. Osteoclasts in pagetic lesions are markedly increased in number and size. A striking feature of osteoclasts from patients with Paget's disease is the characteristic nuclear inclusions that are similar to nucleocapsids of paramyxoviruses. Several groups have demonstrated that these nuclear inclusions cross react with antibodies against respiratory syncytial virus, measles virus, and canine distemper virus. Furthermore, in situ hybridization studies have shown the presence of measles virus nucleocapsid transcripts in pagetic osteoclasts. Recently, Friedrichs and coworkers have reported the full-length sequence of the measles virus nucleocapsid protein from a patient with Paget's disease. Further supporting a potential role of paramyxoviruses in Paget's disease, Kurihara and coworkers transfected normal osteoclast precursors with the measles virus nucleocapsid gene and reported that the osteoclasts that formed were very similar to pagetic osteoclasts. Other groups in Great Britain have reported that canine distemper virus is present in pagetic osteoclasts. However, other investigators have failed to detect paramyxovirus transcripts in pagetic osteoclasts or their precursors. Thus the role that paramyxovirus plays in the cause of Paget's disease is controversial.

In addition to a viral origin for Paget's disease, a strong genetic component exists. Multiple families have been identified that demonstrate vertical transmission of Paget's disease in an autosomal-dominant fashion with variable penetrance. These large kindred links have led to the identification of several chromosomal loci for Paget's disease, including chromosomes 18, 5, 6, and 2. The most common locus that is linked to Paget's disease has been identified on chromosome 5. This gene encodes sequestosome 1, an adapter protein that may be involved in the receptor activator of nuclear factor kappa B ligand (RANKL)-signaling pathway. Mutations in this gene occur in almost 30% of patients with familial Paget's disease and have also been reported in a small proportion of patients with sporadic rather than familial Paget's disease. In one family from Japan with very early-onset Paget's disease, a mutation in the *RANK* gene on chromosome 18 has been reported. RANKL and its receptor, RANK, are critical factors involved in osteoclast formation and survival.

Pathologic and Pathophysiologic Factors

In pagetic lesions, osteoclasts are increased in number and size and have increased rough endoplasmic reticulum and mitochondria, consistent with their increased metabolic activity. Osteoblasts, which are morphologically normal, are also increased in the lesions. Initially, osteoclastic bone resorption is increased, followed by increased numbers of osteoblasts that form large amounts of woven bone (Fig. 76–1). This marked increase in osteoblast activity

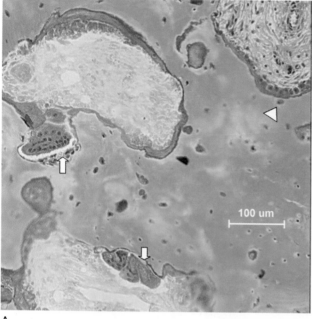

A

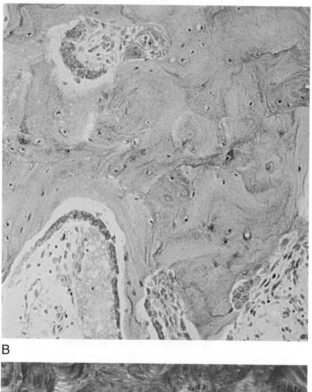

B

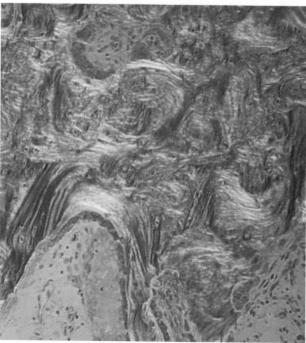

C

Figure 76–1 Typical histologic abnormalities present in bone biopsies from patients with Paget's disease. *A,* Increased numbers of abnormal osteoclasts activity resorbing bone *(arrows).* Increased numbers of osteoblasts are also seen actively forming large amounts of new bone *(arrowhead). B,* Increased numbers of osteoblasts are shown actively forming large amounts of woven bone. *C,* Polarized light view of the specimen shown in *B* demonstrating the highly disorganized woven bone formed by pagetic osteoblasts. Large amounts of sclerotic bone are present. (Photoneurographs courtesy of Dr. David Dempster, Helen Hayes Hospital, Columbia University.)

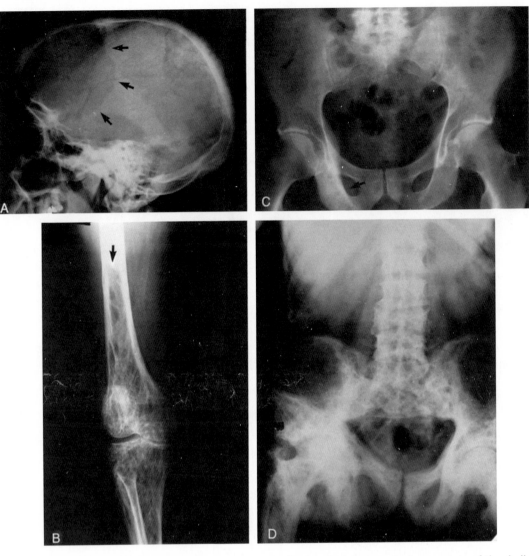

Figure 76–2 Typical radiologic abnormalities in patients with Paget's disease. *A,* Osteoporosis circumscripta of the skull. *B,* Lytic lesions in the femur with the characteristic *blade of grass* lesion. *C,* Blastic involvement of the right ischial ramus of the pelvis with thickening of the medial cortex. *D,* Mixed lytic and blastic disease involving the entire pelvis along with L4 and L5 and both femoral heads. (Courtesy of Dr. Daniel Rosenthal.)

accounts for the sclerotic lesions so typical on radiographic examination (Fig. 76–2), for the increase uptake of radionu-clide on bone scan (Fig. 76–3), and for the increase in serum alkaline phosphatase, the biochemical hallmark of Paget's disease. Ultimately, the pagetic lesions become sclerotic. The vascularity of the abnormal bone is increased.

The increased bone resorption probably results from increased production of cytokines that enhance osteoclast formation. For example, levels of interleukin-6, a potent stimulator of osteoclast formation, are increased in pagetic lesions but not in normal bone. In addition, RANKL levels also are increased in the bones involved with Paget's disease but not in the uninvolved bones from the same patients. The factors that enhance bone formation have not been clearly identified but may include transforming growth factor-β, insulin-like growth factor, and/or fibroblast growth factor, which are present in large quantities in bone and can be released by osteoclastic bone resorption.

Clinical Presentation

Paget's disease may affect any skeletal site. It most commonly involves the pelvis, vertebrae, skull, tibia, and femur. It may be monostotic (affecting only one bone) or more commonly polyostotic (affecting two or more bones) and is often asym-metrical in its distribution. Although progression of the disease may occur at a given site, the appearance of new lesions is rare. As noted previously, the majority of patients with Paget's disease are asymptomatic, and the disease is detected by an increased serum alkaline phosphatase level or unexpectedly on a routine radiograph. Among patients who are symptomatic, bone pain is the most common complaint, with pain in the back, knee, and hip being the classic symp-toms (Table 76–1). Bone pain in Paget's disease can be due to the pagetic lesion itself but more often results from the joint distortion and nerve compression caused by adjacent pagetic bone.

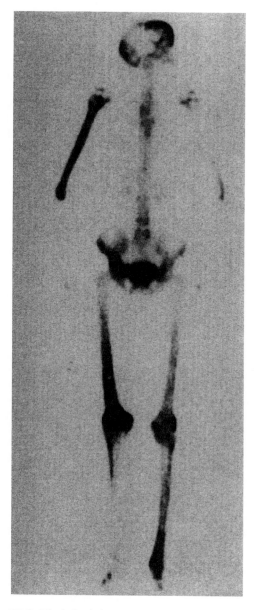

Figure 76–3 Whole-body bone scan demonstrating abnormalities in a patient with polyostotic Paget's disease. Increased radionuclide uptake is seen in the skull, right humerus, pelvis, right femur, and left tibia. (Courtesy of The Paget's Foundation.)

Table 76–1	**Clinical Manifestations of Paget's Disease**

Musculoskeletal pain
Degenerative arthritis in joints near affected areas
Headaches
Skeletal deformity
Pathologic fractures
Enlarged skull
Erythema and warmth over pagetic bones
Hearing loss
Platybasia with or without basilar invagination
Neurologic compression syndromes
Angioid streaks in retina
Increased cardiac output; rarely congestive heart failure
Bone tumors
  Osteogenic sarcoma
  Fibrosarcoma
  Chrondrosarcoma
  Reparative granuloma
  Giant cell tumor
Laboratory abnormalities
  Increased serum alkaline phosphatase (bone fraction)
  Increased urinary hydroxyproline
  Hypercalciuria and hypercalcemia during immobilization
  Hyperuricemia
Characteristic radiographs
Increased uptake on bone scan

Spinal cord or nerve root compression with associated radicular pain and weakness may result from expanding pagetic lesions in the spine. Because pagetic lesions tend to be highly vascular, increased warmth in the skin over affected areas is often present.

Complications and Associated Conditions

Secondary arthritis is a common and often debilitating complication of periarticular Paget's disease. Hyperuricemia and gout may occur with increased frequency in affected persons. Highly vascularized pagetic lesions have been reported to cause a *vascular steal* syndrome, and high-output cardiac failure has been described in severe disease. The most serious complication of Paget's disease is sarcomatous degeneration. This situation occurs most often in the setting of severe polyostotic disease and may be heralded by a sudden increase in pain, a soft tissue mass, an abrupt increase in serum alkaline phosphatase, or a pathologic fracture. Although extremely rare (<1%), osteosarcoma in Paget's patients is approximately 1000-fold greater than in age-matched normal controls. Sarcomatous degeneration is the main cause of death caused by Paget's disease. Although most Paget's-associated tumors are osteosarcomas, fibrosarcomas and chondrosarcomas may also be seen.

Arthritis is often found in joints near areas involved with Paget's disease, particularly when subchondral bone is affected or when the integrity of the joint is compromised by enlarged or distorted bones. Skeletal deformities occur most frequently in affected sites in the skull and long bones of the lower extremities. The skull can become enlarged, and temporal bone involvement may affect hearing and cause other cranial nerve palsies or headaches. Softening of the base of the skull may produce flattening *(platybasia)* with the development of basilar invagination and may lead to cranial nerve and spinal cord compression syndromes. Affected long bones of the lower extremity can become bowed. Fissure fractures along the convex surface of long bones and pathologic fractures in weight-bearing bones are not uncommon.

Diagnostic Evaluation

Paget's disease is most often diagnosed using a combination of biochemical markers of bone turnover and radiologic abnormalities. Biochemical markers of bone formation (such as serum alkaline phosphatase) and bone resorption (such as N-telopeptide cross-links [NTX], C-telopeptide cross-links [CTX] and pyridium cross-links) are usually increased in patients with active disease. For most patients with Paget's disease, serum total alkaline phosphatase is an adequate and sensitive indicator of disease activity. However, serum bone-specific alkaline phosphatase may be a more sensitive marker than serum total alkaline phosphatase for assessing disease in patients with low levels of disease activity. Serum osteocalcin, another marker of bone formation, is often in the normal range and is not a clinically useful marker of disease activity.

A bone scan at the time of diagnosis is the most useful test to define the location and extent of lesions (see Fig. 76–3). Radiographs of the affected areas confirm the presence of Paget's disease and are useful for evaluating complications and local disease progression (see Fig. 76–2). The radiologic abnormalities seen on standard radiographs may reflect one of the three distinctive stages of pagetic lesions. The earliest lesions are osteolytic lesions, which are often observed as *osteoporosis circumscripta* in the skull (see Fig. 76–2A) or as an advancing *blade of grass* in long bones (see Fig. 76–2B). Cortical thickening, coarse trabecular markings, and both lytic and sclerotic lesions in the same bone (see Fig. 76–2C) characterize the second stage of the disease. In the final stage, sclerotic lesions are primarily observed and are often associated with an increase in bone width (see Fig. 76–2D). Bone biopsy is rarely needed to diagnose Paget's disease and should be avoided in weight-bearing areas.

Treatment

The two major goals of therapy are to relieve symptoms and to prevent complications. Potential indications for treatment include the following four situations:

1. In patients with symptoms caused by metabolically active Paget's disease (i.e., bone pain, headache, neurologic complications)
2. In patients planning to undergo elective surgery on a pagetic site to decrease blood flow and minimize intra-operative blood loss
3. In the management of hypercalcemia, which is a rare complication when a patient with severe Paget's disease is immobilized for a prolonged period
4. In patients who may be at high risk of complications if disease progresses locally, such as those at risk for bowing deformities in long bones, for hearing loss as a result of skull enlargement, for neurologic complications resulting from vertebral involvement, and for secondary arthritis where a pagetic lesion is located next to a major joint

Treatment of Paget's disease usually involves a combination of nonpharmacologic therapy (i.e., physical therapy) and pharmacologic therapy. Pharmacologic therapy includes antiresorptive agents (Table 76–2) and analgesics for pain management. The bisphosphonates form the mainstay of therapy for Paget's disease. The bisphosphonates decrease bone resorption at pagetic sites by inhibiting osteoclasts both directly and indirectly. Currently five bisphosphonates have been approved by the U.S. Food and Drug Administration for treating Paget's disease: intravenous pamidronate and oral etidronate, tiludronate, alendronate, and risedronate. In addition, intravenous zoledronate is pending FDA approval. Etidronate and tiludronate are less potent than the other bisphosphonates. Previously, etidronate sodium was the only bisphosphonate available, and although effective, its use was limited because of a tendency to induce mineralization disorders when given at higher doses or for a longer period. Etidronate is rarely used in the United States today.

The introduction of the more potent amino-bisphosphonates—pamidronate, alendronate, risedronate, and zoledronate—represents a significant advance in the treatment of Paget's disease. These agents often induce a biochemical remission in patients with Paget's disease without producing mineralizations defects at the recommended doses. Intra-

Table 76–2	**Treatment of Paget's Disease**		
Drug	**Route**		**Dose**
Bisphosphonates			
Alendronate (Fosamax)	Oral		40 mg/day for 6 months
Risedronate (Actonel)	Oral		30 mg/day for 2 months
Pamidronate (Aredia)	Intravenous		30–60 mg/day for 3 days
Zoledronate (Zometa)*	Intravenous		4 mg single infusion
Etidronate (Didronel)	Oral		400 mg/day for 6 months
Tiludronate (Skelid)	Oral		400 mg/day for 3 months
Other			
Calcitonin (Miacalcisn)	Subcutaneous injection		50–100 U/day

*Not approved in the United States for Paget's disease.

venous pamidronate can be given as two or three 30–60 mg infusions in patients with mild disease. More severe disease may require 60 to 90 mg on a weekly or twice-weekly basis. Cumulative doses of 240 to 480 mg may be required in some patients. Alendronate normalizes markers of bone turnover in most patients with Paget's disease when given in an oral dose of 40 mg/day for 6 months. Fewer than 10% of patients treated with alendronate have a biochemical recurrence within 12 months. Risedronate has similar effects on biochemical indices for bone turnover and is recommended at 30 mg/day for 2 months. Intravenous zoledronate, though not yet approved for the treatment of Paget's disease, is the most potent of the bisphosphonates and may be an alternative in patients with refractory disease. It is given as a 4 to 5 mg single infusion. Calcium and vitamin D supplementation therapy is recommended for patients taking the more potent bisphosphonates to prevent hypocalcemia or secondary hyperparathyroidism. Resistance to individual bisphosphonates can occur. However, patients often respond to an alternate bisphosphonate. Therefore some patients may require the use of more than one medication in the long-term management of the disease. Serum alkaline phosphatase should be measured at baseline and 2 to 3 months after the treatment is completed.

Salmon calcitonin was, at one time, the agent of choice for the treatment of Paget's disease. The usual dose of 50 to 100 U/day by subcutaneous injection has been shown to reduce markers of bone turnover by up to 50%, decrease bone pain, and decrease many of the vascular and neurologic complications associated with Paget's disease. However, secondary resistance to salmon calcitonin is not uncommon. It is not as potent as the bisphosphonates. Use of salmon calcitonin today is limited primarily to patients who are unable to take bisphosphonates.

Pain caused by bone deformity or arthritic changes is often relieved with acetaminophen or nonsteroidal anti-inflammatory drugs.

Orthopedic surgery may be indicated in the management of pagetic lesions when a complete fracture through pagetic bone occurs, to realign a severely arthritic knee, and for total joint arthroplasty in a severely affected hip or knee. Preoperative treatment with a bisphosphonate is recommended when possible in an attempt to decrease the vascularity of the lesion and minimize intra-operative bleeding. Surgical decompression may also be indicated if cranial nerve involvement or spinal nerve root compression is not relieved with medical therapy.

Prospectus for the Future

Although Paget's disease is the second most common bone disease after osteoporosis, for unknown reasons, the incidence appears to be decreasing. Some experts believe this decline may be related to a decrease in the frequency of measles or other paramyxoviral infections with widespread vaccination. The reasons for this decline remain one principal unanswered question in Paget's disease. The second major area of controversy in Paget's disease continues to surround its cause. The contribution of a genetic component versus a viral component remains the largest area of ongoing Paget's research. On the viral side of the argument, although studies over the last 30 years—immunohistochemical, ultrastructural, and in situ hybridization studies—have suggested a paramyxoviral origin for Paget's disease, other investigators have failed to detect paramyxovirus transcripts in pagetic osteoclasts or their precursors. On the genetic side, mutations in the gene that encodes an adaptor protein in the RANKL-signaling pathway occur in almost 30% of patients with familial Paget's disease. In addition, genetic linkage of Paget's disease with chromosomal loci on chromosomes 18, 5, 6, and 2 also exists. Obviously, combined genetic and viral causes are possible and probably likely. Ongoing research in these areas will continue to shed light on this disease of complex origin.

References

Altman RD, Bloch DA, Hochberg MC, et al: Prevalence of Paget's disease of bone in the United States. J Bone Miner Res 15:461–465, 2000.

The Paget Foundation and the NIH Osteoporosis and Related Bone Diseases—National Resource Center: The Management of Paget's Disease of Bone: An Educational Outreach Project of the Paget Foundation for Paget's Disease of Bone and Related Disorders and NIH Osteoporosis and Related Bone Diseases—National Resource Center. New York, The Paget Foundation, 2001.

Proceeding of the 3rd International Symposium on Paget's Disease, Napa, California. J Bone Miner Res 14(Suppl. 2):1–104, 1998.

Roodman GD, Windle JJ: Paget disease of bone. J Clin Invest 115(2): 200–208, 2005.

Siris ES, Roodman GD: Paget's disease of bone. In Favus MJ (ed): Primer on the Metabolic Bone Diseases and Disorders of Mineral Metabolism, 5th ed. Washington DC, American Society for Bone and Mineral Research, 2003, pp 495–506.

Selby PL, Davie MWJ, Ralston SH: Guidelines on the management of Paget's disease of bone. Bone 31(3):366–373, 2002.

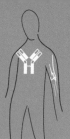

Section XV

Musculoskeletal and Connective Tissue Disease

Approach to the Patient with Rheumatic Disease

Peter A. Merkel

Robert W. Simms

Rheumatic diseases encompass a range of musculoskeletal and systemic disorders that often involve joints and peri-articular tissues and include diseases that are thought to be autoimmune in cause. The causes of arthritis range from local trauma to infection, gout, osteoarthritis, and autoimmune connective tissue diseases, such as rheumatoid arthritis and systemic lupus erythematosus (SLE). Distinguishing localized processes from those that are systemic, executing logical diagnostic procedures, and embarking on appropriate therapeutic courses depend on careful clinical evaluation. As in other areas of medicine, history and physical examination are paramount, and laboratory tests are more confirmatory than diagnostic. The *connective tissue screen* is performed at the bedside, not in the laboratory. The practice of either including or excluding systemic connective tissue disease on the basis of laboratory panels is unreliable and therefore unwise.

Musculoskeletal History and Examination

Features in the medical history that are useful in distinguishing different types of arthritis are listed in Tables 77–1 and 77–2. Appreciating the demographics of different illnesses provides useful information for diagnostic evaluation. Spondyloarthropathies are more commonly diagnosed in predominantly young men, SLE in young women, gout in middle-aged men and postmenopausal women, and osteoarthritis in the older adult population. Asymmetrical pain and swelling in the knees have different connotations in a 70-year-old patient than they do in a 20-year-old patient. The patient's history provides the basis for distinguishing inflammatory from noninflammatory arthropathies. *Inflammatory arthritis* is characterized by pain at rest, morning stiffness, gelling, joint swelling, and joint tenderness. In *osteoarthritis* and *nonarthritic musculoskeletal problems,* pain is generally not present at rest and is precipitated by activity. Occasionally, however, osteoarthritic joints are stiff and are initially improved with activity. In *crystal-induced arthritis* the onset is abrupt, in *septic arthritis* it is less so, and in most other disorders it is slow and insidious. Patterns of joint involvement—symmetry, migratory features, large versus small joints, and locations characteristic of specific diseases—are also key items in the patient's history. Constitutional features such as fatigue, weight loss, and fever are seen in systemic autoimmune disease and infection but not in localized conditions. Many exceptions can be found to these basic demographic and clinical generalizations, but they are often helpful starting points when evaluating a patient for the first time.

On physical examination, active and passive range of motion in all joints should be carefully assessed, and the presence of tenderness, swelling, warmth, erythema, deformity, and joint effusions should be evaluated (Fig. 77–1). Patients are frequently unaware of detectable joint abnormalities, including deformity and effusion, and the presence of either is a sign of joint disease. Reported pain may be referred from another site, and this feature can be elucidated by examination. Thus pain in the knee is often a sign of hip disease and may be reproduced on examination of the hip. The presence of palpable synovitis, or a thickening of the synovial membrane, is helpful in diagnosing inflammatory arthritides such as rheumatoid arthritis. Different diseases have distinctive patterns of joint involvement, which provides critical diagnostic information. For example, prominent disease of distal interphalangeal joints is seen in psoriasis and in inflammatory osteoarthritis. Wrist and metacarpophalangeal involvement are almost universal in rheumatoid arthritis but rare in osteoarthritis. Examination

Table 77–1 Clinical Features Helpful in Evaluation of Arthritis

Age, sex, ethnicity, family history
Pattern of joint involvement
Monoarticular, oligoarticular, polyarticular
Large versus small joints
Symmetry
Insidious versus rapid onset
Inflammatory versus noninflammatory pain (e.g., morning stiffness, gelling, night pain)
Presence of constitutional symptoms and signs (e.g., fever, fatigue, weight loss)
Presence of synovitis, bursitis, tendinitis
Involvement of other organ systems (e.g., rash, mucous membrane lesions, nail lesions)
Presence of arthritis-associated diseases (e.g., psoriasis, inflammatory bowel disease)
Anemia, proteinuria, azotemia
Presence of erosive joint disease

of the axial skeleton may reveal diminished lumbar flexion, decreased rotational motion of the spine, and decreased chest expansion, as well as features of ankylosing spondylitis and other spondyloarthropathies. Patients may report symptoms in only a single joint, but finding additional affected joints on physical examination could change the entire evaluation of a patient.

Rheumatic diseases may involve any organ system, and a full physical examination should be performed on all patients. Funduscopic changes (SLE), uveitis (spondyloarthropathy and juvenile arthritis), conjunctivitis (reactive arthritis), oral and other mucous membrane ulcers (reactive arthritis, SLE, and Behçet's syndrome), lymphadenopathy (SLE and Sjögren's syndrome), and cutaneous lesions (psoriasis, dermatomyositis, scleroderma, SLE, and vasculitides) should be considerations. Lesions of psoriasis in the scalp, umbilicus, and anal crease; thickening of the skin on the fingers in scleroderma; and mucous membrane ulcers are often overlooked. The lung examination may show evidence of interstitial fibrosis (scleroderma, SLE, rheumatoid arthritis, and myositis), and a cardiac evaluation may reveal aortic insufficiency (SLE and spondyloarthropathy), pulmonary hypertension (systemic sclerosis), or evidence of cardiomyopathy (systemic sclerosis, myositis, and amyloidosis). Pleural and pericardial rubs may be present in SLE, rheumatoid arthritis, and scleroderma. Hepatosplenomegaly (SLE and rheumatoid arthritis) and abdominal distention

Table 77–2 Differentiating Features of Common Arthritides

Disease	Demographics	Joints Involved	Special Features	Laboratory Findings
Gout	Men, postmenopausal women	Monoarticular or oligoarticular	Podagra, rapid onset of attack, polyarticular gout, tophi	SF: Crystals, high WBC, >80% PMN
Septic arthritis	Any age	Usually large joints	Fever, chills	SF: High WBC, >90% PMN, culture
Osteoarthritis	Increases with age	Weight-bearing, hands		Noninflammatory SF
Rheumatoid arthritis	Any age, predominantly women ages 20–50 yr	Symmetrical, small joints disease	Rheumatoid nodules, extra-articular	SF: High WBC, >70% PMN
Reactive arthritis (Reiter's syndrome)	Young males	Oligoarticular, asymmetrical	Urethritis, conjunctivitis, skin and mucous membranes	SF: Moderate WBC, >50% PMN
Spondyloarthropathy	Young to middle-aged men	Axial skeleton, pelvis (sacroiliac joints)	Uveitis, aortic insufficiency, enthesopathy	
Systemic lupus erythematosus	Women in childbearing years	Hands, knees	Nonerosive joint disease, autoantibodies, mostly mononuclear; multi-organ disease	SF: Low-to-moderate WBC, almost 100% have antinuclear antibodies

PMN = neutrophils; SF = synovial fluid; WBC = white blood cells.

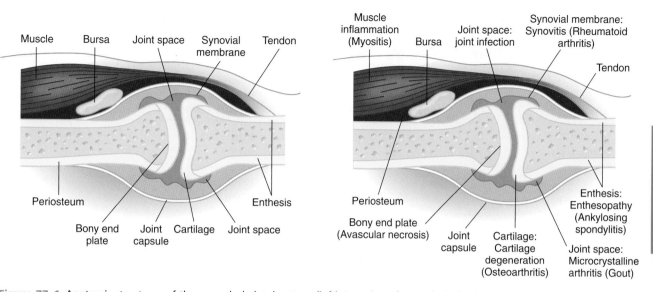

Figure 77–1 Anatomic structures of the musculoskeletal system *(left).* Location of musculoskeletal disease processes *(right).* (From Gordon DA: Approach to the patient with musculoskeletal disease. In Bennett JC, Plum F [eds]: Cecil Textbook of Medicine, 20th ed. Philadelphia, WB Saunders, 1996, p 1440.)

(scleroderma) are also valuable clinical clues. Muscular examination may reveal weakness from myositis, neuropathy (vasculitis and SLE), or myopathy (steroid myopathy). A complete neurologic examination is critical and may reveal carpal tunnel syndrome, peripheral neuropathy such as mononeuritis multiplex (an asymmetrical sensory and/or a motor neuropathy as seen in many vasculitides), and central nervous system disease (SLE and vasculitis).

At the initial evaluation, one important question is whether diagnosis and treatment of the patient's problem require urgent attention. Infectious processes obviously belong in this category. The presence of acute joint inflammation, fever, and systemic signs such as chills, night sweats, and leukocytosis all provide supporting evidence for infection. Gouty arthritis may share some or all of these clinical features, but its onset tends to be more abrupt. Inflammation extending beyond the margins of the joint is characteristic of septic arthritis and is otherwise seen only in crystal disease and rheumatoid arthritis. Nonarticular processes—cellulitis, septic bursitis, tenosynovitis, and phlebitis—may mimic infectious arthritis. Analysis of synovial fluid is the key to diagnosis.

Acute nerve entrapment or spinal cord compression, tendon rupture, and fractures may all occur in the absence of obvious trauma. Spinal cord compression may be the result of a herniated disc or vertebral subluxation. Tendon rupture may occur in inflammatory arthritides, particularly in the wrist in rheumatoid arthritis. Pelvic and other *insufficiency* fractures may be seen in patients with osteoporosis or osteomalacia. Careful musculoskeletal and neurologic examinations help in the detection of these disorders, each of which requires urgent treatment.

In systemic rheumatic diseases, the onset is usually more insidious, and the clinical course is prolonged. Treatment is usually less urgent and can be safely deferred, particularly if the diagnosis is uncertain. However, potential threats to life or the possibility of serious and/or irreversible organ damage may exist in some disorders. In SLE and systemic vasculitis,

patients may have central or peripheral nervous system disease, including brain and peripheral nerve infarcts, glomerulonephritis, inflammatory or hemorrhagic lung disease, coronary artery involvement, intestinal infarcts, and digital infarcts. Threatened digital loss may also be seen in scleroderma and Raynaud's disease. Renal crisis may occur in scleroderma, with vasculopathy leading to renal infarcts, azotemia, micro-angiopathy, and severe hypertension. Urgent therapy to ameliorate or prevent damage may be indicated in these disorders. In giant-cell arteritis, acute blindness is a potential complication, and the diagnosis requires urgent therapy even before confirmatory biopsy. Acute inflammatory myositis should be promptly treated because it may progress rapidly to the involvement of the respiratory musculature. In some cases, major organ involvement may be occult. When systemic disease is suggested, the patient's lung and kidneys should be carefully evaluated.

LABORATORY TESTING

As noted earlier, *synovial fluid analysis* is an important part of the evaluation of arthritis (Table 77–3). It helps distinguish inflammatory from noninflammatory arthritis and can be diagnostic of infectious arthritis or crystal disease. Synovial fluid consists of an ultrafiltrate of plasma into which synovial lining cells secrete hyaluronic acid, which is responsible for the high viscosity of synovial fluid. Evaluation of synovial fluid should include the following: (1) cell count and differential, (2) crystal examination for sodium urate and calcium phosphate dehydrate (CPPD) crystals, and (3) gram stain and culture. Synovial fluid glucose and protein are not diagnostically useful tests. Synovial fluid examination should be performed in the evaluation of all acute arthritides, all situations where joint infection is probable, and ideally should be performed on at least one occasion in the evaluation of chronic inflammatory arthritis. Aspiration and analysis of fluid before therapy are critical to appropriate decision making.

Table 77–3   Classification of Synovial Effusions by Synovial White Cell Count

Group	Diagnosis (Examples)	Appearance	Synovial Fluid White Cell Count (mm³)*	Polymorphonuclear Cells (%)
Normal		Clear, pale yellow	0–200	<10
I. Noninflammatory	Osteoarthritis; trauma	Clear to slightly turbid	50–2000 (600)	<30
II. Mildly inflammatory	Systemic lupus erythematosus	Clear to slightly turbid	100–9000 (3000)	<20
III. Severely inflammatory (noninfectious)	Gout	Turbid	2000–160,000 (21,000)	~70
	Pseudogout	Turbid	500–75,000 (14,000)	~70
	Rheumatoid arthritis	Turbid	2000–80,000 (19,000)	~70
IV. Severely inflammatory (infectious)	Bacterial infections	Very turbid	5000–250,000 (80,000)	~90
	Tuberculosis	Turbid	2500–100,000 (20,000)	~60

*Mean values in parentheses.

Although autoantibodies are often considered the hallmark of rheumatic diseases, their diagnostic utility in individual patients is actually much less than commonly believed. Although almost 100% of patients with SLE have antinuclear antibodies, as do most patients with scleroderma and autoimmune myositis, the proportion of patients with positive tests in other rheumatic diseases is much lower. Conversely, 15% to 25% of healthy persons have antinuclear antibodies when commercial test kits are used, sometimes in high titers. Older persons and patients with nonrheumatic systemic diseases such as malignant disease and nonrheumatic autoimmune diseases such as thyroiditis or hypothyroidism have even higher frequencies. Other specific autoantibodies may be more useful and are discussed in subsequent chapters. *Rheumatoid factor* is found in approximately 80% to 90% of patients with rheumatoid arthritis but also in a variety of other rheumatic diseases, in chronic infection, in neoplasia, and in almost any state that can cause chronic hyperglobulinemia. Neither a positive nor a negative test result is diagnostic, and results should be interpreted only in clinical context. Antibodies to cyclic citrullinated peptides may also be helpful in diagnosing rheumatoid arthritis.

Tests for acute phase proteins, C-reactive protein, and erythrocyte sedimentation rate are nonspecific, but positive results suggest the presence of inflammatory disease. In some cases, such as in patients with giant-cell arteritis and polymyalgia rheumatica, these tests may be useful both in diagnosis and in monitoring the course of disease and therapy. The presence of anemia may suggest chronic disease or hemolytic anemia. Leukopenia, especially lymphopenia, suggests SLE, and thrombocytosis indicates active inflammation. Leukocytosis may also reflect inflammation or infection, and glucocorticoid therapy also elevates the white blood cell count, often dramatically. Urinalysis should always be performed in patients with systemic disease, and proteinuria, red blood cells, and casts should be considered as evidence of occult renal disease. Laboratory tests should always be considered within the context of the clinical presentation.

RADIOGRAPHIC STUDIES

Radiographic evaluation often shows changes characteristic of particular diseases. In established rheumatoid arthritis, patients often have classically erosive disease of the small joints of the wrists, the ulnar styloid, the metacarpophalangeal and proximal interphalangeal joints, and the small joints in the foot. The erosions are bland and nonreactive. In contrast, erosive psoriatic arthritis has sclerotic reaction, and the patient may have characteristic telescoping of joints, the so-called *pencil-in-cup lesions*. Large erosions with overhanging sclerotic margins and even juxta-articular tophi may be seen in gout. In ankylosing spondylitis, sacroiliitis is observed on pelvic films and has high diagnostic specificity. *Syndesmophytes* (calcification of the outer rim of the annulus fibrosis), bridging osteophytes, calcification of spinal ligaments, and a typical bamboo spine in late stages are seen on lumbar and chest radiographs. Joint space narrowing, bony spurs, and sclerosis are seen in osteoarthritis. *Chondrocalcinosis* is a common finding and may be asymptomatic or may lead to crystal arthritis (pseudogout). In acute arthritis, radiographs are much less helpful because bony changes take time to develop; only in septic joint disease is destruction observed in the early stages.

Imaging modalities such as magnetic resonance imaging (MRI), radionuclide scans, ultrasound, and computed tomography (CT) are often useful in assessing diseases of bones, joints, muscle, and soft tissues. Ultrasound may be used to detect synovial cysts, especially Baker's cysts of the knee. MRI is the procedure of choice for evaluating early avascular necrosis of bone, especially the hips, as well as suggested meniscal or rotator cuff disease. MRI is also the preferred procedure for evaluating intervertebral disc disease with suggested radiculopathy and spinal stenosis. MRI is also very useful in evaluating solid lesions of bone and joints, including neoplastic lesions. The sensitivity of MRI for detecting edema (water) makes it useful in evaluating inflammatory muscle disease of both infectious and non-infectious causes. An MRI is a sensitive but not a specific modality for evaluating osteomyelitis, properties shared with radionuclide imaging. MRI should not supplant clinical evaluation or plain radiography.

In many instances, diagnosis can be made with certainty by only pathologic examination of tissue. Muscle biopsy may be necessary to establish a diagnosis of inflammatory muscle disease, and nerve biopsy may be needed to detect vasculitis. Skin biopsy is often quite useful in differentiating the many causes of skin disease in rheumatology. Renal biopsy is often needed for diagnosis, as well as for treatment decisions and prognosis.

Summary

The evaluation of arthritis begins with a careful assessment of the location and pattern of joint involvement, the differentiation of inflammatory from mechanical and other causes, and the consideration of nonarticular systemic features. The patient's age and sex, family history, and medication history, as well as the presence of other medical conditions, are also important; they are often key features. Laboratory and radiographic studies, in particular synovial fluid analysis, provide confirmatory and sometimes diagnostic information.

Prospectus for the Future

- A thorough history and physical examination will remain the basis of rheumatic disease diagnosis.

- Improvement in key laboratory studies, including serologic tests and imaging techniques, will further enhance diagnostic ability.

References

Felson DT: Epidemiology of the rheumatic diseases. In Koopman WJ (ed): Arthritis and Allied Conditions, 13th ed. Baltimore, Williams & Wilkins, 1997, p 3.

Gordon DA: Approach to the patient with musculoskeletal disease. In Goldman L, Bennett JC (eds): Cecil Textbook of Medicine, 21st ed. Philadelphia, WB Saunders, 2000, pp 1472–1475.

Sergent JS: Approach to the patient with pain in more than one joint. In Kelley WN, Harris ED Jr, Ruddy S, et al (eds): Textbook of Rheumatology, 5th ed. Philadelphia, WB Saunders, 1997, p 381.

Chapter 78

Rheumatoid Arthritis

Peter A. Merkel
Robert W. Simms

Rheumatoid arthritis (RA) is a systemic disease characterized by inflammatory polyarthritis, involving small and large joints and constitutional features. It is the prototypic inflammatory arthritis with characteristic clinical features such as morning stiffness, *gelling,* and improvement of symptoms with activity. Most patients have progression to some level of destruction of bone and cartilage, as well as involvement of tendon sheaths; this process leads to deformity and significant loss of function in many patients. Extra-articular manifestations, including nodules and vasculitis, are common; they may involve almost any organ system and may be serious.

Epidemiologic Features and Genetics

RA is among the most common autoimmune diseases, with a prevalence of approximately 1% among the general population. Prevalence is similar in the United States, Europe, and Africa but somewhat lower in Asian populations. It has a female-to-male ratio of 3:1, and onset is most common in the third through fifth decades of life. Human leukocyte antigen (HLA) DR4 is a genetic risk factor, and individuals who are DR4 positive appear to have more serious, seropositive (rheumatoid factor positive) disease. Specific DR4 amino acid sequences in the DR–β molecule antigen-binding site are associated with disease susceptibility. The underlying cause of the disease—that is, the trigger in the susceptible host—is unknown.

Pathologic Features

The hallmark of joint involvement is the *synovial pannus,* a proliferative synovium infiltrated with mononuclear cells, particularly monocytes and T lymphocytes. The pannus *invades* at the bone-cartilage-synovium interface, with progressive destruction of the bone and cartilage. This process is radiographically evident as marginal bony erosions. In other tissues, as well as in the synovium, *rheumatoid nodules* may develop. Rheumatoid nodules are large granulomas with areas of central necrosis that surround mononuclear cells, and they exhibit an outer layer of palisading histiocytes. *Lymphoid aggregates* may be extensive and may assume the appearance of lymphoid follicles.

Pathophysiologic Features

In a joint affected by RA, two related processes are noted (Table 78–1). Symptoms of joint pain and swelling are secondary to an inflammatory process in the synovial space and joint fluid. This inflammation is a result of polymorphonuclear cell chemotaxis and activation, release of prostanoids (prostaglandins and leukotrienes), and concomitant generation of reactive oxygen species, including free radicals, superoxide anion, peroxy nitrite, and peroxy and hydroperoxy acids. Polymorphonuclear cell enzymes, including matrix metalloproteinases such as collagenase, stromelysin, and gelatinases, and cathepsins, promote superficial cartilage erosions. Significantly more important to the destruction of cartilage and bone is the process that occurs in the synovial tissue where proliferative synovial cells are activated by lymphocytes and monocytes. This process (1) elaborates matrix metalloproteinases that directly degrade cartilage and bone matrix, and (2) releases pro-inflammatory prostanoids (Fig. 78–1). The monocyte products interleukin-1 (IL-1) and tumor necrosis factor-α (TNF-α) are central to this process. TNF-α is particularly a key in the activation of matrix metalloproteinases and IL-1 in stimulating prostaglandin E_2 (PGE_2). In addition, TNF-α, IL-1, and lymphotoxin are osteoclast-activating factors; osteoclasts are the central cell in resorption of calcified matrix. The activated pannus of proliferating synovial tissue invades the cartilage and bone and behaves like a locally invasive tumor. Other cytokines such as IL-6, induced by IL-1 and TNF-α, and IL-1 itself play a role in the systemic features of disease, including fever,

Table 78–1   Pathogenesis of Rheumatoid Arthritis

Tissue Phase

Immune cell localization to synovial tissue
T- and B-cell and monocyte recruitment
T-cell activation and proliferation and cytokine release
B-cell elaboration of rheumatoid factor and other antibodies
Monocyte elaboration of inflammatory cytokines: IL-1, TNF-α, IL-6
Synovial cell proliferation and activation by IL-1 and TNF-α
Release of inflammatory eicosanoids (PGE₂)
Synthesis of collagenase and other matrix metalloproteinases
Erosions of bone and cartilage
Osteoclast and chondrocyte activation
Release of proteases
Resorption of bone and cartilage

Fluid Phase

Immune complexes in synovial fluid
Complement activation and release of C3a, C5a
Neutrophil recruitment and activation
Release of prostaglandins, leukotrienes, and reactive oxygen species
Release of lysosomal enzymes
Vasodilation, development of joint effusions, pain, and swelling
Superficial cartilage erosions

IL-1 = interleukin-1; IL-6 = interleukin-6; PGE₂ = prostaglandin E₂; TNF-α = tumor necrosis factor-α.

myalgia, weight loss, and induction of acute phase proteins. B cells and plasma cells in the synovium synthesize rheumatoid factor, an immunoglobulin M (IgM) antibody directed to immunoglobulin G (IgG), as well as other antibodies, including antibodies to matrix degradation products. These enter the synovial fluid and, as complexes, play a role in complement activation, as well as in polymorphonuclear cell activation and chemotaxis.

Clinical Features

RA is a symmetrical polyarthritis typically involving the small joints of the hands and feet, the wrists, and the ankles. Other joints frequently involved include the cervical spine, shoulders, elbows, hips, and knees. Any diarthrodial (synovial) joint may be involved, including the apophyseal, temporomandibular, and cricoarytenoid joints. Involved joints are swollen, warm, and tender, and they may have effusions. The synovium, normally a few cell-layers thick, becomes palpable on examination (*synovitis*). Prolonged *morning stiffness*, usually lasting more than 1 hour and often many hours, is a classic feature in RA and in other inflammatory arthropathies; similarly, gelling occurs after any prolonged inactivity, and symptoms are generally improved with moderate activity (Table 78–2).

Over time, RA progresses to joint destruction and deformity. Erosive lesions of bone and cartilage are radiographically and pathologically visible at the margins of bone and cartilage, the site of synovial attachment. *Tenosynovitis*, or inflammation of tendon sheaths, leads to tendon malalignment, stretching, and/or shortening. Among common deformities are ulnar deviation at the metacarpophalangeal joints

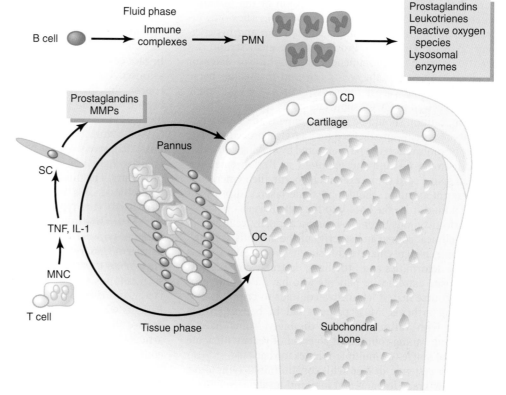

Figure 78–1 Pathogenetic events in rheumatoid arthritis. The proliferative synovial pannus invades at the bone-cartilage interface. Interleukin-1 (IL-1) and tumor necrosis factor-α (TNF) activate synovial cells (SC) to produce prostaglandins and matrix metalloproteinases (MMPs). In the synovial fluid, polymorphonuclear leukocytes (PMN), activated by immune complexes and complement, produce mediators of inflammation and destruction. CD = chondrocyte; MNC = mononuclear cell; OC = osteoclast.

Table 78–2 Clinical Characteristics of Rheumatoid Arthritis

Articular

Morning stiffness, "gelling"
Symmetrical joint swelling
Predilection for wrists, proximal interphalangeal, metacarpophalangeal, and metatarsophalangeal joints
Erosions of bone and cartilage
Joint subluxation and ulnar deviation
Inflammatory joint fluid
Carpal tunnel syndrome
Baker's cyst

Nonarticular

Rheumatoid nodules: Subcutaneous, pulmonary, scleral
Lung disease
Vasculitis, especially skin, peripheral nerves, and bowel
Pleuropericarditis
Scleritis and episcleritis
Leg ulcers
Felty's syndrome

also common. Specific organs other than the musculoskeletal system may be involved (see Table 78–2). Grossly palpable subcutaneous *rheumatoid nodules* can occur almost anywhere but are common along other extensor tendon surfaces, especially at the elbows, and less commonly in the lungs, pleura, pericardium, sclerae, and other sites, including the heart in rare cases. The occurrence of multiple pulmonary nodules in patients with RA and pneumoconiosis is known as *Caplan's syndrome*. Pleuritis, pericarditis, and interstitial lung fibrosis occur in a few patients; pericarditis can be severe and life-threatening, and acute interstitial lung disease can be associated with pulmonary hemorrhage. Vasculitis, associated with circulating complexes of IgG and rheumatoid factor, leads to cutaneous lesions, including ulcers and skin necrosis, mononeuritis multiplex, and intestinal infarction. Secondary *Sjögren's syndrome* (sicca complex) is often present (see Chapter 84). *Felty's syndrome* (splenomegaly, leukopenia, and recurrent pulmonary infections) is a rare complication and is often accompanied by leg ulcers and vasculitis. Extra-articular manifestations of RA are more commonly seen among patients who test positive for rheumatoid factor. Even in patients without vasculitis or pulmonary or pleuropericardial disease, the mortality rate in RA is increased by a variety of causes, including side effects of therapy and infection. Premature and accelerated atherosclerosis is an increasingly recognized problem among patients with RA and is thought, at least, to be partially due to the effects of chronic inflammation.

Diagnosis

RA is a clinical diagnosis. Symmetrical synovitis of small joints—that is, warm, swollen joints with synovial hypertrophy, morning stiffness, and fatigue—is the classic symptom. About 20% to 30% of patients exhibit mono-articular disease, usually in the knee. In such patients the diagnosis cannot be made until the disease evolves. *Systemic lupus erythematosus* can have a similar clinical presentation and may be difficult to differentiate unless other features are present. In rare cases, *Lyme disease* is polyarticular and symmetrical at onset. *Viral arthritis* is best distinguished by its limited course. In the older patient, polymyalgia rheumatica, hypothyroidism, and paraneoplastic syndromes, including hypertrophic osteoarthropathy, should be considered. Crystal arthropathies (gout and pseudogout) can, if left untreated, rarely appear clinically as a chronic polyarthritis.

Examination of joint fluid is the most helpful laboratory procedure. The fluid is inflammatory, with more than 10,000 white blood cells and a predominance of polymorphonuclear leukocytes, typically 80% or more. Rheumatoid factor, an IgM antibody directed to IgG, is found in 80% to 90% of patients with RA. The presence of rheumatoid factor is neither necessary nor sufficient for diagnosis, but its presence labels a patient as being *seropositive*. Other disorders, such as lupus, may be associated with a positive rheumatoid factor, and 10% to 20% of patients with RA are seronegative. Patients who are seropositive are more likely to have severe erosive disease, to have nodules, and to have other extra-articular features. Tests for antibodies to citrullinated-containing cyclic protein (anti-CCP) appear to be of high diagnostic specificity for RA. Antinuclear antibodies are common but not diagnostically helpful.

and volar subluxation at these joints, volar subluxation at the wrists, and flexion and extension contractures in the proximal and distal interphalangeal (DIP) joints of the fingers that lead to characteristic *swan-neck deformity* (flexion contracture at the DIP joint and hyperextension at the proximal interphalangeal joint) or *boutonnière deformity* (flexion contracture at the proximal interphalangeal joint and hyperextension at the DIP joint). Erosions of the ulnar styloid can lead to sharp bony prominences and rupture of extensor tendons. Synovitis at the wrists can lead to median nerve compression and carpal tunnel syndrome. Cervical spine disease may lead to C1-C2 subluxation and spinal cord compression; caution should be taken in moving the neck when the patient is being anesthetized for a surgical procedure. The degree of subluxation can be monitored by looking at the distance between C1 and the odontoid in flexion-extension films. If spinal cord compression does occur, then emergency surgical intervention should be undertaken. Rupture of synovial fluid from the knee into the calf (Baker's cyst) may mimic deep-venous thrombosis or, occasionally, cellulitis.

The clinical course and severity of the arthritis are variable. Some patients have mild, slowly progressive disease with few deformities and little bony destructive change. At the opposite extreme are patients who have a rapidly progressive course that, if left untreated, leads to crippling and deforming arthritis. Most patients fall in between these extremes with various levels of disability; some have a waxing and waning course over a period of years with acute episodes of single- or multiple-joint exacerbations.

RA is a systemic disease with constitutional symptoms: fatigue, low-grade fever, weight loss, and myalgia. Anemia is

Treatment

The goals of treatment for RA are to control pain, preserve maximal function, and prevent deformity and destruction. Aspirin and *nonsteroidal anti-inflammatory drugs* (NSAIDs) are useful in controlling pain and inflammation and may improve daily function; however, they do not affect the underlying disease process, particularly erosions and joint destruction. These agents function largely by inhibiting prostaglandin synthesis, an effect mediated by inhibiting the enzyme cyclo-oxygenase (COX). Aspirin and other nonselective NSAIDs such as ibuprofen and indomethacin inhibit both COX-1 and COX-2, whereas the selective NSAIDs have significant preferential inhibition of COX-2 (the *coxibs*). Anti-inflammatory doses of NSAIDs, as used in RA, are substantially greater than analgesic or antipyretic doses. Although NSAIDs are generally safe, gastrointestinal toxicity (especially bleeding and ulcer perforation), inhibitory effects on platelet function, and decreases in renal blood flow are serious toxicities in some patients. Considering the large number of treated patients, even a small proportion of toxicities amounts to large numbers of serious and even fatal complications of therapy. The introduction of selective COX-2 inhibitors, which do seem to cause less gastrointestinal toxicity compared with nonselective NSAIDs, was heralded as an important pharmaceutical advance, but the initial enthusiasm was abruptly reversed when evidence of increased rates of cardiovascular disease and death were found associated with the coxibs. Anti-inflammatory doses of coxibs are no longer routinely prescribed for patients with RA.

Glucocorticoids remain important in the treatment of RA, especially for acute exacerbations of disease. These agents are usually used sparingly, in low-to-medium doses, and optimally for short periods. Although they are useful for brief exacerbations of the disease or to bide time while waiting for DMARDs to work, many patients require more prolonged use of low doses for optimal control of disease activity, even when other immunomodulatory drugs are also prescribed. The long-term side effects of glucocorticoids can be substantial and particularly devastating in a disease such as RA that is already marked by relative immobility. Side effects include osteoporosis and pathologic fractures, avascular necrosis of bone, obesity, glucose intolerance, and many other problems. Screening, prevention, and treatment for osteoporosis should be considered in all patients who receive long-term therapy with glucocorticoids. Intra-articular glucocorticoids are extremely useful and efficacious in exacerbations involving only a few joints, and intra-articular delivery of these agents is associated with almost no side effects.

Although NSAIDs and glucocorticoids are important for the treatment of RA, they do not control symptoms or alter the disease course for the majority of patients. Current practice is to place most patients with RA on so-called *disease-modifying antirheumatic drugs* (DMARDs) (Table 78–3). Previously, many of these drugs were given only late in the course of disease to patients with severe disease. Recognition of the extent of disability resulting from RA and growing evidence that DMARD use inhibits the progression of erosive disease and disability have led to earlier and more widespread use of these agents.

A wide variety of DMARDs are now available for use in treating RA. Table 78–3 includes several agents of historical interest but almost no current use, including D-penicillamine and gold preparations. Similarly, azathioprine and cyclosporine are now less commonly used, whereas cyclophosphamide is almost only used in extremely severe disease, especially with extra-articular manifestations such as vasculitis. Hydroxychloroquine, minocycline, and sulfasalazine are frequently prescribed for patients with mild-to-moderate disease and/or in combination with other agents. Methotrexate remains the most widely used DMARD for RA; its popularity is due to its high degree of efficacy combined with good tolerability. However, its teratogenicity, as well as liver disease, cytopenias, infections and other problems associated with methotrexate, is important to keep in mind. Leflunomide is a relatively new immunosuppressive drug that is widely used for moderate-to-severe RA and shares several potential toxicities with methotrexate.

TERATOGENICITY

The newest and seemingly most effective therapeutic for RA are DMARDs that are *anticytokine-directed therapies* and

---

Table 78–3	**Treatment of Rheumatoid Arthritis**

Glucocorticoids

Systemic (oral, intravenous, intramuscular)
Intraarticular

Nonsteroidal Anti-Inflammatory Drugs

Aspirin
Nonacetylated salicylates
Nonsalicylate nonselective prostaglandin inhibitors
Selective cyclooxygenase-2 inhibitors1

Disease-Modifying Anti-Rheumatic Drugs

Hydroxychloroquine
Minocycline
Sulfasalazine
Azathioprine
Cyclosporine
Cyclophosphamide
Methotrexate
Leflunomide

Disease-Modifying Anti-Rheumatic Drugs-Biologic Agents

Tumor necrosis factor (TNF) blockers:

Etanercept (soluble TNF receptor)
Infliximab (chimeric anti-TNF antibody)
Adalimumab (fully human anti-TNF antibody)
Anakinra (IL-1–receptor antagonist)
Abatacept (T-cell–costimulation inhibitor)
Rituximab (anti-CD20 B cell–depleting agent)

commonly referred to as *biologics*. Blockers of TNF have demonstrated remarkable benefit for many patients and have set a new standard for efficacy for DMARDs. Three different TNF blockers are now available, and more variants are under development. All of the available TNF blockers are given by intravenous or subcutaneous injection, are quite expensive, and carry risks of reactivation of tuberculosis and increased risk for some other infections; otherwise, they are well tolerated. Other biologic agents now available for treatment of RA include an IL-1 receptor antagonist, anakinra; an inhibitor of T-cell costimulation, abatacept; and a B cell–depleting agent, rituximab. Antagonists or modulators of many other cytokines are under development for RA.

Although methotrexate and the biologic drugs have brought about a remarkable overall improvement in the ability to treat RA, it is important to recognize that many patients still have active disease despite using these drugs, even in combination, and the need for different, safer, and more efficacious treatment options for RA still exists.

Joint replacement surgery plays an extremely important role in patients who have had severe destructive joint disease, particularly in the knee and hip. Early reconstructive surgery in the hand and foot can improve function and sometimes can prevent deformity and tendon rupture. Total joint arthroplasty can have life-changing benefits for patients with RA with destructive joint disease.

Physical therapy and *occupational therapy* also continue to play important roles for many patients with RA. Physical therapy improves muscle strength and conditioning and maintains joint mobility. Splints for the wrists, used at night, may help prevent deformity. Various appliances are available that help protect joints and make daily activities easier, ranging from Velcro "buttons" to special grips for keys and writing implements to raised chairs and toilet seats.

Prognosis

Available data suggest that 50% of patients are disabled in terms of work within 5 years, and the overall mortality rate is increasing, at least in patients with severe RA. Increased mortality is related to infection and gastrointestinal bleeding, as well as pulmonary, renal, and cardiovascular disease; some increase in mortality may also be the result of therapeutic interventions. Early and aggressive use of DMARDs has been beneficial, and most patients respond well to therapy. Studies have shown that DMARDs retard the development of erosive joint disease, control symptoms, improve functional capacity, and may extend the lifespan of patients with RA. The long-term benefits of the newer biologic drugs are not yet clear.

In summary, considerable strides have been made in understanding the pathogenesis and clinical outcomes of RA. Although the underlying cause of RA is unknown, advances in cell biology, immunology, and molecular biology have led to dramatic alterations in therapies available to treat this disease. The development of novel effective biologic agents and the earlier introduction of aggressive therapy should prevent joint deformity and destruction and should improve short- and long-term outcomes. Assessment of efficacy in long-term studies and evaluation of long-term risks and toxicities will determine whether these drugs become the new paradigms for the treatment of RA.

Prospectus for the Future

- Large-scale genetic studies may yield important insights into the pathogenesis of RA and may potentially allow more precise targeting of therapeutic agents.
- An ever-increasing number of biologic agents will be available for the treatment of RA with associated needs for clinical trials to guide the appropriate and safe use of these drugs, especially in combination.
- More rapid and extensive access to effective therapies for RA will, hopefully, significantly reduce the cumulative disability this common systemic disease causes.

References

American College of Rheumatology Subcommittee on Rheumatoid Arthritis Guidelines: Guidelines for the management of rheumatoid arthritis, 2002 update. Arthritis Rheum 46:328–346, 2002.

Arnett FC: Rheumatoid arthritis. In Goldman L, Bennett JC (eds): Cecil Textbook of Medicine, 21st ed. Philadelphia, WB Saunders, 2000, pp 1492–1499.

De Vries-Bouwstra JK, Dijkmans BACC, Breedveld FC: Biologics in early rheumatoid arthritis. Med Clin North Am 31:745–762, 2005.

Harris ED Jr: Clinical features of rheumatoid arthritis. In Kelley WN, Harris ED Jr, Ruddy S, et al (eds): Textbook of Rheumatology, 5th ed. Philadelphia, WB Saunders, 1997, p 898.

Jain R, Lipsky PE: Treatment of rheumatoid arthritis. Med Clin North Am 81:57–84, 1997.

Singh R, Robinson DB, El-Gabalawy HS: Emerging biologic therapies in rheumatoid arthritis: cell targets and cytokines. Curr Opin Rheumatol 17:274–279, 2005.

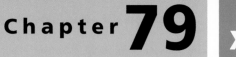

Spondyloarthropathies

Peter A. Merkel

The *seronegative spondyloarthropathies* are a related group of inflammatory disorders with clinical features unique among rheumatic diseases. The four types of spondyloarthropathies in adults are ankylosing spondylitis, reactive arthritis (Reiter's disease), enteropathic arthritis (inflammatory bowel disease), and psoriatic arthritis. The peripheral arthropathies associated with either inflammatory bowel disease or psoriasis are not always associated with spondylitis and can also be considered separate entities. In addition, a juvenile form of spondyloarthropathy exists that is similar to ankylosing spondylitis and generally persists into adulthood. The cardinal features of the spondyloarthropathies are inflammation of the sacroiliac joints *(sacroiliitis)*, spine *(spondylitis)*, tendon insertion sites *(enthesitis)*, and anterior chamber of the eye *(uveitis)*. Other manifestations are present within each type. Because these diseases are so similar, they are best described by first highlighting the features common to all types of spondyloarthropathy and then mentioning the unique manifestations of each type.

Epidemiologic Features

Ankylosing spondylitis is much more common among adolescent boys and young men, but this finding may reflect underdiagnosis in women in whom disease manifestations may be milder than it is in men. *Reactive arthritis* is more common among men when it follows genitourinary *Chlamydia trachomatis* infection, but the sex distribution is even found among patients after dysentery. *Inflammatory arthritis* including spondylitis affects approximately 5% to 8% of patients with psoriasis and 10% to 25% of patients with ulcerative colitis or Crohn's disease. The sex ratio is also apparent among patients with spondylitis associated with psoriasis and inflammatory bowel disease, in which patients commonly exhibit symptoms in young or middle adulthood. The prevalence of spondyloarthropathy also increases in association with rises in infection in populations with human immunodeficiency virus (HIV).

Pathogenesis

Among the most fascinating aspects of the spondyloarthropathies are their strong associations with human leukocyte antigen (HLA)–B27, a specific allele of the B locus of the HLA-encoding class I major histocompatibility complex genes. The frequency of HLA-B27 among whites is approximately 6% to 8%. However, up to 90% of white patients with ankylosing spondylitis and 80% of white patients with reactive arthritis or juvenile spondyloarthropathy are HLA-B27 positive; these percentages are even higher among those patients with uveitis. The rate of HLA-B27 positivity among patients with inflammatory bowel disease or psoriasis and peripheral arthritis is not increased unless spondylitis is present, in which case the frequency of HLA-B27 is 50%. The frequency of HLA-B27 varies widely among other ethnic groups, but it is associated with spondyloarthropathy in many groups. Further, other major histocompatibility complex antigens have been associated with spondylitis among patients who are HLA-B27 negative; these class I antigens are cross-reactive with HLA-B27. Rodents transgenic for HLA-B27 develop inflammatory abnormalities strikingly similar to those seen in B27-associated human diseases.

In addition to the strong genetic links to the spondyloarthropathies, important associations exist between specific bacterial agents and disease pathogenesis. Genitourinary infection with *Chlamydia trachomatis* or diarrheal illness with *Shigella, Salmonella, Campylobacter,* and *Yersinia* species, as well as *Klebsiella pneumoniae* infection, can induce reactive arthritis. These infections appear to trigger an inflammatory response, possibly as a result of persistence of bacterial antigens. However, no one theory of pathogenesis of spondyloarthropathies explains the clinical spectrum of these disorders, and more research is clearly needed to solidify an understanding of their origin.

The complex role of the immune system in the spondyloarthropathies is highlighted by the observation that patients infected with HIV appear more likely to have severe disease, especially psoriatic arthritis. Interestingly, when HIV infection is treated with antiviral agents, the incidence of spondyloarthropathy declines.

Clinical Features

COMMON CLINICAL FEATURES AMONG THE SPONDYLOARTHROPATHIES

As mentioned earlier, the spondyloarthropathies have considerable clinical overlap with one another and are most easily considered as a group of related disorders. Table 79–1 outlines the clinical features of these disorders. Because of the delay in presentation of different clinical manifestations of these chronic diseases, the condition in some patients appears to *evolve* from one type of spondyloarthropathy to another. For example, a patient initially diagnosed with ankylosing spondylitis may subsequently develop inflammatory bowel disease or psoriasis. For this reason, clinicians need to be attuned to possible extra-articular manifestations of disease in patients with spondyloarthropathies.

Spondyloarthropathies are not associated with positive tests for rheumatoid factor, antinuclear antibodies, or any other autoimmune serologies. A family history of spondylitis may be present.

Sacroiliitis and *spondylitis* are the hallmarks of the spondyloarthropathies and are not seen in any other rheumatic diseases. Sacroiliitis may develop in a subtle fashion with low back or gluteal area pain, but it can also cause severe pain. Patients generally have significant morning stiffness, sometimes of many hours' duration, and pain after periods of inactivity. Sacroiliitis may mimic sciatica, with pain radiating into the gluteal and posterior thigh areas. Spondylitis may occur at any area of the spine, but it often progresses first in the lumbar spine and subsequently in the cervical and thoracic regions. The sacroiliac joints and spine become painful and stiff with increasingly reduced range of motion as bony fusion occurs over time. Involvement of the spine and costovertebral joints may result in a restrictive lung physiologic condition. Fusion on the spine increases the risk of vertebral fractures in patients with spondyloarthropathies and, depending on the angle of fusion, may cause significant kyphosis and reduced line of sight. When bony fusion is complete, the pain may be significantly reduced.

Enthesitis may occur in many different anatomic locations. These include spinous processes, costosternal junctions, ischial tuberosities, plantar aponeuroses, and Achilles tendons.

The *peripheral arthritis* of the spondyloarthropathies, when it occurs, begins as an episodic, asymmetrical, oligoarticular process often involving the lower extremities. The arthritis can progress and may become chronic and disabling. A unique feature of spondyloarthropathies is the appearance of fusiform swelling of an entire finger or toe, referred to as *dactylitis* or *sausage digits.*

Uveitis, or inflammatory disease of the anterior chamber of the eye, is a common extra-articular manifestation of the

Table 79–1   Comparison of the Spondyloarthropathies

	Ankylosing Spondylitis	Posturethral Reactive Arthritis	Postdysenteric Reactive Arthritis	Enteropathic Arthritis	Psoriatic Arthritis
Sacroiliitis	+++++	+++	++	+	++
Spondylitis	++++	+++	++	++	++
Peripheral arthritis	+	++++	++++	+++	++++
Articular course	Chronic	Acute or chronic	Acute chronic	Acute or chronic	Chronic
HLA-B27	95%	60%	30%	20%	20%
Enthesopathy	++	++++	+++	++	++
Common extra-articular manifestations	Eye Heart	Eye GU Oral and/or GI Heart	GU Eye	GI Eye	Skin Eye
Other names	Bekhterev's arthritis Marie-Strümpell disease	Reiter's syndrome SARA NGU Chlamydial arthritis	Reiter's syndrome	Crohn's disease Ulcerative colitis	

GI = gastrointestinal; GU = genitourinary; HLA = human leukocyte antigen; NGU = nongonococcal urethritis; SARA = sexually acquired reactive arthritis; + = relative prevalence of a specific feature.
Data from Cush JJ, Lipsky PE: The spondyloarthropathies. In Goldman L, Bennett JC (eds): Cecil Textbook of Medicine, 21st ed. Philadelphia, WB Saunders, 2000, pp 1499–1507.

spondyloarthropathies, especially among patients who are HLA-B27 positive. Bouts of uveitis are usually monocular, acute at onset, painful, and accompanied by eye redness and blurred vision. Recurrent attacks are common. Uveitis may be serious and lead to blindness. Anterior uveitis may be the presenting symptom of spondyloarthropathy; thus all patients with anterior uveitis should be screened for signs and symptoms of these disorders.

Spondyloarthropathies may occasionally involve other organ systems and may cause significant morbidity and mortality. Aortitis, especially occurring in the ascending segment, can result in aortic insufficiency from aortic root dilation, aortic dissection, and cardiac conduction system abnormalities. Pulmonary fibrosis of the apical regions can occur, often in an insidious fashion. Spinal cord compression can result from atlantoaxial joint subluxation, cauda equina syndrome, or vertebral fractures. In rare cases, long-standing spondyloarthropathy is associated with secondary amyloidosis.

SPECIFIC CLINICAL FEATURES OF THE SPONDYLOARTHROPATHIES

Reactive (Reiter's) Arthritis

Among the unique clinical features of reactive (Reiter's) arthritis are *urethritis, conjunctivitis,* and certain dermatologic problems. The urethritis may be secondary to the chlamydial infection that triggers the disease, or it may be a sterile inflammatory discharge also seen in diarrhea-associated disease. Conjunctivitis may be mild in reactive arthritis and is distinct from uveitis. *Keratoderma blennor-rhagicum* is a distinct papulosquamous rash usually found on the palms or soles. *Circinate balanitis* is a rash that may appear on the penile glans or shaft of men with reactive arthritis. Nonpitting *nail thickening* and *oral ulcers* may also occur in patients with reactive arthritis. These lesions can be confused with similar findings in patients with psoriasis and inflammatory bowel disease, respectively.

Psoriatic Arthritis

Five identifiable clinical patterns of psoriatic arthritis are recognized: (1) *distal interphalangeal joint involvement with nail pitting;* (2) *asymmetrical oligoarthropathy* of both large and small joints; (3) *arthritis mutilans,* a severe, destructive arthritis; (4) *symmetrical polyarthritis,* identical to rheumatoid arthritis; and (5) *spondyloarthropathy.* These patterns are not exclusionary, and clinical overlap is significant. Spondylitis or sacroiliitis may occur along with any of the other four patterns. The prevalence of HLA-B27 is increased among the patients with spondylitis or sacroiliitis but not among patients with the other patterns. Little or no temporal association exists between the skin disease and the arthritis in psoriasis, and either can precede the other by many years.

Enteropathic Arthritis (Inflammatory Bowel Disease)

The inflammatory bowel diseases, Crohn's disease, and ulcerative colitis (see also Chapter 37) are frequently associated with both spondyloarthropathy and peripheral arthri-

tis. The peripheral arthritis is typically nonerosive and oligoarticular.

Radiographic Features. The radiographic features of the spondyloarthropathies are highly specific and, in the correct clinical setting, virtually diagnostic of these diseases. These changes progress over many years of illness. Sacroiliitis is usually the earliest radiographic sign of the spondyloarthropathies and results in sclerosis and erosions of the sacroiliac joints with eventual bony fusion (Fig. 79–1A). Bony erosions and osteitis may occur at sites of enthesitis. Many different radiographic changes occur secondary to chronic spinal inflammation, including ossification of the annulus fibrosus, calcification of spinal ligaments, bony sclerosis and *squaring* of vertebral bodies, and ankylosis of apophyseal joints. These changes can lead to vertebral fusion and a bamboo spine appearance (Fig. 79–1B). Magnetic resonance imaging in increasingly being used for research purposes in the spondyloarthropathies because it may provide both diagnostic information and a means of objectively measuring inflammation.

Treatment. No cure has yet been found for any of the spondyloarthropathies, but effective treatment for many of the manifestations is available. *Patient education* regarding the disease is essential and allows for identification of affected family members and early presentation of urgent clinical features such as uveitis. *Physical therapy,* including a daily stretching program, postural adjustments, and strengthening, can be useful in maintaining proper bony alignment, reducing deformities, and maximizing function. Selective use of *orthopedic surgery* may be highly effective in correcting significant spinal deformities or instability.

The most important medical therapy for patients with symptomatic spondylitis and sacroiliitis consists of *nonsteroidal anti-inflammatory drugs* (NSAIDs). NSAIDs can provide significant relief of spinal pain and stiffness, and many patients take these drugs continually for years. No clear evidence indicates that systemic glucocorticoids benefit patients with spondyloarthropathies, and these agents are generally avoided. *Intra-articular glucocorticoid injection* into the sacroiliac or other involved joints may provide temporary relief. Similarly, the role and efficacy of older immunosuppressive agents in the treatment of the axial manifestations of the spondyloarthropathies have not been established. In contrast, the peripheral arthritis of spondyloarthropathies has been shown in clinical trials to improve with *sulfasalazine. Methotrexate* is also regularly used for the peripheral arthritis, but no large clinical trials have been performed with this agent in these diseases.

Tumor necrosis factor (TNF) blockers represent a substantial breakthrough in treatment of the spondyloarthropathies. The efficacy of these agents is now well established, and these drugs have rapidly become the treatment of choice for patients with spondyloarthropathies who do not satisfactorily or fully respond to NSAIDs and physical therapy. TNF blockers can significantly reduce pain, improve function, improve quality of life, and may prevent or slow disease progression and structural damage.

Flares of *uveitis* require care by an ophthalmologist experienced in treating inflammatory eye diseases. Topical or intraocular glucocorticoids may suffice, but systemic therapy with glucocorticoids or immunosuppressive medications

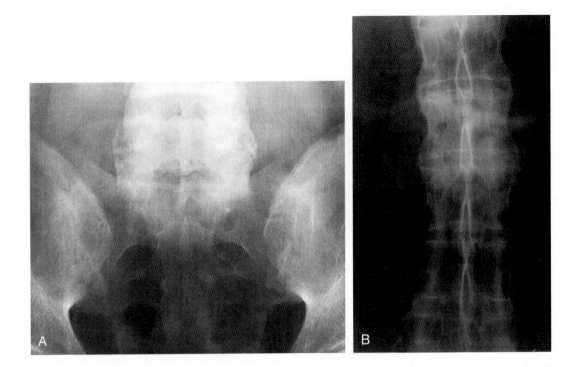

Figure 79–1 *A,* Bilaterally symmetrical sacroiliitis in ankylosing spondylitis. *B,* Lumbar spondylitis in ankylosing spondylitis with symmetrical, marginal bridging syndesmophytes and calcification of the spinal ligament. (From Cush JJ, Lipsky PE: The spondyloarthropathies. In Goldman L, Bennett JC [eds]: Cecil Textbook of Medicine, 21st ed. Philadelphia, WB Saunders, 2000, pp 1499–1507.)

may be necessary to control the inflammation and prevent permanent visual loss.

Specific types of spondyloarthropathy may require different therapies, including that for the underlying associated disease. Evaluation and treatment for *C. trachomatis* and associated sexually transmitted diseases in patients with reactive arthritis and their sex partners are essential. Aggres-

sive medical therapy for the more disabling and destructive forms of psoriatic arthritis is often prescribed in a manner similar to that used for patients with rheumatoid arthritis. Immunosuppressive therapy for the skin disease may also help the arthritis of patients with psoriasis. Treatments for the gastrointestinal manifestations of inflammatory bowel disease may also be beneficial for the rheumatic symptoms.

Prospectus for the Future

- Increased insights into the immunogenetics of the spondyloarthropathies may lead to greater understanding of the pathophysiologic features of these diseases.
- Further research on the use of biologic agents, especially anti-tumor necrosis-α products, in the treatment of spondy-

loarthropathies may help determine whether the structural and functional deterioration these diseases often cause can be prevented with long-term therapy.

References

Arnett FC: Seronegative spondyloarthropathies: B. Reactive arthritis (Reiter's syndrome) and enteropathic arthritis. In Klippel JH (ed): Primer of the Rheumatic Diseases, 12th ed. Atlanta, Arthritis Foundation, 2001, pp 245–250.

Boumpas DT, Illei GG, Tassiulas IO: Psoriatic arthritis. In Klippel JH (ed): Primer of the Rheumatic Diseases, 12th ed. Atlanta, Arthritis Foundation, 2001, pp 233–238.

Cush JJ, Lipsky PE: The spondyloarthropathies. In Goldman L, Bennett JC (eds): Cecil Textbook of Medicine, 21st ed. Philadelphia, WB Saunders, 2000, pp 1499–1507.

Inman RD: Seronegative spondyloarthropathies: D. Treatment. In Klippel JH (ed): Primer of the Rheumatic Diseases, 12th ed. Atlanta, Arthritis Foundation, 2001, pp 255–258.

Keat A: Seronegative spondyloarthropathies: C. Ankylosing spondylitis. In Klippel JH (ed): Primer of the Rheumatic Diseases, 12th ed. Atlanta, Arthritis Foundation, 2001, pp 255–258.

Khan MA: Update on spondyloarthropathies. Ann Intern Med 136:896–907, 2002.

Mease PJ: Psoriatic arthritis therapy advances. Curr Opin Rheumatol 17:426–432, 2005.

Reveille JD: Seronegative spondyloarthropathies: A. Epidemiology, pathology, and pathogenesis. In Klippel JH (ed): Primer of the Rheumatic Diseases, 12th ed. Atlanta, Arthritis Foundation, 1997, pp 239–245.

Zochling J, Braun J: Management and treatment of ankylosing spondylitis. Curr Opin Rheumatol 17:418–425, 2005.

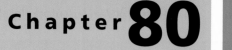

Systemic Lupus Erythematosus

Peter A. Merkel

Systemic lupus erythematosus (SLE, lupus) is a multisystem autoimmune disorder of unknown cause and is strongly associated with various autoantibodies. The clinical course of SLE is characterized by periods of both active disease and remission, with manifestations ranging from mild dermatologic and joint symptoms to life-threatening internal organ failure and cytopenias. The diagnosis is based on a combination of clinical and laboratory findings, and certain clinical subsets have been identified.

SLE can occur at any age, in children and older adults; it can strike both sexes and is found in all ethnic and racial groups. However, it is more common among women and is both more common and often more severe among blacks and Hispanics. The most common age at first presentation is in the second, third, or fourth decade.

Pathogenesis

Although the origin of SLE is not yet known, increasing evidence indicates that it is caused, or at least influenced, by a combination of genetic, immunologic, hormonal, and possibly environmental factors. Both large population studies and animal models of SLE have increased the understanding of disease pathogenesis. The genetic contribution to SLE has been demonstrated in studies of specific ethnicities, families, twin cohorts, and other groups. Certain genes related to the human leukocyte antigen system, various other immune markers, and specific proteins have all been considered possible candidate genes associated with SLE. Many different immune abnormalities have been noted in patients with SLE, a finding implicating dysregulation of both the humoral and cellular immune systems in the pathogenesis of the disease. The established roles of immune complex formation and abnormalities in the complement system in certain manifestations of SLE also support an immunologic origin for SLE. Hormonal influences on SLE are indicated by the

striking differences in disease prevalence between men and women, as well as the variances in disease activity with pregnancy and other physiologic states of sex hormonal changes. Finally, various environmental agents, including microorganisms, may influence lupus activity and may possibly explain observed geographic clustering of cases.

Clinical Manifestations

Virtually any organ system may be involved in SLE, often in multiple ways. Table 80–1 outlines many but not all of the clinical manifestations of SLE. The prognosis for patients with SLE ranges from a chronic, smoldering disease with relatively minor problems to a rapidly progressive, life-threatening illness and early mortality. Among the manifestations that result in critical illness in patients with SLE are lupus nephritis, lupus cerebritis, pulmonary hemorrhage, and small-vessel vasculitis of major organs such as the mesentery or brain. *Lupus nephritis* refers to a spectrum of glomerulopathies that range from minor focal scarring to diffuse proliferative destruction of glomeruli with active inflammation and immune complex deposition. Both the renal disorder and the clinical syndromes are usually classified according to the World Health Organization classification system for renal disease in SLE. This system includes six classes of disorder ranging from normal tissue (class I) to advanced sclerosing glomerulonephritis (class VI). Class V refers to diffuse membranous glomerulopathy, a distinct nephritic syndrome that can be present either in isolation or in conjunction with the other classes. *Lupus cerebritis* is a vague term encompassing a variety of central neurologic deficits, including psychosis, seizures, and coma. The more subtle cognitive and psychologic manifestations of SLE are areas of active current clinical research and should not be overlooked when physicians treat patients. Lupus nephritis, cerebritis, and vasculitis can all develop insidiously and may

Table 80–1 Clinical Manifestations of Systemic Lupus Erythematosus

Systemic and Miscellaneous

Fever
Malaise and/or fatigue
Lymphadenopathy
Recurrent spontaneous abortions
Premature fetal delivery

Vascular

Raynaud's phenomenon
Arterial or venous thrombosis
Vasculitis (almost any location)
Livedo reticularis

Dermatologic

Malar (butterfly) rash*
Discoid lesions*
Photosensitivity*
Oral, genital, nasal ulcers*
Maculopapular rash
Panniculitis
Alopecia
Subacute cutaneous lupus
Urticaria

Renal

Cellular casts or glomerulonephritis*
Proteinuria or membranous nephropathy or nephrotic syndrome*

Gastrointestinal

Pancreatitis
Lupus enteropathy
Peritoneal serositis
Hepatitis and/or hepatomegaly

Serologic Abnormalities

Autoantibodies*
Hypocomplementemia
Elevated acute phase reactants

Hematologic

Hemolytic anemia*
Nonhemolytic anemia
Leukopenia*
Lymphopenia*
Thrombocytopenia*

Musculoskeletal

Arthritis*
Arthralgias
Avascular necrosis
Myositis

Neurologic

Psychosis*
Seizures*
Depression
Cognitive impairment
Headache
Cerebritis
Transverse myelitis
Peripheral neuropathy
Episcleritis or scleritis

Cardiac

Pericarditis*
Myositis
Libman-Sacks endocarditis

Pulmonary

Pleuritis*
Alveolar hemorrhage
Pulmonary hypertension
Shrinking lung syndrome
Interstitial lung disease
Pulmonary emboli

*An item in the American College of Rheumatology diagnostic criteria.

be in advanced stages by the time they become clinically apparent. *Pulmonary hemorrhage* is a rare and potentially catastrophic manifestation of SLE that may result in fulminant hemoptysis and respiratory failure. The *arthritis* of lupus is usually nonerosive, but it can result in significant joint laxity and disability. The *skin manifestations* of SLE are protean and can cause permanent scarring and disfigurement that can be personally devastating to patients. Common cutaneous features of SLE include the classic malar (*butterfly*) rash, discoid lesions, alopecia, photosensitivity, and urticaria.

Pregnancy presents unique problems for patients with SLE. Women with SLE may have severe disease flares during pregnancy. Similarly, underlying organ damage or medications for SLE can cause or worsen maternal pregnancy-related complications. The rates of spontaneous abortions

and fetal prematurity are significantly higher among pregnant women with SLE, and many of these miscarriages are associated with antiphospholipid antibodies (see Chapter 81).

Various *autoantibodies* are found in patients with SLE and are the hallmark laboratory features of the disease (Table 80–2). Virtually all patients with SLE (99%) test positive for antinuclear antibodies when a sensitive assay is used. Although many of the specific antigens to which these antinuclear antibodies are directed have been determined and are useful both diagnostically and clinically in SLE, some antibodies are also seen in other autoimmune diseases. Antibodies to double-stranded DNA and the Smith (Sm) antigen are highly specific for lupus, whereas antibodies to Ro and La antigens are also commonly found in patients with rheumatoid arthritis and are especially common in patients

Table 80–2 **Autoantibodies in Patients with Systemic Lupus Erythematosus***

Test	Sensitivity (%)	Specificity (%)	Predictive Value (%)
ANA	99	80	15–35
dsDNA	70	95	95
ssDNA	80	50	50
Histone	30–80	Moderate	Moderate
Nucleoprotein	58	Moderate	Moderate
Sm	25	99	97
RNP (U1-RNP)	50	87–94	46–85
Ro/SS-A antigen	25–35		
La/SS-B antigen	15		
PCNA	5	95	95

Data from Schur PH: System lupus erythematosus. In Bennett JC, Plum F (eds): Cecil Textbook of Medicine, 21st ed. Philadelphia, WB Saunders, 2000, p 1511.
*Cytoplasm: mitochondria, lysosomes, microsomes, ribosomes. RNA: dsRNA, ssRNA, rRNA. Cell membranes: red blood cells, white blood (T and B) cells, platelets, brain. Other: clotting factors (APL), thyroid, rheumatoid factors, BFP-STS. In SLE, anti-DNA and anti-Sm are associated with renal disease, anti-RNP with Raynaud's disease, and anti-Ro with photosensitivity. Anti-RNP is observed in SLE, rheumatoid arthritis, scleroderma, Sjögren's syndrome, and mixed connective tissue disorders. Anti-Ro (SS-A) is seen in SLE, Sjögren's syndrome, primary photosensitivity, and primary biliary cirrhosis. Anti-La (SS-B) is seen in SLE and Sjögren's syndrome.
ANA = antinuclear antibodies; dsDNA = double-stranded DNA; PCNA = proliferating cell nuclear antigen; RNP = ribonuclear protein; Sm = Smith; ssDNA = single-stranded DNA.

with Sjögren's syndrome. Certain antibodies are associated with specific clinical manifestations of disease. For example, many patients with lupus nephritis have anti–double-stranded DNA antibodies. The relationship between antibodies to ribosomal P or neuronal antigens and lupus cerebritis is still under investigation. Autoantibodies alone are not diagnostic for any autoimmune disease but must be interpreted in the clinical context.

SLE is a clinical diagnosis; no one test or feature is fully diagnostic of the disease. Further, many patients' clinical syndromes *evolve* over time, and only after several years are they recognized as having SLE. To classify patients with SLE more accurately and reproducibly for research purposes, an internationally accepted set of diagnostic criteria was developed (Table 80–3). By design, the diagnostic specificity of these criteria is high, to ensure that all subjects enrolled in research studies truly have SLE. However, although these criteria are valuable for practicing clinicians, patients may have clinical lupus without meeting the criteria. More than one half of the manifestations listed in Table 80–1 are not part of the criteria.

Patients with SLE may exhibit all the features of the *antiphospholipid antibody syndrome,* including multiple thromboses, thrombocytopenia, and recurrent spontaneous miscarriages. Chapter 81 provides details on the antiphospholipid antibody syndrome.

Patients with SLE may also have *secondary Sjögren's syndrome* and may have xerophthalmia, xerosis, and other clinical features of this disease. Chapter 84 provides details on Sjögren's syndrome.

Increasing recognition suggests that patients with SLE are at significantly increased risk for premature atherosclerosis, a disease manifestation that is multifactorial but likely especially related to persistent inflammation. Screening and treating reversible risk factors for coronary disease is now part of the standard of care of patients with SLE.

Clinical Subsets

OVERLAP SYNDROME

Some patients with symptoms consistent with autoimmune disease do not readily fit one diagnosis and have clinical and laboratory features of two or more specific diseases such as SLE, rheumatoid arthritis, Sjögren's syndrome, scleroderma, or inflammatory myositis. Such patients may be considered to have an *overlap syndrome.* For example, patients with erosive arthritis, skin features of lupus, and positive tests for both rheumatoid factor and antibodies to Sm antigen may be referred to as having *rhupus* or an overlap between rheumatoid arthritis and lupus. Similarly, overlaps among scleroderma, lupus, and the myositides are common, with *mixed connective tissue disease* one of several clinical patterns described. Another intriguing overlap disorder is *lupus-sclerosis,* a term used to describe patients with features of both lupus and multiple sclerosis, another idiopathic autoimmune disorder. Autoimmune serologic components may be helpful both diagnostically and prognostically in evaluating patients with these syndromes. Patients with overlap disease are often monitored for development of new features of the *parent* disorders.

DRUG-INDUCED LUPUS ERYTHEMATOSUS

Certain medications may induce a lupus-like syndrome referred to as *drug-induced lupus erythematosus* (DILE). DILE is generally a milder form of SLE with arthritis, serositis, and constitutional symptoms common, whereas renal or central nervous system involvement is rare. The most common and well-studied medications associated with DILE are procainamide and hydralazine, but many other drugs have been implicated, including anticonvulsants,

Table 80–3 Criteria for Classification of Systemic Lupus Erythematosus*

Criterion	Definition
1. Malar rash	Fixed erythema, flat or raised, is observed over the malar eminences, tending to spare the nasolabial folds.
2. Discoid rash	Erythematous raised patches develop with adherent keratotic scaling and follicular plugging; atrophic scarring may occur in older lesions.
3. Photosensitivity	Skin rash occurs as a result of unusual reaction to sunlight by patient history or physician observation.
4. Oral ulcers	Oral or nasopharyngeal ulceration, usually painless, is observed by the physician.
5. Arthritis	Nonerosive arthritis involves two or more peripheral joints, characterized by tenderness, swelling, or effusion.
6. Serositis	a. Pleuritis: Convincing history of pleuritic pain exists or rub is heard by a physician or pleural effusion is in evidence. OR b. Pericarditis: Is documented by electrocardiogram or rub or evidence of pericardial effusion.
7. Renal disorder	a. Persistent proteinuria is >0.5 g/day or >3+ if quantitation is not performed. OR b. Cellular casts: May be red cell, hemoglobin, granular, tubular, or mixed.
8. Neurologic disorder	a. Seizures: Occurs in the absence of offending drugs or known metabolic derangements (e.g., uremia, ketoacidosis, electrolyte imbalance) OR b. Psychosis: Occurs in the absence of offending drugs or known metabolic derangements (e.g., uremia, ketoacidosis, electrolyte imbalance)
9. Hematologic disorder	a. Hemolytic anemia: Develops with reticulocytosis. OR b. Leukopenia: <4000/mm^3 total is documented on two or more occasions. OR c. Lymphopenia: <1500/mm^3 is documented on two or more occasions. OR d. Thrombocytopenia: <100,000/mm^3 develops in the absence of offending drugs.
10. Immunologic disorder	a. Anti-DNA: Antibody to native DNA in abnormal titer. OR b. Anti-Sm: Presence of antibody to Sm nuclear antigen. OR c. Positive finding of antiphospholipid antibodies is based on (1) an abnormal serum level of IgG or IgM anticardiolipin antibodies, (2) a positive-test result for lupus anticoagulant using a standard method, or (3) a false-positive serologic test for syphilis is known to be positive for at least 6 months and is confirmed by *Treponema pallidum* immobilization or fluorescent treponemal antibody absorption test.
11. Antinuclear antibody	An abnormal titer of antinuclear antibody is documented by immunofluorescence or an equivalent assay at any point in time and in the absence of drugs known to be associated with drug-induced lupus syndrome.

Adapted from Schur PH: Systemic lupus erythematosus. In Bennett JC, Plum F (eds): Cecil Textbook of Medicine, 20th ed. Philadelphia, WB Saunders, 1996; and Hochberg MC: Updating the American College of Rheumatology Revised Criteria for the Classification of Systemic Lupus Erythematosus. Arthritis Rheum 40:1725, 1997.
*The classification is based on 11 criteria. For the purpose of identifying patients in clinical studies, a person shall be said to have SLE if any 4 or more of the 11 criteria are present, serially or simultaneously, during any interval of observation.
IgG = immunoglobulin G; IgM = immunoglobulin M.

β-blockers, antimicrobials, and some tumor necrosis factor blockers; new drugs continue to be implicated in DILE. Although these drugs may induce antinuclear antibodies in some patients, only a subset of these patients will actually develop clinical DILE. Although antibodies to histones are found in up to 90% of patients with DILE, only rarely are patients found to have antibodies to double-stranded DNA or other lupus-related antigens. DILE is reversible on drug discontinuation.

NEONATAL LUPUS ERYTHEMATOSUS

Neonatal lupus erythematosus is a rare disorder that exclusively affects some children born to mothers with maternal anti-Ro or anti-La antibodies. These antibodies pass through the placenta and are involved in disease causation. Manifestations include transient rashes, thrombocytopenia, hemolytic anemia, and, the most serious problem, permanent complete heart block. Although the dermatologic and hematologic problems are transient and readily treatable, the conduction system abnormalities are often permanent and are associated with high intrauterine and peripartum mortality. Fewer than 5% of children born to Ro-positive and/or La-positive women will have neonatal lupus erythematosus. The mothers of affected children do not necessarily have SLE or another autoimmune disease themselves. However, some of these women who have no obvious signs or symptoms of SLE will exhibit manifestations years later with a more definable autoimmune disease.

Treatment

No cure for lupus has yet been found, and treatment is aimed at reducing inflammation, suppressing the immune system, and closely clinically monitoring patients to identify disease features as early as possible. Treatment with glucocorticoids and immunosuppressive agents has reduced both the morbidity and the mortality of patients with SLE, although these treatments themselves are associated with extensive toxicity. Many cases of SLE are mild and remain so for the life of the patient. Thus the physician must carefully weigh the benefits of therapy against the known risks of treatment, especially long-term therapy.

Patient education and *prophylactic measures* to prevent disease flares are central to the care of patients with lupus. Sunscreens and protective clothing are effective in avoiding photosensitivity reactions. The use of estrogen-containing oral contraceptives is controversial in SLE, but many centers avoid these medications because of evidence that they are associated with an increase in lupus activity. Protective or warm clothing and avoidance of vasoconstrictive drugs are helpful in treating Raynaud's phenomenon in SLE, and these patients may also benefit from vasodilator therapy. *Low-dose aspirin* is frequently prescribed for patients with positive antiphospholipid antibodies to prevent thrombotic events, but evidence supporting the efficacy of this practice is lacking. Other treatments for antiphospholipid antibody syndrome are discussed in Chapter 81. *Psychological support* is essential for patients with SLE because this chronic disease may cause depression and anxiety in many patients. *Routine immunizations,* such as for influenza and pneumococcus, are recommended in all patients.

Although nonsteroidal anti-inflammatory medications are used for mild arthralgias, *glucocorticoids* remain the main anti-inflammatory agents for SLE. Glucocorticoids are used for almost all manifestations of lupus in doses ranging from extremely small alternate-day doses to huge pulsed intravenous doses. Although glucocorticoids are often effective for lupus, the chronic nature of the disease may lead to prolonged use of these medications and extensive toxicity, including obesity, diabetes mellitus, accelerated atherosclerosis, osteoporosis, avascular necrosis, cataracts, glaucoma, and increased risk of infections. To avoid such toxicities, different immunomodulating agents are used to provide a steroid-sparing effect. In addition, some manifestations, such as nephritis and severe vasculitis, are only partially responsive to glucocorticoids and require other immunosuppressive agents for greater disease control.

Antimalarial medications have been found to be effective agents in SLE and are an important part of treatment for many patients. Hydroxychloroquine and chloroquine are especially effective for the fevers, arthritis, and mucocutaneous manifestations of SLE. Many patients take one of these drugs on a long-term basis because investigators have demonstrated that patients who discontinue the medications, even if they are asymptomatic at the time, experience significantly more flares than do patients who continue the medications. Although retinal toxicity is not common, it is dose dependent; the extent of routine ophthalmologic screening required for patients taking these drugs is controversial, but it is at most biannual.

Azathioprine is an immunosuppressive agent prescribed in patients with lupus either when glucocorticoids alone are not fully effective or to allow for a reduction in the glucocorticoid dose. Toxicities of azathioprine include leukopenia, anemia, and an increased risk of infection. An area of ongoing controversy is whether prolonged use of this drug poses an increased risk of hematologic malignant disease.

Mycophenolate mofetil is an immunosuppressive agent now increasingly being used for treating patients with lupus, including for nephritis. This drug is highly successful in regimens to prevent solid organ transplant rejection and is increasingly replacing azathioprine for this purpose because of its higher efficacy and high tolerability. Toxicity of mycophenolate mofetil includes gastrointestinal disturbance and leukopenia. Several clinical trials have demonstrated the efficacy of mycophenolate for lupus nephritis and, although long-term follow-up data is lacking, mycophenolate mofetil is now regularly prescribed as a first-line agent for lupus nephritis.

Cyclophosphamide is the most potent immunosuppressive agent used to treat SLE. However, because this drug is extremely toxic, especially with long-term use, it is usually reserved for the most severe disease manifestations of lupus. In a series of studies, mostly conducted at the National Institutes of Health, cyclophosphamide by monthly intravenous administration was effective in reducing the rate of progression of lupus nephritis to end-stage renal disease. Patients with severe lupus cerebritis or small-vessel necrotizing vasculitis are often treated with cyclophosphamide, although extensive trials or even case series demonstrating the efficacy of this approach are lacking. Acute toxicities of cyclophosphamide include pancytopenia, alopecia, mucositis, and hemorrhagic cystitis. Long-term use of cyclophosphamide may lead to transitional cell carcinoma, hematologic malignant disease, sterility, premature menopause, and opportunistic infections.

Many other treatments have been suggested for SLE, most of which try to manipulate the immune response in some manner. *Intravenous immunoglobulin* is effective for the thrombocytopenia of SLE but is less well established for other indications. Trials of *plasmapheresis* in lupus nephritis have failed to demonstrate any efficacy, although this therapy continues to be studied for this indication. *Methotrexate* is prescribed for patients with lupus, especially for treatment of arthritis, although no clinical trials have been performed for this medication in SLE. The results of trials of immunoablation with high-dose chemotherapy with or without autologous stem-cell transplant have been disappointing in treating patients with SLE. Investigators have shown long-standing interest in hormonal therapy for SLE, but no consistent effect of such agents has been demonstrated.

Great potential and optimism exist for *"biologic" immunomodulating agents* produced by the biotechnology industry to provide new, effective treatments for SLE. Drugs that block the action of cytokines, complement, and immune cellular functioning are all being investigated in clinical trials. The most promising current biologic agents are those that deplete B cells, particularly rituximab. Several trials are ongoing, testing the efficacy of rituximab for both SLE and lupus nephritis.

Prospectus for the Future

- Advances in the understanding of the immunopathologic features of SLE, providing a logical framework for specific targeting and testing of new biologic therapies
- Increased understanding of the scope and pathologic characteristics of central nervous system disease in SLE
- Clinical trial data to evaluate the efficacy of new biologic agents for the treatment of SLE

References

Buyon JP: Systemic lupus erythematosus: B. Clinical and laboratory features. In Klippel JH (ed): Primer of the Rheumatic Diseases, 12th ed. Atlanta, Arthritis Foundation, 2001, pp 335–346.

Ginzler EM, Dooley MA, Aranow C, et al: Mycophenolate mofetil or intravenous cyclophosphamide for lupus nephritis. N Engl J Med 353:2219–2228, 2005.

Hochberg MC: Updating the American College of Rheumatology Revised Criteria for the Classification of Systemic Lupus Erythematosus. Arthritis Rheum 40:1725, 1997.

Manzi S: Systemic lupus erythematosus: C. Treatment. In Klippel JH (ed): Primer of the Rheumatic Diseases, 12th ed. Atlanta, Arthritis Foundation, 2001, pp 346–352.

Pisetsky DS: Systemic lupus erythematosus: A. Epidemiology, pathology, and pathogenesis. In Klippel JH (ed): Primer of the Rheumatic Diseases, 12th ed. Atlanta, Arthritis Foundation, 2001, pp 329–335.

Schur PH: Systemic lupus erythematosus. In Goldman L, Bennett JC (eds): Cecil Textbook of Medicine, 21st ed. Philadelphia, WB Saunders, 2000, pp 1509–1517.

Sfikakis PP, Boletis, MN, Tsokos GC: Rituximab anti-B-cell therapy in systemic lupus erythematosus: pointing to the future. Curr Opin Rheumatol 17:511–512, 2005.

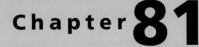

Antiphospholipid Antibody Syndrome

Peter A. Merkel

Antiphospholipid antibody syndrome (APS) is a disorder characterized by any or all of the following three manifestations in the setting of positive tests for antiphospholipid antibodies: (1) recurrent arterial and/or venous thromboses, (2) thrombocytopenia, or (3) recurrent spontaneous abortions. Because APS is a relatively newly described syndrome, the full clinical spectrum is still being defined, and well-accepted diagnostic criteria do not yet exist.

APS is considered *secondary* if it occurs in conjunction with systemic lupus erythematosus (SLE, lupus) or another autoimmune disease and *primary* if it occurs in isolation. The discovery of *antiphospholipid antibodies* and of their clinical associations has improved the understanding of the clinical spectrum of SLE because each manifestation of APS can be seen in SLE (see Chapter 80). The false-positive test results for syphilis found in many patients with SLE are actually caused by antiphospholipid antibodies. In recognition of the importance of these antibodies, the American College of Rheumatology revised the diagnostic criteria for SLE in 1997 to include antiphospholipid antibodies.

Etiologic Factors

Animal studies suggest that antiphospholipid antibodies are directly pathogenic, but the exact mechanism of action is not known. The likely existence of other co-factors for the development of APS could explain why only a subset of people who produce antiphospholipid antibodies eventually exhibit manifestations of APS. Among the more thoroughly studied co-factors for APS is β_2-glycoprotein.

Clinical Features

The clinical features of APS are outlined in Table 81–1. The list of clinical associations with APS continues to grow beyond the original three cardinal manifestations of thrombosis, thrombocytopenia, and recurrent spontaneous abortions. Increasingly, *microthrombotic* disease is being recognized as a manifestation of APS; for example, renal failure may occur as a result of microthrombosis and renal artery thrombosis. A renal biopsy may be necessary to differentiate APS from lupus or other renal pathologic conditions. The association of APS with SLE and the varied sequelae of arterial thromboses, such as strokes, make the assignment of disorders to APS difficult. The term *catastrophic APS* has been coined to describe patients who exhibit multiple thromboses, positive antiphospholipid antibodies, and often a life-threatening illness.

Diagnosis

Combining clinical features with laboratory evidence of antiphospholipid antibodies contributes to the diagnosis of APS. Most authorities agree that the diagnosis should not be made unless at least one of the major features of APS is present. In addition, the patient should repeatedly test positive for either anticardiolipin antibodies or the lupus anticoagulant, and alternative diagnoses must be eliminated. Patients with APS should be screened for possible concomitant SLE or other autoimmune diseases.

Laboratory testing for antiphospholipid antibodies is complex and can be confusing or misunderstood. Although several types of antiphospholipid antibodies are recognized, the two that are used clinically to establish the diagnosis are *anticardiolipin antibodies* and the *lupus anticoagulant*. Lupus anticoagulant is a misnomer that reflects the early observation that it can result in a prolonged partial thromboplastin time. Various methods are used to test for the lupus anticoagulant. The partial thromboplastin time test is *not* a screen for the lupus anticoagulant. When patients are screened for

Table 81–1	**Clinical Features of Antiphospholipid Antibody Syndrome**

Definite Features

Arterial thrombosis
Venous thrombosis
Thrombocytopenia
Recurrent pregnancy loss

Possible and/or Probable Features

Hemolytic anemia
Livedo reticularis
Skin ulcers
Chorea
Transverse myelitis
Vasculitis
Cardiac valvular abnormalities
Other direct manifestations of thrombosis

APS, they should be tested for both anticardiolipin antibodies and the lupus anticoagulant. Further, patients with APS should repeatedly demonstrate positive results for these tests—at a minimum of two points of time, 6 or more weeks apart.

Treatment

Currently, neither a cure for APS nor a single treatment for all its manifestations exists. Rather, treatment is specific to each aspect of APS. For patients with demonstrated hypercoagulability, indefinite anticoagulation is usually prescribed as prophylaxis against recurrence. Warfarin is the usual drug of choice, with the international normalized ratio (INR) often kept in the upper range for anticoagulation (i.e., INR = 3.0 to 4.5). Heparin is also an effective anticoagulant for patients with APS with both unfractionated and low–molecular-weight preparations of heparin used.

The thrombocytopenia of APS does not often need treatment, but it usually responds to glucocorticoids. Intravenous immunoglobulin, danazol, splenectomy, and immunosuppressive agents have also been used for this indication. The approach to treatment of thrombocytopenia in APS is similar to that of idiopathic thrombocytopenic purpura.

The rate of recurrent pregnancy loss in APS has been shown to be significantly reduced after treatment with low-dose aspirin in combination with either heparin or glucocorticoids, with heparin usually the favored option. Although immunosuppression with cyclophosphamide and plasmapheresis has been used for thrombosis in APS and in catastrophic APS, no consensus exists on the use of such regimens.

Prospectus for the Future

- Large cohort studies may provide data for better risk stratification and targeted prophylactic therapy.

- Newer antithrombotic agents may find a role in the treatment of patients with APS.

References

Asherson RA, Cervera R, Piette JC, et al: Catastrophic antiphospholipid syndrome: Clues to the pathogenesis from a series of 80 patients. Medicine (Baltimore) 80:355–377, 2001.

Cervera R, Piette JC, Font J, et al: Antiphospholipid syndrome: Clinical and immunologic manifestations and patterns of disease expression in a cohort of 1,000 patients. Arthritis Rheum 46:1019–1027, 2002.

Harris EN: Antiphospholipid syndrome. In Klippel JH (ed): Primer of the Rheumatic Diseases, 12th ed. Atlanta, Arthritis Foundation, 2001, pp 423–426.

Hochberg MC: Updating the American College of Rheumatology Revised Criteria for the Classification of Systemic Lupus Erythematosus. Arthritis Rheum 40:1725, 1997.

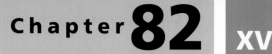

Systemic Sclerosis (Scleroderma)

Robert W. Simms

Peter A. Merkel

Systemic sclerosis (SSc) is a disease characterized by cutaneous and visceral fibrosis, vascular dysfunction (most prominently Raynaud's phenomenon), and immune activation. The term *scleroderma* (thick skin) highlights the most obvious feature of the disorder and is often used synonymously. However, although cutaneous changes can be widespread and disabling, visceral and vascular manifestations are, in most cases, more serious and are the major causes of mortality. These features include inflammatory interstitial lung disease leading to fibrosis, myocardial fibrosis and conduction abnormalities, pulmonary hypertension, renovascular disease, intestinal hypomotility and severe gastroesophageal reflux, as well as digital ischemia, infection, and infarction.

Epidemiologic Factors and Genetics

SSc has an annual incidence of 10 to 20 cases per million and a prevalence that is approximately 10-fold greater. The disease is threefold to fourfold more common in women. Onset before the third decade is unusual, and incidence rises slowly through the fourth through seventh decades of life. Familial occurrence is unusual, and twin studies suggest a mixture of genetic and environmental factors. However, multiple different autoimmune rheumatic diseases may occur in the same family, such as an index case with SSc, a mother with systemic lupus erythematosus (SLE, lupus), and an aunt with rheumatoid arthritis.

Pathologic and Pathophysiologic Considerations

The pathogenesis of scleroderma has three noteworthy aspects: (1) metabolic defect in fibroblast metabolism leading to the overproduction of collagen and other matrix proteins, (2) vascular injury and obliteration, and (3) immune cell activation and autoimmunity (Fig. 82–1). Pathologic examination reflects these processes. In the skin a significant increase in connective tissue matrix is evident with the replacement of subcutaneous fat and secondary skin appendages such as hair follicles and sweat and sebaceous glands. The patient has infiltrates of activated mononuclear cells, T lymphocytes, and monocytes in the dermis. Endothelial damage is probably an early event in SSc. This sign leads at first to functional alterations in blood vessels and subsequent structural disease. Blood vessels in the skin, kidney, heart, and elsewhere demonstrate endothelial cell and smooth muscle cell proliferation, which leads to intimal occlusion, medial thinning, and perivascular cuffing with connective tissue. No vasculitis (i.e., inflammation within the blood vessel wall) exists, per se, and the process has been called *vasculopathy*. In the blood, evidence of immune activation exists, with increased levels of circulating cytokines and T-cell receptor molecules. Finally, autoantibodies are directed at nuclear antigens, including species of antinuclear antibodies that show high specificity for SSc (see later discussion) but with a role in pathogenesis that is not yet established.

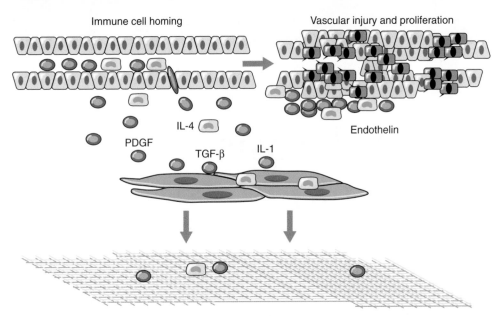

Figure 82–1 Pathogenetic processes in systemic sclerosis. Vascular injury leads to intimal proliferation of both endothelial cells *(in red)* and smooth muscle cells *(in blue)*. Fibroblasts are activated to deposit increased amounts of interstitial matrix. IL = interleukin; PDGF = platelet-derived growth factor; TGF-β = transforming growth factor-β.

Table 82–1	**Clinical Features of Systemic Sclerosis**	
	Diffuse Scleroderma	**Limited Scleroderma**
Skin induration	Widespread; extremities, trunk, face	Fingers, toes, face
Raynaud's phenomenon	80%–90%; ischemia, digital ulcers	95%–100%; ischemia, digital ulcers
Telangiectasia	Common	May be extensive
Calcinosis	Common	Common
Esophageal hypomotility and reflux	80%–90%, may be severe; strictures	90%; may be severe
Malabsorption, intestinal hypomotility	Common, may be severe	Less common, not usually severe
Interstitial lung disease	Common, major cause of death	Uncommon, rarely severe
Pulmonary hypertension	Secondary to pulmonary fibrosis; primary type uncommon	3%–5%; primary type
Cardiac fibrosis, cardiomyopathy	Common	Secondary to pulmonary hypertension
Renal disease	Vasculopathy, renal infarcts	None
Myositis	May be severe	None
Tendon friction rubs	Common	None
Antinuclear antibodies	Common	Common
	30%–40% antitopoisomerase I	50% anticentromere
	5%–10% anticentromere antibodies to RNA polymerase	10% antitopoisomerase

The relationship among vascular, connective tissue, and immune events is unclear. Although immune cells can stimulate fibrosis, fibroblasts from scleroderma-involved skin display abnormalities in connective tissue metabolism even ex vivo, a property that does not depend on continued immune stimulation. The origin of vascular injury is unclear but may include T-cell factors and free radicals. Vascular injury and tissue hypoxia, in turn, may contribute to fibrosis.

Clinical Features

The two distinct subsets of SSc are limited cutaneous SSc (lcSSc) and diffuse cutaneous SSc (dcSSc). Although these entities are identified based on the extent of cutaneous involvement, classification also implies patterns of visceral disease (Table 82–1). Patients with lcSSc, also called *limited scleroderma,* have skin thickening limited to the distal extremities, usually just the fingers and toes and the face. Dermal fibrosis is accompanied by the loss of subcutaneous fat and the atrophy of the overlying epidermis. The result is thickened skin tightly tethered to the underlying fascia. The skin thickening leads to the loss of joint mobility and the development of contractures, as well as decreased pliability of skin in other locations. Replacement of secondary skin structures with fibrosis leads to a loss of hair and sweat glands; the dry skin is prone to fissures and infection.

Raynaud's phenomenon is a triphasic vascular response to cold exposure consisting of pallor, cyanosis, and reactive hyperemia. It is present in more than 90% of patients with scleroderma and may precede other manifestations by years. Raynaud's phenomenon may be severe enough to cause digital ulcerations, ischemia, and infarction. Other vascular features include telangiectasia of the face, hands, and chest; intestinal telangiectasia that may cause bleeding; and dilated nail-fold capillaries. Esophageal hypomotility may lead to dysphagia, and decreased lower esophageal sphincter pressure causes severe gastroesophageal reflux with resultant heartburn and even esophageal ulcers and stricture. The acronym CREST (cutaneous calcinosis, Raynaud's phenomenon, esophageal dysmotility, sclerodactyly, and telangiectasia) has been used to describe this subgroup and highlights the cardinal clinical manifestations. Pulmonary hypertension is a late complication that seriously affects up to approximately 15% of patients with lcSSc and resembles primary pulmonary hypertension. Obliterative disease of the pulmonary vascular tree occurs with interstitial lung disease. The onset is insidious, and patients may have few symptoms until vascular disease is well advanced; lcSSc is the leading cause of death in patients with limited scleroderma.

Patients with *diffuse skin disease* (dcSSc) generally experience rapid and progressive symmetrical induration of the skin of the extremities, face, and trunk. Visceral organ involvement is common, with renovascular disease, interstitial inflammatory lung disease, and cardiac involvement the most serious. Renal involvement commonly appears as severe hypertension, often abrupt in onset, with proteinuria, microangiopathy, and rapidly progressive renal insufficiency; dcSSc has been termed *scleroderma renal crisis*. If it is left untreated, then rapidly progressive renal failure with renal infarcts is the predictable outcome. Interstitial lung disease is common and is accompanied by nonproductive cough, dyspnea, or fatigue. Patients with interstitial lung disease often develop associated pulmonary hypertension. Lung disease is now the leading cause of death in diffuse scleroderma. Cardiac disease is secondary to vascular occlusion and microinfarcts; arrhythmias and cardiomyopathy with congestive heart failure may develop. Pleuritis and pericardial effusions, sometimes large, may be seen especially within the first years of disease onset.

Intestinal involvement includes the esophageal manifestations seen in lcSSc but is more extensive, and hypomotility often affects the length of the intestinal tract. Diarrhea and malabsorption are common and are the result of bacterial overgrowth and deconjugation of bile acids. Abdominal bloating and constipation may be a direct result of hypomotility. With advanced hypomotility and intestinal fibrosis, progressive weight loss and inanition may occur. Colonic involvement includes herniation of mucosa through an atrophic muscular layer with colonic sacculations and severe dilation, which may be mistaken for toxic megacolon. Musculoskeletal manifestations include inflammatory myositis, tendinitis, and polyarthritis resembling rheumatoid arthritis but without erosive arthropathy. Fatigue and malaise are common symptoms.

Diagnosis and Differential Diagnosis

SSc is a clinical diagnosis suggested by the presence of Raynaud's phenomenon, esophageal reflux, and sclerodactyly. Raynaud's phenomenon is a common condition affecting 5% to 10% of the adult population and is more common in women. Although most patients with SSc are idiopathic, defined causes include exposure to vibrating instruments such as jackhammers and chain saws, certain drugs such as β-blockers and ergots, and blood disorders such as cryoglobulinemia and hyperviscosity syndrome. Raynaud's phenomenon is also seen in other connective tissue diseases such as dermatomyositis, SLE, and rheumatoid arthritis. The presence of other clinical features of SSc, such as severe heartburn or telangiectasia and the presence of antinuclear antibodies, particularly specific antibodies in high titer, indicates the risk of developing scleroderma. However, antinuclear antibodies are not specific for scleroderma or other autoimmune diseases, and some patients with SSc do not have autoantibodies.

At presentation, the distinction between lcSSc and dcSSc is not always obvious because many clinical features are common to both subsets. Clues that suggest the development of diffuse SSc include palpable or audible tendon friction rubs resulting from fibrosis around tendons, puffiness and swelling of the hands, and a tightness of the skin proximal to the hands. Most patients have antinuclear antibodies. Of patients with dcSSc, 30% to 50% have antibodies to *topoisomerase* (also called Scl-70); this subgroup and patients with antibodies to RNA polymerases are at a higher risk of renal and lung disease. Approximately 50% of patients with lcSSc have anticentromere antibodies, and these patients appear to be at higher risk of pulmonary hypertension.

A small subset of patients with dcSSc has vascular and visceral manifestations of the disease but without the dermal manifestation of skin thickening; the term *scleroderma sine scleroderma* has been used to describe these patients. In addition, some patients have overlapping features of multiple connective tissue diseases, including scleroderma, SLE, dermatomyositis, and rheumatoid arthritis. Although some investigators have used the term *mixed connective tissue disease* to describe these patients, *undifferentiated connective tissue disease* is the more accurate term. Many of these patients, with time, develop a more classic picture of a single entity, most commonly SSc or SLE. Others patients continue to have this overlap syndrome.

Other entities that may resemble SSc include diffuse morphea, scleroderma, eosinophilic fasciitis and eosinophilia myalgia syndromes, and certain environmental or drug-induced scleroderma syndromes (Table 82–2). *Morphea* is a form of localized scleroderma that occurs more commonly in children. Patients have inflammatory skin infiltrates and dermal fibrosis and atrophy, but no Raynaud's

Table 82–2 Scleroderma-like Syndromes

Other Diseases	Distinguishing Features
Morphea	Patchy or linear distribution
Eosinophilic fasciitis	Sparing of hands
	Biopsy shows involvement extending to fascia and muscle
Scleredema (of Buschke)	Prominent involvement of neck, shoulders, and upper arms; hands spared
	Associated with diabetes
Scleromyxedema	Association with gammopathy; skin lichenoid and thickened but not tethered
	May have Raynaud's phenomenon
Graft-versus-host	Skin changes similar to scleroderma; vasculopathy
Nephrogenic-fibrosing dermopathy	Skin changes similar to scleroderma in patients with chronic renal failure

Environmental Agents and Drugs	Distinguishing Features
Bleomycin	Skin and lung fibrosis similar to scleroderma
L-Tryptophan	Eosinophilia-myalgia; from contaminant or metabolite (described in the 1980s)
	Fever, eosinophilia, neurologic manifestations, pulmonary hypertension
Organic solvents	Trichloroethylene and others implicated
	Clinically indistinguishable from idiopathic systemic sclerosis
Pentazocine	Localized lesions at injection sites
Toxic oil syndrome	Contaminated rapeseed oil (Spanish epidemic 1981)
	Similar to eosinophilia myalgia syndrome
Vinyl chloride disease	Vascular lesions, acro-osteolysis, sclerodactyly
	No visceral disease

phenomenon or systemic manifestations develop. Morphea can occur as a single lesion, as multiple lesions, or in a linear form. The linear form may affect large body parts and often involves tissues down to fascia and muscle. Contractures and deformity may also result. The recently described syndrome of nephrogenic fibrosing dermopathy can exhibit skin thickening that resembles scleroderma, which occurs in the setting of chronic renal failure.

Treatment

No single treatment exists for SSc. However, therapy directed at specific organ involvement is often effective (Table 82–3), and the need for treatment is sometimes urgent. No agent has been proven to retard or reverse skin disease, although some studies suggest that methotrexate and cyclophosphamide may be effective, particularly before significant fibrosis occurs. Several agents that inhibit collagen synthesis or promote its breakdown are under investigation. Avoiding skin trauma to prevent digital ulcers and prompt treatment of ulcers when they do occur may prevent progression to severe infection and/or amputation. Various vasodilating agents are effective in improving symptoms of Raynaud's phenomenon and may also be effective in preventing the development of digital ulcers or in promoting their healing. Bosentan, an endothelin antagonist has been shown to be effective in reducing the development of ischemic digital ulcers, but it does not alter the frequency or severity of Raynaud's phenomenon. Calcium channel blockers are most widely used for the treatment of Raynaud's phenomenon, but drugs such as nitroglycerin ointment or patches and

alpha blockers are also appropriate. Recent studies suggest that phosphodiesterase inhibitors such as sildenafil may be effective in treating patients with severe Raynaud's phenomenon who do not respond to calcium channel blockers. Intravenous prostacyclin analogs appear to be effective in the treatment of severe digital ischemia, a fortunately relatively rare vascular complication of scleroderma.

New hypertension in the setting of scleroderma is a manifestation of renal crisis. Regular blood pressure monitoring allows for early treatment before renal damage becomes extensive. Renal crisis is an emergency and should be aggressively treated with angiotensin-converting enzyme inhibitors, preferably in an inpatient setting, until the patient's blood pressure is controlled. The availability of angiotensin-converting enzyme inhibitors has dramatically altered the course and outcome of renal crisis in SSc. Occasionally, renal *crisis* with proteinuria and microangiopathy occurs without hypertension.

Early recognition of inflammatory interstitial lung disease is important if treatment is to prevent progression to distortion of lung architecture and irreversible fibrosis. Diagnosis is best made by high-resolution computed tomography and bronchoalveolar lavage or biopsy; evaluation with these modalities should be performed before prominent symptoms are present. Cyclophosphamide therapy has been shown to be modestly effective in treating inflammatory lung disease and in arresting the decline in lung function.

Several agents have recently been approved for treatment of pulmonary hypertension in scleroderma, including the prostacyclin analogs, epoprostenol and treprostinil, and the endothelin receptor antagonist, bosentan. Because of the short half-life of prostacyclin analogs, these drugs are

Table 82–3   Therapeutic Approaches to Systemic Sclerosis

Manifestation	Pathophysiologic Features	Treatment
Raynaud's phenomenon	Vascular hyperreactivity	Calcium channel blockers; smoking cessation;
	Vascular obliteration	direct vasodilators
Digital ulcers	Ischemia, infection	Antibiotics
		Treat Raynaud's phenomenon
Swollen puffy hands	Vascular leak, inflammation	Short-term, low-dose corticosteroids
Esophageal reflux	Loss of lower esophageal sphincter function; ischemic damage to myenteric plexus	Proton-pump inhibitors; H_2-blockers; promotility agents: cisapride, metoclopramide
Intestinal hypomotility	Ischemic damage to myenteric plexus; intestinal fibrosis	Promotility agents
Malabsorption	Bacterial overgrowth	Antibiotics
Interstitial lung disease	Inflammation; fibrosis	Cyclophosphamide, corticosteroids
Pulmonary hypertension	Vasospasm; vascular obliteration	Prostacyclin analogs, endothelin-receptor antagonists
Cardiac arrhythmia	Myocardial ischemia and fibrosis	Anti-arrhythmic agents
Renal crisis	Vasculopathy	Angiotensin-converting enzyme inhibitors; angiotensin II–receptor antagonists
Myositis	Inflammatory damage	Corticosteroids; methotrexate
Skin thickening	Fibroblast (defect); inflammation leading to fibrosis	Drugs under investigation
		Inhibitors of TGF-β, CTGF
		Inhibitors of matrix biosynthesis

CTGF = connective tissue growth factor; H_2 = histamine 2; TGF = transforming growth factor-β.

administered parenterally as continuous infusions and are dramatically effective in lowering pulmonary vascular resistance and improving clinical function, even in patients with severe pulmonary hypertension. However, long-term effects on life expectancy are less dramatic. Bosentan is an orally active agent that improves cardiorespiratory function and cardiac hemodynamics. Hepatotoxicity with elevated transaminases occurs in 10% to 14% of patients. The oral phosphodiesterase inhibitor, sildenafil, has recently been approved for the treatment of primary pulmonary hypertension. Several other vasodilating agents are in various stages of investigation.

Gastrointestinal reflux disease, which may progress to stricture, is best treated with proton-pump inhibitors. Diarrhea and malabsorption are usually responsive to antibiotics that suppress bacterial overgrowth. Several drugs may help with intestinal motility. Joint manifestations often respond to nonsteroidal anti-inflammatory drugs, but occasionally short courses of corticosteroids are needed. Caution should

be exercised with glucocorticoids because these agents have been implicated in precipitating renal crisis. Joint symptoms may result from scarring and inflammation around tendons. Mild asymptomatic elevations of muscle enzymes do not require treatment, but inflammatory myositis should be treated with glucocorticoids and/or immunosuppressive agents. A summary of therapeutic approaches is provided in Table 82–3.

Prognosis

Survival in scleroderma improved dramatically in the 1990s. This improvement may be attributed to early aggressive treatment of renal disease, early recognition and treatment of pulmonary interstitial disease, more effective therapies for infection and gastrointestinal involvement, and attention to nutritional needs. Overall survival is approximately 70% at 10 years; patients with lcSSc have higher survival rates unless pulmonary hypertension is present.

Prospectus for the Future

Effective therapy for both vascular and skin disease in scleroderma has been lacking. Studies in the last few years have identified molecular targets for intervening in these areas. It is likely that inhibitors of profibrotic cytokines, such as transforming growth factor-β, will become available. These may be antibodies, receptor inhibitors, or molecules that block cytokine signaling pathways and thus inhibit fibrosis. Blocking fibrosis may also inhibit vascular obliteration and vascular manifestations of scleroderma. Combination therapy of antifibrotic, vascular protective, and immunosuppressive drugs may be needed to combat the multiple aspects of the disease.

References

Medsger TA. Natural history of systemic sclerosis and the assessment of disease activity, severity, functional status, and psychologic well-being. Rheum Dis Clin N Am 29:255–275, 2003

Varga J: Raynaud phenomenon, scleroderma, overlap syndromes and other fibrosing syndromes. Curr Opin Rheumatol 17:735–767, 2005.

Chapter 83

Idiopathic Inflammatory Myopathies

Robert W. Simms

The idiopathic inflammatory myopathies (IIMs) include polymyositis, dermatomyositis, myositis associated with malignancy, myositis associated with other connective tissue disease, and inclusion body myositis. These conditions have in common the clinical features of progressive symmetrical proximal weakness, elevation of muscle enzymes, muscle histologic features demonstrating mononuclear inflammatory cell infiltrates and muscle fiber necrosis, and characteristic electromyographic abnormalities. The IIMs differ in their association with extramuscular manifestations and with certain autoantibody profiles (Tables 83–1 and 83–2).

The IIMs as a group and individually are relatively rare conditions, with estimated prevalence rates of between 2 and 10 cases per million and incidence rates between 0.5 and 8.4 cases per million. The male-to-female ratio is approximately 2:1 for polymyositis and dermatomyositis; inclusion body myositis predominates in men. The age distribution of IIMs is bimodal, with a peak between ages 10 and 15 years in children with dermatomyositis and another peak between ages 40 and 60 years. Both myositis associated with malignancy and inclusion body myositis are more common after the age of 50 years.

Pathologic and Pathophysiologic Features

The hallmark of the IIMs is inflammatory infiltrate within muscle tissue. The infiltrate is primarily lymphocytic, but macrophages, plasma cells, and sometimes eosinophils, basophils, and neutrophils are present. In polymyositis the infiltrate typically clusters in the endomysial area around muscle fibers, whereas in dermatomyositis the infiltrate predominates in the perimysial area around the fascicles and small blood vessels. Perifascicular atrophy occurs more frequently in dermatomyositis (Fig. 83–1). Necrotizing vasculitis is uncommon. Inclusion body myositis is characterized by the presence of intracellular vacuoles, which under electron microscopy appear as intracytoplasmic, intranuclear tubular, or filamentous inclusions.

The association of IIMs with other autoimmune disorders (including Hashimoto's thyroiditis, myasthenia gravis, primary biliary cirrhosis, and connective tissue diseases), in some cases with autoantibodies (see Table 83–2), and the response to corticosteroids suggest an autoimmune pathogenesis. This hypothesis is also supported by the identification of T cells cytotoxic to muscle in biopsy specimens and in the peripheral blood of patients with polymyositis and dermatomyositis. Autoimmunity is also suggested by the finding of immunoglobulin deposition and complement components in the capillaries and small arterioles in dermatomyositis. Additionally, antibodies to autoantigens have been associated with IIMs and their complications. For example, antibodies to Mi 2 (a nuclear helicase) are found in patients with dermatomyositis and skin rash, and antibodies to Jo-1 (a histidine transfer RNA [tRNA] synthetase) are found in patients with polymyositis and interstitial lung disease. Inclusion body myositis probably represents a special case, given its distinctive pathologic features, because amyloid deposits have been identified in the vacuoles that characterize this condition. A wide variety of pro-inflammatory cytokines (e.g. interferon gamma, interleukin-1, tissue necrosis factor α), chemokines (e.g., monocyte chemotactic protein) and cell adhesion molecules (e.g., platelet endothelial cell adhesion molecule-1, vascular cellular adhesion molecule) appear to be upregulated in the inflammatory myopathies. However, the sequence of events involved in the production of these molecules, their targets, and their precise role in muscle fiber damage and repair remain uncertain.

Clinical Presentation

Patients with polymyositis are representative of the IIMs in their presentation and clinical features. The onset of the disease is typically insidious over a period of months, with proximal muscle weakness; in rare cases the presentation is more fulminant, with both proximal and distal muscle weakness. A more indolent onset over years with both proximal and distal involvement suggests inclusion body myositis. The symmetrical proximal muscle weakness often impairs specific tasks such as getting up from a sitting position, getting out of a car, and reaching overhead or combing the hair, and it should be distinguished from conditions that produce a generalized fatigue or loss of energy that rarely interferes with these functions. Approximately one third of patients with polymyositis have upper esophageal involvement, which produces dysphagia and, occasionally, aspiration of oral contents. Myalgia occurs in approximately one half of patients, but it is generally mild, although it may cause confusion with polymyalgia rheumatica among older patients.

The assessment of muscle strength should include active resistive testing; the physician should keep in mind that this testing should also be supplemented by asking the patient to perform specific tasks such as getting up from a low chair without using the arms, raising the arms over the head, and lifting the head from the examining table when in the supine position. The examiner should be aware that assessment of motor power may be confounded by the fatigue or pain of arthritis or myalgia.

In dermatomyositis, a characteristic skin eruption occurs, usually preceding the development of myositis. In rare cases, patients have the classic skin manifestations without the myositis (*dermatomyositis sine myositis* or *amyopathic dermatomyositis*). The rash has several distinctive varieties: Gottron's lesions, the erythematous or poikilodermatous rash, and the heliotrope rash. *Gottron's papules* consist of erythematous, sometimes scaly papules, plaques, or macules (Gottron's sign) over the metacarpophalangeal and proximal interphalangeal joints. The *poikilodermatous eruption* of dermatomyositis consists of an erythematous or violaceous rash on the face, trunk, neck, extremities, or scalp. Occasionally, a characteristic distribution in the shape of a V appears on the anterior chest, or the so-called *shawl sign* (back of neck, upper torso, and shoulders). The *heliotrope (lilac-colored) rash* occurs in 30% to 60% of patients with dermatomyositis and is located characteristically on the upper eyelids, but it may be difficult to detect in dark-skinned patients.

Various nonmuscular and nondermatologic manifestations of the IIM may occur (Table 83–3). Pulmonary involvement in polymyositis and dermatomyositis may take several forms, including respiratory muscle weakness, interstitial lung disease, pulmonary hypertension, pulmonary vasculitis, and aspiration pneumonia. Respiratory muscle

---

Table 83–1   Classification of the Idiopathic Inflammatory Myopathies

Primary idiopathic polymyositis
Primary idiopathic dermatomyositis
Polymyositis or dermatomyositis associated with malignancy
Juvenile dermatomyositis (or polymyositis)
Overlap syndrome of polymyositis or dermatomyositis with another autoimmune rheumatic disease
Inclusion body myositis

Table 83–2   Myositis Syndromes and Associated Autoantibodies

Autoantibody	Clinical Features	Treatment Response
Anti-Jo 1 (also known as antisynthetase)*	Polymyositis or dermatomyositis Acute interstitial lung disease Fever Arthritis Raynaud's phenomenon	Moderate with persistent disease
Anti-SRP†	Polymyositis Abrupt onset Severe weakness Palpitations	Poor
Anti-Mi2‡	Dermatomyositis V sign and shawl sign Cuticular overgrowth	Good

*Anti-Jo 1 is the most common myositis-specific autoantibody. It is known as *antisynthetase* because the putative antibody target is an RNA synthetase. The prevalence of anti-Jo 1 is approximately 20%. Other antisynthetase antibodies include anti-PL-7, anti-PL-12, anti-EJ, and anti-OJ, each of which has a prevalence of less than 3%.
†Prevalence is approximately 5%.
‡Prevalence is approximately 10%.
SRP = signal recognition particle.

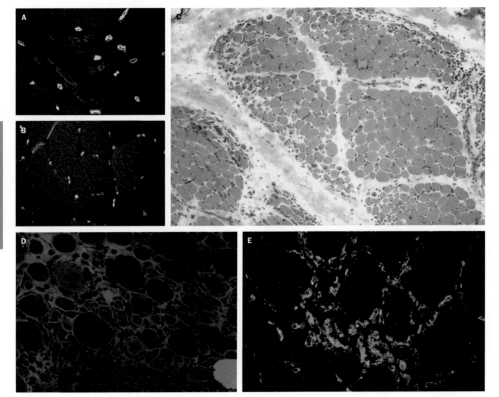

Figure 83–1 Histological findings in polymyositis and dermatomyositis. Depletion of capillaries in dermatomyositis (A) with dilation of the lumen of the remaining capillaries, compared with a normal muscle (B). C, Perifascular atrophy in dermatomyositis. D, Endomysial inflammation in polymyositis and inclusion-body myositis with lymphocytic cells invading healthy fibers. E, MHC-I/CD8 complex in polymyositis and inclusion-body myositis. MHC-I (green) is upregulated on all the muscle fibers, and CD8-positive T cells (orange), which also express MHC-I, invade the fibers. From Dalakas M, Hohlfeld R. Polymyositis and dermatomyositis. Lancet 362, 9388:971–982, 2003.

Table 83–3 Extramuscular Manifestations of Polymyositis and Dermatomyositis

Pulmonary

Respiratory muscle weakness
Aspiration
Interstitial lung disease
Pulmonary vasculitis

Cardiac

Heart block
Arrhythmias
Cardiomyopathy

Gastrointestinal

Esophageal dysmotility
Stomach, small or large bowel dysmotility

Arthritis

Nonerosive, symmetrical, small joint

involvement may include the chest wall musculature and the diaphragm and is clinically significant in approximately 5% of patients. Respiratory failure necessitating ventilatory assistance is fortunately rare. Esophageal and tongue involvement appears to be a risk factor for this complication. Interstitial lung disease occurs in approximately 10% to 30% of patients with either polymyositis or dermatomyositis and in the case of polymyositis is frequently associated with the presence of antisynthetase (Jo-1) antibodies, fever, Raynaud's phenomenon, and arthritis (*the antisynthetase syndrome*) (see Table 83–2). Curiously, the severity of the interstitial lung disease may be independent of the severity of myositis.

Cardiac involvement in IIM may include conduction blocks, arrhythmias, and myocarditis; it appears to be more common than previously estimated (up to 70% in one series) and, as in interstitial lung disease, may be independent of the severity of myositis. Dysphagia, the result of myositis of striated muscle in the upper one third of the esophagus, occurs in up to 30% of patients with IIM. Less common involvement includes cricopharyngeal muscle dysfunction and, in children with dermatomyositis, intestinal vasculitis.

The relationship of IIM with malignant disease has been clarified by population-based studies showing a modest increase in risk (approximate twofold relative risk) within 1 to 2 years of the diagnosis of dermatomyositis and possibly polymyositis. The malignancies associated with dermatomyositis include those that occur most commonly in the general population. They include cancers of the lung, breast, colon, prostate, and ovary. Experts recommend a thorough history, examination, and screening rectal examination;

Table 83–4	**Typical Electromyographic Features of Polymyositis and Dermatomyositis**

Low-amplitude, short-duration motor unit action potentials
Typical myopathic pattern
Polyphasic potentials
Resulting from asynchronous firing of fibers
Increased insertional activity and fibrillation
Attributed to damage to nerve endings or motor end plates
Complex repetitive discharges
Thought to be the result of inflammatory damage to the
  sarcolemma

Papanicolaou's stain in women; urinalysis; blood chemistry studies; chest radiograph; and prostate-specific antigen measurement in men. Serial gynecologic examinations, transvaginal ultrasonography, and serial CA-125 determinations to screen fully for ovarian cancer in women with recently diagnosed dermatomyositis may also be reasonable.

Diagnosis

The diagnosis of IIM is suggested by the typical history and physical examination. Muscle enzymes such as creatine phosphokinase and aldolase are significantly elevated. The diagnosis is confirmed by muscle biopsy, ideally an open biopsy to allow the optimal assessment of muscle architecture, although needle biopsy may be adequate for the diagnosis of polymyositis or dermatomyositis in many cases. The ideal muscle to sample for biopsy is one that is involved but not atrophic. Most commonly, the quadriceps or deltoid muscle is examined by biopsy. Electron microscopy is helpful to establish the diagnosis of inclusion body myositis, and special stains to identify excess glycogen or lipid are useful to exclude metabolic myopathies. With the possible exception of Jo-1 antibodies and the identification of the antisynthetase syndrome (see Table 83–2), the role of myositis-specific antibodies remains limited because they lack sensitivity, and not all are commercially available.

Electromyography alone cannot enable one to establish the diagnosis, but it can indicate muscle involvement in patients with dermatologic or nonmuscular features. Typical electromyographic features are listed in Table 83–4. Magnetic resonance imaging is increasingly used to identify sites of muscle involvement, but it is rarely diagnostic. This technique may be most useful for monitoring the course of IIM.

Differential Diagnosis

Many different conditions should be considered in the differential diagnosis of myositis (Table 83–5). These include other myopathies (infectious myositis, drug-induced disor-

Table 83–5	**Differential Diagnosis of Idiopathic Inflammatory Myositis**

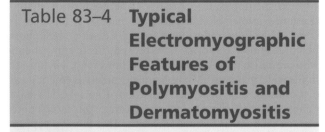

Infectious

Viral myositis:
Retroviruses (HIV, HTLV-1)
Enteroviruses (echovirus, coxsackievirus)
Other viruses (influenza, hepatitis A and B, Epstein-Barr virus)
Bacterial: Pyomyositis
Parasites: Trichinosis, cysticercosis
Fungi: Candidiasis

Idiopathic

Granulomatous myositis (sarcoid, giant cell)
Eosinophilic myositis
Eosinophilia-myalgia syndrome

Endocrine and Metabolic Disorders

Hypothyroidism
Hyperthyroidism
Hypercortisolism
Hyperparathyroidism
Hypoparathyroidism
Hypocalcemia
Hypokalemia

Metabolic Myopathies

Myophosphorylase deficiency (McArdle's disease)
Phosphofructokinase deficiency
Myoadenylate deaminase deficiency
Acid maltase deficiency
Lipid storage diseases
Acute rhabdomyolysis

Drug-Induced Myopathies

Alcohol
D-Penicillamine
Zidovudine
Colchicine
Chloroquine, hydroxychloroquine
Lipid-lowering agents
Cyclosporine
Cocaine, heroin, barbiturates
Corticosteroids

Neurologic Disorders

Muscular dystrophies
Congenital myopathies
Motor neuron disease
Guillain-Barré syndrome
Myasthenia gravis

HIV = human immunodeficiency virus; HTLV-1 = human T-cell lymphotropic virus type 1.

ders, muscular dystrophies, metabolic myopathies, and endocrine disorders) and/or neurologic conditions (e.g., myasthenia gravis, Guillain-Barré syndrome).

Treatment

The mainstay of treatment for the IIMs consists of the corticosteroids. Initially, prednisone is begun at a high dose (e.g., 60 mg/day) until the creatine phosphokinase level has returned to normal or muscle strength has significantly improved. Occasionally, extremely high doses of intravenous corticosteroids are used for severely ill patients. Subsequently, corticosteroids are gradually tapered, depending on the clinical response. Approximately one third to one fourth of patients require additional immunosuppressive agents such as methotrexate or azathioprine because of steroid resistance, intolerable side effects, or inability to taper corticosteroids without inducing a flare-up in disease. Cyclophosphamide and cyclosporine have proved effective in patients who are resistant to steroid therapy; however, their toxicity limits widespread use. Mycophenolate mofetil is emerging as a promising and well-tolerated agent. Clinical trials have established the efficacy and low toxicity of intravenous gamma globulin in dermatomyositis. This therapy appears to work by blocking deposition of activated complement fragments and thereby protecting muscle capillaries from complement-mediated injury. Although intravenous gamma globulin is attractive because of its low toxicity, its long-term efficacy is unknown, and its long-term use is limited by its expense.

Prospectus for the Future

Improved understanding of the sequence of events involving pro-inflammatory cytokines, chemokines, and cell adhesion molecules will allow more precise targeting of therapeutic agents.

References

Dalakas M, Hohlfeld R: Polymyositis and dermatomyositis. Lancet 362(9388):971–982, 2003.

Figarella-Branger D, Civatte M, Bartoli C, et al: Cytokines, chemokines, and cell adhesion molecules in inflammatory myopathies. Muscle Nerve 28:659–682, 2003.

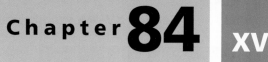

Sjögren's Syndrome

Peter A. Merkel

Sjögren's syndrome is a chronic immune-mediated, inflammatory disorder of exocrine gland dysfunction and exhibits other systemic features. The most common manifestations include inflammation and destruction of the lacrimal and salivary glands, leading to dry eyes (keratoconjunctivitis sicca or xerophthalmia) and dry mouth (xerostomia). Sjögren's syndrome is associated with various autoantibodies and systemic clinical features, including interstitial lung disease, vasculitis, and lymphoma.

Patients are considered to have *secondary* Sjögren's syndrome if they have another immunologic disorder, such as systemic lupus erythematosus, rheumatoid arthritis, systemic sclerosis (scleroderma), or primary biliary cirrhosis, and to have *primary* Sjögren's syndrome if no underlying immunologic disorder is present. Although more common among women, Sjögren's syndrome does affect men and is found among people of all ages, races, and ethnicities.

Clinical Features

The clinical features of Sjögren's syndrome can be divided into those associated with exocrine gland dysfunction (Table 84–1) and those associated with extraglandular manifestations (Table 84–2). Dry eyes and mouth are by far the most common problems and are very troubling to patients. Many of the extraglandular manifestations, although often rare, can be life or organ threatening. For patients with secondary Sjögren's syndrome, differentiating the signs and symptoms of Sjögren's syndrome from those of the underlying disorder can be difficult.

The clinical association with Sjögren's syndrome of most concern is a significant increase in the prevalence of lymphoma. These lymphomas (usually B-cell types) may involve malignant transformation of clinically involved exocrine glands or involve sites not clinically apparent, such as cervi-

Table 84–1	**Clinical Features of Sjögren's Syndrome Associated with Exocrine Gland Dysfunction**
Problems Secondary to Lacrimal Gland Dysfunction	
Dry, irritated eyes with foreign-body sensation	
Corneal abrasions	
Erythematous eyes	
Problems Secondary to Salivary Gland Dysfunction	
Dry mouth	
Oral sores	
Dental caries	
Lingual and labial fissures	
Dysphagia	
Gastroesophageal reflux	
Parotid and/or submandibular gland swelling	
Problems Secondary to Other Exocrine Dysfunction	
Dyspareunia	
Pancreatic malabsorption	

Table 84–2 Extraglandular Clinical Features of Sjögren's Syndrome

Skin and Mucous Membranes

Xerosis

Lower extremity purpura, associated with hyperglobulinemia and/or leukocytoclastic vasculitis on biopsy

Photosensitive lesions, indistinguishable from those of subacute cutaneous lupus erythematosus

Central Nervous System

Focal defects including multiple sclerosis, stroke

Diffuse deficits including dementia, cognitive dysfunction

Spinal cord involvement including transverse myelitis

Pulmonary

Chronic bronchitis secondary to dryness of the tracheobronchial tree

Lymphocytic interstitial pneumonitis, interstitial pulmonary fibrosis, chronic obstructive lung disease, bronchiolitis obliterans organizing pneumonia, pseudolymphoma with intrapulmonary nodules

Peripheral Nervous System

Peripheral sensorimotor neuropathy

Musculoskeletal

Polymyositis

Polyarthralgias, polyarthritis

Reticuloendothelial System

Splenomegaly

Lymphadenopathy and development of pseudolymphoma

Renal

Tubulointerstitial nephritis, type 1 renal tubular acidosis

Liver

Hepatomegaly

Primary biliary cirrhosis

Vascular

Raynaud's phenomenon

Small-vessel vasculitis, with either a mononuclear perivascular infiltrate or leukocytoclastic changes on biopsy

Endocrine

Hypothyroidism caused by Hashimoto's thyroiditis

Other autoimmune endocrinopathies

Data from Hochberg MC: Sjögren's syndrome. In Bennett JC, Plum F (eds): Cecil Textbook of Medicine, 20th ed. Philadelphia, WB Saunders, 1996, p 1488.

cal lymph nodes. Maintaining a low threshold in considering the diagnosis of lymphoma is prudent in patients with Sjögren's syndrome who develop new masses, exhibit constitutional features, or experience persistent glandular swelling that is either resistant to treatment or changes in character.

Diagnosis

A number of different diagnostic criteria sets have been proposed for Sjögren's syndrome without consensus on any one set. Common to each set of criteria is the requirement to demonstrate the following: (1) subjective and objective evidence of both keratoconjunctivitis sicca and xerostomia; (2) presence of at least one of the following four autoantibodies: antinuclear antibodies, rheumatoid factor, anti-Ro antibodies, or anti-La antibodies (these last two autoantibodies are also known as SS-A and SS-B antibodies, respec-

tively, and are so named for Sjögren's syndrome); and (3) exclusion of underlying diseases that may mimic Sjögren's syndrome. Biopsy specimens from salivary glands, which are easily obtainable from the lower lip, may demonstrate characteristic findings of focal lymphocytic infiltration of predominantly CD4 T-cells. These histologic features imply that cell-mediated processes are essential in the pathogenesis of Sjögren's syndrome.

Keratoconjunctivitis sicca can be objectively documented by either measuring decreased tear production with Schirmer's filter paper test (>5 mm of wetting in 5 minutes after placement in the lower eyelid) or viewing corneal abrasions by rose-bengal staining and slit-lamp examination. Reduced salivary production can be demonstrated by provocative sialometry.

The differential diagnosis of Sjögren's syndrome includes a variety of infectious and infiltrative diseases that may cause keratoconjunctivitis sicca symptoms and/or lacrimal and

Table 84–3	Treatment Options for Sjögren's Syndrome

Local Treatment of Exocrine Dysfunction

Xerophthalmia

Artificial tears
Eyeglasses and/or goggles
Punctal occlusion by means of plugs or electrocautery

Xerostomia

Artificial saliva
Fluoride treatments and/or good dental care
Avoid glucose lozenges and/or candies

Dyspareunia

Vaginal lubricants

Systemic Treatment of Exocrine Dysfunction

Pilocarpine or cevimeline
When possible, avoid or discontinue medications with anticholinergic effects

Treatment of Systemic Manifestations

Nonsteroidal anti-inflammatory drugs
Antimalarial agents: hydroxychloroquine or chloroquine
Glucocorticoids
Immunosuppressive agents

salivary gland enlargement. Human immunodeficiency virus causes diffuse infiltrative lymphadenopathy syndrome, which closely mimics Sjögren's syndrome. Diffuse infiltrative lymphadenopathy syndrome, however, involves predominantly CD8 T cells. Additional infections to consider in patients with symptoms of keratoconjunctivitis sicca include hepatitis B and C, human T-cell leukemia virus, syphilis, and infection with mycobacteria. Infiltrative diseases may involve lacrimal and salivary glands and appear in a fashion similar to Sjögren's syndrome. These infiltrative diseases include sarcoidosis, the amyloidoses, and hemochromatosis. Diseases that result in abnormal neural input to exocrine glands, such as multiple sclerosis, must also be considered in a patient with keratoconjunctivitis sicca symptoms.

Many drugs from various pharmaceutical classes have anticholinergic properties that result in clinically significant symptoms of dry eyes and mouth and mimic Sjögren's syndrome. Such medication classes include antidepressants, decongestants, and antihypertensives. The list of medications with anticholinergic side effects is quite long, and all medications, including over-the-counter products, should be carefully reviewed in any patient with signs or symptoms of Sjögren's syndrome.

Treatment

Treatment of Sjögren's syndrome consists of either local measures to counter the exocrine deficiencies or systemic therapy to counter the exocrine and inflammatory disease. Treatment options are outlined in Table 84–3. The interest in the potential therapeutic role of immunomodulatory biologic agents is increasing, especially B cell–depleting agents. Patient education is important, and some measures outlined can be considered prophylactic.

Prospectus for the Future

Increased understanding of the pathophysiologic features of Sjögren's syndrome may lead to disease-modifying therapy rather than just symptomatic relief.

Clinical trials of novel immunomodulator biologic agents in the treatment of Sjögren's syndrome may provide several new options for therapy.

References

Hansen A, Lipskey PE, Dörner T: Immunopathogenesis of primary Sjögren's syndrome: Implications for disease management and therapy. Curr Opin Rheumatol 17:558–565, 2005.

Hochberg MC: Sjögren's syndrome. In Goldman L, Bennett JC (eds): Cecil Textbook of Medicine, 21st ed. Philadelphia, WB Saunders, 2000, pp 1522–1524.

Pillimer SR: Sjögren's syndrome. In Klippel JH (ed): Primer of the Rheumatic Diseases, 12th ed. Atlanta, The Arthritis Foundation, 2001, pp 377–384.

Chapter 85

Vasculitides

Peter A. Merkel

The vasculitides constitute a spectrum of diseases involving inflammation and necrosis of blood vessels with resulting ischemia of those tissues supplied by the affected vessels. Vasculitis can involve virtually any organ system, although each specific syndrome has unique aspects. These diseases are rare with clinical presentations that vary considerably, often leading to delays in diagnosis. Because these disorders can often be life and organ threatening, it is imperative for physicians to have some familiarity with these diseases. Many types of vasculitis exist, and a number of clinical features are common to them. In this chapter the similarities among the vasculitides are emphasized, and then some of the specific syndromes are briefly outlined.

Classification

Because of the wide variation in clinical presentation, anatomic involvement, and overlapping features, both the classification and diagnosis of these disorders are difficult. Multiple classification systems have been proposed, including those that sort the diseases by vessel size, by pathologic lesion, by autoantibodies, or by associated conditions. Table 85–1 outlines the vasculitides as classified by the size of involved vessels. This table provides only a partial listing of vasculitic syndromes, and considerable overlap among the categories is noted, especially between the small- and medium-artery diseases.

The ability of clinicians and researchers to agree on definitions of vasculitides is important for conducting clinical research, deciding on treatment protocols, and determining patients' prognoses.

Pathogenesis

The clinical manifestations of vasculitis result from the disruption of blood flow in vessels, with resulting ischemia.

Inflammation and necrosis of blood vessel walls can cause leakage, stenosis, or total obliteration of the vessel. Stenosis may also be the result of the fibrosis and remodeling that often follow the inflammatory stage of vasculitis. The extent and nature of the damage vary with vessel caliber, thickness, and location.

A number of vasculitides involve inflammatory disease of nonvascular structures, and these may be the most serious aspect of a specific patient's disease. For example, patients with Wegener's granulomatosis (WG) often have destruction of the sinuses and trachea, retro-orbital lesions, and pulmonary nodules. Neural involvement in vasculitis may be the result of vascular insufficiency or the direct destruction of neural tissue by inflammation.

The causes and pathogenesis of most vasculitides are still unknown. However, a great deal of evidence supports the existence of multiple mechanisms for tissue destruction in these diseases. Not only do different vasculitis syndromes have different causes, but more than one triggering process or pathologic mechanism is likely involved even within one type of vasculitis. Evidence suggests that each of the following pathogenic processes is important: immune complex deposition and humoral immune responses, T cell–mediated cellular immunity, autoantibodies, cytokine activation, and toxins.

Infectious causes for a number of the vasculitides have often been proposed, considering the geographic variations in prevalence and the presence of granulomas in some types. Proposed etiologic agents include bacteria, mycobacteria, and viruses. Clear evidence now suggests that hepatitis C virus is the cause of most cases of mixed cryoglobulinemic vasculitis. Hepatitis B and C infections have also long been associated with polyarteritis nodosa, but they are clearly not involved in all cases.

A variety of drugs has been implicated as causative agents for vasculitis. Drugs from most pharmaceutical classes and herbal supplements have been linked to leukocytoclastic

Table 85–1 Classification of the Vasculitides

Large-Vessel Vasculitides

Takayasu's arteritis

Giant-cell arteritis and/or polymyalgia rheumatica

Aortitis associated with an underlying inflammatory disease such as spondyloarthropathy, relapsing polychondritis, or retroperitoneal fibrosis

Medium-Vessel Vasculitides

Polyarteritis nodosa

Churg-Strauss syndrome

Kawasaki disease

Small-Vessel Vasculitides

Wegener's granulomatosis

Henoch-Schönlein purpura

Leukocytoclastic vasculitis

Microscopic polyangiitis

Cryoglobulinemic vasculitis

Primary angiitis of the central nervous system

Vasculitis associated with connective tissue diseases

Table 85–2 Clinical Features of Vasculitis

Constitutional Symptoms	**Gastrointestinal**
Fever	Bowel ischemia and/or
Weight loss	infarction
Fatigue	**Renal**
Skin	Glomerulonephritis
Purpura	Nephrotic syndrome
Livido reticularis	Renovascular involvement
Digital infarction	Hypertension
Musculoskeletal	**Neurologic**
Arthralgia	Mononeuritis multiplex
Arthritis	Visual disturbance
Cardiovascular	Stroke
Pulselessness and/or bruits	Lightheadedness
common in large vessel	**Laboratory**
disease	**Abnormalities**
Claudication	Anemia
Aneurysms	Eosinophilia
Pulmonary	Elevated acute phase
Alveolar hemorrhage	reactants
Nodules	Renal insufficiency
	Active urinary sediment

vasculitis, although definitive proof from large studies or drug rechallenges are lacking for most agents. Systemic vasculitis has also been linked to a variety of agents, including sympathomimetic agents, illegal drugs of abuse, hematopoietic growth factors, and many commonly used medications.

Clinical Features

The clinical manifestations of vasculitis vary widely among the different types of vasculitis and among different patients with the same type. Table 85–2 outlines many of the clinical manifestations that may be seen in patients with vasculitis. However, no one type of vasculitis involves all these features. Determining which features are present often depends on the vessel size involved in a specific type of vasculitis. For example, the large-vessel vasculitides may involve aortic aneurysmal dilation, but they are not associated with purpura, as seen in small- and some medium-vessel diseases. Further, some organ systems can be involved in different ways in the different types of vasculitis. Renal insufficiency, for example, may be seen with involvement of the renal arteries in polyarteritis nodosa and by glomerulonephritis in WG. The features of specific vasculitides are described later in this chapter.

Although vasculitides are rare diseases, the appearance of some of the listed features should always be seen as clinical *red flags* that warrant investigation for vasculitis. Among these features are unexplained hemoptysis, glomerulonephritis, palpable purpura, and mononeuritis multiplex. Some patients with vasculitis may have a chronic smoldering clinical course, whereas other patients may exhibit fulminant disease such as rapidly progressive renal failure or massive pulmonary hemorrhage. Vasculitis may also appear as unexplained multisystemic disease.

The morbidity and mortality rates of vasculitis are variable. Although treatments continue to improve the course of patients with these diseases, the toxic effects of the anti-inflammatory and immunosuppressive agents used are also severe. Some forms of vasculitis are self-limited, but some are rapidly progressive if not treated. With some types of vasculitis, patients are prone to relapse even after long periods of inactive disease.

Specific Types of Vasculitis

A complete description of all of the vasculitides is beyond the scope of this text, but brief reviews of the most common types follow. Whereas many of the clinical features of vasculitis have been previously outlined, each type has its own unique features and pattern of disease presentation. When possible, accurately establishing not only that a vasculitis is present but also which type it is are both quite useful. The clinical patterns of different types of vasculitis allow clinicians to anticipate clinical problems and conduct appropriate testing to prevent more widespread damage. Many of the treatment protocols used vary with the type of vasculitis.

GIANT-CELL ARTERITIS AND POLYMYALGIA RHEUMATICA

Giant-cell arteritis (GCA), also known as temporal arteritis or cranial arteritis, is the most common type of systemic vasculitis. GCA is a large-vessel vasculitis that especially involves branches of the carotid artery. GCA affects patients older than age 50 years and has a female predominance. The most common clinical signs of GCA include headaches, which are often continuous and poorly responsive to analgesics; scalp tenderness; visual disturbance; jaw claudication; malaise; and arthralgias. The most dreaded complication of GCA is monocular blindness, which is almost never reversible. Most patients with GCA (90%) have an elevated erythrocyte sedimentation rate. Anemia and fever are common and may be the presenting features. Any older patient with new onset of headaches or visual changes should be investigated for possible GCA. Rarely, other branches of the aorta or the aorta itself are involved in GCA.

Diagnosis of GCA is confirmed by biopsy of a segment of either or both temporal arteries. Characteristic findings include inflammation and destruction of the internal elastic lamina, often with giant cells present. The pathologic changes may skip segments, necessitating examination of multiple levels.

Polymyalgia rheumatica (PMR) is the name given to the symptom complex that includes pain and stiffness, often profound, of the shoulder and hip girdles and proximal extremities. Occasionally, true synovitis may be seen. PMR occurs in the same population as GCA and is also typically associated with an elevated erythrocyte sedimentation rate and anemia. Diagnosis is made on clinical grounds and rapid response to glucocorticoid treatment. Differentiating PMR from early older patient–onset rheumatoid arthritis can be often difficult.

PMR and GCA are likely part of the same disease spectrum. Both diseases may exhibit in a very indolent fashion or with a fulminant course. Many patients with GCA will have symptoms of PMR either at diagnosis or on tapering of glucocorticoids. Similarly, patients with PMR symptoms alone may progress to frank arteritis. All patients with PMR must be regularly questioned and examined for signs and symptoms of GCA.

Treatment of GCA always involves high-dose glucocorticoids with tapering over 6 to 12 months. PMR is treated with much lower doses of glucocorticoids. A rapid response to glucocorticoids, usually within 1 to 2 days, is normal for both GCA and PMR. Although the toxic effects from glucocorticoids may be considerable, the outcome for patients with GCA or PMR is excellent. It is rare for visual loss to occur while patients are on glucocorticoid therapy, but relapses can occur either during glucocorticoid tapering or months to years after the cessation of treatment.

TAKAYASU'S ARTERITIS

Takayasu's arteritis is a large-vessel vasculitis that predominantly affects young women but can be seen in either men or women up to age 50 years. Also known as the *pulseless disease,* Takayasu's arteritis results in stenosis of the aorta and its main branches, including involvement of the cerebral, brachiocephalic, renal, mesenteric, femoral, and coronary arteries. Stenoses of the proximal aorta and its branches are the most common. Frequent symptoms include limb claudication, lightheadedness, and constitutional findings such as malaise, fever, or arthralgias. Patients may also be asymptomatic with even extremely tight stenoses. A delay in diagnosis, sometimes for many years, is common. The clinical course is quite variable, with long periods of active and inactive disease alternating within a single patient.

Diagnosis is usually made by conventional angiography; serial magnetic resonance angiographic studies can be quite helpful in tracking disease progression. Treatment involves chronic glucocorticoids, with some patients shown to benefit from the use of the immunosuppressive agents methotrexate or cyclophosphamide. Although collateral vessels often develop around the sites of stenosis, vascular surgery and angioplasty play important roles in maintaining proper blood flow to vital organs.

POLYARTERITIS NODOSA

Polyarteritis nodosa (PAN) is a medium-vessel inflammatory vasculitis involving segmental necrotizing lesions, often at arterial branch points, leading to stenoses, aneurysms, thromboses, infarction, or hemorrhage. Virtually any organ system can be affected, but the more commonly involved ones include the renal, gastrointestinal, and peripheral nervous systems. Elevated levels of acute phase reactants are common. A well-established association exists between infection with both hepatitis B and C viruses and PAN, although not all patients are infected with one of these viruses. Diagnosis is usually established by either biopsy or angiography. Because the disease may often be undetected or develop only after a major ischemic event has occurred, examination of surgical specimens may lead to its diagnosis.

Treatment of PAN is based on glucocorticoid therapy, with other immunosuppressive agents used in more severe cases. The use of antiviral therapy in patients with positive serologic studies for hepatitis B or C has gained favor, and reports of this approach are encouraging.

CHURG-STRAUSS SYNDROME

Churg-Strauss syndrome (CSS), also known as allergic granulomatosis and angiitis, is a medium- and small-vessel vasculitis that has a number of extravascular manifestations that distinguish it from other vasculitides. The classic presentation of CSS is that of a middle-aged person with chronic asthma who develops pulmonary infiltrates, vasculitis, and eosinophilia. The vasculitis commonly involves the skin, peripheral nerves, and gastrointestinal system, but other organs may also be affected. Biopsy specimens often show microgranulomas and eosinophilic deposits. The lung infiltrates may be patchy and are extremely responsive to glucocorticoids. Some recent cases report CSS occurring after initiation of treatment with leukotriene inhibitors for asthma. Diagnosis can be made on clinical grounds when most of the manifestations are present, but tissue biopsy is often necessary. Eosinophilia is present in almost all patients at diagnosis but resolves rapidly on administration of glucocorticoids. Antineutrophil cytoplasmic autoantibodies (ANCA) are positive in many patients with CSS, usually of the perinuclear ANCA (p-ANCA)/antimyeloperoxidase (anti-MPO) type (see "Autoantibodies and Vasculitis" section later in this chapter).

Treatment is based on glucocorticoids, but other immunosuppressive agents are sometimes used in an attempt to allow for successful tapering of glucocorticoids.

The prognosis is fairly good for patients with CSS, but relapsing disease is common.

WEGENER'S GRANULOMATOSIS

WG is a small- to medium-vessel vasculitis with many extravascular manifestations. Although any anatomic area can be affected by WG, the three most common sites of involvement are the sinuses and upper airway, the lungs, and the kidneys. Patients may only be diagnosed after months or even years of subtle symptoms. However, WG can also exhibit fulminant alveolar hemorrhage and/or rapidly progressive glomerulonephritis, both of which account for much of the mortality in the disease. Destruction of the nasal and sinus tissues may result in facial deformities. Inflammatory pseudotumors may form anywhere but are common in the lung and retro-orbital spaces. Skin, peripheral nerve, and eye involvement is common.

Diagnosis is usually based on tissue biopsy. Tests for ANCA (see "Autoantibodies and Vasculitis" section later in this chapter) are positive in 90% of patients with renal involvement and 70% of patients without renal disease at presentation. Most patients who test positive for ANCA are of the cytoplasmic ANCA (c-ANCA)/anti-proteinase 3 (anti-PR3) type, but p-ANCA/anti-MPO positivity is also seen.

The mortality of untreated WG approaches 100%. Treatment with glucocorticoids is helpful in stabilizing the acute inflammatory process but is almost always inadequate. Thus patients are treated with a combination of glucocorticoids and immunosuppressive agents, especially cyclophosphamide, azathioprine, or methotrexate. Relapse is common, even many years after remission of disease.

HENOCH-SCHÖNLEIN PURPURA

Henoch-Schönlein purpura (HSP) is a small-vessel vasculitis most commonly affecting children and young adults, although it can develop at any age. The classic clinical triad of palpable purpura, arthritis, and abdominal pain occurs in 80% of patients. Fever and glomerulonephritis are also common manifestations. Immunoglobulin and complement deposition can be seen in affected tissues, and serum immunoglobulin A (IgA) levels are often elevated. IgA deposition in glomerular lesions is characteristic. Diagnosis is usually made on clinical and laboratory grounds. Although HSP can occasionally result in bowel perforation or significant renal disease, the majority of patients have no long-term sequelae. Although most patients remit within weeks of presentation, relapse in the subsequent few months is common. Treatment of HSP is usually supportive, with nonsteroidal anti-inflammatory agents used for arthralgias and arthritis. Glucocorticoids are sometimes used in more symptomatic patients. The treatment of those patients who develop chronic renal disease is controversial, but it may involve glucocorticoids and immunosuppressive agents.

LEUKOCYTOCLASTIC VASCULITIS

Leukocytoclastic vasculitis (LCV) is more a sign of disease than of a unique vasculitis. The term refers to inflammation and fibrinoid necrosis of vessel walls and deposition of cellular debris in the surrounding tissue of the skin. The clinical sign of LCV is palpable purpura that can be seen in most of the medium- and small-vessel vasculitides.

LCV may be the only obvious sign of a systemic vasculitis; thus all patients with LCV must be evaluated extensively for more diffuse disease and for various other infectious diseases. When an isolated finding, LCV is often a manifestation of a drug reaction. Most classes of drugs have been implicated in causing LCV, although proper evidence of causality is often lacking. Discontinuing any nonessential medications, especially those recently instituted, is prudent in patients with newly diagnosed LCV.

Therapy for LCV is directed at the underlying vasculitis or other disease. In cases of presumed drug-induced LCV, drug discontinuation may be sufficient or a short course of glucocorticoids may be administered.

Diagnosis

Combining the clinical presentation with laboratory, radiographic, or pathologic data make up the diagnosis of vasculitis. The *gold standard* for the diagnosis of any vasculitis remains tissue biopsy. Commonly sampled sites include skin, peripheral nerves, lungs, sinuses, kidneys, and temporal arteries. Because the inflammation and necrosis of vasculitis often involve skip lesions, multiple sections from various tissue levels, especially vessels, are sampled from the biopsy material. Understanding that the diagnosis of vasculitis may come from tissue abnormalities that do *not* involve vascular inflammation, per se, is important. For example, a biopsy from a pulmonary nodule in a patient with WG may show granulomas with palisading histiocytes and giant cells but no vascular inflammation or destruction, yet such a biopsy would still be diagnostic for WG.

Angiography can be very useful in diagnosing vasculitis or in evaluating the extent of disease. Vasculitis may cause stenoses, tapering, micro-aneurysms, and other abnormalities that alter flow. However, only those syndromes involving medium or large arteries will show abnormalities on traditional angiography. Magnetic resonance arteriography is evolving into an increasingly useful tool for studying vascular disease, with the resolution of images rapidly improving. However, both catheter-based and magnetic resonance arteriography can be misleading for the diagnosis of vasculitis because vasospasm, atherosclerosis, noninflammatory endothelial diseases, emboli, or thrombi may all cause abnormalities on angiography. Current angiographic techniques cannot detect small-vessel vasculitis.

Certain laboratory studies are useful in diagnosing vasculitis. Urinalysis may show red blood cell casts, providing strong evidence of glomerulonephritis, a common aspect of vasculitis. ANCA (see "Autoantibodies and Vasculitis" section later in this chapter) may be extremely useful in the evaluation of certain types of vasculitis. Other laboratory abnormalities, such as eosinophilia and elevated acute phase reactants, may be suggestive of and consistent with vasculitis, but they are never diagnostic alone.

A variety of pathologic processes may mimic the clinical presentation of vasculitis, leading to misdiagnosis. Table 85–3 outlines some of these processes and provides specific examples. Considering that vasculitis is a rare diagnosis and

Table 85–3   Mimickers of Vasculitis
Infection
Meningococcemia
Sepsis
Syphilis
Neoplasms
Kaposi's sarcoma
Lymphoma
Emboli
Cardiac emboli
Cholesterol emboli
Thrombosis
Cerebral artery
Renal vein
Vasoconstriction
Drugs (e.g., cocaine, vasopressors)
Blood (e.g., subarachnoid hemorrhage)
Fibrosis
Radiation
Previously healed or resolving vasculitis
Atherosclerosis
Carotid disease and strokes
Peripheral vascular disease
Congenital Abnormalities and Anatomic Variants
Fibromuscular dysplasia (e.g., renal arteries)
Ehlers-Danlos syndrome
Aneurysms
Miscellaneous Disorders
Amyloidosis
Sarcoidosis
Calciphylaxis

that the treatment often involves significant toxic effects, it is imperative that clinicians conduct a thorough evaluation to exclude other diagnoses.

Autoantibodies and Vasculitis

The discovery of the association between ANCA and the spectrum of vasculitis that includes WG, microscopic polyangiitis, and CSS (allergic granulomatous vasculitis) has been an important advance in the diagnosis of these diseases. ANCA are detected by both immunofluorescence and enzyme-linked immunosorbent assay. Antibodies to PR3 produce the cytoplasmic immunofluorescence pattern (c-ANCA), and antibodies to MPO produce the perinuclear immunofluorescence pattern (p-ANCA). The combination of positive ANCA by immunofluorescence and enzyme-linked immunosorbent assay provides the most specificity and, in some clinical settings, may allow for the diagnosis of vasculitis to be made. ANCA positivity and frank vasculitis are increasingly being reported in response to exposure to certain medications, including hydralazine and propylthiouracil. Although some reports link ANCA to the pathogenesis of certain vasculitides, more research is needed to establish firmly the roles of these antibodies, if any, in the pathogenesis of these diseases.

Treatment

Treatment of specific vasculitides is described earlier in this chapter, but some general comments apply to most types of vasculitis. These diseases are serious and often life threatening and almost always require medical therapy. Although glucocorticoids and various immunosuppressive agents are mainstays for the treatment of vasculitides, very few large, controlled trials have been conducted in these disorders, and much of the treatment approach is based on expert anecdotal opinion. Cyclophosphamide, despite its serious acute and chronic toxic effects, remains the most widely used agent for serious life-threatening disease. In some cases of drug-induced disease, drug discontinuation alone may result in complete remission of active vasculitis.

In recent years, data from clinical trials and cohort studies have provided support for the use of *step-down* therapy for severe vasculitis. This approach involves inducing disease remission with glucocorticoids and cyclophosphamide over several months, followed by remission maintenance with either azathioprine or methotrexate. This regimen lessens the cumulative dose and toxicity of cyclophosphamide while allowing patients with life- or organ-threatening disease to be treated maximally at treatment initiation. Questions remain regarding precisely which patients to use this approach with and how long to continue immunosuppressive therapy. These issues are being addressed by ongoing clinical trials.

Some other measures can be taken to lessen toxic effects of therapy for vasculitis. Patients who will be treated with an extended course of glucocorticoids should all be evaluated for osteoporosis, with prophylactic therapy initiated early in the treatment. The teratogenicity of methotrexate, cyclophosphamide, and other immunosuppressive drugs must be taken into account when treating women of childbearing age. Infection during immunosuppression is a major cause of morbidity and mortality, and routine or opportunistic infections must be considered when patients have new clinical findings. The standard of care is to prescribe prophylaxis, usually with trimethoprim sulfamethoxazole, for *Pneumocystis carinii* pneumonia in patients receiving glucocorticoids and an immunosuppressive agent. Antivirals and newer immunomodulating agents are being developed and are under investigation for the treatment of systemic vasculitis.

One of the most common treatment errors is the tendency toward overtreatment. Overtreatment may involve either unnecessarily high doses of glucocorticoids or extremely extended courses of medication. The cumulative toxic effects of glucocorticoids must be balanced against the risk of irreversible disease recurrence in patients under regular medical supervision. Physicians experienced in both the clinical course of these rare diseases and the use of immunosuppressive therapies should manage the treatment of vasculitis.

Prospectus for the Future

- Investigations into possible infectious triggers of vasculitis may yield important insights into the epidemiologic features and pathogenesis of these unusual diseases.
- Studies of large patient databases and the use of genetic and autoantibody markers may allow for improved ability to predict clinical outcomes in patients and thus better tailor therapy.
- Significantly improved clinical trial design and conduct will allow for proper testing of new and less toxic therapies, including a variety of biologic agents.

References

Hoffman GS: Vasculitides: B. Wegener's granulomatosis and Churg-Strauss vasculitis. In Klippel JH (ed): Primer of the Rheumatic Diseases, 12th ed. Atlanta, The Arthritis Foundation, 2001, pp 392–396.

Merkel PA, Choi HK, Niles JL: Evaluation and treatment of vasculitis in the critically ill patient. Crit Care Clin 18:321–344, 2002.

Rosenwasser LJ: The vasculitic syndromes. In Goldman L, Bennett JC (eds): Cecil Textbook of Medicine, 21st ed. Philadelphia, WB Saunders, 2000, pp 1524–1527.

Stone JS: Vasculitides: A. Polyarteritis nodosa, microscopic polyangiitis, and the small vessel vasculitides epidemiology. In Klippel JH (ed): Primer of the Rheumatic Diseases, 12th ed. Atlanta, The Arthritis Foundation, 2001, pp 385–391.

Weyand CM, Goronzy JJ: Vasculitides: C. Giant cell arteritis, polymyalgia rheumatica, and Takayasu's arteritis. In Klippel JH (ed): Primer of the Rheumatic Diseases, 11th ed. Atlanta, The Arthritis Foundation, 2001, pp 397–405.

Chapter 86

Crystal Arthropathies

Robert W. Simms

Peter A. Merkel

Gout

Gout is a metabolic disorder first described by Hippocrates approximately 2500 years ago. Its clinical manifestations include acute and chronic arthritis, deposits of uric acid in and around the joints and skin (tophi), renal stones, and, in most patients, hyperuricemia. Uric acid is the metabolic breakdown product of purine metabolism. Accumulation of uric acid can be a result of a primary defect in purine–uric acid metabolism, leading to the overproduction of uric acid and/or the result of a primary defect in renal clearance. Alternatively, secondary or acquired abnormalities of uric acid production or excretion can lead to uric acid accumulation and clinical manifestations of gout.

EPIDEMIOLOGIC FACTORS

Gout is principally a disease of men and, to a lesser extent, postmenopausal women. The prevalence of gout is directly related to the degree of hyperuricemia. Uric acid levels, which are low in childhood, increase at puberty, with the rise being approximately twofold greater in male adolescents than it is in female adolescents. Levels in men and women increase with age, with a sharp increase in women after menopause, but a substantial difference between men and women is maintained. Overall, gout occurs in 2% to 3% of the adult male population. The prevalence is age dependent: 0.24% are younger than age 44 years, and 3.4% are in the 45- to 64-year-old age group, with the prevalence rising to 5% in those older than 65 years of age. In individuals with normal levels of uric acid, the risk is less than 1%, rising to 20% to 30% in those with levels of 2 to 3 mg/dL above normal. For a given level of uric acid, it appears that the risk for women of developing gout is similar; however, because of lower levels of uric acid, the prevalence of gout is much lower in women than it is in men, and gout is rarely noted before menopause. Estrogen may play a role in enhancing urate excretion, and its protective effect on serum urate may then disappear with the onset of menopause. Age-specific prevalence rates in women are less than 0.1% when it occurs in women younger than age 44, 1.4% from ages 45 to 64, and 1.9% in those older than age 65.

URIC ACID METABOLISM

Uric acid is the breakdown product of the purines adenine and guanine. The low solubility of uric acid, which at neutral pH is largely in the form of monosodium urate, and combined with uric acid excretion that normally just keeps pace with production, allows for accumulation of crystals of monosodium urate in the body in susceptible individuals. Total-body uric acid stores are approximately 1800 mg, and turnover is high, about one third daily. Two thirds of daily input comes from de novo purine synthesis, and one third comes from dietary sources. Two thirds of the excretion occurs in the kidney, with the balance largely eliminated in the gastrointestinal tract.

Purine biosynthetic pathways have three basic features: (1) de novo synthesis driven by phosphoribosylpyrophosphate (PRPP) and glutamine, (2) purine interconversion (e.g., adenylic acid-inosinic acid-guanylic acid) and (3) reutilization pathways in which the intermediate breakdown products of adenine, guanine, and hypoxanthine are recaptured by reaction with PRPP rather than undergoing further degradation to xanthine and uric acid. Recapture is catalyzed by the enzyme hypoxanthine-guanine phosphoribosyltransferase (HGPRTase). Abnormalities of this enzyme lead to an overaccumulation of PRPP and drive purine synthesis, resulting in increased serum levels of uric acid. Severe homozygous deficiency of HGPRTase results in the self-mutilation disease Lesch-Nyhan syndrome. This rare, X-linked recessive disorder is associated with hyperuricemia, gout, and tophi and uric acid nephrolithiasis. The defining characteristic of the syndrome is self-mutilation, choreoathetosis, spasticity, dystonia, and developmental retardation, although the cause of these complications is unknown. Heterozygous deficiency of HGPRTase results in both hyperuricemia and gout at an early age without the neurologic complications observed in the homozygotes. Some glycogen storage diseases and abnormalities of pentose shunt metabolism can also lead to the overproduction of uric acid.

Overall, 10% to 20% of patients with primary gout have increased uric acid production, of which less than 2% is due to a defined enzyme deficiency. Diseases with increased cell turnover such as leukemias and lymphomas, disorders of hematopoiesis (i.e., sickle cell disease, thalassemia), and widespread psoriasis can lead to uric acid overproduction and secondary gout (Table 86–1). Clinically, the most important stimulus to uric acid production is alcohol, which can dramatically increase de novo synthesis.

In the kidney, uric acid is filtered at the glomerulus, essentially completely reabsorbed in the proximal tubule, and then actively secreted and reabsorbed in the distal and collecting tubules. More than two thirds of individuals with primary gout and up to 90% in some series have normal production levels of uric acid but have a primary and specific defect in uric acid clearance. Secondary gout may result from any disorder leading to decreased renal function; from decreased urine flow and acidosis, which favor urate reabsorption; or from drugs that compete for organic acid transport. Diuretics (including thiazides and furosemide), aspirin (which at low doses preferentially inhibits urate secretion), dehydration, and acidosis all lead to decreased urate clearance. Lead nephropathy has long been associated with gout (saturnine gout); as a tubular toxin, lead has disproportionate effects on urate clearance.

Table 86–1 Causes of Hyperuricemia

Decreased Urate Excretion	Increased Urate Production
Impaired renal function	Ethanol
Dehydration	Myeloproliferative diseases
Acidosis	Ineffective erythropoiesis (sickle cell, thalassemia)
Low-dose salicylates	Widespread psoriasis
Diuretics	Cytotoxic drugs
Pyrazinamide	Glycogen storage diseases
Cyclosporine	G6PD deficiency
Levodopa	HGPRTase deficiency
Ethambutol	Increased PRPP synthetase activity
Nicotinic acid	
Many other drugs	
Hypothyroidism	

G6PD = glucose-6-phosphate dehydrogenase; HGPRTase = hypoxanthine-guanine phosphoribosyltransferase; PRPP = phosphoribosylpyrophosphate.

PATHOGENESIS OF ACUTE ARTHRITIS

When an imbalance exists between uric acid production and excretion, uric acid accumulates at various sites as both microscopic deposits and grossly visible deposits called tophi. Intra-articular and peri-articular urate crystals are important in the pathogenesis of acute attacks of gout. Attacks of gout are thought to result from either local trauma leading to shedding of crystals from local deposits or de novo precipitation of microcrystals (Fig. 86–1). Trauma to the first metatarsophalangeal joint from weight-bearing activities may underlie its predominant involvement. Increased uric acid synthesis and increased serum levels may also

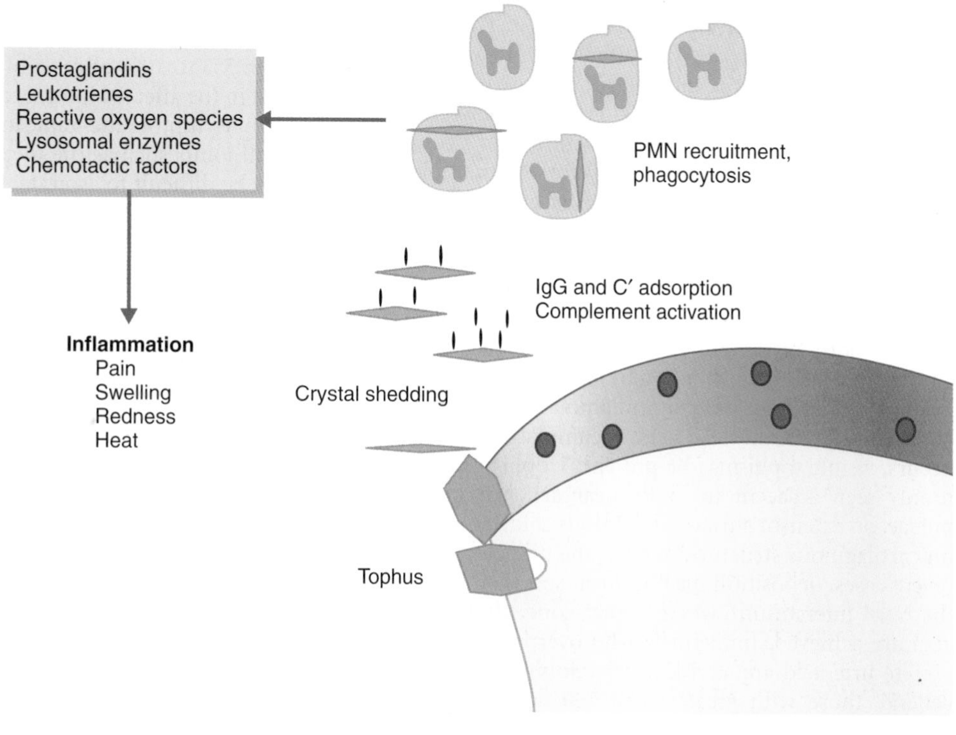

Figure 86–1 Pathogenesis of acute gout. Shedding of crystals leads to leukocyte activation and the release of inflammatory mediators. IgG = immunoglobulin G; PMN = polymorphonuclear leukocyte.

Prostaglandins
Leukotrienes
Reactive oxygen species
Lysosomal enzymes
Chemotactic factors

PMN recruitment, phagocytosis

IgG and C′ adsorption
Complement activation

Inflammation
Pain
Swelling
Redness
Heat

Crystal shedding

Tophus

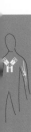

precipitate attacks. For example, dehydration, acidosis, alcohol ingestion, and extensive cell death from chemotherapy all lead to temporary rises in the levels of uric acid in the blood. Rapid lowering in the levels of uric acid (e.g., with allopurinol) sometimes leads to partial solubilization and a breakdown of tophi and crystal shedding. Newly formed or shed uric acid crystals in the synovial fluid or interstitium may activate complement, leading to polymorphonuclear leukocyte (PMN) chemotaxis and crystal phagocytosis. PMN activation leads to the release of inflammatory mediators, including prostaglandins, leukotrienes, and reactive-oxygen species, as well as further PMN accumulation. The latter is mediated by chemotactic leukotrienes (leukotriene B_4) and chemokines, such as interleukin-8, facilitated by increased vascular permeability from the actions of these mediators.

CLINICAL PRESENTATION

Acute gouty arthritis is characterized by a rapid crescendo onset. Typically, the patient goes to sleep without symptoms and is awakened by severe pain, erythema, and swelling in the affected joint. The first metatarsophalangeal joint is the most commonly involved, and this involvement is termed *podagra*. Pain and inflammation extend to the skin, which is often very erythematous and warm. As described by Sydenham in the 1800s, an inability to "bear the weight of bedclothes" develops, and the patient frequently cannot put on a sock or cover the foot with a sheet. Any joint may be involved in acute gout, but the foot, ankle, and knee, followed by the small joints of the hands, wrists, and elbows, follow the toe in frequency. Involvement of the hips, shoulders, and apophyseal joints is unusual. Hydrostatic factors may cause the predominant involvement of lower extremity joints. During the day, with the legs in the dependent position, transudation of plasma into the interstitial space occurs; at night, water is more quickly reabsorbed than uric acid, leading to higher concentrations of uric acid in the interstitial fluid and precipitation of crystals. The lower temperature in joints may also contribute to urate precipitation.

On examination, the affected joint is warm or hot, and any motion is resisted. The overlying skin is red to violaceous and extraordinarily tender; inflammation commonly extends beyond the confines of the joint. For example, when the great toe is involved, inflammation and erythema may extend to the midfoot or proximally. Occasionally, two or more joints are simultaneously involved. A similar process may occur in bursae, particularly the olecranon, and may cause confusion with septic bursitis. At times the process may be both more subdued and widespread, leading to chronic polyarthritis, which may clinically masquerade as rheumatoid arthritis or other inflammatory arthritides.

When significant uric acid accumulation in the body occurs, visible tophi may be present. Trophi are most commonly seen adjacent to joints near articular surfaces, in bursae, on extensor surfaces of tendons, and, less commonly, on cartilaginous structures such as the pinnae of the ear. In severe cases, deposition may occur in soft tissues, including the renal interstitium, where higher concentrations of uric acid are achieved. Individuals who overproduce and overexcrete uric acid are at risk for developing renal stones; in general, those with greater than 700 mg/day of uric acid in the urine are at risk. Stones may be composed of uric acid, or uric acid may form a nidus for calcium and other stones.

DIAGNOSIS

The acute onset of inflammatory monoarthritis in a joint of the lower extremity, particularly in middle-aged and older men, is likely to be gout, particularly when the first metatarsophalangeal joint is affected. The differential diagnosis includes septic arthritis, pseudogout (calcium pyrophosphate dihydrate [CPPD] deposition disease) reactive arthritis (Reiter's disease), mono-articular presentation of rheumatoid arthritis or other inflammatory arthritides, Lyme disease, viral arthritis, and sarcoid. Infectious arthritis is obviously the most important and usually the most difficult to differentiate at presentation. Low-grade fever is common in acute gout, and occasionally the patient's temperature may reach 39°C (102.2°F). Patients with septic joint disease usually have a more insidious onset than patients with gout; they are more systemically ill, have chills and sweats accompanying the fever, and develop peripheral leukocytosis and toxic granulation of peripheral blood PMNs.

The joint fluid in gout is inflammatory, with more than 10,000 white blood cells (sometimes >50,000) and more than 90% PMNs. Polarized light microscopic examination of synovial fluid is the key to diagnosis. Intracellular, needle-shaped, negatively birefringent crystals are both pathognomonic for and essential to the definitive diagnosis of acute gouty arthritis. Viewed under polarized light with a red compensator, urate crystals are yellow when parallel to the compensator axis and blue when perpendicular. Crystals may range in length from 1 to 2 mcm to 15 to 20 mcm, sometimes will appear similar to a lance that has pierced the neutrophil. Extracellular crystals, when typical in size and shape, are helpful but not diagnostic of acute gouty arthritis. Urate crystals may also be seen in the white *cheesy* or toothpaste-like material obtained from tophaceous deposits and occasionally from a joint into which a tophus has ruptured.

In 5% to 10% of cases of gouty arthritis, crystals are not seen in the affected joint; occasionally, crystals may be found in an asymptomatic joint. In other instances, particularly in small joints such as the metatarsophalangeal, synovial fluid may be difficult to aspirate. In a patient with known gout, a presumptive diagnosis is reasonable unless clinical features suggest septic joint disease. Serum uric acid is not helpful; many patients have normal levels at the time of an acute attack, and 15% never have levels outside the normal range, at least with routine testing. Further, elevated levels of uric acid are found in a high proportion of the nongouty population. Radiographs may show tophi or typical *rat bite* marginal joint erosions with sclerotic borders and overhanging edges characteristic of gout. Mild peripheral blood leukocytosis, elevated erythrocyte sedimentation rate, and increased acute phase proteins may be seen but are not diagnostically useful.

CHRONIC POLYARTICULAR GOUT

Gout may develop as chronic polyarthritis with or without acute attacks of arthritis. Patients often have multiple juxta-articular tophi and develop destructive, erosive joint disease.

Table 86–2	**Treatment of Acute Gout**	
Drug	**Route**	**Side Effects**
Colchicine	PO	Diarrhea, cramps
NSAIDs	PO, IV	Gastritis, bleeding, renal insufficiency
Glucocorticoids	PO, IV, IM, Intra-articularly	Increased blood sugar; Mask infection

PO = orally; IV = intravenously; IM = intramuscularly; NSAIDs = nonsteroidal anti-inflammatory drugs.

Table 86–3	**Treatment of Intercritical Gout**	
Drug	**Mechanism of Action**	**Side Effects**
Colchicine	Prophylaxis for attacks No effect on uric acid	Very safe, rare myopathy
NSAIDs	Prophylaxis for attacks No effect on uric acid	Peptic ulcer disease, renal insufficiency
Probenecid	Uricosuric No anti-inflammatory activity	Very safe
Allopurinol	Inhibits uric acid synthesis	Dermatitis, hepatitis, marrow failure

Occasionally, polyarticular gout may appear similar to rheumatoid arthritis, and tophi may be mistaken for rheumatoid nodules. Radiographs in gout typically show sclerotic changes at erosive borders, in contrast to the nonreactive margins in rheumatoid arthritis. Examination of synovial fluid is diagnostic, and every patient with polyarthritis should have the synovial fluid examined for crystals at least once.

TREATMENT

Acute Arthritis

A variety of treatments are effective for acute gouty arthritis (Table 86–2). Joint drainage per se has a therapeutic effect in removing degenerating PMNs and in relieving joint distention. Nonsteroidal anti-inflammatory drugs (NSAIDs) are highly effective when adequate anti-inflammatory doses are used and are often the first drug of choice; however, NSAIDs should be used with caution or not at all in patients with renal insufficiency, a common association with gout. Colchicine prevents the release of PMN chemotactic factors and inhibits phospholipase activation, which is needed for prostaglandin synthesis. It is particularly effective early in a gout attack, resulting in rapid resolution of symptoms, and is much less effective after 24 hours. Colchicine can be given by repeated dosing every 1 to 2 hours with a strict limit to total dosing. The practice of using hourly doses until abdominal cramps or diarrhea supervene is to be discouraged, and extreme caution should be used when the patient has hepatic or renal insufficiency. Intravenous colchicine is effective and rapid in onset, but a few cases of fatal arrhythmia and bone marrow failure have been reported, and its use has been largely abandoned. Intra-articular glucocorticoids have rapid onset of action and are almost free of side effects; they may be instilled at the time of joint aspiration if the diagnosis of gout is fairly certain. Oral glucocorticoids in moderate-to-high doses may be used; however, in patients with underlying diabetes or diabetic susceptibility, hyperglycemia may be triggered. Nonetheless, for many patients, especially when hospitalized for other medical conditions, systemic glucocorticoids are the best treatment option for acute gout. Parenteral adrenocorticotropic hormone and parenteral glucocorticoids are both effective treatments but are more costly. To prevent recurrent attacks, colchicine prophylaxis for several weeks is a reasonable treatment option for patients who have had acute gout (see later discussion).

Intercritical Gout

After a single attack of gout, the physician must decide whether to recommend long-term therapy. A substantial number of patients will have rare attacks, even if left untreated, and little rationale exists for lifelong therapy. In patients who have tophi, erosive joint disease, polyarticular disease, or renal stones, long-term treatment is clearly indicated. Patients with very high levels of serum uric acid or whose first attack occurs at a young age are at greatest risk of frequent attacks and of developing chronic gouty arthritis, tophaceous gout, and/or destructive joint disease. After an attack, when the acute period is over, serum and 24-hour urinary excretion of uric acid should be evaluated. Unless the serum urate is significantly deviated from normal levels, it is reasonable to observe the patient. If patients have frequent recurrent attacks, then prophylactic treatment is advised (Table 86–3). In older patients with mild gout and occasional attacks, prophylaxis with colchicine alone may be sufficient. In patients with frequent attacks or when colchicine alone is ineffective, treatment directed at uric acid is indicated. Probenecid inhibits urate reabsorption in the distal tubule and promotes excretion. Its uricosuric effect depends on normal or near-normal renal function. Probenecid is particularly useful in patients with impaired urate clearance, that is, increased serum levels and low-to-normal daily excretion. In patients who over produce uric acid, or when tissue stores of uric acid (i.e., tophi) are found, a sustained increase in uric acid excretion may develop to a level at which the risk of renal stones is the result.

Allopurinol inhibits xanthine oxidase, the enzyme that catalyzes the formation of xanthine from hypoxanthine and uric acid from xanthine. It is effective in lowering the levels of uric acid whether they are due to impaired clearance or to overproduction. Allopurinol, although generally safe, has greater toxicity than probenecid and has been associated with hepatitis and severe skin reactions.

If allopurinol or probenecid is used, then colchicine prophylaxis should be initiated at the same time and continued for several months. Initiation of allopurinol, in particular, can precipitate gouty attacks; presumably, the rapid lowering of uric acid levels mobilizes tissue deposits and facilitates shedding of preformed crystals. Neither allopurinol nor probenecid should be started in the setting of an acute attack. Recent studies suggest that febuxostat, a nonpurine inhibitor of xanthine oxidase, may be a potential alternative to allopurinol for patients with hyperuricemia and gout.

Dietary purines account for a relatively small proportion of daily uric acid turnover. Anchovies, sweetbreads, organ meats, and cellular leafy vegetables such as spinach are particularly high in purines. Other than avoiding ethanol and perhaps anchovies, little clinical effect will likely occur from drastic dietary alterations.

Patients with chronic arthritis should have pharmacologic therapy directed at lowering the levels of serum uric acid. In addition, chronic use of nonsteroidal agents (other than aspirin) may be required for the control of chronic pain and inflammation. Occasionally, surgical removal of tophi may be beneficial, particularly in locations where they become irritated, inflamed, or infected.

Asymptomatic Hyperuricemia

Little rationale exists in treating asymptomatic elevations of uric acid. In patients who are to receive chemotherapy, short-term prophylaxis with allopurinol may prevent both gout and renotubular precipitation of uric acid.

Calcium Pyrophosphate Deposition Disease

CPPD is due to the deposition of crystals of calcium pyrophosphate dihydrate in articular cartilage and fibrocartilage. Such deposits are common and increase in incidence with advancing age, affecting over 30% of individuals older than the age of 80. In most individuals, an asymptomatic radiographic finding termed *chondrocalcinosis* is observed. The menisci of the knee, the triangular fibrocartilage of the wrist, and the symphysis pubis are most commonly affected. Articular cartilage may be involved anywhere, but the knee, wrist, and ankle are the sites most commonly involved. Acute gout-like attacks of arthritis may result when crystals are shed from such deposits; hence, the disease is often called pseudogout. Occasionally, particularly in middle-aged women, a chronic polyarthritis resembling rheumatoid arthritis may occur with CPPD, involving especially the wrists and fingers; acute hemorrhagic arthritis has also been reported.

CPPD is increased in patients with diabetes, hyperparathyroidism, gout, and hemochromatosis, among other disorders. In patients with hemochromatosis, CPPD occurs at an earlier age, may be the presenting clinical finding, and characteristically involves the second and third metacarpophalangeal joints, areas not usually involved in idiopathic CPPD.

DIAGNOSIS AND TREATMENT

The finding of intracellular, positively birefringent, rhomboid-shaped crystals in synovial fluid aspirates confirms the diagnosis of acute CPPD arthropathy or pseudogout. Crystals may be small and fragmented and are less easily found than are urate crystals. Chondrocalcinosis on a radiograph suggests but does not establish the diagnosis of acute pseudogout. Acute attacks of CPPD are effectively treated with NSAIDs or with intra-articular glucocorticoids.

Other Crystal Disorders

Hydroxyapatite crystals are composed of basic calcium phosphates and deposit at soft tissue sites, particularly tendons and bursae. Calcific tendonitis, especially in the supraspinatus tendon and subacromial bursae, is one such manifestation. Oxalate crystals may deposit in cartilage and intervertebral discs.

Prospectus for the Future

Future studies of long-term use will help define the role of new agents such as febuxostat in the prevention of gout.

References

Hershfield MS: Gout and uric acid metabolism. In Goldman L, Bennett JC (eds): Cecil Textbook of Medicine, 21st ed. Philadelphia, WB Saunders, 2000, pp 1541–1548.

Kelley WN, Wortmann RL: Gout and hyperuricemia. In Kelley WN, Harris ED Jr, Ruddy S, Sledge CB (eds): Textbook of Rheumatology, 5th ed. Philadelphia, WB Saunders, 1997, p 1313.

Ryan LM, McCarty DJ: Calcium pyrophosphate crystal deposition disease, pseudogout and articular chondrocalcinosis. In Koopman WJ (ed): Arthritis and Allied Conditions, 13th ed. Baltimore, Williams & Wilkins, 1997, p 2103.

Schumacher HR Jr: Crystal deposition arthropathies. In Goldman L, Bennett JC (eds): Cecil Textbook of Medicine, 21st ed. Philadelphia, WB Saunders, 2000, pp 1548–1550.

Becker MA, Schumacher HR, Wortmann RL, et al: Febuxostat compared with allopurinol in patients with hyperuricemia and gout. New Engl J Med 353:245–2507, 2005.

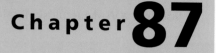

Osteoarthritis

Robert W. Simms

Osteoarthritis (OA) is the most common joint disorder, occurring radiographically in 60% to 90% of individuals older than the age of 65 years and symptomatically in up to approximately 20% of the general population. OA is the most common cause of long-term disability in most populations. It has a large economic impact as the result of both direct medical costs (e.g., physician visits, laboratory tests, medications, surgical procedures) and indirect costs (e.g., lost wages, home care, lost wage-earning opportunities). OA is an increasingly important public health problem whose affect will increase as the population ages.

Pathologic Factors

Also known as degenerative arthritis, OA is characterized by whole joint failure with deterioration in most joint structures, including cartilage, bone, muscle, synovium, and joint capsule. The cardinal feature is progressive loss of articular cartilage with associated remodeling of subchondral bone. OA, however, is a complex disorder with one or more identifiable risk factors, which range from biomechanical, metabolic, and inflammatory processes to age, sex, and genetic factors. OA may result from a variety of biomechanical insults, including repetitive or isolated joint trauma. Certain occupations that involve repeated joint stress, such as to the knees in dockworkers and to the fingers in assembly line workers, predispose an individual to early OA. Sex and race are also prominent risk factors for OA. Whereas OA is equally prevalent in men and women younger than age 45 years, it is more common among women after age 55. Nodal OA, involving the distal and proximal interphalangeal joints, is significantly more common in women and tends to affect female first-degree relatives. Knee OA may be more disabling among black women than it is among white women; but otherwise, no striking racial differences appear to be in prevalence, with the exception of the hip OA prevalence among Asian populations, which seems to be much lower than among other racial and ethnic groups. Certain metabolic disorders such as hemochromatosis and ochronosis are also associated with OA. Mutations in the genes encoding types II, IX, and X collagen have been identified in several kinships, resulting in abnormal collagen and premature OA. Inflammatory joint disease such as rheumatoid arthritis may result in cartilage degradation and biomechanical factors that lead to secondary OA. The destruction of the joint, including wearing away of articular cartilage, is therefore best viewed as the final product of a variety of possible etiologic factors.

OA is classified into two basic forms: primary and secondary (Table 87–1). Primary OA is the idiopathic variety, which may be localized or generalized, and its causes are multifactorial. Secondary OA occurs when a particular cause of OA overwhelms all others and serves as a sole cause of disease. The most common cause of secondary OA is a severe joint injury, but other causes include congenital and developmental disorders (especially in the hip), inflammatory arthritis, and neurologic diseases.

The earliest finding in OA is fibrillation of the most superficial layer of the articular cartilage. With time, the disruption of the articular surface becomes deeper with extension of the fibrillations to subchondral bone, fragmentation of cartilage with release into the joint, matrix degradation, and, eventually, complete loss of cartilage, leaving only exposed bone. Early in this process the cartilage matrix undergoes significant change, with increased water and decreased proteoglycan content. This progression is in contrast to the dehydration of cartilage that occurs with aging. The *tidemark* zone, separating the calcified cartilage from the radial zone, becomes invaded with capillaries. Chondrocytes initially are metabolically active and release a variety of cytokines and metalloproteinases, contributing to matrix degradation, which in the later stages results in the penetration of fissures to the subchondral bone and the release

Table 87–1	**Classification of Osteoarthritis**
Idiopathic	**Secondary**
Localized	Post-traumatic
Hands	Congenital or developmental
Feet	disorders
Knee	Localized
Medial compartment	Generalized
Lateral compartment	Bone dysplasias
Patellofemoral	Metabolic diseases (e.g.,
compartment	hemochromatosis, ochronosis)
Hip	**Calcium Deposition**
Spine	**Disease**
	Calcium pyrophosphate
	deposition disease
	Apatite arthropathy
Generalized	**Other**
Small joint	Inflammatory joint diseases;
(peripheral) and	rheumatoid arthritis; septic
spine	arthritis
Large joint and spine	Neuropathic arthropathy
Mixed and spine	Avascular necrosis

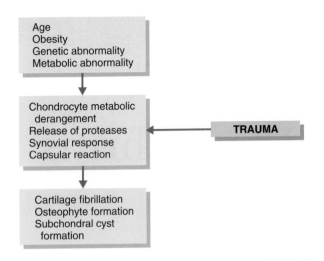

Figure 87–1 Scheme for the production of osteoarthritis (OA).

of fibrillated cartilage into the joint space. An imbalance between tissue inhibitors of metalloproteinases and the production of metalloproteinases may be operative in OA. Subchondral bone increases in density and cystlike bone cavities containing myxoid, fibrous, or cartilaginous tissue occur. Osteophytes, or bony proliferations at the margin of joints at the site of bone-cartilage interface, may also form at capsule insertions. Osteophytes contribute to joint-motion restriction and are thought to be the result of new bone formation in response to the degeneration of articular cartilage, but the precise mechanism for their production remains unknown.

A variety of crystals have been identified in synovial fluid and other tissues from osteoarthritic joints, most notably calcium pyrophosphate dihydrate and apatite. Although these crystals clearly have potent inflammatory potential, their role in the pathogenesis of OA remains uncertain. Frequently, these crystals are asymptomatic and do not correlate with extent or severity of disease.

The diversity of risk factors predisposing to OA suggests that a wide variety of insults to the joints, including biomechanical trauma, chronic articular inflammation, and genetic and metabolic factors, can contribute to or trigger the cascade of events that result in the characteristic pathologic features of OA described earlier (Fig. 87–1). At some point, the cartilage degradative process becomes irreversible, perhaps the result of an imbalance of regulatory molecules such as tissue inhibitors of metalloproteinases. With progressive changes in articular cartilage, joint mechanics become altered, in turn perpetuating the degradative process.

CLINICAL FEATURES AND DIAGNOSIS

Pain is the characteristic feature of OA. Pain is typically deep-aching discomfort, slow in onset, initially aggravated with activity, improved with rest, and localized to the involved joint. Occasionally, pain is referred to a distant site; for example, pain originating in the hip may be referred to the anterior thigh or knee. The pain associated with OA may result from venous engorgement of subchondral bone, accumulation of fluid in the joint, or synovitis. With progressive disease, pain may occur at rest. Stiffness, particularly after prolonged inactivity, is characteristic but is not as prolonged as that associated with rheumatoid arthritis, usually lasting for 20 or 30 minutes. Exacerbation of symptoms with weather changes is a common feature reported by patients with OA. Examination reveals joint-line tenderness and bony enlargement of the joint with or without effusion. Crepitation on motion and limitation of joint motion are additional characteristic features. Several subtypes of generalized OA have been identified. The nodal form of OA, involving primarily the distal interphalangeal joints, is most common in middle-aged women, typically with a strong family history among first-degree relatives. Erosive, inflammatory OA is associated with prominent erosive, destructive changes, especially in the finger joints, and may suggest rheumatoid arthritis, although systemic inflammatory signs and other typical features of rheumatoid arthritis (e.g., nodules, proliferative synovitis, extra-articular features, rheumatoid factor) are absent.

The diagnosis of OA is based on the history, physical examination, and characteristic radiographic features. The physician must distinguish OA from inflammatory joint diseases such as rheumatoid arthritis and identify those patients who have the secondary form of OA. Distinguishing OA from inflammatory joint diseases involves identifying the characteristic pattern of joint involvement and the nature of the individual joint deformity. Joints involved in OA include the distal interphalangeal joints, proximal interphalangeal joints, first carpometacarpal joints, facet joints of the cervical and lumbar spine, hips, knees, and first metatarsophalangeal joints. Involvement of the wrist, elbows, shoulders, and ankles is uncommon, except in the case of trauma, congenital disease, or endocrine or metabolic disease. Joint deformity associated with OA is characteristic in several locations: Heberden's and Bouchard's nodes in the hands and, depending on the compartment of the knee, valgus or varus deformity. Inflammatory signs such as joint warmth, synovial thickening, and fusiform deformity are generally not observed in patients with OA, but effusions, particularly of the knee, are common. The radiographic features of OA include subchondral sclerosis, joint-space narrowing, subchondral cysts, and osteophytes.

TREATMENT

The natural history of OA is quite variable, with periods of relative stability interspersed with rapid deterioration or even improvement. The management of OA should therefore be tailored to the individual patient and may include a variety of modalities such as education, physical measures, pharmacologic therapies, and surgical approaches. Education includes advice on joint protection, exercise, and appropriate use of pharmacologic therapies. Physical modalities encompass strengthening exercises, for example, quadriceps strengthening for knee OA and perhaps grip strengthening for small-joint hand OA. The physical therapist can play an important role in both the teaching and monitoring of specific exercises. Weight loss may retard knee OA progression in obese patients and alleviate symptoms. The use of assistive devices such as a cane provides important joint protection for patients with advanced knee or hip OA. Neoprene knee braces have been shown to be beneficial, perhaps by improving proprioception, and when a varus deformity and medial knee OA exist, valgus braces have been shown to force the knee into a more neutral alignment, relieving pain. Orthotics to provide cushioning and heel wedges to counteract valgus or varus deformities of the knee may provide significant symptomatic improvement. Spinal orthoses may provide benefit to patients with significant cervical or lumbar OA. Local applications such as heat and ultrasound may provide short-term benefit.

Pharmacologic therapy for OA provides symptomatic relief but has not been shown to successfully alter the course of the disease. Although the optimal pharmacologic treatment approach remains undefined, an individualized regimen accounting for potential toxicities and patient comorbidities appears to be the most rational approach. The available pharmacologic therapies include simple analgesics, nonsteroidal anti-inflammatory drugs (NSAIDs), including the newer cyclo-oxygenase (COX)-2 selective agents, intra-articular corticosteroids, *chondroprotective* agents, and antidepressants. Simple analgesics are useful and generally well tolerated in mild-to-moderate OA; stronger narcotic agents may be indicated in patients with more severe disease. Evidence suggests that anti-inflammatory drugs are more efficacious than acetaminophen for knee and hip OA. However, the use of NSAIDs has been controversial in the treatment of OA, largely because of the debate over risks and benefits. NSAIDs clearly provide analgesic benefit, and recent evidence increasingly favors their anti-inflammatory effect in OA. The potential toxicity of NSAIDs, particularly affecting the gastrointestinal tract, has created concern and calls to limit their use in patients with OA. Agents that limit the gastrointestinal toxicity of NSAIDs, such as misoprostol and proton-pump inhibitors used in combination with NSAIDs, have become popular. The COX-2 selective agents such as celecoxib, rofecoxib, and valdecoxib, although initially believed to reduce the risk of gastrointestinal complications, appear to increase the risk of cardiovascular disease. Older nonselective NSAIDs have also been linked in some patients to an increased risk of cardiovascular events. As a result, the U.S. Food and Drug Administration (FDA) has required all marketed prescription NSAIDs, including celecoxib, to revise package insert labeling, highlighting the potential for increased risk of cardiovascular events. The respective manufacturers voluntarily withdrew both rofecoxib (Vioxx) and valdecoxib (Bextra) from the market in 2004 and 2005.

Intra-articular therapies such as corticosteroids appear to provide modest symptomatic benefit, especially in the knee. Synthetic hyaluronate injected intra-articularly appears to have little if any benefit based on current evidence. Chondroprotective agents such as chondroitin sulfate and glucosamine (key constituents of glycosaminoglycans) have been shown in short-term European clinical trials to be of modest symptomatic benefit in the treatment of OA, although no evidence suggests that these agents, which are currently classified as nutritional supplements in the United States, actually repair or retard cartilage degradation. A large, multicenter trial of glucosamine and chondroitin sulphate, sponsored by the National Institutes of Health, compared the effects of glucosamine alone, chondroitin alone, glucosamine and chondroitin in combination, and celecoxib or placebo for 24 weeks in subjects with symptomatic knee OA. Overall, glucosamine and chondroitin sulfate were not significantly better than placebo in reducing knee pain.

Surgical management of OA includes total joint replacement, which for both knees and hips is extremely effective in relieving pain and improving function. Because the resultant artificial joints have limited life spans, however, their use is restricted to patients with end-stage OA of the hip or the knee.

Prospectus for the Future

- Better understanding the molecular events leading to cartilage loss in osteoarthritis will permit the development of novel therapies.

- Studies of biomechanical alterations in OA will allow for more targeted intervention.

References

Clegg DO, Reda DJ, Harris, CL, et al. Glucosamine, chondroitin sulfate, and the two in combination for painful knee osteoarthritis. N Engl J Med 354(8):795–808, 23 Feb 2006.

Dieppe PA, Lohmander S. Pathogenesis and management of pain in osteoarthritis. Lancet 365, 9463:12–18 March, 2005.

Hinz B, Brune K. Pain and osteoarthritis: new drugs and mechanism. Curr Op Rheumatol 16:628–633, 2004.

Chapter 88

Nonarticular Soft Tissue Disorders

Robert W. Simms

The nonarticular soft tissue disorders account for the majority of musculoskeletal complaints in the general population. These disorders include a large number of anatomically localized conditions (bursitis and tendinitis), as well as a more generalized pain disorder, fibromyalgia syndrome. The majority of these nonarticular soft tissue conditions include common syndromes in which the etiologic factors and pathogenesis are poorly understood. Thus the nonarticular soft tissue syndromes are generally best classified according to the anatomic region involved, for example, *shoulder pain*. Once the region is defined, an attempt is made to identify the structure at fault, such as supraspinatus tendon, bicipital tendon, and subacromial bursa, among others. In the case of back pain, precise anatomic delineation of the structure involved (e.g., intervertebral disc, facet joint, ligament, paraspinal muscle) is frequently impossible. Precise data on prevalence or incidence of most nonarticular soft tissue syndromes are not available, but these conditions account for up to approximately 30% of all outpatient visits.

Etiologic Factors and Pathogenesis

The precise pathophysiologic factors of most cases of nonarticular soft tissue disorders remains unknown, although in many cases predisposing factors can be identified, such as *overuse* or repetitive activities (e.g., *tennis elbow,* lateral epicondylitis) or biomechanical factors (e.g., leg-length discrepancy in trochanteric bursitis). The term *tendinitis* implies that an inflammatory process is present in the involved tendon sheath; however, small tendon tears, periostitis, and even nerve entrapment have been postulated as potential mechanisms. Similarly, although bursitis implies bursal inflammation, demonstrable inflammation is difficult to find. In some cases (e.g., acute bursitis of the olecranon or prepatellar bursa), the mechanism is an acute inflammatory response to sodium urate crystals deposited in the soft tissue, an extra-articular manifestation of gout. The favorable response of tendinitis and bursitis syndromes to anti-inflammatory agents, including corticosteroids, supports the view that at least one component of these syndromes is the result of an inflammatory process. In myofascial pain syndrome the causes are even more obscure. Frequently, overuse and trauma are cited as etiologic factors; however, many cases lack antedating mechanical considerations. In the case of fibromyalgia syndrome, which is characterized by pain, muscle spasm, and tender points in muscle or tendon structures, depression may be a predisposing factor.

Classification of Bursae

Many of the soft tissue rheumatic syndromes involve bursae. Bursae are closed sacs lined with mesenchymal cells that are similar to synovial cells, which are strategically located to facilitate tissue gliding. Most bursae develop concurrently with synovial joints during embryogenesis, although new ones can develop in response to mechanical stress or inflammation (e.g., iliopsoas bursa, trochanteric bursa, semimembranous bursa). In general, bursae do not communicate with joints. An exception is the semimembranous or popliteal bursa in the knee that communicates with the anterior knee in approximately 40% of individuals. The subacromial or subdeltoid bursa communicates with the glenohumeral joint only if a complete tear of the rotator cuff tendon occurs. Bursae are anatomically divided into the *superficial* bursae (e.g., suprapatellar, olecranon) and the *deep* bursae (e.g., subacromial, iliopsoas, trochanteric). Although most forms of bursitis involve isolated, local conditions, some may be the result of systemic conditions such as gout.

Table 88–1	**Differentiating Nonarticular Soft Tissue Disorders from Articular Disease**		
	Nonarticular Soft Tissue Disorders		**Articular Disease**
Limitation of motion	Active > passive		Active = passive
Crepitus of articular surfaces (structural damage)	0		+/–
Tenderness			
Synovial (fusiform)	0		+
Local	+		0
Swelling			
Synovial (fusiform)	0		+
Local	+/–		0

Diagnosis of Nonarticular Soft Tissue Disorders

Tendinitis, bursitis, and myofascial disorders should be distinguished from articular disorders. In most cases, this can be accomplished by a careful examination of the involved structure (Table 88–1). General principles of the musculoskeletal examination are as follows:

1. Observation: If deformity or soft tissue swelling is present, then is it fusiform (surrounding the entire joint in a symmetrical fashion) or is it localized? Local rather than fusiform deformity distinguishes nonarticular disorders from articular disorders.
2. Palpation: Is tenderness localized or in a fusiform distribution? Is an effusion present? Local, not fusiform or joint-line, tenderness distinguishes nonarticular disorders from articular disorders. The presence of an effusion almost always indicates an articular disorder.
3. Assessing range of motion: The musculoskeletal examination includes the assessment of both *active* (i.e., the patient attempts to move the symptomatic structure) and *passive* (i.e., the examiner moves the symptomatic structure) range of motion. Articular disorders are generally characterized by equal impairment of both active and passive movements as a result of the mechanical limitation of joint motion resulting from proliferation of the synovial membrane, the presence of an effusion, or the derangement of intra-articular structures. Impairment of active movement characterizes nonarticular disorders to a much greater degree than passive movement.

Bursitis

CLINICAL PRESENTATION

Septic Bursitis

Superficial forms of bursitis, particularly olecranon bursitis and prepatellar and occasionally infrapatellar bursitis, are more frequently infected or involved with crystal deposition than are deep forms of bursitis. Presumably, these infections or involvements are the result of direct extension of organisms through subcutaneous tissues. Most commonly, *Staphylococcus aureus* is isolated from infected superficial bursae. Infectious bursitis should be suggested with surrounding cellulitis, erythema, fever, and peripheral leukocytosis. Definitive diagnosis and especially exclusion of infectious bursitis of subcutaneous bursae generally require aspiration of the distended bursa. The bursal fluid should be assessed for cell count and culture and examined for crystals.

Nonseptic Bursitis

Nonseptic bursitis frequently appears as an overuse condition associated with sudden or unaccustomed repetitive activity of the associated extremity. The two most common types of bursitis are subacromial and trochanteric bursitis (Table 88–2). Subacromial bursitis is the most common overall cause of shoulder pain over the lateral upper arm or deltoid muscle that is exacerbated with abduction of the arm. Nonseptic bursitis is the result of compression of the inflamed rotator cuff tendon between the acromion and humeral head. Because the rotator cuff forms the floor of the subacromial bursa, bursitis in this location actually results from tendinitis of the rotator cuff. Occasionally, subacromial bursitis or rotator cuff tendinitis results from osteophyte compression of the rotator cuff tendon originating from the acromioclavicular joint. The differential diagnosis includes tears of the rotator cuff, intra-articular pathologic mechanisms of the glenohumeral joint, bicipital tendinitis, cervical radiculopathy, and referred pain from the chest.

Trochanteric bursitis is the result of inflammation at the insertion of the gluteal muscles at the greater trochanter and produces lateral thigh pain, which is often worse when lying on the affected side. Women seem to be more prone to develop this condition, perhaps because of increased traction of the gluteal muscles as a result of the relatively broader female pelvis. Other potential risk factors include local trauma, overuse activities such as jogging, and leg-length discrepancies (primarily on the side with the longer leg). These factors are thought to lead to increased tension of the

Table 88–2 Bursitis Syndromes

Location	Symptom	Finding
Subacromial	Shoulder pain	Tender subacromial space
Olecranon	Elbow pain	Tender olecranon swelling
Iliopectineal	Groin pain	Tender inguinal region
Trochanteric	Lateral hip pain	Tender at greater trochanter
Prepatellar	Anterior knee pain	Tender swelling over patella
Infrapatellar	Anterior knee pain	Tender swelling lateral or medial to patellar tendon
Anserine	Medial knee pain	Tender medioproximal tibia (below joint line of knee)
Ischiogluteal	Buttock pain	Tender ischial spine (at gluteal fold)
Retrocalcaneal	Heel pain	Tender swelling between Achilles tendon insertion and calcaneus
Calcaneal	Heel pain	Tender central heel pad

Table 88–3 Tendinitis Syndromes

Location	Symptom	Finding
Extensor pollicis brevis and abductor pollicis longus (deQuervain's tenosynovitis)	Wrist pain	Pain on ulnar deviation of the wrist, with the thumb grasped by the remaining four fingers (Finkelstein's test)
Flexor tendons of fingers	Triggering or locking of fingers in flexion	Tender nodule on flexor tendon on palm over metacarpal joint
Medial epicondyle	Elbow pain	Tenderness of medial epicondyle
Lateral epicondyle	Elbow pain	Tenderness of lateral epicondyle
Bicipital tendon	Shoulder pain	Tenderness along bicipital groove
Patellar	Knee pain	Tenderness at insertion of patellar tendon
Achilles	Heel pain	Tender Achilles tendon
Tibialis posterior	Medial ankle pain	Tenderness under medial malleolus with resisted inversion of the ankle
Peroneal	Lateral midfoot or ankle pain	Tenderness under lateral malleolus with passive inversion

gluteus maximus on the iliotibial band, producing bursal inflammation. The differential diagnosis of trochanteric bursitis includes lumbar radiculopathy (particularly of the L1 and L2 nerve roots), meralgia paresthetica (entrapment of the lateral cutaneous nerve of the thigh as it passes under the inguinal ligament), true hip joint disease, and intraabdominal pathologic processes.

TREATMENT

Septic bursitis is treated with a combination of serial aspirations of the infected bursa and antibiotics, initially directed against *S. aureus* and then adjusted depending on the results of bursal fluid cultures. The approach to nonseptic bursitis should include rest, local heat, and, unless contraindicated (e.g., peptic ulcer disease, renal disease, advanced age), nonsteroidal anti-inflammatory drugs (NSAIDs). Usually, the most effective approach is a local injection of a corticosteroid. Superficial bursae with obvious swelling should be aspirated before the corticosteroid is injected. For deep bursae, such as the subacromial or trochanteric bursae, aspiration yields little if any fluid, and direct injection of a corticosteroid without attempted aspiration is most

comfortable for the patient. Caution is advised in attempted aspiration or injection of the iliopsoas bursa, the ischiogluteal bursa, and the gastrocnemius-semimembranosus bursa (Baker's cyst). These bursae lie close to important neural and/or vascular structures, and only those with extensive experience should attempt aspiration.

Tendinitis

CLINICAL PRESENTATION

Most tendinitis syndromes are the result of inflammation in the tendon sheath. Overuse with microscopic tearing of the tendon is the most common risk factor for tendinitis, but tendon compression by an osteophyte may occur, for example, in the rotator cuff tendon compressed by an osteophyte originating from the acromioclavicular joint.

One of the most common forms of tendinitis is lateral epicondylitis, also known as tennis elbow (Table 88–3). This is a common overuse syndrome among tennis players, but it can be seen in many other settings requiring repetitive extension of the forearm (e.g., painting overhead). The diagnosis is confirmed by exclusion of elbow joint pathologic deterioration and the finding of local tenderness at the lateral epicondyle, which is typically exacerbated by forearm extension against resistance. Achilles tendinitis and peroneal and posterior tibial tendinitis may occur in the setting of an underlying seronegative arthropathy such as Reiter's disease or psoriatic arthritis.

TREATMENT

Therapy for tendinitis—NSAIDs, local heat, and corticosteroid injection—is similar to that for bursitis. Rest, physical therapy, occupational therapy, and occasionally ergonomic modification are useful adjuncts. The goal of corticosteroid injection in tendinitis is to infiltrate the tendon sheath rather than the tendon itself, because direct injection into a tendon may result in rupturing the tendon. Attempted corticosteroid injection of the Achilles tendon should be avoided because of the propensity of this tendon to rupture. Surgical management of tendinitis is indicated only with failures of conservative treatment. For example, chronic impingement of the supraspinatus tendon that is refractory to conservative treatment may require subacromial decompression.

Fibromyalgia Syndrome

Fibromyalgia syndrome, formerly known as fibrositis, is a controversial chronic pain condition characterized by increased tenderness at muscle and tendon insertions; it is therefore considered a form of soft tissue rheumatism. Although it has only recently been the subject of investigation, descriptions of the syndrome exist far back in the medical literature. Controversy persists, however, because of the lack of objective diagnostic or pathologic findings.

PATHOPHYSIOLOGIC FEATURES

Investigators have examined diverse mechanisms in fibromyalgia syndrome, including studies of muscle, sleep physiologic processes, neurohormonal function, and psychological status. Although the pathophysiologic mechanisms remain unknown, an increasing body of literature points to central (central nervous system) rather than peripheral (muscle) mechanisms. Muscle tissue has been a focus of investigation for many years. Initial studies, including histologic and histochemical studies, suggested a possible metabolic myopathy; however, carefully controlled studies indicated that these abnormalities were simply the result of deconditioning. Sleep studies suggested that disruption of deep sleep (stage IV) by so-called alpha-intrusion (the normal awake electroencephalographic pattern) may play a causal role, but this finding was later observed in other disorders, more likely indicating effect rather than cause. In some cases, musculoskeletal injury has been implicated as a trigger for fibromyalgia, but social and legal issues cloud its causative role. Several studies have suggested that subtle hypothalamic-pituitary-adrenal axis hypofunction may occur in fibromyalgia syndrome, although it remains uncertain whether these changes are constitutive or are the result of fibromyalgia. Fibromyalgia has long been linked to psychological disturbance. Most studies have confirmed high

Table 88–4	**American College of Rheumatology Classification Criteria for Fibromyalgia Syndrome**

For classification purposes, patients are said to have fibromyalgia if both criteria are satisfied.

1. *History of chronic, widespread pain:* Pain is considered widespread when present above and below the waist on both sides of the body.
   Chronic: Is defined as greater than 3 months in duration.
2. *Pain in 11 of 18 tender points on digital palpation:* Points include occiput, low cervical, trapezius, supraspinatus, second rib, lateral epicondyle, gluteal, greater trochanter, knee.

lifetime rates of major depression, which range from 34% to 71%, associated with fibromyalgia syndrome. High lifetime rates of migraine, irritable bowel syndrome, and panic disorder have also been associated with fibromyalgia syndrome, suggesting that fibromyalgia may be part of an *affective spectrum* group of disorders.

CLINICAL PRESENTATION AND DIFFERENTIAL DIAGNOSIS

The clinical presentation of fibromyalgia syndrome is generally that of the insidious onset of chronic, diffuse, poorly localized musculoskeletal pain, typically accompanied by fatigue and sleep disturbance. The physical examination shows a normal musculoskeletal examination, with no deformity or synovitis; however, widespread tenderness occurs especially at tendon insertion sites, indicating a general reduction in pain threshold. The American College of Rheumatology has published the results of a multicenter study to identify clinical classification criteria for fibromyalgia syndrome, which were shown to have high sensitivity and specificity (Table 88–4). These criteria have facilitated population-based studies, which suggest that fibromyalgia syndrome affects approximately 2% of the population and up to 7% of women. Approximately 10% of surveyed patients are disabled to varying degrees by their symptoms; therefore the economic impact is large. The prevalence of fibromyalgia appears to be similar in most ethnic and racial groups.

Approximately one third of the patients identify antecedent trauma as a precipitant for their symptoms, one third of patients describe a viral prodrome, and one third have no clear precipitant. A variety of less typical presentations have been described, including a predominantly neuropathic presentation with paresthesias (numbness and tingling) in a nondermatomal distribution, an arthralgic rather than myalgic presentation, and an axial skeletal presentation (resembling degenerative disc disease). Many patients may have undergone invasive diagnostic tests and in some cases inappropriate procedures such as carpal tunnel release or cervical or lumbar laminectomies.

Conditions that should be considered in the differential diagnosis of fibromyalgia syndrome include polymyalgia rheumatica, hypothyroidism, polymyositis, and early systemic lupus erythematosus or rheumatoid arthritis. In general, however, symptoms are exhibited for many months or years, without evidence of other signs or symptoms of an underlying connective tissue disease, make other possible diagnoses unlikely. Laboratory and radiographic studies are usually normal in patients with fibromyalgia syndrome. Exclusion of other conditions, such as osteoarthritis, rheumatoid arthritis, or systemic lupus erythematosus, by radiography, erythrocyte sedimentation rate, assays for rheumatoid factor or antinuclear antibody, and other tests is no longer considered a necessary preliminary to the diagnosis of fibromyalgia syndrome, which should be diagnosed on the basis of positive criteria.

TREATMENT

The treatment of fibromyalgia includes reassurance that the condition is not a progressive, crippling, or life-threatening entity. A combination of treatment options, including medication and physical measures, is helpful in most patients. Medications shown to be helpful in short-term, double-blind, placebo-controlled trials include amitriptyline and cyclobenzaprine. Low doses of these medications (e.g., 10 to 30 mg of amitriptyline, 10 to 30 mg of cyclobenzaprine) are moderately effective and generally well tolerated. Studies have also shown that newer antidepressants of the selective serotonin reuptake inhibitor class are also effective, particularly in combination with low doses of tricyclic antidepressants. Patients should also be encouraged to take an active role in the management of their condition. They should, if possible, begin a progressive, low-level aerobic exercise program to improve muscular fitness and a sense of well being. A combination approach is effective in most patients in alleviating symptoms, although a small minority of patients require more intensive treatment strategies, such as psychiatric or referral to a pain center.

Prospectus for the Future

Improved trial design and outcome measures will facilitate the development of more effective therapies in soft tissue disorders.

References

Goldenberg DL, Burkhardt C, Crofford L: Management of fibromyalgia syndrome. JAMA 292:2388–2395, 2004.

Littlejohn GO: Balanced treatments for fibromyalgia. Arthritis Rheum 50:2725–2729, 2004.

Rheumatic Manifestations of Systemic Disorders

Robert W. Simms

A large number of systemic disorders have musculoskeletal mechanisms, which are frequently the presenting manifestations and may provide clues to the initial and perhaps earlier diagnosis and treatment of systemic conditions associated with rheumatic manifestations (Table 89–1).

Rheumatic Syndromes Associated with Malignancy

HYPERTROPHIC OSTEOARTHROPATHY

Hypertrophic osteoarthropathy (HOA) is a form of long-bone periostitis associated with clubbing of the fingers and toes. Approximately 90% of cases are associated with lung cancer. Other disorders associated with HOA include cystic fibrosis, pulmonary fibrosis, chronic pulmonary infections, pulmonary arteriovenous fistulas, mesothelioma, congenital heart disease, cirrhosis, and inflammatory bowel disease. Isolated digital clubbing (a bulbous deformity of the distal digits with loss of the normal angle between the nail and the nail bed) is associated with pleuropulmonary disease in approximately 80% of patients, but only a small minority of patients has cancer. Chronic digital clubbing does not appear to lead to the development of HOA. The most common long bones involved in HOA are the distal femur, tibia, and radius. The pathogenesis is unknown, and its understanding is complicated by the diversity of conditions associated with HOA. Increased blood flow to the bones and in adjacent connective tissue is a uniform finding, perhaps the result of humoral or neural mechanisms.

HOA typically produces bone and joint pain with swelling that results from peri-articular periostitis. Joints appear swollen, but no proliferative synovium or inflammation develops, and joint fluid is noninflammatory. Radiographic features include periostitis with periosteal new bone formation, especially along the distal and/or proximal fourths of long bones, and these radiographic findings are diagnostic. Treatment of the underlying disorder ameliorates HOA.

Chapter 89

LEUKEMIA AND LYMPHOMA

Leukemia may simulate various rheumatic syndromes by producing synovitis or bone pain resulting from direct invasion of the synovium or marrow expansion. Approximately 6% of adult patients with leukemia exhibit rheumatic manifestations, which precede the diagnosis of leukemia by an average of 3 months. The most common presentation is an asymmetric large-joint oligoarthritis, often accompanied by low back pain. Up to 60% of children with acute leukemia have been diagnosed with either monoarthritis or polyarthritis. Although lymphoma is frequently associated with bone lesions, arthritis is a rare presentation. The combination of nocturnal bone pain, hematologic abnormalities, and radiographic features such as periosteal elevation should suggest the possibility of leukemia. Treatment of the leukemia usually results in resolution of the musculoskeletal manifestations.

CARCINOMATOUS POLYARTHRITIS

In rare cases, metastatic or occult carcinoma may be associated with polyarthritis, which is not the result of direct infiltration of the synovium by tumor. The peak age at onset is in the sixth decade of life, and no sex predisposition exists. Nonintrathoracic malignancies predominate. The differential diagnosis includes HOA, rheumatoid arthritis, and polymyalgia rheumatica. Treatment of the underlying malignancy produces resolution of the arthritis.

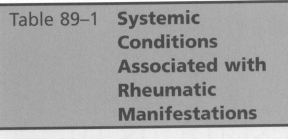

Table 89–1	Systemic Conditions Associated with Rheumatic Manifestations

Malignant Disorders

Hypertrophic osteoarthropathy
Lymphoma
Leukemia
Carcinoma polyarthritis

Hematologic Disorders

Hemophilia
Sickle cell disease
Thalassemia
Multiple myeloma
Amyloidosis

Gastrointestinal Disorders

Spondyloarthropathies
Whipple's disease
Hemochromatosis
Primary biliary cirrhosis

Endocrinopathies

Diabetes
Hypothyroidism
Hyperthyroidism
Hyperparathyroidism
Other

Hematologic Disorders

HEMOPHILIA

Hemarthrosis is the most common bleeding complication of either hemophilia A (factor VIII deficiency) or hemophilia B (factor IX deficiency) and occurs in up to two thirds of patients. Hemarthrosis may occur spontaneously or as the result of minor trauma, and the level of factor deficiency determines its frequency and age at onset. Acute, painful swelling of the knees, elbows, and ankles is the most common presentation. A chronic arthropathy with persistent synovitis may also occur, perhaps as a result of excessive iron deposition in synovial membrane and cartilage. Radiographic findings are those of degenerative joint disease, with joint space narrowing, subchondral sclerosis, and cyst formation. Treatment consists of prompt administration of factor VIII or IX concentrate or recombinant forms, intra-articular corticosteroid injections, local ice application, rest, and later physical therapy. Aspiration is indicated only if concomitant sepsis is suggested or if the joint is unusually tense and only after factor replacement. No evidence suggests that prophylaxis of acute hemarthrosis may reduce the incidence of chronic synovitis and future joint damage.

SICKLE CELL DISEASE

Of the sickle cell hemoglobinopathies, sickle cell (SS) anemia, sickle cell–β-thalassemia, sickle cell–hemoglobin C (SC) disease, and sickle cell–hemoglobin D (SD) disease all produce musculoskeletal complications, which include painful crises, arthropathy, dactylitis, osteonecrosis, osteomyelitis, and gout. SS crises are the most common musculoskeletal features, producing pain in the chest, back, and joints. Involvement of joints may produce a painful arthritis, typically of the large joints. The mechanism of the arthropathy is thought to be an articular reaction to juxta-articular bone infarction or infarction of the synovial membrane. The synovial fluid is typically noninflammatory. Dactylitis resulting from vaso-occlusion in bone may occur in young children, producing acute, painful, nonpitting edema of the hands and feet. Osteonecrosis of the femoral head or shoulder may also result from repeated crises and is most common in SS disease. An increased incidence of septic arthritis and osteomyelitis has been associated with SS disease; *Salmonella* is the bacterial species most frequently isolated in the patient with osteomyelitis.

Gout presumably resulting from the increased marrow turnover and urate production is an uncommon complication of SS disease.

THALASSEMIA

β-Thalassemia major (also known as Cooley's anemia) is one of the most severe forms of congenital hemolytic anemia and may produce musculoskeletal manifestations from significant expansion of the erythroid bone marrow. These include osteoporosis, pathologic fractures, and epiphyseal deformities. Thalassemia minor has been associated with a noninflammatory arthritis, perhaps also the result of articular reaction to chronic marrow expansion.

MULTIPLE MYELOMA AND AMYLOIDOSIS

Multiple myeloma is one of the most common plasma cell dyscrasias and is frequently accompanied by musculoskeletal manifestations, which include bone pain resulting from lytic bone lesions, pathologic fractures, and osteoporosis. The diagnosis of multiple myeloma should be suggested in any of these clinical settings and is confirmed with the finding of a monoclonal gammopathy and sheets of immature neoplastic plasma cells on bone marrow biopsy. Primary (AL) amyloidosis accompanies approximately 15% of patients with myeloma. Alternatively, AL amyloidosis occurs without significant plasma cell proliferation on bone marrow biopsy, but patients have evidence of a plasma cell dyscrasia by virtue of the presence of a serum monoclonal gammopathy. AL amyloidosis results when amyloid protein, consisting of microscopic fibrils derived from monoclonal light chains, is deposited in organs such as the kidneys, heart, peripheral nerves, and gastrointestinal tract. It should be considered in the differential diagnosis of a patient older than 40 years of age who has nephritic syndrome, unexplained heart failure, idiopathic peripheral neuropathy, or hepatomegaly. Infrequently, amyloid joint infiltration produces a symmetric, small-joint polyarthritis–simulating rheumatoid arthritis. Occasionally, significant infiltration of the shoulder joints with amyloid deposits produces an anterior glenohumeral soft tissue deformity known as the *shoulder pad* sign. Macroglossia and submandibular gland infiltration may also occur. The diagnosis of this form of amyloidosis is the most easily established, with the demonstration of apple-green birefringent fluorescence on Congo red staining of an abdominal fat pad aspirate. Additionally, immunoelectrophoresis and immunofixation of serum and urine should be performed. Optimal treatment of AL amyloidosis now consists of high-dose chemotherapy with stem-cell transplantation.

The three other principal systemic forms of amyloidosis are (1) secondary (AA) amyloidosis, (2) heredofamilial (familial amyloid polyneuropathy) amyloidosis, and (3) β_2-microglobulin–associated (β_2M) amyloidosis. AA amyloidosis is a rare complication of chronic inflammatory conditions such as rheumatoid arthritis, inflammatory bowel disease, or familial Mediterranean fever. Certain chronic infections such as leprosy, tuberculosis, and osteomyelitis are also associated with this form of amyloidosis. The amyloid fibrils are derived from the acute phase reactant, serum amyloid A protein. The disease usually exhibits proteinuria or gastrointestinal symptoms because of infiltration of the kidney or gastrointestinal tract. The diagnosis generally requires organ biopsy because the sensitivity of the abdominal fat pad aspirate is considerably lower in AA amyloidosis than it is in the AL form. Treatment consists of controlling the underlying disorder, producing the chronic inflammatory process.

Heredofamilial (familial amyloid polyneuropathy) amyloidosis is the least common form of amyloidosis. This rare autosomal dominant disease is the result of single-point mutations in the gene coding for transthyretin, a thyroid-transport protein. Transthyretin is synthesized principally in the liver. Amyloid fibrils in this disease are composed of fragments of mutant transthyretin that have a propensity to form amyloid fibrils. The condition typically exhibits an axonal and/or autonomic neuropathy late in life. Abdominal fat aspiration has high sensitivity in the diagnosis of this type of amyloidosis. Studies suggest that the optimal treatment is orthotopic liver transplantation, which prevents further production of the mutant transthyretin.

β_2M-associated amyloidosis occurs almost exclusively in patients on long-standing hemodialysis. This disease typically exhibits carpal tunnel syndrome and flexor tendon deposits in the hands or in the rotator cuff. Cystic bone deposits in the carpal bones, hips, shoulders, and cervical spine have also been described. The pathogenesis of β_2M-associated amyloidosis is not completely understood but may in part be the result of altered proteolysis of β_2-microglobulin in long-standing hemodialysis. Treatment includes physical measures such as splinting for carpal tunnel syndrome and physical therapy for shoulder involvement. Anti-inflammatory agents may provide additional symptomatic relief. Surgical removal of carpal or shoulder deposits may be required. Renal transplantation may be the most effective way to halt progression.

Gastrointestinal Diseases

WHIPPLE'S DISEASE

Whipple's disease is a rare, multisystemic disease of late middle-aged to older men and is characterized by the pres-

ence of fever, abdominal pain, steatorrhea with weight loss, lymphadenopathy, and arthritis, the last of which is now known to be the result of infection with *Tropheryma whippleii.* Polyserositis, arterial hypotension, hyperpigmentation, and various central nervous system manifestations, such as personality changes, memory loss, dementia, and spastic paraparesis, may also occur. The organism's DNA can be detected in duodenal biopsy specimens. Biopsy has long been used to detect this unculturable organism in histiocytes of the lamina propria, which show intracytoplasmic inclusions of irregular granular material that is positive on periodic acid-Schiff staining. This last finding is not specific for Whipple's disease, and therefore polymerase chain reaction to detect the organism's DNA is now the preferred technique for diagnosis.

The arthritis of Whipple's disease occurs in 60% to 90% of patients and is the most common prodrome. Classically, the arthritis is an intermittent migratory oligoarthritis lasting from a few hours to days with spontaneous remission. Some patients have only arthralgia, whereas others have a florid polyarthritis. Synovial fluid findings are typically inflammatory with a high percentage of mononuclear cells. Treatment consists of antibiotic therapy with tetracycline, which results in complete resolution within 1 week to 1 month.

HEMOCHROMATOSIS

Hereditary hemochromatosis is an autosomal recessive disorder associated with increased iron absorption and deposition that, via hemosiderin, eventually produces multiorgan damage. Hemochromatosis is among the most common genetic diseases among Europeans, with a homozygous prevalence of 0.3% to 0.5% and a heterozygote frequency of 6.7% to 10%. Approximately 90% of white patients with hereditary hemochromatosis are homozygous for the same mutation (C282Y) in the *HFE* gene. HFE protein forms complexes with the transferrin receptor, which is important in iron transport, and mutations in *HFE* decrease the protein's affinity for the receptor, impairing iron transport and resulting in iron overload.

The classic clinical features of hemochromatosis include hepatic cirrhosis, cardiomyopathy, diabetes mellitus, pituitary dysfunction, skin pigmentation, and sicca syndrome. Symmetric arthropathy of the second and third metacarpal joints is a disabling complication that occurs in approximately 50% of patients. Radiographic manifestations are similar to those of osteoarthritis (see Chapter 87) and often include the presence of chondrocalcinosis. Occasionally, superimposed attacks of pseudogout dominate the clinical picture. Osteoarthritis-like disease occurring in a middle-aged man with involvement of the metacarpophalangeal joints should indicate the possibility of hemochromatosis. Formerly, the diagnosis was suggested by high serum levels of iron, ferritin, and transferrin and confirmed by liver biopsy. Currently, however, the diagnosis may be established with the identification of the mutated gene sequence in DNA obtained from peripheral blood.

PRIMARY BILIARY CIRRHOSIS

Primary biliary cirrhosis is an inflammatory disease of the intrahepatic bile ducts that is frequently associated with other disorders presumed to be autoimmune, including limited scleroderma (see Chapter 82), rheumatoid arthritis (see Chapter 78), Sjögren's syndrome (see Chapter 84), autoimmune thyroiditis, and renotubular acidosis. Approximately 90% of patients have detectable immunoglobulin G–antimitochondrial antibodies, which are rare in other forms of liver disease. Up to 50% of patients with primary biliary cirrhosis have secondary Sjögren's syndrome, which represents the most common rheumatic disorder associated with primary biliary cirrhosis. Other musculoskeletal complications include (1) osteomalacia caused by reduced vitamin D absorption and (2) accelerated osteoporosis. The diagnosis of primary biliary cirrhosis should be suggested in the patient with unexplained pruritus or elevated levels of serum alkaline phosphatase. A positive antimitochondrial antibody test provides strong evidence, which should then be confirmed with a liver biopsy.

Endocrine Disorders

DIABETES

Many musculoskeletal complications of diabetes exist (Table 89–2). One of the most common complications is the so-called diabetic stiff-hand syndrome, which is characterized by waxy thickening of the skin in long-standing type 1 or 2 diabetes. Occasionally, it may develop before the onset of overt diabetes and may create confusion because of the similarity of its appearance to that of scleroderma-like sclerodactyly. These changes are thought to be the result of excess sugar alcohols, such as sorbitol, producing excess water content in the skin and leading to increased stiffness. Joint contractures, flexor tendon contractures (including Dupuytren's contractures), and joint thickening produce a condition known as diabetic cheiroarthropathy, or the syndrome of limited joint mobility; these conditions appear to be related to the duration of diabetes. Although it is most common in the fingers, limited mobility may also occur in the shoulders.

Charcot's joints or neuropathic arthropathy may occur with any neuropathy, but it is most commonly associated with diabetes. Tarsal and tarsometatarsal joints are most commonly involved, and trauma together with diminished pain perception, proprioception, and position sense are major factors in the genesis of this arthropathy. The most common presentation is swelling of the foot with little or no pain. Characteristic radiographic features include the so-called sucked-candy appearance. Treatment consists of avoiding weight-bearing activities, which would result in ankylosis of the affected joints.

HYPOTHYROIDISM

Almost one third of patients with frank hypothyroidism exhibit objective musculoskeletal findings. A rheumatoid, arthritis-like presentation involving especially the large joints is characteristic. Wrists, metacarpophalangeal joints, and proximal interphalangeal joints may also be involved. Joint pain, stiffness, and detectable synovial thickening are present. Synovial fluid is generally noninflammatory. Pseudogout may also be a presenting manifestation of hypothyroidism. Myopathy, especially proximal, is common

Table 89–2	Musculoskeletal Manifestations of Endocrine Disease
Endocrine Disease	**Musculoskeletal Manifestation**
Diabetes mellitus	Carpal tunnel syndrome Charcot's arthropathy Adhesive capsulitis Syndrome of limited joint mobility (cheiroarthropathy) Diabetic amyotrophy Diabetic muscle infarction
Hypothyroidism	Proximal myopathy Arthralgias Joint effusions Carpal tunnel syndrome Chondrocalcinosis
Hyperthyroidism	Myopathy Osteoporosis Thyroid acropachy
Hyperparathyroidism	Myopathy Arthralgias Erosive arthritis Chondrocalcinosis
Hypoparathyroidism	Muscle cramps Soft tissue calcifications Spondyloarthropathy
Acromegaly	Carpal tunnel syndrome Myopathy Raynaud's phenomenon Back pain Premature osteoarthritis
Cushing's syndrome	Myopathy Osteoporosis Avascular necrosis

in hypothyroidism and is often associated with elevated levels of creatine phosphokinase. Muscle biopsy specimens show atrophy of type II fibers but no inflammation. Thyroid replacement results in gradual improvement of both the arthropathy and myopathy of hypothyroidism.

HYPERTHYROIDISM

Four principal rheumatic manifestations occur in thyrotoxicosis: proximal myopathy, shoulder periarthritis, thyroid acropachy (thickened skin with periosteal new bone formation), and osteoporosis. Myopathy is common, occurring in 70% of patients with hyperthyroidism, but it is seldom a presenting manifestation. Peri-arthritis of the shoulder (especially bilateral) occurs in up to 10% of patients. Thyroid acropachy consists of clubbing and soft tissue swelling of the hands and feet. Radiographs show periosteal new bone formation, which is best seen on the radial aspect of the second and third metacarpals. Osteoporosis is produced by increased bone turnover, which accompanies the hyperthyroid state.

HYPERPARATHYROIDISM

Musculoskeletal manifestations are common in hyperparathyroidism and are the initial manifestations in up to 15% of patients. Pseudogout is the most common rheumatic complication, occurring in up to 10% of patients with hyperparathyroidism, although radiographic chondrocalcinosis is seen in up to 40% of patients. A rheumatoid, arthritis-like disorder has also been described with involvement of the knees, wrists, hands, and shoulders, showing radiographic erosions. In contrast to rheumatoid arthritis, however, synovial proliferation is absent, the joint space is preserved, and erosions are characteristically on the ulnar side, as opposed to rheumatoid arthritis, in which the erosions are typically on the radial side.

Secondary hyperparathyroidism is common in patients with chronic renal failure and is a component of renal osteodystrophy. Musculoskeletal features are similar to those described earlier.

Sarcoidosis

Sarcoidosis is a multisystemic inflammatory disorder exhibited by the formation of noncaseating granulomas. It may be associated with both acute and chronic rheumatic manifestations. The acute syndrome is known as Löfgren's syndrome and consists of the classic triad of hilar adenopathy, erythema nodosum, and arthritis. It occurs in approximately 15% of those patients with sarcoidosis. The arthritis is usually symmetric and migratory; it frequently involves the ankles, although it may be difficult to distinguish from erythema nodosum and peri-arthritis of the ankle. Joint effusions are typically noninflammatory. The arthritis is nondeforming, nonerosive, and self-limiting, usually not lasting more than 3 to 4 months. Patients with the nonarticular manifestations of Löfgren's syndrome have an excellent prognosis.

Chronic arthropathy involving the knees, ankles, wrists, and elbows occurs less frequently and is generally associated with active multisystemic disease. Synovial thickening and effusions are common; a synovial biopsy specimen may show the typical noncaseating granulomas. Treatment of acute sarcoid arthropathy includes the use of nonsteroidal anti-inflammatory drugs or, occasionally, a short course of corticosteroids. Treatment of the chronic arthropathy is dependent on the severity of the extra-articular manifestations that usually accompany it. Corticosteroids are generally needed to control the systemic disease.

Prospectus for the Future

Advances in understanding disease mechanisms will facilitate improved recognition and treatment of the rheumatic manifestations of systemic disorders.

References

Cagliero E, Apruzzese W, Perlmutter GS, et al: Musculoskeletal disorders of the hand and shoulder in patients with diabetes mellitus. Am J Med 112:487–490, 2002.

Seldin DC, Anderson JJ, Sanchorawala V, et al: Improvement in quality of life of patients with AL amyloidosis treated with high-dose melphalan and autologous stem cell transplantation. Blood. 104(6):1888–1893, 2004 Sep 15.

Simms RW: Arthropathies associated with hematologic and malignant disorders. In Klippel JH (ed): Primer on the Rheumatic Diseases, 11th ed. Atlanta, Arthritis Foundation, 1997, pp 337–338.

Section XVI

Infectious Disease

Cecil Andreoli and Carpenter's *Essentials* of Medicine

Organisms that Infect Humans

Benigno Rodríguez

Michael M. Lederman

O f diseases afflicting humans, most that are curable and preventable are caused by infectious agents. The infectious diseases that capture the attention of physicians and the public periodically shift—for example, from syphilis to tuberculosis to acquired immunodeficiency syndrome (AIDS)—but the challenges of dealing with these processes endure. To the student, an understanding of infectious diseases offers insights into medicine as a whole. Osler's adage (with updating) remains relevant: "He [or she] who knows syphilis [AIDS], knows medicine."

Viruses

Viruses produce a wide variety of clinical illnesses. A virus consists of either DNA or RNA (in rare cases, both) wrapped within a protein nucleocapsid. An envelope composed of glycoproteins and lipids may cover the nucleocapsid; pathogenic viruses that lack an envelope tend to survive better in the environment and are more often transmitted by the fecal-oral route, whereas those that possess an envelope are more often transmitted by the parenteral route or through the genital or respiratory mucosa. Viral genes can code for only a limited number of proteins, and viruses possess no metabolic machinery; they are entirely dependent on host cells for protein synthesis and replication and are therefore obligate intracellular parasites. Some viruses are dependent on other viruses to replicate or produce active infection. Such is the case with the delta agent, which completes its life cycle only in the presence of hepatitis B infection. All must attach to receptors on the host cell and achieve entry into the cell through mechanisms that include receptor-mediated endocytosis, fusion, pinocytosis, or, in the case of certain nonenveloped viruses, direct penetration of the cell membrane. Once within the cells, the virus uncoats, allowing its nucleic acid to use host cellular machinery to reproduce (productive infection) or to integrate into the host cell (latent infection). Some viruses, such as influenza virus, cause disease by lysis of infected cells. Others, such as hepatitis B virus, do not directly cause cell destruction but may involve the host immune responses in the pathogenesis of

disease. Still others, such as the human T-lymphotropic virus type 1, promote neoplastic transformation of infected cells.

Viruses have developed several mechanisms for evading host defense mechanisms. By multiplying within host cells, viruses can avoid neutralizing antibodies and other extracellular host defenses. Some viruses can spread to uninfected cells by intercellular bridges. Others, especially the herpes group and human immunodeficiency virus (HIV), are capable of persisting latently without multiplication in a metabolically inactive form within host cells for prolonged periods. The influenza virus is capable of extensive gene rearrangements, resulting in significant changes in surface antigen structure. This capability allows new strains to evade host antibody responses directed at earlier strains.

Some viruses, as they exit the host cell during productive infection, may carry antigens of host cell origin, thus providing another potential mechanism for evading host defenses, whereas others block host immune defense mechanisms, such as expression of human leukocyte antigens. HIV induces both specific and nonspecific escape mechanisms by selectively deleting HIV-reactive T-cell clones and coating itself with a host-derived *glycan shield* that hinders neutralizing antibody activity, while also causing profound global immune dysfunction that paralyzes host defenses.

Prions

Prions are a group of host-encoded transmissible proteins devoid of nucleic acid material that cause disease through accumulation of a pathogenic isoform of the prion protein. They are thought to be responsible for a significant number of progressive and ultimately fatal neurologic diseases in humans, including kuru, Creutzfeldt-Jakob disease (CJD), Gerstmann-Straüssler-Scheinker syndrome and familial fatal insomnia, and animal diseases such as scrapie and bovine spongiform encephalopathy *(mad cow disease)*. Although some prion diseases (e.g., familial CJD) are inherited, others, including kuru and new variant CJD, are acquired through consumption of infected neural tissue. No known treatment has been developed for these disorders.

Bacteria

Bacteria are a tremendously varied group of organisms that are generally capable of cell-free growth, although some produce disease as intracellular parasites. Bacteria can be classified in numerous ways, including morphologic mechanisms, ability to retain certain dyes, growth in different physical conditions, ability to metabolize various substrates, and antibiotic sensitivities. Although combinations of these methods are used to identify bacteria in clinical bacteriology laboratories, relatedness for taxonomic purposes is established by DNA homology.

CHLAMYDIAE

Chlamydiae are also obligate intracellular parasites; they always contain both DNA and RNA, divide by binary fission (rather than multiplying by assembly), can synthesize proteins, and contain ribosomes. Although classified as a unique family of bacteria, Chlamydiae are unable to synthesize adenosine triphosphate and thus depend on energy from the host cell to survive. The three chlamydial species known to cause disease in humans are *Chlamydia trachomatis, C. pneumoniae,* and *C. psittaci. C. trachomatis* causes trachoma, the major cause of blindness in the developing world, and a wide variety of sexually transmitted genitourinary disorders, including urethritis, salpingitis, and lymphogranuloma venereum. *C. pneumoniae* is a common cause of atypical pneumonia, bronchitis, and sinusitis. *C. psittaci,* the cause of a common infectious disease of birds, can produce a serious systemic illness with prominent pulmonary manifestations in humans. Chlamydiae are susceptible to tetracyclines, rifampin, macrolides and related compounds, ketolides, and certain quinolones.

RICKETTSIAE AND EHRLICHIAE

Rickettsiae and ehrlichiae are also small bacterial organisms that, similar to chlamydiae, are obligate intracellular parasites. They are primarily animal pathogens that generally produce disease in humans through the bite of an insect vector, such as a tick, flea, louse, or mite. Most of these rickettsiae specifically infect vascular endothelial cells, whereas *Ehrlichichia chaffeensis* and *Anaplasma phagocytophilum* target human monocytes and granulocytes, respectively. With the exception of Q fever and human ehrlichiosis, rash caused by vasculitis is a prominent manifestation of these often disabling febrile illnesses. These organisms are susceptible to tetracyclines and chloramphenicol.

MYCOPLASMAS

Mycoplasmas are the smallest free-living organisms. In contrast to viruses, chlamydiae, rickettsiae, and ehrlichiae, mycoplasmas can grow on cell-free media and produce disease without intracellular penetration. Similar to other bacteria, these organisms have a membrane, but, unlike other bacteria, they have no cell walls. Thus, antibiotics that are active against bacterial cell walls have no effect on mycoplasmas. At least 14 species of *Mycoplasma* may cause disease in humans. *Mycoplasma pneumoniae* is an agent of pharyngitis and pneumonia. Although *Mycoplasma*

hominis, Ureaplasma urealyticum, and the newly described *Mycoplasma genitalium* are primarily agents of genitourinary disease, they may also cause systemic infections, particularly in compromised hosts. Mycoplasmas are sensitive to erythromycin, tetracycline, or a combined regimen of both.

SPIROCHETES

Spirochetes are slender, motile, spiral-shaped organisms that are not readily seen under the microscope unless stained with silver or viewed under darkfield illumination. Many of these organisms cannot yet be cultured on artificial media or in cell culture. Four genera of spirochetes cause disease in humans. *Treponema* species include the pathogens of syphilis and the nonvenereal, endemic, syphilis-like illnesses of yaws, pinta, and bejel. The illnesses caused by these organisms are chronic and characterized by prolonged latency in the host. Penicillin is active against *Treponema. Leptospira* species are the causative agents of leptospirosis, an acute or subacute febrile illness occasionally resulting in aseptic meningitis, jaundice, and (in rare cases) renal insufficiency. *Borrelia* species are arthropod-borne spirochetes that are the causative agents of Lyme disease (see Chapter 94) and relapsing fever. During afebrile periods in relapsing fever, these organisms reside within host cells and emerge with modified cell surface antigens. These modifications may permit the bacterium to evade host immune responses and produce relapsing fever and recurrent bacteremia. *Spirillum minus* is one of the causative agents of rat-bite fever.

ANAEROBIC BACTERIA

Anaerobes are organisms that cannot grow in atmospheric oxygen tensions. Some anaerobes are killed by very low oxygen concentrations, whereas others are relatively aerotolerant. As a general rule, anaerobes that are pathogens for humans are not as sensitive to oxygen as nonpathogens. Anaerobic bacteria are primarily commensals. They inhabit the skin, gut, and mucosal surfaces of all healthy individuals. In fact, the presence of anaerobes may inhibit colonization of the gut by virulent, potentially pathogenic bacteria. Anaerobic infections generally occur in two circumstances:

1. Contamination of otherwise sterile sites with anaerobe-laden contents. Examples include (a) aspiration of oral anaerobes into the bronchial tree, producing anaerobic necrotizing pneumonia, (b) peritonitis and intra-abdominal abscesses after bowel perforation, (c) fasciitis and osteomyelitis after odontogenic infections or oral surgery, and (d) some instances of pelvic inflammatory disease.
2. Infections of tissue with lowered redox potential as the result of a compromised vascular supply. Examples include (a) foot infections in patients with diabetes in whom vascular disease may produce poor tissue oxygenation and (b) infections of pressure sores in which fecal anaerobic flora gain access to tissue whose vascular supply is compromised by pressure.

The pathogenesis of anaerobic infections—that is, soilage by a complex flora—generally results in polymicrobial infections. Thus, the demonstration of one anaerobe in an infected site generally implies the presence of others. In many instances, facultative organisms (organisms capable of anaerobic and aerobic growths) co-exist with anaerobes. Certain anaerobes, such as *Clostridium,* produce toxins that cause well-defined systemic illnesses such as food poisoning, tetanus, and botulism. Other toxins may play a role in soft tissue infections (cellulitis, fasciitis, and myonecrosis) occasionally produced by *Clostridium* species. *Bacteroides fragilis,* the most numerous bacterial pathogen in the normal human colon, has a polysaccharide capsule that inhibits phagocytosis and promotes abscess formation. Clues to the presence of anaerobic infection include (1) a foul odor (the diagnosis of anaerobic pneumonia can, on occasion, be made from across the room), (2) the presence of gas, which may be seen radiographically or manifested by crepitus on examination (although not all gas-forming infections are anaerobic), and (3) the presence of mixed gram-positive and gram-negative flora on a Gram stain of purulent exudate, especially when little or no growth occurs on plates cultured aerobically. Many pathogenic anaerobes are sensitive to penicillin. Exceptions are strains of *Bacteroides fragilis* (usually sensitive to metronidazole, clindamycin, or ampicillin-sulbactam) and *Clostridium difficile,* which is almost always sensitive to metronidazole and vancomycin. Strains of *Fusobacterium* may also be relatively resistant to penicillin. As a general rule, infections caused by anaerobes originating from sites above the diaphragm are more often (but not always) penicillin sensitive, whereas penicillin-resistant organisms, notably *B. fragilis,* often cause infections below the diaphragm.

GRAM-NEGATIVE BACTERIA

The cell walls of gram-negative bacteria, which appear pink on a properly prepared Gram stain, contain lipopolysaccharide, a potent inducer of cytokines such as tumor necrosis factor, and are associated with fever and septic shock. These organisms cause a wide variety of illnesses. Gram-negative bacteria are the most common cause of cystitis and pyelonephritis. *Haemophilus* species are common pathogens of the respiratory tract and cause otitis media, sinusitis, tracheobronchitis, and pneumonia. Lower respiratory tract infections with these organisms are particularly common in adults with chronic obstructive pulmonary disease. *Haemophilus* can be an important cause of meningitis, particularly in children. Except for *Haemophilus* and *Klebsiella* species, gram-negative bacteria are uncommon causes of community-acquired pneumonia but are common causes of nosocomial pneumonia.

Except for the peculiar risk of *Pseudomonas* infection in intravenous drug users, gram-negative organisms are rare causes of endocarditis on natural heart valves but are occasional pathogens on prosthetic valves. The *Enterobacteriaceae* include *Escherichia coli, Klebsiella, Enterobacter, Serratia, Salmonella, Shigella,* and *Proteus.* These organisms are large gram-negative rods. Except for the occasional presence of a clear space surrounding some *Klebsiella* (representing a large capsule), these organisms are not readily distinguished from each other on Gram stain. The *Enterobacteriaceae* can be described as gut-related or genitourinary pathogens. *Salmonella,* a relatively common cause of enteritis, may occasionally infect atherosclerotic plaques or

aneurysms. *Shigella* is an agent of bacterial dysentery. *Proteus* species, which split urea, are the agents associated with staghorn calculi of the urinary collecting system. Increasingly, gram-negative bacteria that are often resistant to multiple antibiotics are important causes of nosocomial infection. The genus *Bartonella* contains a group of emerging pathogens that cause uncommon, unique infections, including Q fever, bacillary angiomatosis, cat-scratch disease, and South American bartonellosis.

Helicobacter pylori, a highly motile, curved microaerophilic gram-negative rod, first isolated from humans in 1982, has subsequently been shown to be the major cause of peptic ulcer worldwide. This subject is discussed in greater detail in Chapter 35.

Gram-negative cocci that cause disease in humans include *Neisseria* and *Moraxella* species. These kidney bean–shaped diplococci are not distinguishable from one another on Gram stain. *Neisseria meningitidis* is an important cause of meningitis, and *Neisseria gonorrhoeae* causes gonorrhea. *Moraxella catarrhalis,* which is part of the normal oral flora, is a cause of lower respiratory tract infection, especially in adults with chronic obstructive pulmonary disease.

GRAM-POSITIVE BACTERIA

Although gram-positive bacteria, which appear deep purple on Gram stain, lack endotoxin, infections with these bacteria also produce fever and cannot be reliably distinguished on clinical grounds from infections caused by gram-negative bacteria.

Gram-Positive Rods

Infections caused by gram-positive rods are relatively uncommon outside certain specific settings. Diphtheria is now unusual in the industrialized world (although epidemics have occurred in recent years), but other corynebacteria produce infections in the immunocompromised host and on prosthetic valves and shunts. Because corynebacteria are regular skin colonizers, they often contaminate blood cultures; in the appropriate setting, however, they must be considered potential pathogens. *Listeria monocytogenes* resembles *Corynebacterium* on initial isolation, and this food-borne pathogen is an increasingly important cause of meningitis and bacteremia in the immunocompromised patient. *Bacillus cereus* is a recognized cause of food poisoning. Serious infections with this and other *Bacillus* species occur among intravenous drug users. Infections with *Clostridium* species are previously discussed.

Gram-Positive Cocci

Staphylococcus aureus is a common pathogen that can infect any organ system. It is a common cause of bacteremia and sepsis. The organism often colonizes the anterior nares, particularly among patients with insulin-treated diabetes, patients on hemodialysis, and intravenous drug users; these populations therefore have an increased frequency of infections with this organism. Hospital workers colonized with *S. aureus* have been responsible for hospital epidemics of staphylococcal disease.

Generally protected by an antiphagocytic polysaccharide capsule, staphylococci also possess catalase, which inactivates hydrogen peroxide—a mediator of bacterial killing by

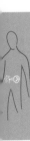

neutrophils. Staphylococci tend to form abscesses; the low pH within an abscess cavity also limits the effectiveness of host defense cells. Staphylococci elaborate several toxins that mediate specific manifestations of disease. A staphylococcal enterotoxin is responsible for staphylococcal food poisoning. Staphylococcal toxins also mediate the scalded skin syndrome and the multisystem manifestations of toxic shock syndrome. Most staphylococci are penicillinase producing, and an increasing proportion are resistant to penicillinase-resistant penicillin analogs. Although commonly referred to as methicillin-resistant *S. aureus* (MRSA), they are resistant to all β-lactams. Vancomycin remains active against most strains, but strains with reduced susceptibility, and even complete resistance to this and other glycopeptides, have recently been isolated from clinical cases. Resistance in these strains is the result of acquisition of mobile genetic elements from *Enterococcus* species, likely in the hospital setting. These strains are still uncommon, but they can cause severe disease, including bloodstream infections.

Other staphylococci are distinguished from *S. aureus* primarily by their inability to produce coagulase. Some of these coagulase-negative staphylococci produce urinary tract infection *(S. saprophyticus)*. Another species, *S. epidermidis,* is part of the normal skin flora and an increasingly important cause of infection on foreign bodies such as prosthetic heart valves, ventriculoatrial shunts, and intravascular catheters. Similar to *Corynebacterium, S. epidermidis* may be a contaminant of blood cultures but in the appropriate setting should be considered a potential pathogen. *S. saprophyticus* is sensitive to a wide variety of antibiotics used in treating urinary tract infection; *S. epidermidis* is usually resistant to all β-lactams but sensitive to vancomycin.

Streptococci are classified into groups according to the presence of serologically defined carbohydrate capsules (Lancefield typing). Group A streptococci produce skin infections, pharyngitis, and systemic infections. These organisms are also associated with the immunologically mediated poststreptococcal disorders—glomerulonephritis and acute rheumatic fever. Streptococci are further classified according to the pattern of hemolysis on blood agar-α for incomplete hemolysis (producing a green discoloration on the agar), β for complete hemolysis, and γ for nonhemolytic strains. An important α-hemolytic strain is *Streptococcus pneumoniae* (pneumococcus), the most common cause of community-acquired pneumonia and an important cause of meningitis and otitis media. Penicillin resistance in pneumococcal isolates is an increasingly important problem and is often associated with concomitant resistance to other agents. Whereas pneumococcal pneumonia caused by strains with intermediate penicillin resistance can still be successfully treated with very high doses of penicillin, other antimicrobial agents must now be used for pneumococcal meningitis (see Chapter 96). Penicillin-resistant *S. pneumoniae* generally remains susceptible to vancomycin. A heterogeneous group of streptococci, often improperly referred to as viridans streptococci (these organisms may show α- or γ-hemolysis), includes several species of *Streptococcus* that are common oral or gut colonists and are important agents of bacterial endocarditis, abscesses, and odontogenic infections.

Formerly classified as members of the *Streptococcus* genus, enterococci, unlike most streptococci, exhibit varying degrees of resistance to penicillins and are uniformly resistant to cephalosporins. Strains of vancomycin-resistant enterococci (VRE) are increasingly prevalent causes of serious hospital-acquired infections, particularly in immunocompromised and postsurgical patients, that are exceedingly difficult to treat.

MYCOBACTERIA

Mycobacteria are a group of rod-shaped bacilli that stain weakly gram positive. These organisms are rich in lipid content and are recognized in tissue specimens by their ability to retain dye after washing with acid alcohol (acid fast). These bacteria are generally slow-growing (some require up to 6 weeks to demonstrate growth on solid media), obligate aerobes. They generally produce chronic disease and survive for years as intracellular parasites of mononuclear phagocytes. Some mycobacteria escape intracellular killing mechanisms by blocking phagosome-lysosome fusion or by disrupting the phagosome. Almost all mycobacteria provoke cell-mediated immune responses in the host, and clinical disease expression may be related in large part to the nature of the host immune response. Tuberculosis is caused by *Mycobacterium tuberculosis*. Other mycobacteria (nontuberculous mycobacteria) can cause diseases resembling tuberculosis. Certain rapid-growing mycobacteria cause infections after surgery or implantations of prostheses, as well as epidemic and sporadic skin and soft tissue infections. *M. avium* complex (MAC) is an important cause of disseminated infection among patients with AIDS. MAC is frequently resistant to drugs usually used in the treatment of tuberculosis. Leprosy is a mycobacterial disease of the skin and peripheral nerves caused by the noncultivatable *M. leprae*.

ACTINOMYCETALES

Nocardia and *Actinomyces* are weakly gram-positive filamentous bacteria. *Nocardia* is acid fast and aerobic; *Actinomyces* is anaerobic and not acid fast. *Actinomyces* inhabits the mouth, gut, and vagina and produces cervicofacial osteomyelitis and abscess, pneumonia with empyema, and intra-abdominal and pelvic abscesses, the last often associated with intrauterine contraceptive devices. *Nocardia* most commonly produces pneumonia and brain abscess. Approximately one half of patients with *Nocardia* infection have underlying impairments in cell-mediated immunity. Infections with either of these slow-growing organisms require long-term treatment. *Actinomyces* is relatively sensitive to many antibiotics; penicillin is the treatment of choice. *Nocardia* infections are treated with high doses of sulfonamides, but serious or resistant infections may require the combinations of carbapenems, aminoglycosides, or cephalosporins.

Fungi

Fungi are larger than bacteria. Unlike bacteria, they have rigid cell walls that contain chitin, as well as polysaccharides. Fungi grow and proliferate by budding, by elongation of hyphal forms, and/or by spore formation. Except for *Candida* and related species, fungi are rarely visible on

Gram-stained preparations but can be stained with Gomori methenamine silver stain or calcofluor white stain. They are also resistant to potassium hydroxide and can often be seen on wet mounts of scrapings or secretions to which several drops of a 10% solution of potassium hydroxide have been added. Fungi are resistant to most antibiotics used in the treatment of bacterial infections and must be treated with drugs active against their unusual cell wall. Most fungi can exist in a yeast form (round to ovoid cells that may reproduce by budding) and a mold form, a complex of tubular structures (hyphae) that grow by branching or extension.

Candida species are oval yeasts that often colonize the mouth, gastrointestinal tract, and vagina of healthy individuals. They may produce disease by overgrowth and/or invasion. *Candida* stomatitis (thrush) often occurs in individuals who are receiving antibiotic or corticosteroid therapy or who have impairments of cell-mediated immunity. Vulvovaginitis caused by *Candida* may occur in these same settings but can also occur in women with no apparent predisposing factors and more commonly in women with diabetes mellitus. *Candida* can also colonize and infect the urinary tract, particularly in the presence of an indwelling urinary catheter. *Candida* species may also gain entry into the bloodstream and produce fungemia with or without seeding of solid tissues, especially in hospitalized patients, in whom *Candida* species are now the fourth leading cause of intravascular infection. This infection most frequently occurs in the setting of neutropenia after chemotherapy, in which the portal of entry is the gastrointestinal tract or in individuals with intravascular catheters, which provide a route for cutaneous *Candida* to enter the systemic circulation (see Chapter 105). Mucosal candidiasis can be treated with topical (e.g., clotrimazole) or systemic (e.g., fluconazole) antifungal drugs; systemic candidiasis is generally treated with parenteral amphotericin B, azoles, or echinocandins.

Histoplasma capsulatum is a fungus endemic to the Ohio and Mississippi River valleys that produces asymptomatic infection or a mild febrile syndrome in most individuals and a self-limited pneumonia in some. In predisposed individuals, *H. capsulatum* can cause cavitary pulmonary disease and mediastinal fibrosis. Infants and immunosuppressed individuals, such as those with AIDS or neutropenia, are susceptible to the progressive disseminated form of the infection, which is potentially fatal (see Chapter 107). Systemic or progressive disease is treated with parenteral amphotericin B followed by itraconazole.

Coccidioides immitis is endemic in the southwestern United States and, similar to *H. capsulatum*, produces a self-limited respiratory infection or pneumonia in most infected individuals. Immunocompromised individuals are at greatest risk for fatal systemic dissemination or meningitis. Fluconazole, in high doses, is used for progressive or extrapulmonary disease (see Chapter 107).

Cryptococcus neoformans is a yeast with a large polysaccharide capsule. It produces a self-limited or chronic pneumonia, but the most common clinical manifestation of infection with this fungus is a form of chronic meningitis. Although patients with impairment in cell-mediated immunity are at risk for cryptococcal meningitis, some patients with this syndrome have no identifiable immunodeficiency. Treatment is with amphotericin B combined with flucyto-

sine. Long-term oral fluconazole therapy is effective in preventing relapse in patients with AIDS (see Chapter 107).

Blastomyces dermatitidis is a yeast also endemic in the Ohio and Mississippi River basins. Acute self-limited pulmonary infection is followed in rare instances by disseminated disease. Skin disease is most common, but bones, the central nervous system and the genitourinary tract may be involved as well. Parenteral amphotericin B is used for treating serious systemic disease; oral itraconazole is appropriate for moderate disease in immunocompetent hosts.

Aspergillus is a mold that produces several clinical illnesses in humans. Acute bronchopulmonary aspergillosis is an immunoglobulin E–mediated hypersensitivity to *Aspergillus* colonization of the respiratory tract. This condition produces wheezing and fleeting pulmonary infiltrates in patients with asthma. Occasionally, *Aspergillus* will colonize a pre-existent pulmonary cavity and produce a mycetoma or fungus ball. Hemoptysis is the most serious complication of such an infection. Invasive pulmonary aspergillosis is a rare cause of a chronic illness of marginally compromised hosts; more often, it is a cause of acute, life-threatening pneumonia or disseminated infection in patients with neutropenia or in recipients of organ transplants. Voriconazole is now the drug of choice for most cases of invasive aspergillosis; amphotericin B and caspofungin remain important alternative or concomitant agents.

The Zygomycetes (Mucorales) are molds with ribbon-shaped hyphae that produce disease in patients with poorly controlled diabetes mellitus or hematologic malignancy or in recipients of organ transplantation. Invasive disease of the palate and nasal sinuses, which may extend intracranially, is the most common presentation, but pneumonia may be seen as well. These infections are generally treated with surgical excision plus high-dose amphotericin B.

Pneumocystis jirovecii (formerly *P. carinii*) was once thought to be a protozoan; genetic analyses have classified *P. jirovecii* as a fungus. This organism causes life-threatening pneumonia in patients with impaired cell-mediated immunity; it is the most common major opportunistic pathogen in persons with AIDS (see Chapter 107).

Protozoans

The protozoal pathogens listed in Table 90–1 are all important causes of disease within the United States. Infections caused by these organisms are diagnosed as indicated in Table 90–1 and are discussed in the relevant disease-oriented chapters.

Helminths

Diseases caused by helminths are among the most prevalent diseases in the developing world but are uncommon causes of illness in North America. In contrast to the pathogens discussed previously, helminths are multicellular parasites. Helminthic diseases found in the United States include ascariasis (maldigestion and obstruction), hookworm (intestinal blood loss), enterobiasis (pinworm and anal pruritus), and strongyloidiasis (gastroenteritis and dissemination in the immunocompromised host). Recognizing the risk of other helminthic diseases in travelers returning from endemic regions is important (see Chapter 109).

Table 90–1   Some Protozoal Diseases of Humans

Protozoan	Clinical Illness	Transmission	Diagnosis
Plasmodium	Malaria: fever, hemolysis	Mosquito, transfusion	Peripheral blood smear
Babesia microti	Fever, hemolysis	Tick, transfusion	Peripheral blood smear
Trichomonas vaginalis	Vaginitis	Sexual contact	Vaginal smear
Toxoplasma gondii *	Fever, lymph node enlargement; encephalitis, brain abscess in compromised host	Raw meat, cat feces	Serologic test, tissue biopsy
Entamoeba histolytica	Colitis, hepatic abscess	Fecal-oral	Stool smear, serologic test
Giardia lamblia	Diarrhea, malabsorption	Fecal-oral	Stool smear, small bowel aspirate
Cryptosporidium *	Diarrhea	Fecal-oral	Sugar flotation, acid-fast stain of stool, biopsy
Isospora belli *	Diarrhea, malabsorption	Fecal-oral	Wet mount or acid-fast stain of stool
Microsporidium *	Diarrhea, malabsorption, dissemination	Fecal-oral	Small bowel biopsy Electron microscopy

*Important opportunistic pathogens in persons with acquired immunodeficiency syndrome (see Chapter 107).

Prospectus for the Future

Clinicians should anticipate the identification of *novel* pathogens causing disease:

- Prevalent microbes not previously recognized as pathogenic
- *Discovery* of prevalent pathogens not previously identified

- Influx into new communities of pathogens prevalent elsewhere
- Increased frequency and different clinical presentations of uncommon pathogens as a consequence of immunosuppressive conditions and treatments

References

Bruckner DA, Colonna P: Nomenclature for aerobic and facultative bacteria. Clin Infect Dis 29:713–723, 1999.

Dermody TS, Tyler KL: Introduction to viruses and viral diseases. In Mandell GL, Bennett JE, Dolin R (eds): Principles and Practice of Infectious Diseases, 6th ed. Philadelphia, Elsevier, 2005, pp 1729–1742.

Summanen P: Microbiology terminology update: Clinically significant anaerobic gram-positive and gram-negative bacteria (excluding spirochetes). Clin Infect Dis 29:724–727, 1999.

Host Defenses Against Infection

Benigno Rodríguez

Michael M. Lederman

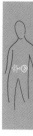

Host Defenses Versus Mechanisms of Microbial Pathogenesis: The Struggle for Survival

As our experience suggests, and as fossil records indicate, life is a continual struggle for survival. Pathogenic and host defense–evasive mechanisms of microbes are countered by multiple and overlapping host-innate and adaptive immune defense mechanisms. In some cases, the pathogen *wins,* with destruction of the host; in others, the host immune response prevails, with eradication of the microbe. In many instances, a standoff ensues characterized by latent infection or colonization without substantial morbidity to the host; sometimes the relationship is actually symbiotic, with both host and pathogen gaining from it. In settings of latent or colonizing pathogens, microbes have the capacity to activate and cause disease if host defenses become impaired. Much of our understanding of host defenses and their relationship to microbial pathogenesis has been derived from recognizing the spectrum of infections experienced by individuals with specific impairments of host defenses. Thus, persons with neutrophil depletion or defects in neutrophil function tend to experience bacterial and fungal infections, those with antibody defects are particularly at risk for infections caused by encapsulated bacteria, and persons with impairments in cell-mediated immunity tend to be at particular risk for infection with pathogens that replicate within host cells. Reflecting the importance of these insights, in the early days of the acquired immunodeficiency syndrome (AIDS) epidemic, astute clinicians recognized immediately that the kinds of infections seen in the first patients with AIDS implicated an acquired impairment of cell-mediated adaptive immune defenses; this insight accelerated research on the pathogenesis and cause of AIDS.

Evolutionary Advantage of Adaptable Organisms

Fundamental to our understanding of evolution is the concept that organisms most capable of adaptation to environmental stresses are most likely to survive, to propagate, and to persist. Thus, random mutations in the germline that confer survival advantage are passed on to adapting, succeeding generations. With this concept in mind, the fact that complex organisms such as humans can compete for survival with microbes much more capable of rapid genetic adaptation to challenge is astounding. The number of germline mutations over time depends on generation time, the number of offspring per generation, and the mistake rate of the DNA or RNA polymerase required for genomic replication. In each of these indices, microbes have the clear adaptive advantage. As an example, humans must survive at least 10 years or more before they are even capable of reproduction and then generate only a small number of offspring before dying. In contrast, bacteria can grow exponentially, with generation times measured in minutes to hours, and viruses express thousands of progeny, with replication cycles that can be completed within hours to days. Human DNA polymerases have an error rate of approximately one base pair per 10^{12} cellular divisions, bacterial DNA polymerases have an error rate of approximately one base pair per 10^6 divisions, and the reverse transcriptase of human immunodeficiency virus type 1 (HIV-1) has an error rate of approximately one base pair per 10^3 to 10^4 replications. These mutations are, to a large extent, random, and most mutations result in decreased function or are incompatible with survival. Because of the limited number of offspring humans produce, a faithful DNA polymerase that maximizes survival of an individual's descendants is important to our species. In contrast, microbes are prepared to generate many defective organisms with null mutations to ensure the emergence of rare mutations conferring survival advantage. The rapid emergence of resistance to antimicrobials is reflective of the genetic flexibility of microbes.

The ability to recognize and respond nonspecifically to foreign organisms has existed for millions of years and can be demonstrated even in relatively primitive life forms. However, to survive in the struggle for the survival against microbes and their seemingly unending ability to replicate and evolve over short intervals of time, more complex species (including humans) with slow and infrequent germline evolution events require a system that can efficiently adjust to protect the individual against the constantly changing onslaught of microbial pathogens. Thus, with the appearance of the gnathostomes, or jawed vertebrates, an adaptable immune defense system emerged that for the first time permitted a rapid *evolution* of host defenses against infectious agents without the need for reproduction or germline mutation. This *real-time evolution* is achieved through rearrangement (and, in the case of B lymphocytes, somatic mutation) of the genes encoding the receptors of T and B lymphocytes and the ability to expand clones of these microbe-specific cells—the directors of adaptive immune recognition.

Categories of Host Defenses and Risks for Infection

Over the course of species development, numerous mechanisms have evolved to protect larger organisms from infection or parasitization by another organism. These mechanisms can be categorized according to the primary defense mechanism as anatomic, humoral, or cellular and according to their specificity as innate or adaptive. Anatomic defenses are primarily innate and nonadaptive, whereas humoral and cellular defenses can be either innate or adaptive. Innate defenses, present in many primitive organisms, comprise a rapid, *already primed* response to microbial invasion, whereas adaptive responses may be more delayed in their onset but ultimately are both more specific in their targets and capable of providing *memory* of prior encounters to protect against recurrence of infection. Although distinguishing between these two kinds of host defenses is important, both innate and adaptive immune mechanisms are intimately interactive, thereby providing, in most instances, remarkable synergistic protection against infection.

ANATOMIC DEFENSES

Anatomic defenses protect directly against microbial colonization and infection and are primarily located at sites with proximate environmental contact. Thus, skin and mucosal surfaces are enriched with defenses ranging from the tightness of epithelial junctions to resist microbial penetration, to the presence of cough and gag reflexes to expel aspirated secretions, and to the presence of chemical agents such as acids and defensins with antimicrobial properties. Permissiveness to colonization of these surfaces by microbes of low pathogenicity prevents colonization and infection by more virulent organisms. In some clinical settings, interference with anatomic defense mechanisms may increase the risk of

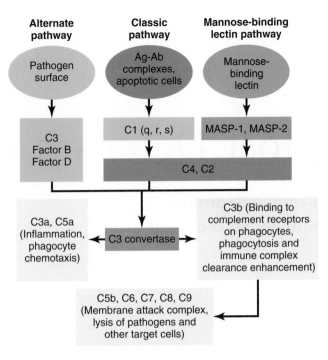

Figure 91–1 Simplified diagram of the complement system. The final effector components are shown in clear symbols at the bottom of the graphic, with a summary of their most important biologic activities. Not all molecular events leading to the final effector components are shown.

infection. Thus, burns with denuding of the epithelial barrier, illnesses or intoxicants that suppress gag and cough reflexes, treatment with agents that decrease gastric pH, and treatment with antibiotics that disturb the commensal mucosal flora can increase the risks of microbial infection.

HUMORAL DEFENSES AGAINST INFECTION
Complement System

Humoral defenses, comprising soluble compounds found in blood plasma and in other extracellular fluids, also play important roles in the defense against microbes. One of the most important of these humoral defenses is the complement system. Complement activity results from the sequential interaction of a large number of plasma and cell membrane proteins. A simplified diagram of the most important steps in the complement cascade is shown in Figure 91–1. The *classic complement pathway* is activated by antibody-coated targets or antigen-antibody complexes through the interaction of the initial protein C1 with the Fc receptor of the antigen-bound antibody molecule. The *alternative pathway* is activated in the absence of antibody by constituents of the microbial surface, including polysaccharides. Finally, the sugar-binding protein *mannose-binding lectin* can also activate the complement cascade after binding to surface mannose residues on viruses and other pathogens. All three pathways converge with the formation of C3 convertase, which leads to the production of the effector components of the complement system. C3b or iC3b deposited on the surface of microbes binds to complement receptors

Table 91–1   Properties of Human Immunoglobulins

	IgG	IgA	IgM	IgD	IgE
H chain class	γ	α	μ	δ	ε
Molecular weight (approximate)	150,000	170,000	900,000	180,000	190,000
Complement fixation	++	0	++++	0	0
Opsonic activity	++++	++	0	0	0
Reaginic activity	0	0	0	0	++++
Serum concentration (mg/dL)	1500	150–350	100–150	2	2
Serum half-life (days)	23	6	5	3	2.5
Major functions	Recall response; opsonization; transplacental immunity	Secretory immunity	Primary response; complement fixation	?	Allergy; anthelmintic immunity

(CR1, CR3, and CR4) on neutrophils and macrophages and promotes phagocytosis. Moreover, C3b furthers clearance of immune complexes by linking them to CR1 on the erythrocyte surface. C5a is a chemotaxin for neutrophils and activates oxidative burst activity. C5a and C3a also stimulate histamine release from mast cells and thus promote inflammation. The ultimate effector element of the complement system is the membrane attack complex, which involves C5 to C9. This complex produces pores in the membrane of microbes and subjects them to osmotic lysis. Thus, the complement system can opsonize microbes, can directly damage them, and can induce inflammation through liberation of chemotactically active fragments. Persons with complement deficiencies, particularly deficiencies in terminal components, are especially at risk for repeated infections with gram-negative encapsulated bacteria, especially *Neisseria* species.

Antibodies

Antibodies are large polypeptides produced by B lymphocytes and plasma cells that are key components of the adaptive immune response (Table 91–1). Antibody molecules recognize structural elements of microbial surfaces and, when bound, may block the ability of that structure to interact with and infect a cell (neutralization), may facilitate ingestion of the microbe by phagocytes (opsonization), or may bind and activate complement, resulting in the killing of certain microbes. Finally, antibodies may recognize microbial or other foreign antigens expressed on a cell surface and facilitate the destruction of that cell by host defense cells with cytolytic capabilities (antibody-dependent cellular cytotoxicity [ADCC]). Distinctive characteristics of the five recognized classes of antibodies are summarized in Table 91–1. Immunoglobulin (Ig) M constitutes the earliest immune response to antigenic challenge and often predominates in response to polysaccharides; IgG is the most prevalent immunoglobulin class in blood; IgA is present both in blood and at mucosal surfaces and is a key element in mucosal immune protection; IgD and IgM may serve as B-lymphocyte surface antigen receptors; and IgE plays an important role in allergic reaction by triggering mast cell activation and is also important in mediating responses to parasitic infestation. As components of the adaptive immune response, antibodies have great diversity in their recognition domains, and the generation of this diversity permits both targeted investment of immune *energy* and the generation of immune *memory*. Antibodies provide protection against microbes primarily when these organisms are in the extracellular space. Once within cells that they infect, microbes are largely (but not always; see ADCC discussed earlier) invisible to antibody-mediated defenses. Persons with defects in antibody formation are at greatest risk for infection with encapsulated bacteria such as the pneumococcus.

CELLULAR DEFENSES AGAINST INFECTION
Phagocytic Cells

Phagocytic cells—neutrophils and macrophages—are rapidly attracted to sites of microbial invasion by the elaboration of chemoattractant cytokines called chemokines and are able to ingest (phagocytose) microbes both directly and even more efficiently when the microbes are opsonized (coated with antibody or complement) through attachment to specific receptors on the phagocyte cell surface. Once ingested, microbes are killed by a system of enzymes and other antimicrobial factors. The phagocytic cells are efficient mediators of defense against many bacteria and fungi; decreases in the numbers or function of neutrophils place persons at risk for bacterial and fungal infections.

Macrophages also serve as *professional antigen-presenting cells* (see later discussion) and can activate cell-mediated immune defenses by presenting digested microbial peptides to T cells.

T Lymphocytes

T lymphocytes are critical effector and helper cells of the adaptive cell-mediated immune response; they are generated through a complex process of selection in the thymus gland. In the thymus, the genes encoding the T-cell antigen receptor are rearranged, generating an enormous diversity of T-cell receptor (TCR) structures. T cells recognize peptide antigen bound by host cell surface human leukocyte antigens (HLAs). T cells with insufficient affinity or too great an affinity for host HLAs fail to survive thymic development; thus, the population of T cells that survive thymic maturation maintains a diverse yet select repertoire of TCRs capable of recognizing a wide array of peptides when bound by cell surface HLA molecules. The TCR of CD4$^+$ T cells recognizes ingested peptides bound by class II HLA molecules, whereas class I HLA molecules bind peptides synthesized within the cell by invading pathogens for recognition by the TCR of CD8$^+$ T cells. Not surprisingly therefore, after TCR engagement, CD8$^+$ T cells destroy infected cells expressing the foreign peptides, whereas CD4$^+$ T cells are activated largely to express T-helper cytokines that enhance the function of other immune cells such as CD8$^+$ T cells, natural killer (NK) cells, macrophages, and B lymphocytes. Destruction of target cells by cytolytic CD8$^+$ T cells can be mediated by receptor-ligand interaction, whereby binding of receptors on the target cell (such as Fas) by ligand on the effector cell results in activation of programmed cell death (apoptosis) of the target. Perhaps more importantly, cytolytic cells are enriched for perforin, which, similar to the terminal components of complement, produces pores in the target cell membrane, and for granzymes that gain entry to target cells through these pores and induce programmed cell death of the target. Therefore, impairments in T cell numbers or function place persons at particular risk for infection with pathogens that replicate within host cells. Because of their central role in mediating immunologic help, decreases in CD4$^+$ T cells or their function also diminishes many other aspects of host defense, such as antibody responses.

Natural Killer Cells

NK cells are large granular lymphocytes that, similar to CD8$^+$ T cells, have cytolytic function. These NK lymphocytes can kill tumor cells or normal cells infected by viruses. They are most active against target cells with low-level expression of class I HLA molecules, which, when present, activate inhibitory molecules on the NK cell surface. Because many viruses decrease host HLA class I expression as a means to evade host cytotoxic T-lymphocyte recognition, NK lymphocytes may serve to identify and lyse cells resistant to antigen-specific T cell–mediated cytotoxicity. As an effector of innate or nonadaptive host defense, NK cells appear to be important also in early responses to viral infections and in defense against malignancy. NK cells also have receptors for the Fc portion of IgG that, when recognizing a foreign antigen on a target cell, promote lysis of that target by the NK cell (ADCC). Rarely, persons with marked decreases in numbers of NK cells experience repeated and severe herpesvirus infections.

How Cells Communicate with Other Cells

Cellular interactions are critical for host defense against microbes. Cells must signal other cells so as to attract them to sites of infection; specific cells can also arm and activate other cells to perform their function more effectively, and cellular interactions are essential to generate and amplify host adaptive immune responses. Cells establish these communications in two basic ways: by direct contact and by the expression of soluble factors—cytokines—that bind to cellular receptors and result in the generation of intracellular signals that affect the function of the cell. Some cytokine receptors are specific for a single cytokine (e.g., the high-affinity interleukin-2 receptor and interleukin-2), whereas others can be triggered by multiple cytokines (as is often the case for chemokine receptors). Chemokines are cytokines that induce cellular movement and play important roles in trafficking cells to appropriate sites. Different cell types may express the same cytokine, and one cytokine may target several cell types, resulting in different effects in each. Thus, the network of cellular interactions in host defense is quite complex.

Interferons

Interferons are antiviral cytokines that can be induced as a response to viral infection; these cytokines also have potent effects on host defense cells. The plasmacytoid dendritic cell (pDC) is the major source of interferon-α—a type 1 interferon that is induced when these professional antigen–presenting cells recognize microbial motifs through toll-like receptors (see later discussion). Type I interferons (α and β) also are induced in virus-infected cells. Type II interferon (interferon-γ) is produced by T cells and NK cells. Interferon binding to the type 1 interferon receptor activates a large number of host genes, including systems of antiviral defenses, thereby attenuating viral replication. Interferon-γ also activates cytolytic activity of T cells and NK cells and activates monocytes.

How Enormous Diversity in Immune Recognition Is Possible

Because enormous diversity exists in the structure and sequence of microbial pathogens, host defenses must have the ability to generate and maintain a diverse repertoire of defenses against potential invaders. Both the humoral (B cell–driven) and cellular (T cell–driven) arms of the adaptive immune response are activated by the specific interaction of foreign antigen with cellular receptors. In the case of B cells, the receptor is a surface Ig (antibody) molecule that recognizes three-dimensional structures; in the case of the T cells, the receptor recognizes short foreign peptides from 8 to 20 amino acids in length that are bound to host HLA

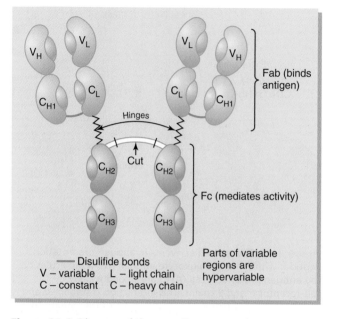

Figure 91–2 Diagram of the overall structure of immunoglobulin G, which is the basic structural pattern for all immunoglobulins (see text), drawn to highlight the various reactive areas and to emphasize the globular domain features of the immunoglobulin molecule. (From Bennett JC: Approach to the patient with immune diseases. In Bennett JC, Plum F [eds]: Cecil Textbook of Medicine, 20th ed. Philadelphia, WB Saunders, 1996, p 1394.)

molecules. The flexibility of T cell– and B cell–receptor rearrangements permits the adaptive immune system to respond to a large number of antigenic structures. B cells and T cells appear to use similar mechanisms to generate and express the diversity required for such a broad range of specific antigenic responses.

Five classes of antibodies (isotypes) are recognized (see Table 91–1). An *IgG antibody* (Fig. 91–2) consists of two light (κ or λ) chains and two heavy chains. Each antibody has constant regions, which are identical in structure to all antibodies of that class, and distinctive antigen-recognition sites whose structures are variable. An IgG_1 molecule has two such antigen-combining sites. The antigen-combining sites of antibody molecules recognize the structure of an antigen and bind to it in a lock-and-key manner through multiple weak, noncovalent interactions. The variable regions consist of the approximately 110 amino-terminal amino acids of each chain. Three short, hypervariable regions are present in each of the light and heavy chains. The six hypervariable regions form the antigen-combining site.

Antibody diversity is generated as B lymphocytes mature and is understood at the molecular level. The variable portion of the heavy chain is encoded by three different genes: V, D, and J; investigators have identified 500 to 1000 different V genes, 10 D genes, and 4 J genes. The variable portions of the light chains are encoded by V and J genes; investigators have identified 200 possible V genes and 6 J genes. During the differentiation of B cells in the bone marrow, somatic translocations randomly select the V, D, and J heavy-chain genes and the V and J light-chain genes that will be transcribed in that cell. The diversity achieved by this means

is enormous. Somatic mutations in B cells as they divide after encountering antigen in lymphoid tissue allow the possibility of improving the fit between antibody and antigen; repeated or sustained exposure to antigen selects B cells capable of producing antibody with the highest binding affinity. These cells circulate as *memory cells*.

T lymphocytes can be divided into two subpopulations based on the polypeptide chains constituting the antigen receptor. The $\alpha\beta$ *T cells*, constituting the larger population (~95%), possess a receptor comprising a heterodimer of α- and β-polypeptide chains. The variable portion of the $\alpha\beta$ TCR is composed of the approximately 100 amino-terminal amino acids. The generation of diversity is by translocation of V, D, and J genes; this process takes place as the cells mature within the thymus. During thymic maturation, T cells are selected for survival and exportation into the periphery according to their affinity for self-HLA molecules. T cells with too great an affinity for self-peptides and HLA molecules and those with too low an affinity for self-HLA do not survive. Thus, T cells that may have *autoimmune* reactivity and those with affinities too low to recognize any peptide bound to host HLA molecules are largely deleted from the circulating T cell pool.

The TCR is directed to foreign peptides bound by cell surface HLA molecules. $\alpha\beta$ T cells can be divided by their surface expression of glycoproteins into CD4 and CD8 subpopulations. CD4 and CD8 cells also differ in their genetic restriction and function. Peptides bound by class I HLA are recognized by CD8[+] T cells, whereas peptides bound by HLA class II molecules are recognized by CD4[+] helper T cells. The TCR recognizes linear peptides of 8 to 20 amino acids in length. Importantly, in addition to crucial roles in recognizing antigens presented in this manner, T cells also provide co-stimulatory signals that enable the maturation and proliferation of naïve B cells as they encounter antigen and thus link the humoral and cellular immune responses (see the section on Antibody Response later in this chapter). Another subpopulation of T lymphocytes, $\gamma\delta$ *T cells*, constitutes fewer than 5% of circulating and lymphoid T cells; these cells do not express CD4 or CD8; their TCRs contain heterodimers of γ and δ chains. Although diversity exists in the rearrangement of these chains, it is far less than that seen among $\alpha\beta$ T cells. $\gamma\delta$ T cells may not respond to peptides bound to major HLA molecules but instead tend to be activated directly by phospholipid antigens, by heat shock proteins, and by minor HLA molecules. Thus, these cells comprise a defense intermediate between the intrinsic and adaptive host defenses.

Host-Microbe Interaction

PRIMARY ENCOUNTER AND ROLE OF INNATE DEFENSES

The skin and mucosal surfaces represent the primary interface with the external world and its microbial flora. At these sites, certain intrinsic defenses such as peptide antimicrobial defensins and occupation of microbial niches by normal nonpathogenic colonists, in addition to secretory antibody, help defend against the development of invasive disease. Mucosal colonization by pathogenic microbes, such as pneumococcal colonization of the oropharynx, can induce an adaptive immune response. If this response develops before tissue invasion takes place, colonization may result in acquisition of a protective antibody response. Factors that disrupt normal host defenses, such as a depressed sensorium blocking gag and cough reflexes, cigarette smoking suppressing ciliary clearance, or intercurrent influenza virus infection denuding the tracheal epithelium, can increase the likelihood that colonization with a pathogenic microbe will result in invasive infection. Once anatomic barriers are breached and an invading microbe gains access to tissues, other intrinsic host defenses come into play rapidly. These rapid responders are phagocytic cells that express *toll-like* receptors that recognize classes of microbial components such as lipopolysaccharide, cell wall constituents, or microbial nucleotide sequences. Activation of these families of toll-like receptors results in activation of phagocytic cells that result in heightened ability of these cells to ingest nearby microbes, to induce expression of interferons that have antiviral activities, and to enhance immune responses and the expression of chemotactic cytokines that facilitate entry of additional inflammatory cells to the site of microbial breach. Some microbes are armed to resist these defenses, as is the case for bacteria with capsules that resist phagocytosis. Host complement can be activated to bind to these capsules, helping to opsonize the bacterium to enhance phagocytosis and to enhance ingress of inflammatory cells to the site. Because several days to a few weeks are generally required for the adaptive immune system to mobilize and generate sufficient effector activity to protect the host, one key role of the innate immune system is to provide a method of limiting microbial replication and pathogenesis until the more potent and specific adaptive immune response can be mobilized. Activation of microbicidal phagocytic cells, activation of complement and NK cell, and induction of antiviral interferons all may play roles in the early innate defense against microbial invasion. Many collaborative interactions occur between innate and adaptive defense mechanisms to ensure optimal arming of host defenses.

GENERATION OF ADAPTIVE IMMUNE RESPONSES

Cell-Mediated (T-Cell) Responses

Skin and mucosal tissue contain large numbers of dendritic cells, such as Langerhans cells, that also express toll-like receptors. These cells ingest foreign antigens and foreign microbes and may ingest dying inflammatory cells that have themselves ingested invading microbes. As they migrate to lymphoid tissues, these dendritic cells mature, degrading the ingested antigens and expressing these microbial peptides on cell surface HLA molecules. At the same time, these cells lose the ability to ingest additional material and begin to express numerous co-receptors that enhance their ability to interact with and activate T lymphocytes. In lymphoid tissues, these professional antigen–presenting cells encounter *naïve* T cells that have undergone TCR gene rearrangement in the thymus, and a small number of these cells will (by chance) express a TCR configuration that recognizes an HLA-bound peptide. What largely *restricts* the breadth of immune recognition is the ability of peptide to bind to that particular HLA molecule. Thus, different HLA molecules can bind different

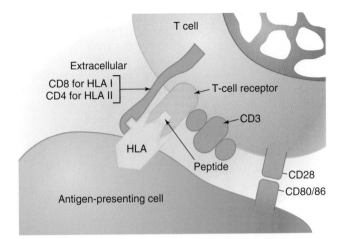

Figure 91–3 The molecular events in antigen presentation. Peptides within human leukocyte antigen (HLA) molecules on the antigen-presenting cell (APC) are bound weakly by T cell–receptor α and β chains. This interaction is stabilized and facilitated by CD4 binding to class II HLA or CD8 binding to class I HLAs. Other accessory molecule interactions between the APC and T cell are as shown.

peptides, and this variable binding ability (and not so much the recognition by the T cell) determines an individual's ability to recognize a foreign peptide and mount an immune response to it. T cells with high affinity for self peptides or too low an affinity for self-HLA molecules have already been deleted within the thymus. The relatively low-affinity interactions between TCR and HLA-bound peptides are supported by multiple co-receptor-ligand and adhesion molecule interactions between the T cell and antigen-presenting cell that also result in activation of the T cell (Fig. 91–3). The naïve T cell is thus activated to divide time and time again, rapidly expanding the number of T cells with the same clonal antigenic specificity. CD4+ T cells thus activated are no longer antigen *naïve* but are now activated to express helper cytokines, and some will develop long-lived *memory* function. Cytokines expressed by these CD4+ T-helper cells enhance the activity of other immune cells such as cytolytic CD8+ T cells and NK cells and are also critical to the development and maturation of B lymphocytes to result in the generation of antibody responses. T-helper cells also interact directly with dendritic cells, affecting their maturation and function. CD8+ T cells also mature to develop effector activity that includes elaboration of cytokines and cytolytic function.

Antibody Response

In lymphoid tissues, more complex antigens, including whole microbes, can be bound in an antigen-specific fashion by B lymphocytes, which have as their antigen receptor membrane-bound immunoglobulins (IgD and IgM). Thus bound, a particle can be ingested by the B cell and degraded, and then these microbial peptides are expressed on the B-cell surface HLA class II molecules. Thus, B lymphocytes may serve as professional antigen-presenting cells for recognition by CD4+ T cells. For most antigens therefore, attraction of CD4+ T cell help is essential to permit B lymphocyte expansion and ultimately antibody synthesis. As is the case for the interaction between the CD4+ T cell and other professional antigen-presenting cells, multiple receptor-ligand interactions stabilize the interaction between the TCR and the peptide-HLA molecule that it recognizes on the B cell surface. At the site of this intimate interaction, the CD4+ T cell is activated to express T-helper cytokines that, in turn, activate the B cell, promoting cellular division and maturation. In this fashion, microbial peptides that are recognized by CD4+ T cells induce the *help* that is needed to result in generation and amplification of an antibody response to that microbe. Recognition of this basic principle has resulted in the development of *conjugate vaccines* that, through linkage of immune help-inducing peptides to microbial sugars, which themselves do not induce T-cell responses, can enhance the antibody responses to these sugars. Conjugate vaccines are now used to prevent *Haemophilus* and pneumococcal infection.

The B lymphocytes thus activated by binding antigen to their surface receptors and helped by their interaction with CD4+ T cells begin clonal replication and maturation. Replication amplifies the *mass* of antigen-reactive B cells, and maturation involves both transformation of B cells into antibody-secreting plasma cells and the induction of *class-switching*, wherein the variable antigen-binding domains of the antibody are *switched* by gene rearrangements onto constant domains of different classes of antibody molecules. Thus, an initial IgM response is followed later by an IgG response with the same specificity in terms of antigen recognition (hence the utility of a high-level IgM response to a microbial antigen as a clinically meaningful indicator of recent infection). These events take place largely in germinal centers within lymphoid tissue that is enriched also with follicular dendritic cells. These follicular dendritic cells trap and hold intact antigens on their surfaces and facilitate B-lymphocyte maturation. During the early course of antibody generation, the affinity of antibody molecules for their antigens can increase. This affinity maturation takes place during the rapid expansion of B lymphocytes and is the consequence of somatic hypermutation of sequences within the hypervariable regions of the antibody genes. Progeny B lymphocytes with greater surface immunoglobulin (receptor) affinity for antigen will be more rapidly activated to divide and will *outcompete* B lymphocytes with lower affinity receptors. The antibodies thereby secreted by progeny plasma cells become increasingly capable of binding microbial antigens with higher affinity. Thus, the humoral immune response *evolves* in real time, selecting for B cells that produce antibodies with progressively higher affinity for microbial pathogens.

Microbial Pathogenesis Versus Host Defenses—The Continuing Drama

RESISTANCE TO EXTRACELLULAR BACTERIA: ENCAPSULATED ORGANISMS

Streptococcus Pneumoniae

The type-specific polysaccharide capsule is a major virulence factor because of its antiphagocytic properties. Antibody to the polysaccharide is itself capable of preventing pneumo-

coccal disease, as reflected by experimental studies and the efficacy of pneumococcal polysaccharide vaccines.

In the absence of immunity, pneumococci reaching the alveoli are not effectively contained by the host. Their phagocytosis by neutrophils is inefficient because organisms must be trapped against a surface to be ingested (*surface phagocytosis*). The pneumococcus does, however, elicit a neutrophilic inflammatory response. The organism activates complement by the alternative pathway and interactions of C-reactive protein in serum with pneumococcal C-polysaccharide. Activated complement fragments (C3a, C5a, and C567) and bacterial oligopeptides are chemotactic for neutrophils. Opsonic complement fragments (C3b) coating pneumococci favor their attachment to neutrophils but are less effective in promoting phagocytosis and killing than specific antibody. Clinical observations also directly support the primal role of antibody in immunity. The development of specific antibody on days 5 to 9 of untreated pneumococcal pneumonia may produce a clinical *crisis*, with dramatic resolution of symptoms. Opsonization of *Streptococcus pneumoniae* by type-specific antipolysaccharide antibody promotes ingestion and oxidative burst activity, with destruction of the organism.

Neisseria Meningitidis

Capsular polysaccharide also represents an important virulence factor for meningococci. In addition, pathogenic *Neisseria* species produce an IgA protease that dissociates the Fc fragment from the Fab portion of secretory and serum IgA and thus interferes with effector properties of the antibody molecule. Antibody-dependent, complement-mediated bacterial killing is the most critical host defense against meningococci. Therefore, the presence of bactericidal antibody is associated with protection against the meningococcus. In epidemic situations, 40% of persons who become colonized with the epidemic strain but who lack bactericidal antibodies develop disease. Protective serum antibody is elicited by colonization with the following: (1) nonencapsulated and encapsulated strains of meningococci of low virulence, which elicit antibodies cross-reactive with virulent strains, and (2) *Escherichia coli* and *Bacillus* species with cross-reacting capsular polysaccharides. The lack of bactericidal activity in the serum of adolescents and adults who exhibit susceptibility to *Neisseria meningitidis* may be due to blocking IgA antibody. Heightened susceptibility of patients lacking C6, C7, or C8 to meningococcal infection provides important evidence that the dominant protective mechanism against this organism involves complement-mediated bacteriolysis.

RESISTANCE TO FACULTATIVE INTRACELLULAR PARASITES: *MYCOBACTERIUM TUBERCULOSIS*

Activation of host phagocytes provides the critical defense mechanism against *Mycobacterium tuberculosis*. Primary infection progresses locally in the nonhypersensitive host because ingested organisms persist and multiply within mononuclear phagocytes. The bacteria escape intracellular digestion by secreting products that inhibit phagolysosomal fusion. Antibody-coated mycobacteria do not evade phagolysosomal fusion but nonetheless resist degradation, probably because of shielding provided by their rich lipid content. The development of cellular immunity leads to T lymphocyte–dependent macrophage activation and to the killing of the intracellular tubercle bacillus organism. The lesions of primary tuberculosis regress. However, latent foci persist, and delayed reactivation remains a threat throughout the lifetime of the host.

RESISTANCE TO OBLIGATE INTRACELLULAR PARASITES: VIRUSES

Host antiviral defense is characterized by overlap and redundancy, which allows an effective response to most viral agents. The key element of the response varies with the virus, the site, and the timing. Initially, infection is limited at the local site by type I interferons, which increase the resistance of neighboring cells to spread of the infection. Complement directly neutralizes some enveloped viruses. NK cells destroy infected cells, a process enhanced by interferons. As specific antibody is produced, IgA may neutralize the virus at mucosal surfaces; IgG may neutralize virus that has spread systemically to extracellular sites and allows uptake and destruction by FcR-bearing effector cells. Later, effector cyto-toxic T lymphocytes are expanded and activated to lyse host cells expressing viral peptides in the context of HLA antigens. The host thus directs several defenses against viral infection. Humoral defenses are active against extracellular viruses and, if neutralizing antibody is present at high enough levels before infection, may prevent clinical infection entirely. The induction of neutralizing antibody is the focus of most effective vaccination strategies against viruses. Cell-mediated defenses largely play more critical roles in attenuating the magnitude of viral replication during chronic infection. Viruses, at the same time, have evolved numerous mechanisms to blunt or block host antiviral defenses. Many viruses can decrease the expression of class I HLA molecules on cells they infect, thereby limiting recognition of these cells by CD8+ cytotoxic T lymphocytes. Certain viruses that cause chronic infection, such as herpesviruses and HIV, can maintain a latent infection whereby, in the absence of viral protein synthesis, no viral peptide targets for recognition by cytotoxic T lymphocytes exist. Other viruses have acquired gene sequences that encode homologues of host cytokine or cytokine receptor genes that may help viruses escape from host immune surveillance or contribute to viral pathogenesis.

Prospectus for the Future

- Increased understanding of the molecular and cellular mechanisms responsible for the establishment and regulation of the immune response
- More accurate and reproducible techniques to quantify and evaluate the different components of the immune response
- Expanding role of genomics and proteomics as techniques to map the biochemical profiles that characterize the immune response to various pathogens
- Application of recent advances in understanding immune responses to develop innovative therapies to enhance or attenuate specific components of the immune response selectively

References

Autran B, Molet L, Lederman MM: Host defenses against viral infection. In Boucher CAB, Galasso GJ (eds): Practical Guidelines in Antiviral Therapy. Amsterdam, Elsevier, 2002, pp 65–94.

Delves PJ, Roitt IM: The immune system (I). N Engl J Med 343:37–49, 2000.

Goronzy JJ, Weyand CM: The innate and adaptive immune systems. In Goldman L, Ausiello D (eds): Cecil Textbook of Medicine, 22nd ed. Philadelphia, Elsevier, 2004, pp 208–217.

Holland SM, Gallin JI: Evaluation of the patient with suspected immunodeficiency. In Mandell GL, Bennett JE, Dolin R (eds): Principles and Practices of Infectious Diseases, 6th ed. Philadelphia, Elsevier, 2005, pp 149–160.

Karp DR, Holer VM: Complement in health and disease. In Goldman L, Ausiello D (eds): Cecil Textbook of Medicine, 22nd ed. Philadelphia, Elsevier, 2004, pp 233–240.

Schwartz RS: Shattuck lecture: Diversity of the immune repertoire and immunoregulation. N Engl J Med 348:1017–1026, 2003.

Von Andrian UH, Mackay CR: T-cell function and migration: Two sides of the same coin. N Engl J Med 334:1020–1034, 2000.

Laboratory Diagnosis of Infectious Diseases

Benigno Rodríguez

Michael M. Lederman

Five basic laboratory techniques can be used in the diagnosis of infectious diseases: (1) direct visualization of the organism, (2) detection of microbial antigen, (3) search for *clues* produced by the host response to specific microorganisms, (4) detection of specific microbial nucleotide sequences, and (5) isolation of the organism in culture. Each technique has its uses and pitfalls. The laboratory can usually provide the clinician with prompt, accurate, and, if used judiciously, inexpensive diagnosis.

Diagnosis by Direct Visualization of the Organism

In many infectious diseases, pathogenic organisms can be directly visualized by microscopic examination of readily available tissue fluids. With the use of Gram or acid-fast stains, bacteria, mycobacteria, and *Candida* can be readily identified. An India ink preparation can often identify *Cryptococcus*, and potassium hydroxide (KOH) preparations can occasionally identify other fungal pathogens.

Because laboratory technicians now generally perform Gram and acid-fast stains, a description of their techniques is not provided in this text. The following three diagnostic procedures are described, however, because they continue to provide simple, inexpensive approaches to bedside diagnosis of clinically important infections.

India Ink Preparation

A drop of centrifuged cerebrospinal fluid (CSF) is placed on a microscope slide next to a drop of artist's India ink. A coverslip is placed over the drops, and the area of mixing of CSF and India ink is examined at 100× magnification. Cryptococci are identified by their large capsules, which exclude the India ink (Fig. 92–1).

Potassium Hydroxide Preparation

A drop of sputum, a skin scraping, or a smear of vaginal or oral exudate is placed on a slide together with one drop of 5% to 40% KOH. A coverslip is placed on the specimen, and the slide is heated for 2 to 5 seconds above a flame. The condenser of the microscope is lowered, and the specimen is examined at 100× magnification when searching for elastin fibers, whose presence in sputum suggests a necrotizing pneumonia, or at 400× magnification when looking for fungal forms. The KOH will partially dissolve host cells and bacteria, sparing fungi and elastin fibers.

Tzanck Preparation

A vesicle suspected of harboring herpesvirus (zoster or simplex) is unroofed with a scalpel, and the base is gently scraped. The scrapings are placed on a glass slide, air dried, and stained with Wright stain, Giemsa stain, or a rapid stain such as methylene blue. The slide is then examined at low power (100×) for the presence of multinucleated giant cells; their characteristic appearance is then confirmed at high power (400×). Although this direct bedside technique identifies the host response to infection and not the organism itself, demonstration of giant cells is diagnostic for herpesvirus infection (Fig. 92–2).

Other more sophisticated techniques can be used. Silver staining using the Gomori methenamine technique can identify most fungi, including *Pneumocystis jiroveci*. Experienced pathologists can also identify *P. jiroveci* on Giemsa-stained specimens of induced sputum. Darkfield microscopy can identify *Treponema pallidum*, and electron microscopy can sometimes detect viral particles in infected cells.

DIAGNOSIS BY DETECTION OF MICROBIAL ANTIGENS

Certain pathogens can be detected by examination of specimens for microbial antigens (Table 92–1). These studies can be performed rapidly, often within 1 hour. The diagnosis of meningitis caused by *Streptococcus pneumoniae*, *Cryptococcus neoformans*, some strains of *Haemophilus influenzae*, and *Neisseria meningitidis* can be made rapidly by detecting specific polysaccharide antigens in the CSF. Although these diagnoses may also be made by Gram stain or India ink

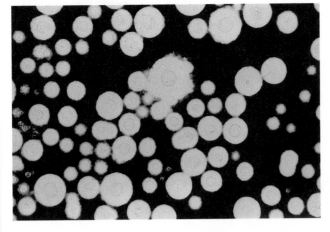

Figure 92–1 India ink preparation of cerebrospinal fluid reveals encapsulated cryptococci. Large capsules surround the smaller organisms.

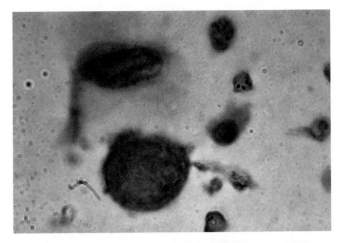

Figure 92–2 Tzanck preparation for diagnosis of herpesvirus infection. Multicolored giant cell *(bottom)* is characteristic of herpes infection.

Table 92–1 Diseases Often Diagnosed by Detection of Microbial Antigens

Disease	Assay	Agent Detected
Meningitis	Latex agglutination Nucleic acid amplification	*Cryptococcus neoformans, Streptococcus pneumoniae, Haemophilus influenzae, Neisseria meningitidis, Mycobacterium tuberculosis*
Encephalitis	Nucleic acid amplification	Herpes simplex virus
Respiratory tract infection	Immunofluorescence Enzyme immunoassay	*Bordetella pertussis, Legionella pneumophila,* influenza virus Respiratory syncytial virus; adenovirus
Genitourinary tract infection	Nucleic acid amplification	*Chlamydia trachomatis, Neisseria gonorrheae*
Hepatitis B	Radioimmunoassay	Hepatitis B surface antigen

preparation, antigen detection is especially helpful when attempts at direct visualization of the pathogen are not diagnostic (e.g., in the patient with partially treated bacterial meningitis). Immunofluorescence techniques using antibodies directed against the organisms identify pathogens such as *Legionella pneumophila* and *Bordetella pertussis* in respiratory secretions. Immunofluorescence can also be used to identify cells infected with influenza virus, respiratory syncytial virus, and adenovirus. Detection of urinary pneumococcal antigen can enhance the diagnostic capabilities of direct visualization and culture techniques in community-acquired pneumonia. Quantitation of cytomegalovirus antigen in blood may help predict the development of active disease in immunocompromised patients. The demonstration of hepatitis B surface antigen in blood establishes the presence of infection by this virus.

DIAGNOSIS BY EXAMINATION OF HOST IMMUNE OR INFLAMMATORY RESPONSES

Histopathologic examination of sampled or excised tissue often shows patterns of the host inflammatory response that can narrow the diagnostic possibilities. As a general rule, a polymorphonuclear leukocytic infiltrate suggests an acute bacterial process. A lymphocytic infiltrate suggests a more chronic process and is characteristically seen in viral, mycobacterial, and fungal infections. Similarly, examination of infected fluids such as CSF will provide etiologic clues. Bacterial infections generally provoke a polymorphonuclear leukocytosis with elevated protein and depressed glucose concentrations. Viral infections most often provoke a lymphocytic pleocytosis; protein elevations are less significant, and glucose levels are usually normal. Eosinophilia commonly occurs in helminthic infestations and is also characteristic of allergic bronchopulmonary aspergillosis. Granuloma formation in a febrile patient suggests mycobacterial infection. Many fungi (commonly *Histoplasma, Cryptococcus,* and *Blastomyces)* and certain helminths (notably *Schistosoma* species) can also lead to granuloma formation. Some diseases, such as syphilis (obliterative endarteritis), cat-scratch disease (mixed granulomatous, suppurative, and lymphoid hyperplastic changes), and lymphogranuloma venereum (stellate abscesses), have fairly characteristic histologic features.

Several viral infections produce characteristic changes in host cells, which are detectable by cytologic examination. Skin or respiratory infection with herpesviruses or pneumonia caused by cytomegalovirus or measles virus, for example, can be diagnosed with reasonable accuracy by cytologic examination (e.g., Tzanck preparation for herpesvirus infection).

Host cell–mediated immune responses can be used to help make certain diagnoses. A positive skin test for delayed-type hypersensitivity to mycobacterial or fungal antigens indicates active or previous infection with these agents. A negative skin test may be seen despite active infection in individuals with depression of cell-mediated immunity (anergy). Control skin tests using commonly encountered antigens (e.g., *Candida*, mumps, *Trichophyton*) have been used in an attempt to exclude global anergy as the reason for a negative skin reaction, but their value as diagnostic tools is questionable; therefore, these tests are not routinely recommended. The QuantiFERON-TB test is an assay for detecting interferon-γ production by *Mycobacterium tuberculosis*–specific lymphocytes and is an example of a clinically useful in vitro diagnostic procedure based on detection of the cellular immune response to a specific pathogen.

Host humoral responses may be used to diagnose certain infections, particularly those caused by organisms whose cultivation is difficult (e.g., *Ehrlichia chaffeensis*) or hazardous to laboratory personnel (e.g., *Francisella tularensis*). In general, two sera are obtained at intervals of at least 2 weeks, and a fourfold or greater rise or fall in antibody titer generally suggests a recent infection. Antibodies of the immunoglobulin M class also suggest recent infection. Depending on the organism, assays may detect either specific (hepatitis viruses) or nonspecific, cross-reactive antibodies (syphilis nontreponemal tests).

ASSAYS THAT DETECT MICROBIAL NUCLEOTIDE SEQUENCES

Detection of microbial nucleotide sequences can provide a sensitive and specific means of identification of pathogens in clinical specimens. These genetic molecular diagnostic techniques can provide rapid speciation of slow-growing microbial isolates. In addition, these techniques can also provide rapid quantitation of pathogens that can sometimes establish the prognosis and also determine the effectiveness of modes of therapy (e.g., cryptococcal antigen in CSF). Finally, genetic analyses can identify genetic determinants of antimicrobial resistance that can guide the selection of therapy.

The exquisite sensitivity and specificity of these techniques are consequences of the specificity of DNA-base

pairing and the dramatic amplifications of signals that can be provided by techniques such as the quantitative polymerase chain reaction, nucleic acid sequence–based amplification, and branched-chain signal amplification analyses.

The sensitivity of these techniques has revolutionized laboratory diagnostics. For example, most standard techniques for detecting microbial antigens cannot reliably detect fewer than 100,000 molecules in clinical samples. In contrast, the genetic techniques discussed in this text are being routinely used to identify as few as 20 to 50 molecules in clinical samples and can be modified to have even greater sensitivity. Table 92–2 lists some examples of diseases in which molecular diagnostic methods have represented a major advance in recent years.

CLINICAL APPLICATIONS OF MOLECULAR DIAGNOSTICS

Speciation

The slow replication of mycobacteria limits rapid speciation of these organisms after their identification in clinical samples. In certain clinical settings, such as those that may occur in patients with human immunodeficiency virus (HIV) infection, the distinction between nontuberculous mycobacteria and *Mycobacterium tuberculosis* may be particularly important. Genetic probes that distinguish among these organisms can provide rapid speciation after only limited growth.

Diagnosis of Infection

In acute HIV infection, detection of genomic HIV-1 RNA in plasma can provide diagnosis of this syndrome 2 to 3 weeks before the development of diagnostic HIV-specific antibodies (see Chapter 107). Nucleic acid amplification techniques (NAAT) are now routine for the diagnosis of gonorrhea and *Chlamydia* infections and can be performed on a single specimen with a rapid turnaround time. Detection of herpes simplex virus sequences within CSF can provide a sensitive and specific diagnosis of herpes simplex encephalitis. Similar assays can be used for the diagnosis of cytomegalovirus, JC virus, Epstein-Barr virus, and *Bartonella henselae* infection. In certain anatomic locations such as the pericardium and central nervous system, nucleic acid amplification may help in the diagnosis of tuberculosis. It is anticipated that numerous infectious diseases will soon be diagnosed with great sensitivity by means of these techniques. The exquisite sensitivity of the NAAT technique may, however, yield false-positive results unless the assays are carefully standardized.

Quantification of Microbial Infection

Molecular diagnostic assays have been refined and standardized to permit reliable quantification of microbial genomic sequences in clinical samples. Quantification of cytomegalovirus DNA, for example, has proved a useful tool in identifying individuals at risk for developing progressive cytomegalovirus disease during chemotherapy-induced or organ transplantation–induced immunosuppression. These quantitative assays have also provided evidence that the magnitude of microbial replication is predictive of disease progression in HIV infection, and sequential application of these

Table 92–2 Diseases in Which Molecular Diagnosis Techniques Are Commonly Used

Pathogen	Test	Clinical Situation
Hepatitis C virus	Quantitative PCR	Confirmation of chronic infection; monitoring of the effectiveness of therapy; documentation of sustained virologic response
Cytomegalovirus	PCR Hybrid capture DNA, NASBA	Diagnosis of CMV encephalitis and myelitis on CSF specimens Prediction of development of clinical disease in immunocompromised patients
Chlamydia trachomatis, Neisseria gonorrheae	PCR, ligase chain reaction	Diagnosis of sexually transmitted diseases on a single specimen (now the standard of care in many centers)
Hepatitis B virus	PCR	Determination of infectiousness
HIV	PCR, branched DNA amplification, NASBA	Quantification of viral replication; monitoring of response to therapy; confirmation of diagnosis in acute infection and mother-to-child transmission
Enteroviruses	Real-time PCR	Etiologic diagnosis of viral meningitis
Herpes simplex virus	PCR	Reliable diagnosis of HSV encephalitis, a life-threatening disease

CMV = cytomegalovirus; CSF = cerebrospinal fluid; HIV = human immunodeficiency virus; HSV = herpes simplex virus; NASBA = nucleic acid-sequenced based amplification; PCR = polymerase chain reaction.

techniques is now routinely used to monitor the activity of therapy for HIV and for hepatitis B and C virus infection.

Detecting Genetic Markers for Antimicrobial Resistance

Microbial resistance to therapeutic interventions is an increasing problem in infectious diseases. When genetic sequences that confer resistance to therapies are known, assays to detect them can be applied rapidly to clinical samples, providing information that can be used to select treatment regimens. Direct analysis of plasma HIV sequences has provided genetic information that can predict the failure of specific modes of therapy; under certain circumstances, routine application of this information is used to guide the selection of antiretroviral treatment regimens (see Chapter 107).

DIAGNOSIS BY ISOLATION OF THE ORGANISM IN CULTURE

Isolation of a single microbial species from an infected site is generally considered evidence that the infection is caused by this particular organism. Information obtained from the culture, however, must be interpreted according to the clinical setting. For example, cultures obtained from ordinarily contaminated sites (e.g., vagina, pharynx) may be overgrown with nonpathogenic commensals, and fastidious organisms such as *Neisseria gonorrhoeae* are difficult to recognize unless cultured on medium that selects for their growth. Similarly,

cultures of expectorated sputum may also be uninterpretable if heavily contaminated with saliva. The culture of an organism from an ordinarily sterile site is reasonable evidence for infection with that organism. Conversely, the failure to culture an organism may simply result from inadequate culture conditions (e.g., *sterile* pus from a brain abscess cultured only on aerobic media). Anaerobic bacteria that do not grow under aerobic conditions cause most brain abscesses. Thus, when submitting samples for culture, the physician must alert the laboratory to the likely pathogens.

Gram stains of specimens submitted for culture are often invaluable aids to the interpretation of culture results. A Gram stain of sputum will readily detect contamination by saliva if numerous squamous epithelial cells are seen. In contrast, a Gram stain revealing many bacteria despite negative cultures suggests infection by fastidious organisms. The presence of an organism in high density and within neutrophils strongly suggests that the corresponding bacterial isolate is causing disease rather than colonizing the patient or contaminating the specimen. Gram staining of the initial clinical specimen may also help determine the relative importance of different isolates when cultures show mixed flora.

Viral Isolation

Because all viral pathogens that can be cultured require eukaryotic cells in which to grow, virus isolation is expensive and often laborious. Throat washings, rectal swabs, or cultures of infected sites should be transported immediately to the laboratory or, if this is not possible, placed in virus transport medium and refrigerated overnight until they can be cultured in the laboratory. Certain viruses such as HIV and cytomegalovirus are often cultivated from whole blood samples. Notifying the laboratory of the suggested pathogens allows selection of the best cell lines or systems for culture. The clinician must be aware of the viruses that the hospital's laboratory can isolate. A fourfold rise in titer of antibody to the isolated virus suggests that it is causing disease.

Isolation of Rickettsiae, Chlamydiae, and Mycoplasmas

Rickettsiae are cultivated primarily in reference laboratories. Diagnosis of rickettsial illness is generally made on clinical grounds and confirmed serologically. Although chlamydiae can be propagated in cell cultures used in most hospital virology laboratories, chlamydial infection is most often diagnosed through antigen detection techniques. Mycoplasmas will grow on selective media; however, the prolonged period of incubation results in little advantage over serologic diagnosis.

Bacterial Isolation

Most hospital laboratories readily achieve isolation of common bacterial pathogens. Specimens should be carried promptly to the laboratory. In instances in which likely isolates may be fastidious (e.g., bacterial meningitis) and immediate processing cannot be ensured, the specimen should be placed directly onto the culture medium with careful attention to sterile techniques. Widespread availability of transport media has minimized the need for this approach. Blood culture is a special case of bacterial isolation technique, for which immediate inoculation into the culture medium is required. Blood cultures are arguably some of the most critical specimen types processed by a microbiology laboratory, and errors in their collection and processing can have major clinical consequences. Common mistakes include insufficient blood volume (30 to 40 mL total is recommended for adults), collection of multiple specimens from the same venipuncture site or intravenous catheter (making it difficult to interpret the significance of normal skin colonizers and to estimate the persistence of the bacteremia), collection after antibiotic initiation and less than meticulous aseptic techniques (resulting in contaminant growth).

Isolation of anaerobic bacteria is often critical for diagnosis. When anaerobes are suggested, the specimen, if pus or liquid, can then be drawn into a syringe, the air expelled, and the syringe capped before transport to the laboratory. Otherwise, specimens must be taken immediately to the laboratory or placed in an anaerobic transport medium appropriate for survival of pathogens. Because of contamination by oral anaerobes, sputum should not be cultured anaerobically unless the sample was obtained by transtracheal or percutaneous lung aspiration.

Isolation of Fungi and Mycobacteria

Specimens for fungal and mycobacterial cultures must be processed and cultured by the microbiology laboratory. Although some fungi and rapid-growing mycobacteria grow readily on standard agars used for routine isolation of bacteria, others, such as *Mycobacterium tuberculosis* and *Histoplasma capsulatum*, must be cultured on special media for as long as several weeks.

Monitoring Antimicrobial Resistance

Historically, phenotypic methods have been used to evaluate the susceptibility of bacteria and fungi to antimicrobial agents. Methods have been standardized to examine the ability of organisms to grow on solid or liquid media in the presence of varying concentrations of drug or on solid medium on which drug-containing disks are placed. These standardized methods help direct antimicrobial resistance patterns for an individual patient's isolate, and summary results are also used throughout hospitals and communities to help guide empiric therapies. Recently, a modification of the phenotypic resistance assay has been used to examine antiviral resistance patterns for HIV. Using polymerase chain reaction techniques, genes targeted by antiviral drugs are amplified from patient plasma and are cloned into expression vectors. The ability of these drugs to inhibit replication of these chimeric viruses in cell lines is tested.

Prospectus for the Future

- Greater use of molecular methods for the diagnosis and monitoring of infectious diseases
- Broader use of molecular methods for the detection of antimicrobial-resistant microbes
- Greater use of rapid bedside tests for the diagnosis of infectious diseases

References

Gill VJ, Fedorko DP, Witebsky FG: The clinician and the microbiology laboratory. In Mandell GL, Bennett JC, Dolin R (eds): Principles and Practice of Infectious Diseases, 6th ed. Philadelphia, Elsevier, 2005, pp 203–241.

Versalovic J, Lupski JR: Molecular detection and genotyping of pathogens: More accurate and rapid answers. Trends Microbiol 10:S15–S21, 2002.

Antimicrobial Therapy

Benigno Rodríguez

Michael M. Lederman

Perhaps the most dramatic advance in medical practice in the 20th century was the development of antimicrobial therapy. Antimicrobials are agents that interfere with microbial metabolism, resulting in inhibition of growth or death of bacteria, viruses, fungi, protozoa, or helminths. Some antimicrobials, such as penicillin, are natural products of other microbes. Others, such as sulfa drugs, are chemical agents synthesized in the laboratory. Still others are semisynthetic, with chemical modifications of naturally occurring substances that result in enhanced activity (e.g., nafcillin) and/or diminished toxic effects.

The most effective antimicrobials are characterized by their relatively selective activity against microbes. Some antimicrobials, such as penicillins and amphotericin B, interfere with the synthesis of microbial cell walls that are absent in human cells. Others, such as trimethoprim and sulfa drugs, inhibit obligate microbial synthesis of essential nucleic acid intermediates, pathways not required by human cells. Still others, such as acyclovir, an antiviral agent, are relatively inactive until metabolized by pathogen-derived enzymes. Antiretroviral agents selectively inhibit viral enzymes that are essential for replication. Antimicrobial agents, although relatively selective in activity against microbes, have varying degrees of toxicity for human cells. Thus, monitoring for toxicity during antimicrobial therapy is always important.

Pathogen

If the pathogen has been clearly identified (see Chapter 92), a drug with a narrow spectrum of activity (i.e., highly selective for the particular pathogen) is usually the most reasonable choice. If the pathogen responsible for the patient's illness has not been identified, then the physician must choose a drug or combination of drugs active against the most likely pathogens in the specific setting. In either instance, the physician must be guided by patterns of antimicrobial resistance common in the community and in the specific hospital. Some pathogens (e.g., group A streptococci) are almost always sensitive to narrow-spectrum antimicrobials such as penicillin. Other pathogens, such as staphylococci, are variably resistant to penicillins but almost always susceptible to vancomycin. Resistance patterns, particularly among hospital-acquired bacteria, may vary widely and are important in devising antimicrobial strategies. Broad-spectrum antimicrobial coverage for all febrile patients (*shotgunning*) must not be substituted for carefully evaluating the clinical problem and pinpointing therapy directed toward the most likely pathogen or pathogens. Widespread use of broad-spectrum antimicrobials almost invariably leads to emergence of resistant strains. However, the greater the severity of a patient's illness and the less certain the physician is of the responsible pathogen, the more important initial, empiric, broad-spectrum coverage becomes. Initial empiric treatment is also frequently indicated in the immunocompromised febrile patient (e.g., the patient with severe neutropenia secondary to chemotherapy). Once the pathogen is isolated and its antimicrobial sensitivities are known, empiric therapy must be scaled down to a definitive regimen with optimal activity against the specific micro-organism.

Site of Infection

The location of the infection is also important in determining the selection and dosage of an antimicrobial. Deep-seated infections and bacteremic infections generally require higher doses of antimicrobials than, for example, superficial infections of the skin, upper respiratory tract, or lower urinary tract. Penetration of antimicrobials into sites such as the meninges, eye, and prostate is quite variable. Thus, treatment of infections at these sites involves selection of an antimicrobial agent that penetrates these tissues in concentrations sufficient to inhibit or kill the pathogen. The meninges are relatively resistant to penetration by most antimicrobials; inflammation renders the meninges somewhat more permeable. Therefore, high doses of antibiotics are the rule when treating meningitis. Bacterial infections of certain sites such as the heart valves or meninges must be treated with antibiotics that kill the microbe (bactericidal) rather than simply inhibiting its growth (bacteriostatic), largely because local host defenses at these sites are inadequate to rid the host of infecting organisms. Infections involving foreign bodies may be impossible to eradicate without removing the foreign material.

Antimicrobials alone are often insufficient in treating large abscesses. Although many drugs achieve reasonable concentrations in abscess walls, the low pH antagonizes the activity of some drugs (e.g., aminoglycosides), and some drugs bind to and are inactivated by white blood cells or their products. The large number of organisms, their depressed metabolism in this unfavorable milieu, and the frequent polymicrobial nature of certain abscesses increase the likelihood that some organisms present may be resistant to antimicrobial therapy. Most extracranial abscesses should be drained whenever anatomically possible.

Characteristics of the Antimicrobial

The physician must know the pharmacokinetics of the drug (i.e., its absorption, its penetration into various sites, its metabolism and excretion) and its toxic effects, as well as its spectrum of antimicrobial activity, before selecting it for use (Table 93–1).

DISTRIBUTION AND EXCRETION

Lipid-soluble drugs, such as chloramphenicol and rifampin, penetrate most membranes, including the meninges, more readily than do more ionized compounds, such as the aminoglycosides. Understanding a drug's distribution, rate and site of metabolism, and route of excretion is essential in selecting the appropriate drug and dose. Drugs excreted unchanged in the urine may be particularly suitable for treating lower urinary tract infection or for treating systemic infection in the presence of renal insufficiency. Some antimicrobials are metabolized in the liver and must be adjusted appropriately in the presence of hepatic dysfunction.

ACTIVITY OF THE DRUG

The physician must understand the spectrum of activity of the drug against microbial isolates, the mechanism of activity of the agent, and whether it is bactericidal or bacteriostatic in achievable concentrations. An important point to remember, however, is that the actual activity of an agent as bacteriostatic or bactericidal may depend on concentration at the anatomic site, the micro-organism involved, or both. As a general rule, cell wall–active drugs are likely to be bactericidal. Bactericidal drugs are necessary for treating infections sequestered from effective host inflammatory responses, such as meningitis and endocarditis. With the exception of aminoglycosides and certain azalide and macrolide antibiotics, agents inhibiting protein synthesis at ribosomal sites are generally bacteriostatic.

The penicillins are the prototype of cell wall–active bacteriocidal drugs, which inhibit the formation of cross-links that bridge peptidoglycan, the final step in assembly of the cell wall of both gram-positive and gram-negative bacteria. Despite sharing a similar mechanism of antibacterial activity, the spectrum of activity differs for each of the β-lactam antibiotics.

The macrolides, including azithromycin, clarithromycin and erythromycin, all bind to the same receptor on the bacterial 50S ribosomal subunit and inhibit RNA-dependent protein synthesis by the same mechanism. However, as with penicillin, each of the macrolides has a distinctive spectrum of antibacterial activity.

Each of the several categories of antifungal agents has a distinct mechanism of action. Of major interest at present because of excellent absorption after oral administration and relative paucity of side effects are the azoles, which block biosynthesis of ergosterol, a critical element in fungal wall stability.

The four currently available classes of antiretroviral agents act at different sites in the life cycle of human immunodeficiency virus, as described in Chapter 107.

TOXIC EFFECTS OF THE DRUG

The physician must have a thorough understanding of the contraindications of the drug, as well as the major toxic effects and their general frequencies. This knowledge will help in evaluating the risks of treatment and will also assist in advising the patient about possible adverse reactions. History of drug hypersensitivity must be elicited before prescribing any antimicrobial. The presence or absence of previous reactions to penicillin should be documented for every patient. Patients with a history suggestive of immediate hypersensitivity to penicillin, such as hives, wheezing, hypotension, laryngospasm, or angioedema at any site, must be considered at risk for anaphylaxis. These patients should not receive penicillins or related drugs (cephalosporins or imipenem) if adequate alternatives are available. The major and minor determinants of penicillin allergy (breakdown products that bind to serum proteins to form haptens) can be used to detect most persons at risk for serious immediate hypersensitivity. If skin test reactivity to these determinants is present and no reasonable alternatives to therapy with penicillin or a related compound are available, these patients may be desensitized to penicillin using a graduated protocol of intracutaneous penicillin administration. Desensitization should be done only in consultation with an expert and may only be justified in cases (such as neurosyphilis, endocarditis caused by enterococcus) in which most alternative treatments are considered suboptimal. Patients with a history of an uncomplicated morbilliform or delayed rash after penicillin therapy are not likely to be at risk for immediate hypersensitivity and may be treated with cephalosporins, for which the risk of cross-hypersensitivity to penicillins is likely to be in the range of 5%.

Route of Administration

Oral administration of antimicrobials can often prevent the morbidity and expense associated with parenteral (intravenous or intramuscular) administration. Although some antimicrobials (e.g., amoxicillin, the fluoroquinolones) are very well absorbed after oral administration, most patients hospitalized with severe infections should be treated, at least initially, with intravenous antibiotics. Gut absorption of antimicrobials can be unpredictable, and the intravenous route often permits administration of greater amounts of drug than can be tolerated orally. Intramuscular administration of some antimicrobials can result in excellent drug absorption but should be avoided in the presence of hypotension (erratic absorption) and coagulation disorders

| Table 93–1 | Characteristics of Commonly Used Antimicrobial Agents | | |

Drug Class	Site of Action	Excretion/ Metabolism	Uses/Activity
Antibacterials			
β-Lactams			
Penicillins	Cell wall	Renal	Streptococci, *Neisseria*, oral anaerobes
β-Lactamase–resistant penicillins (e.g., nafcillin)	Cell wall	Renal and/or hepatic	Methicillin-sensitive staphylococci
Amino penicillins (e.g., ampicillin)	Cell wall	Renal	Gram-positive organisms, not staphylococci, some gram-negative organisms
Extended-spectrum penicillins (e.g., piperacillin)	Cell wall	Renal	Broad-spectrum gram-positive organisms; gram-negative organisms, including *Pseudomonas*, not *Staphylococcus*
β-Lactamase inhibitors (e.g., clavulanic acid)	Inactivate β-lactamase	Renal/metabolic	Used with ampicillin, amoxicillin, piperacillin, or ticarcillin, expand activity to include anaerobes, many gram-negative organisms, and methicillin-sensitive staphylococci
Cephalosporins*			
First generation (e.g., cefazolin)	Cell wall	Renal	Gram-positive organisms, many common gram-negative bacteria
Second generation (e.g., cefuroxime)		Renal	Some with anaerobic activity (e.g., cefoxitin)
Third generation (e.g., ceftriaxone)		Renal or hepatic	Some active against *Pseudomonas* (e.g., ceftazidime)
Fourth generation (e.g., cefepime)		Renal	Broadest spectrum, including resistant nosocomial gram-negative organisms, and gram-positive cocci, including methicillin-sensitive staphylococci
Monobactams			
Aztreonam	Cell wall	Renal	Aerobic gram-negative bacilli
Carbapenems			
Imipenem, cilastatin	Cell wall	Renal	Very broad-spectrum, some enterococci, and methicillin-sensitive staphylococci, anaerobes
Glycopeptides			
Vancomycin	Cell wall	Renal	Coagulase-positive and coagulase-negative staphylococci, other gram-positive bacteria
Streptogramins			
Quinopristin-dalfopristin	Ribosome	Hepatic, fecal	Gram-positive organisms, including methicillin-resistant staphylococci and non-*faecalis* vancomycin-resistant enterococci

| Table 93–1 | **Characteristics of Commonly Used Antimicrobial Agents—cont'd** | | |

Drug Class	Site of Action	Excretion/ Metabolism	Uses/Activity
Lipopeptides			
Daptomycin	Cell membrane (?)	Renal	Coagulase-positive and coagulase-negative staphylococci, other gram-positive bacteria, including glycopeptide-resistant enterococci
Oxazolidinones			
Linezolid	Ribosome	Renal	Coagulase-positive and coagulase-negative staphylococci, other gram-positive bacteria, including glycopeptide-resistant enterococci, certain mycobacteria, *Nocardia*
Sulfonamides, trimethoprim	Inhibit nucleic acid synthesis	Renal	Gram-negative bacilli, *Salmonella*, *Pneumocystis jiroveci*, *Nocardia*
Fluoroquinolones	DNA gyrase	Some hepatic metabolism	Broad spectrum, including *Legionella*; newer agents also active vs. streptococci or anaerobes
Metronidazole	DNA disruption	Hepatic metabolism	Anaerobes, *Clostridium difficile*, amoebas *Trichomonas*, *Giardia*
Rifampin	Transcription	Renal/hepatic metabolism	*Mycobacterium tuberculosis*; meningococcal and *Haemophilus influenzae* prophylaxis
Aminoglycosides	Ribosome	Renal	Gram-negative bacilli; no activity in anaerobic conditions
Chloramphenicol	Ribosome	Renal/hepatic metabolism	Broad spectrum; especially useful for *Salmonella*, anaerobes, *Rickettsia*, *Brucella*, *Bartonella*
Clindamycin	Ribosome	Renal/hepatic metabolism	Anaerobes; gram-positive cocci
Tetracyclines	Ribosome	Renal/hepatic metabolism	Broad spectrum; especially useful for spirochetes, *Rickettsia*
Glycylcyclines			
Tigecycline	Ribosome	Renal/hepatic metabolism	Broad spectrum, including methicillin-resistant staphylococci, anaerobes, gram-negatives
Macrolides/Azalides			
Erythromycin	Ribosome	Hepatic	Gram-positive cocci, *Legionella*, *Mycoplasma*
Azithromycin, clarithromycin	Ribosome	Hepatic	High intracellular levels have enhanced activity against mycobacteria, *Toxoplasma*
Ketolides			
Telithromycin	Ribosome	Renal/hepatic metabolism	Enhanced activity against gram-positives, including methicillin-resistant staphylococci, intracellular respiratory pathogens, macrolide-resistant *Streptococcus pneumoniae*

Continued

Table 93–1 Characteristics of Commonly Used Antimicrobial Agents—cont'd

Drug Class	Site of Action	Excretion/ Metabolism	Uses/Activity
Antifungals			
Polyenes			
Amphotericin B	Binds membrane ergosterol	Tissue breakdown	Most fungi (not *Candida lusitaniae*)
Flucytosine	Blocks DNA synthesis	Renal	Candidiasis; *Cryptococcus* with amphotericin B
Azoles			
Ketoconazole	Block ergosterol biosynthesis	Hepatic	Mucosal candidiasis, pulmonary histoplasmosis (nonmeningeal)
Itraconazole	Block ergosterol biosynthesis	Hepatic	Histoplasmosis, blastomycosis
Fluconazole	Block ergosterol biosynthesis	Renal	Candidiasis, cryptococcosis, coccidioidomycosis
Voriconazole	Block ergosterol biosynthesis	Hepatic	Invasive aspergillosis, *Fusarium* and *Scedosporium* infections, empiric for febrile neutropenia
Echinocandins			
Caspofungin	Inhibit glucan synthesis	Chemical decay and degradation	*Candida* species, invasive aspergillosis
Antivirals			
Acyclovir	DNA polymerase	Renal	Herpes simplex, including encephalitis; herpes zoster
Famciclovir	DNA polymerase	—	Herpes simplex, zoster
Ganciclovir	DNA polymerase	Renal	Cytomegalovirus, herpesviruses
Foscarnet	DNA polymerase	Renal	Cytomegalovirus, herpesviruses, possibly HIV
Cidofovir	DNA polymerase	Renal	Cytomegalovirus, herpesviruses
Amantadine/rimantadine	Endocytosis	Renal	Influenza A treatment and prophylaxis
Zanamavir	Neuraminidase	Renal	Influenzas A and B
Oseltamivir	Neuraminidase	Renal	Influenzas A and B
Ribavirin	RNA synthesis (?)	Renal/hepatic metabolism	RSV, hepatitis C (together with interferon-α)
Interferon-α	Immunomodulator		Hepatitis B, C
Antiretrovirals			
Nucleoside/nucleotide reverse transcriptase inhibitors[†]	Reverse transcriptase	Renal and/or hepatic	HIV-1
Non-nucleoside reverse transcriptase inhibitors[‡]	Reverse transcriptase	Hepatic	HIV-1
Protease inhibitors[§]	HIV-1 protease	Hepatic	HIV-1
Fusion inhibitors[¶]	Viral entry	Catabolism	HIV-1

*As a rule: First-generation cephalosporins have better activity against gram-positive cocci and minimal CNS penetration; second-generation cephalosporins have somewhat better activity against gram-negative bacteria and may penetrate the CNS; third-generation cephalosporins have broader activity against gram-negative bacteria and generally penetrate the CNS, but they are relatively less active against gram-positive cocci; fourth-generation cephalosporins have the broadest spectrum of activity, regaining activity against gram-positive organisms.
[†]These include zidovudine, stavudine, didanosine, lamivudine, emtricitabine, tenofovir, and abacavir.
[‡]These include efavirenz and nevirapine.
[§]These include indinavir, nelfiinavir, ritonavir, saquinavir, fosamprenavir, tipranavir,darunavir, and lopinavir/ritonavir.
[¶]The only currently approved agent is enfuvirtide.
CNS = central nervous system; HIV = human immunodefiiciency virus; RSV= respiratory syncytial virus.

(hematomas). Repeated intramuscular injections are uncomfortable and can also result in the formation of sterile abscesses (e.g., pentamidine).

Duration of Therapy

Antimicrobial therapy should be initiated as part of a treatment plan of defined duration. In a few settings, the duration of optimal antimicrobial therapy is established (e.g., 10 days, but not 7 days, of oral penicillin will consistently prevent rheumatic fever after streptococcal pharyngitis); in many other settings, the duration of treatment is empiric and sometimes can be based on the clinical and bacteriologic courses. Bloodstream infections without endocarditis or other focal infections can generally be treated for 10 to 14 days. Pneumococcal pneumonia can be effectively treated in 7 to 10 days.

Combinations

Combinations of antimicrobials are indicated in serious infection when they provide more effective activity against a pathogen than any single agent. In some instances, combinations of drugs are used to prevent the emergence of resistance (e.g., infections caused by *Mycobacterium tuberculosis*, the human immunodeficiency virus). In other settings, combinations are used because they provide synergistic action against the pathogen (e.g., penicillin, a cell wall–active antibiotic, facilitates uptake of aminoglycosides by enterococci). In still other instances, drug combinations are used in empiric therapies to cover a wide spectrum of potential pathogens when the causative agent is unidentified or when infection is likely to be due to a mixture of organisms (e.g., fecal soilage of the peritoneum). The use of more than one drug increases the likelihood of toxic effects, increases costs, and often increases the risk of superinfection.

Monitoring of Antimicrobial Therapy

The physician and patient should be alert to potential toxic effects and should be prepared to halt the drug in the event of serious toxicity. For some antimicrobials, such as aminoglycosides, the ratio of effective to toxic drug levels is low, often requiring monitoring of serum levels of the drug to ensure appropriate dosing. For certain infections (e.g., infective endocarditis caused by relatively resistant organisms), monitoring of antimicrobial activity in serum shortly after (peak) and just before (trough) drug administration may help guide antimicrobial choices and usage. Although these techniques are not well standardized, clinicians often adjust drugs and doses to maintain serum bactericidal titers of at least 1:8 in treating certain forms of endocarditis (e.g., ente-

rococcal) in which the antimicrobial resistance patterns of the micro-organisms may be quite variable.

Antiviral Agents

As obligate intracellular pathogens, viruses depend on interactions with host cellular machinery for completion of the life cycle. Thus, toxic effects on host cells limit many potential antiviral treatment strategies. Specificity for viruses or virus-infected cells can be obtained by interfering with the function of unique viral elements (e.g., the M2 protein of influenza virus that is the target of amantadine and rimantadine) or by developing drugs such as acyclovir that must be processed by viral enzymes (in this instance, phosphorylated by herpesvirus thymidine kinase) before becoming active. In contrast to antibacterial drugs, however, antiviral agents generally have a limited spectrum of activity, each agent being useful against a small number of viruses. In the 1990s the numbers and types of drugs effective in the treatment of viral infections increased dramatically. This proliferation has been particularly striking in the field of antiretroviral therapies (see Chapter 107), and new agents against influenza, hepatitis B, and cytomegalovirus are now part of the therapeutic armamentarium. Additional developments in therapies for other viruses (e.g., hepatitis C) are anticipated.

Antifungal Agents

A large number of drugs are useful when applied topically or systemically in the treatment of fungal diseases. Most of these drugs target the ergosterol-containing cell membrane either by inhibiting ergosterol synthesis (azoles) or by aggregating in proximity to ergosterol and increasing membrane permeability (polyenes). Flucytosine inhibits fungal DNA synthesis. Echinocandins inhibit glucan synthesis. Increasing resistance to azoles and flucytosine among clinically relevant fungal isolates limits the usefulness of these agents in patients requiring chronic therapy.

Antimicrobial Resistance Testing

As treatment options expand, emergence of antimicrobial resistance to therapies is predictable. Thus, physicians must be prepared to evaluate the resistance patterns of specific microbial isolates. Resistance testing is now routinely provided for bacterial pathogens (see Chapter 92) and is increasingly used in the design of antiretroviral treatment strategies (see Chapter 107). Certain resistance assays are not yet fully standardized, and all require some level of expertise to facilitate their interpretation. Thus, interpretation of resistance assay results to guide treatment decisions, whether for serious bacterial, fungal, or viral infections, should generally involve discussion with an expert in infectious diseases.

Prospectus for the Future

- Newer classes of antiviral medications targeting hepatitis and other viruses
- Newer classes of antiretroviral medications targeting different phases of HIV-1 viral replication
- Newer classes of antibacterials targeting antibiotic-resistant organisms

- Newer, less toxic antifungal agents
- Antimicrobial peptides and other *designer* drugs with innovative mechanisms of action

References

Craig WA: Antibacterial therapy. In Goldman L, Bennett JC (eds): Cecil Textbook of Medicine, 22nd ed. Philadelphia, Saunders, 2005, pp 1753–1764.

Hayden FG: Antiviral drugs (other than antiretrovirals). In Mandell GL, Bennett JE, Dolin R (eds): Principles and Practice of Infectious Diseases, 6th ed. Philadelphia, Elsevier, 2005: pp 514–551.

Moellering RC, Eliopoulos GM: Principles of anti-infective therapy. In Mandell GL, Bennett JE, Dolin R (eds): Principles and Practice of Infectious Diseases, 6th ed. Philadelphia, Elsevier, 2005: pp 242–253.

Chapter 94

Fever and Febrile Syndromes

David B. Blossom

Robert A. Salata

Regulation of Body Temperature

Although normal body temperature ranges vary considerably, oral temperature readings in excess of 37.8°C (100.2°F) are generally abnormal. In healthy individuals, core body temperature is maintained within a narrow range, so that for each individual, daily temperature variations greater than 1° to 1.5°C are distinctly unusual. The hypothalamic nuclei that establish set points for body temperature control this homeostasis. Homeostasis is affected by a complex balance between heat-generating and heat-conserving mechanisms that raise body temperature on the one hand and mechanisms that dissipate heat and lower body temperature on the other. Heat is regularly generated as a by-product of obligate energy use (e.g., cellular metabolism, myocardial contraction, breathing). When an increase in body temperature is needed, shivering—nondirected muscular contractions—generates large amounts of heat. Peripheral vessels constrict to diminish heat lost to the environment. At the same time, the person feels cold; this heat preference promotes heat-conserving behavior, such as wrapping up in a blanket.

Obligate heat loss to the environment occurs through the skin and by evaporation of water through sweat and respiration. When the body must cool down, heat loss is promoted. Vasodilation flushes the skin capillaries, temporarily raising skin temperature but ultimately lowering core body temperature by increasing heat loss through the skin to the cooler environment. Sweating promotes rapid heat loss through evaporation, and at the same time the person feels warm and sheds blankets or initiates other activities to promote heat loss.

Fever and Hyperthermia

Fever is an elevated body temperature that is mediated by an increase in the hypothalamic heat-regulating set point. Although exogenous substances such as bacterial products may precipitate fever, the increase in body temperature is achieved through physiologic mechanisms. In contrast, hyperthermia is an increase in body temperature that over-rides or bypasses the normal homeostatic mechanisms. As a general rule, body temperatures in excess of 41°C (105.8°F) are rarely physiologically mediated and suggest hyperthermia. Hyperthermia may occur after vigorous exercise, in patients with heat stroke, as a heritable reaction to anesthetics (malignant hyperthermia), as a response to phenothiazines (neuroleptic malignant syndrome), and occasionally in patients with central nervous system disorders such as paraplegia (see also Chapter 117). Some patients with severe dermatoses are also unable to dissipate heat and therefore experience hyperthermia.

Fever is usually a physiologic response to infection or inflammation. Monocytes or tissue macrophages are activated by various stimuli to liberate various cytokines with pyrogenic activity (Fig. 94–1). Interleukin-1 is also an essential co-factor in initiating the immune response. Another pyrogenic cytokine, tumor necrosis factor-α, or cachectin, activates lipoprotein lipase and may also play a role in immune cytolysis; tumor necrosis factor-β, or lymphotoxin, has similar properties. A fourth cytokine, interferon-α, has antiviral activity (see Chapter 91). Interleukin-6, a cytokine that potentiates B-cell immunoglobulin synthesis, also has pyrogenic activity. Endogenous pyrogens activate the anterior pre-optic nuclei of the hypothalamus to raise the set point for body temperature. Infection by all types of microorganisms can be associated with fever. Tissue injury with resulting inflammation, as observed in patients with myocardial or pulmonary infarction or after trauma, can produce fever. Certain malignancies such as lymphoma and leukemia, renal cell carcinoma, and hepatic carcinoma are also associated with fever. In some instances, fever is related to the liberation of endogenous pyrogen by monocytes in the inflammatory response surrounding the tumor; in other patients, the malignant cell may release an endogenous pyrogen. Many immunologically mediated disorders, such as connective tissue diseases, serum sickness, and some drug reactions, are characterized by fever. In most patients with drug-induced fevers, the mechanisms are unknown. Virtually any disorder associated with an inflammatory response (e.g., gouty arthritis) can be associated with fever. Certain endocrine disorders such as thyrotoxicosis, adrenal insufficiency, and pheochromocytoma can also produce fever.

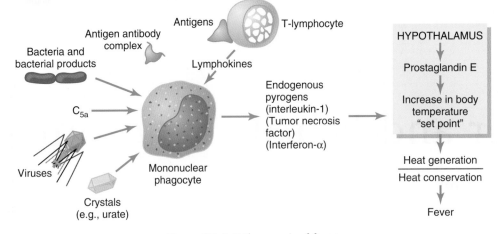

Figure 94–1 Pathogenesis of fever.

The association of fever with infections or inflammatory disorders raises the question of whether fever is beneficial to the host. For example, interleukin-1 (an endogenous pyrogen) is critical for initiating the immune response, elevated temperatures marginally enhance certain in vitro immune responses, and some infectious organisms prefer cooler temperatures. It is not certain, however, that fever is helpful to humans in any infectious disease, with the possible exception of neurosyphilis. Fever is deleterious in certain situations. Among individuals with underlying brain disease and even in healthy older persons, fever can produce disorientation and confusion. Fever and associated tachycardia may compromise patients, especially older individuals with significant cardiopulmonary disease. Fever should be controlled if the patient is particularly uncomfortable or whenever it poses a specific risk to the patient. Fever in patients with severe congestive heart failure or myocardial infarction should be treated with antipyretics.

Heat stroke almost always results from prolonged exposure to high environmental temperatures and humidity, usually associated in otherwise healthy individuals after strenuous exercise. Heat stroke is characterized by a body temperature greater than 40.6°C (105°F) and is associated with altered sensorium or coma and with cessation of sweating. Rapid cooling is critical to the patient's survival. Covering the patient with cold (11°C), wet compresses until the core temperature reaches 39°C is the most effective initial therapeutic approach and should be followed by intravenous infusions of fluids appropriate to correct the antecedent fluid and electrolyte losses.

FEVER PATTERNS

The normal diurnal variation in body temperatures results in a peak temperature in the late afternoon or early evening. This variation often persists when patients have fever. In certain individuals, fever patterns may be helpful in suggesting the cause of fever. Rigors—true shaking chills—often herald a bacterial process (especially bloodstream infection), although they may occur in patients with viral infections, as well as in those with drug or transfusion reactions. Hectic fevers, which are characterized by wide swings in tempera-

ture, may indicate the presence of an abscess, disseminated tuberculosis, or collagen vascular diseases. Patients with nonfalciparum malaria may have a relapsing fever with episodes of shaking chills and high fever, which are separated by 1 to 3 days of normal body temperatures and relative well-being. Medications that may have been recently initiated may cause high, constant fevers. Patients with tuberculosis may be relatively comfortable and unaware of a significantly elevated body temperature. Patients with uremia, diabetic ketoacidosis, or hepatic failure generally have a lower body temperature; thus, normal temperature readings in these settings may indicate infection. Similarly, older patients with infection often fail to mount a febrile response and may experience instead a loss of appetite, confusion, or even hypotension without fever. The administration of anti-inflammatory drugs (NSAIDs) (e.g., aspirin, corticosteroids) also blunts or ablates the febrile response.

Acute Febrile Syndromes

Fever is one of the most common complaints that bring patients to a physician. The challenge is in discerning the few individuals who require specific therapy from among the many with self-limited benign illness. The approach is simplified by considering patients in three groups: (1) those with fever without localizing symptoms and signs, (2) those with fever and rash, and (3) those with fever and lymphadenopathy. This chapter deals only with fever caused by microbial agents. Clearly, autoimmune, neoplastic, and other disease processes may cause fever as well.

FEVER ONLY

Most patients with fever as their sole complaint defervesce spontaneously or exhibit localizing clinical or laboratory findings within 2 to 3 weeks of the onset of illness (Table 94–1). Beyond 3 weeks, the patient can be considered to have a fever of undetermined origin (FUO), a designation with its own circumscribed group of management considerations, as discussed later in this chapter.

Table 94–1	Infections Exhibiting Fever as the Sole or Dominant Feature		
Infectious Agent	**Epidemiologic Exposure and History**	**Distinctive Clinical and Laboratory Findings**	**Diagnosis**
Viral			
Rhinovirus, adenovirus, parainfluenza virus, enterovirus, echovirus	None (adenovirus in epidemics) Summer, epidemic	Often URI symptoms Occasionally, aseptic meningitis, rash, pleurodynia, herpangina	Throat and rectal cultures, serologic findings
Influenza	Winter, epidemic	Headache, myalgias, arthralgias	Throat cultures, serologic findings
EBV, CMV	See text	See text	Monospot test, quantitive PCR
Colorado tick fever	Southwest and northwest tick exposure	Biphasic illness, leukopenia	Blood, CSF cultures, erythrocyte-associated viral antigen (indirect immunofluorescence)
Bacterial			
Staphylococcus aureus	IV drug users, patients with IV plastic cannulas, hemodialysis, dermatitis	Must exclude endocarditis	Blood cultures
Listeria monocytogenes	Depressed cell-mediated immunity	50% have meningitis	Blood, CSF cultures
Salmonella typhi, S. paratyphi	Food or water contaminated by carrier or patient	Headache, myalgias, diarrhea or constipation, transient rose spots	Early blood, bone marrow cultures; late stool culture
Streptococci	Valvular heart disease	Low-grade fever, fatigue, anemia	Blood cultures
After Animal Exposure			
Coxiella burnetii (Q fever)	Infected livestock	Retrobulbar headache, occasionally pneumonitis, hepatitis, culture-negative endocarditis	Serologic findings
Leptospira interrogans	Water contaminated by urine from dogs, cats, rodents, small mammals	Headache, myalgias, conjunctival suffusion Biphasic illness Aseptic meningitis	Serologic findings
Brucella species	Exposure to cattle or contaminated dairy products	Occasionally epididymitis	Blood cultures, serologic findings
Ehrlichia chaffeensis	South and southeast deer or dog tick exposure	Acute onset of headache, fever, myalgias; leukopenia and thrombocytopenia	PCR, serologic findings
Granulomatous Infection			
Mycobacterium tuberculosis	Exposure to patient with tuberculosis, known positive tuberculin skin test	Back pain suggests vertebral infection; sterile pyuria or hematuria suggests renal infection	Liver, bone marrow histology, cultures
Histoplasma capsulatum	Mississippi and Ohio River valleys	Pneumonitis, oropharyngeal lesions	Serologic findings; histologies and cultures on liver, bone marrow, oral lesions

CMV = cytomegalovirus; CSF = cerebrospinal fluid; EBV = Epstein-Barr virus; IV = intravenous; PCR = polymerase chain reaction; URI = upper respiratory infection.

Viral Infections

In young, healthy individuals, acute febrile illnesses generally represent viral infections. The causative agent is rarely established, largely because establishing the precise diagnosis seldom has major therapeutic implications. Rhinovirus, parainfluenza, or adenovirus infections are usually, but not invariably, associated with symptoms of coryza or upper respiratory tract infection (e.g., rhinorrhea, sore throat, cough, hoarseness). Enterovirus and echovirus infections occur predominantly in the summer, usually in an epidemic setting. Undifferentiated febrile syndromes account for the majority of enteroviral infections, but the etiologic features are more likely to be established definitively when a macular rash, aseptic meningitis, pericarditis, or a characteristic syndrome such as herpangina (vesicular pharyngitis caused by coxsackievirus A) or acute pleurodynia (fever, chest wall pain, and tenderness caused by coxsackievirus B) is present. Serologic surveys also indicate that many arthropod-borne viruses (California encephalitis virus; eastern, western, and Venezuelan equine encephalitis viruses; St. Louis encephalitis virus) usually produce mild, self-limited febrile illnesses. West Nile virus, in particular, has recently become a common cause of febrile syndromes (only later associated with neurologic signs and symptoms) during the summer months throughout the United States. Influenza causes sore throat, cough, myalgias, arthralgias, and headache in addition to fever; it most often occurs in an epidemic pattern during the winter months. It is unusual, however, for fever to persist beyond 5 days in uncomplicated influenza.

The mononucleosis syndromes caused by Epstein-Barr virus (EBV), primary human immunodeficiency viral (HIV) infection (see Chapter 107), cytomegalovirus (CMV), and (in rare cases) *Toxoplasma gondii* may sometimes exhibit in a typhoidal manner—that is, with high fever but little or no detectable lymph node enlargement. Diagnosis and management are discussed later in the section, "Generalized Lymphadenopathy: Mononucleosis Syndromes," in keeping with the more typical presentation of these processes. The mononucleosis syndromes are generally self limited. The need to establish a specific diagnosis therefore is usually not urgent with the exception of acute HIV infection. Viral cultures of the throat and rectum and virus-specific antibodies in acute and convalescent serum samples may allow retrospective diagnosis of the specific viral cause. Acute retroviral syndrome (HIV) may require diagnosis through plasma p24 antigen or RNA polymerase chain reaction (PCR) assays because antibodies are frequently not detectable in the early stages (see Chapter 107).

The recognition of other viral syndromes, however, can be critically important. The recent outbreak of severe acute respiratory syndrome (SARS) in Southeast Asia highlights the importance of early recognition. In the spring of 2003, several people in local hospitals exhibited a variety of complaints that typically included fever and dry cough. Only through the combined efforts of the global medical community was the epidemic contained and the SARS coronavirus identified as the causative agent. Avian influenza is the latest in a series of emerging viruses to pose the threat of widespread infection. Fever is an important element in the early stages of this disease, and only by recognizing the threat can the spread of this highly contagious virus be prevented.

Bacterial Infections

Pathogenic bacteria most commonly cause sepsis, or disseminated blood-borne infection (see Chapter 95). *Staphylococcus aureus* (**Web Fig. 94–1**) frequently causes sepsis without an obvious primary site of infection. Fever may be the predominant clinical manifestation of the illness. *S. aureus* sepsis should be considered in patients undergoing intravenous therapy with a plastic cannula, patients on hemodialysis, intravenous drug users, and patients with severe chronic dermatoses. In the patient with *S. aureus* bacteremia, the question of whether intravascular infection exists is key in determining the length of therapy. The following developments are more typical of endocarditis: long duration of symptoms, absence of removable focus of infection (e.g., intravenous cannula, soft tissue abscess), metastatic sites of infection (e.g., septic pulmonary emboli, arthritis, meningitis), younger age, history of injection drug use, and new heart murmur. Transesophageal echocardiogram is frequently necessary to evaluate for an endovascular focus especially in community-acquired *S. aureus* bacteremia (see Chapter 99). *Listeria monocytogenes* septicemia is seen predominantly in patients with depressed cell-mediated immunity. Up to one half of patients with *Listeria* sepsis have meningitis. Occasionally, a relatively indolent clinical syndrome belies the bacterial cause of *S. aureus* and *L. monocytogenes* bacteremia.

Enteric fevers may also present manifestations in a subacute fashion despite the presence of bacteremia. The major species producing this syndrome are *Salmonella typhi*, which has a human reservoir, and *Salmonella paratyphi* A, B, and C. The paratyphoid strains also have their major reservoirs in humans but usually produce less severe disease than *S. typhi*, which is acquired by ingesting food or water contaminated with fecal material from a chronic carrier or a patient with typhoid fever. A large number of bacteria (10^6 to 10^8) must be ingested to cause disease in the normal host. Major host risk factors are achlorhydria, malnutrition, malignancy (particularly lymphomas), sickle cell anemia, and other defects in cellular and humoral immunity. *S. typhi* penetrates the gut wall and enters the lymphoid follicles (Peyer's patches), where it multiplies within mononuclear phagocytes and produces local ulceration. Primary bacteremia occurs with spread to the reticuloendothelial system (liver, spleen, and bone marrow). After further multiplication at those sites, secondary bacteremia occurs and can localize to lesions such as tumors, aneurysms, and bone infarcts. Infection of the gallbladder, particularly in the presence of gallstones, leads to a chronic carrier state. Approximately 2 weeks after exposure, patients develop prolonged fever with chills, headache, and myalgias. Diarrhea or constipation may be present but usually does not dominate the clinical picture. Occasionally, crops of rose spots (2- to 4-mm erythematous maculopapular lesions) appear on the upper abdomen but are evanescent. Typhoid fever usually resolves in about 1 month if left untreated. However, complication rates are high because of bowel perforation, metastatic infection, and general debility of patients, and the mortality rate exceeds 20% in the absence of antibiotic therapy. *S. typhi* may be isolated from blood or stool to confirm the diagnosis. Typhoid fever should be treated with third-generation cephalosporins or fluoroquinolones.

Localized bacterial infection can be clinically occult and develop as an undifferentiated febrile syndrome. Intra-abdominal abscess, vertebral osteomyelitis, streptococcal pharyngitis, urinary tract infection, infective endocarditis, and early pneumonia may all cause fever with surprisingly few clinical clues to the location of the infection. Therefore, urinalysis, throat and blood cultures, and chest radiography should be performed in the patient who is febrile with features suggestive of a bacterial infection.

Eleven cases of inhalational anthrax in the United States in 2001 have highlighted this bacterial infection as an important cause of fever without early localizing signs. Cases were seen in seven men with incubation periods ranging from 5 to 11 days. The illness appeared biphasically with an initial influenza-like illness, followed by sepsis syndrome and severe respiratory distress. All had abnormal chest radiographs, with the majority demonstrating pleural effusions, mediastinal widening, and pulmonary infiltrates, with a high rate of positive blood cultures. Early recognition and initiation of appropriate antimicrobial therapy are essential to survival. Antimicrobial prophylaxis for individuals with credible exposures is critical. The potential use of preventative vaccination is being vigorously pursued.

Febrile Syndromes Associated with Animal Exposure

Q fever, brucellosis, and leptospirosis are diseases associated with exposure to fluids from infected animals and may have similar clinical presentations.

Q Fever. Q fever is an under-recognized cause of acute febrile illness. *Coxiella burnetti*, the causative agent, produces mild infection in livestock. Humans are infected by inhalation of aerosolized particles or by contact with placental and amniotic fluids from infected animals. The source of animal exposure may go unnoticed. For example, in an outbreak of Q fever at the University of Colorado Medical School, 70% of infected individuals lacked direct exposure to infected sheep.

Q fever characteristically begins explosively with severe, often retrobulbar headache, high fever, chills, and myalgias. Pneumonitis and hepatitis may occur but are seldom severe. Although definitive diagnosis is usually based on a fourfold rise in titer of complement-fixing antibodies, DNA amplification using PCR of *C. burnetti*–specific primers may be helpful in rapidly identifying suggested cases. If not treated, then Q fever lasts 2 to 14 days. *C. burneti* is sensitive to doxycycline, which should be used in its treatment (100 mg twice daily for 14 days). Q fever may cause subacute endocarditis, apparently as a form of reactivation of infection. The occurrence of hepatomegaly and thrombocytopenia in a patient with apparently culture-negative endocarditis may be a clue to this diagnosis.

Leptospirosis. Humans are infected with *Leptospira interrogans* by exposure to urine from infected dogs, cats, wild mammals, and rodents. Exposure on the farm, in the slaughterhouse, on camping trips, or during swims in contaminated water is frequent. After an incubation period of approximately 1 week, patients develop chills, high fever, headache, and myalgias. The illness often pursues a biphasic course. During the second phase of illness, fever is less prominent, but headache and myalgias are excruciating;

nausea, vomiting, and abdominal pain become prominent complaints. Aseptic meningitis is the most important manifestation of the second or immune phase of the illness. Suffusion of the bulbar conjunctivae with visible corkscrew vessels surrounding the limbus is a useful early sign of leptospirosis. Lymphadenopathy, hepatomegaly, and splenomegaly may occur. Leptospirosis may also pursue a more severe clinical course characterized by renal and hepatic dysfunction and hemorrhagic diathesis (Weil's syndrome). Darkfield examination will reveal leptospires in body fluids. The diagnosis is made by a fourfold rise in indirect hemagglutination antibody titer. A urine assay for detecting leptospiral antigen has been developed but is not yet commercially available. Early antibiotic treatment shortens the duration of fever and may reduce complications. However, to be effective, antibiotics must be initiated presumptively, before serologic confirmation. Penicillin G, 2.4 to 3.6 million U/day, or doxycycline, 100 twice a day orally, for seven days, is effective therapy.

Brucellosis. *Brucella* species infect the genitourinary tract of cattle (*Brucella abortus*), pigs (*Brucella suis*), sheep, and goats (*Brucella melitensis*). Humans are exposed occupationally or by ingestion of unpasteurized dairy products. Acute disease is characterized by chills, fever, headache, and arthralgias and sometimes by lymphadenopathy, hepatomegaly, and splenomegaly. During the associated bacteremia, any organ may be seeded. Epididymo-orchitis and vertebral (**Web Fig. 94–2**) and sacroiliac involvement are characteristic localized findings. With or without antibiotic treatment of acute infection, brucellosis may relapse or enter a chronic phase. *Brucella* species can be isolated from blood or other normally sterile fluids. However, the organism requires special media and conditions for growth. Otherwise, diagnosis must be made serologically. Treatment consists of doxycycline, 100 mg twice daily, and rifampin, 600 mg/day given orally for 21 days.

Granulomatous Infection

Tuberculosis. Extrapulmonary and miliary tuberculosis (**Web Fig. 94–3**) may develop as febrile syndromes. In disseminated tuberculosis, initial chest radiographs may be normal and tuberculin skin tests are often nonreactive. This finding is particularly true in older patients. Protracted FUO should always suggest this possibility. Liver biopsy and bone marrow biopsy have a high yield in miliary disease. Genitourinary and vertebral tuberculosis may develop as unexplained fever. However, careful history, urinalysis, intravenous pyelography, and radiographs of the spine should reveal the site of tissue involvement. Extrapulmonary tuberculosis should be treated for the first 2 months with isoniazid, 300 mg orally; rifampin, 600 mg orally; ethambutol, 15 mg/kg/day; and pyrazinamide, 15 to 30 mg/kg (maximum 2 g/day) given orally. Thereafter, isoniazid and rifampin are continued for 7 months (longer in patients with skeletal tuberculosis). The ethambutol can be discontinued once the organism is shown to be sensitive to isoniazid. Corticosteroids may be a useful adjunctive measure in the patient with severe systemic toxicity or central nervous system involvement (see Chapter 96). The dose of corticosteroids should be tapered as soon as the patient shows symptomatic improvement.

Histoplasmosis. Most individuals living in endemic areas in the Mississippi and Ohio River valleys who become infected with *Histoplasma* (**Web Fig. 94–4**) have a subclinical, self-limited febrile illness as a manifestation of acute pulmonary histoplasmosis (**Web Fig. 94–5**). Although patients may complain of chest pain or cough, physical examination of the chest is usually unremarkable despite radiographic findings, of infiltrates and mediastinal and hilar adenopathy. Therefore, in the absence of chest radiographs, the lower respiratory tract component of the illness is easily overlooked. Approximately 90% of fungal cultures grow *Histoplasma* within 7 days. A complement fixation titer of at least 1:32 or a fourfold rise in titer is also suggestive of the diagnosis of acute histoplasmosis. Although spontaneous resolution of symptoms is normal, unusually prolonged illness (more than 2 to 3 weeks) may require antifungal treatment with amphotericin B or itraconazole.

Progressive disseminated histoplasmosis may occur as a consequence of reactivation of latent infection in immunosuppressed individuals (e.g., acquired immunodeficiency syndrome) (see Chapter 107) or may reflect an uncontained or poorly contained primary infection. The febrile illness in such patients is protracted. Oropharyngeal nodules and ulcerative lesions are commonly found in disseminated histoplasmosis. Biopsy of such lesions permits rapid diagnosis. Serologic studies are less helpful in disseminated histoplasmosis because they are positive in less than one half of patients; cultures and methenamine silver stains of bone marrow biopsy specimens, however, should establish the diagnosis. *Histoplasma* urine antigen detection is a sensitive predictor of disseminated infection. Disseminated histoplasmosis is treated with amphotericin B, 0.5 to 0.6 mg/kg/day administered intravenously for a total dose of 2 to 3 g. Itraconazole, 400 to 600 mg/day for 6 to 12 months, appears to be an effective alternative for patients who are unable to tolerate amphotericin B and who do not have meningeal disease.

Other Infections. Malaria characteristically produces febrile paroxysms that occur every 48 (*Plasmodium vivax*) to 72 (*Plasmodium malariae*) hours in some patients. However, during the first few days of illness, the fever may be low grade and sustained or intermittent. The diagnosis should therefore be suggested in all febrile travelers who have returned from endemic areas. Malaria may also occur, albeit rarely, in intravenous drug users and recipients of blood transfusions. *Plasmodium falciparum* (**Web Fig. 94–6**) causes a high level of parasitemia and is associated with a high mortality rate unless recognized and treated promptly. Daily fever often occurs in this form of malaria. Although *P. vivax* and *P. malariae* may cause relapsing infection long after primary infection because of latent extra-erythrocytic infection, the course is milder. Demonstration of parasites in blood smears establishes the diagnosis of malaria.

Many, if not most, infectious diseases may exhibit fever as an early finding with subclinical or eventual clinical involvement of specific organ systems. Examples include cryptococcosis, coccidioidomycosis, psittacosis, infection with *Legionella* species, and *Mycoplasma pneumoniae* infections. Pulmonary involvement by these infectious agents often produces few signs on physical examination; chest radiographs often reveal more prominent abnormalities than are clinically suggested.

FEVER AND RASH

Many of the febrile syndromes already discussed may occasionally be associated with a rash (Table 94–2). This section, however, considers diseases in which rash is a prominent feature of the presentation. The most life-threatening infections associated with fever and rash include meningococcemia, staphylococcal toxic shock syndrome (TSS), and Rocky Mountain spotted fever (RMSF).

Bacterial Diseases

Petechial lesions, purpura, and ecthyma gangrenosum are lesions associated with bacteremia (see Chapter 95). Disseminated gonococcemia (**Web Fig. 94–7**) causes sparse vesiculopustular, hemorrhagic, or necrotic lesions on an erythematous base, typically on the extremities and particularly their dorsal surfaces (see Chapter 106). Meningococcemia is also an important cause of fever, and a rash that may range from a few petechiae to, in the most severe cases, purpura fulminans (**Web Fig. 94–8**).

Bacterial toxins produce characteristic clinical syndromes. Pharyngitis or other infections with an erythrogenic toxin-producing *Streptococcus* (**Web Fig. 94–9**) may lead to scarlet fever. Diffuse erythema begins on the upper part of the chest and spreads rapidly, although sparing palms and soles. Small red petechial lesions are found on the palate, and the skin has a sandpaper texture caused by occlusion of the sweat glands. The tongue at first shows a yellowish coating and then becomes beefy red. The rash of scarlet fever (**Web Fig. 94–10**) heals with desquamation.

A streptococcal toxic shock–like syndrome associated with scarlet fever toxin A may also occur as a complication of group A streptococcal soft tissue infections and occasionally after cases of influenza. Major manifestations include cellulitis and/or fasciitis with septicemia, shock, acute respiratory distress syndrome, renal failure, hypocalcemia, and thrombocytopenia. Treatment consists of high-dose penicillin and supportive measures. The mortality remains high (>30%) with optimal current therapy. *Corynebacterium haemolyticum* also produces pharyngitis and rash.

TSS (**Web Figs. 94–11 and 94–12**) was first recognized as a distinct entity in 1978 and became an epidemic in 1980 and 1981, probably because of the extensive marketing of hyperabsorbable tampons. *S. aureus* strains producing TSS toxin (TSST-1) or other closely related exotoxins cause the syndrome. TSST-1 is a potent stimulus of interleukin-1 production by mononuclear phagocytes, which enhances the effects of endotoxin; this property may be important in the pathogenesis of this syndrome. Most patients are 15- to 25-year-old girls and women who use tampons. Other settings include prolonged use of contraceptive diaphragms, vaginal or cesarean deliveries, and nasal surgery. Superficial staphylococcal infections and abscesses usually cause TSS in men. Patients with TSS develop the abrupt onset of high fever (temperature >40°C [104°F]), hypotension, nausea and vomiting, severe watery diarrhea, and myalgias, followed in severe cases by confusion and oliguria. Characteristically, diffuse erythroderma (a sunburn-like rash) with erythematous mucosal surfaces is apparent. Later, intense scaling and desquamation of the skin occur, particularly on the palms and soles. Laboratory abnormalities include elevated levels of liver and muscle enzymes, thrombocytopenia, and

Table 94–2	**Differential Diagnosis of Infectious Agents Producing Fever and Rash**

Maculopapular Erythematous

Enterovirus
EBV, CMV, *Toxoplasma gondii*
Acute HIV infection
Colorado tick fever virus
Salmonella typhi
Leptospira interrogans
Measles virus
Rubella virus
Hepatitis B virus
Treponema pallidum
Parvovirus B19
Human herpesvirus 6

Vesicular

Varicella-zoster virus
Herpes simplex virus
Coxsackievirus A
Vibrio vulnificus

Cutaneous Petechiae

Neisseria gonorrhoeae
Neisseria meningitidis
Rickettsia rickettsii (Rocky Mountain spotted fever)
Rickettsia typhi (murine typhus)
Ehrlichia chaffeensis
Echoviruses
Viridans streptococci (endocarditis)

Diffuse Erythroderma

Group A streptococci (scarlet fever, toxic shock syndrome)
Staphylococcus aureus (toxic shock syndrome)

Distinctive Rash

Ecthyma gangrenosum—*Pseudomonas aeruginosa*
Erythema chronicum migrans—Lyme disease

Mucous Membrane Lesions

Vesicular pharyngitis—coxsackievirus A
Palatal petechiae—rubella, EBV, scarlet fever (group A streptococci)
Erythema—toxic shock syndrome (*Staphylococcus aureus* and group A streptococci)
Oral ulceronodular lesion—*Histoplasma capsulatum*
Koplik's spots—measles virus

CMV = cytomegalovirus; EBV = Epstein-Barr virus; HIV = human immunodeficiency virus.

hypocalcemia. Diagnosis is based on the clinical findings and requires specific exclusion of RMSF, meningococcemia, leptospirosis, and measles. Management of the patient consists of restoring an adequate circulatory blood volume by the administration of intravenous fluids, removal of tampons if present, and treatment of the staphylococcal infection with nafcillin, 12 g/day and clindamycin 600 mg/8 h intravenously. Vancomycin is the alternative therapy for nafcillin-resistant staphylococci. Patients must be advised against using tampons in the future because TSS often recurs within 4 months of the initial episode if tampon use continues.

Rickettsial Diseases

In the United States, three rickettsial diseases are endemic: RMSF (**Web Fig. 94–13**), Q fever, and murine typhus. Rash is not a characteristic of Q fever. "Rocky Mountain spotted fever" is a misnomer because most cases occur in the southeastern United States. The causative organism, *Rickettsia rickettsii*, is transmitted from dogs or small wild animals to ticks and then to humans. Infection occurs primarily during warmer months, the periods of greatest tick activity. About two thirds of patients cite a history of tick exposure. The fulminant onset of severe frontal headache, chills, fever, myalgias, and conjunctivitis occur after 2 to 14 days; cough and shortness of breath develop in one fourth of patients. The diagnosis may be obscure at onset. Rash characteristically begins on the third to fifth day of illness as 1- to 4-mm erythematous macules on the hands, wrists, feet, and ankles. Palms and soles may also be involved. The rash may be transient, but it usually spreads to the trunk and may become petechial. Intravascular coagulopathy develops in some patients who are severely ill. Diagnosis and the institution of appropriate therapy must be based on the clinical and epidemiologic findings; delay in treatment may be fatal. The specific complement fixation test shows a rise in titers and allows retrospective confirmation of the diagnosis. Treatment is with doxycycline, 100 mg twice daily given orally or parenterally, or tetracycline, 25 to 50 mg/kg/day for 7 days administered orally.

Human Ehrlichiosis

Human ehrlichiosis is an acute, febrile illness caused most frequently by *Ehrlichia chaffeensis* (**Web Fig. 94–14**) (human monocytic ehrlichiosis [HME]), or another *Ehrlichia*-like species (anaplasma phagocytophilum) causing human granulocytic ehrlichiosis (HGE). *Ehrlichia chaffeensis*, like *R. rickettsii*, is transmitted by woodland exposure to deer or dog ticks and causes illness with peak incidence in the summer months. Since first recognized in 1986, cases of HME have been identified most frequently in 21 contiguous southeastern states from Maryland to Texas but have been documented in 47 states. The illness characteristically begins with fever, chills, headache, and myalgias, with a maculopapular rash occurring in less than one third of cases. Although a wide spectrum of illness exists, roughly one half of clinically recognized cases are associated with pulmonary infiltrates. Acute respiratory distress syndrome often associated with renal failure may develop, most often occurring in older patients. If left untreated, the mortality rate may exceed 10% in hospitalized patients.

HGE peaks in July and occurs in areas where infected *Ixodes* ticks are found. Nine percent of patients have concurrent Lyme disease or babesiosis because the same tick vector transmits these diseases. HGE usually exhibits a nonspecific influenza-like illness with fever, chills, malaise, headache, nausea and vomiting, leukopenia, and thrombocytopenia. Older patients tend to have more severe disease.

Presumptive diagnosis of HME or HGE is made on clinical grounds in patients with acute febrile illnesses, which are generally associated with decreasing leukocyte and platelet counts, after tick exposure. Peripheral blood smears may show intracellular organisms called *morulae* in infected leukocytes. Serodiagnosis is sensitive but helpful only in retrospective confirmation of diagnosis. A new PCR method for diagnosing *E. chaffeensis* appears to be effective for a timely diagnosis of active infection with this organism. Treatment with doxycycline, 100 mg twice a day, or tetracycline, 500 mg four times a day for 7 days, is effective in decreasing both the duration and severity of illness.

Major clinical distinctions between human ehrlichiosis and RMSF include the earlier, more frequent and more severe cutaneous manifestations of RMSF and the more common pulmonary manifestations and characteristically decreasing leukocyte counts in ehrlichiosis.

Lyme Disease

Lyme disease is a common, multisystem spirochetal infection caused by *Borrelia burgdorferi* (**Web Fig. 94–15**) and is transmitted by the tick *Ixodes dammini*. Initial case reports were clustered in several major foci (the Northeast, Wisconsin and Minnesota, California, and Oregon), but this infection is distributed broadly throughout North America and Western Europe. Between 3 days and 3 weeks after the tick bite, of which most individuals are unaware, patients develop a febrile illness, usually associated with headache, stiff neck, myalgias, arthralgias, and erythema chronicum migrans (**Web Fig. 94–16**). Erythema chronicum migrans begins as a red macule or papule at the site of the tick bite; the surrounding bright red patch expands to a diameter of up to 15 cm. Partial central clearing is often seen. The centers of lesions may become indurated, vesicular, or necrotic. Several red rings may be found within the outer border. Smaller secondary lesions may appear within several days. Lesions are warm but nontender. Enlargement of regional lymph nodes is common. The rash usually fades in approximately 1 month.

Several weeks after the onset of symptoms, important neurologic manifestations occur in more than 15% of patients. Most characteristic is meningoencephalitis with cranial nerve involvement and peripheral radiculoneuropathy. Bell's palsy may occur as an isolated phenomenon; when associated with fever, this finding is strongly suggestive of Lyme disease. The cerebrospinal fluid at this time shows about 100 lymphocytes/mL. Heart involvement may also exhibit as atrioventricular block, myopericarditis, or cardiomegaly.

Joint involvement eventually occurs in 60% of patients. Early in the course, arthralgias and myalgias may be quite severe. Months later, arthritis often develops with significant swelling and little pain in one or two large joints, typically the knee. Episodes of arthritis may recur for months or years; in about 10% of patients the arthritis becomes chronic, and erosion of cartilage and bone occurs. Diagnosis is suggested on clinical grounds and confirmed by the demonstration of immunoglobulin M (IgM) antibody, which peaks by the third to sixth week. Total serum IgM is increased, as are IgM-containing immune complexes and cryoglobulins. The level of IgM is reflective of disease activity and predictive of neurologic, cardiac, and joint involvement. However, serologic studies are not precise. Antibody titers may be negative in early disease, and early antibiotic therapy may blunt the antibody response. Synovial fluid contains an average of 25,000 cells/mL, most of them neutrophils. Synovial fluid polymerase chain reaction provides a moderately sensitive means of diagnosis.

Treatment with doxycycline 200 mg orally within 72 hours of a deer tick bite in an endemic area appears to decrease the subsequent development of Lyme disease. Treatment of the early manifestations of Lyme disease with doxycycline, 100 mg twice daily for 14 to 21 days, usually prevents late complications. Meningitis, cardiac involvement, or arthritis should be treated with aqueous penicillin G, 20 million U/day; or intravenous ceftriaxone, 4 g/day for 14 to 28 days; or prolonged doxycycline therapy. Repeated courses may be necessary if relapses occur.

Viral Infections

The rashes associated with viral infections may be so typical as to establish unequivocally the cause of the febrile syndrome (**Web Table 94–1**). Varicella-zoster requires special consideration because of the availability of effective antiviral drugs. In the normal host, neither chickenpox nor herpes zoster confined within specific dermatomes requires treatment with antiviral agents. Ophthalmic zoster demands antiviral treatment because of its association with potentially severe complications, including orbital compression syndromes and intracranial extension. Acyclovir is also effective in decreasing the severity of chickenpox in immunocompromised children and in limiting the extradermatomal spread of zoster in immunocompromised adults. Acute onset of high fever characterizes viral hemorrhagic fevers and, in some cases, bleeding complications and high mortality rates. Arthropod vectors usually transmit these infections; in other patients, they are acquired by direct contact with the reservoir animal or with infected persons and their body fluids. These illnesses include dengue and Marburg hemorrhagic, Ebola hemorrhagic, and Lassa fevers.

FEVER AND LYMPHADENOPATHY

Many infectious diseases are associated with some degree of lymph node enlargement. However, in some diseases, lymphadenopathy is a major manifestation. Lymph node enlargement can be further divided according to whether the enlargement is generalized or regional.

Generalized Lymphadenopathy: Mononucleosis Syndromes

The mononucleosis syndromes are important causes of fever and generalized lymph node enlargement.

Epstein-Barr Virus Infection. Approximately 90% of American adults have serologic evidence of EBV infection; most infections are subclinical and occur before the age of 5 years or midway through adolescence. EBV causes approximately 80% of clinical cases of infectious mononucleosis.

Table 94–3	**Most Common Infectious Causes of Heterophil-Negative Atypical Lymphocytosis**

Babesiosis
Chickenpox
Cytomegalovirus
Epstein-Barr virus (particularly in children)
Human herpesvirus 6
Human immunodeficiency virus (especially during acute seroconversion)
Infectious mononucleosis
Malaria
Measles
Toxoplasmosis
Varicella
Infectious hepatitis

Table 94–4	**Differential Diagnosis of Monospot-Negative Mononucleosis**

Acute HIV infection
EBV mononucleosis (particularly in children)
Cytomegalovirus
Acute toxoplasmosis
Streptococcal pharyngitis
Acute hepatitis B infection

EBV = Epstein-Barr virus; HIV = human immunodeficiency virus.

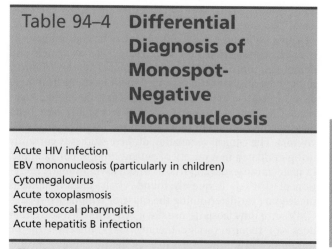

This acute illness usually develops late in adolescence after intimate contact with asymptomatic oropharyngeal shedders of EBV. Patients develop sore throat, fever, and generalized lymphadenopathy and sometimes experience headache and myalgias. Between 5% and 10% of patients have a transient rash that may be macular, petechial, or urticarial. Palatal petechiae are often present, as is pharyngitis, which may be exudative. Cervical lymph node enlargement, particularly involving the posterior lymphatic chains, is prominent, although some involvement elsewhere is common. The spleen is palpably enlarged in about 50% of patients. Autoimmune hemolytic anemia, thrombocytopenia, encephalitis or aseptic meningitis, Guillain-Barré syndrome, hepatitis, or splenic rupture, although rare, may dominate the clinical presentation. The enlarged spleen may be very fragile, which dictates gentleness in palpation of the left upper quadrant. Three fourths of patients exhibit an absolute lymphocytosis. At least one third of their lymphocytes are atypical in appearance: large, with vacuolated basophilic cytoplasm; rolled edges often deformed by contact with other cells; and lobulated, eccentric nuclei. Immunologic studies indicate that some circulating B cells are infected with EBV and that the cells involved in the lymphocytosis are mainly cytotoxic T cells capable of damaging EBV-containing lymphocytes. Atypical lymphocytes may also be seen in other viral illnesses (Table 94–3).

B-cell infection with EBV is a stimulus to the production of polyclonal antibodies. The Monospot rapid diagnostic test is sensitive and specific; false-positive results occur in rare cases in patients with lymphoma or hepatitis. The presence of IgM antibody to viral capsid antigen is diagnostic of acute infectious mononucleosis. The appearance of antibody to EBV nuclear antigen is also indicative of EBV infection.

Infectious mononucleosis usually pursues a benign course even in patients with neurologic involvement. The fever resolves after 1 to 2 weeks, although residual fatigue may be protracted. Occasional patients have a persistent or recurrent syndrome with fever, headaches, pharyngitis, lymphadenopathy, arthralgias, and serologic evidence of chronic active EBV infection. Patients should be managed symptomatically. Acetaminophen may be useful for sore throat. Antibiotics, particularly ampicillin, should be avoided. The use of ampicillin causes a rash in almost all patients with EBV infection, and this phenomenon can also be a diagnostic clue to the occurrence of EBV infection. Corticosteroids are indicated in the rare individual with serious hematologic involvement (i.e., thrombocytopenia, hemolytic anemia) or impending airway obstruction as a result of massive tonsillar swelling.

Acute bacterial superinfections of the pharynx and peritonsillar tissues should be considered when the course is unusually septic.

The differential diagnosis of Monospot-negative mononucleosis is shown in Table 94–4.

Cytomegalovirus. Serologic surveys indicate that most adults have been infected with CMV. The ages of peak incidence of CMV infection are in the perinatal period (transmission by breast milk) and during the second to fourth decades of life. CMV shares the propensity to reactivate, particularly in immunosuppressed patients, with the other *Herpesviridae.*

Two modes of transmission of CMV are particularly important in the development of fever and lymph node involvement in otherwise healthy adults. CMV can be transmitted sexually. Semen is an excellent source for viral isolation. The frequency of antibody to CMV and active viral excretion is particularly high in male homosexuals. Blood transfusions carry a risk of approximately 3% per unit of blood for transmitting CMV infection. This risk becomes substantial in the setting of open-heart surgery or multiple transfusions for other indications.

Primary infection with CMV causes a major proportion of cases of Monospot-negative mononucleosis (see Table 94–4). The distinction between CMV and EBV may be impossible on clinical grounds alone. However, CMV tends to involve older patients (mean age 29) and often produces milder disease, is less likely to cause pharyngitis, and often causes high fever with little or no peripheral lymph node enlargement. The infrequent but serious forms of neurologic

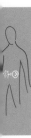

and hematologic involvement that develop in EBV infection occur less commonly with CMV. As with EBV infection, hepatitis (which is usually mild and may be granulomatous) may occur. Isolation of CMV from urine or semen and demonstration of conversion of serologic studies (indirect fluorescent antibody test or complement fixation) from negative to positive are useful in establishing its etiologic features. CMV hybrid capture and PCR techniques have been developed to provide rapid laboratory diagnosis of CMV viremia. The clinical correlation of these studies is currently being evaluated in a variety of patient groups. For example, in male homosexual cohorts, in whom asymptomatic excretion of CMV is frequently found, viral isolation alone is inadequate for determining the cause of lymphadenopathy. CMV mononucleosis is usually a self-limited disease that does not require specific therapy. CMV infection in the immunocompromised host may be life threatening; in this setting it usually responds to long-term therapy with ganciclovir, valganciclovir, or foscarnet.

Primary HIV Infection (acute retroviral syndrome). Typical presenting features of primary HIV infection overlap those of the mononucleosis syndrome (see Chapter 107). Although most patients with the acute retroviral syndrome seek medical attention, the correct diagnosis is missed in a large number of cases because of physician failure to consider HIV infection. Because it is of critical importance to both the patient and his or her sexual partners to establish this diagnosis (see Chapter 107), primary HIV infection must be considered in all patients with mononucleosis syndromes.

Acute Acquired Toxoplasmosis. *Toxoplasma gondii* is acquired by ingesting oocyst-contaminated meat and other foods or by exposure to cat feces. In certain geographic areas such as France, 90% of individuals have serologic evidence of *Toxoplasma* infection. In the United States, the figure is close to 50% by age 50. Between 10% and 20% of infections in normal adults are symptomatic. Presentation may take the form of a mononucleosis-like syndrome, although maculopapular rash, abdominal pain caused by mesenteric and retroperitoneal lymphadenopathy, and chorioretinitis may also occur. Striking lymph node enlargement and involvement of unusual chains (occipital or lumbar) may necessitate lymph node biopsy to exclude lymphoma. More commonly, cervical adenopathy is observed in symptomatic patients. Overall, however, toxoplasmosis accounts for less than 1% of mononucleosis-like illnesses. Histologically, focal distention of sinuses with mononuclear phagocytes, histiocytes blurring the margins of germinal centers, and reactive follicular hyperplasia indicate *Toxoplasma* infection. Acute acquired toxoplasmosis is suggested by the conversion of the indirect fluorescent antibody test from negative to positive or a fourfold increase in titer. Usually the titer is greater than 1:1000 and is associated with increased specific IgM antibody. Acute acquired toxoplasmosis is generally self limited in the immunologically intact host and does not require specific therapy. Significant involvement of the eye is an indication for treatment with pyrimethamine plus sulfadiazine.

Granulomatous Disease. Disseminated tuberculosis, histoplasmosis, and sarcoidosis may be associated with generalized lymphadenopathy, although involvement of certain lymph node chains can predominate. Lymph node biopsy shows granulomas or nonspecific hyperplasia.

Regional Lymphadenopathy

Pyogenic Infection. *S. aureus* and group A streptococcal infections produce acute suppurative lymphadenitis. The most frequently affected lymph nodes are submandibular, cervical, inguinal, and axillary, in that order. Involved nodes are large (>3 cm), tender, and firm or fluctuant. Pyoderma, pharyngitis, or periodontal infection may be present at the presumed primary site of infection. Patients are febrile and have a leukocytosis. Fluctuant nodes should be aspirated. Otherwise, antibiotic therapy should be directed toward the most common pathogens. Penicillin G therapy is appropriate if pharyngeal or periodontal origin implicates a streptococcal or mixed anaerobic infection. Skin involvement suggests possible staphylococcal infection and is an indication for nafcillin (or dicloxacillin) therapy. The dose and route of administration of the drug should be determined by the severity of the infection.

Tuberculosis. Scrofula, or tuberculous cervical adenitis, develops in a subacute to chronic fashion. Fever, if present, is low grade. A large mass of matted lymph nodes is palpable in the neck. If *Mycobacterium tuberculosis* is the causative organism, then other sites of active infection are usually present. The most common causative agent in children in the United States is *Mycobacterium scrofulaceum*. Infection with this and other drug-resistant nontuberculous mycobacteria usually requires surgical excision.

Cat-scratch Disease. Chronic regional lymphadenopathy after exposure to cats or cat scratches should suggest the diagnosis. About 1 week after contact with the cat, a local papule or pustule may develop. One week later, regional adenopathy appears. Lymph nodes may be tender (sometimes exquisitely so) or just enlarged (1 to 7 cm). Fever is low grade if present at all. Lymph node enlargement usually persists for several months. The diagnosis can usually be established on clinical grounds. Lymph node biopsy shows necrotic granulomas with giant cells and stellate abscesses surrounded by epithelial cells. Pleomorphic gram-negative bacilli (*Bartonella henselae*) can be identified in the lymph node biopsy specimens during the first 4 weeks of illness. Serologic testing can confirm the diagnosis. The course is usually self limited and benign in immunocompetent individuals but may be life threatening in persons with severe immunodeficiency. The best approach to the treatment of cat-scratch disease in the immunocompromised patient is not known. Erythromycin or doxycycline may be helpful.

Ulceroglandular Fever. Tularemia is the classic cause of ulceroglandular fever. The syndrome is acquired by contact with tissues or fluids from an infected rabbit or the bite of an infected tick. Patients have chills, fever, ulcerated skin lesion at the site of inoculation, and painful regional adenopathy. When infection is acquired by contact with rabbits, the skin lesion is usually on the fingers or hand, and lymph node involvement is epitrochlear or axillary. In tick-borne transmission, the ulcer is on the lower extremities, perianal region, or trunk, and the adenopathy is inguinal or femoral. Most cases are diagnosed serologically, because Gram-stained preparations are usually negative, and culture of the causative organism, *Francisella tularensis*, is hazardous. A four fold rise in agglutination titer is diagnostic. PCR techniques for diagnosis have also been developed, and their use is becoming more widespread. Patients should be treated presumptively with streptomycin, 15 to 20 mg/kg/day for 10 days.

Oculoglandular Fever. Conjunctivitis with preauricular lymphadenopathy can occur in tularemia, cat-scratch disease, sporotrichosis, lymphogranuloma venereum infection, listeriosis, and epidemic keratoconjunctivitis caused by adenovirus.

Inguinal Lymphadenopathy. Inguinal lymphadenopathy associated with sexually transmitted diseases (see Chapter 106) may be bilateral or unilateral. In primary syphilis, enlarged nodes are discrete, firm, and nontender. Early lymphogranuloma venereum causes tender lymphadenopathy with later matting of involved nodes and sometimes fixation to overlying skin, which assumes a purplish hue. The lymphadenopathy of chancroid is most often unilateral, is very painful, and is composed of fused lymph nodes. Tender inguinal lymphadenopathy also occurs in primary genital herpes simplex virus infection.

Plague. Bubonic plague usually exhibits fever, headache, and a large mat of inguinal or axillary lymph nodes, which go on to suppurate and drain spontaneously. Plague is an important consideration in the acutely ill patient in the southwestern United States with possible exposure to fleas and rodents. If plague is suggested, then blood cultures and aspirates of the buboes should be obtained, and tetracycline, 30 to 50 mg/kg/day, plus streptomycin, 20 to 30 mg/kg/day, should be instituted. Gram-stained preparations of the aspirate reveal gram-negative rods in two thirds of patients. A fluorescent antibody test allows rapid specific diagnosis and is available through the Centers for Disease Control and Prevention.

Fever of Undetermined Origin

Fever of undetermined origin (FUO) is the term applied to febrile illnesses with temperatures exceeding 38.3°C (101°F) that are of at least 3 weeks duration and remain undiagnosed after 3 days in the hospital or after three outpatient visits. Improvements in noninvasive diagnostic testing have resulted in newly proposed categories of FUO (Table 94–5). They include (1) classic FUO, for which the common causes are infections, malignancy, inflammatory diseases, and drug fever; (2) nosocomial FUO; (3) neutropenic (500 neutrophils/mm³) FUO; and (4) HIV-associated FUO (see later discussion). The evaluation of FUO remains among the most challenging problems facing the physician. The majority of illnesses that cause FUO are treatable, making the pursuit of the diagnosis particularly rewarding. No substitute for a meticulous history and physical examination exists; both should be repeated frequently during the patient's hospital course because recurrent questioning of the patient may reveal an important historical clue from the patient and important physical findings may develop while the patient is in the hospital. These clues may direct the next series of diagnostic studies. Patients with FUO should always be offered HIV testing. Directed biopsy specimens of lesions should be stained and cultured for pathogenic microbes. In many instances, however, localizing clues are not present or fail to yield rewarding information. In these patients, bone marrow biopsy can reveal granulomatous or neoplastic disease, even in the absence of clinical evidence of bone

marrow involvement. Similarly, liver biopsy may also reveal the cause of an FUO but seldom in the absence of any clinical or laboratory evidence of liver disease. Exploratory laparotomy is generally not helpful unless signs, symptoms, or laboratory data (most often an isolated elevated level of alkaline phosphatase) point to abdominal pathologic considerations. Computed tomography (CT) may assist in determining the need for laparotomy in patients with FUO. If tuberculosis remains a reasonable possibility after careful work-up fails to establish a diagnosis, then an empiric trial of antituberculous therapy may be initiated while awaiting results of bone marrow, liver, and urine cultures.

Table 94–6 indicates the final diagnoses in a study of over 100 patients with FUO observed in the decade from 1970 to 1980. More recent series of studies have revealed an increasing occurrence of malignancy-associated FUO, decreases in intra-abdominal abscesses because of the increasing sensitivity of CT, and more frequent identification of prolonged viral illnesses, especially CMV, in adolescents and young adults. Table 94–6 simply emphasizes the range of diagnostic possibilities to be considered. Numbers of patients in each category are not presented because regional and temporal

---

Table 94–5	**Fever of Undetermined Origin— Definitions**

Classic FUO

Fever ≥38.3°C (101°F) on multiple occasions
Duration ≤3 wk
Uncertain diagnosis after investigations (3 hospital days or 3 outpatient visits)

Nosocomial FUO

Fever ≥38.3°C (101°F) on multiple occasions in hospitalized patient
Infection not incubating on admission
Uncertain diagnosis after 3-day evaluation, including 2-day microbiologic culture incubation

Neutropenic FUO

Fever ≥38.3°C (101°F) on multiple occasions
Absolute neutrophil count <500/mcL
Uncertain diagnosis after 3-day evaluation, including 2-day microbiologic culture incubation

HIV-Associated FUO

Fever ≥38.3°C (101°F) on multiple occasions
Confirmed diagnosis of HIV infection
Fever 1 mo (outpatients) or >3 days (inpatients)
Uncertain diagnosis after 3-day evaluation, including 2-day microbiologic culture incubation

FUO = fever of undetermined origin; HIV = human immunodeficiency virus.

Table 94–6 Fever of Undetermined Origin: Possible Diagnoses

Infections

Intra-abdominal abscesses
  Subphrenic
  Splenic
  Diverticular
  Liver and biliary tract
  Pelvic
Mycobacterial
Cytomegalovirus
Infection of the urinary tract
Sinusitis
Osteomyelitis
Catheter infections
Other infections

Neoplastic Diseases

Hematologic neoplasms
  Non-Hodgkin's lymphoma
  Leukemia
  Hodgkin's disease
Solid tumors

Collagen Diseases
Granulomatous Diseases
Drug Fever
Factitious Fever

Adapted from Larson EB, Featherstone HJ, Petersdorf RG: Fever of undetermined origin: Diagnosis and follow-up of 105 cases, 1970–1980. Medicine 61:269–292, 1982.

variations in the frequency of specific diagnoses are great. Infectious diseases continue to cause approximately one third of these cases; neoplasms cause another one third; and connective tissue disorders, granulomatous diseases, and other illnesses cause the remainder of cases.

CAUSES OF FEVERS OF UNDETERMINED ORIGIN

Infections

Abscesses account for approximately one third of infectious causes of FUO. Most of these abscesses are intra-abdominal or pelvic in origin because abscesses elsewhere (e.g., lung, brain, superficial abscesses) are more readily identifiable radiographically or as a result of the signs or symptoms they produce.

Intra-abdominal abscesses generally occur as a complication of surgery or leakage of visceral contents, as might occur with the perforation of a colonic diverticulum. Surprisingly, large abdominal abscesses may be present with few localizing symptoms. This development is especially true in the older or immunocompromised patient. Abscesses of the liver (see Chapter 101) occur most often as a consequence of inflammatory disease of the biliary tract or of the bowel; in the latter instance, bacteria reach the liver through portal blood flow. Occasionally, blunt trauma predisposes the liver or spleen to abscesses. Hepatic, perinephric, splenic, or sub-diaphragmatic abscesses are generally readily detected by ultrasonography or a CT scan. However, diagnosis of intra-abdominal abscess may be challenging because even large abscesses in the pericolonic spaces may be difficult to distinguish from fluid-filled loops of bowel on CT. Gallium or tagged white blood cell scanning, ultrasonography, or barium enemas may assist if the diagnosis is probable and a CT scan is not definitive.

Endovascular infections (infective endocarditis, mycotic aneurysms, and infected atherosclerotic plaques) are uncommon causes of FUO because blood cultures are generally positive unless the patient has received antibiotics within the preceding 2 weeks. Infections of intravascular catheter sites are generally also associated with bacteremia unless the infection is limited to the insertion site. Diagnosis of endovascular infection is more difficult to make when blood cultures are negative and infection is with slow-growing or fastidious organisms, such as *Brucella* species, *C. burnetii* (Q fever), or *Haemophilus* species. Diagnosis is especially difficult among patients who have been treated with antimicrobial agents. If endocarditis is suggested, then blood cultures should be repeated for at least 1 week after antimicrobial agents are discontinued, the bacteriologic laboratory should be alerted to the possibility of infection with a fastidious organism, and evidence of valvular vegetations should be sought by transesophageal echocardiography (see Chapter 99). Occasionally, the suggestion of valvular infection is strong enough to warrant empiric antibiotic treatment of a presumed culture-negative endocarditis.

Although most patients with osteomyelitis have pain at the site of infection, localizing symptoms are occasionally absent and patients have only fever. Technetium pyrophosphate bone scans and gallium scans demonstrate uptake at sites of osteomyelitis, but positive scans are not always specific for infection. Magnetic resonance imaging can be especially useful in differentiating between bone and soft tissue infections (see Chapter 100).

Mycobacterial infections, generally with *M. tuberculosis*, remain important causes of FUO. Patients with impaired cell-mediated immunity are at particular risk for disseminated tuberculosis, and occult infection with this organism is seen with particular frequency among older patients, patients after organ transplantation, or those undergoing hemodialysis. Fever may be the only sign of this infection. Among both immunocompromised patients and previously healthy persons with disseminated tuberculosis, purified protein derivative skin tests are often negative. In some patients, careful review of chest radiographs reveals apical calcifications or upper lobe scars suggestive of remote tuberculous infection. A diffuse, often subtle radiographic pattern of *millet seed* densities, which is best visualized on the lateral chest views, is highly suggestive of disseminated tuberculosis. In this setting, transbronchial or open lung biopsy will establish the diagnosis. Similar radiographic patterns may be seen in sarcoidosis, disseminated fungal infection (e.g., histoplasmosis), and some malignancies. Bone marrow or liver biopsy often reveals granulomas, and cultures of these samples are positive in 50% to 90% of patients with disseminated tuberculosis.

Viral infections, especially those caused by CMV or EBV, can produce prolonged fevers. Both infections may be seen in young, healthy adults. Recipients of blood are at risk for acute post-transfusion CMV infection. Recipients of organ transplantation and other immunosuppressed patients may experience reactivation of latent CMV infection producing fever, leukopenia, and pulmonary and hepatic disease. Lymph nodes are often enlarged in EBV infection, and a peripheral blood smear usually reveals a lymphocytosis with increased numbers of atypical lymphocytes. Occasionally, the atypical lymphocytosis is delayed several weeks after the onset of fever. A positive Monospot test result may clarify the diagnosis. Unexplained fever may be a complication of infection with HIV; most such fevers are attributable to complicating opportunistic pathogens (see Chapter 107).

Simple lower urinary tract infections are readily diagnosed by symptoms and urinalysis. Complicated infections such as perirenal or prostatic abscess may be occult and result in an FUO. In general, a history of antecedent urinary tract infection or disorder of the urinary tract is present. In prostatic abscess the prostate is usually tender on rectal examination. In suggested cases of perirenal and prostatic abscesses, the urinalysis should be repeated if it is initially normal because abnormalities of the sediment may be intermittent. Ultrasonography or a CT scan detects most of these lesions (see Chapter 104).

Although most patients with sinusitis have localizing symptoms, infections of the paranasal sinuses may occasionally exhibit fever only, particularly among hospitalized patients who have had nasotracheal and/or nasogastric intubation. Sinus films reveal fluid in the sinuses. Infection of the sphenoidal sinus may be difficult to detect unless special views or CT scans are obtained.

Neoplastic Diseases

Neoplasms account for approximately one third of patients with FUO. Some tumors, particularly those of hematologic origin and hypernephromas, release endogenous pyrogens. In others, the mechanism of fever is less clear but may result from pyrogen release by infiltrating or surrounding inflammatory cells. Lymphomas can cause an FUO; usually enlargement of lymph nodes or the spleen is found. The presentation of some lymphomas is with intra-abdominal disease only. CT scans may be helpful in detecting these tumors. Leukemia may also exhibit an FUO, sometimes with a normal peripheral blood smear. Bone marrow examination reveals an increased number of blast forms. Solid tumors more typically associated with fevers include renal cell carcinoma, atrial myxoma, sarcoma, primary hepatocellular carcinoma, and tumor metastatic to the liver. Liver function abnormalities (predominantly alkaline phosphatase) are common in all these tumors except in atrial myxoma. Myxoma can be suggested in the presence of heart murmur and multisystem embolization (mimicking endocarditis) and is readily diagnosed by echocardiogram. Radiographic studies of the abdomen and retroperitoneum (CT or ultrasonography) generally detect the other tumors. Colon carcinoma must also be considered in the differential diagnosis, because one third or more of patients with this diagnosis

may have low-grade fever; in some this is the only sign of disease.

Other Causes

Collagen vascular diseases account for approximately 10% of patients with an FUO. Systemic lupus erythematosus is readily diagnosed serologically and thus accounts for a small proportion of patients with an FUO. Vasculitis remains an important cause of FUO and should be suggested in febrile patients with *embolization* or *infarctions* or with *multisystem disease.* Giant cell arteritis should be considered in older patients with an FUO, particularly in the presence of polymyalgia rheumatica symptoms (see Chapter 85). Juvenile rheumatoid arthritis, or Still's disease, can exhibit FUO with joint symptoms. An evanescent rash, sore throat, adenopathy, and leukocytosis may occur in this disorder, which is diagnosed on the basis of clinical criteria in the absence of other potential causes of fever.

Granulomatous diseases without a defined cause have been associated with FUO. Sarcoidosis often involves the lungs, skin, and lymph nodes. The majority of patients are anergic to skin test antigens. Diagnosis is based on the exclusion of an infectious cause and the demonstration of discrete, noncaseating granulomas on biopsy of bone marrow, liver, lung, or other tissues. Granulomatous hepatitis can exhibit prolonged fevers, occasionally lasting for years. Serum alkaline phosphatase levels are generally elevated; liver biopsy reveals granulomas, and no underlying cause can be demonstrated.

A number of miscellaneous disorders, including Crohn's disease, familial Mediterranean fever, and hypertriglyceridemia, make up the remainder of FUO cases. In the appropriate setting, drug-related fevers always demand consideration in the differential diagnosis. Fever may be the only manifestation in 4% to 5% of drug sensitivity reactions. The fever may develop months after initiation of the drug. Although relatively more common with anticonvulsants (especially phenytoin and carbamazepine), fever may occasionally result from any class of drug. Another recently appreciated condition is hypergammaglobulinemia immunoglobulin D (IgD) syndrome, which exhibits periodic prolonged fevers, large joint arthritis, skin rash, and highly elevated IgD ($\geq 100\,U/mL$). A significant minority of FUOs (approximately 10%) remains undiagnosed after careful evaluation. Most of these patients have experienced an undefinable but self-limited illness, with fewer than 10% developing an underlying serious disorder after several years' follow-up.

FEVER OF UNDETERMINED ORIGIN IN SPECIAL GROUPS

Besides patients with *classic* FUO, several other groups of patients with fever in whom the diagnosis is not readily apparent deserve special attention. These special groups are encountered more frequently in clinical practice and include patients with nosocomial FUO (see Table 94–6).

Nosocomial Fever of Undetermined Origin

Most patients in this group have significant underlying co-morbidities that lead to hospitalization and complex treatment. The hospital environment, invasive procedures, foreign devices, antibiotic resistance, and alteration of host defenses by diseases or therapy set the stage for potentially unique infectious complications. Bacterial and fungal infections of the urinary tract, surgical wounds, respiratory tract, bloodstream, sinuses, and vascular catheter sites are significant concerns. A frequent cause of nosocomial FUO is *Clostridium difficile*–associated colitis, especially if diarrhea is minimal or absent. This disease is more often encountered in older patients, and a clue to the diagnosis can be an unexplained leukocytosis. Nosocomial FUO in the intensive care unit presents a unique challenge. Disorders to consider in this situation include cholesterol emboli syndrome or CMV postperfusion syndrome after open heart surgery, nosocomial sinusitis, intra-abdominal or pelvic abscess, invasive fungal infection (especially in patients on prolonged steroids), and nosocomial pneumonia. Patients with CMV postperfusion syndrome exhibit a mononucleosis-like syndrome several weeks after open heart surgery. The risk of developing the condition is directly related to the number of blood units transfused during the procedure, and the diagnosis must be differentiated from Dressler's syndrome, which is an autoimmune condition and more likely to occur 2 weeks after the procedure. Other causes of nosocomial FUO that are noninfectious in origin can be loosely divided into those that exceed 102°F and those that are less than 102°F. Possible causes of nosocomial FUO with temperatures less than 102°F include tissue injury or infarction, thromboembolic disease, gastrointestinal hemorrhage, and acute pancreatitis. Noninfectious conditions with temperatures greater than 102°F include adrenal insufficiency and drug fever. Temperatures greater than 106°F are rarely of infectious causes. The most common causes of high fevers of this nature are malignant neuroleptic syndrome, central nervous system trauma, and drug fevers. Most drug fevers are caused by common medications; consequently, a close review of a patient's active medication list is essential to make the diagnosis.

Immune-Deficient Fever of Undetermined Origins

Patients who are immunosuppressed have a higher likelihood of infectious complications. Neutropenic FUO refers to undiagnosed fever in the context of persistent and severe neutropenia. In general, most patients in this category will have received cytotoxic and/or immunosuppressive therapy for their underlying disease. Regardless of the cause, complicating infections are frequently encountered when the absolute neutrophil count (mature neutrophils and bands) falls below 1000/mcL (and especially below 500/mcL). Occult bacterial infections are the most frequent causes of fever, and deterioration may be rapid; empiric broad-spectrum antibiotics are mandated in patients with febrile neutropenia after appropriate cultures are obtained. If the cultures are negative and the patient remains febrile, then the patient is considered to have neutropenic FUO.

In patients with impaired cell-mediated immunity, FUO caused by agents other than bacteria are being increasingly recognized. Populations of patients who are receiving chronic steroids or who are using immunomodulatory agents to control underlying disease processes are growing. In these patients, occult fungal infections and reactivation of viral or mycobacterial diseases need to be considered when they develop unexplained febrile episodes. For example, several recent cases of opportunistic infections have been documented in patients receiving anticytokine therapy for rheumatologic conditions such as rheumatoid arthritis. Other etiologic considerations in these patients should also always include perirectal or periodontal disease, drug-induced fever, relapse of underlying disease (especially lymphoreticular malignancy), and thromboembolic conditions.

HIV-Associated Fever of Undetermined Origin

Fever is one of the most common symptoms in patients infected with HIV. With advanced HIV disease, more frequent causes of FUO include mycobacterial disease (especially disseminated *Mycobacterium avium* complex), CMV (retinitis or colitis) infection, drug reactions, and bacterial line infections (see Chapter 107).

Factitious or Self-Induced Fever

Patients with factitious or self-induced illness present unique ethical and therapeutic problems. Once the possibility of factitious or self-induced illness is considered, the physician-patient relationship is changed. Typically, the physician can rely on the good faith of the patient's history. In the case of factitious or self-induced illness, the physician must assume a more detached role to establish the diagnosis. Patients with factitious fever are typically young and often women. Many have been or are employed in health-related professions. Usually articulate and well educated, these patients are adept at manipulating their family, friends, and physicians. In these instances, a consultant new to the patient may provide a detached and helpful perspective of the problem.

Clues to factitious fever include the absence of a toxic appearance despite high temperature readings, lack of an appropriate rise in pulse rate with fever, and absence of the physiologic diurnal variation in temperature. Suggested factitious readings can be evaluated by immediately repeating the reading with the nurse or physician in attendance. The use of electronic thermometers allows rapid and accurate recording of a patient's temperature (see also Chapter 117).

Self-injection of pyrogen-containing substances, usually bacteria-laden culture medium, urine, or feces, can produce bacteremia and high fever; usually these bacteremic episodes are polymicrobial and intermittent, often suggesting a diagnosis of intra-abdominal abscess. However, patients with self-induced bacteremia may appear remarkably well between episodes of fever. The occurrence of polymicrobial bacteremia in an otherwise healthy person should suggest the possibility of self-induced infection. Illicit ingestion of medications known by the patient to produce fever can also present a difficult diagnostic problem. Clues to the presence of self-induced illness are subtle. The patients are often emotionally immature. Some fabricate unrelated aspects of their history. The most extreme form of factitious or self-induced illness is called the Munchausen syndrome. Some patients are surprisingly stoic about the apparent seriousness of their illness and the procedures used to diagnose or treat them. In some instances, interviewing family members can elicit clues to the possibility of factitious or self-induced illness. Confirming the diagnosis is crucial and, in many instances, requires a search of the patient's hospital room. Although most will deny their role in inducing or feigning illness, the diagnosis must be explained, and psychiatric care is essential. These complicated patients are at risk for inducing life-threatening disease; some respond to psychiatric counseling.

Prospectus for the Future

Advances in medical technology will allow for faster and more accurate diagnosis and treatment of febrile syndromes. For example, new and sophisticated radiographic imaging techniques will provide more detailed identification of internal abnormalities. Highly specific molecular techniques, such as immunohistochemistry, in situ hybridization, and nucleic acid amplification will improve the ability to diagnose infectious causes of fever and FUO. In addition, the sequencing of human and microbial genomes and advances in functional genomics will significantly affect the development of new vaccines and therapies for pathogens associated with febrile syndromes. Nevertheless, medical progress will also change the spectrum of febrile syndromes and FUO. For example, it is likely that the increased numbers and types of compromised hosts created by the expansion of transplantation programs and new immunosuppressive medications will add significant challenges for the diagnosis and management of febrile syndromes. In addition, the creation of new organisms by chance or through bioterrorism and the spread of old organisms to new parts of the world through increased global communication will shape the evolution of this area of medicine.

References

Beutler B, Beutler SM: Pathogenesis of fever. In Goldman L, Ausiello D (eds): Cecil Textbook of Medicine, 22nd ed. Philadelphia, Elsevier, 2004, pp 1730–1733.

Corey L, Boeckh M: Persistent fever in patients with neutropenia. N Engl J Med 346(4):222–224, 2002.

Santos ES, Raez LE, Eckardt P, et al: The utility of a bone marrow biopsy in diagnosing the source of fever of unknown origin in patients with AIDS. J Acquir Immune Defic Syndr 37(5):1599–1603, 2004.

Chapter 95

Bacteremia and Sepsis Syndrome

Gopala K. Yadavalli

Robert A. Salata

Sepsis syndrome, the systemic response to an infectious process, is a leading cause of morbidity and mortality in hospitalized patients. A growing understanding of the pathophysiologic mechanism of sepsis and the recognition of the critical interdependence of the inflammatory and coagulation systems has led to the recent development of the first therapy shown to reduce sepsis-related mortality. Novel therapeutic approaches now being tested in sepsis syndrome are a direct result of the elucidation of the molecular mechanisms of sepsis and the practical applications of modern techniques of biochemistry and molecular biology to rational drug design.

The bases for current definitions of sepsis syndrome and related disorders are presented in Table 95–1 and Figure 95–1. Infection, defined by the presence of microbial pathogens in normally sterile sites, can be symptomatic or inapparent. Bloodstream infection (BSI) implies the presence of organisms that can be cultured from blood. Septicemia implies BSI with greater severity. Sepsis indicates clinical settings in which evidence of infection and a systemic response to infection exists (fever or hypothermia, tachycardia, tachypnea, leukocytosis or leukopenia). Sepsis syndrome emphasizes an increased degree of severity, with evidence of altered organ perfusion with one of the following: hypoxemia, oliguria, altered mentation, or elevated serum lactate level. Severe sepsis represents a more advanced degree of organ compromise and is often associated with multi-organ failure. Septic shock indicates sepsis plus hypotension despite adequate intravenous fluid challenge. Refractory septic shock is defined as shock lasting more than 1 hour that is unresponsive to fluids and/or vasopressors. Noninfectious insults (e.g., thermal burns, severe trauma, severe pancreatitis, certain toxins, therapy with monoclonal antibodies for solid organ transplant rejection) can also be associated with a severe systemic reaction simulating sepsis syndrome. The term *systemic inflammatory response syndrome* (SIRS) encompasses both infectious and noninfectious causes of a profound host inflammatory response with systemic symptoms and signs; sepsis syndrome is the predominant cause of SIRS.

Epidemiologic Factors

The incidence of sepsis and associated deaths has increased dramatically in the United States, and evidence suggests that this rise will continue. Septic shock is the most common cause of death in intensive care units and the thirteenth most common cause of death in the United States. The incidence is approximately 600,000 cases per year.

The National Nosocomial Infection Surveillance System indicates significant increases in the frequency of septicemia caused by gram-positive infections since 1985. Highest rates for hospital-acquired septicemias occur in patients with cancer and burn or trauma victims, as well as individuals in high-risk nurseries. Hospital-acquired BSI is associated with 7.4 extra days of hospitalization and $4000 of extra hospital charges per occurrence. The most commonly identified bloodstream pathogens include staphylococci, streptococci, *Escherichia coli*, *Enterobacter* species, and *Pseudomonas aeruginosa*. Fungal bloodstream isolates are less frequent but increasing over the last decade.

Major epidemiologic factors that have contributed to the increased occurrence of sepsis include the growing number of immunocompromised hosts resulting from more intense chemotherapy regimens, an aging population, and the aggressive employment of increasingly invasive procedures and complex surgery.

Table 95–2 lists organisms important in sepsis syndrome as they relate to host factors. Factors that have negatively influenced survival in the setting of BSI have included severity of underlying disease, delayed initiation of appropriate antimicrobial therapy, virulence of the pathogen (e.g., *P. aeruginosa*), extremes of age, site of infection (respiratory being more common than abdominal, which is more common than urinary), health care–associated infection,

Table 95–1　Definitions of Sepsis and Related Disorders

Disorder	Definition
Infection	Microorganisms in a normally sterile site; subclinical or symptomatic
Bacteremia	Bacteria present in bloodstream; may be transient
Septicemia	Same as bacteremia but greater severity
Sepsis	Clinical evidence of infection plus systemic response to infection (fever/hypothermia, tachycardia, tachypnea, leukocytosis/leukopenia)
Sepsis syndrome	Sepsis plus altered organ perfusion (hypoxemia, oliguria, altered mentation)
Severe sepsis	Sepsis syndrome plus hypotension/hypoperfusion
Septic shock	Sepsis with hypotension despite adequate fluid resuscitation; patients on vasopressors may not be hypotensive at the time hypoperfusion abnormalities are evident
Refractory septic shock	Shock lasting more than 1 hr that is unresponsive to fluid administration and/or vasopressors
Systemic inflammatory response syndrome (SIRS)	Wide variety of insults (infectious response syndrome and noninfectious) that initiate profound systemic responses; sepsis syndrome is a subset of SIRS

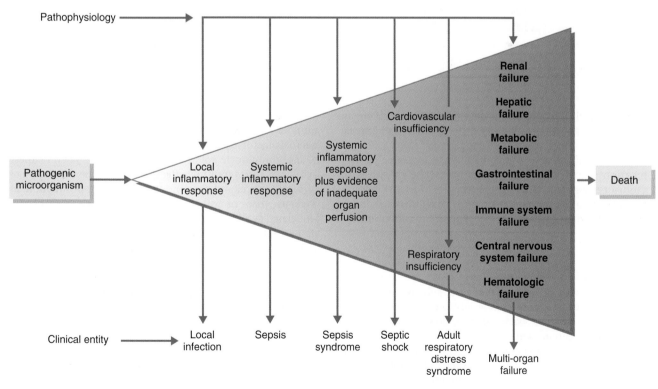

Figure 95–1 Natural history of the sepsis process.

Table 95–2	Micro-organisms Involved in Sepsis Syndrome in Relation to Host Factors	
Host Factors	**Organisms of Particular Importance**	
Asplenia	Encapsulated organisms: *Streptococcus pneumoniae, Haemophilus influenzae, Neisseria meningitidis, Capnocytophaga canimorsus*	
Cirrhosis	*Vibrio, Yersinia,* and *Salmonella* species, other gram-negative rods, encapsulated organisms	
Alcoholism	*Klebsiella* species, *Streptococcus pneumoniae*	
Diabetes	Mucormycosis, *Pseudomonas* species, *Escherichia coli*	
Steroids	Tuberculosis, fungi, herpesviruses	
Neutropenia	Enteric gram-negative rods, *Pseudomonas, Aspergillus, Candida, Mucor* species, *Staphylococcus aureus*	
T-cell dysfunction	*Listeria, Salmonella,* and *Mycobacterium* species, herpesvirus group (herpes simplex virus, cytomegalovirus, varicella-zoster virus)	

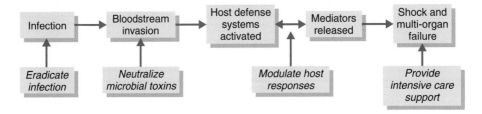

Figure 95–2 The pathogenesis and treatment of sepsis syndrome.

polymicrobial infection, and development of end-organ complications (acute respiratory distress syndrome, anuria, disseminated intravascular coagulation [DIC], bowel ischemia or infarction, and coma). When evidence of dysfunction in two or more systems exists, the diagnosis of multi-organ system failure can be made. Mortality rises in proportion to the number of organ systems involved and is near 100% when four or more systems are dysfunctional.

Pathogenesis

The pathogenesis of sepsis is shaped largely by the infected host's complex response to the invading pathogen (Fig. 95–2). Gram-negative bacterial lipopolysaccharide (LPS), or endotoxin, is representative of a larger class of microbial products causally linked to septic shock syndrome. Cell wall products of gram-positive bacteria, such as teichoic acid and peptidoglycan, induce inflammatory responses similar to those produced by LPS. Indeed, sepsis syndrome may complicate infections with bacteria, viruses, fungi, rickettsiae, mycobacteria, and parasites. The pathogenesis of shock involves a series of events initiated by the invading pathogen or its products, and shock is produced through a causally related sequence of host responses.

Endotoxin induces macrophages to produce a large number of pro-inflammatory cytokines, including tumor necrosis factor-α, interleukin (IL)-1, IL-6, IL-8, interferon-γ, and granulocyte colony-stimulating factor. Each of these cytokines exerts multiple effects related to the development of septic shock, and each modulates its own production, as well as that of other mediators. These macrophage-associated cytokines can also stimulate B and T lymphocytes, natural killer cells, and bone marrow cells (Table 95–3).

Systemic inflammation influences activity of the coagulation system by directly and indirectly modulating production of pro- and anticoagulant molecules. In response to pro-inflammatory cytokines, tissue factor released by endothelium and associated thrombin formation, respectively, activate the extrinsic and intrinsic pathways of coagulation. Simultaneous depletion of endogenous anticoagulant molecules occurs, including antithrombin III, tissue factor pathway inhibitor, protein S and protein C, and inhibition of fibrinolysis via increases in plasminogen activator inhibitor and thrombin-activatable fibrinolysis inhibitor. Endotoxin stimulates membrane phospholipid metabolism, leading to the generation of platelet-activating factor and other bioactive metabolites of arachidonic acid, including prostaglandins and leukotrienes. These compounds, in turn, exert a variety of synergistic and

Table 95–3	**Cytokines with a Potential Role in Systemic Inflammatory Response Syndrome**

Cytokine	Source	Target Cell	Function
Granulocyte-macrophage colony-stimulating factor (GM-CSF)	T cells, macrophages, endothelial cells, fibroblasts	Myeloid precursor cells, neutrophils, eosinophils, macrophages	Proliferation of progenitor cells Differentiation and maturation of neutrophils and macrophages
Granulocyte colony-stimulating factor (G-CSF)	Monocytes, endothelial cells, fibroblasts, neutrophils	Neutrophils, promyelocytes	Proliferation of myeloid progenitor cells Enhanced neutrophil survival and function
Interleukin-1 (IL-1) (α and β)	Macrophages, fibroblasts, T cells, endothelial cells, hepatocytes	Fibroblasts, T cells, monocytes, neutrophils	Induces cytokines (IL-2, IL-3, IL-6, TNF); induces B- and T-cell activation, growth, and differentiation Synthesis of acute phase reaction, induces fever, catabolism
Interleukin-2 (IL-2)	Activated T cells	Activated lymphoid cells	Enhances T- and B-cell immune responses Promotes cytotoxic T cells Induces INF-γ and TNF
Interleukin-4 (IL-4)	Th2 T cells	B and T cells, macrophages, mast cells	Induces B-cell activation, proliferation, and differentiation and IgG1 and IgE production Enhances MHC class I and II receptors
Interleukin-6 (IL-6)	Macrophages, fibroblasts, Th2 T cells	Lymphocytes, monocytes	Stimulates B-cell growth, differentiation, and activation Induces synthesis of acute phase reactants
Interleukin-8 (IL-8)	Monocytes, fibroblasts, endothelial cells	Neutrophils, monocytes	Enhanced neutrophil activity and histamine release
Interleukin-12 (IL-12)	Macrophages, B cells	T cells	Induces differentiation of Th1 cells Initiates production of IFN-α
Interferon-γ (INF-γ)	T cells	Macrophages, monocytes, T and B cells	Pronounced monocyte/macrophage activation Increased MHC class II expression
Tumor necrosis factor (TNF): TNF-α (cachectin), TNF-β (lymphotoxin)	Monocytes, macrophages, lymphocytes, mast cells	Monocytes, macrophages, lymphocytes, neutrophils, fibroblasts	Induces cascade of inflammatory reactions (fever, catabolism, acute phase reactants) Induces multiple cytokines (IL-1, GM-CSF) Increases MHC class I expression Enhances B-cell proliferation and immunoglobulin production

IgE = immunoglobulin E; IgG1 = immunoglobulin G1; MHC = major histocompatibility complex.

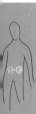

antagonistic effects on vascular endothelium, smooth muscle, platelets, and leukocytes. The resultant, exaggerated, procoagulant state leads to microvascular thrombosis (often in association with DIC) and tissue ischemia and may ultimately cause multiple organ failure.

Endotoxin may also serve as a co-factor to prime granulocytes to produce toxic oxidative radicals. Finally, endotoxin induces the production of β-endorphins, which have been implicated in the pathogenesis of sepsis, as well as counter-regulatory hormones such as cortisol, glucagon, and catecholamines, which may oppose certain shock-producing actions of endorphins and other mediators.

Clinical Manifestations

The clinical manifestations of sepsis syndrome are multiple and often do not point to the specific cause (Table 95–4). The clinician is faced with the challenge of early recognition and sorting through the various possible causes of SIRS so that appropriate therapy can be initiated. Patients with the clinical picture of sepsis of uncertain origin should be presumed to have BSI and treated accordingly. Prompt, thorough cultures of blood and suspicious local sites should be followed immediately by initiation of antibiotics appropriate for the most likely pathogens.

Fever and chills are usually present, but older or debilitated patients (especially those with renal or liver failure or those receiving systemic corticosteroids) may not develop fever. Hypothermia may occur and is associated with a poorer prognosis. One of the early clues to a systemic infectious process is hyperventilation and respiratory alkalosis.

Skin manifestations in sepsis can occur with any infectious agent and at times may represent the earliest sign of sepsis syndrome. Staphylococci and streptococci can be associated with cellulitis or diffuse erythroderma in association with toxin-producing strains. BSI with gram-negative bacteria can be associated with a skin lesion called ecthyma gangrenosum (round or oval 1- to 15-cm lesions with a halo of erythema and usually a vesicular or necrotic central area). Although ecthyma gangrenosum is most commonly associated with *P. aeruginosa*, other invaders such as *Aeromonas* organisms, *Klebsiella* organisms, *E. coli*, *Serratia* species, and fungal organisms may also cause ecthyma gangrenosum (see

also Chapter 100). *Neisseria meningitidis* bacteremia is often heralded by petechial and hemorrhagic skin lesions and followed by rapidly progressive shock.

The sepsis syndrome is characteristically associated with hypotension and oliguria. In many patients, hypotension may initially respond to intravenous fluids. Other patients progress from an initial stage of hypotension, tachycardia, and vasodilation (warm shock) to deep pallor, vasoconstriction, and anuria (cold shock). Of all infectious causes of sepsis syndrome, gram-negative bacilli most often cause shock; up to 35% of patients with gram-negative sepsis develop shock, often with mortality rates between 40% and 70%.

As sepsis syndrome progresses, myocardial function becomes profoundly depressed. This situation greatly complicates fluid management and necessitates continuous cardiopulmonary monitoring in an intensive care setting.

Pulmonary complications of sepsis syndrome are frequent. Acute respiratory distress syndrome, characterized by arterial oxygen tension less than 50 mm Hg despite fractional inspired oxygen greater than 50%, diffuse alveolar infiltrates, and pulmonary capillary wedge pressure less than 18 mm Hg, occurs in 10% to 40% of patients with sepsis syndrome and is most frequently seen in conjunction with gram-negative organisms. Increased pulmonary capillary permeability, resulting from inflammatory cytokines released during sepsis, is a major causative factor in acute respiratory distress syndrome and makes administration of intravenous fluids, often given in an attempt to improve cardiac output, extremely hazardous. Failure of respiratory muscles can also complicate sepsis and contribute significantly to morbidity and mortality.

Most patients with sepsis have a neutrophilic leukocytosis. Leukopenia may occur, most often with overwhelming bacteremias but also with severe systemic viral infections. Alcoholics and the older adults are at increase risk for sepsis-associated neutropenia. A low platelet count and evidence of coagulopathy occur in up to 75% of patients with gram-negative bacillary bacteremia. DIC occurs in roughly 10% of patients with sepsis.

Renal insufficiency in sepsis syndrome is multifactorial and depends to varying degrees on the host, the microbe, and the therapy administered. Most often in sepsis, acute tubular necrosis is the basis for renal dysfunction and may be secondary to hypotension, volume depletion, or cytokines elaborated in sepsis syndrome. Tubulointerstitial disease caused by specific pathogens and/or antimicrobial therapy may also occur.

Upper gastrointestinal tract bleeding may be a life-threatening complication in patients with sepsis who also have coagulopathy and thrombocytopenia. Liver dysfunction may occur with evidence of cholestatic jaundice or of hepatocellular injury. With bacteremia related to gram-negative bacilli, *hyperbilirubinemia of sepsis* often occurs, with little change in the other liver enzymes. Large increases in transaminase values usually indicate ischemia of the liver; these abnormalities usually resolve rapidly with restoration of blood pressure.

Hypoglycemia may complicate sepsis syndrome and can be a correctable cause of mental status change or seizures. Hypoglycemia occurs more frequently in individuals with underlying liver disease.

Table 95–4	Signs and Symptoms Indicative of Sepsis Syndrome

Fever, chills
Hyperventilation
Hypothermia
Mental status changes
Hypotension
Leukopenia, thrombocytopenia
End-organ failure: lung, kidney, liver, heart, disseminated intravascular coagulation

Diagnosis

The initial evaluation of the patient with possible sepsis syndrome ideally begins with a thorough history. However, in patients with fully developed sepsis syndrome, the working diagnosis is made on the basis of physical findings, and the detailed history must necessarily follow correction of hemodynamic problems, obtaining appropriate microbial cultures, and empiric initiation of antimicrobial therapy. Attention should be focused on underlying diseases or predispositions to sepsis, previous infections and antimicrobial therapy, available microbiologic information, and symptoms suggesting localization of infection. A history of travel, environmental exposure, and any contact with infectious agents should be thoroughly explored. Information on the complications of previous treatment (e.g., toxic effects of drugs or drug allergies) can be critical in the selection of therapy.

Physical examination should focus on discovering clues to infection and localizing sites thereof. Appropriate specimens for microbiologic evaluation must be obtained. Two or three sets of blood cultures from patients with bacteremia yield the organism in 89% and 99% of patients, respectively.

The selection of additional laboratory studies should be based on the clinical manifestations. Obtaining appropriate diagnostic studies expeditiously is critical. These studies are usually aimed at delineating the focus of infection (e.g., cerebrospinal fluid examination, computed tomography scans) and determining whether adjunctive surgical therapy (e.g., abscess drainage, foreign body removal) is indicated.

Therapy

The key to managing sepsis is the early recognition of the systemic response and initiation of therapy before hypotension and complications ensue. Patients with sepsis syndrome, especially if hypotensive, are best managed in the intensive care unit. The essential therapies of sepsis syndrome and septic shock include judicious fluid administration, oxygen, vasopressors, and antibiotics.

Early goal-directed therapy focused on optimal oxygen delivery to tissues is associated with improved survival. This therapy includes crystalloid fluid resuscitation, red blood cell transfusion to maintain a hematocrit of at least 30%, careful hemodynamic monitoring, and the use of inotropes in select persons. Antibiotic choices should reflect epidemiologic concerns (see Table 95–2), antibiotic resistance patterns, and potential sites of infection. Time does not allow holding antimicrobial therapy until bacteremia or an infectious source is proved in patients with sepsis syndrome. Until culture results and other diagnostic studies are completed, empiric broad-spectrum antimicrobial therapy (covering both gram-positive and gram-negative pathogens, as well as antifungal therapy in select patients) is necessary in patients with sepsis. Initiation of appropriate empiric antimicrobial therapy has a major impact on survival of these patients. As soon as a specific microbial cause has been established by culture, antibiotics should be changed, if necessary, to target the etiologic agent. Attention should also be directed to serum glucose control because maintenance of glucose between 80 and 110 mg/dL using intensive insulin therapy is associated with reduced mortality.

The limitations of currently available therapy for sepsis and septic shock are demonstrated by the continued high mortality rates associated with this disease, despite improvement in antibiotic therapy and critical care techniques. Standard approaches to therapy for sepsis and septic shock are crucial. Of the various steps in the pathogenesis of septic shock, beginning with tissue invasion by the offending organism and culminating in pathophysiologic phenomena associated with septic shock syndrome, current therapy addresses only the initial and final steps of this process (see Figs. 95–1 and 95–2). Few currently employed therapies target intermediate steps in the pathogenesis of septic shock, even though these steps dominate the disease process in fully developed sepsis syndrome. Newer strategies entail attempts to amplify selectively or modulate the host responses to the invading pathogen or its pathogenic products. Targets include the bacterium, endotoxin (or other bacterial products), host cells that respond to endotoxin, mediators produced by these cells in response to endotoxin, and cells injured by endotoxin-induced mediators (see Fig. 95–2).

Clinical trials of high-dose corticosteroids have failed to show survival benefit and may predispose the treated individual to an increased risk of secondary infections. Trials of lower-dose corticosteroids, especially in patients with adrenal insufficiency, have shown improved results, but the role of steroid therapy has not yet been definitively determined. Numerous trials targeting cytokines in sepsis have failed to demonstrate clinical efficacy. These studies have emphasized that targeting a specific molecule as adjunctive therapy for sepsis may be inadequate, given the complex cascade and temporal relationships of factors involved in the pathophysiologic parameters of SIRS. Indeed, the only adjunctive therapeutic agent to show significant further reduction in mortality in sepsis syndrome is activated protein C. In a multicenter, randomized, double-blinded, placebo-controlled trial for severe sepsis, infusion of activated protein C (drotrecogin-α) resulted in a 6.1% absolute risk reduction for mortality. The major adverse effect in this trial was bleeding, occurring in 3.5% of patients receiving the drug. Although clinical experience with this agent is limited and optimal target populations have not been fully identified, drotrecogin-α is currently the only medication approved by the U.S. Food and Drug Administration specifically for the treatment of severe sepsis in adults.

Prospectus for the Future

The evolving epidemiology of microbes causing BSI and sepsis is a reflection of trends such as the increasing age of inpatients, higher numbers of immunocompromised individuals, and widespread antibiotic use. Technologic advances in microbe identification will therefore have an important role in the management of individuals with sepsis syndrome. The recent explosion in our understanding of microbial recognition by the immune system will lead to more rational immunomodulatory approaches to these patients as well.

Improved Diagnostics

Rapid diagnosis of the microbial cause of BSI and sepsis syndrome is essential to ensure both that antimicrobial therapy is directed against the appropriate pathogen and that coverage is not needlessly broad. Peptide nucleic acid-fluorescence *in situ* hybridization (PNA-FISH) can differentiate *Staphylococcus aureus* from the less pathogenic coagulase-negative staphylococci earlier than conventional methods, allowing for appropri-ate modification of antibiotics. Galactomannan and other markers may better identify fungi such as *Aspergillus* species than currently available techniques.

Immune-Based Therapies

Dysregulation of the immune response has long been the focus of novel therapies for sepsis syndrome. The recent identification of toll-like receptors and other pattern-recognition receptors as key players in host defense and the elucidation of subsequent intracellular signaling pathways have opened up new targets for potential pharmacologic intervention. Furthermore, the fact that immune dysregulation in critical illness exists across a spectrum is increasingly recognized, from heightened immune activation associated with SIRS to severe immunodepression characterized by impairments in antigen presentation and pro-inflammatory cytokine production. Immunostimulatory approaches, including cytokines and growth factors, are under study.

References

Bernard GR, Vincent JL, Laterre PF, et al: Recombinant Human Protein C Worldwide Evaluation in Severe Sepsis (PROWESS) study group: Efficacy and safety of recombinant human activated protein C for severe sepsis. N Engl J Med 344:699–709, 2001.

Martin GS, Mannino AM, Eaton S, et al: The epidemiology of sepsis in the United States from 1979 through 2000. N Engl J Med 348(16):1546–1554, 2003.

Munford RS: Sepsis, severe sepsis and septic shock. In Mandell GM, Bennett JE, Dolin R (eds): Principles and Practice of Infectious Diseases, 6th ed. New York, Elsevier, 2005, pp 906–926.

Rivers E, Nguyen B, Havstad S, et al: Early goal-directed therapy in the treatment of severe sepsis and septic shock. N Engl J Med 345(19):1368–1377, 2001.

Van den Berghe G, Wouters P, Weekers F, et al: Intensive insulin therapy in critically ill patients. N Engl J Med 345(19):1359–1367, 2001.

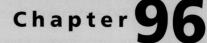

Infections of the Nervous System

Scott A. Fulton

Robert A. Salata

Infections of the central nervous system (CNS) range from fulminant, readily diagnosed septic processes to indolent illnesses requiring exhaustive investigation to identify their presence and define their causes. Neurologic outcome and survival depend largely on the extent of CNS damage before effective treatment begins. Accordingly, it is essential that the physician move quickly to achieve a specific diagnosis and institute appropriate therapy. The initial evaluation must, however, take into account both the urgency of beginning antibiotic treatment in bacterial meningitis and the potential hazard of performing a lumbar puncture in the presence of focal neurologic infection or mass lesions.

Patients with CNS infection usually exhibit some combination of fever, headache, altered mental status, depressed sensorium, seizures, focal neurologic signs, and stiff neck. The history and physical examination, the results of lumbar puncture (Table 96–1), and the neuroradiographic procedures provide the mainstays of diagnosis. The order in which the last two procedures are performed is critical. A subacute history, evolving over 7 days to 2 months, of unilateral headache with focal neurologic signs and/or seizures implies a mass lesion that may or may not be infectious. A brain-imaging procedure should be performed first; lumbar puncture is potentially dangerous because it may precipitate cerebral herniation, even in the absence of overt papilledema. However, patients with fulminating symptoms of fever, headache, lethargy, confusion, and stiff neck should have an immediate lumbar puncture, and if this test proves abnormal, then antibiotics should be instituted for presumed bacterial meningitis. If the distinction between focal and diffuse CNS infection is unclear or evaluation is not adequately possible, as in the comatose patient, then cultures of blood samples and throat and nasopharyngeal swabs should be obtained, antibiotic therapy started, and an emergency scanning procedure performed. If the last is unavailable, then lumbar puncture should be delayed pending evidence that no danger of herniation exists. Inevitably, this approach means that some patients will receive parenteral antibiotics

several hours before a lumbar puncture is performed. In acute bacterial meningitis, 50% of cerebrospinal fluid (CSF) cultures will be negative by 4 to 12 hours after instituting antibiotics; negative CSF cultures are even more likely if the causative organism is a sensitive pneumococcus. Should the CNS infection actually represent acute bacterial meningitis, however, the characteristics of the CSF would still suggest the diagnosis because neutrophilic pleocytosis and hypoglycorrhachia (low CSF glucose) usually persist for at least 12 to 24 hours after antibiotics are instituted. Furthermore, Gram-stained preparation (or assay for microbial antigen in the CSF by latex agglutination) should indicate the causative organism even after antibiotics have rendered the CSF culture negative. Blood and nasopharyngeal cultures obtained before therapy are also likely to be positive in view of the high frequency of isolation of causative organisms from these sites. The approach of treating suggested CNS infections promptly is often life saving and does not significantly compromise management. This approach to the use of scanning procedures is germane only for adults with community-acquired CNS infection. In children, technically adequate computed tomography (CT) requires heavy sedation; therefore, scanning procedures must be reserved for more stringent indications.

Armed with the clinical presentation and the results of the lumbar puncture and CT scan, the clinician must decide on a probable cause and develop a plan for initial management and definitive evaluation. The task is simplified by addressing the following issues:

1. Is the host immunocompetent? The spectrum of CNS diseases and their causes shifts dramatically in the patient who is immunocompromised (**Web Table 96–1**). For example, the possibility of human immunodeficiency viral (HIV) infection must be determined expeditiously by serologic testing. Additional determination of plasma HIV RNA via polymerase chain reaction (PCR) assay may be necessary

Table 96–1   Typical Cerebrospinal Fluid Findings in Central Nervous System Infections

Infection	Cells	Neutrophils	Glucose	Protein
Bacterial meningitis	500–10,000/mcL	>90%	<40 mg/dL	>150 mg/dL
Aseptic meningitis	10–2000/mcL	Early >50%; late <20%	Normal	>100 mg/dL
Herpes simplex virus encephalitis	0–1000/mcL	>50%	Normal	<100 mg/dL
Tuberculous meningitis	50–500/mcL	Early >50%; late <50%	<30 mg/dL	>150 mg/dL
Syphilitic meningitis	50–500/mcL	<10%	<40 mg/dL	<100 mg/dL

if the likelihood is sufficiently high (see Chapter 107), because acute HIV infection may cause CNS signs and symptoms before seroconversion.

2. Are there relevant exposures? Exposure to persons with tuberculosis or HIV infection may be associated with the acquisition of these diseases. Ticks may transmit Lyme disease or spotted fever, and mosquitoes may transmit arboviral encephalitis. Exposure to livestock or unpasteurized dairy products suggests brucellosis. Residence in the Ohio and Mississippi River valleys increases the risk of histoplasmosis and blastomycosis; coccidioidomycosis is endemic to semi-arid regions of the Southwest. Travel and particularly residence in developing countries may suggest cysticercosis, echinococcal cyst disease, tuberculosis, and cerebral malaria.

3. Does the patient have meningitis, encephalitis, or meningoencephalitis? Is the disease acute, subacute, or chronic? These distinctions narrow and modify the differential diagnosis considerably and form the basis for the organization of the sections that follow. The meningitis syndrome consists of fever, headache, and stiff neck. Confusion and a depressed level of consciousness may occur as part of the encephalopathy in patients with acute bacterial meningitis. Seizures are rare and may indicate complicating processes such as cortical vein thrombosis. In contrast, encephalitis characteristically causes confusion, bizarre behavior, depressed levels of consciousness, focal neurologic signs, and seizures (generalized or focal). A presentation suggestive of encephalitis raises a variety of issues quite different from those surrounding a patient with bacterial meningitis.

Meningitis

Meningitis is inflammation of the leptomeninges caused by infectious or noninfectious processes. The causes of infectious meningitis may be bacterial, viral, tuberculous, and fungal. The most common noninfectious causes are subarachnoid hemorrhage, cancer, and sarcoidosis. Infec-

tious meningitis is considered in three categories: acute bacterial meningitis, aseptic meningitis, and subacute to chronic meningitis.

ACUTE BACTERIAL MENINGITIS

Epidemiologic Features

Three fourths of patients with acute bacterial meningitis present before the age of 15 years. *Neisseria meningitidis* causes sporadic disease or epidemics in closed populations. Closed population outbreaks often occur among students in primary and secondary schools and college students residing in dormitories. However, most cases occur in winter and spring and involve children younger than 5 years of age. *Haemophilus influenzae* meningitis is even more selectively a disease of childhood, with most cases developing by the age of 10 years. Infections are sporadic, although secondary cases may occur in close contacts. The incidence of *H. influenzae* meningitis has significantly declined with the widespread use of effective conjugated vaccines. In contrast, pneumococcal meningitis is a disease observed in all age groups. In addition, pneumococcus is becoming increasingly resistant to penicillin, making therapy more challenging (see later discussion). Recent clinical series of hospitalized adults show a relative frequency of 40% to 55% pneumococcal, 3% to 13% meningococcal, 10% to 13% listerial, and 4% to 8% *H. influenzae* for community-acquired meningitis. The use of the conjugated pneumococcal vaccine in early childhood should decrease the incidence of meningitis caused by *Streptococcus pneumoniae*.

Vaccination is particularly important for persons with inherited (e.g., complement deficiency, sickle cell anemia) and acquired immunodeficiency (e.g., HIV infection, splenectomy) (see **Web Table 96–1**).

Close contact with a patient with *N. meningitidis* or *H. influenzae* disease is particularly important in the secondary cases of meningitis and other severe disease manifestations (e.g., sepsis, epiglottitis) as well. For example, the risk of meningococcal disease is 500 to 800 times greater in a close contact of a patient with meningococcal meningitis than it is with no contact. Asymptomatic pharyngeal carriers of

H. influenzae can also spread infection to their contacts. Thus, prophylactic therapy for close contacts is critical to prevent secondary cases (see discussion under "Treatment and Outcome").

Pathogenesis and Pathophysiologic Features

The bacteria that cause most community-acquired meningitis transiently colonize the oropharynx and nasopharynx of healthy individuals. Meningitis may occur in nonimmune hosts after bacteremia from an upper respiratory site (*N. meningitidis* or *H. influenzae*) or pneumonia and by the direct spread from contiguous foci of infection (nasal sinuses or mastoids).

The pathogenesis of acute bacterial meningitis is best understood for meningococcal disease. The carrier state occurs when meningococci adhere to pharyngeal epithelial cells by means of specialized filamentous structures termed *pili*. The production of immunoglobulin A (IgA) protease by pathogenic *Neisseria* species favors adherence by inactivating IgA, a major host barrier to mucosal colonization. Organisms enter and pass through epithelial cells to subepithelial tissues, where they multiply in nonimmune individuals and produce bacteremia. The localization of organisms to the CSF is not well understood but presumably depends on invasive properties of the capsular polysaccharide, which permit penetration of the blood-brain barrier. Immunity is conferred by bactericidal antibody and presumably is acquired by earlier colonization of the pharynx with nonpathogenic meningococci and other cross-reacting bacteria. The presence of blocking IgA antibody may increase susceptibility transiently in some individuals. Bacterial meningitis usually remains confined to the leptomeninges and does not spread to adjacent parenchymal tissue. Focal and global neurologic deficits develop because of involvement of blood vessels coursing in the meninges and through the subarachnoid space. In addition, cranial nerves and cerebral tissue can be damaged by the attendant inflammation, edema, and scarring, as well as by the development of obstructive hydrocephalus.

Gram-negative bacterial meningitis occurs mainly in severely debilitated persons or in individuals whose meninges have been breached or damaged by head trauma or after a neurosurgical procedure or the development of a parameningeal infection or tumor.

Clinical Presentation

Patients with bacterial meningitis may exhibit fever, headache, lethargy, confusion, irritability, and stiff neck. One of three principal modes of onset can occur. (1) Approximately 25% of cases begin abruptly with fulminant illness; mortality is very high in this setting. (2) More often, meningeal symptoms progress over 1 to 7 days. (3) Meningitis may superimpose itself on 1 to 3 weeks of an upper respiratory-type illness; diagnosis is most difficult in this group. Occasionally, no more than a single additional neurologic symptom or sign hints at disease more serious than a routine upper respiratory tract infection. Stiff neck is absent in roughly one half of all patients with meningitis, notably in the very young, the old, and the comatose. A petechial or purpuric rash is found in one half of patients with meningococcemia; although not pathognomonic, palpable purpura is very suggestive of *N. meningitidis* infection. Approximately

20% of patients with acute bacterial meningitis have seizures, and a similar fraction has focal neurologic findings.

Laboratory Diagnosis

In acute bacterial meningitis the CSF usually contains 500 to 10,000 cells/mcL, mostly neutrophils (see Table 96–1). Glucose concentration falls below 40 mg/dL, and the protein level rises above 150 mg/dL in most patients. The Gram-stained preparation of CSF is positive in 80% to 88% of patients. However, certain cautionary notes are appropriate. Cell counts can be lower (occasionally zero) early in the course of meningococcal and pneumococcal meningitis or in patients with neutropenia. In addition, predominantly mononuclear cell pleocytosis may occur in patients who have received antibiotics before the lumbar puncture. A similar mononuclear pleocytosis may be seen in meningitis caused by *Listeria monocytogenes*, *Mycobacterium tuberculosis*, and *Treponema pallidum* (secondary syphilis) (Table 96–2). Gram-stained preparations of CSF may be negative or misinterpreted when meningitis is caused by *H. influenzae*, *N. meningitidis*, or *L. monocytogenes* because Gram-negative diplococci and coccobacilli may be difficult to visualize. In addition, bacteria tend to be pleomorphic in CSF and may assume atypical forms. Compared with patients with acute meningitis caused by other bacterial pathogens, patients with *Listeria* infection have a significantly lower incidence of meningeal signs, and the CSF profile is significantly less likely to have a high white blood cell count or a high protein

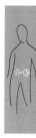

Table 96–2	**Meningitis and Meningoencephalitis in the Immunocompromised Patient**
Abnormality	**Infectious Agent**
Complement deficiencies (C6–C8)	*Neisseria meningitides*
Splenectomy and/or antibody defect	*Streptococcus pneumoniae* *Haemophilus influenzae* Enterovirus *Neisseria meningitidis*
Sickle cell disease	*S. pneumoniae* *H. influenzae*
Impaired cellular immunity (e.g., HIV infection, chemotherapy, and organ transplantation)	*Listeria monocytogenes* *Cryptococcus neoformans* *Toxoplasma gondii* *Histoplasma capsulatum* *Coccidioides immitis* *Mycobacterium tuberculosis* *Treponema pallidum* JC virus Cytomegalovirus

concentration. Gram stain is negative in two thirds of patients with listerial meningitis or meningoencephalitis. If interpretation of the Gram-stained CSF is not clear, then broad-spectrum antibiotics should be instituted while results of cultures are pending. If the initial Gram-stained preparation does not contain organisms, then examining the Gram-stained sediment prepared by concentrating up to 5 mL of CSF with a cytocentrifuge may reveal the causative organism.

Cultures of CSF, blood, fluid expressed from purpuric lesions, and nasopharyngeal swabs have a high yield. The latter is particularly valuable in patients who have received antibiotic therapy before hospitalization because most antibiotics do not achieve substantial levels in nasopharyngeal secretions to eradicate the colonization state.

Recognition of meningitis may be difficult after head trauma or neurosurgery because the symptoms, signs, and laboratory findings of infection can be difficult to separate from those of trauma. A low level of CSF glucose usually indicates infection but can also be seen after subarachnoid hemorrhage. The causative organism, characteristically an enteric Gram-negative bacillus (including *Pseudomonas aeruginosa*), may already have been cultured from an extraneural site such as a wound or urine. The known antibiotic sensitivities of such isolates therefore may provide a valuable guide to the initial treatment of meningitis in patients after neurosurgery.

All patients with meningitis caused by unusual agents or mixed infections and certain patients with meningitis caused by *S. pneumoniae* and *H. influenzae* should undergo radiography of nasal sinuses and mastoids to exclude a parameningeal focus of infection.

Differential Diagnosis

Classic acute bacterial meningitis resembles few other diseases. Ruptured brain abscess should be considered, particularly if the CSF white blood cell count is unusually high and focal neurologic signs are present. Parameningeal infections usually cause fever, headache, and local neurologic signs. CSF characteristically shows modest neutrophilic pleocytosis and moderately increased protein, but the CSF glucose level is usually normal. The CSF may be sterile in patients with bacterial meningitis who have already received antibiotics, but neutrophils commonly are present in CSF and the glucose level is depressed. Early in the evolution of viral or tuberculous meningitis, the pleocytosis may be predominantly neutrophilic. Serial CSF examinations, however, will show a progressive shift to mononuclear cell predominance. Similarly, acute viral meningoencephalitis may be difficult to distinguish clinically from bacterial meningitis; the evolution of CSF findings and the clinical course usually decide the matter.

Treatment and Outcome

Bacterial meningitis requires prompt administration of appropriate antibiotics. If the Gram-stained smear of CSF indicates pneumococcal or meningococcal disease, then penicillin G or a third-generation cephalosporin (e.g., ceftriaxone, 2 g every 12 hours) should be administered intravenously. Because the frequency of intermediate and highly penicillin-resistant *S. pneumoniae* has increased significantly, additional therapy with vancomycin is recommended until

the results of sensitivity testing are available. Alternative drugs for patients with severe penicillin allergy are vancomycin and/or imipenem. Patients with suggested *H. influenzae* meningitis should be treated with ceftriaxone (2 g given intravenously every 12 hours). In a patient with probable community-acquired meningitis, if the Gram-stained preparation of CSF is negative but clinical and laboratory findings suggest bacterial meningitis, then penicillin (or ampicillin) and ceftriaxone therapy should be started. Third-generation cephalosporins are the indicated choice for treating sensitive Gram-negative enteric organisms causing meningitis. Agents such as ceftazidime (2 g given intravenously every 6 to 8 hours) may be effective against *P. aeruginosa*. If the organism is resistant to cephalosporins, then the patient should be treated with meropenem. Regardless of the results of sensitivity testing, chloramphenicol is not an adequate drug for the treatment of Gram-negative bacillary meningitis; its use has been associated with unacceptably high mortality rates. The functional outcome and mortality for adults with acute pneumococcal meningitis are significantly improved by early adjuvant treatment with dexamethasone (10 mg administered with the first dose of antibiotic and repeated at 6 hourly intervals for 4 days).

The management of bacterial meningitis extends beyond the patient. Contacts also must be protected because they are at substantial risk of developing meningococcal meningitis or serious *H. influenzae* disease. At the time when bacterial meningitis is first suggested, respiratory isolation procedures should be initiated. Antibiotic prophylaxis of contacts should begin when the clinical course or Gram-stained preparation of CSF suggests meningococcal or *H. influenzae* meningitis. The recommended drug for household and other intimate contacts of patients with meningococcal meningitis is rifampin, 10 mg/kg (up to 600 mg) twice daily for 2 days. The goal of prophylaxis of contacts of *H. influenzae* type B meningitis is to protect children younger than 4 years of age. Because the organism may be passed from patient to asymptomatic adults to an at-risk child, rifampin, 20 mg/kg (up to 600 mg) daily for 4 days, should be given to all members of the household and day care center of the index case who have contact with children younger than 4 years old. Alternatives to rifampin include intramuscular ceftriaxone or oral ciprofloxacin. Despite parenteral antibiotic therapy, patients with *N. meningitidis* or *H. influenzae* meningitis may have persistent nasopharyngeal carriage and should also receive rifampin treatment before discharge from the hospital. Because *L. monocytogenes* is resistant to cephalosporins, ampicillin for a minimum of 15 to 21 days (with an aminoglycoside for the first 7 days) is the treatment of choice for *Listeria* meningitis.

Although hospital contacts of patients with meningococcal meningitis are at low risk of acquiring the carrier state and disease, secondary cases occasionally occur. Thus, personnel in close contact with the patient's respiratory secretions should receive prophylactic antibiotics. All persons receiving rifampin prophylaxis should be warned that their urine and tears will turn orange and that the antiestrogen effects of the drug will temporarily inactivate oral contraceptives.

Approximately 30% of adults with bacterial meningitis die of the infection. In survivors, deafness (6% to 10%) and other serious neurologic sequelae (1% to 18%) are common.

Table 96–3	**Three Rs of Central Nervous System Infection**	
R	**Deterioration**	**Possibilities**
Recrudescence	During therapy, same bacteria	Wrong therapy
Relapse	3–14 days after stopping treatment, same bacteria	Parameningeal focus
Recurrence	Delayed, same, or other bacteria	Congenital or acquired dural defects

The prognosis in individual cases depends largely on the level of consciousness and extent of CNS damage at the time of the first treatment. Misdiagnosis (50% of patients) and delays in starting antibiotics are factors in morbidity that physicians must try to avoid. Patients with suggested bacterial meningitis should be treated with antibiotics within 30 minutes of reaching medical care. Even after antibiotic therapy and presumed cure, bacterial meningitis may recur. The pattern of recurrence usually suggests a parameningeal infection or dural defect (Table 96–3).

Because more effective protein conjugated vaccines are now available for some strains of *N. meningitidis, S. pneumoniae,* and *H. influenzae* type B, vaccination of susceptible individuals can prevent the most common types of bacterial meningitis.

ASEPTIC MENINGITIS

Leptomeningitis associated with Gram-negative stains of CSF and negative cultures for bacteria has been designated aseptic meningitis, a somewhat unfortunate designation that often implies a benign illness that resolves spontaneously. However, assuming a high level of vigilance with this group of patients is important because they may have a potentially treatable but progressive illness.

Epidemiologic Features

Viral infections are the most frequent cause of aseptic meningitis (Table 96–4). Of those cases in which a specific causal agent can be established, 97% are due to enteroviruses (particularly coxsackievirus B, echovirus, mumps virus, and lymphocytic choriomeningitis virus), herpes simplex virus (HSV), and *Leptospira.* Viral meningitis is most often a disease of children and young adults (70% of patients are younger than 20 years of age). Seasonal variation reflects the predominance of enteroviral infection; most cases occur in summer or early fall. Mumps usually occurs in winter, and lymphocytic choriomeningitis usually occurs in fall or winter.

Pathogenesis and Pathophysiologic Features

Localization to the meninges occurs during systemic viremia. The basis for the meningotropism of viruses that cause aseptic meningitis is not understood. HSV type 2 may cause meningitis during the course of primary genital herpes.

Table 96–4	**Viral Etiologic Features of Encephalitis and Meningoencephalitis**
	Herpes simplex virus
	Epstein-Barr virus
	Varicella-zoster virus
	Cytomegalovirus
	Mumps
	Measles
	La Crosse virus
	West Nile virus
	St. Louis encephalitis virus
	Eastern equine encephalitis virus
	Coxsackievirus
	Echovirus
	Rabies
	Human immunodeficiency virus

Clinical Presentation

The syndrome of aseptic meningitis of viral origin begins with the acute onset of headache, fever, photophobia, and meningismus associated with CSF pleocytosis. The headache is often described as the worst ever experienced and is exacerbated by sitting, standing, or coughing. In typical cases, the course is benign. The development of changes in sensorium, seizures, or focal neurologic signs shifts the diagnosis to encephalitis or meningoencephalitis. Additional clinical features may suggest a particular infectious agent. Patients with mumps may have parotitis or orchitis and usually give a history of appropriate contact. Lymphocytic choriomeningitis often follows exposure to mice, guinea pigs, or hamsters and causes severe myalgias; an infectious mononucleosis-like illness can ensue, with rash and orchitis. Leptospirosis often follows exposure to rats or mice or swimming in water contaminated by their urine; aseptic meningitis occurs in the second phase of the illness. Aseptic meningitis can also be seen in persons with HIV infection, either as a manifestation of the primary infection or as a later complication. The pleocytosis generally is modest, the protein level is only slightly

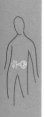

Table 96–5	**Subacute to Chronic Meningitis**
Causative Agent	**Association**
Human immunodeficiency virus	Direct involvement or opportunistic infection
Mycobacterium tuberculosis	May have extraneural tuberculosis
Cryptococcus neoformans	Compromised host
Coccidioides immitis	Southwestern United States
Histoplasma capsulatum	Ohio and Mississippi River valleys
Treponema pallidum	Acute syphilitic meningitis, secondary meningovascular syphilis
Lyme disease	Tick bite, rash, seasonal occurrence

elevated, and the glucose concentration is normal or slightly depressed. HIV serologic findings may be negative during acute HIV infection, but the diagnosis is readily established by detectable plasma HIV RNA (see Chapter 107).

Laboratory Diagnosis

In viral meningitis, the CSF shows a pleocytosis of 10 to 2000 white blood cells/mcL (see Table 96–1). Two thirds of patients have mainly neutrophils in the initial CSF specimen. However, serial lumbar punctures reveal a rapid shift (within 6 to 8 hours) in the CSF differential count toward mononuclear cell predominance. CSF protein is normal in one third of patients and almost always is less than 100 mg/dL. The level of CSF glucose is characteristically normal, although minimal depression occurs in mumps (30% of cases), in lymphocytic choriomeningitis (60%), and, less frequently, in echovirus and HSV meningitis. Serial lumbar punctures show a 95% reduction in cell count by 2 weeks. Stool cultures have the highest yield for enterovirus isolation (40% to 50%), whereas CSF and throat cultures are positive in approximately 15% of patients. Serologic studies also may indicate a specific causative agent; a fourfold rise in antibody titer is helpful in confirming the significance of a virus isolated from the throat or stool. Serologic studies are seldom useful in acute diagnosis, but PCR-based testing detects enteroviral RNA in CSF of approximately 70% of persons with aseptic meningitis.

Differential Diagnosis

Partially treated bacterial meningitis and a parameningeal focus of infection may be particularly difficult to distinguish from aseptic meningitis. Serial lumbar punctures may be helpful in establishing the former, and radiographs of the paranasal sinuses, mastoids, and spine may help confirm the latter. In addition, the differential diagnosis includes infectious agents that are not cultured on routine bacterial media and are considered to be causes of subacute meningitis (see the following discussion). Infective endocarditis may cause aseptic meningitis and is an important diagnostic consideration in the appropriate setting (see Chapter 99).

Treatment and Course

Viral meningitis is generally benign and self limited. HSV meningitis associated with primary genital herpes occasion-ally causes sufficient symptoms to warrant treatment with acyclovir.

SUBACUTE AND CHRONIC MENINGITIS

Certain infectious and noninfectious diseases can develop as subacute or chronic meningitis. Chronic meningitis refers to a clinical syndrome that develops over a course of several weeks, clinically takes the form of meningitis or meningoencephalitis, and is associated with a predominantly mononuclear pleocytosis in the CSF. The infectious causes of this syndrome may develop as a subacute to chronic meningitis (Table 96–5).

At the outset, considering the possible role of HIV as directly causing this syndrome or predisposing the patient to specific opportunistic infections such as cryptococcosis or toxoplasmosis is important; these may develop as subacute meningitis, although the latter most often develops as a mass lesion. However, the incidence of HIV-associated CNS cryptococcal and toxoplasmic infection has diminished greatly in the era of highly active antiretroviral therapy (HAART) (see Chapter 107).

Tuberculous meningitis results from the rupture of a parameningeal focus into the subarachnoid space. The presentation is generally one of subacute meningitis, with a neurologic syndrome being present for less than 2 weeks in over one half of the patients. Headache, fever, meningismus, and altered mental status are characteristic, with papilledema, cranial nerve palsies (II, III, IV, VI, or VII), and extensor plantar reflexes each occurring in about one fourth of patients. The initial CSF sample may show predominance of neutrophils, but the differential shifts to mononuclear cells within the next 7 to 10 days. Acid-fast bacilli are identified in the CSF sediment of 15% to 25% of patients. Because delayed treatment is associated with increased mortality, therapy is initiated before confirmation of the diagnosis by culture in most patients. More rapid diagnosis can be established by CSF PCR in the majority of patients. The clinical suggestion of tuberculous meningitis is heightened by a history of remote tuberculosis in one half of patients. Because concurrent pulmonary disease occurs in approximately one third of patients, smears or cultures of pulmonary secretions may support the diagnosis. Appropriate therapy consists of isoniazid, rifampin, ethambutol, and pyrazinamide. *Vasculitis* related to entrapment of cerebral vessels in inflammatory exudate may lead to stroke syndromes. This rationale has been used for the use of corticosteroids as adjunctive therapy. Although strong evidence of improved outcome is not available, many authorities believe that corticosteroids should be given in tapering doses for 4 weeks when the diagnosis of tuberculosis is established, particularly if cranial palsies appear or stupor or coma supervenes.

Cryptococcal meningitis is the most common fungal meningitis and can occur in apparently normal, as well as immunocompromised, patients. The presentation is of insidious onset, followed by weeks to months of progressive meningoencephalitis, sometimes clinically indistinguishable from the course of tuberculous meningitis. Certain associations are useful in this differential diagnosis. The presence of immunosuppression suggests cryptococcosis, whereas chronic debilitating disease, miliary infiltrates on chest radiograph, or the syndrome of inappropriate secretion of antidiuretic hormone suggests tuberculosis. An India ink preparation of CSF reveals encapsulated yeast in 50% of patients with cryptococcal meningitis. More than 90% of patients have cryptococcal polysaccharide antigen in CSF or serum. Fungal cultures of urine, stool, sputum, and blood should be obtained; they may be positive in the absence of clinically apparent extraneural disease. Initial treatment of cryptococcal meningitis requires amphotericin B. Addition of flucytosine allows use of less amphotericin B. Fluconazole is also effective but causes less rapid sterilization of the CSF. Daily fluconazole is effective for maintenance therapy to prevent relapses in persons with acquired immunodeficiency syndrome (AIDS) and should continue until CD4 counts rise to over 200 cells/mcL after initiation of HAART.

Coccidioides immitis is a major cause of granulomatous meningitis in semi-arid areas of the southwestern United States; *Histoplasma capsulatum* may cause a similar syndrome in endemic areas (Ohio and Mississippi River valleys) (see Chapter 107).

Neurosyphilis reflects the fact that the spirochete causing syphilis (*T. pallidum*) invades the CNS in most instances of systemic infection. The organism then may either be cleared by host defenses or persist to produce a more chronic infection expressed symptomatically only years later. The most common form of neurosyphilis is asymptomatic; patients harbor a few white cells in the CSF and have a positive serologic test for syphilis. Symptomatic neurosyphilis can appear as acute or subacute meningitis (meningitic form), resembling those of other bacterial infections and usually occurring during the stage of secondary syphilis when cutaneous findings are documented as well. Hydrocephalus and cranial nerve (VII and VIII) abnormalities may develop. CSF and serum serologic studies are usually strongly positive, and the disease is responsive to penicillin.

Vascular syphilis begins 2 to 10 years after the primary lesion. The disorder is characterized by both meningeal inflammation and a vasculitis of small arterial vessels, the latter leading to arterial occlusion. Clinically, the disorder produces few signs of meningitis but results in monofocal or multifocal cerebral or spinal infarction. The disorder may be mistaken for an autoimmune vasculitis or even arteriosclerotic cerebrovascular disease (stroke syndrome). The early and prominent spinal cord signs should lead the physician

to expect syphilis, and the findings in the CSF of pleocytosis, elevated gamma globulin, and a positive serologic test for syphilis establish the diagnosis. Patients respond to antibiotic therapy, although recovery from focal abnormalities may be incomplete. Syphilis is more difficult to diagnose and may have an accelerated course in the HIV-infected individual. Meningovascular syphilis may develop within months of primary infection, despite treatment with intramuscular benzathine penicillin (see Chapter 106).

General paresis, once a common cause of admission to mental institutions, is now rare. The disorder results from syphilitic invasion of the parenchyma of the brain and begins clinically 10 to 20 years after the primary infection. Paresis is characterized by progressive dementia, sometimes with manic symptoms and megalomania and often with coarse tremors affecting facial muscles and tongue. The diagnostic clue is the presence of Argyll Robertson pupils. The CSF is always abnormal. The diagnosis is made by serologic tests. Early treatment with antibiotics usually leads to improvement but not complete recovery.

Tabes dorsalis is a chronic infective process of the dorsal nerve roots that appears 10 to 20 years after primary syphilitic infection. Lightning-like pains and a progressive sensory neuropathy affecting predominantly large fibers supplying the lower extremities characterize the disorder. A profound loss of vibration and position sense, as well as areflexia, occurs. Autonomic fibers are also affected, causing postural hypotension, trophic ulcers of the feet, traumatic arthropathy of the joints, and Argyll Robertson pupils. CSF serologic tests are usually positive. The disorder responds only partially to treatment with antibiotics.

Rare complications of syphilis include progressive optic atrophy, gumma (a mass lesion in the brain), congenital neurosyphilis, and syphilitic infection of the auditory and vestibular system.

Lyme disease, a tick-borne spirochetosis (see Chapter 94), is associated in 15% of clinically affected individuals with meningitis, encephalitis, or cranial or radicular neuropathies. Characteristically, the neurologic disease begins several weeks after the typical rash of erythema chronicum migrans. Furthermore, the rash may have been so mild as to go unnoticed and usually has faded by the time neurologic manifestations appear. The diagnosis should be suggested when a patient develops subacute or chronic meningitis during late summer or early fall with CSF changes consisting of a modest mononuclear pleocytosis, protein values below 100 mg/dL, and normal levels of glucose. The diagnosis is established serologically or by PCR analysis of CSF, which provides a sensitive approach to the diagnosis of CNS Lyme disease. Patients with early Lyme disease usually respond to oral doxycycline. Patients with late or disseminated Lyme disease respond less predictably to prolonged (14 to 21 days) courses of intravenous ceftriaxone.

Several noninfectious diseases may develop as subacute or chronic meningitis. Typical of this group is a CSF containing 10 to 100 lymphocytes, elevated protein levels, and a mild-to-severely lower glucose level. Meningeal carcinomatosis represents diffuse involvement of the leptomeninges by metastatic adenocarcinoma, lymphoma, or melanoma. Cytologic analysis often identifies malignant cells. Sarcoidosis may cause basilar meningitis and asymmetric cranial nerve involvement, as well as a low-grade pleocytosis, sometimes associated with borderline low levels of CSF glucose. Granulomatous angiitis and Behçet's disease also belong in this category.

Approach to Diagnosis

Diagnosing the specific cause of subacute or chronic meningitis may be quite difficult. In patients with tuberculous or fungal meningitis, cultures may not become positive for 4 to 6 weeks or longer; moreover, meningitis caused by some fungi (e.g., *H. capsulatum*) is often associated with negative cultures of the CSF.

Because of the uncertainties involved in establishing the diagnosis of infectious diseases and even the question of whether a particular patient has an infectious or noninfectious disease, an organized approach must be taken. Routine laboratory tests (on multiple samples of CSF) should include an India ink preparation and cultures for bacteria, mycobacteria, and fungi. In addition, the patient with chronic meningitis of unknown cause should have the following: Venereal Disease Research Laboratories (VDRL) testing, cryptococcal antigens determined on blood and CSF samples; fluorescent treponemal antibody–absorbed (FTA-abs) and antinuclear antibody (and, when epidemiologically appropriate, antibody to *Borrelia burgdorferi*) on blood samples; *Histoplasma* antigen on urine and CSF samples; antibody to HIV and *H. capsulatum* on serum samples (and, when appropriate, *C. immitis*); and cytologic studies (three times) on CSF samples. A tuberculin skin test (intermediate strength, 5 TU) should be performed. Diagnosis by PCR of specific pathogens in CSF can expedite evaluation of patients with chronic meningitis when available.

The appropriate management is decided by the patient's clinical status and the results of these tests. If the CSF pleocytosis consists of more than 50 to 100 cells/mcL, then an infectious disease is likely. Empiric therapy for tuberculous meningitis is now seldom appropriate, since availability of PCR testing of CSF for mycobacterial, cryptococcal, and histoplasma antigens has minimized the need for empiric treatment. Repeated cytologic and microbiologic studies of the CSF may reveal the diagnosis. If the pleocytosis is low grade (less than 50 cells/mcL), then a noninfectious cause is more likely; the condition may even be self limited, the so-called chronic benign lymphocytic meningitis. The approach to treating such patients must be individualized. Only rarely is brain or meningeal biopsy necessary or helpful. If all CSF studies are nondiagnostic and the patient's clinical condition is stable, then a period of careful observation is almost always preferable to an invasive diagnostic procedure.

Encephalitis

Acute viral and other infectious causes of encephalitis usually produce fever, headache, stiff neck, confusion, alterations in consciousness, focal neurologic signs, and seizures.

EPIDEMIOLOGIC FEATURES

A large number of viral and nonviral agents can cause encephalitis (see Table 96–5). Seasonal occurrence may help limit the differential diagnosis. Arthropod-borne viruses peak in the summer (West Nile virus [WNV]), California encephalitis [La Crosse virus], and western equine encephalitis peak in August; St. Louis encephalitis slightly later). The tick-borne infections (RMSF) occur in early summer, enterovirus infections in late summer and fall, and mumps in the winter and spring. Geographic distribution is also helpful. Eastern equine encephalitis is confined to the coastal states. Serologic surveys indicate that infections by encephalitis viruses are most often subclinical. The reason so few among the many infected patients develop encephalitis is not clear.

HSV is the most frequent, treatable, and devastating cause of sporadic, severe focal encephalitis. Overall, it is implicated in 10% of all patients with encephalitis in North America. No age, sex, seasonal, or geographic preference exists.

PATHOGENESIS

Viruses reach the CNS by the bloodstream or peripheral nerves. HSV presumably reaches the brain by cell-to-cell spread along recurrent branches of the trigeminal nerve, which innervate the meninges of the anterior and middle fossae. Although this would explain the characteristic localization of necrotic lesions to the inferomedial portions of the temporal and frontal lobes, the reason why such spread is so rare is not clear, with one case of HSV encephalitis occurring per one million in the population per annum.

CLINICAL FEATURES

The course of HSV encephalitis is considered in this text in detail because of the importance of establishing the diagnosis of this treatable entity. Patients affected by HSV commonly describe a prodrome of 1 to 7 days of upper respiratory tract symptoms followed by the sudden onset of headache and fever. The headache and fever may be associated with acute loss of recent memory, behavioral abnormalities, delirium, difficulty with speech, and seizures (often focal). Disorders of the sensorium are not, however, always apparent at the time of presentation and are not essential for the working diagnosis of this eminently treatable but potentially lethal infection of the CNS.

LABORATORY DIAGNOSIS

In HSV encephalitis, the CSF can contain 0 to 1000 white blood cells/mcL, predominantly lymphocytes. Protein is moderately high (median 80 mg/dL). CSF glucose is reduced in only 5% of individuals within 3 days of onset but becomes abnormal in additional patients later in the course of the disease. The CSF is normal in approximately 5% of patients. Other laboratory findings at onset are of little help, although focal abnormalities may be present in the electroencephalogram and develop in CT or magnetic resonance imaging brain scan by the third day in most patients. Acyclovir offers such high likelihood of therapeutic benefit in HSV encephalitis with so little risk in this highly fatal and neurologically damaging disease that brain biopsy should not be performed unless an alternative, treatable diagnosis seems very likely. A low level of CSF glucose should increase the suggestion that a granulomatous infection (e.g., tuberculosis, cryptococcosis) is present. If the initial CSF shows a low glucose level, then roughly one third of individuals will have an alternatively treatable infection. If CSF studies and brain imaging remain inconclusive in such circumstances, then biopsy may be appropriate.

Viral cultures of stool, throat, buffy coat, CSF, and brain biopsy specimens, as well as indirect immunofluorescence or immunoperoxidase staining of tissues, may provide a specific diagnosis. However, viral isolation and serologic evidence of a rise in antibody titer usually come too late to guide initial treatment. In the case of HSV encephalitis, serologic studies are particularly helpful in 30% of individuals with a primary infection. In addition, CSF titers of antibody to HSV, which reflect intrathecal production of antibody, may show a diagnostic fourfold rise. CSF HSV DNA detection by PCR is highly sensitive and specific in HSV encephalitis. Additional PCR-based diagnostic tests are available for other viruses and should be considered in the appropriate clinical and epidemiologic settings.

DIFFERENTIAL DIAGNOSIS

Acute (demyelinating) encephalomyelitis, infective endocarditis producing brain embolization, meningoencephalitis caused by *C. neoformans, M. tuberculosis,* or the La Crosse virus, acute bacterial abscess, acute thrombotic thrombocytopenic purpura, cerebral venous thrombosis, vascular disease, and primary and metastatic tumors may all initially simulate HSV encephalitis.

TREATMENT AND OUTCOME

The course of viral encephalitis depends on the etiologic agent. Untreated HSV encephalitis has a high mortality rate (70%), and survival is associated with severe neurologic residua. Acyclovir therapy improves survival and greatly lessens morbidity in patients if initiated early, before deterioration to coma. Prognosis is particularly favorable in young patients (younger than 30 years old) with a preserved mental status at the time of presentation.

West Nile Virus

WNV was first identified in 1937 and recognized as a CNS pathogen as early as 1957 during an outbreak in Israel. Infections in the United States were heralded by an outbreak that occurred in New York City in 1999. WNV infection represents an emerging mosquito-borne infectious disease in the United States. Since the outbreak of WNV meningoencephalitis in New York City, WNV has spread to most states. Similar to most cases of viral meningitis and encephalitis, WNV occurs primarily during the summer months. Culicine mosquitoes that have bitten infected birds (primarily crows and blue jays) transmit the disease. Although direct human-to-human transmission does not occur, WNV can be transmitted through blood products and organs donated from asymptomatic donors. Additional infections in children have resulted from transplacental transmission and through breast-feeding. Although most infections are asymptomatic, symptomatic patients often exhibit (within 3 to 15 days) a range of nonspecific signs and symptoms that include fever, headache, and myalgia, and in some patients acute flaccid paralysis. Seizures have been observed in less than one third of patients. A roseolar or maculopapular rash involving the face and trunk are seen in nearly 50% of patients. CSF fluid examination typically reveals a lymphocytic pleocytosis (3 to 100 cells/mcL, mild protein elevation, and a normal glucose level. Fatal cases of meningoencephalitis have been primarily limited to patients older than 65 years of age in whom autopsy studies reveal neuronal cell death and severe cerebral edema. The diagnosis is made based on clinical grounds and identification of WNV-specific IgM or RNA. Approximately 90% of patients will have positive WNV-specific IgM within 7 to 9 days of infection, whereas detection of viral RNA is more difficult because symptoms usually begin as the viremia wanes.

Recovery is the rule, though chronic fatigue, weakness, memory loss, and depression may follow WNV infections. Specific antiviral therapy is not available, and management is supportive. Both personal protective measures (e.g., insect repellents) and environmental control measures are important in controlling exposure to mosquitoes and limiting outbreaks and disease transmission.

Rabies

Rabies encephalitis is always fatal, requiring major attention on prevention. Currently, zero to six cases of rabies occur each year in the United States, and approximately 20,000 people receive postexposure prophylaxis.

The incubation period for rabies is generally 20 to 90 days, during which the rabies virus replicates locally and then migrates along nerves to the spinal cord and brain. Rabies begins with fever, headache, fatigue, and pain or paresthesias at the site of inoculation; confusion, seizures, paralysis, and stiff neck follow. Periods of violent agitation are characteristic of rabies encephalitis. Attempts at drinking produce laryngospasm, gagging, and apprehension. Paralysis, coma, and death supervene. When rabies is suggested, protective isolation procedures should be instituted to minimize additional exposure of the hospital staff to saliva and other infected secretions. Detecting rabies-neutralizing antibody or isolating the virus from saliva, CSF, and urine sediment confirm the diagnosis. Immunofluorescent rabies antibody staining of a skin biopsy specimen taken from the posterior neck is a rapid means of establishing the diagnosis.

Indications for prophylaxis are based on two central principles. First, the patient must have been exposed. Nonbite exposure is possible if mucous membranes or open wounds are contaminated with animal saliva; exposure to bat urine in heavily contaminated caves has been followed by rabies. Second, small rodents (rats, mice, chipmunks, and squirrels) and rabbits rarely are infected and have not been associated with human disease. Consultation with local or state health authorities is essential because certain areas of the United States are considered rabies free. In other areas, if rabies is present in wild animals, then dogs and cats have the potential to transmit rabies. Domestic dogs and cats should be quarantined for 10 days after biting someone; if they develop no signs of the illness, then no risk of transmission by their earlier bite is possible. Nondomestic animals should be destroyed and their brains examined for rabies virus by direct fluorescent antibody testing. Bites by bats, skunks, and raccoons always require treatment if the animal is not caught. Unusual behavior of animals and truly unprovoked attacks can be signs of rabies.

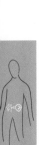

Currently, postexposure management consists of (1) thorough wound cleansing; (2) human rabies immune globulin, 20 IU/kg, one half infiltrated locally in the area of the bite and one half intramuscularly; and (3) human diploid cell rabies vaccine, 1.0 mL given intramuscularly five times during a 1-month period. Individuals at high risk of exposure (e.g., veterinarians, spelunkers) should be vaccinated.

Spectrum of Tuberculous, Fungal, and Parasitic Infections

The spectrum of tuberculous, fungal, and parasitic infections of the CNS is briefly considered. Many, but not all, of these infections are increasing in incidence as the direct result of the increasing prevalence of HIV infection in the population (see Chapter 107).

TUBERCULOSIS

CNS tuberculosis can occur in several forms, sometimes without evidence of active infection elsewhere in the body. The most common form is *tuberculous meningitis*. This disorder is characterized by the subacute onset of headache, stiff neck, and fever. After a few days, affected patients become confused and disoriented. They often develop abnormalities of cranial nerve function, particularly hearing loss as a result of significant inflammation at the base of the brain. Most patients, if left untreated, lapse into coma and die within 3 to 4 weeks of onset. An accompanying arteritis may produce focal signs, including hemiplegia, during the course of the disorder. Tuberculous meningitis must be distinguished from other causes of acute and subacute meningeal infection, a process that is often not easy even after examination of the CSF. The pressure and cell counts are elevated with up to a few hundred cells, a mixture of leukocytes and lymphocytes. The protein level is elevated, usually above 100 mg/dL and often to very high levels, and the glucose concentration is depressed. Smears for acid-fast bacilli are positive in only 15% to 25% of CSF samples. Tuberculosis organisms grow on culture but only after several weeks. Thus, patients with subacutely developing meningitis consistent with tuberculosis should be treated with antituberculous agents before definitive diagnosis, if rapid PCR identification of mycobacterial antigens in CSF is not available. Large samples of CSF should be sent for culture, and a careful search should be made for tuberculosis elsewhere in the body.

Tuberculomas of the brain produce symptoms and signs either of the mass lesion or of meningitis with the tuberculomas being found incidentally. One or multiple lesions are identified on a CT scan, but the scan itself does not distinguish tuberculomas from brain tumor or other brain abscesses. Without evidence of meningeal or systemic tuberculosis, biopsy is necessary for diagnosis. Patients with tuberculomas usually respond well to antituberculous therapy, but brain lesions may remain visible on the CT scan long after the patient has improved clinically; the clinical course, not the scan, predicts the outcome.

Less common manifestations of CNS tuberculosis include chronic arachnoiditis, characterized by a low-grade inflammatory response in the CSF and progressive pain with signs of either cauda equina or spinal cord dysfunction. The diagnosis of arachnoiditis is suggested by a myelogram showing evidence of fibrosis and compartmentalization instead of the usually smooth subarachnoid lining. The disorder responds poorly to treatment. Tuberculous myelopathy probably results from direct invasion of the organism from the subarachnoid space. Patients exhibit a subacutely developing myelopathy, characterized by sensory loss in either the legs or all four extremities, depending on the site of the spinal cord invasion. Many patients have additional signs of meningitis, including fever, headache, and stiff neck. The CSF usually contains cells and tuberculous organisms. The myelogram may show evidence of arachnoiditis and frequently demonstrates an enlarged spinal cord or complete block to the passage of contrast material in the thoracic or cervical region.

FUNGAL AND PARASITIC INFECTIONS

Fungal and parasitic infections of the CNS are less common than viral and bacterial infections and often affect patients who are immunosuppressed. Similar to bacterial infections, fungal and parasitic infections may cause either meningitis or parenchymal abscesses. These meningitides exhibit clinical symptoms that, although similar, are usually less severe and abrupt than those of acute bacterial meningitis. The common fungal causes of meningitis include cryptococcosis, coccidioidomycosis, and histoplasmosis. Cryptococcal meningitis is a sporadic infection that affects both patients who are immunosuppressed (>50%) and those who are nonimmunosuppressed. Headache and sometimes fever and stiff neck characterize the disorder. The clinical symptoms may evolve for periods as long as weeks or months; diagnosis can be made only by identifying the organism or its antigen in the CSF. *Histoplasma* and coccidioidomycosis meningitides occur in endemic areas and often affect individuals who are nonimmunosuppressed. The diagnosis is suggested by a history of residence in appropriate geographic areas and is confirmed by CSF and serologic evaluation. Antifungal treatment, particularly in the nonimmunosuppressed patient, is usually effective.

Parasitic infections of the nervous system usually produce focal abscesses rather than diffuse meningitis. The most common infection to affect the patient who is nonimmunosuppressed is cysticercosis, a disorder caused by the larval form of the *Taenia solium* tapeworm and contracted by ingesting food or water contaminated with parasite eggs. The disorder is common in many resource-restricted regions, as well as in Southern California. The brain may be invaded in as many as 60% of infected persons. Invasion of the brain leads to the formation of either single or multiple cysts, which often lie in the parenchyma but sometimes reside in the ventricles or subarachnoid space. Seizures and increased intracranial pressure are the most common clinical symptoms. A CT scan identifies small intracranial calcifications and hypodense cysts (Fig. 96–1). Serum indirect hemagglutination tests are usually positive and confirm the diagnosis. Where cysts obstruct the ventricular system to cause symptoms, shunting procedures may be necessary. The anthelmintic agent praziquantel is effective therapy.

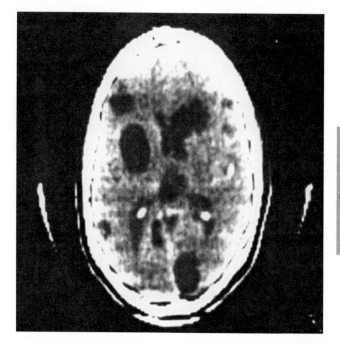

Figure 96–1 Neurocystercosis. A computed tomographic (CT) scan shows multiple confluent cysts.

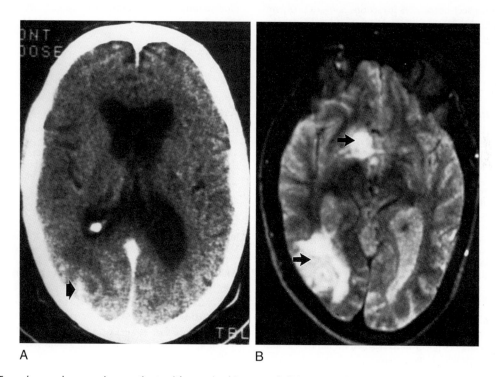

A   B

Figure 96–2 *Toxoplasma* abscesses in a patient with acquired immunodeficiency syndrome. *A,* Computed tomography (CT) scan shows a contrast medium–enhanced mass *(arrow)*. *B,* Magnetic resonance image reveals multiple masses *(arrows)* not visualized with CT scanning, leading physicians to suggest abscesses rather than tumor.

Toxoplasmosis of the brain, when it occurs in the adult, is a manifestation of immunosuppression. Patients with abnormal cellular immunity usually develop single or multiple abscesses, which usually appear as ring-enhancing lesions on a CT scan (Fig. 96–2). The management of CNS toxoplasmosis is discussed in Chapter 107.

Prospectus for the Future

CNS infections (meningitis and encephalitis) may result in permanent loss of cognitive and motor neuron function. Thus, *immunization can reduce the incidence and morbidity and mortality associated with select viral and bacterial infections of the CNS.* This fact has been most evident from the near worldwide eradication of poliomyelitis. *Recent development and use of protein-conjugated vaccines against* Hemophilus influenzae *and* Neisseria meningitidis *have dramatically reduced invasive CNS infections* caused by these respiratory bacterial pathogens. Because these pathogens are transmitted through respiratory droplets and can readily spread from humans in close contact, recognition and treatment of primary infections and prophylactic *treatment of nonimmune contacts are important in controlling outbreaks.* Prevention of outbreaks will be facilitated by immunization of people at risk for developing these infections.

Prevention of insect-borne CNS infections is more problematic. *Environmental control (e.g. insecticides) and personal protective measures (e.g. N,N-diethyl-meta-toluamide [DEET]) are important measures that help reduce insect reservoirs and personal exposure.* However, transmission of WNV to organ transplant recipients and breast-feeding infants has further heightened the awareness that new, often *asymptomatic infections may be transmitted unwittingly* to others. Thus, medical personnel must maintain a high index of suspicion for new and old CNS infections.

In appropriate clinical settings, sensitive molecular diagnostic tests (e.g., PCR) have been used to diagnose infections caused by a wide array of viruses (e.g. HSV, enterovirus, rubella, rabies, measles, mumps, influenza). *Molecular techniques will continue to be developed* and will play a critical role in identifying both old and new emerging pathogens (WNV) associated with CNS infections. Rapid identification of CNS pathogens may limit collateral exposure of *high-risk patients like the older adults* who represent a large proportion of the general population.

References

Bacterial Meningitis

Behlau I, Ellner JJ: Chronic meningitis. In Mandell GL, Bennett JE, Dolin R (eds): Principles and Practice of Infectious Disease, 6th ed. Philadelphia, Elsevier, 2005, pp 1132–1143.

Biluka OO, Rosenstein N: Prevention and control of meningococcal disease. MMWR 54:1–21, 2005.

DeGans J, Van de Beek D: Dexamethasone in adults with bacterial meningitis. N Engl J Med 347:1549–1556, 2002.

Quagliarello VJ, Scheld WM: Treatment of bacterial meningitis. N Engl J Med 336:708–716, 1997.

Sampathkumar P: West Nile virus: Epidemiology, clinical presentation, diagnosis and prevention. Mayo Clin Proc 78:1137–1144, 2003.

Swartz MN: Bacterial meningitis. In Goldman L, Ausiello D (eds): Cecil Textbook of Medicine, 22nd ed. Philadelphia, WB Saunders, 2004, pp 1809–1824.

Thomas KE, Hasbun R, Jakel J, et al: The diagnostic accuracy of Kernig's sign, Briedzenski's sign, and nuchal rigidity in adults with suspected meningitis. Clin Infect Dis 35:46–52, 2002.

Tunkel AR, Scheld WM: Acute meningitis. In Mandell GL, Bennett JE, Dolin R (eds): Principles and Practice of Infectious Disease, 6th ed. Philadelphia, Elsevier, 2005, pp 1083–1126.

Aseptic Meningitis

Hayes EB, Komar N, Nasci RS, et al: Epidemiology and transmission dynamics of West Nile virus disease. Emerg Infect Dis 11:1167–1173, 2005.

Hayes, EB, Sejvar JJ, Zaki SR, et al: Virology, pathology and clinical manifestations of West Nile virus disease. Emerg Infect Dis 11:1174–1179, 2005.

Encephalitis

Johnson RT: Acute encephalitis. Clin Infect Dis 23:219–226, 1996.

Marfin AA, Gubler DJ: West Nile encephalitis: An emerging disease in the United States. Clin Infect Dis 33:1713–1719, 2001.

Whitley RJ, Gnann JW: Viral encephalitis: Familiar infections and emerging pathogens. Lancet 359:507–513, 2002.

Molecular Diagnostics

Cinque P, Bossolasco S, Lunkkvist A: Molecular analysis of cerebrospinal fluid in viral diseases of the central nervous system. J Clin Vir 26:1–28, 2003.

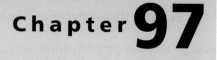
Infections of the Head and Neck

Christoph Lange

Michael M. Lederman

Infections of the Ear

Otitis externa is an infection of the external auditory canal. The process may begin as a folliculitis or pustule within the canal. Staphylococci, streptococci, and other skin flora are the most common pathogens. Some cases of otitis externa have been associated with the use of hot tubs. This infection (swimmer's ear) is usually caused by *Pseudomonas aeruginosa.*

Patients with otitis externa complain of ear pain that is often quite severe, and they may also complain of itching. Examination shows an inflamed external canal; the tympanic membrane may be uninvolved. (Patients with otitis media, in contrast, do not have involvement of the external canal unless the tympanic membrane is perforated.) Otitis externa with cellulitis can be treated with systemic antibiotics such as dicloxacillin or a macrolide and local heat. In the absence of cellulitis or perforation of the tympanic membrane, eardrops (0.3% ofloxacin solution or polymyxin B + neomycin + hydrocortisone) are sufficient. Ointments should not be used in the ear. Patients with diabetes mellitus are at risk for an invasive external otitis (malignant otitis) caused by *P. aeruginosa*. In malignant otitis externa, pain is a presenting complaint, and infection rapidly invades the bones of the skull and may result in cranial nerve palsies, invasion of the brain, and death. Computed tomography or magnetic resonance imaging of the cranial bones can establish the extent of disease. Treatment must include débridement of as much necrotic tissue as is feasible and at least 4 to 6 weeks of treatment with two different drugs active against *Pseudomonas* (a carbapenem, an extended spectrum penicillin or an antipseudomonal cephalosporin, plus ciprofloxacin or an aminoglycoside). *Otitis media* is an infection of the middle ear seen primarily among preschool children but occasionally in adults as well. Infection caused by upper respiratory tract pathogens is promoted by obstruction to drainage through edematous, congested eustachian tubes. *Streptococcus pneumoniae, Haemophilus influenzae,* and *Moraxella catarrhalis* are the most common bacterial pathogens, and viral infection caused by respiratory syncytial virus, influenza virus, enteroviruses, and rhi-

novirus may predispose the patient to acute otitis media. Fever, ear pain, diminished hearing, vertigo, or tinnitus may occur. In young children, however, localizing symptoms may not be present. The tympanic membrane may appear inflamed, but, to diagnose otitis media with certainty, either fluid must be seen behind the membrane or diminished mobility of the membrane must be demonstrated by tympanometry or after air insufflation into the external canal.

Treatment with amoxicillin-clavulanic acid, trimethoprim-sulfamethoxazole, or cefaclor is generally effective; the addition of decongestants or corticosteroids is of no proved value. Complications of otitis media are uncommon but may include infection of the mastoid air cells (mastoiditis), bacterial meningitis, brain abscess, and subdural empyema.

Infections of the Nose and Sinuses

Rhinitis is a common manifestation of numerous respiratory viral infections characterized by a mucopurulent or watery nasal discharge that may be profuse. If rhinitis is caused by respiratory viral infection, then pharyngitis, conjunctival suffusion, and fever may be present. Rhinitis can also be caused by hypersensitivity responses to airborne allergens. Patients with allergic rhinitis often have a history of atopy and often have a transverse skin crease on the bridge of the nose a few millimeters from the tip. The demonstration of eosinophils in a wet preparation of nasal secretions readily distinguishes allergic rhinitis from rhinitis of infectious origin. (Eosinophils can be identified in wet preparations by the presence of large refractile cytoplasmic granules.) Occasionally, after head trauma or neurosurgery, cerebrospinal fluid (CSF) may leak through the nose. *CSF rhinorrhea* places patients at risk for bacterial meningitis. CSF is readily distinguished from nasal secretions by its low protein and relatively high glucose concentrations.

Sinusitis is an infection of the air-filled paranasal sinuses, which are sterile under normal conditions. Allergic rhinitis and structural abnormalities of the nose that interfere with sinus drainage also predispose the patient to sinusitis. Acute bacterial sinusitis is primarily caused by upper respiratory tract bacterial pathogens *S. pneumoniae* and *H. influenzae,* by *Moraxella catarrhalis,* or less often by Gram-negative bacteria, anaerobes and staphylococci. *Staphylococcus aureus* or Gram-negative bacteria may cause nosocomial sinusitis. With chronic sinusitis, anaerobic bacteria play a more important role. Viral infections such as those caused by rhinovirus, influenza virus, parainfluenzavirus, and adenovirus have been associated with sinusitis.

Sinusitis may be difficult to distinguish from a viral upper respiratory tract illness, which, in many instances, precedes sinus infection. Patients may complain of persistent cough, headache, *stuffiness,* a *toothache,* or purulent nasal discharge. Bending over may exacerbate headache. Sinusitis is suggested in a person with a febrile upper respiratory tract illness that lasts more than 7 to 10 days. Tenderness may be present over the involved sinus, and pus may be seen in the turbinates of the nose. Failure of a sinus to light up on transillumination may suggest the diagnosis, but not all sinuses transilluminate, even in healthy states. Computed tomography is more sensitive than sinus radiographs in establishing the diagnosis of sinusitis. Most patients with bacterial sinusitis can be treated with a 10- to 14-day course of amoxicillin-clavulanate, clarithromycin, or trimethoprim-sulfamethoxazole, along with nasal decongestants. Patients who do not respond to antimicrobial therapy or who appear severely ill should undergo sinus puncture for drainage and lavage and further microbiologic evaluation. Sinusitis may be complicated by bacterial meningitis, brain abscess, or subdural empyema. Therefore, patients with sinusitis and neurologic abnormalities must be evaluated carefully for these complications, by computed tomography if a mass lesion is suspected, or by CSF examination if meningitis is suggested (see Chapter 96).

Rhinocerebral mucormycosis is an invasive infection arising from the nose or sinuses and is caused by fungi of the order *Mucorales.* This infection can result in progressive bony destruction and invasion of the brain. Rhinocerebral mucormycosis is seen primarily among persons with poorly controlled diabetes and ketoacidosis, recipients of organ transplants, and in patients with hematologic malignancy and iron overload. Black necrotic lesions of the palate or nasal mucosa are characteristic. Most patients have a depressed sensorium at presentation. Vascular thrombosis and cranial nerve palsies are common. Diagnosis is made by demonstration of the broad, ribbon-shaped, nonseptate hyphae on histologic examination of a scraping or biopsy specimen. Differential diagnosis includes infection caused by *P. aeruginosa* or by fungi such as *Aspergillus* species and cavernous sinus thrombosis. Rhinocerebral mucormycosis is a surgical emergency. Treatment involves correcting the underlying process, if possible, broad surgical débridement, and administration of amphotericin B.

Infections of the Mouth and Pharynx

STOMATITIS

Stomatitis, or inflammation of the mouth, can be caused by a wide variety of processes. Patients with stomatitis may complain of diffuse or localized pain in the mouth, difficulty in swallowing, and difficulty in managing oral secretions. Various nutritional deficiencies (vitamins B_{12} and C, folic acid, and niacin) and cytotoxic chemotherapies, as well as viral infections, can produce stomatitis.

Thrush is an infection of the oral mucosa by *Candida* species. Thrush may be seen among infants and in patients receiving broad-spectrum antibiotics or corticosteroids (systemic or inhaled), among patients with leukopenia (e.g., acute leukemia), among persons with diabetes, and among patients with impairments in cell-mediated immunity (e.g., acquired immunodeficiency syndrome). In its milder form, thrush is exhibited by an asymptomatic white, *cheesy* exudate on the buccal mucosa and pharynx that when scraped leaves a raw surface. In more severe cases, pain and erythema surrounding the exudate may be present. The diagnosis is suggested by the characteristic appearance of the lesions and may be confirmed by microscopic examination of a potassium hydroxide preparation of the exudate, which reveals yeast and the pseudohyphae characteristic of *Candida.* Thrush related to administration of antibiotics and corticosteroids should resolve after the drugs are withdrawn. Otherwise, thrush in the immunocompetent patient can usually be managed with clotrimazole troches. Thrush in the immunocompromised individual, or candidal infection involving the esophagus, should be treated with fluconazole (see Chapter 107). Rarely, when azole resistance has developed, treatment with amphotericin or an echinocandin may be required.

ORAL ULCERS AND VESICLES

Herpes Simplex Virus Infection

Although most recurrences of oral herpes simplex infections occur on or near the vermillion borders of the lips, the primary attack usually involves the mouth and pharynx (Table 97–1). Generalized symptoms of fever, headache, and malaise often precede the appearance of oral lesions by as much as 24 to 48 hours. The involved regions are swollen and erythematous. Small vesicles soon appear; these rupture, leaving shallow, discrete ulcers that may coalesce. Autoinoc-

Table 97–1	**Oral Vesicles and Ulcers**

Primary herpes simplex infection
Aphthous stomatitis
Vincent's stomatitis
Syphilis
Fungi (histoplasmosis)
Behçet's syndrome
Systemic lupus erythematosus
Reiter's syndrome
Crohn's disease
Erythema multiforme
Pemphigus
Pemphigoid

ulation may spread the infection; herpetic keratitis is one of the major infectious causes of blindness in the industrialized world. The diagnosis can be made by scraping the base of an ulcer. Wright or Giemsa stain of this material (Tzanck preparation) may reveal the intranuclear inclusions and multinucleated giant cells characteristic of herpes simplex infection. Viral cultures are more sensitive but more expensive. Diagnosis may also be established by immunoassay for viral antigen or by amplification of viral sequences in the scraping by polymerase chain reaction (PCR). Treatment of the primary infection with acyclovir or valacyclovir will decrease the duration of symptoms but has no effect on the frequency of recurrence.

Aphthous Stomatitis

Aphthae are discrete, shallow, painful ulcers on erythematous bases; they may be single or multiple and are usually present on the labial or buccal mucosa. Attacks of aphthous stomatitis may be recurrent and quite debilitating. The cause of the disease is uncertain, and many experts consider it an autoimmune disorder. Symptoms may last for several days to 2 weeks. Treatment is symptomatic with saline mouthwash or topical anesthetics. Giant aphthous ulcers may occur in persons with the acquired immunodeficiency syndrome and often respond either to systemic corticosteroids or to thalidomide (see Chapter 107).

Vincent's Stomatitis

Vincent's stomatitis is an ulcerative infection of the gingival mucosa caused by anaerobic fusobacteria and spirochetes. The patient's breath is often foul, and the ulcerations are covered with a purulent, dirty-appearing, gray exudate. Gram stain of the exudate reveals the characteristic Gram-negative fusobacteria and spirochetes. Treatment with penicillin is curative. If not treated, the infection may extend to the peritonsillar space (quinsy) and even involve vascular structures in the lateral neck (see later discussion under "Soft Tissue Space Infections").

Syphilis

Syphilis may produce a painless primary chancre in the mouth or a painful mucous patch that is a manifestation of secondary disease. The diagnosis should be considered in the sexually active patient with a large (>1 cm) oral ulceration and should be confirmed serologically, because dark-field examination may be confounded by the presence of nonsyphilitic oral spirochetes.

Fungal Disease

Occasionally, an oral ulcer or nodule may be a manifestation of disseminated histoplasmosis. These ulcers are generally minimally symptomatic and are usually overshadowed by the constitutional symptoms of disseminated fungal illness.

Systemic Illnesses Causing Ulcerative or Vesicular Lesions of the Mouth

Recurrent aphthous oral ulcerations may be part of Behçet's syndrome. Oral ulcerations have been associated with connective tissue diseases, including systemic lupus erythematosus and Reiter's syndrome, and with Crohn's disease. Although isolated oral bullae and ulcerations occur in patients with erythema multiforme, pemphigus, and pem-

phigoid, almost all such patients have an associated rash. The *iris* or *target* lesion of erythema multiforme is characteristic. Otherwise, biopsy will establish the diagnosis. Corticosteroids may be life saving for patients with pemphigus. Corticosteroids are also used in the treatment of erythema multiforme major (Stevens-Johnson syndrome), although proof of their efficacy is not available.

PHARYNGITIS AND APPROACH TO THE PATIENT WITH SORE THROAT

When evaluating a patient with a sore throat, distinguishing between the relatively common and benign sore throat syndromes (viral or streptococcal pharyngitis) and the less common but more dangerous causes of sore throat is an important first step. Patients with viral or streptococcal pharyngitis often give a history of exposure to individuals with upper respiratory tract infections. Symptoms of cough, rhinitis, and hoarseness (indicating involvement of the larynx) suggest a viral upper respiratory tract infection, although an important point to remember is that hoarseness may also be seen with more serious infections, such as epiglottitis.

Examination of the Throat

Two points regarding examination of the throat need emphasis. First, a complete examination of the oral cavity is important. Not only will a thorough examination give clues to the cause of the complaint, but it may also provide early diagnosis of an asymptomatic malignancy at a time when cure is feasible. The second point is that the normal tonsils and mucosal rim of the anterior fauces are generally a deeper red than the rest of the pharynx in healthy individuals. This appearance should not be mistaken for inflammation. Patients with pharyngitis often have a red, inflamed posterior pharynx. The tonsils are often enlarged and red and may be covered with a punctate or diffuse white exudate. Lymph nodes of the anterior neck are often enlarged.

If any of the seven *danger signs* listed in Table 97–2 is present, the clinician must anticipate an illness other than viral or streptococcal pharyngitis. Symptoms persisting longer than 1 week are rarely caused by streptococci or viruses and should prompt consideration of other processes (see later section on Persistent or Penicillin-Unresponsive

Table 97–2 **Seven Danger Signs in Patients with Sore Throat**
1. Persistence of symptoms longer than 1 wk without improvement
2. Respiratory difficulty, particularly stridor
3. Difficulty in handling secretions
4. Difficulty in swallowing
5. Severe pain in the absence of erythema
6. A palpable mass
7. Blood, even in small amounts, in the pharynx or ear

Pharyngitis). Respiratory difficulty, particularly stridor, difficulty in handling oral secretions, or difficulty in swallowing should suggest the possibility of potentially rapidly lethal epiglottitis or soft tissue space infection. Severe pain in the absence of erythema of the pharynx may be seen with some of the *extrarespiratory* causes of sore throat, as well as in cases of epiglottitis or retropharyngeal abscess. A palpable mass in the pharynx or neck suggests a soft tissue space infection, and blood in the ear or pharynx may be an early indication of a lateral pharyngeal space abscess eroding into the carotid artery.

A thorough history and careful examination will distinguish between the common and benign causes of a sore throat and the unusual but often more serious causes.

Pharyngitis

Agents that have been associated with pharyngitis in adults are presented in Table 97–3. More than one half of all cases are caused by respiratory viruses or group A streptococci. Most of the remaining cases are without defined origin. Most cases occur during the winter months. In practice, once a diagnosis of pharyngitis is established clinically, the clinician must distinguish between group A streptococcal infections, which should be treated with penicillin, and viral infections, which should be treated symptomatically (e.g., salicylates, saline gargles). Clinical criteria do not reliably predict streptococcal pharyngitis; however, the presence of fever, tonsillar exudates, no cough, and tender cervical lym-

phadenopathy increases the likelihood of streptococcal infection. In patients with at least two of these findings, a positive rapid streptococcal antigen test will confirm the diagnosis. Some cases may be missed by this test, and, for patients with three or four of these findings, clinicians may prefer to treat empirically with penicillin for 10 days.

Pharyngitis and Respiratory Virus Infections. Many patients with common colds caused by rhinovirus, coronavirus, adenovirus, or influenza virus have an associated pharyngitis. Other signs such as rhinorrhea, conjunctival suffusion, and cough suggest a cold virus; fever and myalgias suggest influenza. Symptoms generally resolve in a few days without treatment.

Infectious mononucleosis caused by Epstein-Barr virus is often associated with pharyngitis. Patients often also complain of malaise and fever. On examination, the pharynx may be inflamed and the tonsils hypertrophied and covered by a white exudate. Cervical lymph node enlargement is often prominent, and generalized lymph node enlargement and splenomegaly are common. Examination of a peripheral blood smear shows atypical lymphocytes, and the presence of heterophil antibodies (e.g., Monospot test) or a rise in antibodies to Epstein-Barr virus viral capsid antigen will confirm the diagnosis. Patients with acute Epstein-Barr virus infection should be advised to abstain from contact sports, because traumatic rupture of the enlarged spleen may be fatal.

Primary human immunodeficiency virus seroconversion illness is often exhibited by fever, pharyngitis, and lymph node enlargement and is sometimes associated with a generalized maculopapular rash. A high index of suspicion is essential, because this diagnosis is often missed in clinical practice. Diagnosis is established by demonstration of human immunodeficiency virus RNA in plasma (see Chapter 107).

Streptococcal Pharyngitis. Streptococcal pharyngitis may produce mild or severe symptoms. The pharynx is generally inflamed, and exudative tonsillitis is common but not universal. Fever may be present, and cervical lymph nodes may be enlarged and tender. Clinical distinction between streptococcal and nonstreptococcal pharyngitis is inaccurate, and patients with pharyngitis should therefore have a swab of the posterior pharynx tested for streptococcal infection. The growth of group A β-hemolytic streptococci or detection of group A streptococcal antigen is an indication for treatment with penicillin (or erythromycin if the patient is penicillin allergic). Antibiotics may shorten the duration of symptoms caused by this infection but are administered for 10 days primarily to decrease the frequency of rheumatic fever, which may follow untreated streptococcal pharyngitis.

Pharyngitis Caused by Other Bacteria. Diphtheria, caused by *Corynebacterium diphtheriae,* is a rare disease in the United States, with five or fewer cases recognized annually since 1980. The gray pseudomembrane bleeds when removed and in rare cases may cause death by means of airway obstruction. Most morbidity and mortality in diphtheria are related to the elaboration of a toxin with neurologic and cardiac effects. Treatment consists of antitoxin plus erythromycin. A self-limited pharyngitis, often associated with a diffuse scarlatiniform rash, may be caused by *Arcanobacterium* (formerly *Corynebacterium*) *haemolyticum.* This infection, when recognized, can be treated with penicillin or erythromycin.

Table 97–3	**Causes of Pharyngitis in Adults**

Viral

Human immunodeficiency virus
Respiratory viruses*
Adenovirus
Herpes simplex
Epstein-Barr virus
Cytomegalovirus

Bacterial

Group A *Streptococcus**
Group C *Streptococcus*
Mixed aerobic and/or anaerobic infections (Vincent's angina, quinsy)
Corynebacterium diphtheriae
Arcanobacterium hemolyticum
Neisseria gonorrhoeae
Yersinia enterocolitica
Chlamydia pneumoniae
Mycoplasma pneumoniae

Fungal

Candida (thrush)

*Most frequent identifiable causes of pharyngitis.

Epiglottitis

Epiglottitis is most often an aggressive disease of young children but occurs in adults as well. Early recognition of this entity is critical because delay in diagnosis or treatment frequently results in death, which may occur abruptly, within hours after the onset of symptoms. This diagnosis must be considered in any patient with a sore throat and *any* of the following key symptoms or signs: (1) difficulty in swallowing; (2) copious oral secretions; (3) severe pain in the absence of pharyngeal erythema (the pharynx of patients with epiglottitis may be normal or inflamed); and (4) respiratory difficulty, particularly stridor.

Patients with epiglottitis often display a characteristic posture; they lean forward to prevent the swollen epiglottis from completely obstructing the airway and resist any attempt at placement in the supine position. The diagnosis can be confirmed by lateral radiographs of the neck or by indirect laryngoscopy with visualization of the swollen, erythematous epiglottis. This examination should be performed with the patient in the sitting position to minimize the risk of laryngeal spasm. Furthermore, the physician must be prepared to perform emergency tracheostomy should spasm occur. Therapy has two major objectives: protecting the airway and providing appropriate antimicrobial coverage. Because the most likely pathogen is *H. influenzae,* which may produce β-lactamase, effective antibiotic choices are a second- or third-generation cephalosporin or ampicillin-sulbactam. Corticosteroids may relieve some inflammatory edema; however, the role of this therapy remains unproved. Patients with respiratory difficulty should have their airway protected by endotracheal intubation or tracheostomy. Patients without respiratory complaints may be monitored continuously in an intensive care setting and intubated at the first sign of respiratory difficulty. Young children who are close contacts of patients with invasive disease caused by *H. influenzae* are themselves at particular risk of serious infection. Children younger than 4 years of age who have not received the complete *H. influenzae* vaccine series and are close contacts of the index patient, as well as all family members in a household with children younger than 4 years of age who have not been completely vaccinated, should receive prophylaxis with rifampin (20 mg/kg given orally, up to 600 mg twice daily for four doses).

Soft Tissue Space Infections

Quinsy. Quinsy is a unilateral peritonsillar abscess or phlegmon that is an unusual complication of tonsillitis. The patient has pain and difficulty in swallowing and often trouble in handling oral secretions. Trismus (inability to open the mouth because of muscle spasm) may be present. Examination shows swelling of the peritonsillar tissues and lateral displacement of the uvula. A mass may be felt on digital examination. In the phlegmon stage, penicillin therapy may be adequate; abscess can be identified by computed tomography and requires surgical drainage (Table 97–4). If untreated, quinsy may result in glottic edema and respiratory compromise or lateral pharyngeal space abscess.

Septic Jugular Vein Thrombophlebitis. An uncommon complication of bacterial pharyngitis or quinsy is septic jugular vein thrombophlebitis (syndrome of postanginal sepsis or Lemierre disease). Several days after a *sore throat,* the patient (most often an adolescent or young adult) will

| Table 97–4 | **Indications for Surgical Drainage: Parapharyngeal Soft Tissue Space Infections** |

Infection	**Indications for Surgery**
Quinsy	Abscess or respiratory compromise
Lateral pharyngeal space abscess	Abscess
Jugular vein septic thrombophlebitis	Febrile after 5–6 days of medical therapy
Retropharyngeal abscess	Abscess or respiratory compromise
Ludwig's angina	Abscess or respiratory compromise

note increasing pain and tenderness in the neck. In many instances, swelling occurs at the angle of the jaw. The patient will have a high fever, bacteremia (usually with *Fusobacterium* species), and often septic pulmonary emboli. Treatment is intravenous penicillin, 10 million U/day, plus metronidazole, 500 mg every 6 hours. Patients with persistent fevers may require surgical excision of the jugular vein.

Lateral Pharyngeal Space Abscess. This rare infection, which may complicate jugular vein thrombophlebitis, is associated with serious morbidity because of its proximity to vascular structures. Extension of lateral pharyngeal space abscess to the carotid artery may result in exsanguination, which may be preceded by small amounts of blood in the ear or pharynx. This infection is generally associated with tenderness and a mass at the angle of the jaw. Prompt surgical intervention may be life saving.

Retropharyngeal Space Abscess. This complication of tonsillitis is rare in adults because, by adulthood, the lymph nodes that give rise to this infection are generally atrophied. Most cases in adults are secondary to trauma (e.g., endoscopic) or to extension of a cervical osteomyelitis. The patient often has difficulty in swallowing and may complain of dyspnea, particularly when sitting upright. Diagnosis may be suspected by the presence of a posterior pharyngeal mass and confirmed by lateral neck films.

Ludwig's Angina. This mixed bacterial-spirochetal cellulitis or phlegmon of the floor of the mouth is generally secondary to an odontogenic infection. The tongue is pushed upward, and firm induration of the submandibular space and neck is often present. Laryngeal edema and respiratory compromise may also occur and necessitate protection of the airway. High-dose ampicillin-sulbactam or penicillin G plus metronidazole are the antibiotics of choice and have resulted in dramatic decreases in mortality rates. Protection of the airway is crucial in this setting, and endotracheal intubation should be provided if any suggestion of airway compromise is present.

Extrarespiratory Causes of Sore Throat

Several extrarespiratory causes of sore throat should be kept in mind. The older patient who complains of soreness in the

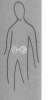

throat when climbing stairs or when upset may have angina pectoris with an unusual radiation. The hypertensive patient with an abrupt onset of a *tearing pain* in the throat may have a dissecting aortic aneurysm. In these patients, swallowing is generally unaffected. Patients with de Quervain's subacute thyroiditis may have fever and pain in the neck radiating to the ears. In patients with thyroiditis, the thyroid is generally tender. Patients with specific vitamin deficiencies may complain of soreness in the mouth and throat (see the previous section on Stomatitis). Examination may reveal a red *beefy* tongue with flattened papillae, resulting in a smooth appearance.

Persistent or Penicillin-Unresponsive Pharyngitis

Most cases of viral or streptococcal pharyngitis are self limited, and symptoms generally resolve within 3 to 4 days. In addition to acute human immunodeficiency virus infection and infectious mononucleosis, as discussed earlier, persistent sore throat should prompt consideration of the following possibilities.

Pharyngeal Gonorrhea. Although most cases of pharyngeal gonorrhea are asymptomatic, mild pharyngitis may be seen occasionally. This infection does not always respond to low-dose penicillin, and the gonococcus is relatively resistant to phenoxymethyl penicillin (Pen-V); high-dose penicillin or tetracycline is generally effective. The gonococcus will not likely be identified on routine culture medium; isolation generally requires culture of a fresh throat swab on a selective medium such as Thayer-Martin (see Chapter 106).

Acute Lymphoblastic Leukemia. Persistent exudative tonsillitis may be a presentation of acute lymphoblastic leukemia (ALL). Diagnosis can be suspected by examination of the peripheral blood smear; however, some experience may be required to distinguish between the blasts of ALL and the atypical lymphocytes of infectious mononucleosis.

Other Leukopenic States. Stomatitis or pharyngitis may be the presenting complaint of patients with *aplastic anemia* or *agranulocytosis*. Because some of these cases are drug induced (e.g., propylthiouracil, phenytoin), a complete medication history on initial presentation may suggest this possibility. Prompt discontinuation of the offending drug may be life saving.

Although sore throat is a common complaint of patients with relatively benign illness, it is sometimes the presenting complaint of a patient with a serious or life-threatening disease. Any of the key signs or symptoms shown in Table 97–2 should alert the clinician to the possibility of an extraordinary process.

Prospectus for the Future

More sensitive imaging procedures, both computed tomography and magnetic resonance imaging, will permit earlier and more precise diagnosis of such potential lethal infections as acute epiglottitis, septic jugular vein thrombophlebitis, and lateral pharyngeal and retropharyngeal space abscesses.

References

Bruce AJ, Rogers RS 3rd: Acute oral ulcers [Review]. Dermatol Clin 21(1):1–15, 2003 Jan.

Del Mar CB, Glasziou PP, Spinks AB: Antibiotics for sore throat. Cochrane Database Syst Rev 2:CD000023, 2004.

Hendley JO: Clinical practice: Otitis media. N Engl J Med 347(15): 1169–1174, 2002 Oct.

Porter S, Scully C: Aphthous ulcers (recurrent). Clin Evid 11:1766–1173, 2004 Jun.

Sack JL, Brock CD: Identifying acute epiglottitis in adults: High degree of awareness, close monitoring are key. Postgrad Med 112(1):81–82, 85–86, 2002 Jul.

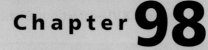

Infections of the Lower Respiratory Tract

Christoph Lange

Michael M. Lederman

Pneumonia is one of the most common causes of admissions to adult medical services in North America and is one of the leading causes of death during the productive years of life. This potentially lethal illness is readily reversible. Every physician must therefore be adept at the rapid diagnosis and management of pneumonia. Viruses, bacteria (including chlamydia, rickettsia, and mycoplasmas), fungi, protozoans, and parasites can all produce serious infections of the lower respiratory tract. A thorough history and physical examination can provide clues to the likely cause of infection. The clinical spectra of pneumonias caused by different pathogens overlap considerably, however. Microscopic examination of respiratory secretions can provide a rapid and useful step in the differential diagnosis of pneumonia.

Pathogenesis

Under normal circumstances, the lower respiratory tract is sterile. Microbes can enter the lung to produce infection by hematogenous spread, by spread from a contiguous focus of infection, by inhalation of aerosolized particles, or, most commonly, by aspiration of oropharyngeal secretions. In the last instance, the organisms colonizing the oropharynx will determine the spectrum of micro-organisms in the aspirated secretions and presumably the nature of the resultant pneumonia. Some organisms such as *Streptococcus pneumoniae* may transiently colonize the oropharynx in healthy individuals. Colonization often results in the development of protective antibodies to that strain. Other organisms, such as Gram-negative bacilli, are more prevalent in the upper respiratory tract of debilitated and hospitalized patients. Aspiration of normal oropharyngeal flora may lead to necrotizing pneumonia caused by mixtures of oral anaerobic bacteria.

Inoculum size (the number of bacteria aspirated) is an important factor in the development of pneumonia. Studies using radioisotopes have shown that up to 45% of healthy men aspirate some oropharyngeal contents during sleep. In most instances, the bacteria aspirated are relatively avirulent, and back-up defenses, including cough, mucociliary clearance, and other innate immune defenses, are adequate to prevent the development of pneumonia. Individuals with structural disease of the oropharynx and lungs or patients with cough reflexes impaired as a result of drugs, alcohol, or neuromuscular disease are at particular risk for developing pneumonia as a result of aspiration. A layer of mucus that traps foreign particles, which are propelled upward by rhythmic beating of the cilia to a point where a cough can expel the particles, covers the specialized ciliated cells of the bronchial mucosa. Impaired mucociliary transport, as seen in persons with chronic obstructive pulmonary disease, predisposes the individual to bacterial infection. Denuding of the respiratory epithelium by infection with the influenza virus is one mechanism by which influenza predisposes a person to bacterial pneumonia. Within the alveoli and smaller airways, alveolar macrophages, granulocytes, lymphocytes, small peptides such as defensins and humoral opsonins, as well as antibody and complement, serve as host defenses against infection.

Infection by *Mycobacterium tuberculosis* is usually acquired through inhalation of aerosolized contaminated droplet nuclei. A primary infection is established in the parenchyma of the lungs and in the draining lymph nodes, which may result in a progressive primary infection, but in most instances it remains clinically silent or produces a mild respiratory illness. The mycobacteria remain alive, sequestered within host macrophages, and are contained by host cell–mediated defenses in granulomas. Reactivation of infection may never occur, may occur without apparent precipitating events, or may occur at times when host cell–mediated immune responses are impaired and granulomas break down. Examples of these impairments include starvation, intercurrent viral infections, administration of corticosteroids or cytotoxic drugs, and illnesses associated with immunosuppression, such as Hodgkin's disease and human immunodeficiency virus (HIV) infection.

Table 98–1	**Important Pathogens Causing Pneumonia**
Population*	**Pathogens**
Young, healthy adult	*Streptococcus pneumoniae*, *Mycoplasma pneumoniae*, *Chlamydia pneumoniae*, respiratory viruses
Older adults	*S. pneumoniae*, influenza virus, *Mycobacterium tuberculosis*
Debilitated	*S. pneumoniae*, influenza virus, oral flora, *M. tuberculosis*, Gram-negative bacilli
Hospitalized	Oral flora, *Staphylococcus aureus*, Gram-negative bacilli, *Legionella* spp.

*See also Chapters 107 and 108.

Table 98–2	**Specific Disorders and Associated Pneumonias**
Disorder	**Pneumonia**
Seizures	Aspiration (mixed anaerobes)
Alcoholism	Aspiration, *Streptococcus pneumoniae*, *Klebsiella pneumoniae*, other Gram-negative bacilli
Diabetes mellitus	Gram-negative bacilli, *Mycobacterium tuberculosis*
Sickle cell disease	*S. pneumoniae*, *Mycoplasma pneumoniae*
Chronic lung disease	*S. pneumoniae*, *Haemophilus influenzae*, *Moraxella catarrhalis*, *Pseudomonas aeruginosa*, *Burkolderia cepacia*, other Gram-negative bacilli
Chronic renal failure	*S. pneumoniae*, *M. tuberculosis*, *Legionella pneumophila*

Table 98–3	**Exposures Associated with Pneumonia**
Source/Location	**Pneumonia**
Cattle, goats, sheep	Q fever, brucellosis, tularemia
Rabbits	Tularemia
Birds	Psittacosis, avian influenza, cryptococcosis, histoplasmosis*
Rodents	Hantavirus
Dog ticks	Ehrlichiosis
Southwestern United States	Coccidioidomycosis
Mississippi and Ohio River valleys	Histoplasmosis, blastomycosis
Developing countries	Tuberculosis

*Exposure to bird and bat droppings.

Epidemiologic Factors

Common pathogens of community-acquired and nosocomial pneumonia are shown in Table 98–1. As a general rule, the pneumococcus is an important pathogen in all age groups, and influenza and tuberculosis become more frequent with increasing age. Although *Mycoplasma* occasionally produces pneumonia in older adults, it is primarily a pathogen of the young. Certain systemic disorders appear to be associated with pneumonias caused by particular organisms (Table 98–2). The exposure history may be helpful in suggesting specific causative agents (Table 98–3). Pneumonias associated with bone marrow suppression and malignant disorders are discussed in Chapter 108.

Differential Diagnosis

A critical historical point in the differential diagnosis of pneumonia is the duration of symptoms. Pneumonia caused by pneumococci, *Mycoplasma*, or virus is usually an acute illness. Symptoms last for hours to a few days, although a longer viral prodrome may occasionally occur before bacterial superinfection. In contrast, symptoms of pneumonia lasting 10 days or more are rarely caused by the common bacterial pathogens and should raise suspicion of mycobacterial, fungal, or anaerobic pneumonia (anaerobes can produce acute or chronic infection), and/or the presence of an anatomic defect such as bronchiectasis or an endobronchial mass.

A history of an unusual exposure or the knowledge of the nature of an underlying immunodeficiency often provides clues to the cause of some less common pneumonias (see Table 98–3). Although these pneumonias are uncommon, they should be considered in the appropriate setting because, if improperly treated, some may be fatal.

A history of rhinitis or pharyngitis suggests respiratory virus or *Mycoplasma* or *Chlamydia* pneumonia. Diarrhea has been associated with *Legionella* pneumonia in some outbreaks. A persistent hacking, nonproductive cough characterizes some *Mycoplasma* infections; an abrupt onset of myalgia, arthralgia, headache, and fever are the typical clinical presentation of a patient with influenza-virus infection and may also be seen with *Mycoplasma* pneumonia. A true rigor is highly suggestive of a bacterial (often pneumococcal) pneumonia. Whereas small pleural effusions may be seen in nonbacterial pneumonias, severe pleuritic pain and/or empyema in a patient with pneumonia is highly suggestive of bacterial infection. Night sweats in the absence of rigors are seen in chronic pneumonias and suggest tuberculosis, fungal disease, or lung abscess.

Most patients with pneumonia have cough, fever, tachypnea, and tachycardia. Fever without a concomitant rise in pulse rate may be seen in legionellosis, *Mycoplasma* infections, and other *nonbacterial* pneumonias. Patients with pulmonary tuberculosis often have high fever that is relatively asymptomatic when compared with patients with acute bacterial pneumonia. Respirations may be shallow in the presence of pleurisy. Increasing tachypnea, cyanosis, and the use of accessory muscles for respiration indicate serious illness. Foul breath suggests anaerobic infection (e.g. lung abscess). Confusion in a patient with pneumonia should immediately raise the suspicion of meningeal involvement, which occurs most commonly in patients with pneumococcal pneumonia. Confusion may, however, be the most prominent clinical feature of pneumonia in older patients in the absence of associated meningitis. Nonetheless, patients with pneumonia who are confused should be evaluated by examination of cerebrospinal fluid.

Physical evidence of consolidation, dullness to percussion, bronchial breath sounds, crackles, increased fremitus, and whispered pectoriloquy suggest bacterial pneumonia. Early in the course of pneumonia, however, the physical examination may not be indicative of consolidation.

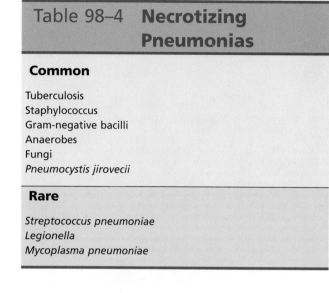

Table 98–4	Necrotizing Pneumonias
Common	
Tuberculosis	
Staphylococcus	
Gram-negative bacilli	
Anaerobes	
Fungi	
Pneumocystis jirovecii	
Rare	
Streptococcus pneumoniae	
Legionella	
Mycoplasma pneumoniae	

RADIOGRAPHIC PATTERNS

Successful interpretation of radiographs requires an integration of clinical data with expert reading of the film. Thus, fever and malaise often help differentiate the miliary pattern of tuberculosis from that of sarcoidosis in which patients may be without symptoms. A clinical-radiographic dissociation is a typical feature of *Mycoplasma* pneumonia, in which the clinical signs of pneumonia may be minimal but extensive infiltrates are detected on the chest radiograph. The converse applies to patients with early *P. jirovecii* pneumonia, in early miliary tuberculosis, or in hypersensitivity pneumonia, in which chest radiographs are often normal despite symptomatic clinical disease. In this instance, a high-resolution computed tomographic scan may demonstrate evidence of pathologic abnormality. Similarly, early in the course of acute bacterial pneumonias, pleuritic chest pain, cough, purulent sputum, and inspiratory crackles may precede specific radiographic findings by many hours. A *negative* radiograph can never rule out the possibility of acute bacterial pneumonia when the patient's symptoms and signs point to this diagnosis. A lobar consolidation suggests a bacterial pneumonia; however, patients with chronic lung disease often fail to exhibit clinical or radiographic evidence of consolidation during the course of bacterial pneumonia. Interstitial infiltrates suggest a nonbacterial process but may also be seen in early staphylococcal pneumonia. Enlarged hilar lymph nodes suggest a concomitant lung tumor but may also be seen in primary tuberculous, viral, or fungal pneumonias. Large pleural effusions should suggest streptococcal pneumonia or tuberculosis. Pneumatoceles are seen in patients after ventilator-mediated barotrauma but occur frequently in the evolution of staphylococcal pneumonia, particularly among children, and may also occur in patients with *P. jirovecii* pneumonia. The presence of cavitation identifies the pneumonia as necrotizing. This finding virtually excludes viruses and *Mycoplasma* and makes pneumococcal

infection unlikely (Table 98–4). Whenever possible, radiographs should be compared with older films.

OTHER LABORATORY FINDINGS

In patients with bacterial pneumonia, the white blood cell count is often (but not invariably) elevated. Among patients with pneumococcal infection, white blood cell counts of 20,000 to 30,000/mcL or more may be seen. A left shift with immature forms is common. Patients with nonbacterial pneumonias tend to have lower white blood cell counts. The C-reactive protein is a useful marker for monitoring both the severity of the bacterial infection and the treatment response. Modest elevations of serum bilirubin (conjugated) level may be noted in many bacterial infections but are particularly common in patients with pneumococcal pneumonia.

Diagnosis

When the patient exhibits abrupt onset of shaking chills, followed by cough, pleuritic chest pain, fever, rusty or yellow sputum, and shortness of breath, and the physical examination shows tachypnea and even minimal signs of alveolar inflammation (e.g., harsh breath sounds at one lung base), the presumptive diagnosis of bacterial pneumonia should be made, sputum should be examined, and appropriate therapy should be begun regardless of radiographic findings. The radiographic abnormalities may lag for several hours after the clinical onset of pneumonia.

Empiric treatment of community-acquired pneumonia without laboratory examination of sputum may be successful in managing many patients. However, this practice promotes indiscriminate use of broad-spectrum antibiotics, with attendant increases in antibiotic resistance. This approach also will result in occasional misdiagnoses and may place nonresponding patients at risk for increased morbidity and death.

Examination of respiratory secretions facilitates prompt diagnosis and proper treatment of pneumonia. When the

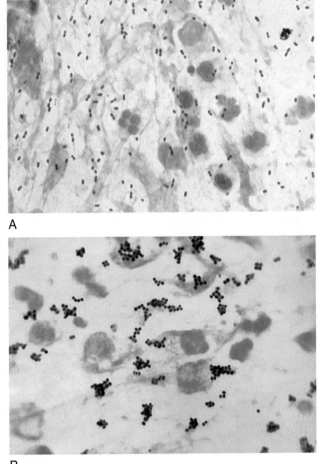

A

B

Figure 98–1 Gram stains of expectorated sputum that demonstrate *(A)* Gram-positive, lancet-shaped diplococci from a patient with pneumococcal pneumonia and *(B)* clusters of Gram-positive cocci in a patient with *Staphylococcus aureus* pneumoniae. Note the presence of alveolar macrophages and virtual absence of squamous epithelial cells, which confirm the lower respiratory tract origin of the specimen. Mandell GL, Bennett JL, Dolin R. Principles and Practice of Infectious Diseases. 6th ed. Philadelphia, Churchill Livingstone, 2005.

history and physical examination suggest pneumonia, a specimen of sputum must be Gram-stained and examined immediately. The adequacy of the specimen can be ascertained by (1) the absence of squamous epithelial cells and (2) the presence of polymorphonuclear leukocytes (10 to 15 per high-power field). The presence of alveolar macrophages and bronchial epithelial cells confirms the lower respiratory tract origin of the specimen. A specimen with many (>5 per high-power field) squamous epithelial cells is of little value for either culture or Gram stain, because it is contaminated with upper respiratory tract secretions (Fig. 98–1A and B).

In some cases, the patient cannot produce an adequate sputum sample, despite vigorous attempts at sputum induction using an aerosolized solution of 3% hypertonic saline. The sicker the patient and the greater the likelihood of a multidrug-resistant pathogen, the more important it is to get an adequate sample of sputum for examination and culture.

This goal can often be achieved by nasotracheal aspiration. The vigorous coughing stimulated by this procedure often produces an additional excellent expectorated specimen. (*Note:* Expectorated sputum and sputum obtained through nasotracheal aspiration cannot be cultured anaerobically because of universal contamination with bacteria from the oropharynx.)

The Gram-stained specimen should be examined using an oil immersion lens. The presence of a predominant organism, particularly if found within white blood cells, suggests that this pathogen is the likely one. In cases of aspiration of mouth flora, a mixture of oral streptococci, Gram-positive rods, and Gram-negative organisms is found. In some cases, inflammatory cells but no organisms may be seen on Gram stain. This finding suggests a large number of possibilities, many of which are *nonbacterial* pneumonias (Table 98–5). The importance of obtaining a good-quality sputum specimen for examination and culture from patients with community-acquired pneumonia has been debated. A good-quality baseline sputum specimen is of value primarily in patients who do not show an expected clinical response to therapy (see later discussion). Because these persons are not readily identifiable at presentation, a good baseline sample is routinely recommended. Unless the diagnosis of acute bacterial pneumonia is clear, an acid-fast stain or fluorescent auramine-rhodamine stain of sputum for mycobacteria should be performed. If legionellosis is suspected, immunofluorescence stains for *Legionella* can be used, although the yield on expectorated sputum is low. The demonstration of elastin fibers in a potassium hydroxide preparation of sputum establishes a diagnosis of necrotizing pneumonia (see Table 98–4). Blood cultures should be obtained routinely and may be positive in 20% to 30% of patients with bacterial pneumonia.

Results of sputum cultures must be interpreted with caution because pathogens causing pneumonia may fail to grow, and sputum isolates may not be the pathogens responsible for infection. Careful screening of sputum specimens with Gram stain increases the accuracy of culture results. A tuberculin skin test should be applied in all cases of pneumonia of uncertain origin. In severely ill patients, a negative tuberculin test may occur despite active pulmonary and/or disseminated tuberculosis. If the tuberculin test is negative but tuberculosis remains a diagnostic possibility, then the patient's blood lymphocytes can be tested for the production of interferon in response to mycobacterial RD-1 proteins. A negative test result makes the diagnosis less likely.

Specific Pathogenic Organisms

VIRAL AGENTS

Respiratory viral infection is usually limited to the upper respiratory tract, and only a small proportion of infected adults develop pneumonia. In children, viruses are the most common cause of pneumonia, and respiratory syncytial virus is the most frequent organism. In adults, viruses are estimated to account only for a minority of pneumonias, and the influenza virus is the most common viral pathogen. Patients at increased risk of influenzal pneumonia include

Table 98–5	**Sputum Gram Stains Showing Inflammatory Cells and No Organisms**		

Possibilities	Clinical Setting	Confirmation of Diagnosis	Treatment
Prior antibiotic treatment	—	—	—
Viral pneumonia	Winter months influenza; may be mild or life threatening	Serologic studies, virus culture, antigen detection	Oseltamivir for influenza A or B, ribavirin for respiratory syncytial virus
Mycoplasma pneumoniae infection	Hacking, nonproductive cough	Cold agglutinins, serologic studies	Doxycycline or macrolide
Legionella pneumophila infection	Chronic lung disease, hospital acquired, summer predominance	Unique antigen test, DFA of sputum or bronchial brush biopsy, culture	Azithromycin or levofloxacin
Chlamydophila psittaci infection	Exposure to birds (e.g., parrots, turkeys)	Serologic studies	Tetracycline or doxycycline
Chlamydophila pneumoniae infection	Hacking cough, sinusitis	Serologic studies, antigen detection	Tetracycline or macrolides
Q fever	Exposure to cattle, South Africa	Serologic studies	Doxycycline or ciprofloxacin

DFA = direct immunofluorescence assay.

older adults; patients with chronic disease of the heart, lung, or kidney; and women in the last trimester of pregnancy. Cytomegalovirus may cause severe pneumonia in immunosuppressed patients, especially in organ transplant recipients. When varicella occurs in adults, some 10% to 20% develop pneumonia, which commonly leaves a pattern of diffuse punctate calcification on chest radiograph. Measles is occasionally complicated by pneumonia. Cases of pneumonia and adult respiratory distress syndrome caused by *Hantavirus* in North America have occurred primarily in the southwestern United States. This rapidly progressive and often fatal infection occurs largely among otherwise healthy young adults who have been exposed to rodent droppings. Treatment is supportive. Although ribavirin has been used in the treatment of this infection, its value is unproved.

Other viral pneumonias, of which influenza is the prototype in adults, typically occur in community epidemics and usually develop 1 to 3 days after the onset of influenza-like symptoms. Major features include a dry cough, dyspnea, generalized discomfort, unremarkable physical examination, and an interstitial pattern on the chest radiograph. Influenza-induced necrosis of respiratory epithelial cells predisposes the patient to bacterial colonization, which may result in superimposed bacterial pneumonia, most often caused by *S. pneumoniae, Staphylococcus aureus,* or *Hemophilus influenzae.* A presumptive diagnosis may be made based on the clinical presentation and the epidemiologic setting. Gram stain of sputum reveals inflammatory cells and

rare bacteria. Detection of viral antigens in sputum can confirm the diagnosis rapidly. Viral isolation or serology cannot establish the diagnosis in time to guide management decisions.

In 2003, pandemic spread of a newly identified coronavirus (severe acute respiratory syndrome–coronavirus [SARS-CoV]) caused clinical illness in more than 8000 persons around the globe, with a mortality of nearly 10%. To date, no effective antiviral treatment is available. Seasonal outbreaks of SARS-CoV and possibly other emerging viral respiratory infections, including those caused by the closely related *Nipah* and *Hendra* viruses, may be anticipated.

Recently, highly pathogenic influenza virus strains (H5N1) emerging from avian reservoirs have caused mortality in over 50% of infected persons in some Southeast Asian nations. When reassortment and/or recombination with currently circulating strains occurs, avian influenza might potentially cause another major influenza pandemic. This potential is of special concern because the high case mortality rate exceeds that observed with the H1N1 strain, which caused the devastating 1918 influenza pandemic, during which over 50 million persons worldwide died within a 12-month period. Although little evidence yet of direct human-to-human transmission of the avian H5N1 strain has been discovered, this possibility has triggered worldwide efforts to develop and produce an effective vaccine on a large scale and to increase production of osaltamivir, an agent that is effective against this viral strain in the rodent model.

BACTERIAL AGENTS

Streptococcus Pneumoniae

The pneumococcus is still the most common bacterial cause of pneumonia in the community. The organism colonizes the oropharynx in up to 25% of healthy adults. An increased predisposition to pneumococcal pneumonia is seen in persons with sickle cell disease, prior splenectomy, chronic lung disease, hematologic malignancy, alcoholism, HIV infection, and renal failure. Clinical features include fever, rigors, chills, pleuritic chest pain, cough, purulent sputum, respiratory distress, signs of pulmonary consolidation, and confusion. By the second or third day of illness, the chest radiograph typically shows lobar consolidation with air bronchograms, but a patchy bronchopneumonic pattern may also be found. Abscess or cavitation rarely occurs. Sterile pleural effusions occur in up to 25% of patients, and empyema occurs in 1%. Typically, a leukocytosis of 15,000 to 30,000 cells/mcL with neutrophilia is found, but leukopenia may be observed with fulminant infection, particularly among alcoholics and persons with HIV infection. Gram-positive cocci in pairs can be seen on microscopic examination of expectorated sputum samples in more than 60% of patients with pneumococcal pneumonia. Positive blood cultures are found in 20% to 25% of patients. In most regions of the world, penicillin G remains the treatment of choice. In regions with a higher frequency of penicillin-resistant pneumococci, or in persons who are severely ill, cephalosporins or vancomycin may be indicated, depending on regional antibiotic sensitivity patterns.

Staphylococcus Aureus

Persistent staphylococcal nasal colonization is observed in 15% to 30% of adults, and 90% of adults display intermittent colonization. *Staphylococcus aureus* infection accounts for 2% to 5% of community-acquired pneumonias, 11% of hospital-acquired pneumonias, and up to 26% of pneumonias following influenza. Initial presentation may be similar to that of pneumococcal pneumonia, but contrasting features include the development of parenchymal necrosis and abscess formation in up to 25% of patients and empyema in 10%. A hematogenous source of infection, such as septic thrombophlebitis, infective endocarditis, or an infected intravascular device, should be anticipated in cases of staphylococcal pneumonia, particularly if the chest radiograph shows multiple or expanding nodular or wedge-shaped infiltrates. Early in staphylococcal pneumonia of hematogenous origin, sputum is rarely available. Blood cultures are usually positive, and associated skin lesions occur in 20% to 40% of patients. When sputum is available, Gram stain shows grapelike clusters of Gram-positive cocci. *Staphylococcus aureus* is recovered easily from mixed culture samples so that its absence in a purulent specimen usually excludes it as a cause of the pneumonia. Treatment requires a penicillinase-resistant agent, such as nafcillin or vancomycin. In hospital-acquired infections or in communities with endemic methicillin-resistant *S. aureus*, vancomycin or linezolid should be used until sensitivity studies indicate that the isolate is sensitive to semisynthetic penicillins.

Streptococcus Pyogenes

Streptococcus pyogenes is now an uncommon cause of pneumonia, probably accounting for less than 1% of all cases. Occasional outbreaks continue to occur, however, in military recruit populations. Carriage rate in the pharynx (approximately 3% in adults) is less than with the other Gram-positive cocci. Presentation is similar to that observed with *S. pneumoniae* and *S. aureus*, except that empyema, often massive, is found in 30% to 40% of patients, and the illness more often shows a rapid progression that can be measured in hours. Gram stain shows Gram-positive cocci in pairs or chains. Penicillin G, 1 million U every 4 hours, remains effective in most patients. However, because of possible resistance to penicillin, some authorities prefer cefotaxime, 1 g every 6 hours, or ceftriaxone, 1 g every 12 hours. Some authorities recommend co-administration of clindamycin. Early decortication is indicated if empyema is present.

Haemophilus Influenzae

Haemophilus influenzae is a Gram-negative coccobacillus often present in the upper respiratory tract, particularly among patients with chronic obstructive pulmonary disease. Confirmation of its role in the pathogenesis of pneumonia depends on isolating the organism in the blood, pleural fluid, or lung tissue. Nevertheless, many cases of pneumonia caused by this organism will not be confirmed using these rigid criteria, and, in a patient with pneumonia, the demonstration of Gram-negative coccobacilli on Gram stain of sputum should prompt institution of treatment with ampicillin plus a β-lactamase inhibitor or a second- or third-generation cephalosporin.

Gram-Negative Bacilli

Gram-negative bacilli have emerged as pulmonary pathogens of major importance with the introduction of potent antibiotics and the proliferation of intensive care units. They are frequently encountered in patients with structural abnormalities of the tracheobronchial tree, such as chronic obstructive pulmonary disease and cystic fibrosis, as well as in the settings of neutropenia, alcoholism, diabetes mellitus, malignancy, and chronic disease of the heart and kidney. Gram-negative bacilli are ubiquitous throughout hospitals, contaminating equipment and instruments, and are the major source of nosocomial pneumonia.

Specific organisms are associated with certain situations; for example, *Klebsiella pneumoniae* is particularly common in chronic alcoholics, *Escherichia coli* pneumonia is associated with bacteremias arising from the intestinal or urinary tract, and *Pseudomonas* species commonly infect the lungs of patients with cystic fibrosis. Precise etiologic diagnosis is confounded by the frequency with which these organisms colonize the upper airways in predisposed patients. Treatment of patients with *Pseudomonas aeruginosa* infection or seriously ill patients generally includes the use of two active agents, such as an extended-spectrum penicillin, a carbapenem, or a third-generation cephalosporin, together with a fluoroquinolone or aminoglycoside.

OTHER CAUSES OF ACUTE PNEUMONIA

Mycoplasma Pneumoniae

Not only is *Mycoplasma pneumoniae* a common cause of pneumonia in young adults, but it also produces a wide range of extrapulmonary features that may be the only findings. Fewer than 10% of infected patients develop symptoms of lower respiratory tract infection. Respiratory findings resemble those of viral pneumonia. Hacking, non-productive cough is characteristic. Nonpulmonary features include myalgias, arthralgias, skin lesions (rashes, erythema nodosum and multiforme, or Stevens-Johnson syndrome), and neurologic complications (meningitis, encephalitis, transverse myelitis, cranial nerve, or peripheral neuritis). The occurrence of acute, multifocal neurologic abnormalities may be helpful in distinguishing *Mycoplasma* pneumonia from that caused by *Chlamydia* or *Legionella*. The neurologic abnormalities characteristically resolve completely as the acute illness subsides.

In some patients, cold agglutinins may be seen at the bedside by observing red blood cell clumping on the walls of a glass tube containing anticoagulated blood incubated on ice for at least 10 minutes; this cold agglutinin test is also occasionally positive in other respiratory infections. Polymerase chain reaction (PCR) performed on a throat swab specimen can provide a rapid and specific diagnosis. Treatment for 7 to 14 days with doxycycline or a macrolide decreases the duration of symptoms and hastens radiographic resolution but does not eradicate the organism from the respiratory tract.

Chlamydophila (Chlamydia) Pneumoniae

Chlamydophila pneumoniae (formerly called the Taiwan acute respiratory [TWAR] agent) causes 5% to 15% of cases of community-acquired pneumonia. Infection is spread presumably through the respiratory route, from person to person, and onset of disease is generally subacute, often demonstrated by pharyngitis, sinusitis, bronchitis, and pneumonia. The radiographic appearance of pneumonia caused by *C. pneumoniae* resembles that of *Mycoplasma* infection. Illness is relatively mild and often prolonged. Diagnosis of this infection is difficult and requires cultivation of the organism in special cell lines or testing of acute and convalescent sera for antibody levels. Although the organism is sensitive to macrolides and tetracyclines, treatment may have little effect on the course of disease.

Legionella Species

Legionella species are fastidious, Gram-negative bacilli that were responsible for respiratory infections long before the well-publicized outbreak of legionnaires' disease in 1976, which led to the recognition of this distinct disease entity and to the identification of the responsible bacillus. (The high mortality rate from this outbreak of a hitherto unrecognized disease among participants at an American Legion convention destroyed the reputation of one of Philadelphia's finest hotels.) These organisms are distributed widely in water, and outbreaks have been related to their presence in water towers, air conditioners, condensers, potable water, and even hospital showerheads. Infection may occur sporadically or in outbreaks. Although healthy individuals can be affected, an increased risk occurs in patients with chronic diseases of the heart, lungs, or kidneys; malignancy; and impairment of cell-mediated immunity. After an incubation period of 2 to 10 days, the illness usually begins gradually with a dry cough, but may then progress rapidly with respiratory distress, fever, rigors, headache, and confusion. The chest radiograph shows alveolar shadowing that may have a lobar or patchy distribution, with or without pleural effusions. The diagnosis is suggested clinically by the combination of a rapidly progressive pneumonia, dry cough, and multiorgan involvement. Microhematuria is often present. Gram stain of sputum shows neutrophils and no predominant organisms.

Diagnosis can be made by four methods:

1. *Legionella* antigen can be detected in urine with a sensitivity of 80% to 95% for *Legionella pneumophila* type 1. Specificity of this test is better than 99%.
2. Direct fluorescence antibody testing of respiratory secretions is technically demanding and has a specificity of 95%, but sensitivity of this method is low when using expectorated sputum.
3. Indirect fluorescent antibody testing of serum is positive in 75% of patients, but up to 8 weeks are required for seroconversion.
4. The organism can be cultured on charcoal yeast extract medium (the laboratory must be informed), but up to 10 days are required for growth.

Levofloxacin for 10 to 14 days or alternatively azithromycin for 7 to 10 days is an effective therapy. Rifampin may be added in the gravely ill patient, but its value is unproved. Prompt treatment results in a fourfold to fivefold reduction in mortality. Patients usually respond within 12 to 48 hours, and for fever, leukocytosis, and confusion to persist beyond 4 days of therapy is unusual.

COMMUNITY-ACQUIRED PNEUMONIA OF UNCERTAIN ORIGIN

Many instances have occurred in which, because of difficulty in obtaining adequate sputum specimens or lack of laboratory facilities, empiric treatment of acute community-acquired pneumonia may be necessary. In such instances, initial therapy should be guided by the patient risk factors, co-morbidities, and the severity of illness. Guidelines for the treatment of community-acquired pneumonia are frequently updated by the Infectious Disease Society of America (IDSA) and American Thoracic Society (ATS) and are available online (see references: *http://www.idsociety.com*, *http://www.ats.org*).

TUBERCULOSIS

Approximately 25,000 new cases of tuberculosis occur in the United States each year, with a worldwide incidence of 7 to 10 million. The worldwide figures are now increasing dramatically because tuberculosis is the major communicable complication of acquired immunodeficiency syndrome (see Chapter 107). In North America, a disproportionately high number of cases occur among the foreign born and the poor.

Mycobacterium tuberculosis is transmitted by the respiratory route from an infected patient with pulmonary tuberculosis to a susceptible host. Primary infection may be documented by the development of a positive tuberculin skin test. Occasionally, the patient develops sufficient symptoms of fever and nonproductive cough to visit a physician, and a chest radiograph is taken; patchy or lobular infiltrates are noted in the anterior segment of the upper lobes (**Web Fig. 98–1**) or in the middle or lower lobes, often with associated hilar adenopathy. Pleurisy with effusion is a less common manifestation of primary tuberculosis. Primary infection usually is self limited, but hematogenous dissemination seeds multiple organs, and latent foci are established and become niduses for delayed reactivation. Overall, 5% to 10% of infected individuals develop disease. Factors associated with progression to clinical disease are age (the periods of greatest biologic vulnerability to tuberculosis being infancy, childhood, and old age); underlying diseases that depress the cellular immune response (see Chapters 107 and 108); diabetes mellitus, gastrectomy, silicosis, and sarcoidosis; and the interval since primary infection, with disease progression most likely in the first few years after infection. Anti-TNFα therapy (e.g., infliximab) for rheumatoid arthritis or inflammatory bowel disease can lead to exacerbation of latent tuberculosis infection. Early progression of infection to disease is known as progressive primary tuberculosis and may exhibit as miliary tuberculosis (**Web Fig. 98–2**), sometimes with meningitis, or as pulmonary disease of the apical and posterior segments of the upper lobes or lower lobe disease.

Most commonly, tuberculosis represents delayed reactivation. Symptoms begin insidiously with night sweats or chills and fatigue; fever is noted by fewer than 50% of patients, and hemoptysis by fewer than 25%. Physical examination may be unremarkable or may show dullness and crackles in the upper lung fields, occasionally with amphoric breath sounds. The chest radiograph may show cavitary disease (**Web Fig. 98–3**) with infiltrates in the posterior segment of the upper lobes or apical segments of the lower lobes.

Extrapulmonary tuberculosis also reflects reactivation of latent foci and accounts for approximately 15% of cases in the industrialized world. Miliary tuberculosis is discussed in Chapter 94, meningeal tuberculosis in Chapter 96, and tuberculosis of bones and joints in Chapter 103.

Because of the growing proportion of older individuals in our society and the growing prevalence of HIV infection, *atypical* presentations of tuberculosis are increasingly common. Older adults and patients with diabetes mellitus are more likely to have lower lobe tuberculosis. In patients infected with HIV, involvement of the lower lobes is frequent, extrapulmonary tuberculosis is almost as common as pulmonary involvement, and tuberculin skin tests are likely to be negative in patients with CD4+ T-cell counts less than 200 cells/mcL. The index of suspicion must be high in these settings.

Before starting antituberculosis drug treatment, two or three sputum samples should be obtained for cultures; bronchoscopy and bronchial washing are indicated only if sputum smears are negative for acid-fast bacilli. Amplification of bacterial sequences by PCR can distinguish between *M. tuberculosis* and nontuberculous mycobacteria. Obtain-

ing a baseline evaluation of liver function is important for individuals who are to receive potentially hepatotoxic drugs (isoniazid, rifampin, or pyrazinamide); color vision, visual fields, and acuity when ethambutol will be used; and audiometry for patients who are to receive streptomycin.

A major principle of chemotherapy for tuberculosis is to avoid resistance by treating with at least two drugs to which the organism is likely to be sensitive. Pulmonary tuberculosis should be treated with daily isoniazid (5 mg/kg, up to 300 mg), rifampin (10 mg/kg, up to 600 mg), ethambutol (15 to 25 mg/kg, up to 2.5 g), and pyrazinamide (15 to 30 mg/kg, up to 2.0 g) for 2 months, followed by isoniazid and rifampin for 4 more months. A longer treatment duration (a total of 9 months) is suggested for persons infected with HIV when cultures are still positive after 2 months of therapy. If reason exists to believe that the patient is infected with multidrug-resistant isolates, then additional or alternative drugs are necessary until drug sensitivities are known. At that point, the regimen can be tailored to include at least two drugs to which the organism is sensitive. Close monitoring during treatment is mandatory to maximize compliance and minimize side effects. The World Health Organization recommends direct observation therapy for all patients with tuberculosis.

Contact tracing is critical because recent infection or additional cases of tuberculosis are likely in some household contacts. Preventive therapy with isoniazid is discussed later.

Treatment and Outcome

BACTERIAL PNEUMONIA

As soon as the causative organism is identified on Gram stain, antibiotics must be administered without delay. If the pathogen is readily identified, the antibiotic choices are straightforward (Table 98–6). Occasionally, a young patient with no underlying disease can also be managed at home, provided that the patient is reliably attended by friends or family and has ready access to a physician or hospital. Patients with *Mycoplasma* and viral pneumonia can, in most cases, be treated on an ambulatory basis. Otherwise, patients with bacterial pneumonia should be hospitalized.

Supplemental oxygen should be provided if the patient is tachypneic or hypoxemic. Patients at risk for the development of respiratory failure should be monitored in a critical care setting. Patients who are not capable of adequately coughing up respiratory secretions should have frequent clapping and drainage; meticulous attention must be paid to suctioning of oral secretions. Patients with suspected pulmonary tuberculosis should be placed in isolation rooms with negative pressure, frequent air exchange, and germicidal lamps to prevent nosocomial transmission of infection.

Patients treated for pneumococcal pneumonia should begin to improve within 48 hours after institution of antibiotics; patients with pneumonia caused by Gram-negative bacilli, staphylococci, *P. carinii,* and oral anaerobes may remain ill for longer periods after initiation of treatment. Several possibilities should be considered among patients who fail to improve or whose condition deteriorates during treatment.

Table 98–6 Initial Antibiotics for Treatment of Pneumonia

Pathogen	Treatment
Streptococcus pneumoniae	Ceftriaxone, 2 g IV*
Mycoplasma pneumoniae	Azithromycin, 500 mg PO day 1; 250 mg PO days 2–7
Chlamydophila pneumoniae	Azithromycin, 500 mg PO day 1; 250 mg PO days 2–7
Haemophilus influenzae	Ampicillin/sulbactam, 500 mg IV every 8 hr, or cefuroxime, 1 g IV every 8 hr
Staphylococcus aureus	Nafcillin, 3 g IV every 6 hr, or vancomycin, 1 g IV every 12 hr
Legionella pneumophila	Levofloxacin, 500 mg IV/PO four times daily, azithromycin, 500 mg PO day 1; 250 mg PO days 2–7
Ehrlichia chaffeensis	Doxycycline, 100 mg PO twice daily
Mixed oral flora (anaerobes)	Ampicillin/sulbactam, 500 mg IV every 8 hr, or clindamycin, 600 mg IV/PO every 8 hr
Gram-negative rods	Extended spectrum penicillin (e.g., piperacillin/tazobactam, 3.375 g IV every 6 hr) or third-generation cephalosporin (e.g., ceftazidime, 2 g IV every 8 hr)† or carbapenem (e.g., meropenem, 1 g IV every 8 hr) plus/or fluoroquinolone (e.g., ciprofloxacin, 200–400 mg IV or 250–750 mg PO twice daily)#
Tuberculosis	Isoniazid/vitamin B6, 300/50 mg PO every day, plus rifampin, 600 mg PO every day, ethambutol, 15–25 mg/kg PO every day, and pyrazinamide, 30 mg/kg PO every day

*Levofloxacin, 500 mg daily, for penicillin-allergic patients. Vancomycin, 1 g IV twice daily, for penicillin-resistant isolates.
†Antibiotics can be adjusted when sensitivity data are available.
IV = intravenously; PO = orally.
#Double coverage always indicated against *Pseudomonas aeruginosa*.

ENDOBRONCHIAL OBSTRUCTION

Physical examination may fail to show sounds of consolidation, and radiographs may show evidence of lobar collapse. Bronchoscopy can establish the diagnosis.

UNDRAINED EMPYEMA

Radiographs may not always distinguish between fluid and consolidation; ultrasonography and computed tomography can identify the fluid and provide direction for its drainage.

PURULENT PERICARDITIS

Purulent pericarditis should be suspected in a very ill patient with pneumonia involving a lobe adjacent to the pericardium. Chest pain, pulsus paradoxus, and electrocardiographic evidence of pericarditis are helpful when present but do not occur in all patients. Similarly, distended neck veins and pericardial friction rubs are present in only a minority of patients. Echocardiography or chest ultrasonography shows fluid in the pericardium. If purulent pericarditis is suggested, emergency pericardiocentesis can be life saving (see Chapter 11).

INCORRECT DIAGNOSIS OR TREATMENT

In cases in which clinical response is poor, a clinician with expertise in the diagnosis and treatment of pneumonia should review the patient's hospital course and admission sputum stains. Pulmonary embolism with infarction, a treatable disease, can prove fatal if misdiagnosed as bacterial pneumonia. Misinterpretation of sputum Gram-stained preparations with either failure to recognize an important pathogen or a treatment decision based on examination of an inadequate specimen is an avoidable pitfall of medical practice. Bronchoscopy should be considered, both to obtain better specimens for diagnosis and to exclude underlying endobronchial obstruction.

PATIENT WITH PLEURAL EFFUSION AND FEVER

The approach to patients with pleural effusion and fever is straightforward: The fluid must be examined. A pleural effusion infected with pneumococcus can often be treated with simple needle aspiration and antibiotics. If a bacterium other than *S. pneumoniae* is seen on Gram stain of pleural fluid or grown in culture, chest tube drainage is required. Pleural

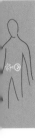

fluids that do not show organisms on Gram stain but are purulent or have a pH of less than 7.1 and/or a glucose concentration below 40 mg/dL may require chest tube drainage for satisfactory resolution. Patients with empyema complicating an aggressive bacterial pneumonia such as that caused by group A streptococci may benefit from early surgical débridement of the pleural space (decortication).

Pleurisy caused by *M. tuberculosis* is often an acute illness. In most patients, pneumonia is not present or readily appreciated. Inflammatory cells—polymorphonuclear leukocytes, mononuclear leukocytes, or both—are present in the pleural fluid. Mesothelial cells are usually sparse (<0.5% of the total cell count). Pleural fluid glucose levels are often low but may be normal. Mycobacteria are rarely seen on stains of pleural fluid. As many as one third of patients do not have positive tuberculin skin tests. Detection of *M. tuberculosis* antigen–specific, interferon-secreting T cells in pleural fluid may confirm a diagnosis of tuberculous pleuritis. Other causes of pleural effusion in this setting may be pulmonary infarction (less than one half of patients produce a hemorrhagic exudate), malignancy (most patients do not have fever), and connective tissue diseases, including systemic lupus erythematosus and rheumatoid arthritis. If the cause of the effusion is not evident, a biopsy of the pleura is needed.

Prevention

Pneumococcal pneumonia may be preventable by immunizing patients at high risk with polyvalent pneumococcal polysaccharide vaccine. The current polyvalent vaccine is 60% to 80% effective for a 5-year period in individuals with normal immune responses. Yearly immunization with influenza vaccine is also advised for many of these patients; by decreasing the attack rate of influenza, immunization also decreases morbidity and mortality resulting from secondary bacterial pneumonia (Table 98–7).

Patients without active tuberculosis but with skin test reactivity to purified protein derivative are at risk for reactivating their infection. The development of active tuberculosis can be prevented in most instances by treatment for 6 to 12 months with isoniazid, 300 mg/day. Indications for prophylaxis are shown in Table 98–8.

Table 98–7 Prevention of Pneumonia: Candidates for Pneumococcal and Influenza Vaccines

Factor	Pneumococcal Vaccine (may be repeated after 5–7 yr)	Influenza Vaccine (yearly)
Patient ≥65 years	Yes	Yes
Chronic lung or heart disease	Yes	Yes
Sickle cell disease	Yes	Consider
Asplenic patients	Yes	No
Hodgkin's disease	Yes	Consider
Multiple myeloma	Yes	Consider
Cirrhosis	Yes	Consider
Chronic alcoholism	Yes	Consider
Chronic renal failure	Yes	Consider
Cerebrospinal fluid leaks	Yes	No
Residents of chronic care facilities	Consider	Yes
Diabetes mellitus	Yes	Yes
Human immunodeficiency virus infection	Yes	Yes
Pregnant women in the second or third trimester during influenza season	No	Yes
Health care workers	No	Yes

Table 98–8   Indications for Prophylaxis with Isoniazid

Documented new skin test conversion to tuberculin over past 2 yr

Tuberculin-positive contacts of patients with active TB

Tuberculin-negative contacts of patients with active TB*

Tuberculin-positive persons with HIV infection

Anergic HIV-infected patients at high risk for TB

Positive tuberculin skin test of unknown duration in patients younger than 35 yr of age

Patients with radiographic evidence of inactive TB who have never received an adequate course of antituberculosis drugs

Consider isoniazid prophylaxis for patients with positive tuberculin skin tests and gastrectomy, diabetes mellitus, organ transplantation, silicosis, or prolonged (>1 mo) administration of corticosteroids or immunosuppressive drugs

*These individuals should have repeat skin tests 3 months after isoniazid is begun. If the repeat test is negative, isoniazid may be discontinued.
HIV = human immunodeficiency virus; TB = tuberculosis.

Prospectus for the Future

- Preservation of clinical skills for the diagnosis and treatment of pneumonia
- Better techniques for the rapid etiologic diagnosis of pneumonia
- Techniques for more rapid evaluation of antimicrobial susceptibility

- An increasing incidence of drug resistance in bacteria causing pneumonia, including pneumococci
- More outbreaks of life-threatening pneumonias caused by newly recognized pathogens

References

American Thoracic Society; Infectious Diseases Society of America: Guidelines for the management of adults with hospital-acquired, ventilator-associated, and healthcare-associated pneumonia. Am J Respir Crit Care Med 171(4):388–416, 2005.

Hansell DM, Armstrong P, Lynch DA, et al: Imaging of Diseases of the Chest. London, Elsevier-Mosby, 2005.

Infectious Diseases Society of America: Update of practice guidelines for the management of community-acquired pneumonia in immunocompetent adults. Clin Infect Dis 37(11):1405–1433, 2003.

Mandell LA, Bartlett JG, Dowell SF, et al; American Thoracic Society: Guidelines for the management of adults with community-acquired pneumonia: Diagnosis, assessment of severity, antimicrobial therapy, and prevention. Am J Respir Crit Care Med 163(7):1730–1754, 2001.

Infections of the Heart and Vessels

Benigno Rodríguez

Michael M. Lederman

Infective Endocarditis

Infective endocarditis (IE) ranges from an indolent illness with few systemic manifestations, readily responsive to antibiotic therapy, to a fulminant septicemic disease with malignant destruction of heart valves and life-threatening systemic embolization. The varied features of endocarditis relate in large measure to the different infecting organisms. *Streptococcus viridans* is the prototype of bacteria that originate in the mouth, infect previously abnormal heart valves, and may initially cause minimal symptoms despite progressive valvular damage. *Staphylococcus aureus,* in contrast, can invade previously normal valves and destroy them rapidly. Universally fatal in the pre-antibiotic era, endocarditis remains a life-threatening but potentially curable disorder.

EPIDEMIOLOGIC FACTORS

The average age of patients with endocarditis has increased in the antibiotic era to the current median of 58 years. This change can be attributed to the decreasing prevalence of rheumatic heart disease, the increasing prevalence of underlying degenerative heart disease, and the increasing frequency of procedures and practices predisposing older patients to bacteremia (genitourinary instrumentation, intravenous catheters, hemodialysis shunts). Rheumatic heart disease is now a predisposing factor in fewer than 25% of patients with IE in industrialized countries. Up to 24% of patients have congenital heart disease (exclusive of mitral valve prolapse). The propensity to develop endocarditis varies with the congenital lesion. For example, infection of a bicuspid aortic valve accounts for one fifth of cases of IE occurring in persons over the age of 60 years; a secundum atrial septal defect, however, rarely becomes infected. Mitral valve prolapse with valvular regurgitation is associated with more than one third of patients with endocarditis of the mitral valve. Intravenous drug users have a unique propensity to develop IE of the tricuspid valve. On long-term follow-up, patients with prosthetic heart valves have a 4% to

17% lifetime risk of IE, and this risk may be higher for those with bioprosthetic valves.

PATHOGENESIS

Endocarditis ensues when bacteria entering the bloodstream from an oral or other source lodge on heart valves that may already bear platelet-fibrin thrombi as a consequence of prior valvular damage or turbulent blood flow. The frequency of bacteremia is quite high after dental extraction (18% to 85%) or periodontal surgery (32% to 88%) but also is significant after everyday activities such as tooth brushing (0% to 26%) and chewing candy (17% to 51%). The ability of certain organisms to adhere to platelet-fibrin thrombi (for example, through production of extracellular dextran by some streptococcal strains), promotes occurrence of endocarditis after bacteremia caused by these organisms. The localization of infection is partly determined by the production of turbulent flow; thus, left ventricular infection is much more common than right ventricular infection, except among intravenous drug users. Vegetations usually are found on the valve surface facing the lower pressure chamber (e.g., atrial surface of the mitral valve), a relative haven for deposition of bacteria from the swift bloodstream. Occasionally, *jet lesions* develop in foci in which the regurgitant stream strikes the heart wall or the chordae tendineae. Once infection begins, bacteria proliferate freely within the interstices of the enlarging vegetation; in this relatively avascular site, they are protected from serum bactericidal factors and leukocytes.

The infection may cause rupture of the valve tissue itself or of its chordal structures, leading to either gradual or acute valvular regurgitation, with resultant congestive heart failure. Some virulent bacterial (e.g., *S. aureus, Haemophilus* species) or fungal vegetations may become large enough to obstruct the valve orifice or create a large embolus. Aneurysms of the sinus of Valsalva may occur and can rupture into the pericardial space. The conducting system may be affected by valve ring or myocardial abscesses. The infection may invade the interventricular septum, causing intramyocardial abscesses or septal rupture that can also damage the conduction system of the heart. Systemic septic emboli often occur with left ventricular endocarditis, and septic pulmonary emboli may occur with right ventricular endocarditis.

CLINICAL FEATURES

Some cases of endocarditis caused by oral streptococci become clinically apparent within 2 weeks of initiating events, such as dental extraction. Diagnosis is usually delayed further, however, because of the paucity of symptoms. If the causative organism is slow growing and produces an indolent syndrome, symptoms may be extremely protracted (6 months or longer) before definitive diagnosis. The symptoms and signs of IE relate to systemic infection, emboli (bland or septic), metastatic infective foci, congestive heart failure, or immune complex–associated lesions. The most common complaints in patients with IE are fever, chills, weakness, shortness of breath, night sweats, loss of appetite, and weight loss. Musculoskeletal symptoms develop in nearly one half of patients and may dominate the presentation. Fever is present in at least 90% of patients. Fever is more often absent in older or debilitated patients or in the setting of underlying congestive heart failure, liver or renal dysfunction, or previous antibiotic treatment. Heart murmurs are frequent (85%); changing murmurs (5% to 10%) and new cardiac murmurs, when observed, suggest the diagnosis of IE. With endocarditis involving the aortic or the mitral valve, congestive heart failure occurs in up to two thirds of patients; it may occur precipitously with perforation of a valve or rupture of chordae tendineae. More common peripheral manifestations of IE are presented in Table 99–1. Certain manifestations of subacute IE (i.e., splenomegaly, clubbing) are now less frequently observed than before, as more patients are diagnosed and treated earlier in the course of the illness. However, cutaneous Janeway lesions, resulting from septic emboli, remain a helpful diagnostic sign, which often occur early in the course of left ventricular endocarditis caused by *S. aureus* (Fig. 99–1). Splenomegaly (25% to 60%) and clubbing (10% to 15%) are more likely when symptoms have been prolonged.

The clinical syndrome of IE differs in intravenous drug users in that the majority do not have an underlying cardiac lesion, and only one third of proved cases have audible murmurs on patient admission. Fever remains the most common manifestation, and tricuspid valve infection is most common in this setting, probably the result of antecedent scarring of the tricuspid valve by injected particulate matter. Some patients exhibit pleuritic chest pain caused by septic pulmonary emboli, and round, cavitating infiltrates may be found on the chest radiograph, especially when *S. aureus* is the pathogen. The infective foci are initially centered in blood vessels; only after they erode into the bronchial system does cough develop, productive of bloody or purulent sputum.

Serious systemic emboli, associated with infection of the aortic or mitral valve, may cause dramatic findings, at times masking the systemic nature of IE. Embolism to the splenic artery may lead to left upper quadrant pain, sometimes radiating to the left shoulder, a friction rub, and/or left pleural effusion. Renal, cerebral, coronary, and mesenteric arteries are frequent sites of clinically important emboli.

Neurologic manifestations occur in up to one third of patients with IE and may be the predominant clinical features in 10% of patients, sometimes delaying the diagnosis. Central nervous system (CNS) embolization is one of the most serious complications, and acute neurologic deterioration is an ominous sign, being associated with a twofold to fourfold increase in mortality. IE must always be considered in the differential diagnosis of stroke in young adults, as well as in all patients with valvular heart disease. In addition to stroke caused by vascular occlusion by an infected embolus, toxic encephalopathy, which may mimic psychosis, and meningoencephalitis may also occur. The aseptic meningitis

Table 99–1 Peripheral Manifestations of Infective Endocarditis (IE)

Physical Finding (Frequency)	Pathogenesis	Most Common Organisms
Petechiae (20–40%) (red, nonblanching lesions in crops on conjunctivae, buccal mucosa, palate, extremities)	Vasculitis or emboli	*Streptococcus, Staphylococcus*
Splinter hemorrhages (15%) (linear, red-brown streaks most suggestive of IE when proximal in nail beds)	Vasculitis or emboli	*Staphylococcus, Streptococcus*
Osler's nodes (10–25%) (2- to 5-mm painful nodules on the pads of fingers or toes, usually with subacute IE)	Vasculitis	*Viridans streptococci*
Janeway lesions (<10%) (macular, red or hemorrhagic, painless patches on palms or soles) (in acute IE)	Emboli	*Staphylococcus*
Roth's spots (<5%) (oval, pale retinal lesions surrounded by hemorrhage)	Vasculitis	*Viridans streptococci*

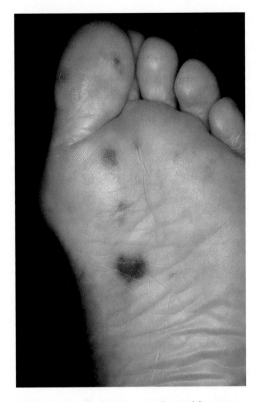

Figure 99–1 Janeway lesions in a patient with acute staphylococcal endocarditis. These intracutaneous lesions result from septic emboli. (From Sande MA, Strausbaugh LJ: Infective endocarditis. In Hook EW, Mandell GL, Gwaltney JM Jr, et al [eds]: Current Concepts of Infectious Diseases. New York, Wiley Press; 1977. Copyright © 1977 Wiley Press. This material is used by permission of John Wiley & Sons, Inc.)

or meningoencephalitis seen in patients with IE is not always clinically distinguishable from viral causes of a similar syndrome.

The consequences of CNS embolization depend on the site of lodging and the bacterial pathogen, and clinical syndromes caused by CNS emboli may be distinctive. Organisms such as *S. viridans* initially produce symptoms entirely attributable to the vascular occlusion; however, damage to the blood vessel can result in formation of a mycotic aneurysm that may leak or rupture at a later date. Resolution of aneurysms may occur after antimicrobial therapy. In many patients, however, surgical clipping is necessary to prevent recurrent hemorrhage; single aneurysms in accessible areas should be considered for prompt surgical clipping. *Staphylococcus aureus,* in contrast, produces progressive infection extending from the site of embolization; brain abscess and purulent meningitis are common sequelae.

The kidney can be the site of abscess formation, multiple infarcts, or immune complex glomerulonephritis. When renal dysfunction develops during antibiotic therapy, drug toxicity is an additional consideration.

LABORATORY FINDINGS

Nonspecific laboratory abnormalities occur in IE and often reflect chronic infection. These abnormalities include anemia (typically normocytic, normochromic in subacute

cases), reticulocytopenia, hypergammaglobulinemia, circulating immune complexes, false-positive serologic tests for syphilis, and rheumatoid factor. The presence of rheumatoid factor may be a helpful clue to diagnosis in patients with culture-negative endocarditis. Urinalysis frequently shows proteinuria (50% to 60%) and microscopic hematuria (10% to 50%). The presence of red blood cell casts is indicative of immune complex–mediated glomerulonephritis. The finding of Gram-positive cocci in the urine of a febrile patient with microscopic hematuria should always prompt consideration of the possibility of IE.

The bacteremia of IE is continuous but often low grade (often 1 to 100 bacteria per milliliter in subacute cases). Thus, in most instances, all blood cultures are positive. With subacute IE, three sets of blood cultures should be obtained in the first 24 hours of hospitalization. However, with acute IE, blood cultures should be obtained more rapidly (over 60 to 90 minutes), and the patient should be placed on appropriate antibiotics as soon as possible. Two or three additional blood cultures are important if the patient has received antibiotic therapy in the preceding 1 to 2 weeks and if initial blood cultures are negative at 48 to 72 hours. Five percent to 10% of patients with the clinical diagnosis of IE may have negative blood cultures, usually because of previous antibiotic therapy or fastidious organisms; cultures are more often negative in fungal endocarditis.

Echocardiography is recommended in all cases of suspected IE. Although transthoracic echocardiography (TTE) may be sufficient when suspicion is low and the patient's body habitus and clinical condition allow optimal imaging quality, transesophageal echocardiography (TEE) is considerably more sensitive, especially for small (less than 10 mm) vegetations; it is also capable of identifying such complications of IE as valve ring abscesses and valvular perforation more readily than TTE. Valvular vegetations can be demonstrated in most (75% to 95%) cases of IE by TEE, but the enhanced detail provided by TEE also mandates caution in interpreting the findings in the presence of other structural abnormalities, such as prosthetic valves, which may produce nonspecific echoes that are easily mistaken for vegetations.

A combination of the clinical, microbiologic, and echocardiographic features discussed previously, known as the Duke criteria, has been shown to be highly predictive of the likelihood of IE in various groups of patients, and recently proposed modifications have increased its specificity. The currently proposed Duke criteria are summarized in Table 99–2.

DIFFERENTIAL DIAGNOSIS

The diagnosis of IE usually is firmly established based on the clinical findings and the results of blood cultures. In some instances, the distinction between IE and nonendocarditis bacteremia may be difficult. Because the bacteremia is usually continuous in IE and intermittent in other bacteremias, the fraction of blood cultures that are positive may be helpful in distinguishing between these entities. The more frequent causative agents of IE are shown in Table 99–3; with increasing numbers of patients acquiring IE after invasive procedures or intravenous drug abuse, the relative importance of staphylococci has increased in recent years. In streptococcal infection, the speciation of the blood culture isolate

Table 99–2   Modified Duke Criteria for the Diagnosis of Infective Endocarditis

Major Criteria

Blood culture positive for IE, defined as (a) typical micro-organisms consistent with IE from two separate blood cultures: *viridans* streptococci, *Streptococcus bovis,* HACEK* group, *Staphylococcus aureus;* or community-acquired enterococci in the absence of a primary focus; (b) micro-organisms consistent with IE from persistently positive blood cultures defined as follows: at least two positive cultures of blood samples drawn >12 hr apart; or all of three or a majority of at least four separate cultures of blood (with first and last samples drawn at least 1 h apart); or (c) single positive blood culture for *Coxiella burnetii* or anti-phase 1 IgG antibody titer >1:800

Evidence of endocardial involvement: echocardiogram positive for IE defined as follows: oscillating intracardiac mass on valve or supporting structures, in the path of regurgitant jets, or on implanted material in the absence of an alternative anatomic explanation; or abscess; or new partial dehiscence of prosthetic valve; new valvular regurgitation (worsening or changing or pre-existing murmur not sufficient)

Minor Criteria

Predisposition, predisposing heart condition, or intravenous drug use
Fever, temperature >38° C
Vascular phenomena, major arterial emboli, septic pulmonary infarcts, mycotic aneurysm, intracranial hemorrhage, conjunctival hemorrhages, and Janeway lesions
Immunologic phenomena: glomerulonephritis, Osler's nodes, Roth's spots, and rheumatoid factor
Microbiologic evidence: positive blood culture but does not meet a major criterion as noted above (excluding single positive cultures for coagulase-negative staphylococci and organisms that do not cause endocarditis) or serologic evidence of active infection with organism consistent with IE

Interpretation

Definite infective endocarditis

Pathologic criteria
Micro-organisms demonstrated by culture or histologic examination of a vegetation, a vegetation that has embolized, or an intracardiac abscess specimen; or
Pathologic lesions; vegetation or intracardiac abscess confirmed by histologic examination showing active endocarditis
Clinical criteria
Two major criteria, or
One major criterion and three minor criteria, or
Five minor criteria

Possible infective endocarditis

One major criterion and one minor criterion, or
Three minor criteria

Infective endocarditis rejected

Firm alternative diagnosis explaining evidence of infective endocarditis, or
Resolution of clinical syndrome with antibiotic therapy for <4 days, or
No pathologic evidence of infective endocarditis at surgery or autopsy, with antibiotic therapy for <4 days, or
Does not meet criteria for possible infective endocarditis as above

Modified from Li JS, Sexton DJ, Mick N, et al: Proposed modifications to the Duke criteria for the diagnosis of infective endocarditis. Clin Infect Dis 30:633–638, 2000.
*HACEK = *Hemophilus sp, Actinobacillus sp, Cardiobacterium sp, Eikenella corrodens,* and *Kingella kingae;* IE = infective endocarditis; IgG = immunoglobulin G.

may provide circumstantial evidence for or against infection of the heart valves (Table 99–4). The identity of the causative organism may be helpful for other bacteria as well; the ratio of IE to non-IE bacteremias is approximately 1:1 for *S. aureus,* 1:7 for group B streptococci, and 1:200 for *Escherichia coli. Streptococcus bovis* bacteremia and endo-carditis are often (<50%) associated with colonic carcinomas or polyps. Isolation of this organism in blood cultures warrants thorough evaluation of the lower gastrointestinal tract.

The initial presentation of IE can be misleading: The young adult may exhibit a stroke, pneumonia, or meningitis; the older patient may show confusion or simply fatigue

Table 99–3   Frequency of Infecting Micro-organisms in Endocarditis

Native Valve (%)		Prosthetic Valve Endocarditis(%)			Endocarditis in IVDU (%)	
			Early	Late		
Streptococci	50	Coagulase-negative staphylococci	33	29	S. aureus	60
Enterococci	10	S. aureus	15	11	Streptococci	13
Staphylococcus aureus	20	Gram-negative bacilli	17	11	Gram-negative bacilli	8
HACEK	5	Fungi	13	5	Enterococci	7
Culture negative	5	Streptococci	9	36	Fungi	5
		Diphtheroids	9	3	Polymicrobial	5
					Culture negative	5

HACEK = Hemophilus, Actinobacillus, Cardiobacterium, Eikenella, Kingella; IVDU = intravenous drug user.
From Levison ME: Infective endocarditis. In Bennett JC, Plum F (eds): Cecil Textbook of Medicine, 20th ed. Philadelphia, WB Saunders, 1996, pp 1596–1605.

Table 99–4   Relative Frequency of Infective Endocarditis (IE) and Non-IE Bacteremias for Various Streptococci

Species	IE:Non-IE
Streptococcus mutans	14:1
Streptococcus bovis	6:1
Streptococcus faecalis	1:1
Group B streptococci	1:7
Group A streptococci	1:32

Modified from Parker MT, Ball LC: Streptococci and aerococci associated with systemic infection in man. J Med Microbiol 9:275, 1976.

or malaise without fever. The index of suspicion for IE therefore must be high, and blood cultures should be obtained in these varied settings if antibiotic use is contemplated.

Major problems in diagnosis arise if antibiotics have been administered before blood is cultured or if blood cultures are negative. Attempts to culture slow-growing organisms, including those with particular nutritional requirements, should be done in consultation with a clinical microbiologist. The HACEK organisms (Hemophilus sp, Actinobacillus sp, Cardiobacterium sp, Eikenella corrodens, and Kingella kingae) collectively account for up to 5% to 8% of patients of endocarditis. These organisms are fastidious Gram-negative organisms, which grow slowly in carbon dioxide–enriched media. Laboratory personnel should be notified when these organisms are suggested. The differential diagnosis of culture-negative endocarditis includes Q fever, acute rheumatic fever, multiple pulmonary emboli,

atrial myxoma, systemic vasculitis, and nonbacterial thrombotic endocarditis. Nonbacterial thrombotic endocarditis (sometimes called marantic endocarditis) occurs in patients with severe wasting, whether caused by malignancy or other conditions. Additionally, patients with systemic lupus erythematosus may develop sterile valvular vegetations, termed Libman-Sacks lesions, on the undersurfaces of the valve leaflets. These diagnoses should be considered and excluded, if possible, before beginning a prolonged course of therapy for presumed culture-negative IE. The absence of vegetations on TEE makes a diagnosis of endocarditis unlikely.

MANAGEMENT AND OUTCOME

The outcome of IE is determined by the extent of valvular destruction, the size and friability of vegetations, the presence and location of emboli, and the choice of appropriate antibiotics. These factors, in turn, are influenced by the nature of the causative organism and delays in diagnosis. The goal of antibiotic therapy is to halt further valvular damage and to cure the infection. Surgery may be necessary for hemodynamic stabilization, prevention of embolization, or control of drug-resistant infection.

Antibiotics should be selected based on the clinical setting (Tables 99–5 and 99–6) and started as soon as blood cultures are obtained if the diagnosis of IE appears highly likely and the course is suggestive of active valvular destruction or systemic embolization. The antibiotics can be adjusted later based on culture and sensitivity data.

Antibiotics

A number of regimens have been advocated for the treatment of IE resulting from each of the causative organisms. Because few of these regimens have been subjected to valid comparative trials, the selection of drugs, dosages, and duration remains somewhat empiric. Similarly, although sophisticated laboratory tests such as serum bactericidal activity may be used to monitor and adjust drug regimens, they have not been standardized or validated adequately. Nonetheless, each regimen must be capable of bactericidal activity against the offending pathogen and must be of sufficient duration, at least 6 weeks in left ventricular endocarditis caused by S. aureus, to sterilize the affected heart valves.

Table 99–5 Syndromes Suggesting Specific Bacteria Causing Infective Endocarditis

Indolent Course (Subacute)

Streptococcus viridans
Streptococcus bovis
Streptococcus faecalis
Fastidious Gram-negative rods

Aggressive Course (Acute)

Staphylococcus aureus
Streptococcus pneumoniae
Streptococcus pyogenes
Neisseria gonorrhoeae

Drug Users

S. aureus and coagulase-negative staphylococci
Pseudomonas aeruginosa
S. faecalis
Candida species
Bacillus species

Intravenous Catheters

S. aureus and coagulase-negative staphylococci
Candida species
Aerobic Gram-negative bacilli

Animal Contact

Bartonella species
Pasteurella species
Capnocytophaga species
Brucella species
Coxiella burnetti

Frequent Major Emboli

Haemophilus species
Bacteroides species

Most, but not all, strains of *S. viridans* and nonenterococcal group D streptococci, such as *S. bovis,* are exquisitely sensitive to penicillin; the serum bactericidal level of penicillin for these organisms is less than 0.1 mcg/mL. Aqueous penicillin G, 12 million U/day given intravenously for 4 weeks, is curative in almost all patients, as is a 2-week course of penicillin G plus gentamicin in younger patients with uncomplicated disease.

Treatment of enterococcal endocarditis and IE caused by other penicillin-resistant streptococci is more difficult because of frequent relapses and high mortality. The recommended regimen for penicillin-sensitive strains is intravenous aqueous penicillin G, 20 million U/day, plus intravenous gentamicin, 3 mg/kg/day. This relatively low dose of aminoglycoside is associated with a low incidence of nephrotoxicity. The aminoglycoside dose should be adjusted according to measured serum levels and the bactericidal activity of serum. Regimens to treat enterococcal infection should be continued for 6 weeks because of high relapse rates with shorter duration of treatment. Culture-negative endocarditis should be treated similarly.

Determination of the minimum inhibitory and bactericidal concentrations (MIC and MBC, respectively) are helpful in the management of IE caused by penicillin-resistant organisms, given that therapeutic success is largely dependent on the ability to achieve a bactericidal effect in the relative sanctuary of the vegetation. Serum bactericidal determinations have been used to assess the appropriateness of antibiotic therapy of IE (especially in enterococcal IE), but systematic reviews of the evidence have failed to show an association between the classically recommended cut-off of a 1:8 dilution and the likelihood of therapeutic success.

S. aureus endocarditis should be treated with intravenous nafcillin, 12 g/day, unless the isolate is penicillin sensitive, in which case penicillin, 12 million U/day, is the treatment of choice. Infection with a methicillin-resistant species of *Staphylococcus* necessitates the use of vancomycin. The addition of an aminoglycoside hastens clearance of bacteremia and is often used during the initial 4 to 7 days of therapy, especially in critically ill patients. The duration of antibiotic therapy for staphylococcal endocarditis of the mitral or aortic valve is a minimum of 6 weeks.

In the patient with streptococcal or staphylococcal IE and a history of serious penicillin allergy, vancomycin can be

Table 99–6 Antibiotic Agents for Treatment of Endocarditis*

Staphylococcus aureus	Nafcillin or cefazolin or vancomycin ± gentamicin
Streptococcus pneumoniae	PCN G or ampicillin
Streptococcus viridans, Streptococcus bovis	PCN G or ampicillin or ceftriaxone + gentamicin
Enterococcus	Ampicillin or PCN G or vancomycin + gentamicin
Enterococcus, vancomycin-resistant	Linezolid or quinupristin-dalfopristin or imipenem ± ampicillin
HACEK organisms	Ceftriaxone, cefotoxime, or ampicillin-sulbactam
Fungal	Amphotericin B + surgery
Pseudomonas	Antipseudomonal penicillin (e.g., ticarcillin) or ceftazidime or cefepime + tobramycin

*See text for details. The choice among the various alternatives presented should be guided by sensitivity results. Therapy for prosthetic valve endocarditis may differ.
PCN G = penicillin G; HACEK = *Hemophilus sp, Actinobacillus sp, Cardiobacterium sp, Eikenella corrodens,* and *Kingella kingae.*

substituted for penicillin. Among patients at risk for complicated disease, consideration should be given to penicillin desensitization.

Pseudomonas endocarditis is a particular problem in intravenous drug users. Therapy should be initiated with tobramycin, 8 mg/kg/day given intravenously, plus an extended-spectrum penicillin such as ticarcillin, 3 g given intravenously every 4 hours, or a third- or fourth-generation cephalosporin with antipseudomonal activity for at least 6 weeks. The unusually high doses of aminoglycosides have improved the outcome of medical therapy of *Pseudomonas* infection of the tricuspid valve in younger patients with little nephrotoxicity. Left ventricular *Pseudomonas aeruginosa* infections, however, most often require surgery for cure. Measuring serum drug levels and adjusting dosages as appropriate is particularly critical when aminoglycosides are used.

Fungal endocarditis is usually refractory to antibiotics and requires surgery for management. Amphotericin B generally is administered to such patients before surgery but is not in itself curative.

Surgery

The indications for early surgery in IE need to be individualized and forged by discussions with the cardiac surgeon. Refractory infection is a clear indication for surgery; the requirement for surgery is predictable in IE caused by certain organisms. Persistence of bacteremia for longer than 7 to 10 days, despite the administration of appropriate antibiotics, frequently reflects paravalvular extension of infection with development of valve ring abscess or myocardial abscesses. Medical cure is not likely in this setting. Intravenous drug users show an increased likelihood of having IE caused by organisms refractory to medical therapy (e.g., *Pseudomonas* species, fungi). Refractory tricuspid endocarditis may be amenable to valve débridement or excision without immediate placement of a prosthetic valve. Tricuspid valvulectomy, however, is often followed by gradual onset of right-ventricular heart failure.

Protracted fever is not unusual in patients undergoing treatment of endocarditis and should not automatically be equated with refractory infection. In fact, 10% of patients remain febrile for more than 2 weeks, and persistent fever is not an independent indication for surgery, particularly when tricuspid endocarditis is complicated by multiple septic pulmonary emboli with necrotizing pneumonia. Delayed defervescence also is common, despite appropriate antimicrobial therapy, with endocarditis caused by *S. aureus* and enteric bacteria, associated with multiple systemic abscesses.

Congestive heart failure refractory to medical therapy is the most frequent indication for early cardiac surgery. The extent of valvular dysfunction may be difficult to gauge clinically, particularly in patients with acute aortic regurgitation; in the absence of compensatory ventricular dilation, classic physical signs associated with aortic regurgitation, such as wide pulse pressure and decrescendo murmur throughout diastole, may not be present. Echocardiography and cardiac catheterization may be necessary to evaluate the extent of aortic regurgitation. When congestive heart failure develops in the patient with *S. aureus* IE, aortic valvular destruction usually is extensive, necessitating early surgery. Delaying surgery to prolong the course of antibiotic therapy is never

appropriate if the patient is hemodynamically unstable or fulfills other criteria for surgical intervention. The incidence of prosthetic valve endocarditis (PVE) is not influenced by duration of preoperative antibiotics.

Recurrent major systemic embolization is another indication for surgery. If valvular function is preserved, vegetations sometimes can be removed without valve replacement. Septal abscess, although often difficult to recognize clinically, and aneurysms of the sinus of Valsalva are absolute indications for surgery.

Prosthetic Valve Endocarditis

PVE complicates 3% to 6% of cardiac valve replacements within 5 years after surgery. Two separate clinical syndromes have been identified. Early PVE occurs within 60 days of surgery and most often is caused by *Staphylococcus epidermidis,* Gram-negative enteric bacilli, *S. aureus,* or diphtheroids. The prosthesis may be contaminated at the time of surgery or seeded by bacteremia from extracardiac sites (e.g., intravenous cannula, indwelling urinary bladder catheter, wound infection, pneumonia). In addition to forming vegetations, which may be bulky and cause obstruction, particularly of mitral valve prostheses, circumferential spread of infection may cause dehiscence and paravalvular leak at the site of an aortic prosthesis. The combination of intravenous vancomycin, 2 g/day, and intravenous gentamicin, 3 mg/kg/day, plus oral rifampin, 900 mg/day, is indicated to treat *S. epidermidis* infection. Other infections should be treated with synergistic bactericidal combinations of antibiotics based on in vitro sensitivity testing. Surgery is mandatory in the presence of moderate to severe congestive heart failure. The rate of mortality from early PVE remains high.

Late PVE is most frequently caused by *S. viridans* bacteremia from an oral site that seeds a re-endothelialized valve surface. Treatment with intravenous aqueous penicillin G, 12 to 20 million U/day, or ceftriaxone, 2 g/day, plus intravenous gentamicin, 3 mg/kg/day, is appropriate. The prognosis for cure with antibiotic therapy alone is improved in patients infected with penicillin-sensitive streptococci. Moderate to severe congestive heart failure is the main indication for surgery. The rate of mortality from late PVE may be as high as 40%.

Prophylaxis of Infective Endocarditis

Patients with prosthetic heart valves or mitral or aortic valvular heart disease are at relatively high risk of developing IE. Mitral valve prolapse associated with a systolic murmur is another risk factor. Neither the value of antibiotic prophylaxis nor the optimal regimens have been definitively established. Conditions that place patients at risk for endocarditis are presented in Table 99–7. Procedures for which prophylaxis is given are listed in Table 99–8, and appropriate prophylactic antibiotic regimens are presented in Tables 99–9 and 99–10.

Administration of antibiotics has become an accepted practice for patients undergoing open-heart surgery, includ-

Table 99–7 Prophylaxis of Infective Endocarditis

Prophylaxis for Specific Procedures Recommended

High-risk category

Prosthetic heart valves
Prior endocarditis
Complex cyanotic congenital heart disease
Surgical systemic pulmonary shunts

Moderate-risk category

Most other congenital cardiac malformations
Acquired valvular dysfunction (e.g., rheumatic heart disease)
Hypertrophic cardiomyopathy
Mitral valve prolapse with regurgitation or thickened leaflets

Prophylaxis *Not* Recommended

Mitral valve prolapse without murmur and without
   regurgitant or myxomatous leaflets on echocardiogram
Physiologic murmurs
Isolated secundum atrial septal defect
Surgically repaired atrial septal defect, ventricular septal
   defect, patent ductus arteriosus (after 6 mo)
Cardiac pacemakers and defibrillators
History of rheumatic fever or Kawasaki's disease without
   valvular dysfunction
Previous coronary artery bypass surgery

Table 99–8 Procedures That Require Antimicrobial Prophylaxis against Infective Endocarditis

Dental Procedures Involving Significant Bleeding from Hard or Soft Tissues

Extractions
Periodontal procedures
Implant placement
Endodontic (root canal) procedures
Subgingival placement of orthodontic bands but not brackets
Intraligamentary local anesthetic injections
Prophylactic cleaning of teeth or implants where bleeding is
   expected

Respiratory Tract Procedures

Tonsillectomy and/or adenoidectomy
Surgical procedures that involve respiratory mucosa
Rigid bronchoscopy

Gastrointestinal Tract Procedures

Sclerotherapy for varices
Dilation of esophageal stricture
Endoscopic retrograde cholangiopancreatography with biliary
   obstruction
Biliary tract surgery
Surgery involving gastrointestinal mucosa

Genitourinary Tract Procedures

Prostatic surgery
Cytoscopy
Urethral dilation

Table 99–9 Prophylactic Regimens Recommended for Dental, Oral, Respiratory Tract, or Esophageal Procedures in Susceptible Patients

Amoxicillin, 2.0 g 1 hr before the procedure
Allergic to penicillin: clindamycin, 600 mg, 1 hr before the
   procedure; or cephalexin or cefadroxil, 2.0 g, 1 hr before
   the procedure; or azithromycin or clarithromycin, 500 mg
   1 hr before the procedure

Table 99–10 Prophylactic Regimens for Genitourinary or Gastrointestinal (Excluding Esophageal) Procedures

High-risk patients: ampicillin, 2.0 g IM/IV, plus gentamicin,
   1.5 mg/kg (not to exceed 120 mg) IM/IV, within 30 min of
   starting the procedure; 6 hr later: ampicillin, 1 g IM/IV, or
   amoxicillin, 1 g by mouth
High-risk patients allergic to penicillin: vancomycin, 1.0 g IV,
   over 1 to 2 hr, plus gentamicin, 1.5 mg/kg (not to exceed
   120 mg) IM/IV, within 30 min of starting the procedure
Moderate-risk patients: amoxicillin, 2 g by mouth, 1 hr before
   the procedure, or ampicillin, 2 g IM/IV, within 30 min of
   starting the procedure

IM = intramuscular; IV = intravenous.

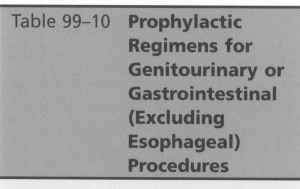

ing valve replacement. Intravenous cefazolin, 2.0 g at induction of anesthesia, repeated 8 and 16 hours later, or intravenous vancomycin, 1.0 g at induction and 0.5 g 8 and 16 hours later, is an appropriate regimen. Cardiac diagnostic procedures (catheterization), pacemaker placement, and coronary artery bypass do not pose sufficient risk to warrant the use of prophylactic antibiotics for IE or PVE.

Devices that are associated with high rates of infection and bacteremia (e.g., intravenous cannulas, indwelling urinary bladder catheters) should be avoided in hospitalized patients at risk for IE, if at all possible; established local infections should be treated promptly and vigorously.

Bacterial Endarteritis and Suppurative Phlebitis

Bacterial endarteritis usually develops by one of three mechanisms: (1) arteries, particularly those with intimal abnormalities, may become infected as a consequence of transient bacteremia; (2) during the course of IE, septic emboli to vasa vasorum may lead to mycotic aneurysms; or (3) blood vessels also may be infected by direct extension from contiguous foci and trauma.

A septic presentation is characteristic of endarteritis caused by organisms such as *S. aureus*. Besides sepsis, the major problem caused by endarteritis is hemorrhage. Between 3% and 4% of patients with IE develop intracranial mycotic aneurysms. Mycotic aneurysms in IE typically are situated peripherally and in the distribution of the middle cerebral artery. Focal seizures, focal neurologic signs, or aseptic meningitis may herald catastrophic rupture of such aneurysms. These premonitory findings therefore indicate the need for evaluation with arteriography; neurosurgical intervention should be considered if accessible lesions are demonstrated.

Infection of an atherosclerotic plaque can occur as a complication of bacteremia, particularly in older patients with bacteremia caused by *Salmonella* species. Traumatic endarteritis with pseudoaneurysm often complicates arterial injection of illicit drugs but rarely complicates arterial catheterizations. Treatment often requires combined medical and surgical management; antibiotic selection should be based on the results of in vitro sensitivity testing.

Suppurative thrombophlebitis usually is a complication of the use of intravenous plastic cannulas. Burn patients, especially those with lower extremity catheterization, are at particular risk. Typically, intravenous cannulas have been left in place 5 days or more. In many instances, the vein is sclerosed and tender, and the surrounding skin is erythematous. The vein should be milked to identify pus. If pus is present, or if bacteremia and fever persist despite antibiotic therapy, involved segments of vein must be excised. Initial presumptive therapy should be selected to ensure coverage of the most common pathogens, *Staphylococcus* species (vancomycin, 2 g/day given intravenously) and Enterobacteriaceae (gentamicin, 5 mg/kg/day given intravenously). When infection of an intravenous cannula is suggested, the catheter should be removed and 2-inch segments rolled across a blood agar plate. The growth of more than 15 colonies suggests infection (see also Chapter 105).

Suppurative phlebitis is preventable. Peripheral intravenous cannulas should be inserted aseptically and replaced at least every 72 hours by well-trained personnel.

Prospectus for the Future

- Refinement in imaging techniques for the diagnosis and management of infectious endocarditis and its complications

- Increased use of molecular microbiology techniques for the diagnosis of culture-negative IE

References

Baddour LM, Wilson WR, Bayer AS, et al: Infective endocarditis: Diagnosis, antimicrobial therapy, and management of complications. AHA scientific statement. Circulation 111:e394–e434, 2005.

Chambers HF: Infective endocarditis. In Goldman L, Bennett JC (eds): Cecil Textbook of Medicine, 22nd ed. Philadelphia, Elsevier, 2005, pp 1794–1803.

Dajani AS, Taubert KA, Wilson W, et al: Prevention of bacterial endocarditis: Recommendations by the American Heart Association. JAMA 277:1794–1801, 1997.

Lederman MM, Sprague L, Wallis RS, et al: Duration of fever during infective endocarditis. Medicine 71:52, 1992.

Moreillon P, Que YA: Infective endocarditis. Lancet 363:139–149, 2004.

Mylonakis E, Calderwood SB: Infective endocarditis in adults. N Engl J Med 345:1318–1330, 2001.

Skin and Soft Tissue Infections

Christoph Lange

Michael M. Lederman

Innate immune defense mechanisms render the normal skin remarkably resistant to infection. Most common infections of the skin are initiated by breaks in the epithelium. Hematogenous seeding of the skin by pathogens is less frequent by comparison.

Some superficial infections, such as folliculitis and furuncles, may be treated with local measures. Other superficial infections (e.g., impetigo, cellulitis) necessitate systemic antibiotics. Deeper soft tissue infections, such as fasciitis and myonecrosis, necessitate surgical débridement. As a general rule, infections of the face and hands should be treated particularly aggressively because of the risks of intracranial spread in the former and the potential loss of function as a result of closed-space infection in the latter.

Superficial Infections of the Skin

CIRCUMSCRIBED INFECTIONS OF THE SKIN

Vesicles, papules, pustules, nodules, and ulcerations are the lesions in this category (Table 100–1).

Folliculitis is a superficial infection of hair follicles. The lesions are crops of red papules or pustules that are often pruritic; careful examination using a hand lens shows hair in the center of most papules. Staphylococci, yeast, and, occasionally, *Pseudomonas* species are the most common pathogens. Local treatment with cleansing and hot compresses is usually sufficient. Topical antibacterial or antifungal agents also may be useful. The skin lesions of disseminated candidiasis seen in neutropenic patients may resemble folliculitis. In this setting, skin biopsy readily distinguishes these two processes; in disseminated disease, yeast is found within blood vessels and not simply surrounding the hair follicle.

Furuncles and carbuncles are subcutaneous abscesses caused by *Staphylococcus aureus*. The lesions are red, tender nodules that may have a surrounding cellulitis, and occur most prominently on the face and back of the neck. They often drain spontaneously. Furuncles may be treated with moist hot compresses. The larger carbuncles necessitate incision and drainage if fluctuant. Anti-staphylococcal antibi-

otics should be given if the patient has systemic symptoms such as fever or malaise, if accompanying cellulitis is present, or if the lesions are on the head.

Impetigo is a superficial infection of the skin caused by group A streptococci, although *S. aureus* may also be found in the lesions. Impetigo is seen primarily among children who initially develop a vesicle on the skin surface; this vesicle rapidly becomes pustular and breaks down, leaving the characteristic dry, golden crust. This pruritic lesion is highly contagious and spreads by the child's hands to other sites on the body or to other children. Gram stain shows gram-positive cocci in chains (streptococci); occasionally, clusters of staphylococci are also seen. Certain strains of streptococci causing impetigo have been associated with the later development of poststreptococcal glomerulonephritis. The differential diagnosis of impetigo includes herpes simplex infection and varicella. These viral lesions may become pustular; Gram stain of an unruptured viral vesicle or pustule should not, however, contain bacteria. A Tzanck preparation (see Chapter 92) (or assay for viral antigens for optimal sensitivity) can establish the diagnosis of herpes simplex or varicella if the differential diagnosis is uncertain. Penicillin remains generally effective for the treatment of impetigo; however, some authorities prefer penicillinase-resistant penicillins (e.g., dicloxacillin) because penicillinase-producing staphylococci are often also present in these lesions. Large bullous lesions, particularly in children, suggest bullous impetigo caused by *S. aureus*. This condition should be treated with penicillinase-resistant penicillins (or a newer macrolide for the penicillin-allergic patient). Antibiotics do not appear to affect the development of poststreptococcal glomerulonephritis, but they will prevent the spread of infection to others.

Ecthyma gangrenosum is a cutaneous manifestation of disseminated gram-negative rod infection, usually caused by *Pseudomonas aeruginosa* in patients with neutropenia. The initial lesion is a vesicle or papule with an erythematous halo. Although generally small (<2 cm), the initial lesion may exceed 20 cm in diameter. In a short time, the vesicle ulcerates, leaving a necrotic ulcer with surrounding erythema or a violaceous rim. Gram stain of an aspirate may show gram-negative rods; cultures of the aspirate are generally positive. Biopsy of the lesion shows venous thrombosis, often with

Table 100–1 Circumscribed Cutaneous Infections (Predominant Organism)

Folliculitis (*Staphylococcus aureus*, *Candida* species)
Furuncles, carbuncles (*S. aureus*)
Impetigo (group A streptococci, *S. aureus*)
Ecthyma gangrenosum (gram-negative bacilli [systemic infection])
Anthrax
Vesicular or vesiculopustular lesions of the skin
  Impetigo
  Folliculitis
  Herpes simplex virus infection
  Varicella-zoster virus infection
  Rickettsialpox
Ulcerative lesions of the skin
  Pressure sores
  Stasis ulcerations
  Diabetic ulcerations
  Sickle cell ulcers
  Mycobacterial infection
  Fungal infection
  Ecthyma gangrenosum
  Syphilis
  Chancroid

bacteria demonstrable within the blood vessel walls. Because these lesions are manifestations of gram-negative rod bacteremia, treatment should be instituted immediately with an aminoglycoside or ciprofloxacin plus a third-generation cephalosporin, piperacillin, or a carbapenem to protect against *P. aeruginosa* until the results of culture and sensitivity studies are known (see also Chapter 95).

Herpes Simplex Virus

Oral infections caused by herpes simplex virus are discussed in Chapter 97, and genital infections are discussed in Chapter 106. On occasion, infection with this virus occurs on extraoral or extragenital sites, usually on the hands. This circumstance is most often the case in health care workers but also may result from sexual contact or from autoinoculation. The virus may produce a painful erythema, usually at the junction of the nail bed and skin (whitlow). The erythema progresses to a vesiculopustular lesion. At both stages of infection, herpetic whitlow can resemble a bacterial infection (paronychia). Distinguishing between herpetic and bacterial infections is important because incision and drainage of a herpetic whitlow are contraindicated. When more than one digit is involved, herpes is highly likely. Puncture of the purulent center of a paronychia and Gram stain of the exudate allow prompt and accurate diagnosis. In the case of herpetic whitlow, bacteria are not present unless the lesion has already drained and become superinfected. In the case of a bacterial paronychia, bacteria are readily seen. Recurrences of herpetic whitlow may be seen but are generally less severe than the primary infection. Treatment with oral acyclovir, famciclovir, or valacyclovir may shorten the duration of symptoms.

Varicella-Zoster Virus

Primary infection with varicella-zoster virus (chickenpox) is thought to occur through the respiratory route but may also occur through contact with infected skin lesions. Viremia results in crops of papules that progress to vesicles and then to pustules, followed by crusting. The lesions are most prominent on the trunk (**Web Fig. 100–1**). Varicella-zoster virus infection is almost always a disease of childhood. Systemic symptoms may precede development of the characteristic rash by 1 or 2 days but are mild, except in the case of an immunocompromised patient or primary infection in the adult. In the immunocompromised patient, chickenpox can produce a fatal systemic illness. In otherwise healthy adults, chickenpox can be a serious illness, with life-threatening pneumonia. Clinical diagnosis is based on the characteristic appearance of the rash. Impetigo and folliculitis are readily distinguished clinically by Gram stain or Tzanck preparation of the pustule contents. Disseminated herpes simplex virus infection is seen only in the immunocompromised host or in patients with eczema. Viral culture or viral antigen detection will distinguish herpes simplex from herpes zoster in these settings. Most patients with rickettsialpox, which, in rare cases, is confused with chickenpox, also have an ulcer or eschar that precedes the generalized rash by 3 to 7 days and represents the bite of the infected mouse mite, which transmits the disease. Although officially eradicated, smallpox must be included in the differential diagnosis of chickenpox when bioterrorism might be an issue. Lesions of smallpox are characteristically larger than those of varicella, are sometimes umbilicated, are more concentrated peripherally than the central lesions of varicella, and all tend to be at the same stage of development.

Immunocompromised children exposed to varicella should receive prophylaxis with zoster immune globulin. Immunocompromised persons and seriously ill patients with varicella should be treated with acyclovir. Prophylaxis within 96 hours of exposure with varicella-zoster immune globulin is recommended for adults at risk for complications (immunodeficiencies, malignancies, pregnancy). Active immunization against varicella-zoster virus infection is now recommended for all children and susceptible adults in the United States.

After primary infection, the varicella-zoster virus persists in a latent state within sensory neurons of the dorsal root ganglia. The infection may reactivate, producing the syndrome of zoster (shingles). Pain in the distribution of the affected nerve root precedes the rash by a few days. Depending on the dermatome, the pain may mimic pleurisy, myocardial infarction, or gallbladder disease. A clue to the presence of early zoster infection is the finding of dysesthesia, an unpleasant sensation when the involved dermatome is gently stroked by the examiner's hand. The appearance of papules and vesicles in a unilateral dermatomal distribution confirms the diagnosis. Herpes zoster infections of certain dermatomes merit special attention. Ramsay Hunt syndrome can be caused by infection involving the geniculate ganglia and produces painful eruption of the ear canal and tympanic membrane, often associated with an ipsilateral seventh cranial nerve (facial nerve) palsy. Infection involving the second branch of the fifth cranial nerve (trigeminal nerve) often produces lesions of the cornea. This infection should be treated promptly with systemic acyclovir to prevent loss of visual acuity. A clue to possible ophthalmic involvement is the presence of vesicles on the tip of the nose.

In most instances, dermatomal zoster is a disease of the otherwise healthy adult. However, immunocompromised patients (e.g., persons with human immunodeficiency virus infection) are at greater risk for re-activation of this virus. Patients with zoster should receive a thorough history and physical evaluation; in the absence of specific suggestive findings or recurrent episodes of zoster, these patients do not require an exhaustive evaluation for a malignancy or immunodeficiency.

In older, nonimmunocompromised patients, postherpetic neuralgia (severe, prolonged burning pain, with occasional lightning-like stabs in the involved dermatomes) may persist for 1 to 2 years and become disabling. A brief course of corticosteroids (40 to 60 mg of prednisone, tapered over 3 to 4 weeks) during the acute episode of zoster shortens the duration of acute neuritic pain but does not prevent postherpetic neuralgia. Initiation of treatment during the first 72 hours with antiviral drugs (e.g., valacyclovir, famciclovir) accelerates the healing of lesions and may decrease the occurrence of postherpetic neuralgia.

Cutaneous Mycobacterial and Fungal Diseases

Mycobacteria and fungi can produce cutaneous infection, exhibiting generally as papules, nodules, ulcers, crusting lesions, or lesions with a combination of these features. *Mycobacterium marinum,* for example, can produce inflammatory nodules that ascend through lymphatic channels of the arm among individuals who keep or are exposed to fish; similar lesions caused by *Sporothrix schenckii* may be seen among gardeners. *Blastomyces dermatitidis* and *Coccidioides immitis* are other fungi that produce skin nodules or ulcerations.

As a general rule, a biopsy should be done on a chronic inflammatory nodule, crusted lesion, or nonhealing ulceration that is not readily attributable to pressure, vascular insufficiency, or venous stasis. Mycobacteria and fungi should be carefully sought, using acid-fast and silver stains, and appropriate cultures should be performed. In specialized laboratories, gene amplification by polymerase chain reaction may be used to identify the causative microbe rapidly.

Ulcerative Lesions of the Skin

A common factor in the pathogenesis of many skin ulcers is the presence of vascular insufficiency. Microbial infection of these lesions is secondary but often extends into soft tissue and bone.

Pressure sores occur at weight-bearing sites among individuals who are incapable of moving. Patients with stroke, quadriplegia, or paraplegia, or patients in a coma who remain supine, rapidly develop skin necrosis at the sacrum, spine, and heels because pressures at these weight-bearing sites can exceed local perfusion pressure. Patients who are kept immobile on their sides will ulcerate over the greater trochanter of the femur. As the skin sloughs, bacteria colonize the necrotic tissues; abetted by further pressure-induced necrosis, the infection extends to deeper structures. Infected pressure sores are common causes of fever and occasional causes of bacteremia in debilitated patients. Not infrequently, a necrotic membrane hides a deep infection. The physician should probe the extent of a pressure sore with a sterile glove; potential sites of deeper infection should be probed with a sterile needle. Necrotic material must be débrided, and the ulceration may be treated with topical antiseptics and relief of pressure. Systemic antibiotics are indicated when bacteremia, osteomyelitis, or significant cellulitis is present. Anaerobes and gram-negative rods are the most frequent isolates. Skin grafting can be used to repair extensive ulceration in patients who can eventually be mobilized. Prevention of pressure sores by frequent turning and by inspecting pressure sites among immobilized patients is far more effective than treatment. The use of specialized beds that distribute pressure evenly may be of particular value among immobilized patients.

Stasis Ulceration

Patients with lower extremity edema are at risk for skin breakdown and formation of stasis ulcers. These ulcers may become secondarily infected, but, unless cellulitis is present, systemic antibiotics are not necessary, and treatment is aimed at reducing the edema.

Diabetic Ulcers

Patients with diabetes mellitus often develop foot ulcers. Peripheral neuropathy may result in the distribution of stress to sites on the foot not suited to weight bearing and may also result in failure to sense foreign objects stepped on or caught in the shoe. The resulting ulceration heals poorly, which is related to micro- and macro-angiopathies and poor metabolic control. Secondary infection with anaerobes and gram-negative bacilli progresses rapidly to involve bone and soft tissue. Prevention of these events requires meticulous foot care, avoidance of walking barefoot, the use of properly fitting shoes, and checking the inside of the shoe before use. Once an ulcer develops, the physician should evaluate the patient promptly. Bed rest and topical antiseptics are always indicated. Systemic antibiotics active against anaerobes and gram-negative bacilli should be employed for all but the most superficial and clean wounds. In most instances, this treatment requires admission to the hospital. Aggressive management is indicated because, if the ulcer is left untreated or improperly treated, then the proximate bones and soft tissues of the entire foot may become involved. Once this involvement occurs, eradication of infection without amputation may be difficult.

Other Ulcerative Lesions of the Skin

Ulcerative lesions of the skin, particularly in the genital region, may be caused by *Treponema pallidum,* the agent of syphilis, or by *Haemophilus ducreyi,* the agent of chancroid (see Chapter 106).

DIFFUSE LESIONS OF THE SKIN
Erysipelas

Erysipelas is an infection of the superficial layers of the skin (Table 100–2); it is usually caused by group A streptococci.

Table 100–2   Diffuse Cutaneous and Subcutaneous Bacterial Infections

Description	Predominant Organisms
Erysipelas	Group A streptococci
Cellulitis	Group A (B, C, and G) streptococci, *Staphylococcus aureus, Haemophilus influenzae, Clostridium perfringens,* other anaerobic organisms, gram-negative bacilli
Erythema migrans (expanding circular erythema after tick bite)	*Borrelia burgdorferi*
Fasciitis	Group A streptococci, *C. perfringens,* other anaerobic organisms, gram-negative bacilli
Myonecrosis	*C. perfringens,* streptococci, mixed anaerobes, gram-negative bacilli

Table 100–3   Processes That May Resemble Cellulitis

Process	Diagnosis
Thrombophlebitis	Tender cord, no lymphangitis, ultrasound
Arthritis	Pain on passive joint movement, joint effusion, joint aspiration
Ruptured Baker's cyst	History of arthritis, joint effusion, arthrogram, MRI
Acute gout (podagra)	Painful inflammation of underlying joint, most often the great toe
Brown recluse spider bite	Exposure history
Fasciitis	MRI, surgical exploration
Myositis	Muscle tenderness, less prominent skin involvement, MRI, surgical exploration

MRI = magnetic resonance imaging.

This infection, seen primarily among children and older adults, most commonly occurs on the face. Erysipelas is a bright red to violaceous raised lesion with sharply demarcated edges. This sharp demarcation distinguishes erysipelas from the deeper tissue infection, cellulitis, the margins of which are not raised and merge more smoothly with uninvolved areas of skin. Fever is generally present, but bacteremia is uncommon; in rare cases, the pathogen can be isolated by aspiration or biopsy of the leading edge of the erythema (clysis culture). Penicillin, 2 to 6 million U/day, is curative, but defervescence is gradual.

Cellulitis

Cellulitis is an infection of the deeper layers of the skin. Cellulitis has a particular predilection for the lower extremities, where venous stasis predisposes the individual to infection. Cellulitis causes recurrent infection, perhaps by impairing lymphatic drainage. A breakdown in normal skin barriers almost always precedes this infection. Lacerations, small abscesses, tick bites (in the instance of erythema migrans caused by *Borrelia burgdorferi*), or even tiny fissures between the toes caused by minor fungal infection antedate the onset of pain, swelling, and fever. Although shaking chills often occur, bacteremia is infrequently documented. Linear streaks of erythema and tenderness indicate lymphatic spread. Regional lymph node enlargement and tenderness are common. Patches of erythema and tenderness may occur a few centimeters proximal to the edge of infection; this circumstance is probably caused by spread through subcutaneous lymphatics. Cellulitis of the calf is often difficult to distinguish from thrombophlebitis. Rupture of a Baker's cyst or inflammatory arthritis may also mimic calf cellulitis (Table 100–3); pain within the joint on passive motion suggests arthritis, whereas, after a Baker's cyst rupture, examination of the joint may be relatively benign. Lymph node enlargement and lymphatic streaking virtually confirm the diagnosis of cellulitis. Most cases of lower extremity cellulitis are caused by group A β-hemolytic streptococci (less frequently group B, C, or G streptococci), but, on occasion, *S. aureus* is responsible. Gram-negative bacilli often cause cellulitis in neutropenic and other immunosuppressed patients. Cellulitis of the face or upper extremities, particularly among children, may be caused by *Haemophilus influenzae*. Among patients with diabetes mellitus, streptococci and staphylococci are the predominant causes of cellulitis. However, if the cellulitis is associated with an infected ulceration of the skin, then anaerobic bacteria and gram-negative rods are also likely involved. After a bite from a cat or dog, cellulitis caused by *Pasteurella multocida* or other facultative anaerobes may develop.

Occupational exposures are often associated with painful cellulitis of the hands. Erysipeloid cellulitis (caused by *Erysipelothrix rhusiopathiae*) most often occurs in fish or meat handlers and responds to high doses of penicillin (12 to 20 million U/day). Freshwater exposures are associated with cellulitis caused by *Aeromonas* species, and saltwater exposures may result in aggressive cellulitis caused by *Vibrio* species, especially *V. vulnificus;* third-generation cephalosporins are usually effective in the treatment of these potentially lethal infections.

As in the case of erysipelas, cultures of blood and clysis cultures of the leading edge of infection rarely yield the pathogen. Patients with cellulitis who appear toxic or who have underlying diseases causing impaired immune response should be hospitalized. Cellulitis should be treated with a semisynthetic penicillin active against *S. aureus,* such as nafcillin (or, in regions where methicillin resistance among *S. aureus* is high, with vancomycin). If *Haemophilus* infection is suggested, then ampicillin-sulbactam is usually effective.

People with diabetes who also have foot ulcers complicated by cellulitis should be treated with agents active against anaerobes and enteric gram-negative rods (e.g., ampicillin-sulbactam); control of diabetes should be optimized. Radiologic studies should be performed on patients with ulcers to determine whether osteomyelitis is present (see Chapter 103). The affected limb should be elevated to enhance venous drainage. Prevention of cellulitis can be achieved by instituting measures aimed at reducing venous stasis and edema. Patients with recurrent cellulitis may benefit from antibiotic prophylaxis and resolution of venous stasis, if present.

Soft Tissue Gas

Crepitus on palpation of the skin indicates the presence of gas in the soft tissues. Although this circumstance often reflects anaerobic bacterial metabolism, subcutaneous gas can also be found after ventilator-induced barotrauma or after application of hydrogen peroxide to open wounds.

In the setting of soft tissue infection, crepitus suggests the presence of gas-forming anaerobes that may include clostridia or facultative bacteria such as streptococci or gram-negative rods. Radiographs will occasionally demonstrate gas before crepitus is detected (Fig. 100–1). Magnetic resonance imaging is more sensitive than other techniques in detecting soft tissue gas. The presence of gas necessitates emergency surgery to determine the extent of necrosis and requirements for débridement. Involvement of the muscle establishes the diagnosis of myonecrosis (see later discussion) and mandates extensive débridement. Despite the often extensive crepitus seen in clostridial cellulitis, exploration shows the muscles to be uninvolved, and proper treatment is limited to débridement of necrotic tissue, open drainage, and antibiotics, usually penicillin G, 10 to 20

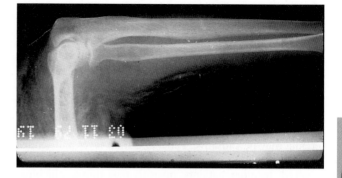

Figure 100–1 Radiograph of patient with clostridial myonecrosis shows gas within tissues. (Courtesy of Dr. J. W. Tomford.)

million U/day, and metronidazole, 500 mg every 6 hours. For streptococcal infection, clindamycin (900 mg every 8 hrs) plus penicillin is often used. Thus, the principles of treatment for necrotizing soft tissue infections are (1) removal of necrotic tissue, (2) drainage, and (3) appropriate antibiotics. These measures apply to superficial necrotizing infections (clostridial cellulitis), deeper anaerobic infections (necrotizing fasciitis [see later discussion]), and deepest infections (necrotizing myonecrosis [see later discussion]).

Deeper Infections of the Skin and Soft Tissue

NECROTIZING FASCIITIS

Necrotizing fasciitis is a deep infection of the subcutaneous tissues that generally occurs after trauma (sometimes minor) or surgery but may occur spontaneously in previously healthy persons. β-Hemolytic streptococci with or without staphylococci cause most cases of necrotizing fasciitis; in some patients, especially among those with diabetes, mixtures of anaerobic organisms and gram-negative bacilli cause the disease. Because fasciitis involves subcutaneous tissues, the skin may appear normal or may have a red or dusky hue. The clue to this diagnosis is pain and the presence of subcutaneous swelling, particularly in the absence of overlying cellulitis. In some instances, crepitus is present. In time, skin necrosis and dark bullae may develop. The patient appears more toxic than expected from the superficial appearance of the skin. Radiographs may show gas within tissues; its absence does not exclude the diagnosis. Men with diabetes mellitus, urethral trauma, or obstruction may develop an aggressive fasciitis of the perineum, called Fournier's gangrene. Perineal pain and swelling may antedate the characteristic discoloration of the scrotum and perineum. Prompt débridement of all necrotic tissue is critical to the cure of these infections. Once the diagnosis is made, the patient must be taken immediately to the operating room, where incision and exploration will determine whether fasciitis is present. Gram stain of necrotic material will guide antibiotic choice. Broad and repeated dissection with removal of infected tissue is required for cure.

INFECTIONS OF MUSCLE

Pyomyositis

Pyomyositis is a deep infection of muscle usually caused by *S. aureus* and occasionally by group A β-hemolytic streptococci or enteric bacilli. Most cases occur in warm or tropical regions, and most occur among children. Nonpenetrating trauma may antedate the onset of symptoms, suggesting that infection of a minor hematoma during incidental bacteremia may be causative. Patients exhibit fever and tender swelling of the muscle; the skin is uninvolved or minimally involved. In older patients, myositis may mimic phlebitis. Diagnosis can be readily made, if suggested, by needle aspiration, ultrasonography, or computed tomography. Early aggressive débridement and appropriate antibiotics are usually curative.

Myonecrosis

Myonecrosis generally occurs after a contaminated injury to muscle. Within 1 or 2 days of injury, the involved extremity becomes painful and begins to swell. The patient appears toxic and is often delirious. The skin may appear uninvolved at first but eventually may develop a bronzed-blue discoloration. Crepitus may be present but is not as prominent as in patients with necrotizing cellulitis (a less aggressive lesion). Most of these infections are caused by clostridial species (gas gangrene); however, streptococci, mixtures of anaerobes, or gram-negative rods cause other infections. In rare cases, clostridial myonecrosis occurs spontaneously in the absence of trauma; most of these patients have an underlying malignancy, usually involving the bowel. Regardless of the cause, this illness progresses rapidly, producing extensive necrosis of muscle. Hypotension, hemolytic anemia caused by clostridial lecithinase, and renal failure can complicate this illness. Gram stain of the thin and watery wound exudate reveals large gram-positive rods and very few inflammatory cells. Emergency surgery with wide débridement is essential. Large doses of penicillin (10 to 20 million U/day) plus clindamycin (900 mg every 8 hours) may prevent further spread of the bacilli. Chloramphenicol may be used in patients with hypersensitivity to penicillin. If gram-negative rods are seen in the exudate, then treatment with an extended-spectrum penicillin that also has excellent anaerobic activity (e.g., piperacillin-tazobactam) is indicated. Hyperbaric oxygen therapy is of uncertain value.

APPROACH TO THE PATIENT WITH THE *RED LEG*

Cellulitis of the leg is a common infection that is generally responsive to antibiotic therapy. A willingness to accept this common diagnosis uncritically can result in missed diagnoses of other treatable diseases, which in some instances are life threatening (see Table 100–3).

The first key issue is to determine whether the process is infectious. The presence of fever does not exclude inflammatory mimics of cellulitis that also may present with a red leg. The presence of ulcers or other wounds that provide entry to bacteria suggests infection; streaks of lymphangitis, tender lymph nodes, and skip areas of skin inflammation are highly suggestive of cellulitis. Thrombophlebitis may occasionally be distinguished by palpation of a tender, inflamed, and clotted vein; this diagnosis may be suggested by elevated fibrin degradation products in plasma and confirmed by ultrasound. Septic or crystal-induced arthritis has findings most prominent around the affected joint and even minimal passive joint motion is painful; aspiration of joint fluid is diagnostic.

For each patient in whom a diagnosis of cellulitis is presumed, the careful clinician must ask: Does this patient also have deeper infection, such as necrotizing fasciitis? Although this disorder is uncommon, it progresses at life-threatening speed, and clues to its presence are often subtle. To miss this diagnosis even for a few hours can place patients at risk for loss of limb or life. Clues to this diagnosis include pain and swelling out of proportion to the degree of inflammation, particularly at sites where no erythema is present (alternatively, some patients may experience topical anesthesia as a sign of skin necrosis), a dusky or bluish appearance of the skin with development of hemorrhagic vesicles or bullae, clinical *toxicity* out of proportion to the degree of fever, and history of rapid clinical progression. Magnetic resonance imaging sometimes will show gas in tissues. If the diagnosis of necrotizing fasciitis or of myonecrosis is presumed, then emergent surgical exploration is required with repeated broad dissection to remove necrotic tissues. Antibiotic therapy plays a supplementary role.

Prospectus for the Future

- Improved treatment for diabetic ulcers by neovascularization
- Better strategies to prevent recurrent cellulitis
- More effective means to prevent stasis ulcerations

References

DiNubile MJ, Lipsky BA: Complicated infections of skin and skin structures: When the infection is more than skin deep. J Antimicrob Chemother 53(Suppl 2):ii37–50, 2004.

Nichols RL, Florman S: Clinical presentations of soft-tissue infections and surgical site infections. Clin Infect Dis 33(Suppl 2):S84–93, 2001.

Raghavan M, Linden PK: Newer treatment options for skin and soft tissue infections. Drugs 64(15):1621–1642, 2004.

Ulbrecht JS, Cavanagh PR, Caputo GM: Foot problems in diabetes: An overview. Clin Infect Dis 39(Suppl 2):S73–82, 2004.

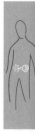

Intra-Abdominal Abscess and Peritonitis

Christoph Lange

Michael M. Lederman

Intra-Abdominal Abscess

Intra-abdominal abscesses are classified under two general categories. The first category is an infection of an intra-abdominal organ, generally arising as a consequence of hematogenous, lymphatic, or enteral spread. The second category includes extravisceral abscesses, which are localized collections of pus within the peritoneal or retroperitoneal space. These abscesses usually follow peritonitis or contamination by rupture or leakage from the bowel. Most patients with an intra-abdominal abscess are febrile. The fever may be recurrent and may be associated with rigors, suggesting intermittent bacteremia. Nausea, vomiting, and paralytic ileus are common with extravisceral abscesses. Clues to the presence of intra-abdominal abscess may be subtle and may include extravisceral gas or air-fluid levels on plain radiographs. Abdominal ultrasound, computed tomography (CT), and magnetic resonance imaging (MRI) have simplified both the diagnosis and the management of these potentially life-threatening infections.

With the exception of amebic abscess, or multiple micro-abscesses of the liver, antibiotic therapy alone is rarely curative. Failure of the antibiotic to penetrate the abscess cavities, inactivation of antibiotics within the abscess by bacterial enzymes, low pH, and low redox potential all contribute to the failure of medical management. Drainage is essential, and antibiotics are important primarily to prevent bacteremia and seeding of other organs.

ABSCESSES OF SOLID ORGANS

Hepatic Abscess

Pyogenic liver abscess is a disease that occurs predominantly among individuals with other underlying disorders, most commonly biliary tract disease. Obstruction to biliary drainage allows infected bile to produce ascending infection of the liver. Inflammatory diseases of the bowel, such as appendicitis and diverticulitis, may also lead to hepatic abscess through spread of infection through portal veins

(Table 101–1). Hepatic abscesses are also recognized complications of liver transplantation. Penetrating or nonpenetrating trauma may also result in pyogenic liver abscess.

Clinical findings in patients with pyogenic hepatic abscess are often nonspecific. Most patients are febrile, but only approximately one half have abdominal pain and tenderness. Two thirds of these patients have palpable hepatomegaly, but fewer than one in four is clinically jaundiced.

The chest radiograph may show an elevated right hemidiaphragm and atelectasis or effusion at the right lung base. The diagnosis is best achieved by contrast-enhanced CT of the abdomen or ultrasonography of the right upper quadrant (Fig. 101–1). Pyogenic abscesses may be single or multiple; multiple abscesses often arise from a biliary source of infection.

Anaerobic bacilli, micro-aerophilic streptococci, and gram-negative bacilli are the predominant micro-organisms in pyogenic liver abscess. Occasionally, *Staphylococcus aureus* causes hepatic abscesses during the course of bacteremic seeding of multiple organs. Positive blood cultures are obtained from approximately one half of the patients with pyogenic liver abscess.

Clinical laboratory studies generally show a moderate elevation of the alkaline phosphatase level, which is disproportionate to the modest elevation in bilirubin level that occurs in approximately one half of the patients. In contrast, patients with the nonspecific jaundice that occasionally accompanies bacterial infection at other sites generally have elevated bilirubin levels of as much as 5 to 10 mg/dL and only slightly elevated alkaline phosphatase levels. In patients with leukemia, multiple hepatic abscesses caused by *Candida* species may exhibit fever and poorly localized abdominal pain, and an elevated serum alkaline phosphatase level may be the only abnormality pointing to the hepatic origin. MRI provides the most sensitive imaging technique for diagnosis.

Hepatic abscess caused by *Entamoeba histolytica* is rare in North America, although it should be anticipated in a patient with fever and right upper quadrant pain who has traveled to or emigrated from the developing world. Amebic abscesses are generally single and are usually located in the

Table 101–1   Intra-Abdominal Abscesses

Site	Predisposing Factors	Likely Pathogens	Diagnosis	Empiric Treatment*
Solid Organs				
Hepatic	Gastrointestinal or biliary sepsis, trauma	Gram-negative bacilli, anaerobes, streptococci, amebae	CT, MRI, ultrasonography	Drainage Piperacillin-tazobactam or Ampicillin-sulbactam
Splenic	Trauma, hemoglobinopathy, endocarditis, injection drug use	Staphylococci, streptococci, gram-negative bacilli	CT, MRI, ultrasonography	Piperacillin-tazobactam or Ampicillin-sulbactam Drainage and/or splenectomy
Pancreatic	Pancreatitis, pseudocyst	Gram-negative bacilli, streptococci	CT, MRI, ultrasonography	Drainage Piperacillin-tazobactam or Ampicillin-sulbactam
Extravisceral				
Subphrenic	Abdominal surgery, peritonitis	Gram-negative bacilli, streptococci, anaerobes	CT	Piperacillin-tazobactam or Ampicillin-sulbactam Drainage
Pelvic	Abdominal surgery, peritonitis, pelvic or gastrointestinal inflammatory disease	Gram-negative bacilli, streptococci, anaerobes	CT	Piperacillin-tazobactam or Ampicillin-sulbactam Drainage
Perinephric	Renal infection or obstruction, hematogenous	Gram-negative bacilli, staphylococci	CT	Piperacillin-tazobactam or Ampicillin-sulbactam Drainage
Psoas	Vertebral osteomyelitis, hematogenous	Staphylococci, gram-negative bacilli, mycobacteria	CT	Piperacillin-tazobactam or Ampicillin-sulbactam Drainage

*Dosages: ampicillin-sulbactam, 2 g/1 g given intravenously (IV) every 8 hr; piperacillin-tazobactam, 3.375 g IV every 6 hr; ampicillin-sulbactam, 3 gm IV every 6 hr.
CT = computed tomography: MRI = magnetic resonance imaging.

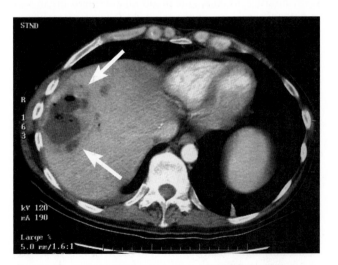

Figure 101–1 Abdominal computed tomography (CT) scan with intravenous contrast demonstrates an irregular hypodense area containing gas bubbles in the right lobe of the liver (*arrows*). *Klebsiella pneumoniae* bacilli were cultured from CT-guided aspirate. (From Goldman L, Ausiello D (eds): Cecil Textbook of Medicine, 22nd ed. Philadelphia, Elsevier, 2004.)

right lobe of the liver. Only a minority of patients with amebic liver abscess have concurrent intestinal amebiasis. Antibody titers against *E. histolytica* are nearly always positive.

The Fitz-Hugh–Curtis syndrome, or gonococcal perihepatitis, may share some clinical manifestations suggestive of hepatic abscess and should be presumed in young, sexually active women with fever and right upper quadrant tenderness. Tumors involving the liver may produce fever and a clinical and radiologic picture that may mimic hepatic abscess. This situation is complicated by the occasional concurrence of malignancy and abscess. Patients with hepatic abscesses generally exhibit a less acute illness than patients with cholecystitis or cholangitis. Ultrasonography, CT, and MRI are all useful in defining liver abscesses; MRI is most effective when the abscesses are less than 1 cm in diameter.

If pyogenic abscess is suggested, then needle aspiration is indicated. With the guidance of ultrasonography or CT, a percutaneous catheter can be inserted into the abscess cavity for both diagnostic and therapeutic purposes. The pus should be Gram stained and cultured aerobically and anaerobically. Unless the Gram stain indicates otherwise, initial therapy for pyogenic liver abscess should include drugs active against enteric aerobic and anaerobic bacteria (see Table 101–1). Antibiotics should be continued for at least 4 to 6 weeks. Surgery is required to relieve biliary tract obstruction and to drain abscesses that do not respond to percutaneous drainage and antibiotics. Patients with pyogenic liver abscess should be evaluated for a primary intra-abdominal source of infection.

Patients with multiple hepatic abscesses caused by *Candida* or *Candida*-like species (e.g., *Torulopsis glabrata*) require long-term therapy with either amphotericin B or fluconazole, as determined by the microbiologic mechanisms of the fungus. Voriconazole may be a feasible alternative treatment option, but clinical evidence for its utility in the treatment of abscesses is not yet available.

If epidemiologic features strongly suggest an amebic abscess, then metronidazole is the drug of choice. Needle aspiration is necessary only to exclude pyogenic infection or, if the abscess is large or close to other viscera, to prevent rupture. In the case of amebic abscess, the *anchovy paste* material obtained by needle drainage is not pus but necrotic liver tissue. Trophozoites of *E. histolytica* are infrequently seen on aspiration of abscesses but are often seen on biopsy of the abscess capsule. Large numbers of white cells suggest pyogenic abscess or bacterial superinfection.

Splenic Abscess

Splenic abscesses are generally the result of hematogenous seeding of the spleen. In the pre-antibiotic era, splenic infarction and abscess were common complications of infective endocarditis. Now the most common predisposing factors are trauma and (in children) sickle cell disease. Patients with splenic abscess most often exhibit left upper quadrant abdominal pain, which may be pleuritic. The left hemidiaphragm may be elevated, and an associated pleural rub or effusion may be present. The diagnostic approach, most likely etiologic agents, and initial antimicrobial therapy are outlined in Table 101–1. Splenectomy is usually the definitive treatment, but ultrasound- or CT-guided percutaneous drainage of large, solitary abscesses may also be successful in select cases.

Pancreatic Abscess

Pancreatic abscess is an uncommon complication of pancreatitis. The symptoms of pancreatic abscess (fever, nausea, vomiting, and abdominal pain radiating to the back) resemble those of pancreatitis. Thus, abscess should be presumed in cases of persistent or recurrent fever after pancreatitis. The inflamed organ becomes colonized and infected with microbes inhabiting the upper gastrointestinal tract. Enterobacteriaceae, anaerobes, and streptococci (including the pneumococci) are likely pathogens. The diagnosis may be made by abdominal ultrasound, CT, or MRI; however, radiographic definition of the pancreatic bed is often difficult. Initial antibiotic therapy (see Table 101–1) should be followed by surgical drainage of the abscess as soon as the patient's condition is stable. The mortality rates range from 12% to 22%.

EXTRAVISCERAL ABSCESSES

Extravisceral abscesses most often arise after peritonitis, after intra-abdominal surgery, as a consequence of rupture of the bowel, or after extension of infection of a viscus, such as diverticulitis or appendicitis. Abscesses may occur in the subphrenic, pelvic, or retroperitoneal spaces. Fever, nausea, vomiting, and paralytic ileus are common. Although fever is almost always present, localizing symptoms may be subtle, making the bedside diagnosis difficult. Predisposing factors, most likely etiologic pathogens, and appropriate initial antimicrobial therapy are outlined in Table 101–1.

When an abscess is suggested, CT, MRI, or ultrasound scans should be obtained. CT can identify abscesses in the retroperitoneal and abdominal spaces and guide percutaneous drainage. Ultrasonography may be more helpful than CT in identifying pelvic fluid collections. Fluid-filled abscesses may be difficult to distinguish from loops of viscera on CT or ultrasonography; review of such studies by an experienced radiologist is essential before they are considered negative. Radionuclide imaging using gallium 67–labeled or indium 111–labeled leukocytes may be useful in localizing collections of pus when other studies are not diagnostic. Drainage of an abscess either by radiologic guidance or by surgery in conjunction with antibiotics is the mainstay of treatment.

Peritonitis

Peritonitis may occur spontaneously (primary peritonitis) or as a consequence of trauma, surgery, or peritoneal soilage by bowel contents (secondary peritonitis). Peritonitis also may be caused by chemical irritation. Patients with peritonitis generally complain of diffuse abdominal pain. They may have nausea and vomiting; some have diarrhea, and others have paralytic ileus. Patients are usually febrile and uncomfortable and prefer to lie quietly in the supine position. Physical examination may reveal diffuse tenderness, diminished bowel sounds, and evidence of peritoneal inflammation, including rebound tenderness and involuntary guarding. In patients with underlying ascites, the signs and symptoms of peritonitis may be subtle, with fever as the only manifestation of infection.

PRIMARY PERITONITIS

Primary or spontaneous peritonitis occurs principally among persons with ascites associated with either chronic liver disease or the nephrotic syndrome. Bacteria may infect ascitic fluid by means of bacteremic spread by transmural migration through the bowel or through the fallopian tubes. In patients with cirrhosis, clearance of portal bacteremia by hepatic reticuloendothelial cells may be impaired by intrahepatic portosystemic shunting. Not surprisingly, therefore, gram-negative rods, especially *Escherichia coli*, are the predominant pathogens in spontaneous bacterial peritonitis; enteric streptococci are isolated in approximately one third of cases. Staphylococci, *Streptococcus pneumoniae*, or anaerobic bacilli are isolated in a smaller proportion of cases (Table 102–2).

In patients with ascites, the presenting symptoms may be nonspecific abdominal pain, nausea, vomiting, diarrhea, or altered mental status. Thus, febrile patients with ascites should undergo paracentesis unless another certain explanation for fever can be found. Inoculation of the culture

Table 101–2   Causes, Diagnosis, and Treatment of Peritonitis

Site	Predisposing Factors	Causative Agent	Clues to Diagnosis	Empiric Treatment*
Primary				
Spontaneous	Cirrhosis, nephrotic syndrome	Gram-negative bacilli, streptococci	>250 neutrophils/mcL of ascites	Cefotaxime or Piperacillin-tazobactam or Ampicillin-sulbactam or if resistant *Escherichia coli* or *Klebsiella*: Carbapenem or Fluoroquinolone
Secondary				
Postoperative	Hemorrhage, visceral rupture	Gram-negative bacilli, streptococci, staphylococci, anaerobes	Postoperative fever, pain, prolonged ileus	Piperacillin-tazobactam or Ampicillin-sulbactam or Carbapenem
Chemical	Abdominal surgery	Bile, starch, talc	Postoperative fever, pain	Biliary drainage when indicated
Visceral rupture	Perforating ulcer, ruptured appendix, bowel infarction	Gram-negative bacilli, anaerobes, streptococci	Polymicrobial gram stain or culture	Piperacillin-tazobactam or Ampicillin-sulbactam or Carbapenem; surgery
Peritoneal dialysis	—	Staphylococci, gram-negative bacilli	Pain, fever, neutrophilic pleocytosis	Vancomycin[†] plus: Third-generation cephalosporin or Piperacillin-tazobactam Consider catheter removal
Periodic peritonitis	Familial	—	Recurrent, familial	Colchicine prophylaxis, 0.6 mg two to three times daily
Tuberculosis	Infection of fallopian tubes or ileum	*Mycobacterium tuberculosis*	Lymphocytic pleocytosis, high protein level (>3 g/dL) in ascitic fluid	Isoniazid, rifampin, pyrazinamide, ethambutol

*Dosages: ampicillin-sulbactam, 2g/L g given intravenously (IV) every 8 hr; piperacillin-tazobactam, 3.375 g IV every 6 hr; imipenem, 0.5 g IV every 6 hr; metronidazole, 500 mg IV every 6 hr; vancomycin, 1 g IV every 12 hr; isoniazid, 300 mg/day; rifampin, 600 mg/day; ethambutol, 15–25 mg/kg/day; pyrazinamide, 25 mg/kg/day (maximum, 2.5 mg/kg/day); ceftazidime, 2g IV every 8 hr; moxifloxacin, 400 mg IV every day.
[†]Intraperitoneal vancomycin, initially 1 g/L dialysate, followed by 25 mg/L dialysate.

media should be performed at the bedside; a white blood cell count in the fluid that exceeds 250/mcL is suggestive of infection. Gram stain may reveal the responsible pathogen. Antibiotic penetration into the peritoneum is excellent, and systemic antimicrobial therapy is the treatment of choice (see Table 101–2). Bacteria may be cultured from ascitic fluid in the absence of clinical findings of peritonitis (bacterascites), and as many as one third of patients with clinical and laboratory findings consistent with peritonitis have sterile ascitic fluid cultures. Empiric antimicrobial treatment is indicated in these settings. Among patients with cirrhosis and ascites, prophylactic administration of norfloxacin or trimethoprim-sulfamethoxazole may decrease the risk of spontaneous peritonitis.

SECONDARY PERITONITIS

If Gram stain or culture reveals a mixed flora, or if anaerobes are anticipated on stain or demonstrated by culture, then secondary peritonitis caused by leakage of bowel contents should be presumed. Secondary peritonitis may follow penetrating abdominal trauma or surgery or may result from visceral rupture (e.g., perforated duodenal ulcer or appendix) or visceral infarction. In the postoperative setting, secondary peritonitis should be presumed in the patient whose abdominal discomfort and fever do not resolve, or even worsen, after the first few postoperative days. If peritonitis is secondary to the leakage of bowel contents, then immediate surgical intervention is mandatory. Despite the use of appropriate antibiotics (see Table 101–2) and intensive support systems, mortality from generalized peritonitis still approaches 50%.

Peritonitis is also a common complication of peritoneal dialysis. Most infections are caused by staphylococci, followed by gram-negative bacilli and yeast. Intraperitoneal antibiotics, administered via the dialysis catheter, are generally effective. Refractory or recurrent peritonitis may necessitate dialysis catheter removal.

TUBERCULOUS PERITONITIS

Tuberculous peritonitis may occur as a result of hematogenous, lymphatic, or local extension of tuberculous infection into the peritoneal cavity. Fever, abdominal pain, and weight loss are common. In patients with underlying ascites, a lymphocytic pleocytosis in the peritoneal fluid should suggest the diagnosis. Laparoscopy, with biopsy of the granulomatous peritoneal nodules, is the most effective approach to diagnosis. Standard antituberculous therapy over 6 months is generally curative (see Table 101–2).

Prospectus for the Future

Increasing diagnostic and therapeutic challenges as a greater proportion of intra-abdominal infections occurs in iatrogenically immunocompromised individuals.

References

Farthmann EH, Schoffel U: Epidemiology and pathophysiology of intraabdominal infections (IAI). Infection 26(5):329–334, 1998.

Levison ME, Bush LM: Peritonitis and other intra-abdominal infections. In Mandell GL, Bennett JE, Dolin R (eds): Principles and Practice of Infectious Diseases, 6th ed. Philadelphia, Elsevier, 2005, pp 927–951.

Marshall JC: Intra-abdominal infections. Microbes Infect 6(11):1015–1025, 2004.

Minton J, Stanley P: Intra-abdominal infections. Clin Med 4(6):519–523, 2004.

Chapter 102

Infectious Diarrhea

Christoph Lange

Michael M. Lederman

Acute diarrheal illnesses caused by bacterial, viral, protozoal, and parasite pathogens vary from mild bowel dysfunction to fulminant, life-threatening diseases. Worldwide, acute diarrheal illnesses are the most common cause of death in childhood. With the best techniques available, a specific causative agent can be identified in 70% to 80% of patients (Table 102–1).

Pathogenesis and Pathophysiologic Features: General Concepts

In general, pathogens or microbial toxins that produce acute diarrhea must be ingested. Therefore, socioeconomic conditions that result in crowding, poor sanitation, and contaminated water sources lead to increased risk of diarrheal illnesses. Normally, the low pH of the stomach, the rapid transit time of the small bowel, and antibody produced by cells in the lamina propria of the small bowel are adequate to keep the jejunum and proximal ileum free of pathogenic micro-organisms (although not sterile). Furthermore, the ileocecal valve inhibits retrograde migration of the huge numbers of bacteria that reside in the large bowel.

Pathogenic micro-organisms can pass through the hostile environment of the stomach if (1) they are acid resistant (e.g., *Shigella*) or (2) they are ingested with food and are therefore partially protected in the neutralized environment. People with decreased gastric acidity are at increased risk of acute diarrheal disease.

In the small bowel, the organisms either colonize (e.g., *Vibrio cholerae, Escherichia coli*) or invade (e.g., *Rotavirus, Norovirus*) the mucosa. Small bowel peristalsis deters colonization of most organisms. Special colonization factors such as fimbria (hair-like projections from the cell wall) or lectins (proteins that attach to mucosal cell–surface carbohydrates) facilitate adherence of successful colonists to mucosal cell surfaces.

Organisms that do not have special colonization properties pass into the terminal ileum and colon, where they may compete with the naturally residing micro-organisms. These resident intestinal bacteria produce substances that prevent intraluminal proliferation of most newly introduced bacterial species (*Bacteroides* produces inhibitory fatty acids; other enteric bacteria produce inhibitory colicins). The ability of the colonic enteropathogens (e.g., *Shigella dysenteriae*) to invade intestinal mucosa allows these micro-organisms to multiply preferentially.

Types Of Microbial Diarrheal Diseases

Microbes can cause diarrhea either directly by invasion of the gut mucosa or indirectly through elaboration of one of three classes of microbial toxins: secretory enterotoxins, cytotoxins, or neurotoxins. Toxins may be elaborated after microbial replication in the gut or, in some patients, are preformed and ingested directly.

SECRETORY TOXIN-INDUCED DIARRHEAS

Patients infected with secretory toxin-producing pathogens seldom have fever or other major systemic symptoms, and little or no inflammatory response occurs. Characteristically, large numbers of bacteria (10^5 to 10^8) must be ingested with grossly contaminated food or water (although a smaller inoculum may produce disease in individuals with achlorhydria). The enterotoxin-producing bacteria then colonize but do not invade the small bowel. After multiplying to large numbers (10^8 to 10^9 organisms per milliliter of fluid), the bacteria produce enterotoxins that bind to mucosal cells, causing hypersecretion of isotonic fluid at a rate that overwhelms the reabsorptive capacity of the colon. The diarrhea is watery with a low protein concentration and an electrolyte content that reflects its source. Rapid loss of this diarrheal fluid results in predictable saline depletion, base-deficit acidosis, and potassium deficiency. The amount and rate of fluid loss determine the severity of the illness. Certain of the secretory diarrheas, such as those caused by *V. cholerae* or *E. coli* enterotoxins, can result in massive intestinal fluid losses, sometimes exceeding 1 L/hr in adults. The *V. cholerae* enterotoxin rapidly binds to monosialogangliosides of the gut mucosa and causes sustained stimulation of cell-bound

Table 102–1	Major Etiologic Agents in Acute Diarrheal Illnesses

Invasive and Destructive Pathogens

*Shigella**

Salmonella

Campylobacter jejuni

*Vibrio parahaemolyticus**

Yersinia enterocolitica

Enterohemorrhagic *Escherichia coli* (EHEC)*

Clostridium difficile[†]

Rotavirus

Other viruses

Entamoeba histolytica

Noninvasive Pathogens

Enterotoxigenic *E. coli* (ETEC)[†]

Vibrio cholerae[†]

Giardia lamblia

Isospora belli

Cryptosporidium parvum

Cyclospora cayetanensis

Bacterial Causes of Toxin-Induced Food Poisoning

Staphylococcus aureus (short incubation, 2–6 hr)

Clostridium perfringens (longer incubation, 8–14 hr)

Bacillus cereus (short and longer incubations)

*Mucosal destruction mediated by a toxin.
[†]Diarrhea mediated by a secretory enterotoxin.

adenylate cyclase. This results, through both increased secretion and decreased absorption of electrolytes, in net movement of large quantities of isotonic fluid into the gut lumen. In the absence of antibiotic treatment, the disease runs its course in 2 to 7 days, during which time continued fluid and electrolyte repletion is of critical importance.

Enterotoxigenic *E. coli* (ETEC), probably the major cause of traveler's diarrhea worldwide, produces two major types of plasmid-encoded bacterial enterotoxins. The labile toxin (LT) of *E. coli* is identical in mode of action to cholera enterotoxin. The *E. coli* stable toxin (ST) causes gut fluid secretion through activation of guanylate cyclase. Other enteropathogenic bacteria that cause diarrhea primarily through direct invasion (e.g., *Salmonella typhimurium, S. dysenteriae*) may also produce secretory enterotoxins.

CYTOTOXIN-INDUCED DIARRHEAS

Cytotoxins are soluble factors that directly destroy mucosal epithelial cells. *Shigella dysenteriae* elaborates a toxin (Shiga toxin) that causes the destructive colitis observed in patients with shigellosis. A closely related cytotoxin is produced by enterohemorrhagic *E. coli* (EHEC) strains that are associated

with hemorrhagic colitis and hemolytic uremic syndrome. Other bacteria that can produce cytotoxins include *Clostridium perfringens* and *Vibrio parahaemolyticus*. *Clostridium perfringens*, often ingested in contaminated meat or poultry, replicates within the small bowel and produces a secretory enterotoxin that also has cytotoxin activity. Toxin-induced diarrhea caused by *C. perfringens*, similar to that caused by *Staphylococcus aureus* and *Bacillus cereus*, has a short incubation period and brief duration (<36 hours). *Clostridium difficile* can colonize the large bowel and, in the presence of antibiotic therapy that limits the growth of naturally occurring bacteria, can produce cytotoxins that can cause severe mucosal damage, producing a colitis that may have a pseudomembranous appearance or may resemble the diffuse colitis observed in shigellosis.

FOOD POISONING CAUSED BY CYTOTOXINS, SECRETORY ENTEROTOXINS, AND/OR NEUROTOXINS

Some toxins are ingested directly in food, as with *S. aureus* and *B. cereus* food poisoning. These organisms grow to a high concentration in the food, and ingestion of the toxins they produce causes the symptoms of food poisoning. Distinctive features of acute food poisoning include a short incubation period (2 to 6 hours), high attack rates (up to 75% of the population at risk), and prominent vomiting (probably caused by the effect of absorbed neurotoxins on the central nervous system).

Organisms ingested in food that produce toxins during replication in the bowel can cause food poisoning syndromes of somewhat longer incubation (8 to 16 hours). In this setting, *B. cereus* produces an enterotoxin similar to *E. coli* LT. Thus, the longer incubation food poisoning syndrome caused by some strains of *B. cereus* (often associated with ingestion of contaminated rice) may resemble the diarrhea caused by ETEC. *Clostridium perfringens* can produce both secretory and cytotoxic enterotoxins after ingestion and replication in the bowel, also producing a longer incubation food poisoning. Nausea and vomiting are less prominent than diarrhea in these food poisoning syndromes with longer incubation times.

DIARRHEAS CAUSED BY INVASIVE PATHOGENS

Diarrheas caused by invasive pathogens are usually accompanied by fever and other systemic symptoms, including headache and myalgia. Cramping abdominal pain may be prominent, and small amounts of stool are passed at frequent intervals, often associated with tenesmus. The invasive micro-organisms often induce a significant inflammatory response; as a result, the stool contains pus cells, large amounts of protein, and often gross blood. Significant dehydration rarely results from this kind of diarrhea in adults, because the diarrheal fluid volume is small, seldom exceeding 750 mL/day, although critical dehydration may occur in children. Although certain clinical features are statistically more frequent in invasive diarrheas caused by specific enteropathogens (e.g., more severe myalgias with shigellosis, higher temperature spikes with salmonellosis), epidemiologic characteristics are more helpful than are signs or

Table 102–2 Epidemiologic Characteristics of Common Invasive Enteric Pathogens

Microorganisms	Epidemiologic Features	Antibiotics
Shigella species	Outbreaks in child-care centers or custodial institutions; person-to-person transmission	Yes
Nontyphoidal *Salmonella* species	Zoonosis; survives desiccation in processed foods	Only in the severely ill and immunocompromised patients
Campylobacter jejuni	Zoonosis; worldwide distribution; transmitted in dairy products	Early treatment for severely ill patients
Yersinia enterocolitica	Zoonosis; occasionally transmitted in dairy products	Maybe
Vibrio parahaemolyticus	Coastal salt waters; transmitted by inadequately cooked shrimp and shellfish	No
Clostridium difficile	Almost always follows antimicrobial therapy	Yes
Rotavirus	Outbreaks among children; worldwide distribution; unusual and mild in adults	No
Norovirus	Microepidemic pattern; no specific age predilection	No
Entamoeba histolytica	Person-to-person transmission; very rare in the United States, Canada, and Western Europe	Yes

symptoms in determining the etiologic agent in invasive diarrheal illnesses (Table 102–2).

Acute Shigellosis

Acute shigellosis occurs when susceptible individuals ingest fecal-contaminated water or food. The bacteria are relatively resistant to killing by gastric acid; shigellosis can therefore occur after ingestion of only 10 to 100 micro-organisms. Largely for this reason, direct person-to-person transmission (e.g., in day care centers) is more common with shigellosis than it is with other bacterial enteric infections. The organism initially multiplies in the small intestine, producing watery, noninflammatory diarrhea. Later the organisms invade the colonic epithelium, causing the characteristic bloody stool. Unlike *Salmonella*, *Shigella* rarely causes bacteremia. The disease usually resolves spontaneously after 3 to 6 days, but antimicrobial agents can shorten the clinical course (see Table 102–2).

Acute Salmonellosis

Acute salmonellosis usually results from ingestion of contaminated meat, dairy, or poultry products. In the industrialized world, nontyphoidal *Salmonella* is often transmitted by means of commercially prepared dried, processed food (e.g. spices). Unlike *Shigella*, *Salmonella* is remarkably resistant to desiccation. The nontyphoidal salmonellae invade primarily the distal ileum. The organisms typically cause a short-lived

(2 to 3 days) illness characterized by fever, nausea, vomiting, and diarrhea. (This presentation is in marked contrast to typhoid fever, a 3- to 4-week febrile illness that is caused by *Salmonella typhi*; typhoid fever is not usually associated with diarrhea.)

Campylobacter Jejuni Infection

Campylobacter jejuni may be responsible for up to one third of acute febrile diarrheal illnesses in North America. This organism may invade both the small intestine and the colon. Thus, the range of symptoms is broad, ranging from an acute *Shigella*-type syndrome to a milder but more protracted diarrheal illness.

Other Invasive Enteropathogens

Three other organisms—*Yersinia enterocolitica, V. parahaemolyticus,* and enteroinvasive *E. coli*—also cause tissue invasion and acute diarrheal illnesses that may be clinically indistinguishable from those caused by the more commonly recognized invasive bacterial enteropathogens (see Table 102–2).

Another distinct *E. coli* strain, 0157:H7 EHEC, produces bloody diarrhea without evidence of mucosal inflammation (grossly bloody stool with few or no leukocytes), usually with little or no fever. The intestinal mucosal damage is caused by a Shiga-like toxin, which is also thought to be responsible for the hemolytic uremic syndrome, which develops in 2% to

5% of patients. In the last two decades, EHEC have been responsible for several multistate outbreaks of acute diarrheal illness, most often associated with ingestion of inadequately cooked hamburger meat.

Although most diarrhea-causing pathogens produce either invasive or enterotoxic diarrhea, both processes contribute to the illness in some situations. Certain strains of *Shigella*, nontyphoidal *Salmonella*, *Y. enterocolitica*, and *C. jejuni* both invade and produce secretory enterotoxins in vitro. Such enterotoxins may play a contributory role in the acute disease process. The invasive capacity of these organisms is, however, of paramount importance in their ability to produce disease.

Viral Causes of Diarrhea

Both *Rotavirus* and *Norovirus* (formerly Norwalk agent) invade and damage villous epithelial cells, with the degree of injury ranging from modest distortion of epithelial cells to sloughing of villi. Presumably, both *Rotavirus* and *Norovirus* cause diarrhea by interfering with the absorption of normal intestinal secretions, which may occur through selective destruction of absorptive villous tip cells with the sparing of secretory crypt cells. Affected patients may have low-grade fever and mild-to-moderate cramping abdominal pain. The stool is usually watery, and its contents resemble those of a noninvasive process, with few inflammatory cells, probably because of a lack of damage to the colon.

Protozoan Causes of Diarrhea

In North America, Rocky Mountain water sources are frequent origins of *Giardia lamblia* microepidemics. As is the case in shigellosis, ingestion of only a few organisms is required to establish infection. The organisms multiply in the small bowel, attach to and occasionally invade the mucosa, but do not cause gross damage to the mucosal cells. Clinical manifestations span the spectrum from an acute, febrile diarrheal illness to chronic diarrhea with associated malabsorption and weight loss. Diagnosis may be made by identifying the organism in either the stool or the duodenal mucus or by small bowel biopsy. *Entamoeba histolytica* may cause intestinal syndromes ranging from mild diarrhea to fulminant amebic colitis with multiple bloody stools, fever, and severe abdominal pain. Although *E. histolytica* has a worldwide distribution, it is an uncommon cause of diarrhea in the United States. Three other protozoa, *Cryptosporidium parvum*, *Isospora belli*, and *Cyclospora cayetanensis* occasionally cause self-limited acute diarrheal illness in otherwise healthy individuals; but they may cause voluminous, life-threatening diarrheal disease in patients with immunodeficiencies. Stool examination will often distinguish *Giardia*, *Entamoeba*, *Isospora*, *Cryptosporidium*, and *Cyclospora* (see Chapter 107); occasionally, biopsy may be needed for diagnosis.

General Epidemiologic Considerations

In developing countries where sanitation is inadequate, young children (up to 2 years of age) contract multiple episodes of diarrhea, a process that engenders intestinal immunity to the majority of enteropathogens in their environment. Most of these diarrheal episodes are mild, but some are life threatening. In these areas, ETEC and rotavirus together cause the large majority of diarrheal illnesses. *Shigella* infections are less common during early childhood.

Infants and small children in industrialized countries have fewer episodes of diarrhea than do those in developing countries, and the most common etiologic agent is the rotavirus. Most episodes are mild. ETEC and *Shigella* infections are infrequent except in a few defined population groups (e.g., individuals in custodial institutions).

Throughout the world, clinically significant diarrhea is relatively unusual in adults except in specifically defined epidemics or common-source outbreaks caused by contaminated food or water. However, diarrhea is the most common illness to affect travelers. More than 20% of travelers to Latin America, Africa, South Asia, and the Middle East develop *traveler's diarrhea*. When immunologically inexperienced adults from the developed world visit developing countries, the organisms responsible are the same ones as those causing most childhood diarrhea in the country visited.

In addition to the pathogens listed earlier, certain sexually transmissible pathogens cause acute diarrheal illnesses among sexually active homosexual men; these illnesses differ from those that most commonly occur in the general population (see Chapter 106).

Diagnosis

In managing life-threatening diarrheal illnesses, determining the specific etiologic agent is not as important as prompt repletion of lost electrolytes. Fluid losses represent the chief causes of serious morbidity and mortality in acute diarrheal illness. Moreover, antimicrobial therapy has proved of value in only a minority of cases (see Table 102–2). Discerning the epidemiologic features of the illness is often more helpful than are laboratory techniques in identifying patients in which antimicrobial therapy is likely to be helpful! Figure 102–1 provides a schematic approach to diagnosis and management.

The examination of a methylene blue-stained stool preparation for erythrocytes and pus cells may help distinguish acute diarrheal illnesses caused by invasive pathogens from those caused by noninvasive pathogens. This preparation is easily accomplished by adding one drop of methylene blue dye to one drop of liquid stool or mucus, allowing the preparation to air dry and examining the specimen under the high dry microscope lens. Few, if any, leukocytes or erythrocytes are seen in the stools of patients with diarrhea caused by noninvasive organisms (e.g., ETEC). Varying numbers of leukocytes and erythrocytes are present in diarrheas secondary to invasive bacteria (e.g., *Shigella*) or cytopathic toxins (*C. difficile* toxin).

The precise diagnosis of any diarrheal illness lasting longer than 4 to 5 days is important because these illnesses (e.g., giardiasis) may be responsive to specific antimicrobial therapy. Furthermore, among patients with negative stool examinations and cultures, endoscopy may yield a diagnosis of a noninfectious disease (e.g., ulcerative colitis, Crohn's disease).

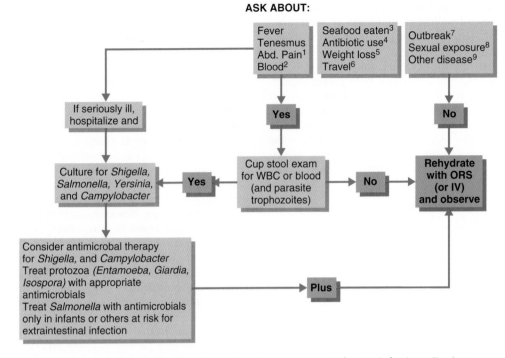

ASK ABOUT:

Figure 102–1 Approach to the diagnosis and management of acute infectious diarrhea.

1. If unexplained abdominal pain and fever suggest an appendicitis-like syndrome, then culture substance for *Yersinia enterocolitica* should be prepared.
2. Bloody diarrhea, in the absence of fecal leukocytes, suggests enterohemorrhagic *Escherichia coli* or amebiasis (where leukocytes are destroyed by the parasite).
3. Ingestion of inadequately cooked seafood prompts consideration of *Vibrio infections* or *Norovirus.*
4. Associated antibiotics should be stopped, and *Clostridium difficile* should be considered.
5. Persistence of diarrhea (>10 days) with weight loss prompts consideration of giardiasis, cryptosporidiosis, or inflammatory bowel disease.
6. Travel to tropical areas increases the chance of enterotoxic *E. coli* (ETEC), as well as viral, protozoal (e.g., *Giardia, Entamoeba, Cryptosporidium*), and invasive bacterial pathogens if fecal leukocytes are present.
7. Outbreaks should prompt consideration of *Staphylococcus aureus, Bacillus cereus, Clostridium perfringens,* ETEC, *Vibrio, Salmonella, Campylobacter,* or *Shigella* infection.
8. Sigmoidoscopy in symptomatic homosexual men should distinguish proctitis in the distal 15 cm (caused by herpesvirus, gonococcal, chlamydial, or syphilitic infection) from colitis (*Campylobacter, Shigella,* or *C. difficile* infection).
9. Immunocompromised patients should have a wide range of viral (e.g., cytomegalovirus, herpes simplex virus, rotavirus), bacterial (e.g., *Salmonella, Mycobacterium avium complex, C. difficile*), protozoal (e.g., *Cryptosporidium, Isospora, Microsporidia, Entamoeba, Giardia*) and parasitic (e.g., strongyloides hyperinfection syndrome) agents considered.

IV = intravenous; ORS = oral rehydration solution; WBC = white blood cell. (Adapted from Guerrant RL, Shields DS, Thorson SM, et al: Evaluation and diagnosis of acute infectious diarrhea. Am J Med 78:91–98, 1985.)

Management: General Principles of Electrolyte Repletion Therapy

INTRAVENOUS FLUIDS

All acute diarrheal diseases respond to a similar fluid repletion regimen because voluminous infectious diarrhea in adults consistently produces the same pattern of electrolyte loss. The fluid losses of massive diarrhea can rapidly be corrected by infusing fluids intravenously that approximate those that have been lost. Lactated Ringer's solution is readily available and provides uniformly good results. With patients who are hypotensive, the intravenous fluids should be initially infused rapidly. Subsequent maintenance fluid administration can be guided by the patient's clinical appearance, including vital signs, appearance of neck veins, and skin turgor. Clinical evaluation alone provides an adequate guide to fluid replacement in most acute diarrheal illnesses. If intravenous fluids are administered in adequate quantities throughout the diarrheal illness, then virtually every patient with diarrhea caused by toxigenic bacteria should be restored to health. Complications (e.g., acute renal failure secondary to hypotension) are exceedingly rare if these principles are followed.

ORAL FLUIDS

In most patients with acute diarrheal illness, fluid repletion can also be achieved through the oral route, using isotonic glucose-containing electrolyte solutions. A uniformly effective solution can be easily prepared by the addition of 2

Table 102–3   Rehydration and Eating in Cases of Diarrhea

Rehydration

1 L boiled (drinking) water
2 T sugar (or honey)
$^1/_4$ teaspoon salt (NaCl)
$^1/_4$ teaspoon baking soda (NaHCO$_3$)

BRAT Diet

Banana, rice, applesauce, toast

tablespoons of sugar, one-quarter teaspoon of salt (NaCl), and one-quarter teaspoon of baking soda (NaHCO$_3$) into boiled drinking water (Table 102–3). These fluids should be administered initially in large quantities, 250 mL every 15 minutes in adults, until clinical observations indicate that fluid balance has been restored. Thereafter, fluids should be administered in quantities sufficient to maintain normal balance; if stool output is measured, then approximately 1.5 L of glucose-electrolyte solution should be given orally for each liter of stool. The oral glucose-electrolyte fluid does not decrease the volume of fluid lost through the intestinal tract but rather facilitates absorption of adequate fluid to counterbalance the toxin-induced fluid secretion.

Patients with fluid depletion caused by invasive microbial agents (e.g., rotavirus, *Salmonella*) also respond well to oral glucose-electrolyte therapy, although the pathogenesis of diarrheal disease caused by invasive microbes is quite different from that caused by enterotoxigenic bacteria.

ANTIMICROBIAL THERAPY

Most acute infectious diarrheas do not require antibiotic therapy (see Table 102–2). Of the noninvasive bacterial diarrheas, antibiotics dramatically decrease the volume of diarrhea only in cholera. Doxycycline, 300 mg in a single dose, is the drug of choice.

Of the invasive bacterial diarrheas, short-term antimicrobial treatment significantly decreases the duration and severity of shigellosis. A quinolone such as ciprofloxacin, 500 mg twice daily for 5 days, is effective; trimethoprim-sulfamethoxazole, one double-strength tablet given twice daily, may be used if the organism is recognized as sensitive.

Antimicrobial therapy may also be helpful in decreasing the duration and severity of enteritis caused by *Yersinia* and *Campylobacter*. Ciprofloxacin, 500 mg twice daily for 5 days, is useful against these pathogens as well. Antimicrobial agents are of no known value in *V. parahaemolyticus* infections. In uncomplicated nontyphoidal *Salmonella* enteritis, antibiotics may prolong the fecal shedding of salmonellae. Treatment of nontyphoidal salmonella gastroenteritis is, however, indicated in certain settings to prevent bacteremia and its complications (e.g., meningitis, endovascular infec-

tion, infections of joint or vascular prostheses). Treatment until defervescence with a third-generation cephalosporin or a quinolone is therefore indicated for patients who are septic, for those ill enough to be hospitalized, for immunocompromised patients, and for patients with advanced atherosclerotic disease, sickle cell disease, or bone or vascular prostheses.

Antimicrobial therapy is indicated, paradoxically, for the treatment of antibiotic-associated diarrhea. Antibiotic-associated diarrhea develops in 1% to 15% of patients who receive broad-spectrum antimicrobial agents and is caused by cytotoxins produced by *C. difficile*, which proliferate in the colonic mucosa when the colonization of bacteria that naturally live in the gut is disturbed. Although generally characterized by mild diarrhea, antibiotic-associated diarrhea may result in a potentially lethal pseudomembranous colitis. In all patients, the responsible antibiotic should be stopped. In moderately ill patients (i.e., those with fever, mucosal ulceration, and/or pseudomembranes), metronidazole, 500 mg every 8 hours for 7 days, should be started on the basis of strong clinical probability before the diagnosis is confirmed by stool assay for *C. difficile* toxins. Oral vancomycin should be used only in patients who are severely ill. Empiric treatment with these agents should be avoided in patients with mild diarrhea because it may result in the emergence of antibiotic-resistant bacteria, such as vancomycin-resistant enterococci.

Antimicrobial agents decrease the duration and severity of giardiasis. In adults, metronidazole, 250 mg every 8 hours for 3 days, and quinacrine, 300 mg/day for 7 days, appear to be equally effective in adults. Acute intestinal amebiasis demands antimicrobial therapy. Metronidazole, 750 mg every 8 hours for 5 days, is the drug of choice in adults. The duration of diarrhea caused by *I. belli* is significantly shortened with the administration of trimethoprim-sulfamethoxazole, twice daily for 5 days.

ANTIMICROBIAL PROPHYLAXIS

Prophylactic antimicrobial agents are effective in preventing traveler's diarrhea, which is caused most often by ETEC. Doxycycline, trimethoprim-sulfamethoxazole, and a quinolone such as ciprofloxacin are each effective when taken once daily for up to 3 weeks. However, because of the rapid response of most patients to early treatment with any of these three agents, the advantages of prophylactic drugs are, in many instances, outweighed by their potential risks (adverse reactions).

SYMPTOMATIC THERAPY

Adjuvant symptomatic therapy is not essential but may provide modest symptomatic relief in acute infectious diarrheas associated with cramping abdominal pain. Bismuth subsalicylate, 0.6 g every 6 hours, may ameliorate symptoms of traveler's diarrhea. Agents that decrease intestinal motility (e.g., codeine, diphenoxylate, loperamide) also relieve the cramping abdominal pain associated with many acute diarrheal illnesses but are potentially hazardous because they may enhance the severity of illness in shigellosis, the prototype of invasive bacterial diarrheas.

Prospectus for the Future

- Continuing increase in the prevalence of acute diarrheal illnesses as the result of further migration of populations to urban areas with inadequate clean water supply and waste disposal systems.

- Further increase in bacterial resistance to currently effective antimicrobial agents.

References

Casburn-Jones AC, Farthing MJ: Management of infectious diarrhea. Gut 53(2):296–305, 2004 Feb.

Al-Abri SS, Beeching NJ, Nye FJ: Traveller's diarrhea. Lancet Infectious Dis 5:(6):349–360, 2005.

Spira AM: Assessment of travelers who return home ill. Lancet 361: 1459–1469, 2003.

Infections Involving Bones and Joints

Christoph Lange

Michael M. Lederman

Arthritis

In adults, almost all cases of infective arthritis of natural joints occur through hematogenous seeding. In rare cases, intra-articular trauma can result in septic arthritis. Causative agents for infective arthritis include bacteria, viruses, mycobacteria, and fungi. In addition, certain viruses such as human parvovirus B-19, rubella, and hepatitis B and C viruses can produce a polyarthritis through the direct infection of joint synovial tissue or immune complex deposition. Immune mechanisms also underlie arthritis syndromes that have developed after diarrhea caused by *Salmonella*, *Shigella*, *Yersinia*, and *Clostridium difficile* infections; the majority of patients with postdysenteric arthritis syndrome share the human leukocyte antigen B27 (see Chapter 79).

ACUTE ARTHRITIS

Underlying joint disease, particularly rheumatoid arthritis, predisposes the patient to septic arthritis. Many patients with septic arthritis have a history of joint trauma antedating symptoms of infection. Conceivably, disruption of capillaries during an unrecognized and transient bacteremia allows bacteria to spill into hemorrhagic and traumatized synovium or joint fluid, resulting in the initiation of infection.

Microbiology

Staphylococcus aureus is the most common cause of septic arthritis (Table 103–1). Patients with underlying joint disease and intravenous drug users are at particular risk for infection with this organism. *Pseudomonas aeruginosa* is another important cause of septic arthritis among intravenous drug users.

Other gram-negative bacilli are infrequent causes of septic arthritis and are found primarily among older debilitated patients with chronic arthritis. In adults younger than 30 years of age, *Neisseria gonorrhoeae* is the most likely pathogen. Isolates causing disseminated gonococcal infec-

tion with arthritis are generally resistant to killing by normal serum.

Chapter 103

Clinical Presentation

Symptoms of septic arthritis are generally present for only a few days before the patient seeks medical attention. Fever is usual; shaking chills may occur. The knee is the most commonly affected joint and is generally painful and swollen. Fluid can be found in most infected joints, and a limitation of motion is significant. In some patients, however, physical findings indicating infection may be subtle, particularly among patients with underlying rheumatoid arthritis who are receiving corticosteroids. In these individuals, who are at particular risk for septic arthritis, superimposed infection may be difficult to distinguish from a flare-up of underlying disease. Symmetric symptoms in multiple joints are more indicative of a rheumatoid flare-up. Approximately 10% of patients with septic arthritis, however, involve more than one joint.

Differential Diagnosis of Acute Monoarticular or Oligoarticular Arthritis

Infections, crystal deposition (uric acid gout or calcium pyrophosphate pseudogout), trauma, osteoarthritis, ischemic necrosis, foreign bodies, tumors, and systemic diseases like systemic lupus erythematosus can produce acute monoarticular arthritis. Radiographs may show evidence of osteoarthritis, gouty tophi, or the linear densities of chondrocalcinosis, which are characteristic of pseudogout. All red, warm, tender joints must be aspirated. The synovial fluid should be cultured anaerobically and aerobically. A Gram-stained preparation should be examined, and a wet mount of fluid should be examined using a polarized microscope to look for crystals. Synovial fluid leukocyte counts and chemistries are of limited value in the differential diagnosis of a probable septic joint. As a general rule, however, synovial fluid white blood cell counts in excess of 100,000/mcL suggest either infection or crystal-induced

Table 103–1   Infective Arthritis—Acute

	Etiologic Agents	Characteristics
Bacterial	*Staphylococcus aureus*	Most common overall
		Usually monoarticular, large joint involvement
	Streptococcus spp.	Second most common overall
		Groups B, F, and G
		Associated with diabetes mellitus, malignancy, and genitourinary tract abnormalities
	Neisseria gonorrhoeae	Most common in young, sexually active adults
		Commonly polyarticular in onset
		Often associated with skin lesions
	Pseudomonas aeruginosa	Largely restricted to intravenous drug users
		Often involves sternoclavicular joint
Viral	Hepatitis B, rubella, mumps, parvovirus	Usually polyarticular, with minimal joint effusions
		Normal peripheral white blood cell count

disease (see Table 77–3). Blood cultures should be obtained in all patients with probable septic arthritis.

Treatment

The two major modalities for treatment of acute septic arthritis are drainage and antibiotics. The first needle aspiration of a septic joint should remove as much fluid as possible. Initial antibiotic choice should be based on the clinical presentation and the results of the Gram stain. Staphylococcal infection can be treated with penicillinase-resistant penicillin or, if the organism is resistant, with vancomycin. Gonococcal infections should be treated with ceftriaxone, 1 g every 24 hours for 10 days. Arthritis caused by gram-negative rods should initially be treated with an aminoglycoside or a quinolone, such as ciprofloxacin, plus another drug active against *Pseudomonas aeruginosa*, either a third generation cephalosporin or piperacillin. Arthritis caused by *S. aureus* or gram-negative bacilli should be treated with antibiotics for 4 to 6 weeks. Otherwise, 2 to 3 weeks of antibiotic treatment are usually sufficient to eradicate infection.

Septic joints (with the notable exception of joints infected with the gonococcus) generally reaccumulate fluid after treatment is initiated. These reaccumulations must be removed by repeated needle aspirations as often as is necessary. Indications for open surgical drainage of the joint include failure of the synovial fluid white blood cell count to fall after 5 days of antibiotic treatment with repeated needle aspirations and the presence of loculated fluid within the joint. Septic arthritis of the hip is generally drained surgically because of the difficulty and potential hazard of repeated needle aspirations of this joint. Early surgical drainage also should be considered for joint infections with gram-negative rods or with *S. aureus*. Untreated or inadequately treated septic arthritis may be complicated by osteomyelitis. In patients in whom the diagnosis and treatment have been delayed, radiographs of the involved joint should be obtained at the beginning and end of treatment.

POLYARTICULAR ARTHRITIS

Arthritis involving multiple joints is infrequently attributable to direct microbial invasion. In many patients, a polyarticular arthritis represents an immunologically mediated process. Acute rheumatic fever, a delayed immune-mediated response to group A streptococcal infection, may develop as a migratory, asymmetric arthritis of the knees, ankles, elbows, and wrists. Heart involvement, subcutaneous nodules, or erythema marginatum is present in a minority of individuals. Most patients have serologic evidence of recent streptococcal infection. Antistreptolysin O, anti-deoxyribonuclease (anti-DNase), and antihyaluronidase antibodies are usually present. The importance of making this diagnosis lies primarily in the requirement for long-term prophylaxis against streptococcal infection and the clinical response of this process to salicylates.

Viral infections including hepatitis B and C, rubella, parvovirus B-19, and mumps may be associated with polyarthritis. In mumps and rubella, the arthritis results from direct infection of articular tissue; with hepatitis viruses, the joint inflammation is a secondary result of the host immune response. Serum sickness, polyarticular gout, sarcoidosis, rheumatoid arthritis, and other connective tissue disorders must be considered in the differential diagnosis. Chronic essential mixed cryoglobulinemia induced by hepatitis B and C viruses can cause arthralgias, although severe arthritis is rare. Because approximately 10% of the cases of septic arthritis involve more than one joint, acutely inflamed joints containing fluid should be tapped to exclude bacterial infection.

Disseminated gonococcal infection (see Chapter 106) may exhibit fever, tenosynovitis, or arthritis involving several joints and a characteristic rash. The rash may be petechial but more often consists of a few to a few dozen pustules on an erythematous base. Cultures of the joint fluid are usually negative at this stage, but blood cultures are often positive; Gram stain of a pustule may reveal the pathogen. Ceftriaxone, 1 g/day for 10 days, is curative.

Table 103–2	Causes of Infective Arthritis—Chronic

Nontuberculous mycobacteria
Tuberculosis
Fungi
Lyme disease (oligoarticular)

Table 103–3	Factors Predisposing to Hematogenous Osteomyelitis	
Setting	**Likely Pathogens**	
Intravenous drug use	*Staphylococcus aureus*	
	Pseudomonas aeruginosa	
Intravenous catheters	*S. aureus*	
	Staphylococcus epidermidis	
	Candida species	
Urinary tract infection	Enterobacteriaceae	

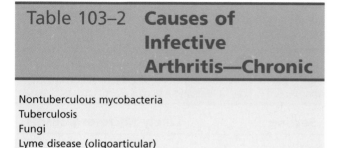

CHRONIC ARTHRITIS

Mycobacteria and fungi may produce an indolent, slowly progressive arthritis, usually involving only one joint or contiguous joints, such as those of the wrists and hands (Table 103–2). Fever may be low grade or absent. Cultures of joint fluid may be negative. Some patients with tuberculous arthritis have no evidence of active disease in the lungs. As a general rule, patients with inflammatory chronic monoarticular arthritis should have a synovial biopsy for culture and histology. Granulomas indicate the likelihood of fungal or mycobacterial infection. Cultures should confirm the diagnosis.

Fungal arthritis should be treated surgically by arthroscopic débridement and drainage and medically with amphotericin B. Voriconazole and caspofungin are better-tolerated alternatives to amphotericin B, but their efficacy in this setting is uncertain. Mycobacterial arthritis must be treated for 18 months with at least two drugs active against the isolate. Because some mycobacterial isolates causing joint disease are nontuberculous, extensive susceptibility testing may be needed to guide antimicrobial therapy.

A spirochete, *Borrelia burgdorferi*, is the pathogen responsible for Lyme disease. Several months to years (mean 6 months) after the bite of the *Ixodes* tick and the characteristic expanding rash of erythema chronicum migrans, some patients develop an intermittent arthritis with large effusions involving one or more joints, usually including the knees. This chronic arthritis may result in joint destruction, but fever is unusual. Treatment with intravenous ceftriaxone, 4 g/day for 14 to 21 days, will halt the progression of disease in the majority of patients, but appropriate antibiotic treatment during the acute stage, usually associated with erythema migrans, will prevent the later development of arthritis (see Chapter 94).

Septic Bursitis

In more than 80% of patients, *S. aureus* causes septic bursitis, which involves predominantly the olecranon or the prepatellar bursa. In most patients a history of antecedent infection or irritation of the skin overlying the bursa has been documented. The skin over the bursa is red and often peeling, the bursa has a doughy consistency, and fluid may be present on thorough examination. Daily needle aspiration until sterile fluid is obtained, along with antibiotics that are selected according to the Gram stain, culture, and sensitivity findings, are generally curative.

Osteomyelitis

Infections of the bone occur either as a result of hematogenous spread or through the extension of local infection.

HEMATOGENOUS OSTEOMYELITIS

Hematogenous osteomyelitis occurs most commonly in the long bones or vertebral bodies (Table 103–3). The peak age distributions are in childhood and old age. Individuals predisposed to hematogenous osteomyelitis include intravenous drug users, who are especially at risk for infections with *S. aureus* and *P. aeruginosa,* and patients with hemoglobinopathy, in whom nontyphoidal salmonellae often infect infarcted regions of bone. *Staphylococcus epidermidis* has emerged as an important nosocomial pathogen among patients with infected intravenous catheters. Similar to patients with septic arthritis, patients with hematogenous osteomyelitis often give a history of trauma antedating symptoms of infection, suggesting that transient, unrecognized bacteremia might result in infection of traumatized tissue.

Patients with acute hematogenous osteomyelitis generally exhibit acute onset of pain, tenderness, and fever; soft tissue swelling may also be observed over the affected bone. In most patients, physical examination distinguishes acute osteomyelitis from septic arthritis because range of joint motion is preserved in osteomyelitis. In the first 2 weeks of illness, radiographs may be negative or show only soft tissue swelling. Magnetic resonance imaging (MRI) demonstrates bone erosion, with decreased signal intensity on T1-weighted images and generally increased signal intensity on T2-weighted images, before it is apparent on plain films (Fig. 103–1). If MRI imaging is excluded by hardware, then technetium or gallium scans, which are now the standards of care, are almost always positive, but technetium scans may also be positive in the setting of increased vascularity or increased bone formation of any cause. After 2 weeks of infection, plain radiographs generally show some abnormality, and untreated osteomyelitis may produce areas of periosteal elevation or erosion followed by increased bone formation (sclerosis). The white blood cell count is usually but not always elevated.

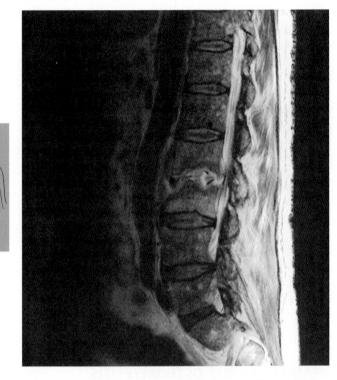

Figure 103–1 T-1 weighted magnetic resonance image (MRI) show an abnormal signal in the disc between L2 and L3 with associated vertebral osteomyelitis. Fluid collection is mild in the posterior parts of L2 and L3 with elevation of the posterior ligament. A computed tomography–guided aspirate grew *Staphylococcus aureus*. (From Mandell GL, Bennett JE, Dolin R: Principles and Practice of Infectious Diseases, 6th ed. Philadelphia, Elsevier, 2004, p. 1326.)

A patient with back pain and fever must be considered to have a serious infection until proved otherwise. Spasm of the paravertebral muscles is common but nonspecific in patients with vertebral osteomyelitis. Point tenderness over bone suggests the presence of local infection. A thorough history should be obtained and a careful neurologic examination performed. Abnormalities of bowel or bladder or of strength or sensation in the lower extremities suggest the possibility of spinal cord involvement by means of spinal epidural abscess with or without osteomyelitis. Acute spinal epidural abscess is a surgical emergency. The challenge is to make the diagnosis before neurologic signs appear (see Chapter 127). MRI provides excellent definition of epidural or paravertebral abscess and is the diagnostic procedure of choice. Demonstration of an epidural abscess mandates immediate intervention, either by surgical intervention or, in select patients, by computed tomography–guided drainage. Although most patients with hematogenous osteomyelitis have an acute presentation, some may have an indolent course. These patients may have an illness of more than 1 year's duration characterized by pain and low-grade fever. Radiographs are abnormal but may show only collapse of a vertebral body. This collapse most often occurs in infections with *P. aeruginosa*, but *Candida* species and *S. aureus* infections may also develop in this manner.

Blood cultures may be positive in up to one half of patients with acute osteomyelitis. Patients with acute

Table 103–4	Osteomyelitis Secondary to Contiguous Spread
Setting	**Likely Micro-organisms**
Surgery, trauma	*Staphylococcus aureus*
	Aerobic gram-negative bacilli
Cat or dog bites	*Pasteurella multocida*
Human bites	Mixed anaerobic infections
Periodontal infections	Mixed anaerobic infections
Cutaneous ulcers	Mixed aerobic and anaerobic organisms

osteomyelitis should have a needle biopsy and culture of the involved bone unless blood culture results are known beforehand. Antibiotic treatment directed against the causative pathogen for 4 to 6 weeks is usually sufficient for native bone and joint infections. (Rifampin is often added in prosthetic joint infections.)

OSTEOMYELITIS SECONDARY TO EXTENSION OF LOCAL INFECTION

Local infection predisposes the patient to osteomyelitis in several major settings (Table 103–4). The first is after penetrating trauma or surgery where local infection gains access to traumatized bone. In postsurgical infections, staphylococci and gram-negative bacilli predominate. Generally, wound infection with erythema, swelling, increased postoperative tenderness, and drainage are evident. A traumatic incident often associated with osteomyelitis is either a human or an animal bite. Human bites, if deep enough, may result in osteomyelitis caused by anaerobic mouth bacteria. Cat bites notoriously result in the development of osteomyelitis because the cat's thin, sharp, long teeth often penetrate the periosteum. *Pasteurella multocida* is a frequent pathogen in this setting. A 4- to 6-week course of ampicillin-sulbactam, 3 g every 8 hours, is recommended.

The intimate relationship of the teeth and periodontal tissues to the bones of the maxilla and mandible may predispose patients to osteomyelitis after local infection. Débridement of necrotic tissue and ampicillin-sulbactam, 3 g every 6 hours, is usually an effective treatment because mixed anaerobic infections are usually present.

The third setting in which local infection predisposes patients to osteomyelitis is that of an infected sore or ulcer. Pressure sores of the sacrum or femoral region may erode into contiguous bone and produce an osteomyelitis (see Chapter 100) caused by several bacterial species including anaerobic organisms. Patients with diabetes mellitus often develop traumatic vascular ulcerations of their toes and feet, with eventual development of osteomyelitis. Anaerobes, streptococci, staphylococci, and gram-negative bacilli are often involved in these infections (see Chapter 100). Treatment involves débridement (often amputation in the case of patients with diabetes) and antibiotics active against the pathogens involved for at least 6 weeks. Optimizing metabolic control and correction of macrovasculopathy if possible (e.g., angioplasty) will improve wound healing. Of far greater importance than treatment in the patient with diabetes, however, is early education of the patient about the need to wear appropriate footwear, to see podiatrists at regular intervals, and to have periodic pedicures if possible. A large proportion of osteomyelitis in the feet of patients with diabetes can be avoided by such simple, although demanding, prophylactic measures.

CHRONIC OSTEOMYELITIS

Untreated or inadequately treated osteomyelitis results in avascular necrosis of bone and the formation of islands of nonvascularized and infected bone called *sequestra*. Patients with chronic osteomyelitis may tolerate their infection reasonably well, with intermittent episodes of disease activity exhibited by increased local pain and the development of drainage of infected material through a sinus tract. Some patients have tolerated chronic osteomyelitis for decades. A normochromic, normocytic anemia of chronic disease is common in this setting. Occasionally amyloidosis and, in rare cases, osteogenic sarcoma complicate this disorder.

Staphylococcus aureus is responsible for the great majority of cases of chronic osteomyelitis; the major exception is among patients with sickle cell anemia, in whom nontyphoidal salmonellae may cause chronic infection of the long bones.

Cultures of sinus tract drainage do not reliably reflect the pathogens involved in the infection. Diagnosis and cure are best affected by surgical débridement of necrotic material, followed by long-term administration of antibiotics active against the organism found in the surgical specimens.

Mycobacteria, most often *Mycobacterium tuberculosis*, can produce a chronic osteomyelitis. The anterior portions of vertebral bodies are the most common sites of infection. Hematogenous dissemination and lymphatic spread are the usual routes of infection. Paravertebral abscess (often termed *cold abscess* because of the lack of signs of acute inflammation) may complicate this infection. Diagnosis is usually confirmed by histologic examination and culture of biopsy material. Treatment against skeletal tuberculosis involves at least 6 to 12 months of standard therapy and, often, surgical débridement.

Prospectus for the Future

- More consistent and effective approaches to prevent pedal osteomyelitis in individuals with diabetes
- Improved multidisciplinary treatment of chronic osteomyelitis with a major focus on limb-sparing modalities for diabetic osteomyelitis

References

Baker DG, Shumacher HR: Acute monoarthritis. N Engl J Med 329: 1013–1020, 1993.
Lew DP, Waldvogel FA: Osteomyelitis. Lancet 364:369–379, 2004.
Ohl CA: Infectious arthritis of native joints. In Mandell GL, Bennett JR, Dolin R (eds): Principles and Practice of Infectious Diseases, 6th ed. 2005, Elsevier, Philadelphia, pp 1311–1322.
Pinals RS: Polyarthritis and fever. N Engl J Med 330:769–774, 1994.

Infections of the Urinary Tract

Christoph Lange

Michael M. Lederman

The urethra, bladder, kidneys, and prostate are all susceptible to infection. Most urinary tract infections (UTIs)
cause local symptoms, yet clinical manifestations do not always
pinpoint the site of infection. The purpose of this chapter is to
simplify the clinical and laboratory approaches to the diagnosis and treatment of UTIs. Infections associated with indwelling
urinary catheters are discussed in Chapter 105.

Urethritis

Urethritis is predominantly an infection of sexually active
individuals, usually men. The symptoms are pain and
burning of the urethra during urination, and some discharge
generally occurs at the urethral meatus. Urethritis may be
gonococcal in origin. However, nongonococcal urethritis is
now increasingly frequent in North America. Nongonococcal urethritis may be caused by *Chlamydia trachomatis* or
Ureaplasma urealyticum and less commonly by *Trichomonas
vaginalis* or herpesviruses. Diagnosis and management of
urethritis are considered in Chapter 106.

Cystitis and Pyelonephritis

EPIDEMIOLOGIC FACTORS

Bacterial infections of the bladder (cystitis) and kidney
(pyelonephritis) are more frequent in women than men, and
the incidence of infection increases with age. Factors that
predispose an individual to UTI include instrumentation
(e.g., catheterization, cystoscopy), pregnancy, anatomic
abnormalities of the genitourinary tract, and diabetes
mellitus.

PATHOGENESIS

Although some infections of the kidney may arise as the
result of hematogenous dissemination, most UTIs ascend
through a portal of entry in the urethra. Most pathogens
responsible for community-acquired UTIs are bacterial
species that naturally live in the human bowel. *Escherichia
coli* is the most common isolate; in women, colonization of
the vaginal and periurethral mucosa may antedate infection
of the urinary tract. Bacteria with fimbriae capable of adherence to epithelial cells are increasingly likely to cause UTIs,
and persons whose epithelial cells bind these fimbriae may
be at increased risk for infection. The longer and protected
male urethra may account for the decreased incidence of
UTIs in men. Motile bacteria may swim upstream, and reflux
of urine from the bladder into the ureters may predispose
the individual to the development of kidney infection.

CLINICAL FEATURES

Suprapubic pain, discomfort, or burning sensation on urination and frequency of urination are common symptoms
of infection of the urinary tract. Back or flank pain or the
occurrence of fever suggests that infection is not limited to
the bladder (cystitis) but involves the kidney (pyelonephritis or extrarenal or perinephric abscess) or prostate as well.
However, clinical presentation often fails to distinguish
between simple cystitis and pyelonephritis. If perinephric
abscess is suggested, then diagnosis can usually be established by either ultrasound (Fig. 104–1) or computed
tomography with contrast (Fig. 104–2). Approximately one
half of infections that appear clinically to involve the bladder
can be shown by instrumentation and other specialized techniques to affect the kidneys. Older or debilitated patients
with infection of the urinary tract may have no symptoms
referable to the urinary tract and may exhibit only fever,
altered mental status, or hypotension.

LABORATORY DIAGNOSIS

Analysis of a midstream urine sample obtained from
patients with infection of the bladder or kidney shows white
blood cells (WBCs) and may also reveal red blood cells and
slightly increased amounts of protein. The presence of at
least 10 WBCs/mm^3 of midstream urine by counting
chamber is defined as pyuria. The vast majority of patients
with symptomatic or asymptomatic bacteriuria have pyuria.
The presence of WBC casts in an infected urine sample indicates the presence of pyelonephritis. Bacteria may be seen in
sedimented urine and can be readily identified by Gram
stain.

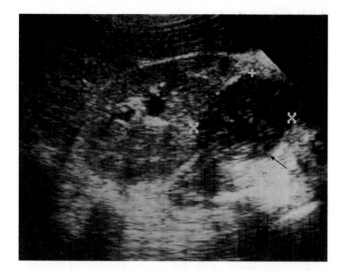

Figure 104–1 Ultrasound examination revealing a perinephric abscess *(arrow)*. (Courtesy of M. Bergeron, MD; from Mandell GL, Bennett JE, Dolin R: Principles and Practice of Infectious Diseases, 6th ed. Philadelphia, Churchill Livingstone, 2004, p 896.)

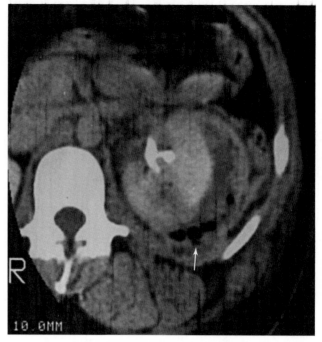

Figure 104–2 Computed tomography with contrast material demonstrating a large left perinepheric abscess containing gas *(arrow)*. (From Mandell GL, Bennett JE, Dolin R: Principles and Practice of Infectious Diseases, 6th ed. Philadelphia, Churchill Livingstone, 2004, p 896).

At present, many clinical laboratories consider bacterial growth of greater than 10^5 colony-forming units/mL to be indicative of infection. Studies have indicated that smaller numbers of bacteria (as few as 10^2 colony-forming units/mL) also can be indicative of UTIs, and this lower level cut-off should be used in persons with symptoms suggestive of UTI. A hazard in interpreting results of urine culture is that, if the sample is allowed to stand at room temperature for a few hours before being cultured, bacteria can multiply. This growth results in spuriously high bacterial counts. For this reason, urine for culture should not be obtained from a catheter bag. Specimens that are not plated immediately should be refrigerated. Biochemical tests to detect bacteriuria are not reliable when numbers of bacteria are low.

TREATMENT AND OUTCOME

All symptomatic patients with UTI should be treated with antimicrobials. Whereas most women with lower urinary tract infections are cured by a single dose of antibiotic, for example, amoxicillin, 3 g, or a double-strength trimetroprim-sulfamethoxazole (TMP-SMZ) tablet, a 3-day *(short course)* treatment with ciprofloxacin, 250 mg twice daily, or TMP-SMZ, 160 and 800 mg, respectively, twice daily, provides increased cure rates and is now generally recommended. (Note that, in some regions, more than 20% of *E. coli* are resistant to TMP-SMZ, and regional variations exist in the resistance patterns of all common urinary tract pathogens.) Short-course therapy is not recommended for women with a history of UTI owing to a resistant bacterium or when the duration of symptoms is longer than 1 week or for any UTI in men. In these patients, 7 to 10 days of treatment are recommended. Culture and sensitivity confirm the diagnosis and determine whether the antibiotic is active against the pathogen, but these tests are not essential in persons with uncomplicated cystitis unless treatment fails. Because of the difficulty in clinical distinction between cystitis and upper urinary tract disease, some patients treated for cystitis may experience relapse because of unrecognized upper tract disease. Recurrent UTIs in men should always raise the suspicion for an anatomic alteration of the urinary tract.

Occasionally, urine cultures obtained from a patient with symptoms of UTI and pyuria are reported as exhibiting *no growth* or *insignificant growth*. This situation has been labeled the *urethral syndrome*. Low numbers of bacteria (as few as 100 bacteria/mL of urine) may produce such infections of the urinary tract. In other instances, the urethral syndrome may be caused by *Chlamydia* or *Ureaplasma*, which will not grow on routine culture media. Thus, if a patient with the urethral syndrome has responded to antibiotics, the course should be completed; otherwise, if symptoms and pyuria persist, then the patient should receive doxycycline 100 mg twice daily for 7 days, or azithromycin 1 gm in a single dose, either of which is usually effective. Other considerations for patients with lower urinary tract symptoms and no or *insignificant* growth on cultures of urine include vaginitis, herpes simplex infection, and gonococcal infection. (*Neisseria gonorrhoeae* will not grow on routine media used for urine culture.) Thus, a pelvic examination and culture for gonococci may be indicated in this setting if the patient is sexually active. Men with urethral discomfort and discharge should be evaluated for urethritis (see Chapter 106). Men with suprapubic pain, frequency, and urgency should be evaluated for cystitis, as discussed earlier.

The presence of fever suggests that infection involves more than just the bladder. Young, otherwise healthy, febrile patients with UTIs may be treated on an ambulatory basis with a fluoroquinolone for 2 weeks, provided that (1) they

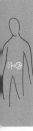

do not appear toxic, (2) they are able to take oral fluids and medications, (3) they have friends or family at home, (4) they have good provisions for follow-up, and (5) they have no potentially complicating features such as diabetes mellitus, history of renal stones, obstructive disease of the urinary tract, or sickle cell disease. Gram stain of urine in patients hospitalized for pyelonephritis will guide initial therapy. Initial therapy with TMP-SMZ for pyelonephritis can no longer be routinely recommended in the United States because of high levels of resistance in *E. coli* in many areas. In ill patients with community-acquired pyelonephritis, parenteral treatment for a gram-negative rod infection should be initiated with a fluoroquinolone, ampicillin-sulbactam, piperacillin-tazobactam, or a third-generation cephalosporin. An aminoglycoside may be added if drug resistance is presumed or if the patient is very ill. The aminoglycoside should be promptly discontinued if antibiotic sensitivity studies indicate that it is not essential. The finding of gram-positive cocci in chains suggests that enterococci are the pathogens. This infection should be treated, at least initially, with ampicillin plus an aminoglycoside. Gram-positive cocci in clusters may indicate staphylococci. *Staphylococcus saprophyticus* is a likely agent in otherwise healthy women and is sensitive to most antibiotics used in the treatment of UTI. In the older patient, *Staphylococcus aureus* should be considered, and this infection may be treated with a penicillinase-resistant penicillin, such as nafcillin. Gram-positive cocci in the urine may be indicative of endocarditis with septic embolization to the kidney.

Therapy should be simplified when reports of antimicrobial susceptibility are available. A repeat urine culture after 2 days of effective treatment should show sterilization or a marked decrease in the urinary bacterial count. If the patient fails to demonstrate some clinical improvement after 2 to 3 days of treatment or exhibits the clinical picture of sepsis and has been febrile for more than 1 week, then a complicating feature should be presumed. Intranephric or perinephric abscess or obstruction caused by a stone or an enlarged prostate may underlie this presentation. Ultrasonography is a good first-diagnostic procedure in this setting, which will generally detect obstruction and collections of pus and will also detect stones greater than 3 mm in diameter. If ultrasonography is negative in this setting, then computed tomography is indicated. Obstruction must be relieved and abscesses drained to result in cure. Computed tomography–guided percutaneous drainage is usually successful because of the proximity of the abscess to the flank wall; this approach is the procedure of choice whenever possible.

All patients with complicated UTIs should have repeat urine cultures 1 to 2 weeks after treatment is completed to check for relapse. If relapse occurs, then the patient may have pyelonephritis, prostatitis, or neuropathic or structural disease of the urinary tract. If a 6-week course of antibiotics active against the bacterial isolate is not effective in eradicating infection, then the possibility of structural abnormalities or prostatic infection should be investigated. Urologic evaluation should be performed for all men with UTI (except those with urethritis) because of the high frequency of correctable anatomic lesions in this population.

Some women have frequent episodes of UTI that are caused by different bacterial isolates. In some instances, these reinfections are related to sexual activity. Prompt voiding and a single dose of an active antibiotic (100 mg nitrofurantoin, 80 and 400 mg TMP-SMZ. or 100 mg ciprofloxacin) just after sexual contact can decrease the reinfection rate in these women. In other women, in whom no precipitating factor can be found and infections are frequent, prophylaxis with one half of a tablet of trimethoprim-sulfamethoxazole nightly has been effective.

On occasion, urine cultures show bacterial growth in the absence of symptoms. If the sample has been obtained properly and repeat culture reveals the same organism, then the condition is termed *asymptomatic bacteriuria*. This condition is generally observed in older or middle-age individuals and, in the absence of structural disease of the urinary tract or diabetes mellitus, does not require treatment. Asymptomatic bacteriuria occurring during pregnancy or in immunocompromised patients should be treated because of the high risk of pyelonephritis in these settings.

The occurrence of pyuria in the absence of bacterial growth on culture of urine ($<10^2$ colonies/mL) may be termed *sterile pyuria*. If this condition occurs in the patient with lower urinary tract symptoms, then chlamydial or gonococcal infection, vaginitis, or herpes simplex infection should be considered. In the absence of lower urinary tract symptoms, sterile pyuria may be seen among patients with interstitial nephritis of numerous causes or with tuberculosis of the urinary tract. Patients with renal tuberculosis often have nocturia and polyuria; more than one half of male patients also have involvement of the genital tract, most commonly the epididymis. Diagnosis can be made by biopsy of genital masses, when present, and by three morning cultures of urine for mycobacteria.

Prostatitis

Although prostatic fluid has antibacterial properties, the prostate can become infected, usually by direct invasion through the urethra. Symptoms of back or perineal pain and fever are common. Some patients have pain with ejaculation. Rectal examination usually shows a tender prostate. Patients with acute prostatitis generally have abnormal urinary sediment and pathogenic bacteria (usually gram-negative enteric rods) in cultures of urine.

Acute prostatitis may be caused by the gonococcus but is most often caused by gram-negative bacilli. Treatment is directed against the pathogen observed on Gram stain of urine and is generally effective. Therapy should be continued for a minimum of 4 weeks. Parenteral therapy is required rarely. Prostatic abscesses can be drained with ultrasound guidance. Chronic prostatitis may be asymptomatic and should be suggested in men with recurrent UTI. The urine sediment may be relatively benign in patients with chronic prostatitis. In this instance, comparison of the first part of the urine sample, midstream urine, excretions expressed by massage of the prostate, and postmassage urine should reveal bacterial counts more than 10-fold greater in the prostatic secretions and postmassage urine samples than in first-void and midstream samples. Treatment of chronic prostatitis is hampered by poor penetration of the prostate by most antimicrobial agents. Long-term (6 to 12 weeks) treatment with a fluoroquinolone or TMP-SMZ is indicated and is effective in a 60% to 70% of cases.

Prospectus for the Future

- More precisely targeted antimicrobial therapy to limit the spread of drug resistance
- More sensitive assays to identify low-level bacterial infection in symptomatic patients
- Antimicrobials that provide more effective treatment for chronic infection of the prostate
- More effective prophylaxis against recurrent UTIs

References

Miller LG, Tang AW: Treatment of uncomplicated urinary tract infections in an era of increasing antimicrobial resistance. Mayo Clin Proc 79(8):1048–1053, 2004.

Sobel JD, Kaye D: Urinary tract infections. In Mandell GL, Bennett JR, Dolin R (eds.): Principles and Practice of Infectious Diseases, 6th ed. Philadelphia, Elsevier, 2005, pp 875–905.

Chapter 105

Nosocomial Infections

Michelle V. Lisgaris
Robert A. Salata

A nosocomial or hospital-acquired infection is an infection that was not present or incubating at the time of hospital admission. In most patients, infections appearing after 48 to 72 hours of hospitalization are considered to be nosocomially acquired. A patient admitted to the hospital in the United States has a 5% to 10% chance of developing a nosocomial infection. These infections result in significant morbidity and mortality. Eighty-eight thousand deaths are attributable to nosocomial infections annually. The medical costs of nosocomial infections in the United States are estimated at ~$10 billion per year. To encompass infections acquired while residing in a nursing home environment or rehabilitation facility, the term *health care–associated infection* is often used when describing these situations.

Factors associated with an increased risk of nosocomial infection that are not avoidable by optimal medical practice include advanced age and severity of underlying illnesses. Contributing factors that can be minimized by thoughtful patient management include prolonged duration of hospitalization, the inappropriate use of antibiotics, the prolonged use of indwelling catheters, and the failure of health care personnel to wash their hands.

Infection Control

Surveillance of nosocomial infections and the implementation of practices to prevent and control them are the responsibility of infection control personnel. Practices used to limit the spread of infection include isolating patients with potentially transmissible diseases (e.g., tuberculosis, influenza, methicillin-resistant *Staphylococcus aureus*), isolating patients at increased risk for acquiring infections (e.g., patients with neutropenia and cancer), and instituting mandatory hand washing and *Universal Precautions* with all patient contact. Universal Precautions consider all blood and certain body fluids (e.g., cerebrospinal, amniotic, peritoneal, seminal, vaginal, blood contaminated) as potentially infectious. Gloves must be worn when exposure to these fluids, nonintact skin, or mucosal surfaces is expected. Additionally, masks and gowns are worn when splashes are expected.

Approach to the Hospitalized Patient with Possible Nosocomial Infection

The development of a nosocomial infection is often heralded by a rise in temperature. The only sign of infection, particularly in the older or demented patient, may be a change in mental status (Table 105–1). Confusion or alterations in vital signs may be the only sign of serious underlying infection. Respiratory alkalosis or metabolic acidosis (caused by lactate accumulation), either with or without hypoxia, may be present.

When evaluating a patient with a new fever or suggested nosocomial infection, the physician should first assess the stability of the patient; hypotension, tachypnea, or new obtundation mandates rapid evaluation and treatment. The patient's problem list and hospital course must be reviewed. The physician should elicit a history directed at possible causes of the fever, given that the patient often has a specific complaint that helps identify the source. Possible causes for nosocomial infections by anatomic site are listed in **Web Table 105–1**. Special attention should be given to examination of the skin for rash (e.g., drug eruption, ecthyma gangrenosum, disseminated candidiasis), wounds, or pressure sores; in addition, the physician must examine the sinuses (especially with nasogastric or nasotracheal tubes in place), mouth (for candidiasis or herpes infections), lungs (for pneumonia or thromboembolism), abdomen (e.g., for *Clostridium difficile*–associated colitis, postoperative abscess, biliary sepsis), catheters, joints (for septic arthritis, gout, and pseudogout), and extremities (for deep-venous thrombosis). The patient's medications should also be reviewed carefully for agents likely to produce fever (antibiotics and anticonvulsants especially). With drug fever, associated eosinophilia and/or rash is present in fewer than 25% of patients. Occasionally, a source of fever cannot be identified despite extensive evaluation. The classic definition of fever of unknown origin has recently been adapted to include the diagnosis of fever of unknown origin acquired nosocomially (see Chapter 94).

Table 105–1	**Signs of Infection in the Hospitalized Patient**

Fever or hypothermia
Change in mental status
Tachypnea and respiratory alkalosis
Hypotension
Oliguria
Leukocytosis

Nosocomial Pneumonia

Pneumonia comprises 15% to 20% of all nosocomial infections, making it the second most frequent hospital-acquired infection. The vast majority of instances arise from aspiration of oropharyngeal contents. Aerobic Gram-negative bacilli and often staphylococci, typically after the first 5 days of hospitalization, rapidly replace the normal oropharyngeal flora of the patient admitted to the hospital. The administration of broad-spectrum antibiotics, severe underlying illness (e.g., chronic lung disease), respiratory intubation, advanced age, and prolonged duration of hospitalization predispose individuals to colonization with these organisms.

Sedation, loss of consciousness, and factors that depress gag and cough reflexes place the colonized patient at increased risk for aspiration and the development of pneumonia. The development of a new pulmonary infiltrate in a hospitalized patient may represent pneumonia, atelectasis, aspiration of gastric contents, drug reaction, or pulmonary infarction. If pneumonia is suggested, then prompt identification of the pathogen and appropriate treatment are critical because nosocomial pneumonia carries a 20% to 50% risk of mortality. If the patient cannot produce a sputum specimen adequate for interpretation (<10 epithelial cells, >25 neutrophils per low-power [×100] field), then nasotracheal aspiration or bronchoscopic evaluation should be performed (see Chapter 98). Ventilator-associated pneumonia (VAP) accounts for up to 80% of nosocomially acquired respiratory infections, thus the intubated patient in the intensive care unit should be monitored carefully for signs of pneumonia. Many patients are paralyzed to facilitate ventilator-dependent respiration. These patients have ineffective gag reflexes and often depressed cough as well and are therefore entirely dependent on suctioning to prevent aspiration. Patients whose airways are simply colonized but whose lower respiratory tracts are not infected should not be treated with antibiotics, despite positive sputum cultures. Premature treatment of colonization results in replacement of the initial colonists by more resistant organisms, whereas delay in treatment of nosocomial pneumonia can result in death from overwhelming infection. The physician must therefore be able to distinguish accurately between colonization and infection. The development of new fever, leukocytosis, pulmonary infiltrates, or deterioration of oxygenation suggests pneumonia rather than colonization. A Gram stain of sputum should be performed to identify the predominant

Diagnostic Criterion	Results	Points
Temperature (°C)	≥ 36.5 and ≤ 38.4	0
	≥ 38.5 and ≤ 38.9	1
	≤ 36.0 and ≤ 39.0	2
Leukocyte count (/μL)	≥ 4000 and ≤ 11,000	0
	< 4000 or > 11,000	1
	≥ 500 band forms	1
Tracheal secretions	Absent	0
	Nonpurulent	1
	Purulent	2
PaO$_2$/FiO$_2$ (mm/Hg)	> 240 or ARDS	0
	≤ 240 and no evidence of ARDs	2
Pulmonary radiographic findings	No infiltrate	0
	Diffuse or patchy infiltrate	1
	Localized infiltrate	2
Progression of pulmonary infiltrate	No radiographic progression	0
	Radiographic progression after excluding CHF/ARDS	2
Tracheal aspirate Gram stain and culture	No pathologic bacteria cultured	0
	Pathologic bacteria cultured	1
	Some pathologic bacteria on Gram stain	1

Figure 105–1 With use of these diagnostic criteria, a Clinical Pulmonary Infection Score of 6 or greater has better than 90% sensitivity in detecting pulmonary infection.

organism or organisms, but initial antimicrobial therapy in these critically ill patients should include all likely pathogens because the high frequency of colonization makes interpretation of Gram stain results difficult. The use of clinical tools to assist in the distinction between colonization and infection, primarily in ventilated patients, is helpful in determining when antimicrobial treatment is needed (Fig. 105–1). The clinical pulmonary infection score (CPIS) assigns a numeric value to readily available clinical variables and assists in the determination of the presence of VAP. A CPIS of 6 or greater suggests pneumonia rather than simple colonization of the tracheobronchial tree. A CPIS score greater than 6 has greater than 90% sensitivity in detecting pulmonary infection. Epidemics of nosocomial pneumonia are most often caused by transmission of pathogenic bacteria from the hands of medical personnel.

The results of Gram stain and culture of the sputum and aspirate or the results of bronchoscopy specimens both guide antibiotic therapy. Gram-negative rods have been the predominant pathogens in this setting over the past 3 decades; these infections should be treated with a fluoroquinolone or aminoglycoside plus an extended-spectrum penicillin or cephalosporin until results of culture and sensitivity testing are known. Recent data from the National Nosocomial Infection Surveillance System indicates that *Staphylococcus aureus* is the most common cause of nosocomial pneumonia in critically ill patients in the United States and that the prevalence of methicillin resistance is on the rise among these organisms. Thus, if Gram-positive cocci in clusters are seen, then vancomycin or linezolid should be administered until sensitivities are known. A mixed flora suggestive of aspiration of oral anaerobes should prompt treatment with clindamycin or a penicillin–β-lactamase inhibitor combination. In certain hospitals, nosocomial pneumonia caused by *Legionella* species is a consideration, and, if suggested, then a fluoroquinolone or macrolide should be included in the initial treatment regimen until specific testing can be performed. Selection of an appropriate antimicrobial agent is critical because initial treatment with an antibiotic to which the causative organism is not sensitive is associated with a greater than twofold increase in mortality. Patients with nosocomial pneumonia should also receive aggressive respiratory therapy to promote coughing and expectoration of secretions.

Nosocomial pneumonias are best prevented in ventilated and nonventilated patients by (1) avoiding excessive sedation, (2) providing frequent suctioning and respiratory therapy, (3) positioning the patient in the semirecumbent position, (4) weaning the patient from mechanical respiratory support as soon as possible, (5) initiating early enteral nutrition, (6) encouraging frequent hand washing by all health care personnel, and (7) avoiding injudicious use of broad-spectrum or high-dose antibiotics.

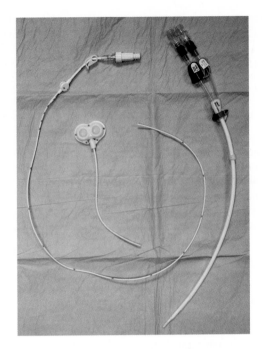

Figure 105–2 Long-term catheters.

Intravascular Catheter-Related Blood-Stream Infections

Greater than 200,000 nosocomial bloodstream infections occur annually in the United States, the vast majority of which can be attributed to the presence of an intravascular catheter (catheter-related bloodstream infection [CRBSI]).

Infections related to intravascular catheters may occur by means of bacteremic seeding or through infusion of contaminated material, but the vast majority of these infections occur through bacterial invasion at the site of catheter insertion. Catheters in frequent use today differ in their indications for use and their risk for CRBSI, thus familiarization of appropriate selection may go a long way toward preventing CRBSI (Table 105–2; **Web Fig. 105–1**).

Bacteria migrating through the catheter insertion site may colonize the catheter and then produce a septic phlebitis or bacteremia without evidence of local infection. Factors associated with a greater risk of intravenous CRBSI are shown in Table 105–3. Coagulase-negative staphylococci are the predominant pathogen in this setting, followed in equal frequency by *S. aureus* and enterococci. *Candida* species have now surpassed individual Gram-negative rods as the third leading cause of CRBSI. The rising incidence of candidemia and enterococcal bacteremia is a reflection of the increasing proportion of immunocompromised and severely ill patients being admitted to acute care facilities. As a group, Gram-negative enteric bacilli are the fourth most common cause of nosocomial bacteremia. Patients receiving parenteral nutrition are at particular risk for systemic infection with *Candida* species and Gram-negative bacilli.

If nosocomial bacteremia is suggested, then at least two sets of blood cultures should be obtained, one of which should be drawn from a peripheral vein and the other or others through the catheter of concern.

Management of CRBSI varies according to the type of catheter involved and whether bacteremia-associated complications (e.g., septic thrombosis, endocarditis, osteomyelitis, metastatic seeding of bacteria) are present (see Table 105–2 and **Web Fig. 105–1**).

A peripheral catheter (and all readily removable foreign bodies) should be replaced if bacteremia occurs and no other primary site of infection is found. The catheter should also be removed if fever without an obvious source occurs or if local phlebitis develops. Once the catheter is removed, the site should be compressed in an attempt to express pus from the catheter entry site. If septic thrombophlebitis is documented, then surgical exploration may be required. The value of culturing a peripheral catheter tip is limited unless semiquantitative techniques are used (e.g., isolation of >15 colony-forming units of bacteria by the roll plate method). Routine replacement of peripheral indwelling intravascular catheters every 72 hours decreases the risk of CRBSI.

Central venous catheters are of the nontunneled, tunneled, or implanted device variety (**Web Fig. 105–1**). These catheters may be kept in place for prolonged periods with a lower infection risk than peripheral catheters. However, because they typically remain in place for prolonged periods of time, central venous catheters are associated with a greater overall rate of infection. Special microbiologic techniques can be employed to assist in the diagnosis of catheter-related bacteremia. When the diagnosis is confirmed, assessment for infection-related complications (e.g., port abscess, tunnel infection, endocarditis, septic thrombosis) should be performed to devise an appropriate management strategy. Consideration of catheter removal should be given with any nontunneled, central venous catheter–related bacteremia and is generally recommended. Removal of tunneled catheters or implanted devices is generally required when

Table 105–2 Catheters Used for Vascular Access

Catheter Type	Entry Location	Size	Replacement	Comments
Peripheral Catheters				
Venous catheter (IV)	Peripheral veins	<3 inches	72 hr is recommended; 96 hr is safe if IV site is not indicative for thrombosis or phlebitis.	Risk of phlebitis exists with prolonged use; CRBSI is rare.
Arterial catheter	Primarily used in radial artery	<3 inches	Routine replacement is not supported unless malfunction or signs and symptoms of systemic complications exist.	CRBSI is rare; overall infection risk is low.
Midline catheters	Distal tip lies in proximal basilic or cephalic veins.	3–8 in	Same as for arterial catheters	Phlebitis occurs less often with midline catheters than with standard IV catheters; anaphylactoid reactions have occurred with elastomeric hydrogel–containing catheters.
Central Catheters (see Web Fig. 105–1 for images)				
Nontunneled venous catheters (Fig. 105–2A and C)	Subclavian, internal jugular, or femoral veins	≥8 cm*	Routine replacement is not supported unless malfunction or signs and symptoms of systemic complications are exhibited.	Is the leading cause of CRBSI; placement in upper torso is preferred. Replacement of catheter over a guidewire is *only* acceptable in cases of catheter malfunction. In the presence of bacteremia, the source of infection is typically the bacteria colonizing the tract formed by the catheter as it traverses the skin into the venous system.
Peripherally inserted central venous catheters (PICC) (Fig. 105–2B)	Basilic, cephalic, or brachial veins into the SVC	≥20 cm*	Same as nontunneled venous catheters	Lower rate of infection occurs with PICCs than with the nontunneled catheters; can be associated with thrombosis.
Tunneled venous catheter (Broviac, Hickman) (Fig. 105–2D)	Subclavian, internal jugular, or femoral veins	≥8 cm*	Is the same as nontunneled venous catheters.	Lower rates of infection occur with tunneled venous catheters than with nontunneled catheters; cuff inhibits the migration of bacteria into the catheter tract or *tunnel*.

Continued

Table 105–2   Catheters Used for Vascular Access—cont'd

Catheter Type	Entry Location	Size	Replacement	Comments
Implanted venous catheters (Mediport) (Fig. 105–2E)	Tunneled beneath skin into internal jugular or subclavian vein; accessed with needle placement into a subcutaneous port; needle may remain in place for up to six months, barring infection	≥8 cm*	Is the same as nontunneled venous catheters.	Carries lowest risk for CRBSI; no local care is required for maintenance; is a cosmetically appealing option for patients; requires surgery for removal.
Pulmonary artery catheters (Fig. 105–2F)	Enters central circulation through a Teflon-coated introducer placed in subclavian, internal jugular, or femoral veins.	≥30 cm*	No recommendations for replacement of catheters that are required for >7 days	Typically heparin bonded; carries same risk for CRBSI as central venous catheters; subclavian vein is insertion site of choice to reduce risk of CRBSI.

*Length depends on patient size.
Adapted from O'Grady NP, Alexander M, Patchen Dellinger E, et al: Guidelines for the management of intravascular catheter-related infections. Clin Infect Dis 35:1281–1307, 2002.
CRBSI = catheter-related bloodstream infection.

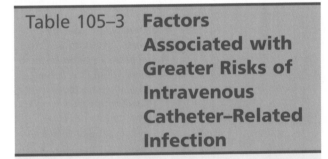

Table 105–3   Factors Associated with Greater Risks of Intravenous Catheter–Related Infection

Failure of staff to wash hands
Duration of catheterization >72 hr for peripheral intravenous catheters
Lower extremities and groin are at greater risk than upper extremities
Cutdown presents a greater risk than percutaneous insertion
Emergency insertion results in a greater risk than elective insertion
Breakdown in skin integrity (e.g., burns)
Insertion by physician is a greater risk than intravenous therapy teams

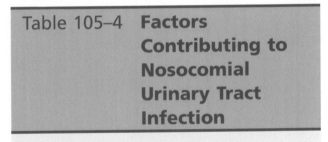

Table 105–4   Factors Contributing to Nosocomial Urinary Tract Infection

Indwelling catheters
Duration of catheterization
Open drainage (vs. closed-bag drainage)
Interruption of closed drainage system
Use of broad-spectrum antibiotics (Candida)

Nosocomial Urinary Tract Infection

Urinary tract infections are the most common nosocomial infections and result in 900,000 additional hospitalization days at a cost well over $615 million annually. They are accountable for 15% of nosocomial bacteremias. Approximately 80% of patients with nosocomial urinary tract infections are associated with the use of indwelling urinary catheters. Placement of an indwelling catheter into the urethra of a hospitalized patient facilitates access of pathogens to an ordinarily sterile site. Factors that predispose the patient to infection are shown in Table 105–4. The most common pathogens are enteric Gram-negative rods; however, Candida and Enterococcus species are also impor-

infectious complications occur. In situations in which the infected tunneled catheter or port cannot be removed, an antibiotic lock technique may be employed as an attempt to salvage the catheter. In cases of central venous catheter infections involving Candida species or other fungi, attempts at catheter salvage have been largely unsuccessful.

tant causes of infection. Prophylactic antibiotics, irrigation, urinary acidification, and use of antiseptics are of no value in preventing infection in this setting. Using indwelling catheters only when necessary can reduce nosocomial urinary tract infections; studies have observed that 21% to 50% of all urinary catheters placed were for inappropriate indications. Urinary incontinence and routine fluid balance monitoring are not sufficient indications. Thrice-daily straight (in-and-out) catheterization, with the use of aseptic technique, is less likely to produce infection than indwelling catheters, and many patients with dysfunctional bladders have used this technique for years without developing significant urinary tract infections.

If the use of an indwelling catheter is unavoidable, then the catheter drainage system should remain closed and unobstructed and kept securely fastened, with the collection bag remaining below the level of the bladder. The catheter should not be disconnected from the bag because specimens can be collected aseptically by inserting a needle through the distal catheter wall. Most important, the catheter should be removed as soon as possible. Additional strategies to reduce the incidence of urinary catheter–related infections have been the use of silver-coated or antibiotic-impregnated catheters; several studies have been performed and show either conflicting results or benefit only in select populations, respectively. As such, implementation of their use as routine practice has not been widely recommended.

Asymptomatic bacterial colonization of the catheterized bladder need not be treated. *Candida* infection of the bladder often resolves once broad-spectrum antibiotics are discontinued and the indwelling catheter has been removed. If *Candida* infection persists, then oral fluconazole or single-dose intravenous amphotericin B will often eradicate the organism, although recurrence rates are high, and the long-term benefit of this approach has not been demonstrated.

The best way to prevent catheter-related infections of the urinary tract is to avoid catheterization unless absolutely necessary.

Clostridium Difficile–Associated Diarrhea

Clostridium difficile–associated diarrhea (CDAD) is the most clinically significant cause of hospital-acquired diarrheal disease and is often accompanied by fever. It is a cause of significant morbidity and mortality and becoming increasingly difficult to control and eradicate. For full description of this important clinical condition, the reader is referred to Chapter 102.

Surgical Site Infections

Infections at the operative incision that develop within 30 days of a surgical procedure account for approximately 15% of all nosocomial infections and are the most common nosocomial infection among surgical patients. The pathogenesis of these infections involves inoculation of skin bacteria at the time of the surgical incision. Nonantibiotic prevention measures, such as minimizing preoperative length of stay, nonirritative hair removal techniques, and appropriate preoperative skin cleansing, are of great importance. If possible, pre-existing infections must be treated before surgery to decrease the risk of bacterial seeding of the surgical site. Antibiotic therapy directed at staphylococci and streptococci, administered no later than 2 hours before the time of incision, markedly reduces but does not eliminate the risk of infection for select surgical procedures.

Prospectus for the Future

Antimicrobial-resistant bacteria (methicillin-resistant *Staphylococcus aureus,* vancomycin-resistant enterococci, lactamase-producing Gram-negative bacilli), brought about by injudicious use of broad-spectrum antimicrobial agents, will continue to offer greater challenges in the treatment of nosocomially acquired infections. With continued medical advances, such as organ and bone marrow transplantations, the emergence of additional opportunistic nosocomial pathogens will undoubtedly occur. Additionally, monitoring and controlling infections in chronic care facilities will be increasingly important because of the emergence and transmission of antibiotic-resistant bacteria in this patient population and the risk of introducing these strains into the hospital environment. As medical professionals, we must share with infection control practitioners the burden of recognizing individuals who are at risk for developing nosocomial infections and instituting appropriate measures to prevent these infections.

References

American Thoracic Society; Infectious Disease Society of America: Guidelines for the management of adults with hospital-acquired, ventilator-associated, and healthcare-associated pneumonia. Am J Respir Crit Care Med 162:505–511, 2005.

O'Grady NP, Alexander M, Patchen Dellinger E, et al: Guidelines for the management of intravascular catheter-related infections. Clin Infect Dis 35:1281–1307, 2002.

Poutanen SM, Simor AE: *Clostridium difficile*-associated diarrhea in adults. CMAJ 171(1):51–58, 2004.

Chapter 106

Sexually Transmitted Diseases

Keith B. Armitage
Robert A. Salata

Sexually transmitted diseases (STDs) comprise a diverse group of infections caused by multiple microbial pathogens. These infections have common epidemiologic and clinical features. Since the mid-1980s, the field of STDs has evolved from one emphasizing the traditional venereal diseases of gonorrhea and syphilis to one concerned also with infections associated with *Chlamydia trachomatis,* herpes simplex virus (HSV), human papillomavirus (HPV), and human immunodeficiency virus (HIV).

Changes in sexual attitudes and practices have contributed to a resurgence of some, but not all, venereal infections. Gonorrhea, for example, has increased in incidence in the United States since 1963; approximately 2 million cases now occur each year, a higher incidence than in any nation in Western Europe. In contrast, the number of new cases of syphilis has decreased since peaking in the early 1990s. Chlamydia remains the most commonly reported STD, with an estimated 3 million cases in 2004. Adolescents make up approximately 40% of new cases of gonorrhea and chlamydia.

At the outset, two common errors in approaching the patient with STD should be avoided. The first error is failing to consider that an individual is at risk for STD. All sexually active persons are at risk, not only because of their own sexual behavior, but because of their sexual partner's behavior as well. Failure to consider risk factors often results in mistakes in diagnosis, inappropriate treatment, poor follow-up of infected sexual contacts, and, ultimately, recurrent or persistent infection. A second error with STDs is failing to recognize and diagnose co-infection. The most serious co-infection is with HIV. The worldwide epidemic of STDs fuels the global spread of HIV. STDs, most of which can be readily diagnosed and treated, may greatly enhance the transmission of HIV infection. HIV, in turn, may alter the natural history of other STDs.

STDs can be considered in broad groups according to whether major initial manifestations are (1) genital ulcers; (2) urethritis, cervicitis, and pelvic inflammatory disease (PID); or (3) vaginitis. All patients with any STD should be strongly encouraged to undergo screening for HIV infection (see Chapter 107). Updated information on STDs can be found on the Centers for Disease Control and Prevention website at *www.cdc.gov/std.*

Genital Sores

Six infectious agents cause most genital lesions (Table 106–1). The appearance of the lesions, natural history, and laboratory findings allow a clear-cut distinction among the possible causes in most instances. The two most common and significant infections in North America are HSV infection and syphilis.

HERPES SIMPLEX VIRUS INFECTION

Genital herpes infection has reached epidemic proportions, causing a corresponding increase in public awareness and concern. Genital herpes differs from other STDs in its tendency for spontaneous recurrence. Its importance stems from the morbidity, both physical and psychological, of the recurrent genital lesions and the danger of transmission of a fulminant, often fatal, disease to newborns.

Epidemiologic Factors

HSV has a worldwide distribution. Humans are the only known reservoir of infection, which is spread by direct contact with infected secretions. Of the two types of HSV, HSV-2 is the more frequent cause of genital infection. The major risk of infection is in the 14- to 29-year-old cohort and varies with sexual activity. Seroprevalence rates for HSV-2 infection are 22% in the general population and are as high as 40% to 50% in some North American populations. Many patients with serologic evidence of infection remain asymptomatic.

After exposure, HSV replicates within epithelial cells and lyses them, producing a thin-walled vesicle. Multinucleated cells are formed with characteristic intranuclear inclusions. Regional lymph nodes become enlarged and tender. HSV also migrates along sensory neurons to sensory ganglia, where it assumes a latent state. Exactly how viral reactivation occurs is uncertain. During reactivation, the virus appears to migrate back to skin along sensory nerves.

Table 106–1 Differentiation of Diseases Causing Genital Sores

Disease	Primary Lesion	Adenopathy	Systemic Features	Diagnosis/Treatment
Herpes genitalis primary (20% of sexually active adults, caused by HSV-2)	Incubation 2–7 days; multiple painful vesicles on erythematous base; persists 7–14 days	Tender, soft adenopathy; often bilateral	Fever	Tzanck smear positive; tissue culture isolation, HSV-2 antigen; fourfold rise in antibodies to HSV-2 Rx: acyclovir
Recurrent	Grouped vesicles on erythematous base; painful; lasts 3–10 days	None	None	Tzanck HSV-2 antigen; tissue culture positive; titers not helpful Rx: acyclovir
Syphilis (90,000 cases in United States per year, caused by *Treponema pallidum*)	Incubation 10–90 days (mean, 21); chancre: papule that ulcerates; painless, border raised, firm, ulcer indurated, base smooth; usually single; may be genital or almost anywhere; persists 3–6 wk, leaving thin, atrophic scar	1 wk after chancre appears; bilateral or unilateral; firm, discrete, movable, no overlying skin changes; painless, nonsuppurative; may persist for months	Later stages	Cannot be cultured; positive darkfield; VDRL test positive, 77%; FTA-abs positive, 86% (see Table 106–2) Rx: see Table 106–3
Chancroid (2000 cases in United States per year, caused by *Haemophilus ducreyi*)	Incubation 3–5 days; vesicle or papule to pustule to ulcer; soft, not indurated; very painful	1 wk after primary in 50%; painful, unilateral (two thirds), suppurative	None	Organism in Gram stain of pus; can be cultured (75%) but direct yields highest from lymph node Rx: ceftriaxone, 250 mg IM once, or ciprofloxacin, 500 mg twice daily for 3 days
Lymphogranuloma venereum (600–1000 cases per year in the United States, caused by *Chlamydia trachomatis*)	Incubation 5–21 days; painless papule, vesicle, ulcer, evanescent (2–3 days), noted in only 10–40%	5–21 days after primary; one third bilateral, tender, matted iliac/femoral *groove sign;* multiple abscesses; coalescent, caseating, suppurative, sinus tracts; thick yellow pus; fistulas; strictures; genital ulcerations	Fever, arthritis, pericarditis, proctitis, meningoencephalitis, keratoconjunctivitis, preauricular adenopathy, edema of eyelids, erythema nodosum	LGV CF positive 85–90% (1–3 wk); must have high titer (>1:16), cross-reacts with other *Chlamydia;* also positive STS, rheumatoid factor, cryoglobulins Rx: doxycycline, 100 mg twice daily for 7 days

Continued

| Table 106–1 | **Differentiation of Diseases Causing Genital Sores—cont'd** | | | |

Disease	Primary Lesion	Adenopathy	Systemic Features	Diagnosis/Treatment
Granuloma inguinale (50 cases in United States per year, caused by *Calymmatobacterium granulomatis*)	Incubation 9–50 days; at least one painless papule that gradually ulcerates; ulcers are large (1–4 cm), irregular, nontender, with thickened, rolled margins and beefy red tissue at base; older portions of ulcer show depigmented scarring, white; advancing edge contains new papules	No true adenopathy; in one fifth, subcutaneous spread through lymphatics leads to indurated swelling or abscesses of groin *(pseudobuboes)*	Metastatic infection of bones, joints, liver	Scraping or deep curetting at actively extending border; Wright or Giemsa stain reveals short, plump, bipolar staining; *Donovan's bodies* in macrophage vacuoles Rx: tetracycline, 2 g/day for 21 days
Condyloma acuminatum (genital warts, frequent, caused by human papillomavirus)	Characteristic large, soft, fleshy, cauliflower-like excrescences around vulva, glans, urethral orifice anus, perineum	None	None per se; association with cervical dysplasia/neoplasia	Chief importance is distinction from syphilis and chancroid Rx: topical podophyllin ± cryosurgery, laser resection

CF = complement fiixation; FTA-abs= flluorescent treponemal antibody absorption; HSV= herpes simplex virus; LGV = lymphogranuloma venereum; Rx = prescription; STS = serologic test for syphilis; VDRL = Venereal Disease Research Laboratory.

Clinical Presentation

Genital lesions that develop 2 to 7 days after contact with infected secretions are the manifestations of the clinical illness. In men, painful vesicles usually appear on the glans or penile shaft; in women, they occur on the vulva, perineum, buttocks, cervix, or vagina. A vaginal discharge is frequently present, usually accompanied by inguinal adenopathy, fever, and malaise. Sacroradiculomyelitis or aseptic meningitis can complicate primary infection. Perianal and anal HSV infections are especially common in male homosexuals; tenesmus and rectal discharge often are the main complaints.

The precipitating events associated with genital relapse of HSV infection are poorly understood. In individual cases, stress or menstruation may be implicated. Overall, genital recurrences develop in approximately 60% of patients infected with HSV. The frequency of clinically apparent recurrences is increased. The frequency of asymptomatic cervical recurrence in women is not known. Many patients describe a characteristic prodrome of tingling or burning for 18 to 36 hours before the appearance of lesions. Recurring HSV genital lesions are decreased in number, are usually stereotyped in location, are often restricted to the genital region, heal more quickly, and are associated with few systemic complaints.

Laboratory Diagnosis

The appearance of the characteristic vesicles is strongly suggestive of HSV infection. However, diagnosis should be confirmed by a Tzanck smear (66% sensitive) (see Chapter 92), Papanicolaou smear, immunofluorescent assay for viral antigen, or viral isolation. Serologic studies for HSV can be useful in the diagnosis of primary infection. Culture remains the *gold standard* for diagnosis. Direct antigen detection, by means of an enzyme immunoassay test, shows greater sensitivity than culture for later-stage HSV lesions and is equivalent to culture for early-stage infection and is generally the diagnostic test of choice.

Treatment

Topical or oral administration of acyclovir shortens the course of primary genital HSV infection. Intravenous or oral administration is recommended for severe cases with fever, systemic symptoms, and extensive local disease. Antiviral agents do not, however, prevent the latent stage of virus and cannot prevent recurrence. Prophylactic oral acyclovir decreases the frequency of symptomatic recurrences by 60% to 80% when used over a 4- to 6-year period, but asymptomatic viral shedding may occur despite prophylaxis. Oral acyclovir also hastens recovery from severe recurrent episodes; valacyclovir and famciclovir appear equally efficacious.

Shedding of HSV from active cervical or vulvar lesions late in pregnancy is an indication for cesarean section. Neonates exposed to asymptomatic shedding of HSV during parturition may also rarely acquire neonatal HSV. Primary HSV infection of the mother during pregnancy carries the greatest risk of neonatal infection.

SYPHILIS

Syphilis is of unique importance among the venereal diseases because early lesions heal without specific therapy; however, serious systemic sequelae pose a major risk to the patient, and transplacental infections can occur.

Epidemiologic Factors

Primary syphilis occurs mostly in sexually active 15- to 30-year-old individuals, and the incidence of primary syphilis increased sharply in North America during the early 1990s but has decreased in most risk groups in the early 2000s, with the exception of men who have sex with men (MSM). Approximately 50% of the sexual contacts of a patient with primary syphilis become infected. The long incubation period of syphilis becomes a key factor in designing strategies for contact tracing and management. Unless successful follow-up seems certain, contacts of proved cases must be treated with penicillin. HIV co-infection is on the increase, which poses a serious problem because the mucosal lesions of primary syphilis facilitate transmission of HIV infection (see Chapter 107). In turn, HIV appears to accelerate the course of syphilis, with more rapid and frequent involvement of the neurologic system.

Pathogenesis

Treponema pallidum penetrates intact mucous membranes or abraded skin, reaches the bloodstream by means of the lymphatics, and disseminates. The incubation period for the primary lesion depends on inoculum size, with a range of 3 to 90 days.

Natural History and Clinical Presentation

Primary syphilis is considered in Table 106–1. If the primary chancre is not treated, secondary syphilis may develop 6 to 8 weeks later. This time period can be accelerated in persons infected with HIV. Skin, mucous membranes, and lymph nodes are involved. A variety of skin lesions may occur, including macular, papular, papulosquamous, pustular, follicular, or nodular. Most commonly, they are generalized, symmetric, and of like size and appear as discrete, erythematous, macular lesions of the thorax or as red-brown hyperpigmented macules on the palms and soles. In moist intertriginous areas, large, pale, flat-topped papules coalesce to form highly infectious plaques or condylomata lata; darkfield microscopy reveals that they are teeming with spirochetes. Mucous patches are painless, dull erythematous patches or grayish-white erosions. They, too, are infectious and darkfield positive.

Systemic manifestations of secondary syphilis include malaise, anorexia, weight loss, fever, sore throat, arthralgias, and generalized, nontender, discrete adenopathy. Specific organ involvement also may develop: gastritis (superficial, erosive), hepatitis, nephritis, or nephrotic syndrome (immune-complex mediated), and symptomatic or asymptomatic meningitis. One fourth of patients have relapses of the mucocutaneous syndrome within 2 years of onset. Thereafter, infected patients become asymptomatic and noninfectious except through blood transfusions or transplacental spread.

Late syphilis, now relatively rare in the United States, develops after 1 to 10 years in 15% of untreated patients. Gummas are nonspecific granulomatous lesions once common in late syphilis but are rarely seen today. The skin gumma is a superficial nodule or deep granulomatous lesion that may develop punched-out ulcers. Superficial gummas respond dramatically to therapy. Gummas also may involve bone, liver, and the cardiovascular or central nervous system. Deep-seated gummas may have serious pathophysiologic consequences; treatment of the infection often does not reverse organ dysfunction.

Gradually progressive cardiovascular syphilis begins within 10 years in more than 10% of untreated patients, most frequently men. Patients develop aortitis with medial necrosis secondary to an obliterative endarteritis of the vasa vasorum.

Central nervous system syphilis develops in 8% of untreated patients 5 to 35 years after primary infection and includes meningovascular syphilis, tabes dorsalis, and general paresis (see Chapter 96). Late central nervous system syphilis may be asymptomatic despite cerebrospinal fluid (CSF) abnormalities indicating active inflammation. The natural history of syphilis may be altered by co-infection with HIV; such patients may develop signs and symptoms of secondary syphilis more rapidly, sometimes even before healing of the primary chancre (see Chapter 107).

Diagnosis and Treatment

Serologic studies are the primary method for diagnosis, but diagnosis may also be made by darkfield examination of clinical specimens. Spirochetes are seen in darkfield preparations of chancres or moist lesions of secondary syphilis. Serologic diagnosis is considered in Table 106–2. The differential diagnosis of a primary chancre includes herpes simplex and three conditions that are relatively rare in the United States: chancroid, lymphogranuloma venereum, and granuloma inguinale. The characteristics of these diseases are presented in Table 106–1.

The presence of neurosyphilis requires modifying the standard antibiotic treatment of syphilis. For this reason, a lumbar puncture should be considered in all patients with latent syphilis (positive Venereal Disease Research

Table 106-2 Serologic Studies in Syphilis

	VDRL	FTA-abs
Technique	Standard nontreponemal test; antibody to cardiolipin-lecithin	Standard treponemal test; antibody to Nichol's strain of *Treponema pallidum* after absorption on nontreponemal spirochetes
Indications	Screening and assessing response to therapy; should be quantified by diluting serum	Confirmation of specificity of positive VDRL test; remains reactive longer than VDRL test; useful for late syphilis, particularly neurosyphilis

Percent Positive in Syphilis

	VDRL	FTA-abs
Primary	77%	86%
Secondary	98%	100%
Early latent	95%	99%
Late latent and late	73%	96%
False positives	Weakly reactive VDRL test is common (~30% of normals); positive VDRL test should be repeated and, if confirmed, FTA-abs performed; relative frequency of false positives determined by prevalence of syphilis in the population	Borderline positive is frequent (80%) in pregnancy; should be repeated

FTA-abs = flluorescent treponemal antibody absorption; VDRL= Venereal Disease Research Laboratory.

Table 106-3 Treatment for Syphilis in the Normal Patient

Clinical Category	Regimen of Choice	History of Penicillin Allergy
Primary Secondary Early latent Healthy contact*	Benzathine penicillin, 2.4 MU IM	Tetracycline or erythromycin, 2 g/day for 15 days
Late latent or late	Benzathine penicillin, 2.4 MU IM per week for 3 weeks	No regimen adequately evaluated; tetracycline or erythromycin, 2 g/day for 30 days
Neurosyphilis	Aqueous penicillin G, 20 MU IV per day for 10 days	Same as for late latent or late

*Contact of patient with active skin or mucous membrane lesions.
IM = intramuscular.

Laboratory [VDRL] test at least 1 year after primary syphilis) or syphilis of unknown duration. An elevated CSF white blood cell count, elevated protein, and positive VDRL test on diluted samples of CSF establish the diagnosis of neurosyphilis. A patient with a persistent positive blood VDRL test and a positive CSF VDRL test should be considered to have neurosyphilis and treated accordingly. However, the sensitivity of the CSF VDRL test in proved cases of neurosyphilis is only 40% to 50%. Treatment of neurosyphilis is therefore indicated in patients with a consistent neurologic syndrome, characteristic CSF changes, and a positive serum VDRL test. Because the VDRL test may be negative in late syphilis, the presence of a positive serum fluorescent treponemal antibody absorption (FTA-abs) test in a patient with a neurologic syndrome consistent with syphilis is a sufficient indication for treatment. A small proportion (2% to 3%) of patients with neurosyphilis may undergo abrupt deterioration after treatment with penicillin; this Jarisch-Herxheimer reaction, thought to represent a systemic response to penicillin-induced lysis of spirochetes, may be ameliorated by concomitant treatment with corticosteroids. This reaction is especially important in secondary syphilis with meningeal involvement. Treatment protocols are shown in Table 106–3.

Serologic studies for syphilis must be followed after treatment. With the recommended treatment schedules, 1% to 5% of patients with primary syphilis will develop relapse or be reinfected. In adequately treated primary syphilis, the VDRL test should become negative by 2 years after therapy (usually by 6 to 12 months). The FTA-abs test, however, often remains positive for life. Seventy-five percent of adequately treated patients with secondary syphilis will have a negative serum VDRL test by 2 years. If the VDRL test does not become negative or achieve a low fixed titer, lumbar puncture should be performed to evaluate the possibility of asymptomatic neurosyphilis, and the patient should be re-treated with penicillin. Two percent to 10% of patients with central nervous system syphilis will experience relapse after treatment. However, asymptomatic patients rarely develop symptomatic disease after penicillin therapy; the only major exception is the patient infected with HIV, in whom meningovascular syphilis can develop within months of the standard treatment for primary syphilis. Every patient who is treated for syphilis should be seronegative or *serofast* with a low fixed titer before termination of follow-up. If not, therapy should be repeated.

Because of the documented progression to neurosyphilis in some individuals infected with HIV who have received treatment for primary syphilis, the following approach is suggested. All patients with syphilis should be tested for HIV infection. All individuals infected with HIV should be tested for syphilis. If dual infection is likely or documented, a lumbar puncture is indicated regardless of the stage or activity of the syphilis. Any CSF abnormality warrants a 10- to 14-day course of intravenous penicillin to treat neurosyphilis. If the CSF is unremarkable, three weekly doses of benzathine penicillin plus a 10-day course of amoxicillin may be appropriate. In any event, careful clinical and laboratory follow-ups are essential.

Urethritis, Cervicitis, and Pelvic Inflammatory Disease

These syndromes can be considered broadly as gonococcal and nongonococcal in origin.

GONORRHEA

Neisseria gonorrhoeae is second only to *C. trachomatis* as a cause of sexually transmitted diseases in the United States.

Epidemiologic Factors

The incidence of gonorrhea reached a plateau in the United States between 1975 and 1980, possibly reflective of a decrease in the size of the at-risk cohort. Re-infection is common, and for one sexually active patient to have 20 or more discrete infections is not unusual. Particular risk factors are urban habitat, low socioeconomic status, unmarried status, and large numbers of unprotected sexual contacts. Fifty percent of women having intercourse with a man with gonococcal urethritis will develop symptomatic infection. The risk for men is 20% after a single sexual contact with an infected woman. Orogenital contact and anal intercourse also transmit infection. Asymptomatic infection of men is an important factor in transmission. Forty percent of male contacts of symptomatic women have asymptomatic urethritis. Such patients may remain culture positive and asymptomatic but capable of transmitting infection for periods of up to 6 months. Co-infection with *C. trachomatis* is observed in up to 30% to 40% of patients with gonorrhea.

Pathogenesis

Neisseria gonorrhoeae is a gram-negative, kidney bean–shaped diplococcus. Specialized projections from the organism (pili) aid in attachment to mucosal surfaces, contribute to resistance to killing by neutrophils, and constitute an important virulence factor. In women, several factors alter susceptibility to infection. Group B blood type increases susceptibility, whereas vaginal colonization with normal flora, immunoglobulin (Ig) A content of vaginal secretions, and high progesterone levels may be protective. Spread from the cervix to the upper genital tract is associated with menstruation, because changes in the pH and biochemical constituents of cervical mucus lead to increased shedding of gonococci; cervical dilation, reflux of menses, and binding of the gonococcus to spermatozoa may be additional factors in ascending genital infection and dissemination. Intrauterine contraceptive devices increase the risk of endometrial spread of infection twofold to ninefold (oral contraceptives are associated with a twofold decrease).

Clinical Presentation

In men who develop symptomatic urethritis, symptoms of purulent discharge and severe dysuria usually occur 2 to 7 days after sexual contact. Prompt treatment usually follows, so that more extensive genital involvement is uncommon.

In women, cervicitis is the most frequent manifestation and results in copious yellow vaginal discharge. Overall, 20% of women with gonococcal cervicitis develop PID, usually beginning at a time close to the onset of menstruation. PID exhibits as endometritis (abnormal menses and midline abdominal pain), salpingitis (bilateral lower abdominal pain and tenderness), or pelvic peritonitis. Salpingitis can cause tubal occlusion and sterility. Gonococcal perihepatitis (Fitz-Hugh–Curtis syndrome) also may complicate PID and produce right upper quadrant pain.

Women also may develop urethritis with dysuria and frequency. In certain populations of sexually active women, one fourth of those complaining of urinary tract symptoms and 60% of those with symptoms but no bacteriuria have urethral cultures positive for *N. gonorrhoeae*.

Anorectal gonorrhea occurs in both homosexual men and heterosexual women. In men, the resultant rectal pain, tenesmus, mucopurulent discharge, and bleeding may represent the only signs of infection. In women, asymptomatic anorectal involvement is a frequent complication of symptomatic genitourinary disease even in the absence of anal intercourse (44%); isolated anorectal infection (4%), as well as acute or chronic proctitis (2% to 5%), is rare. Treatment failures are frequent in anorectal gonorrhea (7% to 35%).

Because of the frequency of asymptomatic infection in each of the potential sites, patients with symptoms suggestive of gonococcal infection should have cultures from the urethra, anus, pharynx, and (when applicable) cervix.

Pharyngeal gonorrhea occurs in homosexual men or heterosexual women after oral sex and is less frequent in heterosexual men. The pharynx is rarely the sole site of gonococcal infection (5% to 8%).

Extragenital dissemination occurs in approximately 1% of men and 3% of women with gonorrhea. Strains of *N. gonorrhoeae* causing dissemination differ from other gonococci in several respects. They are generally more penicillin

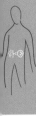

sensitive but resist the normal bactericidal activity of antibody and complement. The latter finding may result from their binding of a naturally occurring blocking antibody. Complement deficiency states can predispose patients to disseminated gonorrhea. Dissemination of gonococcal infection may take the form of the arthritis-dermatitis syndrome, with 3 to 20 papular, petechial, pustular, necrotic, or hemorrhagic skin lesions usually found on the extensor surfaces of the distal extremities. An associated finding is an asymmetric polytenosynovitis, with or without arthritis, that predominantly involves wrists, fingers, knees, and ankles. Joint fluid cultures usually are negative in arthritis-dermatitis syndrome, leading to speculation that circulating immune complexes, demonstrable in most patients, are important in its pathogenesis. Synovial biopsies may yield positive cultures. Biopsy of skin lesions reveals gonococcal antigens (by immunofluorescent antibody staining) in two thirds of patients. Blood cultures are positive in 50% of patients. Septic arthritis is another manifestation of dissemination; *N. gonorrhoeae* is the most frequent cause of septic arthritis in 16- to 50-year-old persons. The joint fluid cultures are positive (particularly when the leukocyte count in joint fluid exceeds 80,000/mcL) in less than 50% of instances, and blood cultures are positive in less than 25%; the diagnosis is most often confirmed by extra-articular cultures (usually genital sites). Gonococcemia may in rare cases lead to endocarditis, meningitis, myopericarditis, or toxic hepatitis.

Laboratory Diagnosis and Management

Gram stain of the urethral discharge will determine the cause of urethritis in most men with gonorrhea because typical intracellular diplococci are diagnostic (**Web Fig. 106–1**). The finding of only extracellular gram-negative diplococci is equivocal. The absence of gonococci on a smear of urethral discharge from a man virtually excludes the diagnosis. Diagnosis by Gram staining of cervical exudates is relatively specific but insensitive (<60%). Modified Thayer-Martin medium contains antibiotics that inhibit the growth of other organisms and increase the yield of gonococci from samples likely to be contaminated; Thayer-Martin culture of normally sterile fluids, such as joint fluid, blood, and CSF, is not necessary. Specimens from these sites should be cultured on chocolate agar. Other important considerations for isolating gonococci include using synthetic swabs (unsaturated fatty acids in cotton may be inhibitory), introducing a very thin calcium alginate swab or a loop 2 cm into the male urethra, and avoiding vaginal douching (12 hours), urination (2 hours), and vaginal speculum lubricants before culture. In all suggested cases of gonorrhea, the urethra, anus, and pharynx should be cultured. In women, 20% of cases in which initial cervical cultures were negative yield *N. gonorrhoeae* when cultures are repeated. Gene probes are less sensitive than culture in diagnosis.

Gonococcal resistance to penicillin is increasing worldwide. The current recommendation for the treatment of uncomplicated gonorrhea is ceftriaxone, 125 mg given intramuscularly once. This step should always be followed by a course of doxycycline (100 mg orally twice daily for 7 days) or azithromycin (1 g orally as single dose) to treat concurrent chlamydial infection. Alternative therapies include cefixime, 400 mg once orally; ciprofloxacin, 500 mg once orally; or levofloxacin, 500 mg once. Resistance among gonococci to quinolones is increasing in Southeast Asia, Hawaii, California, and Washington, as well as among MSM. The Centers for Disease Control and Prevention no longer recommends quinolones for patients from these geographic areas and for MSM. Practitioners should be aware of the possibility of the emergence of quinolone resistance in new geographic areas and among new risk groups. In patients with severe β-lactam allergies, spectinomycin, 2 g intramuscularly, can be used; this therapy is inadequate for pharyngeal infection. PID should be treated with cefoxitin, 2 g given intramuscularly, followed by doxycycline, 100 mg twice daily administered orally for 10 days. Seriously ill women with PID should be hospitalized. Evaluation by ultrasonography for the presence of a pelvic abscess or peritonitis is indicated in this setting. Surgery may be indicated to drain a tubo-ovarian or pelvic abscess.

Disseminated gonococcal infection should be treated with ceftriaxone, 1 g every 24 hours for 10 days. If history suggests an IgE-mediated allergy to penicillin (anaphylactoid reaction, angioedema, or urticaria), then ciprofloxacin, 500 mg twice daily for 7 days, is an effective alternative in areas of low quinolone resistance.

A VDRL test should be performed in all patients with gonorrhea. If negative, no further follow-up is necessary because ceftriaxone in the dosage used is probably effective in treating incubating syphilis. If alternative drugs are used, the VDRL test should be repeated after 4 weeks. Anal cultures for *N. gonorrhoeae* should be part of the routine follow-up of women because persistent anorectal carriage may be a source of relapse. Postgonococcal urethritis occurs in 30% to 50% of men 2 to 3 weeks after penicillin therapy if this treatment is not followed by doxycycline. It usually is caused by *C. trachomatis* or *Ureaplasma urealyticum*.

NONGONOCOCCAL URETHRITIS, CERVICITIS, AND PELVIC INFLAMMATORY DISEASE

The diagnosis of nongonococcal urethritis (NGU) requires the exclusion of gonorrhea because considerable overlap exists in the clinical syndromes.

Epidemiologic Factors

At least as many cases of urethritis are nongonococcal as gonococcal. Typically, NGU predominates in higher socioeconomic groups. *Chlamydia trachomatis* causes 30% to 50% of NGU and can be isolated from 0% to 11% of asymptomatic, sexually active men. *Chlamydia trachomatis* also can be isolated from 30% of men with gonorrhea and presumably represents a concurrent infection. Some cases of *Chlamydia*-negative NGU are caused by *U. urealyticum* or *Trichomonas vaginalis*.

Clinical Syndromes

NGU is less contagious than gonococcal infection. The incubation period is 7 to 14 days. Characteristically, patients complain of urethral discharge, itching, and dysuria. Importantly, the discharge is not spontaneous but becomes apparent after milking the urethra in the morning. The mucopurulent discharge consists of thin, cloudy fluid with

Table 106–4 Vaginitis

Disease	Epidemiology/ Pathogenesis	Clinical Findings	Laboratory Diagnosis	Treatment
Candidiasis	Yeast is part of normal flora; overgrowth favored by broad-spectrum antibiotics, high estrogen levels (pregnancy, before menses, oral contraceptives), diabetes mellitus, may be early clue to HIV infection	Itching, little or no urethral discharge, occasional dysuria; labia pale or erythematous with satellite lesions; vaginal discharge thick, adherent, with white curds; balanitis in 10% of male contacts	Vaginal pH = 4.5 (normal), negative whiff test, yeast seen on wet mount in 50%, culture positive	Miconazole, butoconazole, terconazole, or clotrimazole cream or suppositories for 3–7 days; fluconazole, 150 mg orally as a single dose
Trichomonas vaginalis infection	STD; incubation 5–28 days; symptoms begin or exacerbate with menses	Discharge, soreness, irritation, mild dysuria, dyspareunia; copious loose discharge, one fifth yellow-green, one third bubbly	Elevated pH; wet mount shows large numbers of WBCs, trichomonads; positive whiff test (10% KOH causes fishy odor)	Metronidazole, 2 g as single dose; treat sexual contacts
Bacterial vaginosis	Synergistic infection, *Gardnerella vaginalis* and anaerobes *Mobiluncus* sp.	Vaginal odor, mild discharge, little inflammation; grayish, thin, homogeneous discharge with small bubbles	Elevated pH; positive whiff test; wet prep contains clue cells (vaginal epithelial cells with intracellular coccobacilli), few WBCs	Metronidazole, 500 mg twice daily for 7 days; alternatives include metronidazole gel (0.75%), 5 g intravaginally twice daily for 7 days, or clindamycin cream (2%) 5 g intravaginally daily at night for 7 days; do not treat contacts unless recurrent vaginitis

HIV = human immunodeficiency virus; KOH = potassium hydroxide; STD = sexually transmitted disease; WBCs = white blood cells.

purulent specks; these characteristics do not always allow clear distinction from gonococcal disease. *Trichomonas vaginalis* causes a typically scanty discharge.

Chlamydia trachomatis also is a common cause of epididymitis in men younger than 35 years of age and can produce proctitis in men and women who practice receptive anal intercourse.

Chlamydial infections are also more common than gonococcal infections in women but frequently escape detection. Two thirds of women with mucopurulent cervicitis have chlamydial infection. Similarly, many women with the acute onset of dysuria, frequency, and pyuria, but sterile bladder urine, have *C. trachomatis* infection. *Chlamydia trachomatis* is at least as common a cause of salpingitis as is the gonococcus.

Laboratory Diagnosis

Ordinarily, the distinction between gonococcal and non-gonococcal infections relies mainly on Gram-stained prepa-rations of exudates and cultures. In a man with urethritis and typical gram-negative diplococci associated with neutrophils, the diagnosis of gonococcal urethritis is clear-cut, and the culture is unnecessary. Coincident NGU cannot be excluded, however. Whenever interpretation of the Gram stain is not straightforward in men, and in all women, culture on Thayer-Martin medium is appropriate. Techniques for isolation and detection (DNA probes) of chlamydiae should be used routinely in evaluating genital infection.

Treatment

The patient and all sexual contacts should be treated with azithromycin, 1 g orally as a single dose, or doxycycline, 100 mg orally twice daily for 7 days. Recurrence may occur and requires longer periods (2 to 3 weeks) of treatment. In pregnancy, erythromycin base, 500 mg orally four times daily for 7 days, is an alternative acceptable regimen. Patients who fail to respond to doxycycline may be infected with *U. urealyticum*, given that 30% of strains are doxycycline resistant.

Patients who fail to respond to doxycycline and azithromycin may have a syndrome of NGU caused by *T. vaginalis,* and consideration should be given to therapy with metronidazole.

Proctocolitis in Men Who Have Sex with Men

Men who practice receptive anal intercourse may exhibit with proctitis or proctocolitis, causing anorectal pain, mucoid or bloody discharge, tenesmus, diarrhea, or abdominal pain. Sigmoidoscopy should be performed, with culture and Gram stain of the discharge. The potential causative organisms are diverse (**Web Table 106–1**). The diarrheal syndromes are considered in Chapter 102. Ten percent of patients harbor two or more pathogens. Proctitis also may occur without a definable pathogen (42%). Diarrhea in the patient infected with HIV has an entirely different set of implications (see Chapter 107).

Vaginitis

Table 106–4 considers salient features in the diagnosis and management of patients with vaginitis.

Prospectus for the Future

Effective treatment of STDs will be increasingly important in worldwide efforts to counter the HIV epidemic. More extensive treatment for STDs may lead to increasing resistance of gonococci and other genital pathogens to currently available antimicrobial agents. Treatment guidelines will necessarily evolve in response to the changing patterns of antimicrobial resistance.

References

Centers for Disease Control and Prevention: 2002 Sexually transmitted diseases treatment guidelines. MMWR Morb Mortal Wkly Rep 51(RR-6):1–82, 2002 (see also *http://www.cdc.gov/mmwr*).

Corey L, Handsfield HH: Genital herpes and public health. JAMA 283:791–794, 2000.
Rein M, et al: Sexually transmitted diseases. In Goldman L, Ausiello D (eds): Cecil Textbook of Medicine, 22nd ed. Philadelphia, WB Saunders, 2004, pp 1914–1933.

Human Immunodeficiency Virus Infection and Acquired Immunodeficiency Syndrome

Charles C. J. Carpenter

Curt G. Beckwith

Benigno Rodríguez

Michael M. Lederman

Two and one half decades after acquired immunodeficiency syndrome (AIDS) was recognized as a new disease entity in 1981, over 75 million individuals worldwide have been infected by the causative human immunodeficiency virus-1 (HIV-1). Of these individuals, more than 90% live in the developing world, and the vast majority have acquired the infection through heterosexual intercourse. The worldwide incidence of HIV-1 infection has increased steadily until the present time.

A second human immunodeficiency virus (HIV-2) was identified in West Africa in the mid-1980s. HIV-2 infection may also result in AIDS but has a considerably longer clinically latent period than HIV-1. Although HIV-2 shares many genetic characteristics with HIV-1, each of the two viruses has regulatory and structural genes that are unique. Whereas HIV-1 is closely related to the simian immunodeficiency virus (SIV) isolated from a subspecies of chimpanzee (SIV$_{cpz}$), HIV-2 is more closely related to an SIV that is commonly found in the sooty mangaby monkey (SIV$_{sm}$). HIV-2 infections have infrequently been identified in the United States to date. Throughout this chapter, the abbreviation *HIV* refers to HIV-1.

Epidemiologic Factors

Available data suggest that humans first became infected with HIV in the 1930s or 1940s, in the process of slaughtering chimpanzees for human consumption in the African *bushmeat* market. In retrospect, HIV infection had spread extensively in Central Africa by the early 1970s; the significant wasting of advanced HIV disease was then reflected by the descriptive eponym *slim disease,* which was applied to the unexplained illness that was occurring in large numbers of young adults in Uganda at that time.

AIDS was first recognized in 1981 as a distinct clinical entity in several major North American cities in previously healthy young men who had sex with men. These men exhibited serious infections caused by unusual opportunistic pathogens (OIs), most frequently *Pneumocystis jirovecii* pneumonia (PCP), an illness previously observed only among patients with severe cellular immunodeficiency. Studies confirmed profound immunodeficiency in these individuals, leading to the name *acquired immunodeficiency syndrome.* When similar OIs were observed in intravenous drug users and in men with hemophilia and their female sexual partners, the fact became clear that this syndrome was caused by an agent transmitted either through sexual contact or by blood or blood products. The *human immunodeficiency virus* was identified in 1983 and confirmed in 1984 as the causative agent of AIDS.

Based on the recognition of several thousand individuals with advanced disease in 1981 and 1982, and current knowledge that the average lag period between initial infection by HIV and the clinical manifestations of severe immunodeficiency (AIDS) is 8 to 10 years, HIV infection was likely introduced into North America in the early 1970s.

The Centers for Disease Control and Prevention (CDC) surveillance criteria for the diagnosis of AIDS, as modified in 1987, included a large number of OIs (Table 107–1) indicative of defects in cellular and/or humoral immunity, as well as certain neoplasms and other conditions associated with severe immunodeficiency (Table 107–2). The occurrence of any one of these conditions in an individual with no other cause of immunosuppression constituted the surveillance diagnosis of AIDS. In 1992, the CDC broadened the

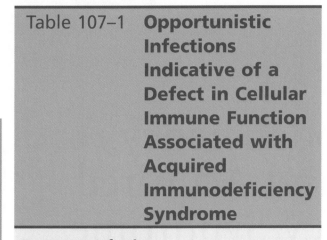

Table 107–1 **Opportunistic Infections Indicative of a Defect in Cellular Immune Function Associated with Acquired Immunodeficiency Syndrome**

Protozoan Infection

Toxoplasma gondii encephalitis
Cryptosporidium parvum enteritis (>1 mo)
Isospora belli enteritis (>1 mo)

Fungal Infection

Candida esophagitis
Cryptococcus neoformans meningitis
Disseminated *Histoplasma capsulatum*
Disseminated *Coccidioides immitis*
Pneumocystis jirovecii pneumonia

Bacterial Infection

Disseminated Mycobacterium avium-intracellulare
Active Mycobacterium tuberculosis infection
Recurrent Salmonella septicemia
Recurrent bacterial pneumonia*

Viral Infection

Chronic (>1 mo) mucocutaneous or esophageal herpes simplex infection
Cytomegalovirus retinitis, esophagitis, or colitis
Progressive multifocal leukoencephalopathy (JC virus)

*Requires laboratory evidence of HIV infection.

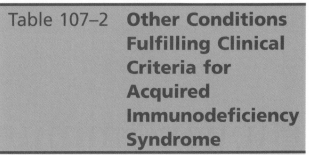

Table 107–2 **Other Conditions Fulfilling Clinical Criteria for Acquired Immunodeficiency Syndrome**

Neoplasms

Kaposi's sarcoma (in a person <60 yr of age)
High-grade, B-cell non-Hodgkin's lymphoma*
Primary brain lymphoma*
Immunoblastic sarcoma*
Invasive carcinoma of the cervix*

Systemic Illness

HIV-wasting syndrome (unintentional loss of >10% of body weight)*

HIV = human immunodeficiency virus.
*Requires laboratory evidence of HIV infection.

definition of AIDS to include all persons infected with HIV with severely depressed levels of cell-mediated immunity as indicated by CD4 + T-lymphocyte counts (CD4 counts) less than 200 cells/mm^3.

By 1993, AIDS had become the leading cause of death of American adults ages 25 to 44 (Fig. 107–1). By the year 2006, over 1 million persons in the United States were living with HIV infection; over 400,000 persons had died with AIDS. From 1998 through 2005, 40,000 to 45,000 individuals acquired HIV infection annually in the United States.

Retrospective analysis of stored serum revealed that HIV infection had been present in parts of Central Africa for 2 decades before recognition of the clinical syndrome of AIDS. Since the early 1980s, HIV infection has become a major worldwide pandemic. HIV infection continues to spread, albeit at strikingly different rates, throughout all continents. Since the late 1990s, transmission of HIV has been most rapid throughout Southern Africa, India, Southeast Asia, Eastern Europe, and the former Soviet Union.

Because of the latency between HIV infection and development of AIDS-associated illnesses, the clinically recognized epidemic has lagged 6 to 8 years behind the spread of HIV into new populations. Heterosexual intercourse has been the dominant mode of HIV transmission throughout most of the world. The virus is present in semen and cervicovaginal secretions of infected individuals and can be transmitted by either partner during vaginal or anal intercourse. The concurrent presence of other sexually transmitted diseases (STDs), especially those associated with genital ulcerations, strongly facilitates sexual transmission of HIV (see Chapter 106). In the United States, HIV infection has increased rapidly in women in the last decade; in several rural areas in the Southeast, women accounted for over one half of new cases in 2005.

A disproportionate number of North American men and women infected with HIV are economically disadvantaged African-American or Hispanic individuals. Transmission by injection drug use (IDU) has been a major factor in this imbalance, given that IDU transmission has occurred most commonly in impoverished inner-city areas. Differences in regional patterns of IDU have been a major factor in the greater than 100-fold regional variation in prevalence of AIDS cases in the United States. Since 2003, IDU transmission has significantly declined in the United States, whereas heterosexual transmission has continued to increase (Fig. 107–2).

Vertical transmission of HIV from infected mother to child may occur in utero, during labor, or through breastfeeding. In the absence of antiretroviral treatment, HIV infects 25% to 30% of infants born to HIV-infected mothers. The rate of vertical transmission can be reduced to less than 2% by prenatal and perinatal treatment of the mother and postnatal treatment of the infant with effective antiretroviral drugs.

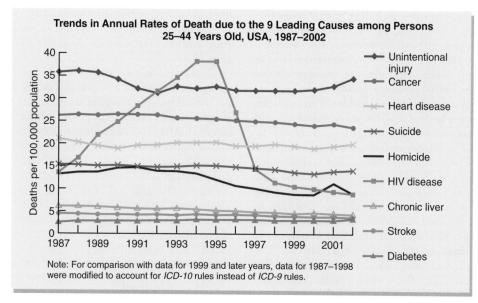

Figure 107–1 Trends in annual death rates in persons ages 25 to 44, United States, 1987–2002. In 1993, AIDS became the leading cause of death of Americans in this age group. Since the widespread adoption of effective ART in 1996, AIDS-related death rates have fallen sharply. By 2001, AIDS ranked sixth among the causes of death in this age group. (Data from the Centers for Disease Control and Prevention, *http://www.cdc.gov/hiv/graphics/htm.*)

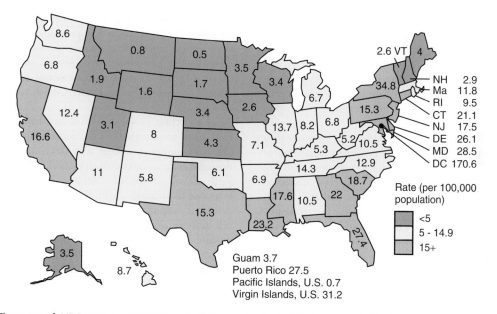

Figure 107–2 The rates of AIDS cases per 100,000 population in the United States, reported in 2003. The rates show tremendous regional variation, from 170.6 in the District of Columbia to 0.5 in North Dakota. Overall rates for men are roughly three times those of women. (Data from the Centers for Disease Control and Prevention, *http://www.cdc.gov/hiv/graphics/htm.*)

HIV is universally present in the blood of infected patients in the absence of effective antiretroviral therapy. Thus, before nationwide implementation of a blood-screening test in late 1985, infection by transfused blood or blood products accounted for nearly 3% of AIDS cases in the United States. Since 1985, all blood products in North America have been screened for HIV. The risk of transfusion-acquired HIV infection in North America and Western Europe is now exceedingly small but not absent.

HIV infection may occur after accidental parenteral exposures of health care workers. After injury by a HIV-contaminated hollow needle, the risk of infection is approximately 0.3%. This risk can be reduced at least tenfold by prompt postexposure prophylaxis.

Pathophysiologic Factors

HIV is a member of the lentivirus family of retroviruses, which includes the agents of visna, equine infectious anemia virus, and the SIVs. The core of HIV contains two single-stranded copies of the viral RNA genome, together with several virus-encoded enzymes, including reverse transcriptase, proteases, and integrases, as well as certain other accessory proteins (Fig. 107–3). Surrounding the structural proteins (*p24* and *p18*) is a lipid bi-layer derived from the host cell, through which protrude the transmembrane (*gp41*) and surface (*gp120*) envelope glycoproteins.

The HIV envelope glycoproteins have high affinity for the CD4 molecule on the surface of T-helper lymphocytes and other cells of monocyte and macrophage lineage. After HIV binds to CD4, the envelope undergoes a conformational change that facilitates binding to another cellular co-receptor (the most important of these are the chemokine receptors CCR5 and CXCR4). This second binding event promotes a major conformational change that causes approximation of the viral and cellular membranes; fusion of these membranes is effected by insertion of the newly exposed fusion domain of the envelope *gp41* into the host cell membrane. As a result, the HIV nucleoprotein complex enters the cytoplasm. The RNA viral genome undergoes reverse transcription by the virally encoded reverse transcriptase. The resulting double-stranded viral DNA enters the nucleus, where integration of the DNA provirus into the host chromosome is catalyzed by the retroviral integrase, as well as certain other accessory proteins (see Fig. 107–3). In some lymphocytes, after integration within the host genome, the provirus may remain in a latent state for years, without detectable transcription of RNA or synthesis of viral protein. Latently infected resting memory CD4 lymphocytes serve as reservoirs of persistent infection for the life of infected patients even in the presence of effective antiretroviral therapy (see later discussion). The bulk of viral replication takes place, however, in activated T cells that are both more susceptible to HIV infection and more capable of supporting productive HIV replication.

When a CD4 lymphocyte is activated (e.g., by recognition of antigenic peptides or by binding of pro-inflammatory cytokines), the viral promoter-enhancer region (the long terminal repeat) increases expression of HIV messenger RNA (mRNA). Virus-encoded regulatory proteins *tat* and *rev* facilitate mRNA expression and cytoplasmic transport, respectively. The gag, pol, and env genes of HIV encode core proteins, viral enzymes, and envelope proteins, respectively. *Gag*- and *pol*-encoded polyproteins are cleaved by viral proteases (see Fig. 107–3), whereas the envelope protein is cleaved and glycosylated by host proteases and glycosylases. Viral particles are assembled, each containing two copies of unspliced mRNA within the core as the viral genome, and virions then are released from the cell by budding. Productive viral replication is lytic to infected CD4 cells. A large number of other host cells, including macrophages and certain dendritic cells, are also infected by HIV, but viral replication does not appear to be lytic to these cells.

IMMUNE DEFICIENCY IN HUMAN IMMUNODEFICIENCY VIRAL INFECTION

After HIV infection, high-level viral multiplication occurs in lymphatic tissue, and plasma HIV RNA levels (plasma viral load [PVL]) often exceed 1 million copies per milliliter during the second to fourth weeks after infection. During subsequent weeks, the PVL decreases, often rapidly. The decrease in viremia results largely from a partially effective, but incomplete, immune response. After 6 to 12 months, the PVL generally stabilizes at a level often called the viral *set point* and may remain roughly at this level for several years (Fig. 107–4).

During the initial burst of viral replication shortly after infection, the majority of patients develop an acute retroviral syndrome (see Sequential Clinical Manifestations of Human Immunodeficiency Virus Infection, later in this chapter). After spontaneous recovery from the acute retroviral syndrome, the patient may feel entirely well for several years. During this period of *clinical latency*, however, rapid viral multiplication continues in multiple organs. In the asymptomatic infected individual, over 100 billion new virions may be produced daily while an equal number are removed from circulation. Rapid production and turnover of circulating CD4 cells also occur throughout the course of HIV infection. Although a highly dynamic and complex equilibrium between HIV and CD4 cells may be maintained for several years, a progressive decline in circulating CD4 cells eventually occurs in the great majority of individuals; as disease progresses, an increasingly dramatic CD4-cell decline is often observed following a sharp increase in PVL (see Fig. 107–4).

An HIV-specific immune response contributes to the decrease in the rate of viral replication during the initial weeks after acute HIV infection. During the years of clinical latency, virions are present in large numbers in the follicular dendritic processes of the germinal centers of the lymph nodes and spleen, which undergo intense hyperplasia. As HIV disease progresses over several years, the lymphatic tissue atrophies, and plasma viremia intensifies. In later-stage HIV disease, persistent high-level viremia often occurs (see Fig. 107–4).

The decline in CD4 cells is accompanied by profound functional impairment of the remaining lymphocyte populations. Cutaneous anergy may develop early in HIV infection and eventually occurs in virtually all persons with AIDS. With development of anergy, CD4-cell proliferation in response to antigenic stimuli is dramatically impaired. T cell cytotoxic responses are also diminished, and natural killer cell activity against virus-infected cells is greatly impaired, despite normal or increased numbers of these cells. Decrease in function, as well as number of CD4 cells, is central to the immune dysfunction; this impairment likely underlies the concomitant failure of B-lymphocyte function, as measured by impaired capacity to synthesize antibody in response to new antigens. Profound impairment of multiple arms of the immune system underlies the enhanced risk of acquiring the OIs that are characteristic of AIDS.

INADEQUATE HOST DEFENSE MECHANISMS

HIV continues to replicate despite brisk initial antibody responses to many components of the virus, as well as cell-mediated immune responses to several HIV-derived proteins. Several possible explanations can be given for the inability of host responses to control HIV infection. Integrated provirus persists in the host genome in a transcriptionally latent state, in which it is not recognized by either humoral or cellular immune mechanisms (see Fig. 107–3). Conserved domains of the HIV envelope are relatively

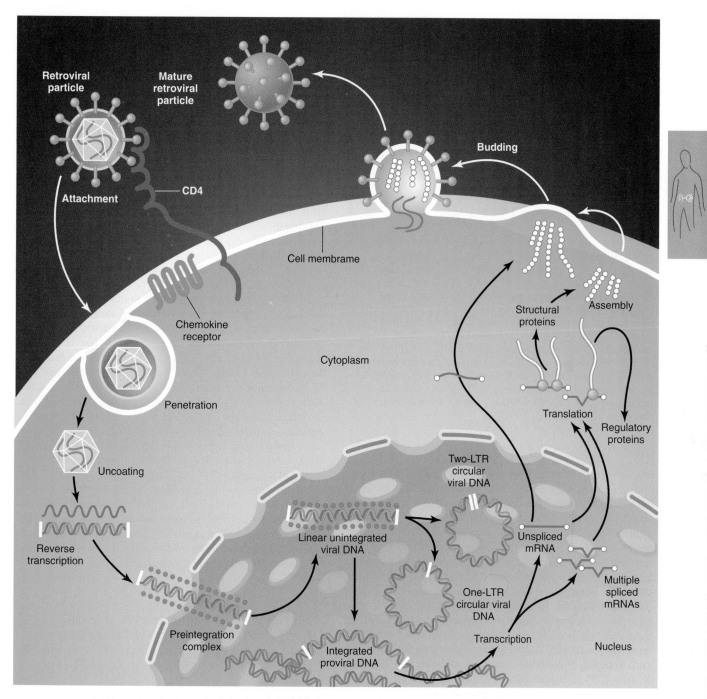

Figure 107–3 Essential steps in the life cycle of HIV-1. The first step is the attachment of the virus particle to the CD4 and chemokine (CCR4 or CXCR5) receptors on the surface of the lymphocyte (site of action of viral entry inhibitors, see text). The HIV-1 RNA genome then enters the cytoplasm as part of a nucleoprotein complex. The viral RNA genome is reverse-transcribed into a DNA duplex (site of action of *nucleoside nucleotide* and non-nucleotide reverse transcriptase inhibitors; see text). Once the viral DNA has been synthesized, the linear viral DNA molecule is incorporated into a pre-integration complex that enters the nucleus. In the nucleus, unintegrated viral DNA is found in both linear and circular forms. The linear unintegrated viral DNA is the precursor of integrated proviral DNA (site of action of integrase inhibitors; see text), which remains indefinitely in the host-cell genome and serves as a template of viral transcription. Transcription of the integrated DNA template and alternative messenger RNA (mRNA) splicing creates spliced viral mRNA species encoding the viral accessory proteins, including *tat, rev,* and *nef,* and the unspliced viral mRNA encoding the viral structural proteins, including the *gag-pol* precursor protein. (Cleaving of the precursor proteins is prevented by protease inhibitors; see text.) All the viral transcripts are exported into the cytoplasm, where translation, assembly, and processing of the retroviral particle take place. The cycle is completed by the release of infectious retroviral particles from the cell. (Modified from Furtado MR, Callaway DS, Phair JP, et al: Persistence of HIV-1 transcription in patients receiving potent ART. N Engl J Med 340:1614–1622, 1999, with permission.)

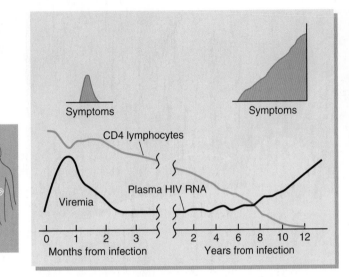

Figure 107–4 Natural history of HIV-1 infection in the untreated adult. Note the extended mean period of clinical latency between the acute retroviral syndrome and AIDS-related disease. Note also the relative stability of the plasma HIV RNA level for several years after recovery from the initial burst of viremia, followed by an increase before the onset of AIDS-related symptoms. (Modified from Shaw GW: Biology of human immunodeficiency viruses. In Goldman L, Ausiello D [eds]: Cecil Textbook of Medicine, 22nd ed. Philadelphia, Saunders, 2004, p 2142.)

inaccessible for generation of neutralizing antibody responses, and extensive glycosylation of the viral envelope hinders antibody formation and binding. Other envelope regions vary among different isolates. Selective pressure (e.g., the development of antibodies against a nonconserved region of the envelope) results in the emergence of viral mutants that are resistant to neutralizing activity of specific antibody species. Similarly, though CD8 lymphocyte responses are key to the control of retroviral replication in established infection, evidence can be found of both CD8-cell dysfunction and the emergence of escape mutations in sequences targeted by these cells. These escape mutations are facilitated by the high error rate of the HIV reverse transcriptase that replicates the viral genome. Preferential infection and deletion of HIV-specific CD4 T helper cells additionally hamper development of an effective anti-HIV immune response.

Diagnosis and Testing for Human Immunodeficiency Viral Infection

Because HIV transmission is preventable, antiretroviral therapy is effective, and prophylaxis against major OIs can be achieved, persons at any risk for HIV infection must undergo serologic testing. Testing should *not* be confined to individuals at highest risk (e.g., injecting drug users) but should be strongly recommended for all sexually active persons. HIV testing should be routinely offered as an integral component of primary care. All individuals should be counseled regarding safe sexual practices. Injecting drug users should strongly be advised to avoid sharing needles.

Positive test results should be given in a face-to-face meeting, during which the patient is given assurance that, with adherence to current therapy, he or she may live asymptomatically with HIV infection for decades. All seropositive patients should be encouraged to notify their sexual partners and persons with whom they may have shared needles. This precaution is often difficult; regional health authorities may be of great assistance in confidential notification of persons at risk. All pregnant women should routinely be offered HIV testing because antiretroviral therapy will dramatically reduce mother-to-child transmission.

Diagnosis of HIV infection is established by detection of serum or salivary antibody to HIV by enzyme-linked immunosorbent assay (ELISA), usually confirmed by Western blot. These techniques are highly sensitive in detecting HIV antibody, but individuals who have been infected recently may be antibody negative. If the suggestion of infection is high during this *window period*, typically 1 to 3 weeks after exposure, then diagnosis can be confirmed by the presence of HIV RNA or core *p24* antigen in plasma. Such newly infected persons have very high levels of virus in plasma and are especially infectious to their sexual partners. For recently exposed individuals whose initial ELISA test is negative, repeat ELISA tests at 6 weeks and 3 months are indicated. False-positive ELISA tests rarely occur because the HIV ELISA test has been calibrated to achieve maximum sensitivity; all positive ELISA tests must therefore be confirmed by Western blot. In a person at high risk for HIV exposure, an indeterminate Western blot reaction pattern often represents early seroconversion; in such instances, plasma HIV RNA (>10,000 copies/mL) or *p24* antigen is indicative of acute HIV infection.

Rapid and readily accessible testing methods play an increasingly important role in the diagnosis and confirmation of HIV infection. Salivary testing offers a noninvasive approach, and rapid test kits can provide preliminary positive test results within 30 minutes; positive rapid tests must be confirmed by Western blot testing.

Sequential Clinical Manifestations of Human Immunodeficiency Virus–1 Infection

ACUTE HUMAN IMMUNODEFICIENCY VIRAL INFECTION AND THE ACUTE RETROVIRAL SYNDROME

Over one half of persons infected with HIV experience a mononucleosis-like syndrome (acute retroviral syndrome) from 2 to 6 weeks after initial infection. Acute symptoms may include fever, sore throat, lymph node enlargement, rash, arthralgias, and headache and usually persist for several days to 3 weeks (Table 107–3). A maculopapular rash is common, is short lived, and most often affects the trunk or face. Acute, self-limited aseptic meningitis, documented by cerebrospinal fluid (CSF) pleocytosis and isolation of HIV from CSF, is the most common clinical neurologic presentation and occurs in up to 10% of patients.

The acute retroviral syndrome is sufficiently severe that a large proportion of patients seek medical attention. In the

Table 107–3	Acute Human Immunodeficiency Virus Retroviral Syndrome: Common Signs and Symptoms

Sign/Symptom	Frequency (%)
Fever	98
Lymph node enlargement	75
Sore throat	70
Myalgia or arthralgia	60
Rash	50
Headache	35

absence of a high index of suspicion, these symptoms are often mislabeled as *acute viral syndromes.* Such misdiagnoses have serious implications because a very high plasma HIV RNA level during this period results in a high likelihood of HIV transmission to sexual or needle-sharing partners, or from mother to infant. Within 3 to 12 weeks after HIV infection, specific antibodies develop that are directed against the three main gene products of HIV: *gag, pol,* and *env.*

ASYMPTOMATIC PHASE

Untreated HIV infection usually results in a slow, nonlinear progression to severe immunodeficiency. Roughly 50% of untreated adults develop AIDS within 10 years after HIV infection (see Fig. 107–4); an additional 30% have milder symptoms related to immunodeficiency, and less than 20% are entirely asymptomatic 10 years after infection. Progression of disease varies greatly among individuals. Adolescents progress to AIDS at a slower rate than older persons, and fewer than 30% develop AIDS within 10 years after HIV infection. The rate of progression of immunodeficiency is not influenced by route of HIV transmission and does not appear to differ by gender. Although persistent lymph node enlargement is often present early in the course of asymptomatic HIV infection, it is not significantly associated with either rate of progression of immunodeficiency or subsequent development of lymphoma. Thrombocytopenia, probably caused by autoimmune platelet destruction, often occurs as a transient phenomenon during early HIV infection. The majority of individuals infected with HIV remains undiagnosed during acute retroviral syndrome and are unaware of their infection and asymptomatic, often until their CD4 counts fall below 200 cells/mm^3.

EARLY SYMPTOMATIC PHASE

Mucocutaneous lesions may be the first manifestations of immune dysfunction, especially polydermatomal varicella-zoster infection (shingles), recurrent genital herpes simplex virus (HSV) infections, oral or vaginal candidiasis, or oral

hairy leukoplakia. Patients with only moderate immuno-deficiency (CD4 counts between 200 and 500 cells/mm^3) exhibit diminished antibody response to protein and poly-saccharide antigens, as well as decreased cell-mediated immune function. These functional impairments are identi-fied clinically by a threefold to fourfold increase in incidence of bacteremic pneumonias caused by common pulmonary pathogens (especially *Streptococcus pneumoniae* and *Haemo-philus influenzae*), as well as a marked increase in incidence of active pulmonary tuberculosis in endemic areas.

ADVANCED SYMPTOMATIC PHASE: MAJOR OPPORTUNISTIC INFECTIONS

With advanced immunodeficiency, indicated by CD4 counts below 200 cells/mm^3, patients are at high risk of developing major OIs (Table 107–4). For example, in the late 1980s, in the absence of specific prophylaxis and before the availabil-ity of effective antiretroviral drugs, 60% of North American men infected with HIV developed PCP.

CD4 counts less than 50 cells/mm^3 indicate profound immunosuppression and, in the absence of effective anti-retroviral therapy, are associated with a high mortality within the subsequent 12 to 24 months. Cytomegalovirus (CMV) retinitis and disseminated *Mycobacterium avium-intracellulare* (MAI) infections occur frequently. These infec-tions respond adequately to specific therapy only when accompanied by effective antiretroviral therapy.

Management of Human Immunodeficiency Viral Infection

Because patients are asymptomatic during the early course of HIV-1 infection (see Fig. 107–4), and even seriously immunocompromised individuals may function produc-tively between bouts of OIs, the ambulatory management of persons with HIV infection deserves major emphasis.

INITIAL EVALUATION

Once HIV infection is recognized, the physician should discuss, in an unhurried manner, the clinical course and treatment of HIV infection and the use of immunologic and virologic studies (e.g., CD4 counts, PVL assays) to guide therapy. The physician should emphasize that most patients, even without antiviral therapy, live for 10 to 12 years after acquiring HIV infection and are asymptomatic during most of that time. The physician should then emphasize that, with effective currently available antiretroviral therapy, HIV disease progression can be prevented indefinitely.

Prevention of further transmission through unprotected sex and sharing of needles must be discussed not only at the first visit, but also periodically thereafter. Emphasizing that these activities place both the *contact* and the patient at risk is important because they may lead to transmission to the patient of new HIV strains that may be resistant to current or future medications used in his or her treatment.

Initial evaluation should include both an HIV-oriented review of systems and a complete physical examination

Table 107–4 **Relation of CD4 Lymphocyte Counts to the Onset of Certain Human Immunodeficiency Virus–Associated Infections and Neoplasms in North America**

CD4 Count (cells/mm^3)*	Opportunistic Infection or Neoplasm	Frequency (%)†
>500	Herpes zoster, polydermatomal	5–10
200–500	*Mycobacterium tuberculosis* infection	4–20
	Bacterial pneumonia, recurrent	15–20
	Kaposi's sarcoma, mucocutaneous	15–25 (M)
	Oral hairy leukoplakia	25–40
	Candida pharyngitis (thrush)	20–35
	Cervical neoplasia	1–2 (F)
100–200	*Pneumocystis jirovecii* pneumonia	20–60
	Histoplasma capsulatum, disseminated	0–20
	Kaposi's sarcoma, visceral	3–8 (M)
	Lymphoma, non-Hodgkin's	3–5
	Progressive multifocal leukoencephalopathy	2–3
≤100	*Candida* esophagitis	15–20
	Cytomegalovirus retinitis, esophagitis or colitis	10–20
	Mycobacterium avium-intracellulare, disseminated	20–35
	Toxoplasma gondii encephalitis	5–25
	Cryptococcus neoformans meningitis	10–20
	Histoplasma capsulatum, disseminated	2–20
	Cryptosporidium parvum enteritis	2–8
	Mucocutaneous herpes simplex ulcers, extensive	4–8
	Lymphoma, central nervous system	3–6

*CD4 count at which specific infections or neoplasms may begin to appear. Each infection may recur or progress during the subsequent course of human immunodeficiency virus disease.
†Even within North America, great regional differences in the incidence of specific opportunistic infections are apparent. For example, disseminated histoplasmosis is relatively common in the Mississippi River drainage area, but is rare in individuals who have lived exclusively on the east or west coast.
F = exclusively in women; M = usually in men.

(Table 107–5). The skin must be examined for HIV-associated rashes and Kaposi's sarcoma. Examination of the oral cavity may reveal thrush, gingivitis, hairy leukoplakia, superficial ulcers caused by HSV, aphthous ulcers, or lesions characteristic of Kaposi's sarcoma. The optic fundi may have hemorrhagic lesions characteristic of CMV retinitis. Hepatomegaly, splenomegaly, and any genital lesions should all be carefully noted. Neurologic examinations for both peripheral neuropathy and decreased global cognition deserve close attention. Pelvic examination with Papanicolaou (Pap) smear should be routine.

Purified protein derivative (PPD) testing should be performed early in the course of HIV infection. Induration of 5 mm or more should be considered positive. Any patient with a positive PPD test should be evaluated for the presence of active tuberculosis; if no active disease is present, then the patient should receive 1 year of prophylaxis with isoniazid or combination drug therapy for a shorter time period (see Chapter 98). If active tuberculosis is identified, then multidrug therapy should be initiated after careful consideration of possible interactions with antiretroviral medications.

Routine initial serologic testing for *Toxoplasma gondii* infection is important in the event that a person subsequently develops an intracerebral lesion (see later discussion). Serologic testing for syphilis should be followed by prompt treatment if confirmed positive (see Chapter 106). Pneumococcal vaccine is indicated at an early visit because antibody responses to pneumococcal polysaccharides are increased among patients with elevated CD4 counts.

Because of common routes of transmission, persons infected with HIV have a much greater prevalence of hepatitis B (HBV) and C (HCV) infection than the general population, and HIV infection results in an increasingly rapid progression of liver disease in HIV-HCV co-infected individuals. Patients infected with HIV should be screened for hepatitis A, B, and C, and hepatitis A and B vaccine should be given to those who are seronegative for these viruses. Individuals who have HIV-HCV co-infection should be evaluated for possible treatment of this entity (see Chapter 41).

The CD4 count and the PVL should be obtained at the first visit and repeated at intervals of 3 to 4 months in asymptomatic individuals. The patient should understand that the CD4 count and the PVL are rough guides to the degree of immunodeficiency and the rate of viral replication, respectively, and that modest fluctuations in these measurements may not indicate a change in clinical course. A helpful approach for the physician is to use graphic illustrations of the interaction between PVL and CD4 count as predictors of the course of illness in the absence of treatment, as well as a guide to initiating and monitoring of antiretroviral therapy (Table 107–6).

Table 107–5 Management of Early Human Immunodeficiency Virus Disease

Monitoring

Confirm positive HIV test
Complete baseline history and physical examination: HIV-specific interval interview and examination every 3–4 mo

Laboratory Evaluation

Baseline plasma HIV RNA level and CD4 cell count with repeat every 3–4 mo
Baseline purified protein derivative (PPD)
Baseline *Toxoplasma* antibody; syphilis serology; hepatitis A, B, and C antibodies; liver function tests; and chest radiograph
Consider baseline resistance testing if recently infected and initiation of antiretroviral treatment anticipated

Health Care Maintenance

Assessment for ongoing counseling needs and/or psychosocial problems
Pneumococcal vaccine, hepatitis A and B vaccines (if seronegative)
Yearly influenza vaccine

HIV = human immunodeficiency virus.

GOAL OF ANTIRETROVIRAL THERAPY

The goal of antiretroviral therapy (ART) is to ensure that persons living with HIV infection lead symptom-free productive lives. Currently available therapy makes achieving this goal possible in almost all individuals with early, asymptomatic HIV infection who have not acquired major resistance mutations as the result of earlier suboptimal ART. This circumstance is in stark contrast to the situation only 15 years earlier, when progression to marked immunodeficiency was almost inevitable, and such devastating health consequences as blindness caused by CMV retinitis and crippling neurologic deficits as the result of *Toxoplasma encephalitis* were common preterminal events.

PRINCIPLES OF ANTIRETROVIRAL THERAPY

Treatment of HIV infection is exceptional among infectious diseases because specific therapy is not initiated as soon as the diagnosis has been established. Principles underlying this approach include the following:

1. Antiretroviral treatment is not curative but suppressive; because HIV infection cannot be eradicated, treatment will be lifelong with currently available drugs.
2. All effective treatment regimens may be associated with toxicities; occasionally, these may be life threatening.
3. The risk for developing resistance to individual antiretroviral drugs is increased in persons who adhere irregularly to therapy.
4. Although damage to the host immune system occurs throughout the course of HIV infection, loss of protective immune response to the most serious OIs occurs only with advanced HIV disease.

ART should therefore be initiated at a time when the benefit of halting replication of the virus exceeds the risks of sustained treatment with available drugs and at a time when the patient is prepared to adhere closely to the treatment regimen.

Table 107–6 Guidelines for the Initiation of Antiretroviral Therapy*

Clinical Category	CD4 + T-Cell Count	Recommendation
Symptomatic (e.g., thrush)	Any value	Treat
Asymptomatic	CD4 + T cells ≤200/mm³	Treat
Asymptomatic	CD4 + T cells >200 mm³, but <350/mm³	Treatment should be offered and decision should be individualized and made only after careful discussion with the patient (see text).
Asymptomatic	CD4 + T cells >350/mm³	Treatment should generally be deferred.

*These guidelines should be used only in conjunction with the text. No absolute laboratory thresholds have been established on which the initiation of therapy can be based. This decision must always be made jointly by the informed patient and the physician.

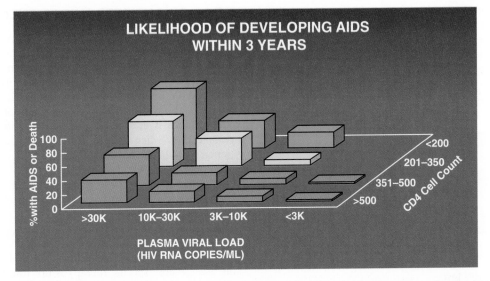

Figure 107–5 Relationship of CD4 cell count and PVL to likelihood of developing symptomatic AIDS or death within 3 years in the absence of treatment. Values in the red zone (CD4 cell count <200/mm³) indicate a high likelihood of disease progression over the next 3 years. ART should *always* be initiated before the CD4 count has reached this zone. Values in the yellow zone indicate a 6% to 24% likelihood of disease progression within 3 years. ART should be offered to all patients when values fall in this zone, with the exact time of initiation of treatment determined by patient-physician discussion (see text). Values in the green zone indicate small likelihood of 3-year progression to symptomatic AIDS.

WHEN TO INITIATE THERAPY

Initiation of therapy must be based on a joint decision by the informed patient and the physician. ART in an asymptomatic patient is not an urgent issue, and the physician should spend whatever time is necessary (e.g., three patient visits over a 12-week period) for the patient to understand both the potential benefits and the risks of the specific regimens. Graphs such as that shown in Figure 107–5 can be effective in helping the patient understand the importance of the CD4 count in determining when to initiate therapy. Therapy should be individualized to the extent possible (e.g., a patient with recurrent nephrolithiasis should generally avoid a protease inhibitor [PI] that crystalizes in urine). Because inadequate adherence to any antiretroviral regimen will result, over time, in resistance to the antiretroviral drugs, the patient absolutely must have as full an understanding of the regimen as possible before initiating ART.

Symptomatic Patients

All patients with symptomatic AIDS (with active or past OIs) should receive ART. Without effective ART, patients with symptomatic AIDS have a high risk of death within 6 to 18 months.

Some experts recommend treatment of patients in whom the acute retroviral syndrome is recognized, but data to date cannot support a definitive recommendation in this regard.

Asymptomatic Patients

Whenever possible, treatment should be initiated before the patient becomes symptomatic. The CD4 count is the major determinant of when to start antiviral treatment. Although the optimal time to initiate therapy in a given asymptomatic patient cannot be precisely defined, all available data indicate that patients should begin effective ART before the CD4 count falls below 200 cells/mm³ (see Table 107–6). For patients with CD4 counts greater than 350 cells/mm³, the disadvantages of initiating ART (short- and long-term toxicities and development of antiretroviral resistance) generally outweigh the advantage (prevention of progressive immunologic damage). The optimal timing for treatment initiation in asymptomatic individuals with CD4 levels between 200 and 350 cells/mL is uncertain. For patients in this category, the overall risk of clinical progression to symptomatic disease over a 3-year period is less than 25% (see Fig. 107–5). The option of treatment should be offered to all such patients, but the decision must be individualized through careful discussion with the patient and evaluation of the clinical circumstances. Current guidelines for treatment are summarized in Table 107–6.

ANTIRETROVIRAL DRUG REGIMENS

Clarification of the mechanisms of HIV replication has identified several potential sites at which retroviral replication might be limited or blocked (see Fig. 107–3). The drugs that have proved effective for the treatment of HIV infection include six nucleoside analogues (nucleoside reverse transcriptase inhibitors [NRTIs]) and one nucleotide analog (nucleotide reverse transcriptase inhibitor [NtRTI]) that inhibit HIV reverse transcriptase, two nonnucleoside reverse transcriptase inhibitors (NNRTIs), nine HIV protease inhibitors (PIs), and one viral entry inhibitor (Table 107–7). Additional agents in each of these categories are currently in clinical trials; several will likely be approved soon.

The goal of ART is to ensure that the patient has the highest possible quality of life for as long as possible. In general, this approach requires therapy that durably suppresses the PVL below levels that are detectable by available

Table 107–7   Drugs Recommended for Use in Highly Active Antiretroviral Therapy Regimens

Nucleoside/Nucleotide Reverse Transcriptase Inhibitors (RTIs)	Non-nucleoside Reverse Transcriptase Inhibitors (non-RTIs)	Protease Inhibitors (PIs)	Viral Entry Inhibitor
Abacavir	Efavirenz	Atazanavir	Enfuvirtide
Didanosine	Nevirapine	Fosamprenavir	
Emtricitabine		Indinavir	
Lamivudine		Lopinavir	
Stavudine		Nelfinavir	
Zidovudine		Ritonavir[†]	
Tenofovir*		Saquinavir	
		Tipranivir	
		Darunavir	

*Nucleotide RTI; other agents in the column are nucleoside RTIs.
[†]Used in low doses to boost plasma levels of other protease inhibitors (see text).

assays (<75 copies of HIV RNA per milliliter). Achievement of this objective currently demands that the patient take combination ART with a minimum of three antiretroviral drugs.

Currently recommended initial regimens that predictably provide profound and durable suppression of viral replication include a potent NNRTI plus two NRTIs or a ritonavir-boosted PI plus two NRTIs. Each of these regimens can result in prompt durable suppression of PVL associated with gradual recovery of immunologic competence. Each regimen has specific advantages and potential toxicities of which the patient must be aware.

Because the long-term effectiveness of any regimen depends on the patient's ability to adhere closely to it, the physician and the informed patient should jointly choose the regimen. Ease of administration and lack of adverse effects are critical to adherence; thus, each regimen must be tailored, as much as possible, to the individual patient. Once-a-day regimens are preferable when possible, especially for patients with rigorous occupational schedules (see U.S. Department of Health and Human Services HIV Treatment Guidelines at *http://www.aidsinfo.nih.gov/guidelines* for regularly updated treatment information). The recent development of a coformulation of efavirenz, tenofovir, and emtricitabine in a single tablet, taken once daily, represents a major step forward in providing an effective regimen which does not interfere with normal activities of daily living.

WHEN TO CHANGE THERAPY

When an effective antiretroviral regimen is initiated in an asymptomatic patient with no previous ART, the PVL should decrease sharply, generally by tenfold in 2 weeks and to an undetectable level (>75 copies/mL) within 12 to 24 weeks. If reduction of this magnitude is not achieved, then the physician should, with the patient, assess whether adherence has been adequate. If adherence has been nearly complete (>95%), then the physician should test for resistance mutations, followed, if indicated, by changing to another regimen.

If a given regimen achieves a sustained reduction of PVL below detectable limits, then the patient can anticipate effective viral suppression for many years and possibly indefinitely. The PVL should be monitored at 3- to 4-month intervals throughout the course of therapy. If, after months or years of adequate viral suppression, the viral load again becomes detectable on two consecutive determinations, then testing for resistance mutations is indicated, a change in therapy if indicated by testing results (see regularly updated International AIDS Society-USA resistance guidelines at *http://www.IASUSA.org/pub/index.html*).

Available data do not precisely define the threshold at which a change in therapy is indicated. Some experts recommend change as soon as the PVL is above detectable limits on two determinations. Others would not change until the viral load exceeded an arbitrary figure of 3000 to 5000 copies/mL. At this point, results of resistance testing should be used to define a second effective regimen. The most durable second regimen usually requires a change in at least two antiretroviral drugs (e.g., efavirenz-zidovudine-lamivudine might be changed to lopinavir-ritonavir-tenofovir-emtricitabine).

After failure of a second antiretroviral regimen, change becomes difficult because the remaining options are reduced. Antiviral resistance testing is critical in the choice of the third regimen because viral isolates will demonstrate a significant number of resistance mutations at this time, making the choice of the third regimen considerably more difficult.

Many treated patients continue to do well clinically, with stable CD4 counts, for months to years after viral *escape*, indicated by increasing PVL. In such patients, stopping ART generally results in clinical deterioration. The basis for continued clinical well being, despite increasing PVL, during long-term ART is uncertain but may reflect diminished *pathogenicity* of viruses with multiple drug-resistance mutations and/or ongoing antigenic stimulation in the setting of partially controlled viremia, resulting in improved immunologic control of viral replication. Thus, many patients receive

Table 107–8	Preferred Prophylaxis against Certain Opportunistic Infections (OIs) in Human Immunodeficiency Virus–Infected Adults*			
Pathogen	**Indication**	**First Choice**	**Alternatives**
Pneumocystis jirovecii[†]	CD4 count >200/mm³, or history of thrush	Trimethoprim-sulfamethoxazole (TMP-SMZ), 1 tablet daily	Dapsone, 100 mg/day Atovaquone, 1500 mg/day Pentamidine, aerosolized, 300 mg/mo
Mycobacterium tuberculosis[†] Isoniazid sensitive	TST (t) reaction >5 mm, or prior positive TST without treatment, or contact with case of active tuberculosis	Isoniazid, 300 mg PO, plus pyridoxine, 50 mg/day for 9 mo	Rifampin, 600 mg, and pyrizinamide, 800 mg/day for 2 mo
Isoniazid resistant	Same as above	Rifampin, 600 mg/day, plus pyrizinamide, 800 mg/day for 2 mo	Pyrizinamide, 15–20 mg/kg/day for 2 mo, plus rifabutin, 300 mg/day for 2 mo
Toxoplasma gondii[†]	IgG antibody to Toxoplasma and CD4 count <100	TMP-SMZ, 1 double-strength tablet daily	Dapsone, 50 mg PO daily, plus pyrimethimine, 50 mg PO every wk
Mycobacterium avium intracellulare[†]	<50	Azithromycin, 1200 mg every week	Clarithromycin, 500 mg PO two times/day

*Department of Health and Human Services recommendations for prophylaxis against OIs are updated regularly and are available at http://www.aidsinfo.nih.gov/guidelines.
[†]Strongly recommended as standard of care in all patients.
IgG = immunoglobulin G; TST (t) = tuberculosis skin test.

clinical and immunologic benefits from continued ART despite diminishing control of viral replication. Continued administration of the ART maintains selection pressure which results in drug-resistant viruses that tend to be less *fit* in terms of replicative capacity and possibly also less pathogenic. How long the clinical benefit will be sustained in such patients is unknown; clearly, these patients do not maintain CD4 cell numbers as well as do patients with more complete suppression of HIV replication.

PROPHYLAXIS AGAINST OPPORTUNISTIC INFECTIONS

During the first 15 years of the HIV pandemic, the most effective medical interventions for HIV infection were prophylactic measures against OIs. The greatest success was the prevention of PCP for individuals with CD4 counts less than 200 cells/mm³; routine use of prophylaxis resulted in a greater than fourfold (from 60% to >15%) decrease in the frequency of PCP as the initial OI in North American men with HIV infection. Specific antimicrobial prophylaxis (Table 107–8) is also effective for prevention of *T. gondii* encephalitis in patients with anti-*Toxoplasma* antibodies and with CD4 counts less than 100 cells/mm³ and for prevention of active tuberculosis in patients with positive tuberculin skin tests at any CD4 level (see Table 107–8). Prophylaxis

against disseminated MAI infection is recommended at lower CD4 counts (<50 cells/mm³). Prophylaxis against CMV retinitis may be effective in patients with CD4 counts less than 50 cells/mm³; the value of prophylaxis must be carefully weighed against potential toxicities of the prophylactic agents. Prophylaxis is highly effective against recurrent HSV-2 infection (acyclovir, famciclovir, or valacyclovir) and against recurrent *Candida* esophagitis (fluconazole) but should generally be reserved for patients with recurrent symptomatic disease.

Management of Specific Clinical Manifestations of Immunodeficiency

In the course of HIV infection, OIs vary considerably in time of onset (see Table 107–4). For example, some patients may develop multidermatomal herpes zoster with CD4 counts greater than 500 cells/mm³ and then have no other OIs until they develop PCP pneumonia with CD4 counts less than 200 cells/mm³. Conversely, some patients may remain entirely asymptomatic until their CD4 counts are below 50 cells/mm³, at which time they may develop major life-threatening OIs, such as *T. gondii* encephalitis. Life-threatening OIs seldom occur with CD4 counts greater than 200 cells/mm^3 (see Table 107–4).

In general, OIs that occur with higher CD4 counts respond to routine therapy for the specific infection (e.g., appropriate β-lactam antibiotic for pneumococcal pneumonia, standard multidrug therapy for pulmonary tuberculosis), whereas OIs occurring with CD4 counts less than 200 cells/mm^3 require chronic suppressive therapy after treatment of acute infection (e.g., PCP pneumonia, *Cryptococcus neoformans* meningitis).

Effective ART has had a dramatic impact on the incidence of OIs. Although the impact on specific OIs has varied, with decreases greater than 85% in CMV retinitis and PCP pneumonia, all recognized OIs have greatly decreased in frequency in North America and Western Europe since 1996. Furthermore, after partial restoration of immunologic function in response to effective therapy, withdrawal of prophylaxis against specific OIs is generally safe. Current data support withdrawal of prophylaxis against PCP, MAI, CMV, and *T. gondii* and *Cryptococcus neoformans* infections after two consecutive CD4 counts greater than 200 cells/mm^3 at an interval of 3 months in patients receiving effective ART.

Because of the great reduction in OIs associated with effective ART, rates of hospitalization and mortality for AIDS-related illnesses have dropped sharply since 1996, with decreases of as much as 80% in major North American and Western European cities.

CONSTITUTIONAL SYMPTOMS

Nonspecific symptoms may be the initial clinical manifestations of severe immunodeficiency. Patients may develop unexplained fever, night sweats, anorexia, weight loss, or diarrhea. These symptoms may last for months before development of identifiable OIs in patients who do not receive effective ART. These constitutional symptoms may represent manifestations of specific, but unidentified, OIs.

CUTANEOUS DISEASE

Cutaneous infections ultimately occur in most patients with untreated HIV disease. Most patients respond to specific therapy as outlined in Table 107–9.

MUCOSAL DISEASE

Oral *Candida* stomatitis, or thrush, is often the earliest recognized OI. Early thrush may be entirely asymptomatic; as infection becomes more extensive, it causes pain on eating. The characteristic cheesy white exudate on the mucous membranes can easily be scraped off. The underlying mucosa may be normal or inflamed.

Oral hairy leukoplakia (OHL) is a white, lichenified, plaquelike lesion, most commonly seen on the lateral surfaces of the tongue and likely caused by Epstein-Barr virus (EBV). Unlike thrush, the lesions of OHL cannot be scraped off with a tongue depressor. OHL may also be an early manifestation of severe immunodeficiency. OHL is painless, may remit spontaneously, and almost always responds to effective ART.

Patients may develop painful ulcers in the mouth. HSV-1 or -2 may cause these sores, but often they represent aphthous lesions of uncertain origin. Small oral aphthous ulcers may respond to topical corticosteroids, whereas giant oral or esophageal ulcers require systemic administration of thalidomide or corticosteroids. Obtaining cultures for HSV and CMV is important to exclude a viral origin before initiating corticosteroid or thalidomide therapy. Thalidomide should be used, if at all, only when birth control can be ensured in women with childbearing potential because of its well-documented adverse effects on fetal development.

Kaposi's sarcoma has a predilection for the oral cavity and skin. Oral lesions may be purple, red, or blue and may be raised or flat. Usually painless, these lesions cause symptoms when they enlarge, bleed, or ulcerate.

ESOPHAGEAL DISEASE

Symptomatic esophageal disease seldom occurs with CD4 counts greater than 100 cells/mm^3. Pain on swallowing, substernal burning, and rapid weight loss are common symptoms and most often indicate *Candida* esophagitis, usually associated with oral thrush. Diagnostic esophagoscopy with biopsy, cytology, and culture should be performed if symptoms do not rapidly respond (within 3 to 4 days) to antifungal therapy. If esophagoscopy shows ulcerative lesions, then they are usually caused by CMV (50%), aphthae (45%), or HSV (5%). Because each of these lesions is responsive to appropriate therapy, definitive etiologic diagnosis is essential (Table 107–10). CMV esophageal ulcers respond well to intravenous ganciclovir or foscarnet therapy for 2 to 3 weeks or until resolution is confirmed endoscopically. Esophageal ulcerations caused by HSV usually respond well to intravenous acyclovir (see Table 107–10).

GENITAL DISEASE

Recurrent genital ulcers are most often caused by HSV. Viral culture or specific immunofluorescence of ulcer scrapings confirms the diagnosis. Primary syphilis also occurs with increased frequency (see Chapter 106). Chancroid is unusual in North America.

All vaginal mucosal inflammatory diseases appear to enhance both acquisition and transmission of HIV infection. This consideration makes prompt and definitive treatment of vaginal mucosal infections imperative.

Candida species, most often *Candida albicans,* can cause an irritating vulvovaginitis in women with HIV infection, as well as among healthy HIV-seronegative women. A potassium hydroxide preparation of the cheesy white exudate will reveal budding yeast or pseudohyphae.

Bacterial vaginosis and trichomoniasis are common, and both respond well to specific treatment (see Chapter 106).

Infection with HPV is associated not only with genital warts in both men and women, but also with a greater frequency of cervical dysplasia in women infected with HIV and anal dysplasia in both men and women. Pap smears indicative of cervical dysplasia should be followed by prompt colposcopy, biopsy when indicted, and appropriate treatment of any dysplastic lesions. Similarly, anal Pap smears indicative of high-grade dysplasia should be followed by definitive evaluation and treatment. With this approach, progression of dysplasia to invasive cervical or anal cancer is exceedingly rare.

Table 107–9	**Dermatologic Conditions Common in Human Immunodeficiency Virus Infection**	
Condition	**Description**	**Treatment**
Herpes simplex	Clear or crusted vesicles with an erythematous base; ulceration common when chronic; location: oral or genital mucous membranes, face, and hands	Acyclovir, 200 mg five times/day, *or* famciclovir, 250 mg three times/day, or valacyclovir, 1000 mg three times/day, each for 7–10 days
Herpes zoster (shingles)	Cluster of vesicles in a dermatomal distribution; usually involve adjacent dermatomes, but may disseminate	Acyclovir, 800 mg five times/day, *or* famciclovir, 500 mg three times/day, or valacyclovir, 1000 mg three times/day, each for 7 days; if disseminated or involvement of ophthalmic branch of trigeminal nerve, IV acyclovir, 10 mg/kg every 8 hr
Staphylococcal folliculitis	Erythematous pustules on face, trunk, and groin, often pruritic	Dicloxacillin, 500 mg four times/day, or erythromycin, 500 mg four times/day for 1 week
Bacilliary angiomatosis	Friable vascular papules or subcutaneous nodules on skin; may involve liver, spleen, and lymph nodes	Clarithromycin, 500 mg two times/day, or doxycycline, 100 mg two times/day for 4 to 8 weeks
Molluscum contagiosum	Chronic, flesh-colored papules, often umbilicated, on face or anogenital area	Cryotherapy and curettage
Seborrheic dermatitis	White scaling or erythematous patches on scalp, eyebrows, face, trunk, axilla, and groin	Hydrocortisone cream 2.5% and ketoconazole cream
Psoriasis	Scaling, marginated patches on elbows, knees, and lumbosacral areas	Triamcinolone acetonide cream 0.1%
Candidal dermatitis	Urticarial scaling or erythematous patches on face, trunk, axilla, and groin	Hydrocortisone cream 1% and ketokonazole cream

Table 107–10	**Human Immunodeficiency Virus–Associated Esophagitis**	
Condition	**Characteristics**	**Treatment**
Candida infection	Thrush usual, esophageal plaques	Fluconazole, 400 mg/day
CMV infection	Large, shallow esophageal ulcers on endoscopy	Ganciclovir, 5 mg/kg two times/day
Herpes simplex	Deep ulceration on endoscopy	Acyclovir, 800 mg five times/day
Aphthae	Giant ulcers on endoscopy; no virus on biopsy	Prednisone, 40–60 mg/day, or thalidomide, 200 mg/day*

*Thalidomide must *never* be given during pregnancy.
CMV = cytomegalovirus.

Table 107–11	**Major Clinical Manifestations of Acquired Immunodeficiency Syndrome–Associated Dementia Complex**		
	Early		**Late**
Cognition	Inattention, reduced concentration, forgetfulness.		Global dementia
Motor performance	Slowed movements, clumsiness, ataxia		Ataxia, paraplegia
Behavior	Apathy, altered personality, agitation		Mutism

NERVOUS SYSTEM DISEASES

Nervous system complications ultimately occur in most untreated persons infected with HIV. These complications range from mild cognitive disturbances or peripheral neuropathy to severe dementia and life-threatening central nervous system (CNS) infections. As with other lentiviruses, HIV enters microglial cells of the CNS early in the course of HIV infection. Both direct neuronal destruction and effects of viral proteins on neuronal cell function may contribute to nervous system disease in AIDS.

Cognitive Dysfunction

Intellectual impairment rarely occurs early in HIV infection, but subtle changes (decreased learning accuracy and learning speed) may be present in patients with only moderate immunodeficiency, and more striking changes often occur with advanced immunodeficiency. AIDS-associated dementia is characterized by poor concentration, diminished memory, slowing of thought processes, motor dysfunction, and occasionally behavioral abnormalities characterized by social withdrawal and apathy (Table 107–11). Symptoms of clinical depression overlap many of the characteristics of early AIDS-associated dementia and must be considered carefully in differential diagnosis and therapy. Computed tomography (CT) of the head in AIDS-associated dementia reveals only atrophy, with enlarged sulci and ventricles. Examination of CSF is most often normal.

Motor abnormalities may include a progressive gait ataxia. As disease progresses, patients may develop focal neurologic complications characterized by spastic weakness of the lower extremities and incontinence secondary to vacuolar myelopathy.

Focal Lesions of the Central Nervous System

Serious neurologic problems often complicate later stages of untreated HIV infection. A neuro-anatomic classification of these manifestations is presented in Table 107–12. Several of the more frequent or treatable problems are discussed here.

Several opportunistic infections produce focal CNS lesions. Patients with focal neurologic signs, seizures of new onset, or recent onset of rapidly progressive cognitive impairment should undergo magnetic resonance imaging (MRI) and/or CT of the brain. Toxoplasmosis, CNS lymphoma, and progressive multifocal leukoencephalopathy (PML) are the most common causes of CNS focal lesions in this setting (Table 107–13).

Table 107–12	**Neuro-anatomic Classification of the Common Complications of Human Immunodeficiency Virus Infection**

Meningitis and Headache

Aseptic meningitis
Cryptococcal meningitis
Tuberculous meningitis

Diffuse Brain Diseases

With preservation of consciousness
  AIDS dementia complex
With concomitant depression of arousal
  Toxoplasma encephalitis
  Cytomegalovirus encephalitis

Focal Brain Diseases

Cerebral toxoplasmosis
Primary central nervous system lymphoma
Progressive multifocal leukoencephalopathy
Tuberculous brain abscess (*Mycobacterium tuberculosis*)

Myelopathies

Subacute, progressive vacuolar myelopathy
Cytomegalovirus myelopathy

Peripheral Neuropathies

Predominantly sensory polyneuropathy
Toxic neuropathies (didanosine, stavudine)
Autonomic neuropathy
Cytomegalovirus polyradiculopathy

Myopathies

Noninflammatory myopathy
Zidovudine myopathy

AIDS = acquired immunodeficiency syndrome.

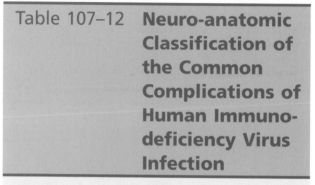

Table 107–13	**Comparative Clinical and Radiologic Features of Cerebral Toxoplasmosis, Primary Central Nervous System Lymphoma, and Progressive Multifocal Leukoencephalopathy**

	Clinical Onset		Neuroradiologic Features			
Condition	Temporal Profile	Level of Alertness	Fever	Number of Lesions	Characteristics of Lesions	Location of Lesions
Cerebral toxoplasmosis	Days	Reduced	Common	Usually multiple	Spheric, ring-enhancing on CT	Basal ganglia or cortex
Primary CNS lymphoma	Days to weeks	Variable	Absent	One or few	Irregular, weakly enhancing on CT	Periventricular or cortex
Progressive multifocal leukoencephalopathy	Weeks to months	Variable	Absent	Usually extensive	Multiple lesions, seen on MRI only	White matter

CNS = central nervous system; CT = computed tomography; MRI = magnetic resonance imaging.

In the absence of ART, *T. gondii* encephalitis occurs in up to one third of patients infected with HIV who have serologic evidence of *T. gondii* infection and CD4 counts less than 100 cells/mm³; it is rare in individuals who have no such antibodies. Patients often exhibit progressive headache and focal neurologic abnormalities, usually associated with fever. CT with contrast dye usually shows multiple ring-enhancing lesions. MRI is a more sensitive technique than CT and often shows multiple small lesions in the basal ganglia that are not apparent on CT (see Fig. 96–2). Management of symptomatic, ring-enhancing brain lesions in persons with AIDS includes initiation of empiric therapy with pyrimethamine, sulfadiazine, and folinic acid. Brain biopsy should be reserved for patients with atypical presentations, those with no serum antibodies to *T. gondii*, or those whose lesions do not respond after 10 to 14 days of antiprotozoal treatment. After the initial response, patients must remain on chronic suppressive therapy until a sustained rise in CD4 count above 200 cells/mm³ is achieved with effective ART.

Primary CNS lymphoma complicates advanced HIV infection in 3% to 6% of patients (see Table 107–13). Lesions may be single or multiple and are often weakly ring enhancing. Irradiation often provides remission, which may be sustained as immune function is restored by effective antiviral therapy.

PML is a demyelinating disease caused by a papovavirus (JC virus, named derived from the initials of the patient in whom it was first discovered). Symptoms may include progressive dementia, visual impairment, seizures, and/or hemiparesis. MRI usually shows multiple lesions predominantly involving the white matter. These lesions are usually less visible on CT than they are with MRI and are not ring enhancing, which helps distinguish PML from other mass lesions of the CNS. No consistently effective treatment for PML has been established; the disease often, but not always, regresses in response to effective ART.

Central Nervous System Diseases without Prominent Focal Signs

Evaluation of the patient infected with HIV who exhibits fever and headache is difficult because of the often subtle manifestations of serious CNS lesions in immunocompromised patients. Patients with bacterial meningitis (see Chapter 96) are managed the same as noncompromised patients. Meningeal diseases in patients infected with HIV often, however, fall into the broad categories of aseptic meningitis, chronic meningitis, and meningoencephalitis.

Aseptic Meningitis. Patients with aseptic meningitis, which may be a manifestation of the acute retroviral syndrome, complain most often of headache; the sensorium is generally intact, and the neurologic examination is normal (see Chapter 96). In the person with established HIV infection, aseptic meningitis may result from several potentially treatable causes (see Chapters 96 and 106).

Chronic Meningitis. Patients with chronic meningitis characteristically exhibit headache, fever, difficulty in concentrating, and/or changes in sensorium. CSF examination shows low glucose concentration, elevated protein level, and mild to modest lymphocytic pleocytosis. Cryptococcal meningitis is the most common cause. The presence of cryptococcal antigen in serum or CSF or a positive CSF India ink preparation establishes the diagnosis (see Chapter 96). Treatment with amphotericin B for at least 2 weeks followed by high-dose fluconazole is usually effective. Serial lumbar punctures, with removal of CSF to decrease intracranial pressure, may be necessary in the early management of cryptococcal meningitis.

Mycobacterium tuberculosis is an eminently treatable cause of subacute meningitis in the patient infected with HIV, although rare in North America. Antituberculosis therapy should be considered in the setting of chronic meningitis if the CSF cryptococcal antigen test is negative (see Chapter 96).

Table 107–14 Pulmonary Disease Associated with Human Immunodeficiency Virus Infection

Condition	Characteristics	Chest Radiograph	Diagnosis	Treatment
Pneumocystis jirovecii pneumonia	Subacute onset, dry cough, dyspnea	Interstitial infiltrate most common	Sputum or bronchoalveolar lavage for organism by stain	Trimethoprim-sulfamethoxazole, clindamycin-primaquine, or atovaquone
Bacterial (pneumococcus, *Haemophilus* most common)	Acute productive cough, fever, chest pain	Lobar or localized infiltrate	Sputum Gram stain and culture, blood culture	Cefuroxime or alternative antibiotics
Mycobacterial (*Mycobacterium tuberculosis* or *M. kansasii*)	Chronic cough, weight loss, fever	Localized infiltrate, lymphadenopathy	Sputum acid-fast stain and mycobacterial culture	Isoniazid, rifampin, pyrazinamide, ethambutol
Kaposi's sarcoma	Cough, often hemoptysis cough	Pulmonary nodules, pleural effusion	Open lung biopsy	Chemotherapy

Coccidioides immitus and *Histoplasma capsulatum* may cause subacute or chronic meningitis in patients residing in, or with a travel history to, endemic regions (desert Southwest and Ohio and Mississippi River drainage areas, respectively) (see Chapter 96).

Meningoencephalitis. Patients with HIV meningoencephalitis exhibit headache and alterations in sensorium varying from mild lethargy to coma. Patients may be febrile, and neurologic examination often shows evidence of diffuse CNS involvement. MRI may show only nonspecific abnormalities, whereas electroencephalography often is consistent with diffuse disease of the brain.

CMV encephalitis is rare and difficult to diagnose. Patients may show confusion, cranial nerve abnormalities, or long tract signs. CSF findings may resemble bacterial meningitis, and MRI may reveal peri-ventricular abnormalities. Many patients have associated CMV retinitis. PCR detection of CMV antigens in CSF appears to be a sensitive and specific method for the diagnosis of CMV encephalitis and polyradiculopathy.

Meningoencephalitis caused by HSV is unusual in HIV infection (see Chapter 96).

PULMONARY DISEASES

Pulmonary infections are common in persons living with HIV and range from nonspecific interstitial pneumonitis to life-threatening pneumonias (Table 107–14).

Patients infected with HIV have a threefold to fourfold increased risk of bacterial pneumonia, often associated with bacteremia, generally caused by encapsulated bacteria, including *S. pneumoniae* and *H. influenzae*. The increased risk begins with modest degrees of immunodeficiency (CD4 counts of 200 to 500 cells/mm³). The onset is often abrupt, and the response to prompt initiation of therapy is usually good; however, delay in appropriate antimicrobial therapy may result in a fulminant downhill course. Initial therapy is guided by the results of Gram stain of sputum (see Chapter 98).

PCP remains a life-threatening infection in North American persons with AIDS and now occurs most often in severely immunocompromised individuals who are not receiving PCP prophylaxis because they are not aware that they have HIV infection. Patients usually complain of gradual onset of nonproductive cough, fever, and shortness of breath with exertion; a productive cough suggests another process. In contrast to the acute onset of PCP in other immunocompromised patients, patients with AIDS and PCP often have pulmonary symptoms for weeks before presentation to a physician. Arterial hypoxemia rapidly worsens with slight exertion; the chest radiograph often shows a subtle interstitial pattern but may be entirely normal. The patient often appears sicker than the radiograph would suggest.

If PCP is suggested clinically, then treatment should be started immediately; treatment for several days does not interfere with the ability to make a specific diagnosis. Confirmation of PCP is essential; delay in establishing a correct diagnosis of another treatable condition may be lethal. Some experienced centers, by Giemsa or direct fluorescent-antibody stain of induced sputum, may confirm the diagnosis. Alternatively, bronchoalveolar lavage, with Gomori's methenamine silver or immunofluorescent staining of specimens, is adequate to diagnose PCP in more than 95% of patients.

Table 107–15	Diarrhea in Advanced Human Immunodeficiency Virus Infection		
Cause	**Characteristics**	**Diagnosis**	**Treatment**
Frequent			
Cryptosporidium parvum	Varies from increased frequency to large-volume diarrhea	Acid-fast stain of stool	Antiretroviral therapy
Clostridium difficile	Abdominal pain, fever common	*C. difficile* toxin in stool or endoscopy	Metronidazole or vancomycin
Cytomegalovirus	Small bowel movements with blood or mucus (colitis)	Colonoscopy and biopsy	Ganciclovir
Mycobacterium avium-intracellulare	Abdominal pain, fever, retroperitoneal lymphadenopathy	Blood culture or endoscopy with biopsy	Multidrug regimen, including clarithromycin; ethambutol
Less Frequent			
Salmonella or *Campylobacter*	Sometimes with blood or mucus in bowel movements (colitis)	Stool culture	Norfloxacin (check sensitivities)
Isospora belli	Watery diarrhea	Acid-fast stain of stool	Trimethoprim-sulfamethoxazole

Treatment with high-dose trimethoprim-sulfamethoxazole for 3 weeks is usually effective (see Table 107–14). Patients with advanced PCP and arterial hypoxemia (oxygen tension of 75 mm on breathing room air) benefit from administration of corticosteroids (40 mg of prednisone twice daily, with tapering of the drug over a 3-week period).

As with acute bacterial pneumonia, active pulmonary tuberculosis may develop at a time when the CD4 count remains well above 200 cells/mm^3 (see Table 107–4). Chest radiographs in patients infected with HIV may show features of primary tuberculosis, including hilar adenopathy, lower or middle lobe infiltrates, miliary pattern, or pleural effusions, as well as classic patterns of reactivation. Extrapulmonary *M. tuberculosis* infection, especially involving cervical or intraabdominal lymph nodes, also occurs with increased frequency with advanced immunodeficiency. Specific blood cultures may yield *M. tuberculosis* in the severely immunocompromised patient.

Both pulmonary and extrapulmonary tuberculosis generally respond well to standard antituberculosis therapy. Treatment therefore should begin with four antituberculosis drugs (see Chapter 98).

Disseminated histoplasmosis and coccidioidomycosis each occur with significantly increased frequency in persons with HIV infection. Either fungal infection may be demonstrated with nodular infiltrates or with a miliary pattern on chest radiograph. Histoplasmosis usually involves bone marrow, as well as skin; bone marrow examination often shows the organism. Standard initial treatment of disseminated mycoses in patients with AIDS is high-dose amphotericin. Because relapse is common, oral azole therapy (fluconazole for coccidioidomycosis, itraconazole for histoplasmosis) must be continued after resolution of signs and symptoms until two successive CD4 counts above 200 cells/mm^3 have been obtained at an interval of at least 3 months.

GASTROINTESTINAL DISEASES

HIV affects the gastrointestinal tract early in infection, with profound depletion of memory CD4 T cells in gut-associated lymphoid tissue within the first few weeks of infection. Symptomatic disease of the gut is, however, unusual in the early stage of infection.

Abnormalities of hepatic enzymes and/or liver function tests are common but often nonspecific. Elevations of serum alanine aminotransferase and aspartate aminotransferase often represent chronic active hepatitis B or C but may reflect hepatic toxicity caused by medications, including trimethoprim-sulfamethoxazole and/or antiretroviral agents. In patients with HCV-HIV co-infection, progression to advanced cirrhosis is accelerated and is now a major cause of death in this population. Marked elevations in serum alkaline phosphatase levels may reflect infiltrative disease of the liver (e.g., MAI, *Mycobacterium tuberculosis* infection) but also may occur with acalculous cholecystitis, cryptosporidiosis, or AIDS-associated sclerosing cholangitis.

DIARRHEA

Diarrhea occurs, at least intermittently, in many persons with advanced immunodeficiency and may be caused by a variety of micro-organisms (Table 107–15) or by certain antiviral medications. In many instances, no clear cause is found. Stool specimens should be cultured for *Salmonella*, *Campylobacter*, and *Yersinia* species; patients usually respond to standard antimicrobial therapy (see Chapter 102). Patients may also have recurrent episodes of diarrhea associated with *Clostridium difficile* toxin; this probably reflects the frequent use of broad-spectrum antibiotics.

In cases of persistent diarrhea, a fresh stool specimen should be examined for parasites using a modified acid-fast stain for *Cryptosporidium parvum, Microsporidia,* and *Isospora belli,* the most common enteric protozoal infections in patients with AIDS. Although cryptosporidiosis is generally self limited in persons with CD4 counts over 200 cells/mm^3, massive diarrhea (up to 10 L/day) may occur in patients with CD4 counts under 100 cells/mm^3. Isosporiasis responds to oral trimethoprim-sulfamethoxazole. All symptoms of both cryptosporidiosis and isosporiasis resolve following immune reconstitution in response to effective ART.

If stool diagnostic studies are negative and diarrhea persists, then patients should undergo endoscopy (see Chapter 33). Biopsy of the duodenum or small bowel may show histologic evidence of cryptosporidial, microsporidial, MAI, or CMV infection, or villous atrophy characteristic of HIV enteropathy. Biopsy of the colon may be indicative of HSV proctitis, CMV colitis, or MAI infection. For patients with refractory diarrhea, symptomatic treatment may improve the quality of life.

With advanced immunodeficiency (CD4 count >50 cells/mm^3), gastrointestinal disease evidenced by dysphagia (see Table 107–10), diarrhea, or colitis is common. Each process may contribute to inadequate nutrition, compounding the weight loss associated with advanced HIV disease.

UNEXPLAINED FEVER

Most persistent fevers late in the course of HIV infection reflect a definable OI.

The most common cause of unexplained fever and anemia in patients with CD4 counts less than 50 cells/mm^3 is disseminated MAI infection. *Blood* cultures are positive in over 90% of patients. Specific treatment (see Table 107–8) usually results in resolution of fever and weight gain.

Aggressive non-Hodgkin's lymphoma may also cause unexplained fever and weight loss. A rapidly enlarging spleen or asymmetric lymph node enlargement may suggest the diagnosis. CT-guided biopsy of enlarged intra-abdominal nodes may provide the diagnosis.

WASTING

Cachexia may be prominent in advanced HIV disease. In some instances, an intercurrent infectious process may be causing the wasting. Heightened production of tumor necrosis factor may contribute to fever, cachexia, and hypertriglyceridemia in advanced HIV disease.

If orthostatic hypotension occurs, especially if associated with hyperkalemia, then the possibility of adrenal insufficiency, which rarely can result from CMV adrenalitis, should be investigated (see Chapter 66).

Most patients with AIDS-associated cachexia gain weight and achieve a sense of well being after initiation of effective ART. Weight gain is sometimes enhanced by administration of recombinant growth hormone, nonmethylated androgens, or megestrol, but definitive indications for hormone therapy have not been established.

ACQUIRED IMMUNODEFICIENCY SYNDROME–ASSOCIATED MALIGNANCIES

Among homosexual men infected with HIV, the frequency of Kaposi's sarcoma, caused by human herpesvirus-8, has fallen from 40% at the outset of the epidemic to less than 15% in 1999. In many patients, lesions resolve after institution of effective ART. Systemic chemotherapy can provide remissions in many patients with symptomatic visceral disease.

Non-Hodgkin's B-cell lymphomas occur roughly 200 times more often in persons infected with HIV than in the general population. Up to 40% of AIDS-related systemic lymphomas, and almost all of those isolated to the CNS, are related to EBV. Most AIDS-associated lymphomas are of small noncleaved or immunoblastic histologic factors. Extranodal presentation of these tumors is the rule, with a high frequency of gastrointestinal or intracranial presentation. Chemotherapy for systemic disease or radiation therapy for CNS disease generally provides a clinical remission, which may be maintained if accompanied by effective ART.

RENAL DISORDERS

Renal insufficiency in patients with AIDS may be a consequence of nephrotoxic drug administration, heroin injection, or HIV-associated nephropathy (HIVAN). Certain histologic features (e.g., focal and segmental glomerulosclerosis) may distinguish HIVAN from renal failure associated with intravenous heroin use. In the United States, HIVAN occurs most commonly in African Americans and usually produces heavy proteinuria and progressive renal insufficiency. Without treatment, most patients develop end-stage renal disease within several months. The incidence of this complication appears to have been decreased by effective ART.

Prevention of Human Immunodeficiency Viral Infection

Three approaches—behavior modification, treatment of STDs, and ART of seropositive pregnant women—can have major impacts on HIV transmission.

In a large number of communities at increased risk for HIV (e.g., homosexually active men in the United States and Western Europe, young adults in Uganda), adoption of safe sexual practices have been associated with a decrease in incidence of HIV infection. Sustaining these behavioral changes over long periods requires ongoing reinforcement.

Studies in Africa have demonstrated that periodic community-wide STD treatment programs may result in significant reductions in HIV transmission in some communities.

Antiretroviral treatment of pregnant women who are infected with HIV, and of their infants, for 6 weeks has decreased maternal-child transmission from 25% to less than 2% in North America, without harm to the newborn child.

The use of universal blood and body fluid precautions is routinely recommended to protect health care workers. Meticulous attention to proper use and disposal of sharp instruments is critical because most nosocomial HIV infections have occurred through accidental needlesticks. Prompt administration of antiretroviral drugs decreases the risk of HIV infection after needlestick injuries. Current recommendations by the U.S. Public Health Service for prophylaxis after high-risk occupational exposure include a combination regimen of three effective antiretroviral drugs initiated as soon as possible after exposure and continuing for 4 weeks (see ***http://www.cdc.gov/mmwr*** for more information).

The development of an effective prophylactic vaccine is the target of active research. Clinical trials of vaccine candidates are ongoing.

Prospectus for the Future

- New treatment strategies targeting additional stages of the viral life cycle
- Antiviral agents effective against strains of HIV resistant to currently available regimens
  - Increased once-daily treatment regimens with few long-term toxicities
- Effective approach to eradication of HIV from resting T lymphocytes
- Testing of potential prophylactic and therapeutic vaccines

References

Aberg JA, Gallant JE, Anderson J, et al: Primary care guidelines for the management of persons infected with human immunodeficiency virus: Recommendations of the HIV Medicine Association of the Infectious Diseases Society of America. Clin Infect Dis 39:609–629, 2004.

Castro KG, Ward JW, Slutsker L, et al: 1993 revised classification system for HIV infection and expanded surveillance case definition for AIDS among adolescents and adults. Morb Mortal Wkly Rep 41(RR-17): 1–19, 1992 (available at: *http://www.cdc.gov/mmwr*).

Centers for Disease Control and Prevention: Guidelines for preventing opportunistic infections among HIV-infected persons–2002: Recommendations of the U.S. Public Health Service and the Infectious Diseases Society of America. Morb Mortal Wkly Rep 51:1–52, 2002 (available at: *http://www.cdc.gov/mmwr/INDRR_2002*).

Department of Health and Human Services: DHHS Panel on Clinical Practices for Treatment of HIV Infection. Guidelines for the Use of Antiretroviral Agents among HIV-Infected Adults and Adolescents. Bethesda,

Department of Health and Human Services, April 7, 2005 (updated quarterly at: *http://aidsinfo.nih.gov/guidelines*).

Egger M, May M, Chene G, et al: Prognosis of HIV-1 infected patients starting highly active ART: A collaborative analysis of prospective studies. Lancet 360:119–129, 2002.

Hammer SM, Saag M, Schechter M, et al: Treatment for adult HIV infection: 2006 recommendations of the International AIDS Society-USA Panel. JAMA 296:827–843, 2006.

Hirsch M, Brun-Vizinet F, D'Aquila RT, et al: Antiretroviral drug testing in adult HIV-1 infection. JAMA 283:2417–2426, 2002.

Mellors J, Munoz AM, Giorgi VJ, et al: Plasma viral load and CD4 lymphocytes as prognostic markers of HIV-1 infection. Ann Intern Med 126:946–954, 1997.

Scheld WM, et al: HIV and the acquired immunodeficiency syndrome. In Goldman L, Ausiello DA (eds): Cecil Textbook of Medicine, 22nd ed. Philadelphia, Elsevier, 2004, pp 2136–2195.

Skiest DJ: Focal neurological disease in patients with acquired immunodeficiency syndrome. Clin Infect Dis 34:103–115, 2002.

Infections in the Immunocompromised Host

David A. Bobak

Robert A. Salata

Immunosuppression is an increasingly common by-product of diseases and modern approaches to their treatment. The immunocompromised host suffers from increased susceptibility to *opportunistic infection,* defined as infection caused by organisms of low virulence that constitute normal mucosal and skin flora or by pathogenic microbial agents that are usually maintained in a latent state. Compromised hosts include patients with congenital immunodeficiencies, those infected with human immunodeficiency virus (HIV), and those who are immunocompromised as a consequence of cancer and its treatment, bone marrow failure, or treatment with steroids, cytotoxic therapy, or other immunosuppressive agents.

Immunocompromise is not an all-or-none phenomenon. The extent of immunosuppression varies with the underlying cause and must exceed a threshold to predispose the individual to opportunistic infections. Analysis of the type of immunosuppression can help predict the spectrum and types of agents likely to cause infections in an individual patient. Accordingly, opportunistic infections are usually considered in categories that reflect the nature of the immune deficiency. An important point to remember, however, is that most patients have several interacting risk factors that may cause combinations of defects affecting several different aspects of host defense and immune function.

Disorders of Cell-Mediated Immunity

Cell-mediated immunity is the major host defense against facultative and some obligate intracellular pathogens (see also Chapter 91). A partial list of diseases and conditions that impair cell-mediated immunity is presented in Table 108–1. However, only a certain number of these conditions result in increased susceptibility to infection with intracellular pathogens. Several forms of congenital immunodeficiencies are associated with severe infections early in childhood (Table 108–2). Foremost among the acquired immunodeficiencies are HIV infection, Hodgkin's disease and other lymphomas, hairy cell leukemia, and disseminated solid tumors. Severe malnutrition, as well as treatment with high-dose corticosteroids, cytotoxic drugs, or radiation therapy, can produce a similar predilection to infections. Patients with impaired cell-mediated immunity are especially susceptible to the types of organisms shown in Table 108–3 (**Web Figs. 108–1 to 108–8**).

The relative frequency of infection varies with the underlying disease (e.g., *Mycobacterium avium* complex is common in HIV infection, whereas *Listeria* is not), the geographic area (*Mycobacterium tuberculosis* is more common in developing countries than in developed countries), and the extent and type of immunosuppression (*M. tuberculosis* is an early, and *M. avium* complex a late, complication of HIV infection). Immunosuppressive medications vary greatly in their potency and mechanisms of action. In addition, the duration of immunosuppressive therapy is as important as the potency of the medication in assessing potential risk for opportunistic infection. For example, a patient receiving relatively high doses of corticosteroids for a short period (e.g., for an allergic reaction) is at much less risk for infection compared with a patient with an autoimmune disease receiving much lower doses of the same agent for a prolonged period.

Depression of cell-mediated immunity also permits organisms ordinarily constituting the normal flora, such as *Candida* species, to act as virulent opportunistic pathogens capable of causing aggressive infections. Latent viruses, fungi, mycobacteria, and parasites can reactivate to cause locally progressive or disseminated disease. In many instances, the signs, symptoms, and laboratory abnormalities indicating an infection are subtle and nonspecific, an important distinction to the clinical presentations commonly observed in immunocompetent patients.

In some instances, treatment of the underlying disease causing the immunodeficiency, or progression of the disease itself, produces an increased severe and generalized compro-

Table 108–1   Conditions Causing Impaired Cell-Mediated Immunity

Infectious Diseases

Measles
Chickenpox
Human immunodeficiency virus
Typhoid fever
Tuberculosis
Leprosy
Histoplasmosis

Malignant Diseases

Hodgkin's disease
Lymphomas
Advanced solid tumors

Vaccinations

Measles
Mumps
Rubella

Drugs

Corticosteroids
Cytotoxic drugs
Antirejection drugs and antilymphocyte antibodies used for
 organ transplant patients
Monoclonal antibodies targeting tumor necrosis factor-α
 (e.g., infliximab, etanercept)

Miscellaneous

Congenital immunodeficiency states
Sarcoidosis
Uremia
Diabetes mellitus
Malnutrition

Table 108–2   Examples of Congenital Immunodeficiency Syndromes

Severe combined immunodeficiency (SCID)
X-linked SCID
Adenosine deaminase deficiency
Purine-nucleosidase phosphorylase deficiency
Zeta-associated protein (ZAP)-70 kinase deficiency
Wiskott-Aldrich syndrome
DiGeorge syndrome
Ataxia telangiectasia

Table 108–3   Agents Commonly Causing Infections in Patients with Impaired Cell-Mediated Immunity

Viruses

Varicella-zoster virus
Herpes simplex virus
Cytomegalovirus **(Web Fig. 108–8)**
Epstein-Barr virus
JC virus
Human herpesvirus 6
Human herpesvirus 8
Respiratory viruses (e.g., influenza, parainfluenza, adenovirus,
 respiratory synctial virus)

Bacteria

Listeria monocytogenes
Salmonella species
Legionella species
Nocardia species
Mycobacterium tuberculosis
Nontuberculous mycobacteria

Fungi

Pathogenic: *Histoplasma, Coccidioides, Blastomyces*
 (Web Fig. 108–4)
Saprophytic: *Cryptococcus* **(Web Fig. 108–5)**, *Candida,*
 Pneumocystis jirovecii **(Web Fig. 108–6)**; less commonly,
 Aspergillus **(Web Fig. 108–2)**, *Zygomycetes* **(Web Fig. 108–2**
 and **Web Fig. 108–3)**

Protozoa

Cryptosporidium parvum
Leishmania donovani
Toxoplasma gondii **(Web Fig. 108–7)**

Helminths

Strongyloides stercoralis

mised state, one that predisposes the individual to infection by additional types of micro-organisms. For example, during chemotherapy for lymphoma, bacterial infections initially predominate. Disease progression may also alter other factors that favor bacterial infections, such as mucosal breakdown and obstruction by tumor masses of the bronchi, the ureters, or the biliary tract. The result is a marked increase in severe bacterial infection and sepsis syndrome, often caused by multiple-resistant pathogens, late in the course of many diseases associated with impaired cell-mediated immunity.

Disorders of Humoral Immunity

The acquired disorders of antibody production associated with increased frequency of infection in adults are common variable immunodeficiency, chronic lymphocytic leukemia, lymphosarcoma, multiple myeloma, nephrotic syndrome, major burns, and protein-losing enteropathy. The paraproteinemic states belong in this category because of secondary decreases in levels of functioning antibody. Therapy with cytotoxic drugs may produce similar immunocompromised states.

Infections with pneumococci, *Haemophilus influenzae,* streptococci, and staphylococci predominate early in the course of the humoral immunodeficiency. As the underlying disease itself progresses, infections with gram-negative bacilli become increasingly frequent. Treatment of the underlying condition with corticosteroids and cytotoxic drugs causes additional defects in cell-mediated immunity and provides susceptibility to infections with the group of pathogens presented in Table 108–3. Some agents predicted to alter humoral immunity may have unexpected effects. For example, the monoclonal antibody rituximab used for treating certain types of lymphoma profoundly depletes B lymphocytes but causes increased risk of hepatitis B reactivation, rather than increased infectious risk by the bacterial pathogens outlined previously.

In sickle cell anemia, heat-labile opsonic activity is diminished. Complement depletion by erythrocyte stroma impairs opsonization of pneumococci and *Salmonella* species and leads to frequent infections with these organisms. Impaired reticuloendothelial system function resulting from erythrophagocytosis and functional asplenia also predisposes patients with sickle cell disease to other serious bacterial infections. The predisposition to infection is related to age; once children with sickle cell disease develop antibodies to pneumococcal capsular polysaccharide, they lose their thousandfold increased susceptibility to severe pneumococcal infection.

Splenectomy results in a loss of mechanisms for the clearing of opsonized organisms. Splenectomy therefore predisposes patients to fulminant infections caused by encapsulated bacteria. Over a period of years, the liver may partially compensate for certain aspects of splenic function. The splenic tissue also represents a major source of production of antibody, as well as other opsonic factors such as tuftsin, which opsonizes staphylococci. Splenectomized patients are also predisposed to severe and overwhelming infection with *Capnocytophaga* species and additionally have an increased risk for acquiring babesiosis. Pneumococcal and meningococcal vaccines should be administered to adult patients who will be undergoing splenectomy or who suffer from diseases likely to produce functional asplenia. The newer protein conjugate forms of the pneumococcal and meningococcal vaccines, when available, may offer increased response rates for splenectomized or functionally asplenic patients. Fever in a patient with asplenia should immediately raise concern for possible underlying sepsis, and such a patient should be immediately treated with empiric antibiotics while awaiting results of cultures and laboratory tests.

Impaired Neutrophil Function

Many types of inherited or acquired diseases impair neutrophil function. The defect may be extrinsic or intrinsic to the neutrophil itself. For example, impaired chemotaxis predisposes patients with inherited C3 and C5 deficiencies to frequent bacterial infections (see also Chapter 91). Corticosteroid therapy is generally associated with defective cell-mediated immunity (see previous discussion) but may also interfere with neutrophil chemotaxis. Even though circulating neutrophil counts are frequently normal or increased in patients receiving corticosteroids, these cells do not localize normally to the site of infection. Many other illnesses and conditions are associated with impaired neutrophil function, including myelodysplasia, paroxysmal nocturnal hemoglobinuria, radiation therapy, and cytotoxic drug therapy.

Inherited intrinsic defects in neutrophils are rare but have provided insights into understanding the microbicidal mechanisms of these cells. Neutrophils from patients with chronic granulomatous disease (CGD) cannot develop an oxidative burst. Catalase-negative organisms produce sufficient hydrogen peroxide to facilitate their own killing by CGD neutrophils via the myeloperoxidase pathway. Catalase-producing organisms such as staphylococci, *Serratia, Nocardia,* and *Aspergillus,* however, scavenge hydrogen peroxide. These organisms therefore cannot be killed effectively by neutrophils from patients with CGD and can result in serious recurrent infections.

The most severe intrinsic neutrophil defects occur in the Chédiak-Higashi syndrome. The neutrophils of patients with this syndrome have giant and abnormal granules and also exhibit defective microtubule assembly. These defects together cause impaired chemotaxis, abnormal phagolysosomal fusion, and delayed bacterial killing, predisposing the patients to recurrent infections. Other phenotypic abnormalities often associated with this rare syndrome include partial albinism, depigmentation of the iris, peripheral neuropathies, and nystagmus.

Neutropenia

Neutropenia is one of the most common and most important risk factors for serious infection in the compromised host. Other alterations in host defense mechanisms frequently co-exist with neutropenia, and these additional alterations often further increase the risk of infection. Most data regarding the incidence of fever and risk of infection associated with neutropenia come from studies of patients with leukemia undergoing cytotoxic chemotherapy. As the neutrophil count falls below 500/mcL, an exponential increase occurs in both the frequency and severity of associated infections. Neutrophil counts between 100 and 500/mcL are frequently associated with infections, whereas with neutrophil counts below 100/mcL, fever and some form of infection, are almost universal. The duration of neutropenia is also important in determining the level of risk and types of infections in an individual patient.

Chemotherapy-associated neutropenia in acute leukemia is usually profound and sustained and occurs in conjunction with other predisposing factors for infection such as

Table 108–4	**Agents That Frequently Cause Infections in Neutropenic Patients**

Viruses

Cytomegalovirus (**Web Fig. 108–8**)
Herpesviruses

Bacteria

Pseudomonas aeruginosa
Serratia
Enterobacter
Escherichia coli
Klebsiella
Staphylococcus aureus (including methicillin-resistant staphylococci)
Coagulase-negative staphylococci
Corynebacterium group JK
Viridans group streptococci (e.g., *Streptococcus mitis*)
Enterococci (including vancomycin-resistant enterococci)

Fungi

Candida
Pneumocystis jirovecii (**Web Fig. 108–6**)
Aspergillus (**Web Fig. 108–1**)
Zygomycetes (**Web Fig. 108–2** and **Web Fig. 108–3**)

mucositis and the presence of indwelling central venous catheters. These patients therefore become susceptible to organisms that are ubiquitous in the environment and are part of the normal flora (Table 108–4). In contrast, in patients with chronic or cyclic neutropenias, the susceptibility to infection varies inversely with the monocyte count because these cells help substitute for some of the antibacterial capacity of the missing neutrophils.

Diagnostic Problems in the Compromised Host

PULMONARY INFILTRATES

Pneumonia and bloodstream infections represent the most serious forms of infection for most immunocompromised patients. The immunocompromised patient with pulmonary infiltrates presents a particularly difficult diagnostic problem. Pulmonary infiltrates can represent infection, extension of underlying tumor, complication of chemotherapy, fluid overload, pulmonary infarction, hemorrhage, or any combination of these conditions. Because of the seriousness of the condition and the variety of possible causes, obtaining a specific diagnosis is essential. Unfortunately, noninvasive serodiagnostic tests are rarely helpful in this setting, and accurate diagnosis can often be made only by direct sampling and examination of lung tissue by bronchoalveolar lavage and/or biopsy.

The clinical setting and radiographic appearance of the pulmonary infiltrate will influence the decision about whether to proceed with lung biopsy. For example, in patients with leukemia, parenchymal infiltrates occurring before or within 3 days of initiating chemotherapy are usually caused by infection from common bacterial pathogens. Major efforts should be directed first at collecting adequate sputum samples to stain and culture for bacterial, mycobacterial, and fungal pathogens. The course of pneumonitis following initial antibiotic therapy indicates whether to proceed with lung biopsy.

In contrast, diffuse infiltrates occurring *after* treatment of leukemia are suggestive of infection by opportunistic micro-organisms. *Pneumocystis jirovecii* (**see Web Fig. 108–6**), for example, is an important preventable, treatable cause of diffuse infiltrates and occurs most often after treatment of acute lymphocytic leukemia or in patients with an acquired deficiency of cell-mediated immunity (see Chapter 107). In these settings, the diagnosis should be established by examination of induced sputum, by bronchoalveolar lavage, or by transbronchial biopsy. If these diagnostic approaches are not helpful, empiric therapy with trimethoprim-sulfamethoxazole may be initiated. Importantly, the clinical presentation of *Pneumocystis* pneumonia (PCP) frequently differs in HIV-negative immunocompromised hosts compared with HIV-infected individuals. PCP in HIV-negative patients is often more acute, more severe, and more frequently associated with other concurrent pathogens. In addition, the diagnostic sensitivity of bronchoalveolar lavage for detecting *Pneumocystis* organisms is considerably reduced in HIV-negative patients, and lung biopsy may be needed to obtain the correct diagnosis.

The indication and timing for lung biopsy must be individualized. Delay in proceeding with biopsy may reduce the chances of favorably affecting the outcome of the infection, even if the biopsy shows a potentially treatable disease. Thrombocytopenia and/or coagulopathies frequently coexist in compromised patients with pulmonary infiltrates and need to be corrected to minimize bleeding risk of a biopsy. If a decision has been made to perform a biopsy, several technical options are available. Transbronchial biopsy by fiberoptic bronchoscopy will often provide adequate tissue samples for diagnosis, particularly in the evaluation of diffuse pulmonary lesions. Open-lung biopsy has an additional yield of 50% to 75% in the patient with a nondiagnostic transbronchial biopsy and should be performed without delay if progression of the patient's illness mandates immediate diagnosis. Early treatment of most pulmonary infections in immunocompromised hosts, even aspergillosis (Fig. 108–1), can be associated with an initially favorable outcome.

DISSEMINATED MYCOSES

Disseminated mycoses represent another major diagnostic problem in the immunocompromised host. Fungal infections are found postmortem in more than one half of patients with leukemia or lymphoma; usually, the nature of the infection has not been established antemortem. Culture of a saprophytic organism such as *Candida* from superficial

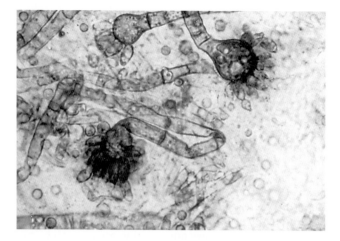

Figure 108–1 Fruiting head of *Aspergillus fumigatus* on a lung biopsy **(see Web Fig. 108–1)**. Aspergillosis usually causes an expanding perihilar pulmonary infiltrate with a characteristic *halo* sign noted on a computed tomographic scan of the lungs. Prompt institution of potent antifungal therapy is essential in attempting to achieve a good clinical response.

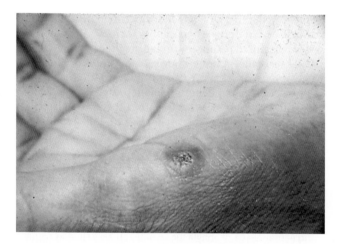

Figure 108–2 Skin lesion in a 76-year-old woman treated with corticosteroids and cytotoxic drugs for chronic lymphocytic leukemia and exhibiting nodular pulmonary infiltrates and lymphocytic meningitis. Fluid expressed from the lesion contained encapsulated yeast seen on India ink preparation and yielded *Cryptococcus neoformans* on culture **(see Web Fig. 108–5)**.

sites does not establish pathogenicity. Even in patients with widespread infection, detectable fungemia may be a late event.

How, then, can the diagnosis of fungal infection be established early, at a time when the infection is potentially curable? The physician should search for superficial lesions accessible to scraping, aspiration, or biopsy (Fig. 108–2). Dissemination of *Candida tropicalis* frequently causes hyperpigmented macular or pustular skin lesions that show the organisms within blood vessel walls on punch skin biopsy. Hepatosplenic candidiasis is most frequently encountered in patients with fever after recovery from neutropenia. The presence of bull's-eye lesions on computed tomographic

scans of the liver and spleen suggests hepatosplenic candidiasis. Cryptococcal polysaccharide antigen is usually present in the serum and/or cerebrospinal fluid of the patient with disseminated cryptococcosis **(see Web Fig, 108–5)**. Serodiagnosis for other fungi has, in general, been disappointing.

Acute invasive pulmonary aspergillosis occurs most often in patients with prolonged, profound neutropenia who complain of fever and pleuritic chest pain during or after broad-spectrum antibacterial therapy. Accurate diagnosis of invasive disease caused by *Aspergillus* species usually requires examination of affected tissue obtained from a biopsy **(see Web Fig. 108–1)**. The diagnosis of pneumonia caused by *Aspergillus,* or other molds, is also strongly suggested by the appearance of a distinctive *halo* sign visible on a computed tomographic scan of the lungs in at-risk patients. Recent studies further indicate that serially elevated levels of *Aspergillus* galactomannan in the serum can be useful in the presumptive diagnosis of invasive disease and may also aid in determining the efficacy of treatment.

In the absence of a definitive diagnosis, empiric use of antifungal drugs is generally indicated in the immunocompromised host with a moderate to high clinical suggestion of invasive fungal disease (e.g., in the febrile patient with neutropenia for more than 3 days despite empiric broad-spectrum antibacterial therapy). Several new antifungal agents have become available over the last few years (e.g., the echinocandins) and have widened our choices for immunocompromised patients with fungal infection. Current efforts focus on improved strategies for prophylaxis (see later discussion), as well as studying potential synergistic combinations of antifungal agents.

Prevention and Treatment of Infections in the Patient with Neutropenia

PREVENTION

Acute bacterial infections and sepsis caused by organisms comprising the gut flora occur frequently in patients with neutropenia and may have fever as their sole clinical sign. Prophylactic nonabsorbable antibiotics and protective isolation have generally failed to prevent such infection. Certain antibiotics, given prophylactically, may decrease the number of infections and bacteremic episodes in some patients with neutropenia. Prophylactic trimethoprim-sulfamethoxazole also decreases the risk of pneumonia caused by *P. jirovecii* (see Chapter 107). However, the bone marrow toxicity of this drug and selection of resistant organisms decreases the suitability for widespread prophylactic use in patients with neutropenia. Quinolones, such as ciprofloxacin, may be equally effective in preventing bacterial infections and generally have reduced toxicity. Quinolones have no activity against *P. jirovecii*, however, and have also been associated with an increased risk of severe streptococcal (including *Streptococcus viridans* group) infection in some patients. Prophylactic administration of agents to prevent systemic fungal infections is not routine for all patients with neutropenia but is generally used for patients with hematologic malignancies or those undergoing bone marrow or stem cell transplantation.

Adherence to strict hand-washing procedures by all hospital personnel remains the single best approach preventing infection in patients with neutropenia.

TREATMENT

Empiric antibiotic therapy is indicated in febrile patients with granulocytopenia because at least two thirds have an underlying infection. Selection of two drugs with activity against gram-negative enteric bacilli and *Pseudomonas* is usually necessary (e.g., use of an antipseudomonal β-lactam and an aminoglycoside). Initial empiric therapy for staphylococci is indicated when clinical concern exists about infections of vascular catheters or of skin or soft tissue. Methicillin-resistant *Staphylococcus aureus* (MRSA) has become a major pathogen in this clinical situation. Antibiotic coverage for MRSA, though, is generally reserved for documented infection, given that empiric addition of an agent such as vancomycin does not affect short-term outcomes in neutropenic febrile patients without a documented source of infection. Despite the early use of empiric antibiotics, the clinical outcome of patients with both neutropenia and bacterial infections is poor unless the initial neutrophil count exceeds 500/mcL, the count rises during treatment, or the pathogen is a gram-positive organism. Adjunctive treatment with granulocyte colony-stimulating factors may result in shorter duration of neutropenia and fewer infectious complications in certain situations. Use of these biologics may also be beneficial in cases of documented or suggested invasive fungal disease (e.g., *Aspergillus* pneumonia) or refractory infection with gram-negative bacilli.

The appropriate duration of antimicrobial therapy of febrile patients with neutropenia is uncertain. If a specific diagnosis is made, narrowing antimicrobial coverage is sometimes appropriate to target the isolated organism, assuming that the neutrophil counts recover. If no etiologic agent is identified, many physicians continue to administer the empiric antibiotic regimen until the neutropenia resolves. The empiric addition of antifungal therapy is indicated in the patient with neutropenia who remains febrile for at least 3 days despite broad-spectrum antibacterial therapy. In this setting, the best approach is often to continue broad-spectrum antibiotics for the duration of the neutropenia unless the cause of the patient's fever can be clearly defined. Whereas the management of a patient with neutropenic fever has generally required hospital-based treatment, recent studies have attempted to identify a subset of low-risk patients who can be managed as outpatients. In some centers, certain relatively low-risk patients with neutropenia and fever (e.g., highly dependable individuals with absolute neutrophil counts ≥ 500/mcL) are initially managed at home using outpatient intravenous or oral combinations of highly active antibiotics.

With ever-increasing numbers of patients receiving a variety of potent and novel immunosuppressive agents, the number and variety of infections occurring in susceptible individuals can only be expected to increase. In addition to newly recognized pathogenic organisms, increases in antimicrobial resistance among known pathogens will also likely be observed. Newer strategies for dealing with infections in immunocompromised hosts include expanded use of targeted forms of prophylaxis, development of molecular assays permitting diagnosis at an earlier stage, and the evolution of combination therapies for particularly resistant organisms.

Prospectus for the Future

- The increasing use of immunosuppressive drugs with novel modes of action will predispose patients to infections by additional opportunistic pathogens.

- Increased use of prophylactic antimicrobials will lead to parallel increases in antibiotic resistance, increasing the demand for novel antimicrobial agents.

References

Giles JT, Bathon JM: Serious infections associated with anticytokine therapies in the rheumatic diseases. J Intensive Care Med 19:320–334, 2004.

Kotloff RM, Ahya VN, Crawford SW: Pulmonary complications of solid organ and hematopoietic stem cell transplantation. Am J Respir Crit Care Med 170:22–48, 2004.

Ramphal R: Changes in the etiology of bacteremia in febrile neutropenic patients and the susceptibilities of the currently isolated pathogens. Clin Infect Dis 39(Suppl. 1):S32–37, 2004.

Singh N, Paterson DL: Aspergillus infections in transplant recipients. Clin Microbiol Rev 18:44–69, 2005.

Sipsas NV, Bodey GP, Kontoyiannis DP: Perspectives for the management of febrile neutropenic patients with cancer in the 21st century. Cancer 103:1103–1113, 2005.

Wingard JR: The changing face of invasive fungal infections in hematopoietic cell transplant recipients. Curr Opin Oncol 17:89–92, 2005.

Chapter 109

Infectious Diseases of Travelers: Protozoal and Helminthic Infections

Keith B. Armitage

Robert A. Salata

Medical advice for overseas travelers, some common clinical symptoms that may develop on their return, and the diagnosis and treatment of common parasitic diseases endemic in the United States and abroad are reviewed in this chapter.

Preparation of Travelers

More than 12 million Americans travel to developing countries each year. Major increases in international travel and the resurgence of malaria, dengue fever, and other infectious diseases worldwide bring the issues of prevention and management of health problems in travelers into the office of every physician.

Risks associated with international travel are dependent on the destination, duration of the trip, underlying health and age of the traveler, and activities while abroad. In general, destinations within the industrialized world require no specific health precautions. In contrast, travelers to developing areas, especially the tropics, can occasionally be exposed to life-threatening infections. Major issues to be addressed in the pretravel period include required and recommended immunizations, malaria prophylaxis, travelers' diarrhea, and other problems that can be avoided or prevented. Information about health risks in specific geographic areas, updated weekly, can be obtained from the Centers for Disease Control and Prevention (CDC) through its publications or by calling the International Travelers' Hotline (1-877-394-8747; website: *http://www.cdc.gov/travel*).

IMMUNIZATIONS

Only yellow fever vaccination may be required by law for international travel. Both polio and meningococcal meningitis vaccinations may be required during outbreak situations, and the meningococcal vaccine is required for religious pilgrimages (Hajj) to Saudi Arabia. Although some immunizations are not generally considered *travel* immunizations, many Americans have allowed routine diphtheria-tetanus immunizations to lapse or may not have been fully immunized against measles and polio. Finally, other immunizations are often strongly recommended, depending on the type and duration of travel. With a few exceptions, vaccines can be given simultaneously. Before immunization, a thorough history should be obtained to determine allergies to eggs or chick embryo cells. Pregnant women and individuals immunocompromised by human immunodeficiency virus (HIV), malignancy, or chemotherapy pose specific and important challenges; most live virus vaccines are contraindicated in these patients.

Yellow Fever

Yellow fever is a live, attenuated virus vaccine that is highly effective and recommended for persons traveling to areas in South America and Africa where yellow fever is endemic. Vaccination is generally safe and lasts for 10 years, but it must be given at designated vaccination centers.

Cholera

Cholera is endemic in parts of Asia and Africa and has returned to South and Central America, where it is a major concern to travelers. The currently available vaccine is not highly effective and is not routinely recommended for travel into endemic areas. Health education on likely sources of transmission is far more effective in preventing disease than is vaccination.

Measles

Up to 20% of first-year college students have no serologic evidence of prior measles infection or immunization and must be presumed to be susceptible. Individuals born after

1956 with no physician-documented record of immunization are at greatest risk for measles. In addition, a single immunization with measles vaccine at 15 months of age may permit breakthrough infection as a young adult. A second measles vaccination after age 5 is now recommended; international travelers born after 1956 who have not received a booster after early childhood should have a one-time booster.

Diphtheria-Tetanus

Tetanus is a ubiquitous problem and is most prevalent in tropical countries. A booster within the previous 5 years is recommended. This precaution eliminates the need for a tetanus booster if the traveler sustains a tetanus-prone injury overseas. This recommendation is made primarily because of the uncertainty of obtaining sterile, disposable needles in many overseas locations. Given the resurgence of diphtheria in countries of the former Soviet Union and the occurrence of disease in travelers to these areas, diphtheria toxoid should be co-administered with tetanus toxoid.

Polio

Polio remains endemic in some regions of Asia and Africa, and small, geographically restricted, vaccine-associated outbreaks have occurred in the Western Hemisphere. Most young adults have been immunized with at least four doses of trivalent oral poliovirus vaccine (OPV). Many adults (>18 years of age) cannot remember, however, whether they received OPV; such individuals should be given inactivated poliovirus vaccine. The live oral vaccine is no longer recommended for adults.

Hepatitis A

Hepatitis A is a major risk for travelers to areas of poor sanitation, affecting an estimated 1 in 500 to 1000 travelers per 2- to 3-week trip in some areas. Therefore, hepatitis A is the most frequent and important vaccine-preventable infection for travelers. Hepatitis A vaccine should be given at least 2 weeks before departure. A single dose provides protection for 1 to 2 years; a booster 6 to 18 months later is required for long-lasting immunity (>15 years).

Meningococcal Meningitis

Meningococcal meningitis is a worldwide disease, but cases in international travelers are infrequent except with prolonged contact with the local population. Vaccination with the quadrivalent polysaccharide vaccine (A, C, Y, and W-135) is recommended for travel to northern India, Nepal, and Saudi Arabia during the Hajj; certain parts of sub-Saharan Africa; and other locations where travel advisories have been issued (*http://www.cdc.gov/travel/*). A new quadrivalent A/C/Y/W-135 meningococcal conjugate vaccine was licensed in the United States in 2005 for preferred use among persons 11 to 55 years of age.

Typhoid

American international travelers are at greatest risk of contracting typhoid in the Indian subcontinent, Central America, western South America, and sub-Saharan Africa. Vaccination is recommended for travel to endemic areas where exposure to contaminated food and water is likely. Vaccination is also strongly indicated for travelers with achlorhydria, immunosuppression, or sickle cell anemia and for those taking broad-spectrum antibiotics. Both an oral vaccine (four enteric-coated capsules given over 7 days) and an injectable vaccine (one dose) are available and are essentially equivalent in effectiveness.

Other Vaccines

Some travelers, including missionaries, physicians, and anthropologists, need special consideration. These individuals live for prolonged periods in developing countries or are at special risk for contracting certain highly contagious diseases. Consideration should be given to immunization with hepatitis B, Japanese B encephalitis, plague, and rabies vaccines. In general, such travelers should be referred to a qualified travelers' clinic.

MALARIA PROPHYLAXIS

Malaria prophylaxis is a major problem for international travelers because of the high and increasing prevalence of drug resistance by the parasite. The need for, as well as the type of, prophylaxis is dependent on the exact itinerary within a given country because transmission risk is quite regional. Recommended chemoprophylactic regimens have changed frequently within the last few years. In general, travelers to areas where chloroquine-sensitive *Plasmodium falciparum* strains are exclusively found (Central America, the Caribbean, North Africa, and the Middle East) should take chloroquine phosphate (300-mg base or 500-mg salt) weekly starting 1 week before, continuing during, and for 4 weeks after leaving areas in which malaria is endemic. Travelers to areas where chloroquine-resistant *P. falciparum* is common may take mefloquine (Lariam), atovaquone-proguanil (Malarone), or doxycycline. These areas currently include Southeast Asia, sub-Saharan Africa, South America, and South Asia. Mefloquine, 250 mg/wk starting a week before travel, continuing during travel, and for 4 weeks after, is effective and convenient but may be associated with minor neurologic side effects (dizziness and vivid dreams) and rarely significant neuropsychiatric side effects. Mefloquine is not completely effective in Myanmar, rural Thailand, or some parts of East Africa, where resistance is a growing problem. Atovaquone-proguanil and doxycycline are effective in Southeast Asia and may be used in other areas of chloroquine resistance. Atovaquone-proguanil is well tolerated but must be taken every day and is relatively expensive. Doxycycline is inexpensive but must also be taken every day and is associated with photosensitivity and occasionally vaginal candidiasis. Although the sickle cell trait provides significant protection from death caused by falciparum malaria, this protection is not absolute and does not alter recommendations for prophylaxis. Emphasis must also be given to the use of mosquito netting, screens, and insect repellents, as well as to the prompt diagnosis and treatment of any febrile episodes (temperature >102° F [39° C]) in malaria-endemic areas.

TRAVELERS' DIARRHEA

Between 20% and 50% of individuals traveling to developing countries will develop diarrhea during or shortly after their trip. The average duration of an episode of travelers' diarrhea is 3 to 6 days. Approximately 10% of episodes last longer than 1 week. The diarrhea may be accompanied by abdominal cramping, nausea, headache, low-grade fever, vomiting, or bloating. Fewer than 5% of persons have fever greater than 101°F (38°C), bloody stools, or both. Travelers with these symptoms may not have simple travelers' diarrhea and should see a physician at once (see Chapter 102).

Diarrheal illness (including cholera) can be avoided through precautions with food and beverages. All water should be presumed to be unsafe. Salads are often contaminated by protozoal cysts and, along with street vendor foods, are the most dangerous foods encountered by most travelers. Food should be well cooked, including meat, seafood, and vegetables. Dairy products should be avoided.

Bismuth subsalicylate (Pepto-Bismol) can be used as a prophylactic measure (two tablets four times a day) or used to treat acute bouts of diarrhea (1 oz every 30 minutes for eight doses). Diphenoxylate (Lomotil) and loperamide (Imodium) may give symptomatic relief of diarrhea but should be avoided if the diarrhea is severe, fever exists, or blood is present in the stool. Trimethoprim-sulfamethoxazole, doxycycline, or one of the newer fluoroquinolones can be taken orally for 3 days to reduce the duration of symptoms and is effective against a wide variety of bacterial pathogens, including most *Shigella* and *Salmonella* species. Prophylactic antibiotics are not generally recommended. An exception is rifaxim, a nonsystemic, gastrointestinal-selective oral antibiotic approved for the treatment of travelers' diarrhea in 2004. Some authorities recommend this luminal agent for prophylaxis in high-risk travelers. Rifaxim is also an alternative to therapy of travelers' diarrhea caused by *Escherichia coli* (the most commonly pathogen) but has limited actively against other common pathogens.

GENERAL HEALTH INFORMATION

Other potentially dangerous activities overseas include exposure to dogs and cats (rabies), swimming in fresh water (schistosomiasis or leptospirosis), walking barefoot (hookworm or strongyloidiasis), and insect bites. In addition to malaria, many diseases, including dengue, sleeping sickness, and yellow fever, are transmitted by insects bites, and avoidance measures should be stressed when applicable. Travelers should also be reminded to use seat belts.

SPECIAL PROBLEMS
Pregnant Women

Live virus vaccines are contraindicated in women during pregnancy, which greatly complicates pretravel preparations. Chloroquine probably can be used safely. Travel to areas of chloroquine-resistant malaria should be strongly discouraged. No drug regimen to prevent or treat chloroquine-resistant malaria is safe in pregnant women, and malaria during pregnancy is a medical emergency for both the mother and her fetus.

Acquired Immunodeficiency Syndrome

Many countries, including the United States, now bar entry to patients with the acquired immunodeficiency syndrome (AIDS). Several countries require HIV serologic testing for all travelers applying for more than a 3-month visa, which requires official documentation well in advance of travel. Patients with HIV infection need special preparation before travel to developing countries because of their increased susceptibility to certain illnesses (e.g., pneumococcal infection, tuberculosis).

Most international travelers are concerned about the risk of acquiring HIV infection while abroad. Most concerns center on untested blood or nonsterile needles, which might be used in an emergency. Issues of HIV infection and other sexually transmitted diseases should be discussed, especially with young, sexually active adults.

Returning Traveler

With the exception of skin testing for tuberculosis, asymptomatic returning travelers generally do not need screening tests. The clinical problems that most often arise in travelers soon after return are fever and diarrhea, whereas eosinophilia is the most common cause for later referral. Fever is most important because delay in the diagnosis of *P. falciparum* malaria is often fatal. Fever should always prompt consideration of malaria until proved otherwise in travelers returning from countries where malaria is endemic, even if they are still taking prophylactic drugs. Determining the malaria species with a blood film is important because this finding affects therapy. Chloroquine-sensitive *P. falciparum* is treated with 1 g of chloroquine given orally, followed by 500 mg at 6, 24, and 48 hours. For *P. vivax* and *P. ovale* (also generally chloroquine sensitive), this regimen is followed by primaquine daily for 14 days to eradicate latent hepatic forms. Resistant *P. falciparum* is treated with atovaquone-proguanil, four full-strength pills a day for 3 days; or quinine sulfate, 650 mg given orally every 8 hours for 3 days, and doxycycline, 100 mg orally twice daily for 7 days. Intravenous quinidine is used in patients with severe malaria. Artemisinin compounds are used in many parts of the world to treat chloroquine-resistant malaria but may be associated with a high rate of relapse. All patients with possible resistant malaria infection should be hospitalized. If fever is not caused by malaria, then dengue, tuberculosis, typhoid fever, and amebic liver abscess, among other conditions, should be considered.

Persistent travelers' diarrhea that is unresponsive to empiric antibiotics is often due to *Giardia lamblia*. Three stool specimens for ova and parasites and a stool culture are warranted (**Web Fig. 109–1**). Unfortunately, *G. lamblia* may be missed in up to one third of patients even after this workup. Assessment of stool *Giardia* antigen by enzyme-linked immunosorbent assay is more sensitive than culture. If clinical suggestion is high, an empiric course of metronidazole (500 mg orally three times a day for 7 days) is usually justified. Antibiotic-resistant bacteria, amebiasis, temporary lactose intolerance, bacterial overgrowth, and tropical sprue should also be considered.

Eosinophilia in a returning traveler usually exhibits weeks or months after travel. It is usually caused by one of a wide variety of helminth infections. A stool specimen for ova and parasites is indicated but may be negative during the tissue-migrating phase of many intestinal worms or in tissue nematode infections, such as filariasis or onchocerciasis. Management of the more common parasitic infections encountered in travelers is included in the next section.

Protozoal and Helminthic Infections

PROTOZOAL INFECTIONS IN THE UNITED STATES

More than 2 billion people worldwide are infected with helminths. The incidence of protozoan parasitic infections is increasing in part because of the emergence of antimicrobial resistance (e.g., malaria) and an increasing number of susceptible hosts, especially those with HIV infection. Protozoal infections in the United States occur more frequently in immunocompromised hosts than in the general population (Table 109–1) (see Chapter 108). Babesiosis is very severe in asplenic individuals, and *Toxoplasma* encephalitis primarily affects patients with AIDS.

GIARDIASIS AND AMEBIASIS

Giardiasis is a common cause of persistent, nonbloody diarrhea in returning travelers. *Giardia lamblia* is prevalent throughout much of the developing world. Latin America is the most common site of *Giardia* acquisition by North American travelers. Men who have sex with men also have a high prevalence of infection because of specific sexual practices. Persons who work in day care centers are also at increased risk for giardiasis because of its relatively high prevalence in young children. The diagnosis and treatment are described previously in the "Returning Traveler" section.

As with *Giardia*, *Entamoeba histolytica* is transmitted by the fecal-oral route; the vast majority of infected individuals are asymptomatic. When *E. histolytica* causes acute illness, it is generally identified by bloody diarrhea. In the United

Table 109–1 Protozoal Infections

Protozoan	Setting	Vectors	Diagnosis	Special Considerations	Treatment
Endemic in the United States					
Babesia microti	New England	Ixodid ticks, transfusions	Thick or thin blood smear	Severe disease in asplenic persons	Quinine and clindamycin
Giardia lamblia	Mountain states	Humans, small mammals	Microscopic examination of stool or duodenal fluid	Common in homosexual men, travelers, children in day care centers	Quinacrine, nitazoxanide, or metronidazole
Toxoplasma gondii	Ubiquitous	Domestic cats, raw meat	Clinical; serologic confirmation	Pregnant women, immunosuppressed host (AIDS)	Pyrimethamine and sulfadiazine
Entamoeba histolytica	Southeast	Human	Microscopic examination of stool or *touch prep* from ulcer	Common in homosexual men, travelers, institutionalized persons	Metronidazole
Cryptosporidium sp.	Ubiquitous	Human	Acid-fast stain of stool	Severe in immunosuppressed hosts (AIDS)	Nitazoxanide
Trichomonas vaginalis	Ubiquitous	Human	*Wet prep* of genital secretions	Common cause of vaginitis	Metronidazole
Primarily Seen in Travelers and Immigrants					
Plasmodium sp.	Africa, Asia, South America	*Anopheles* mosquito	Thick and thin blood smears	Consider in returning travelers with fever	Dependent on regional resistance pattern (see text)
Leishmania donovani	Middle East	Sandfly	Tissue biopsy	Consider in immigrants with fever and splenomegaly	Pentostam
Trypanosoma sp.	Africa, South America	Reduviid bugs, transfusion	Direct examination of blood or CSF	Very rare in travelers, transfusion associated	Supportive

AIDS = acquired immunodeficiency syndrome; CSF = cerebrospinal fluid.

States, amebic dysentery is occasionally misdiagnosed as ulcerative colitis or Crohn's disease, and the administration of corticosteroids may cause significant worsening and toxic megacolon. Stool examination for ova and parasites is generally diagnostic, but sigmoidoscopy may be required. Serologic testing is useful to exclude amebiasis in individuals from industrialized countries because the background antibody positivity is quite low. Extraintestinal amebiasis generally exhibits as hepatic liver abscess (see Chapter 101).

PROTOZOAL INFECTIONS COMMON IN TRAVELERS AND IMMIGRANTS

Leishmaniasis

Cutaneous and mucocutaneous leishmaniasis (see Table 109–1) should be considered in any traveler returning from the Middle East or endemic areas of Latin America who has a persistent skin or mucous membrane lesion. Diagnosis is made by tissue biopsy. Visceral leishmaniasis should be anticipated in immigrants with fever and splenomegaly. Diagnosis is made by bone marrow biopsy and culture. Cutaneous leishmaniasis is generally self limited. Other types are treated with sodium stibogluconate (Pentostam), 20 mg/kg/day for up to 20 days.

African Trypanosomiasis

African trypanosomiasis is a protozoal infection, endemic in Africa, that causes sleeping sickness. Rarely imported into developed countries, it should be presumed in systemically ill patients from Africa who exhibit fever, headache, and confusion (see Table 109–1). Many patients will remember a painful chancre at the site of an insect bite (**Web Fig. 109–2**). Diagnosis is made by direct examination of the blood, lymph aspirate, or cerebrospinal fluid (**Web Fig. 109–3; Web Fig. 109–4**). Treatment should be supervised by an expert in the field.

Chagas' Disease (American Trypanosomiasis)

Trypanosoma cruzi is the most common cause of heart failure in Brazil. Transmission is through contact with feces from infected reduviid bugs (kissing bugs) (**Web Fig. 109–5**), and cases of transfusion-associated *T. cruzi* infection have been recognized in the United States (see Table 109–1). Most patients are asymptomatic for decades and then exhibit as cardiomegaly, megaesophagus, or megacolon. Diagnosis of acute disease is made by direct examination of the blood (**Web Fig. 109–6**). Early diagnosis is critical because patients may respond to nitrofuran or nitroimidazole derivatives. Treatment of chronic Chagas' disease is largely supportive.

HELMINTHIC INFECTIONS COMMON IN THE UNITED STATES

Pinworm

Enterobiasis is common in the United States (Table 109–2), particularly among children. Perianal pruritus is the major clinical presentation. Infection is maintained by fecal-oral contamination. Diagnosis is made by the application of cellophane tape to the anus and subsequent microscopic examination for ova. Treatment is with mebendazole, 100 mg given once. In heavy or recurrent infection, treating all family members is advisable.

Other Intestinal Nematodes

Ascaris (giant roundworm), *Ancylostoma duodenale* and *Necator americanus* (hookworm), and *Trichuris* (whipworms), still endemic in the United States, are extremely common in immigrants and are ubiquitous in the developing world (see Table 109–2). Most individuals are asymptomatic. Ascariasis and hookworm may cause transient pulmonary infiltrates with eosinophilia during the tissue

Table 109–2	**Helminthic Infections**			
Helminth	**Setting**	**Vectors**	**Diagnosis**	**Treatment**
Endemic in the United States				
Pinworm (enterobiasis)	Ubiquitous	Human	Direct examination for ova	Mebendazole, albendazole
Ascaris lumbricoides	Southeast	Human	Stool examination for ova	Mebendazole, albendazole
Trichuris trichiura	Southeast	Human	Stool examination for ova	Mebendazole, albendazole
Hookworm	Southeast	Human	Stool examination for ova	Mebendazole, albendazole
Common in Travelers and Immigrants				
Strongyloides stercoralis	Developing world	Human	Stool examination for larvae	Thiabendazole, ivermectin
Schistosoma sp.	Developing world	Snails	Stool examination for ova	Praziquantel
Wuchereria sp.	Asia	Mosquitoes	Nocturnal blood examination	Ivermectin
Onchocerca volvulus	Africa, South and Central Americas	Black fly	Biopsy	Ivermectin
Loa Loa	Africa	Mosquitoes	Blood examination, clinical setting	Ivermectin

migratory phase of infection. Heavy *Ascaris* infection may cause intestinal, biliary, or pancreatic obstruction. Hookworm infection can be associated with iron deficiency. Diagnosis is made based on stool examination for ova and parasites (**Web Fig. 109–7; Web Fig. 109–8**). Each of these worms can be eradicated with appropriate anthelmintic therapy such as mebendazole, 100 mg orally twice daily for 3 days.

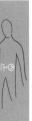

HELMINTH INFECTIONS COMMON IN TRAVELERS AND IMMIGRANTS

Strongyloidosis

Strongyloides stercoralis is a common cause of eosinophilia in returning long-term travelers and immigrants, particularly those from Southeast Asia (see Table 109–2). Infection can persist for years; many men who served in the Pacific theater during World War II or in Vietnam still harbor infections. *Strongyloides stercoralis* is unique in its ability to complete its life cycle in the host and produce persistent infection. Although usually asymptomatic, infection can cause diarrhea, abdominal pain, and malabsorption. This helminth can cause life-threatening disseminated infection in individuals who are immunosuppressed by cancer chemotherapy, corticosteroids, or HIV infection. Diagnosis may be made by stool examination (**Web Fig. 109–9**), but this is not a very sensitive technique. Treatment with thiabendazole, 25 mg/kg (maximum 3 g/day) orally twice daily for 2 days, is curative in more than 90% of immunocompetent hosts. Ivermectin (200 mcg/kg/day) may be more effective than thiabendazole and is preferred in immunocompromised hosts.

Schistosomiasis

Schistosoma mansoni (Africa, South America, and the Caribbean), *S. japonicum* (Philippines, China, and Indonesia), and *S. mekongi* (Cambodia, Laos, and Vietnam) are the most common causes of hepatosplenic enlargement in the world (see Table 109–2). Chronic infection can lead to periportal hepatic fibrosis, obstruction of portal blood flow, and bleeding esophageal varices. Patients in the United States are often misdiagnosed as having hepatitis B or alcohol-induced liver disease. A clue to the correct diagnosis is that the liver is enlarged, in contrast to the small, shrunken liver of alcoholic cirrhosis. *Schistosoma haematobium* (Africa) commonly causes hematuria and leads to urinary obstruction. Diagnosis is made by examination of stool or urine for ova and parasites. Praziquantel is the drug of choice.

Lymphatic Filariasis

Wuchereria bancrofti and *Brugia malayi* cause elephantiasis throughout the tropics (see Table 109–2). Patients may exhibit acute lymphadenitis or asymptomatic eosinophilia. Some patients have pulmonary symptoms, infiltrates, and marked eosinophilia (tropical pulmonary eosinophilia). The diagnosis is made by finding microfilariae in blood specimens obtained at midnight. Treatment currently consists of a single oral dose of ivermectin, 100 to 400 mcg/kg.

Loa Loa

Eyeworm is endemic in West and Central Africa (see Table 109–2). Patients exhibit transient pruritic subcutaneous swellings. Eosinophilia is universal. In the United States, patients are often misdiagnosed for years as having chronic urticaria. In rare instances, the adult worm can be visualized as it crosses the anterior chamber of the patient's eye, giving this worm its common name. Diagnosis is generally suggested on clinical grounds and is confirmed by biopsy. Loasis can be treated with diethylcarbamazine.

River Blindness

Infection from *Onchocerca volvulus* occurs in West and Central Africa, as well as in South and Central America (see Table 109–2). Although the most severe manifestations occur in the eye, the most common clinical presentation in the United States is recurrent pruritic dermatitis. The diagnosis can be made by direct examination of skin snips for microfilariae; a specific serologic test is also available. Ivermectin, 150 mcg/kg orally for one dose, is the treatment of choice. Ivermectin should be repeated after 6 months to suppress cutaneous and ocular microfilariae.

Clonorchiasis

The Chinese liver fluke, *Clonorchis sinensis,* is important to diagnose in Asian immigrants. Symptoms may be confused with those of biliary tract disease. If untreated, infection can lead to cholangiocarcinoma. Praziquantel is curative.

Cysticercosis

The invasive larval form of pork tapeworm (*Taenia solium*) is the most common cause of seizures throughout the world, as well as in young adults in Los Angeles, chiefly among immigrants from Mexico. Typically, patients exhibit new onset of seizures or severe headache. A single ring-enhancing lesion is the characteristic finding on computed tomographic scan. The diagnosis may be confirmed by an immunoblot assay using peripheral blood. Praziquantel (50 mg/kg/day in three divided doses for 15 days) or albendazole (for 30 days, dosed by weight: >60 kg, 400 mg orally twice daily; <60 kg, 15 mg/kg/day in divided doses twice daily) is curative but may precipitate focal cerebral edema and seizures by killing other cysticercariae within the central nervous system. An expert should be consulted before treatment.

Intestinal Tapeworms

Three intestinal tapeworms commonly infect humans: *Taenia saginata* from raw beef, *Taenia solium* from raw pork, and *Diphyllobothrium latum* from raw fish. Most individuals are asymptomatic, but *T. solium* can cause invasive disease (cysticercosis) if humans ingest ova of the adult worm. *Diphyllobothrium latum* is associated with vitamin B_{12} deficiency. All three infections are treated with praziquantel.

Hydatid Disease

Hydatid disease commonly produces a cystic liver mass in emigrants from sheep-raising parts of the world. Early diagnosis is important because rupture of the cyst can lead to dissemination. Diagnosis is often suggested from the appearance of the cyst (calcified wall and dependent hydatid *sand*) on abdominal computed tomographic scan. Serologic testing can be helpful but is occasionally negative if the cyst has not leaked. Currently, primary therapy is the surgical removal of the cyst without spillage of its contents.

Prospectus for the Future

- Treatment guidelines for malaria will continue to evolve in response to patterns of drug resistance.
- Increased international cooperative efforts, coupled with promising basic research advances, suggest that an effective malaria vaccine may become available over the next decade.
- Significant drug resistance in helminths has not been seen, but surveillance for the development of resistance is gaining support.

- Antimicrobial resistance among enteric pathogens may complicate the management of travelers' diarrhea.
- Changing patterns of established infections and new and emerging pathogens will continue to challenge travelers and health care providers.

References

Arguin PM, Navin AW; Centers for Disease Control and Prevention: Health Information for International Travel 2005–2006. Washington, DC: Department of Health and Human Services, 2005 (available at: *http://www.cdc.gov/travel/yb/*).

Greenwood BM, Bojang K, Whitty CJ, et al: Malaria. Lancet 365(9469): 1487–1498, 2005.

Newman RD, Parise ME, Barber AM, et al: Malaria-related deaths among U.S. Travelers, 1963–2001. Ann Int Med 141(7):547–558, 2004.

Pearson RD: Advice to travelers. In Goldman L, Ausiello D (eds): Cecil Textbook of Medicine, 22nd ed. Philadelphia, Saunders, 2004, pp 1749–1752.

Section XVII

Bioterrorism

Bioterrorism

Robert W. Bradsher, Jr.

Introduction

Bioterrorism returned to the consciousness of physicians in the days after the attack on the World Trade Center and Pentagon on September 11, 2001. Before a month had passed, the first case of inhalational anthrax in more than 50 years was diagnosed in the United States when a man was hospitalized and rapidly died in Florida. Soon thereafter, cases of cutaneous and inhalational anthrax were reported in New York; Washington, D.C.; New Jersey; Virginia; and Connecticut. The nation's attention was galvanized on the topics of anthrax, the U.S. Postal Service, gas masks, and antibiotic stockpiling, as well as with other bioterrorism concerns. Since then, bioterrorism has been a major topic of medical concern. The need to review bioterrorism is obvious; health professionals are unfamiliar with disease manifestations from these biologic agents used as weapons because they no longer occur or occur only rarely in nature. Those health care professionals on the frontline will likely be emergency department personnel, primary care physicians, pediatricians, and nurse practitioners rather than experts from the Centers for Disease Control and Prevention (CDC) or even traditional first responders, public health officers, or military officials. The purpose of this chapter is to highlight the recognition of these weapons that are designed for use in terrorism.

Definition and Categorization

Bioterrorism is the intentional use of biologic agents to cause disease in humans or animals to provoke terror. The agents can cause disease either by specific infection or by action of a toxin produced by micro-organisms. Depending on the microbe or toxin, resulting disease may or may not be contagious. The CDC has categorized bioterrorism agents into three categories (Table 110–1).

Category A includes agents that can be easily transmitted to humans and that can cause substantial mortality and morbidity. These agents have been most strongly considered as bioweapons and would lead to panic and social disruption. Category A agents have been the major focus for public health officials in preparation for bioterrorism episodes. These agents include anthrax, botulism, plague, smallpox, tularemia, and viral hemorrhagic fevers.

Category B agents (see Table 110–1) are moderately easy to transmit with moderate morbidity and mortality. These agents are not well known, and the CDC considers that increased awareness and surveillance are required. In addition, agents associated with water safety threats and food safety threats are included in Category B.

Category C agents include emerging pathogens that could be engineered because of their availability and potential for having a major health impact.

Chemical weapons (see Table 110–1) are divided by the CDC into biotoxins, vesicants, blood agents, caustics, long-acting anticoagulants, metals, organic solvents, toxic alcohols, choking or pulmonary agents, and nerve agents, as well as vomiting, riot control, and incapacitating agents. Finally, the CDC website for bioterrorism provides links to radiation emergencies. This listing of potential biologic, chemical, and radiation weapons is likely to change substantially. Websites from federal agencies or universities will be the most likely sources for up-to-date information in the event of terrorist attacks, rather than textbooks or journal articles (Table 110–2 and **Web Table 110–1**).

History

Biologic weapons are part of the history of warfare. The Roman army is said by historians to have poisoned the wells

Table 110–1 **Biological and Chemical Weapons**

Biological Weapons

Category A	Category B	Category C
Anthrax (*Bacillus antracis*)	Brucellosis (*Brucella* spp.)	Nipah virus
Botulism (*Clostridium botulinum* toxin)	Epsilon toxin—*Clostridium perfringens*	Hantavirus
Plague (*Yersinia pestis*)	Glanders (*Burkholderia mallei*)	
Smallpox (variola major)	Melioidosis (*Burkholderia pseudomallei*)	
Tularemia (*Francisella tularensis*)	Psittacosis (*Chlamydia psittaci*)	
Viral hemorrhagic fevers (Ebola, Marburg, Lassa, Machupo)	Q fever (*Coxiella burnetii*)	
	Ricin toxin—castor beans	
	Enterotoxin B—*Staphylococcus aureus*	
	Typhus fever (*Rickettsia prowazelii*)	
	Viral encephalitis (Venezuelan equine, Eastern equine, Western equine)	
	Water safety—*Virbrio cholerae, Cryptosporidium parvum*	
	Food safety—*Salmonella, Escherichia coli* 0157:H7, *Shigella*	

Chemical Weapons

Vesicants	Blood and Pulmonary Agents	Nerve Agents	Other
Distilled mustard	Arsenic	G–	Vomiting agent
Nitrogen mustard	Cyanide	Sarin	Riot-control agent
Lewisite	Nitrogen oxide	Soman	
Phosgene oxime	Chlorine	Tabun	Incapacitating agent
Ethyldichloroarsine	Phosgene	GF	
Methyldichloroarsine	Diphosgene	GE	Benzene
Diphosgene	Perflurorisobutylene	V–	Super warfarin
Phenodichloroarsine	Red phosphorous	VX	Arsenic, barium, mercury, thallium
Sesqui mustard	Sulfur trioxide-chlorosulfonic acid	VM	
	Titanium tetrachloride	VE	
		VG	
		V-gas	

Modified from the Centers for Disease Control and Prevention (CDC) website: *www.bt.cdc.gov/Agent/Agentlist.asp*

of their enemies to shorten their military campaigns. The Tartar's siege of Kaffa in the Crimea in the Middle Ages included the use of cadavers who had died from plague being tossed over the walls of the city, presumably along with fleas that were the source of transmission of *Yersinia pestis*. In the twentieth century, German and Japanese troops investigated the distribution of biologic weapons before and during World Wars I and II. The United States began investigating biologic warfare at Fort Dietrich in 1942 and later at the Pine Bluff, Arkansas, arsenal before President Nixon ended all offensive efforts in biologic warfare in 1969 (micro-organisms) and 1970 (toxins). After the termination of these investigative programs, the U.S. Army Medical Research Institute of Infectious Diseases (USAMRIID) was started to conduct research for medical defense against biologic weapons.

The former Soviet Union had multiple sites for the production of biologic weapons. Even after signing the 1972 treaty on prohibition of biologic weapon development, 55,000 employees in six separate sites were reported to be working on bioweapons under the name *Biopreparate*. An unintentional release of a relatively minute number of spores at the Sverdlovsk bioweapon production site caused anthrax to infect humans and animals over a 2-month period with an estimated 100 deaths resulting in as many as 250 individuals. Iraq is one of a number of nations considered to have a modern biologic warfare program. Between 1985 and the end of Operation Desert Storm of the Persian Gulf War, Iraq developed anthrax, botulinum toxin, and aflatoxin for warfare use. In 1990, 200 bombs were produced with one half containing botulinum toxin and one fourth containing anthrax. The more recent war in Iraq was started, in large part, because of the concern regarding the existence of weapons of mass destruction including bioweapons, although none were identified.

These biologic agents are clearly weapons of mass destruction. It has been estimated that 100 kg of anthrax would lead to the death of up to 3 million individuals if released near a major metropolitan area. Evans and associ-

Table 110–2 Websites Related to Biological, Chemical, and Radiologic Weapons

1. *www.bt.cdc.gov/* the Centers for Disease Control and Prevention's (CDC's) Bioterrorism Preparedness and Response Network
2. *www.umn.edu/cidrap/* University of Minnesota through the Center for Infectious Disease Research and Policy (CIDRAP)
3. *bioterrorism.slu.edu/* Study of Bioterrorism and Emerging Infections; St. Louis University, School of Public Health
4. *www.usamriid.army.mil/* U.S. Army Medical Research Institute of Infectious Diseases Fort Detrick, Maryland
5. *www.whitehouse.gov/homeland/* Department of Homeland Security
6. *www.cbiac.apgea.army.mil/* Chemical and Biological Defense Information Analysis Center (CBIAC)
7. *www.state.gov/s/ct/* Interagency Working Group on Counterterrorism and the State Department's terrorism task forces
8. *www.idsociety.org/BT/ToC.htm* Collaboration between Infectious Diseases Society of America and the CIDRAP
9. *www.acponline.org/bioterro/* American College of Physicians/American Society of Internal Medicine (ACP/ASIM)
10. *www.stimson.org* Henry L. Stimson Center, an independent, nonprofit, public policy institute on security issues
11. *www.emergency.com/cntrterr.htm* "Counter-Terrorism Archive," Emergency Response and Research Institute (ERRI)
12. *telemedicine.org/BioWar/biologic.htm* Document to dispel mystery: History and origins of biological weapons
13. *www.nbc-med.org/SiteContent/HomePage/WhatsNew/MedAspects/contents.htm* Surgeon General is office
14. *www.foodsafety.gov/~fsg/bioterr.html* Food safety information from the United States Department of Agriculture (USDA), the CDC, and the Canadian Food Inspection Agency
15. *www.who.int/pcs/en* International Programme on Chemical Safety (IPCS)
16. *www.bt.cdc.gov/Radiological.asp* Information from the Radiation Emergency Assistance Center
17. *www.who.int/peh/Radiation/radaccidents.htm* World Health Organization (WHO) coordinates response to weapons of mass destruction (WMD) incidents

ates estimate that 62,000 individuals would be killed with the release of 5 pounds of anthrax powder in St. Louis. This amount compares with the 2 to 3 g of powder estimated to be used in terrorist mailings in 2001. Further, it has been suggested that the release of 100 kg of anthrax spores would cause a comparable number of deaths as would a hydrogen bomb. However, the agents have also been dubbed "weapons of mass disruption." To illustrate this fact, in October through November of 2001 when anthrax was delivered through the U.S. Postal Service, only 22 confirmed or probable cases of infection were discovered, but the nation was almost paralyzed by the event. Holloway and colleagues have reported that the idea of infection caused by invisible agents is particularly frightening. Feelings of horror, anger, panic, magical thinking about microbes, fear of contagion, scapegoating and xenophobia, paranoia, social isolation, helplessness, and demoralization are considered to be results of terrorist acts such as the discovery of bioterrorism agents.

Biologic Agents

ANTHRAX

These bacteria, named for the appearance of the black eschar of the cutaneous lesions (Gr: *anthrakos:* coal), are primarily diseases of grazing animals. The organism exists in a spore form in soil as the reservoir. Humans become infected after contact either with soil or animal material infected with the organisms. The cutaneous form is the most common with approximately 95% of cases of anthrax. After 1 to 7 days of incubation, a small papule develops into an ulcer. Edema and erythema surround the ulcer, which develops a blackened eschar that will dry and fall off within 1 to 2 weeks (see **Web Table 110–1**: links 1, 3, 8, 9 for clinical photographs). This form is not as highly lethal as are other forms; response to antimicrobials is prompt. Gastrointestinal anthrax is very rare and follows the ingestion of contaminated meat. Progression to toxemia is thought to be common with a high mortality rate. Inhalation anthrax follows respiratory inhalation of spores, although the incubation period may be significantly longer (up to 60 days) than the cutaneous form. Symptoms include fever, malaise, myalgia, substernal pressure, and discomfort with progression over days to high fever, dyspnea, cyanosis, progressive shock, and death. Hemorrhagic meningitis develops in this stage in approximately one half of patients. Hemorrhagic mediastinitis and pleural effusion are also common in this stage (see **Web Table 110–1**: links 1, 3, 8, 9 for clinical photographs).

The pathogenesis of anthrax involves ingestion of spores by macrophages, followed by sporulation to vegetative organisms in lymph nodes, which drains the initial site of infection. Toxins known as lethal toxin and edema factor lead to the death. This toxin mediation of the disease explains why the mortality is high despite effective antimicrobial therapy.

Penicillin used to be the treatment of choice of anthrax infection; however, because of the production of β-lactamase by the organisms, either doxycycline or a quinolone (ciprofloxacin) is now considered as the first-line treatment. The earlier the treatment is started, the more likely a response to the antimicrobial therapy will occur because the late manifestations are due to toxin rather than replication of the organism. Either ciprofloxacin or doxycycline for a total of 60 days has been used as postexposure prophylaxis.

The only human vaccine for anthrax is the supernatant from culture of an attenuated strain and is not available for the general population. The U.S. military uses the vaccine for troops; however, some controversy has developed regarding the safety and efficacy of this immunization. It appears to protect against cutaneous disease and possibly inhalational anthrax. A very effective animal vaccine program is used in agricultural settings.

SMALLPOX

The smallpox virus is one of the most feared organisms that could be considered as a biologic weapon because of its 30% mortality rate (with a range toward 100% with certain forms of the disease) and because of it ability to spread person to person with a multiplier effect of 10 to 20. Another reason for the fear of smallpox relates to one of the greatest successes of the twentieth century. The organism was eliminated in the 1970s from natural infection after a worldwide public health vaccination effort. The elimination effort was successful because smallpox has a single, stable serotype, and only human hosts were infected (no animal reservoir). Other factors included the observation that prompt antibody response occurred with vaccination; even exposed individuals were protected if vaccinated early. The disease was easily recognized clinically, which enabled exposed persons to be immunized promptly, and no carrier or subclinical state was observed with smallpox. However, diagnosis of a patient may very likely be missed because smallpox has not been seen anywhere in the world since 1978. In the last decade shortages of smallpox vaccine were reported; since the events of 2001, however, an adequate vaccine supply is available.

The virus of variola major and variola minor causes smallpox, named in the fifteenth century to differentiate it from the Great Pox, or syphilis. After an incubation of approximately 2 weeks, smallpox has a prodrome of fever, nausea, headache, and backache, followed by a transient erythematous rash. The typical exanthem then occurs, beginning on the head and upper extremities and spreading to the trunk and lower extremities. The number of lesions on the head and extremities remain greater than those on the trunk for the duration of the rash (see **Web Table 110–1**: links 1, 3, 8, 9 for clinical photographs). The lesions begin as macules, which develop into vesicles and then pustules. The pustules dry and shrink in approximately 12 days with a hard crust or scab that then falls off, leaving a sunken scar. The variants of flat smallpox and hemorrhagic smallpox do not have the typical appearance and have a mortality rate approaching 100%. Except for the lesions on the skin and mucous membranes, other organs are not thought to be involved. Secondary bacterial infection is uncommon. Toxemia from the virus is considered to be the most likely cause of death. Complications include encephalitis and blindness from panophthalmitis and keratitis. Cough is not particularly prominent, but it is considered a key element in the transmission of the virus to others.

The differential diagnosis for smallpox includes a number of illnesses with rash. However, the most likely illness to be confused with smallpox is the primary varicella zoster viral infection (chickenpox), which produces crops of lesions, resulting in various stages of papule, vesicle, and pustule that can be observed at the same time in different areas of the body. In addition, chickenpox is more likely to be concentrated on the trunk than it is on the face and extremities as is smallpox.

Smallpox is spread by respiratory droplet nuclei or contaminated clothing or bedding material and is not transmitted during the incubation period but only during the initial fever and through the first week of the rash illness. Cough may transmit the virus in a widespread area. An example reviewed by Henderson is a patient admitted to a first floor hospital room with subsequent transmission to individuals located on the third floor of the building.

Treatment of patients with smallpox centers on preventing transmission with respiratory isolation and possibly instituting quarantine in the setting of a large epidemic. Studies are underway to examine antiviral agents. Cidofovir is licensed for cytomegalovirus and has activity for smallpox; some benefit has been recognized in animals with monkeypox and vaccinia infection, but obviously no trials have been performed.

Prevention of infection with smallpox has been accomplished with vaccinia vaccination. The cutaneous inoculation of this modified virus (cowpox) leads to local infection (Fig. 110–1A, B) with immunity, which should persist for at least a decade or longer. Even when given during the early incubation period, the vaccine can attenuate or abolish the manifestations of smallpox. The National Vaccination Program for the Smallpox Response Plan was ordered in December 2002; a total of 38,440 vaccinations were administered to civilian health care workers and first responders, and the number of adverse events was smaller than

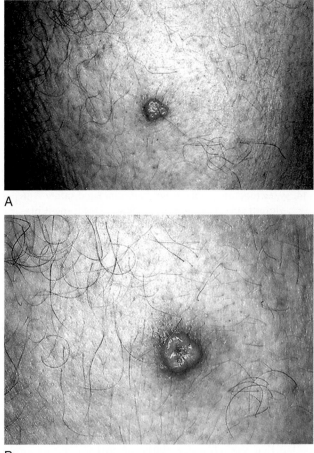

A

B

Figure 110–1 *A,* Vaccinia vaccination day 3. *B,* Vaccinia vaccination day 7.

predicted. The complications of vaccine that occurred included skin lesions that range from accidental vaccination to generalized vaccinia to eczema vaccinatum. These complications included 29 reports of generalized vaccinia, 3 patients with potential eczema vaccinatum, and 7 individuals with potential progressive vaccinia. The voluntary vaccination program was placed on hold after 21 cases of potential myocarditis or pericarditis were identified (see **Web Table 110–1**: link 1 for further discussion). Vaccinia immune globulin (VIG) can modify or ameliorate the complications. Pregnant women, those with eczema, and individuals who are immunosuppressed should not receive vaccinia vaccination.

PLAGUE

Yersinia pestis is the cause of plague, which occurs at a rate of 10 to 12 patients per year in the United States, predominately in the western states. This organism was used by Japan in bioterrorism attempts in the 1940s but with infected fleas rather than airborne distribution. The infection either occurs as the bubonic form or septicemic form usually with pneumonia; unlike anthrax, this organism can be spread from person to person with the pneumonic form. The incubation period is from 2 to 8 days after inoculation, followed by the sudden onset of high fever, chills, generalized weakness, and tender regional lymphadenitis, known as *buboes.* Inguinal, axillary, or cervical lymphadenopathy is most commonly found (see **Web Table 110–1**: links 1, 3, 8, 9 for clinical photographs). With late-stage disease, purpuric lesions develop and may be the source of the name *black plague* in the Middle Ages. The septicemic form can either follow cutaneous disease in a secondary manner or pneumonic infection as a primary disease. The systemic inflammatory response syndrome follows the severe endotoxemia with subsequent multiorgan dysfunction syndromes exhibited as acute respiratory distress syndrome (ARDS), disseminated intravascular coagulation (DIC), shock, and death. The pneumonic form has sudden onset with headache, malaise, fever, myalgia, and prominent cough, and the pneumonia progresses rapidly with pronounced dyspnea, cyanosis, and hemoptysis. Death results either from respiratory collapse or sepsis. Because secondary transmission is possible and likely, contact and droplet isolation precautions should be maintained for at least 48 hours after sputum cultures are negative or pneumonic plague is excluded. Antibiotic therapy with a quinolone, aminoglycoside, or doxycycline is warranted as is supportive therapy. Prophylaxis with ciprofloxacin, doxycycline, or trimethoprim-sulfamethoxazole is used in contacts of patients with pneumonic plague. In the event of a bioterrorism event, federal authorities will give recommendations regarding the definition of the exposure that should prompt prophylaxis.

BOTULINUM TOXIN

Botulism is caused by toxin from *Clostridium botulinum,* which is a ubiquitous micro-organism found in soil. The toxin types A, B, and E are most commonly associated with human disease of which about 100 cases per year are reported in the United States. This toxin is the most potent lethal substance known to man with a lethal dose of 1 ng/kg.

No person-to-person transmission is observed with this toxin.

The clinical manifestations of botulism occur after an incubation of 18 to 36 hours in a dose-dependent fashion. The patient will be afebrile, alert, and oriented with a normal sensory examination, and the hallmark symptoms of the disease are cranial nerve abnormalities, such as ptosis, blurry or double vision, difficulty swallowing or talking, and decreased salivation. Progressive motor symptoms then develop with bilateral descending flaccid paralysis and resultant respiratory paralysis (see **Web Table 110–1**: link 1 for clinical photographs). Death rates of 60% are documented in untreated patients, whereas fewer than 5% of patients who are treated will die.

The treatment of botulism includes ventilatory assistance and supportive care. Botulinum antitoxin with the trivalent equine product against types A, B, and E, currently available only from the CDC, is recommended. It is most effective if administered early in the course of the illness. Antibiotic therapy with penicillin is used for infant and wound botulism. The recovery period may be prolonged with supportive care, including mechanical ventilation, necessary for weeks to months. After antitoxin, no new nerve endings are affected, but recovery is dependent on the generation of new motor end plates at the neuromuscular junction. Vaccine for botulism is only investigational and not available for clinical use.

VIRAL HEMORRHAGIC FEVERS

A number of viruses cause hemorrhagic fever. These include several different viral families of *Filoviruses* (Ebola, Marburg), *Arenaviruses* (Lassa, Junin, Machupo, Sabia, Guanarito), *Bunyaviruses* (Rift Valley fever), and *Flaviviruses* (yellow fever). Each of these has virus-dependent natural vectors of rodents, mosquitoes, or ticks. These viruses have no natural occurrence in the United States; consequently, identification of a patient with this illness will likely be a bioterrorism event.

The findings of viral hemorrhagic fevers include symptoms of fever, headache, malaise, dizziness, myalgias, nausea, and vomiting. Initial signs of infection would be flushing, conjunctival injection, and periorbital edema. A positive tourniquet test with petechiae is an indication of the bleeding propensity. Hypotension from blood loss and intra-abdominal hemorrhage is a marker of the end stages of this infection. Progressive disease is also indicated by prostration, pharyngeal, chest, or abdominal pain discomfort, mucous membrane bleeding, and skin ecchymosis. Shock and multiorgan dysfunction follow. Usually the patient is either improving or moribund within a week. Clinical bleeding, central nervous system involvement, and significant elevation of hepatic enzymes are indicators of a poor prognosis. The mortality rate is dependent on the infectious agent and ranges from 10% to 90%.

The viruses that cause hemorrhagic fevers are thought to be spread by contact with infected body fluids and not by aerosol or droplet transmission. Therefore, standard infection control procedures will prevent the spread of infection to others. The patient should be in a private room with an adjoining anteroom, if available. Particular attention should be placed to strict adherence to hand washing, using an adequate facility with decontamination solution such as

Betadine-containing or other hand-washing agents. Negative air pressure rooms should be used, although aerosol transmission is not believed to occur. Strict barrier precautions including protective eyewear and a face shield should be followed. Disposable equipment should be used with "sharps" being disposed of in rigid containers with disinfectant stored inside and then autoclaved or incinerated. All body fluids should be disinfected because they are believed to be responsible for transmission.

Chemical Agents and Radiation

Chemical weapons are primarily either vesicants similar to nitrogen mustard or nerve agents, although terrorists could use vomiting agents and incapacitating agents such as mace as weapons. As would be expected, a substantial number of individuals would simultaneously exhibit the same symptoms and likely be from the same location. Individuals exposed to chemical warfare would exhibit ocular findings, upper airway symptoms such as rhinorrhea or wheezing or dyspnea, skin complaints of itching to necrosis, and central nervous system findings from headache to confusion to seizures (see **Web Table 110–1**: links 1, 6, 15 for further discussion).

Illness caused by radiation exposure would initially exhibit as acute radiation sickness. The severity and timing of the symptoms would depend on the dose of radiation. Bone marrow, gastrointestinal, vascular, neurologic, or cutaneous manifestations would be found, once again depending on the source and total dose. Suppression of blood elements might result in infection and sepsis. Gastrointestinal injury would result in diarrhea, gastrointestinal hemorrhage, and electrolyte abnormalities. Nervous system radiation might lead to ataxia, central nausea, or seizures. Other effects of blindness, pneumonitis, and cutaneous burns would be observed with acute radiation injury (see **Web Table 110–1**: links 1, 16, 17 for further discussion).

The major difference in chemical weapons or intentional radiation injury from "dirty" bombs and biologic weapons is in the incubation time required for the latter. Illness cause by biologic warfare would not be seen until days to weeks after the release of the weapon. In contrast, chemical weapons would likely cause symptoms within minutes to hours in individuals located near the weapon and would likely be recognized by the traditional first responders. Likewise, radiation from a nuclear device would be immediately obvious. The CDC and other links from that website provide recognition and treatments for these conditions.

Prospectus for the Future

- Development of rapid detection systems for environmental monitoring for biologic, chemical, and radiologic weapons
- Development of newer vaccines and consideration of vaccine strategies to prevent bioterrorism outbreaks
- Construction of local, state, and federal plans to control and manage bioterrorism events
- Upgrading of the local, state, and federal public health infrastructures
- Re-education of physicians in practice and in training regarding infectious diseases that are extremely rare or no longer occur but which might be used as biologic weapons

References

General

Bartlett JG, Inglesby TV Jr, Borio L: Management of anthrax. Clin Infect Dis 35:851–858, 2002.

Christopher GW, Cieslak TJ, Pavlin JA, et al: Biologic warfare: A historical perspective. JAMA 298:412–417, 1997.

Evans RG, Crutcher JM, Shadel B, et al: Terrorism from a public health perspective. Am J Med Sci 323:291–298, 2002.

Greenfield RA, Brown BR, Hutchins JB, et al: Microbiological, biological, and chemical weapons of warfare and terrorism. Am J Med Sci 323:326–340, 2002.

Hogan DE, Kellison T: Nuclear terrorism. Am J Med Sci 323:341–349, 2002.

Holloway HC, Norwood AE, Fullerton CS, et al: The threat of biological weapons: Prophylaxis and mitigation of psychological and social consequences. JAMA 278:425–427, 1997.

Vellozzi C, Lane JM, Averhoff G, et al: Generalized vaccinia, progressive vaccinia, and eczema vaccinatum are rare following smallpox (vaccinia) vaccination: United States surveillance, 2003. Clin Infect Dis 41:689–697, 2005.

Anthrax

Bush LM, Abrams BH, Beall A, et al: Index case of fatal inhalational anthrax due to bioterrorism in the United States. N Engl J Med 345:1607–1610, 2001.

Jernigan JA, Stephens DS, Ashford DA, et al: Bioterrorism related inhalational anthrax: The first 10 cases reported in the United States. Emerg Infect Dis 7:933–944, 2001.

Swartz MN: Recognition and management of anthrax. N Engl J Med 345:1621–1626, 2001.

Smallpox

Breman JG, Henderson DA: Current concepts: Diagnosis and management of smallpox. N Engl J Med 346:1300–1308, 2002.

Frey SE, Couch RB, Tacket CO, et al: Clinical responses to undiluted and diluted smallpox vaccine. N Engl J Med 346:1265–1274, 2002.

Henderson DA: Bioterrorism as a public health threat. Emerg Infect Dis 4:488–492, 1998.

Consensus Papers on Bioterrorism Agents

Arnon SS, Schechter R, Inglesby TV, et al: Botulinum toxin as a biological weapon: Medical and public health management. JAMA 285:1059–1070, 2001.

Borio L, Inglesby T, Peters CJ, et al: Hemorrhagic fever viruses as biological weapons: Medical and public health management. JAMA 287:2391–2405, 2002.

Dennis DT, Inglesby TV, Henderson DA, et al: Tularemia as a biological weapon: Medical and public health management. JAMA 285:2763–2773, 2001.

Henderson DA, Inglesby TV, Bartlett JG, et al: Smallpox as a biological weapon: Medical and public health management. JAMA 281:2127–2137, 1999.

Inglesby TV, Dennis DT, Henderson DA, et al: Plague as a biological weapon: Medical and public health management. JAMA 283:2281–2290, 2000.

Inglesby TV, O'Toole T, Henderson DA, et al: Anthrax as a biological weapon. 2002. JAMA 287:2236–2252, 2002.

Andreoli and Carpenter's

cecil Essentials of Medicine

Neurologic Evaluation of the Patient

Frederick J. Marshall

To arrive at an accurate neurologic diagnosis, the clinician must generate and test hypotheses about both the location and the mechanism of injury to the nervous system. Hypotheses are refined as the clinician progresses from the interview to the physical examination to the laboratory assessment of the patient. The focus is first placed on those entities that are common, serious, and treatable. Typical presentations of common diseases account for 80% of all cases, unusual presentations of common diseases account for 15%, typical presentations of rare diseases account for 5%, and unusual presentations of rare diseases account for less than 1%.

Taking a Neurologic History

The clinician must determine the location, quality, and timing of symptoms. He or she must avoid hearsay and ask the patient to report the progression of actual symptoms rather than a litany of diagnostic procedures and specialty evaluations. Establishing when the patient last felt perfectly normal is important. Ambiguous descriptors such as *dizzy* should be rejected in favor of evocative descriptors such as *light-headed* (which might implicate cardiovascular insufficiency) or *off balance* (which might implicate cerebellar or posterior column dysfunction).

Family members and other witnesses must corroborate historical information when appropriate. Historical information should include the medical and surgical histories; current medications; allergies; family history; review of systems; and social history, including the patient's level of education, work history, possible toxin exposures, substance use, sexual history, and current life circumstance.

Clues to localization are sought during the interview. For example, pain is generally due to a lesion of the peripheral nervous system, whereas aphasia (disordered language processing) indicates an abnormality of the central nervous system. Because sensory and motor functions are anatomically relatively distant in the cerebral cortex but progressively closer together as fibers converge in the brainstem, spinal cord, roots, and peripheral nerves, the co-existence of sensory loss and motor dysfunction in a limb implies either a large lesion at the level of the cortex or a smaller lesion lower down in the neuraxis. Small lesions in areas of *high traffic* such as the spinal cord or brainstem can result in widespread neurologic dysfunction, whereas small lesions elsewhere may be asymptomatic.

Table 111–1 lists the potential localizing values of common neurologic symptoms to help settle the issue of lesion localization. Tables 111–2 and 111–3 list symptoms that are commonly associated with lesions at specific locations in the nervous system. Some symptoms can result from a lesion at any of several levels of the nervous system. For example, double vision can result from a focal lesion in the brainstem, peripheral nerves (cranial nerve III, IV, or VI), neuromuscular junction, or extraocular muscles; or it can be nonfocal from an increase in intracranial pressure. Associated symptoms (or the lack thereof) may lead the interviewer to reject certain hypotheses that at first seemed most likely. Table 111–4 lists the most important types of neuropathologic conditions and provides examples of diseases in each category.

Some neuropathologic locations point to a specific diagnosis or a limited number of diagnoses. For example, an autoimmune process—myasthenia gravis (common) or Eaton-Lambert myasthenic syndrome (uncommon)—usually causes disease of the neuromuscular junction. The exceptions—botulism and congenital myasthenic disorders—are rare. Alternatively, some areas of the nervous system (e.g., the cerebral hemispheres) are vulnerable to practically any of the categories of disease outlined in Table 111–4.

The pace and temporal order of symptoms are important. Degenerative diseases generally progress gradually, whereas vascular diseases (e.g., stroke, aneurysmal subarachnoid hemorrhage) progress rapidly. Certain symptoms such as double vision almost invariably develop abruptly, even if the

Table 111–1 Potential Localizing Value of Common Neurologic Symptoms

Potential Localizing Value	Symptom
High	Focal weakness, sensory loss, or pain
	Focal visual loss
	Language disturbance
	Neglect or anosognosia
Medium	Vertigo
	Dysarthria
	Clumsiness
Low	Fatigue
	Headache
	Insomnia
	Dizziness
	Anxiety, confusion, or psychosis

underlying disorder has been developing gradually over days to weeks.

Neurologic Examination

Although the performance of the main elements of a general screening neurologic examination is imperative (Table 111–5), the examination should be tailored to confirm or disprove the clinical hypotheses generated from the patient's history. Unexpected signs must be explained (often with a return to the history for further clarification).

The examination is approached as if only one of two possible injuries has occurred: either the *final common pathway* to a structure is disrupted or the input to that pathway is disrupted (Fig. 111–1). In the case of the motor system, the *final common pathway* includes the anterior horn cells giving rise to axons in a nerve, the nerve itself, neuromuscular junctions, and the muscle. Injury to any of these structures will result in dysfunction of the muscle. Conversely, if these structures are intact, observing the muscle function may be

Table 111–2 Clues to Symptom Localization in the Central Nervous System

Symptom	Location
Cerebral Hemispheres	
Unilateral weakness or sensory complaints	Contralateral cerebral hemisphere
Language dysfunction	Left hemisphere (frontal and temporal)
Spatial disorientation	Right hemisphere (parietal and occipital)
Anosognosia (lack of insight into deficit)	Right hemisphere (parietal)
Hemivisual loss	Contralateral hemisphere (occipital, temporal, and parietal)
Flattening of affect or social disinhibition	Bihemispheric (frontal and limbic)
Alteration of consciousness	Bihemispheric (diffuse)
Alteration of memory	Bihemispheric (hippocampus, fornix, amygdala, and mammillary bodies)
Cerebellum	
Limb clumsiness	Ipsilateral cerebellar hemisphere
Unsteadiness of gait or posture	Midline cerebellar structures
Basal Ganglia	
Slowness of voluntary movement	Substantia nigra and striatum
Involuntary movement	Striatum, thalamus, and subthalamus
Brainstem	
Contralateral weakness or sensory complaints in the body with ipsilateral weakness or sensory complaints in the face	Midbrain, pons, and medulla
Double vision	Midbrain and pons
Vertigo	Pons and medulla
Alteration of consciousness	Midbrain, pons, medulla (reticular formation)
Spinal Cord	
Weakness and spasticity (ipsilateral) and anesthesia (contralateral) below a specified level	Corticospinal and spinothalamic tracts
Unsteadiness of gait	Posterior columns
Bilateral (can be asymmetric) weakness and sensory complaints in multiple contiguous radicular radicular distributions	Central cord

Table 111-3   Clues to Symptom Localization in the Anterior Horn Cell and the Peripheral Nervous System

Symptom	Location
Anterior Horn Cell	
Weakness and wasting with muscle *twitching* (fasciculation) but no sensory complaints	Anterior horn of spinal cord (diffuse or segmental)
Spinal Root	
Weakness and sensory loss confined to a known radicular distribution (pain, a common feature, may spread)	Cervical, thoracic, lumbar, and sacral
Plexus	
Pain, weakness, and sensory loss in a limb; not limited to a single radicular or peripheral nerve distribution	Brachial and lumbosacral (may also be caused by polyradiculopathy)
Nerve	
Pain, distal weakness, and/or sensory changes confined to a single peripheral nerve distribution	Peripheral nerves (mononeuropathy)
Pain, distal weakness, and/or sensory changes affecting both sides symmetrically (generally starting in feet)	Peripheral nerves (polyneuropathy)
Pain, distal weakness, and/or sensory changes affecting scattered single peripheral nerve distributions	Peripheral nerves (mononeuropathy multiplex)
Unilateral special sensory loss	Cranial nerves I, II, V, VII, VIII, and IX
Unilateral facial weakness involving entire one half of face	Cranial nerve VII (ipsilateral)
Neuromuscular Junction	
Progressive weakness with repeated use of a muscle; no sensory complaints	Ocular, pharyngeal, and skeletal
Muscle	
Proximal weakness; no sensory complaints	Diffuse and various patterns

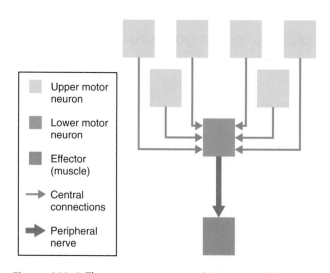

Figure 111–1 The nervous system can be conceptually reduced to a series of higher order inputs that converge on final common pathways. For example, upper motor neurons converge on lower motor neurons, whose axons form the final common pathway to an effector muscle.

possible under the right circumstances. If all modes of engaging the final common pathway fail to elicit a response, then the clinician can conclude that the lesion is located somewhere within the final common pathway.

For example, a man with paralysis of facial movement on one side that is caused by a lesion of cranial nerve VII cannot smile voluntarily, close his eye, or wrinkle his forehead on the affected side. Spontaneous laughter or smiling as an automatic response to a joke also fails to be evident on the paretic side. If the problem is central, however, then facial movement with involuntary (spontaneous) smiling may be preserved or even increased. This observation is common in patients with facial weakness caused by a stroke.

Central input to a final common pathway in the nervous system is usually tonically inhibitory. Damage to this input typically results in overactivity of the involved muscle group. Signs of damage to central inhibitory systems include (1) spasticity and hyperreflexia (motor cortex, subcortical white matter, or corticospinal pathways in the brainstem and spinal cord); (2) dystonia, rigidity, tremor, and tic (basal ganglia or extrapyramidal systems); and (3) ataxia and dysmetria (cerebellum). An exception is hypotonia caused by cerebellar disease.

Table 111–4	Categories of Neurologic Disease

Disease Category	Example
Genetic	
Autosomal dominant	Huntington's disease
Autosomal recessive	Friedreich's ataxia
Sex-linked recessive	Duchenne's muscular dystrophy
Sporadic	Down syndrome
Neoplastic	
Intrinsic	Glioblastoma
Extrinsic	Metastatic melanoma
Paraneoplastic	Cerebellar degeneration
Vascular	
Stroke	Thrombotic, embolic, lacunar, hemorrhagic
Structural	Arteriovenous malformation
Inflammatory	Cranial arteritis
Infectious	
Bacterial	Meningococcal meningitis
Viral	Herpes encephalitis
Protozoal	Toxoplasmosis
Fungal	Cryptococcal meningitis
Helminthic	Cysticercosis
Prion	Creutzfeldt-Jakob disease
Degenerative	
Central	Parkinson's disease
Central and peripheral	Amyotrophic lateral sclerosis
Autoimmune	
Central demyelinating	Multiple sclerosis
Peripheral demyelinating	Guillain-Barré syndrome
Neuromuscular junction	Myasthenia gravis
Toxic and Metabolic	
Endogenous	Uremic encephalopathy
Exogenous	Alcoholic neuropathy
Other Structural	
Trauma	Spinal cord injury
Hydrodynamic	Normal pressure hydrocephalus
Psychogenic	Hysterical paraparesis

Technologic Assessment

Laboratory investigations and special testing should be used to confirm a clinical suggestion and to finalize the diagnosis. Testing should be selectively performed because of expense, risk, and discomfort to the patient. Frequently helpful tests are discussed in this text; diagnostic tests should never be ordered without a specific differential diagnosis firmly in mind. Many neurodiagnostic tests disclose *diagnoses* unrelated to a patient's symptomatic disease process.

LUMBAR PUNCTURE

Investigation of the cerebrospinal fluid (CSF) is indicated in a small number of specific circumstances (usually meningitis and encephalitis) (Table 111–6). A CSF specimen should be routinely sent for laboratory testing to determine cell and differential counts, protein and glucose levels, and bacterial cultures. The CSF should be also be examined for its color and clarity. Cloudy or discolored CSF should be centrifuged and examined for xanthochromia in comparison with water. Special studies may be supplemented as appropriate, including Gram stain; fungal, viral, and tuberculous cultures; cryptococcal and other antigens; tests for syphilis; Lyme titers; malignant cytologic patterns; or oligoclonal bands. Polymerase chain reaction for specific viruses holds promise for many conditions. Recording the opening and closing pressures is important. Tissue infection in the region of the puncture site is an absolute contraindication to lumbar puncture. Relative contraindications include known or probable intracranial or spinal mass lesion, increased intracranial pressure as a result of mass lesions, coagulopathy caused by thrombocytopenia (usually correctable), anticoagulant therapy, or bleeding disorders. Rare but severe complications include transtentorial or foramen magnum herniation, spinal epidural hematoma, spinal abscess, herniated or infected disc, meningitis, and adverse reaction to a local anesthetic agent. More common and relatively benign complications include headache and backache.

TISSUE BIOPSIES

In select specialty centers, a diagnostic biopsy is performed on various tissues, including brain, peripheral nerve (see Chapter 129), muscle (see Chapter 130), and skin. On occasion, biopsy provides the only means of arriving at a definitive diagnosis.

ELECTROPHYSIOLOGIC STUDIES

Electrophysiologic studies include electroencephalography, electromyography, nerve conduction studies, and evoked potentials. These studies are helpful in situations in which the patient cannot be examined or interviewed adequately.

Electroencephalography is most often used to investigate seizures (see Chapter 125). It can document encephalopathy, in which case the background electrical activity of the brain is slowed, and it is also used in the evaluation of brain death.

Electromyography is useful in the differential diagnoses of muscle disease, neuromuscular junction disease, peripheral nerve disease, and anterior horn cell disease (see Chapters 129 and 130). Nerve conduction studies (see Chapters 129 and 130) may show decreased amplitude (characteristic of axonal neuropathy) or decreased velocity (characteristic of demyelinating neuropathy).

Visual-evoked potential studies are commonly used in the evaluation of probable multiple sclerosis (see Chapter 128). Asymmetric slowing of the cortical response to visual

Table 111–5 Elements of a General Screening Neurologic Examination

General Systemic Physical Examination

Head (trauma, dysmorphism, and bruits)
Neck (tone, bruits, and thyromegaly)
Cardiovascular (heart rate, rhythm, and murmurs; peripheral pulses and jugular venous distention)
Pulmonary (breathing pattern and cyanosis)
Abdomen (hepatosplenomegaly)
Back and extremities (skeletal abnormalities, peripheral edema, and straight-leg raising)
Skin (neurocutaneous stigmata and hepatic stigmata)

Mental Status

Level of consciousness (awake, drowsy, and comatose)
Attention (coherent stream of thought, serial 7s)
Orientation (temporal and spatial)
Memory (short- and long-term)
Language (naming, repetition, comprehension, fluency, reading, and writing)
Visuospatial skills (clock drawing and figure copying)
Judgment, insight, thought content (psychotic)
Mood (depressed, manic, and anxious)

Cranial Nerves

Olfactory (smell in each nostril)
Optic (afferent pupillary function, funduscopic examination, visual acuity, visual fields, and structural eye findings)
Oculomotor, trochlear, and abducens (smooth pursuit and saccadic eye movements, nystagmus, efferent pupillary function, and eyelid opening)
Trigeminal (jaw jerk, facial sensation, afferent corneal reflex, and muscles of mastication)
Facial (efferent corneal reflex, facial expression, eyelid closure, nasolabial folds, and power and bulk)
Vestibulocochlear (nystagmus, speech discrimination, Weber's test, and Rinne's test)
Glossopharyngeal and vagus (afferent and efferent gag reflex and uvula position)
Spinal accessory (power and bulk of sternocleidomastoid and trapezii muscles)
Hypoglossal (position, bulk, and fasciculations of tongue)

Motor Examination

Pronator drift (subtle corticospinal lesion)
Tone and bulk of muscles (basal ganglia lesion yields rigidity, cerebellar lesion yields hypotonia, corticospinal lesion yields spasticity, nonspecific bihemispheric disease yields paratonia, hypertrophy indicates dystonia, pseudohypertrophy indicates muscle disease, and atrophy indicates lower motor neuron disease)
Adventitious movements (tremor, tic, dystonia, and chorea indicate disease of the basal ganglia; asterixis and myoclonus may indicate toxic metabolic process)
Power of major muscle groups (scale 0–5)
Upper extremities: deltoids, biceps, triceps, wrist extension and flexion, finger extension and flexion, and interossei
Lower extremities: hip flexion, extension, abduction, and adduction; knee extension and flexion; ankle dorsiflexion, plantar flexion, inversion, and eversion; toe extension and flexion

Sensory Examination

Light touch (posterior columns)
Pinprick (spinothalamic tract)
Temperature (spinothalamic tract)
Joint position sense (posterior columns)
Vibration (posterior columns)
Graphesthesia (cortical sensory)
Double simultaneous stimulation (cortical sensory)
Two-point discrimination (posterior columns and cortical sensory)

Continued

Table 111–5	**Elements of a General Screening Neurologic Examination—cont'd**

Reflex Examination

Standard reflexes (grades 0–4)
Biceps
Triceps
Brachioradialis
Knee jerk
Ankle jerk
Pathologic reflexes
Babinski sign (if present)
Myerson sign (if present)
Snout (if present)
Jaw jerk (if brisk)
Palmomental (if present)
Hoffmann sign (if brisk)

Coordination and Gait

Finger-nose-finger (intention tremor suggesting cerebellar disease)
Rapid alternating movements (dysdiadochokinesia suggesting cerebellar disease)
Fine motor movements (slowness and small amplitude suggesting basal ganglia or corticospinal tract abnormalities)
Heel-to-shin (ataxia suggesting cerebellar disease)
Arising from chair with arms folded across chest (inability in advanced basal ganglia, cerebellar, corticospinal, or muscle disease)
Walking naturally (look for decreased arm swing, spasticity, broad base, festination, waddle, footdrop, start hesitation, and dystonia)
Tandem gait (look for ataxia)
Walking with feet everted or inverted (look for latent dystonia)
Hopping on each foot separately (look for latent dystonia)
Stand with feet together and eyes open, eyes closed (sensory ataxia and cerebellar disease)
Response to retropulsive stress (loss of postural righting mechanisms)

Table 111–6	**Indications for Lumbar Puncture**

Urgent (do not wait for brain imaging):
Acute central nervous system infection in the absence of focal neurologic signs
Less urgent (wait for brain imaging):
Vasculitis, subarachnoid hemorrhage, or cryptic process
Increased intracranial pressure in the absence of mass lesion on magnetic resonance imaging or computed tomography
Intrathecal therapy for fungal or carcinomatous meningitis
Symptomatic treatment for headache from idiopathic intracranial hypertension or subarachnoid hemorrhage

pattern stimulation suggests demyelination in the optic nerve or central optic pathways. Brainstem auditory-evoked potential studies are useful in the diagnoses of diseases affecting cranial nerve VIII or its central projections. Lesions at the cerebellopontine angle and the brainstem cause abnormal delay in conduction. Brainstem auditory-evoked potentials are helpful in the diagnosis of deafness in infants. Somatosensory-evoked potentials are used to identify a slowing of central sensory conduction that results from demyelinating disease, compression, or metabolic derangements. They are also used to evaluate spinal cord–mediated sensory abnormalities.

IMAGING STUDIES

Magnetic resonance imaging (MRI) and computed tomography (CT) are high-resolution imaging techniques that provide extraordinary diagnostic precision for central nervous system lesions. Most neurologic diseases, however, can have normal CT and MRI findings. Moreover, many abnormal findings on CT and MRI bear no relation to the diagnosis responsible for the patient's symptoms. Table 111–7 compares CT with MRI. MRI is used for most purposes, although CT has the advantage of wider accessibility, greater speed of acquisition, and better tolerability by the patient. CT detects acute hemorrhage and is preferred for emergencies. MRI provides more detail and simultaneously obtains images in the horizontal, vertical, and coronal planes. Contrast media for CT or MRI are useful in the diagnosis of tumors, abscesses, and other processes that derange the blood-brain barrier. MRI can now be used for functional imaging and spectroscopy; both techniques have great promise for the evaluation of cognitive and metabolic disorders, epilepsy, multiple sclerosis, and many other conditions.

Table 111–7	**Magnetic Resonance Imaging (MRI) versus Computed Tomography (CT)**

MRI

Resolution 1–2 mm
Gadolinium contrast relatively safe
Unaffected by bone
Multiple planes of imaging available
Functional (physiologic) imaging capacity

CT

Resolution >5 mm
Iodine contrast associated with anaphylaxis and rash
Faster acquisition than an MRI
Metallic objects such as pacemaker or aneurysm clip preclude MRI
Acute hemorrhage well visualized
Better tolerated by patients who are severely ill or claustrophobic

Table 111–8	**Some Neurologic Conditions for Which Genetic Tests Are Available**

Peripheral neuropathies (Charcot-Marie-Tooth 1A, Kennedy's syndrome)
Neuromuscular diseases (myotonic dystrophy, Duchenne's muscular dystrophy, Becker's muscular dystrophy, spinal muscular atrophy, MELAS, MERRF, familial amyotrophic lateral sclerosis)
Movement disorders (spinocerebellar ataxia, multiple types; Friedreich's ataxia; dystonia DYT1; Huntington's disease)
Mental retardation (fragile X)

MELAS = mitochondrial encephalomyelopathy, lactic acidosis, and stroke-like symptoms (syndrome); MERRF = myoclonus epilepsy with ragged red fibers (syndrome).

Magnetic resonance angiography allows noninvasive visualization of the major vessels of the head and neck. Conventional angiography with an intra-arterial injection of contrast agent is used for evaluation of many intracranial vascular abnormalities—small aneurysms and arteriovenous malformations and inflammation of small blood vessels.

Noninvasive ultrasonography of the carotid and vertebral arteries can define stenotic vessels and has been supplemented by transcranial Doppler technology, which allows characterization of blood flow in intracranial arteries.

Single-photon emission CT is useful for the evaluation of intracranial blood flow. Moreover, the development of new radioligands makes it possible to visualize the dopamine transporter on nigral-striatal dopaminergic projection neurons by using a ligand (β-CIT) to follow cell loss in patients with Parkinson's disease. As the techniques of neural transplantation for Parkinson's disease improve, it may be possible to image restoration of function.

Positron-emission tomography (PET) is an extremely useful functional imaging technology that can demonstrate specific metabolic derangements. It remains a largely investigational method but is particularly useful for evaluating local abnormalities of glucose and oxygen metabolism. The high cost of the cyclotron technology needed to generate the radioactive ligands limits its clinical use to specialized centers. PET is of particular value in defining the site of origin of focal seizures.

GENETIC AND MOLECULAR TESTING

Many more neurologic diseases exist than diseases of all other systems combined. Continuing scientific discoveries have yielded a revolution in the diagnostic approach to many of these diseases, and new genetic tests are added to the armamentarium with each passing year. Table 111–8 outlines a number of tests that are now commercially available. The use of a genetic test for a given disorder requires that the clinician perform a thoughtful and caring evaluation of the patient, usually with input from and evaluation of the patient's family. Many important ethical issues surround the use of genetic tests, including the ability to ensure privacy, to ensure adequate psychological and social support for patients who may be given devastating news, and to address adequately the appropriateness of prenatal screening or presymptomatic testing when no treatment is available.

Prospectus for the Future

Functional imaging (PET and functional magnetic resonance imaging [fMRI]) is now being used for the study of acute coma and/or stupor in the emergency department and the intensive care unit. These techniques will provide a better understanding of the metabolic derangements occurring in acute brain dysfunction. As specific ion channels of brain neurons are characterized, targeted molecular therapies will enter clinical trials.

References

Hackney D: Radiologic imaging procedures. In Goldman L, Ausiello DA (eds): Cecil Textbook of Medicine, 23rd ed. Philadelphia, Saunders, 2007.

Samuels MA, Feske S (eds): Office Practice of Neurology, 2nd ed. New York, Churchill Livingstone, 2002.

Chapter 112

Disorders of Consciousness

Roger P. Simon

Coma is a sleeplike state in that the eyes are closed even when the person is vigorously stimulated. A poorly responsive state in which the eyes are open, or an agitated confused state, or delirium, is not coma, but it may represent early stages of the same disease processes and should be investigated in the same manner.

Consciousness requires an intact and functioning brain stem reticular activating system and its cortical projections. The reticular formation begins in the midpons and ascends through the dorsal midbrain to synapse in the thalamus; it then innervates higher centers through thalamocortical connections. Knowledge of this anatomic substrate provides the short list of regions to be investigated in the search for a structural cause of coma; brain stem or bihemispheric dysfunction must satisfy these anatomic requirements; otherwise, it is not the cause of the patient's unconsciousness. In addition to structural lesions, meningeal inflammation, metabolic encephalopathy, and seizures diffusely affect the brain and complete the differential diagnosis for the patient in a coma.

Pathophysiologic Factors

Meningeal irritation caused by infection or blood in the subarachnoid space is an essential early consideration in coma evaluation because its cause requires immediate attention (especially with purulent meningitis) and may not be diagnosed by computed tomography (CT).

Hemispheric mass lesions result in coma either by expanding across the midline laterally to compromise both cerebral hemispheres or by impinging on the brain stem to compress the rostral reticular formation. These processes—*lateral herniation* (lateral movement of the brain) and *transtentorial herniation* (vertical movement of the brain)—most commonly occur together. At the bedside, clinical signs of an expanding hemispheric mass evolve in a level-by-level, rostral-caudal manner (Fig. 112–1). Hemispheric lesions of adequate size to produce coma are readily seen on CT.

Brain stem mass lesions produce coma by directly affecting the reticular formation. Because the pathways for lateral eye movements (the pontine gaze center, medial longitudinal fasciculus, and oculomotor—third nerve—nucleus) tra-

verse the reticular activating system, impairment of reflex eye movements is often the critical element of diagnosis. A comatose patient without impaired reflex lateral eye movements does not have a mass lesion compromising brain stem structures in the posterior fossa. CT is not able to show some lesions in this region. Posterior fossa lesions may block the flow of cerebrospinal fluid from the lateral ventricles and result in the dangerous situation of *noncommunicating hydrocephalus.*

Metabolic abnormalities are caused by deficiency states (e.g., thiamine, glucose), by derangements of metabolism (e.g., hyponatremia), or by the presence of *exogenous toxins* (drugs) or *endogenous toxins* (organ system failure). Metabolic abnormalities result in diffuse dysfunction of the nervous system and therefore produce, with rare exceptions, no localized signs such as hemiparesis or unilateral pupillary dilation. The diagnosis of *metabolic encephalopathy* means that the examiner has found no focal anatomic features on examination or neuroimaging studies to explain coma, but it does not state that a specific metabolic cause has been established. Drugs have a predilection for affecting the reticular formation in the brain stem and producing paralysis of reflex eye movement on examination. *Multifocal structural disorders* may simulate metabolic coma (Table 112–1).

In the late stages of status epilepticus, motor movements may be subtle even though *seizure activity* is continuing throughout the brain (nonconvulsive status epilepticus). Once seizures stop, the so-called *postictal state* can also cause unexplained coma.

Diagnostic Approach

The history and examination are essential in the diagnosis and are not replaced by brain imaging (Table 112–2). History of a premonitory headache supports a diagnosis of meningitis, encephalitis, or intracerebral or subarachnoid hemorrhage. A preceding period of intoxication, confusion, or delirium points to a diffuse process such as meningitis or endogenous or exogenous toxins. The sudden apoplectic onset of coma is particularly suggestive of ischemic or hemorrhagic stroke affecting the brain stem or of subarachnoid hemorrhage or intracerebral hemorrhage with intraventricular rupture. Lateralized symptoms of hemiparesis or

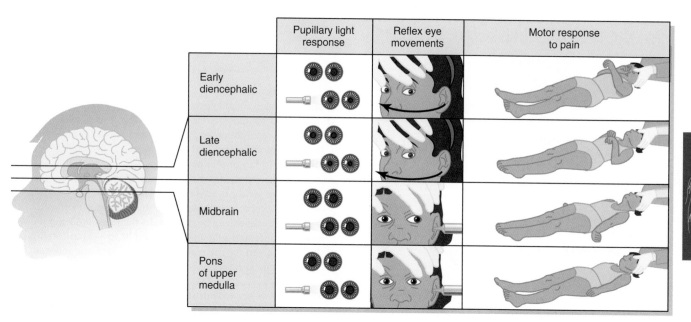

	Pupillary light response	Reflex eye movements	Motor response to pain
Early diencephalic			
Late diencephalic			
Midbrain			
Pons of upper medulla			

Figure 112–1 The evolution of neurologic signs in coma from a hemispheric mass lesion as the brain becomes functionally impaired in a rostral-caudal manner. Early and late diencephalic refer to levels of dysfunction just above (early) and just below (late) the thalamus. (From Aminoff MJ, Greenberg DA, Simon RP: Clinical Neurology. Stamford, CT, Appleton and Lange, 1996.)

Table 112–1 Multifocal Disorders Indicating Metabolic Coma

Disseminated intravascular coagulopathy
Sepsis
Pancreatitis
Vasculitis
Thrombotic thrombocytopenic purpura
Fat emboli
Hypertensive encephalopathy
Diffuse micrometastases

aphasia before coma occur in patients with hemispheric masses or infarctions.

The physical examination is critical, quickly accomplished, and diagnostic. The issues are three: (1) Does the patient have meningitis? (2) Are signs of a mass lesion present? (3) Is this condition a diffuse syndrome of exogenous or endogenous metabolic cause? Emergency management should then be instituted (Table 112–3).

IDENTIFICATION OF MENINGITIS

Although signs of meningeal irritation are not invariably present and have differing sensitivity in regard to cause (extremely common with acute pyogenic meningitis and subarachnoid hemorrhage, less common with indolent, fungal meningitis), the presence of these signs on examination is the central clue to the diagnosis. Missing these signs results in time-consuming additional tests such as brain imaging and the potential loss of a narrow therapeutic window of opportunity. Passive neck flexion should be carried out (Fig. 112–2) in all comatose patients unless a history of head trauma exists. When the neck is passively flexed, by attempting to bring the chin within a few fingerbreadths of the chest, patients with irritated meninges reflexively flex one or both knees. This sign (*Brudzinski's reflex*) is usually asymmetric and not dramatic, but any evidence of knee flexion during passive neck flexion requires that the cerebrospinal fluid be examined. Is CT required before lumbar puncture in this setting? In the absence of lateralized signs (such as hemiparesis) supporting a superimposed mass lesion, a spinal puncture should be performed immediately. Although rare cases of herniation after lumbar puncture have been reported in children with bacterial meningitis, the urgency of diagnosis and treatment at the point of coma is paramount. The time needed for CT may result in a fatal therapeutic delay. An alternative approach involves obtaining blood cultures and immediately initiating antibiotic therapy with subsequent lumbar puncture; cerebrospinal fluid cell count, glucose determination, and protein content are unchanged, and Gram stain and culture often remain positive despite a short period of antibiotic treatment. Bacterial antigens in the cerebrospinal fluid or blood can also be obtained.

SEPARATION OF STRUCTURAL FROM METABOLIC CAUSES OF COMA

The goal of separation is achieved by neurologic examination. Because the evaluation and potential treatments for structural and metabolic coma are widely divergent and the disease processes in both categories are often rapidly progressive, initiating the evaluation medically or surgically may be life saving. This task is accomplished by focusing on three features of neurologic examination: the *motor response*

Table 112–2 Causes of Coma with Normal Computed Tomography Scan

Meningeal Disorders

Subarachnoid hemorrhage (uncommon)
Bacterial meningitis
Encephalitis
Subdural empyema

Exogenous Toxins

Sedative drugs and barbiturates
Anesthetics and γ-hydroxybutyrate*
Alcohols
Stimulants
Phencyclidine[†]
Cocaine and amphetamine[‡]
Psychotropic drugs
Cyclic antidepressants
Phenothiazines
Lithium
Anticonvulsants
Opioids
Clonidine[§]
Penicillins
Salicylates
Anticholinergics
Carbon monoxide, cyanide, and methemoglobinemia

Endogenous Toxins, Deficiencies, Derangements

Hypoxia and ischemia
Hypoglycemia
Hypercalcemia
Osmolar
Hyperglycemia
Hyponatremia
Hypernatremia
Organ system failure
Hepatic encephalopathy
Uremic encephalopathy
Pulmonary insufficiency (carbon dioxide narcosis)

Seizures

Prolonged postictal state
Spike-wave stupor

Hypothermia or Hyperthermia

Brain Stem Ischemia

Basilar Artery Stroke

Pituitary Apoplexy

Conversion or Malingering

*General anesthetic, similar to γ-aminobutyric acid; recreational drug and body building aid. Rapid onset, rapid recovery often with myoclonic jerking and confusion. Deep coma (2–3 hr; Glasgow Coma Scale score = 3) with maintenance of vital signs.
[†]Coma associated with cholinergic signs: lacrimation, salivation, bronchorrhea, and hyperthermia.
[‡]Coma after seizures or status (i.e., a prolonged postictal state).
[§]An antihypertensive agent active through the opiate receptor system; frequent overdose when used to treat narcotic withdrawal.

Table 112–3 Emergency Management

Ensure airway adequacy.
Support ventilation and circulation.
Obtain blood for glucose, electrolytes, hepatic and renal function, prothrombin and partial thromboplastin times, complete blood count, and drug screen.
Administer 100 mg of thiamine IV.
Administer 25 g of dextrose IV (typically 50 mL of 50% dextrose) to treat possible hypoglycemic coma.*
Treat opiate overdose with naloxone (0.4–1.2 mg IV).
The specific benzodiazepine antagonist flumazenil (0.2 mg IV repeated once and followed by 0.1 mg IV to 1–3 mg total) should be given for the reversal of benzodiazepine-induced coma or conscious sedation.[†]

*The glucose level is poorly correlated with the level of consciousness in hypoglycemia; stupor, coma, and confusion are reported with blood glucose concentrations ranging from 2 to 60 mg/dL.
[†]Not recommended in coma of unknown origin because seizures may be precipitated in patients with polydrug overdoses containing benzodiazepines with tricyclic antidepressants or cocaine.

to a painful stimulus, *pupillary function*, and *reflex eye movements*.

Motor Response

Asymmetric or reflex function of the motor system provides the clearest indication of a mass lesion. Elicitation of a *motor response* requires that a painful stimulus be applied to which the patient will react. The patient's arms should be placed in a semiflexed posture, and a painful stimulus should be applied to the head or trunk. Strong pressure on the supra-orbital ridge or pinching of the skin on the anterior chest or inner arm is the most useful method; finger nail bed pressure is also used, but it makes the interpretation of upper limb movement difficult.

The neurologic examination of a patient with an expanding hemispheric mass lesion is shown in Figure 112–1. Hemispheric masses at their early stage (*early diencephalic,* i.e., compromising the brain above the thalamus) produce appropriate movement of one upper extremity, that is, toward the painful stimulus. The attenuated contralateral arm movement reflects a hemiparesis. This lateralized motor movement in a comatose patient establishes the working diagnosis of a hemispheric mass. As the mass expands to involve the thalamus (*late diencephalic*), the response to pain becomes reflex arm flexion associated with extension and internal rotation of the legs (*decorticate posturing*); asymmetry of the response in the upper extremities is seen. With further brain compromise at the midbrain level, the reflex posturing changes in the arms such that both arms and legs respond by extension (*decerebrate posturing*); at this level, the asymmetry tends to be lost. At this point, the pupils become midposition in size, and the light reflex is lost, first unilaterally and then bilaterally. With further progression to the level of the pons, no response to painful stimulation is the most frequent finding, although spinal mediated movements of leg flexion may occur. The classic postures illustrated in

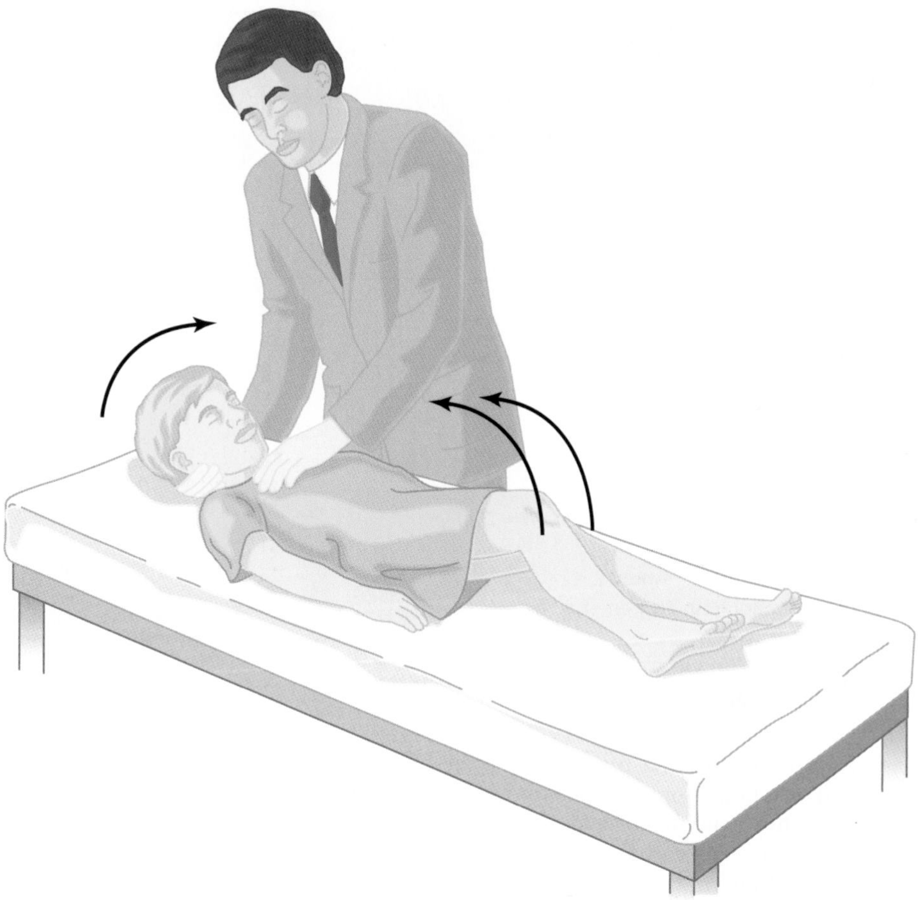

Figure 112–2 Elicitation of Brudzinski's sign of meningeal irritation as seen in infectious meningitis or subarachnoid hemorrhage. (From Aminoff MJ, Greenberg DA, Simon RP: Clinical Neurology. Stamford, CT, Appleton and Lange, 1996.)

Figure 112–1, and particularly their asymmetry, strongly support the presence of a mass lesion. These motor movements, especially early in coma, are, however, most frequently seen as fragments of the abnormal, asymmetric flexion or extension of the arms illustrated as decorticate and decerebrate postures in Figure 112–1. A small amount of asymmetric flexion or extension of the arms in response to painful stimulus carries the same implications as the full-blown postures of decortication or decerebration.

Metabolic lesions do not compromise the brain in a progressive, level-by-level manner as do hemispheric masses, and they rarely produce the asymmetric motor signs typical of masses. Reflex posturing may be seen, but it lacks the asymmetry of decortication from a hemispheric mass and is not associated with the loss of pupillary reactivity at the stage of decerebration.

Pupillary Reactivity

In metabolic coma, one feature is central to the examination: Pupillary reactivity is present. This reactivity is seen both early in coma, when an appropriate motor response to pain may be retained, and late in coma, when no motor responses can be elicited. The pupillary reaction is lost only when coma is so deep that the patient requires ventilatory and blood pressure support.

Reflex Eye Movements

The presence of inducible lateral eye movements reflects the integrity of the pons and midbrain. These reflex eye movements (see Fig. 112–1) are brought about by passive head rotation to stimulate the semicircular canal input to the vestibular system (so-called doll's eyes maneuver) or by inhibiting the function of one semicircular canal by infusion of ice water against the tympanic membrane (caloric testing).

In metabolic coma, reflex eye movements may be lost or retained. Lack of inducible eye movements with the doll's eyes maneuver, in the setting of preserved pupillary reactivity, is virtually diagnostic of drug toxicity. With metabolic coma of non–drug-induced origin, such as organ system failure, electrolyte disorders, or osmolar disorders, reflex eye movements are preserved.

Brain stem mass lesions are most commonly caused by hemorrhage or infarction. Reflex lateral eye movements, the pathways for which traverse the pons and midbrain, are particularly affected, and the reflex postures of decortication and decerebration typical of brain stem injury are common. Lesions restricted to the midbrain (e.g., embolization from the heart to the top of the basilar artery) are exhibited by sluggish pupillary reflexes or their absence, with or without impaired medial eye movements (both are controlled by the third cranial nerve). With lesions restricted to the pons (e.g., intrapontine hypertensive hemorrhage), pupils are reactive but very small (pinpoint or pontine pupils), which reflects focal impairment of sympathetic innervation; pinpoint pupils are rare. Ocular bobbing (spontaneous symmetric or asymmetric rhythmic vertical ocular oscillations) is more often seen as a manifestation of a pontine lesion.

Table 112–4	Percentage of Patients Recovering Independent Function from Coma After Cardiac Arrest (Predicted by Signs on Examination at 0, 1, 3, and 7 Days)			
	Days After Cardiac Arrest			
Sign	**0**	**1**	**3**	**7**
No verbal response	13	8	5	6
No eye opening	11	6	4	0
Unreactive pupils	0	0	0	0
No spontaneous eye movements	6	5	2	0
No caloric response	5	6	6	0
Extensor posturing	18	0	0	0
Flexor posturing	14	3	0	0
No motor response. From Levey et al. (*N* = 210)	4	3	0	0
No eye opening to pain	31	8	0	0
Absent or reflex motor response	25	9	0	0
Unreactive pupils. From Edgren et al. (*N* = 131)	17	7	0	0

Data from Levey DE, Caronna JJ, Singer BH: Predicting the outcome from hypoxic coma. JAMA 523:1420–1426, 1985; and from Edgren E, Hedstrand U, Kelsey S: Assessment of neurological prognosis in comatose survivors of cardiac arrest. Lancet 343:1055–1059, 1994.

Seizures occurring in a patient with acute brain injury (e.g., that resulting from encephalitis, hypertensive encephalopathy, hyponatremia or hypernatremia, hypoglycemia or hyperglycemia) or chronic brain injury (e.g., dementia, mental retardation) often result in prolonged postictal coma. The examination shows reactive pupils and inducible eye movements (in the absence of overtreatment with anticonvulsants) and often up-going toes or focal signs (Todd's paresis). Nonconvulsive seizures, particularly spike-wave stupor, may occur in a patient without a history of epilepsy. The diagnosis is made by electroencephalogram (see Chapter 125).

Prognosis in Coma

In coma after cardiac arrest, the prognosis for meaningful recovery can be assessed from clinical signs. Return of pupillary reactivity within 24 hours and purposeful motor movements within the first 72 hours after cardiac arrest are highly correlated with a favorable outcome (Table 112–4). Rare late recoveries, however, have been reported.

Coma-like States

Locked-in patients are those in whom a lesion (usually a hemorrhage or an infarct) transects the brain stem at a point below the reticular formation (therefore sparing consciousness) but above the ventilatory nuclei of the medulla (therefore maintaining cardiopulmonary function) (Table 112–5). Such patients are awake, with eye opening and sleep-wake cycles, but the descending pathways through the brain stem necessary for volitional vocalization or limb movement have been transected. Voluntary eye movement, especially vertically, is preserved, and patients open and close their eyes or produce appropriate numbers of blinking movements in answer to questions. The electroencephalographic data are usually normal, reflecting normal cortical function.

Table 112–5	Locked-in Syndrome

Clinical Features

Eye opening
Reactive pupils
Volitional vertical eye movements to command
Mute
Quadriparesis
Sleep-wake cycles

Causes

Pontine vascular lesions (common)
Head injury, brain stem tumor, pontine myelinolysis (rare)

Recovery Possible

Onset 1–12 weeks (vascular)* *or*
Onset 4–6 months (nonvascular)*
Prognosis favorable
Normal CT scan*
Early recovery of lateral eye movements*

*Implications for care.
CT = computed tomography.

Psychogenic unresponsiveness is a diagnosis of exclusion. The neurologic examination shows reactive pupils and no reflex posturing in response to pain. Eye movements during the doll's eyes maneuver show volitional override rather than the smooth, uninhibited reflex lateral eye movements of coma. Ice water caloric testing either arouses the patient because of the discomfort produced or induces cortically mediated nystagmus rather than the tonic deviation typical of coma. The slow, conjugate roving eye movements of metabolic coma cannot be imitated and therefore rule out psychogenic unresponsiveness. In addition, the slow, often asymmetric and incomplete eye closure seen after passive eye opening of a comatose patient cannot be feigned. These signs therefore rule out psychogenic coma. In contrast, conscious patients usually exhibit some voluntary muscle tone in the eyelids during passive eye opening. The electroencephalogram in psychogenic unresponsiveness is that of normal wakefulness with reactive posterior rhythms on eye opening and eye closing. In patients with catatonic stupor, lorazepam administration may produce awakening.

In *persistent vegetative states* (PVSs), patients have awakened from coma but have not regained awareness. Wakefulness is exhibited by eye opening and sleep-wake cycles. The reticular activating system of the brain stem is intact to produce wakefulness, but the connections to the cortical mantle are interrupted, precluding awareness.

Clinical features do not differ by cause (Table 112–6). Patients in PVS open their eyes diurnally and in response to loud sounds; blinking occurs with bright lights. Pupils react and eye movements occur both spontaneously and with the doll's eyes maneuver. Yawning, chewing, swallowing, and, uncommonly, guttural vocalizations and lacrimation may be preserved. Spontaneous roving eye movements (very slow, constant velocity) are particularly characteristic and distressing to the patient's visitors because the patient appears to be looking about the room. The brain stem origin of the eye movements is documented by their being readily redirected by the oculocephalic (doll's eyes) reflex. The limbs may move, but motor responses are only primitive; pain usually produces decorticate or decerebrate postures or fragments of these movements.

A vegetative state is termed *persistent* after 3 months if the brain injury was medical and after 12 months if the brain injury was traumatic. The determination as to when *persistent* equals *permanent* cannot be stated absolutely; to predict which patients early in the vegetative state will remain persistently vegetative is particularly difficult in trauma. Lesions of the corpus callosum and dorsolateral brain stem seen on magnetic resonance images between 6 and 8 weeks after trauma correlated with persistence of the vegetative state at a year. In rare cases, patients show late improvement, but none of these patients returns to normal.

Brain imaging studies depict the sequelae of the causative injury but are not diagnostic of PVS. Magnetic resonance spectroscopy has shown a decrease in the neuronal marker of *N*-acetylaspartate. Positron-emission tomographic studies have shown decreased glucose usage and cerebral blood flow, but such studies are rarely diagnostic. Bilateral absence of somatosensory-evoked responses in the first week predicts death or vegetative state.

Brain death characterizes the *irreversible cessation* of brain function. Therefore, death of the organism can be determined based on death of the brain. Although local laws may dictate some details, the standard definition permits a diagnosis of brain death based on documentation of irreversible cessation of all brain function, including function of the brain stem (Table 112–7).

Documentation of *irreversibility* requires that the cause of the coma be known, that the cause be adequate to explain the clinical findings of brain death, and that exclusionary criteria are absent (Table 112–8). Confirmatory tests are sometimes used but are not required for diagnosis (Table 112–9).

Brain death results in asystole, usually within days (mean = 4) even if ventilatory support is continued. Recovery after appropriate documentation of brain death has never been reported. Removal of the ventilator results in terminal rhythms (most often complete heart block without ventricular response), in junctional rhythms, or in ventricular tachycardia. Purely spinal motor movements may occur in the moments of terminal apnea (or during apnea testing in the absence of passive administration of oxygen): arching of the back, neck turning, stiffening of the legs, and upper extremity flexion.

Table 112–6 Persistent Vegetative State: Common Causes*

Trauma (diffuse axonal injury)
Cardiac arrest and hypoperfusion (laminar necrosis of cortical mantle and/or thalamic necrosis)
Bihemispheric infarctions
Purulent meningitis or encephalitis (cortical injury)
Carbon monoxide
Prolonged hypoglycemic coma

*A vegetative state may not necessarily begin with coma but can also develop as the end stage of neurodegenerative diseases (e.g., Alzheimer's disease) of adults or children or also accompany severe congenital developmental abnormalities of the brain such as anencephaly.

Table 112–7 Criteria for Cessation of Brain Function*

Anatomic Region Tested	Confirmatory Sign
Hemispheres	Unresponsive and unreceptive to sensory stimuli including pain[†]
Midbrain	Unreactive pupils[‡]
Pons	Absent reflex eye movements[§]
Medulla	Apnea[‖]

*Sequential testing is necessary for a clinical diagnosis of brain death; at least 6 hr for all cases and at least 24 hr in the setting of anoxic-ischemic brain injury.
[†]The patient does not rouse, groan, grimace, or withdraw limbs; purely spinal reflexes (deep tendon reflexes, plantar flexion reflex, plantar withdrawal, and tonic neck reflexes) may be maintained.
[‡]Most easily assessed by the bright light of an ophthalmoscope viewed through its magnifying lens when focused on the iris; unreactive pupils may be either midposition (as they will be in death) or dilated, as they often are in the setting of a dopamine infusion.
[§]No eye movement toward the side of irrigation of the tympanic membrane with 50 mL of ice water; the oculocephalic response (doll's eyes) will always be absent in the setting of absent oculovestibular testing.
[‖]No ventilatory movements in the setting of maximum CO_2 stimulation (≥60 mm Hg; with apnea, PCO_2 will passively rise 2–3 mm Hg/min); disconnect the ventilator from the endotracheal tube and insert cannula with 6 L/min O_2.
CO_2 = carbon dioxide; PCO_2 = partial pressure of carbon dioxide.

Table 112–8	**Exclusionary Criteria for Brain Death**

Seizures
Decorticate or decerebrate posturing
Sedative drugs
Hypothermia (<32.2° C)
Neuromuscular blockade
Shock

Table 112–9	**Confirmatory Tests for Brain Death**

EEG isoelectricity: Deep coma from sedative drugs or hypothermia below 20° C can produce EEG flattening; patients clinically brain dead may have residual EEG activity for a significant number of days following a brain death diagnosis
No cerebral blood flow at angiography
The most definitive confirmatory test (the role of transcranial Doppler is still unclear)

EEG = electroencephalogram.

Prospectus for the Future

Functional imaging (positron-emission tomography and functional magnetic resonance imaging) is now being employed for study of acute coma and stupor in the emergency room and the intensive care unit. These techniques will provide a better understanding of the metabolic derangements occurring in acute brain dysfunction. As specific ion channels of brain neurons are characterized, targeted molecular therapies will enter clinical trials.

References

Bernat JL: Chronic disorders of consciousness. Lancet 367:1181–1192, 2006.

Plum F, Posner JB: The Diagnosis of Stupor and Coma (Contemporary Neurology Series), 3rd ed, vol 19. Philadelphia, FA Davis, 1980.

Quality Standards Subcommittee of the American Academy of Neurology: Practice parameters: Assessment and management of patients in the persistent vegetative state. Neurology 45:1015–1018, 1995.

Wijdicks EFM: The diagnosis of brain death. N Engl J Med 344:1215–1221, 2001.

Wijdicks EFM: Neurologic Complications of Critical Illness (Contemporary Neurology Series), 2nd ed, vol 64. New York, Oxford University Press, 2002.

Wijdicks EFM, Hijdra A, Young GB, et al: Practice parameter: Prediction of outcome in comatose survivors after cardiopulmonary resuscitation (an evidence-based review). Neurology 67:203–210, 2006.

Young GB, Ropper AH, Bolton CF: Coma and Impaired Consciousness: A Clinical Perspective. New York, McGraw-Hill, 1998.

Zandbergen EGJ, Hijdra A, Koelman JHTM, et al: Prediction of poor outcome within the first three days of postanoxic coma. Neurology 66:62–68, 2006.

Zeman A: Persistent vegetative state. Lancet 350:795–799, 1997.

Disorders of Sleep

Roger P. Simon

Maria J. Sunseri

Neurobiology of Sleep

The precise function of *sleep* is not completely understood. Rest periods are known throughout all biologic systems. Sleep occurs in reptiles and birds, and nearly all mammals sleep and dream. Sleep is necessary for life; deprivation in the rat results in death in about 1 month. Endogenous sleep-inducing factors have been isolated but not fully characterized. Wakefulness is under the control of the reticular-activating system of the rostral brainstem, which projects to the thalamus and cortex. The pons contains the rapid eye movement (REM) sleep generator, which may play a role in the random imagery of dreaming.

Sleep stages (Table 113–1), defined by electroencephalogram (EEG) and by behavior, are associated with specific sleep disorders. In phasic *REM sleep,* the EEG is similar to that seen in waking and is characterized by low-voltage mixed frequencies and abrupt REMs, penile erections, and an absence of electromyographic (EMG) activity (muscular atonia). In tonic REM, sleep is interspersed with short bursts of phasic REM with increased EMG activity, which may be associated with a body twitch. REM sleep occupies 20% to 25% of sleep time. Patients awakening during REM sleep report vivid dream imagery. *Non-REM (NREM) sleep* lacks these special features and is associated with EEG slowing.

Insomnia

Insomnia is the perception of inadequate sleep, either in amount or quality, and is usually not associated with daytime sleepiness. The normal duration of sleep in a given person can vary from as little as 4 hours to as many as 11 hours a day.

Diagnosis and treatment of insomnia are based on the patient's history. Is the problem of recent onset, or is it chronic? Does the patient have associated psychological, medical, or medication changes (Tables 113–2 and 113–3)? Is the symptom impairment of sleep onset, multiple awak-enings during sleep (arousal), early awakenings, or normal but nonrefreshing sleep? Does the patient have partial arousal (history often elicited from the bed partner), breathing abnormalities, or involuntary movements? Each of these forms of insomnia has different differential diagnoses. *Situational insomnia* may be associated with exogenous events: life stresses, death of a family member, stress at work, a new sleeping location or partner, work shift, jet lag, or endogenous depression. *Depression* suppresses stage 4 sleep and REM latency (although the percentage of REM may be increased). These changes are restored after nonpharmacologic treatment and, to a lesser extent, after pharmacologic treatment of depression. *Chronic behavioral insomnia* occurs in persons with a characteristic personality inducing rumination, emotional arousal, and increased autonomic activity. The focus on the inability to fall asleep becomes self-perpetuating.

The treatment of insomnia (Table 113–4) includes an optimal sleep environment, supplemented with a brief use of sedatives as needed. For patients with persistent insomnia, specific causes should be sought such as sleep apnea or abnormal arousal including periodic limb movements.

Abnormal Arousal

Abnormal arousal results in the perception of inadequate sleep. *Restless leg syndrome* (RLS), a disagreeable sensation causing a need to move the legs or a deep sensory complaint in the lower extremities, typically occurs nocturnally or at rest, interfering with sleep onset; it is briefly relieved by walking or by rubbing or moving the limbs. Sinemet (carbidopa, levodopa) (beginning with 25/100 mg 30 minutes before bedtime) is effective. The dopamine agonists ropinirole (Requip), 0.25 to 1 mg, the first U.S. Food and Drug Administration (FDA)–approved drug for RLS, pramipexole (Mirapex), 0.375 to 0.75 mg/day, or pergolide (Permax), 0.5 mg 2 hours before sleep, are now the preferred treatments. RLS is occasionally symptomatic of an underlying neuropathic condition, but most cases are idiopathic. A

Table 113–1 Sleep Stages, their Characteristics, and Disorders Associated with Them

Sleep Stage	Electroencephalogram*	Eye Movements	Electromyographic Activity	Imagery	Sleep Disorder
Wakefulness	Alpha and beta activity (low voltage fast)	Random, rapid	Active, spontaneous	Vivid, external	Insomnia
Presleep	Reduction of alpha rhythms	Reduced	Reduced	External	Restless legs syndrome; sleep onset myoclonus
Non-REM Sleep (NREM):					
Stage 1 (drowsiness, sleep)	Theta activity / Sleep spindles, K complexes	Slow, rolling / Slow or absent	Attenuated, episodic / Attenuated	Dulled / Nonvivid	Periodic limb movements of sleep; sleep myoclonus
Stages 3 and 4 (slow-wave sleep)	Delta activity	Absent	Attenuated		Sleepwalking; sleep terrors
REM sleep	Low-amplitude, irregular	Abrupt, REMs	Absent (REM atonia)	Vivid, bizarre	Nightmares; REM behavioral disorder
Sleep-wake transition	Disappearance of slowing	Random	Active	Dream recall	Sleep paralysis; hypnopompic hallucinations

*Alpha activity: 8–13 Hz (cycles/sec); beta: >13 Hz; theta: 4–7 Hz; delta: <4 Hz.
REM = rapid eye movement.

Table 113–2 Drug-Related Insomnia

Caffeine or caffeine-containing over-the-counter drugs (in susceptible patients)
Alcohol (hastens sleep onset but increases sleep-related breathing abnormalities, sleep fragmentation, and early awakening)
Corticosteroids
Antidepressants
Bronchodilators
Central nervous system stimulants
Short-acting sedatives (on withdrawal)

Table 113–3 Medical or Neurologic Conditions Associated with Insomnia

Pain (especially skeletal pain and arthritis)
Shortness of breath and congestive heart failure (paroxysmal nocturnal dyspnea)
Bowel hypermotility disorders and nocturnal diarrhea
Eating disorders and hunger
Neurologic disorders that impair normal movement during sleep (stroke, multiple sclerosis, or Parkinson's disease)
Nocturnal headaches (cluster and hypnic headaches)
Aging (increased awakenings between non-REM and REM sleep; daytime napping shortens nocturnal sleep; sundowning)
Arrival at high altitude (hypoxia, altered ventilatory drive, periodic breathing, and multiple awakenings)

REM = rapid eye movement.

family history of RLS is common with a young onset of symptoms.

Periodic limb movements often accompany RLS. The movements are brief and consist of repetitive dorsiflexion of the great toe or plantar flexion of the foot during sleep stages 1 to 2. Clonazepam may be useful. Myoclonus involving body or limb jerking at the onset of sleep has been reported in nearly 80% of healthy persons. The prolongation of these fragments of myoclonus during NREM sleep constitutes sleep myoclonus, which does not usually require treatment.

Table 113–4	**Treatment of Insomnia**

Treat depression

Eliminate stimulant drugs

Provide an optimal sleep environment (optimal temperature, light, and ambient noise; a regular sleep and wake-up time; increased daytime exercise; *winding down* before sleep (e.g., quiet, reading)

Avoid drugs and alcohol

Medications (prescribe only briefly because tolerance develops within weeks). Lunesta 1–3 mg (nonbenzodiazepine hypnotic) has been approved for long-term use

Triazolam (Halcion) or zolpidem (Ambien) (rapid acting, short half-life for sleep onset)

Flurazepam (Dalmane) or quazepam (Doral) (longer acting for sleep maintenance)

Zaleplon (Sonata) (ultra short-acting nonbenzodiazepine for nocturnal awakening)

Trazodone or zolpidem (for sundowning)

Sleep Apnea

Obstructive sleep apnea occurs in 2% to 5% of the adult population of the United States and affects primarily middle-aged or older men. The classic presentation is the obese patient with loud snoring and daytime sleepiness who may have multiple arousals or awakenings during the night, with gasping for breath. Approximately 35 events over 6 to 7 hours of sleep are sufficient for the diagnosis. Up to 100 or more events lasting between less than 10 to 30 seconds per night may occur. The resultant sleep fragmentation produces daytime sleepiness and impaired occupational performance. Episodes are exacerbated by alcohol use at bedtime, as well as by sedative-hypnotic drugs. The supine position typically exacerbates sleep disordered breathing because of the additional gravitational factor contributing to anteroposterior oropharyngeal collapse. The diagnosis should be confirmed in a sleep laboratory; the presence or absence of respiratory effort separates obstructive from central causes. Preventive treatments include weight loss and alcohol avoidance. Continuous positive airway pressure during sleep results in symptomatic improvement in most patients.

Parasomnias

Parasomnias are sleep-related motor disorders, with or without autonomic features, that induce brief partial arousals not associated with daytime sleepiness. They are most common in childhood but may occur in adults. *Sleep-walking* occurs in more than 10% of children, many of whom have a family history of the condition. The behavior occurs during sleep stages 3 and 4 and may be fragmentary, such as merely sitting up in bed. Patients are difficult to arouse during the event and do not recollect it. Events usually occur in the first few hours of sleep and are brief (<10 minutes), but they may be recurrent. *Sleep terrors* are often associated; they also occur in NREM sleep and include intense autonomic arousal, significant vocalization and movements, difficulty in arousing the patient, and minimal recall of the episode. The spells may be attenuated by benzodiazepines. *Nightmares* are distinct from sleep terrors as they occur in REM sleep; thus motor movements are limited, vocalization is much less intense, the patient is relatively easily aroused, and vivid dream recall is evident. *REM behavioral disorder* is an uncommon parasomnia affecting middle-aged or older men or patients with degenerative disease of the central nervous system. The absence of the usual muscle paralysis characteristic of REM (resulting from the absence of EMG activity during this sleep stage, known as *REM atonia*) allows for REM motor behaviors that are often violent and may injure the patient or the bed partner. Vivid imagery is reported on awakening. Clonazepam is an effective treatment.

Narcolepsy

Narcolepsy, a disorder of excessive daytime sleepiness, is associated with abnormalities in REM sleep. A reduction in the sleep modulatory hypocretin peptide-containing neurons in the hypothalamus and decreased cerebrospinal fluid hypocretin concentrations are found in patients with narcolepsy. A degenerative cause has been proposed: postnatal immune-mediated gliosis of the hypocretin neurons in the lateral hypothalamus. It may be associated with cataplexy or with hypnagogic hallucinations and sleep paralysis. The onset of narcolepsy is between the second and fifth decades. *Narcoleptic hypersomnia* occurs in settings of sedentary activity and boredom but also during conversation, during meals, and while driving. The induced sleep episodes are brief, and their frequency is little changed in patients after the first months of the disorder. The diagnosis is made on the history of excessive daytime sleepiness, the absence of underlying nocturnal sleep disorders on nocturnal polysomnography, two or more sleep-onset REM periods, and a mean sleep latency of less than 8 minutes on multiple sleep-latency testing performed in a sleep laboratory. False-positive results occur in patients with depression, drug withdrawal, and sleep deprivation.

Treatment of narcolepsy should begin with a short nap of 15 to 30 minutes in the morning and a longer nap of 1 hour in the afternoon, 180 degrees out of phase with the midpoint of their nocturnal sleep. Pharmacologic therapy with stimulants (methylphenidate, 10 to 60 mg, or dextroamphetamine, 5 to 50 mg/day) rarely achieves complete relief of daytime sleepiness. Modafinil (an α-adrenergic agonist), 200 to 400 mg every morning, is the first-line treatment.

Cataplexy is eventually associated with narcolepsy in 70% of patients. A reduction in hypocretin activation of brainstem monoaminergic neurons has been postulated. The cataplectic phenomenon is that of emotion-induced, brief, reflex muscular atonia (partial or generalized), which spares respiratory muscles. Laughter is the most common inducer. Cataplectic attacks can be attenuated by tricyclic antidepressants such as clomipramine (10 to 150 mg/day) and/or γ hydroxybutyrate (Xyrem) 4.5 to 9 g nightly in two divided doses.

Prospectus for the Future

Advances in imaging will soon identify the pathogenesis and pathophysiologic patterns of sleep disorders, paving the way for specific pharmacotherapies of these once mysterious conditions.

References

Earley CJ: Restless legs syndrome. N Engl J Med 348:2103–2109, 2003.

Espie CA: Insomnia: Conceptual issues in the development, persistence and treatment of sleep disorders in adults. Ann Rev Psychol 53:215–243, 2002.

Pack AI, Dinges DF, Gehrman PR, et al: Risk factors for excessive sleepiness in older adults. Ann Neurol 59:893–904, 2006.

Scammell TE: The neurobiology, diagnosis, and treatment of narcolepsy. Ann Neurol 53:154–166, 2003.

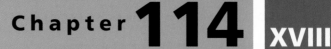

Cortical Syndromes

Timothy J. Counihan

Anatomy

The paired cerebral hemispheres are connected by a large band of white matter fibers, the *corpus callosum.* Each hemisphere has four anatomically and functionally distinct regions: (1) frontal, (2) temporal, (3) parietal, and (4) occipital lobes. The two cerebral hemispheres supplement each other functionally in a variety of behavioral and sensorimotor tasks; however, certain functions, particularly language, manual dexterity, and visuospatial perception, are strongly lateralized to one hemisphere. Language function, for instance, is lateralized to the left hemisphere in 95% of the population; although 15% of the population is left handed, only a minority of persons possess a right hemisphere that is dominant for language. Visuospatial functions are largely subserved by the right (nondominant) hemisphere.

The Rolandic fissure separates the motor cortex (precentral gyrus) from the sensory cortex (postcentral gyrus). In these regions, cortical representation of the different parts of the body is arranged as the motor (in the frontal lobe) and sensory (in the parietal lobe) homunculi.

Regional Syndromes

Because many neurologic disorders affect the cerebral hemispheres in a regionally specific or focal manner, a thorough history and clinical examination that includes the Mini-Mental State Examination (see Table 115–4) is helpful not only in localizing brain lesions, but also in establishing the cause. Tables 114–1 to 114–4 summarize some of the core clinical features involved with damage to individual hemispheres. The rate of onset of symptoms and the tempo of progression influence the extent of the clinical deficit. The homuncular arrangement of cortical motor and sensory representation may allow for more precise localization of a lesion. For instance, motor or sensory signs confined to the lower extremities may suggest a parasagittal lesion, whereas signs involving the face and upper limbs may be found in laterally placed cortical lesions.

APHASIA

Aphasia or *dysphasia* refers to a loss or impairment of language function as a result of damage to the specific language centers of the dominant hemisphere. This condition is distinct from dysarthria, which is a disturbance in the articulation of speech. The principal types of aphasia are summarized in Table 114–5. An effective bedside screening test for aphasia is to have the patient read and write a sentence; writing is almost invariably affected in patients with disturbances of language. An exception to this circumstance occurs in the syndrome of *alexia without agraphia;* this syndrome results from a vascular lesion of the dominant hemisphere's posterior cerebral artery, in which the patient's language center is *disconnected* from the contralateral (unaffected) visual cortex. Such patients can write a sentence but are unable to read what they have written. Clinical assessment for aphasia requires testing of fluency, comprehension, repetition, naming, reading, calculation, and writing. *Anomia* (difficulty in recalling the names of objects) in isolation has little localizing value.

Broca's aphasia is characterized by a severe disruption in the fluency of speech, with profound impairments in expression in both speech and writing. Comprehension may be mildly affected. The language disturbance is almost invariably accompanied by contralateral facial and arm weakness as a result of the proximity of the motor homunculus to Broca's speech area.

Wernicke's aphasia is characterized by an inability to comprehend spoken or written language. Affected patients speak fluently but the content is meaningless; they may use words that are close in meaning to the intended word (semantic paraphasia) or words that sound similar to the intended word (literal paraphasia). Some patients with Wernicke's aphasia have an associated contralateral, usually right, homonymous hemianopia.

Conduction aphasia is characterized by an inability to repeat a spoken phrase such as *no ifs, ands, or buts,* although patients have normal comprehension. The responsible lesion lies in the arcuate fasciculus connecting Broca's and Wernicke's areas. *Global aphasia* results from large lesions of

Table 114–1 Frontal Lobe Syndromes

Symptom and Sign	Site of Lesion
Contralateral spastic weakness	Primary motor, premotor cortex
Broca's aphasia	Dominant inferior frontal lobe
Forced eye deviation	Frontal eye fields
Executive dysfunction, poor sequencing	Dorsolateral prefrontal lobe
Akinetic mutism, urinary incontinence	Medial frontal cortex
Disinhibition, emotional lability	Orbitofrontal cortex

Table 114–3 Temporal Lobe Syndromes

Symptom and Sign	Lesion Site
Anomic/sensory aphasia	Lateral temporal lobe (dominant)
Contralateral superior quadratic anopsia	Superior lateral temporal lobe
Amnesia	Hippocampus
Oral-exploratory behavior, passivity, hypersexuality (Klüver-Bucy syndrome)	Amygdala (bilateral)
Visual and olfactory hallucinations; delusions (déjà vu, jamais vu)	Inferomedial temporal lobe

Table 114–2 Parietal Lobe Syndromes

Symptom and Sign	Site of Lesion
Contralateral sensory loss	Postcentral gyrus
Contralateral sensory neglect	Postcentral gyrus (nondominant)
Wernicke's aphasia, apraxia	Inferior parietal, superior temporal cortex
Acalculia, finger agnosia, right-left confusion, agraphia (Gerstmann's syndrome)	Angular gyrus

Table 114–4 Occipital Lobe Syndromes

Symptom and Sign	Lesion Site
Contralateral homonymous hemianopia	Striate cortex
Alexia without agraphia	Primary visual cortex (dominant) and splenium of corpus callosum
Visual agnosia, denial of blindness (Anton's syndrome), visual hallucinations	Medial occipital lobe
Optic apraxia, absent optokinetic nystagmus	Lateral (visual association) cortex

Table 114–5 Principal Types of Aphasia

Type	Lesion Site	Fluency	Comprehension	Repetition	Naming	Other Signs
Broca's	Inferior frontal lobe	↓	Good	↓	↓	Contralateral weakness
Wernicke's	Posterior superior temporal lobe	Good	↓	↓	↓	Homonymous hemianopia
Conduction	Supramarginal gyrus	Good	Good	↓	↓	None
Global	Frontal lobe (large)	↓	↓	↓	↓	Hemiplegia

the frontal lobe, in which all aspects of language are affected. Lesions of the nondominant hemisphere language areas result in *dysprosody*. For instance, patients with lesions in the inferior frontal lobe of the nondominant (usually right) hemisphere, analogous to Broca's area, speak with a monotonous voice, losing the natural cadence of speech.

In *dysarthria*, language function is intact, which can be confirmed by having the patient write a sentence, but patients have difficulty articulating speech. Dysarthria results from supranuclear, nuclear, or peripheral lesions of the lower cranial nerves or from lesions of the bulbar musculature or neuromuscular junction.

AGNOSIA AND APRAXIA

Agnosia is the inability to recognize a specific sensory stimulus despite preserved sensory function. For instance, visual agnosia is the inability to recognize a visual stimulus despite normal visual acuity. Similar syndromes include the inability to recognize sounds (auditory agnosia), color (color agnosia), and familiar faces (prosopagnosia). In most instances, the responsible lesions are located in the occipitotemporal region.

Apraxia refers to an inability to perform learned motor tasks despite sufficient memory and sensorimotor function to understand the command. The responsible lesions are usually in the dominant inferior parietal lobe. Lesions of the right parietal lobe often result in hemispatial neglect: The patient does not attend to stimuli in the left visual field or on the left side of the body. In a milder form of neglect, called *extinction*, patients can attend to stimuli contralateral to the side of the brain with the lesion (and the lesion is usually on the right side), but, when presented with bilateral stimuli simultaneously, they respond only on the ipsilateral (right) side. Anosognosia, or the lack of awareness of the person's own deficit, frequently accompanies hemispatial neglect.

AMNESIA

Memory and mechanisms for recall are located in the hippocampus of the temporal lobe. The common memory disorders are summarized in Table 114–6. Degeneration of the hippocampus or its connections results in the inability to form new memories and is a central accompaniment of Alzheimer's disease. Concussion injuries typically induce severe retrograde amnesia (the inability to recall events that occurred before the injury) and mild anterograde amnesia (the inability to recall events that occur after the injury).

Transient global amnesia typically affects persons older than 65 years and consists of abrupt onset of amnesia for time, place, and recent memory and lasts less than 12 hours. Patients are distressed and repeatedly require reorientation to their environment. They are, however, able to carry out

Table 114–6	Common Disorders of Memory

Benign forgetfulness of aging
Mild cognitive impairment (MCI), Alzheimer's disease, other dementias
Head trauma
Transient global amnesia
Korsakoff's syndrome (thiamine deficiency)
Encephalitis (herpes simplex)
Stroke (posterior cerebral artery)
Temporal lobe seizures
Psychogenic disorders

complex, previously learned tasks such as driving. Although the cause is not known, hippocampal abnormalities are detectable by imaging in most patients.

Korsakoff's syndrome is the end result of untreated or partially treated *Wernicke's encephalopathy* caused by thiamine deficiency. Patients (many of whom are alcoholic or malnourished) exhibit confusion, gait ataxia, nystagmus, and ophthalmoparesis. The condition may be precipitated by the administration of glucose unless thiamine is given in advance. If Korsakoff's syndrome is untreated, a profound inability to form new memories results, with devastating consequences for the patient. In the chronic phase, patients confabulate freely in an attempt to fill the memory void.

Psychogenic amnesia often affects long-term memory, as well as recent memory, and patients are occasionally unable to recall their own names. This condition is in contrast to most organic amnestic states, in which only short-term memory is affected and disorientation is greatest for time and place, but never for self.

Prospectus for the Future

Cortical localization of neurologic disease once required neuropathologic study by biopsy or autopsy. Novel imaging methods are making it possible to localize disease reliably in vivo—often with exquisite detail—permitting study of the earliest biochemical and metabolic changes in diseases of the central nervous system.

Reference

Knopman D: Regional cerebral dysfunction. In Goldman L, Ausiello DA (eds): Cecil Textbook of Medicine, 23rd ed. Philadelphia, Elsevier, 2006.

Chapter 115

Dementia and Memory Disturbances

Frederick J. Marshall

Major Dementia Syndromes

Dementia is defined as the progressive loss of intellectual function. Memory loss is the central feature, and specific dementia syndromes characteristically show particular forms of memory impairment. Dementia syndromes also produce specific abnormalities of cognition: language, spatial processing, *praxis* (learned motor behavior), and *executive function* (the ability to plan and sequence events). *Cortical dementia* and *subcortical dementia* subdivide the dementias (Table 115–1). Table 115–2 provides the differential diagnosis of neurodegenerative causes of dementia, and Table 115–3 outlines other causes of dementia. Neurodegeneration is the most common underlying cause of dementia and is seen in Alzheimer's disease (AD), frontotemporal dementia, and diffuse Lewy body disease, among others. Most causes of dementias are untreatable. Potentially correctable causes account for less than 10% of all cases of dementia. Structural processes or infections must be considered along with metabolic and nutritional diseases. Every patient with dementia should have tests of serum electrolytes and vitamin B_{12}, as well as assessments of liver, renal, and thyroid function; serologic studies for syphilis should be done if risk factors are identified. Chronic infections (see Chapter 127) and normal-pressure hydrocephalus should be considered. Magnetic resonance imaging (MRI) of the brain should be performed.

Neuropsychological testing characterizes the pattern of cognitive and memory impairments and is helpful in the differential diagnosis. The Mini-Mental State Examination (Table 115–4) is a standard test that should be used as a bedside or office screening tool for identifying patients with dementia. This examination emphasizes memory and language and is better than other tests for detecting cortical rather than subcortical dementia. In addition to the Mini-Mental State Examination, patients with dementia should have tests of visuospatial processing (clock drawing), praxis *(show how you would comb your hair; show how you would blow out a match)*, and verbal fluency *(name as many animals as you can in 60 seconds)*.

ALZHEIMER'S DISEASE

AD accounts for approximately 70% of all cases of dementia in older adults. Nearly 5 million persons in the United States are affected, and this number will double by 2020 as the population ages. AD places enormous burdens on the patient, on the family, and on society; annual direct and indirect expenditures are estimated to exceed $100 billion. The incidence of AD increases with age, and the disease occurs in up to 30% of persons older than 85 years of age.

AD has many causes, but none are fully defined. All causes, however, produce similar clinical and pathologic findings. Pathologically, the disease is characterized by the progressive loss of cortical neurons and the formation of amyloid plaques and intraneuronal neurofibrillary tangles. β-Amyloid (Aβ) is the major component of the plaques, whereas hyperphosphorylated *tau* protein is the major constituent of the neurofibrillary tangles. The process starts in the hippocampus and entorhinal cortex and spreads to involve diffuse areas of association cortex in the temporal, parietal, and frontal lobes. The relative deficiency of cortical acetylcholine (resulting from the loss of neurons in the nucleus basalis) provides the rationale for symptomatic treatment of the disease with centrally acting acetylcholinesterase inhibitors.

Pathogenesis

AD is often categorized into two forms: (1) a young-onset hereditary or familial form, which is extremely uncommon and for which three specific genetic abnormalities have been determined, and (2) a more common, sporadic form that typically occurs in persons older than 65 years of age (Table 115–5).

The autosomal-dominant, early-onset forms of AD have provided clues to the molecular pathogenesis of sporadic AD. Progressive dementia and pathologic changes characteristic of AD are almost universal in older patients with Down syndrome (trisomy 21). This observation suggested that chromosome 21 harbors a gene responsible for AD. Aβ is a cleavage product of the amyloid precursor protein, the

Table 115–1 Distinguishing Characteristics of Cortical and Subcortical Dementias

Cortical Dementia

Symptoms: major changes in memory, language deficits, perceptual deficits, praxis disturbances

Affected brain regions: temporal cortex (medial), parietal cortex, and frontal lobe cortex

Examples: Alzheimer's disease, diffuse Lewy body disease, vascular dementia, frontotemporal dementias

Subcortical Dementia

Symptoms: behavioral changes, impaired affect and mood, motor slowing, executive dysfunction, less severe changes in memory

Affected brain regions: thalamus, striatum, midbrain, striatofrontal projections

Examples: Parkinson's disease, progressive supranuclear palsy, normal-pressure hydrocephalus, Huntington's disease, Creutzfeldt-Jakob disease, chronic meningitis

Table 115–2 Etiologic Diagnosis of Neurodegenerative Dementia in Adults

Alzheimer's disease*

Parkinson's disease*

Diffuse Lewy body disease*

Progressive supranuclear palsy

Corticobasal-ganglionic degeneration

Multisystem atrophy

Striatonigral degeneration

Olivopontocerebellar degeneration

Shy-Drager syndrome

Huntington's disease

Frontotemporal dementias

Pick's disease

Frontotemporal dementia without characteristic neuropathology

Frontotemporal dementia with motor neuron disease

Hallervorden-Spatz disease

*Denotes conditions for which symptomatic treatment is available.

Table 115–3 Other Causes of Progressive Dementia in Adults

Structural Disease or Trauma

Normal-pressure hydrocephalus[†]

Neoplasms[†]

Dementia pugilistica (multiple concussions in boxers)

Vascular Disease

Vascular dementia*

Vasculitis[†]

Heredometabolic Disease

Wilson's disease[†]

Neuronal-ceroid lipofuscinosis (Kufs' disease)

Other late-onset lysosomal storage diseases

Demyelinating or Dysmyelinating Disease

Multiple sclerosis*

Metachromatic leukodystrophy

Infectious Disease

Human immunodeficiency virus, type 1[†]

Tertiary syphilis[†]

Creutzfeldt-Jakob disease

Progressive multifocal leukoencephalopathy

Whipple's disease[†]

Chronic meningitis[†]

Cryptococcal meningitis[†]

Others

Metabolic or Nutritional Disease

Vitamin B_{12} deficiency[†]

Thyroid hormone deficiency or excess[†]

Thiamine deficiency[†] (Wernicke-Korsakoff syndrome)

Alcoholism*

Psychiatric Disease

Pseudodementia from depression[†]

*Denotes conditions for which symptomatic treatment is available.
[†]Denotes conditions for which preventive or corrective treatment is available.

gene for which is on chromosome 21. Abnormal processing of amyloid precursor protein into the amyloidogenic fragment $A\beta_{42}$ may be important in the pathogenesis of AD. The *apolipoprotein E (ApoE)* gene was found to be a susceptibility locus for sporadic AD in late-onset familial AD pedigrees. The gene is polymorphic (ϵ2/3/4), and persons who inherit one or both ϵ4 alleles are at increased risk of developing AD. ApoE-ϵ4 interacts selectively with $A\beta$ and with *tau* protein, but how ApoE-ϵ4 increases the risk of AD is still unknown.

Table 115–4   Elements of the Mini-Mental State Examination*

Cognitive Domain	Items	Score
Attention, concentration	Spell *world* backward (or perform *serial 7s* subtraction)	5
Memory and Orientation		
Temporal	Indicate year, season, month, day, date	5
Spatial	Indicate state, country, city, building, floor	5
Learning		
Immediate recall	Register three words *(apple, table, penny)*	3
Delayed recall	Recall three words *(apple, table, penny)*	3
Language		
Naming	Name two objects *(pen, watch)*	2
Repetition	Repeat phrase *(no ifs, ands, or buts)*	1
Comprehension	Follow three-step verbal command	3
	Follow one-step written command	1
Writing	Write original sentence	1
Visuospatial processing	Copy intersecting pentagons	1
	Total possible score	30

*Based on data from Folstein M, Folstein S, McHugh P: "Mini-mental state"—A practical method for grading the cognitive state of patients for the clinician. J Psychiatr Res 12:189–198, 1975.

Table 115–5   Familial Versus Sporadic Alzheimer's Disease

Chromosome/Gene	Age at Onset (yr)	% of All FAD Cases	% of All AD Cases
Familial Alzheimer's Disease: Early Onset, Autosomal Dominant			
1/presenilin 2	40–80	5–10	<0.5
14/presenilin 1	30–60	70	<1
21/amyloid precursor protein	35–65	5	<0.5
Sporadic Alzheimer's Disease: Late Onset, Possibly Polygenetic ± Possibly Environmental			
No single determinant gene†	Usually >60	—	98

AD = Alzheimer's disease; FAD = familial Alzheimer's disease.
†Apolipoprotein E-ε4 allele on chromosome 19 yields increased risk compared with ε2 or ε3 allele.

Clinical Features

AD begins gradually and affects multiple cognitive functions: memory, orientation, language, visuospatial processing, praxis, judgment, and insight. Depression is frequent early in AD; frank psychosis with agitation and behavioral disinhibition often occur in advanced stages. Patients become dependent on others for all activities of daily living. The rate of progression of AD is variable, usually taking 5 to 15 years to progress from presentation to advanced illness. Diagnostic criteria are outlined in Table 115–6. Although a definitive diagnosis of AD requires biopsy (rarely done) or autopsy confirmation, these diagnostic criteria establish the diagnosis with more than 85% specificity in moderately demented patients.

Treatment

Treatments for AD have been developed. Although their benefits are modest, the cholinesterase-inhibiting drugs tacrine (Cognex), donepezil (Aricept), rivastigmine (Exelon), and galantamine (Reminyl/Razadyne) represent important advances. Tacrine can be hepatotoxic and must be given four times a day; donepezil is given once a day and has fewer side effects than tacrine. In clinical trials, cholinesterase inhibitors benefited fewer than 50% of patients. The glutamate

Table 115–6 Diagnostic Criteria for Probable Alzheimer's Disease

Progressive functional decline and dementia established by clinical examination and mental status testing and confirmed by neuropsychological assessment

Cognitive deficits in two or more domains (including memory impairment)

Normal level of consciousness at presentation

Not developmentally acquired; onset between 40 and 90 yr

Absence of other illnesses capable of causing dementia

antagonist memantine (Namenda) has been shown to prolong daily function in patients with moderate-to-advanced AD.

Nursing services provide oversight of hygiene, nutrition, and medication compliance. Antipsychotics, antidepressants, and anxiolytics are useful for patients with behavioral disturbances, which are the most common cause of nursing home placement. Acetylcholinesterase inhibition may also benefit the behavioral disorder.

DIFFUSE LEWY BODY DISEASE

Lewy bodies are pathologic inclusions that are the hallmark of Parkinson's disease when they are restricted to the brainstem (see Chapter 121). Patients with diffuse Lewy body disease have clinical parkinsonism (slow movement, rigidity, and balance problems) combined with early and prominent dementia. Pathologically, Lewy bodies are found in the brain-stem, limbic system, and cortex. Visual hallucinations and cognitive fluctuations are common, and patients are increasingly sensitive to the adverse effects of neuroleptic medication. Diffuse Lewy body disease may represent the second most common cause of dementia after AD. However, the common concurrence of the pathologic features of diffuse Lewy body disease with the classic neuritic plaques and neurofibrillary tangles of AD complicates the identification of the cause of dementia in a given patient.

VASCULAR DEMENTIA

Approximately 10% to 20% of older patients with dementia have radiographic evidence of focal stroke on MRI or computed tomography, combined with focal signs on the neurologic examination. When the dementia syndrome begins with the stroke, and when the progression of the illness is stepwise (suggesting recurrent vascular events), the diagnosis of *vascular dementia* is likely. Patients typically develop early incontinence, gait disturbances, and flattening of affect. A subcortical dementing process attributed to small vessel disease in the periventricular white matter has been referred to as *Binswanger's disease,* but it may merely be a radiographic finding rather than a true disease. Appropriate treatment of risk factors for vascular disease—blood pressure control, smoking cessation, diet modification, and anticoagulation (in select settings such as atrial fibrillation)—is clearly mandatory and may be of benefit.

FRONTOTEMPORAL DEMENTIAS

Unlike AD, in which the presenting symptom is typically memory loss, frontotemporal dementia often begins with significant behavioral disturbances. Patients with *Pick's disease,* the classic form of frontotemporal dementia, are frequently irascible and socially disinhibited. As in AD, the illness progresses for years; no intervention slows the inevitable decline of these patients. Approximately 50% of patients have a family history of the disease; for some families, a mutation in the *tau* protein gene on chromosome 17 is the cause.

PARKINSON'S DISEASE

Nearly 50% of patients with Parkinson's disease (see Chapter 121) become demented by the time they reach the age of 85 years. The dementia of Parkinson's disease affects executive function out of proportion to its impact on language and visuospatial processing. Thought processes appear to slow down (*bradyphrenia*), analogous to the slowing of movement (*bradykinesia*). Because dementia occurs relatively late in the progression of Parkinson's disease, most patients are taking drugs to improve their movement disorder by enhancing dopaminergic neurotransmission. These drugs can induce psychosis. Dose reductions should be attempted before the diagnosis of underlying dementia in these patients is made. Acetylcholinesterase inhibition has recently been shown to be helpful in patients with dementia caused by Parkinson's disease.

NORMAL-PRESSURE HYDROCEPHALUS

The triad of dementia (typically subcortical), gait instability, and urinary incontinence suggests *normal pressure hydrocephalus.* These patients walk with their *feet stuck to the floor,* without lifting up the knees and with a broad base. Symptoms evolve over the course of weeks to months, and brain imaging reveals ventricular enlargement out of proportion to the amount of cortical atrophy. Numerous diagnostic tests have been described, including radionuclide cisternography and MRI flow studies. The most important test remains a therapeutic lumbar puncture with removal of a large amount of cerebrospinal fluid, followed by examination of the patient's gait and cognitive function. Neurosurgical placement of a ventriculoperitoneal shunt may correct the problem. Patients likely to benefit from shunt placement have a clear response to the removal of 30 to 40 mL of spinal fluid, with improved gait and alertness within minutes to hours of the procedure. The cause of normal-pressure hydrocephalus is a derangement of the cerebrospinal fluid hydrodynamics. Shunt placement is most likely to be effective if normal-pressure hydrocephalus occurs after severe head trauma or subarachnoid hemorrhage.

PRION INFECTION, CHRONIC MENINGITIS, DEMENTIA RELATED TO ACQUIRED IMMUNODEFICIENCY SYNDROME

Creutzfeldt-Jakob disease (CJD) is a subacute, dementing, transmissible illness with typical onset between 40 and 75 years of age and an incidence of 1 in 1,000,000 (see Chapter 127). The disease causes spongiform degeneration and gliosis in widespread areas of the cortex. Clinical variants of the disorder are differentiated by the relative predominance of cerebellar symptoms, extrapyramidal hyperkinesias, or visual agnosia and cortical blindness (*Heidenhain's variant*). Ninety percent of patients with CJD have myoclonus, compared with 10% of patients with AD. Patients with all forms of the disease share a relentlessly progressive dementia and disruption of personality over weeks to months. The electroencephalogram develops characteristic abnormalities, including diffuse slowing and periodic sharp waves or spikes. The transmissible agent, a prion protein, is invulnerable to routine modes of antisepsis. Cerebrospinal fluid can be tested for the 14-3-3 protein, although this test is not 100% sensitive or specific for CJD (see Chapter 127).

Certain *infectious agents* can cause the subacute or chronic development of subcortical dementia. These chronic meningitides are discussed in Chapter 127.

Human immunodeficiency virus accesses the central nervous system through monocytes and the microglial system and causes associated neuronal cell loss, vacuolization, and lymphocytic infiltration. The dementia associated with this infection is characterized by bradyphrenia and bradykinesia. Patients have executive dysfunction, impaired memory, poor concentration, and apathy. Treatment of the underlying viral infection with protease inhibitors and reverse transcriptase inhibitors may slow the progression of the dementia (see Chapter 127).

Other Memory Disturbances

STRUCTURE OF MEMORY

Memory function is divided into introspective processes (declarative, explicit, aware memories) and those that are not accessible to introspection (nondeclarative, implicit, procedural memories). Short-term memory (e.g., for words on a list) is a form of *declarative memory*. Other forms include the conscious recall of episodes from personal experience (*episodic memory*), factual knowledge (*semantic memory*) that can be consciously recalled and stated (declared), and the ability to remember (*prospective memory*). Thus, declarative memories involve consciously *knowing that. . . .* Patients with amnesia resulting from lesions of the medial temporal lobes or midline diencephalic structures have deficits of declarative memory.

Nondeclarative memory encompasses several distinct and neuroanatomically less clearly localized functions related to the performance of specific learned motor, cognitive, or perceptual tasks. Nondeclarative (procedural) memories involve unconsciously *knowing how. . . .* Deficits in nondeclarative memory may involve various areas of association neocortex, depending on the nature of the task (e.g., parieto-occipital cortex for visual perceptual tasks, frontal association cortex for motor tasks). Patients with amnesia resulting from lesions of the medial temporal lobes tend to perform normally on tests of nondeclarative memory.

Anterograde amnesia refers to the inability to learn new information. It commonly occurs after brain injury or in association with dementia. The inability to recollect prior information is known as *retrograde amnesia*. Both types of amnesia usually occur together in brain injury syndromes, although the extent of one type or the other may vary.

ISOLATED DISORDERS OF MEMORY FUNCTION

Memory can be impaired in relative isolation as a consequence of head injury, thiamine deficiency (Korsakoff's syndrome), benign forgetfulness of aging, transient global amnesia, or psychogenic disease.

Head injury typically results in retrograde amnesia in excess of anterograde amnesia, with both forms stretching out in time away from the discrete event. As time passes, these disrupted memories generally gradually return, although rarely to the point at which the events immediately surrounding the trauma are recalled.

Korsakoff's syndrome is characterized by the near-total inability to establish new memory. Patients often confabulate responses when they are asked to convey the details of their current circumstance or to relay the content of a recently presented story. Deficiency of thiamine and other nutritional deficiencies in the context of chronic alcoholism are the most common underlying causes. Thiamine is a necessary co-factor in the metabolism of glucose, and for this reason, thiamine must be replenished at the same time glucose is administered whenever a comatose patient is presented to the emergency department.

Aging is associated with mild loss of memory, exhibited by difficulty in recalling names and forgetfulness for dates. Population-based assessments of neuropsychological function have demonstrated that poor performance on delayed-recall tasks is the most sensitive indicator of cognitive change with advancing age. Verbal fluency, in contrast, remains intact with advancing age, and vocabulary may increase with time, even into old age.

Transient global amnesia is a dramatic memory disturbance that affects older patients (>50 years). Patients usually have only one episode; occasionally, episodes recur over the course of several years. Patients have complete temporal and spatial disorientation; orientation for person is preserved. Near-total retrograde and anterograde amnesia persists for variable periods, typically 6 to 12 hours. Patients are often anxious and may repeat the same question over and over again. Transient global amnesia may be confused with psychogenic amnesia, fugue state, or partial complex status epilepticus. Transient global amnesia is thought to reflect underlying vascular insufficiency to the hippocampus or midline thalamic projections.

Unlike patients with organic memory disturbances, patients with *psychogenic amnesia* typically have inconsistent loss of recent and remote memory, relatively more loss of emotionally charged memory (rather than relatively less loss of such memory in organic disease), and an apparent indifference to their own plight—they ask few questions. Most characteristically, patients with psychogenic amnesia tend to express disorientation to person (asking, *Who am I?*), a phenomenon seldom seen in organic memory disturbance.

Patients with *severe depression* may exhibit *pseudodementia*. Vegetative signs, including changes in appetite, weight, and sleep pattern, are common, whereas signs of cortical impairment, such as aphasia, agnosia, and apraxia, are rare. Memory and bradyphrenia improve with antidepressant therapy. Depression often co-exists with other causes of dementia: AD, Parkinson's disease, and vascular dementia.

Prospectus for the Future

Molecular Genetics and the Future of the Diagnosis and Treatment of Dementia

Breakthroughs in the fields of proteomics, information processing of megadata sets, and messenger-RNA expression profiling promise to improve the diagnosis and treatment of dementia in the future. In all likelihood, AD will be subcategorized into more precise etiologic categories, and patients will be offered selective treatments based on their particular pharmacogenetic background. Drug development will be enhanced by emerging knowledge about the molecular mechanisms of Aβ deposition, synaptic loss, and *tau* protein hyperphosphorylation. Treatment strategies currently in clinical trials include decreasing Aβ peptide production by blocking α-secretase or β-secretase or upregulating cleavage of the amyloid precursor protein at the α-secretase site. In addition, studies of active and passive immunization designed to lower brain Aβ levels are ongoing. Although acetylcholinesterase inhibition has not been shown to be effective in the treatment of mild cognitive impairment (considered to be a precursor condition to AD), these novel molecular and immunologic approaches continue to hold promise for disease modifying treatments in the future.

References

Cummings JL: Alzheimer's disease. N Engl J Med 351:56–67, 2004.

Doody RS, Stevens JC, Beck C, et al: Practice parameter: Management of dementia (an evidence-based review). Report of the Quality Standards Subcommittee of the American Academy of Neurology. Neurology 56:1154–1166, 2001.

Jacobsen JS, Reinhar P, Pangalos MN: Current concepts in therapeutic strategies targeting cognitive decline and disease modification in Alzheimer's disease. NeuroRx 2:612–626, 2005.

Knopman DS, DeKosky ST, Cummings JL, et al: Practice parameter: Diagnosis of dementia (an evidence-based review). Report of the Quality Standards Subcommittee of the American Academy of Neurology. Neurology 56:1143–1153, 2001.

Mendez MF, Cummings JL: Amnesia and aphasia. In Goldman L, Bennett JC (eds): Cecil Textbook of Medicine, 21st ed. Philadelphia, WB Saunders, 2000, pp 2038–2042.

Selkoe DJ: American College of Physicians, American Physiological Society: Alzheimer disease: Mechanistic understanding predicts novel therapies. Ann Intern Med 140:627–638, 2004.

Troster AI (ed): Memory in Neurodegenerative Disease: Biological, Cognitive, and Clinical Perspectives. Cambridge, UK, Cambridge University Press, 1998.

Disorders of Mood and Behavior

Frederick J. Marshall

The major disorders of mood and behavior are outlined in Tables 116–1 through 116–3, adapted from the fourth edition of the *Diagnostic and Statistical Manual of Mental Disorders* (DSM-IV). The DSM-IV uses a multi-axial classification system for psychiatric illness, medical illness, personality structure, and social and environmental factors. This approach provides an integrated picture of the impediments to an individual's functional adaptation. Table 116–4 outlines the multi-axial diagnostic approach of the DSM-IV.

Psychotic Disorders

Psychosis is a disordered pattern of thought, perception, emotion, and behavior. The psychotic person has a bizarre sense of reality, with emotional and cognitive impairment, leading to loss of function in the environment. Some primary features of psychosis are outlined in Table 116–5. Psychotic disorders may be *functional* (without known biologic cause) or *organic* (resulting from medical or neurologic illness). Drug intoxication and withdrawal may cause psychosis. Clues to the possible organic basis of psychosis include the following: substantial memory loss, clouding of consciousness, absence of a family or personal history of psychiatric illness, presence of a serious underlying medical or neurologic condition, acute onset of symptoms, visual rather than auditory hallucinations, and presence of myoclonus or asterixis.

Schizophrenia, the most common form of psychosis, affects 1% to 2% of people worldwide. The illness places an enormous burden on individuals, families, and society, leads to pervasive dysfunction, and causes downward social mobility. Schizophrenia is more prevalent among individuals in the lower socioeconomic strata than the general population. Between psychotic episodes, patients show social withdrawal, odd manners, flat or inappropriate affect, and eccentric thinking. Patients may be diagnosed with a personality disorder (schizoid, borderline, schizotypal, or antisocial) before their first acute psychotic episode, which typically occurs between the ages of 15 and 35 years.

Although schizophrenia has a strong genetic component, its cause remains poorly understood. The risk of developing schizophrenia is 10% to 15% if one parent is affected and 30% to 40% if both parents are affected. Earlier theories about *schizophrenogenic* parenting styles are poorly supported. Abnormal family dynamics may be the result of (rather than the cause of) a child with schizophrenia.

Schizophrenia is a chronic disorder for which no cure exists. *Positive symptoms* include delusions and hallucinations; *negative symptoms* include emotional withdrawal and apathy. Psychotropic medications are useful to control positive symptoms, but they offer little benefit for negative symptoms.

Evidence for the dopamine hypothesis of schizophrenia (an imbalance of central dopaminergic neurotransmission) includes the following: the antipsychotic activity of dopamine receptor-blocking neuroleptic medications, the propsychotic activity of levodopa in patients with Parkinson's disease, and the propsychotic activity of amphetamines known to cause the central release of dopamine.

Antipsychotic agents are the mainstay of drug treatment during acute psychotic episodes and should usually be continued during periods of relative remission. These medications may cause drug-induced movement disorders and blunting of affect, as well as other side effects. Many patients and unwary physicians discontinue medications during times of relative remission. This practice generally hastens the return of active psychosis; long-acting depot formulations may be used to ensure compliance. Newer generations of atypical antipsychotic agents have reduced side effects; they hold promise for the management of formerly intractable negative symptoms.

The other psychiatric disorders characterized by psychosis and listed in Table 116–1 differ from schizophrenia in several important respects. *Schizophreniform disorder* is characterized by an increased rapid onset and remission of symptoms, by improved premorbid adjustment and subsequent functioning, and by a negative family history. *Schizoaffective disorder* is an overlap syndrome of schizophrenia and major affective disorder with depressed mood. Prognosis is worse

Table 116–1 Major Disorders of Mood and Behavior

Psychotic Disorders

Schizophrenia
Schizophreniform disorder
Schizoaffective disorder
Mood disorder with psychotic features
Delusional disorder

Mood Disorders

Major depressive disorder
Dysthymic disorder
Bipolar disorder
Cyclothymic disorder

Anxiety Disorders

Panic disorder
Phobic disorder
Obsessive-compulsive disorder
Post-traumatic stress disorder
Generalized anxiety disorder

Somatoform Disorders

Somatization disorder
Conversion disorder
Pain disorder
Hypochondriasis
Body dysmorphic disorder

Factitious Disorders

Dissociative disorder
Dissociative amnesia
Dissociative fugue
Dissociative identity disorder
Depersonalization disorder

Data from the American Psychiatric Association: Diagnostic and Statistical Manual of Mental Disorders, 4th ed. Washington, DC, American Psychiatric Association, 1994.

Table 116–2 Personality Disorders

Paranoid
Schizoid
Schizotypal
Antisocial
Borderline
Histrionic
Narcissistic
Avoidant
Dependent
Obsessive-compulsive

Data from the American Psychiatric Association: Diagnostic and Statistical Manual of Mental Disorders, 4th ed. Washington, DC, American Psychiatric Association, 1994.

Table 116–3 Substance-Related Disorders

Substance	Symptoms
Sedatives: alcohol, barbiturates, benzodiazepines	Acute lethargy, stupor, coma, aware memory loss, apathy
Hallucinogens: cannabis, opioids, mescaline, phencyclidine	Hallucinations
Stimulants: amphetamine, caffeine, cocaine	Agitation, paranoia

Table 116–4 Multi-axial Approach to Diagnosis

Axis I	Clinical psychiatric disorders
Axis II	Personality disorders, mental retardation
Axis III	General medical conditions
Axis IV	Psychosocial and environmental problems
Axis V	Global assessment of functioning

Data from the American Psychiatric Association: Diagnostic and Statistical Manual of Mental Disorders, 4th ed. Washington, DC, American Psychiatric Association, 1994.

than in those with pure affective illness. Patients with *delusional disorder* have isolated delusions (generally of persecution, grandeur, or a spouse's infidelity), without other positive or negative symptoms of schizophrenia.

Depression and Bipolar Disorder

Disorders of mood include *depression* and *mania*. Classification is based on severity, underlying cause, and whether depression and mania occur together or in isolation. Mood disorders affect up to 30% of the U.S. population. Certain medical conditions are strongly associated with depression: carcinoma of the pancreas, lung cancer, brain tumors

(particularly those affecting the frontal lobes), Cushing's disease (and exogenous steroid use), hypothyroidism, aftermath of myocardial infarction, Parkinson's disease, stroke, and Huntington's disease. Table 116–6 outlines important features of depression, and Table 116–7 outlines features of mania.

Depression occurs when sadness or grief lasts longer than usual and causes dysfunction. *Dysthymia* is prolonged but relatively minor depression. *Cyclothymia* is minor depression alternating with hypomania. *Major depression* causes severe and chronic depressive symptoms with vegetative signs

Table 116–5   Common Features of Psychosis

Disruption of the Form and Flow of Thought and Speech

Flight of ideas (disconnected ideas, incoherent speech, loose associations)

Pressured speech (rapid and unrelenting speech)

Thought blocking (speech halted for variable intervals)

Clanging (rhyming speech without meaningful content)

Echolalia (sing-song repetition of recently heard words or phrases)

Neologisms (idiosyncratic or newly coined words)

Alogia (paucity of speech, mutism)

Disruption of the Content of Thought and Perception

Delusions (false beliefs about reality that are not amenable to revision by fact)

Persecutory delusions (others intend the person harm)

Delusions of grandeur (person is famous or all powerful)

Delusions of reference (events or others' actions are directed at the person)

Thought broadcasting (the person's thoughts can be sensed by others)

Thought insertion (others' thoughts are invading the person's mind)

Loss of insight (unawareness of the person's illness)

Hallucinations (typically auditory > visual in schizophrenia; visual > auditory in organic psychoses)

Disruption of Emotions

Blunting of affect

Inappropriate affect

Labile affect

Disruption of behavior

Ritual behavior

Aggressiveness

Sexual inappropriateness

Posturing or grimacing

Mimicking

Withdrawal

Data from Tomb DA: Psychiatry, 5th ed. Baltimore, Williams & Wilkins, 1995.

Table 116–6   Clinical Features of Depression

Emotional Content

Interpersonal withdrawal

Anhedonia

Sadness

Irritability

Anxiety

Thought Content

Guilt

Self-criticism, worthlessness

Pessimism, hopelessness

Distractibility

Indecision

Delusions and hallucinations

Memory complaints

Physical Content (Vegetative Features)

Fatigue

Insomnia

Hypersomnia

Anorexia

Overeating

Weight loss

Weight gain

Poor libido

Somatic complaints

Psychomotor retardation

Psychomotor agitation

Data from Tomb DA: Psychiatry, 5th ed. Baltimore, Williams & Wilkins, 1995.

(sleep disturbance, change of appetite or weight, loss of libido). Patients vary widely in the duration and pattern of recurrence of these signs and symptoms. Patients may have associated psychotic thought content, generally of self-blame or persecution. Memory may be severely impaired; the distinction between depression and dementia is particularly challenging in elderly patients, in whom both conditions often co-exist. Major depression is more common in women than in men. Most young people with one attack of major depression will have another during their lifetime; approximately 10% develop lifelong dysthymia. An episode of major depression comes on gradually over the course of months and may last up to 3 years or more.

Abnormalities of the neurotransmitters norepinephrine and serotonin play a major role in mood disorders: their levels or effects are underactive in depression and are overactive in mania. Treatments that affect these neurotransmitters include tricyclic antidepressants, monoamine oxidase inhibitors, and selective serotonin reuptake inhibitors (SSRIs). All patients with major depression and most patients with chronic minor depressions merit a trial of antidepressant medication (typically starting with an SSRI or tricyclic antidepressant). Adequate trials require increasing doses over the course of 4 to 6 weeks. Therapeutic counseling should also be offered. Electroconvulsive therapy is useful in patients with refractory depression, acute suicide ideation, or concomitant psychosis that is unresponsive to antipsychotic drugs.

Bipolar disorder shows 70% concordance in monozygotic twins. Men and women are equally at risk. First-degree relatives have a 5% to 10% lifetime risk (compared with

Table 116–7	**Clinical Features of Mania**

Emotional Content

Euphoria
Emotional lability
Irritability

Thought Content

Egocentric
Grandiose
Poor judgment
Pressured speech
Delusions
Hallucinations

Physical Content

Insomnia
Hyperarousal
Loss of appetite
Psychomotor agitation

Data from Tomb DA: Psychiatry, 5th ed. Baltimore, Williams & Wilkins, 1995.

Table 116–8	**Clinical Features of Anxiety**

Emotional Content

Tension
Irritability
Apprehension
Fear

Thought Content

Obsessions
Ruminations
Distractibility

Physical Content

Psychomotor agitation
Insomnia
Loss of appetite
Loss of libido
Palpitations
Diarrhea
Sweating
Urinary frequency

Table 116–9	**Medical Illnesses that Can Indicate Anxiety**

Neurologic

Encephalitis
Meniere's disease

Cardiac

Angina
Mitral valve prolapse

Pulmonary

Chronic obstructive pulmonary disease
Asthma

Metabolic or Endocrine

Acute intermittent porphyria
Hyperthyroidism
Hypoglycemia
Pheochromocytoma
Carcinoid tumor

Gastrointestinal

Bleeding ulcer
Ulcerative colitis

Data from Tomb DA: Psychiatry, 5th ed. Baltimore, Williams & Wilkins, 1995.

1% to 2% in the general population). More than 90% of patients have periods of depression. Attacks of mania and depression are usually separated by years, but some patients have *rapid cycling* (four or more episodes per year). Rapid cycling is more common in women than in men. Lithium, carbamazepine, and valproate are used alone or in combination with antidepressants to prevent recurrence of symptoms. Acute mania may require treatment with neuroleptic agents.

Anxiety Disorders

Common clinical features of anxiety disorders are outlined in Table 116–8. *Chronic generalized anxiety* is a familial trait, with depression developing in up to one half of all patients at some point in life. Treatment is challenging. Benzodiazepines provide short-term benefit, but they are associated with a risk of long-term addiction. Buspirone (BuSpar) and tricyclic antidepressants are useful, especially in patients with concomitant depression.

Panic disorder involves episodic, acute-onset, overwhelming anxiety accompanied by autonomic symptoms (e.g., palpitations, sweating) and a feeling of impending doom. Medical conditions that may produce panic are outlined in Table 116–9.

Phobic disorders involve irrational fear of specific objects or events. The fear may be overwhelming and may result in reclusive, eccentric behavior. *Agoraphobia*, the fear of being in public situations from which escape may be difficult (typically new situations or wide-open spaces), is named for the ancient Greek open marketplace *(agora)*. This phobia is common in elderly patients or in persons with chronic medical illness; it can occur with or without associated panic attacks. *Specific phobias* (formerly known as simple phobias) include discrete, irrational fears of specific objects or situations. Common specific phobias include fear of flying, fear of enclosed spaces, and fear of snakes. Treatment of the phobic disorders often involves desensitization with behavioral therapy.

Obsessive-compulsive disorder has a strong genetic component, but its underlying origin remains unknown. *Obsessions* are recurrent unwanted thoughts (e.g., self-deprecatory preoccupations, fears of contamination); *compulsions* are repetitive unwanted *(ego-dystonic)* behaviors (e.g., hand washing, double-checking whether appliances have been turned off). Treatment with SSRIs may alleviate symptoms in some patients.

Somatoform Disorders

The somatoform disorders involve psychological preoccupation with physical symptoms. Patients with *somatization disorder* have numerous physical symptoms involving several organ systems. Symptoms tend to be migratory (both in time and space) and are exhibited with dramatic flair. The patient insists on complete medical attention. Symptoms include ill-defined pains, pseudoneurologic symptoms (often poorly described alterations of consciousness), and gastrointestinal, genitourinary, and sexual dysfunction. The disorder is more common in women than it is in men and is frequently associated with concomitant psychiatric illness, including depression, unsuccessful suicide attempts, anxiety, and irritability.

Conversion disorder involves an obvious loss of neurologic function in the absence of organic neurologic disease. Patients do not consciously realize the nonorganic basis of the illness, yet they frequently demonstrate lack of concern for the deficit *(la belle indifférence)*. Clues to the nonorganic nature of common conversion symptoms are outlined in Table 116–10. Patients often have an antecedent psychosocial stressor, as well as unconscious secondary gain (e.g., extra attention from the spouse, relief from onerous work obligations).

Factitious Disorder

Patients with *factitious disorder* intentionally feign physical or psychological symptoms to assume the sick role. Once the condition is diagnosed, patients may disappear, only to present their symptoms to another physician. Patients may change their symptoms once the initial complaints have been thoroughly evaluated. Patients with *Munchausen syndrome* inflict real physical harm on themselves (e.g., ingesting anticoagulants to cause hematuria, injecting contaminated fluids to cause abscesses or fever). Rarely, a parent may provoke symptoms in a child; such *Munchausen syndrome by proxy* can lead to recurrent unexplained pediatric sickness and should raise the physician's suspicion under appropriate circumstances.

In *malingering*, a person consciously feigns disease for concrete personal goals, rather than for psychological goals. The malingerer may intentionally feign disease or may

Table 116–10	**Clues to the Nonorganic Basis of Common Conversion Symptoms**

Pseudoseizures

These episodes are often bizarre, without associated loss of bladder continence or self-injury (tongue biting, lacerations). Patients with pseudoseizures commonly also suffer from true epileptic seizures.

Pseudocoma

The coma is light, with responsiveness to noxious stimulation and subtle avoidance of physical threat (e.g., arm suspended above face and dropped does not strike face, patient shifts to avoid falling from table).

Pseudoparalysis

Weakness is variable, with little resistance to passive movement but intact resistance to gravity. Contraction of antagonist muscles is inappropriate when the patient is asked to engage agonist muscles.

Pseudosensory Loss

This loss may include blindness, deafness, or anesthesia. Blindness may be total but is commonly tunnel loss. If the examiner defines the perimeter of the tunnel by drawing it on a target paper held close to the patient, the tunnel remains the same size when the examiner subsequently steps back (this does not obey fundamental rules of optics). Sensory loss may not respect the midline or may deviate from known anatomic distributions of roots and nerves.

Pseudoataxia

The patient may have swooping dives and thrusts, sustained monopedal postures, and clutching to surfaces. The patient rarely falls. This style of gait is also known as *astasia-abasia* or *stasibasiphobia*.

provoke real (although usually not life-threatening) illness to avoid some unwanted task (e.g., military service).

Dissociative Disorders

Dissociative disorders disrupt the coherent sense of self, and several variants are recognized. In *dissociative amnesia*, patients are unable to recall traumatic personal events, despite intact cognition and memory in other domains. *Dissociative fugue* involves acting in complex ways, such as traveling away from home, without having personal memory of the events or of details of the person's own past. *Dissociative identity disor-*

der (also known as *multiple personality disorder*) involves switching from one internally coherent personality to another; sometimes several distinct personalities are involved. Patients fail to recall important elements of personal history, and transitions among identities are triggered by stress. In *depersonalization disorder,* patients have persistent or recurrent episodes of feeling outside their body or of dispassionately observing their mental processes. The differential diagnosis of the dissociative disorders includes complex partial seizures, factitious disorder, malingering, and psychosis.

Personality Disorders and Substance Abuse

The major personality disorders are listed in Table 116–2. These disorders are generalized styles of behavior that persevere over time and interfere with a person's social functioning. Common classes of abused substances are listed in Table 116–3, along with symptoms of intoxication or addiction.

Prospectus for the Future

Advances in understanding of disease pathogenesis and origin will no doubt occur as ongoing epidemiologic and genetic studies are completed. Pharmacogenomics and proteomics will facilitate customized treatment for patients based on their genetic profiles. Deep brain stimulation with implantable programmable electrodes may provide new therapeutic advantages in cases of refractory obsessive-compulsive disorder or other affective disorders.

References

American Psychiatric Association: Diagnostic and Statistical Manual of Mental Disorders, 4th ed. Washington, DC, American Psychiatric Association, 1994.

Brust J: Nutritional and alcohol related neurologic disorders. In Goldman L, Ausiello DA (eds): Cecil Textbook of Medicine, 23rd ed. Philadelphia, WB Saunders, 2007.

Samet JH: Drug abuse and dependence. In Goldman L, Ausiello DA (eds): Cecil Textbook of Medicine, 22nd ed. Philadelphia, Saunders, 2003.

Schiffer RB: Psychiatric disorders in medical practice. In Goldman L, Ausiello DA (eds): Cecil Textbook of Medicine, 23rd ed. Philadelphia, Saunders, 2007.

Tomb DA: Psychiatry, 5th ed. Baltimore, Williams & Wilkins, 1995.

Disorders of Thermal Regulation

Roger P. Simon

Hypothermia

Hypothermia (core body temperature <35° C [95° F]) may result from disorders that depress the sensorium directly (drug overdose and alcohol abuse), from disorders that affect the anterior hypothalamus directly (Wernicke's encephalopathy and hypoglycemia), or from environmental cold exposure (Table 117–1). Alcohol predisposes the individual to hypothermia by inducing vasodilation and attenuating peripheral vasoconstriction; neuroleptic drugs vasodilate and suppress shivering as well. Because the body's ability to vasoconstrict and shiver diminishes with age, older adults are at greatest risk.

In mild or early hypothermia, shivering appears and muscle tone increases, coordination is poor, speech becomes slurred, and judgment is impaired; in severe cases, the patient may be presumed dead because of barely detectable pulse or respiration and unmeasurable blood pressure. Patients' bodies are cold to the touch. Mental function remains normal to 34° C (93° F). Major deviations from the neurologic signs and vital sign changes outlined in Table 117–2 should prompt a search for factors other than hypothermia that are responsible for nervous system dysfunction.

Physiologic responses to hypothermia (see Table 117–2) reflect three responses to progressive temperature reduction:

1. Shivering, which doubles or triples muscle heat output above 30° to 32° C.
2. Decreasing metabolism (blood pressure, pulse, and respiration) at 32° to 28° C.
3. Poikilothermia below 28° C. The electroencephalogram shows diffuse slowing and is isoelectric below 20° C.

The severity of the underlying disease, not the features of the neurologic examination or the degree of hypothermia, predicts survival. Hypothyroidism causing hypothermia is an exception because the degree of thyroid dysfunction is related to outcome. Hypothermia-induced neurologic abnormalities are fully reversible with rewarming.

Treatment begins with passive external rewarming, suitable for mild hypothermia. For more severe hypothermia, active external and core rewarming may be required. A number of methods such as heating lamps, hot tubs, warm fluid lavage of body cavities, and cardiopulmonary bypass have been recommended. Warmed (42° to 45° C), humidified inhaled oxygen should be part of any regimen. All patients with hypothermia are hypovolemic and require intravenous fluids.

Hyperthermia

Hyperthermia (core body temperature >41° C [105.8° F]) results from environmental heat exposure with or without exertion (heat stroke or heat exhaustion), from anesthesia in persons with an inherited defect of calcium transport in skeletal muscle (malignant hyperthermia), or as an idiosyncratic reaction to neuroleptics involving blockade of central dopamine receptors (neuroleptic malignant syndrome). The features of these three forms of hyperthermia are compared in Table 117–3.

Heat stroke or *heat exhaustion* occurs in young persons, who overexert themselves in a hot, humid climate (e.g., military recruits); in older adults, who cannot dissipate heat generated at rest (sometimes as a result of drugs with anticholinergic properties, such as tricyclic antidepressants and antihistamines; phenothiazine, butyrophenone, and thioxanthene use also predisposes older adults to heat stroke); and in patients with schizophrenia medicated with anticholinergics or neuroleptics. In the most severe form (heat stroke), core temperature rises very rapidly to 40.4° C (105° F) or greater. Altered consciousness ranges from confusion to coma. Patients may, but more often do not, sweat. Tachycardia is universal. More protracted symptoms of dizziness, fatigue, and weakness developing over a few days, constitute heat exhaustion. Rapid reduction in body temperature is mandatory. Evaporative cooling (water spray plus fans) to reduce temperatures to 38.0° to 38.8° C is effective; antipyretics and dantrolene are not.

Hyperthermia and diffuse muscle rigidity *(malignant hyperthermia)* occur most often with the use of halothane and succinylcholine. Rigidity of limb, chest, or jaw muscles occurs within 30 minutes of anesthesia. Hyperthermia may be delayed

Table 117–1   Causes of Hypothermia*

Alcohol abuse	43%
Wernicke's encephalopathy	18%
Age >70	26%
Sepsis or shock	25%
Exposure without other causes	14%
Hypoglycemia	12%
Sedative overdose	10%
Hepatic encephalopathy, uremia	8%
Structural brain disorder, head trauma, hypothyroidism, diabetic ketoacidosis, renal failure, ethylene glycol poisoning	5% or less

*N = 148: more than one factor occurred in 35 patients.
Data from Fischbeck KH, Simon RP: Neurological manifestations of accidental hypothermia. Ann Neurol 10:384–387, 1981.

in onset. Treatment is drug discontinuation and dantrolene (1 to 10 mg/kg IV until muscular relaxation occurs, followed by 4 to 8 mg/kg every 6 hours for 24 to 48 hours).

Neuroleptic malignant syndrome causes hyperthermia, rigidity, and altered mental status; rhabdomyolysis is frequent. Haloperidol is responsible in most cases, but other neuroleptic drugs and withdrawal from levodopa have been implicated. Symptoms begin within 1 to 3 days of drug initiation or dose change. All patients have elevated temperatures (average 39.9° C). Dysphagia, dysarthria, tremors, and altered mental status (agitation to coma) occur early. Treatment is with dantrolene (as discussed earlier) and dopamine agonists (bromocriptine, 2.5 to 10 mg three times daily).

Experimental studies show that elevation of body temperature to 42° C causes a rise in cerebral oxygen consumption, but a subsequent fall occurs at higher temperatures. The electroencephalograph slows above 42° C. Neurologic abnormalities resolve with temperature reduction except for

Table 117–2   Effects of Hypothermia*

	Mild (90°–95° F; 32°–35° C)	Moderate (82°–90° F; 28°–32° C)	Severe (<82° F; <28° C)
Blood pressure and pulse	Normal	Normal to decreased; atrial fibrillation frequent	Decreased; ventricular fibrillation may occur
Respiration	Normal	Normal	Normal to decreased
Level of consciousness	Alert or lethargic	Lethargic	Nonverbal but purposively responsive
Pupils	Normal	Normal to sluggish	Sluggish to fixed
Tendon reflexes	Normal	Normal	Normal to decreased
Muscle tone	Normal or increased	Increased	Increased
Eye movements, posturing, plantar reflexes	No correlation with temperature	—	—

*N = 97.
Data from Fischbeck KH, Simon RP: Neurological manifestations of accidental hypothermia. Ann Neurol 10:384, 1981.

Table 117–3   Comparative Features of Neuroleptic Malignant Syndrome (NMS), Malignant Hyperthermia, and Heat Stroke

	NMS	Malignant Hyperthermia	Heat Stroke
Hyperthermia	+	+	+
Muscle rigidity	+	+	Rare
Sweating	+	+	Rare
Tachycardia	+	+	+
Acidosis	+	+	+
Coagulopathy	+	+	+
Myoglobinuria	+	+	+
Impaired mental status	+	+	+
Genetic predisposition	−	+*	−
Precipitant	Neuroleptics	Halothane, succinylcholine	Heat exposure, exercise
Onset	Hours–days	Minutes–hours	Minutes–hours
Treatment	Dantrolene, dopa agonists	Dantrolene	Rapid external cooling

*MHS1 mutation associated with the *RYR1* gene, chromosome 19, most common.
Modified from data from Lazarus A, Mann SC, Caroff SN: The Neuroleptic Malignant Syndrome and Related Conditions. Washington, DC, American Psychiatric Press, 1989.

a persistent neuropathy in one third of patients. Mortality rises with temperature extremes, but the underlying cause is a better predictor of outcome than the degree of hyperthermia. Temperatures up to 42° C are usually tolerated.

Prospectus for the Future

Hypothermia is now a beneficial treatment for infants with anoxic brain injury and adult patients with coma following cardiac arrest. As this treatment becomes routine, more will be learned about the effect of hypothermia on systemic and brain metabolism.

References

Bouchama A, Knochel JP: Heat stroke. N Engl J Med 346: 1978–1988, 2002.

Danzl DF, Pozos RS: Accidental hypothermia. N Engl J Med 331:1756–1760, 1994.

Litman RS, Rosenberg H: Malignant hyperthermia: Update on susceptibility testing. JAMA 293(23):2918–2924, 2005.

Headache, Neck Pain, and Other Painful Disorders

Timothy J. Counihan

Headache

PAIN-SENSITIVE INTRACRANIAL STRUCTURES

Headache is caused by irritation of pain-sensitive intracranial structures, including the dural sinuses; the intracranial portions of the trigeminal, glossopharyngeal, vagus, and upper cervical nerves; the large arteries; and the venous sinuses. Many structures are insensitive to pain, including the brain parenchyma, the ependymal lining of the ventricles, and the choroid plexuses. That the brain parenchyma itself is insensitive to pain accounts for the not infrequent clinical observation of patients who have large intracerebral lesions, such as intracerebral hematomas or malignant brain tumors, but little or no headache. Painful stimuli arising from brain tissue above the tentorium cerebelli are conveyed by means of the trigeminal nerve, whereas the glossopharyngeal, vagus, and first two cervical nerves convey impulses from the posterior fossa. The term *cervicogenic* headache is sometimes used to indicate that the source of headache (usually occipital in location) emanates from an abnormality in the cervical spine.

EVALUATION OF THE PATIENT WITH HEADACHE

Distinguishing benign from ominous causes of headache is important. A detailed history helps the examiner decide which patients have a symptomatic structural intracranial lesion. The physician should ask about the quality, location, duration, and time course of the headache. What exacerbates or relieves it? Pain intensity is not of much diagnostic value, except for the patient who complains of the acute onset of the worst headache of his or her life. This headache suggests subarachnoid hemorrhage (SAH). The quality of pain *(throbbing, pressure, jabbing)* and the location may also be helpful, especially if the pain is of extracranial origin, such as the temporal location of temporal arteritis. Posterior fossa lesions cause occipitocervical pain, occasionally associated with unilateral retro-orbital pain. Multifocal pain usually implies a benign cause. Clarifying the acuity of onset of the headache is most important; patients who describe the onset of pain as being *like being struck across the head by a bat* suggests the sentinel headache of subarachnoid headache. Equally important is to establish the time course of the headache: Is this a paroxysmal, nonprogressive headache (typical of migraine or tension type headache), or is the headache daily persistent (such as temporal arteritis) or progressive (suggesting the presence of a structural brain lesion)? Patients should be asked about any known triggers for the headache, such as menses, particular foods, caffeine, alcohol, or stress. Positional headache (that is maximal in the upright position and disappears rapidly after lying down) is characteristic of intracranial hypotension (low-pressure headache). Diurnal variation in headache severity may give a clue to its origin; morning headache or headache that awakens a patient from sleep may indicate raised intracranial pressure or sleep apnea as a cause. The presence of associated symptoms such as visual disturbances, nausea, or vomiting should be noted. The history should include inquiries about medications, especially analgesics and over-the-counter remedies. Information regarding the patient's medical history, as well as family history, should also be taken into consideration. In the majority of patients with headache, the physical and neurologic examination is normal, although special attention may be directed toward examination of the eyes for papilledema, as well as the temporal arteries for a palpable nonpulsatile artery.

HEADACHE SYNDROMES

Migraine

Clinical Features. Migraine is an episodic headache disorder characterized by various combinations of neurologic, gastrointestinal, and autonomic changes. The diagnosis is based on the headache's characteristics and associated symptoms. Results of the physical examination, as well as the laboratory studies, are usually normal.

The prevalence of migraine is up to 16% in women and 8% in men. Estimates indicate that 28 million Americans have disabling migraine headaches. All varieties of migraine may begin at any age, from early childhood, although peak ages at onset are adolescence and early adulthood.

Several varieties of migraine are described (Table 118–1), of which the two most common are migraine without aura (formerly known as *common migraine*) and migraine with aura *(classic migraine);* migraine without aura accounts for 80% of patients. Migraine auras are focal neurologic symptoms that precede, accompany, or (rarely) follow an attack. The aura usually develops over 5 to 20 minutes, lasts less than 60 minutes, and can involve visual, sensorimotor, language, or brain stem disturbances. The most common aura is typified by positive visual phenomena (e.g., scintillating scotomata) that precede the headache; they resemble the effect of being too close to a photographer with a flash camera *(phosphenes).* The pain of migraine is often pulsating, unilateral, frontotemporal in distribution, and is often accompanied by anorexia, nausea, and, occasionally, vomiting. In characteristic attacks, patients are intolerant of light (photophobia) and seek rest in a dark room; they may also be intolerant to sound (phonophobia) and occasionally to odors (osmophobia). The diagnosis of migraine requires the presence of at least one of these features, particularly in the absence of gastrointestinal symptoms (Table 118–2). The presence of these symptoms results in a syndrome that is invariably disabling for the patient to the extent that, for the duration of the attack, they are unable to function normally. In children, migraine is often associated with episodic abdominal pain, motion sickness, and sleep disturbances. Onset of typical migraine late in life (older than age 50 years) is rare, although recurrence of migraine that had been in remission is not uncommon. Recurrent migraine headache associated with transient hemiparesis or hemiplegia occurs rarely as a clearly genetically determined disease (familial hemiplegic migraine).

Other rare types of migraine include recurrent ophthalmoplegia and basilar migraine, which occur primarily in childhood and in which severe episodic headache is preceded, or accompanied by, signs of bilateral occipital lobe, brain stem, or cerebellar dysfunction (e.g., diplopia, bilateral visual field abnormalities, ataxia, dysarthria, bilateral sensory or motor disturbances, other cranial nerve signs, occasionally coma). The term *complicated migraine* refers to migraine attacks with major neurologic dysfunction (e.g., migraine with hemiplegia or coma) separate from the visual aura; in these patients, neurologic dysfunction outlasts the headache by hours to 1 or 2 days. Acute severe headache can reflect serious central nervous system disease (Table 118–3). Certain symptoms raise suspicion for a structural brain lesion (Table 118–4).

Causes. A migraine attack is the end result of the interaction of a significant number of factors of varying importance in different individuals. These factors include a genetic predisposition, a susceptibility of the central nervous system to certain stimuli, hormonal factors, and a sequence of neurovascular events. A positive family history is reported in up to 65% to 91% of patients. Familial hemiplegic migraine is associated with mutations in a gene for *P/Q* type calcium channel on chromosome 19 and a gene encoding a sodium-potassium ion pump on chromosome 1. Thus, mutations of diverse channels result in a common phenotype. The cause in the majority of patients is still unknown.

The traditional view has been that the neurologic phenomena of migraine were caused by spasm of cerebral

Table 118–1	Classification of Migraine

Migraine without aura (common migraine)
Migraine with aura (classic migraine)
Complicated migraine
Hemiplegic migraine
Confusional migraine
Ophthalmoplegic migraine
Basilar migraine

Table 118–2	Clinical Features Distinguishing Migraine from Tension Headache		
	Migraine with Aura	**Migraine without Aura**	**Tension Headache**
Aura	Focal neurologic deficit (visual, sensory, language) Onset >4 min Lasts <60 min	No focal neurologic deficit	No focal neurologic deficit
Headache	Unilateral Throbbing and/or pulsating Aggravated by activity Inhibits or prohibits activity Onset within 60 min of aura	Unilateral Throbbing/pulsating Aggravated by activity Inhibits/prohibits activity	Bilateral Nonpulsating (*pressure*) Not aggravated by activity May inhibit but not prohibit activity
Associated symptoms	Nausea ± vomiting Photophobia Phonophobia	Nausea ± vomiting Photophobia Phonophobia	No nausea/vomiting Minimal photophobia

Table 118–3 Differential Diagnosis of Acute Headache—Major Causes

Migraine
Cluster headache
Stroke
Subarachnoid hemorrhage
Intracerebral hemorrhage
Cerebral infarction
Arterial dissection (carotid or vertebral)
Acute hydrocephalus
Meningitis, encephalitis
Giant cell arteritis (often chronic)
Tumor (usually chronic)
Trauma

Table 118–4 Clinical Features of Headaches Suggesting a Structural Brain Lesion

Symptoms

Worst of the patient's life
Progressive
Onset >50 years of age
Worse in early morning—awakens patient
Marked exacerbation with straining
Focal neurologic dysfunction

Signs

Nuchal rigidity
Fever
Papilledema
Pathologic reflexes or reflex asymmetry
Altered state of consciousness

vessels, and the pain was caused by subsequent dilation of extracranial arteries. Good evidence indicates that diminished cerebral blood flow accompanies the aura of the migraine attack. One of the key structures in the mechanism of pain in all migraine is the trigeminal vascular system. Stimulation of the trigeminal nerve or its ganglion can activate serotonin receptors and nerve endings on small dural arteries and result in a state of neurogenic inflammation. The theory asserts that, in migraine, these processes, in turn, stimulate perivascular nerve endings, with resultant orthodromic stimulation of the trigeminal nerve and pain referred to its distribution. The precise role of other factors such as female sex hormones, environmental triggers, and stress in the pathogenesis of migraine remains unclear.

Treatment. The goals of treatment are (1) making an accurate and confident diagnosis of migraine to reassure the patient that no more sinister cause exists for the headache, (2) relieving acute attacks, and (3) preventing pain and associated symptoms of recurrent headaches. The first step is to inform the patient that he or she has a migraine. The benign nature of the disorder and the patient's central role in the treatment plan should be emphasized. The patient must keep a headache diary.

Acute Migraine Attack. Acute attacks are alleviated with single agents or varying combinations of drugs (Fig. 118–1), as well as with behavioral modification therapy. Many attacks of migraine respond to simple analgesics, such as acetaminophen, aspirin, or nonsteroidal anti-inflammatory agents. Opioid drugs have a limited use in the migraine attack. Overuse of analgesics is particularly frequent in patients with headache; one of the most important aspects of therapy of patients with migraine therefore is the monitoring of amounts of analgesic used. In patients who are nauseated, prescribing an antiemetic agent early in an attack is often helpful. Phenothiazine drugs have anti-emetic, prokinetic, and useful sedative properties, but they can produce involuntary movements as an acute adverse effect (acute dystonic reaction).

A large number of *migraine-specific* serotonin agonist drugs have become available (see Fig. 118–1). Although many of these drugs are highly effective in alleviating migraine, patients must be carefully instructed in their appropriate use. Moreover, a response to these medications does not confirm a diagnosis of migraine.

Migraine Prevention. A number of drugs have been used in the prevention of migraine (Table 118–5). The use of these agents should be restricted to patients who have frequent attacks (usually more than four per month) and who are willing to take daily medication. With any of the medications, an adequate trial period should be given, using adequate doses, before it is declared ineffective. Combination therapy is occasionally required but is not routinely prescribed. For a preventative drug to be considered successful, it should reduce the headache frequency rate by 50%. Magnesium supplementation, feverfew, and high-dose riboflavin (vitamin B_2) have been effective in some patients.

Future of Migraine Treatment. Given the increasing experimental evidence that neurogenic inflammation is the principal cause of migraine pain, a predictable increase has occurred in the use of anticonvulsant medication (see Table 118–5) for prevention. Clinical trials are currently underway of an antagonist to calcitonin gene–related peptide (CGRP) as a potentially viable target for the treatment of acute migraine.

Cluster Headache

Clinical Features. Cluster headache comprises a group of symptoms with a relatively specific temporal course. It is uncommon, accounting for less than 10% of all headache sufferers. Unlike migraine, cluster headache is much more common in men than women, and its mean age at onset is

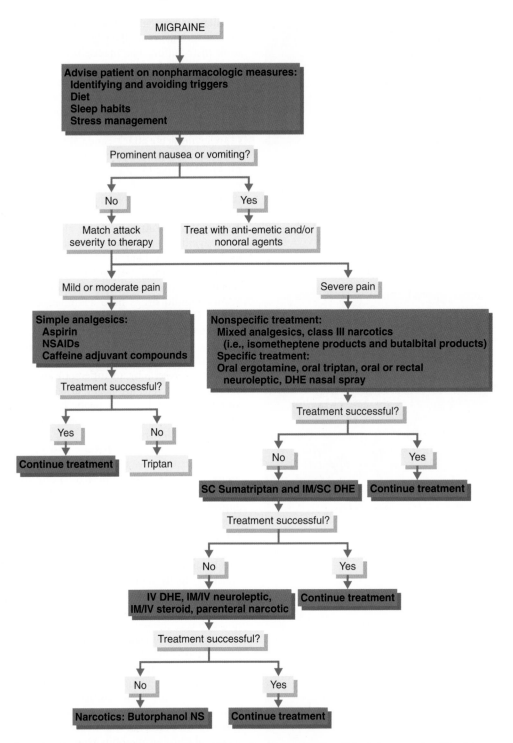

Figure 118–1 Algorithm for the treatment of migraine. DHE = dihydroergotamine; IM = intramuscular; IV = intravenous; NS = normal saline; NSAIDs = nonsteroidal anti-inflammatory drugs; SC = subcutaneous. (Data from Silberstein SD, Young WB, Lipton RB: Migraine and cluster headaches. In Johnson RT, Griffin JW, McArthur JC [eds]: Current Therapy in Neurologic Disease, 6th ed. St. Louis, CV Mosby, 2001.)

later in life than migraine. Also, unlike migraine, cluster headache rarely begins in childhood, and a family history is found less often. Cluster headache has been classified as one of a large number of *trigeminal autonomic cephalgias*. The pain in cluster headache pain is of extreme intensity, is unilateral, and is associated with congestion of the nasal mucosa and injection of the conjunctiva on the side of the pain.

Increased sweating of the ipsilateral side of the forehead and face may occur. Associated ocular signs of Horner's syndrome may be present: miosis, ptosis, and the additional feature of eyelid edema. The pain is usually steady, nonthrobbing, and invariably localized retro-orbitally on one side of the head; it may occasionally spread to the ipsilateral side of the face or neck. Attacks often awaken patients,

Table 118–5   Preventive Therapy for Migraine

Drug Class	Agent	Dose	Adverse Effects
β-Adrenergic receptor blockers	Propranolol	40–160 mg/day	Contraindicated in asthma; nightmares,
	Nadolol	40–160 mg/day	fatigue, syncope
Tricyclic antidepressants	Amitriptyline	10–75 mg once a day at bedtime	Dry mouth, confusion, palpitations
Serotonin reuptake inhibitors	Paroxetine	10–50 mg/day	Insomnia, somnolence, sexual dysfunction
	Sertraline	50–200 mg/day	
Calcium channel blockers	Verapamil	120–900 mg/day	Constipation, edema, hypotension
	Flunarizine*	5 mg/day	Parkinsonism
Serotonin antagonists	Methysergide	2–8 mg/day	Prolonged use associated with fibrotic
	Pizotifen*	0.5–1.5 mg/day	reactions
Anticonvulsants	Divalproex sodium	500–1000 mg/day	Weight gain, tremor
	Gabapentin	300–900 mg/day	Somnolence
	Topiramate	50–200 mg/day	Renal calculi

*Not licensed in the United States.

usually 2 to 3 hours after the onset of sleep. In contrast to migraineurs, resting in a dark, quiet area does not relieve the pain; on the contrary, patients sometimes seek an activity that can distract them.

As the name implies, cluster attacks frequently recur over a period of several days or weeks. These periods of frequent headaches are separated by headache-free periods of varying duration, often several months or years. Attacks have a striking tendency to be precipitated by even small amounts of alcohol. Rare variants of cluster headache include a *chronic variety* in which remissions are brief (less than 14 days), *chronic paroxysmal hemicrania* in which attacks are shorter and strikingly more prevalent in women than men, and *hemicrania continua* in which continuous, moderately severe, unilateral headache occurs. The cause of all these syndromes is unknown, although the distribution of the pain suggests dysfunction of the trigeminal nerve.

Treatment. Therapy for cluster headache may be abortive for acute headache or prophylactic to prevent headache. Acute headache may respond to oxygen by mask (7 to 10 L/min for 15 min), which is effective within several minutes in 70% of patients. Sumatriptan and dihydroergotamine are also effective. Preventative medications include lithium, divalproex sodium, verapamil, methysergide, and corticosteroids. Paroxysmal hemicrania and related syndromes are often strikingly sensitive to indomethacin.

Tension-Type Headache

In contrast to migraine, tension-type headache is featureless. The pain is usually not throbbing but rather steady and often described as a *pressure feeling* or a *vicelike* sensation. It is usually not unilateral and may be frontal, occipital, or generalized. Frequently, pain occurs in the neck area, unlike in migraine. Pain commonly lasts for long periods (e.g., days) and does not rapidly appear and disappear in attacks. No *aura* is present. Photophobia and phonophobia are usually absent (see Table 118–2). Although the patient may indicate that tension-type headache occurs or is exacerbated in times of particular emotional stress, the pathophysiologic factors may relate to sustained craniocervical muscle contraction;

hence a more appropriate term for this syndrome is *muscle-contraction headache.*

A thorough evaluation should be made of the patient's life situations and the presence of anxiety or depression. The tricyclic antidepressant drugs in low doses have proved the most useful for preventing tension-type headache; although the best documented is amitriptyline, newer agents with fewer side effects may be equally effective. Nonpharmacologic therapies such as relaxation therapy, massage, physiotherapy, or acupuncture may be useful in refractory cases. Intramuscular botulinum toxin injections have been used both in migraine and in tension-type headaches.

Other Defined Headache Syndromes

A wide variety of acute headache syndromes need to be differentiated from migraine, cluster, or tension headache. These headaches include *thunderclap* headache, *ice cream* headache, and coital headache. The last of these forms may be indistinguishable from the headache of SAH and requires computed tomography (CT) and lumbar puncture to exclude SAH. All three headache syndromes are common in migraineurs.

Headache Secondary to Structural Brain Disease

Headache may be a manifestation of underlying structural brain disease (Table 118–6). Headache can be found in all forms of cerebrovascular disease: infarction, transient ischemic attacks, and intracerebral and subarachnoid hemorrhage. The headache in SAH is usually extremely severe and often described by the patient as *"the worst headache of my life."* Nuchal rigidity, third nerve palsy (usually involving the pupil), and retinal, preretinal, or subconjunctival hemorrhages may be found. CT of the head usually shows subarachnoid, intraventricular, or intracerebral blood.

The patient with headache and fever presents a common diagnostic problem in the emergency department. Neck stiffness is a common symptom. Meningismus is confirmed by eliciting Brudzinski's (flexion at the hips when the head is flexed chin to chest) and Kernig's signs (neck pain induced

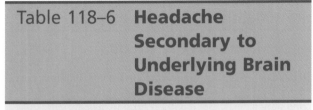

Table 118–6	**Headache Secondary to Underlying Brain Disease**

Cerebrovascular Disease

Ischemic stroke
Intracerebral hemorrhage
Subarachnoid hemorrhage

Inflammatory Disease

Cranial arteritis
Isolated central nervous system vasculitis
Tolosa-Hunt syndrome
Systemic lupus erythematosus

Infectious Disease

Meningitis
Abscess
Encephalitis
Sinusitis
Post-traumatic
Subdural hematoma
Empyema

Neoplastic Disease

Malignant brain tumor
Benign brain tumor
Metastasis

Other

Idiopathic intracranial hypertension

on attempted knee extension with hips flexed). Vomiting occurs in approximately 50% of patients. Suspicion for meningitis should prompt further investigation, including a lumbar puncture. If the patient shows focal signs, papilledema, or profound alteration in level of consciousness, then CT scan of the head before lumbar puncture is required to rule out focal disease such as an abscess or subdural empyema. These lesions, however, are rare.

Acute Sinusitis. Head and face pain is the most prominent feature of sinusitis. Malaise and low-grade fever are usually present. The pain is dull, aching, nonpulsatile, and is exacerbated by movement, coughing, or straining and improved with nasal decongestants. The pain is most pronounced on awakening or after any prolonged recumbency and is diminished after maintaining an upright posture.

The location of the pain depends on the sinus involved. Maxillary sinusitis provokes ipsilateral malar, ear, and dental pain, with significant overlying facial tenderness. Frontal sinusitis produces frontal headache that may radiate behind the eyes and to the vertex of the skull. Tenderness to frontal palpation may be present, with point tenderness on the

undersurface of the medial aspect of the superior orbital rim. In ethmoidal sinusitis, the pain is between or behind the eyes, with radiation to the temporal area. The eyes and orbit are often tender to palpation, and, in fact, eye movements themselves may accentuate the pain. Sphenoidal sinusitis causes pain in the orbit and at the vertex of the skull and occasionally in the frontal or occipital regions. Chronic sinusitis is seldom a cause of headache.

Brain Tumors. Posterior fossa tumors (particularly of the cerebellum) frequently produce headache, especially if hydrocephalus occurs because cerebrospinal fluid (CSF) flow is partially obstructed. Supratentorial tumors, however, are less likely to cause headache than posterior fossa tumors and are more frequently heralded by altered mental status, focal deficits, or seizures. Although increased intracranial pressure is often associated with headache, it is usually not the primary mechanism because uniform pressure elevations do not usually produce distortions of pain-sensitive structures.

Idiopathic Intracranial Hypertension (IIH). This syndrome, also called benign intracranial hypertension, is defined as a syndrome of elevated intracranial pressure without evidence of focal lesions, hydrocephalus, or frank brain edema. IIH occurs usually between the ages of 15 and 45 and frequently occurs in obese women. The disorder is characterized by headache with features suggestive of raised intracranial pressure. The headache is usually insidious in onset, is typically generalized, is relatively mild in severity, and is often increased in the morning or after exertion (e.g., straining, coughing). At times, patients have visual disturbances, such as restricted peripheral visual fields, enlarged blind spots, slight visual blurring, or diplopia secondary to abducens nerve palsies. Funduscopic examination shows papilledema, which is often more impressive than the clinical picture. IIH can be a benign and self-limited disorder, but it may lead to visual loss, including blindness.

The condition has been associated with drugs—vitamin A intoxication, nalidixic acid, danazol (Danocrine), and isotretinoin (Accutane)—as well as corticosteroid withdrawal and with systemic disorders such as hypoparathyroidism and systemic lupus erythematosus.

CT results are usually normal but can show small ventricles and an *empty sella* in some patients. CSF opening pressure is elevated, usually in the range of 250 to 450 mm of water, with the pressure fluctuating markedly when monitored over a prolonged period.

Treatment. After eliminating secondary causes of IIH, the patient should have dietary counseling for weight loss. Carbonic anhydrase inhibitors (acetazolamide) and corticosteroids have proved useful in headache control. As a second-line agent, furosemide also acts to lower CSF production. Serial lumbar punctures are understandably unpopular with patients, even though transient headache relief is obtained. CSF shunting procedures (ventriculoperitoneal shunt) are occasionally necessary. For patients with progressive visual loss, optic nerve sheath fenestration has been shown to preserve or restore vision in 80% to 90% of patients and to provide headache relief in a majority of patients.

Idiopathic Intracranial Hypotension. Also known as low-pressure headache, intracranial hypotension is commonly encountered as a sequel to lumbar puncture owing to leakage of CSF through the dural sac. Low-pressure headaches also occur spontaneously after rupture of subarachnoid cysts. The headache is initially characteristically positional, being severe after standing but relieved rapidly after lying down. Occasionally, the headache is associated with focal or *false localizing* signs, such as abducens nerve palsy.

Post-Traumatic Headache. Headache in individuals with post-traumatic headache has no specific quality and is associated with irritability, impaired concentration, insomnia, memory disturbance, and light-headedness. Anxiety and depression may be present. Amitriptyline and nonsteroidal anti-inflammatory agents may be useful. Occasionally, muscle relaxants and anxiolytics are beneficial.

Giant-Cell Arteritis. Headache occurs in 60% of patients with giant-cell arteritis, a granulomatous vasculitis of medium and large arteries. More than 95% of patients are over 50 years of age. Malaise, fever, weight loss, and jaw claudication occur early, in addition to headache. Polymyalgia rheumatica, a syndrome of painful stiffness of the neck, shoulders, and pelvis, is found in one half the patients. Visual impairment secondary to ischemic optic neuritis may occur. The headache is usually described as aching and is exacerbated at night and after exposure to cold. The superficial temporal artery is frequently swollen, tender, and may be pulseless. The erythrocyte sedimentation rate is usually elevated; the mean is 100 mm/hr. Anemia is frequently present. Temporal artery biopsy usually confirms the diagnosis, but, because the arteritis is segmental, pathologic examination requires multiple sections of a long segment. Prednisone therapy is often dramatically effective and must be given promptly to preserve vision on the affected side.

HEADACHE IN SYSTEMIC DISEASE

A wide variety of systemic diseases have headache as a prominent symptom; some of the more prevalent disorders are summarized in Table 118–7.

Cranial Neuralgias

Neuralgias are differentiated from other head pains by the brevity of the attacks (usually 1 to 2 seconds or less) and by the distribution of the pain.

Trigeminal Neuralgia. In trigeminal neuralgia (tic douloureux), paroxysmal, excruciating pain occurs unilaterally in one of the divisions of the trigeminal nerve. It lasts seconds, but it may occur many times a day for weeks at a time. Trigeminal neuralgia is characteristically induced by even the lightest touch to particular areas of the face or mouth, such as the lips, gums, or teeth. Trigeminal neuralgia is the most frequent neuralgia in older adults and is usually caused by compression of the trigeminal nerve root exiting the pons by an aberrant arterial loop. A small minority of cases are caused by multiple sclerosis, cerebellopontine angle tumors, aneurysms, or arteriovenous malformations, although in these patients (unlike trigeminal neuralgia), objective signs of neurologic deficit are usually present, such as areas of diminished sensation. In these cases of *symptomatic* or secondary neuralgia, the pain is often atypical. Magnetic resonance imaging (MRI) is indicated in patients who have sensory loss, who are under 40 years of age, and who exhibit bilateral or atypical symptoms. Trigeminal neuralgia may be life threatening when it interferes with eating.

Table 118–7 Headaches Secondary to Systemic Disease

Endocrine/Metabolic

Malignant hypertension (e.g., pheochromocytoma)
Acromegaly
Cushing's disease
Carcinoid
Hyperparathyroidism
Paget's disease

Pulmonary

Hypercapnea
Sleep apnea

Pharmacologic

Alcohol
Nitrates
Caffeine withdrawal
Analgesic withdrawal *(rebound)* headache
Others: dipyridamole, cyclosporine, tacrolimus, calcium channel antagonists

Neuralgic pain is often responsive to treatment with standard doses of an anticonvulsant such as phenytoin, carbamazepine, gabapentin, pregabalin, and, occasionally, baclofen. Antidepressant drugs such as amitriptyline and, more recently, duloxetine, may also be useful. The combination of an antidepressant, anticonvulsant, and opiate analgesic has synergistic benefit.

If medical treatments are unsuccessful, then a wide variety of surgical procedures are used, including microvascular decompression and radiofrequency lesioning of the sensory portion of the trigeminal nerve.

Glossopharyngeal Neuralgia. Glossopharyngeal neuralgia is much less common than trigeminal neuralgia. Brief paroxysms of severe, stabbing, unilateral pain radiate from the throat to the ear or vice versa and are frequently initiated by stimulation of specific *trigger zones* (e.g., tonsillar fossa, pharyngeal wall). Swallowing occasionally provokes an attack; yawning, talking, and coughing are other potential triggers. Microvascular decompression is necessary if medical treatment is ineffective.

Postherpetic Neuralgia. Herpes zoster produces head pain by cranial nerve involvement in one third of patients. In some instances, a persistent intense burning pain follows the initial acute illness. The discomfort may subside after several weeks or persist (particularly in older adults) for months or years. The pain is localized to the distribution of the affected nerve and associated with exquisite tenderness to even the lightest touch. The first division of the trigeminal nerve is the most frequent cranial nerve involved (ophthalmic herpes) and is occasionally associated with keratoconjunctivitis. When the seventh nerve is affected *(geniculate herpes)*, the pain involves the external auditory meatus and pinna.

Occasionally, concomitant facial paralysis may occur (Ramsay Hunt syndrome).

Occipital Neuralgia. This syndrome includes occipital pain starting at the base of the skull and is often provoked by neck extension. Physical examination shows tenderness in the region of the occipital nerves and altered sensation in the C2 dermatome. Treatment includes the use of a soft collar, muscle relaxants, physical therapy, and local injections of analgesics and anti-inflammatory agents.

Complex Regional Pain Syndrome

Complex regional pain syndrome (CRPS), formerly known as reflex sympathetic dystrophy, denotes a syndrome that consists of pain and hyperesthesia and autonomic changes. Almost any type of injury can lead to CRPS, including blunt trauma, lacerations, and burns.

The symptoms of CRPS usually develop gradually over days or weeks and are divided into three stages, the duration of which may vary considerably. The *acute stage* is characterized by spontaneous aching or burning pain that is restricted to a particular vascular, peripheral nerve, or root territory. Hyperpathia (pain characterized by overreaction and *aftersensation* to a stimulus) may occur with dysesthesia. The *dystrophic stage* usually begins 3 to 6 months after the injury and is characterized by spontaneous burning pain and more marked hyperpathia than in the acute stage. The nails become cracked, grooved, or ridged, and hair growth is decreased. In addition, range of joint motion is decreased, and muscle wasting, osteoporosis, and edema are present. *Atrophy* (the third stage) usually occurs more than 6 months after the injury. Irreversible trophic changes occur in the skin and subcutaneous tissues and result in smooth, glossy skin, with subcutaneous atrophy, tapering of digits, and fixed joints with contractures. CRPS often is associated with behavioral changes: emotional instability, anxiety, and social withdrawal.

The mechanisms by which the signs and symptoms of CRPS develop have not been fully elucidated. Sympathetic blockade by anesthetic block of the sympathetic ganglia innervating the painful part or by systemic α-adrenergic blockade relieves the pain in many patients, suggesting that the pain is sympathetically maintained. Sympathetic blockade is the mainstay of treatment.

Neck and Back Pain

Most patients with acute neck or back pain have a musculoskeletal disorder that is self limited and does not require specific therapy. The pain may originate from a number of sources, including the vertebrae and intervertebral discs, facet joints, and muscles and ligaments of the vertebral column.

Because the thoracic spine is designed for rigidity rather than mobility, thoracic disc rupture is exceedingly rare. Dissection of the aorta or anterior spinal artery thrombosis may be the cause of acute-onset pain in the thoracic region.

CERVICAL SPONDYLOSIS

Cervical spondylosis is a degenerative disorder of the cervical intervertebral discs, leading to osteophyte formation and hypertrophy of adjacent facet joints and ligaments. In contrast to the lumbar spine, herniation of cervical intervertebral disks (nucleus pulposus) accounts for only 20% to 25% of cervical root irritation. Cervical spondylosis is present radiographically in over 90% of the population older than 60 years of age. However, the degree of radiographic abnormality does not correlate with the clinical signs and symptoms. Clinical disease may represent a combination of normal, age-related, degenerative changes in the cervical spine and a congenital or developmental stenosis of the cervical canal; the process may be aggravated by trauma. It may present as a painful stiff neck, with or without symptoms or signs of cervical root irritation or spinal cord compression. Patients with root irritation (cervical radiculopathy) complain of pain and paresthesias radiating down the arm. Typically, the pain radiates in a myotomal pattern, whereas numbness and paresthesias follow a dermatomal distribution. Discrete sensory loss is uncommon and certainly less prominent than symptoms (Table 118–8). For relief, patients

---

Table 118–8 **Common Root Syndromes of Intervertebral Disc Disease**

Disc Space	Root Affected	Muscles Affected	Distribution of Pain	Distribution of Sensory Symptoms	Reflex Affected
C4–5	C5	Deltoid/biceps	Medial scapula; shoulder	Shoulder	Biceps
C5–6	C6	Wrist extensors	Lateral forearm	Thumb, index finger	Triceps
C6–7	C7	Triceps	Medial scapula	Middle finger	Brachioradialis
C7–T1	C8	Hand intrinsics	Medial forearm	Fourth and fifth fingers	Finger flexion
L3–4	L4	Quadriceps	Anterior thigh	Across knee joint	Knee jerk
L4–5	L5	Peronei	Great toe/dorsum of foot	Great toe	
L5–S1	S1	Gastrocnemius, glutei	Calf	Lateral sole of foot	Ankle jerk

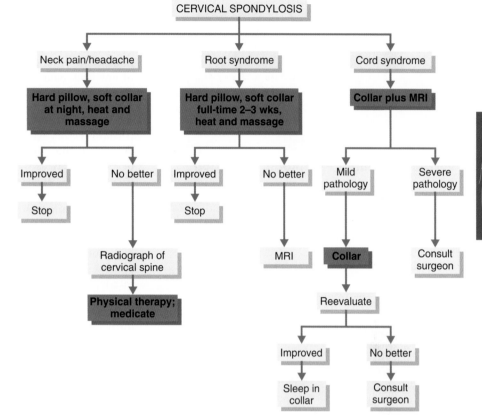

Figure 118–2 Algorithm for the treatment of cervical spondylosis. MRI = magnetic resonance imaging. (Data from Ronthal M, Rachlin JR: Cervical spondylosis. In Johnson RT, Griffin JW, McArthur JC [eds]: Current Therapy in Neurologic Disease, 6th ed. St. Louis, CV Mosby, 2001.)

often adopt a position with the arm elevated and flexed behind the head. Turning the head, ear down, to the side of the pain (Spurling maneuver) will exacerbate the pain. Objective neurologic findings may be limited to reflex asymmetry because weakness may be obscured by pain. Patients who have some degree of spinal cord compression exhibit gait and bladder disturbances and evidence of spasticity on examination of the lower extremities. These patients require investigation with an imaging study, ideally MRI or CT myelography. Plain radiographs of the cervical spine add little information except in patients with rheumatoid arthritis in whom basilar invagination or atlantoaxial subluxation is suggested.

Cervical spondylosis is so common in the general population that it may be present coincidentally in a patient with another disease of the spinal cord. Among other diseases that may mimic cervical spondylosis are multiple sclerosis, amyotrophic lateral sclerosis, and subacute combined system disease (vitamin B_{12} deficiency). Conservative treatment includes the use of anti-inflammatory medication, cervical immobilization, and physical therapy for isometric strengthening of neck muscles once pain has subsided (Fig. 118–2). Surgery should be considered if progression of the neurologic deficit occurs, especially the emergence of signs of cervical cord compression.

ACUTE LOW BACK PAIN

Low back pain without sciatica (radiating radicular pain) is common, with a reported point prevalence of up to 33%.

Acute low back pain lasting several weeks is usually self limited, with a low risk for serious permanent disability. Risk factors for prolonged disability include psychological distress, compensation conflict over work-related injury, and other co-existent pain syndromes. The evaluation of patients with acute low back pain should focus on distinguishing pain of mechanical origin from neurogenic pain caused by nerve root irritation (Table 118–9). The same pathologic changes that affect the cervical spine may also affect the lumbar spine. Because the spinal cord ends at the level of the first lumbar vertebra (L1), lumbar canal stenosis from intervertebral disc disease and degenerative spondylosis will affect the roots of the *cauda equina*. The most common levels for lumbar degenerative disc disease are at L4–L5 and L5–S1, resulting in the common complaint of sciatica caused by irritation of the lower lumbar roots. Pain tends to improve with sitting or lying down, in contrast to the pain from spinal or vertebral tumors, which is aggravated by prolonged recumbency. Examination shows loss of the normal lumbar lordosis, paraspinal muscle spasm, and exacerbation of pain with straight leg-raising, owing to stretching of the lower lumbar roots. Approximately 10% of disc herniations occur lateral to the spinal canal, in which case the more rostral root is compressed. Percussion of the spine may cause focal tenderness of one of the vertebrae, suggesting bony infiltration by infection or tumor.

Spinal stenosis of the lumbar region may exhibit as *neurogenic claudication,* which is usually described as unilateral or bilateral buttock pain worse on standing or walking and relieved by rest or flexion at the waist. Patients may have pain

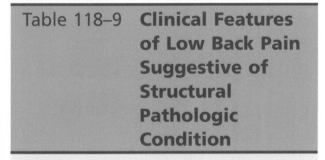

Table 118–9 Clinical Features of Low Back Pain Suggestive of Structural Pathologic Condition

Vertebral Column Pathologic Condition

Pain maximal at rest or at night
Worsening pain over time
Constitutional symptoms
Focal vertebral tenderness
History of recent trauma
History of cancer (especially breast, bronchial, renal cell, prostate, myeloma)

Nerve Root Pathologic Condition

Radicular pain (sciatica)
Dermatomal sensory loss
Absent/asymmetric reflexes
Positive straight leg raise test (S1 root compression)
Urinary or bowel incontinence
Perineal sensory loss
Cauda equina syndrome

that is exacerbated when walking downhill, in contrast to patients with vascular claudication, whose pain is maximal walking up an incline.

MRI in many patients with isolated low back pain shows nonspecific findings; MRI early in the course of an episode of low back pain does not improve clinical outcome. MRI should be performed in patients with back pain who have associated neurologic symptoms or signs, especially new-onset disturbances of bladder or bowel continence or perineal sensory symptoms suggestive of a *cauda equina syndrome*. Patients with risk factors for malignancy, infection, or osteoporosis, as well as those with pain maximal at rest (or nocturnal pain), require imaging (see Table 118–9).

Treatment strategies for lumbar pain are similar to those for cervical pain, with surgery reserved for patients with neurologic signs and clear pathologic processes seen on imaging studies. Most cases of acute low back pain, even with rupture of an intervertebral disc, can be treated conservatively with a short period of rest, muscle relaxants, and analgesics. Prolonged bed rest is no longer recommended except for patients in severe pain. Patient education regarding proper posture and appropriate back exercises is helpful, as is a formal physical therapy program. Chiropractic manipulation should be reserved for patients who have no evidence of neurologic injury or spine instability.

Prospectus for the Future

As the pathogenesis of the headache syndromes are defined, increasingly specific treatments will be developed for migraine, cluster, and tension-type headaches. Some rare headache disorders have been shown to be ion channelopathies. The episodic nature of all of these disorders reflects the occurrence of *triggers* that precipitate the headache. Such triggers are now targets for therapeutic intervention.

References

Carette S, Fehlings MG: Cervical radiculopathy. N Engl J Med 353:392–399, 2005.
Carragee EJ: Persistent low back pain. N Engl J Med 352:1891–1898, 2005.
Cutrer FM, Moskowitz MA: Headaches and other head pain. In Goldman L, Ausiello DA (eds): Cecil Textbook of Medicine, 23rd ed. Philadelphia, Elsevier, 2006.

Jarvic JG, Deyo RA: Diagnostic evaluation of low back pain with emphasis on imaging. Ann Intern Med 137:586–597, 2002.
Silberstein SD: Migraine. Lancet 363:381–391, 2004.
Silberstein SD: Practice parameter: Evidence-based guidelines for migraine headache (an evidence-based review). Report of the Quality Standards Subcommittee of the American Academy of Neurology. Neurology 55:754–762, 2000.

Disorders of Vision and Hearing

Timothy J. Counihan

Disorders of Vision and Eye Movements

EXAMINATION OF THE VISUAL SYSTEM

Acuity

The clinical examination of visual function should begin with the testing of visual acuity. Patients should wear their corrective lenses, if available, and, if possible, testing should be performed with a Snellen chart at a distance of 20 feet to minimize the influence of pupil size and lens accommodation on visual acuity. When errors of refraction are responsible for decreased visual acuity, vision may be improved by having the patient look through a pinhole. Corrected vision in one eye of less than 20/40 suggests damage to the lens (cataract) or retina or a disorder of the anterior visual (prechiasmal) pathway. Color vision in each eye should also be tested; even when visual acuity is normal, patients with lesions of the optic nerve may complain that colors appear *washed out* in the affected eye.

Visual Fields

Thorough examination of the visual fields (Fig. 119–1) can often localize lesions that interrupt the afferent visual system. Comparing the patient's field with that of the examiner (confrontation) will test the visual fields in all four quadrants. Asking the patient to count the number of the examiner's extended fingers is more sensitive than presenting moving objects in detecting visual field deficits. The field should be tested first unilaterally and then bilaterally because uncovering a defect (particularly in the left hemifield) with bilateral testing only (extinction) suggests a lesion in the contralateral parietal lobe.

Partial or complete visual loss in one eye implies damage only to the retina or optic nerve anterior to the optic chiasm, whereas a visual field abnormality involving both eyes implies a defect at or posterior to the optic chiasm. Scotomas are areas of partial or complete visual loss and may be central or peripheral; central scotomas severely disrupt vision as a result of damage to macular fibers. A scotoma impairing one half of a visual field is known as a hemianopia. A homonymous hemianopia implies a postchiasmal lesion. Quadrantanopias are smaller defects in the visual field and may be superior, which suggests a temporal lobe lesion, or inferior, which suggests a parietal lobe lesion. Bitemporal hemianopia implies a lesion at the chiasm, such as a pituitary tumor. An altitudinal hemianopia occurs with vascular damage to the optic nerve. Scintillating scotomas refer to hallucinations of flashing lights. If they are monocular, then they may be caused by retinal detachment; binocular scintillations suggest occipital oligemia (as in migraine) or seizure. Any suggested findings on bedside confrontation testing warrant formal visual field testing.

Chapter 119

Pupils

Pupil constriction results from stimulation of the parasympathetic division of the oculomotor (third cranial) nerve, whereas dilation is mediated by the sympathetic system. If the balance of these systems is upset, then pupillary inequality (anisocoria) results. The pupils should be examined in both dim and bright light; if the anisocoria increases going from dim to bright light, then a lesion of the parasympathetic system is likely (Fig. 119–2). *Physiologic anisocoria* is characterized by a difference in pupil size that appears less in bright light and has no associated pathologic findings.

Both the direct and the consensual light responses should be noted for each eye; in the latter response, when the light is shone in one eye, both pupils should constrict. This response is best tested using the *swinging light test,* in which the light is moved quickly from one eye to the other. If one pupil is dilated as the light is moved to it from the other side, then an abnormality of the optic nerve in that eye is suggested. This abnormality is referred to as an *afferent pupillary defect.* Asking patients to look first in the distance and then at their own or the examiner's finger, held 12 inches away, will test the accommodative pupillary response. The pupils should constrict symmetrically and rapidly.

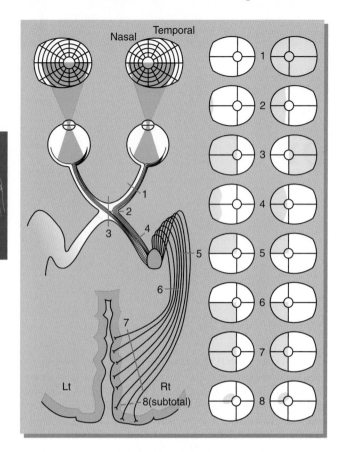

Figure 119–1 Visual fields that accompany damage to the visual pathways: *1,* Optic nerve: unilateral amaurosis. *2,* Lateral optic chiasm: grossly incongruous, incomplete (contralateral) homonymous hemianopia. *3,* Central optic chiasm: bitemporal hemianopia. *4,* Optic tract: incongruous, incomplete homonymous hemianopia. *5,* Temporal (Meyer's) loop of optic radiation: congruous partial or complete (contralateral) homonymous superior quadrantanopia. *6,* Parietal (superior) projection of the optic radiation: congruous partial or complete homonymous inferior quadrantanopia. *7,* Complete parieto-occipital interruption of optic radiation: complete congruous homonymous hemianopia with psychophysical shift of foveal point often sparing central vision, giving *macular sparing. 8,* Incomplete damage to visual cortex: congruous homonymous scotomas, usually encroaching at least acutely on central vision. (From Baloh RW: Neuro-ophthalmology. In Goldman L, Bennett JC [eds]: Cecil Textbook of Medicine, 21st ed. Philadelphia, WB Saunders, 1998, p 2236.)

The presence of ptosis should be noted. A large, unreactive pupil with ptosis indicates a lesion of the oculomotor nerve *(third cranial nerve palsy)* interrupting the parasympathetic nerve supply to the pupil. The associated paralysis of the medial and inferior rectus and inferior oblique muscles (see later discussion) results in disturbed eye position (inferolaterally, *down and out*) and a complaint of double vision by the patient. Common causes of a third cranial nerve palsy include compression by an aneurysm of the posterior communicating artery, by transtentorial herniation, or from ischemia, usually in the setting of diabetes or vasculitis. Third cranial nerve palsy can be assumed to be caused by ischemia only when the pupil is completely spared

and complete paralysis of the oculomotor and eyelid levator muscles occurs.

A small, unreactive pupil with associated ptosis is known as *Horner's syndrome* and results from damage to the sympathetic fibers to the pupil. Associated unilateral anhidrosis resulting from damage to sympathetic fibers may occur. Horner's syndrome may result from lesions of the hypothalamus, brain stem, cervical spinal cord, or sympathetic fibers to the pupil. Horner's syndrome may be the first sign of an apical lung tumor (Pancoast's tumor) or may occur in diseases affecting the carotid artery.

Argyll-Robertson pupils are small, irregular pupils that constrict to near vision but not in response to light. They are often associated with neurosyphilis and occasionally diabetes. This so-called *light-near dissociation* may also occur in rostral dorsal midbrain lesions, in which abnormalities of vertical gaze, eyelid retraction, and convergence retraction nystagmus are present.

Tonic (Adie's) pupils constrict slowly and incompletely in response to light; this is usually an incidental finding on examination but may be associated with loss of quadriceps and gastrocnemius reflexes (Adie's syndrome). Theories suggest that the disorder is a result of parasympathetic denervation.

Hippus refers to pupillary unrest with synchronous oscillation of the pupil size; it is considered a normal phenomenon.

Eye Movements

Elements in the history help in evaluating the patient with diplopia. Is the diplopia primarily horizontal or vertical, or is it greater looking to the right or to the left? Double vision that varies during the day suggests myasthenia gravis. Is the diplopia maximal with near or distant vision? Greater difficulty with near vision suggests impairment of the medial rectus, oculomotor nerve, or convergence system, whereas abducens nerve weakness results in horizontal diplopia when viewing objects at a distance. Monocular diplopia is usually caused by diseases of the retina or lens and often corrected by having the patient look through a pinhole, unless the cause is psychogenic.

The examination should begin by determining the position of the patient's head and eyes with the eyes in primary gaze. Both smooth pursuit and (voluntary) saccadic eye movements in horizontal and vertical directions are checked to determine whether the movements are conjugate or disconjugate. Disconjugate eye movements suggest a disorder of the brain stem (at the level of the ocular motor nuclei or their connections), the peripheral nerves (cranial nerves III, IV, or VI), individual eye muscles (ocular myopathy), or the neuromuscular junction (myasthenia gravis or botulism). A large deficit in the range of eye movements may provide sufficient diagnostic information. However, in many cases, although the patient complains of diplopia, no clear misalignment is visible on testing eye movements. The corneal reflection test may help identify misalignment in these patients. The patient is instructed to look at a light shining directly at the eyes. If the eyes are normally aligned, then the light reflection will be approximately 1 mm nasal to the center of the cornea. If one eye is deviated medially, then the reflection will be displaced outward; the reflection will be displaced inward if the eye is deviated outward.

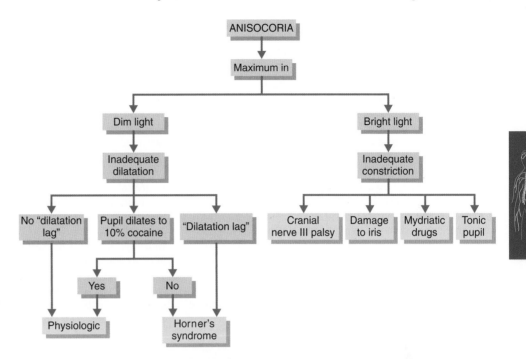

Figure 119–2 Algorithm for the approach to unequal pupils (anisocoria).

The abducens (sixth cranial) nerve supplies the lateral rectus muscle. The trochlear (fourth cranial) nerve subserves the superior oblique muscle, which intorts the eye and depresses the eye in adduction (such as when a patient tries to look downstairs). All other muscles are innervated by the oculomotor nerve. Other signs, such as weakness, ataxia, or dysarthria, usually accompany abnormalities of the cranial nerves in the brain stem. The abducens nerve has a long ascending course through the posterior fossa, where it is prone to compression at multiple sites and as a result of raised intracranial pressure; hence a sixth cranial nerve palsy may be a false localizing sign. Table 119–1 lists the major causes of acute ophthalmoplegia.

Supranuclear pathways from the cerebral hemisphere to the medial longitudinal fasciculus in the brain stem regulate conjugate eye movement. A lesion in the cerebral hemisphere resulting from hemorrhage, infarction, or tumor disrupts conjugate gaze to the contralateral side such that the eyes *look away* from the hemiplegia. Lesions of the brain stem cause conjugate paralysis to the ipsilateral side (eyes looking toward the side of the hemiplegia). Lesions of the medial longitudinal fasciculus, which connect the nuclei of the oculomotor and abducens nerves, lead to *internuclear ophthalmoplegia*. In this instance, horizontal gaze results in failure of adduction in one eye and nystagmus in the abducting eye. The lesion is on the side of failed adduction; bilateral lesions are frequently seen in multiple sclerosis.

Funduscopy

The retina should be carefully examined in each patient by direct ophthalmoscopy, which provides a magnified view of the fundus without the necessity for dilation of the pupil.

UNILATERAL VISUAL LOSS

Lesions of the cornea, lens, vitreous, retina, or optic nerve may cause loss of vision in one eye. A thorough funduscopic examination will usually detect ocular and retinal lesions,

Table 119–1	**Major Causes of Acute Ophthalmoplegia**
Condition	**Diagnostic Features**
Bilateral	
Botulism	Contaminated food, high-altitude cooking; pupils involved
Myasthenia gravis	Fluctuating degree of paralysis; responds to edrophonium chloride (Tensilon) IV
Wernicke's encephalopathy	Nutritional deficiency; responds to thiamine IV
Acute cranial polyneuropathy	Antecedent respiratory infection; elevated CSF protein level
Brain stem stroke	Other brain stem signs
Unilateral	
P Comm aneurysm	Third cranial nerve; pupil involved
Diabetic-idiopathic	Third or sixth cranial nerve; pupil spared
Myasthenia gravis	As above
Brain stem stroke	As above

CSF = cerebrospinal fluid; IV = intravenous; P Comm = posterior communicating artery.

but acute lesions of the optic nerve (optic neuritis) may not be associated with abnormalities of the optic nerve head. *Optic neuritis* is a condition characterized by inflammation of the optic nerve accompanied by nonhomonymous defects in vision. The term *papillitis* refers to ophthalmoscopically observable changes in the optic nerve; *retrobulbar neuritis* refers to this condition without observable changes in the funduscopic examination.

The patient with optic neuritis complains of difficulty with vision in the affected eye. Loss of vision may be insidious and recognized only when the unaffected eye is accidentally occluded. The evolution of visual loss is highly variable, progressing over a period ranging from less than one day to several weeks, although most patients will have reached their maximal visual deficit in 3 to 7 days. Patients may describe their vision as blurred or dim, and colors may appear less bright than usual or gray. At the time the patient is first examined, visual acuity may range from almost 20/20 to the extreme of total blindness. Examination of the visual field shows defects within the central 25 degrees, with central and paracentral scotomas being the most common types. An afferent pupillary defect is frequently present. The funduscopic examination is abnormal in only approximately one half of patients. The disc may appear hyperemic with blurred margins, and hemorrhages, when present, are few and found only on the disc or in the area immediately surrounding the disc. By far the most common cause of optic neuritis is multiple sclerosis.

Ischemic optic neuropathy occurs in two forms. The *atherosclerotic* variety occurs mostly between the ages of 50 and 70, and no evidence of systemic disease is present. The *arteritic* form is usually a manifestation of giant-cell arteritis in which systemic manifestations of the disease may be present, including headache, scalp tenderness, and generalized myalgias. Laboratory evaluation shows anemia and elevated erythrocyte sedimentation rate in almost every case. Patients with arteritis should be treated with high doses of corticosteroids to prevent permanent loss of vision.

The optic nerve may be compressed by tumors that originate in the nerve itself or in the region of the optic chiasm. Pathologic processes that appear acutely as optic disc edema frequently result in a secondary optic atrophy, including papilledema, optic neuritis, and ischemic optic neuropathy. Glaucoma is responsible for more cases of optic atrophy in the adult population than any other cause. In young patients with inherited optic atrophy, Leber's hereditary optic neuropathy, which is usually bilateral, should be kept in mind.

Acute transient monocular blindness is usually the result of embolization to the central retinal artery from an atheromatous plaque in the carotid artery *(amaurosis fugax)*. Any complaint of transient visual loss constitutes an emergency, and steps must be taken to prevent permanent loss of vision by making a prompt diagnosis and initiating appropriate therapy. Examples of sight-saving procedures include corticosteroid therapy for cranial arteritis, reduction of intraocular pressure for acute glaucoma, and carotid surgery, anticoagulation, or antiplatelet therapy for severe cerebrovascular disease.

BILATERAL VISUAL LOSS

Gradual bilateral visual loss caused by optic nerve lesions is rare but may be from Leber's hereditary optic neuropathy or a toxic–nutritional deficiency state. Acute transient bilateral visual loss (visual obscuration) may be a symptom of raised intracranial pressure caused by a brain tumor or pseudotumor cerebri; papilledema is often severe. Lesions of the optic chiasm or postchiasmal optic pathways lead to specific patterns of partial visual loss, as summarized in Figure 119–1. Bilateral damage to the optic radiations or visual cortex results in *cortical blindness.* The pupillary light reflex is normal, as is the funduscopic examination, and the patient may occasionally be unaware that he or she is blind (Anton's syndrome). Patients are often misdiagnosed as having a conversion reaction. Transient cortical blindness occurs most often in basilar artery insufficiency but is also seen in hypertensive encephalopathy. Positive visual phenomena (e.g., phosphenes, scintillating scotomas) are characteristic of migrainous aura and probably reflect oligemia to the occipital lobes from vasoconstriction. Arteriovenous malformations, tumors, and seizures may produce similar symptoms and should be distinguished from migraine with aura by a thorough history and examination, as well as by imaging, in appropriate cases.

Visual hallucinations are visual sensations independent of external light stimulation; they may be either simple or complex, may be localized or generalized, and may occur in patients with a clear or clouded sensorium. Visual illusions are alterations of a perceived external stimulus in which some features are distorted. The simplest visual phenomena consist of flashes of light (photopsias), blue lights (phosphenes), or scintillating zigzag lines, which last a fraction of a second and recur frequently or which appear to be in constant motion. These phenomena can arise from dysfunction within the optic pathways at any point from the eye to the cortex. Glaucoma, incipient retinal detachment, retinal ischemia, or macular degeneration can cause simple visual hallucinations based on dysfunction in the eye. Lesions of the occipital lobe are often associated with simple hallucinations; classic migraine is by far the most common condition of this type. Complex visual hallucinations such as seeing objects as people, animals, landscapes, or various indescribable scenes occur most frequently with temporal lobe lesions or parieto-occipital association areas.

Hearing and Its Impairments
SYMPTOMS OF AUDITORY DYSFUNCTION

The main symptoms of lesions within the auditory system are hearing loss and tinnitus. Hearing loss can be classified as conductive, sensorineural, or central based on the anatomic site of pathology (Fig. 119–3). Tinnitus can be either subjective or objective. Conductive hearing loss results from lesions involving the external or middle ear. Patients with conductive hearing loss can hear speech in a noisy background better than in a quiet background because they can understand loud speech as well as anyone can. The ear often feels full, as if it is blocked. The Weber's test localizes to the deaf ear, if the deafness is unilateral.

Sensorineural hearing loss results from lesions of the cochlea or the auditory division of the vestibulocochlear (eighth cranial) nerve. Patients with sensorineural hearing loss often have difficulty hearing speech that is mixed with background noise and may be annoyed by loud speech. They hear low tones better than high-frequency ones. Distortion of sounds is common with sensorineural hearing loss. Central hearing disorders are rare and result from bilateral lesions of the central auditory pathways, including the

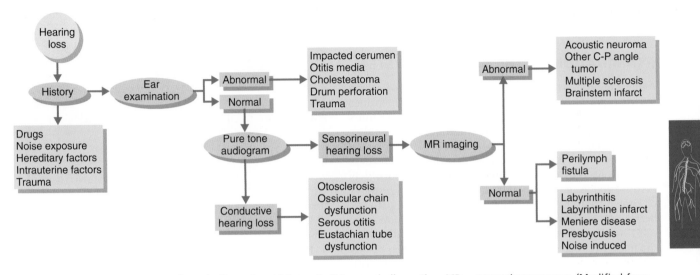

Figure 119–3 Evaluation of deafness (unilateral and bilateral). C-P = cerebellopontine; MR = magnetic resonance. (Modified from Baloh RW: Hearing and equilibrium. In Goldman L, Bennett JC [eds]: Cecil Textbook of Medicine, 21st ed. Philadelphia, WB Saunders, 1998, p 2250.)

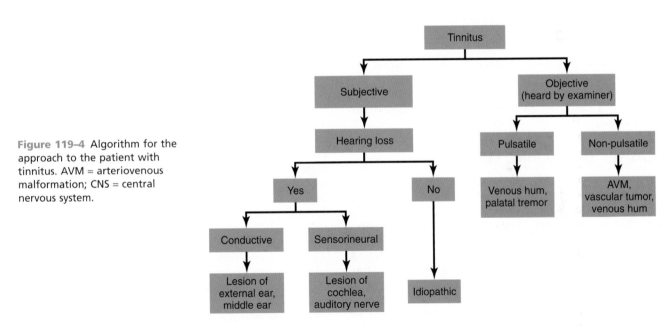

Figure 119–4 Algorithm for the approach to the patient with tinnitus. AVM = arteriovenous malformation; CNS = central nervous system.

cochlear and dorsal olivary nuclear complexes, inferior colliculi, medial geniculate bodies, and auditory cortex in the temporal lobes. Damage to both auditory cortices may result in pure word deafness, in which patients are selectively unable to discriminate language but may be able to hear nonverbal sounds.

Tinnitus is a noise or ringing in the ear that is usually audible only to the patient (subjective), although, rarely, an examiner can hear the sound as well. The latter, so-called objective tinnitus, can be heard when the examining physician places a stethoscope against the patient's external auditory canal. Tinnitus that is pulsatory and synchronous with the heartbeat suggests a vascular abnormality within the head or neck (Fig. 119–4). Aneurysms, arteriovenous malformations, and vascular tumors can produce this type of tinnitus.

Subjective tinnitus, heard only by the patient, can result from lesions involving the external ear canal, tympanic membrane, ossicles, cochlea, auditory nerve, brain stem, and cortex. The character of the tinnitus does not usually aid in determining the site of the disturbance. For this reason, the examiner must rely on associated symptoms and signs. Tinnitus that results from a lesion of the external or middle ear is usually accompanied by a conductive hearing loss. The patient may complain that his or her voice sounds hollow and that other sounds are muffled. Because the masking effect of ambient noise is lost, the patient may be disturbed by normal muscular sounds such as chewing, tight closure of the eyes, or clenching of the jaws. The characteristic tinnitus associated with Ménière's syndrome is low pitched and continuous, although fluctuating in intensity. In many instances, the tinnitus becomes loud immediately preceding an acute attack of vertigo and then may disappear after the attack. Tinnitus resulting from lesions within the central nervous system is usually not associated with hearing loss but is nearly always associated with other neurologic symptoms and signs. Salicylate toxicity frequently results in tinnitus.

EXAMINATION OF THE AUDITORY SYSTEM

A quick test for hearing loss in the speech range is to observe the response to spoken commands at different intensities (whisper, conversation, and shouting). The examiner must be careful to prevent the patient from reading the examiner's lip movement. A high-frequency stimulus such as a watch tick should also be used because sensorineural disorders often involve only the higher frequencies. Tuning fork tests permit a rough assessment of the hearing level for pure tones of known frequency. The Rinne test compares the patient's hearing by air conduction with that by bone conduction. A 512-cycles-per-second tuning fork is first held against the mastoid process until the sound fades. It is then placed 1 inch from the ear. Normal patients can hear the fork approximately twice as long by air conduction as by bone conduction. If hearing by bone conduction is longer than by air conduction, a conductive hearing loss is suggested. Weber's test compares the patient's hearing by bone conduction in the two ears. The fork is placed at the center of the forehead, and the patient is asked where he or she hears the tone. Normal individuals hear it in the center of the head, patients with unilateral conductive loss hear it on the affected side, and patients with unilateral sensorineural loss hear it on the side opposite the loss. Otoscopic examination may reveal impacted cerumen as a cause of conductive hearing loss.

CAUSES OF HEARING LOSS

The bilateral hearing loss commonly associated with advancing age is called *presbycusis*. Presbycusis is not a distinct disease entity but rather represents multiple effects of aging on the auditory system (Table 119–2). Presbycusis may include conductive and central dysfunction, although the most consistent effect of aging is on the sensory cells and neurons of the cochlea; as a result, higher tones are lost early.

Otosclerosis is a disease of the bony labyrinth that is usually exhibited by immobilizing the stapes and thereby producing a conductive hearing loss. Seventy percent of patients with clinical otosclerosis notice hearing loss between the ages of 11 and 30. A family history of otosclerosis can be found in approximately 50% of patients.

A lesion of the cerebellopontine angle, such as an acoustic neuroma, often causes unilateral hearing loss that progresses slowly. Acoustic neuromas (vestibular schwannomas) usually begin on the vestibular nerve in the internal auditory canal; they cause symptoms by compressing the nerve in the narrow confines of the canal. By far the most common symptoms associated with acoustic neuromas are slowly progressive hearing loss and tinnitus from compression of the cochlear nerve. Vertigo occurs in fewer than 20% of patients, but approximately 50% complain of imbalance or disequilibrium. Next to the auditory nerve, the most common cranial nerves involved by compression are the seventh (facial weakness) and fifth (facial numbness). Treatment in most patients is surgical removal.

Ménière's syndrome (endolymphatic hydrops) is characterized by fluctuating hearing loss and tinnitus, episodic

Table 119–2	**Features Distinguishing Conductive versus Sensorineural Hearing Loss**	
	Conductive	**Sensorineural**
Improved by increasing volume	Yes	No
Improved in quiet background	No	Yes
Only certain frequencies affected	No	Yes
Examples	Cerumen	Labyrinthitis
	Otosclerosis	Presbycusis
	Otitis media	Ménière's disease
	Trauma	Acoustic neuroma

vertigo, and a sensation of fullness or pressure in the ear. Typically, the patient develops a sensation of fullness and pressure along with decreased hearing and tinnitus in one ear. Vertigo rapidly follows, reaching a maximum intensity within minutes and then slowly subsiding over the next several hours. The patient usually has a sense of unsteadiness and dizziness for days after the acute vertiginous episode. In the early stages, the hearing loss is completely reversible, but in later stages, a residual hearing loss remains. Patients with idiopathic Ménière's syndrome frequently have a positive family history (in some reports as high as 50%), which suggests genetic predisposing factors. The key to the diagnosis of Ménière's syndrome is to document fluctuating hearing levels in a patient with the characteristic clinical history. The mainstay of medical therapy for endolymphatic hydrops is dietary sodium restriction and oral diuretics.

Acute unilateral deafness usually results from damage to the cochlea and may be caused by viral or bacterial labyrinthitis or vascular occlusion in the territory of the anterior inferior cerebellar artery. Perilymphatic fistulas may also cause abrupt unilateral deafness, usually in association with tinnitus and vertigo.

A large number of drugs may cause acute irreversible bilateral hearing loss; these include aminoglycosides, cisplatin, and furosemide. Salicylates may cause reversible hearing loss and tinnitus.

TREATMENT OF HEARING LOSS

The best treatment is prevention, particularly by the appropriate use of earplugs for persons working in a noisy environment. Hearing aids help patients with conductive hearing loss, and developments with cochlear implants may help patients with sensorineural hearing loss.

Prospectus for the Future

Because of better understanding of neuronal development and connectivity, transplanting neurons into the visual pathways to restore vision lost to ischemic or inflammatory diseases may become feasible.

References

Baloh RW: Dizziness, Hearing Loss, and Tinnitus. Philadelphia, FA Davis, 1998.

Baloh RW: Hearing and equilibrium. In Goldman L, Ausiello DA (eds): Cecil Textbook of Medicine, 23rd ed. Philadelphia, WB Saunders 2006, p 2236.

Dizziness and Vertigo

Roger P. Simon

izziness is a nonspecific term that includes not only *vertigo* (definite rotational sensation), but also *presyncope* (lightheadedness, impending fainting, and dimming of vision), instability, and *disequilibrium* (impaired balance or gait). These symptoms can be caused by peripheral or central vestibular disorders (vertigo), systemic or cardiovascular disorders producing impaired cerebral blood flow (presyncope), neurologic disorders producing disordered sensory input into the brain (disequilibrium), or by hyperventilation (Table 120–1).

Chapter 120

Approach to the Diagnosis

Separate vestibular from nonvestibular disorders. Presyncope is diagnosed by history and examination, and its cause may be cardiac arrhythmia, outflow obstruction, or orthostatic hypotension. Symptoms are wooziness or giddiness, disequilibrium without true vertigo, global weakness, and, finally, dimming of vision. Cardiac causes are suggested by events occurring when the patient is in the recumbent position and/or during exercise. Orthostatic hypotension is established by positional blood pressure examinations. Disequilibrium of a nonvestibular nature requires a neurologic examination and a neurologic diagnosis (e.g., peripheral neuropathy, gait apraxia, Parkinsonism; see Table 120–1). The diagnosis of hyperventilation can be excluded by asking the patient to compare the symptoms of dizziness with those induced by hyperventilation (3 minutes).

Vestibular Disorders

NYSTAGMUS

The sign of vestibular dysfunction is nystagmus. If the vertigo is peripheral in origin, then nystagmus is invariably present; the fast phase is directed away from the affected ear. Thus, if the patient has the symptom of vertigo at the moment of the examination and has no nystagmus, then the cause of such vertigo is central. If nystagmus is present but a disassociation of nystagmoid movements exist between the two eyes or if the nystagmus is purely vertical, then a central cause is again determined.

VERTIGO

The symptom of vestibular disorders is vertigo, an illusory sense of unidirectional rotational movement. With eyes open, the patient sees the environment move (in a direction opposite the slow component of nystagmus); and with the eyes closed, the patient feels a turning or whirling sensation in space. Both vertigo and nystagmus have characteristics that point to a central or a peripheral cause (Tables 120–2 and 120–3). Peripheral (i.e., vestibular) disorders may be disabling (e.g., severe vertigo with vomiting), but they are rarely life threatening. Central nervous system disorders may produce only mild symptoms, but these symptoms may progress to central nervous system dysfunction (e.g., multiple sclerosis) or even death (e.g., basilar artery stroke).

PERIPHERAL VERTIGO

Acute peripheral vestibular disorders produce acute vertigo, nausea, and vomiting. The patient appears ill, typically lies on one side with the affected ear upward, and is reluctant to move the head. Horizontal nystagmus with the fast phase directed away from the affected ear is always present.

Vestibular neuronitis refers to repetitive attacks of peripheral vertigo without auditory dysfunction. *Labyrinthitis* is the phenomenon of severe acute vertigo, with autonomic symptoms, in the setting of otitis or viremia. *Peripheral vestibulopathy* refers to recurrent attacks of vertigo in any age group without other neurologic symptoms and with a normal neurologic examination. These various terms are based on unverifiable inferences about the site of disease and pathogenetic mechanism.

Positional vertigo is extremely common and is most often described as severe vertigo induced by the maneuver of moving from an upright to a recumbent posture and/or rolling over in bed. The diagnosis is confirmed when the symptom of vertigo and the sign of nystagmus are reproduced by the Nylen-Bárány or Dix-Hallpike maneuver (Fig. 120–1, **Web video 120-1**). The syndrome is caused by freely moving debris within the semicircular canals of the vestibular system; repositioning maneuvers are used for

Table 120–1   Common Causes of Dizziness

Cause	Frequency (%)
Peripheral vestibular disorders*	38
Hyperventilation	23
Multiple sensory deficits†	13
Psychiatric disorders	9
Uncertain	9
Brain stem stroke	5
Other neurologic disorders‡	4
Cardiovascular disorders	4
Multiple sclerosis	2
Visual disorders	2
Other	2

N = 104.
*Benign positional vertigo most common.
†Gait apraxia, Parkinson's disease, temporal lobectomy.
‡Peripheral neuropathy, cervical spondylosis, vestibular abnormalities, visual impairment.
Data from Drachman DA, Hart CW: An approach to the dizzy patient. Neurology 22:323, 1972.

Table 120–2   Symptoms Suggestive of Central Versus Peripheral Vertigo

Symptom or Sign	Peripheral	Central
Severity	4+	1–4+
Onset	Sudden	Nonparoxysmal
Nausea and vomiting	Common	Uncommon
Nystagmus	*Always* present	Present or absent
Tinnitus and hearing loss	Often present	Very rare
Visual fixation	Inhibits	No effect

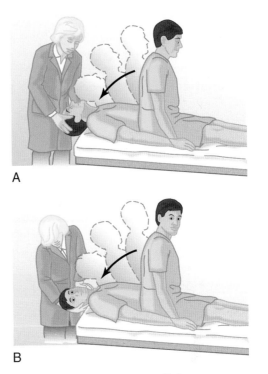

A

B

Figure 120–1 Nylen-Bárány or Dix-Hallpike maneuver to test for positional nystagmus. The patient is seated on an examining table with head and eyes directed forward (A) and is then quickly lowered to the supine position with the head over the table edge, 45 degrees below the horizontal. The patient is instructed to keep the eyes open; the examiner observes for nystagmus, and the patient is asked to report vertigo. The test is repeated with the patient's head turned to the right (B) and again to the left. (From Simon RP, Aminoff MJ, Greenberg DR: Clinical Neurology, 4th ed. Stamford, CT, Appleton & Lange, 1999.)

treatment (Fig. 120–2). *Positional nystagmus* occurs when the head is placed in the provocative position. This condition must be differentiated from the exacerbation of vertigo by head movement (head movements make all vertigo symptoms worse).

The most common positional nystagmus, termed *benign paroxysmal positional nystagmus,* usually has a 3- to 10-second latency before onset and rarely lasts longer than 15 seconds. The nystagmus is always rotational and is prominent in only one head-hanging position (see Fig. 120–1). Another key feature is fatigability, in which the vertigo and nystagmus disappear with repeated positioning. In most patients, benign paroxysmal positional vertigo occurs as an isolated symptom of unknown cause; it may also follow head

injury, viral labyrinthitis, or occlusion of the vasculature to the inner ear. The diagnosis is made clinically, with the typical history of abrupt-onset positional vertigo, nausea, and disequilibrium.

Other causes of peripheral vertigo include *Ménière's disease,* an uncommon disorder of vertiginous spells on the background of progressive unilateral hearing loss and tinnitus. *Acoustic neuromas* are extremely rare causes of vertigo; they most often produce hearing loss, tinnitus, and unsteadiness.

CENTRAL VERTIGO

Cerebrovascular Disease

Vertigo can be the presenting sign of *vertebral basilar ischemia,* but vertiginous episodes continuing for more than 6 weeks without other symptoms or signs of a nervous system dysfunction are rarely caused by cerebral ischemia. Cerebral ischemia, producing vertigo, is in the vertebral basilar distribution. Therefore, carotid Doppler studies are not indicated for this symptom in isolation. Computed tomographic scan of the brain is rarely useful because the brain stem is poorly seen with this technique. Magnetic resonance imaging may show areas of ischemic injury in the

Table 120–3	Characteristics of Central Versus Peripheral Nystagmus	
Characteristic	**Peripheral**	**Central**
Direction	Usually horizontal, may have rotary component	Any direction (pure vertical is always central)
Symmetry between eyes	Always symmetric	Dissociation between eyes possible
Lesion side	Fast component away from injured labyrinth	No relation between direction and lesion location
Duration of problem	Minutes to weeks	Days to years
Visual fixation	Decreases	No effect

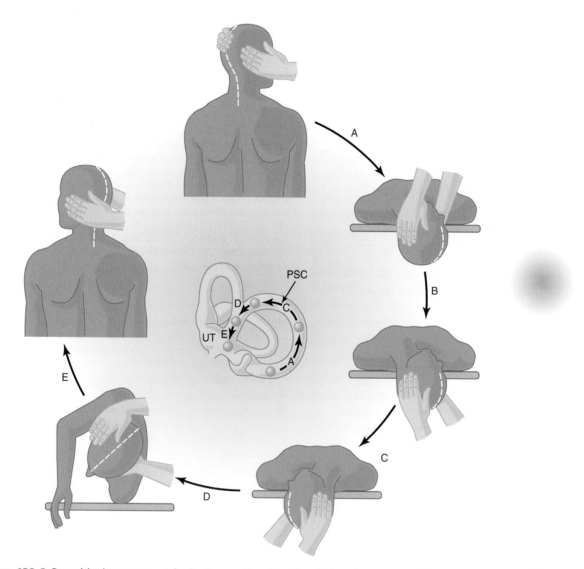

Figure 120–2 Repositioning treatment for benign positional vertigo designed to move endolymphatic debris out of the posterior semicircular canal (PSC) of the right ear and into the utricle (UT). The patient is seated, and the patient's head is turned 45 degrees to the right *(A)*. The head is then lowered rapidly to below the horizontal *(B)*. The examiner shifts hand positions *(C)*, and the patient's head is rotated rapidly 90 degrees in the opposite direction, so it now points 45 degrees to the left, where it remains for 30 seconds *(D)*. The patient then rolls onto the left side without turning the head in relation to the body and maintains this position for another 30 seconds *(E)* before sitting up. The treatment is repeated until nystagmus is abolished. The procedure is reversed for treating the left ear. The patient must avoid the supine position for 2 days. (Adapted from Foster CA, Baloh RW: Episodic vertigo. In Rakel RE [ed]: Conn's Current Therapy. Philadelphia, WB Saunders, 1995.)

brain stem or cerebellum or low flow through the vertebral basilar system.

The sudden onset of dizziness with vomiting, disequilibrium, and truncal ataxia is a common manifestation of *cerebellar hemorrhage* or *infarction*. Nystagmus is uncommon. Computed tomography enables the examiner to make the diagnosis. *Cerebellar swelling* can produce brain stem compression and death. Surgical decompression is a life-saving procedure.

Vertigo is a common symptom in patients with infarction of the lateral brain stem, which is supplied by the posterior inferior cerebellar artery *(Wallenberg's syndrome)*. Characteristic findings include vertigo, ipsilateral facial pain, diplopia, dysphagia, and dysphonia. The diagnosis is confirmed by the neurologic examination, which discloses unilateral Horner's syndrome, ipsilateral facial hypesthesia with contralateral sensory loss, and nystagmus.

Other Conditions

Demyelinating disease, mass lesions, and basilar migraine are additional considerations for central vertigo. Epilepsy may produce brief episodic episodes of disequilibrium or a sensation of rotation with *absences*.

Treatment

The treatment of vertigo depends on the cause. Ménière's disease is treated with diuretics; spontaneous remissions are common. Surgical ablation is indicated only in severe persistent cases. Vertigo in patients with migraine responds to antimigrainous therapy (see Chapter 118). Vertebrobasilar insufficiency should be treated with an antiplatelet agent: aspirin, clopidogrel, or aspirin with dipyridamole. For peripheral vertigo, vestibular suppressant drugs may be helpful (Table 120–4), or the patient may respond to desensitization techniques (repetitive body and head rotations and tilts, adequate to produce dizziness, performed two to three times daily).

Table 120–4　**Treatment of Vertigo**
Vestibular Suppressants (Peripheral)*
Meclizine (12.5–25.0 mg every 6 hr)   Dimenhydrinate (50 mg every 6 hr)   Promethazine (25 mg every 6 hr)
Vestibular Suppressants (Central)*
Low-dose diazepam (2 mg every 4–6 hr) or oxazepam   (10–15 mg every 6 hr)   Anti-emetics (as needed)
*May be more effective in combination.

Prospectus for the Future

The key factor in the vertigo and dizziness syndromes is the distinction between brain stem disease and labyrinthine disease. Imaging studies, particularly magnetic resonance imaging and now positron emission tomography, should go a long way toward facilitating this differential diagnosis.

References

Baloh RW: Vestibular neuritis. N Engl J Med 348:1027–1032, 2003.
Radtke A, von Brevern M, Tiel-Wilck K, et al: Self-treatment of benign paroxysmal positional vertigo: Semont maneuver vs. Epley procedure. Neurology 63:150–152, 2004 (and accompanying editorial by Furman JM, Hain TC).
Sloane PD, Coeytaux RR, Beck RS, et al: Dizziness: State of the science. Ann Intern Med 134:823–832, 2001.
Tusa RJ: Vertigo. Neurol Clin 19:23–55, 2001.

Disorders of the Motor System

Frederick J. Marshall

The human voluntary motor system originates in the motor areas of the frontal lobe cortex, which send their output caudally in the corticospinal tract. The basal ganglia and cerebellum have additional integrating, postural, reinforcing, and coordinating influences (Fig. 121–1). Descending influences from the red nuclei, vestibular nuclei, and brainstem reticular formation converge with descending corticospinal pathways on bulbospinal motor neurons to activate integrated, functionally automatic motor programs. At every level, afferent feedback provides input from muscle, nerves, the spinal segment, brainstem, cerebellum, basal ganglia, and cortex to guide the efferent messages from the motor cortex. Figures 121–2 and 121–3 indicate the corticobasal ganglia connections and corticocerebellar loops that unconsciously precede movement.

Disease can selectively affect every level of the motor system from brain to muscle. Table 121–1 lists the anatomic locations of diseases affecting the motor system.

Symptoms and Signs of Motor System Disease

The patient with motor system disease usually complains of difficulty with accomplishing specific tasks. Patients with central nervous system (CNS) disorders (see Table 121–1) typically have difficulty with coordination, balance, and rapid movements. Muscle strength is frequently normal, and muscle atrophy (wasting) is usually lacking. Muscle tone is usually increased, characterized by spasticity or rigidity. Patients with peripheral nervous system (PNS) disorders (see Table 121–1) usually complain of difficulty with tasks; if weakness is proximal, then this weakness includes activities such as climbing or descending stairs, rising from a chair, or lifting heavy objects above the head. If this weakness is distal, then the patient complains of stumbling and tripping or of having problems fastening buttons or opening locks or doors with the hands.

The patient with weakness of gradual onset may not recognize it, emphasizing the useful axiom that "signs of muscle weakness precede symptoms of weakness." A patient with weakness who is unfamiliar with what is taking place may use words such as *numbness, deadness, tiredness,* or *fatigue.*

In contrast, when a patient complains of *weakness,* it often results from systemic rather than neurologic disease. In such patients, strength is often normal or only mildly reduced because the complaint is usually a loss of stamina and endurance. The patient with a complaint of fatigue should be asked to distinguish between true weakness and the less specific symptoms of lassitude and asthenia. If the patient is unable to perform a specific normal activity, then true weakness is suggested. Objective evidence of weakness is established if symptoms exceed the boundaries of normal variation (e.g., double vision, drooping eyelids, difficulty in swallowing, repeated aspiration of food or liquids into the airway), as opposed to the more subjective complaints of inability to lift, carry, or push an object.

CNS motor disorders (see Table 121–1) can result from focal brain or spinal cord diseases such as those that occur with stroke, tumor, or inflammatory or demyelinating disease, each of which is covered in specific chapters elsewhere in this text. CNS motor disorders can also be the result of a widespread, nonfocal *system* degeneration, which is considered in this chapter. Focal brain disease usually produces abnormalities on neuroimaging procedures. System degeneration, in contrast, seldom produces detectable abnormalities on neuroimaging and other neurodiagnostic tests until long after patients first report symptoms and have signs of abnormal function on examination.

Corticospinal diseases from system degeneration are uncommon and are characterized by upper motor neuron signs (spasticity and hyperreflexia). The most common is amyotrophic lateral sclerosis, which differs from other CNS motor diseases by the prominent involvement of both the CNS and PNS. The hereditary spastic paraplegias are rare, usually hereditary diseases with only upper motor neuron signs.

Movement Disorders and Ataxia

Central motor systems are divided into three constituents: pyramidal, extrapyramidal, and cerebellar. The pyramidal system (named for the pyramidal cross-section of fiber tracts in the medulla) is the major outflow from motor cortex to

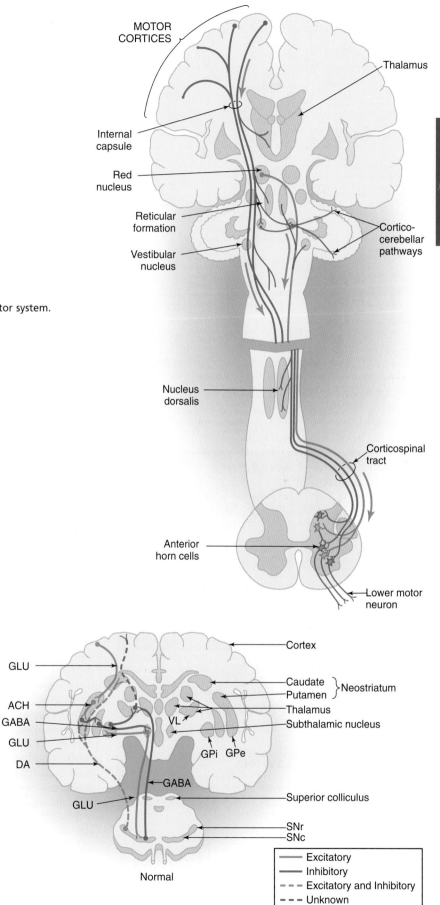

Figure 121–1 Normal human voluntary motor system.

Figure 121–2 Anatomy of the basal ganglia and their connections. The feedback loop proceeds from cerebral prefrontal areas to the basal ganglia and eventually back from the basal ganglia to the thalamus to the motor cortex. This ultimately regulates the descending corticospinal motor system. ACH = acetylcholine; DA = dopamine; GABA = γ-aminobutyric acid; GLU = glutamate; GP = globus pallidum (e = external, i = internal); SN = substantia nigra (c = compacta, r = reticulate); VL = ventrolateral. (From Jankovic J: The extrapyramidal disorders: Introduction. In Goldman L, Bennett JC [eds]: Cecil Textbook of Medicine, 21st ed. Philadelphia, WB Saunders, 2000, p 2078.)

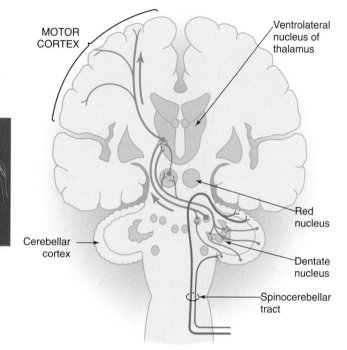

Figure 121–3 Corticocerebellar loop. The major cerebellar input is from the spinocerebellar tract. Outflow is to the motor cortex via the mesencephalon and thalamus.

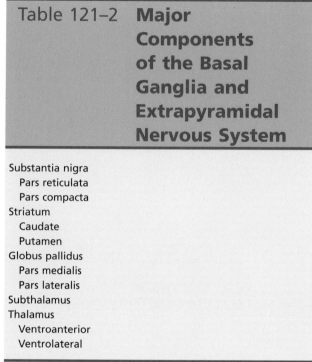

Table 121–2	**Major Components of the Basal Ganglia and Extrapyramidal Nervous System**

Substantia nigra
  Pars reticulata
  Pars compacta
Striatum
  Caudate
  Putamen
Globus pallidus
  Pars medialis
  Pars lateralis
Subthalamus
Thalamus
  Ventroanterior
  Ventrolateral

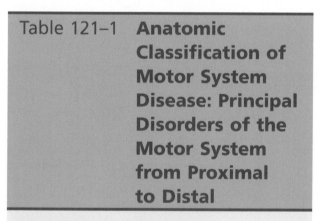

Table 121–1	**Anatomic Classification of Motor System Disease: Principal Disorders of the Motor System from Proximal to Distal**

Central Nervous System

Corticospinal diseases (disorders of the upper motor neuron)
Extrapyramidal movement disorders
Cerebellar ataxias
Spinal cord diseases

Peripheral Nervous System

Radiculopathies and lower motor neuron diseases
Peripheral nerve disorders
Polyneuropathy
Focal neuropathy
Neuromuscular junction
Myasthenia
Lambert-Eaton myasthenic syndrome
Botulism
Muscular

spinal cord. Lesions of the pyramidal system cause motor weakness (paresis), spasticity, and hyperreflexia. Although lesions of this system disturb motor function, they are not considered *movement disorders.* Movement disorders are caused by extrapyramidal or cerebellar dysfunction. The term *extrapyramidal* refers to the basal ganglia and their projections. The main components of the extrapyramidal system are noted in Table 121–2, and their major interconnections are depicted in Figure 121–4.

The basal ganglia receive input from the cortex and give feedback to the cortex through projections from the thalamus. Multiple neurotransmitters are involved in complex feedback loops. The basal ganglia modulate not only motor cortical activity but also the activity of association cortex, particularly in the frontal lobes. Many movement disorders therefore involve complex neurobehavioral symptoms (e.g., dementia in Huntington's disease, attentional deficits and obsessive-compulsive behavior in Tourette's disorder, depression in Parkinson's disease). Clinicoanatomic correlations between lesions in a component of the system and development of a characteristic movement disorder or neurobehavioral syndrome remain elusive. An exception is hemiballismus, a dramatic flailing movement of the extremities on one side of the body usually caused by a lesion of the contralateral subthalamic nucleus. Neurosurgical interventions designed to ablate or stimulate specific nuclei and neuropharmacologic treatments designed to modulate selective receptor systems are increasingly widespread.

Movement disorders entail either too little movement (hypokinesia) or too much movement (hyperkinesia). Table 121–3 outlines the hypokinetic disorders in the differential diagnosis of akinetic-rigid syndrome. The disorders listed in Table 121–3 cause progressive immobility. Rigidity refers to increased muscular tone throughout the range of motion. It does not vary with passive acceleration of the limb by the examiner. Lead-pipe rigidity connotes the ductile quality of metal being passively bent. Cogwheel rigidity is the super-imposition of tremor on underlying rigidity. Paratonic rigidity or paratonia refers to a velocity-dependent resistance to passive movement. Such resistance increases as the speed of passive limb displacement increases. Patients with paratonic rigidity demonstrate *gegenhalten,* an inability to fully relax a limb for passive range-of-motion testing. This group of patients also demonstrates *mitgehen,* the tendency to *help out* as the examiner attempts to move the limb passively. Paratonia is clinically nonspecific; it is common in patients with diminished cerebral function resulting from a variety of causes. True rigidity always implies basal ganglia dysfunction on the contralateral side.

Many different hyperkinetic movements may be exhibited (Table 121–4). Accurate identification of these movements is required for proper diagnosis and treatment of extrapyramidal diseases. For example, chorea occurring in successive generations is most likely caused by Huntington's disease (hereditary chorea). Parkinson's disease is most likely the cause of resting tremor in an older patient with rigidity and bradykinesia (slow movement). Essential tremor (a common, often inherited disorder) is most likely the cause of action tremor in a patient without rigidity or bradykinesia).

Table 121–5 outlines a number of signs commonly associated with lesions of the cerebellar system. Disorders of proprioceptive function may result in *sensory* ataxia caused by impairment of the spinocerebellar inputs.

Hypokinetic Movement Disorders

IDIOPATHIC PARKINSON'S DISEASE

James Parkinson, a London physician, first described the clinical triad of tremor, bradykinesia, and postural

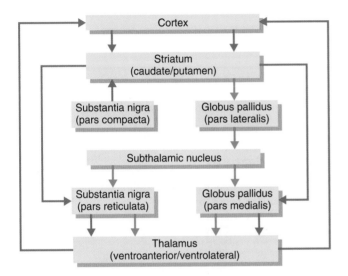

Figure 121–4 In this simplified version of the basal ganglia wiring diagram, information flows in one of two ways, either facilitating motor output by means of the direct pathway *(red lines)* or inhibiting motor output by means of the indirect pathway *(blue lines).* In Parkinson's disease, loss of neurons in the pars compacta of the substantia nigra shifts the balance away from the direct pathway and toward the indirect pathway, resulting in hypokinesia. Conversely, in Huntington's disease, loss of select neurons in the striatum shifts the balance away from the indirect pathway and toward the direct pathway, resulting in hyperkinesia.

Table 121–3	**Differential Diagnosis of the Akinetic-Rigid Syndrome**

Idiopathic Parkinson's disease
Drug-induced parkinsonism
Diffuse Lewy body disease
Progressive supranuclear palsy
Multisystem atrophy: parkinsonian type, cerebellar type, mixed type
Vascular parkinsonism
Other hereditary neurodegenerative disorders: Huntington's disease; Hallervorden-Spatz disease
Toxic parkinsonism: carbon monoxide; manganese; MPTP
Catatonia (psychosis)

MPTP = methyl-phenyl-tetrahydropyridine.

Table 121–4　Descriptive Terms of the Hyperkinesias

Asterixis	Transitory loss of motor tone resulting in rapid movement of a joint (the conceptual opposite of myoclonus) **(Web Video 121–2)**
Athetosis	Slow writhing movement
Ballism	Flailing movement (typically unilateral—hemiballism)
Chorea	Irregular flicking, dancelike movement **(Web Video 121–3)**
Choreoathetosis	The combination of chorea and athetosis
Dystonia	Sustained contortion resulting from excess muscular activity across a joint: generalized, segmental, or focal **(Web Video 121–4)**
Dyskinesia	Nonspecific term for hyperkinesia (generally chorea, athetosis, and dystonia, alone or in combination)
Myoclonus	Rapid jerking muscular movement: multifocal or segmental; rhythmic or irregular **(Web Video 121–5)**
Tic	Semi-suppressible motor or vocal gestural movement (may be simple, such as eye blinking or throat clearing, or complex, such as hopping or swearing)
Tremor	Rhythmic oscillating movement: predominantly at rest or with action

Table 121–5	**Signs of Cerebellar System Impairment**
Ataxia	Poorly coordinated, broad-based, lurching gait
Ataxic dysarthria	Abnormal modulation of speech velocity and volume
Dysmetria	Irregular placement of voluntary limb or ocular movement
Hypometria	Movement falling short of the intended target
Hypermetria	Movement overshooting the intended target
Dysdiadochokinesis	Breakdown in precision and completeness of rapid alternating movements (as with a pronation-supination task)
Dysrhythmokinesis	Irregularity of the rhythm of rapid alternating movements or planned movement sequences
Dyssynergia	Inability to perform movement as a coordinated temporal sequence
Hypotonia	Decreased resistance to passive muscular extension (seen immediately after injury to the lateral cerebellum)
Intention tremor	Tremor orthogonal to the direction of intended movement (tends to increase in amplitude as the target is approached)
Titubation	Rhythmic rocking tremor of the trunk and head

instability in 1817. Later, physicians recognized that muscular rigidity was also a fundamental aspect of the illness. These four signs remain the diagnostic criteria for Parkinson's disease. Parkinson's disease affects 750,000 to 1 million people in the United States and is a leading cause of neurologic disease in individuals older than 65 years of age. Premature death of pigmented dopaminergic neurons in the pars compacta of the substantia nigra is the underlying basis of the disease, but the cause remains unclear. Neuronal loss occurs in the substantia nigra, with characteristic eosinophilic hyaline intraneuronal inclusions called Lewy bodies. Dopamine-containing neurons with cell bodies in the substantia nigra project to the striatum (caudate and putamen), where they synapse on a variety of cell types. Early in the course of the disease, dopamine receptors in the striatum are upregulated in response to decreased dopaminergic input from the substantia nigra. This compensatory ability of the striatum is eventually overwhelmed, and progressive clinical dysfunction ensues.

Symptoms and signs of Parkinson's disease are listed in Table 121–6. The patient typically notes unilateral symptoms initially: characteristically hand tremor, decreased arm swing, foot dragging, or micrographia. Symptoms and signs subsequently spread to involve both sides. Gradually worsening postural instability ultimately results in wheelchair confinement. Symmetric onset of symptoms and early falls caused by postural instability are atypical of idiopathic Parkinson's disease, whereas they are common in other causes of the akinetic-rigid syndrome (see Table 121–3). Tremor may be a prominent feature of idiopathic Parkinson's disease, but it is not usually a prominent feature of other akinetic-rigid disease states (**Web Video 121–1**).

Treatment of Parkinson's disease is outlined in Table 121–7. Carbidopa-levodopa (Sinemet) remains the mainstay of treatment for advanced Parkinson's disease. Failure of bradykinesia and rigidity to improve in response to a trial of levodopa treatment raises the possibility of another disease (see Table 121–3) because these diseases typically involve primary pathologic deterioration at the level of the striatum rather than the substantia nigra.

Levodopa requires enzymatic conversion to dopamine within substantia nigra neurons. The dopamine agonists do

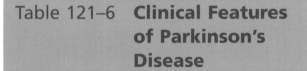

Table 121–6	**Clinical Features of Parkinson's Disease**

Primary Features

Bradykinesia; rest tremor; rigidity; postural instability; therapeutic response to levodopa

Secondary Features

Masked facies (facial hypomimia)
Dysphagia; hypophonia/palilalia; micrographia; stooped posture; festinating gait; start hesitation; dystonic cramps
Autonomic dysfunction: orthostatic hypotension; urinary incontinence; constipation
Behavioral alterations: depression; dementia; sleep disorders including restless legs syndrome
Sensory complaints: aching; numbness; tingling

not compete with other amino acids to cross the blood-brain barrier; they require no enzymatic conversion and act directly at the level of the striatum, bypassing the substantia nigra. Concern has been expressed that treatment with levodopa may eventually provoke motor complications, such as *on-off* fluctuations and dyskinesias. Initiating therapy with dopamine agonists allows the physician to reserve levodopa treatment for later stages of the illness. The co-administration of a dopamine agonist in the later stages of illness may reduce the amount of levodopa required.

Selegiline delays the need for levodopa treatment in patients with early Parkinson's disease. Selegiline inhibits monoamine oxidase type B, an enzyme that breaks down dopamine. Toxic-free radicals generated in the normal catabolism of dopamine may damage dopaminergic neurons in the substantia nigra, which may cause Parkinson's disease in patients who are vulnerable as a result of a combination of inherited risk and as yet undetermined environmental exposures. It has been postulated that selegiline may act as a

Table 121–7	**Medications for Parkinson's Disease**

Anticholinergic Agents

Trihexyphenidyl (Artane)
Benztropine (Cogentin)

Dopamine Precursors (Combined with Peripheral Aromatic Amino Acid Decarboxylase Inhibitors)

Carbidopa/levodopa (Sinemet, Sinemet-CR) (regular and controlled-release forms)
Benserazide/levodopa (Madopar) (marketed in Europe)

Dopamine Agonists

Bromocriptine (Parlodel)
Pergolide (Permax)
Pramipexole (Mirapex)
Ropinirole (Requip)

Monoamine Oxidase Type B (MAO-B) Inhibitors

Selegiline (deprenyl) (Carbex, Eldepryl)
Rasagiline (Azilect)

Catechol-O-Methyltransferase (COMT) Inhibitors

Tolcapone (Tasmar)
Entacapone (Comtan)

Table 121–8	**Drugs Causing Bradykinesia or Rigidity**

Established

Neuroleptics (virtually all phenothiazines, butyrophenones, others)
Metoclopramide
Reserpine

Reported

Lithium
Phenytoin
Angiotensin-converting enzyme inhibitors

neuroprotective agent if the formation of free radicals is inhibited. Rasagiline, the newest medication for PD, was recently approved by the FDA. It is also a selective monoamine oxidase type B inhibitor. Patients may tolerate it better because it is not metabolized to amphetamine.

Similar to aromatic amino acid decarboxylase, the catechol-O-methyltransferase (COMT) inhibitors catalyze the catabolism of levodopa. Co-administration of levodopa with carbidopa and a COMT inhibitor suppresses its peripheral catabolism, maximizing the amount available to cross the blood-brain barrier and prolonging its effective half-life. Tolcapone has been associated with rare but potentially lethal liver toxicity; the hepatic function of patients undergoing treatment with this drug must be monitored closely. Entacapone has no adverse effect on liver function and is now in widespread use.

Because enhancing dopaminergic neurotransmission is the underlying rationale of drug treatments for Parkinson's disease, most antiparkinsonian drugs have unwanted dopaminergic side effects. These include nausea, orthostatic hypotension, hallucinations, psychosis, and dyskinesia (i.e., abnormal involuntary hyperkinetic movements such as chorea and dystonia). Management of progressive Parkinson's disease requires a careful balance between the potential beneficial effects of medication and these potential side effects.

In the past decade, great advances have been made in the surgical treatment of Parkinson's disease. Most centers of excellence in the care of Parkinson's disease now offer deep-brain stimulation (DBS) of the subthalamic nuclei (STN) as a treatment option. This procedure is performed with the patient awake, using the combined expertise of the stereotactic neurosurgeon, an electrophysiologist, and a clinical neurologic assessment. Parameters such as the frequency of pulse, pulse width, amplitude, and electrical port can be modulated to achieve dynamic suppression of output from the STN to the thalamus. This procedure can be performed bilaterally. Documented benefits in rigidity, tremor, and bradykinesia can occur; gait and postural instability are relatively refractory to treatment. Although dyskinesia increases initially, overall dyskinesia is reduced in a majority of patients with DBS by improving other symptoms, which subsequently reduces the levodopa and dopamine agonist doses. The ideal patient is young, free of dementia or neuropsychiatric complications, and highly responsive to medications for Parkinson's disease. Patients with a poor response to levodopa are less likely to benefit from DBS surgery.

DRUG-INDUCED PARKINSONISM

The most common cause of drug-induced parkinsonism is treatment with neuroleptic medication. A number of other agents may provoke a bradykinetic-rigid syndrome (Table 121–8).

DIFFUSE LEWY BODY DISEASE

Lewy body disease may be classified into three types based on the pathologic distribution of underlying Lewy bodies: brainstem, transitional, and diffuse. When Lewy bodies are restricted to the brainstem, no clinical or pathologic difference between Lewy body disease and Parkinson's disease is recognized. In the transitional phase, Lewy bodies spread to involve the limbic system. In diffuse Lewy body disease, clinical parkinsonism combined with early and prominent dementia occurs. Visual hallucinations are common, patients may be extremely sensitive to the adverse effects of neuroleptic medication, and cognitive fluctuations occur (see Chapter 115).

PROGRESSIVE SUPRANUCLEAR PALSY

In the early 1960s, Steele, Richardson, and Olszewski described a series of patients who exhibited gait disturbance, unheralded falls, bradykinesia, and rigidity. Unlike patients with idiopathic Parkinson's disease, patients with progressive supranuclear palsy typically do not have tremor. A progressive loss of voluntary eye movements occurs with the preservation of oculocephalic reflex eye movements (the hallmark of a supranuclear eye movement abnormality). Patients develop dementia, pseudobulbar affect (i.e., affective lability without normal underlying emotional content), and frontal release signs. Progression is faster than it is in patients with idiopathic Parkinson's disease, and symptomatic response to dopaminergic agents is poor. The cause of progressive supranuclear palsy remains unknown. Neurofibrillary tangles develop with neuronal loss and gliosis involving the globus pallidus, subthalamic nucleus, substantia nigra, pons, oculomotor complex, medulla, and dentate nucleus of the cerebellum.

MULTISYSTEM ATROPHY

Three entities are included under the rubric *multisystem atrophy* (see Table 121–3). A group of abnormal glial cytoplasmic inclusions containing alpha-synuclein is the pathologic hallmark of the disorder, with progressive loss of neurons—in particular brain nuclei—determining the particular clinical presentation. All eventually progress to a profoundly akinetic-rigid state. In olivopontocerebellar atrophy, the predominant early symptoms are cerebellar dysmetria and ataxia, with abnormalities of vocal modulation, appendicular coordination, and smooth pursuit eye movements. A dramatic and progressive loss of neurons occurs in the olivary nucleus of the medulla, pons, and cerebellum, giving rise to characteristic atrophy of these regions on computed tomography (CT) or magnetic resonance imaging (MRI). In striatonigral degeneration, predominant bradykinesia, symmetric rigidity, and postural instability develop relatively early, typically without prominent resting tremor. These symptoms are relatively refractory to levodopa treatment—a clue to differentiating these from similar symptoms caused by idiopathic Parkinson's disease. In Shy-Drager syndrome, bradykinesia, rigidity, and postural instability are combined with early and prominent loss of autonomic function. Severe orthostatic hypotension results in syncopal events. Cardiac arrhythmias, urinary incontinence, constipation, diarrhea, sudomotor instability, and disordered central temperature regulation may occur.

VASCULAR PARKINSONISM

Vascular parkinsonism is a controversial entity because its findings are varied and its pathogenesis is ill defined. Patients have signs of Parkinson's disease and have microangiopathic changes in the basal ganglia that cause periventricular high T2-weighted signals on MRI. However, such changes are commonly seen on MRI in older individuals, regardless of whether they have bradykinesia and rigidity. Vascular parkinsonism is often diagnosed whenever vascular risk factors are known and periventricular white matter lesions that are evident on MRI accompany clinical evidence of parkinsonism. A lack of improvement with levodopa therapy or the overt evidence of stroke involving the basal ganglia supports this diagnosis.

TOXIC PARKINSONISM

Carbon monoxide intoxication may cause bilateral necrosis of the basal ganglia, leading to an akinetic-rigid state. Chronic exposure to manganese has also been associated with the development of parkinsonism. An intriguing clue to a possible toxic basis for idiopathic Parkinson's disease was discovered in the 1970s with the report of a series of formerly asymptomatic individuals who developed bradykinesia, postural instability, tremor, and rigidity after exposure to the designer street drug methyl-phenyl-tetrahydropyridine (MPTP). Selective uptake of this agent into pigmented cells of the substantia nigra, with conversion by monoamine oxidase type B to the toxic-free radical MPP(+), accounts for selective cell death of dopaminergic neurons. MPTP has been widely studied in animal models of Parkinson's disease.

Hyperkinetic Movement Disorders

ESSENTIAL TREMOR

The most common cause of tremor is *essential tremor*. This condition is inherited and ranges in severity from cosmetic to disabling. Unlike the tremor of Parkinson's disease, essential tremor typically affects both sides of the body symmetrically and is more prominent with action than it is at rest. The frequency of the tremor oscillation is relatively constant, but the amplitude may vary. As with all forms of tremor, stress, sleep deprivation, and stimulants (e.g., caffeine) make the condition worse. Alcohol often relieves essential tremor. When essential tremor occurs in the context of a dominant family history, it is called *familial tremor*. Essential tremor starts somewhat earlier than it does with Parkinson's disease and may affect the neck and head muscles and the voice, as well as the arms and hands. The most useful medications for essential tremor include propranolol (Inderal), primidone (Mysoline), and topiramate (Topamax). DBS surgery with electrode placement in either the ventral intermediolateral nucleus of the thalamus or the subthalamic nucleus is also effective.

OTHER CAUSES OF TREMOR

Parkinson's disease tremor is worst at rest, is somewhat slower than essential tremor, and responds best to anticholinergic treatment rather than to medications for essential tremor. Cerebellar tremor has a more irregular rhythm, is coarser than either essential tremor or the tremor of Parkinson's disease, and is more significant as the limb approaches a target (action tremor). So-called *rubral tremor* is an extremely coarse tremor with significant intention dysmetria that occurs with lesions in the area of the red nucleus in the mesencephalon. Numerous drugs can provoke tremor, including stimulants (e.g., theophylline, methylphenidate), dopamine receptor–blocking drugs, lithium, tricyclic antidepressants, anticonvulsants (e.g., valproate, phenytoin, carbamazepine), cardiac agents (e.g., amiodarone, calcium channel blockers, procainamide), and immunosuppressive agents (e.g., cyclosporin A, corticosteroids).

DYSTONIA

Dystonia consists of sustained muscle contractions that result in abnormal postures and contortions. It may occur as a primary process or as a secondary symptom of an underlying neurologic disease (e.g., Wilson's disease, Huntington's disease, cerebral anoxia). Derangements in the physiologic makeup of the dopamine synapse may lead to acute drug-induced dystonic reactions. Such reactions can be life threatening if respiratory function is compromised, but they generally respond to emergent treatment with anticholinergic medication. Metoclopramide (Reglan), commonly prescribed for nausea and vomiting, may induce dystonia. DBS with implantable electrodes remains experimental for this indication.

Although the primary dystonias presumably involve basal ganglia dysfunction, no underlying pathologic structure has been convincingly documented. Mutations of the *DYT* gene on chromosome 9 have been defined in some families with generalized dystonia. Between 5% and 10% of patients with primary generalized dystonia are responsive to treatment with levodopa (i.e., dopa-responsive dystonia as a result of mutations of the GTP-cyclohydrolase gene), and all patients with symptoms of generalized dystonia should receive a therapeutic trial of levodopa.

A large number of common focal dystonias that were once considered emotional disorders include writer's cramp, spasmodic dysphonia, and torticollis (Table 121–9). Intramuscular injection of botulinum toxin is the treatment of choice for symptomatic control of focal dystonia.

WILSON'S DISEASE

Wilson's disease is a rare (approximately 1 per 40,000 births) but treatable autosomal recessive disorder that is debilitating and eventually fatal if left untreated. It should be considered in the differential diagnosis of new-onset hyperkinesia or parkinsonism in the young adult. Wilson's disease almost never develops after the age of 50 years. Wilson's disease may also exhibit neuropsychiatric manifestations. Psychosis is

common. The disease is a systemic disorder of copper metabolism. In addition to the neurologic signs and symptoms, hepatic dysfunction (including death from fulminant hepatic failure) occurs at variable degrees. All young adult patients with a movement disorder should be screened for Wilson's disease by means of a ceruloplasmin level. In patients with suggested Wilson's disease, slit lamp examination for Kayser-Fleischer rings (i.e., characteristic depositions of copper pigment in the limbus of the iris), 24-hour urine collection for copper, determination of serum copper level, and hepatic biopsy are indicated. Treatment with copper chelation and zinc can arrest further neurologic decline and can occasionally improve neurologic deficits. Mobilization of copper from liver stores can result in neurologic worsening during initial treatment with standard chelation regimens. Patients should be referred to experienced centers for initiation of treatment.

HUNTINGTON'S DISEASE

Huntington's disease is an inexorably progressive autosomal dominant neurodegenerative disorder affecting motor function, cognition, and behavior. The mean age at onset is 40 (10% of cases begin in childhood), and the mean duration of illness is 20 years. In the adult-onset form, chorea affects the limbs and trunk. Other movement abnormalities commonly occur, including dystonia, rigidity, postural instability, and myoclonus. Bradykinesia and rigidity predominate in the juvenile-onset form. Eye movements are often abnormal early in the disease, with slowing of saccadic initiation and velocity and eventual breakdown of smooth pursuit movements. The disease involves premature death of select neurons in the caudate and putamen.

An abnormal expansion in the number of trinucleotide CAG repeat sequences occurs in a *350-kD* gene on chromosome 4, coding for the protein *huntingtin*. Excessive CAG sequences encode an overly expanded number of polyglutamine repeats in the protein. CAG expansion in excess of 37 repeats is diagnostic of the disease. On average, the higher

Table 121–9 Features of the Primary Dystonias

Feature	Description
Generalized (usually childhood onset, autosomal dominant with variable penetrance)	
Idiopathic torsion dystonia	Intorsion of a foot, followed by progressive spread of dystonia to involve the muscles of the limbs, trunk, neck, and face
Dopa-responsive dystonia	As above, with bradykinesia and rigidity common and hyperreflexia in 25%. Dramatic response to low-dose levodopa (50–200 mg)
Focal (usually adult onset, sporadic)	
Spasmodic torticollis	Involuntary contraction of neck musculature resulting in various combinations of twisting, tilting, extension, or flexion
Meige's syndrome	Lower facial/mandibular dystonia with dyskinetic movements of the tongue and lips
Blepharospasm	Involuntary forced eyelid closure
Spasmodic dysphonia	Dystonic vocal cord contraction resulting in hoarse or breathy whisper
Writer's cramp	Task-specific contortion of the hand/forearm when attempting to write

the CAG-repeat expansion, the earlier the age at onset. Despite this inverse correlation between CAG expansion length and age at onset, the variability in age at onset for a given CAG expansion is too high to enable precise prognostication regarding onset for individual patients. No treatment currently exists that slows the progression of Huntington's disease. Downregulation of dopaminergic neurotransmission by means of neuroleptic agents may suppress chorea but often worsens underlying postural instability and rigidity. Treating depression and psychosis may enhance the patient's quality of life. Use of antenatal diagnosis and presymptomatic genetic testing of adult patients at risk for the disease raises ethical and personal questions. Presymptomatic testing of at-risk children is not indicated.

OTHER CAUSES OF CHOREA

Sydenham's chorea occurs in childhood as a postinfectious complication of group A β-hemolytic streptococcal pharyngitis. The illness is usually self limited, but prolonged chorea may occur, as may other neuropsychiatric symptoms. The caudate and STN are affected, presumably on an autoimmune basis. Some patients respond to a short course of corticosteroids. Treatment with intravenous immunoglobulin is also an option.

A number of drugs occasionally cause chorea, including isoniazid, lithium, oral contraceptives, and reserpine. Metabolic causes include thyrotoxicosis, hypoparathyroidism, and hypomagnesemia. Hemichorea may result from stroke or tumor, and autoimmune or vascular mechanisms may underlie the chorea sometimes observed in patients with lupus erythematosus.

MYOCLONUS

Myoclonus occurs in many neurologic disorders, but it may also occur in isolation. *Physiologic (hypnagogic) myoclonus* occurs in healthy individuals as they fall asleep. *Essential myoclonus* is a nonprogressive, generalized disorder that can occur as an autosomal dominant trait. Patients suffer from multifocal, large-amplitude lightning jerks that are provoked by action and are disabling, or they may have mild, small-amplitude jerks that do not disrupt their function. Patients with essential myoclonus almost always also have some degree of underlying dystonia. Myoclonus also occurs in generalized epilepsy syndromes that are not inherently progressive (e.g., benign myoclonus of infancy, juvenile myoclonic epilepsy) or in tonic-clonic epilepsy and progressive encephalopathy (e.g., progressive myoclonic encephalopathy). Static myoclonic encephalopathy occurs most commonly as a consequence of severe anoxia (Lance-Adams syndrome) or head trauma and may be spontaneous or action induced, multifocal, or generalized. Secondary causes of focal or multifocal myoclonus include underlying structural lesions of the nervous system (e.g., stroke, arteriovenous malformation, demyelinating disease, tumor, abscess, other infectious processes) or toxic-metabolic conditions (e.g., hypoxia, uremia, hepatic encephalopathy, sepsis, electrolyte disturbances, hormonal abnormalities). Treatment should be directed to the underlying cause. Valproate or clonazepam is commonly prescribed for symptomatic treatment of myoclonus.

TOURETTE'S DISORDER

In 1885, Gilles de la Tourette described a series of patients with motor and vocal tics, some of whom had coprolalia (foul language). For most of the ensuing century, Tourette's disorder was considered a rare curiosity, existing on the border zone of neurology and psychiatry. Although coprolalia is an uncommon manifestation, Tourette's disorder and its related primary tic disorders (e.g., chronic motor tics, chronic vocal tics, transient tic disorder) have been increasingly recognized in the past decade as common entities. A substantial proportion of children with learning disorders have Tourette's disorder.

Transitory tics are a normal part of child development. Tourette's disorder is defined as the history of both motor and vocal tics (for more than 1 year) with onset before the age 18 years. The tics are associated with obsessions and compulsive behavior in 50% of patients and are accompanied by attention-deficit disorder in 50% of patients. Tourette's disorder is probably an autosomal dominant condition with variable penetrance.

Treatment focuses on the most functionally incapacitating aspect of the disorder (not necessarily the tics), and patients and families should be reassured that the disorder is not progressive or fatal. Approximately two thirds of patients outgrow their tics (but not necessarily the other neuropsychiatric manifestations of the illness) by adulthood. Useful medications are outlined in Table 121–10. Strategies to reduce stress on the patient, including education of parents, peers, and teachers, are frequently preferable. Treatment of attention deficit with stimulants may exacerbate tics; treatment of tics with neuroleptic drugs may blunt affect, disrupt learning, provoke depression, and lead to unwanted weight gain.

OTHER CAUSES OF TICS

Tics may be drug induced (i.e., stimulants or neuroleptic medications causing tardive tics), or they may be symptomatic of developmental, degenerative, toxic-metabolic, or infectious neurologic disorders. Patients with chromosomal abnormalities (e.g., Down and fragile X syndromes) frequently have tics, as do those with pervasive developmental delay, anoxic encephalopathy, and autism. Tics occasionally occur in patients with Huntington's disease, progressive supranuclear palsy, Creutzfeldt-Jakob disease, and encephalitis, as well as those with sequelae of carbon monoxide poisoning or hypoglycemia.

Cerebellar Ataxias

The cerebellum receives input from the spinal cord (spinocerebellar tracts), from the vestibular nuclei in the brainstem, and from pontine relays, carrying information from the motor and premotor cortex. The cerebellar cortex is made up of four main neuronal types. Granule cells input onto Purkinje cells, whose axons form the sole output of the cerebellar cortex, terminating in cerebellar nuclei or select brainstem nuclei. Golgi cells and stellate-basket cells function as inhibitory interneurons within the cerebellar cortex. The cerebellar cortex is organized into three main sagittal zones. The most medial (vermal) zone projects to the fastigial nuclei, which in turn project to the vestibulospinal and reticulospinal tracts. Injuries to this zone or its projections lead to abnormal stance and gait, truncal titubation, and disturbances of extraocular movement. The intermediate (paravermal) zone projects to the interposed nuclei, which in turn project to the red nucleus and the thalamus. Isolated injuries to this zone are rare, and clinical manifestations generally overlap with medial or lateral cerebellar syndromes. The lateral zone projects to the dentate nuclei, which in turn project to the thalamus and cerebral cortex. Injuries to this zone or its projections result in abnormal stance and gait, appendicular dysmetria, eye movement dysmetria, dysdiadochokinesia, dysrhythmokinesia, intention tremor, ataxic dysarthria, and hypotonia.

NONHEREDITARY ATAXIAS

Lesions of the cerebellum, its inflow tracts, or its outflow tracts may all be associated with ataxia. The rapid onset of ataxia suggests an underlying structural condition, an immune-mediated process, drug intoxication, or conversion disorder. Structural lesions of the cerebellum or its connecting tracts include tumors, demyelinating plaques, abscesses, and vascular events such as vertebrobasilar occlusion, cerebellar parenchymal hemorrhage, traumatic hematoma, and arteriovenous malformation. Immune-mediated processes include acute postinfectious cerebellitis or myoclonic encephalopathy with neuroblastoma in children, and paraneoplastic cerebellar degeneration in adults. Migraine headaches, particularly in childhood, may be accompanied by ataxia. Radiographic studies, drug screening, and cerebrospinal fluid analysis will clarify the diagnosis in most patients with acute-onset ataxia.

Chronic or progressive ataxia may result from slow-growing brain tumors (e.g., cerebellar astrocytoma, hemangioblastoma, ependymoma, medulloblastoma, supratentorial tumors), congenital malformations (e.g., basilar impression, Dandy-Walker malformation, Chiari malformation), drug effects (e.g., alcoholic cerebellar vermian degeneration, chronic phenytoin toxicity), or hereditary ataxias.

HEREDITARY ATAXIAS

Progressive ataxia is a feature of numerous hereditary neurologic diseases (Table 121–11). Determining which

Table 121–10	**Medications Used in the Management of Incapacitating Tourette's Disorder**

Tics

Neuroleptics (haloperidol, pimozide, others)
Clonidine (oral or transdermal patch)
Calcium channel blockers (diltiazem, verapamil)
Benzodiazepines (clonazepam, others)
Guanfacine

Obsessive-Compulsive Behavior

Selective serotonin reuptake inhibitors (fluoxetine, sertraline, others)
Clomipramine

Attention-Deficit Disorder

Stimulants (methylphenidate, pemoline)
Clonidine
Selegiline
Tricyclic antidepressants

Table 121–11 Hereditary Ataxias

Disease	Onset	Associated Signs
Autosomal Recessive Inheritance		
Ataxia-telangiectasia	Childhood	Telangiectasia, recurrent sinus and pulmonary infections, choreoathetosis, mental retardation in 30%, neoplasms (lymphoma, lymphocytic leukemia)
Abetalipoproteinemia (Bassen-Kornzweig syndrome or acanthocytosis)	Childhood	Absent serum apolipoprotein B leads to fat malabsorption with decreased vitamins A, E, and K; retinitis pigmentosa; nystagmus
Friedreich's ataxia	Childhood	Scoliosis, cardiomyopathy, dysarthria, areflexia, Babinski signs, loss of joint position and vibration sense in legs, dysmetria
Autosomal Dominant Inheritance		
Spinocerebellar ataxia types 1–8, 10–17, 19–22, and 25	Adulthood	Variable combinations of long-tract signs, parkinsonism, dementia
Dentatorubral-pallidoluysian atrophy		Sensory loss, myoclonus, chorea
Other forms of olivopontocerebellar atrophy		Dystonia and seizures

hereditary disease is responsible depends on a thorough assessment of the familial pattern of inheritance and knowledge of the typical age at onset and progression of symptoms and signs associated with these conditions.

Molecular tests for a number of specific hereditary ataxias have become available within the past decade, but caution should be used to ensure adequate informed consent, support services, and follow-up before such tests are used to determine a potentially fatal diagnosis, especially in presymptomatic individuals. Genetic test results have immediate implications for the risk status of extended family members. Definitive therapies are generally lacking, genetic

testing is expensive, and few mechanisms can ensure against genetic testing results being used by insurers or employers to the disadvantage of the patient or family.

Similar to Huntington's disease, several of the autosomal dominant spinocerebellar ataxias are caused by abnormal expansions in the number of repeated CAG codons within unique genes. These diseases display the phenomenon of *anticipation:* the age at onset is progressively younger in successive generations of a family. This phenomenon occurs because the CAG repeat length of the abnormal genes is upwardly unstable during gametogenesis, and higher CAG repeat burden results in younger age at onset.

Prospectus for the Future

Advances in molecular genetics, gene profiling, stem cell research, and fetal tissue transplant techniques are all proceeding rapidly and promise to improve the diagnosis and therapy of many movement disorders in the coming decade. Initial studies of fetal nigral tissue transplantation in patients with Parkinson's disease have been controversial. A number of patients developed disabling dyskinesias after receiving fetal nigral grafts. Nonetheless, the fact that these grafts survived, developed connections to target structures in the striatum, and had a functional impact on patients' parkinsonian symptoms is

encouraging. More work will need to be done in animal models of parkinsonism in which dyskinesia develops. Great interest exists in developing gene therapy for Parkinson's disease because creating viral vectors with relative tropism for the striatum, specifically targeting the molecular biochemistry of dopamine production and metabolism, is possible. Experimental gene therapy in animal models (e.g., rodents, primates) is promising. Studies of co-affected siblings with Parkinson's disease have revealed new genetic loci of interest. Similar approaches hold promise in most other motor system disorders.

References

Gasser T, Bressman S, Durr A, et al: State of the art review: Molecular diagnosis of inherited movement disorders. Movement Disorders Society task force on molecular diagnosis. Mov Disord 18:3–18, 2003.

Kurlan RM: Treatment of Movement Disorders. Philadelphia, JB Lippincott, 1995.

Lang A: Other Movement Disorders. In Goldman L, Ausiello DA (eds): Cecil Textbook of Medicine, 23rd ed. Philadelphia, Saunders, 2007.

Miyasaki J, Shannon K, Voon V, et al: Practice parameter: Evaluation and treatment of depression, psychosis and dementia in Parkinson's disease. Neurology 66(7):996–1002, 2006.

Mouradian AM: Recent advances in the genetics and pathogenesis of Parkinson disease. Neurology 58:179–185, 2002.

Pahwa R, Factor S, Lyons K, et al: Practice parameter: Treatment of Parkinson's disease with motor fluctuations and dyskinesia (an evidence-based review). Neurology 66(7):983–995, 2006.

Suchowersky O, Gronseth G, Perlmutter J, et al: Practice parameter: Neuroprotective strategies and alternative therapies for Parkinson's disease (an evidence-based review). Neurology 66(7):976–982, 2006.

Suchowersky O, Reich S, Perlmutter J, et al: Practice parameter: Diagnosis and prognosis of new onset Parkinson's disease (an evidence-based review). Neurology 66(7):968–975, 2006.

Developmental and Neurocutaneous Disorders

Robert C. Griggs

Computed tomography and magnetic resonance imaging detect many congenital and developmental diseases that were previously unrecognized. Subarachnoid cysts and ventricular asymmetries, as well as many of the more minor malformations and anomalies described here, usually have no symptoms and need no treatment.

Spinal Malformations

Developmental anomalies of the vertebral bodies are frequent and may result in pain and neurologic symptoms if they cause scoliosis or lead to accelerated degenerative changes of the spine. Neurologic disability is likely if associated cord anomalies are present or if they compress neural structures or alter cerebrospinal fluid flow.

Chiari Malformations

A Chiari I malformation is defined as ectopia of the cerebellar tonsils more than 5 mm below the foramen magnum. The condition is usually asymptomatic but occasionally causes headaches worsened by straining or cough, lower cranial neuropathies, downbeat nystagmus, ataxia, or sensory loss. The malformation is congenital, but symptoms often exhibit in the third decade or later.

Chiari II malformations (also called Arnold-Chiari malformations) are characterized by elongation of the cerebellum and lower brainstem through the foramen magnum. A myelomeningocele and hydrocephalus are usually present. Brainstem dysfunction may develop from malformation or compression of neural structures. Treatment is surgical: repair of the myelomeningocele, relief of hydrocephalus, and cervical bony decompression.

Tethered Spinal Cord

In tethered spinal cord, the filum terminale is anomalous, resulting in either a lack of normal ascent of the conus medullaris to the L1 vertebral level or an ischemic or metabolic disturbance of the caudal spinal cord. Associated spinal anomalies are common: diastematomyelia (split cord), spinal lipomas, dermal sinuses, and fibrolipomas of the filum terminale. Patients exhibit bladder and sexual dysfunction and lower extremity weakness and spasticity. Symptoms typically develop in childhood or adolescence. Focal hypertrichosis, hemangiomas, and nevi occur in the skin over the lumbar spine. Treatment involves surgical release of the tethered cord.

Syringohydromyelia

In syringohydromyelia, the central canal of the spinal cord (hydromyelia), the substance of the spinal cord (syringomyelia), or the brainstem (syringobulbia) is expanded by the presence of fluid under pressure. Symptoms of syringohydromyelia begin in late adolescence or early adulthood and alternate with long periods of stability. The syrinx usually affects the cervical spinal cord. Patients exhibit asymmetric weakness, atrophy, and decreased reflexes of the hands and arms; dissociated sensory loss (impaired perception of pain and temperature, but preservation of light touch and proprioception) in the neck, arms, and upper trunk; and increased muscle tone and reflexes in the legs. Extension into the medulla may cause nystagmus or lower cranial neuropathies. A syrinx can occur 20 or more years after cord trauma. Diagnosis is made by magnetic resonance imaging, which may show an associated craniocervical junction lesion or tumor. Treatment is directed at the cause of the syrinx. In patients with Chiari II malformations, adequate shunting of the lateral ventricles may result in collapse of the syrinx. Syringohydromyelia in patients with spinal tumors is treated by surgery. Focal areas with slight (2- to 3-mm) dilations of the spinal cord central canal are occasionally discovered incidentally; the prognosis without treatment is believed to be good.

Malformations of Cortical Development

Malformations of cortical development are caused by intrauterine infection, intrauterine ischemia, and gene mutations. When small areas of the brain are involved, patients typically develop epilepsy in the first or second decade and have minor static neurologic dysfunction but normal intellect. Persons with involvement of larger areas of the brain often have mental retardation and severe neurologic dysfunction in addition to epilepsy. Diagnosis is established by magnetic resonance imaging. Table 122–1 lists common malformations.

Developmental and Neurocutaneous Disorders

Neurocutaneous syndromes are congenital, usually hereditary, disorders characterized by lesions involving both the nervous system and skin. Often termed the *phacomatoses* (from the Greek *phakoma*, meaning *birthmark*), over 40 syndromes have been described. The most important of these syndromes are neurofibromatosis (types 1 and 2), tuberous sclerosis, Sturge-Weber syndrome, and von Hippel-Lindau disease.

NEUROFIBROMATOSIS TYPE 1

Neurofibromatosis type 1 (NF1) is the classic disorder described by von Recklinghausen, with a prevalence of 1 in 3000 births. Transmission is autosomal dominant, but one half of the cases are sporadic. NF1 causes many types of skin and central nervous system (CNS) tumors: in the skin, neurofibromas and plexiform neurofibromas; and in the CNS, optic nerve gliomas, meningiomas, and astrocytomas of the brain and spinal cord. The NF1 gene is located on chromosome *17q* and expresses a protein designated as neurofi-

bromin (a tumor-suppressor protein). Pathogenic mutations in the NF1 gene are identified in approximately 75% of clinical cases, but no correlation exists between a particular genotype and phenotype. Although NF1 is a congenital disease, most manifestations appear during childhood and adult life. The criteria for the diagnosis include two or more of the following: (1) six or more café au lait macules larger than 5 mm in prepubertal patients and more than 15 mm in postpubertal individuals, (2) two or more neurofibromas of any type or one plexiform neurofibroma, (3) axillary or inguinal freckling, (4) sphenoid bone dysplasia, (5) optic nerve glioma, (6) Lisch nodules, and (7) a family history of NF1. Diagnosis is based on clinical criteria, supplemented by neuroimaging findings. Other manifestations include developmental delay and epilepsy. Important complications include scoliosis, gastrointestinal neurofibromas, pheochromocytomas, and renal artery stenosis. The majority of patients with NF1 do not require treatment. Subcutaneous neurofibromas may be painful and can be excised surgically. Many intraspinal and intracranial tumors are benign and treated surgically. Genetic counseling must be provided in all patients and families in which NF1 is present. Many new mutations occur in the germline of an unaffected parent; siblings of sporadic patients with new mutations may therefore be at risk for the disease.

NEUROFIBROMATOSIS TYPE 2

Neurofibromatosis type 2 (NF2) is also called central neurofibromatosis and, similar to NF1, is transmitted by an autosomal-dominant mechanism. NF2 occurs less frequently than NF1 (approximately 1 in 50,000 individuals). The usual manifestation of NF2 is bilateral eighth nerve schwannomas. However, multiple meningiomas and multiple other schwannomas are also common features. The NF2 gene is located on chromosome *22q*. The gene product (merlin) is a cytoskeletal protein. Skin lesions are present in up to 30% of patients with NF2, but the diagnosis is based

Table 122–1	**Malformations of Central Nervous System Cortical Development Recognized by Magnetic Resonance Imaging**		
Malformation	**Clinical Features**	**Cause(s)**	**Treatment**
Focal cortical dysplasia	Epilepsy (usual); developmental delay (if extensive)	Multiple	Seizure control*
Lissencephaly (smooth brain)	Epilepsy	Genes: 17q13.3 and Xq22	Usually unsatisfactory
Band heterotopia	Women > men; epilepsy; variable developmental delay	Gene: *Xq22*	Seizure control*
Subependymal nodular heterotopia	Men > women; epilepsy; variable developmental delay	Gene: *Xq28*	Seizure control*
Polymicrogyria-schizencephaly	Severe central nervous system dysfunction; epilepsy	Multiple	Seizure control*

*Treatment of seizures with medication is often unsuccessful. Surgical excision of an epileptogenic focus can be curative.

on the following criteria: (1) bilateral eighth nerve tumors detected by magnetic resonance imaging, (2) a family member with either NF2 or unilateral eighth nerve lesions (neurofibroma, meningioma, or schwannoma), and (3) juvenile posterior subcapsular lens opacities. Symptoms of NF2 begin in the second to fourth decades. Surgical treatment of schwannomas and meningiomas is usually indicated, and early recognition is important for successful treatment of eighth nerve tumors. Family members should be screened regularly with hearing tests and magnetic resonance imaging.

TUBEROUS SCLEROSIS

Tuberous sclerosis complex (TSC) causes hamartomatous lesions involving multiple organs at different stages in the course of the disease. Transmission is autosomal dominant, but sporadic cases are frequent because of spontaneous mutations. The incidence of TSC is 1 in 10,000 to 50,000. TSC affects tissues from different embryonic germ layers: cutaneous lesions include adenoma sebaceum, hypomelanotic skin macules (ash leaf spots), shagreen patches, and subungual fibromas; visceral lesions include cardiac and renal tumors; and CNS lesions include hamartomas of the cortex and ventricular walls and subependymal giant cell tumors. At least three TSC gene loci have been found. In *TSC-1*, the gene abnormality is localized on chromosome *9q34,* and the protein product is called hamartin; its function is not known. In *TSC-2*, the gene abnormalities are on chromosome *16p.* This gene encodes tuberin, a guanosine triphosphatase-activating protein. Hereditary cases not linked to these two loci also occur.

The diagnostic clinical triad is mental subnormality, epilepsy, and skin lesions. CNS imaging reveals multiple calcified subependymal nodules, as well as cortical tubers. Retinal hamartomas occur in one half of patients. The diagnosis is usually clinical, with confirmation by identification of hamartomas on imaging studies. Treatment is directed at controlling epilepsy and correcting hydrocephalus. Serial cardiac studies and renal ultrasound evaluation may be indicated in some patients.

STURGE-WEBER SYNDROME

Sturge-Weber syndrome is usually sporadic, without an established hereditary pattern. The incidence and prevalence are not defined; it occurs in less than 1 in 20,000 births. Usual clinical manifestations include facial vascular nevus (portwine stain), epilepsy, cognitive deficits, and, less frequently, hemiparesis or hemiplegia, hemianopia, or glaucoma. The facial lesion suggests the presence of venous angiomatosis of the pia mater. Most patients have epilepsy. The diagnosis is usually made by the facial nevus and imaging confirmation of intracranial abnormality (ipsilateral cerebral cortical calcifications). The treatment is that of the associated epilepsy. If anti-epileptic drugs do not control seizures, then surgical excision of epileptogenic areas is often successful.

VON HIPPEL-LINDAU DISEASE (CENTRAL NERVOUS SYSTEM ANGIOMATOSIS)

Von Hippel-Lindau disease is an autosomal-dominant disorder caused by a defective tumor suppressor gene at chromosome *3p25–p26.* It is characterized by retinal angiomas, brain and spinal cord hemangioblastomas, renal cell carcinomas, pheochromocytomas, angiomas of the liver and kidney, and cysts of the pancreas, kidney, liver, and epididymis. Both sexes are affected equally. The diagnosis is established if patients have more than one CNS hemangioblastoma, one hemangioblastoma with a visceral manifestation of the disease, or one manifestation of the disease and a known family history. Symptoms typically begin during the third or fourth decade. Retinal inflammation with exudates, hemorrhage, and retinal detachment typically antedate cerebellar complaints. Headache, vertigo, and vomiting result from the cerebellar tumor. Cerebellar findings such as incoordination, dysmetria, and ataxia are common.

Retinal detachments and tumors are treated by laser therapy. Brain tumors, renal cell carcinomas, pheochromocytomas, and epididymal tumors are treated surgically. Small CNS tumors may be treated by gamma knife. Early evaluation and repeated imaging studies are indicated once the diagnosis is made, and at-risk individuals should be evaluated.

Prospectus for the Future

Understanding the neurocutaneous disorders associated with tumor development is increasing. As the molecular signals causing tumors are clarified, novel genetic treatment strategies will enter trial. Improved imaging and surgical techniques are already making it possible to treat neurofibromatosis and many other neurocutaneous disorders.

References

Barkovich AJ, Kuzniecky RI: Congenital, developmental, and neurocutaneous disorders. In Goldman L, Ausiello DA (eds): Cecil Textbook of Medicine, 23rd ed. Philadelphia, Saunders, 2007.

Barkovich AJ, Kuzniecky RI, Jackson GD et al: A developmental and genetic classification for malformations of cortical development. Neurology 65:1873–1887, 2005.

Cerebrovascular Disease

Timothy J. Counihan

The term *cerebrovascular disease* refers to disorders of the arterial or venous circulatory systems of the central nervous system. The term *stroke* is used when the symptoms begin abruptly, as a result of either inadequate blood flow (ischemic stroke) or hemorrhage into the brain tissue (parenchymal hemorrhage) or surrounding subarachnoid space (subarachnoid hemorrhage). Approximately 80% of strokes are ischemic in origin. *Focal* ischemic stroke is caused by either thrombotic or embolic occlusion of a major artery, whereas *global* ischemia usually results from inadequate cerebral perfusion such as that which occurs after cardiac arrest or ventricular fibrillation. Rarely is isolated cerebral hypoxia (such as occurs in carbon monoxide poisoning or asphyxiation) a cause of stroke.

Chapter 123

Epidemiologic Factors

Stroke remains the third leading medical cause of death and the second most frequent cause of morbidity in developed countries. Since 1990, the incidence of stroke in the United States has declined by approximately 1.5% annually to approximately 0.5 to 1.0 per 1000 population, accounting for approximately 1 in every 15 deaths. The belief is that this steady decrease is the result of improvements in general public health and is coincident with the decline of cardiovascular deaths and better control of hypertension and other risk factors (Table 123–1). Rates of stroke among men and women are similar, although the incidence and rate of mortality from stroke are higher in blacks than in whites.

Although the reasons for the decline in the incidence of stroke remain unclear, a greater understanding of the importance of controlling risk factors in stroke prevention may be partly responsible. The increasingly successful management of hypertension and the reduction in smoking habits have been major factors in reducing the incidence of stroke. In addition, the increasing public awareness of the warning symptoms of stroke as constituting a *brain attack* (analogous to chest pain as a warning of a *heart attack*) is beginning to improve primary stroke prevention.

Anatomy

Two pairs of major arteries, the carotid (anterior circulation) and vertebral (posterior circulation) arteries supply the brain (Fig. 123–1).

ANTERIOR CIRCULATION

The common carotid artery bifurcates into an internal and an external branch at the level of the thyroid cartilage in the neck. The internal carotid artery (ICA) enters the skull through the carotid canal and passes through the cavernous sinus as the carotid siphon. It gives off the ophthalmic, anterior choroidal, and posterior communicating arteries before bifurcating into the anterior cerebral artery (ACA) and middle cerebral artery (MCA). The ACA supplies the medial surfaces of the cerebral hemispheres, and the MCA supplies the lateral surface (convexity), in addition to much of the basal ganglia and subcortical white matter.

POSTERIOR CIRCULATION

The vertebral arteries (VAs) course upward within the transverse processes of the cervical vertebrae. The intracranial VA gives off a branch to form the anterior spinal artery, as well as the posterior inferior cerebellar arteries (PICAs), before the two arteries unite to form the basilar artery (BA) at the pontomedullary junction. The BA supplies the cerebellum via the anterior inferior cerebellar artery (AICA) and superior cerebellar artery (SCA) before bifurcating into the posterior cerebral arteries (PCAs) at the level of the pontomesencephalic junction.

CIRCLE OF WILLIS

The circle of Willis is formed at the base of the brain by the union of both ACAs via the anterior communicating artery and the union of the ICA with the PCA via the posterior communicating artery (see Fig. 123–1). Hence communication exists between both anterior circulations, as well as

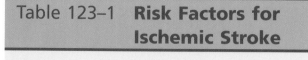

Table 123–1	**Risk Factors for Ischemic Stroke**

Diabetes
Hypertension
Smoking
Family history of premature vascular disease
Hyperlipidemia
Atrial fibrillation
History of transient ischemic attack
History of recent myocardial infarction
History of congestive heart failure (left ventricular ejection fraction >25%)
Drugs (sympathomimetics, oral contraceptives, cocaine)

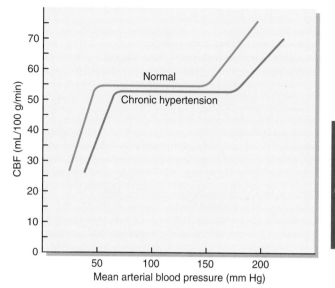

Figure 123–2 Autoregulatory cerebral blood flow (CBF) response to changes in mean arterial pressure in normotensive and chronically hypertensive persons. Note the shift of the curve toward higher mean pressures with chronic hypertension. (From Pulsinelli WA: Cerebrovascular diseases: principles. In Goldman L, Bennett JC [eds]: Cecil Textbook of Medicine, 21st ed. Philadelphia, Saunders, 2000, p 2097.)

Physiologic Factors

Unlike other body tissues, the brain has few energy stores but relies on a sizable and reliable cerebral blood flow (CBF) to meet its energy demands. CBF averages 60 mL/100 g of brain tissue per minute. A complex system of neural pathways regulates CBF in a process known as *autoregulation,* which maintains CBF at a constant level despite wide fluctuations in cerebral perfusion pressure (Fig. 123–2). CBF remains relatively constant when the mean arterial pressure remains between 50 and 150 mm Hg. In the case of chronic systemic hypertension, however, both the upper and the lower levels of autoregulation are raised, which indicates a higher tolerance of hypertension but a greater susceptibility to the effects of hypotension.

Ischemic Stroke

PATHOGENESIS

Cerebral ischemia may result from thrombotic or embolic occlusion of a major vessel that reduces blood flow within the involved vascular territory, or it may be a consequence of diminished systemic perfusion. Prolonged brain ischemia results in infarction, characterized histologically by necrosis of neurons, glia, and endothelial cells. Cerebral infarcts are classified as either *pale* (anemic) or *hemorrhagic* (in areas of endothelial necrosis). In transitional zones between normally perfused tissue and the infarcted central core is a rim of moderately ischemic tissue known as the *ischemic penumbra,* which is the target area for treatment trials of neuroprotective agents.

Global cerebral ischemia usually results from cardiac arrest or ventricular fibrillation. Some neuronal populations

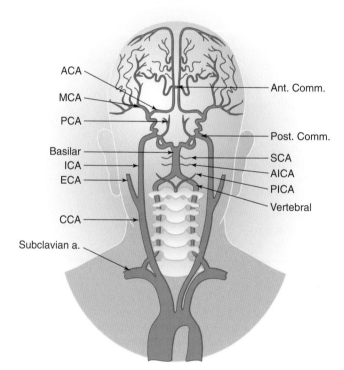

Figure 123–1 Coronal view of the extracranial and intracranial arterial supply to the brain. Vessels forming the circle of Willis are highlighted. a. = artery; ACA = anterior cerebral artery; AICA = anterior inferior cerebellar artery; Ant. Comm. = anterior communicating artery; CCA = common carotid artery; ECA = external carotid artery; ICA = internal carotid artery; MCA = middle cerebral artery; PCA = posterior cerebral artery; PICA = posterior inferior cerebellar artery; Post. Comm. = posterior communicating artery; SCA = superior cerebellar artery. (Modified from Lord R: Surgery of Occlusive Cerebrovascular Disease. St. Louis, Mosby, 1986.)

between the posterior and anterior circulations on each side. Congenital anomalies of the circle are frequent; they include hypoplasia or atresia of a posterior communicating artery or ACA, which may reduce collateral blood supply if an adjacent vessel becomes occluded.

are selectively vulnerable to transient global ischemia, particularly neurons of the hippocampus, cerebellar Purkinje cells, and the deeper layers of the cerebral cortex (inducing so-called laminar necrosis). Pure hypoxia causes cerebral dysfunction (exhibited clinically as lethargy and confusion) but rarely produces irreversible brain injury unless accompanied by other factors such as hypoglycemia. When neurons are rendered ischemic, a significant number of biochemical changes take place. Intracellular membranes are no longer able to control ion fluxes, which leads to increased intracellular concentrations of calcium and arrest of mitochondrial function. Activation of membrane lipases further compromises cell membrane integrity and leads to release of excitatory neurotransmitters, which, in turn, may further exacerbate tissue injury. If blood flow is restored within 15 minutes, then the effects of these events may be reversible.

CEREBRAL EDEMA

Cerebral edema may be intracellular (cytotoxic) or interstitial (vasogenic). Intracellular edema develops rapidly in ischemic neurons as energy-dependent ion-channel pumps fail, whereas vasogenic edema occurs as a result of damage to endothelial cells, disrupting the blood-brain barrier and allowing macromolecules such as plasma proteins to enter the interstitial space. Fluid accumulates over 3 to 5 days after an ischemic stroke and can increase brain water content by as much as 10%; such large volume increases can lead to transtentorial herniation and death.

ETIOLOGIC FACTORS

Table 123–2 lists the major causes of acute cerebral ischemia. Atherosclerosis of the cerebral vasculature accounts for approximately two thirds of strokes, either through embolization of plaque to distal vessels (artery-to-artery embolus) or by in situ thrombosis. Certain sites of the cerebral vasculature are increasingly prone to the development of atheromatous plaques (Fig. 123–3). Cardiogenic emboli make up the majority of the remaining third of ischemic strokes, arising most commonly as a result of atrial fibrillation. Mural thrombi, valvular vegetations, and atrial myxomas are also potential sources of embolus, as are *paradoxical emboli* (emboli of venous origin passing through a patent foramen ovale).

Certain conditions predispose younger patients to stroke (Table 123–3).

TRANSIENT ISCHEMIC ATTACK VERSUS STROKE

A transient ischemic attack (TIA) is a brief episode of neurologic dysfunction caused by focal brain or retinal ischemia, with clinical symptoms typically lasting less than 1 hour and without evidence of acute cerebral infarction. Figure 123–4 provides an algorithm for the evaluation and treatment of patients with TIA. Given that most deficits resolve within 1 hour, symptoms that last longer should prompt a search for an alternative explanation. The previous time window of 24 hours has largely been abandoned, although the importance of performing imaging in the acute setting to exclude infarction has been emphasized. A *completed stroke* indicates that

Table 123–2 Causes of Cerebral Ischemia

Focal

Mural abnormalities

Atherosclerosis
Vasculitis
Vasospasm (migraine, subarachnoid hemorrhage)
Compression (by tumor, aneurysm)
Fibromuscular dysplasia, moyamoya disease
Dissection (spontaneous, traumatic)

Embolism

Cardiogenic (atrial fibrillation, mural thrombus, myxoma, valvular vegetations)
Artery-to-artery
Fat
Air
Paradoxical

Hematologic

Hypercoagulable state
Sickle cell disease
Homocystinuria
Antiphospholipid antibodies (lupus anticoagulant, anticardiolipin antibodies)
Protein C or protein S deficiency

Global

Hypoperfusion
Cardiac arrest
Ventricular fibrillation

infarction has taken place. In most instances, the maximal clinical deficit occurs at the onset of symptoms, with variable recovery over time thereafter. Several factors may contribute to symptom progression (often referred to as a *stroke in evolution*), including propagation of a thrombus or progression of cerebral edema or hemorrhage into an infarcted area. Co-existent medical conditions such as systemic hypotension, fever, hyperglycemia, or hypoxemia may further adversely affect the outcome.

LACUNAR STROKE

A *cerebral lacuna* is a small, deep infarction involving a penetrating branch of a large cerebral artery. Lacunae are usually associated with chronic hypertension, although they are occasionally found in normotensive patients, presumably as a result of micro-atheroma of penetrating arteries, especially of the basal ganglia, thalamus, and white matter of the internal capsule and pons.

Probably the most common clinical syndrome caused by a lacunar stroke is *pure motor hemiparesis*, resulting from a

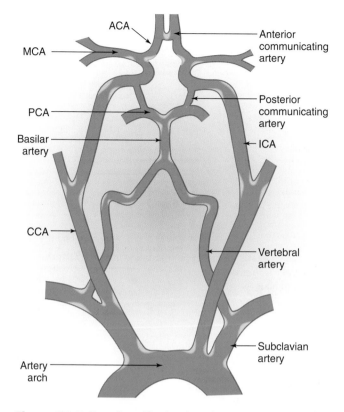

Figure 123–3 Site of predilection for atheromatous plaque. ACA = anterior cerebral artery; CCA = common carotid artery; ICA = internal carotid artery; MCA = middle cerebral artery; PCA = posterior cerebral artery. (From Caplan LR: Stroke—A Clinical Approach. Boston, Butterworth-Heinemann, 1993.)

lesion in the internal capsule. In some patients with lacunar infarction, the clinical picture includes both weakness and ataxia and is known as *ataxic hemiparesis;* the responsible lesion may be in the internal capsule or pons.

BRAINSTEM SYNDROMES

A large number of other brainstem syndromes have been described with a combination of contralateral hemiplegia and cranial nerve dysfunction: *Weber's syndrome,* caused by a midbrain lesion, is associated with a cranial nerve III palsy and contralateral weakness; and *Claude's syndrome,* caused by a lesion in the red nucleus, consists of a cranial nerve III palsy with a contralateral *rubral* tremor. In the lateral medulla, a syndrome involving cranial nerves IX and X, Horner's syndrome, cerebellar ataxia, and crossed hemibody pain and temperature loss is known as *Wallenberg's syndrome.* This last syndrome is most often the result of occlusion of the ipsilateral vertebral artery with resulting ischemia in the territory of the PICA.

Major Stroke Syndromes

The clinical manifestations of ischemic stroke are summarized in Table 123–4.

Table 123–3 **Causes of Stroke in Young Adults**
Migraine
Arterial dissection
Drugs (cocaine, heroin, oral contraceptive pill)
Premature atherosclerosis (homocystinuria, hyperlipidemia)
Postpartum angiopathy
Cardiac factors
Atrial septal defect
Patent foramen ovale
Mitral valve prolapse
Endocarditis
Hematologic factors
Deficiency states (antithrombin III, protein S, protein C)
Disseminated intravascular coagulation
Thrombotic thrombocytopenic purpura
Inflammatory factors
Systemic lupus erythematosus
Polyarteritis nodosa
Neurosyphilis
Cryoglobulinemia
Other factors
Fibromuscular dysplasia
Moyamoya disease

Table 123–4 **Clinical Manifestations of Ischemic Stroke**	
Occluded Vessel	**Clinical Signs**
ICA	Ipsilateral blindness (variable)
	MCA syndrome
MCA	Contralateral hemiparesis, hemisensory loss (face/arm > leg)
	Aphasia (dominant) or anosognosia (nondominant)
	Homonymous hemianopsia (variable)
ACA	Contralateral hemiparesis, hemisensory loss (leg > arm)
	Abulia (especially if bilateral)
VA/PICA	Ipsilateral facial sensory loss, hemiataxia, nystagmus, Horner's syndrome
	Contralateral loss of temperature/pain sensation
	Dysphagia
SCA	Gait ataxia, nausea, vertigo, dysarthria
BA	Quadriparesis, dysarthria, dysphagia, diplopia, somnolence, amnesia
PCA	Contralateral homonymous hemianopsia, amnesia, sensory loss

ACA = anterior cerebral artery; BA = basilar artery; ICA = internal carotid artery; MCA = middle cerebral artery; PCA = posterior cerebral artery; PICA = posterior inferior cerebellar artery; SCA = superior cerebellar artery; VA = vertebral artery.

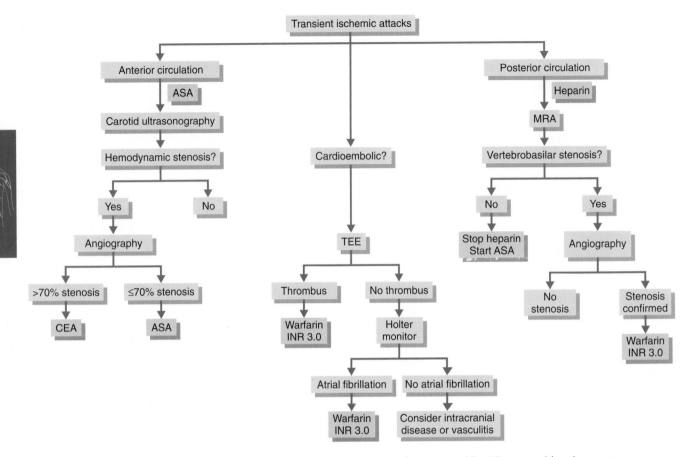

Figure 123–4 Algorithm for the treatment of transient ischemic attacks (TIAs). ASA = aspirin; CEA = carotid endarterectomy; INR = International Normalized Ratio; MRA = magnetic resonance angiography; TEE = transesophageal echocardiography. (Modified from Morgenstern LB, Grotta JC: Transient ischemic attacks. In Johnson RT, Griffin JW [eds]: Current Therapy in Neurologic Disease, 5th ed. St. Louis, Mosby, 1997, p 188.)

INTERNAL CAROTID ARTERY

TIAs that occur in the anterior circulation most frequently affect either the retinal artery or MCA distribution. Symptoms of retinal artery involvement consist of several seconds of a *graying out* of vision in one eye or monocular blindness *(amaurosis fugax)*. An important finding on retinoscopy is the presence of bright, refractile arterial lesions, which represent cholesterol crystals (Hollenhorst plaques) that have become detached from an upstream cholesterol plaque. Most anterior circulation TIAs occur in the setting of significant stenosis or ulceration of the ICA (>75%); cardiogenic embolism accounts for the remainder. Other causes of retinal TIA include traumatic or spontaneous arterial *dissection*.

Acute occlusion of a previously widely patent ICA usually results in contralateral hemiplegia and hemisensory loss, reflecting ischemia to the MCA territory. Headache frequently accompanies ICA occlusion. The extent of the deficit depends on the availability of collateral circulation; in the case of occlusion of a previously severely stenotic ICA, little or no clinical deficit may be apparent because of extensive collateral circulation. Severe bilateral ICA stenosis may occasionally cause *border zone (watershed)* ischemia (between the ACA and MCA) in the setting of systemic hypotension; this results in a well-recognized clinical syndrome comprising bilateral proximal limb weakness *(man-in-a-barrel* syn-

drome). The clinical recognition of ICA stenosis or occlusion may be unreliable because, although the presence of a bruit in the region of the angle of the jaw suggests significant extracranial vascular disease, it does not distinguish the external carotid artery from the ICA.

ANTERIOR CEREBRAL ARTERY

Occlusion of the ACA distal to the anterior communicating artery causes weakness and sensory loss in the contralateral leg. Other clinical manifestations include urinary incontinence and *abulia,* a state of akinetic mutism reflecting bilateral frontal lobe dysfunction.

MIDDLE CEREBRAL ARTERY

Embolism accounts for the majority of MCA occlusions. Emboli may be either cardiogenic or artery-to-artery from the extracranial ICA. Occlusion of the main MCA trunk results in contralateral hemiplegia, hemianesthesia, and homonymous hemianopsia, with a gaze preference away from the side of the hemiplegia. A global aphasia occurs with dominant hemisphere lesions, and anosognosia occurs with nondominant hemisphere involvement. Occasionally, selective occlusion of the lenticulostriate branches from the proximal MCA causes capsular infarction without evidence of cortical infarction, as a result of collateral filling of the distal MCA. Occlusion of the superior division of the MCA causes faciobrachial weakness; an expressive (Broca's) aphasia results from dominant hemisphere lesions, or a motor neglect (characterized by motor impersistence and spatial disorientation) results from lesions in the nondominant side. Inferior division occlusion usually produces impairment of sensory perception (astereognosis) and occasionally a visual field disturbance. Dominant hemisphere lesions result in a fluent (Wernicke's) aphasia.

VERTEBROBASILAR ISCHEMIA

Vertebrobasilar ischemia produces various combinations of symptoms such as dizziness (vertigo), diplopia, ataxia, bilateral sensory or motor symptoms, and fluctuating episodes of drowsiness. Scintillations or transient visual field deficits may indicate ischemia in the PCA distribution. Distinguishing the vertigo of vertebrobasilar ischemia from labyrinthine vertigo can be difficult, although isolated positional vertigo is more likely to be of labyrinthine origin.

OCCLUSION OF VERTEBRAL ARTERY OR BASILAR ARTERY

Occlusion of these arteries and their branches (PICAs, AICA, and SCA) results in discrete syndromes (see Table 123–4). Acute infarction of the cerebellum from occlusion of any of its three supplying vessels may result in its swelling within the posterior fossa, causing obstruction of the fourth ventricle and obstructive hydrocephalus. Such patients require close monitoring and occasionally neurosurgical intervention.

BA occlusion produces massive brainstem dysfunction and is often fatal. If the medulla is spared, a significant number of syndromes can occur, including the *locked-in syndrome,* in which patients are quadriplegic and can communicate only by means of vertical eye movements.

POSTERIOR CEREBRAL ARTERY OCCLUSION

Proximal PCA occlusions cause contralateral hemiparesis (from damage to the cerebral peduncle), hemisensory loss (thalamus), amnesia (medial temporal lobe), and hemianopsia. Macular (central) vision may be spared because of collateral vessels from the MCA.

CEREBRAL VENOUS THROMBOSIS

Occlusion of the sagittal sinus may occur in several settings, often in the setting of a hyperviscosity or hypercoagulable state. The condition is particularly common in pregnancy. The clinical picture varies; patients may complain of headache and papilledema or seizures. The diagnosis frequently rests on imaging findings; bilateral hemorrhagic infarctions in a parasagittal distribution are common; magnetic resonance angiography (MRA) or contrast computed tomography (CT) often shows the sinus-filling defect.

Diagnosis

Evaluation of the patient with a possible stroke should seek to answer two questions: *what* the mechanism is

(focal ischemic—thrombotic or embolic; global ischemia or hypoperfusion or hemorrhage) and *where* the lesion is. Some useful bedside pointers that may be elicited from the history and help define the stroke mechanism include the time of symptom onset and the temporal course and progression of symptoms. The type of activity and the presence of accompanying symptoms, such as headache, vomiting, or syncope, are also useful to determine from the history, as is the presence or absence of stroke risk factors.

The physical examination determines lesion localization, as well as identifies clues to pathogenesis. A thorough cardiovascular examination, including measurements of blood pressure and cardiac rhythm, is essential. Palpation of the facial artery occasionally discloses reversal of flow, which indicates ICA occlusion. Ophthalmoscopy can detect platelet and cholesterol emboli, as well as giving information about the chronicity and severity of systemic hypertension. Papilledema may accompany cerebral venous thrombosis.

Ancillary blood tests include a complete blood count, sedimentation rate, glucose, coagulation screen, and lipid profile. In young patients and in patients with unexplained venous sinus thrombosis, a search for a hypercoagulable state is necessary (see Table 123–3).

Brain imaging with CT is the most reliable test for differentiating ischemic stroke from hemorrhage, but it has limitations in the acute setting in that only 5% of acute ischemic strokes are readily visible on CT scan in the first 12 hours. Magnetic resonance imaging (MRI) may be used to verify infarction if the diagnosis remains in doubt.

The anterior circulation can be assessed with duplex ultrasonography or MRA. Cerebral angiography is reserved for specific indications to investigate possible cerebral vasculitis and carotid dissection or before carotid endarterectomy.

Differential Diagnosis

TIAs need to be distinguished from other paroxysmal events affecting the nervous system. In rare cases, patients with migraine headache have weakness contralateral to the side of the headache (*hemiplegic migraine*). Some generalized seizures are followed by a transient hemiparesis (*Todd's paralysis*).

The acute onset of a stroke generally distinguishes it from other brain lesions, although hemorrhage into a primary or metastatic tumor may manifest in a strokelike fashion. Strokes and seizures may co-exist, and 10% of strokes are associated with seizure at the time of onset. As a general rule, stroke rarely produces an alteration of consciousness unless other signs of brain dysfunction exist.

Primary Stroke Prevention

The identification and reduction of stroke risk factors (see Table 123–1), including therapy for hypertension, cessation of smoking, and treatment of diabetes and hyperlipidemia, is largely responsible for the decline in the incidence of stroke. As a primary preventive measure, antiplatelet agents do not reduce the risk of ischemic stroke in patients without vascular risk factors.

Table 123–5	Guidelines for Treatment of Atrial Fibrillation
Characteristic	**Recommended Therapy**
Age <60, no risk factors*	ASA 325 mg/day or no therapy
Age <60 with heart disease	ASA 325 mg/day
Age 60–75, with heart disease but no risk factors*	ASA 325 mg/day
Age >60 with risk factors*	Warfarin (INR 2.0–3.0)
Prosthetic heart valves	Warfarin (INR 2.5–3.5)
Previous thromboembolism	Warfarin (INR 2.5–3.5)

*Risk factors include moderate (diabetes, coronary heart disease) and high risk (heart failure, left ventricular dysfunction, hypertension).
INR = International normalized ratio.

ATRIAL FIBRILLATION

Atrial fibrillation occurs in approximately 5% of people over 70 years of age. The most devastating complication of atrial fibrillation is thromboembolic stroke. Twenty percent of ischemic strokes are cardioembolic in origin. The risk of stroke in patients with atrial fibrillation depends on a wide variety of factors, including age, sex, and the presence of co-morbid conditions. Table 123–5 summarizes appropriate treatment strategies based on the presence of risk factors. Patients with paroxysmal (self-terminating) atrial fibrillation appear to have the same risk of stroke as patients in permanent atrial fibrillation. Patients with an episode lasting less than 48 hours may be candidates for electrical cardioversion without the need for anticoagulation. In general, the presence of valvular heart disease increases the yearly risk of stroke 17-fold. For these patients, anticoagulation with warfarin to an international normalized ratio (INR) of 2 to 3 is recommended. Patients with nonvalvular atrial fibrillation in whom no other risk factors for stroke are present may be treated with aspirin, 325 mg/day. All patients with atrial fibrillation require investigation with electrocardiography, thyroid function tests, and transthoracic echocardiography. Patients with prosthetic heart valves require long-term anticoagulation. Patients with bacterial endocarditis should not receive warfarin because of the risk of cerebral hemorrhage from septic embolization. New direct thrombin inhibitors such as ximelagatran are being evaluated as alternatives to warfarin for the future.

TRANSIENT ISCHEMIC ATTACK

The occurrence of a TIA or stroke is a significant risk factor for recurrent stroke, with an average 5% risk per year, although the annual risk of stroke after an episode of amaurosis fugax is only 1% to 2%.

Patients with a significant risk for cardiogenic thromboembolism should be treated with warfarin. Hospital admission is advisable for new-onset and recurrent TIAs unless a confident diagnosis of the cause of the event can be made. Imaging studies (carotid Doppler ultrasound or MRA of the neck) should be performed and a decision made promptly to treat the patient either medically or surgically.

CAROTID STENOSIS

For patients with extracranial carotid stenoses of more than 70% (with or without symptoms of ischemia in that vascular distribution), *carotid endarterectomy* reduces the risk of stroke. In high-risk patients, carotid artery stenting has emerged as a treatment alternative to endarterectomy. For patients with moderate (60% to 70%) asymptomatic carotid stenosis, evidence that early endarterectomy is superior to deferred surgery is increasing. In patients with an asymptomatic bruit or extracranial carotid stenosis of less than 60%, treatment with antiplatelet therapy may be effective.

Management of Acute Stroke

GENERAL MEASURES

Specific medical and nursing measures should be initiated in cases of acute stroke, with particular emphasis on reducing the risk of complications from immobility, such as pneumonia, deep venous thrombosis, and urinary tract infection. The early introduction of physical, occupational, and speech therapy and a thorough evaluation of swallowing ability reduce morbidity. Judicious treatment of hypertension and hyperglycemia and correction of dehydration should be instituted. Prevention and prompt treatment of hyperthermia with antipyretics may reduce the extent of the deficit. Early awareness of poststroke depressive symptoms is especially important in preparing patients for rehabilitation.

USE OF ANTICOAGULANTS

No evidence has been found to support the use of anticoagulation (heparin) in the management of acute stroke. Although heparin might reduce the risk of recurrent stroke in the short term, any benefit is offset by the increased risk of intracranial hemorrhage. Antiplatelet therapy remains the treatment of choice to prevent recurrent thromboembolism in the majority of patients with stroke. Anticoagulation may be appropriate in select patients in cases of suggested propagation of thrombus or of stroke in evolution. Cranial CT is necessary before institution of heparin to confirm or rule out intracerebral or subarachnoid hemorrhage. Baseline prothrombin time, partial thromboplastin time, and platelet count, as well as tests for hypercoagulable states, should be obtained before initiation of therapy. A history of active peptic ulceration or uncontrolled hypertension (systolic blood pressure consistently >200 mm Hg) precludes the use of anticoagulants, unless the benefits clearly outweigh the risks.

THROMBOLYSIS

Patients who are diagnosed within 3 hours of the onset of ischemic stroke should be considered for intravenous recombinant tissue-type plasminogen activator (rt-PA). A thorough clinical evaluation is essential to determine whether the patient is an appropriate candidate for the treatment

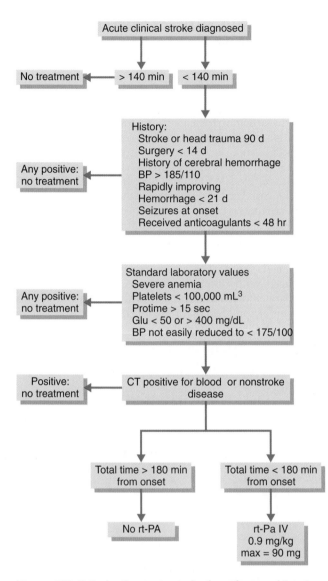

Figure 123–5 Evaluating acute stroke for safe recombinant tissue-type plasminogen activator (rt-PA) therapy. BP = blood pressure; CT = computed tomography; Glu = glucose; IV = intravenous. (From the National Institute of Neurological Disorders and Stroke rt-PA Stroke Study Group: Tissue plasminogen activator for acute ischemic stroke. N Engl J Med 333:1581–1587, 1996.)

(Fig. 123–5). The risks (6% risk of symptomatic intracranial hemorrhage) and benefits (50% chance of little or no disability at 3 months, compared with 38% chance without rt-PA) must be fully explained to the patient and family so that an informed decision can be made rapidly. The odds for a favorable outcome at 3 months improve the earlier the treatment is administered within the 3-hour window. Careful monitoring of blood pressure and avoidance of anticoagulants and aspirin are required for 24 hours after rt-PA administration.

Although preliminary results are promising, intra-arterial thrombolysis remains under investigation as an alternative therapy. A potential future development of thrombolytic therapy may be combination therapy with neuroprotective agents (such as glutamate antagonists), which may extend the therapeutic time window beyond 3 hours. Use of antiplatelet agents, such as platelet glycoprotein IIb/IIIa complex antagonists, is also under study.

MANAGEMENT OF HYPERTENSION

In the setting of acute stroke, care must be taken regarding control of blood pressure. Antihypertensive therapy is instituted if the blood pressure persistently exceeds 220 mm Hg systolic or 120 mm Hg diastolic (except in patients being treated with rt-PA in whom more stringent guidelines apply). Less marked elevations of blood pressure should not be treated acutely.

MANAGEMENT OF CEREBRAL EDEMA

Only in large hemispheric infarction is ischemic cerebral edema sufficient to cause brain shift and transtentorial herniation. If signs of herniation appear, intubation and hyperventilation produce transient cerebral vasoconstriction and may reduce intracranial pressure. Mannitol reduces the volume of the surrounding unaffected brain, but its effects are also transient. Corticosteroids are of no benefit in cytotoxic edema.

HYPERTENSIVE ENCEPHALOPATHY

The term *hypertensive encephalopathy* refers to the diffuse cerebral effects of severe hypertension that are not caused by infarction or hemorrhage and that are potentially reversible with control of blood pressure. Patients experience headache, visual blurring (obscurations), confusion, and drowsiness. Seizures may develop. The blood pressure is typically very high (250/150 mm Hg), and papilledema and retinal hemorrhages are usually apparent on funduscopic examination. CT and MRI show diffuse cerebral edema with a predilection for the occipital lobes.

Hypertensive encephalopathy is a medical emergency. Treatment should be directed to the prompt but controlled lowering of blood pressure (e.g., with sodium nitroprusside), with care taken to avoid hypotension. The condition is clinically and pathophysiologically analogous to eclampsia.

REHABILITATION

The majority of stroke-related deaths result from medical complications (e.g., pneumonia, myocardial infarction, sepsis) rather than the neurologic deficit. Appropriate rehabilitation optimizes functional recovery and minimizes medical complications. Early placement of percutaneous enterostomy feeding tubes does not improve long-term outcome in patients after a stroke.

SECONDARY PREVENTION OF ISCHEMIC STROKE

Recent multicenter clinical trials have shown that aggressive control of stroke risk factors reduces the rate of recurrence.

Antiplatelet Therapy

Prophylactic antiplatelet therapy with aspirin, ticlopidine, clopidogrel, or dipyridamole has been shown to prevent recurrent events. Aspirin, which inhibits platelet aggregation by blocking platelet cyclooxygenase and thus preventing formation of thromboxane, is the first-line therapy for preventing recurrent stroke. Combination therapy using aspirin and dipyridamole is an alternative strategy. Ticlopidine and clopidogrel block platelet aggregation by increasing levels of cyclic adenosine monophosphate (cAMP) and are indicated in patients with aspirin resistance. Ticlopidine is associated with a risk of leukopenia that has limited its use. The addition of aspirin to clopidogrel may increase the risk of intracranial hemorrhage.

Anticoagulation

Table 123–5 outlines the appropriate use of anticoagulants in secondary prevention of stroke. In patients with atrial fibrillation, diabetes and severe myocardial dysfunction, long-term anticoagulation with warfarin reduces the risk of recurrent stroke.

Hypertension

Hypertension is a well-recognized risk factor for ischemic stroke. A target blood pressure of less than 140/90 mm Hg is considered appropriate. Recent studies have identified that the use of angiotensin-converting enzyme inhibitors in combination with a thiazide diuretic reduces the rate of stroke recurrence, even in normotensive patients.

Lipid-Lowering Agents

Increasing evidence suggests that agents used to treat hyperlipidemia, particularly the hydroxymethylglutaryl–coenzyme A (HMG-CoA) reductase inhibitors (statins) have anti-inflammatory and endothelial properties that may confer vascular protection independent of their lipid-lowering effects. All patients with prior TIA or ischemic stroke should be treated with a statin, irrespective of their serum cholesterol level.

Intracerebral Hemorrhage

Intracerebral hemorrhage (ICH) may be diffuse (subarachnoid hemorrhage) or focal (intraparenchymal) and accounts for 20% of all strokes. Table 123–6 lists the causes of spontaneous ICH. The acute rise in intracranial pressure from arterial rupture frequently results in loss of consciousness at the outset; some patients die from herniation.

HYPERTENSIVE INTRACEREBRAL HEMORRHAGE

Hypertensive ICH often occurs at the same sites that are affected in lacunar infarction. Pathologically, micro-aneurysms known as *Charcot-Bouchard aneurysms* have been identified in some patients. The most common sites for hypertensive hemorrhage are the putamen (40%), thalamus (12%), lobar white matter (15% to 20%), caudate (8%), pons (8%), and cerebellum (8%). Although CT readily identifies the hemorrhage, several clinical findings may help localize the site (Table 123–7). In general, severity of headache correlates with the size of the lesion. Diminished level of alertness is caused by mass effect, increased intracranial pressure, or direct involvement of the brainstem reticular–activating system. Seizures are slightly more frequent during the acute phase in ICH than in ischemic stroke. Both basal ganglia and thalamic hemorrhages may rupture into the adjacent ventricle and result in secondary hydrocephalus; cerebellar hemorrhage may cause obstructive hydrocephalus as a result of compression of the fourth ventricle.

Table 123–6	Causes of Spontaneous Intracerebral Hemorrhage

Intraparenchymal Hemorrhage

Hypertension
Amyloid (congophilic) angiopathy
Arteriovenous malformation
Bleeding diathesis
Drugs (amphetamines, cocaine, anticoagulants, thrombolytics)
Tumors

Subarachnoid Hemorrhage

Congenital saccular aneurysm (85%)
Mycotic aneurysm
Arteriovenous malformation
Unknown (10%)

Table 123–7	Clinical Manifestations Related to Site of Intracerebral Hemorrhage

	Site		Manifestation		
	Headache	**Pupils**	**Eye Movements**	**Sensorimotor Signs**	**Other**
Basal ganglia	Severe	Normal	Normal	Hemiparesis	Confusion, aphasia
Thalamus	Moderate	Small, poorly reactive to light	Hyperconvergence Absent vertical gaze	Hemisensory > motor loss	Hypersomnolence
Pons	Severe	Small, reactive	Horizontal gaze paresis	Quadriplegia	Coma
Cerebellum	Severe, occipital	Normal	Normal	Ataxia	Early vomiting

With intracerebral hematoma, the patient's level of consciousness often deteriorates during the first 24 to 48 hours after the initial symptoms, usually because of the development of edema around the lesion. Edema that is sufficient to cause significant brain shift results in herniation of brain tissue. In addition to causing direct pressure on vital brainstem structures, herniation may cause compression of adjacent blood vessels (particularly the PCAs and ACAs), resulting in infarction.

LOBAR HEMORRHAGE

Lobar hemorrhages occur in a peripheral distribution of the cerebral white matter. They are usually smaller than hypertensive ICHs and have a more benign prognosis. In young persons, lobar hemorrhages may be secondary to arteriovenous malformations or ingestion of sympathomimetic drugs. In elderly persons, they are usually secondary to amyloid angiopathy. As in anticoagulant-associated hemorrhage, signs tend to develop insidiously in amyloid angiopathy. The diagnosis of amyloid angiopathy is suggested by the finding of multiple *microbleeds* on gradient echocardiographic MRI.

DIAGNOSIS, MANAGEMENT, AND PROGNOSIS

CT remains the diagnostic test of choice in the diagnosis of ICH, which acutely shows as a hyperintense area with mass effect and (later) hypointense surrounding edema. MRI is less sensitive than CT for detecting hemorrhage in the early stages. The management of ICH depends on the size and location of the lesion. In the acute phase, the mass effect of a cerebral hematoma is far greater than in a large cerebral infarction, with a greater risk of herniation and death. In the chronic phase, however, the prognosis for recovery in patients who survive is much better for those with hemorrhage than for those with ischemic stroke. Thus, therapy for acute hemorrhage is directed at reducing mass effect either by medical decompression with controlled hyperventilation or mannitol or, in rare cases, by surgical decompression. This latter option should be considered urgently in cases of cerebellar hemorrhage in which patients are especially at risk of sudden deterioration either through acute obstructive hydrocephalus (because of compression of the fourth ventricle) or as a result of direct pressure on the caudal brainstem.

Intracranial Aneurysms

Intracranial aneurysms occur in three forms: fusiform, mycotic, and saccular (congenital *berry*) aneurysms.

Fusiform aneurysms represent ectatic dilations of large arteries, usually the basilar or intracranial carotid arteries. They rarely rupture but may compress adjacent brain tissue or cranial nerves and cause local neurologic dysfunction. Fusiform aneurysms are rarely accessible to surgical repair.

Mycotic aneurysms occur in the context of bacterial endocarditis when septic emboli lodge in a peripheral vessel. They are often multiple and located distally in the arterial tree, and thus they are accessible to surgical repair should they fail to respond to antibiotic therapy.

Saccular aneurysms form at arterial bifurcations (Fig. 123–6); 80% are located in the anterior circulation. They are

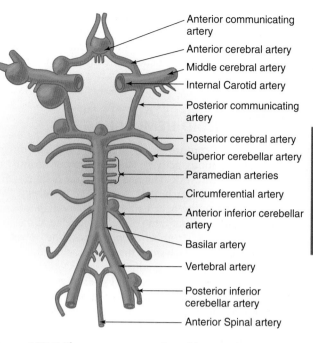

Figure 123–6 The more common sites of berry aneurysms. The diagrammatic size of the aneurysm at the various sites is directly proportional to its frequency at that locus.

thought to arise from a combination of a congenital defect in the arterial media and elastic lamina and gradual deterioration from hemodynamic stress. Higher incidences are found among patients with polycystic kidney disease and Marfan syndrome.

Approximately 1% of the population harbors an unruptured saccular aneurysm; 25% of patients have multiple aneurysms. Fortunately, the annual incidence of rupture is only approximately 10 per 100,000. The risk of rupture is 1%/year. Of those that do rupture, 33% of these individuals die before reaching a hospital, and another 20% die in the hospital. Overall, only 30% of patients recover without significant disability.

Incidental aneurysms of the anterior circulation less than 7 mm have a very low risk of rupture (<0.05%/yr); the risk of rupture increases with the size of the aneurysm and location within the posterior circulation.

Within families, aneurysms tend to be at the same site and to rupture during the same decade. The risk of an unruptured aneurysm in a first-degree relative of a patient with subarachnoid hemorrhage is 4% to 5% with one affected relative, 8% to 10% with two or more affected relatives.

The natural history of aneurysms is unknown. Whether they pose an early high risk after formation or whether a constant risk of rupture exists over time is unknown.

Treatment of Unruptured Intracranial Aneurysms

Aneurysms may be treated by open surgical clipping or by endovascular coiling. The latter procedure has emerged as the treatment of choice in the majority of patients and has a low morbidity and mortality. In aneurysms over 7 mm, the risk-benefit ratio of treatment depends greatly on life expectancy. In persons over 60 years of age, these aneurysms are best untreated, given the low probability of rupture in the patient's natural lifetime. Hypotensive therapy is a useful therapeutic option in patients who are not suitable for coiling or clipping.

CLINICAL MANIFESTATIONS OF SUBARACHNOID HEMORRHAGE

Aneurysms may rupture at any time but especially during periods of strenuous activity, such as exercise, coitus, or strenuous physical work. The most common manifestation is sudden severe headache *(the worst headache of my life)*, often accompanied by neck pain and rigidity. Loss of consciousness and vomiting are common sequelae. Occasionally, with so-called *sentinel hemorrhages,* the onset of symptoms is less cataclysmic than subarachnoid hemorrhage, and the headache gradually resolves over 24 to 48 hours. Aneurysms may also exhibit by compression of adjacent cranial nerves, such as compression of cranial nerve III by an aneurysm of the posterior communicating artery. *Giant aneurysms* (>2.5 cm) may compress cranial nerves III, IV, and VI in the cavernous sinus. In rare instances, aneurysms may produce a TIA as a result of embolization from a thrombus within an aneurysm.

DIAGNOSIS

CT of the brain shows subarachnoid hemorrhage in 95% of patients, and its location may suggest a site of rupture. A normal CT scan does not totally rule out subarachnoid hemorrhage and mandates a lumbar puncture in patients with symptoms. Care must be taken to centrifuge cerebrospinal fluid to detect true xanthochromia, the yellow coloration that develops by 6 hours after subarachnoid hemorrhage. Contrast CT or MRI identifies aneurysms larger than 5 mm, as well as arteriovenous malformations. Cerebral angiography remains the *gold standard* for diagnosing intracranial aneurysms, and it is usually performed when surgery is being contemplated and deferred in severe cases in which significant risk of vasospasm exists. A small group of patients with predominantly peri-mesencephalic hemorrhage on CT have normal cerebral angiograms and a more benign outcome. The electrocardiogram may show deep, symmetric T-wave inversion. Once the diagnosis of subarachnoid hemorrhage has been made (or if clinical suspicion persists, even with inconclusive testing), the patient should be managed under the guidance of a neurosurgical team.

MANAGEMENT AND PROGNOSIS

An essential part of managing patients with subarachnoid hemorrhage is to prevent any one of several complications

Table 123–8	**Complications of Subarachnoid Hemorrhage**

Hypertension (systemic and intracranial)
Vasospasm
Hemorrhage (rebleeding)
Hydrocephalus
Hyponatremia (syndrome of inappropriate antidiuretic hormone; cerebral salt wasting)

(Table 123–8). To reduce the risk of rebleeding, patients are placed on bed rest with analgesics for pain relief, mild sedation, and the use of laxatives to reduce straining. Management of hypertension requires balancing the need to maintain a steady cerebral perfusion pressure in the context of raised intracranial pressure and possible vasospasm and, in contrast, the risk of rebleeding. The peak timing for vasospasm is between 5 and 9 days after the hemorrhage, and it may be accompanied by an alteration in the neurologic status.

Vascular Malformations

Vascular malformations of the brain and spinal cord are grouped according to vessel size and composition. *Venous angiomas* are the most common malformations and tend to lie close to the brain surface. Malformations composed of capillaries are called *capillary telangiectases* and are typically located within the brainstem. *Cavernous angiomas* are composed of dilated sinusoidal channels, are readily detectable by CT, and rarely bleed.

Arteriovenous malformations are composed of tangles of arteries connected directly to veins without intervening capillaries. They may produce headache, seizures, or hemorrhage, accounting for 1% of all strokes. The initial hemorrhage typically occurs before the fourth decade, with a 7% risk of rebleeding within the first year afterward. Hemorrhage may occur into the brain parenchyma, subarachnoid space, or intraventricular space.

Treatment of arteriovenous malformations is guided by individual factors, such as the age of the patient, location and composition of the lesion, and manifestations. In general, arteriovenous malformations in older patients (>55 years) are treated conservatively, whereas younger patients are treated either by surgical excision or, less commonly, by irradiation combined with embolization of the arterial feeding vessel.

Prospectus for the Future

Both ischemic and hemorrhagic strokes can be prevented by risk factor modification. Additional progress can be expected in this area, particularly in defining genetic factors that lead to stroke susceptibility. Treatment of acute ischemic stroke requires improved thrombolytic agents and the development of neuro-protective strategies; a large number are in active clinical trials. Hemorrhagic stroke is just beginning to receive the attention needed to define optimal acute treatment—blood pressure management, surgical drainage, osmotic therapy—and all demand large-scale randomized controlled clinical trials.

References

Adams HA Jr, Adams RJ, Brott T, et al: Guidelines for the early management of patients with ischemic stroke. Stroke 34:1056–1083, 2003.

Barnett HJ, Mohr JP, Stein BM, et al (eds): Stroke: Pathophysiology, Diagnosis and Management. New York, Churchill Livingstone, 1998.

Easton JD: Redefining transient ischemic attack. Neurology 62:(Suppl 6):S1–S2, 2004.

Kizer JR, Devereux RB: Patient foramen ovale in young adults with unexplained stroke. N Engl J Med 353:2361–2372, 2005.

Mitchell P, Gholkar A, Vindlacheruvu R: Unruptured intracranial aneurysms: Benign curiosity or ticking bomb? Lancet Neurol 3:85–92, 2004.

Page RL: Newly diagnosed atrial fibrillation. N Engl J Med 351:2408–2416, 2004.

Pearson TA, Blair SN, Daniels SR, et al: AHA guidelines for primary prevention of cardiovascular disease and stroke: 2002 update: Consensus Panel Guide to Comprehensive Risk Reduction for Adult Patients Without Coronary or Other Atherosclerotic Vascular Diseases. American Heart Association Science Advisory and Coordinating Committee. Circulation 106:388–391, 2002.

Powers WJ: Oral anticoagulant therapy for the prevention of stroke. N Engl J Med 345:1493–1495, 2001.

Rothwell PM, Eliasziw M, Gutnikov SA, et al: Analysis of pooled data from the randomised controlled trials of endarterectomy for symptomatic carotid stenosis. Lancet 361:107–116, 2003.

Sacco RL: Extracranial carotid stenosis. N Engl J Med 345:1113–1118, 2001.

Savitz S, Caplan L: Vertebrobasilar disease. N Engl J Med 352:2618–2626, 2005.

Zivin JA: Approach to cerebrovascular disease. In Goldman L, Ausiello DA (eds): Cecil Textbook of Medicine, 23rd ed. Philadelphia, Saunders, 2007.

Chapter 124

Trauma to Head and Spine

Roger P. Simon

*T*raumatic injury is the third most common cause of death in the United States; one half of the deaths result from head injury, and most deaths occur before patients reach the hospital. Men younger than 30 years of age account for two thirds of these cases; one half of these incidents involve alcohol intoxication. Spinal injury is less likely to be fatal than head injury and therefore results in long-term residual disability. Injury of the head and spine may co-exist; spinal injury should be assumed in unconscious patients or in any patient who has sustained trauma and complains of neck or back pain.

Head Injury

SKULL FRACTURES

Cutaneous signs that suggest *basilar skull fracture* are those resulting from seepage of blood from the fracture site: mastoid *(Battle's sign),* periocular *(raccoon eye),* and conjunctival blood extending from the posterior orbit. These signs occur 24 to 72 hours after injury. Clear fluid, leaking from the auditory canal or nose, should be assumed to be cerebrospinal fluid; it demonstrates a potential portal of entry for infection and mandates close observation, although prophylactic antibiotics are not recommended. The presence of β-2 transferrin demonstrates a cerebrospinal fluid source of rhinorrhea. Fractures of the base of the skull may also result in cranial nerve injury, particularly olfactory, ocular, oculomotor, or facial nerve injury. Bruits over the orbits occur in patients with traumatic carotid-cavernous fistulas and predict the development of pulsating exophthalmos during the next 24 to 48 hours.

FOCAL BRAIN INJURY

In the extracerebral space, *venous bleeding in the subdural compartment* or *arterial bleeding in the epidural space* produces expanding masses; these lesions are readily seen on noncontrast computed tomography. The symptoms and signs are variable (Table 124–1), but altered consciousness, with or without a *lucid interval,* predominates. Emergency neurosurgical evaluation is mandatory. *Parenchymal hemorrhage* occurs in cortical regions adjacent to the skull base or falx, such as the frontal or occipital pole, temporal tip, cerebellar hemispheres, or parasagittal convexity. Bleeding into a contused brain may be delayed. Blood is frequently found in the *subarachnoid space,* which may occasionally cause confusion among primary head trauma, an aneurysmal origin of bleeding, or secondary head injury from a fall after loss of consciousness.

DIFFUSE BRAIN INJURY

Diffuse brain injury results from angular head motion; it causes the immediate phenomenon of *concussion* (brief unconsciousness) and is responsible for prolonged traumatic coma. The pathologic correlate is *diffuse axonal injury,* which is the result of widespread axonal disruption by shearing forces produced as inertia causes the brain to lag behind the skull during head acceleration-deceleration movements.

ACUTE MANAGEMENT

Maintenance of oxygenation and, especially, of blood pressure is essential because cerebral blood flow falls and the protective mechanisms of cerebral blood flow autoregulation are impaired in brain trauma. Systemic hypotension doubles mortality and, in adults, is not the consequence of the intracranial bleeding itself. Blood pressure needs to be adjusted in proportion to intracranial pressure; this *cerebral perfusion pressure* (mean blood pressure minus intracranial pressure) should be initially maintained at over 60 to 70 mm Hg. Hyperventilation decreases intracranial pressure but worsens the outcome because of the induced cerebral vasoconstriction and possibly also by removing the hydrogen ion block of the postsynaptic glutamate (N-methyl-D-aspartate) receptor. Osmotic agents such as mannitol may be effective briefly in reducing intracranial pressure. Anti-edema agents such as corticosteroids have not been shown to improve outcome and may be associated with increased death and severe disability. Moderate (whole-body) hypothermia, 32°

Table 124–1	**Clinical Features of Subdural Hematoma**		
	Acute* (82 Patients) (%)	**Subacute† (91 Patients) (%)**	**Chronic‡ (216 Patients) (%)**
Symptoms			
Depression of consciousness	100	88	47
Vomiting	24	31	30
Weakness	20	19	22
Confusion	12	41	37
Headache	11	44	81
Speech disturbance	6	8	5
Seizures	6	3	9
Vertigo	0	4	5
Visual disturbance	0	0	12
Signs			
Depression of consciousness	100	88	59
Pupillary inequality	57	27	20
Motor asymmetry	44	37	41
Confusion and memory loss	17	21	27
Aphasia	6	12	11
Papilledema	1	15	22
Hemianopia	0	4	3
Facial weakness	0	3	3

*Within 3 days of trauma.
†At 4–20 days after trauma.
‡Greater than 20 days after trauma.
Data from McKissock W, Richardson A, Bloom WH: Subdural hematoma: A review of 389 cases. Lancet 1:1365–1370, 1960.

to 33° C for 24 hours or longer, may increase recovery in patients with severe traumatic brain injury.

QUANTIFYING INJURY

Prognosis

The Glasgow Coma Scale (GCS) (Table 124–2) allows for serial assessment of the head-injured patient and is an excellent guide to the severity of injury. The GCS categorizes injury as mild (13 to 15), moderate (9 to 12), or severe (3 to 8), with motor response being the most sensitive. A patient's GCS score correlates with outcome, as follows:

> Death or vegetative state: GCS score 3 to 4 (80%), 5 to 7 (54%), 8 to 10 (27%), 11 to 15 (6%).
> Residual cognitive disability: CGS score 9 to 12 (62%), less than 8 (80%).
> Approximately 90% of recovery is determined at 6 months, and 95% is determined at 1 year.

Apolipoprotein E

The putative Alzheimer's susceptibility gene, apolipoprotein E *(apo E)* ε4, may also predict the duration of post-traumatic coma and eventual outcome, a concept that suggests a degree of genetic susceptibility to the effects of traumatic brain injury. Patients recovering from traumatic brain injury may be at risk of earlier onset of Alzheimer's disease if they are predisposed to this condition.

Table 1.24–2	**Glasgow Coma Scale***	
Eye Opening	**Best Motor Response**	**Best Verbal Response**
Spontaneous	6: Obeys commands	5: Oriented
3: To voice	5: Localizes pain	4: Confused
2: To pain	4: Withdraws to pain	3: Inappropriate vocalization
1: None	3: Reflex flexion	2: Incomprehensible
	2: Reflex extension	1: No vocalization
	1: Flaccid	

*Glasgow Coma Scale score is the sum of best scores in eye opening and motor and verbal performance (e.g., normal = 15; flaccid, mute, eyes closed = 3).

CHRONIC SEQUELAE

Postconcussive syndrome often follows relatively minor trauma. The symptom constellation nearly always includes headache of almost any clinical pattern, from tension to migraine. Additional symptoms include dizziness, weakness, gait instability, inability to concentrate, memory loss, personality changes, and problems with sleep regulation.

Resolution occurs over many months. In patients with more severe injury, cognitive impairment may be permanent.

Focal or *generalized seizures* may develop immediately (in the first week) or in a delayed fashion after head injury, and they occur in proportion to the severity of injury. Prophylactic anticonvulsants are routinely administered and decrease the incidence of early seizures; the incidence of *posttraumatic epilepsy* is not reduced.

Spinal Cord Injury

Possible spinal cord injuries should be considered in all patients with head injury. Patients who are responsive may complain of neck and back pain, suggesting cervical or thoracolumbar fractures. If evidence of injury is noted in an awake patient, or if the patient is unconscious, then immobilization of the neck must be the first step in treatment. Attention is next focused on maintaining blood pressure and oxygenation so as to preclude secondary injury because blood pressure control will be impaired with injury of descending sympathetic pathways. Bladder catheterization is essential in spinal cord injury because the patient's awareness of bladder filling is impaired or absent.

On examination of patients with severe spinal cord injury, deep tendon reflexes are usually absent below the level of the lesion (ankle, S1-S2; knee, L3-L4; biceps, C5-C6; and triceps, C7-C8). A sensory level to pinprick may be found on the chest. The pattern of motor impairment dictates the focus of imaging studies. High cervical lesions (C3, C4, and C5) affect all arm muscles and ventilation; patients with midcervical lesions are able to flex at the elbow but are unable to extend. Patients with low cervical lesions may preserve elbow flexion and extension but not hand muscle function. Thoracic injury results in paraplegia.

Partial spinal cord injuries may be seen particularly with acute neck extension (e.g., falling and striking the forehead and thereby forcing the neck into hyperextension); typically, a *central spinal cord syndrome* or anterior spinal artery syndrome results, producing bilateral arm weakness with normal leg strength (Fig. 124–1).

IMAGING

Radiographs of the cervical spine should be obtained with portable equipment to decrease the need to move the patient. Lateral radiographs must include all seven cervical vertebrae and the odontoid. In a patient with neck pain, further assessment for cervical spine stability may be indicated even if plain radiographs are normal. Extension and flexion radiographs should be obtained. *The patient moves his or her own neck,* first in extension (usually reducing subluxations) and, if results are normal, then in flexion. Com-

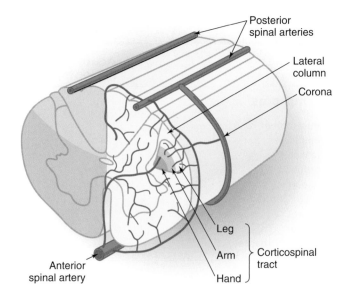

Figure 124–1 Blood supply to the cervical spinal cord. *Left,* Major territories supplied by the anterior spinal artery *(dark shading)* and the posterior spinal artery *(light shading).* *Right,* Pattern of supply by the intramedullary arteries. Both the anterior and the posterior spinal arteries supply the descending motor fibers of the corticospinal tract, with the fibers supplying arm movement in a watershed area susceptible to hypoperfusion. (From Simon RP, Aminoff MJ, Greenberg DA: Clinical Neurology. Stamford, CT, Appleton & Lange, 1999.)

puted tomography should be used in follow-up of patients with subluxations or fractures and is indicated if plain radiographs are normal but a neurologic abnormality is present. Magnetic resonance images bone poorly but readily demonstrates spinal cord hemorrhage or contusion.

TREATMENT

In controlled trials, only methylprednisolone was effective in improving motor outcome. All patients with spinal cord injury should receive 30 mg/kg within 8 hours of injury, followed by 5.4 mg/kg/hr over the next 23 hours. GM_1 gangliosides appear to increase the rate, but not the ultimate degree, of recovery.

Whiplash

Neck-wrenching injuries such as those that occur in *rear end* automobile collisions result in neck and head pain in approximately one half these patients. Most symptoms should resolve in a few weeks to 1 month, and all symptoms should resolve by 1 year.

Prospectus for the Future

Advancement in supportive care has already improved the prognosis in brain and spinal cord injuries, and room still exists for improvements in defining acute management strategies. Restoration of spinal cord function months to years following injury is a focus of intense investigation. Harnessing the regenerative potential of stem cells and designing a strategy to have these cells *home* to the correct location provide hope for the thousands of young people with fixed neurologic deficits.

References

Edwards P, Arango M, Balica L, et al: Final results of MRC CRASH, a randomized placebo-controlled trial of intravenous corticosteroid in adults with head injury—outcomes at six months. Lancet 365:1957–1959, 2005.

Haydel MJ: Clinical decision instruments for CT scanning in minor head injury. JAMA 294(12):1551–1553, 2005.

McDonald JW, Sadowsky C: Spinal cord injury. Lancet 359:417–425, 2002.

White RJ, Likavec MJ: The diagnosis and initial management of head injury. N Engl J Med 327:1507–1511, 1992.

Epilepsy

Robert C. Griggs

Definition

Epilepsy is a chronic condition with the major clinical manifestation of seizures characterized by sudden and usually unprovoked attacks of subjective experiential phenomena, altered consciousness, or involuntary movements. The diagnosis of epilepsy indicates that a patient has recurrent seizures, but not all seizures imply epilepsy. Seizures result from abnormal brain electrical activity and are a common sign of brain dysfunction. They occur during the course of many medical or neurologic illnesses in which brain function is temporarily deranged (*symptomatic* seizures) (Table 125–1). Such seizures are usually self limited and do not persist if the underlying disorder can be corrected. Seizures can also occur as a reaction of the brain to physiologic stress, such as sleep deprivation, fever, and withdrawal from alcohol or sedative drugs. Occurrence of such seizures suggests an increased seizure susceptibility (lowered seizure threshold). Genetic factors or unrecognized previous central nervous system injury may account for such susceptibility. Isolated seizures may also occur for no discoverable reason as unprovoked events in apparently healthy people. These types of seizures are not epilepsy.

Incidence and Etiologic Factors

Seizures can begin at any time of life. In developed countries, 2% to 4% of all persons have recurrent seizures at some time during their lives. Developing countries, as well as inner-city areas, show increased incidence rates. The incidence is highest among young children and older adults, and men are affected more often than women (1.5:1). Epilepsy results from many conditions and mechanisms (Fig. 125–1). Approximately 70% of adults and 40% of children with new-onset epilepsy have partial (focal) seizures. In many of these individuals, identifying a specific cause is not possible, although focal seizures imply a cerebral injury or lesion. The most common specific lesions are hippocampal sclerosis, gangliogliomas and glial tumors, cavernous malformations, neuronal migrational defects (cortical dysplasia) and hamartomas, encephalitis, cerebral trauma, and hemorrhage. Not all patients with cerebral lesions develop epilepsy; how a particular lesion becomes epileptogenic is poorly understood.

Many specific genetic disorders cause epilepsy, but these disorders are uncommon causes. However, a growing number of epilepsies are recognized to be caused by specific gene lesions. Most other epilepsies have clear hereditary influences, but the genetic factors have not yet been defined. At least 10 of the genetic epilepsies are known to be channelopathies. Channel dysfunction will likely cause many of the others. Neuronal migration defects (see Chapter 122) identified by magnetic resonance imaging (MRI) are a common cause of genetic and acquired epilepsies.

Classification and Clinical Manifestations

The most widely used classification scheme is that of the International League Against Epilepsy (Table 125–2). Seizures are classified by their clinical symptoms and signs. The manifestations of a seizure depend on whether most or only a part of the cerebral cortex is involved at the beginning, the functions of the cortical areas where the seizure originates, and the subsequent pattern of spread within the brain. Seizures are of two types: (1) those with onset limited to part of the cerebral hemisphere (*partial* or *focal* seizures) and (2) those that involve the cerebral cortex diffusely from the beginning (*generalized* seizures). Seizures are dynamic and evolve; a patient's seizure pattern varies depending on the extent and manner of spread of the electrical discharge. Thus, *simple* partial seizures may evolve into *complex* partial seizures, and partial seizures can evolve into *secondarily generalized* tonic-clonic convulsions.

PARTIAL SEIZURES

The onset of a seizure, as described by the patient and observers, often indicates if a seizure begins focally. Simple partial seizures result when the epileptic electrical discharge remains limited to a focal area of cortex. Patients can interact normally with their environment except for limitations imposed by the seizure on specific localized brain functions. Simple partial seizures include subjective sensory and psychological phenomena. These auras affect approximately

Table 125–1 Causes of Symptomatic Seizures

Acute electrolyte disorders
Acute hyponatremia (<120 mEq/L)
Acute hypernatremia (>155 mEq/L)
Hyperosmolality (>310 mOsm/L)
Hypocalcemia (<7 mg/dL)
Hypoglycemia (<30 mg/dL)
Drugs
Isoniazid, penicillins
Theophylline, aminophylline, ephedrine,
    phenylpropanolamine, terbutaline
Lidocaine, meperidine
Tricyclic antidepressants
Cyclosporine
Cocaine (crack), phencyclidine, amphetamines; alcohol
    withdrawal
Central nervous system disease
Hypertensive encephalopathy, eclampsia
Hepatic encephalopathy, renal failure
Sickle cell disease, thrombotic thrombocytopenic purpura
Systemic lupus erythematosus
Meningitis, encephalitis, brain abscess
Acute head trauma, stroke, brain tumor

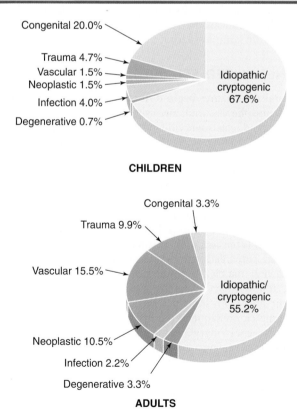

CHILDREN

ADULTS

Figure 125–1 Causes of epilepsy, according to age, in all newly diagnosed cases in Rochester, Minnesota, 1935–1984. (Modified from Hauser WA, Annegers JF, Kurland LT: Incidence of epilepsy and unprovoked seizures in Rochester, Minnesota: 1935–1984. Epilepsia 34:453, 1994.)

Table 125–2 International League Against Epilepsy Classification of Epileptic Seizures and Syndromes

Classification of Seizures

Partial (focal) seizures

Simple partial seizures (consciousness not impaired)
With motor signs
With sensory signs
With psychiatric symptoms
With autonomic symptoms
Complex partial seizures (consciousness is impaired)
Simple partial onset followed by impaired consciousness
With impairment of consciousness at onset
With automatisms
Partial seizures evolving to secondarily generalized seizures

Generalized seizures of nonfocal origin

Absence seizures
Myoclonic seizures; myoclonic jerks (single or multiple)
Tonic-clonic seizures
Tonic seizures
Atonic seizures

Classification of Epileptic Syndromes

Idiopathic epilepsy syndromes (focal or generalized)

Benign neonatal convulsions
Benign partial epilepsy of childhood
Childhood absence epilepsy
Juvenile myoclonic epilepsy
Idiopathic epilepsy, otherwise unspecified

Symptomatic epilepsy syndromes (focal or generalized)

West's syndrome (infantile spasms)
Lennox-Gastaut syndrome
Partial continuous epilepsy
Temporal lobe epilepsy
Frontal lobe epilepsy
Post-traumatic epilepsy

Other epilepsy syndromes of uncertain or mixed classification

Neonatal seizures
Febrile seizures
Reflex epilepsy
Adult nonconvulsive status epilepticus

Table 125–3	Localization of Seizures by Symptoms and Ictal Manifestations
Locus	**Manifestation**
Temporal Lobe	
Uncus/amygdala	Foul odor
Middle/inferior temporal gyrus	Visual changes: micropsia, macropsia
Parahippocampal-hippocampal area	Déjà vu; jamais vu
Parahippocampal-septal area	Fear, pleasure, anger, dreamy sensation
Auditory association cortex	Voices, music
Insular, anterior temporal cortex	Lip smacking, abdominal symptoms, cardiac arrhythmia
Frontal Lobe	
Motor cortex	Clonic movements of the face, fingers, hand, foot
Premotor cortex	Arm extension
Language areas	Speech arrest, aphasia
Parietal lobe cortex	Sensory symptoms
Occipital lobe cortex	Visual: teichopsias, metamorphopsias

60% of patients with focal epilepsy. Specific symptoms often localize the epileptogenic focus (Table 125–3). The location of the focus is important for diagnosis: The location often predicts the nature of the abnormality and directs diagnostic testing. Moreover, both medical and surgical treatments are determined by focus location.

Simple partial seizures with motor signs begin with clonic (rhythmic jerking) or tonic (stiffening) movements of a discrete body part (**Web video 125-1**). Because of their large cortical representation, muscles of the face and hands are involved often. When the seizure discharge begins in the primary motor cortex and spreads to involve the rest of the precentral gyrus, clonic movements progress in an orderly sequence (*jacksonian march*) that reflects the motor cortex homunculus representation (e.g., thumb to fingers to face to leg). More often, however, ictal discharges involve supplementary or other secondary motor areas of the frontal lobe and produce contralateral flexion and elevation of the arm, contralateral turning of the head and eyes, and tonic extension of the ipsilateral arm (*fencer's posture*). Other simple partial motor signs include speech arrest, vocalizations, and eye blinking.

Simple partial seizures may be followed by a transient neurologic abnormality reflecting postictal depression of the epileptogenic cortical area. Thus, focal weakness may follow a simple partial motor seizure, 3or numbness may follow a sensory seizure. These reversible neurologic deficits are referred to as Todd's paralysis and rarely last for more than 48 hours. Examination of a patient immediately after a seizure may show transient focal abnormalities that indicate the site of seizure origin.

Complex partial seizures impair consciousness and produce unresponsiveness. In temporal lobe seizures, loss of consciousness results when the ictal discharge spreads bilaterally to involve both hippocampal and amygdala areas, the parahippocampal gyri, and, to some extent, the entorhinal cortex and subfrontal, especially septal, regions. Seventy to 80% of complex partial seizures arise from the temporal lobe, and more than two thirds of these originate in mesial temporal lobe structures, especially the hippocampus, amygdala, and parahippocampal gyrus. Remaining cases of complex partial seizures arise mainly from the frontal lobe, with smaller percentages originating in parietal and occipital lobes. Many complex partial seizures evolve from simple partial seizures; consciousness becomes impaired as the seizure progresses. Complex partial seizures preceded by an olfactory aura are referred to as *uncinate fits* because of their origin in or near the uncus of the medial temporal lobe. Table 125–3 lists other symptoms and signs of limbic and temporal lesions.

Psychomotor, temporal lobe, and *limbic seizures* are all terms that have been used in the past to describe many of the ictal behaviors now classified as complex partial seizures, but they are not synonymous. Not all complex partial seizures arise from the temporal lobe, nor do all involve the limbic system. Some temporal lobe and limbic phenomena reflect unilateral ictal discharges and may not be associated with the significant alteration in awareness that invariably occurs with complex partial seizures.

GENERALIZED SEIZURES

Generalized seizures begin diffusely and involve both cerebral hemispheres simultaneously from the outset. They lack clinical and electroencephalographic (EEG) features that indicate a localized cerebral origin. Generalized seizures are subdivided based mainly on the presence or absence and character of ictal motor manifestations. They must be distinguished from focal seizures that spread to cause *secondary generalized seizures*.

Generalized tonic-clonic seizures (grand mal convulsions) are characterized by abrupt loss of consciousness with bilateral tonic extension of the trunk and limbs (tonic phase), often accompanied by a loud vocalization as air is forcefully expelled across tightly contracted vocal cords (the *epileptic cry*), followed by bilaterally synchronous muscle jerking (clonic phase). In some patients, a few clonic jerks precede the tonic-clonic sequence; in others, only a tonic or a clonic phase is seen. Urinary incontinence is common; fecal incontinence is rare. The actual ictus does not usually last more than 90 seconds. The postictal phase is marked by transient deep stupor, followed in 15 to 30 minutes by a lethargic, confused state with automatic behavior. As recovery progresses, many patients complain of headache, muscle soreness, mental dulling, lack of energy, or mood changes lasting as long as 24 hours.

Generalized tonic-clonic seizures result in a significant number of striking, but transient, physiologic changes, including blood hypoxia and lactic acidosis, elevated plasma catecholamine levels, and increased concentrations of serum creatine kinase, prolactin, corticotropin, cortisol, β-endorphin, and growth hormone. Complications include oral trauma, vertebral compression fractures, shoulder dislocation, aspiration pneumonia, and sudden death, which may be related to acute pulmonary edema, cardiac arrhythmia, or suffocation.

Absence seizures (petit mal seizures) occur mainly in children and are characterized by sudden, momentary lapses in awareness (the absence attack), staring, rhythmic blinking, and, often, a few small clonic jerks of the arms or hands. Behavior and awareness return to normal immediately. No postictal period occurs, and the individual usually has no recollection that a seizure has occurred. Most absence seizures last less than 10 seconds.

Compared with those of absence seizures, lapses of awareness that have a more gradual onset, do not resolve as abruptly, and are accompanied by autonomic features or loss of muscle tone are referred to as *atypical absence seizures.* These lapses occur most often in children with mental retardation, and they do not respond as well to anti-epileptic drug treatment.

Myoclonic seizures exhibit as rapid, recurrent, brief muscle jerks that can occur bilaterally, synchronously or asynchronously, or unilaterally without loss of consciousness. The myoclonic jerks range from small movements of the face or hands to massive bilateral spasms that simultaneously affect the head, limbs, and trunk. Repeated myoclonic seizures may seem to crescendo and terminate in a generalized tonic-clonic convulsion. Although they can occur at any time, myoclonic seizures often cluster shortly after waking or while falling asleep.

Atonic seizures (drop attacks) occur most often in children with diffuse encephalopathies and are characterized by sudden loss of muscle tone that may result in falls with self injury. *Reflex seizures* are attacks precipitated by a specific stimulus, such as touch, a musical tune, a particular movement, reading, stroboscopic light patterns, or complex visual images.

FEBRILE SEIZURES

Fever is the most common cause of convulsions in children. Febrile seizures affect between 3% and 5% of all children in the United States and Europe younger than the age of 5 years. Most febrile seizures occur between the ages of 6 months and 4 years, although they sometimes occur in children as old as 6 or 7 years. Approximately 30% of children have more than one attack; the chance of recurrence is greatest if the first seizure occurs before 1 year of age or if a family history of febrile seizures is present. Although most affected children have no long-term consequences, febrile seizures increase the risk of developing epilepsy later. This risk is low for most children (2% to 3%), but 10% to 13% in those who have had prolonged or focal seizures, who have a family history of afebrile seizures, or who were neurologically abnormal before the first febrile seizure. Febrile seizures do not cause mental retardation, poor school performance, or behavioral problems.

BENIGN PARTIAL EPILEPSY OF CHILDHOOD WITH CENTRAL-MIDTEMPORAL SPIKES (ROLANDIC EPILEPSY)

Rolandic epilepsy is a common epileptic syndrome of childhood that represents approximately 15% of all pediatric epilepsies. Seizures usually begin between the ages of 4 and 13 years; affected children are otherwise normal. Most of these children have seizures principally or only at night. Because sleep promotes secondary generalization, parents report only tonic-clonic convulsions; the focal signature is usually missed. In contrast, seizures occurring during the day are typically focal: twitching of one side of the face, speech arrest, drooling, and paresthesias of the face, gums, tongue, and inner cheeks. These seizures may be so minor as to escape notice. Seizures may progress to include hemiclonic movements or hemitonic posturing. EEGs show distinctive, stereotyped epileptiform discharges over the central and midtemporal regions. Prognosis is invariably good, and seizures disappear by mid to late adolescence. Outcome is not affected by treatment, but carbamazepine prevents recurrent attacks.

JUVENILE MYOCLONIC EPILEPSY

Juvenile myoclonic epilepsy is a frequently encountered type of idiopathic generalized epilepsy. It begins most often between the ages of 8 and 20 years in otherwise healthy individuals. When fully developed, the syndrome is characterized by morning myoclonic jerks, generalized tonic-clonic seizures that occur just after awakening, normal intelligence, and a family history of similar seizures.

LENNOX-GASTAUT SYNDROME

The term *Lennox-Gastaut syndrome* is used for a heterogeneous group of early childhood epileptic encephalopathies that have in common physical brain abnormalities, mental retardation, and uncontrolled seizures.

TEMPORAL LOBE EPILEPSY

Temporal lobe epilepsy is the most common epileptic syndrome of adults, accounting for at least 40% of epilepsy cases. Seizures begin in late childhood or adolescence, and a history of febrile seizures is often present. Virtually all patients have complex partial seizures, some of which secondarily generalize. Temporal lobe epilepsy arises most often from mesial temporal limbic structures, typically in association with a characteristic lesion known as hippocampal sclerosis. In 20% of patients, temporal lobe epilepsy is caused by other structural lesions such as cavernous malformations, hamartomas, cortical dysplasia, glial tumors, and scars related to previous head injuries or encephalitis.

POST-TRAUMATIC EPILEPSY

The chance of developing post-traumatic epilepsy relates directly to the severity of the head injury. After penetrating wounds and other severe head injuries, for example, approximately one third of patients develop seizures within 1 year. Severe head injuries are defined by the presence of a cerebral contusion, intracerebral or intracranial hematoma, unconsciousness or amnesia lasting more than 24 hours, or persistent abnormalities on neurologic examination, such as hemiparesis or aphasia. Although the majority of patients develop seizures within 1 to 2 years of injury, new-onset seizures may still appear 5 or more years later. Two thirds of patients with post-traumatic epilepsy have partial or secondarily generalized seizures. Mild head injuries (uncomplicated brief loss of consciousness, no skull fracture, absence of focal neurologic signs, and no contusion or hematoma) do not increase the risk of seizures.

Diagnosis

Accurate diagnosis is the cornerstone of treatment. The diagnostic evaluation has three objectives: (1) to determine if the patient has epilepsy, (2) to classify the seizures and type of epilepsy accurately and determine if the clinical data fit a particular epilepsy syndrome, and (3) to identify, if possible, a specific underlying cause. The patient's description of the experience or a witness's accurate observation of an attack is essential for diagnosis. The setting of the attack often suggests acute causes such as drug withdrawal, central nervous system infection, trauma, or stroke; a history of recent-onset seizures in an adult suggests a new intracranial lesion, and a more chronically sustained or remote history of attacks suggests chronic epilepsy. Any focal feature reported either as an aura or during or after the seizure suggests a structural brain lesion, demanding appropriate investigation. The pattern of an attack, as well as the patient's age, suggests the possible types and causes.

The physical examination is normal in most patients with epilepsy. Physical findings that should be sought include café au lait spots, a facial angioma, hypopigmented macules, axillary freckling, and a shagreen patch on the skin; pigmentary abnormalities or hamartomas in the retina; and focal neurologic signs that indicate localized cerebral abnormality. Asymmetry in the size of the hands, feet, or face signifies a long-standing abnormality of the cerebral hemisphere contralateral to the smaller side. Absence seizures can be triggered in untreated patients by having them hyperventilate for 2 or 3 minutes.

LABORATORY TESTS

EEG is the most important diagnostic test for epilepsy. EEG findings are useful and sometimes essential for establishing the diagnosis, classifying seizures correctly, identifying epileptic syndromes, and making therapeutic decisions. In combination with appropriate clinical findings, *epileptiform* EEG patterns termed *spikes* or *sharp waves* strongly support a diagnosis of epilepsy (Fig. 125–2). In patients with seizures, focal epileptiform discharges indicate focal epilepsy, whereas generalized epileptiform activity indicates a generalized form of epilepsy. However, most EEGs are obtained between seizures, and interictal abnormalities alone can never prove or eliminate a diagnosis of epilepsy. Epilepsy can be definitively established only by recording a characteristic ictal discharge during a representative clinical attack, which is uncommon during routine EEG recordings. A further factor that can confound interpretation of interictal EEGs is the occurrence of similar epileptiform abnormalities in approximately 2% of normal people; many of these abnormalities, especially in children, are asymptomatic markers of a genetic trait. Finally, normal epileptiform-like waveforms or artifacts can be misinterpreted and erroneously considered to be evidence of seizure susceptibility.

Forty to 50% of patients with epilepsy show epileptiform abnormalities on their initial EEG. The chance of capturing epileptiform activity is enhanced by sleep deprivation for 24 hours before the test so that the patient sleeps during a portion of the EEG recording. Serial EEGs increase the yield of positive tracings. A small proportion of persons with epilepsy, however, continue to have normal interictal EEGs despite all efforts to record an abnormality.

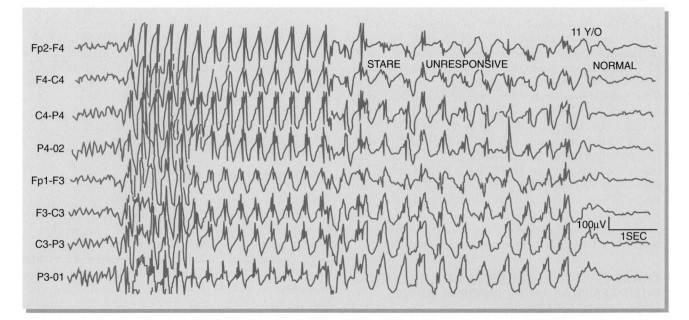

Figure 125–2 Absence (petit mal) epilepsy. The electroencephalogram shows the typical pattern of generalized 3-Hz spike-wave complexes associated with a clinical absence seizure. (From Pedley TA: The epilepsies. In Goldman L, Bennett JC [eds]: Cecil Textbook of Medicine, 21st ed. Philadelphia, WB Saunders, 2000, p 2155.)

NEUROIMAGING STUDIES

Brain MRI complements EEG findings by identifying structural brain conditions that may be causally related to the development of epilepsy. MRI can detect the vast majority of epileptogenic cerebral lesions: hippocampal sclerosis, defects of neuronal migration, and cavernous malformations. Obtaining a complete imaging study that includes both T1- and T2-weighted images in coronal and axial planes is important. Imaging in the coronal plane perpendicular to the long axis of the hippocampus has improved detection of hippocampal atrophy and gliosis, findings that correlate with the pathologic picture of mesial temporal sclerosis and an epileptogenic temporal lobe.

An MRI should be obtained in all patients over the age of 18 years who are suspected of having epilepsy and in all children with partial seizures (except those with benign focal epilepsy of childhood), abnormal neurologic findings, or focal slow-wave abnormalities on EEG.

Positron-emission tomography (PET) and single-photon emission computed tomography (SPECT) offer functional views of the brain. These techniques use physiologically active, radiolabeled tracers to image the brain's metabolic activity (PET) or blood flow (SPECT). For example, approximately 70% of patients with temporal lobe epilepsy show focal hypometabolic areas on interictal PET scans that correspond to the epileptogenic focus. Abnormalities using PET or SPECT are often seen even when MRIs are normal. Functional MRI is beginning to be developed for similar uses.

OTHER TESTS

Routine blood tests rarely offer diagnostic assistance in otherwise healthy patients with epilepsy. Serum electrolytes, liver function tests, and an automated blood cell count are useful as baseline studies before anti-epileptic drug therapy is begun. Blood tests are necessary in older patients with acute or chronic systemic disease. Adolescents and young adults with unexplained generalized seizures should be screened for substance abuse (especially cocaine) with blood or urine studies.

Lumbar puncture is indicated only if meningitis or encephalitis is suspected; it is otherwise unnecessary. Repeated generalized seizures and status epilepticus can increase cerebrospinal fluid protein content slightly and produce a pleocytosis of up to 100 white blood cells/mm^3 for 24 to 48 hours, but *cerebrospinal fluid pleocytosis should be attributed to seizures only in retrospect.* An intracranial inflammatory process should always be excluded first.

An electrocardiogram should be obtained in any young person with a first generalized seizure if there is a family history of arrhythmia, sudden unexplained death, or episodic unconsciousness. An electrocardiogram should also be obtained in any patient with a history of cardiac arrhythmia or valvular disease.

Differential Diagnosis

Not every paroxysmal event is a seizure, and misidentification of other conditions as epilepsy leads to ineffective, unnecessary, and potentially harmful treatment. Misdiagnosis accounts for a substantial portion of patients who have not responded to anti-epileptic drug treatment. A wide variety of

Table 125–4	**Nonepileptic Episodic Disorders That May Resemble Seizures**

Movement disorders: myoclonus, paroxysmal choreoathetosis, episodic ataxias, hyperekplexia (startle disease)
Migraine: confusional, vertebrobasilar
Syncope
Behavioral and psychiatric: psychogenic seizures, hyperventilation syndrome, panic disorder, dissociative states
Cataplexy (usually associated with narcolepsy)
Transient ischemic attack
Alcoholic blackouts
Hypoglycemia

conditions can be confused with epilepsy, depending on the age of the patient and the nature and circumstances of the attacks (Table 125–4). Nonepileptic paroxysmal disorders have in common the occurrence of sudden, discrete events characterized by abnormal behavior, variable responsiveness, changes in muscle tone, and various postures or movements. These conditions are far more common and variable in their presentation in children than in adults.

Syncope (see Chapter 120) refers to the symptom complex that results when a transient, global reduction in cerebral perfusion occurs. Loss of consciousness lasts only a few seconds, uncommonly a minute or more, and recovery is rapid. If the cerebral ischemia is sufficiently severe, the syncopal episode may include brief tonic posturing of the trunk or a few clonic jerks of the arms and legs (*convulsive syncope*). Similarly, some forms of *migraine* can be mistaken for seizures, especially if the headache is atypical or mild. Basilar artery migraine, a variant noted most often in adolescents and young adults, can include lethargy, mood changes, confusion and disorientation, vertigo, bilateral visual disturbances, and alteration or loss of consciousness.

Psychogenic seizures frequently cause intractable *epilepsy* in adults. Some patients with psychogenic seizures have epilepsy as well. Definitive diagnosis requires video-EEG documentation, although a history of atypical and nonstereotyped attacks, emotional or psychological precipitants, psychiatric illness, complete lack of response to anti-epileptic drugs, and repeatedly normal interictal EEGs suggest the possibility of psychogenic seizures. *Panic attacks* and anxiety attacks with hyperventilation can superficially resemble partial seizures with affective, autonomic, or special sensory symptoms. Prolonged hyperventilation results in muscle twitching or spasms (tetany); affected patients may faint.

Treatment

If the cause of symptomatic seizures is corrected, anti-epileptic drugs are usually unnecessary. Adults with a single, unprovoked seizure and normal clinical and laboratory findings frequently do not have subsequent seizures; thus, anti-epileptic treatment is not necessarily indicated. However, patients with focal neurologic findings on clinical, radiologic, or EEG examinations are more likely to have repeated seizures by comparison. In individual patients, social considerations may dictate treatment after a single seizure. However, in otherwise normal patients who are likely to be poorly compliant with medications, treatment after a single seizure is seldom justified.

If seizures are recurrent, the goal of treatment is to stop attacks completely. Anti-epileptic drugs should be used for their indicated conditions (Table 125–5) and according to the following guidelines:

1. The type of seizure should be defined and the preferred medication should be given in usual doses and then increased until seizure control is complete or side effects occur (Table 125–6).

2. Seizures that are infrequent require slow changes in medication doses.
3. If seizures persist at toxic levels, or if major side effects occur, then another agent should be selected.
4. One agent should not be discontinued until another has been added. Otherwise, status epilepticus may result.
5. If seizures persist after two agents have been given to toxic levels, referral to a specialized center for complex combination therapy and seizure monitoring should be considered.
6. Toxic levels of some anti-epileptics (particularly phenytoin and carbamazepine) can cause seizures.

EPILEPSY SURGERY

In the majority of patients, epilepsy is controlled with medication. When seizures cannot be controlled by adequate trials of two appropriate single agents or by the combination of two agents, the epilepsy is termed *medically intractable.* In approximately 20% of patients, the epilepsy cannot be fully controlled. Such patients are at considerable risk for the consequences of seizures: inability to drive; stigmatization by schools, employers, and families; and threats to personal educational and occupational goals. In appropriately selected patients, surgery can abolish seizures with restoration of normal neurologic function. The accurate localization of a small, resectable seizure focus requires intensive investigation before surgery.

SPECIAL TREATMENT CONCERNS
Status Epilepticus

In *major generalized motor status epilepticus,* seizures follow one another so rapidly that new attacks begin before the patient has recovered from the previous one. Status epilepticus can occur with partial or generalized epilepsy. Generalized continuous epileptic activity can damage the brain permanently. The most frequent cause is abrupt withdrawal

Table 125–5	**Drugs Used for Different Types of Seizures**
Type of Seizure	**Drugs**
Simple and complex partial	Carbamazepine, phenytoin, valproate, gabapentin, lamotrigine, topiramate, levetiracetam
Secondarily generalized	Carbamazepine, phenytoin, valproate, gabapentin, lamotrigine, topiramate, levetiracetam
Primary Generalized Seizures	
Tonic-clonic	Valproate, carbamazepine, phenytoin, lamotrigine, levetiracetam
Absence	Ethosuximide, valproate, lamotrigine
Myoclonic and tonic	Valproate, clonazepam

Table 125–6	**Frequently Prescribed Antiepileptic Drugs**		
Drug	**Total Dose/Day**	**Dose Frequency (hr)**	**Therapeutic Concentrations**
Carbamazepine	*Adult:* 800–1600 mg *Child:* 10–40 mg/kg/day	6–8	6–12 mcg/mL
Ethosuximide	*Adult:* 750–1500 mg *Child:* 10–75 mg/kg/day	8–12	40–100 mcg/mL
Gabapentin	*Adult:* 900–3600 mg	8	2–12 mcg/mL
Lamotrigine	*Adult:* 100–600 mg *Child:* 1–5 mg/kg	12	4–15 mcg/mL
Levetiracetam	*Adult:* 500–3000 mg	12	Uncertain
Phenobarbital	*Adult:* 60–240 mg *Child:* 2–6 mg/kg/day	24	15–40 mcg/mL
Phenytoin	*Adult:* 200–600 mg *Child:* 4–12 mg/kg/day	24	10–20 mcg/mL
Topiramate	50–600 mg	12	2–20 mcg/mL
Valproate	*Adult:* 500–6000 mg	8	50–120 mcg/mL

Table 125–7	**Treatment of Status Epilepticus**

Time (min)	Steps
0–5	Give oxygen; ensure adequate ventilation. Monitor: vital signs, electrocardiography, oximetry. Establish intravenous access; obtain blood samples for glucose level, complete blood cell count, electrolytes, toxins, and anticonvulsant levels.
6–9	Give glucose (preceded by thiamine in adults).
10–20	Intravenously administer either 0.1 mg/kg of lorazepam at 2 mg/min or 0.2 mg/kg of diazepam at 5 mg/min. Diazepam can be repeated if seizures do not stop after 5 min; if diazepam is used to stop the status, then phenytoin should be administered promptly to prevent recurrence of status.
21–60	If status persists, administer 15–20 mg/kg of phenytoin intravenously no faster than 50 mg/min in adults and 1 mg/kg/min in children.
>60	If status does not stop after 20 mg/kg of phenytoin, give additional doses of 5 mg/kg to a maximal dose of 30 mg/kg. If status persists, then give 20 mg/kg of phenobarbital intravenously at 100 mg/min. When phenobarbital is given after a benzodiazepine, ventilatory assistance is usually required. If status persists, then give general anesthesia (e.g., pentobarbital). Vasopressors or fluid volume are usually necessary. Electroencephalogram should be monitored. Neuromuscular blockade may be needed.

of anticonvulsant medications from a known epileptic. Other precipitants include withdrawal of alcohol or drugs in a habitual user, cerebral infection, trauma, hemorrhage, and neoplasm. However, merely observing that a patient is in the midst of a seizure does not indicate that he or she should be treated for status epilepticus. If status epilepticus is documented, treatment is urgent (Table 125–7). Identification of the cause must be undertaken as soon as possible after seizures stop.

Partial motor status is also known as partial continuous epilepsy. It is uncommon, occurs in several forms, and can last for hours, days, or longer. The seizure frequency can range from one every 3 seconds to several per second. The motor attacks range from highly focal, myoclonic, repetitively localized twitches to jerks that involve most of the limb or one half of the body. In general, cerebral lesions cause partial motor seizures in the face or distal upper extremity, whereas brainstem or spinal lesions tend to cause proximal myoclonic activity. Causes include stroke, trauma, neoplasms, and encephalitis. In some instances, the cause never becomes clear. Partial continuous epilepsy often resists all efforts at treatment. Severe hyperglycemia can produce partial motor and complex partial status; seizures stop once hyperglycemia is corrected.

Partial complex status produces a sustained state of confusion associated with stereotyped motor and autonomic automatisms. Some attacks produce abrupt-onset schizophreniform or other bizarre activity, whereas others are marked by a stuporous state. Patients may resist assistance in their abnormal state, which can last for hours or even days. The EEG usually shows continuous slow-wave and spike activity predominating over one or both temporal areas, commonly asymmetrically. Occasionally, surface recordings may be only mildly abnormal, but epileptiform activity can be detected by nasopharyngeal leads or from electrodes placed deep in the brain. Treatment should be initiated promptly because the effects of prolonged seizures can permanently impair memory and intellect.

Absence status (petit mal status) occurs in two forms. The more common form resembles partial complex status and consists of confused automatic behavior accompanied by closely spaced or continuous runs of 3- to 4-Hz spike-and-wave activity on the EEG. The condition occurs in adolescents or occasionally young adults with known petit mal seizures. Most episodes last less than 30 minutes. Similar attacks of prolonged (days to months) automatisms associated with confusion, EEG abnormality, and sometimes gradual interictal mental deterioration can occur in older persons with no history of epilepsy. Most of these attacks can be halted with intravenous diazepam.

Genetic Counseling and Pregnancy

Over 90% of women taking anti-epileptic drugs have healthy infants. However, persons with seizure disorders should be advised about the hereditary risks to the fetus. Four percent to 10% of the children of patients with generalized primary epilepsy will have one or more seizures. This number compares with a risk of approximately 1.5% in the general population. Women with epilepsy have a 1.5- to 3-fold increased rate of complications of pregnancy, including bleeding, toxemia, abruptio placentae, and premature labor. Anticonvulsant medication dosage often requires adjustment during pregnancy because blood volume increases and drug pharmacokinetics change. Blood level monitoring during the latter half of pregnancy is essential. During pregnancy, giving vitamins and supplements, including calcium, is advisable. Women of childbearing age should take 1 mg of folic acid daily to protect against developmental defects. Vitamin K, 5 mg twice weekly, should be given orally during the final 6 weeks, with a parenteral supplement administered to the mother and infant at the time of delivery. Breast-feeding is not contraindicated in women taking anti-epileptic drugs.

Children of both mothers and fathers taking anti-epileptic medication have a birth defect risk two to three times that of the general population. Seizures, however, pose a greater risk to the mother and fetus than does the generally low rate of birth defects associated with anti-epileptic drugs. Two agents, valproate and carbamazepine, have been implicated in neural tube defects. Phenytoin, phenobarbital, and trimethadione use during pregnancy have all been associated with neurodevelopmental abnormalities. Use of two or more drugs increases the risk. Discontinuation of medication before conception should be considered only if clear reasons exist to believe that seizures will not recur (see later discussion). Medications should not be discontinued during pregnancy.

Psychosocial Problems

The presence of incompletely controlled epilepsy and its frequent association with other neurologic limitations often create major emotional problems for the patient. In addition, disorders that cause partial complex seizures often cause aberrant personality traits that intensify isolation. Outbreaks of frustration, depression, and suicide are more frequent among patients with epilepsy than in the general population. A reduced libido and hyposexuality have been noted in men with partial complex seizures. However, in the absence of associated brain damage, most persons with epilepsy have normal intelligence.

Patients with seizure disorders are helped most by bringing the attacks under complete control, but reassurance and optimistic social guidance aid immeasurably. Once seizures are under control, affected persons should be encouraged to live normal lives, using common sense as their guide. Body contact and high-risk sports are best avoided unless seizures have been completely controlled for over a year; high diving, deep-water or underwater swimming, high alpine climbing, boxing, and head-contact football should be avoided. All states grant automobile driver's licenses to patients with epilepsy provided that no seizures have occurred for specified periods. Life and health insurance policies can generally be obtained. The Epilepsy Foundation of America can assist patients' social-vocational considerations.

Prognosis

Sixty percent to 70% of people with epilepsy achieve a 5-year remission of seizures within 10 years of diagnosis. Approximately one half of these patients eventually become seizure free without anticonvulsant drugs. Factors favoring remission include an idiopathic form of epilepsy, a normal neurologic examination, and an onset in early to middle childhood (excluding neonatal seizures).

Thirty percent of patients, usually those with severe epilepsy starting in early childhood, continue to have seizures and never achieve a remission. In the United States, the prevalence of intractable epilepsy cases is 1 to 2 per 1000 population.

Discontinuing Anti-Epileptic Drugs

Many patients with epilepsy become seizure free on medication for an extended period. Some patients can discontinue anti-epileptic drugs without a relapse. Successful drug withdrawal is most likely if initial seizure control was readily achieved using monotherapy, relatively few seizures were occurring before remission, and the EEG and neurologic examination are normal just before drugs are discontinued. In addition, seizure-free intervals of 4 years reduce the likelihood of relapse. Conversely, risk of relapse is high if seizure control was difficult to establish and required polytherapy, if generalized tonic-clonic seizures were frequent before control was achieved, and if the EEG demonstrates moderate or severe disturbances of background activity or active epileptiform activity at the time drug withdrawal is considered.

Prospectus for the Future

The molecular pathogenesis of many genetic epilepsies has been defined. These still rare disorders will provide insights and targets for novel anti-epileptic treatments that correct ion channel dysfunction. The molecular cause or causes of the common epilepsies will be defined.

Improved imaging techniques will further facilitate cortical localization and selective ablation of the epileptic focus resulting in more patients becoming seizure-free and returning to normal life.

References

Bleck TP: Refractory status epilepticus. Curr Opin Crit Care 11:117–120, 2005.

Gutierrez-Delicado E, Serratosa J: Genetics of the epilepsies. Curr Opin Neurol 17:147–153, 2004.

Hirtz D, Berg AT, Bettis D, et al: Practice parameter: Treatment of the child with a first unprovoked seizure. Report of the QSS of the AAN and the Practice Committee of the CNS. Neurology 60:166–175, 2003.

Central Nervous System Tumors

Jennifer J. Griggs

Central nervous system (CNS) tumors produce devastating effects and are associated with high mortality rates. Even histologically benign tumors may be unresectable and thus incurable because of their location. Malignant tumors are considered malignant because they cannot be removed completely, and they recur within the CNS. CNS tumors rarely metastasize to other organs.

In childhood, brain tumors are the second most common cancers. The incidence of CNS tumors is low in young adults but increases with advancing age and reaches a plateau between the ages of 65 and 74 years. The incidence of primary CNS lymphoma is increasing, attributable only in part to acquired immunodeficiency syndrome (AIDS).

The cause of most CNS tumors is unknown. With the exception of gliomas associated with vinyl chloride and various tumors that occur after CNS irradiation, no environmental agents are known to be causative. Moreover, no evidence supports a viral origin of CNS tumors. Hereditary syndromes associated with an increased risk of CNS tumors, including von Hippel-Lindau disease, tuberous sclerosis, Li-Fraumeni syndrome, and neurofibromatosis, account for less than 1% of primary CNS tumors. Although the chromosomal abnormality associated with many of these syndromes is known, the specific mechanisms leading to CNS neoplasia have not been defined. The genetic heterogeneity of CNS tumors suggests alternative pathways in tumor progression.

Classification

The World Health Organization has classified primary CNS tumors based on cell of origin. Most primary CNS tumors are of neuroepithelial origin and result from malignant transformation of astrocytes, ependymocytes, and oligodendrocytes. Gliomas, which arise from astrocytes, are the most common. In a patient with a known systemic malignant disease, metastases to the CNS are more likely than a primary CNS tumor.

Clinical Manifestations

Symptoms caused by intracranial tumors result from either (1) compression of the brain by tumor and the presence of associated edema or (2) infiltration and destruction of brain parenchyma by tumor cells. Because of the uncompromising rigidity of the cranial vault, both histologically benign and malignant tumors may cause symptoms even when these tumors are small. Symptoms caused by primary brain tumors tend to be slowly progressive, rather than acute. In contrast, metastatic tumors are more likely to produce acute symptoms because they grow more rapidly and are associated with edema. Moreover, hemorrhage into metastatic tumors, particularly renal cell cancer, melanoma, lung tumors, and choriocarcinomas, causes acute symptoms.

Patients with brain tumors may have generalized symptoms that arise from increased intracranial pressure or with focal symptoms resulting from specific areas of compromise. Among the generalized symptoms, *headache* is the most common and is the first symptom in over one third of adults with brain tumors. Headaches from intracranial tumors are often worse in the morning than at other times of day and are provoked by maneuvers that increase intracranial pressure. The pain may localize to the side of the tumor in patients with supratentorial tumors; patients with infratentorial tumors frequently describe pain in the retro-orbital, retroauricular, or occipital regions. Other generalized symptoms include changes in mood or personality, a decrease in appetite, and nausea. Projectile vomiting, common in children, is rare in adults. Generalized or focal seizures occur in up to 90% of patients, with the incidence of seizures varying with cancer type.

Other focal symptoms of brain tumors depend on the location of the tumor. *Tumors of the frontal lobe* may grow to massive proportion before symptoms prompt the patient or the patient's family to seek medical help. Progressive difficulty with concentration and memory, personality changes, and lack of spontaneity may occur with a frontal lobe tumor.

Urinary incontinence and gait disorder may appear. Bifrontal disease, most commonly seen with gliomas (the *butterfly glioma*) or lymphomas, may cause spasticity of the extremities and the appearance of primitive reflexes (grasp, snout).

Parietal lobe tumors produce subtle sensory signs or hemianesthesia. Tumors of the right parietal lobe may produce spatial disorientation or left homonymous hemianopia, whereas left parietal lobe tumors cause receptive aphasia or right homonymous hemianopia.

Involvement of the *temporal lobes* by tumor can lead to behavioral changes, olfactory hallucinations, complex partial seizures, and quadrantanopia. If tumors are large enough, they can cause herniation of the uncus through the tentorial notch *(uncal herniation)*.

Metastatic spread of primary CNS tumors to sites outside the CNS is exceedingly rare. Spread along the neuraxis to the meninges and spinal cord, however, can occur with most malignant CNS tumors.

Evaluation of the Patient

RADIOGRAPHIC EVALUATION

A thorough neurologic examination helps in localizing the site of a suspected brain tumor. All patients should have either a magnetic resonance imaging (MRI) scan (Fig. 126–1) or a contrast-enhanced computed tomography (CT) scan. MRI, which should be done with and without gadolinium contrast, is superior to CT scanning in almost all patients because it is more useful in imaging the posterior fossa and is more sensitive in detecting parenchymal invasion by a tumor. If MRI is not available, then a contrast-enhanced CT scan should be done. CT scans done without contrast enhancement are not adequate for evaluating either

primary tumors or metastatic tumors. Cerebral angiography is indicated only when an understanding of tumor blood supply is deemed necessary before surgical resection, such as in patients with highly vascularized meningiomas. Positron-emission tomography (PET) scanning reveals areas of increased glucose metabolism and may demonstrate greater extent of tumor than suggested on CT or MRI scanning. PET scans are particularly useful in assessing response to treatment or providing evidence of recurrent disease after primary therapy.

BIOPSY

Biopsy of a suspected brain tumor is essential to make an accurate histologic diagnosis and to detect nonneoplastic disease such as abscess. Exceptions include brainstem tumors with radiographic characteristics of astrocytomas. Tissue may be obtained either by open craniotomy or with MRI-guided or CT-guided stereotactic techniques. Because the histologic features of the tumor may be mixed, small biopsy specimens can be misleading. When the suggestion of a primary brain tumor is high, the tissue diagnosis may be made at the time of surgical resection. This approach yields the greatest amount of tissue for pathologic examination. In 20% of patients with metastatic tumors to the CNS, the primary tumor site is not evident; biopsy can be helpful in identifying the most likely primary site.

OTHER DIAGNOSTIC TESTS

Lumbar puncture is helpful only if leptomeningeal involvement with tumor is suggested; this procedure is generally contraindicated when an intracranial mass lesion is present. Electroencephalography is not routinely performed in patients with brain tumors unless seizures are anticipated.

Treatment

SURGICAL RESECTION

Surgical resection is attempted in most patients with primary brain tumors and in many patients with solitary brain metastases. Even when surgical cure is unlikely, resection of a large portion of the tumor may relieve symptoms for many months. Such *debulking* of primary brain tumors may improve survival, but a clear correlation between extent of resection and survival time has not been established. Tumor resection is seldom possible in patients with brainstem tumors. Additionally, radical resection is not recommended for tumors that lie in language or sensorimotor areas, the basal ganglia, or the corpus callosum because of the risk of permanent and debilitating neurologic dysfunction. Surgical resection is not recommended for patients with CNS lymphomas because these tumors are often multifocal and respond to a combination of chemotherapy and radiation therapy.

ACUTE TREATMENT OF INCREASED INTRACRANIAL PRESSURE

Most patients with CNS tumors have brain edema. Some patients benefit from the use of glucocorticoids. Dexamethasone is usually given because of its long half-life and

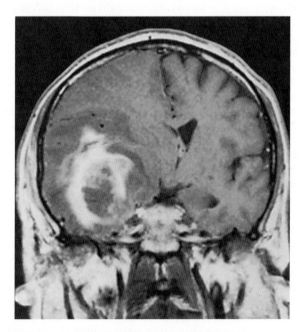

Figure 126–1 Temporal lobe glioblastoma. This T1 gadolinium-enhanced MRI scan shows a typical ring configuration of contrast with central necrosis and marked mass effect. (From Goldman L, Ausiello D. Cecil Textbook of Medicine, 22nd ed., Philadelphia, WB Saunders, 2004.)

minimal mineralocorticoid effect. Doses used for the treatment of tumor-related edema range from 16 to 40 mg/day given in divided doses (two to four times daily). Dexamethasone can be given orally because it is well absorbed from the gastrointestinal tract. Patients with symptoms related to edema often have an improvement in symptoms within 48 hours.

In patients with life-threatening edema with signs of brain herniation, mannitol can be given in an intravenous dose of 0.5 to 2 g/kg to reduce intracranial pressure. Dexamethasone should be given concurrently.

ANTICONVULSANTS

Patients who develop seizures and many patients who are at risk of developing seizures are given anticonvulsants before they undergo biopsy or surgical procedures. Long-term prophylactic use of anticonvulsants is not necessary.

RADIATION THERAPY

Radiation therapy is offered to most patients following resection of a primary brain tumor. Radiation therapy can be delivered in three ways: (1) as external beam (conventional) radiation therapy, (2) as brachytherapy, or (3) as *radiosurgery.* *External beam radiation therapy* uses x-rays directed either at the whole brain or to the focal area involved by tumor. Whole-brain radiation therapy is associated with long-term toxicity, exhibited as dementia and gait disturbance. Although rates of such toxicity are low in people who die within 1 to 2 years of treatment, long-term survivors have a high rate of these complications over time. *Brachytherapy* involves the implantation of either permanent or temporary radiation *seeds* within the tumor. This approach allows increased doses of radiation therapy to be delivered to the tumor while the surrounding normal tissue is protected. The third approach, *radiosurgery,* involves converging more than 200 beams of radiation onto a small, well-defined area. This procedure can be done either with cobalt-60 (the so-called *gamma knife*) or with linear accelerators. Radiosurgery is indicated for treating small tumors that are not surgically accessible.

CHEMOTHERAPY

Chemotherapy is not used as sole therapy for primary CNS neoplasms but rather as part of multimodality therapy. Fewer than 10% of patients with glioblastomas benefit from therapy. The major obstacle to the effective use of chemotherapy is the blood-brain barrier, often disrupted by large tumors but not to the extent that would allow treatment of the entire tumor. Attempts to overcome the blood-brain barrier by giving intra-arterial chemotherapy have not been successful. In addition, CNS tumor cells are often drug resistant. Carmustine is the drug that has been most extensively studied. Temozolomide, an oral agent, is active in the treatment of all types of gliomas. Medulloblastomas may respond to the platinum agents cisplatin and carboplatin.

Oligodendrogliomas are unusually sensitive to chemotherapy. The combination of procarbazine, vincristine, and lomustine (CCNU) produces responses in up to 80% of patients treated with this regimen. CNS lymphomas are treated with a combination of chemotherapy and radiation therapy (see later discussion).

Specific Tumors
MALIGNANT ASTROCYTOMAS

The term *malignant astrocytoma* refers to a group of heterogenous tumors and includes glioblastoma multiforme, anaplastic astrocytoma, and anaplastic oligodendroglioma. Some patients with these types of tumors have mixed histologic features with both high-grade and low-grade characteristics.

Of the anaplastic gliomas, *glioblastoma multiforme* is associated with the worst prognosis, with a median survival of less than 12 months. Surgery and radiation therapy are used together to improve symptoms and quality of life. In young patients and in persons with good function, chemotherapy may prolong survival, but studies showing such prolongation may merely reflect the effects of selection bias. When disease relapse occurs in patients with glioblastoma multiforme, surgical resection, brachytherapy, radiosurgery, and chemotherapy are all occasionally helpful, but, in general, benefit is short lived.

In contrast, *anaplastic astrocytomas* and *anaplastic oligodendrogliomas* are associated with median survival times of 4 to 5 years. Patients with anaplastic oligodendrogliomas or tumors with mixed histologic features benefit most from chemotherapy given after surgical resection. Both carmustine (BCNU) and the combination of procarbazine, CCNU, and vincristine have been used in this setting. Patients with recurrent tumors are treated with the same approach as those with recurrent glioblastoma multiforme.

MENINGIOMAS

Meningiomas arise outside the brain and generally grow slowly; they may be found incidentally during the evaluation of unrelated symptoms. These tumors are histologically benign in 90% of patients and tend to arise along the dorsal surface of the brain, along the falx cerebri, on the sphenoid ridge, within the lateral ventricles, at the base of the skull, or close to the optic nerves.

Complete resection of meningiomas should be attempted; the risk of recurrent disease is inversely proportionate to the extent of resection. For example, in patients who do not have resection or coagulation of dural attachments, the risk of recurrent disease within the subsequent two decades is approximately 20%. In these patients and in those who have only partial resection of the tumor, postoperative radiation therapy should be given. In the patient with malignant meningioma, radiation therapy should be recommended regardless of the extent of resection. Chemotherapy is not used in the treatment of meningiomas.

CENTRAL NERVOUS SYSTEM LYMPHOMA

Primary CNS lymphomas are increasing in incidence among both immunocompromised and immunocompetent people. These lymphomas may arise from lymphocytes that travel into and out of the CNS. By definition, a patient with primary CNS lymphoma has no evidence of lymphoma outside the CNS. Primary CNS lymphomas most often occur deep within the frontal lobe and are therefore less likely to produce seizures than other primary and metastatic CNS neoplasms. Headache, personality changes, and focal symptoms corresponding to the location of the tumor are usual presenting complaints. Forty percent of immunocompetent patients and nearly 100% of patients with AIDS have multifocal lymphoma at the time of diagnosis. More than 40% of patients have involvement of the leptomeninges, but such involvement is rarely symptomatic. Ocular involvement in one or both eyes occurs in 20% of patients.

Treatment of primary CNS lymphomas requires first that the correct diagnosis be made. Because the disease is often multifocal, it may be confused with metastatic disease from other solid tumors. Surgical resection is not indicated in the management of CNS lymphoma. Corticosteroids have cytotoxic effects on lymphoma cells and can result in dramatic responses. Treatment with steroids is not sufficient, however, and most patients are treated with systemic chemotherapy followed by whole-brain radiation therapy. The chemotherapy combinations used are the same as those used in the treatment of systemic non-Hodgkin's lymphoma. The 5-year survival rates associated with combined modality therapy are as high as 30%. In some patients who have a complete response to chemotherapy, whole-brain radiation therapy may be deferred to avoid the late effects associated with brain radiation.

METASTATIC TUMORS TO THE BRAIN

Most intracranial tumors are metastatic from other sites. The tumors that commonly metastasize to the brain are lung cancer, breast cancer, and melanoma, but nearly any solid tumor can metastasize to the CNS. Patients complain of headache, seizures, and focal symptoms reflecting the area of involvement, as well as depression and changes in mental status. Metastases are usually multifocal, although non–small-cell lung cancer and renal-cell cancer often produce solitary metastases. Rapidly growing tumors cause massive edema.

Treatment of metastases is usually with corticosteroids and radiation therapy. Symptomatic improvement may be seen within hours of giving dexamethasone in patients with brain edema. Surgical resection is indicated in select patients with solitary or easily resectable tumors if the systemic malignant disease is well controlled and if the patient is otherwise doing well. Because most chemotherapeutic agents do not cross the blood-brain barrier, CNS metastases other than small-cell lung cancer do not usually respond to systemic chemotherapy. Leptomeningeal metastases are described in Chapter 56.

SPINAL CORD TUMORS

Much less common than tumors of the brain, spinal cord tumors are described as *extradural* (outside of the dural sac) or *intradural.* Most extradural tumors are metastases from other sites, including lung, breast, and prostate cancers. Intradural tumors are further described as either extramedullary (arising outside the spinal cord) or intramedullary (arising within the spinal cord). Examples of extramedullary tumors are schwannomas and meningiomas. Ependymomas and astrocytomas are the most common intramedullary tumors. The most common location for spinal tumors is the thoracic region.

Patients with spinal cord tumors usually develop symptoms as a result of compression of normal structures by the tumor or impairment of the vascular supply, rather than by invasion of the parenchyma by tumor. Back pain and distal paresthesias are among the earliest symptoms, followed by loss of sensation and weakness below the level of the tumor and loss of bowel and bladder control.

MRI is the most useful tool for evaluating the patient with suggested spinal cord tumor and has replaced myelography in most cases. In patients with progressing deficits, urgent evaluation and treatment are indicated.

Treatment of primary spinal tumors is with surgical resection. Resection of high-grade astrocytomas is followed by radiation therapy; the usefulness of radiation therapy for other tumors is not clear. Patients with epidural metastatic tumors are treated with high doses of corticosteroids and surgery or radiation. Although radiation therapy is probably as effective as surgery in many patients, surgical decompression is recommended in patients with an acute onset of symptoms and in those in whom the pathologic features of the tumor have not yet been identified.

Prospectus for the Future

Recent advances in molecular biology have yielded information about brain tumor development and offer the promise of targeted therapies. For example, 70% of glioblastoma multiforme tumors have a specific receptor for interleukin 13 (IL-13), a naturally occurring immune-system regulatory protein. Normal cells, in contrast, lack the IL-13 receptor. In animal models, molecules directed against the IL-13 receptor lead to selective disruption of the malignant cells. A second emerging therapeutic strategy is the development in a mouse model of a vaccine against EphA2, a receptor tyrosine kinase expressed in primary glioblastoma multiforme and anaplastic astrocytoma tissues. A third example of a molecular target in primary brain tumors is the Fos-related antigen 1 (Fra-1), a transcription factor overexpressed in 60% of glioblastoma multiforme tumors and a potent regulator of glioma cell morphology. Cells transfected with antisense Fra-1 exhibit significantly diminished tumorigenic potential. Such knowledge about tumorigenesis and tumor cell regulation may translate into therapies that are effective in the treatment of primary CNS malignancies.

References

Combs SE, Gutwein S, Thilmann C: Stereotactically guided fractionated re-irradiation in recurrent glioblastoma multiforme. J Neurooncol 74:167–171, 2005.

DeAngelis LM: Tumors of the central nervous system and intracranial hypertension and hypotension. In Goldman L, Ausiello DA (eds): Cecil Textbook of Medicine, 23rd ed. Philadelphia, Saunders, 2007.

Shah GD, DeAngelis LM: Treatment of primary CNS lymphoma. Hematology Oncol Clin NA 19:611–627, 2005.

Infectious Diseases of the Nervous System

Robert C. Griggs

Roger P. Simon

The central nervous system can be infected with the same spectrum of infectious agents as the rest of the body. Specific bacterial, fungal, parasitic, and viral infections are covered in Section XVI. In this chapter, we focus on brain and spinal cord infections that are localized to the central nervous system, either as abscesses within the parenchyma itself or as parameningeal infections. Also discussed are the central nervous system manifestations of infections elsewhere in the body. Finally, a category of infections with clinical signs confined to the brain and spinal cord—prion diseases—is considered.

Brain Abscess

Brain abscesses produce symptoms and findings similar to those of other space-occupying lesions, such as brain tumors, but often progress more rapidly and affect meningeal structures more frequently than tumors. They originate or extend from extracerebral locations, resulting from (1) blood-borne metastases from unknown sources, lungs, or heart, and (2) direct extension from parameningeal sites of infection (otitis, cranial osteomyelitis, and sinusitis), sites of recent or remote head trauma or neurosurgical procedures, and infections associated with cyanotic congenital heart disease. The most commonly isolated pathogens are aerobic and microaerobic streptococci and gram-negative anaerobes such as *Bacteroides* and *Prevotella*. Less common are gram-negative aerobes and *Staphylococcus. Actinomyces, Nocardia,* and *Candida* are less frequently found by comparison. Infection is often polymicrobial. Culture-negative abscesses from surgical specimens occur in 30% of antibiotic-treated patients and in 5% of patients undergoing surgery before antibiotic administration.

DIAGNOSIS

Systemic signs of infection may be minimal or absent. Almost one half of patients do not have fever or leukocyto-

sis. Neck stiffness is rare unless increased intracranial pressure is present. The presenting features are, instead, those of an expanding intracranial mass (Table 127–1). A headache of recent onset is the most common symptom. If the process is untreated, then headache increases in severity and focal signs appear, such as hemiparesis or aphasia, followed by obtundation and coma. The period of evolution may be as brief as hours or as long as days to weeks with more indolent organisms. Seizures may occur with abscesses involving the cortical gray matter. Cerebrospinal fluid (CSF) examination should not be performed for diagnosis; it is seldom diagnostic and can be normal and may aggravate impending transtentorial herniation. Contrast-enhanced computed tomography (CT) and magnetic resonance imaging (MRI) are used for diagnosis and for monitoring the response to therapy. MRI is superior to CT for detecting multiple and posterior fossa abscesses; also, with intravenous gadolinium contrast, MRI is superior to CT in demonstrating cerebritis, the extent of mass effect, associated venous thrombosis, and the response to therapy.

Chapter 127

TREATMENT

Pyogenic abscesses are treated with antibiotics alone or with antibiotics combined with surgical aspiration or excision. Surgery is required if a major mass effect is present or if the abscess adjoins the ventricular surface (raising the possibility of catastrophic rupture into the ventricular system). In addition, if the lesion is in the posterior fossa (with the potential of brainstem compression), is large (>3 cm diameter), or is refractory to medical therapy, then surgery is indicated. Antibiotics alone are appropriate for a surgically inaccessible abscess, multiple abscesses (seen in 10% of patients), or those in the early cerebritis stage. If the causal organism is not identified, then antibiotics should cover the most likely organisms (streptococci and anaerobes). If methicillin-resistant *Staphylococcus aureus* is presumed (e.g., postoperative infection or intravenous drug use), then

Table 127–1	Brain Abscess: Diagnostic Features in 43 Patients	
Feature		**%**
Headache		72
Lethargy		71
Fever		60
Nuchal rigidity		49
Nausea, vomiting		35
Seizures		35
Ocular palsy		27
Confusion		26
Visual disturbance		21
Weakness		21
Dysarthria		12
Stupor		12
Papilledema, dysphasia, hemiparesis, dizziness		10 or less

Data from Chun CH, Johnson JD, Hofstetter M, et al: Brain abscess: A study of 45 consecutive cases. Medicine 65:415, 1986.

vancomycin, 1 g intravenously every 12 hours, should be added.

The resolution of abscesses can be followed by serial CT or MRI. With aspiration or surgery, treatment with antibiotics directed at the isolated organism should be given for 4 to 6 weeks. If medical therapy is used without surgery, then treatment should be extended to 6 to 8 weeks. Improvement usually occurs, but not resolution of scan abnormalities, especially in medically treated patients. The presence of enhancement at the end of therapy may identify a group at risk for relapse that should be monitored carefully with scans after therapy is completed. The outcome correlates inversely with the abscess size and the degree of neurologic dysfunction at presentation but less well with age, cause, number of abscesses, or corticosteroid use.

Subdural Empyema

Subdural empyema refers to infection in the space separating the dura and arachnoid. It is responsible for one fifth of localized intracranial infections and results from direct or indirect extension from infected paranasal sinuses through a retrograde thrombophlebitis or, less frequently, from untreated chronic otitis. Unilateral empyema is most common because the falx prevents passage across the midline, but bilateral or multiple empyemas can occur. Cortical venous thrombosis or brain abscess develops in approximately one fourth of patients.

Symptoms initially reflect those of chronic otitis or sinusitis, on which lateralized headache (a universal feature), fever, and obtundation become superimposed. Vomiting, meningeal signs, and focal neurologic abnormalities (hemiparesis or seizures) usually follow. If the disease remains untreated, then obtundation progresses and the septic mass and swollen underlying brain soon lead to venous thrombosis or death from herniation. The major differential diagnosis is that of meningitis. Nuchal rigidity and obtundation occur in both, but papilledema and lateralizing deficits are more common in empyema. Contrast-enhanced CT or MRI can be diagnostic of empyema, showing an extra-axial, crescent-shaped mass with an enhancing rim lying just below the inner table of the skull over the cerebral convexities or in the interhemispheric fissures. MRI, compared with CT, better detects underlying parenchymal edema, as well as the infection itself. Treatment requires both prompt surgical drainage of the empyema cavity and high-dose intravenous antibiotics directed toward organisms found at the time of craniotomy.

Malignant External Otitis

Malignant external otitis occurs in older patients with diabetes and is caused by *Pseudomonas aeruginosa*. An external otitis progresses rapidly, with ear pain, facial swelling, osteomyelitis of the base of the skull, and purulent meningitis accompanied by multiple cranial nerve palsies. Urgent treatment with an antipseudomonal penicillin or a third-generation cephalosporin combined with an aminoglycoside or ciprofloxacin, as well as surgical débridement and drainage, is essential. The mortality rate is high.

Spinal Epidural Abscess

Infection within the epidural space around the spinal cord usually responds to treatment but can cause paralysis and death. Its incidence is 0.5 to 1.0 per 10,000 hospital admissions in the United States, but the frequency is increased in intravenous drug users. Patients are usually febrile (38° to 39° C [100.4° to 102.2° F]) and have acute or subacute neck or back pain, with focal percussion tenderness being a prominent sign; stiff neck and headache are common. The pain can be mistaken for sciatica, a visceral abdominal process, chest wall pain, or cervical disc disease. If the condition goes unrecognized at this stage, then the symptoms can rapidly evolve, over a few hours to a few days, to produce weakness and finally paralysis occurring distal to the spinal level of the infection. In this clinical setting, spinal epidural abscess should be assumed, systemic antibiotics begun, and urgent neuroradiologic confirmatory diagnostic procedures pursued. The differential diagnosis includes compressive and inflammatory processes involving the spinal cord (transverse myelitis, intervertebral disc herniation, epidural hemorrhage, and metastatic tumor), which can usually be detected by MRI.

PATHOPHYSIOLOGIC FACTORS

Infections of the epidural space originate from contiguous spread or through hematogenous routes from a distant source. Cutaneous sites of infection are the most common remote sources, especially in intravenous drug users. Abdominal, respiratory tract, and urinary sources are also common. The anatomy of the epidural space dictates the location of the abscess, the frequency of epidural infections being proportional to the volume of the epidural space. Because the size of the intravertebral canal remains relatively constant while the circumference of the spinal cord changes, abscess formation is maximal in the thoracic and lumbar regions and minimal at the cervical spine enlargement.

BACTERIOLOGIC FACTORS

Causative organisms can be identified by culture or Gram stain from pus obtained at exploration (90% of patients), blood cultures (60% to 90% of patients), or CSF (20% of patients). *Staphylococcus aureus* accounts for most infections, followed by streptococci and gram-negative anaerobes. Tuberculous abscesses remain common, representing as many as 25% of patients in high-risk populations.

TREATMENT

Unless culture and sensitivities dictate otherwise, penicillinase-resistant penicillin should be started empirically as anti-staphylococcal treatment for presumed bacterial infection. If methicillin resistance is suggested, then vancomycin should be used. Considering the severity of the disease, most authorities would provide additional gram-negative coverage with a third-generation cephalosporin or a quinolone. Surgical decompression was once thought to be mandatory in all cases; now, early diagnosis by MRI allows for effective medical therapy alone before the occurrence of neurologic complications.

Septic Cavernous Sinus Thrombosis

Septic cavernous sinus thrombosis produces headache or lateralized facial pain, followed in a few days to weeks by fever and involvement of the orbit, which produces proptosis and chemosis secondary to obstruction of the ophthalmic vein. Paralysis of oculomotor nerves follows rapidly. In some instances, sensory dysfunction occurs in the first and second divisions of the trigeminal nerve and a decrease in the corneal reflex. Further involvement of the contiguous orbital contents follows, with mild papilledema and decreased visual acuity, sometimes progressing to blindness. Extension to the opposite cavernous sinus or to other intracranial sinuses with cerebral infarction or increased intracranial pressure secondary to impaired venous drainage can result in stupor, coma, and death. The CSF is abnormal in almost all patients, sometimes with a profile resembling that of purulent meningitis or parameningeal infection. The most common causative organism is *S. aureus,* with streptococci and pneumococci being less common; anaerobic infection has been reported. Radiologic evaluation includes sinus imaging, with attention to the sphenoidal and ethmoidal sinuses. MRI (with and without intravenous gadolinium) can often show venous thrombosis by illustrating the lack of the normal *flow void* within a vascular structure. Treatment requires early diagnosis and consists of prompt drainage of infected paranasal sinuses, as well as specific anti-staphylococcal agents, such as nafcillin or oxacillin, given intravenously.

Lateral Sinus Thrombosis

Septic thrombosis of the lateral sinus results from acute or chronic infections of the middle ear. The symptoms include ear pain followed over several weeks by fever, headache, nausea, vomiting, and vertigo. Results of otologic examination are abnormal; mastoid swelling may be seen. Sixth cranial nerve palsies and papilledema can occur, but other focal neurologic signs are rare. Treatment includes intravenous antibiotics to cover staphylococci and anaerobes (nafcillin or oxacillin with penicillin or metronidazole), but surgical drainage (mastoidectomy) may be required.

Septic Sagittal Sinus Thrombosis

Septic sagittal sinus thrombosis is uncommon and occurs as a consequence of purulent meningitis, infections of the ethmoidal or maxillary sinuses spreading through venous channels, infected compound skull fractures, or, rarely, neurosurgical wound infections. Symptoms include manifestations of elevated intracranial pressure (headache, nausea, and vomiting) that evolve rapidly to stupor and coma.

Neurologic Complications of Infectious Endocarditis

Neurologic complications occur in one third of patients with bacterial endocarditis and triple the mortality rate of the disease. Most of these complications derive from valvular vegetations. Cerebral (but not systemic) emboli are increasingly common from mitral valve endocarditis. Most emboli, regardless of the bacterial cause of the infection, occur before or early in the course of treatment. By 2 weeks of therapy, the risk of embolization decreases dramatically. Cerebral emboli are distributed in the brain in proportion to cerebral blood flow. Therefore, most emboli lodge in the branches of the middle cerebral artery peripherally, with resultant hemiparesis. Focal seizures may result.

Mycotic aneurysms complicate endocarditis in 2% to 10% of patients and are more common in acute than subacute disease. The middle cerebral artery is most commonly involved, with the aneurysms being located distally in the vessel, differentiating them from congenital berry aneurysms. Small brain abscesses may complicate the course of endocarditis, but macroscopic abscesses are rare, with most occurring in the setting of acute, rather than subacute, endocarditis. Multiple micro-abscesses, however, can result in a diffuse encephalopathy similar to that seen in sepsis. Such lesions may escape detection on CT scan and are not amenable to surgical drainage. Antibiotic treatment of the primary disease is indicated. The CSF is abnormal in 70% of patients and may be the same as with purulent meningitis (polymorphonuclear predominance, elevated protein level, and low glucose level) or with a parameningeal infection (lymphocytic predominance, modest protein elevation, and normal glucose level).

Prion Diseases

Several human diseases have been attributed to a unique infectious protein—the prion. Prion illnesses include Creutzfeldt-Jakob disease (CJD) (also called *subacute spongiform encephalopathy*), kuru, Gerstmann-Sträussler-Scheinker syndrome, and familial fatal insomnia. Prion-related illnesses are unique in that they may be hereditary, may occur spontaneously, or may be acquired by contamination with the agent. The appearance of *variant CJD* in Great Britain, in association with the outbreak of bovine spongiform encephalopathy and the contamination of beef, has greatly increased interest in this group of illnesses.

Creutzfeldt-Jakob Disease

Illness from CJD is seen worldwide, with an incidence of 0.5 to 1.0 cases per 1 million population per year. Most cases are sporadic; 5% to 15% are inherited in an autosomal-dominant pattern. Higher rates of familial disease occur in descendants of Jewish populations from Libya and North Africa, where the annual incidence is as high as 31.3 per million. The illness may also be iatrogenic, as seen in recipients of growth hormone prepared from pooled human pituitary glands, may occur after cadaver corneal and dura mater transplants, and may follow use of stereotactic intracerebral depth electrodes.

CJD is frequently diagnosed incorrectly initially. Prodromal symptoms include altered sleep patterns and appetite, weight loss, changes in sexual drive, and impaired memory and concentration. Disorientation, hallucinations, and emotional lability are early signs, and the patient then develops a rapidly progressive dementia associated with myoclonus (in approximately 90% of patients). Myoclonus is generally provoked by tactile, auditory, or visual startle stimuli. CJD has an apopleptic, abrupt onset in 10% to 15% of patients. Other distinctive presentations include seizures, autonomic dysfunction, and lower motor neuron disease suggesting amyotrophic lateral sclerosis. Cerebellar ataxia occurs in one third of patients.

The clinical tetrad supporting the diagnosis of CJD consists of a subacute progressive dementia, myoclonus, typical periodic complexes on electroencephalography, and normal CSF. Brain imaging is typically normal until late in the disease, when progressive brain atrophy occurs. Routine CSF study is generally normal. A CSF test for the protein 14-3-3, in the appropriate clinical context, is highly specific and sensitive for CJD. No effective therapy has been developed. The disease is inexorably progressive. Death typically occurs within 1 year of the onset of symptoms (range 1 to 130 months).

Although the illness is not communicable in the conventional sense, a risk exists in handling materials contaminated with the prion protein. Gloves should be worn when handling blood, CSF, and other body fluids. Instruments must be disinfected by steam autoclaving for 1 hour at 132° C, by steam autoclaving for 4.5 hours at 121° C (1.5 psi), or by immersion in 1 N sodium hydroxide for 1 hour at room temperature.

Prospectus for the Future

The availability of animal models of prion diseases has paved the way for large-scale screening for agents that can prevent progression of the diseases. Concerns about the transmission of variant CJD via food and transfusions have prompted intense study of techniques to identify prions in blood and other tissues.

References

Castellani RJ, Colucci M, Xie Z, et al: Sensitivity of 14-3-3 protein test varies in subtypes of sporadic Creutzfeldt-Jakob disease. Neurology 63:436–442, 2004.

Ladogana A, Puopolo M, Croes EA, et al: Mortality from Creutzfeldt-Jakob disease and related disorders in Europe, Australia, and Canada. Neurology 64:1586–1591, 2005.

Nath A: Brain abscess and parameningeal infections. In Goldman L, Ausiello DA (eds): Cecil Textbook of Medicine, 23rd. Philadelphia, Saunders, 2007.

Tsai YD, Chang WN, Shen CC, et al: Intracranial suppuration: A clinical comparison of subdural empyemas and epidural abscesses. Surg Neurol 59:191–196, 2003.

Yang SY, Zhao CS: Review of 140 patients with brain abscess. Surg Neurol 39:290, 1993.

Demyelinating and Inflammatory Disorders

Robert C. Griggs

Demyelination refers to the process in which the myelin of the central or peripheral nervous systems is injured. Diseases of peripheral nerve myelin are discussed in Chapter 129. Diseases of central nervous system (CNS) myelin are either acquired or hereditary. Multiple sclerosis (MS) is the most common acquired disease of myelin. Hereditary diseases of myelin often involve problems with formation of myelin and are usually referred to as *dys*myelinating, rather than *de*myelinating. Table 128–1 lists common disorders of myelin.

Multiple Sclerosis

MS is defined clinically by typical symptoms, signs, and disease progression. The annual incidence rate for MS ranges in different populations from 1.5 to 11 per 100,000. The incidence rate may be increasing. The first symptoms of MS usually occur between the ages of 15 and 50 years, and the disease is more frequent in women than in men. Individual bouts of inflammatory demyelination may be accompanied by clinical symptoms, termed *relapses,* followed in most cases by some degree of recovery, producing the typical *relapsing-remitting* course seen early in the disease. Diagnosis requires intermittent or progressive CNS symptoms supported by evidence of two or more CNS white matter lesions occurring in an appropriately aged patient who lacks an alternative explanation, such as recurrent strokes or systemic lupus erythematosus. The diagnosis is based on clinical features; laboratory tests support the diagnosis but cannot be diagnostic.

ETIOLOGIC FACTORS

The initiating cause or causes of MS is unknown, but pathogenesis clearly includes autoimmune-mediated inflammatory demyelination and axonal injury. Pathologic examination of MS brain tissue shows perivascular infiltration by lymphocytes and monocytes; class II major histocompatibility complex (MHC) antigen expression by cells in the lesions; and chemokines, lymphokines, and monokines secreted by activated cells. Also present are immunologic abnormalities in blood and cerebrospinal fluid (CSF), an association with certain MHC class II allotypes, and a response of patients with MS to immunomodulation. Patients may improve with immunosuppressive drugs and worsen with treatment with interferon (IFN)-γ. Moreover, similarities can be found between MS and experimental allergic encephalomyelitis, which is an animal model induced by inoculating susceptible animals with myelin proteins. Both environmental and genetic factors are clearly involved. Certain populations in northern latitudes have a very high incidence of MS. No infectious cause has been found, but theories suggest that one or more ubiquitous viruses may lead to an autoimmune process in susceptible individuals. A genetic influence is well established by the higher concordance in monozygotic compared with dizygotic twins, the clustering of MS in families, racial variability in risk, and associations with class II MHC allotypes.

The earliest event in the MS lesion is breakdown of the blood-brain barrier, followed by perivenular mononuclear infiltrates, and then circumscribed areas of myelin breakdown. Macrophages are necessary for myelin loss, and B lymphocytes and plasma cells surround small CNS blood vessels. T lymphocytes and monocytes infiltrate CNS parenchyma. Products of the immune response, including immunoglobulins, interleukins, IFNs, and tumor necrosis factor, accompany the acute MS lesion. MS also injures CNS neuronal axons; this injury may account for the brain atrophy and permanent damage that occur as the disease progresses.

DIAGNOSIS

A diagnosis of MS is established by clinical criteria, and laboratory tests are useful in supporting the diagnosis. Symptoms can arise from MS involvement of virtually any part of the CNS, but certain presentations are typical of the disease (Table 128–2). Sudden, unilateral visual loss, double vision, vertigo, pins-and-needles sensation, and loss of balance are particularly common. Fever often worsens symptoms. The majority of patients have resolution of their initial symp-

Table 128–1   Demyelinating Disorders

Unknown Cause

Multiple sclerosis
Devic's disease
Optic neuritis
Acute transverse myelopathy

Parainfectious Disorders

Acute disseminated encephalomyelitis
Acute hemorrhagic leukoencephalopathy

Viral Infections

HIV-1–associated myelopathy
Progressive multifocal leukoencephalopathy
Subacute sclerosing panencephalitis

Nutritional Disorders

Combined systems disease (vitamin B_{12} deficiency)
Demyelination of the corpus callosum (Marchiafava-Bignami
    disease)
Central pontine myelinolysis

Anoxic-Ischemic Sequelae

Delayed postanoxic cerebral demyelination
Progressive subcortical ischemic encephalopathy

HIV = human immunodeficiency virus.

Table 128–2   Symptoms and Signs of Multiple Sclerosis Listed in Declining Order of Frequency

Symptoms

Unilateral visual impairment
Double vision
Paresthesias
Ataxia or unsteadiness
Vertigo
Fatigue
Muscle weakness
Urinary disturbance
Dysarthria
Mental disturbance

Signs

Optic neuritis
Internuclear ophthalmoplegia
Nystagmus
Spasticity or hyperreflexia
Babinski sign
Absent abdominal reflexes
Dysmetria or intention tremor
Impairment of central sensory pathways
Labile or changed mood

toms. The criteria for diagnosis of relapsing-remitting MS (Table 128–3) are based on documentation of two or more episodes affecting two or more locations in the CNS. In younger patients, the disease usually starts with a subacute or acute onset of focal neurologic symptoms and signs, most often reflecting disease in the optic nerves, pyramidal tracts, posterior columns, cerebellum, central vestibular system, or medial longitudinal fasciculus. Older individuals commonly exhibit insidiously progressive myelopathy: progressive spastic leg weakness, axial instability, and bladder impairment.

LABORATORY CONFIRMATION

Neurologic imaging is the first step. The computed tomographic (CT) brain scan sometimes shows hypodense regions in white matter, but CT is relatively insensitive and usually shows no abnormalities. Magnetic resonance imaging (MRI) has largely supplanted CT. Head MRI shows abnormalities in more than 85% of clinically definite MS patients. Typical lesions (Fig. 128–1) are multifocal, appear hyperintense on intermediate and T2-weighted MRIs, and occur predominantly in the periventricular cerebral white matter, corpus callosum, cerebellum, cerebellar peduncles, brainstem, and spinal cord. MRI usually shows many more hyperintense lesions than were clinically anticipated. Intravenous gadolinium enhances acute lesions, which appear hyperintense on T1-weighted images. CSF examination is helpful in instances in which MRI is not confirmatory. Routine analysis of CSF is usually normal except for slight elevations of protein and occasional slight pleocytosis (<50 mononuclear cells). Most patients with MS have evidence of increased immunoglobulin G (IgG) production in the CNS: *oligoclonal* bands, increased IgG levels, and antibodies to myelin basic protein. Sensory-evoked potentials, measuring conduction velocity along the optic, auditory, and somatosensory nerves, are often delayed and can confirm multifocal CNS disease.

TREATMENT

The major challenge in the treatment of patients with MS is to halt the progressive disability that occurs with repeated acute attacks of relapsing-remitting MS or with the less common chronic progressive MS. Treatment of acute attacks with corticosteroids is of short-term benefit but has not had a major effect on long-term disability. However, three agents have recently been found to be of benefit in modifying the course of MS (Table 128–4). Two forms of recombinant IFN-β—IFN-β-1a (Avonex and Rebif) and IFN-β-1b

Table 128–3	**Washington Committee Criteria for the Diagnosis of Multiple Sclerosis (MS)**				
Category	**Attacks**	**Clinical Evidence**		**Paraclinical Evidence***	**CSF OB/IgG**
Clinically Definite MS					
1	2	2			
2	2	1	*and*	1	
Laboratory-Supported Definite MS					
1	2	1	*or*	1	+
2	1	2			+
3	1	1	*and*	1	+
Clinically Probable MS					
1	2	1			
2	1	2			
3	1	1	*and*	1	
Laboratory-Supported Probable MS					
1	2				+

CSF = cerebrospinal fluid; IgG = immunoglobulin G; OB = oligoclonal bands.
*Magnetic resonance imaging or evoked potential studies.
Data from Poser CM, Paty DW, Scheinberg L, et al: New diagnostic criteria for multiple sclerosis: Guidelines for research protocols. Ann Neurol 13:227, 1983.

Table 128–4	**Treatment of Multiple Sclerosis**

Specific

Acute exacerbations: IV methylprednisolone,
    500–1000 mg/day for 3 days
Relapsing-remitting attack prevention:
Interferon-β-1a
Interferon-β-1b
Glatiramer acetate

Symptomatic

Antispasticity agents: baclofen, benzodiazepines
Antipyretics for intercurrent infection
Fatigue: amantadine, pemoline
Pain (uncommon): carbamazepine

(Betaseron)—are approved for use in relapsing-remitting MS. IFN-β therapy reduces the frequency and severity of MS relapses, slows disability progression, reduces the number and volume of new lesions seen on MRI, and slows the progressive accumulation of lesions seen on T2-weighted MRI. Based on controlled clinical trials, the individual products are administered at different doses (higher for Betaseron and Rebif compared with Avonex), frequencies (weekly for Avonex, three times weekly for Rebif, and every other day for Betaseron), and routes of administration (intramuscular for Avonex and subcutaneous for Betaseron and Rebif). Adverse effects include transient influenza-like symptoms after each injection with all preparations and inflammatory reactions at the injection sites with Betaseron. Glatiramer acetate (Copaxone) is also used for patients with relapsing-remitting MS. Glatiramer acetate is a myelin-like polypeptide that may inhibit cellular immune reactions to myelin. It is given daily by subcutaneous injection and reduces the relapse rate; its principal side effect is swelling and redness at the injection site. The effect of immunomodulatory therapy on the long-term disability of MS is under study.

Acute attacks are treated with intravenous methylprednisolone, which shortens acute exacerbations. The dosage is 500 or 1000 mg/day for 3 days, followed by prednisone, 60 mg in a single morning dose for 3 days, tapering off over 12 days.

The differential diagnosis of MS (Table 128–5) includes a large number of diseases and is different for relapsing-remitting MS than for the less-frequent progressive disease. Alternative diagnoses must be considered initially and again with each subsequent new symptom. With the initial episode, MS is always a diagnosis of exclusion.

Neuromyelitis Optica (Devic's Disease)

Neuromyelitis optica is a syndrome characterized by partial or complete transverse myelopathy and optic neuritis. Loss of vision and paraplegia may occur, and the two major components of the disease may be widely separated in time. The syndrome of neuromyelitis optica may occur as the result of

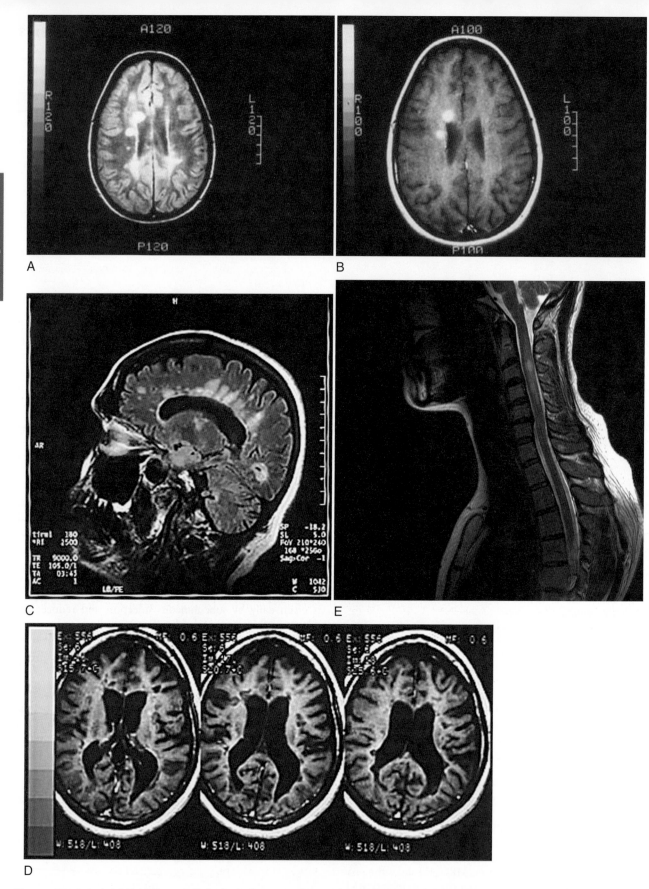

Figure 128–1 *A,* Axial FLAIR image of the brain from a patient with MS revealing classic multiple periventricular and deep white matter high signal lesions. *B,* Axial T1-weighted image post-gadolinium contrast from the same patient shows that two of the lesions are actively inflamed and enhance with contrast. *C,* Sagittal FLAIR image of the brain from a patient with MS revealing classic periventricular lesions radiating outward from the ventricles. *D,* Three consecutive axial T1-weighted images showing numerous areas of T1 low signal *(black holes)* and ventricular enlargement and diffuse atrophy. *E,* Sagittal T2-weighted image of the brain and cervical spine from a patient with multiple sclerosis showing a high signal plaque from C3–C5 in the spinal cord. (From Calabresi P: Multiple sclerosis and demyelinating conditions of the central nervous system. In Goldman L, Ausiello DA [eds]: Cecil Textbook of Medicine, 23rd ed. Philadelphia, Saunders, 2007.)

Table 128–5	Differential Diagnosis of Multiple Sclerosis

Relapsing-Remitting

Vascular disease: strokes, vasculitis
Behçet's syndrome
Systemic lupus erythematosus
Sarcoidosis

Chronic Progressive

Vascular: multiple strokes
Degenerative: spinocerebellar ataxias, spine disease
Infections: HTLV-1-, HIV-related
Neoplastic: lymphoma
Metabolic: adrenomyeloleukodystrophy

HIV = human immunodeficiency virus; HTLV-1 = human T-cell lymphotropic virus type 1.

acute disseminated encephalomyelitis, systemic lupus erythematosus, or sarcoidosis, as well as during the course of typical MS or in isolation without apparent cause. In the latter case, it is considered a variant of MS.

Optic Neuritis

Optic neuritis denotes partial or complete loss of vision in one or both eyes; it is usually acute and due to inflammation. Most patients with optic neuritis have pain in, around, or behind the affected eye, followed within 1 or 2 days by visual loss that progresses for as long as a week. Optic neuritis is termed *retrobulbar neuritis* when the lesion is in the posterior two thirds of the optic nerve and *papillitis* when the lesion is in the anterior portion of the optic nerve. The ophthalmoscopic appearance of papillitis is similar to that of acute papilledema from increased intracranial pressure but differs from papilledema by the markedly reduced visual acuity in papillitis. Visual function almost always recovers to some degree, usually within weeks. Blindness as the result of optic nerve demyelination seldom occurs. The syndrome of optic neuritis can be caused by several diseases, of which MS is by far the most common. Other causes include tobacco-nutritional amblyopia, Leber's hereditary optic neuropathy, vasculitis, optic nerve compression on any basis, neurosyphilis, ischemic optic neuropathy, pernicious anemia, or sarcoidosis. Many patients with idiopathic isolated optic neuritis eventually develop MS; the reported frequency in several series varies from 13% to 85%, according to the length of follow-up.

An increasingly rapid but not necessarily a total visual recovery occurs by treating optic neuritis with intravenous methylprednisolone. A 3-day course of intravenous methylprednisolone followed by a prednisone taper within 8 days of the onset appears to reduce by approximately 50% the likelihood of conversion from idiopathic optic neuritis to MS during 2 years of follow-up.

Acute Transverse Myelitis

Acute transverse myelitis denotes rapidly developing paraparesis or paraplegia as the result of spinal cord dysfunction. If the cervical cord is involved, then quadriparesis and respiratory failure can occur. Abrupt or rapidly developing back or radicular pain may be followed by ascending paresthesias and weakness that begin in the feet. Urinary and fecal retention or incontinence is common. Progression varies from minutes, resembling infarction, to steady or stepwise progression over several days. Progression over days may occur with both spinal cord compression resulting from a tumor and from transverse myelitis. Distinguishing idiopathic transverse myelitis from compressive myelopathy is difficult; acute transverse myelitis demands immediate diagnostic evaluation.

Several disorders can produce an acute transverse myelopathy. The most important disorders to exclude immediately are compressive lesions, including spinal or epidural abscess, tumor, herniated intervertebral disc; vascular occlusion resulting from arteritis, aortic dissection, aortic surgery, or arteriovenous malformation; varicella-zoster infection; and autoimmune disease, including MS. The evaluation must include an immediate imaging procedure such as MRI, with attention to the level of involvement to rule out spinal cord compression. Cord compression from a metastatic tumor may present acutely even though the tumor has been present for weeks or longer. Central herniated intervertebral discs may cause acute cord compression without producing local pain. Rapidly progressing myelopathy in a previously healthy person should always raise the question of spontaneous epidural, subdural, or intraparenchymal abscess or bleeding, the latter occurring from an arteriovenous malformation or as a complication of anticoagulation or blood dyscrasia. Approximately one third of patients with idiopathic transverse myelitis have a history of an antecedent upper respiratory or influenza-like illness. Transverse myelitis may also follow other infectious illnesses such as *Mycoplasma* or measles.

Transverse myelitis and slowly progressive myelopathy are common manifestations of MS, either as a first clinical manifestation or a later development. However, a syndrome suggesting complete cord transection rarely occurs. The treatment for idiopathic transverse myelitis is intravenous methylprednisolone. With severe disease, bladder catheterization, ventilatory support, and proper protection from compression neuropathies are necessary. Prognosis varies widely, with recovery ranging from almost none at all to complete, depending on the degree of acute necrosis.

Acute Disseminated Encephalomyelitis

Acute disseminated encephalomyelitis (ADEM) is a monophasic demyelinating inflammatory disorder that can appear after viral infections or immunizations. ADEM usually produces multifocal brain and spinal cord symptoms, but it may be restricted to one area, particularly the optic nerve (acute optic neuropathy) or spinal cord (acute transverse myelopathy). When related to an antecedent viral infection, ADEM usually occurs 6 to 10 days after the appearance of systemic symptoms. When it follows immunization, it usually begins 10 days to 3 weeks after injection. ADEM can appear in the absence of any identifiable exposure. The pathogenesis is believed to comprise an antibody response, the antigen being either the injected protein or the infecting virus. Clinically, ADEM typically produces acute headache, fever, and multifocal neurologic signs. Severely affected patients may develop delirium, stupor, or coma. Seizures are relatively common. The CSF is usually abnormal, showing pleocytosis (20 to 200 lymphocytes/mm³) and an elevated gamma globulin with slight protein elevation. Glucose concentration is usually normal. The electroencephalogram is usually diffusely abnormal, with widespread slowing, but it does not have the characteristic focal slow and sharp wave activity of herpes simplex encephalitis. ADEM produces clinical and CSF manifestations similar to those of acute viral encephalitis and cannot be distinguished from that disorder by clinical findings. Despite its presumed immune mechanism, neither corticosteroids nor other immunosuppressive agents have been effective in treating ADEM. Anecdotal reports suggest that intravenous immunoglobulin may be of benefit. The most important similar disorder to consider is herpes simplex encephalitis (see Chapter 96).

Acute hemorrhagic leukoencephalitis is a fatal, rare variant of ADEM. The illness usually occurs after an upper respiratory tract infection and is characterized by sudden headache, seizures, and rapid progression to coma. Patients often die within a few days. The CSF often shows more polymorphonuclear leukocytes than lymphocytes. At autopsy, the brain is swollen, with bilateral and asymmetric hemorrhages scattered throughout the white matter. No treatment has been developed.

Prospectus for the Future

The prognosis of MS has improved over the last two decades. However, despite progress in both diagnosis and treatment, the cause of MS remains unknown. Neither autoimmune nor infectious causes are proved or disproved. The highly promising agent natalizumab caused or contributed to the development of progressive multifocal leukoencephalopathy shortly after its approval by the U.S. Food and Drug Administration. It was so effective in preventing MS relapses that either it or a related agent merits further study.

References

Goodin DS, Frohman EM, Garmany GP Jr, et al; Therapeutics and Technology Assessment Subcommittee of the American Academy of Neurology and the MS Council for Clinical Practice Guidelines: Disease modifying therapies in multiple sclerosis: Report of the Therapeutics and Technology Assessment Subcommittee of the American Academy of Neurology and the MS Council for Clinical Practice Guidelines. Neurology 58:169–178, 2002.

Lublin FD: Clinical features and diagnosis of multiple sclerosis. Neurol Clin 23(1):1–15, 2005.

Polman CH, Reingold SC, Edan G, et al: Diagnostic criteria for multiple sclerosis: 2005 revisions to the "McDonald Criteria." Ann Neurol 58(6):840–846, 2005.

Neuromuscular Diseases: Disorders of the Motor Neuron and Plexus and Peripheral Nerve Disease

Robert C. Griggs

The neuromuscular diseases are disorders of the motor unit and of the sensory and autonomic peripheral nerves. Each motor unit consists of (1) the motor neuron cell body, located in either the spinal cord anterior horn (for muscles innervated by the spinal cord) or a cranial nerve nucleus (for ocular, facial, and bulbar musculature), (2) the axon of the motor neuron in the peripheral or cranial nerve, (3) the neuromuscular junction, and (4) the muscle fibers innervated by the motor neuron. The sensory peripheral nerves comprise (1) the sensory neuron cell body in the posterior (dorsal) root ganglion, (2) the central axon passing to the spinal cord in the posterior root, (3) the distal axon in the peripheral nerve, and (4) the sensory nerve terminal in skin, muscle, joint capsule, and other structures. The autonomic nerves are divided into sympathetic and parasympathetic fiber systems. The sympathetic preganglionic fibers arise from cell bodies in the intermediolateral column of the spinal cord and enter the sympathetic ganglia, where postganglionic fibers arise to innervate blood vessels or viscera. The parasympathetic preganglionic neurons lie in the brain stem and sacral portion of the spinal cord, and axons terminate in the viscera, special sensory organs, or skin, which contain the postganglionic neurons and their nerve terminals. Neuromuscular diseases are classified into four groups, according to which portion of the motor unit is involved (Table 129–1). Motor neurons and peripheral nerve diseases are considered in this chapter; myopathies are considered in Chapter 130, and neuromuscular junction diseases are considered in Chapter 131.

The symptoms and signs of the neuromuscular diseases are at times indistinguishable. However, some useful general rules apply (Table 129–2).

The peripheral nerves exiting from the spinal cord can be injured by intervertebral disc or bony compression within the spinal foramina, producing nerve root disease (radiculopathy; see Chapter 118). The roots within the cervical, lumbar, and sacral regions organize into the cervical, lumbar, and sacral plexuses before giving rise to individual peripheral nerves. Diseases of these plexuses (plexopathies) tend to be *focal* in symptoms and signs, whereas many diseases of the peripheral nerves and muscles are *generalized* and widespread in many nerves or muscles.

The major symptoms of diseases of the motor unit are muscle weakness, wasting, fatigue, cramps, pain, and stiffness. Symptoms of peripheral nerve disease also include decreased sensation (hypesthesia or hypalgesia), abnormal sensation (paresthesias), or painful sensations (dysesthesias). Symptoms and signs of autonomic nervous system disease include postural dizziness; abnormal cardiac, visceral, and ocular function; and changes in sweating. The symptoms of neuromuscular disease, particularly those of weakness or sensory disturbance, do not necessarily distinguish disorders of the peripheral nervous system from those of the central nervous system. Most neuromuscular diseases are relatively symmetric, in contrast to the asymmetry of many focal central nervous system diseases.

Diagnostic Tests

BLOOD TESTS

Creatine kinase (CK) is present in high concentrations in the sarcoplasm of muscle and may leak into blood to serve as a sensitive indicator of muscle damage. In patients with active muscle destruction, the serum CK is invariably elevated, and lactate dehydrogenase (LDH), aspartate aminotransferase (AST), and alanine aminotransferase (ALT) levels may be elevated. Because several of these enzymes are used for screening for abnormalities of organs other than muscle, identifying a muscle disease first by an unexpected elevation in one of these enzymes is not uncommon. The clue to the muscle origin of the increased enzyme levels is that the degree of abnormality decreases in the following order: CK > LDH > AST > ALT. The serum CK level is the most sensitive indicator and may be very high (more than tenfold above normal) in patients with diseases with muscle fiber necrosis, such as the muscular dystrophies. It frequently is slightly elevated in patients with spinal muscular atrophy, amyotrophic lateral sclerosis (ALS), and other motor neuron disorders but is usually normal in patients with peripheral neuropathies and neuromuscular junction disorders.

ELECTROMYOGRAPHY

The measurement of electrical activity arising from muscle fibers is performed by inserting a needle electrode percutaneously into a muscle. Normal muscle is electrically silent at rest. Spontaneous activity during complete relaxation occurs in myotonic disorders, in inflammatory myopathies, and in denervated muscles. Spontaneous activity of a single muscle fiber is called a *fibrillation,* and such activity of part of or an entire motor unit is called a *fasciculation.* In myotonia, repeated muscle depolarization and contraction occur despite voluntary relaxation. Abnormalities in motor unit potentials occur during the course of denervation; with the development of reinnervation, the remaining motor units increase in amplitude and become longer in duration and polyphasic (Fig. 129–1). Conversely, in muscle diseases such as the muscular dystrophies and other diseases that destroy scattered fibers within a motor unit (see Fig. 129–1), the motor unit action potentials are of lower amplitude and shorter duration and are polyphasic. A reduced recruitment (interference) pattern from maximum voluntary effort occurs in denervation. Conversely, in patients with primary muscle disease, submaximal voluntary effort produces a full recruitment pattern despite marked weakness.

Nerve conduction is studied by stimulating a peripheral nerve (e.g., the ulnar) with surface electrodes placed over the nerve. The resulting action potential is recorded by electrodes placed over the nerve more proximally in the case of large sensory nerve fibers and over the muscle distally in the case of motor nerve fibers in a mixed motor sensory nerve. For sensory nerves, the sensory nerve action potential (SNAP) is quantitated, and for motor nerves, the compound muscle action potential (CMAP) is quantitated.

REPETITIVE STIMULATION TESTS

In neuromuscular junction disorders, the size of the initial CMAP evoked by electrical stimulation may be normal. However, after a few stimuli at rates of 2 to 3 Hz, the amplitude of the CMAP declines. It then increases again after the fourth or fifth stimulus. This pattern of decrement followed by increment is characteristic of myasthenia gravis.

Table 129–1	Classification of Neuromuscular Disease
Site of Involvement	**Typical Examples**
Anterior Horn Cell	
Without upper motor neuron involvement	Spinal muscular atrophy, poliomyelitis, West Nile virus
With upper motor neuron involvement	Amyotrophic lateral sclerosis
Peripheral Nerve	
Unifocal	Carpal tunnel syndrome
Multifocal	Mononeuritis multiplex (e.g., polyarteritis nodosa)
Diffuse	Diabetic neuropathy, Charcot-Marie-Tooth disease
Neuromuscular junction	Myasthenia gravis
Muscle	Duchenne's muscular dystrophy, dermatomyositis

Table 129–2	Clinical Features of the Neuromuscular Diseases			
Clinical Feature	**Anterior Horn Cell**	**Peripheral Nerve**	**Neuromuscular Junction**	**Muscle**
Distribution of weakness	Asymmetric limb or bulbar	Symmetric distal	Extraocular, bulbar, proximal limb	Symmetric proximal limb (bulbar in some; distal rarely)
Atrophy	Marked and early	Moderate	None (or very late)	Slight early; marked later
Sensory involvement	None	Paresthesias, hypesthesia	None	None (except for myasthenic syndrome)
Characteristic features	Fasciculations, cramps	Combined sensory and motor abnormality	Diurnal fluctuation	Usually painless
Reflexes	Variable (depending on degree of upper motor neuron involvement)	Decreased out of proportion to weakness	Normal in myasthenia gravis, depressed in myasthenic syndrome	Decreased in proportion to weakness

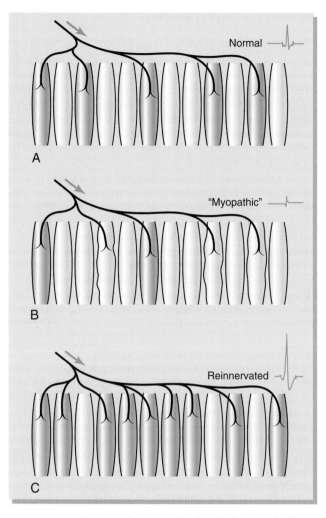

Figure 129–1 Motor unit potentials. The shaded muscle fibers are functional members of one motor unit; the axon, which enters from the upper left, branches terminally to innervate the appropriate muscle fibers. The motor unit action potential produced by each motor unit is seen at the upper right; its duration is measured between the two small vertical lines. The normal-appearing but unshaded fibers belong to other motor units. *A,* The normal situation, with five muscle fibers in the active unit. *B,* In this myopathic unit, only two fibers remain active; the other three (shrunken and unshaded) have been destroyed by a muscle disease. *C,* Four fibers that belonged to other motor units and had been denervated have now been reinnervated by terminal axon sprouting from the healthy motor unit. Both the motor unit and its action potential are now larger than normal. Note that only under these abnormal circumstances do fibers in the same unit lie next to one another. (From Griggs RC, Bradley WG: Approach to the patient with neuromuscular disease. In Isselbacher KJ, Braunwald E, Wilson JD, et al [eds]: Harrison's Textbook of Internal Medicine, 13th ed. New York, McGraw-Hill, 1994, p 2364.)

Diseases of the Motor Neuron (Anterior Horn Cell)

Lower motor neurons are located in the brain stem and in the ventral spinal cord and when diseased produce decreased strength, tone, and reflexes accompanied by fasciculations and atrophy (Table 129–3). The most common *acquired*

Table 129–3	Diseases of the Anterior Horn Cells

Hereditary

Autosomal dominant

Familial amyotrophic lateral sclerosis
Amyotrophic lateral sclerosis with frontotemporal dementia (many cases are sporadic)

Autosomal recessive

Spinal muscular atrophy
Type I: acute, infantile (Werdnig-Hoffmann disease)
Type II: late infantile
Type III: juvenile and adult types (Kugelberg-Welander disease)

X-linked

Bulbospinal muscular atrophy (Kennedy's syndrome)

Acquired

Acute: anterior poliomyelitis, West Nile virus
Chronic
Sporadic amyotrophic lateral sclerosis (ALS)
Post-poliomyelitis syndrome
ALS-like syndromes
Motor neuron disease with paraproteinemia
Hexosaminidase A deficiency
Primary lateral sclerosis

motor neuron disease, *amyotrophic lateral sclerosis,* includes dysfunction of both upper and lower motor neurons. If only the lower motor neuron is affected, the term *spinal muscular atrophy* (SMA) is used. The SMAs are hereditary, progressive motor neuron disorders that begin in utero, infancy, childhood, or adult life. SMA types 1, 2, and 3 represent the first class of neurologic disorders in which a developmental defect in neuronal apoptosis most likely produces the disease. Two genes are involved in SMA: the neuronal apoptosis inhibitor protein *(NAIP)* and survival motor neuron *(SMN)* genes. *Bulbospinal muscular atrophy* (BSMA) is a trinucleotide repeat disorder (see Chapter 1) with a *CAG* expansion encoding for a polyglutamine tract in the first exon of the androgen receptor gene, on chromosome *Xq11–12.* The mechanism by which disruption of the androgen receptor gene alters the function of bulbar and spinal motor neurons is not known. BSMA is an X-linked recessive disorder. The mean age at onset of BSMA is 30 years; the range is from 15 to 60 years. Gynecomastia occurs in 50% of affected individuals, who exhibit facial, tongue, and proximal weakness. Dysphagia and dysarthria are common, and fasciculations are widespread.

Sporadic ALS accounts for approximately 80% of all cases of acquired motor neuron disease; the remaining 20% of patients have either only lower motor neuron signs or a familial form of ALS (FALS). The 80% of patients who have sporadic ALS exhibit spasticity and hyperreflexia (upper motor neuron signs) in the setting of progressive muscle wasting and weakness (lower motor neuron signs). Autosomal-dominant FALS is an adult-onset disease that is clinically and pathologically indistinguishable from sporadic ALS. FALS is caused by missense mutations in the superoxide dismutase gene (SOD1) in a sizable minority of patients. Other genetic causes are also being identified (see Table 129–3). Painless, progressive weakness is the usual presenting sign of ALS. Usually focal in onset, weakness then spreads to contiguous muscle groups. Weakness is accompanied by muscle atrophy. ALS is a relentlessly progressive disease that culminates in respiratory muscle paralysis; the drug *riluzole* delays progression slightly.

Plexopathy

BRACHIAL PLEXOPATHY

The brachial plexus is constructed by mixed nerve roots from C5 to T1 that fuse into upper, middle, and lower trunks above the level of the clavicle and redistribute into lateral, posterior, and medial cords below that landmark. Symptoms include weakness, pain, and sensory loss in the shoulders or arms. Brachial plexopathy occurs with severe neck trauma, with malignant tumor invasion, as a result of radiation therapy, and most commonly with the autoimmune or postinfectious inflammatory disorder brachial neuritis (brachial amyotrophy).

ACUTE AUTOIMMUNE BRACHIAL NEURITIS

Acute autoimmune brachial neuritis is characterized by the abrupt onset of severe pain, usually over the lateral shoulder but at times extending into the entire arm. Young males are predominantly affected. The acute pain generally subsides after a few days to a week; by this time, weakness of the proximal arm becomes apparent. The serratus anterior and supraspinatus are the most commonly paralyzed muscles, but other muscles of the shoulder girdle may also be paralyzed. In rare cases, most of the patient's arm and even the ipsilateral diaphragm are paralyzed. Sensory loss is usually slight. Weakness may last weeks to months and be accompanied by severe atrophy of the shoulder girdle. Total recovery occurs in most patients within several months to 2 years. The disorder frequently follows an upper respiratory infection or an immunization, but in many instances, no antecedent illness occurs. It is occasionally bilateral and may sometimes recur; in rare instances, it occurs within families.

LUMBOSACRAL PLEXOPATHY

The lumbosacral plexus is constructed by mixed spinal roots from T12 to S3. Predominant contributions go to femoral, sciatic, and obturator nerves. Clinical expression includes proximal pain and weakness in anterior thigh muscles (femoral) or posterior thigh muscles and the buttocks. Diabetes, malignancy, radiation therapy, and hemorrhage are the most common causes. An autoimmune form is much less frequent than brachial neuritis.

Peripheral Nerve Disease

Peripheral neuropathies are among the most prevalent neurologic conditions. They range in severity from the mild sensory abnormalities, found in up to 70% of patients with long-standing diabetes, to fulminant, life-threatening paralytic disorders such as the Guillain-Barré syndrome (GBS). Peripheral neuropathies can involve single nerves (mononeuropathy), such as the median nerve in the carpal tunnel syndrome, or multiple nerves, as in metabolic neuropathies such as diabetic or uremic neuropathy.

Normal function of myelinated nerve fibers depends on the integrity of both the axon and its myelin sheath. The simplest type of nerve injury is transection of the axon. The axon distal to the site of transection degenerates, whereas the axon proximal to the injury survives and has the potential for regeneration. As the axon degenerates, the myelin in the distal stump is also broken down and cleared by various cellular mechanisms. Axonal degeneration caused by a focal nerve injury occurs, for example, in severe compression and in focal ischemic injury to nerves. In the symmetric polyneuropathies, the underlying illness is usually a slowly evolving type of axonal degeneration that involves the ends of long nerve fibers first and preferentially. With time, the degenerative process involves more proximal regions of long fibers, and shorter fibers are affected. This pattern of distal axonal degeneration or *dying back* of nerve fibers results from a wide variety of metabolic, toxic, and heritable causes. The resulting clinical picture includes early loss of muscle stretch reflexes at the ankle and weakness that initially involves the intrinsic muscles of the feet, the extensors of the toes, and the dorsiflexors at the ankle; the motor signs are accompanied by distally predominant loss of large-fiber sensory modalities such as vibratory sensibility in the toes. With progression, the hands are similarly involved, and the process may spread proximally up the legs and arms. The resulting pattern of sensory loss is frequently termed a *stocking-and-glove pattern*. Recovery from axonal degeneration requires nerve regeneration, a process that often requires 2 to 3 years.

Demyelination of a peripheral nerve at even a single site can block conduction, resulting in a functional deficit identical to that seen after axonal degeneration. In contrast to repair by regeneration, however, repair by remyelination can be quite rapid. Autoimmune attack on the myelin sheath occurs in the inflammatory demyelinating neuropathies and some neuropathies associated with paraproteinemias. Inherited disorders of myelin comprise the other major category of demyelinating neuropathy. Other causes include some toxic, mechanical, and physical injuries to nerve. Although these examples have nearly pure demyelination, many neuropathies have both axonal degeneration and demyelination. This mixed pathologic abnormality reflects the mutual interdependency of the axons and the myelin-forming Schwann cells.

In general, axonal degeneration decreases the amplitude of the CMAP out of proportion to the degree of reduction in peripheral nerve conduction velocity, whereas demyelination produces prominent reduction in conduction velocities.

Table 129–4 gives a classification of peripheral neuropathies with many of their causes. The symptoms of peripheral neuropathies depend on their anatomic location and on their pathophysiologic mechanisms. *Mononeuropathies* produce sensory loss or weakness (or both) in the

Table 129–4	Classification and Causes of Peripheral Neuropathy

Type of Neuropathy	Examples
Mononeuropathies	
Compression	Median: carpal tunnel syndrome
Hereditary	Familial liability to pressure palsies
Inflammation, infection	Facial: Bell's palsy; herpes simplex
Multiple mononeuropathies (mononeuritis multiplex)	Vasculitis, diabetes, leprosy
Polyneuropathy	
Hereditary	Charcot-Marie-Tooth disease(s)
Metabolic	Diabetes, uremia, porphyria
Infections	Leprosy, diphtheria
Postinfectious (autoimmune)	Guillain-Barré syndrome, chronic inflammatory demyelinating polyneuropathy
Toxic	Lead, arsenic
Drug	Amiodarone, pyridoxine, toluene toxicity

Table 129–5	Common Nerve Entrapments

Median nerve
  Carpal tunnel: wrist
  Pronator muscle: elbow
Ulnar nerve
  Elbow
  Wrist
Radial nerve: humeral groove
Peroneal nerve: behind knee; compression by synovial cysts
Lateral femoral cutaneous nerve: inguinal ligament
Cervical and lumbar roots: intervertebral foramina

territory of the nerve. *Polyneuropathies,* if demyelinating, produce distal weakness and loss of sensation in the modalities served by large myelinated peripheral nerve fibers: vibration and proprioception. Axonal neuropathies produce distal disturbance of pain and temperature perception and may be extremely painful. Motor and sensory functions served by large myelinated fibers, including reflexes, are relatively preserved. Neuropathies generally produce distal symptoms. Exceptions include the acute and chronic inflammatory demyelinating neuropathies, GBS, and chronic inflammatory demyelinating neuropathy (CIDP), which often cause proximal weakness.

Common Mononeuropathies

CARPAL TUNNEL SYNDROME

Carpal tunnel syndrome is a major cause of disability claims (Table 129–5). The median nerve is pathologically compressed at the wrist as it passes beneath the flexor retinaculum. Symptoms include numbness, tingling, and burning sensations in the palm and in the fingers supplied by the median nerve: the thumb, index, middle, and medial one half of the ring finger. Some patients complain that all fingers become numb. Pain and paresthesias are most prominent at night and often interrupt sleep. The pain is prominent at the wrist but may radiate to the forearm and occasionally to the shoulder. Shaking the hand relieves both pain and paresthesias. In some patients, symptoms may persist for years

without objective signs of median nerve damage. In others, sensory loss may appear over the tips of the fingers, and weakness can develop in the median nerve–innervated thumb muscles in association with atrophy of the lateral aspect of the thenar eminence. Percussion of the median nerve at the wrist often provokes paresthesias in a median nerve distribution (Tinel's sign). Flexion of the wrist for 30 to 60 seconds may provoke pain or paresthesias (Phalen's sign). Precipitating factors include activities that require repetitive wrist movements: mechanical work, gardening, house painting, meat wrapping, and typing. Predisposing causes include pregnancy, myxedema, acromegaly, rheumatoid arthritis, and primary amyloidosis.

The diagnosis is based on clinical symptoms and signs and the demonstration of a conduction block at the wrist by motor nerve conduction velocity studies and electromyography. If rest and splinting fail, surgical treatment by section of the transverse carpal ligament decompresses the nerve. Neither hand and arm pain nor electrodiagnostic findings alone establish the diagnosis; both findings should be present.

ULNAR PALSY

The ulnar nerve may be entrapped at the elbow or at the wrist. Injury may also occur years after a malunited supracondylar fracture of the humerus with bony overgrowth. Contrary to the findings in carpal tunnel syndrome, muscle weakness and atrophy characteristically predominate over sensory symptoms and signs. Patients notice atrophy of the first dorsal interosseous muscle and difficulty performing fine manipulations of the fingers. Numbness of the small finger, the contiguous one half of the ring finger, and the ulnar border of the hand may be present.

MERALGIA PARESTHETICA

Meralgia paresthetica is the most common pure sensory mononeuropathy. It results from compression of the lateral cutaneous nerve of the thigh as it passes under or through the inguinal ligament. Numbness or burning sensations occur over the lateral thigh; sometimes prolonged standing or walking provokes the symptoms. Patients are often obese, and weight reduction may help; however, in many patients, the condition subsides spontaneously. If electrophysiologic evidence indicates conduction block at the inguinal ligament, then surgical decompression is often helpful. A similar sensory syndrome can affect the dorsal aspect of the thumb when a tight watchband compresses a cutaneous branch of the radial nerve.

MONONEURITIS MULTIPLEX

Mononeuritis multiplex is a common syndrome that usually occurs in patients who have an underlying symmetric peripheral neuropathy (polyneuropathy): diabetes, rheumatoid arthritis, leprosy, or polyarteritis nodosa or other vasculitic disorders. Onset of a focal deficit such as foot drop or ulnar palsy, usually painful, is abrupt. Although evidence now points to ischemia of an entire cervical or lumbosacral plexus as the site of the pathologic abnormality, the patient clinically appears to have two or more single nerves affected. This phenomenon reflects the fact that individual peripheral nerves are already constituted within the proximal plexuses.

Polyneuropathies

GUILLAIN-BARRÉ SYNDROME (ACUTE INFLAMMATORY DEMYELINATING POLYNEUROPATHY)

GBS is characterized by weakness or paralysis affecting the limbs, usually symmetrically, in association with loss of muscle stretch reflexes and with increased spinal fluid protein without pleocytosis. Since the advent of polio vaccination, GBS has become the most frequent cause of acute flaccid paralysis throughout the world.

GBS is almost certainly an immune-mediated disorder. It follows an identifiable infectious disorder in approximately 60% of patients. The best-documented antecedents include infection with *Campylobacter jejuni*, infectious mononucleosis, cytomegalovirus, herpes viruses, and mycoplasma. *Campylobacter jejuni* is often associated with more severe *axonal* cases and most likely sensitizes the immune system to antigens shared between the organism and the peripheral nerve *(epitopic mimicry)*.

Clinical Manifestations

The initial symptoms of GBS often consist of tingling and *pins-and-needles* sensations in the feet and may be associated with dull low-back pain. By the time of presentation, which occurs hours to 1 to 2 days after the first symptoms, weakness has usually developed. The weakness is usually most prominent in the legs, but the arms or cranial musculature may be involved first. Muscle stretch reflexes are lost early, even in regions where strength is retained. Because the spinal roots are usually prominently involved, GBS can involve short nerves (axial and intercostal nerves, as well as cranial nerves), as well as long nerves. Weakness progresses, and the nadir is reached within 30 days, usually by 14 days. Progression can be alarmingly rapid to the extent that critical functions such as respiration can be lost within a few days or even a few hours. Respiratory insufficiency, as well as swallowing difficulty and autonomic dysregulation, can be life threatening in GBS.

Treatment

Two treatments are of benefit. Plasmapheresis—the exchange of the patient's plasma for albumin—was the first treatment definitively shown to shorten the time to recovery. Infusion of high doses of human immunoglobulin (Ig) intravenously also produces benefit. These treatments are equally effective, and combining them provides no added benefit. In patients with limited venous access, Ig is relatively easy to administer.

GUILLAIN-BARRÉ SYNDROME VARIANTS

Two other acute, immune polyneuropathies resemble GBS in their relatively rapid onset, their relationship to antecedent minor illnesses, and their symmetry of involvement. Ataxic-ophthalmoplegic neuropathy (Miller-Fisher syndrome) predominantly affects oculomotor nerves, other cranial nerves, and proprioceptive sensory nerves arising from the lower limbs.

The other, much more severe, variant causes an acute, noninflammatory axonal neuropathy. The timing of onset and progression resembles that of classic GBS. Prompt immune therapy appears to halt the process, but, once severe paralysis occurs, it often remains for long periods and, sometimes, permanently. Epidemiologic studies have found a close linkage to preceding *Campylobacter* infection.

CIDP, sometimes referred to as chronic GBS, has similarities to the clinical, pathologic, and laboratory pictures seen in acute GBS. It differs primarily in the time course and in the infrequency of identifiable antecedent events. The differences in response to therapy, however, suggest that the precise immunopathogenic mechanisms may differ. CIDP can occur at any age. The usual picture is one of slowly evolving weakness beginning in the legs, with widespread areflexia and loss of large-fiber (vibratory) sensibility on examination. Controlled trials have shown that, unlike GBS, most patients with CIDP respond to corticosteroids alone. Some patients with CIDP respond to plasmapheresis and intravenous Ig. In most instances, the first choice of therapy is with corticosteroids, at first in high doses but subsequently with the lowest dosage needed to maintain an adequate response. Plasmapheresis, although simple and safe, is expensive and usually must be repeated every 4 to 6 weeks to maintain benefit.

MULTIFOCAL MOTOR NEUROPATHY

An uncommon related disorder, multifocal motor neuropathy, occurs as *pure motor* multiple mononeuropathy. A patient may describe, for example, development of unilateral wristdrop (radial nerve involvement) followed by footdrop on the other side (peroneal nerve involvement). In addition, muscle stretch reflexes may be lost outside the distribution of weakness, but the sensory examination is normal even in weak limbs. The pathologic characteristic, inflammatory demyelination, resembles that seen in CIDP but is highly focal and largely spares sensory nerve fibers. The characteristic electrodiagnostic feature is the presence of motor nerve conduction block, a reflection of the focal demyelination. Multifocal motor neuropathy responds favorably to intravenous Ig, as well as to cytotoxic therapy, but not to corticosteroids or plasmapheresis. It is often mistaken for ALS.

NEUROPATHIES ASSOCIATED WITH MONOCLONAL GAMMOPATHIES

Peripheral neuropathy can complicate most monoclonal gammopathies. Monoclonal proteins of IgM, IgG, and IgA types, with both kappa and lambda light chains, are all associated with neuropathy. In some instances, the monoclonal protein has a role in causing the neuropathy. For example, some IgM-kappa monoclonal proteins react with sugars found on a specific Schwann cell protein, the myelin-associated glycoprotein (MAG).

The clinical picture of the neuropathy varies. The IgM-kappa monoclonal antibodies with *anti-MAG* reactivity typically produce neuropathy with prominent large-fiber sensory loss and sensory ataxia, as well as milder weakness. Electrodiagnostic tests indicate demyelination but with nerve fiber loss. In other cases with IgM monoclonal proteins, a distinctive picture is formed that includes scleroderma-like skin changes, hepatomegaly, and endocrine abnormalities, as well as neuropathy (the POEMS syndrome, described in the next paragraph). Other patients with monoclonal proteins have a clinical picture identical to that of CIDP, and still others have distally predominant axonal degeneration.

Three disorders should be specifically sought in patients with paraproteins and neuropathy: First, a special association of neuropathy with solitary plasmacytomas can be found, often osteosclerotic. The POEMS syndrome—*p*olyneuropathy, *o*rganomegaly, *e*ndocrinopathy (hirsutism, testicular atrophy), *m*onoclonal IgM protein, and *s*kin pigmentation—is usually associated with osteosclerotic myeloma. A skeletal radiographic survey is essential in patients with monoclonal proteins and neuropathy. Second, cryoglobulinemia, with or without monoclonal gammopathy, can produce neuropathy. Third, the monoclonal proteins may result in amyloid deposition in nerve and thus produce neuropathy indirectly.

IMMUNE-MEDIATED ATAXIC NEUROPATHIES

This category contains three disorders: carcinomatous sensory neuropathy, sensory ganglionitis associated with features of Sjögren's syndrome, and idiopathic sensory ganglionitis. All three disorders are characterized clinically by subacute or slowly developing proprioceptive sensory loss leading to gait ataxia and inability to localize the limbs. The possibility of occult carcinoma underlying an immunogenic (paraneoplastic) ataxic neuropathy adds urgency to differential diagnosis. The most frequent associations include small cell lung, breast, and ovarian carcinomas. In addition to clinical screening for these neoplasms, serologic tests, particularly the anti-Hu antibody, are helpful.

HEREDITARY NEUROPATHIES

Heritable neuropathies are among the most prevalent inherited neurologic diseases. Because many of these neuropathies occur in midlife, and because the family history is often previously unrecognized, the heritable disorders constitute an important aspect of differential diagnosis of any chronic polyneuropathy.

Charcot-Marie-Tooth Disease

The eponym Charcot-Marie-Tooth (CMT) identifies a group of heritable disorders of peripheral nerves that share clinical features but differ in their pathologic mechanisms

and the specific genetic abnormalities, as shown in Table 129–6. One group of disorders, classed together as CMT type I (CMT I), is characterized pathologically by abnormalities of peripheral myelination and, at a molecular level, by abnormalities of specific proteins found in the myelin sheaths or Schwann cells. The CMT II group is characterized by axonal degeneration. All forms of CMT disease tend to appear during the second to fourth decades with insidiously evolving footdrop. Examination reveals distal weakness and wasting of the intrinsic muscles of the feet, the peroneal muscles, the anterior tibial muscles, and the calves. A variable degree of impaired large-fiber sensory function is reflected in elevated vibratory thresholds in the toes. Muscle stretch reflexes are lost, first at the ankles. Typically, a foot deformity exists, with high arches (pes cavus) and hammer toes, reflecting long-standing muscle imbalance in the feet. Most patients with CMT disease have nearly normal occupational and daily activities, and they have a normal life span. Although no specific treatment has been developed, the footdrop can be relieved by appropriate bracing of the ankle with ankle-foot orthoses. Genetic counseling and education of affected patients and their families are important, both for reassurance and to preclude unnecessary diagnostic evaluation of affected members in future generations.

A variant of CMT is *hereditary neuropathy with liability to pressure palsies* (see Table 129–6). Recurrent mononeuropathies occur, especially in the upper limbs (particularly ulnar); the autosomal-dominant hereditary pattern is seldom recognized initially.

Amyloid Neuropathies

Amyloid neuropathy is caused by extracellular deposition of the fibrillary protein amyloid in peripheral nerve and sensory and autonomic ganglia, as well as around blood vessels in nerves and other tissues. In all forms of amyloidosis, the initial and major abnormalities affect the small sensory and autonomic fibers. Involvement of small fibers responsible for pain and temperature sensibilities leads to loss of the ability to perceive mechanical and thermal injuries and to an increased risk of tissue damage. As a result, painless injuries present a major hazard of this disorder; in advanced stages, they can lead to chronic infections or osteomyelitis of the feet or hands and the necessity for amputation.

DIABETIC NEUROPATHIES

Diabetes is the most frequent cause of peripheral neuropathy worldwide. Incidence figures depend on the definition used; at least some peripheral nerve abnormalities can be detected in approximately 70% of patients with long-standing diabetes, and symptomatic neuropathy affects 5% to 10% of patients. The diabetic neuropathies take many clinical forms, including symmetric polyneuropathies and a wide variety of individual plexus or nerve disorders (Table 129–7).

DIABETIC POLYNEUROPATHY

Diabetic polyneuropathy is symmetric and usually begins distally with sensory loss in the feet. It is the most common of the diabetic neuropathies. Diabetic polyneuropathy is

Table 129–6 Major Hereditary Neuropathies

Disorder	Locus/Gene	Inheritance	Protein	Mutation (Frequency)	Testing Method
Hereditary Motor and Sensory Neuropathies					
CMT1A	17p11.2/PMP22	AD	Peripheral myelin protein 22	Duplication (98%)	Pulse-field gel electrophoresis, FISH, Southern blot
				Point mutation (2%)	Sequencing, mutation scanning, mutation analysis
HNPP	17p11.2/PMP22	AD	Peripheral myelin protein 22	Deletion (80%)	Mutation analysis, FISH, Long PCR-RFLP, Southern blot
				Point mutation/ small deletion (20%)	Sequencing
CMT1B	1q22/MPZ	AD	Myelin protein zero	Point mutation	Sequencing, mutation scanning, mutation analysis
CMT1C	16p13.1–p12.3/LITAF	AD	SIMPLE	—	—
CMT1D	10q21.1–q22.1/EGR2	AD	Early growth response protein 2	Point mutation	Sequencing, mutation scanning, mutation analysis
CMT2A	1p36.2/KIF1B	AD	Kinesin-like protein KIF1B	Point mutation	Direct DNA, linkage analysis
CMT2B	3q21/RAB7	AD	Ras-related protein Rab-7	Point mutation	Direct DNA, linkage analysis
CMT2C	12q23–24/unknown	AD	Unknown		Direct DNA, linkage analysis
CMT2D	7p15/GARS	AD	Glycyl-tRNA Synthetase	Point mutation	Direct DNA, linkage analysis
CMT2E	8p21/NEFL	AD	Neurofilament triplet L protein	Point mutation	Sequencing
CMT2F	7q11–21/unknown	AD	Unknown	—	Linkage
CMT4A	8q13–q21.1/GDAP1	AR	Ganglioside-induced differentiation protein-1	Point mutation	Sequencing
CMT4B1	11q22/MTMR2	AR	Myotubularin-related protein 2	Point mutation	—
CMT4BB2	11p15/CMT4B2	AR	SET binding factor 2	Point mutation	—
CMT4C	5q32/KIAA1985	AR	KIAA1985	Point mutation	—
CMT4D	8q24.3/NDRG1	AR	NDRG1 protein	Point mutation	—
CMT4E	10q21.1–q22.1/EGR2	AR	Early growth response protein 2	Point mutation	Mutation analysis, sequencing
CMT4F	19q13.1–q13.2/PRX	AR	Periaxin	Point mutation	Mutation analysis, sequencing
CMTX	Xq13.1/GJB1	X-linked	Gap junction β-1 protein (Connexin 32)	Point mutations, deletions (rare)	Sequencing, mutation scanning, mutation analysis
Familial Amyloidosis	**(Four Subtypes)**				
Porphyria					
Others (Rare)					
Fabry's disease					
Leukodystrophies					
Refsum's disease					
Tangier disease					
Abetalipoproteinemia					
Mitochondrial neuropathies					

AD = autosomal dominant; AR = autosomal recessive; FISH = fluorescent in situ hybridization; PCR-RFLP = polymerase chain reaction–restriction fragment length polymorphism.

Table 129–7 Major Diabetic Neuropathies

Diabetic Polyneuropathies

Rapidly reversible physiologic dysfunction associated with hyperglycemia
Symmetric polyneuropathy
  Sensorimotor neuropathy
  "Small-fiber" neuropathy, with autonomic dysfunction, reduced pain sensibility, spontaneous burning pain

Diabetic Mononeuropathies and Plexopathies

Diabetic third nerve palsy
Diabetic fourth nerve palsy
Diabetic truncal neuropathy
Diabetic lumbosacral plexopathy (proximal diabetic neuropathy)

uncommon at the time of diagnosis of diabetes, but its prevalence increases with duration of diabetes. The precise pathogenesis is not defined, but, similar to the ocular and renal complications, diabetic neuropathy can be reduced in incidence and in severity by maintaining blood glucose levels close to normal. This effect of tight control is consistent with the hypothesis that hyperglycemia itself contributes to nerve damage. The effect of hyperglycemia that injures nerves may include one or more of the following: abnormalities of nerve vasculature and blood flow, metabolic effects of abnormalities in polyol pathways, and nonenzymatic glycosylation of nerve proteins.

Clinical Manifestations

The neuropathy is usually asymptomatic at the onset, but abnormalities in sensation and reflexes may be detected on routine examination. The symptoms usually begin insidiously, but some cases have an abrupt onset, and in a small percentage of patients, abrupt onset appears to be precipitated by the institution of insulin treatment. In contrast to most other neuropathies, small-fiber sensibility, as well as large-fiber sensation, are typically reduced in patients with diabetes, resulting in elevated pain and thermal and vibratory thresholds. The small-fiber dysfunction often produces spontaneous neuropathic pain. This pain includes dysesthesias, which are unpleasant sensations evoked by normally innocuous stimuli, such as the bed sheets on the toes at night. Continuous burning or throbbing pain may occur, and prolonged walking is often distressing.

The diagnosis of diabetic polyneuropathy is straightforward in a patient with established diabetes with a typical clinical picture. Electrodiagnostic studies can document neuropathy. Conversely, diabetic neuropathy is often overdiagnosed. In general, the diagnosis of diabetic neuropathy should be made only in the setting of long-standing diabetes, usually insulin requiring. If only mild hyperglycemia that developed recently is present, then the diagnosis of diabetic polyneuropathy should be regarded as suggestive. Diabetic polyneuropathy seldom causes severe weakness unless it is associated with the severe pain of an associated mononeuritis multiplex.

Treatment

Correction of blood sugar to as near normal values as possible is important for both primary prevention and slowing of the progression of diabetic neuropathy (see Chapter 68). The painful symptoms of diabetic neuropathy often respond to anticonvulsants such as gabapentin or to tricyclic antidepressants such as desipramine.

ALCOHOL-NUTRITIONAL NEUROPATHY

Polyneuropathy in persons with chronic alcoholism usually occurs in a setting of associated nutritional deficiencies. Most persons with alcoholic neuropathy have evidence of multifactorial nutritional deficiency. Occasionally, the nutritional background seems adequate, and the direct contribution of alcohol cannot be excluded. The pathologic mechanism of alcohol-nutritional neuropathy is that of a *dying back* axonal disorder affecting both sensory and motor fibers. The initial symptoms are pain and paresthesias, beginning in the soles of the feet, sometimes evolving to burning sensations in the feet and severe hyperpathia and often associated with aching and tenderness of the calves. Weakness is seldom severe and invariably distal, and muscle stretch reflexes are lost first at the ankles. Treatment with nutritional supplementation, including thiamine and multivitamins, and cessation of alcohol ingestion are highly beneficial in the early stages of the disease. In advanced cases, the disease may continue to progress for a period after initiation of therapy, and recovery may be incomplete.

Prospectus for the Future

The discovery of the cause of some cases of FALS has not yet translated into treatment strategies, nor has it shed light on the more common, clinically identical sporadic disease. Additional genetic causes are being defined, and with this identification comes the hope that novel treatments will be suggested. In the meantime, many innovative clinical trials are being conducted involving ALS. The molecular cause of the peripheral neuropathies has suggested genetic approaches to treatment. Encouraging preliminary data already exist on the benefit of growth factor treatment for CMT disease.

References

Dyck PJ, Thomas PK (eds): Peripheral Neuropathy, 4th ed. Philadelphia, Saunders, 2005.

Feldman EL: Amyotrophic lateral sclerosis and other motor neuron diseases. In Goldman L, Ausiello DA (eds): Cecil Textbook of Medicine, 23rd ed. Philadelphia, Saunders, 2007.

Shy M: Peripheral neuropathies. In Goldman L, Ausiello DA (eds): Cecil Textbook of Medicine, 23rd ed. Philadelphia, Saunders, 2007.

Muscle Diseases

Robert C. Griggs

Skeletal muscle diseases (myopathies) are disorders in which a primary structural or functional impairment of muscle occurs. Myopathies can be broadly classified into hereditary and acquired disorders (Table 130–1).

Organization and Structure Of Muscle

Muscle comprises many motor units. The number of muscle fibers innervated by a single motor unit varies from muscle to muscle. Muscles subserving finely coordinated movements, such as an ocular muscle, can have fewer than 10 muscle fibers in a motor unit. Powerful proximal limb muscles have large motor units with 1000 to 2000 fibers innervated by a single motor neuron.

The muscle fibers consist of thick and thin filaments (myofibrils). The myofibrils are surrounded by the sarcolemmal membrane and basal lamina. A large number of muscular dystrophies are now known to be caused by genetic defects in this region (Fig. 130–1). The sarcolemmal components are known as the dystrophin-glycoprotein complex (DGC). The DGC is a trans-sarcolemmal complex of proteins and glycoproteins that links the subsarcolemmal cytoskeleton to the extracellular matrix. Dystrophin was the first well-characterized protein in the DGC. Other DGC components include the dystroglycan complex (α and β), the sarcoglycan complex (α, β, γ, and δ), and the syntrophin complex (α, $\beta1$, and $\beta2$). Closely adherent to the extracellular portion of the sarcolemma is the basal lamina, components of which are known as laminins.

Assessment

The most important aspect of evaluating a patient with a myopathy is the history. The most common symptom of a patient with muscle disease is weakness. If the weakness is in the legs, then patients complain of difficulty climbing stairs and rising from a low chair or toilet or from the floor. When the arms are involved, patients notice trouble lifting objects (especially over their heads) and washing or brushing their hair. These symptoms point to proximal weakness, the most common site of weakness in a myopathy. In rare instances, patients first complain of poor hand grip (difficulty opening jar tops and turning door knobs) or tripping as a result of ankle weakness from distal muscle weakness, or they may exhibit a change in speech or swallowing, droopy eyelids, and double vision from weakness of cranial nerve–innervated muscles.

The tempo of the disease course is important. Weakness may be present all of the time (fixed) or intermittently (episodic). Myopathies can produce either fixed or episodic weakness. Muscle disorders can be *acute* (<4 weeks), *subacute* (4 to 8 weeks), or *chronic* (>8 weeks). Examples include (1) acute or subacute inflammatory myopathies (dermatomyositis [DM] and polymyositis [PM]), (2) chronic slow progression over years (most muscular dystrophies), or (3) fixed weakness with little change over decades (congenital myopathies). Patients with channelopathies or metabolic myopathies have recurrent attacks of weakness over many years, whereas a patient with acute muscle destruction caused by a toxin such as cocaine may have a single acute episode.

Patients who complain of a generalized global *weakness* or *fatigue* seldom have a myopathy, particularly if the neurologic examination is normal. Fatigue is a complaint of the patient with myasthenia gravis but otherwise is usually a nonspecific symptom. Muscle pain (myalgia) is also a nonspecific complaint that infrequently accompanies some myopathies. Myalgias may be episodic (e.g., metabolic myopathies) or nearly constant (e.g., occasional inflammatory myopathies). However, muscle pain is surprisingly uncommon in most muscle diseases, and limb pain is more likely to be caused by bone or joint disorders. Rarely is a muscle disease responsible for vague aches and discomfort in muscle if strength is normal. The involuntary muscle cramp is localized to a single muscle and lasts from seconds to minutes. In most instances, cramps are benign and normal; they do not reflect myopathy. Cramps occur with dehydration, hyponatremia, azotemia, and myxedema and in nerve disease such as amyotrophic lateral sclerosis. Muscle contractures are rare and resemble a cramp. They last longer than cramps and occur with exercise

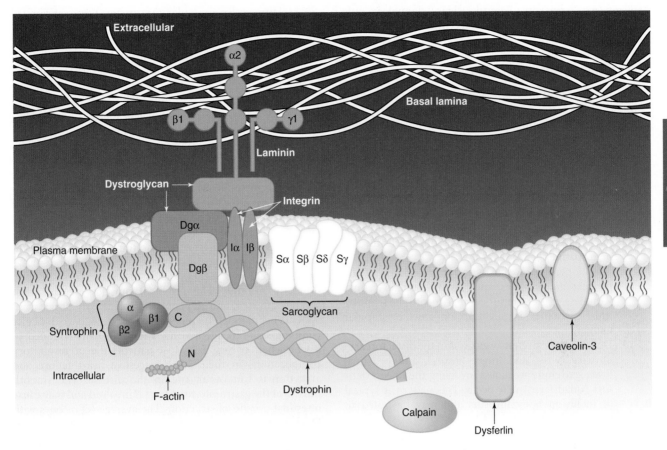

Figure 130–1 The dystrophin-glycoprotein complex and related proteins.

Table 130–1	**Classification of Myopathies**

Hereditary

Muscular dystrophies
Congenital
Myotonias and other channelopathies
Metabolic
Mitochondrial

Acquired

Inflammatory
Endocrine/metabolic
Associated with systemic illness
Drug induced/toxic

in glycolytic enzyme defects. On electromyographic (EMG) examination, contractures are electrically silent, whereas cramps have rapidly firing motor unit discharges. Muscle contracture should not be confused with fixed tendon contracture. Myotonia is the phenomenon of impaired relaxation of muscle after forceful voluntary contraction. Patients report muscle stiffness or persistent contraction in almost any muscle group but particularly the hands and eyelids. Exercise-induced weakness and myalgias may be accompanied by dark or red urine (myoglobinuria). Myoglobinuria follows rapid muscle destruction.

EXAMINATION

Specific muscle function should be tested. Muscle strength is quantitated by the Medical Research Council of Great Britain (MRC) grading scale of 0 to 5:

5: Normal power
4: Active movement against gravity and resistance
3: Active movement against gravity
2: Active movement only with gravity eliminated
1: Trace contraction
0: No contraction

Muscles should be inspected for atrophy or hypertrophy. Atrophy of proximal limb muscles is usual in longstanding myopathies. Muscles can also become diffusely hypertrophic in dystrophic or myotonic conditions. In Duchenne's and Becker's dystrophies, the calves enlarge as a result of pseudohypertrophy from replacement with connective tissue and fat. The sensory examination should be normal in muscle disease. Reflexes are preserved early in the disease process, but, when muscles become extremely weak, reflexes become hypoactive or unelicitable. Evidence of upper motor neuron damage (e.g., spasticity, Babinski signs, clonus) is only present in myopathies if coincidental central nervous system disease exists.

PATTERNS OF WEAKNESS

Six broad patterns of muscle weakness occur in myopathies:

1. The most common is in proximal muscles of the arms and legs: a limb-girdle distribution. Neck flexor and extensor muscles can also be affected. The reason why most myopathies begin in proximal muscles is unknown.
2. Distal weakness may occur in the upper extremities (extensor muscle group) or lower extremities (anterior or posterior compartment muscle groups). Such selective distal weakness is often a feature of neuropathies.
3. Scapuloperoneal weakness includes weakness of the periscapular muscles and distal lower extremity weakness of the anterior compartment. The scapular muscle weakness is usually accompanied by scapular winging.
4. Distal upper extremity weakness in the distal forearm muscles (wrist and finger flexors), and proximal lower extremity weakness involving the knee extensors (quadriceps) may occur. This pattern is typical of inclusion body myositis and may be noted in myotonic dystrophy.
5. Involvement of ocular or pharyngeal muscles may be predominant.
6. Neck extensor weakness (the *dropped head syndrome*) may be prominent.

These six patterns of myopathy are useful in differential diagnosis, but neuromuscular diseases other than myopathies can also exhibit one of these weakness patterns. For example, whereas proximal greater than distal weakness is characteristic of myopathies, patients with acquired demyelinating neuropathies (Guillain-Barré syndrome and chronic inflammatory demyelinating polyneuropathy) often have proximal, as well as distal, muscle involvement. Such neuropathies are additionally accompanied by sensory and reflex loss. Ocular, pharyngeal, and proximal limb weakness is characteristic of neuromuscular junction transmission disorders such as myasthenia gravis. However, these patients also have diplopia, weakness that fluctuates, and additional laboratory features that lead to the correct diagnosis.

MUSCLE BIOPSY

Fixed muscle is of little value for diagnosis. Examination of muscle tissue under light microscopy is primarily performed using frozen specimens. The muscle biopsy can establish if evidence of either a neuropathic or a myopathic disorder is present; it can also provide specific diagnosis of many hereditary and acquired myopathies.

Muscular Dystrophies

Muscular dystrophies are inherited myopathies characterized by progressive muscle weakness and degeneration and subsequent replacement by fibrous and fatty connective tissue. Historically, muscular dystrophies were categorized by their distribution of weakness, age at onset, and inheritance pattern. Advances in the molecular understanding of the muscular dystrophies have defined the genetic mutation and abnormal gene product for most of these disorders (Table 130–2).

Dystrophinopathies are X-linked disorders resulting from mutations of the large dystrophin gene located at Xp21. Dystrophin is a large subsarcolemmal cytoskeletal protein that, along with the other components of the DGC, provides support to the muscle membrane during contraction. Mutations disrupting the translational reading frame of the gene result in near-total loss of dystrophin (Duchenne's dystrophy), whereas in-frame mutations result in the translation of semifunctional dystrophin of abnormal size or amount (Becker's dystrophy). The incidence of Duchenne's dystrophy is 1 in 3500 male births; one third of the cases result from a new mutation. Duchenne's dystrophy presents as early as age 2 to 3 years as delays in motor milestones and difficulty running. The proximal muscles are the most severely affected, and the course is relentlessly progressive. Patients begin to fall frequently by age 5 to 6, have difficulty climbing stairs by age 8 years, and are usually confined to a wheelchair by age 12. Most patients die of respiratory complications in their 20s. Congestive heart failure and arrhythmias can occur late in the disease. The smooth muscle of the gastrointestinal tract is involved and may cause intestinal pseudo-obstruction. The average IQ of boys with Duchenne's dystrophy is low, suggesting central nervous system involvement. Becker's dystrophy is a milder form of dystrophinopathy and varies in severity depending on the gene lesion. It is less common than the Duchenne form, with an incidence of 5 per 100,000.

Myotonic dystrophy occurs in two forms: DM-1 and DM-2. Both dystrophies are autosomal-dominant multisystem disorders that affect skeletal, cardiac, and smooth muscle and other organs, including the eyes, the endocrine system, and the brain. DM-1 is the most prevalent muscular dystrophy, with an incidence of 13.5 per 100,000 live births. DM-1 can occur at any age, with the usual onset of symptoms in the late second or third decade. However, some affected individuals may remain symptom free their entire lives. A severe form of DM-1 with onset in infancy is known as congenital myotonic dystrophy. The severity of DM-1 generally worsens from one generation to the next (anticipation). Typical patients exhibit facial weakness with temporalis muscle wasting, frontal balding, ptosis, and neck flexor weakness. Extremity weakness usually begins distally and progresses slowly to affect the proximal limb-girdle muscles. Percussion myotonia can be elicited on examination in most patients, especially in thenar and wrist extensor muscles.

Associated manifestations in DM-1 include cataracts, testicular atrophy and impotence, intellectual impairment, and hypersomnia associated with both central and obstructive sleep apnea. Respiratory muscle weakness may be severe, with impairment of ventilatory drive. Cardiac conduction defects are common and can produce sudden death. Pacemakers may be necessary, and annual electrocardiographic examinations are recommended. Chronic hypoxia can lead to cor pulmonale. The molecular defect of myotonic dystrophy (DM-1) is an abnormal expansion of CTG repeats in chromosome 19q13.2. The second myotonic dystrophy locus (DM-2) has been mapped to chromosome 3q and is an

Table 130–2　Major Muscular Dystrophies

Disease	Mode of Inheritance	Gene Mutation Location	Gene Defect/Protein
X-Linked MD			
Duchenne's, Becker's	XR	Xp21	Dystrophin
Emery-Dreifuss	XR	Xq28	Emerin
Limb-Girdle MD			
LGMD 1A	AD	5q22–34	Myotilin
LGMD 1B	AD	1q11–21	Lamin A/C
LGMD 1C	AD	3p25	Caveolin-3
LGMD 2A	AR	15q15	Calpain-3
LGMD 2B*	AR	2p12	Dysferlin
LGMD 2C	AR	13q12	γ-Sarcoglycan
LGMD 2D	AR	17q12	α-Sarcoglycan
LGMD 2E	AR	4q12	β-Sarcoglycan
LGMD 2F	AR	5q33	δ-Sarcoglycan
LGMD 2G	AR	17q11	Telethonin
LGMD 2H	AR	9q31	E3-ubiquitin-ligase
LGMD 2I	AR	19q13.3	Fukutin-related protein 1
LGMD 2J	AR	2q31	Titin
Congenital MD With CNS Involvement			
Fukuyama CMD	AR	9q31–33	Fukutin
Walker-Warburg CMD	AR	9q31–33	Fukutin
Muscle-eye-brain CMD	AR	1p	Glycosyltransferase
Without CNS Involvement			
Merosin-deficient classic type	AR	6q2	Laminin-2 (merosin)
Merosin-positive classic type	AR	Unknown	Not known
Integrin-deficient CMD	AR	12q13	Integrin α7
Rigid spine syndrome	AR	1p3	Selenoprotein NI
Distal MD			
Late adult-onset 1A (Welander)	AD	2p15	Unknown
Late adult-onset 1B (Udd)	AD	2q31	Titin
Early adult-onset 1A (Nonaka)	AR	9p1–q1	GNE
Early adult-onset 1B (Miyoshi)†	AR	2q12–14	Dysferlin
Early adult-onset 1C (Laing)	AD	14	MPD1
Other MD			
Facioscapulohumeral	AD	4q35	Deleted chromatin
Oculopharyngeal	AD	14q11	Poly(A) binding protein 2
Myotonic dystrophy type 1	AD	19q13	RNA accumulation
Myotonic dystrophy type 2	AD	3q	RNA accumulation
Myofibrillar myopathy	AD	11q21–23	β-Crystallin
Myofibrillar myopathy	AD	2q35	Desmin
Bethlem myopathy	AD	21q22	Collagen VI

*Probably the same condition as Miyoshi distal MD.
†Probably the same condition as LGMD 2B.
AD = autosomal dominant; AR = autosomal recessive; CMD = congenital muscular dystrophy; CNS = central nervous system; GNE = UDP-N-acetylglucosamine 2-epimerase/N-acetylmannosamine kinase; LGMD = limb-girdle muscular dystrophy; MD = muscular dystrophy; XR = X-linked recessive.

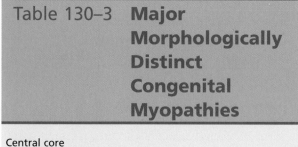

Table 130–3	Major Morphologically Distinct Congenital Myopathies

Central core
Nemaline
Centronuclear (myotubular)
Congenital fiber type disproportion
Sarcotubular
Reducing body
Myofibrillar

Table 130–4	Metabolic and Mitochondrial Myopathies

Glycogen Metabolism Deficiencies

Type II	$\alpha_{1,4}$-Glucosidase (acid maltase)
Type III	Debranching enzyme
Type IV	Branching enzyme
Type V	Phosphorylase* (McArdle's disease)
Type VII	Phosphofructokinase* (Tarui's disease)
Type VIII	Phosphorylase β kinase*
Type IX	Phosphoglycerate kinase*
Type X	Phosphoglycerate mutase*
Type XI	Lactate dehydrogenase*

Lipid Metabolism Deficiencies

Carnitine palmitoyl transferase*
Primary systemic/muscle carnitine deficiency
Secondary carnitine deficiency

Mitochondrial Myopathies

Pyruvate dehydrogenase complex deficiencies
Progressive external ophthalmoplegia (PEO)
Autosomal dominant with multiple mitochondrial DNA deletions:
Adenine nucleotide translocator 1 *(ANT1)*
Twinkle (mitochondrial protein)
Polymerase gamma
Kearns-Sayre syndrome
Myoclonic epilepsy and ragged-red fibers (MERRF)
Mitochondrial encephalopathy with lactic acidosis and strokelike episodes (MELAS)
Mitochondrial neurogastrointestinal encephalomyopathy (MNGIE)
Mitochondrial depletion syndrome
Leigh's disease and neuropathy, ataxia, retinitis pigmentosa (NARP)
Succinate dehydrogenase deficiency*

*Deficiency can produce exercise intolerance and myoglobinuria.

abnormal expansion of a tetranucleotide repeat. The precise pathomechanisms of DM-1 and DM-2 are unknown but probably relate to abnormal RNA transcribed by the pathologic repeats. DM-2 resembles DM-1. However, weakness is often proximal; patients may complain of myotonia and myalgias. Patients with DM-2 may have less severe cardiac and other organ involvement than those with DM-1.

Congenital Myopathies

Congenital myopathies are defined by their appearance on biopsy (Table 130–3). They are usually present at birth with hypotonia and subsequent delayed motor development. Because most congenital myopathies are relatively nonprogressive, patients are commonly seen as adults and may not be diagnosed until the second or third decade. Clinical findings common in the congenital myopathies are reduced muscle bulk, slender body build, and a long, narrow face, with skeletal abnormalities (high-arched palate, pectus excavatum, kyphoscoliosis, dislocated hips, and pes cavus) and absent or reduced muscle stretch reflexes. The molecular genetic defects of many congenital myopathies are now known, and these disorders, as well as the muscular dystrophies, are being reclassified.

Metabolic Myopathies

Metabolic myopathies (Table 130–4) include (1) glucose and glycogen metabolism disorders, (2) lipid metabolism disorders, and (3) mitochondrial disorders.

GLUCOSE AND GLYCOGEN METABOLISM DISORDERS

Glucose, and its storage form glycogen, is essential for the short-term, predominantly anaerobic energy requirements of muscle. Disorders of glucose and glycogen metabolism (called glycogenoses) have two distinct syndromes: (1) dynamic symptoms of exercise intolerance, pain, cramps, and myoglobinuria; and (2) static symptoms of fixed weakness without exercise intolerance or myoglobinuria. Of the 11 glycogenoses, only glucose 6-phosphate (type I) and liver phosphorylase (type VI) deficiencies spare muscle.

Glycogenoses with Exercise Intolerance (Myoglobinuria)

Exercise intolerance (see Table 130–4) begins in childhood with exertional muscle pain, cramps, and myoglobinuria appearing in the second or third decade. Many patients note a *second wind* phenomenon after a period of brief rest so that they can continue the exercise at the previous level of activity. The muscle cramps are caused by electrically silent contractures. Strength, blood creatine kinase (CK) levels, and EMG findings between attacks are usually normal early in the disease, but they may become abnormal with advancing age. After episodes of severe myoglobinuria, EMG shows myopathic units and fibrillations. EMG performed during a *cramp* (contracture) shows electrical silence. In the forearm exercise test, the venous lactate level fails to rise in myophosphorylase, phosphofructokinase, and phosphoglycerate kinase deficiencies and rises subnormally in phosphorylase β kinase, phosphoglucomutase, and lactate dehydrogenase deficiencies. Diagnosis is made by muscle biopsy study of the enzymes or by defining specific genetic mutations.

Glycogenoses with Fixed Weakness and No Exercise Intolerance

Glycogenoses with fixed weakness and no exercise intolerance (see Table 130–4) produce a syndrome of progressive proximal weakness. Diagnosis requires muscle biopsy or genetic mutation definition. Acid maltase deficiency can now be treated with enzyme replacement.

DISORDERS OF FATTY ACID METABOLISM

Lipids are essential for the aerobic energy needs of muscle during sustained exercise. Serum long-chain fatty acids are the primary lipid fuel for muscle metabolism. They are transported into the mitochondria as carnitine esters and are metabolized by means of beta-oxidation. Carnitine palmitoyl transferase (CPT) I converts cytoplasmic acyl coenzyme A (CoA) to acylcarnitine, which is then transported into the mitochondria by carnitine acyltransferase in exchange for carnitine. CPT II on the inner mitochondrial membrane reconstitutes acyl CoA. A deficiency of carnitine, CPT, or the enzymes of beta-oxidation can lead to impaired muscle lipid metabolism.

As with glycogen pathway defects, abnormal fatty acid metabolism causes exercise intolerance with myoglobinuria or static weakness with a lipid storage myopathy. In addition, some disorders of lipid metabolism can produce multiorgan metabolic crises, with hepatic failure and altered mental status. Most lipid disorders are believed to be autosomal recessive (see Table 130–4).

MITOCHONDRIAL MYOPATHIES

Mitochondrial myopathies (see Table 130–4) produce slowly progressive weakness of proximal limbs or external ocular and other cranial muscles and abnormal fatigability on sustained exertion. Some of these myopathies affect multiple organs or systems, in addition to muscle. In many mitochondrial myopathies, some muscle fibers contain abnormal mitochondria. These fibers appear *ragged red* on biopsy stains (trichrome) and may fail to react for cytochrome *c* oxidase. Serum lactic acid levels are often elevated at rest in mitochondrial myopathy. Mitochondrial diseases are caused by mutations in either nuclear or mitochondrial DNA. During fertilization, all of the mitochondria are contributed by the mother; thus all mutations of mitochondrial DNA are either maternally transmitted or arise de novo in the maternal ovum or in early embryonic life. However, because the majority of mitochondrial proteins (95%) are encoded from nuclear genes, mitochondrial disorders can also have autosomal-dominant or X-linked heredity. Mitochondrial disorders produce biochemical defects proximal to the respiratory chain (involving substrate transport and utilization) or within the respiratory chain.

SPECIFIC MITOCHONDRIAL DISORDERS AFFECTING MUSCLE

Progressive External Ophthalmoplegia

Severe ptosis and progressive external ophthalmoplegia (PEO) are clinical hallmarks of mitochondrial disease. Ptosis is often the presenting symptom and is generally first noted in childhood. Patients and their physicians often overlook both ptosis and PEO (lack of eye movements). Patients usually do not note double vision. Slight proximal weakness may occur. PEO caused by mitochondrial disease is associated with single or multiple mitochondrial DNA deletions. Patients with single mitochondrial deletions have Kearns-Sayre syndrome, which exhibits before age 20 years and includes a wide variety of multisystem abnormalities: retinitis pigmentosa, heart block, hearing loss, short stature, ataxia, delayed puberty, peripheral neuropathy, and impaired ventilatory drive. Kearns-Sayre syndrome is caused by single large mitochondrial deletions; it is sporadic with no family history of the disorder. Patients with PEO who have multiple mitochondrial deletions have an autosomal-dominant inheritance pattern. Many of the responsible genes have been identified (see Table 130–4).

Myoclonic Epilepsy and Ragged Red Fibers

Patients with myoclonic epilepsy and ragged red fibers (MERRF) have varying symptoms of myoclonus, generalized seizures, ataxia, dementia, sensorineural hearing loss, and optic atrophy, as well as limb-girdle weakness. Some patients also have a peripheral neuropathy, cardiomyopathy, and cutaneous lipomas. Ptosis and PEO are usually not present.

Mitochondrial Encephalomyopathy with Lactic Acidosis and Strokelike Episodes

Patients with mitochondrial encephalomyopathy with lactic acidosis and strokelike (MELAS) episodes have normal early development, experience migraine-like headaches and strokes before age 40 years, and have chronic lactic acidosis. Other features can include dementia, hearing loss, and episodic vomiting, ataxia, and coma, as well as diabetes. Ptosis and PEO are uncommon.

Channelopathies (Nondystrophic Myotonias and Periodic Paralyses)

The myotonias are categorized into dystrophic and nondystrophic disorders. The nondystrophic myotonias and the periodic paralyses are caused by mutations of various ion channels in muscle (Table 130–5). The term *channelopathies* is often used to describe this group of disorders.

CHLORIDE CHANNELOPATHIES

Myotonia congenita is caused by point mutations in the muscle chloride channel gene. Autosomal-dominant and -recessive forms are allelic. The autosomal-dominant form (Thomsen's disease) and the autosomal-recessive form (Becker's myotonia congenita) are both benign and are associated with muscle hypertrophy and action, percussion, and electrical myotonia. Cold increases the myotonia, and exercise improves it. The heart or other organs are not involved. Patients with Thomsen's disease are not weak, but patients with Becker's myotonia congenita have fluctuations in strength and may develop persistent limb-girdle weakness. Many patients do not require treatment, but drugs such as quinine, procainamide, phenytoin, and mexiletine reduce myotonia and may improve strength.

Table 130–5	**Channelopathies and Related Disorders**			
Disorder	**Clinical Features**	**Inheritance**	**Chromosome**	**Gene**
Chloride Channelopathies				
Myotonia congenita				
Thomsen's disease	Myotonia	Autosomal dominant	7q35	CLC-1
Becker's disease	Myotonia and weakness	Autosomal recessive	7q35	CLC-1
Sodium Channelopathies				
Paramyotonia congenita	Paramyotonia	Autosomal dominant	17q13.1–13.3	SCNA4A
Hyperkalemic periodic paralysis	Periodic paralysis, myotonia, and paramyotonia	Autosomal dominant	17q13.1–13.3	SCNA4A
Hypokalemic periodic paralysis (<10% of cases)	Periodic paralysis	Autosomal dominant	17q13.1–13.3	SCNA4A
Calcium Channelopathies				
Hypokalemic periodic paralysis	Periodic paralysis (most cases)	Autosomal dominant	1q31–32	Dihydropyridine receptor
Malignant hyperthermia (some cases)	Anesthetic-induced delayed relaxation	Autosomal dominant	19q13.1	Ryanodine receptor
Potassium channelopathy (Andersen-Tawil syndrome)	Periodic paralysis, cardiac arrhythmia, skeletal abnormalities	Autosomal dominant	17q23	KCNJ2
Rippling muscle disease **(Web video 130-1)**	Muscle mounding/stiffness	Autosomal dominant	1q41	Caveolin-3

SODIUM CHANNELOPATHIES

Several autosomal-dominant disorders are caused by point mutations in the voltage-dependent sodium channel gene. All of these disorders have symptoms beginning in the first decade. Paramyotonia congenita has paradoxic myotonia in that myotonia *increases* with exercise. Myotonia is worsened by cold temperature. The myotonia can be treated with sodium channel blockers such as mexiletine.

In hyperkalemic periodic paralysis, attacks of weakness last 1 to 2 hours and are precipitated by fasting, by rest after exercise, or by ingesting potassium-rich foods. During attacks, patients are hyporeflexic with normal sensation, and no ocular or respiratory muscle weakness is present. The serum potassium level may be normal during the attack, and therefore a more appropriate term may be *potassium-sensitive periodic paralysis*. Episodes of weakness rarely necessitate acute therapy; oral carbohydrates or glucose improve weakness. Treatments to prevent attacks include thiazide diuretics, β-agonists, and a low-potassium, high-carbohydrate diet, with avoidance of fasting, strenuous activity, and cold.

In a small proportion of patients, hypokalemic periodic paralysis results from mutations in the sodium channel (see **Web video 130-2**).

CALCIUM CHANNELOPATHIES

The majority of cases of hypokalemic periodic paralysis are caused by mutations in the muscle calcium channel. Attacks begin by adolescence and are triggered by exercise, sleep, stress, or meals rich in carbohydrates and sodium. Attacks last from 3 to 24 hours. A vague prodrome of stiffness or heaviness in the legs can occur, and, if the patient performs mild exercise, then a full-blown attack may be aborted. Ocular, bulbar, and respiratory muscles are rarely involved. Early in the disease, patients have normal interattack examinations except for eyelid myotonia (approximately 50%). Later, attack frequency can lessen, but many patients have proximal weakness. Preventive measures include a low-carbohydrate, low-sodium diet and carbonic anhydrase inhibitors. Acute attacks are treated with oral potassium. Patients with hypokalemic periodic paralysis and mutations in the sodium channel are often worsened by carbonic anhydrase inhibitors.

Thyrotoxic periodic paralysis resembles hypokalemic periodic paralysis and is common in male Asian young adults. β-Adrenergic blocking agents reduce the frequency and severity of attacks, but the ultimate treatment is directed against the thyrotoxicosis. A channel defect has not yet been identified.

Malignant hyperthermia is characterized by severe muscle rigidity, fever, tachycardia precipitated by depolarizing muscle relaxants, and inhalational anesthetic agents such as halothane. The symptoms usually occur during surgery but can first be noticed in the postoperative period. Patients may have had previous anesthesia without symptoms. During attacks, the CK level is markedly elevated, and myoglobinuria develops. The disorder is caused by excessive calcium release by the sarcoplasmic reticulum calcium channel, the ryanodine receptor. Some patients have mutations in the ryanodine receptor gene on chromosome 19q13, which is the same gene mutated in central core disease. The symptoms are treated with dantrolene, and at-risk patients should not be given known provocative anesthetic agents. The occurrence of malignant hyperthermia in one member of a family should prompt consideration as to whether other family members might also be at risk.

OTHER FORMS OF MUSCLE STIFFNESS

Neuroleptic malignant syndrome with muscular rigidity, altered mental status, and hyperthermia is caused by central dopaminergic blockade from neuroleptics. The muscle rigidity can produce myoglobinuria.

Stiff-person syndrome is an acquired autoimmune condition that produces severe muscle stiffness of proximal, and especially paraspinous, muscles. Excess motor unit activity caused by autoantibodies to glutamic acid decarboxylase is present, which is a major enzyme in the synthesis of δ-aminobutyric acid, and this circumstance results in disinhibition in the central nervous system. Some patients also have antibodies to islet cells and develop diabetes mellitus. Symptomatic treatment consists of diazepam; immunosuppressive treatment can improve the condition.

Inflammatory Myopathies

Inflammatory myopathies are acquired, nonhereditary disorders (Table 130–6) that are characterized by muscle weakness and inflammation on muscle biopsy. Most have elevated

Table 130–6	**Major Inflammatory Myopathies**

Idiopathic

Polymyositis
Dermatomyositis
Inclusion body myositis
Overlap syndromes with other connective tissue disease
   (e.g., systemic lupus erythematosus)
Sarcoidosis
Inflammatory myopathies with eosinophilia
Eosinophilic polymyositis
Diffuse fasciitis with eosinophilia
Myositis ossificans

Infections

Bacterial (e.g., *Staphylococcus, Streptococcus,* gas gangrene
   Clostridium welchii)
Viral: acute myositis after influenza or other viral infections;
   retrovirus-related myopathies (HIV, HTLV-1)
Parasitic; toxoplasmosis, trypanosomiasis, cysticercosis,
   trichinosis
Fungal

HIV = human immunodeficiency virus; HTLV-1, human T-cell leukemia virus type 1.

CK levels, myopathic EMG findings, and a limb-girdle distribution of weakness. Occasionally, inflammatory myopathies have distal, focal, or other selective involvement of particular muscles.

IDIOPATHIC INFLAMMATORY MYOPATHY

The three major categories of idiopathic inflammatory myopathy are DM, PM, and inclusion body myositis (IBM) (Table 130–7). PM and DM are both characterized by the onset of symmetric weakness subacutely over weeks or several months. Myalgias can occur, but muscle pain and tenderness are rarely chief complaints. Patients complaining of myalgia who do not have demonstrable weakness are more likely to have polymyalgia rheumatica or fibromyalgia than PM. Esophageal muscles are affected in up to 30% of both PM and DM cases, leading to dysphagia.

The rash of DM may accompany or precede the onset of muscle weakness. This rash can be a heliotrope rash (purplish discoloration of the eyelids often associated with periorbital edema); Gottron's sign (papular, erythematous, scaly lesions over the knuckles); a macular erythematous, sun-sensitive rash on the face, neck, and anterior chest, shoulders, upper back, elbows, and knees; or periungual erythema caused by dilated capillary loops with thrombi or hemorrhage.

IBM presents as an insidious onset of slowly progressive proximal and distal weakness typically after age 50 years. It is the most common inflammatory myopathy in older adults. These patients have a distinctive pattern of muscle involvement, with early weakness and atrophy of the quadriceps (knee extensors), volar forearm muscles (wrist and finger flexors), and tibialis anterior (ankle dorsiflexors).

Cardiac involvement, resulting in congestive heart failure and conduction defects, and interstitial lung disease can develop in a minority of patients with PM and DM (but not IBM). Vasculitis of the gastrointestinal tract, kidneys, lungs, and eyes can complicate DM (but not PM), particularly in children. The incidence of malignancy in older adults with DM is increased.

The EMG in DM, PM, and IBM demonstrates brief myopathic motor units, increased recruitment, and fibrillation potentials. The serum CK level is usually increased. The erythrocyte sedimentation rate is normal in most patients. An elevated erythrocyte sedimentation rate suggests a different or coincidental disease. A muscle biopsy should be performed in all patients with suspected inflammatory myopathy to establish the diagnosis (see Table 130–7).

Histologic features and immunologic studies suggest that DM is a humorally mediated micro-angiopathy. The micro-angiopathy leads to ischemic damage of muscle fibers. PM is likely to be a cell-mediated disorder. The cause of IBM is unknown.

Corticosteroids and other immunotherapies can improve strength and function in patients with DM and PM. In contrast, IBM is usually refractory to immunosuppressive therapy.

INFECTIOUS MYOSITIS

An acute viral myositis can occur in the setting of an influenza viral upper respiratory tract infection. In addition to typical influenza-associated myalgias, these patients develop proximal weakness, elevated CK levels, and a

Table 130–7	Idiopathic Inflammatory Myopathies: Clinical and Laboratory Features					
Myopathy	**Sex**	**Typical Age at Onset**	**Pattern of Weakness**	**Creatine Kinase**	**Muscle Biopsy**	**Response to Immunosuppressive Therapy**
Dermatomyositis	Women > men	Childhood and adult	Proximal > distal	Increased (up to 50 × normal)	Perifascicular atrophy, MAC, immunoglobulin, complement deposition on vessels	Yes
Polymyositis	Women > men	Adult	Proximal > distal	Increased (up to 50 > normal)	Endomysial inflammation	Yes
Inclusion body myositis	Men > women	Elderly (>50 yr)	Proximal and distal; predilection for finger/ wrist flexors, knee extensors	Increased (<10 × normal)	Endomysial inflammation, rimmed vacuoles; amyloid deposits; electron microscopy: 15- to 18-nm tubulofilaments	No

MAC = membrane attack complex.

myopathic EMG finding. The disorder is self limited, but when severe, it is often associated with myoglobinuria and occasionally with renal failure. A similar syndrome can complicate infections with other viruses.

An inflammatory myopathy can occur in the setting of human immunodeficiency virus infection, either in early or in later acquired immunodeficiency syndrome. The clinical presentation is similar to that of patients with PM. Patients may improve with corticosteroid therapy. The disorder must be distinguished from the toxic myopathy caused by zidovudine, which responds to dose reduction.

Myopathies Caused by Endocrine and Systemic Disorders

Excess corticosteroids can result from endogenous Cushing's disease or can be caused by exogenous glucocorticoid administration. Iatrogenic corticosteroid myopathy (or atrophy) is the most common endocrine-related myopathy. However, muscle weakness is rarely the presenting manifestation of Cushing's disease, and, in virtually all instances of corticosteroid myopathy, other factors contributing to weakness are also present. Therapy consists of reducing the corticosteroid dose to the lowest possible level. Exercise and adequate nutrition prevent and may improve weakness.

Patients with hyperthyroidism often have some degree of proximal weakness, but this is rarely the presenting manifestation of thyrotoxicosis. Hypothyroid myopathy is associated with proximal weakness and myalgias, muscle enlargement, slow relaxation of the reflexes, and marked (up to 100-fold) increase of the serum CK level.

Progressive, painless proximal weakness in a patient with diabetes is seldom the result of diabetes-related myopathy. Chronic inflammatory demyelinating neuropathy should be suspected. Asymmetric, usually painful, proximal leg weakness can occur from an ischemic radiculoplexopathy. In rare cases, acute muscle infarction can develop in quadriceps or hamstring muscles. These patients complain of severe pain, tenderness, and swelling. Magnetic resonance imaging of the thigh shows changes consistent with a muscle infarct. The syndrome resolves spontaneously over weeks.

Toxic Myopathies

Many drugs have been associated with muscle damage; common ones are listed in Table 130–8. Most of these drugs can produce proximal weakness, elevated CK levels, myopathic EMG readings, and abnormalities on muscle biopsy. Symptoms generally improve on stopping the medication. Some drugs can produce acute, rapidly progressive muscle destruction and myoglobinuria, particularly the hypocholesterolemic drugs clofibrate, gemfibrozil, lovastatin, simvastatin, pravastatin, and niacin. An acute necrotizing myopathy associated with myoglobinuria occurs in chronic alcoholics after heavy drinking. Hypokalemia caused by sweating, vomiting, diarrhea, and renal wastage may be causative.

Also known as critical illness myopathy (CIM), acute quadriplegic myopathy develops in a patient in the intensive

Table 130–8   **Toxic Myopathies**

Inflammatory: cimetidine, D-penicillamine

Noninflammatory necrotizing or vacuolar: cholesterol-lowering agents, chloroquine, colchicine

Acute muscle necrosis and myoglobinuria: cholesterol-lowering drugs, alcohol, cocaine

Malignant hyperthermia: halothane, ethylene, others; succinylcholine

Mitochondrial: zidovudine

Myosin loss: nondepolarizing neuromuscular blocking agents; glucocorticoids

care setting and is often discovered when a patient is unable to be weaned off a ventilator. The cause of the diffuse weakness is the prolonged daily use of either (often both) high-dose intravenous glucocorticoids (usually methyl-prednisolone) or nondepolarizing neuromuscular blocking agents (e.g., vecuronium). Patients often have had sepsis and multiorgan failure. The diagnosis of CIM can be confirmed on muscle biopsy, which shows the loss of myosin thick fil-aments on electron microscopic examination. Treatment is supportive after discontinuing the offending agents. Strength returns over a period of weeks or months; patients can usually be weaned off the ventilator. Many patients with CIM develop plexopathies that cause focal weakness, with evidence of denervation by EMG studies. These plexopathies may result from compression by swollen muscles; they resolve slowly over many months.

Myoglobinuria

Acute muscle destruction can produce a brown discoloration of urine by myoglobin. Myoglobin, a 17,000-D molecular-weight protein that contains the heme moiety, is present in high concentration in muscle. The visible discoloration of urine by myoglobin indicates both massive and acute muscle destruction and warns of impending renal damage. The pigment has to be distinguished from hemoglobin. If no hematuria is present, then a positive urine test for blood strongly suggests myoglobinuria.

Muscle pain, swelling, and weakness precede overt myo-globinuria by a few hours. In addition to myoglobin, phosphate, potassium, creatine, and muscle enzymes are released into the circulation. Serum CK levels can be over 1000 times normal. The heme pigment in the glomerular fil-trate and casts in the tubules cause proteinuria, hematuria, and tubular necrosis. Renal failure is more likely if hypoten-sion, acidosis, and hypovolemia co-exist. With increasing renal insufficiency, hyperphosphatemia, hypocalcemia, tetany, and life-threatening hyperkalemia appear. Death may result from renal or respiratory failure.

Myoglobinuria is caused by massive ischemia of muscle from any cause: crush injuries, prolonged pressure, or per-sistent contraction and rigidity (such as from status epilep-ticus, malignant hyperthermia, or neuroleptic malignant syndrome). Infectious causes include viral and bacterial infections. The acute episode is treated by rest, maintenance of adequate urine flow by hydration and diuretics, and alka-linization of the urine with sodium bicarbonate. Other mea-sures consist of treating the renal insufficiency, as required, and removing the offending cause, if possible.

Prospectus for the Future

With the discovery of the molecular defects in nearly all of the inherited muscle diseases, gene therapy strategies are under development. Vectors are available for potential correction of the defects arising from mutations in small genes. The very large dystrophin gene mutated in Duchenne's dystrophy poses tech-nical challenges. Strategies to correct muscle gene abnormali-ties via arterial administration with viral vectors that target muscle have greater appeal than intramuscular administration into multiple skeletal (and cardiac) muscles.

References

Barohn RJ: Muscle Diseases. In Goldman L, Ausiello DA (eds): Cecil Text-book of Medicine, 23rd ed. Philadelphia, Saunders, 2007.

Hirano M, DiMauro S: ANT1, Twinkle, POLG, and TP: New genes open our eyes to ophthalmoplegia. Neurology 57:2163–2165, 2001.

Karpati G, Hilton-Jones D, Griggs RC (eds): Walton's Disorders of Volun-tary Muscle, 7th ed. Cambridge, UK, Cambridge University Press, 2001.

Neuromuscular Junction Disease

Robert C. Griggs

Disorders of the neuromuscular junction interfere with the transmission of electrical impulses from peripheral nerve to muscle. They can be acquired or inherited and are associated with weakness and fatigability on exertion (Table 131–1). In each disorder, the safety margin of neuromuscular transmission is compromised by one or more specific defects: acetylcholine (ACh) synthesis or packaging of ACh quanta into synaptic vesicles, the release of ACh quanta from the nerve terminal by nerve impulses, and the efficiency of the released ACh quanta to generate a postsynaptic depolarization.

Myasthenia Gravis

Myasthenia gravis (MG) is an acquired autoimmune disorder. Pathogenic autoantibodies induce acetylcholine receptor (AChR) deficiency at the motor end plate. Circulating AChR antibodies are present in 70% to 80% of patients, and immunoglobulin G and complement components are deposited on the postsynaptic membrane. AChR deficiency results from lysis of the junctional folds and destruction of AChRs cross-linked by antibodies that block the binding of ACh to the AChR. The incidence is 2 to 5 per year per 1 million population and the prevalence is 13 to 64 per million. The female-to-male ratio is 6:4. The disease may occur at any age, but the incidence in women peaks in the third decade and in men in the sixth or seventh decade.

CLINICAL FEATURES

MG can involve either the external ocular muscles selectively (ocular MG) or the general voluntary muscle system (generalized MG). The symptoms usually fluctuate, tending to be worse later in the day (diurnal fluctuation). They are provoked or worsened by exertion, intercurrent infections, menses, and excitement. Ocular muscle involvement is usually bilateral, asymmetric, and typically associated with ptosis and diplopia. Weakness of other muscles innervated by cranial nerves results in loss of facial expression, a smile that resembles a snarl, nasal regurgitation of liquids, choking on foods and secretions, and slurred, nasal speech. Abnormal fatigability of the limb muscles causes difficulty in combing the hair, lifting objects repeatedly, climbing stairs, walking, and running. On examination, fatigue is most reliably demonstrated in the eyes: the *curtain sign* of worsening ptosis with upgaze or asymmetric nystagmus on extremes of lateral and medial gaze. Proximal limb muscles are affected more than distal ones, but in advanced cases, weakness is widespread. Initially, the symptoms are ocular in 40%, are generalized in 40%, involve only the extremities in 10%, and involve only the bulbar or bulbar and eye muscles in another 10%. Ocular muscles are affected in nearly all patients after a year of disease. The symptoms remain ocular in only 15% of patients. When the disease becomes generalized, usually it does so within the first year of onset. Two thirds of patients with MG have thymic hyperplasia, and 10% to 15% have thymoma. In approximately 10% of patients, the MG is associated with another autoimmune disease. Circulating AChR antibodies can be detected in most infants born to mothers with MG, but only 12% of such children develop MG, usually during the first few hours of life. The disease is caused by the transfer of AChR antibodies.

DIAGNOSIS

Anticholinesterase Tests

Edrophonium given intravenously acts within a few seconds and lasts for a few minutes. Two milligrams of the drug are injected intravenously over 15 seconds. If no response occurs in 30 to 45 seconds, an additional 8 mg is injected. The evaluation of the response requires objective assessment of one or more signs not easily influenced by motivation, such as degree of ptosis and range of ocular movements. Possible cholinergic side effects of the drug include fasciculations, flushing, lacrimation, abdominal cramps, nausea, vomiting, and diarrhea. The drug must be given cautiously to patients with cardiac disease because it may cause sinus bradycardia, atrioventricular block, and, rarely, cardiac arrest. It should not be given to patients having respiratory difficulty.

Table 131–1 Disorders of the Neuromuscular Junction

Autoimmune

Myasthenia gravis
Lambert-Eaton myasthenic syndrome

Congenital

Presynaptic defects in ACh resynthesis, packaging, or release
Synaptic defect: congenital end plate AChE deficiency
Postsynaptic defects: slow-channel syndromes
Postsynaptic defects: decreased response to ACh
Fast-channel syndromes
AChR deficiency without kinetic abnormality
Familial limb-girdle myasthenia

Toxic

Botulism
Drug induced
Organophosphate intoxication

ACh = acetylcholine; AChE = acetylcholinesterase; AChR = acetylcholine receptor.

Electromyography

Supramaximal stimulation of a motor nerve at 2 or 3 Hz results in a 10% or greater decrement of the amplitude of the evoked compound muscle action potential from the first to the fifth response. The test is positive in most patients with generalized MG, provided that two or more distal and two or more proximal muscles are examined.

Blood Tests and Radiography

The AChR antibody test measures the binding of antibody to AChR labeled with radioactive α-bungarotoxin. The antibody-binding test is positive in nearly all adults with moderately severe or severe MG, in 80% with mild generalized MG, and in 50% with ocular MG. Some patients without AChR have abnormal antibodies to muscle-specific tyrosine kinase (MuSK) with a role in aggregation of AChR and the end plate. Striated muscle antibodies also occur in patients with MG. Their role is unknown, but they are often associated with thymoma. Because of the frequency of thymomas, chest x-ray and chest CT scanning are indicated.

TREATMENT

Anticholinesterases, thymectomy, alternate-day prednisone, azathioprine, cyclosporine, plasmapheresis, and intravenous immunoglobulin are used to treat patients with MG. Anticholinesterases are useful in all forms of the disease. Pyridostigmine bromide (60-mg tablets) acts for 3 to 4 hours, and neostigmine bromide, 15 mg, acts for 2 to 3 hours. Pyridostigmine bromide has fewer muscarinic side effects and is therefore more widely used than neostigmine bromide. One-

half to four tablets are given every 4 hours in the daytime. This medication is also available in 180-mg *time-span* tablets for use at bedtime and as a syrup for children and patients requiring nasogastric feeding. In critically ill patients or postoperatively, intramuscularly injectable pyridostigmine bromide (the dose is one thirtieth of the oral dose) and neostigmine methylsulfate (the dose is one fifteenth of the oral dose) can be used. Patients who have difficulty with respiration, feeding, or handling secretions and who are not responding to relatively high doses of anticholinesterases are best treated by anticholinesterase withdrawal, tracheal intubation, and ventilator support.

In patients with generalized disease not responding adequately to anticholinesterases, other forms of therapy must be used. Thymectomy has been believed to improve the clinical course of MG, but a controlled clinical trial of the procedure is now in progress. On the other hand, thymoma is an indication for thymectomy because the tumor is often locally invasive. Alternate-day prednisone treatment induces remission or improves the disease in more than one half patients. Azathioprine in doses of 2 to 3 mg/kg/day also induces remissions or improvement in more than one half of patients treated. The time required for improvement is 12 to 15 months. Surveillance for side effects (pancytopenia, leukopenia, and hepatocellular injury) must be maintained during therapy. Azathioprine as an adjunct to alternate-day prednisone reduces the maintenance dose of prednisone and is associated with reduced side effects. Mycophenolate, cyclosporine, and other immunosuppressants are sometimes justified. Plasmapheresis is helpful in patients with sudden worsening of MG and is indicated in severe generalized MG refractory to other forms of treatment. Three to five daily exchanges of 2 L of plasma often result in objective improvement and lower the AChR antibody titer in a few days. Plasmapheresis is expensive and not usually suitable for long-term treatment. Intravenous immunoglobulin, 2 g/kg divided over 2 to 5 days, may improve patients with severe MG. The mean duration of the response is 9 weeks in patients also treated with corticosteroids and 5 weeks in those who are not.

Lambert-Eaton Myasthenic Syndrome

Lambert-Eaton myasthenic syndrome is an acquired autoimmune disease in which pathogenic autoantibodies cause a deficiency of voltage-sensitive calcium channels at the motor nerve terminal. Among patients older than age 40 years, 70% of men and 30% of women have an associated carcinoma, usually a small-cell carcinoma of the lung. Lambert-Eaton myasthenic syndrome may predate tumor detection by up to 3 years. Non-neoplastic Lambert-Eaton myasthenic syndrome has an association with other autoimmune disorders, HLA-B8 and DRw3 antigens, and organ-specific autoantibodies. Patients have weakness and fatigability of proximal limb and trunk muscles with relative sparing of extraocular and bulbar muscles. The lower limbs are more severely involved than the upper ones. On maximal voluntary contraction, the force produced by a weak muscle increases for a few seconds and then again decreases. Tendon reflexes are usually hypoactive or absent. Autonomic manifestations (dry mouth, impotence, decreased sweating, orthostatic hypotension, and altered pupillary reflexes) occur in 50% of patients. On electromyography, the amplitude of the compound muscle action potential evoked by a single nerve stimulus from rested muscle is abnormally small. Repetitive stimulation at 2 Hz induces a further decrement, but stimulation at frequencies higher than 10 Hz or voluntary exercise for a brief period facilitates the response to normal amplitude. Treatment strategies include corticosteroids, azathioprine, and intravenous immune globulin. 3,4-Diaminopyridine is helpful but is not widely available in the United States; it can cause seizures and other side effects.

Drug-Induced Myasthenic Syndromes

Aminoglycoside antibiotics, antiarrhythmic agents (procainamide and quinidine), β-adrenergic blockers (propranolol and timolol), phenothiazines, lithium, trimethaphan, methoxyflurane, and magnesium given parenterally or in cathartics reduce the safety margin of neuromuscular transmission. However, overt myasthenic symptoms do not usually appear unless an overdose of the drug is administered or the renal or hepatic elimination of the drug is impaired. The drugs may worsen MG or Lambert-Eaton myasthenic syndrome.

Succinylcholine, a depolarizing blocking drug, is used to induce muscle relaxation during anesthesia. A single dose of the drug sufficient to cause transient apnea is eliminated by plasma pseudocholinesterase in 10 to 20 minutes. In approximately 1 in 2500 patients receiving the drug, prolonged apnea occurs and persists for up to several hours. Most of these patients have an autosomal-recessive abnormality of the plasma pseudocholinesterase. Curare and related agents used during surgery and in critically ill patients to induce muscle relaxation produce blockade of the neuromuscular junction. Their use in patients with MG and other myasthenias is associated with profound and prolonged weakness.

Organophosphate Intoxication

Organophosphate insecticides irreversibly inhibit cholinesterases. Ingestion is associated with alterations in sensorium, convulsions, coma, severe muscarinic side effects, cramps, fasciculations, and muscle weakness from a depolarization block.

Prospectus for the Future

A multicenter, randomized, controlled trial of thymectomy in MG began in early 2006. This trial may provide long-needed answers about the value of this procedure. Randomized, controlled trials of other treatments (e.g., mycophenolate mofetil) are also in progress.

References

Engel AG, Hohfeld R: Acquired autoimmune myasthenia gravis. In Engel AG, Franzini-Armstrong C (eds): Myology, 3rd ed. New York, McGraw-Hill, 2004, 1755–1790.

Engel AG, Ohno K, Sine S: Congenital myasthenic syndromes. In Engel AG, Franzini-Armstrong C (eds): Myology, 3rd ed. New York, McGraw-Hill, 2004, 1801–1844.

Gronseth GS, Barohn RJ: Practice parameter: Thymectomy for autoimmune myasthenia gravis (an evidence-based review). Report of the Quality Standards Subcommittee of the American Academy of Neurology. Neurology 55:7–15, 2000.

Vincent A: Disorders of neuromuscular transmission. In Goldman L, Ausiello DA (eds): Cecil Textbook of Medicine, 23rd ed. Philadelphia, Elsevier, 2007.

Cecil

Andreoli and Carpenter's
Essentials of Medicine

The Aging Patient

Leslie E. Sutton

Hal H. Atkinson

Geriatrics is the field of medicine specializing in the study of aging and illness in the older adult patient. Traditionally, this patient population has been defined as individuals ages 65 years and older. In the United States the percentage of people over 65 years of age rose from approximately 4% in 1900 to 12.4% in 2000, representing an increase in the total number of older individuals from 3.1 million to 35 million. By the year 2030, conservative estimations predict that at least 20% of Americans will be older than 65 years. The largest projected increases are expected to occur among persons over the age of 85 (Fig. 132–1). Key factors in this expansion were declines in infant and maternal mortality rates in the first half of the twentieth century followed by a decline in the birth rate in the late twentieth century.

Current understanding of the physiologic mechanisms of aging and disease in older adults is limited; however, the field of aging research is growing. The expansion in research on aging along with the growth of the older population have created a demand for physicians with expertise in geriatric medicine. This chapter reviews salient topics in geriatrics: theories on aging, techniques of comprehensive assessment, select clinical syndromes, and health care financing for older adults.

Aging Process

Aging is associated with a limited ability to maintain homeostasis in response to stress and an increased susceptibility to disease and mortality. The mechanisms for these changes are uncertain but are considered to be multifactorial. A central question in the study of aging drives much of current scientific thought. Is aging primarily the result of a programmed genetic plan or the consequence of random cellular damage? Though this fundamental issue continues to be debated, scientists have proposed various theories in an attempt to understand the complex aging process. These theories may be divided into two broad categories: evolutionary and molecular.

EVOLUTIONARY THEORIES OF AGING

Two theories, *antagonistic pleiotropy* and *disposable soma*, explain aging based on evolutionary principles. Pleiotropy is the ability of one gene, or a group of genes, to control multiple and seemingly unrelated phenotypes. These traits are termed antagonistic if they have opposing consequences on survival fitness. The *antagonistic pleiotropy* theory proposes that certain genes exhibit characteristics that are advantageous in youth and unfavorable in old age. The physical changes of aging may result from these late-acting genes. According to natural selection, any gene with a detrimental phenotype would be eliminated from the genetic pool. However, the late-acting aging genes escape the pressures of natural selection because of their linkage to the early-acting, beneficial genotype. Reproduction has already occurred by the time the unfavorable age-related traits appear. The tumor suppressor gene *p53* is a potential example of a gene with antagonistic pleiotropy. This gene causes programmed cell death in response to DNA damage. The actions of *p53* confer an early survival advantage by decreasing the incidence of cancer. However, *p53* activity accelerates the aging process by destroying cells that are minimally damaged, though potentially viable. According to the *antagonistic pleiotropy* theory, *p53* is maintained in the genetic code because of its early protective effects, despite its late-acting and potentially adverse consequences.

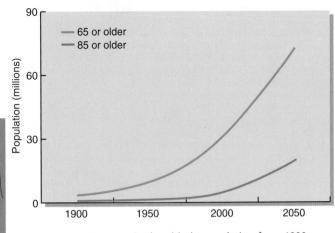

Figure 132–1 Increase in the elderly population from 1900 projected through 2050 based on data from the U.S. Census Bureau.

According to the *disposable soma* theory, aging occurs because limited energy resources are shared between various cellular activities. Intrinsic and extrinsic forces damage somatic cells continually. The body must repair these defects to ensure its existence until successful reproduction. These repairs require large amounts of energy and diminish the energy supply available for reproduction. From an evolutionary perspective, maximum energy resources should be allocated for reproduction. To conserve energy for reproduction, sacrifices are made in somatic maintenance, and some cellular damage is not repaired. These errors do not cause significant dysfunction in the young; however, their mass accumulation may have detrimental effects in older adults, exhibited as the aging phenotype.

MOLECULAR THEORIES OF AGING

Molecular theories of aging involve the effects of truncated telomeres, mitochondrial free radicals, somatic mutations, and altered proteins. Telomeres, nucleotide base pairs positioned at each end of a chromosome, are necessary for successful cell division. The terminal segment of a telomere is lost during each cell cycle until, eventually, mitosis becomes impossible. Cellular senescence then occurs, causing an irreversible arrest to the cell cycle. According to the telomere attrition theory, these senescent cells contribute to aging by decreasing tissue mass and causing organ dysfunction. Leonard Hayflick discovered this physiologic principle while studying fibroblasts grown in tissue culture. He observed that senescence occurred after approximately 50 cell divisions. This replicative limit is thought to protect against uncontrolled cellular division. In fact, cancerous cells escape this limit with the help of an enzyme called *telomerase*, which adds back telomere segments so that a cell may divide infinitely. Therefore, by escaping the Hayflick phenomenon, these cells avoid aging and divide without limit.

Cellular energy production is also implicated as a factor in aging. The mitochondrial reactions of oxidative phosphorylation create energy, but generate free radicals as a by-product. These reactive oxygen species may alter the structure and function of cellular macromolecules, resulting

in the aging phenotype. Free radicals may also directly damage mitochondria. A mitochondrion contains its own genetic code in mitochondrial DNA (mtDNA). As free radicals react with mtDNA, the genetic code for oxidative phosphorylation may be altered. Consequently, energy production occurs in a chaotic fashion, creating even more free radicals. Animal studies have demonstrated some slowing of the aging process by restricting caloric intake, which may partly be attributable to decreasing free-radical production.

Intrinsic and extrinsic forces continually damage DNA. The capacity for DNA repair correlates directly with life expectancies in mammalian species. This principle forms the basis for the somatic mutation theory of aging. According to this theory, the aging phenotype occurs because the DNA repair mechanisms are unable to keep pace with the rate of DNA damage. Genetic repair mechanisms that may be involved in this process include mismatch repair, nucleotide-excision repair, and base-excision repair. The accumulation of these mutations leads to genetic instability, and cellular viability is threatened. The somatic mutation theory attributes aging to the accumulation of these dysfunctional cells.

Intrinsic and extrinsic forces also damage cellular proteins. Young cells have efficient mechanisms for eliminating these denatured proteins; one such system is the ubiquitin-proteasome pathway. In this pathway, abnormal proteins are recognized by the cell and tagged with an ubiquitin polymer. The ubiquitin-protein complex is directed toward a proteasome so that enzymatic destruction of the abnormal protein can occur. The efficacy of this system declines with aging, either because of the proteasome's inability to recognize ubiquitin or its incapacity to degrade the ubiquitin-protein complex. As a result, aged cells tend to accumulate abnormal proteins. These denatured proteins may impair normal cellular function and contribute to the aging phenotype. Cataracts are an age-related consequence of abnormal protein accumulation and may represent evidence for the altered protein theory of aging.

CLINICAL ASSOCIATIONS OF AGING

Longitudinal studies that follow cohorts of individuals from birth to death represent the most reliable method for studying the aging process. However, studies of this design require prohibitive amounts of time and resources. Because of these limitations, current understanding of the clinical associations of aging is based mostly on cross-sectional or short-term longitudinal studies. These studies consistently demonstrate that, for an age-defined cohort, the mean score on tests of physiologic capacity declines as the cohort ages. However, the variability in performance among members within the cohort increases with age. A summary of age-related changes in specific organ systems is shown in Table 132–1.

Aging is associated with increased susceptibility to disease. However, distinguishing *normal aging* from the diseases associated with the aging process is often difficult. Diseases such as hypertension, atherosclerotic disease, congestive heart failure, cancer, infection, and osteoporosis are common among older patients. However, older patients often exhibit these common medical conditions in an atypical manner (Table 132–2).

Table 132–1	Changes in Physiologic Function with Age

Organ System	Age-Related Decline in Function
Special senses	Presbyopia
	Lens opacification
	Decreased hearing
	Decreased taste, smell
Cardiovascular	Impaired intrinsic contractile function
	Decreased conductivity
	Decreased ventricular filling
	Increased systolic blood pressure
	Impaired baroreceptor function
Respiratory	Decreased lung elasticity
	Decreased maximal breathing capacity
	Decreased mucus clearance
	Decreased arterial Po_2
Gastrointestinal	Decreased esophageal and colonic motility
Renal	Decreased glomerular filtration rate
Immune	Decreased cell-mediated immunity
	Decreased T-cell number
	Increased T-suppressor cells
	Decreased T-helper cells
	Loss of memory cells
	Decline in antibody titers to known antigens
	Increased autoimmunity
Endocrine	Decreased hormonal responses to stimulation
	Impaired glucose tolerance
	Decreased androgens and estrogens
	Impaired norepinephrine responses
Autonomic nervous	Impaired response to fluid deprivation
	Decline in baroreceptor reflex
	Increased susceptibility to hypothermia
Neurologic	Decreased vibratory sense
	Decreased proprioception
Musculoskeletal	Decreased muscle mass

Po_2 = partial pressure of oxygen.

Table 132–2	Atypical Disease Presentations in Older Adults

Diagnosis	Potential Presenting Symptoms and Signs
Myocardial infarction	Altered mental status
	Fatigue
	Fever
	Functional decline
Infection	Altered mental status
	Functional decline
	Hypothermia
Hyperthyroidism	Altered mental status
	Anorexia
	Atrial fibrillation
	Chest pain
	Constipation
	Fatigue
	Weight gain
Depression	Cognitive impairment
	Failure to thrive
	Functional decline
Electrolyte disturbance	Altered mental status
	Falls
	Fatigue
	Personality changes
Malignancy	Altered mental status
	Fever
	Pathologic fracture
Pulmonary embolus	Altered mental status
	Fatigue
	Fever
	Syncope
Vitamin deficiency	Altered mental status
	Ataxia
	Dementia
	Fatigue
Fecal impaction	Altered mental status
	Chest pain
	Diarrhea
	Urinary incontinence
Aortic stenosis	Altered mental status
	Fatigue

Note: This table represents only a limited list of select disease processes and presentations; it is not meant to serve as an exhaustive reference for use during patient care activities.

Geriatric Assessment

Comprehensive geriatric assessment (CGA) is an evaluation of the medical, functional, cognitive, and psychosocial factors affecting the health of older patients. This concept was developed in response to the recognition that the complex needs of older adults are best addressed in an interdisciplinary fashion, using the expertise of not only geriatricians, but also other health professionals, including nurses, pharmacists, social workers, occupational and physical therapists, psychologists, audiologists, ophthalmologists, dentists, and nutritionists. Early research documented morbidity reductions and cost savings under this approach to care, but more recent studies have been inconclusive. Formal, interdisciplinary CGAs are not performed in most institutions today. Factors that have limited widespread implementation of CGA include difficulty in identifying appropriate patients, limitations in provider compensation, and a shortage of staff trained in performing CGAs. However, primary care physicians may incorporate the core principles of CGA into patient care to optimize outcomes for their older patients.

MEDICATION ASSESSMENT

Although older adults constitute only 12.4% of the population, they account for over a third of all prescription drugs used in the United States. This level of medication use creates a high potential for adverse drug events. To minimize this risk, each medication from a patient's list should be matched with the diagnosis that necessitates its use, and unnecessary drugs should be eliminated. Additionally, the patient and/or caregiver should understand the appropriate doses, frequencies, and indications for each medicine.

The clinician should be aware of basic pharmacokinetics and pharmacodynamics of drugs in older adults. Though aging diminishes the intestinal surface area available for absorption of medications, typically this effect is clinically insignificant. However, the decline in total body water with aging is clinically relevant. This effect increases the systemic drug concentration in older patients taking water-soluble medications. An additional body composition change that occurs with aging is the increase in the proportion of body mass attributed to fat. Increased fat concentrations result in increased volumes of distribution for lipophilic medications. Therefore fat-soluble drugs may accumulate and produce systemic effects for prolonged periods.

Serum albumin concentrations decrease slightly in healthy older adults and significantly in older patients with malnutrition or acute systemic illness. Hypoalbuminemia produces elevated levels of unbound, chemically active drug in patients who take medications that are highly protein bound. Hepatic metabolism of many drugs may also be reduced with aging. Various physiologic changes of aging contribute to this phenomenon, including decreased liver mass, hepatic blood flow, cytochrome P-450 activity, and first-pass metabolism.

Renal elimination is also decreased in most older patients. The serum creatinine may overestimate renal function; therefore, creatinine clearance should be estimated by taking into account other factors such as age, body mass, and gender. From the creatinine clearance, safe medication doses can be determined. Some useful methods for calculating creatinine clearance are described in Chapter 26.

Pharmacodynamics is the study of medication effects based on drug-receptor interactions, post-receptor modifications, and adaptive homeostatic responses. Medications with altered pharmacodynamic properties in older patients include pulmonary, cardiovascular, and psychiatric medications. Both pharmacodynamic and pharmacokinetic properties are available in package inserts for all medications approved by the U.S. Food and Drug Administration (FDA).

The traditional definition of polypharmacy (many drugs) has been expanded in recent years to include any indiscriminate use of medications. A significant number of medications may be considered irrational because of either pharmacokinetic or pharmacodynamic properties. Examples of potentially inappropriate drugs include those with central nervous system side effects, long half-lives, or anticholinergic properties such as confusion, constipation, and urinary retention. Guidelines regarding undesirable medications for older adults have been published to aid clinicians in preventing and reducing polypharmacy. The *Beers criteria* is one such listing (**Web Table 132–1**).

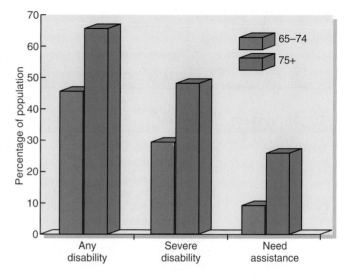

Figure 132–2 Percentage of the elderly population with disabilities and need for assistance, stratified according to age. (Adapted from Health United States: 2001: Current Population Reports, "Americans with Disabilities, 1997" 2001, pp 70–73; data from the United States Census Bureau, National Center on Health Statistics, and Bureau of Labor Statistics.)

FUNCTIONAL ASSESSMENT

Many older adults are affected by functional impairments. Limited mobility is a risk factor for dependency and institutionalization (Fig. 132–2). For this reason, geriatric assessment should focus on a patient's functional capabilities. The initial component of a functional assessment involves an evaluation of a patient's ability to perform routine daily activities. The activities of daily living (ADLs) include transferring from bed to chair, toileting, bathing, dressing, and feeding. The instrumental ADLs (IADLs) consist of advanced functions, including driving, cooking, shopping, managing medications and finances, using the telephone, and performing light housework. Approximately 28% of individuals 65 to 74 years of age and 78% of those 85 and older have difficulty with IADLs or one or more ADLs. The ability to perform these skills correlates well with the capacity for independent living, and an inability to complete these tasks is a risk factor for nursing home placement. Approximately 1.4% of individuals between the ages of 65 and 74 and 20% of those 85 and older live in nursing homes because of these disabilities. Physical and occupational therapists are trained in functional assessment and can help determine a patient's need for assistive devices such as a walker, cane, or shower bench.

The *get up and go* test provides an objective measure of lower extremity strength and coordination by timing a patient in rising from a chair, walking 10 feet, turning around, returning to the chair, and sitting down once again. Individuals who take longer than 10 seconds to complete this sequence have been shown to be at increased risk for falls. However, the examiner should not focus solely on the time required for this task; observing the relative ease or difficulty with which the patient performs this test can provide clues to underlying medical ailments or guide rehabilitative interventions (see **Web Text 132–1**).

SENSORY ASSESSMENT

Vision and hearing impairments often contribute to limited mobility in older adults. The Jaeger eye chart is a tool used to screen for decreased visual acuity. Abnormalities uncovered with this test should prompt a referral to an optometrist or ophthalmologist for further evaluation and consideration of visual aids or eyeglasses. A hand-held audiometer or a screening questionnaire can be used to gauge auditory skills. If limitations in hearing are noted, an audiologist should be consulted so that the deficit can be quantified and potentially corrected with assistive devices such as hearing aids.

COGNITIVE ASSESSMENT

Patients and families should be questioned about problems with cognitive function, particularly short-term memory. Practical questions with safety implications include whether the patient has had difficulty remembering to take medications, missing appointments, or getting lost while driving. The most common screening test for cognitive impairment is the Folstein Mini-Mental State Examination (MMSE). More information on the MMSE can be found in Chapter 115. The MMSE requires several minutes to perform, and its diagnostic value may be limited by educational or language barriers. Recognition of limitations in the MMSE has led to the development of shorter cognitive screening instruments. One such test, the Mini-Cog, was developed to screen for dementia among educationally and linguistically diverse patients. This test includes a three-item recall task and a clock-drawing test. This Mini-Cog test takes an average of 3 minutes to perform and has a sensitivity of 99% in distinguishing demented from nondemented adults. Any abnormalities on the Mini-Cog should prompt a more thorough cognitive evaluation (**Web Fig. 132–1**).

PSYCHOLOGICAL ASSESSMENT

Depression and anxiety are common in older patients and are associated with significant morbidity. The most sensitive question for identifying depression is "Do you often feel sad or depressed?" Clinicians should also ask about the more subtle symptoms of depression such as fatigue, sleep or appetite disturbances, and social withdrawal. With the help of the Geriatric Depression Scale, the physician can formally screen a patient for depression (**Web Table 132–2**).

Anxiety in older patients is common and may produce insomnia, agitation, excessive worry, or physical symptoms. Cognitive behavioral therapy with or without adjunctive treatment with selective serotonin reuptake inhibitors is a relatively safe strategy to treat anxiety in older adults. Benzodiazepines are not ideal medications to use as maintenance therapy in older adults patient because of the increased risk with these drugs of cognitive side effects and falls. For more information on anxiety and depression, the reader is referred to Chapter 116.

SOCIAL AND LEGAL ASSESSMENT

The geriatric social history investigates both the human support and the financial resources available to a patient. For a patient with functional limitations, the physician should determine who is providing assistance to the patient. A patient may rely on sporadic help from neighbors or friends, or he or she may have increased consistent support from nearby family members or paid assistants. For patients requiring assistance, the clinician must be sensitive to the needs of the primary caregivers. These caregivers experience significant stress and are prone to *caregiver burnout.* Additionally, the physician must recognize the potential for elder abuse and neglect; any suspicions of abusive treatment should be conveyed to local investigational agencies. An equally concerning situation is the patient who performs ADLs or IADLs inadequately, placing his or her health and finances in danger. In this situation, a social worker can investigate eligibility for community or governmental assistance and connect family members with home health agencies, assisted living facilities, or nursing homes.

Older patients may experience periods of altered sensorium or cognitive impairment and become unable to participate in their financial or health care decisions. In such situations a surrogate must intervene on behalf of the patient. Powers of attorney, living wills, advance directives, and guardianship documents become important in these situations. These documents are usually drafted with the help of a legal professional and, with the exception of guardianship, may be created by competent adults only.

A power of attorney is a document that lists a surrogate who is authorized to manage a patient's financial affairs. Trust in this representative is important because the surrogate has the right to spend the patient's money and incur debt in the patient's name. A health care power of attorney designates a representative to make health care choices for the patient. If either of these two preceding documents is termed *durable,* the document can be used when the patient becomes incapacitated or incompetent. For patients who have not created a durable health care power of attorney, typically the spouse or other first-degree relative is the default surrogate decision maker. The surrogate's decisions are honored as long as they are in accord with the patient's best interest. However, if the surrogate makes choices in opposition to the patient's best interest, or if no next-of-kin is available, guardianship may be obtained. Guardianship is a legal proceeding whereby the court appoints a surrogate decision maker.

Two related documents are the living will and advance directive. A living will helps instruct the surrogate decision maker of a patient's health care choices regarding terminal and incurable medical conditions or a persistent vegetative state. An advance directive may accompany a living will, providing specific details about a patient's precise health care preferences. Advanced directives often list specific medical interventions, such as dialysis, surgery, and artificial nutrition or hydration, which a patient may request or refuse in writing. These documents are a useful resource for surrogate decision makers. (The reader is referred to *http://www.caringinfo.org* for Caring Connections to view a state-by-state listing of living wills for the United States.)

All primary care physicians should address these legal and ethical issues with each older adult patient. Discussing these matters before an urgent illness arises, and while the patient still has the capacity to understand the implications of these choices, helps ensure that his or her wishes are enacted. These decisions require time and contemplation on the part of the patient, and the opportunity to discuss these decisions with family members is particularly valuable.

Selected Geriatric Syndromes

Although geriatrics encompasses all of internal medicine, certain common problems have been identified to which the clinician should devote particular attention. Three of these geriatric syndromes are described in subsequent paragraphs. Other key issues include osteoporosis, osteoarthritis, and dizziness. These topics are covered in this text in Chapters 75, 87, and 120, respectively.

COGNITIVE DISORDERS: DEMENTIA AND DELIRIUM

Disorders of cognition are increasingly common with advanced age; however, abnormal cognition is not an inevitable consequence of aging. Permanent, progressive impairments of memory and other domains of cognition characterize dementia. The three most common causes of dementia are Alzheimer's disease, dementia with Lewy bodies, and multi-infarct dementia. Alzheimer's disease is characterized by a gradual, insidious loss of cognitive functioning over a period of years. Dementia with Lewy bodies exhibits with parkinsonism, vivid hallucinations, and cognitive deficits. Multi-infarct dementia classically progresses in a stepwise fashion with acute deteriorations in cognition separated by periods of relatively stable cognitive function. For a more detailed discussion of dementia, please refer to Chapter 115.

Delirium is an acute state of confusion characterized by a fluctuating level of consciousness. Accompanying symptoms often include disorientation, memory loss, and hallucinations. A specific trigger for delirium can usually be identified, such as infection, pain, electrolyte disorders, adverse medication effects, surgery, or other acute illness. Table 132–3 lists contrasting features of delirium and dementia.

Successful treatment of delirium requires the diagnosis and treatment of the underlying illness. Other interventions should focus on nonpharmacologic, environmental modifications. Additional measures such as ensuring close nursing supervision, providing recreational activities, and increasing social interactions can help minimize agitation. Physical restraints should be avoided because they increase patient morbidity and raise serious ethical concerns.

If environmental modification is inadequate in controlling severe agitation, pharmacologic interventions may be necessary. However, all of the available medications for behavioral control have potentially serious side effects, and efficacy may be questionable. Small oral doses of atypical antipsychotics can be given (e.g., risperidone, olanzapine, quetiapine); however, recent studies have demonstrated increased cardiovascular mortality among older patients with cognitive impairment who take these medications. These drugs have traditionally been preferred over the typical antipsychotics because they are believed to have less potential for extrapyramidal side effects. However, if intravenous or intramuscular administration is needed, a low dose of the typical antipsychotic haloperidol can be consid-

Table 132–3	Features of Delirium Versus Dementia	
Feature	**Delirium**	**Dementia**
Onset	Acute	Insidious
Course	Fluctuating, lucid at times	Generally stable
Duration	Hours to weeks	Months to years
Alertness	Abnormally low or high	Usually normal
Perception	Illusions and hallucinations common	Usually normal
Memory	Immediate and recent impaired	Recent and remote impaired
Thought	Disorganized	Impoverished
Speech	Incoherent, slow or rapid	Word-finding difficulty
Physical illness or medication causative	Frequently	Usually absent

ered. Both typical and atypical antipsychotics can cause increased agitation, drowsiness, or the life-threatening neuroleptic malignant syndrome. Small doses of short-acting benzodiazepines can be considered as adjuncts for severe behavioral problems. However, benzodiazepines may cause a paradoxic increase in agitation in the confused patient. All of these medications should be used only on an as-needed basis, and they should be discontinued as soon as they are no longer required to control severe symptoms.

Although delirium should never be attributed solely to aging or dementia, delirium is increasingly common in older patients with baseline cognitive impairment. Limited daily mental status examinations and nursing observations are helpful in tracking the course of delirium. Once the acute delirium has resolved, a full mental status examination should be performed to assess the patient's baseline cognitive status.

FALLS AND GAIT INSTABILITY

Falls contribute significantly to morbidity and mortality among older patients. Approximately 30% to 40% of community-dwelling older patients and 50% of long-term care residents fall each year. Up to one half of the patients with a fall requiring hospitalization will not survive more than one year after the fall. The cause of a fall is often multifactorial, including impaired sensation, decreased vestibular function, diminished muscle strength, environmental hazards, postural hypotension, and adverse drug events. Though syncope should be considered as a possible cause for a fall, syncope is a relatively uncommon cause in older patients.

Once a fall has occurred, health care providers should investigate the factors that contributed to the fall so that the

Table 132–4 **Causes, Types, and Treatment of Urinary Incontinence**

Type	Definition	Cause	Treatment
Stress	Leakage associated with increased intra-abdominal pressure (coughing, sneezing)	Hypermobility of the bladder base frequently caused by lax perineal muscles	Pelvic muscle exercise, timed voiding, α-adrenergic drugs, estrogens, surgery
Urge	Leakage associated with a precipitous urge to void	Detrusor hyperactivity (outflow obstruction, bladder tumor, detrusor instability), idiopathic (poor bladder), compliance (radiation cystitis), hypersensitive bladder	Bladder training, pelvic muscle exercise, bladder-relaxant drugs (anticholinergics, oxybutynin, tolterodine, imipramine)
Overflow	Leakage from a mechanically distended bladder	Outflow obstruction, enlarged prostate, stricture, prolapsed cystocele, acontractile bladder (idiopathic, neurologic [spinal cord injury, stroke, diabetes])	Surgical correction of obstruction, intermittent catheter drainage
Functional	Inability or unwillingness to void	Cognitive impairment, physical impairment, environmental barriers (physical restraints, inaccessible toilets), psychological problems (depression, anger, hostility)	Prompted voiding, garment and padding, external collection devices

treatment can be tailored to the specific situation. A multidisciplinary approach with physical and occupational therapy provides the best outcomes. Patients with significant cognitive impairment often cannot participate effectively in rehabilitation. For this group, the best intervention may be environmental modification and close supervision for safety.

URINARY INCONTINENCE

Up to 30% of community-dwelling older patients and at least 50% of those living in long-term care facilities have urinary incontinence. Incontinence may lead to significant morbidity, including perineal irritation, cellulitis, and pressure ulcers. Incontinent older adults may ambulate less for fear of incontinence with movement. Limited ambulation contributes to deconditioning and the loss of functional independence. Additionally, the psychological strain caused by incontinence can contribute to social withdrawal and depression.

Four distinct mechanisms cause urinary incontinence. The most common type of incontinence in older adults is urge incontinence. Detrusor overactivity produces urge incontinence and the associated symptoms of frequency, nocturia, and an uncontrollable urge to void. Stress incontinence occurs as the pelvic muscles and urethral sphincter lose tone. Activities that increase intra-abdominal pressure, such as coughing, sneezing, or straining, precipitate urine leakage in stress incontinence. Overflow incontinence is caused by urinary retention. This type of incontinence occurs as bladder volume increases beyond a critical level, creating a pressure sufficient for urine loss. Patients complain of frequent leakage of small amounts of urine with overflow incontinence. Functional incontinence is the physical inability to get to the bathroom in time to void and is caused by mobility limitations, cognitive impairment, depression, or physical restraints. Table 132–4 outlines the mechanisms, causes, and treatment considerations for the specific types of urinary incontinence. In many instances, more than one mechanism may contribute to a patient's incontinence; this entity is termed mixed incontinence. Mixed incontinence requires a multifaceted treatment approach that addresses the unique combination of etiologic factors.

Evaluation of urinary incontinence must focus on a thorough history and a detailed physical focusing on the pelvic, rectal, and prostate examinations. A urinalysis should be performed to assess for infection, hematuria, or glucosuria. Measurement of postvoid residual bladder volume should be performed in patients with suggested obstruction. Referral to a genitourinary specialist should be considered in patients with recurrent urinary tract infections, increased postvoid residual volumes, hematuria, pelvic prolapse, or prostate mass. Gynecologists, urologists, and some primary care physicians often perform formal urodynamic testing. These tests help elucidate the cause of incontinence by monitoring pressure inside the bladder as it relates to bladder volume, intra-abdominal pressure, stress activities, urge symptoms, and urinary leakage.

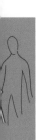

Treatment of all types of incontinence includes correcting underlying medical problems that contribute to incontinence and modifying offending agents that aggravate incontinence. Patients should avoid caffeine and alcohol and, if nocturia is a problem, avoid fluid intake within 2 hours of bedtime. If possible, patients should avoid medications that may aggravate incontinence, such as diuretics. Pelvic muscle exercises can be part of the treatment strategy for stress and urge incontinence. The use of biofeedback may help ensure that patients perform these exercises effectively. Scheduled voiding every 2 hours, with assistance if necessary, can minimize urge, stress, and functional incontinence. Patients with urge incontinence sometimes require the use of anticholinergic agents such as oxybutynin, tolterodine, or trospium to decrease detrusor activity. Because of their anticholinergic side effects, these agents should be prescribed with caution in older adults. Overflow incontinence can be treated with surgical correction or with medications to reduce symptoms of benign prostatic hypertrophy (see Chapter 71). In all types of incontinence, chronic indwelling catheters should be avoided if at all possible because of the increased risk for infection and the functional limitation imposed by the catheter itself.

Health Care Financing for Older Adults

Approximately 34% of public health care funds are spent on older adults. Private insurance and out-of-pocket expenditures for older patients are also substantial. Familiarity with the system for health care financing is essential for physicians who care for older patients. The major insurance provider for the geriatric population in the United States is the Medicare program. The average health care expenditure for Medicare beneficiaries in 2004 was $7542 per person. With the changes in population demographics and the addition of the new prescription drug plan, Medicare costs are predicted to exceed $15,000 per person by 2014. A brief explanation of the current Medicare system follows.

Medicare Part A covers health care costs for hospitals, post-acute care (including short-term skilled nursing facilities), and hospice. All Americans 65 years of age and older are eligible for Medicare Part A; those who worked (or whose spouse worked) for 10 years can receive these benefits without the expense of a monthly premium. Qualified patients are required to pay only a small portion of their bill for inpatient hospitalizations and brief skilled nursing home stays. Home hospice services and inpatient hospice stays are paid entirely by Medicare Part A, with no cost to the patient. Part B carries the additional expense of a monthly premium and typically covers 80% of the cost for durable medical equipment and outpatient services such as clinic visits and diagnostic tests. A newer alternative to the traditional Medicare system of Parts A and B is the managed care system of Part C, or Medicare Advantage. Under Medicare Advantage, private health insurance companies can contract with the federal government to offer Medicare Parts A and B services to patients who choose to enroll in the managed care system. These companies agree to pay the Part A and Part B health care expenses for their enrollees in return for a capitated, or per patient, reimbursement from the federal government. Medicare Part D, new in 2006, provides limited coverage for outpatient prescription medications.

Private companies have the authority to offer supplemental insurance packages to Medicare beneficiaries under the Medigap system. As of 2006, 12 Medicare-sanctioned Medigap policies are available. Medigap policies cover *gaps* in Parts A and B of Medicare, for example, the deductibles and co-payments for Parts A and B benefits.

One area of health care that is not covered by either Medicare or Medigap is the long-term care of stable patients in nursing homes. Long-term care insurance is available through private companies. However, few patients can afford these policies because many plans charge high premiums and offer only limited benefits. Most older adult patients who require long-term care are forced to pay nursing home expenses out of pocket. These patients typically exhaust their personal assets in paying for medical and personal care assistance services. Once they have *spent down* to the poverty level, Medicaid may begin to pay some of the nursing home expenses. Medicaid is a government-sponsored health care financing system for low-income individuals. State governments administer Medicaid programs, so variability exists in the services provided from state to state. (The reader is referred to *http://www.medicare.gov* to access more information on Medicare.)

Prospectus for the Future

The volume of older adult patients in the upcoming decades will create new demands on the United States health care system. With Medicare as the primary payer for most older adults, the federal government will be forced to use health care dollars as efficiently as possible to maintain a high quality of care for older adults. One potential measure to improve efficiency and quality is the implementation of principles of geriatric assessment into medical and surgical ambulatory and inpatient practices. As medical and surgical specialists join in the care of older people, they will need to view patients in terms of physiologic, rather than chronologic, age. This change in philosophy will need to occur as the expanding older population begins to require interventions that have been routine for younger patients but that may have been withheld from older patients in the past because of ageism.

More research into the biologic mechanisms of aging will be needed to better clarify the physiologic from the pathologic changes of aging. Research into preventive medicine will be necessary to prevent, delay, or minimize the disability related to chronic medical conditions so that healthy life years can be extended and quality of life can be enhanced. Enrollment of older adults into clinical trials will be necessary so guidelines that have been developed in younger patients can be tested for applicability in older adults.

References

Armbrecht HJ: The biology of aging. J Lab Clin Med 138:220–225, 2001.

Borson S, Scanlan JM, Chen P, Ganguli M: The Mini-Cog as a screen for dementia: Validation in a population-based sample. J Am Geriatr Soc 51:1451–1454, 2003.

Centers for Medicare and Medicaid Services: Medicare and You 2006. Washington, DC, U.S. Department of Health and Human Services, 2006 (also available at: *http://www.medicare.gov*).

Cole MG: Delirium in elderly patients. Am J Geriatr Psychiatry 12(1)7–21, 2004.

Hill K, Schwarz J: Assessment and management of falls in older people. Intern Med J 34:557–564, 2004.

Kirkwood T: Understanding the odd science of aging. Cell 120:437–447, 2005.

O'Keeffe ST, Mulkerrin EC, Nayeem K, et al: Use of serial Mini-Mental State Examinations to diagnose and monitor delirium in elderly hospital patients. J Am Geriatr Soc 53:867–870, 2005.

Ouslander JG: Management of overactive bladder. N Engl J Med 350:786–799, 2004.

Section XX

Substance Abuse

133 Alcohol and Substance Abuse – LANGE * HILLIS

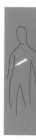

Alcohol and Substance Abuse

Richard A. Lange
L. David Hillis

Alcohol Dependence and Abuse

Alcohol dependence and abuse are major public health problems. An estimated 11 million Americans are considered to be *alcoholics,* and another 7 million are designated as *alcohol abusers.* In the United States, alcohol use is the third leading preventable cause of death—exceeded only by cigarette smoking and obesity—and claims over 100,000 lives annually. Alcohol-related liver disease is responsible for more than 25,000 deaths per year. Alcohol use contributes to approximately 30% of all fatalities caused by motor vehicle accidents and is a major contributor to domestic violence, homicide, and suicide. The total cost to society of alcohol-related property damage or loss, loss of productivity, and criminal interdiction is estimated to be approximately $250 billion annually.

Definitions of Alcohol Abuse and Dependence

The American Psychiatric Association has specific criteria for the diagnoses of *alcohol abuse* and *alcohol dependence;* these criteria are described in the *Diagnostic and Statistical Manual of Mental Disorders,* fourth edition, and are listed in Table 133–1. The so-called *binge drinker* is defined as one who typically consumes five or more drinks in rapid succession. The terms *tolerance* and *dependence* are used to describe a continuum in the adaptation of the central nervous system (CNS) to drug usage. Tolerance may enable the alcoholic to maintain sobriety even in the setting of markedly elevated blood alcohol concentrations. Alcohol dependence describes the physical requirement for repeated alcohol intake to maintain neuronal adaptive changes or to prevent the appearance of symptoms of withdrawal that are associated with alcohol cessation (see Table 133–1).

Epidemiologic Factors

Alcohol-related morbidity and mortality affect twice the number of men as women. Estimates indicate that approximately 40% of 8th graders and 80% of high school seniors and college students use alcohol, and more than one half of all college students admit to heavy episodic drinking. Although the prevalence of ethanol use is highest in individuals younger than 30 years of age, survey data suggest that approximately two thirds of persons over age 30 consume ethanol.

Pharmacologic and Metabolic Factors

Following oral ingestion, alcohol is absorbed predominantly in the small intestine, and its rate of absorption is accelerated by the simultaneous ingestion of carbohydrates and carbonated beverages. Once in the blood, it equilibrates rapidly across all membranes, including the blood-brain barrier, thereby accounting for the prompt onset of its euphoric effects.

The liver metabolizes approximately 90% of ethanol to acetaldehyde via the alcohol dehydrogenase pathway; subsequently, acetaldehyde is converted by aldehyde dehydrogenase to acetate, which enters the Krebs cycle. At low or moderate serum concentrations of ethanol, the alcohol dehydrogenase pathway functions almost exclusively in metabolizing ethanol. At high concentrations, the microsomal ethanol oxidizing system contributes to metabolism. Less than 10% of ethanol is excreted unchanged through the

Table 133–1 Criteria for the Diagnosis of Alcohol Abuse and Dependence in a 12-Month Period

Alcohol Abuse (One or More of the Following)	Alcohol Dependence (Three or More of the Following)
1. Failure to meet obligations at home, school, or work 2. Inappropriate or recurrent use of alcohol in harmful or hazardous situations 3. Evidence of legal problems 4. Concerns related to alcohol consumption are ignored or minimized	1. Alcohol tolerance: increased consumption as a result of decreased effects of alcohol 2. Symptoms or signs of alcohol withdrawal 3. Alcohol consumption increases for long periods 4. Attempts to quit typically fail 5. More time is diverted to obtain, use, and recover from use of alcohol 6. Withdrawal from customary social, occupational, and recreational contacts 7. Alcohol abuse continues despite knowledge of psychophysical dependence

Adapted from the American Psychiatric Association: Diagnostic and Statistical Manual of Mental Disorders, 4th ed. Washington, DC, American Psychiatric Press, 2000.

skin, kidneys, and lungs. Variability among individuals in the efficiency of the alcohol dehydrogenase system has been observed, with some individuals from South Asia having a genetically determined slow alcohol dehydrogenase pathway.

Mechanisms of Alcohol-Induced Organ Damage

The major organs that are susceptible to damage by alcohol are the liver, pancreas, heart, brain, and bone (Table 133–2). Several alcohol-related medical disorders are caused by various nutritional deficiencies, considering that ethanol is deficient in proteins, minerals, and vitamins. Therefore, the initial management of the alcoholic must attend to suggested dietary deficiencies (e.g., thiamine) and electrolyte imbalances, including potassium, magnesium, calcium, and zinc.

Alcohol-related liver disease is the leading preventable cause of hepatic failure in the industrialized world. Genetic factors are thought to play a role in susceptibility to this disorder because alcoholic liver disease is more prevalent in whites than other ethnic groups, despite a similar magnitude of ethanol consumption. The histopathologic features of alcoholic liver disease include fatty infiltration, hepatitis, fibrosis, and end-stage cirrhosis.

Clinical Manifestations of Alcohol Ingestion

ACUTE ALCOHOL INTOXICATION

Mild ethanol intoxication produces slurred speech, ataxia, irregular eye movements, and poor coordination. Signs of CNS depression and associated cerebellar or vestibular dysfunction include dysarthria, ataxia, and nystagmus. At blood levels approaching 400 mg/dL, stupor and coma usually develop, and blood levels of 500 mg/dL often are

fatal. However, understanding that death may occur even when the blood alcohol concentration is as low as 300 mg/dL is important.

WITHDRAWAL SYNDROME (CONVULSIONS)

Alcohol withdrawal occurs in three stages. The signs of minor withdrawal usually appear 6 to 12 hours after the discontinuation of ethanol and are caused by central adrenergic hyperexcitability; they consist of tremors, sweating, tachycardia, diarrhea, and insomnia. Additional evidence of autonomic nervous system hyperactivity often appears within 12 to 24 hours and includes increased startle response, nightmares, and visual hallucinations. Alcohol withdrawal seizures (so-called *rum fits*), which occur 12 and 48 hours after the discontinuation of ethanol, are estimated to occur in 2% to 5% of alcoholics.

DELIRIUM TREMENS

Delirium tremens (DTs) is characterized by delirium (a confused state with varying levels of consciousness), tremor (caused by marked autonomic nervous system overactivity), and agitation. It occurs in approximately 5% of alcoholics, most often in chronic heavy abusers with underlying neurologic damage. If unrecognized and untreated, the in-hospital mortality rate of DTs approaches 25%.

Management and Treatment

Intervention strategies in alcohol abusers are designed to modify the individual's attitudes, knowledge, and skills to prevent alcohol misuse. In the outpatient setting, increased frequency of contact between the primary care physician and the patient increases the likelihood of detection, intervention, and prevention of heavy alcohol consumption. All scheduled office visits should include alcohol screening, assessment, and possible brief attempts at intervention. The

Table 133–2　Medical Complications of Alcohol Abuse

Neurologic

Encephalopathy (Wernicke's with oculomotor dysfunction, gait ataxia)
Cognitive dysfunction
Amnesia (i.e., Korsakoff's syndrome)
Dementia
Cerebellar degeneration
Peripheral neuropathy

Hematologic

Anemia (often with macrocytosis)
Leukopenia
Thrombocytopenia

Gastrointestinal

Esophagitis
Esophageal varices
Gastritis
Gastrointestinal bleeding
Pancreatitis
Hepatitis
Cirrhosis
Splenomegaly

Cardiovascular

Hypertension
Cardiomyopathy
Stroke
Arrhythmias (especially atrial fibrillation)

Electrolyte/Nutritional

Thiamine deficiency
Hypokalemia
Hypomagnesemia
Ketoacidosis
Hypoglycemia
Hypertriglyceridemia
Malnutrition

Endocrine

Diabetes mellitus
Gynecomastia

Musculoskeletal

Myopathy
Osteoporosis
Testicular atrophy
Amenorrhea
Infertility

Miscellaneous

Spontaneous abortion
Fetal alcohol syndrome
Increased risk of cancer (breast, oropharyngeal, esophageal, hepatocellular)
Accidents, trauma, violence, suicide

Table 133–3　CAGE: An Alcoholism Screening Test

1. Have you ever felt you should **C**UT down on your drinking?
2. Have people **A**NNOYED you by criticizing your drinking?
3. Have you felt **G**UILTY about your drinking?
4. Have you ever had a drink first thing in the morning to steady your nerves or to get rid of a hangover (i.e., as an **E**YE-OPENER)?

physician must be proactive in his or her initial evaluation of the patient and in the plan to modify drinking behavior.

SCREENING AND INTERVENTION STRATEGIES

The National Institute on Alcohol Abuse and Alcoholism (NIAAA) provides several web-based guidelines for alcohol screening during routine health examination (see *http://www.niaaa.nih.gov*). A four-step plan exists with which physicians can (1) screen patients for alcohol use, (2) assess for the presence of alcohol-related problems, (3) provide advice concerning appropriate action, and (4) monitor the patient's progress. For the current drinker, the physician should inquire about the number of drinks consumed per day, number of days per week on which ethanol is consumed, and total number of drinks consumed per month. Alcohol consumption that exceeds 14 drinks per week or three drinks per day should trigger an in-depth assessment of alcohol-related problems. The physician should ascertain if the individual is at risk for alcohol-related problems, has an existing problem, or may be alcohol dependent. The CAGE questionnaire (Table 133–3) is a useful screening tool for identifying alcohol-dependent individuals. A positive response to two or more of the four questions is indicative of a potential alcohol problem. Difficulties with work-related, interpersonal, and family relationships and/or evidence of high-risk behavior despite self-reported low-risk consumption indicate that the individual is at risk for alcohol dependence. To assess for alcohol dependence, the individual should be queried about blackouts, depression, abdominal pain, hypertension, sexual dysfunction, trauma, and problems with sleep. The patient with alcohol dependence exhibits a compulsion (e.g., a preoccupation) to drink, lack of control once drinking has started, symptoms of withdrawal, drinking to relieve symptoms, and increased tolerance. On physical examination, evidence of alcoholic liver disease may be exhibited as jaundice, hepatomegaly, palmar erythema, male gynecomastia, spider angiomata, and ascites. The serum γ-glutamyltransferase concentration typically is elevated in individuals who drink excessively.

LOW-RISK DRINKING

A standard drink contains 12 g of alcohol, an amount similar to that found in one 12-ounce bottle of beer or wine cooler, one 5-ounce glass of wine, or 1.5 ounces of distilled spirits. In younger men, moderate drinking is defined as no more than two drinks per day; in all women and men over age 64 years, the limit for moderate drinking is one drink per day. For the same amount of ingested ethanol, women and older adult men achieve a higher blood ethanol concentration than younger men, owing to their smaller volume of body water. A reasonable blood alcohol level should not exceed 50 mg/dL.

A blood alcohol level as low as 80 mg/dL may exceed the legal definition for driving under the influence (DUI) or driving while intoxicated (DWI). In national surveys, the strategy of the *designated driver* appears to be effective at preventing unsafe driving by drinkers at risk of DWI. Complete abstinence is recommended for people with a history of alcohol dependence, other serious medical conditions (e.g., liver disease), and pregnancy.

NONPHARMACOLOGIC THERAPIES

For the foreseeable future, pharmacologic agents will remain complementary and adjunctive to the traditional approaches of abstinence, group therapy, coping mechanisms, and behavior modification. The most widely employed behavioral approach is the 12-step program administered by Alcoholics Anonymous (AA), with which the recovering alcoholic moves through 12 specific steps aided by his or her attendance at regular meetings within a self-help peer group. Cognitive behavioral therapy, though not widely used, is based on the principle that the alcoholic first must identify the internal and external cues to drinking so that he or she can develop effective countermeasures for drinking behavior. Motivation enhancement therapy is another program that encourages self awareness and behavioral changes in the alcoholic.

CONSIDERATIONS FOR DRUG INTERVENTIONS

Behavioral modification has proved to be effective in alcoholics, and medications have not been shown to reduce the chance of relapse. If desired, medications can be administered in conjunction with behavioral modification.

Disulfiram (Antabuse) inhibits aldehyde dehydrogenase (i.e., the enzyme that converts acetaldehyde to acetate), but it is rarely prescribed. *Naltrexone,* an opioid antagonist used for the treatment of opiate addiction, is the first medication to be approved by the U.S. Food and Drug Administration (FDA) for the treatment of alcoholism in over 50 years. In clinical trials, a combination of naltrexone and psychosocial intervention reduced the number of drinking days, induced a longer period of abstinence from ethanol, and decreased the relapse rate in heavy drinkers when compared with psychosocial intervention alone. Naltrexone is administered in a dose of 50 mg daily for 12 weeks, although larger doses (i.e., 100 to 150 mg daily) and a longer duration of administration may improve its success in preventing relapse. Some recovering alcoholics develop nausea when it is initiated. Because hepatic toxicity may occur at high doses (300 mg), periodic testing of liver function is recommended. Naltrexone is contraindicated in patients receiving opioids, given that opiate withdrawal is an unintended adverse effect of the drug.

Nalmefene, an opiate antagonist, has a mechanism of action similar to that of naltrexone, but the FDA has yet to approve nalmefene for the treatment of alcohol abuse. In placebo-controlled trials, nalmefene was substantially better than placebo at reducing the rate of relapse in heavy drinkers. In comparison with naltrexone, hepatotoxicity occurs less often. *Acamprosate,* which interacts with the glutamate neurotransmitter, is approved for the treatment of alcoholism in most European countries. In placebo-controlled trials involving more than 4600 alcoholic patients, acamprosate reduced relapse rates and increased abstinence from ethanol. In comparative trials, it did not appear to be as efficacious as naltrexone. Because the liver does not metabolize acamprosate, it is safe in persons with alcoholic liver disease.

Because the serotonergic system appears to play an important role in drinking behavior, medications that target this pathway have been developed for the treatment of people with alcoholism. *Ondansetron,* a selective serotonin reuptake inhibitor, reduces craving for alcohol and increases its sedative effects. Following 11 weeks of therapy with this agent, *early-onset* alcoholics consumed fewer drinks per day and had more days of abstinence from alcohol than did *late-onset* alcoholics, suggesting that pharmacologic treatment may be particularly beneficial in persons with a reversible serotonergic abnormality.

FETAL ALCOHOL SYNDROME

Despite increased awareness of the dangers of alcohol, new cases of fetal alcohol syndrome (FAS) continue to occur. Recognition by physicians is crucial to improving outcomes in children affected by this condition. The quantity or pattern of alcohol use resulting in FAS has not been clearly defined. Theories suggest that the harmful by-products of ethanol cause cellular damage to the developing tissues of the fetus. FAS is characterized by a specific pattern of four findings:

1. Maternal alcohol exposure
2. Facial anomalies including short palpebral fissures, ptosis, smooth philtrum, and thin upper lip
3. Growth retardation
4. CNS neurodevelopmental findings that include structural abnormalities of the corpus callosum and cerebellum, poor gait coordination, and sensorineural hearing loss

The diagnosis of FAS is relatively easy in the early school years, when the facial features are still prominent and the behavioral and cognitive deficiencies emerge. Impulsiveness, anxiety, and poor social interactions are common behavioral manifestations of this syndrome. Recent studies have estimated that the social abilities of a child who has FAS levels off at 6 years of age and may not progress beyond this point. As a result, adults with FAS are often isolated, with poor adaptive living skills. They often require structured living facilities.

The early recognition of FAS clearly benefits infants and children. Interventions such as evaluation of nutrition, management of medical issues related to birth defects, and speech therapy can enhance their quality of life. Early recognition can also benefit the impaired mother, resulting in access to alcohol treatment and a better social situation for the entire family.

The diagnosis of FAS is important, but prevention is the answer. Given that no safely established level of alcohol consumption in pregnancy exists, recommendations suggest that pregnant women maintain abstinence. In addition, pregnant women must be counseled about the effects of the alcohol on the fetus.

MEDICAL MANAGEMENT OF ALCOHOL WITHDRAWAL AND DELIRIUM TREMENS

For the patient with probable alcohol withdrawal, co-morbid conditions that may co-exist or mimic the symptoms of withdrawal (e.g., infection, trauma, hepatic encephalopathy, meningitis, drug overdose, metabolic derangements) should be excluded. Once these conditions are excluded, the patient should be placed in a quiet and protective environment and receive parenteral thiamine and multivitamins to decrease the risk of Wernicke's encephalopathy or Korsakoff's amnestic syndrome. Benzodiazepines are the only medications proved to ameliorate symptoms and to decrease the risk of seizures and DTs in patients with alcohol withdrawal. Typically, diazepam (5 to 20 mg), chlordiazepoxide (50 to 100 mg), or lorazepam (1 to 2 mg) is administered every 5 to 10 minutes until symptoms subside, with the last of these medications preferred in patients with advanced cirrhosis, considering that the liver minimally metabolizes it. Continued administration of a benzodiazepine with a fixed-interval approach (i.e., administered even if symptoms are absent) or a symptom-driven approach typically continues for 24 to 72 hours. All benzodiazepines appear to be similarly efficacious in treating alcohol withdrawal, but long-acting agents may be more effective in preventing withdrawal seizures and are associated with fewer rebound symptoms. Conversely, short-acting agents may offer a lower risk of oversedation. For the patient who is resistant to benzodiazepines, intravenous phenobarbital (130 to 260 mg administered every 15 minutes) may be given.

Prescription Drug Abuse

SEDATIVES AND HYPNOTICS

Benzodiazepines and barbiturates are the major sedative-hypnotic drugs among the commonly abused drugs that are listed in Table 133–4. The patient with sedative-hypnotic intoxication may have slurred speech, incoordination, unsteady gait, impaired attention or memory, stupor, and coma. The psychiatric manifestations of intoxication include inappropriate behavior, labile mood, and impaired judgment and social functioning. On physical examination, the person may have respiratory depression or even arrest, nystagmus, and hyperreflexia. Although benzodiazepines rarely depress respiration to the extent that barbiturates do (and, as a result, have a much wider margin of safety), the effects of these drugs are additive with other CNS depressants, such as ethanol. Chronic use may produce physical and psychological dependence and a potentially dangerous withdrawal syndrome.

Benzodiazepines potentiate the effects of γ-aminobutyric acid (GABA), which inhibits neurotransmission. They are available as short-acting agents (temazepam [Restoril] and

triazolam [Halcion]), intermediate-acting agents (alprazolam [Xanax], chlordiazepoxide [Librium], estazolam [ProSom], lorazepam [Ativan], and oxazepam [Serax]), and long-acting agents (clorazepate [Tranxene], clonazepam [Klonopin], diazepam [Valium], flurazepam [Dalmane], and quazepam [Doral]). Flunitrazepam (Rohypnol, also known as *roach, roofies,* or *rope*) is a popularly abused benzodiazepine that is not legally available in the United States but is often smuggled here from other countries. Flunitrazepam has been implicated in cases of *date rape* and is known as a *club drug* because adolescents and young adults often use it at nightclubs and bars or during all-night parties called *raves.*

In persons with an acute benzodiazepine overdose, respiratory depression is the major danger. Flumazenil (Romazicon), a competitive antagonist of benzodiazepines, can be given intravenously for acute overdose. Although it reverses the sedative effects of benzodiazepines, flumazenil may not completely reverse respiratory depression, and it may cause seizures in patients with physical dependence or concurrent tricyclic antidepressant poisoning.

Benzodiazepine cessation may precipitate withdrawal symptoms, depending on the half-life of the benzodiazepine, the duration of use, and the dose. Such withdrawal is characterized by intense anxiety, insomnia, irritability, perceptual changes, hypersensitivity to light and sound, psychosis, hallucinations, palpitations, hyperthermia, tachypnea, diarrhea, muscle spasms, tremors, and seizures. Withdrawal symptoms usually peak 2 to 4 days after the discontinuation of a short-acting agent and 5 to 6 days after discontinuation of a longer-acting one; however, panic attacks and nightmares may recur for months. In general, agents with shorter half-lives produce more intense withdrawal symptoms compared with agents with longer half-lives. Detoxification requires a change to a longer-acting benzodiazepine (e.g., clonazepam, diazepam) and a tapering regimen of 7 to 10 days for short-acting agents or 10 to 14 days for longer-acting ones. Propranolol can be given to decrease tachycardia, hypertension, and anxiety.

Barbiturates may be short acting (pentobarbital and secobarbital), intermediate acting (amobarbital, aprobarbital, and butabarbital), or long acting (mephobarbital and phenobarbital). The symptoms of acute intoxication and withdrawal with barbiturates are similar to those of benzodiazepines. For acute barbiturate overdose, oral charcoal and alkalinization of the urine (to a pH >7.5) with forced diuresis are effective in lowering the blood concentration. The effective treatment of withdrawal symptoms requires estimating the daily dose of the abused drug and substituting an equivalent phenobarbital dose to stabilize the patient, after which the dose of phenobarbital is tapered over 4 to 14 days, depending on the half-life of the abused drug. Benzodiazepines may also be used for detoxification, and propranolol and clonidine may help reduce symptoms.

γ-Hydroxybutyrate (GHB) abuse has increased substantially over the last decade in the United States. This drug is abused for its sedative, euphoric, and bodybuilding effects. GHB is a metabolite of the neurotransmitter GABA, and it also influences the dopaminergic system. It potentiates the effects of endogenous or exogenous opiates. The ingestion of GHB results in immediate drowsiness and dizziness, with the feeling of a *high.* These effects can be potentiated by the concomitant use of alcohol or benzodiazepines. Similar to flunitrazepam and ketamine, GHB is a popular club drug,

Table 133–4 Commonly Abused Drugs

Substance: Category and Name	Examples of Commercial and Street Names	How Administered*	Intoxication Effects/Potential Health Consequences
Cannabinoids			Euphoria, slowed thinking and reaction time, drowsiness, inattention, confusion, impaired balance and coordination, enhanced perception; cough, frequent respiratory infections; impaired memory and learning; increased heart rate, anxiety; panic attacks; tolerance, addiction
Hashish	Boom, chronic, gangster, hash, hash oil, hemp	Smoked, swallowed	
Marijuana	Blunt, dope, ganja, grass, herb, joints, Mary Jane, pot, reefer, sinsemilla, skunk, weed	Swallowed, smoked	
Sedative-Hypnotics (CNS Depressants)			Reduced pain and anxiety, feeling of well being, lowered inhibitions, labile mood, impaired judgment, poor concentration; fatigue, confusion, impaired coordination and memory, respiratory depression and arrest, addiction
Benzodiazepines (other than flunitrazepam)	Restoril, Halcion, Xanax, Librium, ProSom, Ativan, Serax, Tranxene, Klonopin, Valium, Dalmane, Doral; candy, downers, sleeping pills, tranks	Swallowed	Sedation, drowsiness, dizziness
Flunitrazepam[†]	Rohypnol; forget-me pill, Mexican Valium, R2, Roche, roofies, roofinol, rope, rophies	Swallowed, snorted	Visual and gastrointestinal disturbances, urinary retention, amnesia while under drug's effects
Barbiturates	Amytal, Nembutal, Seconal, phenobarbital; barbs, reds, red birds, phennies, tooies, yellows, yellow jackets	Injected, swallowed	Sedation, drowsiness; depression, unusual excitement, fever, irritability, poor judgment, slurred speech, dizziness
GHB[†]	γ-Hydroxybutyrate; G, Georgia home boy, grievous bodily harm, liquid ecstasy	Swallowed	Drowsiness, dizziness, nausea/vomiting, headache, loss of consciousness, hallucinations, peripheral vision loss, nystagmus, loss of reflexes, seizures, coma, death

Table 133–4 Commonly Abused Drugs—cont'd

Substance: Category and Name	Examples of Commercial and Street Names	How Administered*	Intoxication Effects/Potential Health Consequences
Dissociative Anesthetics			Increased heart rate and blood pressure, impaired function, memory motor loss, numbness, nausea/vomiting
PCP and analogues	Phencyclidine; angel dust, boat, hog, love boat, peace pill	Injected, swallowed, smoked	Possible decrease in blood pressure and heart rate; panic, aggression, violence, suicidal ideation; loss of appetite, depression
Ketamine*	Ketalar SV; cat Valiums, K, Special K, vitamin K	Injected, snorted, smoked	At high doses: delirium, depression, respiratory depression and arrest, amnesia while under drug's effects
Hallucinogens			Altered states of perception and feeling; nausea; chronic mental disorders, persisting perception disorder (flashbacks)
LSD	Lysergic acid diethylamide; acid, blotter, boomers, cubes, microdot, yellow sunshines	Swallowed, absorbed through mouth tissues	Also, for LSD and mescaline: increased body temperature, heart rate, blood pressure; loss of appetite, sleeplessness, numbness, weakness, tremors
Mescaline	Buttons, cactus, mesc, peyote	Swallowed, smoked	
Opioids and Morphine Derivatives			Pain relief, euphoria, drowsiness; respiratory depression and arrest, pinpoint pupils, nausea, confusion, constipation, sedation, unconsciousness, seizures, coma, tolerance, addiction
Codeine/oxycodone	Empirin with Codeine, Fiorinal with Codeine, Robitussin A–C, Tylenol with Codeine, OxyContin, Roxicodone, Vicodin; Captain Cody, Cody; schoolboy (with glutethimide), doors and fours, loads, pancakes and syrup	Injected, swallowed	Less analgesia, sedation, and respiratory depression than morphine
Fentanyl	Actiq, Duragesic, Sublimaze; Apache, China girl, China white, dance fever, friend, goodfella, jackpot, murder 8, TNT, Tango and Cash	Injected, smoked, snorted	
Heroin	Diacetylmorphine; brown sugar, dope, H, horse, junk, skag, skunk, smack, white horse	Injected, smoked, snorted	Staggering gait
Morphine/meperidine	Roxanol, Duramorph, Demerol; M, Miss Emma, monkey, white stuff	Injected, swallowed, smoked	
Opium	Laudanum, paregoric; big O, black stuff, block, gum, hop	Swallowed, smoked	

Continued

Table 133–4 Commonly Abused Drugs—cont'd

Substance: Category and Name	Examples of Commercial and Street Names	How Administered*	Intoxication Effects/Potential Health Consequences
Stimulants			Increased heart rate, blood pressure, metabolism; feelings of exhilaration, energy, increased mental alertness, rapid or irregular heart beat; reduced appetite, weight loss, heart failure, seizures, coma
Amphetamine	Adderall, Biphetamine, Dexedrine; bennies, black beauties, crosses, hearts, LA turnaround, speed, truck drivers, uppers	Injected, swallowed, smoked, snorted	Rapid breathing, paranoia, hallucinations; tremors, loss of coordination; irritability, anxiety, restlessness, delirium, panic, paranoia, impulsive behavior, aggressiveness, Parkinson's disease, tolerance, addiction
Methamphetamine	Desoxyn; chalk, crank, crystal, fire, glass, go fast, ice, meth, speed	Injected, smoked, snorted	Aggression, violence, psychotic behavior; memory loss, cardiac and neurologic damage; impaired memory and learning, tolerance, addiction
Methylphenidate	Ritalin; JIF, MPH, R-ball, Skippy, the smart drug, vitamin R	Injected, swallowed, snorted	Increase or decrease in blood pressure, psychotic episodes; digestive problems, loss of appetite, weight loss
Cocaine	Cocaine hydrochloride; blow, bump, C, candy, Charlie, coke, crack, flake, rock, snow, toot	Injected, smoked, snorted	Increased temperature, chest pain, respiratory failure, nausea, abdominal pain, stroke, seizures, malnutrition
MDMA† (methylenedioxymethamphetamine)	DOB, DOM, MBDB, MDA; Adam, clarity, ecstasy, Eve, lover's speed, peace, Methyl-J, Eden, STP, X, XTC	Swallowed	Mild hallucinogenic effects, hallucinations, paranoia, increased tactile sensitivity, empathic feelings, nystagmus, ataxia, tremor, hyperthermia; impaired memory and learning
Other Compounds			Stimulation, loss of inhibition, headache, nausea or vomiting, slurred speech, loss of motor coordination, wheezing, unconsciousness, cramps, weight loss, muscle weakness, depression, memory impairment, damage to cardiovascular and nervous systems, sudden death
Inhalants	Solvents (paint thinners, gasoline), glues, gases (butane, propane, aerosol propellants, nitrous oxide) nitrites (isoamyl, isobutyl, cyclohexyl); laughing gas, poppers, snappers, whippets	Inhaled through nose or mouth	

*Taking drugs by injection can increase the risk of infection through needle contamination with staphylococci, human immunodeficiency virus, hepatitis, and other organisms.
†Associated with sexual assaults (e.g., *date rapes*).
CNS = central nervous system.

and it has been implicated in cases of date rape. Adverse effects that may occur within 15 to 60 minutes of its ingestion include headache, nausea, vomiting, hallucinations, loss of peripheral vision, nystagmus, hypoventilation, cardiac dysrhythmias, seizures, and coma. In rare instances, these adverse effects have led to death. The withdrawal from GHB becomes clinically apparent within 12 hours and may last up to 12 days.

OPIOIDS

Opioids include the natural and semisynthetic alkaloid derivatives of opium, as well as the purely synthetic drugs that mimic heroin. They bind to opioid receptors in the brain, spinal cord, and gastrointestinal tract; in addition, they act on several other CNS neurotransmitter systems, including dopamine, GABA, and glutamate, to produce analgesia, CNS depression, and euphoria. With continued opioid use, tolerance and physical dependence develop. As a result, the user must use larger amounts of the drug to obtain the desired effect, and withdrawal symptoms may occur if use is discontinued. The commonly abused opioids include heroin, morphine, codeine, oxycodone (OxyContin or Roxicodone), meperidine (Demerol), propoxyphene (Darvon), hydrocodone (Vicodin), hydromorphone (Dilaudid), and fentanyl (Sublimaze). Intravenous heroin use, particularly when combined with cocaine (a so-called *speedball*), is increasing in the United States. The controlled-release pain reliever OxyContin was made available for use in 1995. By 2001, OxyContin was the most prescribed brand-name narcotic and was frequently diverted for illicit use, where it was ingested orally, inhaled, or dissolved in water and administered intravenously to obtain an immediate high.

Acute opioid overdose produces pulmonary congestion, with resultant cyanosis and respiratory distress, and changes in mental status that may progress to coma. Other manifestations include fever, pinpoint pupils, and seizures. Unsterile intravenous practices can lead to skin abscesses, cellulitis, thrombophlebitis, wound botulism, meningitis, rhabdomyolysis, endocarditis, hepatitis, or human immunodeficiency virus (HIV) infection. Neurologic complications from intravenous heroin use include transverse myelitis, inflammatory polyneuropathy, and peripheral nerve lesions.

For acute opioid overdose, the patient's respiratory status must be assessed and supported. Naloxone should be administered intravenously and repeated at 2- to 3-minute intervals, often in escalating doses. The patient should respond within minutes with increases in pupil size, respiratory rate, and level of alertness. If no response occurs, opioid overdose is excluded, and other causes of somnolence and respiratory depression must be considered. Naloxone should be titrated carefully because it may precipitate acute withdrawal symptoms in opioid-dependent patients.

Withdrawal symptoms may appear as early as 6 to 10 hours after the last injection of heroin. Initially, the individual often has feelings of drug craving, anxiety, restlessness, irritability, rhinorrhea, lacrimation, diaphoresis, and yawning; these signs are followed by dilated pupils, piloerection, anorexia, nausea, vomiting, diarrhea, abdominal cramps, bone pain, myalgias, tremors, muscle spasms, and, in rare cases, seizures. These symptoms and signs peak at 36 to 48 hours and then subside over 5 to 10 days, if untreated.

A protracted abstinence syndrome characterized by bradycardia, hypotension, mild anxiety, sleep disturbance, and decreased responsiveness may occur for up to 5 months.

Withdrawal from opioids can be managed with methadone, a long-acting synthetic agonist drug, with which withdrawal symptoms develop more slowly and are less severe than those caused by heroin. Methadone can be given twice daily and tapered over 7 to 10 days. Alternatively, *l*-α-acetylmethadol (LAAM), a long-acting agonist, or buprenorphine, a partial agonist, can be given three times a week. Clonidine reduces autonomic hyperactivity and is particularly effective if combined with a benzodiazepine.

Patients with repeated relapses can be maintained on methadone or LAAM. Buprenorphine may also be used as maintenance therapy. Naltrexone is a long-acting opioid antagonist that blocks impulsive opioid use. It can be given daily or two to three times weekly but only after the patient is thoroughly detoxified because it may precipitate withdrawal. Pharmacotherapy must be combined with psychotherapy and structured rehabilitation to achieve an optimal outcome.

AMPHETAMINES

Amphetamines have been used therapeutically for weight reduction, attention-deficit disorder, and narcolepsy. Similar to cocaine, they cause a release of monoamine neurotransmitters (dopamine, norepinephrine, and serotonin) from presynaptic neurons. Additionally, however, they have neurotoxic effects on dopaminergic and serotonergic neurons. Their euphoric and reinforcing effects are mediated through dopamine and the mesolimbic system, whereas their cardiovascular effects are caused by the release of norepinephrine. Chronic use leads to neuronal degeneration in dopamine-rich areas of the brain, which may increase the risk for the eventual development of Parkinson's disease.

Amphetamines can be abused orally, intranasally, intravenously, or by smoking. The most frequently used drugs are dextroamphetamine, methamphetamine, and methylphenidate (Ritalin). Methamphetamine is known on the street as *ice*. Recently, the illicit use of amphetamines has increased substantially, in part because (1) it is easily and quickly synthesized from ephedrine or pseudoephedrine (Fig. 133–1), and (2) its psychotropic effects persist for up to 24 hours. The anorexiants, phenmetrazine and phentermine, which are structurally and pharmacologically similar to amphetamine, also have been used illicitly.

Tolerance to the stimulant effects of amphetamines develops rapidly, and toxic effects can occur with higher doses. Acute amphetamine toxicity is characterized by excessive sympathomimetic effects, including tachycardia, hypertension, hyperthermia, cardiac arrhythmias, tremors, seizures, and coma. The patient may experience irritability, hypervigilance, paranoia, stereotyped compulsive behavior, and tactile, visual, or auditory hallucinations. The clinical picture may simulate an acute schizophrenic psychosis. The symptoms of withdrawal are similar to those seen with cocaine (described in the next section), but the acute psychosis and paranoia are often significantly pronounced.

The treatment of amphetamine abuse centers on a quiet environment, benzodiazepines for anxiety, and sodium nitroprusside for severe hypertension. Antipsychotics, such

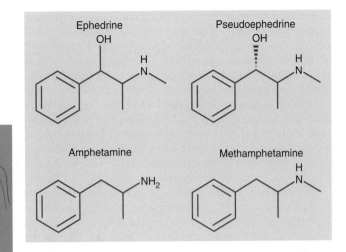

Figure 133–1 The chemical structures of amphetamine and methamphetamine, which can be easily manufactured from ephedrine or pseudoephedrine given that they are structurally similar and widely available.

as haloperidol, can reduce the agitation and psychosis by blocking dopamine's effects on the CNS receptor. Urine acidification with ammonium chloride accelerates amphetamine excretion.

Illicit Drug Abuse

COCAINE

Cocaine use has increased dramatically among adolescents and young adults. It is a frequent cause of drug-related visits to emergency rooms. Cocaine can be taken orally or intravenously; alternatively, because it is well absorbed through all mucous membranes, abusers may achieve a high blood concentration after intranasal, sublingual, vaginal, or rectal administration. Its freebase form—called *crack* because of the popping sound it makes when heated—is heat stable so that it can be smoked. Crack cocaine is considered to be the most potent and addictive form of the drug. Euphoria occurs within seconds after crack cocaine is smoked and is short lived. Compared with smoking of crack cocaine or the intravenous injection of the drug, mucosal administration results in a slower onset of action, a later peak effect, and a longer duration of action. The blood half-life is approximately 1 hour. The drug's major metabolite is benzoylecgonine, which can be detected in the urine for 2 to 3 days after a single dose.

An intense, pleasurable reaction lasting 20 to 30 minutes occurs following cocaine use, after which rebound depression, agitation, insomnia, and anorexia occur, which are then followed by fatigue, hypersomnolence, and hyperphagia (the *crash*). This crash usually lasts 9 to 12 hours but occasionally may last up to 4 days. Users often ingest the drug repetitively at relatively short intervals to recapture the euphoric state and to avoid the crash. On occasion, sedatives or alcohol are ingested concomitantly to reduce the intensity of anxiety and irritability associated with *the crash*. The combination of cocaine and intravenously administered heroin (so-called *speedball*) is frequently ingested so that the abuser can experience the cocaine-induced euphoria and then *float* down on the opiate. Unfortunately, this combination has been reported to cause sudden death. People who use

cocaine in temporal proximity to the ingestion of ethanol produce the metabolite cocaethylene, which has also been implicated in cocaine-related deaths.

Cocaine blocks the presynaptic reuptake of norepinephrine and dopamine, producing an excess of these neurotransmitters at the site of the postsynaptic receptor. Thus, cocaine acts as a powerful sympathomimetic agent, resulting in tachycardia, hypertension, tachypnea, hyperthermia, agitation, pupillary dilation, peripheral vasoconstriction, and seizures. Cocaine causes potent vasoconstriction of cerebral arteries and therefore may result in a stroke. It is associated with myocardial ischemia and arrhythmias and, in rare cases, with myocardial infarction in young persons with normal or nearly normal coronary arteries. The principal mechanisms of ischemia and infarction are coronary arterial vasoconstriction, thrombosis, platelet aggregation, tissue plasminogen activator inhibition, increased myocardial oxygen demand, and accelerated atherosclerosis (Fig. 133–2).

For patients with cocaine-induced hypertension or tachycardia, labetalol and benzodiazepines are usually effective in lowering systemic arterial pressure and heart rate. Patients with acute myocardial infarction should receive aspirin, heparin, nitroglycerin, and, if indicated, reperfusion therapy (with a thrombolytic agent or primary coronary intervention). β-Adrenergic blockers should be avoided because ischemia may be worsened by unopposed α-adrenergically mediated coronary arterial vasoconstriction. Patients with a normal electrocardiographic reading or nonspecific changes can be managed safely with observation.

The immediate treatment of acute cocaine intoxication includes obtaining vascular and airway access, if needed, and careful electrocardiographic monitoring. Benzodiazepines can be given to control CNS agitation, and haloperidol or risperidone can be used in the severely agitated patient. A supportive environment is needed, but detoxification is not required, given that few physical signs of true dependence are present.

Most chronic cocaine abusers have psychological dependence and an intense craving for cocaine. Personal and group therapies are important adjuncts to pharmacologic treatment, but relapse is common and is difficult to manage. Treatment has centered on the short-term use of dopamine agonists (bromocriptine), tricyclic antidepressants (primarily desipramine), or the selective serotonin reuptake inhibitors to diminish the craving for cocaine, as well as the fatigue and depression that follow. More recent research is focused on so-called *vaccine strategies,* whereby protein-conjugated analogues of cocaine would be administered to produce anticocaine antibodies that bind cocaine, thereby preventing its passage across the blood-brain barrier.

CANNABIS

The cannabinoid drugs include marijuana (the dried flowering tops and stems of the hemp plant) and hashish (a resinous extract of the hemp plant). They are among the most commonly used drugs by adolescents, with 46% of 12th graders admitting that they have used marijuana or hashish at least once, and 21% reporting that they are current users. Most of their pharmacologic effects come from metabolites of δ-9-tetrahydrocannabinol, which bind to specific cannabinoid receptors located in the CNS, spinal cord, and peripheral nervous system. The primary mode of

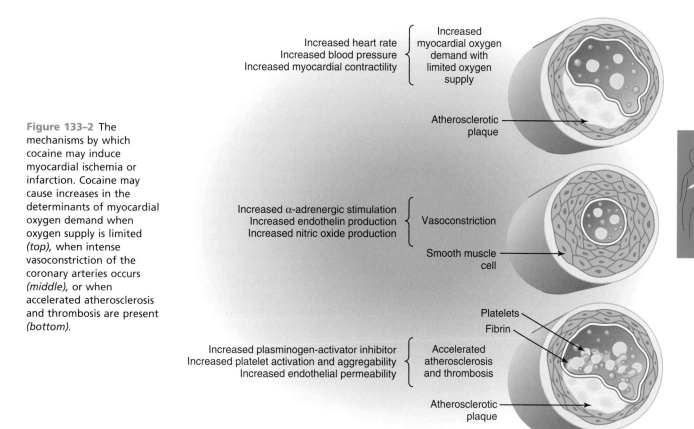

Increased heart rate
Increased blood pressure
Increased myocardial contractility
} Increased myocardial oxygen demand with limited oxygen supply

Atherosclerotic plaque

Figure 133–2 The mechanisms by which cocaine may induce myocardial ischemia or infarction. Cocaine may cause increases in the determinants of myocardial oxygen demand when oxygen supply is limited *(top)*, when intense vasoconstriction of the coronary arteries occurs *(middle)*, or when accelerated atherosclerosis and thrombosis are present *(bottom)*.

Increased α-adrenergic stimulation
Increased endothelin production
Increased nitric oxide production
} Vasoconstriction

Smooth muscle cell

Platelets
Fibrin

Increased plasminogen-activator inhibitor
Increased platelet activation and aggregability
Increased endothelial permeability
} Accelerated atherosclerosis and thrombosis

Atherosclerotic plaque

ingestion is smoking, with mood-altering and intoxicating effects noted within 3 minutes and peak effects in approximately 1 hour. The acute physiologic effects are dose related and often include increased heart rate, conjunctival congestion, dry mouth, fine tremor, muscle weakness, and ataxia. Psychoactive effects include euphoria, enhanced perception of colors and sounds, drowsiness, inattentiveness, and inability to learn new facts. Tolerance and physical dependence occur, and chronic users may experience mild withdrawal symptoms of irritability, restlessness, anorexia, insomnia, or mild hyperthermia. Rarely, acute psychosis with panic reactions occurs. The treatment of withdrawal is supportive and includes reassurance; benzodiazepines may be used in severely agitated patients. Cannabinoids have been used as anti-emetic agents in patients with cancer receiving chemotherapy, for weight stimulation (in patients with cancer or HIV infection), and in the treatment of glaucoma.

HALLUCINOGENS AND DISSOCIATIVE DRUGS

Hallucinogens (drugs that cause hallucinations) include lysergic acid diethylamide (LSD), mescaline, psilocybin, and ibogaine. Dissociative drugs distort perceptions of sight and sound and produce feelings of detachment—dissociation—without causing hallucinations. They include phencyclidine (PCP), ketamine, and dextromethorphan (a widely available cough suppressant).

LSD is the most potent of the hallucinogenic drugs. Although it is known to interact with serotonin receptors in the cerebral cortex and locus ceruleus, the precise psychoactive mechanism is unknown. Within 30 minutes of its oral ingestion, sympathomimetic effects appear, includ-

ing mydriasis, hyperthermia, tachycardia, elevated blood pressure, diaphoresis, dry mouth, increased alertness, tremors, and nausea. Within 2 hours, the psychoactive effects become apparent, with heightened perceptions (highly intensified colors, smells, sounds, and other sensations), body distortions, mood variations, and visual hallucinations. An acute panic reaction may occur, sometimes leading to self injury or suicide. After approximately 12 hours, the syndrome begins to subside, but fatigue and tension may persist for another day. Flashbacks (brief recurrences of the hallucinations) may occur days or even weeks after the last dose but tend to disappear without treatment. Acute panic reactions are best treated in a supportive environment; benzodiazepines can be given to severely agitated patients.

PCP is a potent addictive hallucinogen that produces a prompt stimulant effect similar to that of amphetamines, with feelings of euphoria, power, and invincibility. Patients may have hypertension, tachycardia, hyperthermia, bidirectional nystagmus, slurred speech, ataxia, hallucinations, extreme agitation, and rhabdomyolysis. With more severe reactions, patients may be brought to medical attention in a coma-like state, with open eyes and pupils that are partially dilated, a decreased pain response, brief periods of excitation, and muscle rigidity. On occasion, patients may have hypertensive urgency, seizures, and bizarre (often violent) behavior, which lead to suicide or extreme violence toward others. Tolerance and mild withdrawal symptoms have been seen in daily users, but the major problem is drug craving. Treatment entails a quiet environment, sedation with benzodiazepines, hydration, haloperidol for terrifying hallucinations, and suicide precautions. Continuous gastric suction and acidification of the urine with intravenous ammonium chloride or ascorbic acid may aid in the drug's excretion, but acidification may increase the risk of renal failure if rhabdomyolysis is present.

Ketamine is a rapidly acting general anesthetic; unlike most anesthetics, it produces only mild respiratory depression and appears to stimulate the cardiovascular system. Adverse effects, including delirium and hallucinations, limit the use of ketamine as a general anesthetic in humans. Similar to PCP, ketamine is a dissociative anesthetic. In addition, it has both analgesic and amnestic properties and is associated with less confusion, irrationality, and violent behavior than PCP. Ketamine is one of the club drugs that has been implicated in date rape.

INHALANTS

The inhalants may be classified as (1) *organic solvents,* including toluene (airplane glue), paint thinners, kerosene, gasoline, carbon tetrachloride, shoe polish, and degreasers (dry cleaning fluids); (2) *gases,* such as butane, propane, aerosol propellants, and anesthetics (ether, chloroform, halothane, and nitrous oxide); and (3) *nitrites,* such as cyclohexyl nitrite, amyl nitrite, and butyl nitrite. These drugs are most often inhaled by children or young adolescents, after which they produce dizziness and intoxication within minutes. Prolonged exposure or daily use may lead to hearing loss, bone marrow depression, cardiac arrhythmias, cerebral degeneration, peripheral neuropathies, and damage to the liver, kidneys, or lungs. In rare instances, death may occur, most likely from hypoxemia or cardiac arrhythmias. Detoxification is rarely required for the patient who has abused these substances, but psychiatric treatment may be needed to prevent relapse.

DESIGNER DRUGS

The term *designer drugs* refers to illicit synthetic drugs, many of which have increased potency in comparison with their parent compounds. The most common designer drugs include analogs of fentanyl, meperidine, and methamphetamines. The best-known fentanyl derivatives are α-methyl fentanyl *(China white)* and 3-methyl fentanyl. Because these drugs are approximately 1000 times as potent as heroin, the fact that fatal overdoses from respiratory depression have been reported is not surprising.

The major meperidine derivatives are 1-methyl-4-phenyl-4-propionoxypiperidene (MPPP) and 1-methyl-4-phenyl-1,2,3,6-tetrahydropyridine (MPTP). These drugs produce euphoria similar to that caused by heroin. In some users, MPTP causes neuronal degeneration in the substantia nigra, which produces an irreversible form of Parkinson's disease.

The methylenedioxy synthetic derivatives of amphetamine and methamphetamine are generally referred to as *ecstasy* and include 3,4-methylenedioxy methamphetamine (MDMA, also known as *Adam*); 3,4-methylenedioxyethylamphetamine (MDEA, also known as *Eve*); and N-methyl-1-(3,4-methylenedioxyphenyl)-2-butanamine (MBDB, also known as *Methyl-J* or *Eden*). These drugs have CNS stimulant and hallucinogenic properties. They produce elevated mood and increased self esteem and may cause acute panic, anxiety, paranoia, hallucinations, tachycardia, nystagmus, ataxia, and tremor. Deaths in some users have been attributed to cardiac arrhythmias, hyperthermia with seizures, or intracranial hemorrhage.

Prospectus for the Future

The elucidation of ligands to psychotropic drugs is being used to provide molecular clues for the derivation of structural analogs that have therapeutic benefits. For example, recent studies have identified the receptors to which tetrahydrocannabinoid binds to mediate its effects. In the brain, activation of the cannabinoid-1 receptor causes the psychotropic effects associated with marijuana use. Cannabinoid-1 receptors also are found in adipose tissue and the gastrointestinal tract, where they regulate food intake and glycemic control. A cannabinoid-1 receptor antago-nist, rimonabant, has been shown to be effective in suppressing the reinforcing and rewarding properties of different agents that are often abused (i.e., cocaine, nicotine, alcohol) and reducing food intake and body weight. This agent appears to be effective in treating drug addiction and obesity-related disorders, for which it is currently being tested in clinical trials. The identification of other receptors and signaling pathways may permit the development of other agonists or antagonists that will serve as effective pharmacotherapeutic agents.

References

Banken JA: Drug abuse trends among youth in the United States. Ann NY Acad Sci 1025:465–71, 2004.

Check E: Psychedelic drugs: The ups and downs of ecstasy. Nature 429:126–128, 2004.

Chen CY, O'Brien MS, Anthony JC: Who becomes cannabis dependent soon after onset of use? Epidemiological evidence from the United States: 2000–2001. Drug Alcohol Depend 79:11–22, 2005.

Cone EJ, Fant RV, Rohay JM, et al: Oxycodone involvement in drug abuse deaths. II. Evidence for toxic multiple drug-drug interactions. J Anal Toxicol 28:616–24, 2004.

Cone EJ, Fant RV, Rohay JM, et al: Oxycodone involvement in drug abuse deaths: A DAWN-based classification scheme applied to an oxycodone postmortem database containing over 1000 cases. J Anal Toxicol 27:57–67, 2003.

Government Accounting Office: OxyContin abuse and diversion and efforts to address the problem. Publication GAO-04-110, 2003.

Hanson GR, Rau KS, Fleckenstein A: The methamphetamine experience: A NIDA partnership. Neuropharm 47:92–100, 2004.

Lange RA, Hillis LD: Cardiovascular complications of cocaine use. N Engl J Med 345:351–358, 2001.

McCabe SE, Teter CJ, Boyd CJ, et al: Nonmedical use of prescription opioids among US college students: Prevalence and correlates from a national survey. Addict Behav 30:789–805, 2005.

McCabe SE, Knight JR, Weschler H: Nonmedical use of prescription stimulants among US college students: Prevalence and correlates from a national survey. Addiction 100:96–106, 2005.

Morton J: Ecstasy: Pharmacology and neurotoxicity. Curr Opin Pharmacol 5:79–86, 2005.

Saitz R: Unhealthy alcohol use. N Engl J Med 352:596–607, 2005.

Sulzer D, Sonders MS, Poulsen NW, et al: Mechanisms of neurotransmitter release by amphetamines: A review. Prog Neurobiol 75:406–433, 2005.

Teter CJ, Guthrie SK: A comprehensive review of MDMA and GHB: Two common club drugs. Pharmacotherapy 21:1486–1513, 2001.

Appendix

Commonly Measured Laboratory Values

This appendix lists basic serum and urinary laboratory values measured commonly in clinical medicine. The values are presented in conventional units (CUs) and standard international (SI) units. The table also includes conversion factors (CFs) for interchanging conventional and standard international units using the following formula:

$$\text{SI units} = \text{CU} \times \text{CF}$$

This collection of laboratory values is not intended to be exhaustive. Laboratory values found in this appendix are from the clinical laboratories of University Hospital, University of Arkansas for Medical Sciences, Little Rock, Arkansas.

Commonly Measured Laboratory Values

Test	Conventional Units	Conversion Factor	Standard International Units
Arterial Blood Gases			
pH (37° C)	—	—	7.35–7.45
Oxygen (Po_2)	80–100 mmHg	0.133	11–14.4 kPa (kilopascal)
Oxygen saturation	94–100%	—	Fraction: 0.94–1.00
Carbon dioxide (Pco_2)	35–45 mmHg	1	23–29 mmol/L
Serum Electrolytes			
Sodium	135–145 mEq/L	1	135–145 mmol/L
Potassium	3.5–5.0 mEq/L	1	3.5–5.0 mmol/L
Chloride	100–108 mEq/L	1	100–108 mmol/L
Bicarbonate	22–31 mEq/L	1	22–31 mmol/L
Anion gap [Na − (Cl + HCO_3)]	7–14 mEq/L	1	7–14 mmol/L
Total Calcium	8.7–10.5 mg/dL	0.25	2.18–2.63 mmol/L
Ionized Calcium	4.7–5.2 mg/dL	0.25	1.18–1.3 mmol/L
Magnesium	1.6–2.6 mEq/L	0.50	0.8–1.3 mmol/L
Phosphorus	2.5–4.5 mg/dL	0.323	0.81–1.45 mmol/L
Commonly Measured Serum Nonelectrolytes			
Urea nitrogen	6–20 mg/dL	0.357	2.14–7.14 mmol/L
Creatinine	0.5–1.2 mg/dL	88.4	44.2–97.2 mcmol/L
Uric acid	M: 3.5–7 mg/dL	0.059	0.21–0.41 mmol/L
	F: 2.5–6.0 mg/dL	0.059	0.15–0.35 mmol/L
Glucose (non fasting)	70–110 mg/dL	0.055	3.9–6.1 mmol/L
Osmolality	—	—	289–305 mOsm/kg

Commonly Measured Laboratory Values—cont'd

Test	Conventional Units	Conversion Factor	Standard International Units
Serum Endocrine Tests			
ACTH	9–52 pg/mL	1	9–52 ng/L
Aldosterone	Supine: <1.6–6 ng/dL	0.0277	<0.04–0.44 nmol/L
	Upright: 4–31 ng/dL	0.0277	0.11–0.86 nmol/L
β-Human chorionic gonadotropin (non-pregnant)	<1.0 mU/mL	1	<10 mIU/L
Cortisol	0800 h: 4.3–22.4 mcg/dL	27.6	119–618 nmol/L
	1600 h: 3.1–16.7 mcg/dL	27.6	85.6–461 nmol/L
C-peptide (fasting)	1.1–4.6 ng/mL	0.328	0.36–1.5 nmol/L
Estrogens, total	M: 29–127 pg/mL	1	29–127 ng/L
	F: Late follicular phase, 200–650 pg/mL	1	200–650 ng/mL
	Luteal phase, 50–350 pg/mL	1	50–350 ng/L
	Postmenopausal, <73 pg/mL	1	<73 ng/L
Follitropin (FSH)	M: 1.27–19.26 mIU/mL	1	1.27–19.26 IU/L
	F: Follicular phase, 3.85–8.78 mU/mL	1	3.85–8.78 U/L
	Ovulatory peak, 4.54–22.52 mU/mL	1	4.54–22.52 U/L
	Luteal phase, 1.79–5.12 mU/mL	1	1.79–5.12 U/L
	Postmenopausal, 16.74–113.59 mU/mL	1	16.74–113.59 U/L
Gastrin	<100 pg/mL	1	<100 ng/L
Growth hormone	0.1–5 ng/mL	1	0.1–5 mcg/L
Hemoglobin A_{1c}	4–6% of total Hgb (whole blood)	0.001	Fraction: 0.056–0.075
Insulin (12-hr fasting)	1.5–20.5 mcIU/mL	7.0	10.5–143.5 pmol/L
Luteinizing hormone (LH)	M: 1.5–9.3 mU/mL	1	1.5–9.3 U/L
	F: Follicular phase, 1.9–12.5 mU/mL	1	1.9–12.5 U/L
	Midcycle, 8.7–76.3 mU/mL	1	8.7–76.3 U/L
	Luteal, 0.5–16.9 mU/mL	1	0.5–16.9 U/L
	Postmenopausal, 15.9–54 mU/mL	1	15.9–54 U/L
Progesterone	M: 0.1–0.84 ng/mL	3.2	0.32–2.7 nmol/L
	F: Follicular phase, 0.31–1.52 ng/mL	3.2	0.99–4.9 nmol/L
	Luteal phase, 5.16–18.56 ng/mL	3.2	16.5–59.4 nmol/L
	Postmenopausal, 0–0.78 ng/mL	1	0–0.78 mcg/L
Renin activity	Supine: 0.2–1.6 ng/mL/hr	1	0.2–1.6 mcg/L/hr
	Standing: 0.5–4 ng/mL/hr	1	0.5–4 mcg/L/hr
Testosterone (Free)	M: 47–244 pg/mL	3.5	164.5–854.6 pmol/L
	F: 0.6–6.8 pg/mL	3.5	2.1–23.8 pmol/L
Testosterone (Total)	M: 241–827 ng/dL	0.035	8.4–28.9 nmol/L
	F: 14–76 ng/dL	0.035	0.49–2.7 nmol/L
Thyrotropin (TSH)	0.35–5.5 mcU/mL	1	0.35–5.5 mcU/L
Free Thyroxine (FT_4)	0.58–1.64 ng/dL	13	7.5–21.3 pmol/L
Total Thyroxine (T_4)	4.5–10.9 mcg/dL	13	58.5–141.7 nmol/L
Triiodothyronine resin uptake (T_3RU)	22.5–37%	1	22.5–37 AU (arbitrary units)
Urine Endocrine Tests			
Epinephrine	24 hr: ≤25 mcg/day	0.059	≤1.5 nmol/day
Norepinephrine	24 hr: ≤100 mcg/day	0.059	≤5.91 nmol/day
5-Hydroxyindole-acetic acid	24 hr: ≤15 mg/day	5.2	≤78 mcmol/day
Metanephrines (metanephrine + normetanephrine)	24 hr: ≤0.7 mcg/mg creatinine	0.58	≤0.41 mmol/mol creatinine
Vanillylmandelic acid (VMA)	24 hr: ≤7 mg/day	5.05	≤35.4 mcmol/day
17-Hydroxycorticosteroids	24 hr: 4–14 mg/day	2.76	11.04–38.6 mcmol/day
17-Ketosteroids	24 hr: M: 8–20 mg/day	3.44	27.5–68.8 mcmol/day
	F: 6–15 mg/day	3.44	21–52 mcmol/day

Commonly Measured Laboratory Values—cont'd

Test	Conventional Units	Conversion Factor	Standard International Units
Serum Markers of Gastrointestinal Absorption			
β-Carotene	60–200 mcg/dL	0.0186	1.1–3.72 mcmol/L
Vitamin B$_{12}$	211–911 pg/mL	0.74	156–674 pmol/L
Folate			
Serum	≥3.5 ng/mL	2.27	≥7.9 nmol/L
Red blood cells (RBCs)	145–500 ng/mL packed cells	2.27	329–1135 nmol/L
Serum Lipids			
Cholesterol	Recommended: <200 mg/dL	0.026	<5.18 mmol/L
	Moderate risk: 200–239 mg/dL	0.026	5.18–6.19 mmol/L
	High risk: ≥240 mg/dL	0.026	≥6.22 mmol/L
Fatty acids, free	2.8–16.9 mg/dL	0.0356	0.10–0.60 mmol/L
HDL-cholesterol	Desirable >60 mg/dL	0.026	>0.75 mmol/L
	High risk <35 mg/dL	0.026	>0.91 mmol/L
LDL-cholesterol	Recommended: <130 mg/dL	0.026	<3.37 mmol/L
	Moderate risk: 130–159 mg/dL	0.026	3.37–4.12 mmol/L
	High risk: ≥160 mg/dL	0.026	≥4.14 mmol/L
Triglycerides (fasting)	Desirable <200 mg/dL	0.011	<2.2 mmol/L
	Borderline 200–300 mg/dL	0.011	2.2–3.3 mmol/L
	High risk >300 mg/dL	0.011	>3.3mmol/L
Serum Liver/Pancreatic Tests			
Alanine aminotransferase (ALT, SGPT)	—	—	5–40 U/L
Aspartate aminotransferase (AST, SGOT)	—	—	10–40 U/L
γ-Glutamyltransferase (GGT)	—	—	5–70 U/L
Alkaline phosphatase	—	—	40–120 U/L
Total bilirubin	0.1–1.2 mg/dL	17.1	1.71–20.5 mcmol/L
Conjugated bilirubin	0–0.24 mg/dL	17.1	0–6.84 mcmol/L
Amylase	—	—	25–125 U/L
Lipase	—	—	7–59 U/L
Serum Markers for Cardiac or Skeletal Muscle Injury			
Aldolase	—	—	1.5–8.1 U/L
Lactate dehydrogenase (LDH)	—	—	100–250 U/L
Isoenzymes (%)	Fraction 1: 14–27	—	0.14–0.27
	Fraction 2: 29–42		0.29–0.42
	Fraction 3: 16–22		0.16–0.22
	Fraction 4: 8–15		0.08–0.15
	Fraction 5: 6–23		0.06–0.23
Creatine kinase (CK)	—	—	M: 50–260 U/L
			F: 30–235 U/L
CK Isoenzymes (%)	Fraction 2 (MB): <2.4% of total	—	<0.024
Myoglobin	3–70 mcg/mL	1	3–70 mg/L
Troponin I	0.01–0.03 ng/mL	1	0.01–0.03 mcg/L
β-Natriuretic peptide	0–100 pg/mL	1	0–100 ng/L

Commonly Measured Laboratory Values—cont'd

Test	Conventional Units	Conversion Factor	Standard International Units
Serum Markers for Neoplasia			
Acid phosphatase	—	—	<4.3 U/L
Carcinoembryonic antigen (CEA)	Nonsmokers: 0.5–2.5 ng/mL	1	0.5–2.5 mcg/L
	Smokers: 0.5–10 ng/L	1	0.5–10 mcg/mL
α-Fetoprotein	<8 ng/mL	1	<8 mcg/L
Prostate-specific antigen (PSA)	0–4 ng/mL	1	0–4 mcg/L
Serum Proteins			
Albumin	3.5–5.5 g/dL	10	35–55 g/L
Immunoglobulins (Ig)	IgA: 115–425 mg/dL	10	1150–4250 mg/L
	IgD: 0–10 mg/dL	10	0–100 mg/L
	IgE: 0–180 IU/mL	1	0–180 KIU/L
	IgG: 840–1640 mg/dL	0.01	8.4–16.4 g/L
	IgM: 60–410 mg/dL	10	660–4100 mg/L
Protein			
Total	6.5–8.5 g/dL	10	65–85 g/L
Electrophoresis	α_1-Globulin: 0.1–0.4 g/dL	10	1–4 g/L
	α_2-Globulin: 0.5–0.8 g/dL	10	5–8 g/L
	β-Globulin: 0.5–1 g/dL	10	5–10 g/L
	γ-Globulin: 0.7–1.7 g/dL	10	7–17 g/L
Complete Blood Cell Count			
Hemoglobin (Hb)	M: 13.5–17.5 g/dL	0.155	2.09–2.71 mmol/L
	F: 11.5–16 g/dL	0.155	1.78–2.48 mmol/L
Hematocrit (Hct)	M: 40–52%	—	0.4–0.52
	F: 34–47%	—	0.34–0.47
Mean corpuscular Hb concentration (MCHC)	30–36% Hb/cell, or gHb/dL TBC	0.155	4.65–5.58 mmol Hb/L
Mean corpuscular volume (MCV)	—	—	M: 79–96 fL
			F: 79–102 fL
Leukocyte count	$3–12 \times 10^3$ cells/mcL	—	$3–12 \times 10^9$ cells/L

Differential Count	%	Cells/mcL	Fraction	Cells $\times 10^6$/L
Granulocytes	40–75	1200–9000	0.40–0.75	1200–9000
Lymphocytes	10–60	300–7200	0.10–0.6	300–7200
Monocytes	0–12	0–1440	0–0.12	0–1440
Eosinophils	0–4	0–450	0–0.04	0–450
Basophils	0–3	0–360	0–0.03	0–360
CD_4 (T_H) count	36–54	660–1500	0.36–0.54	660–1500
CD_8 (T_S) count	19–33	360–850	0.19–0.33	360–850
T_H/T_S ratio	1.1–2.9	—	—	—
Platelet count	—	150–500	—	150–500

Commonly Measured Laboratory Values—cont'd

Anemia Tests

Reticulocyte count	0.5–2% of erythrocytes	—	0.005–0.02
Iron (total)	M: 49–189 mcg/dL	0.179	8.77–33.8 mcmol/L
	F: 37–170 mcg/dL	0.179	6.62–30.4 mcmol/L
Ferritin	M: 22–322 ng/mL	1	22–322 mcg/L
	F: 10–291 ng/mL	1	10–291 mcg/L
Total iron-binding capacity	250–450 mcg/dL	0.179	44.8–80.6 mcmol/L
Hemoglobin electrophoresis	HbA: 95–98%	—	0.95–0.98
	HbF: 0–2%	—	0–0.02
	HbS: 0%		0

Coagulation Tests

Prothrombin time (PT)	11.5–14.7 sec
Activated Partial thromboplostintine	23–36.9 sec
INR	Nml <1.4

Bleeding Time

Ivy	—	—	Normal: 2–10 min

Disseminated Intravascular Coagulation Tests

Fibrinogen	197–447 mg/dL	0.01	1.97–4.47 g/L
D-dimer	0–0.5 mcg/mL	1	0–0.5 mg/L

Hemolysis Tests

Haptoglobin	75–350 mg/dL	10	750–3500 mg/L

ACTH = corticotropin; Cl = chlorine; F = female; FSH = follicle-stimulating hormone; HCO_3 = bicarbonate; HDL = high-density lipoprotein; INR = international normalized ratio; LDL = low-density lipoprotein; M = male; MB = myocardial band; Na = sodium; PCO_2 = partial pressure of carbon dioxide; PO_2 = partial pressure of oxygen; SGOT = serum glutamic-oxaloacetic transaminase; SGPT = serum glutamate pyruvate transaminase.

Index